Drug Compatibility Chart

Column headers (left to right):
1. hydrocortisone sodium succinate
2. insulin (regular)
3. isoproterenol
4. lactated Ringer's
5. lidocaine
6. methylprednisolone sodium succinate
7. mezlocillin
8. multiple vitamin infusion
9. nafcillin
10. netilmicin
11. norepinephrine
12. normal saline solution
13. ondansetron
14. oxacillin
15. oxytocin
16. penicillin G potassium
17. phenytoin
18. phytonadione
19. piperacillin
20. potassium chloride
21. procainamide
22. ranitidine
23. sodium bicarbonate
24. thiamine
25. ticarcillin
26. tobramycin
27. vancomycin
28. verapamil
29. vitamin B complex with C

Row drug	1	2	3	4	5	6	7	8	9	10	11	12	13	14	15	16	17	18	19	20	21	22	23	24	25	26	27	28	29
acyclovir	4			4		4		4	4			■		4		4			4	4			4	4		4	4	4	4
albumin																													
amikacin	24			24								24	24	4	8		8	■	24		4		24	24				24	24
amino acid injection	24	24	24			24	24	?	?	24	24	24			24		24	■	24	?	4		12			24	24		
aminophylline	24	■		24	24	?				24	2		24			■					4		24	24				■	
ampicillin	?	2				24					8					3			4		?	?						4	■
bretylium		48	3	48	24						48								48	24	24	48						48	
calcium gluconate			24	24				2			24								4					1		48	4		
cefamandole		■				■			■		12										■			24					
cefazolin		2		24			24				24	4							?					24	4				
cefoxitin		24		24			24				24	4								24			24		24	24			
ceftazidime											24	4							?	6									
cimetidine	24	24		24	24						48	4			24		24		24					24	24	48			
ciprofloxacin	■			48	24				■									24	24		24			24	24				
clindamycin	24		24		24		24			24		4			24			48	24		?	24		48	24	24			
corticotropin																													
dexamethasone sodium phosphate	4										4				4			24	4						24	4			
dextrose 5% in water (D5W)	48		24		24	?	24	24	24	24		48	6	6	24	■	24	24	24	48	24	24	24	24	24	24			
D5W in lactated Ringer's	24		24		24		24				24			24		24		24			24			24				24	
D5W in normal saline solution	48		24		24	?		24	24			48	?		24		24	24		24	24		48		24				
diazepam				■																	?							24	
diphenhydramine	24							72				4			24			4		1								24	
dobutamine		24	24	24						24	24							?		24	48							24	
dopamine	18		48	24	18						48	24		■				24		48								24	4
epinephrine	4		24								24				3		4		24		■							24	4
erythromycin lactobionate	■		18			24					22							24	24									24	
esmolol	24		24			24					24		24	24		24	24		24				24	24	24				
gentamicin		2		24			24	■			24	4							24					24				24	
heparin sodium	?	2	24		24	?					4	4	4	?		4	6	24	4	24	24		6	■		24	24		
hydrocortisone sodium succinate		4	4	24		?		■			24	4	4		4	24		4		24							24		
insulin (regular)	4			24								2				4		24	3		2	2	2	48	4				
isoproterenol	4		■	24							24							24					24					24	
lactated Ringer's	24		24		24	?	72	24	24			24			24		24			24	24				24	24	24		24
lidocaine		24		24					48			24							24	24	24							48	
methylprednisolone sodium succinate	?		?								?				24			?		48	2					24	?		
mezlocillin		72									48														■				
multiple vitamin infusion		24					24				24								24							24			
nafcillin	■		24	48							24								24			24						?	
netilmicin			24				24				24								24									24	
norepinephrine											24										?	■						24	
normal saline solution	24		24		24	?	48	24	24	24		48	24		24			24	24	24	48	24	24	24	48	24	24		
ondansetron	4		24			24					48							4		4			4		4	4			
oxacillin	4		24			24					24													4				24	4
oxytocin	■	2																		4			24				24	4
penicillin G potassium			24		24				24			24							24					24				24	
phenytoin										■	24								24					24				48	
phytonadione	4		24								24								4					4				24	4
piperacillin	24		24								24							24			24	4						24	
potassium chloride	4		24		?		24				24	4		4			4	24		4	48	24						24	
procainamide	4		24				24				24							4				24						48	24
ranitidine		24	24		24	48				?	48	4		24			4	48	24				24	24	24				
sodium bicarbonate	24	3	■	24	2		24	24			24			24		24	24	24					■			■			?
thiamine		24									24																	24	
ticarcillin		2		24							24	4		4							24							24	
tobramycin		2		24							48								24									24	
vancomycin		2		24							24	4							24									24	
verapamil	24	48	24	24	48	24		24			24	24					24	24	48		24	24	48			24	24	24	24
vitamin B complex with C		4			?			?							4	4		4			24		?					24	

SPRINGHOUSE

NURSE'S DRUG GUIDE

T H I R D   E D I T I O N

Springhouse Corporation
Springhouse, Pennsylvania

Staff

Publisher
Donna O. Carpenter, ELS

Clinical Director
Ann M. Barrow, RN, MSN, CCRN

Editorial Director
William J. Kelly

Art Director
John Hubbard

Drug Information Editor
Lisa Truong, RPh, PharmD

Senior Editor
Naina Chohan

Editors
Kevin D. Dodds, Rita M. Doyle, Carol H. Munson,
Patricia Nale

Clinical Editors
Eileen Cassin Gallen, RN, BSN; Nancy Laplante, RN,
BSN; Lori Musolf Neri, RN, MSN, CCRN; Kimberly A.
Zalewski, RN, MSN, CEN

Copy Editors
Karen C. Comerford (manager), Colleen P. Coady,
Leslie Dworkin, Caryl Knutsen, Dolores Matthews,
Jane R. Smith

Designers
Arlene Putterman (associate art director), Elaine
Kasmer Ezrow, Joseph John Clark, Donald G. Knauss

Typographers
Diane Paluba (manager), Joyce Rossi Biletz

Manufacturing
Deborah Meiris (director), Patricia K. Dorshaw (manager), Otto Mezei (book production manager)

Editorial Assistants
Carrie R. Cameron, Carol A. Caputo

Indexer
Deborah K. Tourtlotte

A member of the Reed Elsevier plc group

SNDG3– D   N   O   S   A   J   J   M   A   M
02 01 00   10 9   8   7   6   5   4   3   2
ISSN 1088-8063
ISBN 1-58255-022-0

Contents

Advisors, consultants, and contributors

At the time of publication, the advisors, consultants, and contributors held the following positions.

Advisors

Mary Bobbie
RN, MSN, CCRN
Instructor of Nursing
Thomas Jefferson University
College of Health Professions
Philadelphia

Margaret A. Burns
RN, DNSc
Associate Professor of Nursing
Loma Linda (Calif.) University
School of Nursing

Peggy DeStefanis
RN, MN
Chair, Nursing and Health
Technology
Charles County Community
College
La Plata, Md.

Kathy Lauer
RN, PhD
Associate Chairperson,
Adult Health Nursing
Rush University College of
Nursing
Chicago

Sue Ann Lopez
RN, MSN
Chair, Allied Health
Department
Director, ADN and LVN
Programs
South Plains College
Levelland, Tex.

Pamela M. Mammano
RN, MSN
Nursing Instructor
Illinois Valley Community
College
Oglesby

Diane J. Mancino
RN, EdD, CAE
Executive Director
National Student Nurses'
Association, Inc.
New York

Cheryl K. Schmidt
RN, PhD
Clinical Assistant Professor
College of Nursing
University of Arkansas for
Medical Sciences
Little Rock

Sharon J. Tanner
RN, MSN
Dean of Nursing
Roane State Community
College
Harriman, Tenn.

Consultants

Bonnie F. Angel
RN, EdD
Clinical Associate Professor
University of North Carolina at
Chapel Hill

Michael Paul Atkins
RN, BSN
Nurse Consultant
Fairbanks, Alaska

Marcella M. Atwater
MSN, RN,C
Nursing Instructor
North Carolina Central
University
Durham

Linda J. Avillo
RN, MS
Assistant Professor
Department of Nursing
York College of Pennsylvania
York

Debra K. Bailey
MS, RN,C, NNP, FNP
Assistant Professor of Nursing
Mesa State College
Grand Junction, Colo.

Diana Baker
MSN, RN,C
Director of Nursing Programs
College of Eastern Utah
Price

Paula Cleanthous
RN, MN
Nursing Instructor
North Idaho College
Coeur d'Alene

Dorothy Clough
RN, PhD
Professor
College of Nursing
University of New Mexico
Albuquerque

Frank J. delaRama
RN, BSN, BS Genetics
Imprint Editor,
Board of Directors
National Student Nurses'
Association, Inc.
New York

Nancy Fairchild
RN, MS, CAES
Associate Professor
Boston College School of
Nursing
Chestnut Hill, Mass.

Sharon Sweeney Fee
RN, BSN
Registry Nurse
Nurses Network, Inc.
Prescott Valley, Ariz.

Karin Freas Gapper
RN, MSN
Associate Professor
Department of Nursing
Queensborough Community
College
Bayside, N.Y.

Diane J. Gold
RN, MS
Nursing Instructor
Normandale Community
College
Bloomington, Minn.

Bonnie L. Hammack
RN, MSN, ARNP
Professor of Nursing
Miami Dade Community
College
Medical Center Campus
Miami

Barry Adam Harris
SN
Charles E. Gregory School of
Nursing
Perth Amboy, N.J.

Lorrie N. Hegstad
RN, PhD, CS, ANP
Associate Professor
School of Nursing
University of Texas at
Arlington

Opal S. Hipps
RN, EdD, CS-FWP, FAAN
Professor
Clemson (S.C.) University

Byron T. Jackson
SN
Regents College
Albany, N.Y.

Elizabeth U. Kupczyk
RN, MSN
Nursing Instructor
St. Xavier University School
of Nursing
Chicago

Jeremy Lawrence
RN, BSN
Staff Nurse
Medical Intensive Care Unit
University of Mississippi
Medical Center
Jackson

Wisti M. Lemons
SN
Regents College
Albany, N.Y.

William F. McCreary
SN
Valencia Community College
Orlando, Fla.

Maryann B. McDonough
RN, MS
Assistant Professor of Nursing
Castleton (Vt.) State College

Debbie Moore
RN, MSN, FNP
Nursing Faculty
Northwestern State University
of Louisiana
Shreveport

Frances T. Mosser
MSN, RN,C
Associate Professor
Northern Kentucky University
Highland Heights

Anthony P. Paterniti
RN, PhD
Assistant Professor
Texas Woman's University
Dallas

Thomas H. Pepler, IV
RN
RN—Case Manager
Visiting Health Services of
New Jersey, Inc.
Totowa

Judith L. Pulito
RN, MSN
Assistant Professor
Lorain County Community
College
Elyria, Ohio

Donna Reeves
RN, BSN, MEd
Program Chair, Associate of
Science in Nursing
Ivy Tech State College
Sellersburg, Ind.

Barbara J. Wright
RN, MS
Assistant Professor
Hampton (Va.) University
School of Nursing

Contributors
Paul Amato
BS Pharmacy
Adjunct Professor
University of Connecticut
Drug Information Specialist
Hartford Hospital
Hartford

Lawrence Carey
RPh, PharmD
Clinical Pharmacist
Coordinator
Jefferson Home Infusion
Service
Philadelphia

Alan Caspi
PharmD, MBA, FASHP
Director of Pharmacy
Lenox Hill Hospital
New York

Mary Jo Gerlach
RN, MSNEd
Assistant Professor,
Adult Nursing
Medical College of Georgia
School of Nursing, Athens

James A. Koestner
PharmD
Clinical Pharmacist—
Trauma/Critical Care
Vanderbilt University Medical
Center
Nashville, Tenn.

Luana Martindale
RN, MSN
Associate Professor
University of Arkansas at
Little Rock

Gary Smith
RPh, PharmD
Pharmacotherapy Specialist;
Asthma, Allergy and
Pulmonary Disease
Express Scripts/Value Rx
Plymouth, Minn.

Joseph F. Steiner
PharmD
Professor and Director of
Pharmacy Practice
University of Wyoming School
of Pharmacy
Laramie

Foreword

Recently, a surgeon asked if he could borrow my drug book. "I have to look up a drug before I telephone a patient," he said, "and I need a book that can quickly give me accurate drug information." He then confided that he had used my book before, and it had all the information he wanted.

I smiled as I realized that the surgeon had just discovered what I, as a nurse, have known for a long time: *Springhouse Nurse's Drug Guide* is an indispensable reference that provides necessary drug information in a reader-friendly, accessible manner for practicing health care professionals.

This new edition of *Springhouse Nurse's Drug Guide* builds on the features that have made it so successful, adding 35 recently approved drugs to its already extensive list. The alphabetical presentation of drugs by their generic names allows the reader to quickly locate a drug and its most essential information.

Each drug entry follows a consistent, yet comprehensive, format that includes its pronunciation; trade names; pharmacologic and therapeutic classes; controlled substance schedule, when applicable; pregnancy risk category; description of how the drug is supplied; pharmacokinetics, including a useful chart showing the onset, peak, and duration of action for each administration route; pharmacodynamics; indications and dosages; adverse reactions organized five ways for safety; interactions classified by drug, food, and lifestyle; contraindications and precautions; and nursing considerations.

I believe that this last section is one of the most important features of the book because it uses the nursing process as its organizational framework. It also reflects the contributors' solid understanding of the use of drugs in nursing practice today. *Springhouse Nurse's Drug Guide,* Third Edition, includes new upfront chapters on dosage calculations and drug administration methods. Useful examples and step-by-step illustrations give students the help they need to more fully comprehend these critical areas. Also, an easy-to-follow chart on I.V. drug compatibility is wisely located in the front of the book for easy access.

To keep up with the increasing use of herbal medicines, this edition also includes a new section that summarizes key information on commonly used herbs.

The appendices on selected topical, ophthalmic, and otic drugs have been updated, and new, useful ones added, including a table of equiv-alents, a nomogram for estimating body surface area in children, and a new list of drug imprint codes to help nurses identify commonly prescribed pills. The comprehensive index includes generic and brand drug names, drug classifications, diseases, herbal medicines, and drugs appearing in the full-color photoguide.

Springhouse Nurse's Drug Guide, Third Edition, also comes with a free mini-sized CD-ROM, a valuable aid designed to promote an understanding of drugs and their use. It includes 100 frequently asked pharmacology questions, a dosage calculator, and a fun (yes, *fun*) interactive quiz on drug classes.

Springhouse Nurse's Drug Guide, Third Edition, is officially endorsed by the National Student Nurses' Association. Designed for heavy use, the book has an attractive layout, readable print, and a sturdy cover that can be cleaned easily.

These days, it is not possible to remember all the essential information about each drug. To provide patients with the best possible care, the health care professional must have a thorough knowledge of medications and be able to swiftly access current, accurate drug information. Nurses and nursing students must understand and be able to administer medications and have the expertise to teach patients and families about their proper use.

The new edition of *Springhouse Nurse's Drug Guide* is an invaluable resource for nurses, nursing students, and, yes, surgeons, to help us practice knowledgeably and safely. No one and no clinical unit should be without it.

Carol Toussie Weingarten
RN, PhD
Associate Professor, College of Nursing
Villanova University
Villanova, Pennsylvania

How to use *Springhouse Nurse's Drug Guide*

Springhouse Nurse's Drug Guide is a perfect companion for all students, beginning to advanced, learning the basics of pharmacology. The tightly organized entries and clear and consistent writing style help beginning students understand more easily the material. The comprehensive pharmacokinetics and pharmacodynamics information and the route-onset-peak-duration charts help advanced students grasp a drug's actions. The nursing process organization helps students formulate knowledgeable care plans for assigned patients. Students will find the *Springhouse Nurse's Drug Guide* to be the premier resource for all aspects of drug information.

Chapter 1 discusses drug therapy as it relates to the nursing process. Chapter 2 explains how to calculate dosages and provides examples for each step in the calculation. Chapter 3 discusses how to administer drugs by commonly used routes and includes illustrations to guide students through the steps of each procedure.

Drug classifications

Springhouse Nurse's Drug Guide provides complete entries on 40 pharmacologic and therapeutic classifications, from alkylating drugs to xanthine derivatives. The class name is followed by an alphabetical list of all drugs in that class appearing in this book; the drug highlighted in color represents the prototype drug for this class. The text then provides class-specific information on action, indications, adverse reactions, contraindications and precautions (including special information for geriatric, pediatric, and breast-feeding patients), and nursing considerations.

Alphabetical listing of drugs

Drug entries in this text appear alphabetically by generic name for quick reference. The generic name is followed by its phonetic spelling and an alphabetical list of brand (trade) names. Brands that do not require a prescription are designated with a dagger (†); those available only in Canada with a closed diamond (♦); those available only in Australia with an open diamond (◊); those containing alcohol, with a single asterisk (*); and those containing tartrazine, with a double asterisk (**). The mention of a brand name in no way implies endorsement of that product or guarantees its legality.

Each entry then identifies the drug's pharmacologic and therapeutic classifications; that is, chemical category and its major clinical use. Listing both classifications helps the reader grasp the multiple, varying, and sometimes overlapping uses of drugs within a single pharmacologic class and among different classes. (For detailed coverage of 40 pharmacologic and therapeutic classifications, see *Drug classifications,* pages 31-88.) Newly approved drugs appear alphabetically.

Controlled substance schedule

If applicable, the text then identifies whether the drug is a controlled substance. Drugs regulated under the Controlled Substances Act of 1970 are divided into the following schedules:

● Schedule I (C-I): High abuse potential and no accepted medical use—for example, heroin, marijuana, and LSD.
● Schedule II (C-II): High abuse potential with severe dependence liability—for example, narcotics, amphetamines, dronabinol, and some barbiturates.
● Schedule III (C-III): Less abuse potential than schedule II drugs and moderate dependence liability—for example, nonbarbiturate sedatives, nonamphetamine stimulants, anabolic steroids, and limited amounts of certain narcotics.
● Schedule IV (C-IV): Less abuse potential than schedule III drugs and limited dependence liability—for example, some sedatives, antianxiety agents, and nonnarcotic analgesics.
● Schedule V (C-V): Limited abuse potential. Primarily small amounts of narcotics, such as codeine, used as antitussives or antidiarrheals. Under federal law, limited quantities of certain C-V drugs may be purchased without a prescription directly from a pharmacist if allowed under specific state statutes. The purchaser must be at least age 18 and must provide suitable identification. All such transactions must be recorded by the dispensing pharmacist.

Pregnancy risk category

Each systemically absorbed drug has been assigned a pregnancy risk category based upon available clinical and preclinical information. The Pregnancy Risk Category parallels the five Pregnancy Categories (A, B, C, D, and X) assigned by the FDA to reflect a drug's potential to cause birth defects. Although drugs are best avoided during pregnancy, this rating system permits rapid assessment of the risk-benefit ratio should drug administration to a pregnant woman become necessary. Drugs in category A are generally considered safe to use in pregnancy; drugs in category X are generally contraindicated.

• A: Adequate studies in pregnant women have failed to show a risk to the fetus.

• B: Animal studies have not shown a risk to the fetus, but controlled studies have not been conducted in pregnant women; or animal studies have shown an adverse effect on the fetus, but adequate studies in pregnant women have not shown a risk to the fetus.

• C: Animal studies have shown an adverse effect on the fetus, but adequate studies have not been conducted in humans. The benefits from use in pregnant women may be acceptable despite potential risks.

• D: The drug may cause risk to the human fetus, but the potential benefits of use in pregnant women may be acceptable despite the risks (such as in a life-threatening situation or a serious disease for which safer drugs can't be used or are ineffective).

• X: Studies in animals or humans show fetal abnormalities, or adverse reaction reports indicate evidence of fetal risk. The risks involved clearly outweigh potential benefits.

• NR: Not rated.

How supplied

This section lists all available preparations for each drug (for example, tablets, capsules, solutions for injection) and all available dosage forms and strengths. As with the brand names discussed above, over-the-counter dosage forms and strengths are marked with a dagger (†), those available only in Canada with a closed diamond (♦); and those available only in Australia with an open diamond (◊).

Pharmacokinetics

This section describes absorption, distribution, metabolism, and excretion, along with the drug's half-life when known. It also provides a quick reference chart highlighting onset, peak, and duration for each route of administration. Values for half-life, onset, peak, and duration are for patients with normal renal function, unless specified otherwise.

Pharmacodynamics

This section explains the drug's chemical and therapeutic actions. For example, although all antihypertensives lower blood pressure, they don't all do so by the same pharmacologic process.

Indications and dosage

This section provides dosage information for adults, children, and elderly patients, as applicable. Dosage instructions reflect current clinical trends in therapeutics and can't be considered as absolute or universal recommendations. For individual application, dosage instructions must be considered in light of the patient's clinical condition.

Adverse reactions

This section lists adverse reactions to each drug by body system. The most common adverse reactions (those experienced by at least 10% of people taking the drug in clinical trials) are in *italic* type; less common reactions are in roman type; life-threatening reactions are in **bold italic** type; and reactions that are common *and* life-threatening are in **BOLD CAPITAL LETTERS.**

Interactions

This section lists each drug's confirmed, *clinically significant* interactions with other drugs (additive effects, potentiated effects, and antagonistic effects); foods, with specific suggestions for avoiding dangerous drug or food interactions (for example, by reducing doses or monitoring food intake); or lifestyle (such as alcohol use or smoking). Drug interactions are listed under the drug that is adversely affected. For example, magnesium trisilicate, an ingredient in antacids, interacts with tetracycline to cause decreased absorption of tetracycline. Therefore, this interaction is listed under tetracycline. To check on the possible effects of using two or more drugs simultaneously, refer to the interaction entry for each of the drugs in question.

Contraindications and precautions

This section specifies conditions in which the drug should not be used and details recommendations for cautious use. For example, a drug that can be given safely to most people may be contraindicated or require cautious use in pregnant or breast-feeding women, in elderly or pediatric patients, in those already allergic to it, or in those with a disorder that precludes safe administration.

Nursing considerations

This section uses the nursing process as its organizational framework.

• *Assessment* focuses on observation and monitoring of key patient data, such as vital signs, weight, intake and output, and laboratory values.

• *Nursing diagnoses* represent those most commonly applied to drug therapy. In actual use, nursing diagnoses must be relevant to an individual patient; therefore, they may not include the listed examples and may include others not listed.

• *Planning and implementation* offers detailed recommendations for drug administration, including full coverage of I.V., I.M., S.C., and other routes. *Patient teaching* focuses on explaining the drug's purpose, promoting compliance, and ensuring proper use and storage of the drug. It also includes instructions for preventing or minimizing adverse reactions.

• *Evaluation* identifies the expected patient outcomes that correlate with the listed nursing diagnoses.

Because nursing considerations in this text emphasize drug-specific recommendations, they do not include standard recommendations that apply to all drugs, such as "assess the five rights of drug therapy before administration" or "teach the patient the name, dose, frequency, route, and strength of the prescribed drug."

Photoguide to tablets and capsules

To make drug identification easier for nurses and to enhance patient safety, *Springhouse Nurse's Drug Guide* offers a full-color photoguide to the most commonly prescribed tablets and capsules. Shown in actual size, the drugs are arranged alphabetically for quick reference, along with their most common dosage strengths. Page references to the drugs appear in boldface type in the Index.

Herbal medicines

Herbal medicine entries appear alphabetically by name, followed by a phonetic spelling and an alphabetical list of common names.

Common forms

This section lists the available preparations for each herbal medicine as well as dosage forms and strengths.

Actions

This section describes the agent's chemical and therapeutic actions.

Reported uses

This section lists reported uses of the herbal medicine. Some of these uses are based on anecdotal claims; other uses have been studied. However, a listing in this section should not be considered as a recommendation.

Dosages

This section lists the routes and general dosage information for each form of the herb and, where available, in accordance with its reported use. This information has been gathered from the herbal literature, anecdotal reports, and available clinical data. However, not all uses have specific dosage information; often, no consensus exists. Dosage notations reflect current clinical trends and should not be considered as recommendations by the publisher.

Adverse reactions

This section lists undesirable effects that may follow use of the herbal medicine. Some of these effects have not been reported but are theoretically possible, given the chemical composition or action of the agent. Overdose and treatment information is also included, as appropriate.

Interactions

This section lists each herbal agent's clinically significant interaction with other drugs or foods. The interaction is followed by the effect of the interaction and then a specific suggestion for avoiding the interaction itself. As with adverse reactions, some interactions have not been proven but are theoretically possible.

Contraindications and precautions

This section lists any condition, especially a disease, in which the use of the herbal agent is undesirable, and provides recommendations for cautious use, as appropriate.

Nursing considerations

This section offers helpful information, such as monitoring techniques and methods for the prevention and treatment of adverse reactions. Patient-teaching tips that focus on educating the patient about the herb's purpose, preparation, administration, and storage are also included, as are suggestions for promoting patient compliance with the therapeutic regimen and steps the patient can take to prevent or minimize the risk or severity of adverse reactions.

Appendices and index

The appendices include three quick-reference charts on topical, ophthalmic, and otic drugs; a table of equivalents; a nomogram for estimating body surface area in children; and a comprehensive list of drug imprint codes. The comprehensive index lists drug classifications, all generic drugs, brand names, disorders, and herbal medicines included in this book.

PharmDisk 3.0

The CD-ROM included with this book (inside the back cover) offers three exciting Windows-based software programs. "Pharmacology Review" tests your knowledge with 100 multiple-choice questions. "Dosage Calculator" first teaches you the basics and then lets you perform a virtually unlimited number of calculations. And a challenging interactive game helps you learn drug classifications. *PharmDisk 3.0* also provides a link to eDrugInfo.com, the Springhouse Web site for drug imformation.

Common abbreviations

ACE	angiotensin-converting enzyme		LD	lactate dehydrogenase
ADH	antidiuretic hormone		M	molar
AIDS	acquired immunodeficiency syndrome		m^2	square meter
			MAO	monoamine oxidase
ALT	alanine transaminase		mcg	microgram
AST	aspartate transaminase		mEq	milliequivalent
AV	atrioventricular		mg	milligram
b.i.d.	twice daily		MI	myocardial infarction
BPH	benign prostatic hyperplasia		ml	milliliter
BUN	blood urea nitrogen		mm^3	cubic millimeter
cAMP	cyclic adenosine monophosphate		Na	sodium
CBC	complete blood count		NaCl	sodium chloride
CK	creatine kinase		NG	nasogastric
CMV	cytomegalovirus		NSAID	nonsteroidal anti-inflammatory drug
CNS	central nervous system		OTC	over-the-counter
COPD	chronic obstructive pulmonary disease		PABA	para-aminobenzoic acid
			PCA	patient-controlled analgesia
CSF	cerebrospinal fluid		P.O.	by mouth
CV	cardiovascular		P.R.	by rectum
CVA	cerebrovascular accident		p.r.n.	as needed
DIC	disseminated intravascular coagulation		PT	prothrombin time
			PTT	partial thromboplastin time
D_5W	dextrose 5% in water		PVC	premature ventricular contraction
DNA	deoxyribonucleic acid		q	every
ECG	electrocardiogram		q.i.d.	four times daily
EEG	electroencephalogram		RBC	red blood cell
EENT	eyes, ears, nose, throat		RDA	recommended daily allowance
FDA	Food and Drug Administration		REM	rapid eye movement
g	gram		RNA	ribonucleic acid
G	gauge		RSV	respiratory syncytial virus
GFR	glomerular filtration rate		SA	sinoatrial
GGT	gamma-glutamyltransferase		S.C.	subcutaneous
GI	gastrointestinal		SIADH	syndrome of inappropriate antidiuretic hormone
gtt	drops			
GU	genitourinary		S.L.	sublingual
G6PD	glucose-6-phosphate dehydrogenase		T_3	triiodothyronine
H	histamine		T_4	thyroxine
HIV	human immunodeficiency virus		t.i.d.	three times daily
h.s.	at bedtime		U	units
I.D.	intradermal		USP	United States Pharmacopeia
I.M.	intramuscular		WBC	white blood cell
INR	international normalized ratio			
IPPB	intermittent positive-pressure breathing			
IU	international unit			
I.V.	intravenous			
kg	kilogram			

1

Drug therapy and the nursing process

Springhouse Nurse's Drug Guide integrates the nursing process into its organizational framework for good reason. The nursing process guides nursing decisions about drug administration to ensure the patient's safety and meet medical and legal standards. This process provides thorough assessment, appropriate nursing diagnoses, effective planning and implementation, and constant evaluation.

Assessment

Data collection begins with questions about the patient's background, including allergies; use of prescription and OTC drugs and herbal medicines; medical history; habits; socioeconomic status; lifestyle and beliefs; sensory deficits; and cognitive status. Evaluate also the patient's knowledge and understanding of the drug therapy that he is about to receive. After taking his history, perform a thorough physical examination.

Allergies

Specify the drug or food to which the patient is allergic. Describe the reaction; its situation, time, and setting; and the contributing factors, such as concurrent use of stimulants, tobacco, alcohol, or illegal drugs or a significant change in nutritional patterns.

Drugs and herbal medicines

Explore the patient's reason for using the drug or herbal medicine and his knowledge of its use. Note special procedures that he must perform, such as blood glucose monitoring, and make sure he's performing them correctly. Finally, discuss the effects of therapy to determine whether new symptoms or unpredicted reactions have developed.

Medical history

Note chronic disorders; record the date of diagnosis, the prescribed treatment, and the name of the doctor in charge. Careful attention to this part of the history can uncover one of the most important problems with drug therapy—conflicting and incompatible drug regimens.

Habits

Ask about the patient's diet. Certain foods can influence the efficacy of many drugs. Also inquire about use of alcohol, tobacco, caffeine, and illegal drugs such as marijuana, cocaine, and heroin. Note the substance and the amount and frequency of use.

Socioeconomic status

Note the patient's age, educational level, occupation, and insurance coverage. These factors help determine the plan of care, the likelihood of compliance, and the possible need for financial assistance and counseling.

Lifestyle and beliefs

Ask about the patient's support systems, marital status, childbearing status, attitudes toward health and health care, and daily patterns of activity; they all affect the plan of care and patient compliance.

Sensory deficits

Assess the patient for sensory deficits that will influence the plan of care. For example, impaired vision or paralysis can hinder the patient's ability to administer a subcutaneous injection, break a scored tablet, or open a medication container. Hearing impairment can complicate effective patient instruction.

Cognitive status

Note whether the patient is alert, oriented, and able to interact appropriately with people; whether he can think clearly; and whether his conversation is appropriate. Check his short-term and long-term memory because he needs both to follow a prescribed regimen. Also, determine whether the patient is able to read and at what level.

Physical examination

Examine the patient closely for expected drug effects and for adverse reactions. Every drug has a desired effect on one body system but it may also have an undesired effect on another. For example, chemotherapeutic drugs destroy cancer cells, but they also affect normal cells and typically cause hair loss, diarrhea, or nausea.

Knowledge and understanding of drug therapy

A patient is more likely to comply if he understands the reason for the drug therapy.

Nursing diagnosis

Using information gathered during assessment, define potential or actual drug-related problems by formulating each in a relevant nursing diagnosis. The most common problem statements related to drug therapy are "Knowledge deficit," "Noncompliance," and "Altered health maintenance." Nursing diagnoses provide the framework for planning interventions and outcome criteria (patient goals).

Planning and implementation

Make sure that your outcome criteria state the desired patient behaviors or responses that should result from nursing care. Such criteria should be measurable, objective, concise, realistic for the patient, and attainable by nursing management; express patient behavior in terms of expectations; and specify a time frame. A typical outcome statement is

"Before discharge, the patient verbalizes major adverse effects related to his chemotherapy."

After developing the outcome criteria, determine interventions needed to help the patient reach the desired goals. Appropriate interventions may include administration procedures and techniques, legal and ethical concerns, patient teaching, and concerns related to geriatric, pediatric, pregnant, or breast-feeding patients. Such interventions may be independent nursing actions, such as turning a bedridden patient every 2 hours, or actions that require a doctor's order.

Evaluation

The final component of the nursing process, evaluation, is a formal and systematic process for determining the effectiveness of nursing care. This process enables you to determine whether outcome criteria were met and thereby to make informed decisions about subsequent interventions.

For example, if a patient experiences relief of headache within 1 hour after receiving an analgesic, the outcome criterion was met. If the headache was the same or worse, the outcome criterion was not met and requires a new assessment, which may result in a new plan of care or may yield new data that invalidate the nursing diagnosis or suggest new nursing interventions that are more specific or more acceptable to the patient. This assessment could lead to a higher dosage, a different analgesic, or a reevaluation of the cause.

Evaluation enables you to design and implement a revised plan of care, to continuously reevaluate outcome criteria, and to plan again until each nursing diagnosis is successfully completed.

Essentials of dosage calculations

Nurses perform drug and I.V. fluid calculations frequently, so they need to know and understand drug weights and measures, how to convert between systems and measures, and how to compute drug dosages.

Systems of drug weights and measures

Prescribers use several systems of measurement when ordering drugs, three in particular: the metric, household, and apothecaries' systems. The metric and household systems are so widely used that most brands of medication cups for liquid measurements are calibrated in both systems. The apothecary system isn't widely used but may still be encountered in clinical practice. A fourth system, the avoirdupois system, is rarely used. This system uses solid units of measure, such as the ounce and the pound.

Metric system

The metric system is the international system of measurement; it is the system most widely used and is the system used by the U.S. Pharmacopoeia. It has units for both liquid and solid measures. Among its many advantages, the metric system enables accuracy in calculating small drug dosages, it uses Arabic numerals, which are commonly used by health care professionals worldwide, and most manufacturers calibrate newly developed drugs in the metric system.

Liquid measures
In the metric system, one liter (L) is approximately equal to 1 quart in the apothecaries' system. Liters are often used when ordering and administering I.V. solutions. Milliliters are frequently used in the administration of parenteral and some oral drugs. A milliliter (ml) equals $\frac{1}{1,000}$ of a liter.

Solid measures
The gram (g) is the basis for solid measures or units of weight in the metric system. One milligram (mg) equals $\frac{1}{1,000}$ of a gram. Drugs are frequently ordered in grams, milligrams, or an even smaller unit, the microgram (mcg), depending on the drug. The microgram is equal to $\frac{1}{1,000}$ of a milligram. Body weight is usually recorded in kilograms (kg). One kilogram equals 1,000 g.

The following are examples of drug orders using the metric system:
- 1 L D_5W I.V. every 8 hours
- 30 ml milk of magnesia P.O. at bedtime
- Ancef 1 g I.V. every 6 hours
- Lanoxin 0.125 mg P.O. daily.

Household system

Most food products, recipes, OTC drugs, and home remedies use the household system. Health care professionals seldom use the household system for drug administration; however, knowledge of household measures may be useful to nurses in some clinical situations.

Liquid measures
Liquid measurements in the household system that might be used in the clinical setting include teaspoons (tsp) and tablespoons (tbs). The teaspoon and tablespoon, when used for clinical purposes, have been standardized to equal 5 ml and 15 ml, respectively. Using those standardized amounts, 3 teaspoons equal 1 tablespoon, 6 teaspoons equal 1 ounce, and so forth. Patients who have been pre-

scribed medications to be taken in dosages of teaspoons or tablespoons should obtain clinical equipment calibrated in these measures to receive the exact prescribed dosage. They should not use an ordinary spoon to measure a teaspoonful of a medication, because the measurement will most likely be inaccurate. Teaspoon sizes may vary from 4 to 6 ml or more.

The following are examples of drug orders using the household system:
• 2 tsp Bactrim P.O. twice a day
• Riopan 2 tbs P.O. 1 hour before meals and at bedtime.

Apothecaries' system

Two unique features distinguish the apothecaries' system from other systems: the use of Roman numerals and the placement of the unit of measurement before the Roman numeral. For example, a measurement of 5 grains would be written as *grains v*. In the apothecaries' system, equivalents among the various units of measure are close approximations of one another. By contrast, equivalents in the metric system are exact.

When using apothecaries' equivalents for calculations and conversions, the calculations, although not precise, must fall within acceptable standards.

The apothecaries' system is the only system of measurement that uses both symbols and abbreviations to represent units of measure.

Although the use of the apothecaries' system is becoming less common in health care, nurses must still be able to read dosages that have been written in the apothecaries' system and convert them to the metric system.

Liquid measures

The smallest unit of liquid measurement in the apothecaries' system is the minim (℔) and is about the size of a drop of water. Fifteen to sixteen minims equal about 1 ml.

Solid measures

The grain (gr) is the solid measure or unit of weight in the apothecaries' system.

The following are examples of drug orders using the apothecaries' system:
• Multivitamin elixir ℔ xii P.O.
• Robitussin f℥ (fluidrams) iv P.O. q6h
• Mylanta f℥ (fluidounce) i P.O. 1 hour after meals
• Tylenol gr (grains) X P.O. q4h as needed for headache.

Other systems

Some drugs require special systems developed by the manufacturers for measuring their quantities. Three of the most common special systems of measurement are units, international units, and milliequivalents.

Units

Insulin is one of several drugs measured in units (U). Although many types of insulin exist, all are measured in units. The international standard of U-100 insulin means that 1 ml of insulin solution contains 100 U of insulin, regardless of type. Heparin, an anticoagulant, is also measured in units, as are several antibiotics, available in liquid, solid, and powder forms for oral or parenteral use. Each manufacturer of drugs made available in units provides specific information about the measurement of each drug.

The following are examples of drug orders using units:
• Inject 14 U NPH insulin S.C. this a.m.
• Heparin 5,000 U S.C. q12h
• Nystatin 200,000 U P.O. q6h.

The unit is not a standard measure. Different drugs, although measured in units, might have no relationship to one another in quality or activity.

International units

International units (IU) are used to measure biologicals, such as vitamins, enzymes, and hormones. For instance, the activity of calcitonin, a synthetic hormone used in calcium regulation, is expressed in international units.

The following are examples of drug orders using international units:
- 100 IU calcitonin (salmon) S.C. daily
- 8 IU somatropin S.C. three times a week.

Milliequivalents

Electrolytes may be measured in milliequivalents (mEq). Drug manufacturers provide information about the number of metric units required to provide a prescribed number of milliequivalents. Potassium chloride, for example, is usually ordered in milliequivalents.

The following are examples of drug orders using milliequivalents:
- 30 mEq KCl P.O. b.i.d.
- 1 L dextrose 5% in normal saline solution with 40 mEq KCl to be run at 125 ml/hour.

Conversions between systems of measurement

It is sometimes necessary to make conversions from one system of drug measurement to another. Conversions are necessary when a drug is ordered in one system but is available only in another system. To perform conversion calculations, the nurse needs to know the equivalent measurements for the different systems of measurement. One of the most commonly used methods for converting drug measurements is the fraction method.

Fraction method

The fraction method for converting measurements between systems involves an equation consisting of two fractions. The first fraction is set up by placing the ordered dosage over X units of the available dosage.

For example, a doctor orders 7.5 ml of acetaminophen elixir to be given by mouth. To find the equivalent in teaspoons, first set up a fraction in which the ml dosage represents the ordered dosage

and the teaspoon dosage represents the unknown (X) available dosage:

$$\frac{7.5 \text{ ml}}{X \text{ tsp}}$$

Then, set up the second fraction, which appears to the right of the equation. This fraction consists of the standard equivalents between the ordered and the available measures. Because milliliters must be converted to teaspoons, the right side of the equation appears as:

$$\frac{5 \text{ ml}}{1 \text{ tsp}}$$

The same unit of measure should appear in the numerator of both fractions. Likewise, the same unit of measure should appear in both denominators. The entire equation should appear as:

$$\frac{7.5 \text{ ml}}{X \text{ tsp}} = \frac{5 \text{ ml}}{1 \text{ tsp}}$$

To solve for X, cross multiply.

$$X \text{ tsp} \times 5 \text{ ml} = 7.5 \text{ ml} \times 1 \text{ tsp}$$

$$X \text{ tsp} = \frac{7.5 \text{ ml} \times 1 \text{ tsp}}{5 \text{ ml}}$$

$$X \text{ tsp} = \frac{7.5 \times 1 \text{ tsp}}{5}$$

$$X \text{ tsp} = 1.5 \text{ tsp}$$

The patient should receive 1.5 teaspoons of acetaminophen elixir.

Computing drug dosages

Computing drug dosages, performed after verifying a drug order, is a two-step process. First, determine whether the drug ordered is available in units within the same system of measurement. If not, then convert the measurement for the ordered drug to the system used for the available drug.

If the ordered units of measurement are available, calculate how much of the available dosage form should be administered. For example, if the prescribed dose is 250 mg, determine the quantity of tablets, powder, or liquid that would equal 250 mg. To determine that quantity, use one of the methods described below.

Fraction method

When using the fraction method to compute a drug dosage, write an equation consisting of two fractions. First, set up a fraction showing the number of units to be given over X, which represents the quantity of the dosage form.

On the other side of the equation, set up a fraction showing the number of units of the drug in its dosage form over the quantity of dosage forms that supply that number of units. The number of units and the quantity of dosage forms are specific for each drug. In most cases, the stated quantity equals 1. Information provided on the drug label should supply the details needed to form the second fraction.

For example, if the number of units to be administered equals 250 mg, the first fraction in the equation would appear as:

$$\frac{250 \text{ mg}}{X \text{ tab}}$$

The drug label states that each tablet contains 125 mg, so the second fraction would appear as:

$$\frac{125 \text{ mg}}{1 \text{ tab}}$$

Note that the same units of measure appear in the numerators and the same units appear in the denominators. Note also that the units of measure in the denominators differ from the units in the numerators.

The entire equation would appear as:

$$\frac{250 \text{ mg}}{X \text{ tab}} = \frac{125 \text{ mg}}{1 \text{ tab}}$$

Solving for X determines the quantity of the dosage form—2 tablets, in this example.

Desired-available method

The nurse can also use the desired-available method, also known as the dose-over-on hand (D/H) method. The desired-available method converts ordered units into available units and computes the drug dosage all in one step. The desired-available equation appears as:

$$\begin{array}{l} X \\ \text{quantity} \\ \text{to give} \end{array} = \frac{\begin{array}{c}\text{ordered}\\\text{units}\end{array}}{1} \times \frac{\text{conversion}}{\text{fraction}} \times \frac{\begin{array}{c}\text{quantity}\\\text{of dosage}\\\text{form}\end{array}}{\begin{array}{c}\text{stated}\\\text{quantity of}\\\text{drug within}\\\text{each dosage}\\\text{form}\end{array}}$$

For example, the doctor orders gr x of a drug. The drug is available only in 300-mg tablets. To determine the number of tablets to give the patient, substitute gr x (the ordered number of units) for the first element of the equation. Then use the conversion fraction as the second portion of the formula. The conversion factor is:

$$\frac{60 \text{ mg}}{1 \text{ gr}}$$

The measure in the denominator must be the same as the measure in the ordered units. In this case, the doctor ordered gr x. As a result, grains appear in the denominator of the conversion fraction.

The third element of the equation shows the dosage form over the stated drug quantity for that dosage form. Because the drug is available in 300-mg tablets, the fraction appears as:

$$\frac{1 \text{ tab}}{300 \text{ mg}}$$

The dosage form—tablets—should always appear in the numerator, and the quantity of drug in each dosage form should always appear in the denominator. The completed equation is:

$$X \text{ tab} = 10 \text{ gr} \times \frac{60 \text{ mg}}{1 \text{ gr}} \times \frac{1 \text{ tab}}{300 \text{ mg}}$$

Solving for X shows that the patient should receive 2 tablets.

The desired-available method has the advantage of requiring only one equation.

However, it requires memorizing an equation more elaborate than the one used in the fraction method. Relying on memorization of a more complicated equation may increase the chance of error.

Special computations

The fraction and desired-available methods can be used to compute drug dosage when the ordered drug and the available form of the drug occur in the same units of measure. The two methods can also be used when the quantity of a particular dosage form differs from the units in which the dosage form is administered.

For example, if a patient is to receive 1,000 mg of a drug available in liquid form and measured in milligrams, with 100 mg contained in 6 ml, how many milliliters should the patient receive? Because the ordered and the available dosages occur in milligrams, no initial conversions need to be made. The fraction method would be used to determine the number of milliliters the patient should receive, in this case, 60 ml.

Because the drug is to be administered in ounces, the number of ounces needed should be determined using a conversion method. For the fraction method of conversion, the equation would appear as:

$$\frac{60 \text{ ml}}{X \text{ oz}} = \frac{30 \text{ ml}}{1 \text{ oz}}$$

Solving for X indicates that the patient would receive 2 oz of the drug.

To use the desired-available method, change the order of the elements in the equation to correspond with the situation. The revised equation should appear as:

$$\frac{X}{\substack{\text{quantity} \\ \text{to give}}} = \frac{\substack{\text{ordered} \\ \text{units}}}{1} \times \frac{\substack{\text{quantity} \\ \text{of dosage} \\ \text{form} \\ \text{stated} \\ \text{quantity of} \\ \text{drug within} \\ \text{each dosage} \\ \text{form}}}{} \times \substack{\text{conversion} \\ \text{fraction}}$$

Placing the given information into the equation results in:

$$X \text{ oz} = \frac{1,000 \text{ mg}}{1} \times \frac{6 \text{ ml}}{100 \text{ mg}} \times \frac{1 \text{ oz}}{30 \text{ ml}}$$

Solving for X indicates that the patient should receive 2 oz of the drug.

Inexact nature of dosage computations

Converting drug measurements from one system to another and then determining the amount of a dosage form to give can easily produce inexact dosages. A rounding error made during computation or discrepancies in the dosage to give may occur, depending on the conversion standard used in calculation. The nurse may determine a precise amount to be given, only to find that administering that amount is impossible. For example, precise computations may indicate that a patient should receive 0.97 tablet. Administering such an amount is impossible.

The following general rule helps avoid calculation errors and discrepancies between theoretical and real dosages: *No more than 10% variation should exist between the dosage ordered and the dosage to be given.* Following this simple rule, a nurse who determines that a patient should receive 0.97 tablet could permissibly give 1 tablet.

Computing parenteral dosages

The methods for computing drug dosages can be used not just for oral but also for parenteral routes. The following example shows how to determine drug dosages to be given by a parenteral route.

A doctor orders 75 mg of Demerol. The package label reads: meperidine (Demerol), 100 mg/ml. Using the fraction method to determine the number of milliliters the patient should receive, the equation should appear as:

$$\frac{75 \text{ mg}}{X \text{ ml}} = \frac{100 \text{ mg}}{1 \text{ ml}}$$

To solve for X, cross multiply:

$$X \text{ ml} \times 100 \text{ mg} = 75 \text{ mg} \times 1 \text{ ml}$$

$$X \text{ ml} = \frac{75 \text{ mg} \times 1 \text{ ml}}{100 \text{ mg}}$$

$$X \text{ ml} = \frac{75 \times 1 \text{ ml}}{100}$$

$$X \text{ ml} = 0.75 \text{ ml}$$

The patient should receive 0.75 ml.

Reconstituting powders for injection

Although the pharmacist usually reconstitutes powders for parenteral use, nurses sometimes perform this function. When reconstituting powders for injection, consult the drug label for the needed information. The label gives the total quantity of drug in the vial or ampule, the amount and type of diluent to be added to the powder, and the strength and expiration date of the resulting solution.

When diluent is added to a powder, the powder increases the fluid volume. Therefore, the label will call for less diluent than the total volume of the prepared solution. For example, a label may call for adding 1.7 ml of diluent to a vial of powdered drug to obtain a 2-ml total volume of prepared solution. Reconstituting a powdered drug requires following the directions on the drug label.

To determine the amount of solution to administer, use the manufacturer's information about the concentration of the solution. For example, to administer 500 mg of a drug and the concentration of the prepared solution is 1 g (1,000 mg)/10 ml, the following equation applies:

$$\frac{500 \text{ mg}}{X \text{ ml}} = \frac{1,000 \text{ mg}}{10 \text{ ml}}$$

The patient would receive 5 ml of the prepared solution.

I.V. drip rates and flow rates

A nurse must know the difference between I.V. drip rate and flow rate and also how to calculate each rate. I.V. drip rate refers to the number of drops of solution to be infused per minute. Flow rate refers to the number of milliliters of fluid to be infused over 1 hour.

To calculate I.V. drip rate, first set up a fraction showing the volume of solution to be delivered over the number of minutes in which that volume is to be infused. For example, if a patient is to receive 100 ml of solution within 1 hour, the fraction would be written as:

$$\frac{100 \text{ ml}}{60 \text{ min}}$$

Multiply the fraction by the drip factor (the number of drops [gtt] contained in 1 ml) to determine the number of drops per minute to be infused, or the drip rate. The drip factor varies among different I.V. sets and should appear on the package containing the I.V. tubing administration set.

Following the manufacturer's directions for drip factor is a crucial step. Standard administration sets have drip factors of 10, 15, or 20 drops/ml. A microdrip, or minidrip, set has a drip factor of 60 drops/ml.

Use the following equation to determine the drip rate of an I.V. solution:

$$\text{gtt/min} = \frac{\text{total no. of ml}}{\text{total no. of min}} \times \frac{\text{drip}}{\text{factor}}$$

The equation applies to I.V. solutions that infuse over many hours or to small-volume infusions such as those used for antibiotics, usually administered in less than 1 hour. For example, if an order requires 1,000 ml of 5% dextrose in normal saline solution to infuse over 12 hours and the administration set delivers 15 gtt per ml, what should the drip rate be?

$$X \text{ gtt/min} = \frac{1,000 \text{ ml}}{720 \text{ min}} \times 15 \text{ gtt/ml}$$

$$X \text{ gtt/min} = 20.83 \text{ gtt/min}$$

The drip rate would be rounded to 21 gtt per minute.

Flow rate calculations are used when working with I.V. infusion pumps to set the number of milliliters to be delivered in 1 hour. To perform this calculation, the nurse should know the total volume in milliliters to be infused and the amount of time for the infusion. Use the following equation:

$$\text{flow rate} = \frac{\text{total volume ordered}}{\text{number of hours}}$$

Quick methods for calculating drip rates

There are quicker methods for computing I.V. solution administration rates. To administer I.V. solutions through a microdrip set, adjust the flow rate (number of milliliters per hour) to equal the drip rate (number of drops per minute).

If the nurse used the above method, the flow rate would be divided by 60 minutes and then multiplied by the drip factor, which also equals 60. Because the flow rate and the drip factor are equal, the two arithmetic operations cancel each other out. For example, if 125 ml/hour represented the ordered flow rate, the equation would be:

$$\text{drip rate (125)} = \frac{125 \text{ ml}}{60 \text{ min}} \times 60$$

Rather than spend time calculating the equation, the nurse can use the number assigned to the flow rate as the drip rate.

For I.V. solution administration sets that deliver 15 drops/ml, the flow rate divided by 4 equals the drip rate. For sets with a drip factor of 10, the flow rate divided by 6 equals the drip rate.

Critical care calculations

Many drugs given on the critical care unit are used to treat life-threatening problems; nurses must be able to swiftly and accurately do the calculations, prepare the drug for infusion, administer it, and then observe the patient closely to evaluate the drug's effectiveness.

Three calculations must be performed before administering critical care drugs:
• establish the concentration of the drug in the I.V. solution
• determine the flow rate required to deliver the desired dose

• figure the number of micrograms needed, based on the patient's weight in kilograms. This calculation is done if the drug is ordered in micrograms per kilogram of body weight per minute. *To convert milligrams to micrograms, multiply by 1,000.*

Calculating concentration

To calculate the drug's concentration, use the following formula:

$$\text{concentration in mg/ml} = \frac{\text{mg of drug/ml}}{\text{of fluid}}$$

To express the concentration in mcg/ml, multiply the answer by 1,000.

Figuring flow rate

To determine the I.V. flow rate per minute, use the following formula:

$$\frac{\text{dose/min}}{X \text{ ml/min}} = \frac{\text{concentration of solution}}{1 \text{ ml of fluid}}$$

To calculate the hourly flow rate, first multiply the ordered dose, given in milligrams or micrograms per minute, by 60 minutes to determine the hourly dose. Then use the following equation to compute the hourly flow rate:

$$\frac{\text{hourly dose}}{X \text{ ml/hr}} = \frac{\text{concentration of solution}}{1 \text{ ml of fluid}}$$

Determining the dosage

To determine the dosage in milligrams per kilogram of body weight per minute, first determine the concentration of the solution in milligrams per milliliter. To determine the dose in milligrams per hour, multiply the hourly flow rate by the concentration using the formula:

$$\text{Dose in mg/hr} = \text{hourly flow rate} \times \text{concentration}$$

Then calculate the dose in milligrams per minute. Divide the hourly dose by 60 minutes:

$$\text{dose in mg/min} = \frac{\text{dose in mg/hr}}{60 \text{ min}}$$

Divide the dose per minute by the patient's weight, using the following formula:

$$mg/kg/min = \frac{mg/min}{patient's\ weight\ in\ kg}$$

Finally, make sure that the drug is being given within a safe and therapeutic range. Compare the amount in milligrams per kilogram per minute to the safe range shown in a drug reference book.

The following examples show how to calculate an I.V. flow rate using the different formulas.

Example 1

A patient has frequent runs of ventricular tachycardia that subside after 10 to 12 beats. The doctor orders 2 g (2,000 mg) of lidocaine in 500 ml of D_5W to infuse at 2 mg/minute. What is the flow rate in milliliters per minute? In milliliters per hour?

First, find the solution's concentration by setting up a proportion with the unknown concentration in one fraction and the ordered dose in the other fraction:

$$\frac{X\ mg}{1\ ml} = \frac{2,000\ mg}{500\ ml}$$

Cross multiply the fractions:

$$X\ mg \times 500\ ml = 2,000\ mg \times 1\ ml$$

Solve for X by dividing each side of the equation by 500 ml and canceling units that appear in both the numerator and denominator:

$$\frac{X\ mg \times \cancel{500\ ml}}{\cancel{500\ ml}} = \frac{2,000\ mg \times 1\ \cancel{ml}}{500\ \cancel{ml}}$$

$$X = \frac{2,000\ mg}{500}$$

$$X = 4\ mg$$

The solution's concentration is 4 mg/ml. Next, calculate the flow rate per minute needed to deliver the ordered dose of 2 mg/minute. To do this, set up a proportion with the unknown flow rate per minute in one fraction and the solution's concentration in the other fraction:

$$\frac{2\ mg}{X\ ml} = \frac{4\ mg}{1\ ml}$$

Cross multiply the fractions:

$$X\ ml \times 4\ mg = 1\ ml \times 2\ mg$$

Solve for X by dividing each side of the equation by 4 mg and canceling units that appear in both the numerator and denominator:

$$\frac{X\ ml \times \cancel{4\ mg}}{\cancel{4\ mg}} = \frac{1\ ml \times 2\ \cancel{mg}}{4\ \cancel{mg}}$$

$$X = \frac{2\ ml}{4}$$

$$X = 0.5\ ml$$

The patient should receive 0.5 ml/minute of lidocaine. Because lidocaine must be administered through an infusion pump, compute the hourly flow rate. Set up a proportion with the unknown flow rate per hour in one fraction and the flow rate per minute in the other fraction:

$$\frac{X\ ml}{60\ min} = \frac{0.5\ ml}{1\ min}$$

Cross multiply the fractions:

$$X\ ml \times 1\ min = 0.5\ ml \times 60\ min$$

Solve for X by dividing each side of the equation by 1 minute and canceling units that appear in both the numerator and denominator:

$$\frac{X\ ml \times 1\ \cancel{min}}{1\ \cancel{min}} = \frac{0.5\ ml \times 60\ \cancel{min}}{1\ \cancel{min}}$$

$$X = 30\ ml$$

Set the infusion pump to deliver 30 ml/ hour.

Example 2

A 200-lb patient is to receive an I.V. infusion of dobutamine at 10 mcg/kg/minute. The package insert says to dilute 250 mg of the drug in 50 ml of D_5W.

Because the drug vial contains 20 ml of solution, the total to be infused is 70 ml (50 ml of D_5W plus 20 ml of solution). How many micrograms of the drug should the patient receive each minute? Each hour?

First, compute the patient's weight in kilograms. To do this, set up a proportion with the weight in pounds and the unknown weight in kilograms in one fraction and the number of pounds per kilogram in the other fraction:

$$\frac{200 \text{ lb}}{X \text{ kg}} = \frac{2.2 \text{ lb}}{1 \text{ kg}}$$

Cross-multiply the fractions:

$$X \text{ kg} \times 2.2 \text{ lb} = 1 \text{ kg} \times 200 \text{ lb}$$

Solve for X by dividing each side of the equation by 2.2 lb and canceling units that appear in both the numerator and denominator.

$$\frac{X \text{ kg} \times \cancel{2.2 \text{ lb}}}{\cancel{2.2 \text{ lb}}} = \frac{1 \text{ kg} \times 200 \cancel{\text{ lb}}}{2.2 \cancel{\text{ lb}}}$$

$$X = \frac{200 \text{ kg}}{2.2}$$

$$X = 90.9 \text{ kg}$$

The patient weighs 90.9 kg. Next, determine the dose in micrograms per minute by setting up a proportion with the patient's weight in kilograms and the unknown dose in micrograms per minute in one fraction and the known dose in micrograms per kilogram per minute in the other fraction:

$$\frac{90.9 \text{ kg}}{X \text{ mcg/min}} = \frac{1 \text{ kg}}{10 \text{ mcg/min}}$$

Cross-multiply the fractions:

$$X \text{ mcg/min} \times 1 \text{ kg} = 10 \text{ mcg/min} \times 90.9 \text{ kg}$$

Solve for X by dividing each side of the equation by 1 kg and canceling units that appear in both the numerator and denominator:

$$\frac{X \text{ mcg/min} \times \cancel{1 \text{ kg}}}{\cancel{1 \text{ kg}}} = \frac{10 \text{ mcg/min} \times 90.9 \cancel{\text{ kg}}}{\cancel{1 \text{ kg}}}$$

$$X = 909 \text{ mcg/min}$$

The patient should receive 909 mcg of dobutamine every minute. Finally, determine the hourly dose by multiplying the dose per minute by 60:

$$909 \text{ mcg/min} \times 60 \text{ min/hr} = 54{,}540 \text{ mcg/hr}$$

The patient should receive 54,540 mcg of dobutamine every hour.

Pediatric dosage considerations

To determine the correct pediatric dosage of a drug, doctors, pharmacists, and nurses usually use two computation methods. One is based on the child's weight in kilograms; the other uses the child's body surface area. Other methods are less accurate and are not recommended.

Dosage range per kilogram of body weight

Currently, many pharmaceutical companies provide information on the safe dosage ranges for drugs given to children. The companies usually provide the dosage ranges in milligrams per kilogram of body weight and, in many cases, give similar information for adult dosage ranges. The following example and explanation indicate how to calculate the safe pediatric dosage range for a drug, using the company's suggested safe dosage range provided in milligrams per kilogram.

For a pediatric patient, a doctor orders a drug with a suggested dosage range of 10 to 12 mg/kg of body weight/day. The child weighs 12 kg. What is the safe daily dosage range for the child?

The nurse must calculate the lower and upper limits of the dosage range provided by the manufacturer. The nurse first calculates the dosage based on 10 mg/kg of body weight, then calculates the dosage based on 12 mg/kg of body weight. The answers represent the lower and upper limits of the daily dosage range, expressed in mg/kg of the child's weight.

Body surface area

A second method for calculating safe pediatric dosages uses the child's body surface area as a factor. This method may provide a more accurate calculation because the child's body surface area is thought to parallel the child's organ growth and maturation and metabolic rate.

The nurse determines the body surface area of a child by using a three-column chart called a nomogram (see *Estimating surface area in children* in the appendix section). The nurse marks the child's height in the first column and the child's weight in the third column, then draws a line between the two marks. The point at which the line intersects the vertical scale in the second column indicates the estimated body surface area of the child in square meters. To calculate the child's approximate dose, the nurse uses the body surface area measurement in the following equation:

$$\frac{\text{body surface area of child}}{\substack{\text{average adult} \\ \text{body surface area} \\ (1.73 \text{ m}^2)}} \times \text{average adult dose} = \text{child's dose}$$

The following example illustrates the use of the equation. Using a nomogram, the nurse finds that a 25-lb (11.3-kg) child who is 33 inches (84 cm) tall has a body surface area of 0.52 m². To determine the child's dose of a drug with an average adult dose of 100 mg, the equation would appear as:

$$\frac{0.52 \text{ m}^2}{1.73 \text{ m}^2} \times 100 \text{ mg} = \frac{30.06 \text{ mg}}{\text{(child's dose)}}$$

The child should receive 30 mg of the drug.

Other rules

Clark's rule, Fried's rule, and Young's rule are other methods used to calculate a pediatric dosage. These rules are based on the average adult dose, and their results are approximate. Thus, calculating with equations other than those involving dosage ranges per kilogram of body weight or body surface area is not recommended for determining dosages.

Many institutions have guidelines that determine the acceptable calculation method. Nurses in pediatric settings must familiarize themselves with their institutional policy about pediatric dosages.

3

Drug administration

Whenever a drug is administered, observe the following precautions to ensure that the right drug is given in the right dose to the right patient at the right time by the right route. Use standard precautions, as appropriate, to each patient and type of drug.

Check the order
Check the order on the patient's medication record against the doctor's order.

Check the label
Check the label on the drug three times before administering it to be sure the prescribed drug is being administered in the prescribed dose:
1. Check the label when the container is taken from the shelf or drawer.
2. Check the label right before pouring the drug into the medication cup or drawing it into the syringe.
3. Check the label before returning the container to the shelf or drawer.

If a unit-dose drug is being administered, check the label for the third time immediately after pouring the drug and again before discarding the wrapper. (Unit-dose drug containers should be opened at the patient's bedside.)

Confirm the patient's identity
Before giving the drug, ask the patient his name and confirm his identity by checking his name, room number, and bed number on his wristband. Check again that you have the correct drug.

Always explain the procedure to the patient, and provide privacy.

Have a written order
Make sure there is a written order for every drug given. Verbal orders should be signed by the doctor within the specified time period.

Give labeled drugs
Don't administer a drug from a poorly labeled or unlabeled container. Also, don't attempt to label or reinforce drug labels; this must be done by a pharmacist.

Monitor drugs
• Never give a drug poured or prepared by someone else.
• Never allow the medication cart or tray out of your sight.
• Never leave a drug at the patient's bedside.
• Never return unwrapped or prepared drugs to stock containers; instead, dispose of them, and notify the pharmacy.

Respond to patients' questions
If the patient questions you about his drug or the dosage, check his medication record again. If the drug is correct, reassure him. Tell the patient about changes in his drug or dosage. Instruct him, as appropriate, about possible adverse reactions. Ask him to report anything that he feels may be an adverse reaction.

Topical administration
Topical drugs, such as lotions and ointments, are applied directly to the skin. They're commonly used for local, rather than systemic, effects. Typically, they must be applied two or three times a day for full therapeutic effect.

Equipment
Gather the patient's medication record and chart, prescribed drug, sterile tongue blades, gloves, sterile gloves for open lesions, sterile 4″ × 4″ gauze pads, trans-

parent semipermeable dressing, adhesive tape, solvent (such as cottonseed oil), cotton-tipped applicators, cotton gloves, and terry cloth scuffs, if necessary.

Implementation
• Explain the procedure to the patient because, after discharge, he may have to apply the drug by himself.
• Wash your hands to prevent cross-contamination, and glove your dominant hand.
• Help the patient to a comfortable position, and expose the area to be treated. Make sure the skin or mucous membrane is intact (unless the drug has been ordered to treat a skin lesion). Application of drug to broken or abraded skin may cause unwanted systemic absorption and result in further irritation.
• If necessary, clean the skin of debris. You may have to change the glove if it becomes soiled.

To apply paste, cream, or ointment
• Open the container. Place the cap upside down to avoid contaminating its inner surface.
• Remove a tongue blade from its sterile wrapper, and cover one end of it with drug from the tube or jar. Then transfer the drug from the tongue blade to your gloved hand.
• Apply the drug to the affected area with long, smooth strokes that follow the direction of hair growth, at top right. This technique avoids forcing drug into hair follicles, which can cause irritation and lead to folliculitis. Avoid excessive pressure when applying the drug because it could abrade the skin or cause the patient discomfort.
• When applying drug to the patient's face, use cotton-tipped applicators for small areas, such as under the eyes. For larger areas, use a sterile gauze pad.
• To prevent contamination of the drug, use a new sterile tongue blade each time you remove drug from the container.
• Remove gloves and wash hands.

To remove ointment
• Wash hands and put on gloves. Gently swab ointment from the patient's skin using a sterile 4″ × 4″ gauze pad saturated with a solvent such as cottonseed oil.
• Remove any remaining oil by wiping the area with a clean sterile gauze pad. Don't wipe too hard because you could irritate the skin.
• Remove gloves and wash hands.

Nursing considerations
• To prevent skin irritation from an accumulation of drug, never apply drug without first removing previous applications.
• Always wear gloves to prevent absorption by your skin.
• Never apply ointment to the eyelids or ear canal unless ordered. The ointment may congeal and occlude the tear duct or ear canal.
• Inspect the treated area frequently for any adverse (for instance, allergic) reaction.

Oral administration
Because oral drug administration is usually the safest, most convenient, and least expensive, most drugs are administered by this method. Drugs for oral administration are available in many forms: tablets, enteric-coated tablets, capsules, syrups, elixirs, oils, liquids, suspensions, powders, and granules. Some require special preparation before administration, such as mixing with juice to make them more palatable.

Oral drugs are sometimes prescribed in higher dosages than their parenteral equivalents, because after absorption through the GI system, they are broken down by the liver before they reach the systemic circulation.

Equipment
Gather the patient's medication record and chart, prescribed drug, and medication cup. Other materials that may be used include an appropriate vehicle (such as jelly or applesauce) for crushed pills common-

ly used with children or elderly patients, or juice, water, or milk for liquid drugs; and mortar and pestle for crushing pills.

Implementation
• Wash your hands.
• Assess the patient's condition, including level of consciousness and vital signs, as needed. Changes in the patient's condition may warrant withholding the drug.
• Give the patient the drug and, as needed, an appropriate vehicle or liquid to aid swallowing, minimize adverse effects, or promote absorption. If appropriate, crush the drug to facilitate swallowing.
• Stay with the patient until he has swallowed the drug. If he seems confused or disoriented, check his mouth to make sure he has swallowed it. Return and reassess the patient's response within 1 hour after giving the drug.

Nursing considerations
• To avoid damaging or staining the patient's teeth, give acid or iron preparations through a straw. An unpleasant-tasting liquid can usually be made more palatable if taken through a straw because the liquid contacts fewer taste buds.
• If the patient can't swallow a whole tablet or capsule, ask the pharmacist if the drug is available in liquid form or if it can be administered by another route. If not, ask the pharmacist if the tablet can be crushed or if capsules can be opened and mixed with food.
• Do not crush buccal or sublingual tablets. Do not crush enteric-coated or sustained-action drugs.

Buccal and sublingual administration
Certain drugs are given buccally (between the patient's cheek and teeth) or sublingually (under the patient's tongue) to bypass the digestive tract and facilitate their absorption into the bloodstream.

Drugs given buccally include erythrityl tetranitrate. Drugs given sublingually include ergotamine tartrate, erythrityl

tetranitrate, isoproterenol hydrochloride, isosorbide dinitrate, and nitroglycerin. When using either administration method, observe the patient carefully to ensure that he doesn't swallow the drug or suffer mucosal irritation.

Equipment
Gather the patient's medication record and chart, prescribed drug, medication cup, and gloves.

Implementation
• Wash your hands. Put on gloves if you are placing the drug into the patient's mouth.
• For buccal administration, place the tablet in the patient's buccal pouch, between the cheek and teeth.

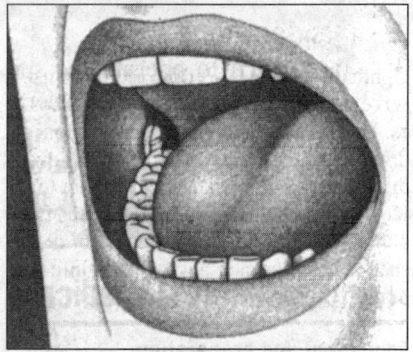

• For sublingual administration, place the tablet under the patient's tongue.

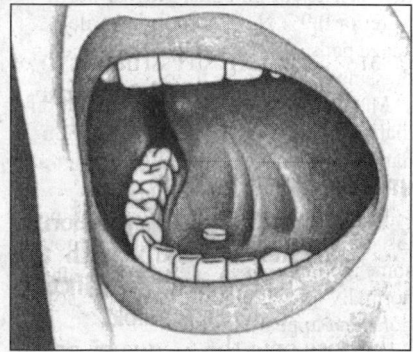

• Remove gloves and wash hands.
• Instruct the patient to keep the drug in place until it dissolves completely to ensure absorption. Caution the patient against chewing the tablet or touching it with his tongue to prevent accidental swallowing.
• Tell the patient not to smoke before the drug has dissolved because the vasoconstrictive effects of nicotine slow absorption.

Nursing considerations
• Don't give liquids because some buccal tablets may take up to 1 hour to be absorbed.
• Tell the patient with angina to wet the nitroglycerin tablet with saliva and to keep it under his tongue until it's fully absorbed.

Ophthalmic administration

Ophthalmic drugs—drops or ointments—serve diagnostic and therapeutic purposes. During an ophthalmic examination, drugs can be used to anesthetize the eye, dilate the pupil, and stain the cornea to identify anomalies. Therapeutic uses include eye lubrication and treatment of such conditions as glaucoma and infections.

Equipment and preparation
Gather the patient's medication record and chart, prescribed ophthalmic medication, sterile cotton balls, gloves, warm water or 0.9% NaCl solution, sterile gauze pads, and facial tissue. An ocular dressing may also be used.

Make sure the drug is labeled for ophthalmic use. Then check the expiration date. Remember to date the container after first use.

Inspect ocular solutions for cloudiness, discoloration, and precipitation, although some medications are suspensions and normally appear cloudy. Don't use solutions that appear abnormal.

Implementation
• Make sure you know which eye to treat because different drugs or doses may be ordered for each eye.
• Put on gloves.
• If the patient has an eye dressing, remove it by pulling it down and away from his forehead. Avoid contaminating your hands. Do not apply pressure to the area around the eyes.
• To remove exudates or meibomian gland secretions, clean around the eye with sterile cotton balls or sterile gauze pads moistened with warm water or 0.9% NaCl solution. Have the patient close his eye; then gently wipe eyelids from the inner to outer canthus. Use a fresh cotton ball or gauze pad for each stroke and use a different cotton ball or pad for each eye.
• Have the patient sit or lie in the supine position. Instruct him to tilt his head back and toward his affected eye so that excess drug can flow away from the tear duct, minimizing systemic absorption through nasal mucosa.
• Remove the dropper cap from the drug container, and draw the drug into it.
• Before instilling eyedrops, instruct the patient to look up and away. This moves the cornea away from the lower lid and minimizes the risk of touching it with the dropper.

To instill eyedrops
• Steady the hand that's holding the dropper by resting it against the patient's forehead. With your other hand, gently pull down the lower lid of the affected eye and instill the drops in the conjunctival sac. Never instill eyedrops directly onto the eyeball.
• When teaching elderly patients how to instill eyedrops, keep in mind that they may have difficulty sensing drops in the eye. Suggest chilling the drug slightly so that the cold drops enhance placement sensation.

To apply eye ointment

• Squeeze a small ribbon of drug on the edge of the conjunctival sac from the inner to the outer canthus. Cut off the ribbon by turning the tube. Do not touch the eye with the tip of the tube.

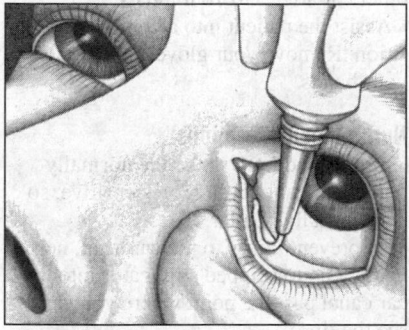

• After instilling eyedrops or applying ointment, instruct the patient to close his eyes gently, without squeezing the lids shut. If drops were instilled, tell the patient to blink. If ointment was applied, tell him to roll his eyes behind closed lids to help distribute the drug over the eyeball.
• Use a clean tissue to remove any excess drug leaking from the eye. Use a fresh tissue for each eye to prevent cross-contamination.
• Apply a new eye dressing, if necessary.
• Remove and discard gloves. Wash your hands.

Nursing considerations

• When administering an eye medication that may be absorbed systemically, gently press your thumb on the inner canthus for 1 to 2 minutes after instillation while the patient closes his eyes. Avoid applying pressure around the eye.
• To maintain the drug container's sterility, do not put the cap down once opening the container and never touch the tip of the dropper or bottle to the eye area. Discard any solution remaining in the dropper before returning it to the bottle. If the dropper or bottle tip has become contaminated, discard it and use another

sterile dropper. Never share eye drops from patient to patient.

Otic administration

Eardrops may be instilled to treat infection and inflammation, to soften cerumen for later removal, to produce local anesthesia, or to facilitate removal of an insect trapped in the ear.

Equipment and preparation

Gather the patient's medication record and chart, prescribed eardrops, gloves, light source, and facial tissue or cotton-tipped applicator. Cotton balls and a bowl of warm water may be needed.

First, warm the drug to body temperature in the bowl of warm water, or carry the drug in your pocket for 30 minutes before administration. If necessary, test the temperature of the drug by placing a drop on your wrist. (If the drug is too hot, it may burn the patient's eardrum.) To avoid injuring the ear canal, check the dropper before use to make sure it's not chipped or cracked.

Implementation

• Wash your hands and put on clean gloves.
• Confirm the patient's identity by asking his name and checking the name and room and bed number on his wristband.
• Have the patient lie on the side opposite the affected ear.

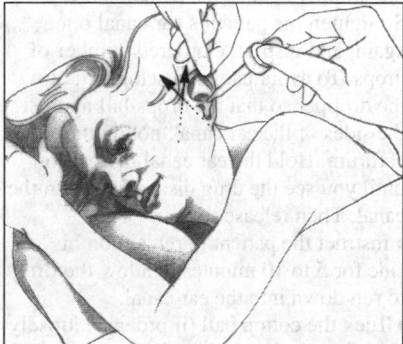

• Straighten the patient's ear canal. For an adult, pull the auricle up and back. For an infant or child younger than age 3 years, gently pull the auricle down and back, because the ear canal is straighter at this age.

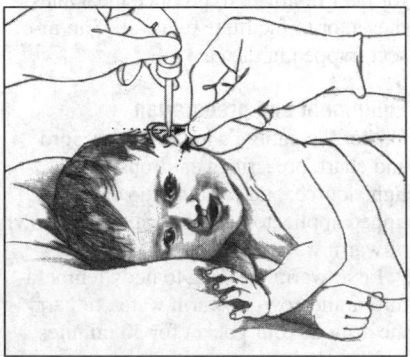

• Using a light source, examine the ear canal for drainage. If there is drainage, gently clean the canal with the tissue or cotton-tipped applicator because drainage can reduce the effectiveness of the drug. Never insert the applicator past the point where it can be seen.

• Compare the label on the eardrops to the order on the patient's medication record. Check the label again while drawing the drug into the dropper. Check the label for the final time before returning the eardrops to the shelf or drawer.

• To avoid damaging the ear canal with the dropper, gently rest the hand holding the dropper against the patient's head. Straighten the patient's ear canal once again, and instill the ordered number of drops. To avoid patient discomfort, aim the dropper so that the drops fall against the sides of the ear canal, not on the eardrum. Hold the ear canal in position until you see the drug disappear down the canal. Then release the ear.

• Instruct the patient to remain on his side for 5 to 10 minutes to allow the drug to run down into the ear canal.

• Tuck the cotton ball (if ordered) loosely into the opening of the ear canal to prevent the drug from leaking out. Be care-

ful not to insert it too deeply into the canal because this would prevent drainage of secretions and increase pressure on the eardrum.

• Clean and dry the outer ear.

• If ordered, repeat the procedure in the other ear after 5 to 10 minutes.

• Assist the patient into a comfortable position. Remove your gloves, and wash your hands.

Nursing considerations

• Some conditions make the normally tender ear canal even more sensitive, so be especially gentle.

• To prevent injury to the eardrum, never insert a cotton-tipped applicator into the ear canal past the point where you can see the tip.

• After applying eardrops to soften cerumen, irrigate the ear as ordered to facilitate its removal. If the patient has vertigo, keep the side rails of his bed up and assist him as necessary during the procedure. Also, move slowly and unhurriedly to avoid exacerbating his vertigo.

• If necessary, teach the patient to instill the eardrops correctly so that he can continue treatment at home. Review the procedure and let the patient try it himself while you observe.

Respiratory administration

Hand-held oropharyngeal inhalers include the metered-dose inhaler and the turbo-inhaler. These devices deliver topical drugs to the respiratory tract, producing local and systemic effects. The mucosal lining of the respiratory tract absorbs the inhalant almost immediately. Examples of inhalants are bronchodilators, used to improve airway patency and facilitate mucous drainage, and mucolytics, which liquefy tenacious bronchial secretions.

Equipment

Gather the patient's medication record and chart, metered-dose inhaler or turbo-inhaler, prescribed drug, and 0.9% NaCl solution.

Implementation

To use a metered-dose inhaler, follow the instructions given below:

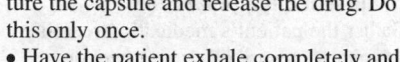

• Shake the inhaler bottle. Remove the cap and insert the stem into the small hole on the flattened portion of the mouthpiece, as shown.
• Have the patient exhale. Place the inhaler about 1″ (2.5 cm) in front of his open mouth.
• As you push the bottle down against the mouthpiece, instruct the patient to inhale slowly through his mouth and to continue inhaling until his lungs feel full. Compress the bottle against the mouthpiece only once.
• Remove the inhaler and tell the patient to hold his breath for several seconds. Then instruct him to exhale slowly through pursed lips to keep distal bronchioles open, allowing increased absorption and diffusion of the drug.
• Have the patient gargle with 0.9% NaCl solution, if desired, to remove drug from the mouth and back of the throat.

To use a turbo-inhaler

• Hold the mouthpiece in one hand. With the other hand, slide the sleeve away from the mouthpiece as far as possible, as shown.
• Unscrew the tip of the mouthpiece by turning it counterclockwise.
• Press the colored portion of the drug capsule into the propeller stem of the mouthpiece. Screw the inhaler together again.
• Holding the inhaler with the mouthpiece at the bottom, slide the sleeve all the way down and then up again to puncture the capsule and release the drug. Do this only once.
• Have the patient exhale completely and tilt his head back. Instruct him to place the mouthpiece in his mouth, close his lips around it, and inhale once. Tell him to hold his breath for several seconds.
• Remove the inhaler from the patient's mouth and tell him to exhale as much air as possible.
• Repeat the procedure until all the drug in the device is inhaled.
• Have the patient gargle with 0.9% NaCl solution, if desired.

Nursing considerations

• Teach the patient how to use the inhaler so that he can continue treatments after discharge, if necessary. Explain that overdosage can cause the drug to lose its effectiveness. Tell him to record the date and time of each inhalation and his response.
• Be aware that some oral respiratory drugs may cause restlessness, palpitations, nervousness, and other systemic effects. They can also cause hypersensitivity reactions, such as rash, urticaria, or bronchospasm.
• Administer oral respiratory drugs cautiously to patients with heart disease because these drugs may potentiate coronary insufficiency, cardiac arrhythmias, or hypertension. If paradoxical bronchospasm occurs, discontinue the drug and call the doctor to prescribe another drug.
• If the patient is ordered a bronchodilator and a steroid, give the bronchodilator first to open the air passages for maximum effectiveness.

Nasogastric administration

Besides providing an alternate means of nourishment, the nasogastric (NG) tube allows direct instillation of drug into the GI system of patients who can't ingest it orally.

Equipment and preparation

Gather the patient's medication record and chart, prescribed drug, towel or linen-saver pad, 50- or 60-ml piston-type catheter-tip syringe, feeding tubing, two 4″ × 4″ gauze pads, stethoscope, gloves, diluent (juice, water, or a nutritional supplement), cup for mixing drug and fluid, spoon, 50-ml cup of water, and rubber band. Pill-crushing equipment and a clamp (if not already attached to tube) also may be needed.

Gather equipment for use at bedside. Liquids should be at room temperature to avoid abdominal cramping. Make sure the cup, syringe, spoon, and gauze are clean.

Implementation

• Wash your hands and put on gloves.
• Unpin the tube from the patient's gown. To avoid soiling the sheets during the procedure, fold back the bed linens and drape the patient's chest with a towel or linen-saver pad.
• Help the patient into Fowler's position, if his condition allows.
• After unclamping the tube, auscultate the patient's abdomen about 3″ (8 cm) below the sternum, as you gently insert 10 ml of air into the tube with the 50- or 60-ml syringe. You should hear the air bubble entering the stomach. Gently draw back on the piston of the syringe. The appearance of gastric contents implies that the tube is patent and in the stomach.
• If no gastric contents appear or if you meet resistance, the tube may be lying against the gastric mucosa. Withdraw the tube slightly, or turn the patient to free it.
• Clamp the tube, detach the syringe, and lay the end of the tube on the 4″ × 4″ gauze pad.
• If the drug is in tablet form, crush it before mixing with the diluent. (Make sure the particles are small enough to pass through the eyes at the distal end of the tube.) Open capsules and pour them into

the diluent. Pour liquid drugs into the diluent and stir well.
• Reattach the syringe, without the piston, to the end of the tube. Holding the tube upright at a level slightly above the patient's nose, open the clamp and pour in the drug slowly and steadily, as shown below.

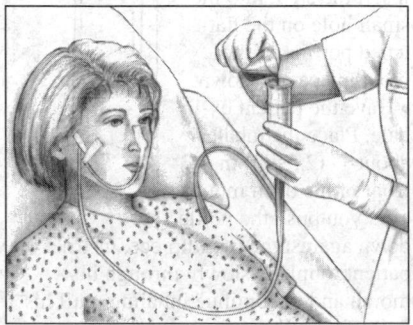

• To prevent air from entering the patient's stomach, hold the tube at a slight angle and add more drug before the syringe empties. If the drug flows smoothly, slowly give the entire dose. If it doesn't flow, it may be too thick. If so, dilute it with water. If you suspect tube placement is inhibiting flow, stop the procedure, and reevaluate the placement.
• Watch the patient's reaction. Stop immediately if she shows signs of discomfort.
• As the last of the drug flows out of the syringe, start to irrigate the tube by adding 30 to 50 ml of water (15 to 30 ml for a child). Irrigation clears drug from the tube and reduces the risk of clogging.
• When the water stops flowing, clamp the tube. Detach the syringe, and discard it properly.
• Fasten the tube to the patient's gown and make the patient comfortable.
• Leave the patient in Fowler's position, or on her right side with her head partially elevated, for at least 30 minutes to facilitate flow and prevent esophageal reflux.
• Remove and discard gloves and wash your hands.

Nursing considerations

• If you must give a tube feeding as well as instill drug, give the drug first to ensure that the patient receives it all.
• Know that certain drugs such as dilantin bind with tube feeding, decreasing the availability of the drug. Tube feeding should be stopped for 2 hours before and after dose, according to institutional policy.
• If residual stomach contents exceed 150 ml, withhold the drug and feeding, and notify the doctor. Excessive contents may indicate intestinal obstruction or paralytic ileus.
• Never crush buccal, sublingual, enteric-coated, or sustained-release action drugs.
• If the NG tube is on suction, turn it off for 20 to 30 minutes after giving drug.

Vaginal administration

Vaginal drugs can be inserted as topical treatment for infection, particularly *Trichomonas vaginalis* and vaginal candidiasis or inflammation. Suppositories melt when they contact the vaginal mucosa, and the drug diffuses topically.

Vaginal drugs usually come with a disposable applicator that enables placement of drug in the anterior and posterior fornices. Vaginal administration is most effective when the patient can remain lying down afterward to retain the drug.

Equipment

Gather the patient's medication record and chart, prescribed drug and applicator (if needed), gloves, water-soluble lubricant, and a small sanitary pad.

Implementation

• If possible, plan to give vaginal drugs at bedtime when the patient is recumbent.
• Wash your hands, explain the procedure to the patient, and provide privacy.
• Ask the patient to void.
• Ask the patient if she would rather insert the drug herself. If so, provide appropriate instructions. If not, proceed with the following steps.

• Help her into the lithotomy position. Drape the patient. Expose only the perineum.
• Remove the suppository from the wrapper and lubricate it with water-soluble lubricant.
• Put on gloves, and expose the vagina by spreading the labia. If discharge is observed, wash the area with several cotton balls soaked in warm, soapy water. Clean each side of the perineum and then the center, using a fresh cotton ball for each stroke. While the labia are still separated, insert the suppository about 3″ to 4″ (7.6 to 10 cm) into the vagina.

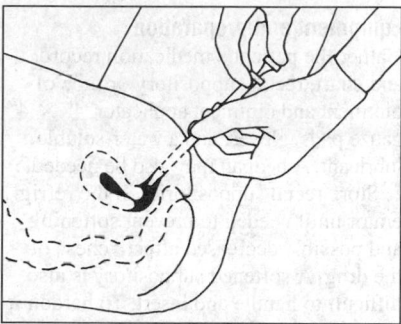

• After vaginal insertion, wash the applicator with soap and warm water and store or discard it, as appropriate. Label it so it will be used only for the same patient.
• Remove and discard your gloves.
• To prevent the drug from soiling the patient's clothing and bedding, provide a sanitary pad.
• Help the patient return to a comfortable position, and advise her to remain in bed as much as possible for the next several hours.
• Wash your hands thoroughly.

Nursing considerations

• Refrigerate vaginal suppositories that melt at room temperature.
• If possible, teach the patient how to insert vaginal drug. She may have to administer it herself after discharge. Give her a patient teaching sheet if one is available.

• Instruct the patient not to wear a tampon after inserting the drug vaginally because it would absorb the drug and decrease its effectiveness.

Rectal administration

A rectal suppository is a small, solid, medicated mass, usually cone shaped, with a cocoa butter or glycerin base. It may be inserted to stimulate peristalsis and defecation or to relieve pain, vomiting, and local irritation. An ointment is a semisolid drug used to produce local effects. It may be applied externally to the anus or internally to the rectum.

Equipment and preparation

Gather the patient's medication record and chart, rectal suppository or tube of ointment and ointment applicator, 4″ × 4″ gauze pads, gloves, and a water-soluble lubricant. A bedpan may also be needed.

Store rectal suppositories in the refrigerator until needed to prevent softening and possible decreased effectiveness of the drug. A softened suppository is also difficult to handle and insert. To harden it again, hold the suppository (in its wrapper) under cold running water.

Implementation

To insert a rectal suppository, follow the instructions given below:
• Wash your hands.
• Place the patient on his left side in Sims' position. Drape him with the bedcovers, exposing only the buttocks.
• Put on gloves. Unwrap the suppository, and lubricate it with water-soluble lubricant.
• Lift the patient's upper buttock with your nondominant hand to expose the anus.
• Instruct the patient to take several deep breaths through his mouth to relax the anal sphincter and reduce anxiety during drug insertion.
• Using the index finger of your dominant hand, insert the suppository—tapered end first—about 3″ (8 cm) until

you feel it pass the internal anal sphincter, as shown.

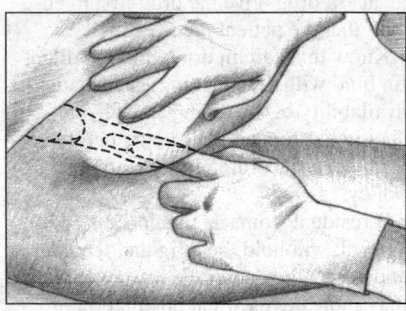

• Direct the suppository's tapered end toward the side of the rectum so it contacts the membranes.
• Encourage the patient to lie quietly and, if applicable, to retain the suppository for the correct length of time. Press on the anus with a gauze pad, if necessary, until the urge to defecate passes.
• Discard the used equipment and gloves. Wash your hands.

To apply an ointment

• Wash your hands.
• For external application, apply gloves and use a gauze pad to spread the drug over the anal area. To apply internally, attach the applicator to the tube of ointment, and coat the applicator with water-soluble lubricant.
• Expect to use about 1″ (2.5 cm) of ointment. To gauge how much pressure to use during application, try squeezing a small amount from the tube before you attach the applicator.
• Lift the upper buttock with your nondominant hand to expose the anus.
• Tell the patient to take several deep breaths through his mouth to relax the anal sphincter and reduce discomfort during insertion. Then gently insert the applicator, directing it toward the umbilicus.
• Squeeze the tube to eject drug.
• Remove the applicator, and place a folded 4″ × 4″ gauze pad between the patient's buttocks to absorb excess ointment.

• Disassemble the tube and applicator, Recap the tube. Clean the applicator with soap and warm water. Remove and discard gloves. Then wash your hands thoroughly.

Nursing considerations
• Because the intake of food and fluid stimulates peristalsis, a suppository for relieving constipation should be inserted about 30 minutes before mealtime to help soften the stool and facilitate defecation. A medicated retention suppository should be inserted between meals.
• Tell the patient not to expel the suppository. If retaining it is difficult, put the patient on a bedpan.
• Make sure that the patient's call button is handy, and watch for his signal because he may be unable to suppress the urge to defecate.
• Inform the patient that the suppository may discolor his next bowel movement.

Subcutaneous administration
S.C. injection allows slower, more sustained drug administration than I.M. injection. Drugs and solutions for S.C. injections are injected through a relatively short needle, using meticulous sterile technique.

Equipment and preparation
Gather the patient's medication record and chart, gloves, prescribed drug, needle of appropriate gauge and length, gloves, 1- to 3-ml syringe, and alcohol sponges. Other materials may include an antiseptic cleaning agent, filter needle, insulin syringe, and insulin pump.
Inspect the drug to make sure it's not cloudy and doesn't contain precipitates. Wash your hands. Select a needle of the proper gauge and length. An average adult patient requires a 25G ⅛" needle; an infant, a child, or an elderly or thin patient usually requires a 25G to 27G ½" needle.

For single-dose ampules
Wrap the neck of the ampule in an alcohol sponge and snap off the top. If de-

sired, attach a filter needle to the needle and withdraw the drug. Tap the syringe to clear air from it. Cover the needle with the needle sheath. Before discarding the ampule, check the label against the patient's medication record. Discard the filter needle and the ampule. Attach the appropriate needle to the syringe.

For single-dose or multidose vials
Reconstitute powdered drugs according to the label's instructions. Clean the vial's rubber stopper with an alcohol sponge. Pull the syringe plunger back until the volume of air in the syringe equals the volume of drug to be withdrawn from the vial. Insert the needle into the vial. Inject the air, invert the vial, and keep the needle's bevel tip below the level of the solution as you withdraw the prescribed amount of drug. Cover the needle with the needle sheath. Tap the syringe to clear any air from it. Check the drug label against the patient's medication record before returning the multidose vial to the shelf or drawer or before discarding the single-dose vial.

Implementation
• Select the injection site from those shown, and tell the patient where you'll be giving the injection.

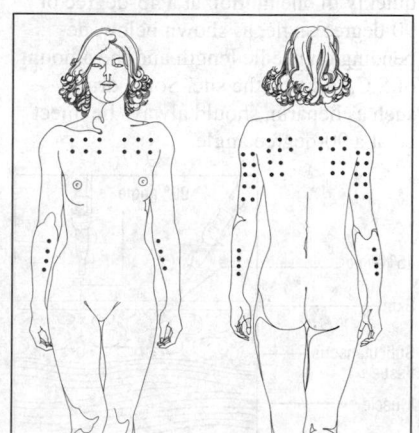

• Put on gloves. Position and drape the patient if necessary.
• Clean the injection site with an alcohol sponge. Loosen the protective needle sheath.
• With your nondominant hand, pinch the skin around the injection site firmly to elevate the S.C. tissue, forming a 1″ (2.5 cm) fat fold, as shown.

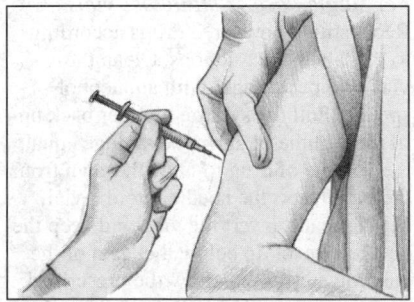

• Holding the syringe in your dominant hand (while pinching the skin around the injection site with the index finger and thumb of your nondominant hand), grip the needle sheath between the fourth and fifth fingers of your nondominant hand, and pull back to uncover the needle. Don't touch the needle.
• Position the needle with its bevel up.
• Tell the patient she'll feel a prick as the needle is inserted. Insert the needle quickly in one motion at a 45-degree or 90-degree angle, as shown below, depending on needle length and the amount of S.C. tissue at the site. Some drugs, such as heparin, should always be injected at a 90-degree angle.

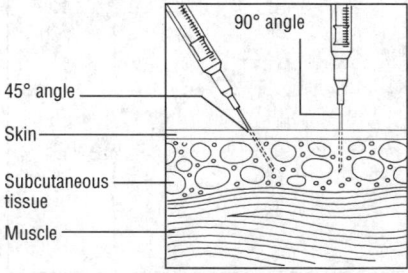

• Release the skin to avoid injecting the drug into compressed tissue and irritating the nerves. Pull the plunger back slightly to check for blood return. If none appears, slowly inject the drug. If blood appears upon aspiration, withdraw the needle, prepare another syringe, and repeat the procedure.
• After injection, remove the needle at the same angle used for insertion. Cover the site with an alcohol sponge, and massage the site gently.
• Remove the alcohol sponge, and check the injection site for bleeding or bruising.
• Do not recap the needle. Follow institutional policy to dispose of injection equipment.
• Remove and discard gloves. Wash hands.

Nursing considerations
• Don't aspirate for blood return when giving insulin or heparin. It's not necessary with insulin and may cause a hematoma with heparin.
• Don't massage the site after administering heparin.
• Repeated injections in the same site can cause lipodystrophy, a natural immune response. This complication can be minimized by rotating injection sites.

Intramuscular administration
I.M. injections deposit drug deep into well-vascularized muscle for rapid systemic action and absorption of up to 5 ml.

Equipment and preparation
Gather the patient's medication record and chart, prescribed drug, diluent or filter needle, if needed, 3- to 5-ml syringe, 20G to 25G 1″ to 3″ needle, gloves, and alcohol sponges.
The prescribed drug must be sterile. The needle may be packaged separately or already attached to the syringe. Needles used for I.M. injections are longer than subcutaneous needles because they reach deep into the muscle. Needle

length also depends on the injection site, the patient's size, and the amount of S.C. fat covering the muscle. A larger needle gauge accommodates viscous solutions and suspensions.

Check the drug for abnormal changes in color and clarity. If in doubt, ask the pharmacist.

Wipe stopper of vial with alcohol, and draw up the prescribed amount of drug.

Provide privacy and explain the procedure to the patient. Position and drape him appropriately, making sure that the site is well lit and exposed.

Implementation
● Wash your hands.
● Select an appropriate injection site. Avoid a site that is inflamed, edematous, or irritated, or that contains moles, birthmarks, scar tissue, or other lesions. Dorsogluteal or ventrogluteal muscles are used most commonly, as shown.

Dorsogluteal muscle

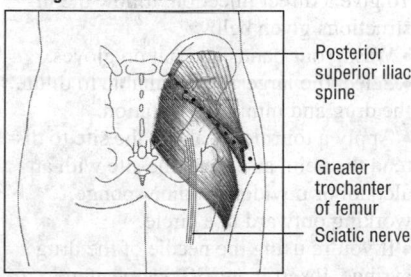

Posterior superior iliac spine

Greater trochanter of femur

Sciatic nerve

Ventrogluteal muscle

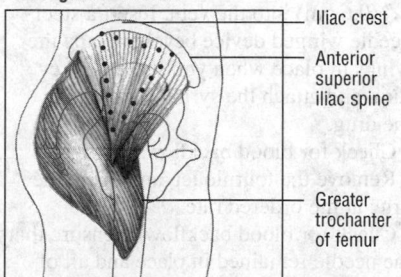

Iliac crest

Anterior superior iliac spine

Greater trochanter of femur

● The deltoid muscle may be used for injections of 2 ml or less, as shown above right.

Deltoid muscle

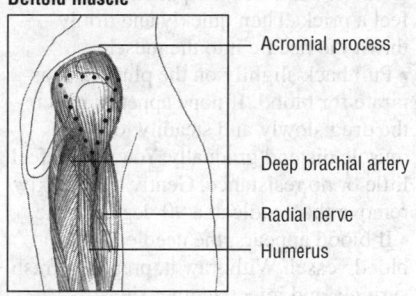

Acromial process

Deep brachial artery

Radial nerve

Humerus

● The vastus lateralis is used most often in children; the rectus femoris may be used in infants, as shown.

Vastus lateralis and rectus femoris muscles

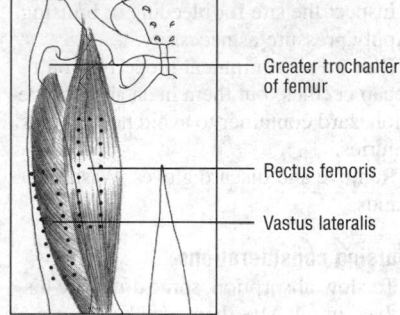

Greater trochanter of femur

Rectus femoris

Vastus lateralis

● Rotate injection sites for patients who require repeated injections.
● Position and drape the patient appropriately.
● Loosen, but don't remove, the needle sheath.
● Gently tap the site to stimulate nerve endings and minimize pain.
● Clean the site by moving an alcohol sponge in circles increasing in diameter to about 2″ (5 cm). Allow the skin to dry; alcohol stings in the puncture.
● Put on gloves.
● With the thumb and index finger of your nondominant hand, gently stretch the skin.
● With the syringe in your dominant hand, remove the needle sheath with the free fingers of the other hand.
● Position the syringe perpendicular to the skin surface and a couple of inches

from the skin. Tell the patient that he will feel a prick. Then quickly and firmly thrust the needle into the muscle.
• Pull back slightly on the plunger to aspirate for blood. If none appears, inject the drug slowly and steadily to let the muscle distend gradually. You should feel little or no resistance. Gently but quickly remove the needle at a 90-degree angle.
• If blood appears, the needle is in a blood vessel. Withdraw it, prepare a fresh syringe, and inject another site.
• Using a gloved hand, apply gentle pressure to the site with the alcohol sponge. Massage the relaxed muscle, unless contraindicated, to distribute the drug and promote absorption.
• Inspect the site for bleeding or bruising. Apply pressure as necessary.
• Discard all equipment properly. Don't recap needles; put them in an appropriate biohazard container to avoid needle-stick injuries.
• Remove and discard gloves. Wash hands.

Nursing considerations
• To slow absorption, some drugs are dissolved in oil. Mix them well before use.
• Never inject into the gluteal muscles of a child who has been walking for less than 1 year.
• If the patient must have repeated injections, consider numbing the area with ice before cleaning it. If you must inject more than 5 ml, divide the solution and inject it at two sites.
• Urge the patient to relax the muscle to reduce pain and bleeding.
• I.M. injections can damage local muscle cells and elevate serum enzyme levels (creatine kinase), which can be confused with elevated levels caused by MI. Diagnostic tests can be used to differentiate between them.

I.V. bolus administration
This method allows rapid I.V. drug administration to quickly achieve peak levels in the bloodstream. It may also be used for drugs that can't be given I.M. because they're toxic or the patient has reduced ability to absorb them. And it may be used to deliver drugs that can't be diluted.

Bolus doses may be injected directly into a vein or through an existing I.V. line.

Equipment and preparation
Gather the patient's medication record and chart, prescribed drug, 20G needle and syringe, diluent, if necessary, tourniquet, povidone-iodine sponge, alcohol sponge, sterile 2″ × 2″ gauze pad, gloves, adhesive bandage, and tape. Other materials may include a steel needle-winged device primed with 0.9% NaCl solution and second syringe (and needle) filled with 0.9% NaCl solution.

Draw the drug into the syringe, and dilute it if necessary.

Implementation
To give a direct injection, follow the instructions given below:
• Wash your hands and put on gloves.
• Select the largest vein suitable to dilute the drug and minimize irritation.
• Apply a tourniquet above the site to distend the vein, and clean the site with an alcohol or povidone-iodine sponge, working outward in a circle.
• If you're using the needle of the drug syringe, insert it at a 30-degree angle with the bevel up. The bevel should reach ¼″ (0.6 cm) into the vein. Insert a steel needle winged device bevel up, tape the wings in place when you see blood return, and attach the syringe containing the drug.
• Check for blood backflow.
• Remove the tourniquet, and inject the drug at the ordered rate.
• Check for blood backflow to ensure that the needle remained in place and all of the injected drug entered the vein.
• For a steel needle winged device, flush the line with 0.9% NaCl solution from

the second syringe to ensure complete delivery.
• Withdraw the needle, and apply pressure to the site with the sterile gauze pad for at least 3 minutes to prevent hematoma.
• Apply an adhesive bandage when the bleeding stops.
• Remove and discard gloves. Wash hands.

To inject through an existing I.V. line
• Wash your hands and put on gloves.
• Check the compatibility of the drug.
• Close the flow clamp, wipe the injection port with an alcohol sponge, and inject the drug as you would a direct injection.
• Open the flow clamp and readjust the flow rate.
• Remove and discard gloves. Wash hands.
• If the drug isn't compatible with the I.V. solution, flush the line with 0.9% NaCl solution before and after the injection.

Nursing considerations
• If the existing I.V. line is capped, making it an intermittent infusion device, verify patency and placement of the device before injecting the drug. Then flush the device with 0.9% NaCl solution, administer the drug, and follow with the appropriate flush.
• Immediately report signs of acute allergic reaction or anaphylaxis. If extravasation occurs, stop the injection, estimate the amount of infiltration, and notify the doctor.
• When giving diazepam or chlordiazepoxide hydrochloride through a steel needle winged device or I.V. line, flush with bacteriostatic water to prevent precipitation.

I.V. administration through a secondary I.V. line
A secondary I.V. line is a complete I.V. set connected to the lower Y-port (sec-

ondary port) of a primary line instead of to the I.V. catheter or needle. It features an I.V. container, long tubing, and either a microdrip or a macrodrip system, and it can be used for continuous or intermittent drug infusion. When used continuously, it permits drug infusion and titration while the primary line maintains a constant total infusion rate.

A secondary I.V. line used only for intermittent drug administration is called a piggyback set. In this case, the primary line maintains venous access between drug doses. A piggyback set includes a small I.V. container, short tubing, and usually a macrodrip system, and it connects to the primary line's upper Y-port (piggyback port).

Equipment and preparation
Gather the patient's medication record and chart, prescribed I.V. drug, diluent, if necessary, prescribed I.V. solution, administration set with secondary injection port, 22G 1″ needle or a needleless system, alcohol sponges, 1″ (2.5 cm) adhesive tape, time tape, labels, infusion pump, extension hook, and solution for intermittent piggyback infusion.

Wash your hands. Inspect the I.V. container for cracks, leaks, or contamination. Check compatibility with the primary solution. Determine whether the primary line has a secondary injection port.

If necessary, add the drug to the secondary I.V. solution. To do so, remove any seals from the secondary container and wipe the main port with an alcohol sponge. Inject the prescribed drug and agitate the solution to mix the drug. Label the I.V. mixture. Insert the administration set spike, and attach the needle or needleless system. Open the flow clamp and prime the line. Then close the flow clamp.

Some drugs come in vials for hanging directly on an I.V. pole. In this case, inject diluent directly into the drug vial. Then spike the vial, prime the tubing, and hang the set.

Implementation

• If the drug is incompatible with the primary I.V. solution, replace the primary solution with a fluid that's compatible with both solutions, and flush the line before starting the drug infusion.

• Hang the container of the secondary set and wipe the injection port of the primary line with an alcohol sponge.

• Insert the needle or needleless system from the secondary line into the injection port, and tape it securely to the primary line.

• To run the container of the secondary set by itself, lower the primary set's container with an extension hook. To run both containers simultaneously, place them at the same height.

• Open the clamp and adjust the drip rate.

• For continuous infusion, set the secondary solution to the desired drip rate; then adjust the primary solution to the desired total infusion rate.

• For intermittent infusion, wait until the secondary solution is completely infused; then adjust the primary drip rate, as required.

• If the secondary solution tubing is being reused, close the clamp on the tubing and follow the hospital's policy: Either remove the needle or needleless system and replace it with a new one, or leave it taped in the injection port and label it with the time it was first used.

• Leave the empty container in place until you replace it with a new dose of drug at the prescribed time. If the tubing won't be reused, discard it appropriately with the I.V. container.

Nursing considerations

• If institutional policy allows, use a pump for drug infusion. Put a time tape on the secondary container to help prevent an inaccurate administration rate.

• When reusing secondary tubing, change it according to institutional policy, usually every 48 to 72 hours. Inspect the injection port for leakage with each use; change it more often if needed.

• Except for lipids, don't piggyback a secondary I.V. line to a total parenteral nutrition line because it risks contamination.

Drug
Classifications

DRUG CLASSIFICATIONS

Alkylating drugs

altretamine
busulfan
carboplatin
carmustine
chlorambucil
cisplatin
cyclophosphamide
dacarbazine
ifosfamide
lomustine
mechlorethamine hydrochloride
melphalan
streptozocin
thiotepa

Action

Alkylating drugs appear to act independently of a specific cell-cycle phase. They are polyfunctional compounds that can be divided chemically into five groups: nitrogen mustards, ethylenimines, alkyl sulfonates, triazenes, and nitrosoureas. Highly reactive, they primarily target nucleic acids and form covalent linkages with nucleophilic centers in many different kinds of molecules. Their polyfunctional character allows them to cross-link double-stranded DNA, preventing strands from separating for replication, which appears to contribute more to the cytotoxic effects of these drugs than other results of alkylation.

Indications

▶ Treatment of various tumors, especially those having large volume and slow cell-turnover rate. See individual drugs for specific uses.

Adverse reactions

The most frequent adverse reactions include bone marrow depression, leukopenia, thrombocytopenia, fever, chills, sore throat, nausea, vomiting, diarrhea, flank or joint pain, anxiety, swelling of feet or lower legs, hair loss, and redness or pain at injection site.

Contraindications and precautions

• Contraindicated in patients with hypersensitivity to drug. See individual drugs for additional contraindications.
• Use with caution in those receiving other cytotoxic drugs or radiation therapy. See individual drugs for additional precautions.
• **Geriatric use:** Elderly patients are at increased risk for adverse reactions. Monitor closely.
• **Pediatric use:** Safety and efficacy of many alkylating drugs have not been established in children. See individual drugs for guidelines.
• **Breast-feeding:** Alkylating drugs are distributed in breast milk. Breast-feeding should be avoided.

NURSING CONSIDERATIONS

⚕ Assessment
• Perform a complete assessment before therapy begins.
• Monitor for adverse reactions throughout therapy.
• Monitor BUN, hematocrit, platelet count, ALT, AST, LD, serum bilirubin, serum creatinine, uric acid total and differential leukocyte, and other levels as required.
• Monitor vital signs and patency of catheter or I.V. line throughout administration.

⊞ Key nursing diagnoses
• Altered protection related to thrombocytopenia
• Risk for infection related to immunosuppression

• Risk for fluid volume deficit related to adverse GI effects

⬢ **Planning and implementation**
• Follow established procedures for safe and proper handling, administration, and disposal of chemotherapeutic drugs.
• Treat extravasation promptly.
• Have epinephrine, corticosteroids, and antihistamines available during carboplatin or cisplatin administration. Anaphylactoid reactions may occur.
• Administer ifosfamide with mesna, as prescribed, to prevent hemorrhagic cystitis.
• Give lomustine 2 to 4 hours after meals. Nausea and vomiting usually last less than 24 hours although loss of appetite may last for several days.
• Administer adequate hydration before and for 24 hours after cisplatin treatment.
• Be aware that allopurinol may be prescribed to prevent drug-induced hyperuricemia.
Patient teaching
• Caution patient to avoid exposure to those with bacterial or viral infections (chemotherapy can increase susceptibility). Urge him to report signs of infection promptly.
• Review proper oral hygiene, including cautious use of toothbrush, dental floss, and toothpicks.
• Advise patient to complete dental work before therapy begins or to delay it until blood counts are normal.
• Warn patient that he may bruise easily because of drug's effect on blood count.

☑ **Evaluation**
• Patient does not develop serious bleeding complications.
• Patient remains free from infection.
• Patient maintains adequate hydration.

Alpha-adrenergic blockers
dihydroergotamine mesylate
doxazosin mesylate
ergotamine tartrate
phentolamine mesylate
prazosin hydrochloride
tamsulosin hydrochloride
terazosin hydrochloride
tolazoline hydrochloride

Action

Selective alpha antagonists (dihydroergotamine, doxazosin, prazosin, and terazosin) have readily observable effects and are currently the only alpha-adrenergic drugs with known clinical uses. They decrease vascular resistance and increase venous capacitance, thereby lowering blood pressure and causing pink warm skin, nasal and scleroconjunctival congestion, ptosis, postural and exercise hypotension, mild to moderate miosis, and interference with ejaculation. They also relax nonvascular smooth muscle, notably in the prostate capsule, thereby reducing urinary symptoms in men with BPH. Because $alpha_1$ blockers do not block $alpha_2$ receptors, they do not cause transmitter overflow.

Nonselective alpha antagonists (ergotamine, phentolamine, and tolazoline) antagonize both $alpha_1$ and $alpha_2$ receptors. Generally, alpha blockade results in tachycardia, palpitations, and increased renin secretion because of abnormally large amounts of norepinephrine (transmitter overflow) released from adrenergic nerve endings as a result of the concurrent blockade of $alpha_1$ and $alpha_2$ receptors. Norepinephrine's effects are clinically counterproductive to the major uses of nonselective alpha blockers.

Indications

▶ Peripheral vascular disorders (Raynaud's disease, acrocyanosis, frostbite, acute atrial occlusion, phlebitis, diabetic gangrene), vascular headaches, dermal necrosis, mild to moderate urinary obstruction in men with BPH, hypertension, pheochromocytoma.

Adverse reactions

Selective alpha antagonists may cause severe postural hypotension and syncope, especially with first dose; most common reactions of alpha$_1$ blockade are dizziness, headache, and malaise.

Nonselective alpha antagonists typically cause orthostatic hypotension, tachycardia, palpitations, fluid retention (from excess renin secretion), nasal and ocular congestion, and aggravation of respiratory infection.

Contraindications and precautions

• Contraindicated in patients with MI, coronary insufficiency, or angina.
• Use with caution in pregnant women.
• **Geriatric use:** Hypotensive effects may be more pronounced in elderly patients.
• **Pediatric use:** Safety and efficacy of many alpha-adrenergic blockers have not been established in children. Use with caution.
• **Breast-feeding:** Use with caution in breast-feeding women.

NURSING CONSIDERATIONS

⚞ Assessment
• Monitor vital signs, especially blood pressure.
• Monitor closely for adverse reactions.

⊞ Key nursing diagnoses
• Decreased cardiac output related to hypotension
• Pain related to headache
• Fluid volume excess related to fluid retention

⧉ Planning and implementation
• Administer at bedtime to minimize dizziness or light-headedness.
• Begin therapy with small dose, as ordered, to avoid first-dose syncope.

Patient teaching
• Warn patient to avoid moving suddenly from a lying or sitting position.
• Urge patient to avoid driving and other hazardous tasks that require mental alertness until drug's effects are known.
• Advise patient that alcohol, excessive exercise, prolonged standing, and heat exposure will intensify adverse effects.
• Tell patient to report dizziness or irregular heartbeat promptly.

☑ Evaluation
• Patient maintains adequate cardiac output.
• Patient's headache is relieved.
• Patient does not have edema.

Aminoglycosides
amikacin sulfate
gentamicin sulfate
kanamycin sulfate
neomycin sulfate
netilmicin sulfate
streptomycin sulfate
tobramycin sulfate

Action

Aminoglycosides are bactericidal. They bind directly and irreversibly to 30S ribosomal subunits, inhibiting bacterial protein synthesis. They are active against many aerobic gram-negative and some aerobic gram-positive organisms.

Susceptible gram-negative organisms include *Acinetobacter*, *Citrobacter*, *Enterobacter*, *Escherichia coli*, *Klebsiella*, indole-positive and indole-negative *Proteus*, *Providencia*, *Pseudomonas aeruginosa*, *Salmonella*, *Serratia*, and *Shigella*. In addition, streptomycin is active against *Brucella*, *Calymmatobacterium granulomatis*, *Pasteurella multocida*, and *Yersinia pestis*.

Susceptible gram-positive organisms include *Staphylococcus aureus* and *S. epidermidis*. In addition, streptomycin is active against *Nocardia, Erysipelothrix,* and some mycobacteria, including *Mycobacterium tuberculosis, M. marinum,* and certain strains of *M. kansasii* and *M. leprae.*

Indications

▶ Septicemia; postoperative, pulmonary, intra-abdominal, and urinary tract infections; infections of skin, soft tissue, bones, and joints; aerobic gram-negative bacillary meningitis (not susceptible to other antibiotics); serious staphylococcal, *P. aeruginosa,* and *Klebsiella* infections; enterococcal infections; nosocomial pneumonia; anaerobic infections involving *Bacteroides fragilis;* tuberculosis; initial empiric therapy in febrile, leukopenic compromised host.

Adverse reactions

Ototoxicity and nephrotoxicity are the most serious complications. Neuromuscular blockade also may occur. Oral drugs most commonly cause nausea, vomiting, and diarrhea. Parenteral drugs may cause vein irritation, phlebitis, and sterile abscess.

Contraindications and precautions

• Contraindicated in patients with known hypersensitivity to aminoglycosides.
• Use with caution in pregnant women and in those with a neuromuscular disorder or renal impairment.
• **Geriatric use:** Elderly patients are at greater risk for nephrotoxicity; they often require lower drug dosages and longer dosing intervals. They are also susceptible to ototoxicity and superinfection.
• **Pediatric use:** The half-life of aminoglycosides is prolonged in neonates and premature infants because of their immature renal systems. Dosage alterations may be necessary in infants and children.
• **Breast-feeding:** Safety has not been established in breast-feeding women.

NURSING CONSIDERATIONS

🔬 Assessment
• Obtain patient's history of allergies.
• Monitor for adverse reactions.
• Obtain results of culture and sensitivity tests before first dose, and check tests periodically to assess drug efficacy.
• Monitor vital signs, electrolyte levels, hearing ability, and renal function studies before and during therapy.
• Draw blood for peak level 1 hour after I.M. injection (30 minutes to 1 hour after I.V. infusion); for trough level, draw sample just before next dose. Time and date all blood samples. Do not use heparinized tube to collect blood samples; it interferes with results.

🔲 Key nursing diagnoses
• Risk for injury related to nephrotoxicity and ototoxicity
• Risk for infection related to drug-induced superinfection
• Risk for fluid volume deficit related to adverse GI reactions

▷ Planning and implementation
• Keep patient well hydrated to minimize chemical irritation of renal tubules.
• Do not add or mix other drugs with I.V. infusions, particularly penicillins, which inactivate aminoglycosides. If other drugs must be given I.V., temporarily stop infusion of primary drug.
• Refer to manufacturer's instructions for reconstitution, dilution, and storage of drugs; check expiration dates.
• Shake oral suspensions well before administering.
• Administer I.M. dose deep into large muscle mass (gluteal or midlateral thigh); rotate injection sites to minimize tissue injury. Apply ice to injection site to relieve pain.
• Too rapid I.V. administration may cause neuromuscular blockade. Infuse I.V. drug continuously or intermittently over 30 to 60 minutes for adults, 1 to 2 hours for in-

fants; dilution volume for children is determined individually.

Patient teaching
• Teach signs and symptoms of hypersensitivity and other adverse reactions. Urge patient to report unusual effects promptly.
• Emphasize importance of adequate fluid intake.

✓ Evaluation
• Patient maintains pretreatment renal and hearing function.
• Patient is free from infection.
• Patient maintains adequate hydration.

Angiotensin-converting enzyme (ACE) inhibitors
benazepril hydrochloride
captopril
enalapril maleate
fosinopril sodium
lisinopril
moexipril hydrochloride
quinapril hydrochloride
ramipril

Action

ACE inhibitors prevent conversion of angiotensin I to angiotensin II, a potent vasoconstrictor. Besides decreasing vasoconstriction and thus reducing peripheral arterial resistance, inhibition of angiotensin II decreases adrenocortical secretion of aldosterone. This reduces sodium and water retention and extracellular fluid volume.

Indications

▶ Hypertension, heart failure.

Adverse reactions

The most common adverse effects of therapeutic doses are headache, fatigue, hypotension, tachycardia, dysgeusia, proteinuria, hyperkalemia, rash, cough, and angioedema of face and extremities.

Severe hypotension may occur at toxic drug levels.

Contraindications and precautions

• Contraindicated in patients with known hypersensitivity to ACE inhibitors.
• Use with caution in patients with impaired renal function or serious autoimmune disease and in those taking other drugs known to depress WBC count or immune response.
• **Geriatric use:** Elderly patients may need lower doses because of impaired drug clearance.
• **Pediatric use:** Safety and efficacy in children have not been established; use only if potential benefit outweighs risk.
• **Breast-feeding:** Some ACE inhibitors are distributed into breast milk. An alternative feeding method is recommended during therapy.

NURSING CONSIDERATIONS

Assessment
• Observe for adverse reactions.
• Monitor vital signs regularly and WBC counts and serum electrolyte levels periodically.

Key nursing diagnoses
• Risk for trauma related to orthostatic hypotension
• Altered protection related to hyperkalemia
• Pain related to headache

Planning and implementation
• Discontinue diuretic therapy 2 to 3 days before beginning ACE inhibitor therapy, as ordered, to reduce risk of hypotension; if drug does not adequately control blood pressure, diuretics may be reinstated.
• Use lower dosage, as ordered, for patient with impaired renal function.
• Use potassium supplements with caution. ACE inhibitors may cause potassium retention.
• Discontinue ACE inhibitors, as ordered, if pregnancy occurs. Drugs can cause

Prototype drug

birth defects or fetal death during second or third trimester.

Patient teaching

• Tell patient that drugs may cause a dry, persistent, tickling cough; it is reversible when therapy is discontinued.

• Urge patient to report light-headedness, especially in first few days, so the dose can be adjusted; signs of infection, such as sore throat and fever, because drugs may decrease WBC count; facial swelling or difficulty breathing because drugs may cause angioedema; and loss of taste, which may necessitate discontinuation.

• Advise patient to avoid sudden position changes to minimize orthostatic hypotension.

• Warn patient to seek medical approval before taking self-prescribed cold preparations.

• Tell female patient to report pregnancy at once.

☑ **Evaluation**

• Patient does not experience injury from orthostatic hypotension.

• Patient's WBC counts remain normal throughout therapy.

• Patient's headache is relieved with mild analgesic.

Antacids

aluminum carbonate
aluminum hydroxide
calcium carbonate
magaldrate
magnesium hydroxide
magnesium oxide
sodium bicarbonate

Action

Antacids reduce total acid load in GI tract and elevate gastric pH to reduce pepsin activity. They also strengthen the gastric mucosal barrier and increase esophageal sphincter tone.

Indications

▶ Ulcer pain.

Adverse reactions

Aluminum-containing antacids may cause aluminum intoxication, constipation, hypophosphatemia, intestinal obstruction, and osteomalacia. Magnesium-containing antacids may cause diarrhea or hypermagnesemia (in renal failure). Calcium carbonate, magaldrate, magnesium oxide, and sodium bicarbonate may cause milk-alkali syndrome or rebound hyperacidity.

Contraindications and precautions

• Calcium carbonate, magaldrate, and magnesium oxide are contraindicated in severe renal disease. Sodium bicarbonate is contraindicated in patients with hypertension, renal disease, edema, or vomiting; during concurrent diuretic administration or continuous GI suction; and with sodium-restricted diets.

• Use magnesium oxide with caution in elderly patients and in those with mild renal impairment. Use aluminum preparations, calcium carbonate, and magaldrate with caution in elderly patients; in those receiving antidiarrheals, antispasmodics, or anticholinergics; and in those with dehydration, fluid restriction, chronic renal disease, or suspected intestinal absorption.

• **Geriatric use:** Elderly patients are at greater risk for adverse reactions. Monitor closely.

• **Pediatric use:** Serious adverse effects are more likely to develop in infants from a change in fluid and electrolyte balance. Monitor closely.

• **Breast-feeding:** Antacids may be given to breast-feeding women.

NURSING CONSIDERATIONS

☲ **Assessment**

• Assess patient's condition before therapy and regularly thereafter.

- Record number and consistency of stools.
- Observe for adverse reactions.
- Monitor patient receiving long-term, high-dose aluminum carbonate and hydroxide for fluid and electrolyte imbalance, especially if patient is on sodium-restricted diet.
- Monitor serum phosphate levels in patient receiving aluminum carbonate or hydroxide.
- Watch for signs of hypercalcemia in patient receiving calcium carbonate.
- Monitor serum magnesium levels in patient who has mild renal impairment and is taking magaldrate.

⊕ Key nursing diagnoses
- Constipation related to adverse effects of aluminum-containing antacid
- Diarrhea related to adverse effects of magnesium-containing antacid
- Altered protection related to drug-induced electrolyte imbalance

❯ Planning and implementation
- Manage constipation with laxatives or stool softeners, or check with doctor about switching patient to magnesium preparations.
- Obtain order for antidiarrheal, as needed, and check with doctor about switching patient to aluminum-containing antacid.
- Shake container well and give with small amount of water or juice to facilitate passage. When administering through nasogastric tube, ensure that tube is patent and placed correctly; after instilling, flush tube with water to ensure passage to stomach and to clear tube.

Patient teaching
- Warn patient not to use antacids indiscriminately or to switch antacids without doctor's consent.
- Tell patient not to take calcium carbonate with milk or other foods high in vitamin D.

- Warn patient not to take sodium bicarbonate with milk to prevent hypercalcemia.

☑ Evaluation
- Patient regains normal bowel pattern.
- Patient states diarrhea is relieved.
- Patient maintains normal electrolyte balance.

Antianginals
Beta blockers
  nadolol
  propranolol hydrochloride
Calcium channel blockers
  amlodipine besylate
  bepridil hydrochloride
  diltiazem hydrochloride
  nicardipine hydrochloride
  nifedipine
  verapamil hydrochloride
Nitrates
  erythrityl tetranitrate
  isosorbide dinitrate
  isosorbide mononitrate
  nitroglycerin

Action

Beta blockers block catecholamine-induced increases in heart rate, blood pressure, and myocardial contraction. Calcium channel blockers inhibit influx of calcium through muscle cells, dilating coronary arteries and decreasing afterload. Nitrates decrease left ventricular end-diastolic pressure (preload) and systemic vascular resistance (afterload) and increase blood flow through collateral coronary vessels.

Indications

▶ Moderate to severe angina (beta blockers); classic, effort-induced angina and Prinzmetal's angina (calcium channel blockers); recurrent angina (long-acting nitrates and topical, transdermal, transmucosal, and oral extended-release nitroglycerin); acute angina (S.L. nitroglycerin and S.L. or chewable isosorbide dinitrate); unstable angina (I.V. nitroglycerin).

Adverse reactions

Beta blockers may cause bradycardia, heart failure, cough, diarrhea, disturbing dreams, dizziness, dyspnea, fatigue, fever, hypotension, lethargy, nausea, peripheral edema, and wheezing. Calcium channel blockers may cause bradycardia, confusion, constipation, depression, diarrhea, dizziness, edema, elevated liver enzymes (transient), fatigue, flushing, headache, hypotension, insomnia, nervousness, and rash. Nitrates may cause ethanol intoxication (from I.V. preparations containing ethanol), flushing, headache, orthostatic hypotension, reflex tachycardia, rash, syncope, and vomiting.

Contraindications and precautions

• Beta blockers are contraindicated in patients with cardiogenic shock, sinus bradycardia, heart block greater than first degree, bronchial asthma, known hypersensitivity to beta blockers, or heart failure unless failure is caused by tachyarrhythmia treatable with propranolol. Calcium channel blockers are contraindicated in those with severe hypotension or heart block greater than first degree (except with functioning pacemaker). Nitrates are contraindicated in patients with severe anemia, cerebral hemorrhage, head trauma, glaucoma, or hyperthyroidism.
• Use beta blockers with caution in pregnant or breast-feeding women and in patients with nonallergic bronchospastic disorders, diabetes mellitus, or impaired hepatic or renal function. Use calcium channel blockers with caution in elderly patients and in those with hepatic or renal impairment, bradycardia, heart failure, or cardiogenic shock. Use nitrates with caution in patients with hypotension or recent MI.

• **Geriatric use:** Elderly patients have an increased risk of adverse reactions.
• **Pediatric use:** Safety and efficacy have not been established in children. Check with doctor before administering to children.
• **Breast-feeding:** Recommendations for breast-feeding vary with individual drugs.

NURSING CONSIDERATIONS

⚏ Assessment
• Monitor vital signs. With I.V. nitroglycerin, monitor blood pressure and pulse rate every 5 to 15 minutes while titrating dosages and every hour thereafter.
• Monitor effectiveness of prescribed drug.
• Observe for adverse reactions.

⚏ Key nursing diagnoses
• Risk for injury related to adverse reactions
• Fluid volume excess related to adverse CV effects of beta blockers or calcium channel blockers
• Pain related to headache

⚏ Planning and implementation
• With first dose of nitrate, have patient sit or lie down; take pulse rate and blood pressure before giving dose and at onset of action.
• Do not administer beta blockers or calcium channel blockers to relieve acute angina. Withhold dose and notify doctor if heart rate is below 60 beats/minute or systolic blood pressure is below 90 mm Hg.
Patient teaching
• Warn patient not to discontinue drug abruptly without doctor's approval.
• Teach patient to take his pulse before taking a beta blocker or calcium channel blocker. Tell him to withhold dose and alert doctor if pulse rate is below 60 beats/minute.
• Instruct patient taking nitroglycerin S.L. to go to the emergency department if

three tablets taken 5 minutes apart do not relieve anginal pain.
• Tell patient to report serious or persistent adverse reactions.

☑ **Evaluation**
• Patient does not experience injury from adverse reactions.
• Patient maintains normal fluid balance.
• Patient's headache is relieved with mild analgesic.

Antiarrhythmics

Class I
  moricizine hydrochloride
Class Ia
  disopyramide
  procainamide hydrochloride
  quinidine bisulfate
  quinidine gluconate
  quinidine polygalacturonate
  quinidine sulfate
Class Ib
  lidocaine hydrochloride
  mexiletine hydrochloride
  phenytoin
  phenytoin sodium
  tocainide hydrochloride
Class Ic
  flecainide acetate
  propafenone hydrochloride
Class II (beta blockers)
  acebutolol
  esmolol hydrochloride
  propranolol hydrochloride
  sotalol hydrochloride
Class III
  amiodarone hydrochloride
  bretylium tosylate
  ibutilide fumarate
Class IV (calcium channel blocker)
  verapamil hydrochloride

Action

Class I drugs reduce the inward current carried by sodium ions, stabilizing neuronal cardiac membranes. Class Ia drugs depress phase O, prolong the action potential, and have cardiac membrane-stabilizing effects. Class Ib drugs depress phase O, shorten the action potential, and have cardiac membrane-stabilizing effects. Class Ic drugs block the transport of sodium ions, decreasing conduction velocity but not repolarization rate. Class II drugs decrease heart rate, myocardial contractility, blood pressure, and AV node conduction. Class III drugs prolong the action potential and refractory period. Class IV drugs decrease myocardial contractility and oxygen demand by inhibiting calcium ion influx; they also dilate coronary arteries and arterioles.

Indications

▶ Atrial and ventricular arrhythmias.

Adverse reactions

Most antiarrhythmics can aggravate existing arrhythmias or cause new ones. They also may produce hypersensitivity reactions; hypotension; GI problems, such as nausea, vomiting, or bowel elimination changes; and CNS disturbances, such as dizziness or fatigue. Some antiarrhythmics may exacerbate heart failure. Class II drugs may cause bronchoconstriction.

Contraindications and precautions

• Contraindicated in patients with hypersensitivity to drug.
• Many antiarrhythmics are contraindicated or require cautious use in patients with cardiogenic shock, digitalis toxicity, and preexisting second- or third-degree heart block in absence of pacemaker. See individual drugs for specific contraindications and precautions.
• **Geriatric use:** Elderly patients exhibit physiologic alterations in CV system. Use with caution.
• **Pediatric use:** Children have an increased risk of adverse reactions. Monitor closely.
• **Breast-feeding:** Many antiarrhythmics are distributed into breast milk.

Recommendations for breast-feeding vary with individual drugs.

NURSING CONSIDERATIONS

⚕ Assessment
• Monitor ECG continuously during initiation of therapy and dosage adjustments.
• Monitor patient's vital signs frequently and assess for signs of toxicity and adverse reactions.
• Measure apical pulse rate before administering drug.
• Monitor serum drug levels as indicated.

⊞ Key nursing diagnoses
• Decreased cardiac output related to arrhythmias or myocardial depression
• Altered protection related to adverse reactions
• Noncompliance related to long-term therapy

⊳ Planning and implementation
• Don't crush sustained-release tablets.
• Take safety precautions if adverse CNS reactions occur.
• Notify doctor of adverse reactions.
Patient teaching
• Stress importance of taking drug exactly as prescribed.
• Teach patient to take his pulse before each dose. Advise him to notify doctor if pulse is irregular or slower than 60 beats/minute.
• Instruct patient to avoid activities that require mental alertness if adverse CNS reactions occur.
• Tell patient to limit fluid and salt intake if his prescribed drug causes fluid retention.

☑ Evaluation
• Patient maintains adequate cardiac output, as evidenced by normal vital signs and adequate tissue perfusion.
• Patient does not experience serious adverse reactions.
• Patient states importance of compliance with therapy.

Antibiotic antineoplastics
bleomycin sulfate
dactinomycin
daunorubicin hydrochloride
doxorubicin hydrochloride
idarubicin hydrochloride
mitomycin
mitoxantrone hydrochloride
plicamycin
procarbazine hydrochloride
streptozocin

Action

Although classified as antibiotics, these drugs exert cytotoxic effects, ruling out their use as antimicrobials. They interfere with proliferation of malignant cells through several mechanisms. Their action may be cell-cycle-phase nonspecific, cell-cycle-phase specific, or both. Some exhibit activity resembling alkylating drugs or antimetabolites; for example, streptozocin is considered an alkylating drug because of its therapeutic activity. By binding to or complexing with DNA, antineoplastic antibiotics directly or indirectly inhibit DNA, RNA, and protein synthesis.

Indications

▶ Treatment of various tumors. See individual drugs for specific uses.

Adverse reactions

The most frequent adverse reactions include nausea, vomiting, diarrhea, fever, chills, sore throat, anxiety, confusion, flank or joint pain, swelling of feet or lower legs, hair loss, redness or pain at injection site, bone marrow depression, and leukopenia.

Contraindications and precautions

• Contraindicated in patients with known hypersensitivity to drug.
• Additional contraindications and precautions vary. See individual drugs for complete listings.

• **Geriatric use:** Elderly patients are at increased risk for adverse reactions. Monitor closely.
• **Pediatric use:** Safety and efficacy of some drugs have not been established in children. See individual drugs for specific guidelines.
• **Breast-feeding:** Breast-feeding is contraindicated in women receiving cancer chemotherapy, including antibiotic antineoplastic drugs.

NURSING CONSIDERATIONS

⚖ Assessment
• Perform a complete assessment before therapy begins.
• Monitor for adverse reactions.
• Monitor vital signs and patency of catheter or I.V. line.
• Monitor BUN, hematocrit, platelet count, ALT, AST, LD, serum bilirubin, serum creatinine, uric acid, and total and differential leukocyte counts, as ordered.
• Monitor pulmonary function tests in a patient receiving bleomycin. Assess lung function regularly.
• Monitor ECG before and during treatment with daunorubicin and doxorubicin.

⊕ Key nursing diagnoses
• Altered protection related to thrombocytopenia
• Risk for infection related to immunosuppression
• Risk for fluid volume deficit related to adverse GI effects

❯ Planning and implementation
• Follow established procedures for safe and proper handling, administration, and disposal of chemotherapeutic drugs.
• Treat extravasation promptly.
• Have epinephrine, corticosteroids, and antihistamines available during bleomycin therapy. Anaphylactoid reactions may occur.
• Ensure adequate hydration during idarubicin therapy.

• Discontinue procarbazine and notify doctor if patient becomes confused or neuropathies develop.
• Try to ease anxiety in patient and family before treatment.
Patient teaching
• Warn patient to avoid close contact with persons who have taken oral poliovirus vaccine.
• Caution patient to avoid exposure to persons with bacterial or viral infections (chemotherapy increases susceptibility). Urge him to report signs of infection immediately.
• Review proper oral hygiene, including cautious use of toothbrush, dental floss, and toothpicks. Chemotherapy can increase incidence of microbial infection, delayed healing, and bleeding gums.
• Urge patient to complete dental work before therapy begins or to delay it until blood counts are normal.
• Warn patient that he may bruise easily.
• Tell patient to report redness, pain, or swelling at injection site immediately. Local tissue injury and scarring may result if I.V. infiltration occurs.
• Warn patient taking procarbazine to avoid hazardous activities that require alertness until drug's CNS effects are known. Also advise him to take procarbazine at bedtime and in divided doses to reduce nausea and vomiting.
• Advise patient taking daunorubicin, doxorubicin, or idarubicin that his urine may turn orange or red for 1 to 2 days after therapy begins.

☑ Evaluation
• Serious bleeding complications do not develop.
• Patient remains free from infection.
• Patient maintains adequate hydration.

Anticholinergics

atropine sulfate
belladonna leaf
benztropine mesylate
dicyclomine hydrochloride
glycopyrrolate
propantheline bromide
scopolamine
scopolamine butylbromide
scopolamine hydrobromide

Action

Anticholinergics competitively antagonize the actions of acetylcholine and other cholinergic agonists at muscarinic receptors.

Indications

▶ Prevention of motion sickness, preoperative reduction of secretions and blockage of cardiac reflexes, adjunct treatment of peptic ulcers and other GI disorders, blockage of cholinomimetic effects of cholinesterase inhibitors or other drugs, and (for benztropine) various spastic conditions, including acute dystonic reactions, muscle rigidity, parkinsonism, and extrapyramidal disorders.

Adverse reactions

Therapeutic doses commonly cause dry mouth, decreased sweating or anhidrosis, headache, mydriasis, blurred vision, cycloplegia, urinary hesitancy and retention, constipation, palpitations, and tachycardia; these reactions usually disappear on discontinuation. Toxicity can cause signs resembling psychosis (disorientation, confusion, hallucinations, delusions, anxiety, agitation, and restlessness); dilated, nonreactive pupils; blurred vision; hot, dry, flushed skin; dry mucous membranes; dysphagia; decreased or absent bowel sounds; urine retention; hyperthermia; tachycardia; hypertension; and increased respirations.

Contraindications and precautions

• Contraindicated in patients with known hypersensitivity to drug, narrow-angle glaucoma, renal or GI obstructive disease, reflux esophagitis, or myasthenia gravis.
• Use with caution in patients with coronary heart disease, GI infection, open-angle glaucoma, prostatic hypertrophy, hypertension, hyperthyroidism, ulcerative colitis, autonomic neuropathy, or hiatal hernia associated with reflux esophagitis. Patients older than age 40 may be more sensitive to these drugs.
• **Geriatric use:** Use with caution in elderly patients. Lower doses are usually indicated.
• **Pediatric use:** Safety and efficacy have not been established in children.
• **Breast-feeding:** Anticholinergics may decrease milk production, and some may be excreted in breast milk, possibly resulting in infant toxicity. Breast-feeding women should avoid these drugs.

NURSING CONSIDERATIONS

⚕ Assessment

• Monitor regularly for adverse reactions.
• Monitor vital signs at least every 4 hours.
• Monitor urine output; check for urine retention.
• Monitor for changes in vision and for signs of impending toxicity.

⊕ Key nursing diagnoses

• Urine retention related to adverse effect on bladder
• Constipation related to adverse effect on GI tract
• Pain related to headache

▶ Planning and implementation

• Administer drug 30 minutes to 1 hour before meals and at bedtime to maximize therapeutic effects. In some instances, drug should be administered with meals; follow dosage recommendations.
• Provide ice chips, cool drinks, or hard candy to relieve dry mouth.
• Relieve constipation with stool softeners or bulk laxatives.
• Administer mild analgesic for headache.

• Notify doctor of urine retention, and be prepared for catheterization.
Patient teaching
• Teach patient how and when to take his drug; caution him not to take other drugs unless prescribed.
• Warn patient to avoid driving and other hazardous tasks if he experiences dizziness, drowsiness, or blurred vision. Inform him that drug may cause increased sensitivity to or intolerance of high temperatures, resulting in dizziness.
• Advise patient to avoid alcohol; it can cause additive CNS effects.
• Urge patient to drink plenty of fluids and to eat a high-fiber diet to prevent constipation.
• Tell patient to notify doctor promptly if he experiences confusion, rapid or pounding heartbeat, dry mouth, blurred vision, skin rash, eye pain, significant change in urine volume, or pain or difficulty on urination.
• Advise female patient to report planned or suspected pregnancy.

☑ **Evaluation**
• Patient maintains normal voiding pattern.
• Patient regains normal bowel patterns.
• Patient is free from pain.

Anticoagulants
Coumarin derivative
  warfarin sodium
Heparin derivatives
  dalteparin sodium
  danaparoid sodium
  enoxaparin sodium
  heparin calcium
  heparin sodium

Action

Heparin derivatives accelerate formation of an antithrombin III-thrombin complex. This inactivates thrombin and prevents conversion of fibrinogen to fibrin. The coumarin derivative, warfarin, inhibits vitamin K-dependent activation of clotting factors II, VII, IX, and X, which are formed in the liver.

Indications

▶ Pulmonary emboli, deep vein thrombosis, thrombus, blood clotting, disseminated intravascular coagulation.

Adverse reactions

Anticoagulants commonly cause bleeding and may cause hypersensitivity reactions. Warfarin may cause agranulocytosis, alopecia (long-term use), anorexia, dermatitis, fever, nausea, tissue necrosis or gangrene, urticaria, and vomiting. Heparin derivatives may cause thrombocytopenia and elevated liver enzyme levels.

Contraindications and precautions

• Contraindicated in patients with aneurysm, active bleeding, CV hemorrhage, hemorrhagic blood dyscrasias, hemophilia, severe hypertension, pericardial effusions, or pericarditis; in pregnant women or those with threatened or complete abortion; and in neurosurgery, ophthalmic surgery, or major surgery.
• Use with caution in patients with severe diabetes, renal impairment, severe trauma, ulcerations, or vasculitis.
• **Geriatric use:** Elderly patients are more susceptible to anticoagulants and are at greater risk for hemorrhage because of altered hemostatic mechanisms or age-related deterioration of hepatic and renal functions.
• **Pediatric use:** Infants, especially neonates, may be more susceptible to anticoagulants because of vitamin K deficiency.
• **Breast-feeding:** Women should avoid breast-feeding during therapy, if possible.

Prototype drug

Assessment
• Monitor closely for bleeding and other adverse reactions.
• Monitor PT, INR, PTT, or activated PTT, as ordered.
• Monitor vital signs, hemoglobin level, and hematocrit value.
• Check patient's urine, stools, and emesis for blood.

Key nursing diagnoses
• Altered protection related to drug's effects on body's normal clotting and bleeding mechanisms
• Risk for fluid volume deficit related to bleeding
• Noncompliance related to long-term warfarin therapy

Planning and implementation
• Don't administer heparin I.M., and avoid I.M. injections of any anticoagulant, if possible.
• Have protamine sulfate available to treat severe bleeding caused by heparin. Have vitamin K available to treat frank bleeding caused by warfarin.
• Notify doctor of serious or persistent adverse reactions.
• Maintain bleeding precautions throughout therapy.
Patient teaching
• Urge patient to take his drug exactly as prescribed. If he's taking warfarin, tell him to take it at night and to have blood drawn for PT or INR in the morning for accurate results.
• Advise patient to consult his doctor before taking any other drug, including OTC medications.
• Review bleeding precautions to take in everyday living. Urge him to make repairs and to remove potential safety hazards from home to reduce potential for injury.
• Caution patient not to increase his intake of green, leafy vegetables (vitamin K may antagonize anticoagulant effects).

• Instruct patient to report bleeding or other adverse reactions promptly.
• Encourage patient to keep appointments for blood tests and follow-up examinations.
• Advise female patient to report pregnancy or intent to conceive.

Evaluation
• Patient does not experience adverse change in health status.
• Patient does not exhibit signs and symptoms of bleeding.
• Patient demonstrates compliance with therapy, as evidenced by normal bleeding and clotting parameters.

Anticonvulsants

acetazolamide sodium
carbamazepine
clonazepam
clorazepate dipotassium
diazepam
divalproex sodium
ethosuximide
gabapentin
lamotrigine
magnesium sulfate
methsuximide
phenobarbital
phenobarbital sodium
phensuximide
phenytoin
phenytoin sodium
phenytoin sodium (extended)
primidone
tiagabine hydrochloride
topiramate
valproate sodium
valproic acid

Action

Anticonvulsants comprise six classes of drugs: selected hydantoin derivatives, barbiturates, benzodiazepines, succinimides, iminostilbene derivatives (carbamazepine), and carboxylic acid derivatives. Two miscellaneous anticonvulsants are acetazolamide and magnesium sulfate. Selected hydantoin derivatives and carbamazepine inhibit the spread of seizure activity in the motor cortex. Selected barbiturates and succinimides limit seizure activity by increasing the threshold for motor cortex stimuli. Selected benzodiazepines and carboxylic acid derivatives are thought to increase the inhibiting action of gamma-aminobutyric acid in brain neurons. Acetazolamide inhibits carbonic anhydrase. Magnesium sulfate interferes with the release of acetylcholine at the myoneural junction.

Indications

▶ Seizure disorders; acute, isolated seizures not caused by seizure disorders; status epilepticus; prevention of seizures after trauma or craniotomy.

Adverse reactions

Anticonvulsants can cause adverse CNS effects, such as confusion, somnolence, tremor, and ataxia. Many anticonvulsants also cause GI effects, such as vomiting; CV disorders, such as arrhythmias and hypotension; and hematologic disorders, such as leukopenia and thrombocytopenia.

Contraindications and precautions

• Contraindicated in patients with hypersensitivity to anticonvulsants.
• Additional contraindications and precautions vary. See individual drugs for complete listings.
• **Geriatric use:** Elderly patients are sensitive to CNS effects and may require lower doses. They also may show prolonged elimination of some anticonvulsants because of decreased renal function. Parenteral use is more likely to cause apnea, hypotension, bradycardia, and cardiac arrest.
• **Pediatric use:** Children, especially young ones, are sensitive to CNS depres-

sant effects of some anticonvulsants. Use with caution.
• **Breast-feeding:** Safety of many anticonvulsants has not been established in breast-feeding women. See individual drugs for guidelines.

NURSING CONSIDERATIONS

⚕ Assessment
• Monitor patient's response to prescribed drug and serum levels as indicated.
• Monitor for adverse reactions.
• Assess patient's compliance with therapy at each follow-up visit.

🔑 Key nursing diagnoses
• Risk for trauma related to adverse reactions
• Impaired physical mobility related to sedation
• Noncompliance related to long-term therapy

❯ Planning and implementation
• Administer oral preparations with food to reduce GI irritation.
• Be aware that phenytoin binds with tube feedings, thus decreasing absorption of drug. Turn off tube feedings 2 hours before and until 2 hours after administering phenytoin according to institutional policy.
• Expect to adjust dosage according to patient's response.
• Use safety precautions if patient exhibits adverse CNS reactions.
Patient teaching
• Instruct patient to take drug exactly as prescribed. Warn him not to discontinue drug without medical supervision.
• Urge patient to avoid activities that require mental alertness if adverse CNS reactions occur.
• Advise patient to carry medical identification at all times.

☑ Evaluation
• Patient does not experience trauma from adverse reactions.
• Patient maintains physical mobility.
• Patient complies with therapy and is free from seizure activity.

Antidepressants, tricyclic

amitriptyline hydrochloride
amitriptyline pamoate
amoxapine
clomipramine hydrochloride
desipramine hydrochloride
doxepin hydrochloride
imipramine hydrochloride
imipramine pamoate
maprotiline hydrochloride
nortriptyline hydrochloride
trimipramine maleate

Action

Tricyclic antidepressants (TCAs) may inhibit reuptake of norepinephrine and serotonin in CNS nerve terminals (presynaptic neurons), enhancing concentration and activity of neurotransmitters in the synaptic cleft. TCAs also exert antihistaminic, sedative, anticholinergic, vasodilatory, and quinidine-like effects.

Indications

▶ Depression (all TCAs), anxiety (doxepin hydrochloride), obsessive-compulsive disorder (clomipramine), enuresis in children older than age 6 (imipramine).

Adverse reactions

Adverse reactions include sedation, anticholinergic effects, and orthostatic hypotension. Tertiary amines (amitriptyline, doxepin, imipramine, and trimipramine) exert strongest sedative effects; tolerance usually develops in a few weeks. Maprotiline and amoxapine are most likely to cause seizures, especially with overdose.

Contraindications and precautions

• Contraindicated in patients with urine retention, narrow-angle glaucoma, or known hypersensitivity to TCAs.
• Use with caution in pregnant or breast-feeding women and in patients with suicidal tendencies, CV disease, or impaired hepatic function.
• **Geriatric use:** Elderly patients are more sensitive to therapeutic and adverse effects and require lower doses.
• **Pediatric use:** TCAs are not recommended for children under age 12.
• **Breast-feeding:** Safety in breast-feeding women has not been established.

NURSING CONSIDERATIONS

☷ Assessment
• Observe patient for mood changes to monitor drug effectiveness; benefits may not appear for 3 to 6 weeks.
• Check vital signs regularly for decreased blood pressure or tachycardia; observe patient carefully for other adverse reactions and report changes. Check ECG in patients older than age 40 before initiating therapy.
• Monitor for anticholinergic adverse reactions (urine retention or constipation), which may require dosage reduction.

⊕ Key nursing diagnoses
• Altered thought processes related to adverse effects
• Risk for injury related to sedation and orthostatic hypotension
• Noncompliance related to long-term therapy

▷ Planning and implementation
• Make sure patient swallows each dose; as depressed patient begins to improve, he may hoard pills for suicide attempt.
• Do not withdraw drug abruptly; gradually reduce dosage over several weeks, as ordered, to avoid rebound effect or other adverse reactions.

• Follow manufacturer's instructions for reconstitution, dilution, and storage of drugs.

Patient teaching

• Explain to patient the rationale for therapy and anticipated risks and benefits. Inform patient that full therapeutic effect may not occur for several weeks.

• Teach patient how and when to take his drug. Warn him not to increase his dosage, discontinue drug, or take any other drug (including OTC products) without medical approval.

• Because overdosage with TCAs is commonly fatal, entrust a reliable family member with the medication, and warn him to store drug safely away from children.

• Advise patient not to take drug with milk or food to minimize GI distress; suggest taking full dose at bedtime if daytime sedation is troublesome.

• Tell patient to avoid beverages and other products containing alcohol.

• Advise patient to avoid tasks that require mental alertness until drug's effects are known.

• Warn patient that excessive exposure to sunlight, heat lamps, or tanning beds may cause burns and abnormal hyperpigmentation.

• Urge a diabetic patient to monitor blood glucose (drug may alter blood glucose levels).

• Recommend sugarless gum or hard candy, artificial saliva, or ice chips to relieve dry mouth.

• Advise patient to report adverse reactions promptly.

☑ **Evaluation**

• Patient regains normal thought processes.

• Patient does not experience injury from adverse reactions.

• Patient complies with therapy, and his depression is alleviated.

Antidiarrheals
bismuth subgallate
bismuth subsalicylate
calcium polycarbophil
diphenoxylate hydrochloride and
    atropine sulfate
kaolin and pectin mixtures
loperamide
octreotide acetate
opium tincture
opium tincture, camphorated

Action

Bismuth preparations may have a mild water-binding capacity; they also may absorb toxins and provide protective coating for intestinal mucosa. Kaolin and pectin mixtures decrease the stool's fluid content by absorbing bacteria and toxins that cause diarrhea. Opium preparations increase smooth muscle tone in the GI tract, inhibit motility and propulsion, and diminish digestive secretions.

Indications

▶ Mild, acute, or chronic diarrhea.

Adverse reactions

Bismuth preparations may cause salicylism (with high doses) or temporary darkening of tongue and stools. Kaolin and pectin mixtures may cause constipation and fecal impaction or ulceration. Opium preparations may cause dizziness, light-headedness, nausea, physical dependence (with long-term use), and vomiting.

Contraindications and precautions

• Contraindicated in patients with known hypersensitivity to drug.

• Additional contraindications and precautions vary with the prescribed drug. See individual drugs for specific recommendations.

• **Geriatric use:** Use with caution when administering antidiarrheal drugs, especially opium preparations.

• **Pediatric use:** Consult doctor before giving bismuth subsalicylate to children or teenagers recovering from flu or chicken-pox. Do not administer kaolin and pectin mixtures to children younger than age 2.
• **Breast-feeding:** Some antidiarrheal drugs may be excreted in breast milk. Check individual drugs for specific rec-ommendations.

NURSING CONSIDERATIONS

▣ Assessment
• Assess patient's condition before thera-py and regularly thereafter.
• Monitor fluid and electrolyte balance.
• Monitor patient for adverse reactions.

▣ Key nursing diagnoses
• Constipation related to adverse effect of bismuth preparations on GI tract
• Risk for injury related to adverse CNS reactions
• Risk for fluid volume deficit related to GI upset

▣ Planning and implementation
• Administer drug exactly as prescribed.
• Take safety precautions if patient expe-riences adverse CNS reactions.
• Do not substitute opium tincture for paregoric.
• Notify doctor of serious or persistent adverse reactions.
Patient teaching
• Instruct patient to take drug exactly as prescribed; inform him that excessive use of opium preparations can result in de-pendence.
• Instruct patient to notify doctor if diar-rhea lasts for more than 2 days and to re-port adverse reactions.
• Warn patient to avoid activities that re-quire alertness if CNS depression occurs.

▣ Evaluation
• Patient does not experience constipa-tion.
• Patient remains free from injury.
• Patient maintains adequate hydration.

Prototype drug

Antihistamines
astemizole
azatadine maleate
brompheniramine maleate
buclizine hydrochloride
chlorpheniramine maleate
clemastine fumarate
cyclizine hydrochloride
cyclizine lactate
cyproheptadine hydrochloride
dimenhydrinate
diphenhydramine hydrochloride
fexofenadine hydrochloride
loratadine
meclizine hydrochloride
promethazine hydrochloride
promethazine theoclate
tripelennamine citrate
tripelennamine hydrochloride
triprolidine hydrochloride

Action

Antihistamines are structurally related chemicals that compete with histamine for histamine H_1-receptor sites on smooth muscle of bronchi, GI tract, uterus, and large blood vessels, binding to cellular receptors and preventing ac-cess to and subsequent activity of hista-mine. They do not directly alter hista-mine or prevent its release.

Indications

▶ Rhinitis, urticaria, pruritus, vertigo, nausea and vomiting, sedation, dyskine-sia, parkinsonism.

Adverse reactions

Most antihistamines cause drowsiness and impaired motor function during ini-tial therapy. They also can cause dry mouth and throat, blurred vision, and constipation. Some antihistamines, such as promethazine, may cause cholestatic jaundice (thought to be a hypersensitivity reaction) and may predispose patients to photosensitivity.

Contraindications and precautions

• Contraindicated in patients with known hypersensitivity to drug and in breast-feeding women.
• Use with caution in patients with narrow-angle glaucoma, stenosing peptic ulcer, pyloroduodenal obstruction, or bladder neck obstruction.
• **Geriatric use:** Elderly patients are usually more sensitive to adverse effects of antihistamines, especially dizziness, sedation, hypotension, and urine retention.
• **Pediatric use:** Children, especially those younger than age 6, may experience paradoxical hyperexcitability with restlessness, insomnia, nervousness, euphoria, tremors, and seizures. Administer cautiously.
• **Breast-feeding:** Antihistamines should not be used during breast-feeding; many of these drugs are excreted in breast milk, exposing the infant to unusual excitability; neonates, especially premature infants, may experience seizures.

NURSING CONSIDERATIONS

⚕ Assessment
• Monitor patient for adverse reactions.
• Monitor blood counts during long-term therapy; watch for signs of blood dyscrasia.

⊕ Key nursing diagnoses
• Risk for injury related to sedation
• Altered oral mucous membrane related to dry mouth
• Constipation related to anticholinergic effect of antihistamines

⊠ Planning and implementation
• Reduce GI distress by giving antihistamines with food.
• Provide sugarless gum, hard candy, or ice chips to relieve dry mouth.
• Increase fluid intake (if allowed) or humidify air to decrease adverse effect of thickened secretions.

Patient teaching
• Advise patient to take drug with meals or snacks to prevent gastric upset and to use warm water rinses, artificial saliva, ice chips, or sugarless gum or candy to relieve dry mouth. Tell him to avoid overusing mouthwash, which may exacerbate dryness and destroy normal flora.
• Warn patient to avoid hazardous activities, such as driving a car or operating machinery, until drug's CNS effects are known.
• Caution patient to seek medical approval before using alcohol, tranquilizers, sedatives, pain relievers, or sleeping medications.
• Advise patient to stop taking antihistamines 4 days before diagnostic skin tests to preserve accuracy of test results.

☑ Evaluation
• Patient does not experience injury from sedation.
• Patient maintains normal mucous membranes by using preventive measures throughout therapy.
• Patient regains normal bowel function.

Antihypertensives

ACE inhibitors
    benazepril hydrochloride
    captopril
    enalaprilat
    enalapril maleate
    fosinopril sodium
    moexipril hydrochloride
    quinapril hydrochloride
    ramipril
Alpha-adrenergic blockers
    doxazosin mesylate
    phentolamine mesylate
    prazosin hydrochloride
    terazosin hydrochloride
Angiotension II receptor blockers
    candesartan cilexetil
    irbesartan
    losartan potassium
    telmisartan

Beta blockers
  acebutolol
  atenolol
  betaxolol hydrochloride
  carteolol hydrochloride
  carvedilol
  labetalol hydrochloride
  metoprolol tartrate
  nadolol
  penbutolol sulfate
  pindolol
  propranolol hydrochloride
  timolol maleate
Calcium channel blockers
  amlodipine besylate
  diltiazem hydrochloride
  felodipine
  isradipine
  nicardipine hydrochloride
  nifedipine
  nisoldipine
  verapamil hydrochloride
Centrally acting sympatholytics
  clonidine hydrochloride
  guanabenz acetate
  guanfacine hydrochloride
  methyldopa
Rauwolfia alkaloid
  reserpine
Vasodilators
  diazoxide
  hydralazine hydrochloride
  minoxidil
  nitroprusside sodium

Action

Antihypertensives reduce blood pressure through various mechanisms, depending on the drug used. For information on the action of ACE inhibitors, alpha-adrenergic blockers, angiotension II receptor blockers, beta-adrenergic blockers, calcium channel blockers, and diuretics, see their drug class entries. Centrally acting sympatholytics stimulate central alpha-adrenergic receptors, reducing cerebral sympathetic outflow, thereby decreasing peripheral vascular resistance and blood pressure. Rauwolfia alkaloids bind to and gradually destroy the norepinephrine-containing storage vesicles in central and peripheral adrenergic neurons. Vasodilators act directly on smooth muscle to reduce blood pressure.

Indications

▶ Essential and secondary hypertension.

Adverse reactions

Most antihypertensives commonly cause orthostatic hypotension, changes in heart rate, headache, nausea, and vomiting. Other reactions vary greatly among different drug types. Centrally acting sympatholytics may cause constipation, depression, dizziness, drowsiness, dry mouth, headache, palpitations, severe rebound hypertension, and sexual dysfunction; methyldopa may also cause aplastic anemia and thrombocytopenia. Rauwolfia alkaloids may cause anxiety, depression, drowsiness, dry mouth, hyperacidity, impotence, nasal stuffiness, and weight gain. Vasodilators may cause heart failure, ECG changes, diarrhea, dizziness, palpitations, pruritus, and rash.

Contraindications and precautions

• Contraindicated in patients with hypotension or known hypersensitivity to drug.
• Use with caution in patients with hepatic or renal dysfunction and in pregnant or breast-feeding women.
• Additional contraindications and precautions exist. See individual drugs for complete listings.
• **Geriatric use:** Elderly patients are more prone to adverse reactions and may require lower maintenance doses. Monitor closely.
• **Pediatric use:** Safety and efficacy of many antihypertensives have not been established in children. Administer cautiously and monitor closely.

• **Breast-feeding:** Some antihypertensives are excreted in breast milk. See individual drugs for recommendations.

NURSING CONSIDERATIONS

≈ Assessment
• Obtain baseline blood pressure and pulse rate and rhythm; recheck regularly.
• Monitor patient for adverse reactions.
• Monitor patient's weight and fluid and electrolyte status.
• Monitor patient's compliance with treatment.

⊞ Key nursing diagnoses
• Risk for trauma related to orthostatic hypotension
• Risk for fluid volume deficit related to GI upset
• Noncompliance related to long-term therapy or adverse reactions

⊠ Planning and implementation
• Administer drug with food or at bedtime, as indicated.
• Follow manufacturer's guidelines when mixing and administering parenteral drugs.
• Take steps to prevent or minimize orthostatic hypotension.
• Maintain patient's nonpharmacologic therapy, such as sodium restriction, calorie reduction, stress management, and exercise program.
Patient teaching
• Instruct patient to take drug exactly as prescribed. Warn him not to discontinue drug abruptly.
• Review adverse reactions associated with drug, and urge patient to notify doctor of serious or persistent reactions.
• Advise patient to avoid sudden changes in position to prevent dizziness, lightheadedness, or fainting.
• Caution patient to avoid driving or performing hazardous activities until drug's effects are known and to avoid physical exertion, especially in hot weather.

• Advise patient to consult doctor before taking any OTC medications; serious drug interactions can occur.
• Encourage patient to comply with therapy.

☑ Evaluation
• Patient does not experience trauma from orthostatic hypotension.
• Patient maintains adequate hydration.
• Patient demonstrates compliance with therapy, as evidenced by normal blood pressure.

Antilipemics
cerivastatin sodium
cholestyramine
clofibrate
colestipol hydrochloride
fenofibrate
fluvastatin sodium
gemfibrozil
lovastatin
pravastatin sodium
simvastatin

Action

Antilipemics lower elevated blood levels of lipids. Bile-sequestering drugs (cholestyramine, colestipol) lower blood levels of low-density lipoproteins by forming insoluble complexes with bile salts, triggering cholesterol to leave the bloodstream and other storage areas to make new bile acids. Fibric acid derivatives (clofibrate, gemfibrozil) reduce cholesterol formation, increase sterol excretion, and decrease lipoprotein and triglyceride synthesis. Cholesterol synthesis inhibitors (fluvastatin, lovastatin, pravastatin, simvastatin) interfere with enzymatic activity that generates cholesterol in the liver.

Indications

▶ Hyperlipidemia, hypercholesterolemia.

Prototype drug

Adverse reactions

Antilipemics commonly cause GI upset. Bile-sequestering drugs may cause cholelithiasis, constipation, bloating, and steatorrhea. Fibric acid derivatives may cause cholelithiasis and GI or CNS effects. Concomitant use of gemfibrozil with lovastatin is associated with myopathy. Cholesterol synthesis inhibitors may affect liver function or cause rash, pruritus, increased CK levels, and myopathy.

Contraindications and precautions

• Contraindicated in patients with known hypersensitivity to drug. Also, bile-sequestering drugs are contraindicated in patients with complete biliary obstruction; fibric acid derivatives in patients with significant hepatic or renal dysfunction or primary biliary cirrhosis and in breast-feeding women; and cholesterol synthesis inhibitors in patients with active liver disease or persistently elevated serum transaminase levels and in pregnant or breast-feeding women.
• Use bile-sequestering drugs with caution in patients with constipation and in pregnant or breast-feeding women. Use fibric acid derivatives with caution in patients with peptic ulcer and in pregnant women. Use cholesterol synthesis inhibitors with caution in patients with high alcohol consumption or history of liver disease.
• **Geriatric use:** Elderly patients are at greater risk for development of severe constipation. Monitor closely.
• **Pediatric use:** Safety of antilipemic drugs has not been established in children.
• **Breast-feeding:** Fibric acid derivatives and cholesterol synthesis inhibitors should not be used in breast-feeding women; bile-sequestering drugs require cautious use.

NURSING CONSIDERATIONS

☰ Assessment
• Monitor blood cholesterol and lipid levels before and periodically during therapy.
• Monitor CK levels when therapy begins and every 6 months thereafter. Also monitor during therapy with a cholesterol synthesis inhibitor if patient complains of muscle pain.
• Monitor patient for adverse reactions.

🔟 Key nursing diagnoses
• Risk for fluid volume deficit related to adverse GI reactions
• Constipation related to adverse effect on bowel
• Noncompliance related to long-term therapy

▶ Planning and implementation
• Mix powder form of bile-sequestering drugs with 120 to 180 ml of liquid. Never administer dry powder alone because patient may inhale it accidentally.
• Administer daily fibric acid derivative according to times prescribed.
• Administer lovastatin with evening meal, simvastatin in the evening, and fluvastatin and pravastatin at bedtime.
Patient teaching
• Instruct patient to take his drug exactly as prescribed. If he's taking a bile-sequestering drug, warn him never to take it in its dry form.
• Stress importance of diet in controlling serum lipid levels.
• Advise him to drink at least 2 to 3 L of fluid daily and to report persistent or severe constipation.

☑ Evaluation
• Patient maintains adequate fluid volume.
• Patient does not experience severe or persistent constipation.
• Patient complies with therapy, as evidenced by normal serum lipid and cholesterol levels.

Antimetabolite antineoplastics

cytarabine
floxuridine
fludarabine phosphate
fluorouracil
hydroxyurea
mercaptopurine
methotrexate
thioguanine

Action

Antimetabolites are structural analogues of normally occurring metabolites and can be divided into three subcategories: purine analogues, pyrimidine analogues, and folinic acid analogues. Most of these drugs interrupt cell reproduction at a specific phase of the cell cycle. Purine analogues are incorporated into DNA and RNA, interfering with nucleic acid synthesis (via miscoding) and replication. They also may inhibit synthesis of purine bases through pseudo-feedback mechanisms. Pyrimidine analogues inhibit enzymes in metabolic pathways that interfere with biosynthesis of uridine and thymine. Folic acid antagonists prevent conversion of folic acid to tetrahydrofolate by inhibiting the enzyme dihydrofolic acid reductase.

Indications

▶ Treatment of various tumors. See individual drugs for specific uses.

Adverse reactions

The most frequent adverse effects include nausea, vomiting, diarrhea, fever, chills, hair loss, flank or joint pain, redness or pain at injection site, anxiety, bone marrow depression, leukopenia, and swelling of feet or lower legs.

Contraindications and precautions

• Contraindicated in patients with known hypersensitivity to drug.

• Additional contraindications and precautions exist. See individual drugs for complete listings.
• **Geriatric use:** Elderly patients are at increased risk for adverse reactions. Monitor closely.
• **Pediatric use:** Safety and efficacy of some drugs have not been established in children. See individual drugs for specific guidelines.
• **Breast-feeding:** Breast-feeding is contraindicated in women receiving chemotherapy, including antimetabolite antineoplastic drugs.

NURSING CONSIDERATIONS

⚖ Assessment
• Perform a complete assessment before therapy begins.
• Monitor patient for adverse reactions.
• Monitor vital signs and patency of catheter or I.V. line throughout administration.
• Monitor BUN, hematocrit, platelet count, ALT, AST, LD, serum bilirubin, serum creatinine, uric acid, total and differential leukocyte, and other values as required.

🔢 Key nursing diagnoses
• Altered protection related to thrombocytopenia
• Risk for infection related to immunosuppression
• Risk for fluid volume deficit related to adverse GI effects

❯ Planning and implementation
• Follow established procedures for safe and proper handling, administration, and disposal of drugs.
• Treat extravasation promptly.
• Give an antiemetic before administering drug, as ordered, to lessen nausea.
• Administer cytarabine with allopurinol, as ordered, to decrease risk of hyperuricemia; promote high fluid intake.

● Provide diligent mouth care to prevent stomatitis with cytarabine, fluorouracil, or methotrexate therapy.
● Anticipate need for leucovorin rescue with high-dose methotrexate therapy.
● Attempt to alleviate or reduce anxiety in patient and family before treatment.
● Have patient avoid immunizations if possible.
● Anticipate diarrhea, possibly severe, with prolonged fluorouracil therapy.
Patient teaching
● Teach patient proper oral hygiene, including cautious use of toothbrush, dental floss, and toothpicks. Chemotherapy can increase incidence of microbial infection, delayed healing, and bleeding gums.
● Advise patient to complete dental work before therapy begins or to delay it until blood counts are normal.
● Warn patient that he may bruise easily because of drug's effect on platelets.
● Advise patient to avoid close contact with persons who have taken oral poliovirus vaccine and to avoid exposure to persons with bacterial or viral infection (chemotherapy may increase susceptibility). Urge him to notify doctor promptly if he experiences signs or symptoms of infection.
● Instruct patient to report redness, pain, or swelling at injection site. Local tissue injury and scarring may result from tissue infiltration at infusion site.

☑ Evaluation
● Patient does not develop serious bleeding complications.
● Patient remains free from infection.
● Patient maintains adequate hydration.

Antiparkinsonian drugs
amantadine hydrochloride
benztropine mesylate
biperiden hydrochloride
biperiden lactate
bromocriptine mesylate
carbidopa-levodopa
levodopa
pergolide mesylate
pramipexole dihydrochloride
ropinirole hydrochloride
selegiline hydrochloride
tolcapone
trihexyphenidyl hydrochloride

Action

Antiparkinsonian drugs include synthetic anticholinergic and dopaminergic drugs and the antiviral drug amantadine. Anticholinergics are thought to prolong dopamine's action by blocking its reuptake into presynaptic neurons in the CNS and by suppressing central cholinergic activity. Dopaminergic drugs act in the brain by increasing dopamine availability, thus improving motor function. Amantadine is thought to increase dopamine release in the substantia nigra.

Indications
▶ Parkinson's disease.

Adverse reactions

Anticholinergic drugs typically cause decreased sweating or anhidrosis, dry mouth, headache, mydriasis, blurred vision, cycloplegia, urinary hesitancy and urine retention, constipation, palpitations, and tachycardia. Dopaminergic drugs may cause vomiting, orthostatic hypotension, confusion, arrhythmias, and disturbing dreams. Amantadine commonly causes irritability, insomnia, and livedo reticularis (with prolonged use).

Contraindications and precautions
● Contraindicated in patients with known hypersensitivity to drug.

• Use with caution in patients with prostatic hyperplasia or tardive dyskinesia and in elderly or debilitated patients.
• Additional contraindications and precautions exist. See individual drugs for complete listings.
• **Geriatric use:** Elderly patients are at higher risk for adverse reactions. Monitor closely.
• **Pediatric use:** Safety and efficacy of drugs have not been established in children.
• **Breast-feeding:** Antiparkinsonian drugs may be excreted in breast milk; avoid using in breast-feeding women.

NURSING CONSIDERATIONS

⚏ Assessment
• Obtain baseline assessment of patient's impairment, and reassess regularly to monitor drug effectiveness.
• Monitor patient for adverse reactions.
• Monitor vital signs, especially during dosage adjustments.

⚏ Key nursing diagnoses
• Risk for injury related to adverse CNS effects
• Urine retention related to anticholinergic effect on bladder
• Sleep pattern disturbance related to amantadine-induced insomnia

⚏ Planning and implementation
• Administer drug with food to prevent GI irritation.
• Adjust dosage, as ordered, according to patient's response and tolerance.
• Never withdraw drug abruptly.
• Institute safety precautions.
• Provide ice chips, drinks, or hard sugarless candy to relieve dry mouth. Increase fluid and fiber intake to prevent constipation, as appropriate.
• Notify doctor of urine retention, and be prepared to catheterize patient.

Patient teaching
• Instruct patient to take drug exactly as prescribed, and warn him not to stop drug suddenly.
• Advise patient to take drug with food to prevent GI upset.
• Teach patient how to manage anticholinergic effects, if appropriate.
• Caution patient to avoid driving and performing hazardous tasks if adverse CNS effects occur, and warn him to avoid alcohol during therapy.
• Encourage patient to report severe or persistent adverse reactions.

☑ Evaluation
• Patient remains free from injury.
• Patient has no change in voiding pattern.
• Patient's sleep pattern is not altered during amantadine therapy.

Antivirals
acyclovir sodium
amantadine hydrochloride
cidofovir
delavirdine mesylate
didanosine
efavirenz
famciclovir
foscarnet sodium
ganciclovir
indinavir sulfate
nelfinavir mesylate
nevirapine
ribavirin
rimantadine hydrochloride
ritonavir
saquinavir mesylate
stavudine
valacyclovir hydrochloride
zalcitabine
zidovudine

Action

Acyclovir, cidofovir, didanosine, famciclovir, ganciclovir, valacyclovir, and zalcitabine interfere with DNA synthesis and replication. Amantadine prevents the release of infectious viral nucleic acid into the host cell and possibly interferes with viral penetration into the cells. Foscarnet blocks the pyrophosphate binding site. Ribavirin's mechanism of action is unknown. Rimantadine prevents viral uncoating. Indinavir, ritonavir, saquinavir, and stavudine inhibit the activity of HIV protease. Delavirdine, efavirenz, nevirapine, and zidovudine inhibit reverse transcriptase.

Indications

▶ Viral infections.

Adverse reactions

Antiviral drugs may cause anorexia, chills, confusion, depression, diarrhea, dry mouth, edema, fatigue, hallucinations, headache, nausea, and vomiting. Additional adverse reactions exist. See individual drugs for complete listings.

Contraindications and precautions

• Contraindicated in patients with known hypersensitivity to drug.
• Additional contraindications and precautions exist. See individual drugs for complete listings.
• **Geriatric use:** Elderly patients are at greater risk for adverse reactions. Monitor closely.
• **Pediatric use:** Recommendations vary, depending on the antiviral prescribed. See individual drugs for specific guidelines regarding use in infants and children.
• **Breast-feeding:** Some antiviral drugs are contraindicated in breast-feeding women; others require cautious use. See individual drugs for specific guidelines.

NURSING CONSIDERATIONS

🔖 Assessment
• Obtain baseline assessment of patient's viral infection, and reassess regularly to monitor drug's effectiveness.

• Monitor renal and hepatic function, CBC, and platelet count regularly. Monitor electrolytes (calcium, phosphate, magnesium, potassium) in patients receiving foscarnet.
• Inspect patient's I.V. site regularly for signs of irritation, phlebitis, inflammation, or extravasation.
• Monitor a patient with a history of heart failure for exacerbation or recurrence of heart failure during amantadine therapy.
• Monitor patient's cardiac status during ribavirin therapy.

🔁 Key nursing diagnoses
• Altered protection related to adverse hematologic reactions
• Risk for fluid volume deficit related to GI upset
• Noncompliance related to long-term therapy

▶ Planning and implementation
• Adjust dosage of selected antiviral drugs, as ordered, for patient with decreased renal function, especially during parenteral therapy.
• Follow manufacturer's guidelines for reconstituting and administering antiviral drugs.
• Obtain an order for an antiemetic or antidiarrheal drug, if needed.
• Institute safety precautions if patient experiences adverse CNS reactions. For example, place bed in low position, raise bed rails, and supervise ambulation and other activities.
• Notify doctor of serious or persistent adverse reactions.
Patient teaching
• Instruct patient to take drug exactly as prescribed, even if he feels better.
• Urge patient to notify doctor promptly of severe or persistent adverse reactions.
• Encourage patient to keep appointments for follow-up care.
• Provide additional teaching as indicated by individual drug.

☑ **Evaluation**
• Patient does not experience serious adverse hematologic effects.
• Patient maintains adequate hydration.
• Patient complies with therapy, and viral infection is eradicated.

Barbiturates
amobarbital
amobarbital sodium
aprobarbital
butabarbital
mephobarbital
pentobarbital sodium
phenobarbital
phenobarbital sodium
primidone
secobarbital sodium

Action

Barbiturates act throughout the CNS, particularly in the mesencephalic reticular activating system, which controls the CNS arousal mechanism. They decrease both presynaptic and postsynaptic membrane excitability, exerting their effects by facilitating the actions of gamma-aminobutyric acid (GABA). Barbiturates also exert a central effect, which depresses respiration and GI motility. The principal anticonvulsant mechanisms of action are reduction of nerve transmission and decreased excitability of the nerve cell. Barbiturates also raise the seizure threshold.

Indications

▶ Insomnia, seizure disorders.

Adverse reactions

Drowsiness, lethargy, vertigo, headache, and CNS depression are common with barbiturates. After hypnotic doses, a hangover effect, subtle distortion of mood, and impaired judgment and motor skills may continue for many hours; after dosage reduction or discontinuation, re-bound insomnia or increased dreaming or nightmares may occur. Barbiturates cause hyperalgesia in subhypnotic doses. They also can cause paradoxical excitement at low doses, confusion in elderly patients, and hyperactivity in children. High fever, severe headache, stomatitis, conjunctivitis, or rhinitis may precede potentially fatal skin eruptions. Withdrawal symptoms may occur after as little as 2 weeks of uninterrupted therapy.

Contraindications and precautions

• Contraindicated in patients with known hypersensitivity to drug and in those with bronchopneumonia or other severe pulmonary insufficiency.
• Use with caution in patients with blood pressure alterations, pulmonary disease, or CV dysfunction.
• **Geriatric use:** Elderly patients may experience hyperactivity, excitement, or hyperalgesia. Use with caution.
• **Pediatric use:** Premature infants are more susceptible to depressant effects of barbiturates because of immature hepatic metabolism. Children may experience hyperactivity, excitement, or hyperalgesia.
• **Breast-feeding:** Barbiturates are excreted in breast milk and may result in infant CNS depression. Use with caution.

NURSING CONSIDERATIONS

☑ **Assessment**
• Assess patient's level of consciousness and sleeping patterns before and during therapy to evaluate drug effectiveness. Monitor neurologic status for alteration or deterioration.
• Assess vital signs frequently, especially during I.V. administration.
• Monitor seizure character, frequency, and duration for changes, as indicated.
• Observe patient to prevent hoarding or self-dosing, especially if patient is depressed, suicidal, or drug dependent.

⊞ Key nursing diagnoses
• Risk for injury related to sedation
• Altered thought processes related to confusion
• Impaired adjustment related to drug dependence

▶ Planning and implementation
• When administering parenteral drug, avoid extravasation, which may cause local tissue damage and tissue necrosis; inject I.V. or deep I.M. only. Do not exceed 5 ml per I.M. injection site to avoid tissue damage.
• Have resuscitative measures available. Too rapid I.V. administration may cause respiratory depression, apnea, laryngospasm, or hypotension.
• Institute seizure precautions, as necessary.
• Institute safety measures to prevent falls and injury. Raise side rails, assist patient out of bed, and have call light within reach.
• Discontinue drug slowly, as ordered. Abrupt discontinuation may cause withdrawal symptoms.
Patient teaching
• Instruct patient to take drug exactly as prescribed. Caution him not to change the dosage or take other drugs, including OTC preparations, without doctor's approval.
• Reassure patient that a morning hangover is common after therapeutic use of barbiturates.
• Advise patient to avoid driving and other hazardous tasks that require alertness, and review other safety measures to prevent injury.
• Explain that barbiturates can cause physical or psychological dependence.
• Instruct patient to report skin eruption or other significant adverse effects.

☑ Evaluation
• Patient does not experience injury from sedation.
• Patient maintains normal thought processes.

• Patient does not sustain physical or psychological dependence.

Beta blockers
Beta₁ blockers
  acebutolol
  atenolol
  betaxolol hydrochloride
  bisoprolol fumarate
  esmolol hydrochloride
  metoprolol tartrate
Beta₁ and beta₂ blockers
  carteolol hydrochloride
  carvedilol
  labetalol hydrochloride
  nadolol
  penbutolol sulfate
  pindolol
  propranolol hydrochloride
  sotalol hydrochloride
  timolol maleate

Action

Beta blockers are chemicals that compete with beta agonists for available beta-receptor sites; individual drugs differ in their ability to affect beta receptors. Some drugs are considered nonselective; that is, they block beta₁ receptors in cardiac muscle and beta₂ receptors in bronchial and vascular smooth muscle. Several drugs are cardioselective and in lower doses primarily inhibit beta₁ receptors. Some beta blockers have intrinsic sympathomimetic activity and simultaneously stimulate and block beta receptors, decreasing cardiac output; still others also have membrane-stabilizing activity, which affects cardiac action potential.

Indications

▶ Hypertension (most drugs), angina pectoris (propranolol, atenolol, nadolol, and metoprolol), arrhythmias (propranolol, acebutolol, sotalol, and esmolol), glaucoma (betaxolol and timolol), prevention of myocardial infarction (timolol,

Prototype drug

propranolol, atenolol, and metoprolol), prevention of recurrent migraine and other vascular headaches (propranolol and timolol), pheochromocytomas or essential tremors (selected beta blockers).

Adverse reactions

Therapeutic doses may cause bradycardia, fatigue, and dizziness; some may cause other CNS disturbances, such as nightmares, depression, memory loss, and hallucinations. Toxic doses can produce severe hypotension, bradycardia, heart failure, or bronchospasm.

Contraindications and precautions

• Contraindicated in patients with known hypersensitivity to drug, cardiogenic shock, sinus bradycardia, heart block greater than first degree, bronchial asthma, and heart failure unless failure is caused by tachyarrhythmia treatable with propranolol.
• Use with caution in pregnant women and in patients with nonallergic bronchospastic disorders, diabetes mellitus, or impaired hepatic or renal function.
• **Geriatric use:** Elderly patients may require lower maintenance doses because of increased bioavailability or delayed metabolism; they also may experience enhanced adverse effects.
• **Pediatric use:** Safety and efficacy of beta-adrenergic blockers in children have not been established; use only if potential benefit outweighs risk.
• **Breast-feeding:** Beta-adrenergic blockers are distributed into breast milk. See individual drugs for specific recommendations.

NURSING CONSIDERATIONS

⚕ Assessment
• Check apical pulse rate daily; alert doctor if extremes occur (for example, a pulse rate slower than 60 beats/minute).
• Monitor blood pressure, ECG, and heart rate and rhythm frequently; be alert

for progression of AV block or bradycardia.
• Weigh patients with heart failure regularly; watch for gains of more than 2.25 kg (5 lb) per week.
• Observe diabetic patients for sweating, fatigue, and hunger. Signs of hypoglycemic shock are masked.

⊞ Key nursing diagnoses
• Risk for injury related to adverse CNS effects
• Fluid volume excess related to edema
• Decreased cardiac output related to bradycardia or hypotension

⊠ Planning and implementation
• Discontinue beta-adrenergic blocker, as ordered, before surgery for pheochromocytoma. Before any surgical procedure, notify anesthesiologist that patient is taking a beta-adrenergic blocker.
• Keep glucagon readily available in case doctor prescribes it to reverse beta blocker overdose.
Patient teaching
• Teach patient to take drug exactly as prescribed, even when he's feeling better.
• Warn patient not to discontinue drug suddenly; abrupt discontinuation can exacerbate angina or precipitate MI.
• Advise patient to seek doctor's approval before taking nonprescription cold preparations.
• Explain potential adverse reactions, and stress importance of reporting unusual effects.

☑ Evaluation
• Patient remains free from injury.
• Patient does not exhibit signs of edema.
• Patient maintains normal blood pressure and heart rate.

Calcium channel blockers

amlodipine besylate
bepridil hydrochloride
diltiazem hydrochloride
felodipine
isradipine
nicardipine hydrochloride
nifedipine
nimodipine
nisoldipine
verapamil hydrochloride

Action

The main physiologic action of calcium channel blockers is to inhibit calcium influx across the slow channels of myocardial and vascular smooth muscle cells. By inhibiting calcium influx into these cells, calcium channel blockers reduce intracellular calcium concentrations. This, in turn, dilates coronary arteries, peripheral arteries, and arterioles and slows cardiac conduction.

When used to treat Prinzmetal's variant angina, calcium channel blockers inhibit coronary spasm, increasing oxygen delivery to the heart. Peripheral artery dilation leads to a decrease in total peripheral resistance; this reduces afterload, which, in turn, decreases myocardial oxygen consumption. Inhibition of calcium influx into the specialized cardiac conduction cells (specifically, those in the sinoatrial and atrioventricular nodes) slows conduction through the heart. Of the calcium channel blockers, verapamil and diltiazem have the greatest effect on the AV node, slowing the ventricular rate in atrial fibrillation or flutter and converting supraventricular tachycardia (SVT) to normal sinus rhythm.

Indications

▶ Prinzmetal's variant angina, chronic stable angina, unstable angina, mild to moderate hypertension, arrhythmias.

Adverse reactions

Adverse reactions vary according to the drug used. Verapamil, for instance, may cause bradycardia, various degrees of heart block, exacerbation of heart failure, and hypotension after rapid I.V. administration. Prolonged oral verapamil therapy may cause constipation. Nifedipine may cause hypotension, peripheral edema, flushing, light-headedness, and headache. Diltiazem most commonly causes anorexia and nausea and may also induce various degrees of heart block, bradycardia, heart failure, and peripheral edema.

Contraindications and precautions

• Contraindicated in patients with known hypersensitivity to drug.
• Use with caution in pregnant women.
• **Geriatric use:** The half-life of calcium channel blockers may be increased in elderly patients as a result of decreased clearance. Use with caution.
• **Pediatric use:** Adverse hemodynamic effects of parenteral verapamil have been observed in neonates and infants. Safety and efficacy of other calcium channel blockers have not been established.
• **Breast-feeding:** Calcium channel blockers may be excreted in breast milk. To avoid possible adverse effects in infants, breast-feeding should be discontinued during therapy.

NURSING CONSIDERATIONS

⬚ Assessment
• Monitor cardiac rate and rhythm and blood pressure carefully when therapy is initiated or dosage is increased.
• Monitor fluid and electrolyte status.
• Monitor patient for adverse reactions.

⬚ Key nursing diagnoses
• Decreased cardiac output related to adverse CV reactions
• Constipation related to oral verapamil therapy
• Noncompliance related to long-term therapy

⧁ Planning and implementation

• Do not administer calcium supplements while patient is taking a calcium channel blocker; they may decrease the drug's effectiveness.

• Expect to decrease dosage gradually; calcium channel blockers should not be discontinued abruptly.

Patient teaching

• Teach patient to take drug exactly as prescribed, even when he's feeling better.

• Instruct patient to take a missed dose as soon as possible, unless it's almost time for his next dose. Warn him never to take a double dose.

• Caution patient not to discontinue drug suddenly; abrupt discontinuation can produce serious adverse effects.

• Urge patient to report irregular heartbeat, shortness of breath, swelling of hands and feet, pronounced dizziness, constipation, nausea, or hypotension.

☑ Evaluation

• Patient maintains adequate cardiac output throughout therapy, as evidenced by normal blood pressure and pulse rate.

• Patient regains normal bowel pattern.

• Patient complies with therapy, as evidenced by absence of symptoms related to underlying disorder.

Cephalosporins

First generation
  cefadroxil monohydrate
  cefazolin sodium
  cephalexin monohydrate
  cephradine
Second generation
  cefaclor
  cefmetazole sodium
  cefonicid sodium
  cefotetan disodium
  cefoxitin sodium
  cefprozil
  cefuroxime axetil
  cefuroxime sodium
  loracarbef

Third generation
  cefixime
  cefdinir
  cefepime hydrochloride
  cefoperazone sodium
  cefotaxime sodium
  cefpodoxime proxetil
  ceftazidime
  ceftibuten
  ceftizoxime sodium
  ceftriaxone sodium

Action

Cephalosporins are chemically and pharmacologically similar to penicillin; they act by inhibiting bacterial cell wall synthesis, causing rapid cell lysis. Their sites of action are enzymes known as penicillin-binding proteins (PBPs). The affinity of certain cephalosporins for PBPs in various microorganisms helps explain the differing spectra of activity in this class of antibiotics. Cephalosporins are bactericidal; they act against many aerobic gram-positive and gram-negative bacteria and some anaerobic bacteria; they do not kill fungi or viruses.

First-generation cephalosporins act against many gram-positive cocci, including penicillinase-producing *Staphylococcus aureus* and *Staphylococcus epidermidis; Streptococcus pneumoniae,* group B streptococci, and group A beta-hemolytic streptococci; susceptible gram-negative organisms include *Klebsiella pneumoniae, Escherichia coli, Proteus mirabilis,* and *Shigella.*

Second-generation cephalosporins are effective against all organisms attacked by first-generation drugs and have additional activity against *Branhamella catarrhalis, Haemophilus influenzae, Enterobacter, Citrobacter, Providencia, Acinetobacter, Serratia,* and *Neisseria. Bacteroides fragilis* is susceptible to cefotetan and cefoxitin.

Third-generation cephalosporins are less active than first- and second-generation drugs against gram-positive bacteria, but more active against gram-negative organisms, including those resistant to first- and second-generation drugs; they have the greatest stability against beta-lactamases produced by gram-negative bacteria. Susceptible gram-negative organisms include *E. coli, Klebsiella, Enterobacter, Providencia, Acinetobacter, Serratia, Proteus, Morganella,* and *Neisseria;* some third-generation drugs are active against *Bacteroides fragilis* and *Pseudomonas.*

Indications

▶ Infections of the lungs, skin, soft tissue, bones, joints, urinary and respiratory tracts, blood, abdomen, and heart; CNS infections caused by susceptible strains of *N. meningitidis, H. influenzae,* and *S. pneumoniae;* meningitis caused by *E. coli* or *Klebsiella;* infections that develop after surgical procedures classified as contaminated or potentially contaminated; penicillinase-producing *N. gonorrhoeae;* otitis media and ampicillin-resistant middle ear infection caused by *H. influenzae.*

Adverse reactions

Many cephalosporins share a similar profile of adverse effects. Hypersensitivity reactions range from mild rashes, fever, and eosinophilia to fatal anaphylaxis and are more common in patients with penicillin allergy. Hematologic reactions include positive direct and indirect antiglobulin (Coombs' test), thrombocytopenia or thrombocythemia, transient neutropenia, and reversible leukopenia. Adverse renal effects may occur with any cephalosporin; they are most common in older patients, those with decreased renal function, and those taking other nephrotoxic drugs. GI reactions include nausea, vomiting, diarrhea, abdominal pain, glossitis, dyspepsia, and tenesmus; minimal elevation of liver function test results occurs occasionally.

Local venous pain and irritation are common after I.M. injection; such reactions occur more often with higher doses and long-term therapy. Disulfiram-type reactions occur when cefoperazone or cefotetan are administered within 72 hours of alcohol ingestion. Bacterial and fungal superinfections result from suppression of normal flora.

Contraindications and precautions

• Contraindicated in patients with known hypersensitivity to drug.
• Use with caution in patients with renal or hepatic impairment, history of GI disease, or allergy to penicillins.
• **Geriatric use:** Elderly patients are susceptible to superinfection and coagulopathies. They commonly have renal impairment and may require lower dosage. Use with caution.
• **Pediatric use:** Serum half-life is prolonged in neonates and infants.
• **Breast-feeding:** Cephalosporins are excreted in breast milk; use with caution in breast-feeding women.

NURSING CONSIDERATIONS

Assessment
• Review patient's history of allergies. Try to determine whether previous reactions were true hypersensitivity reactions or merely adverse effects (such as GI distress) that patient has interpreted as allergy.
• Monitor continuously for possible hypersensitivity reactions or other untoward effects.
• Obtain results of culture and sensitivity tests before administering first dose; check test results periodically to assess drug effectiveness.
• Monitor renal function studies; dosages of certain cephalosporins must be lowered in patients with severe renal impairment. In decreased renal function, monitor BUN levels, serum creatinine levels, and urine output for significant changes.
• Monitor PT and platelet counts and assess patient for signs of hypoprothrombinemia, which may occur (with or with-

out bleeding) during therapy with cefoperazone, cefonicid, or cefotetan, usually
in elderly, debilitated, or malnourished
patients.
• Monitor patients on long-term therapy
for possible bacterial and fungal superinfection, especially elderly and debilitated
patients and those receiving immunosuppressants or radiation therapy.
• Monitor susceptible patients receiving
sodium salts of cephalosporins for possible fluid retention (consult individual
drug entry for sodium content).

🔂 Key nursing diagnoses
• Altered protection related to hypersensitivity
• Risk for infection related to superinfection
• Risk for fluid volume deficit related to
adverse GI reactions

⟩ Planning and implementation
• Administer cephalosporins at least 1
hour before bacteriostatic antibiotics
(tetracyclines, erythromycins, and chloramphenicol); the latter drugs inhibit bacterial cell growth, decreasing cephalosporin uptake by bacterial cell walls.
• Refrigerate oral suspensions (stable for
14 days); shake well before administering to ensure correct dosage.
• Follow manufacturer's directions for reconstitution, dilution, and storage of
drugs; check expiration dates.
• Administer I.M. dose deep into large
muscle mass (gluteal or midlateral thigh);
rotate injection sites to minimize tissue
injury.
• Do not add or mix other drugs with I.V.
infusions, particularly aminoglycosides,
which will be inactivated if mixed with
cephalosporins; if other drugs must be
given I.V., temporarily stop infusion of
primary drug.
• Ensure adequate dilution of I.V. infusion and rotate site every 48 hours to help
minimize local vein irritation; using a
small-gauge needle in a larger available
vein may be helpful.

Patient teaching
• Make sure patient understands how and
when to take drug. Urge him to comply
with instructions for around-the-clock
dosage and to complete the prescribed
regimen.
• Advise patient to take oral drug with
food if GI irritation occurs.
• Review proper storage and disposal of
drug, and remind him to check drug's expiration date.
• Teach signs and symptoms of hypersensitivity and other adverse reactions, and
emphasize importance of reporting unusual effects.
• Teach signs and symptoms of bacterial
and fungal superinfection, especially if
patient is elderly or debilitated or has low
resistance from immunosuppressants or
irradiation; emphasize importance of reporting signs and symptoms promptly.
• Warn patient not to ingest alcohol in
any form within 72 hours of treatment
with cefoperazone or cefotetan.
• Advise patient to add yogurt or butter-
milk to diet to prevent intestinal superinfection resulting from suppression of normal intestinal flora.
• Advise diabetic patient to monitor urine
glucose level with Diastix and not to use
Clinitest.
• Urge patient to keep follow-up appointments.

☑ Evaluation
• Patient does not exhibit signs and
symptoms of hypersensitivity.
• Patient is free from infection.
• Patient maintains adequate hydration.

Corticosteroids

betamethasone
betamethasone sodium phosphate
cortisone acetate
dexamethasone
dexamethasone acetate
dexamethasone sodium phosphate
fludrocortisone acetate
hydrocortisone
hydrocortisone acetate
hydrocortisone cypionate
hydrocortisone sodium phosphate
hydrocortisone sodium succinate
methylprednisolone
methylprednisolone acetate
methylprednisolone sodium succinate
prednisolone
prednisolone acetate
prednisolone sodium phosphate
prednisolone steaglate
prednisolone tebutate
prednisone
triamcinolone
triamcinolone acetonide
triamcinolone diacetate
triamcinolone hexacetonide

Action

Corticosteroids suppress cell-mediated and humoral immunity by reducing levels of leukocytes, monocytes, and eosinophils; decreasing immunoglobulin binding to cell-surface receptors; and inhibiting interleukin synthesis. They reduce inflammation by preventing hydrolytic enzyme release into the cells, preventing plasma exudation, suppressing polymorphonuclear leukocyte migration, and disrupting other inflammatory processes.

Indications

▶ Hypersensitivity; inflammation, particularly of eye, nose, and respiratory tract; induction of immunosuppression; replacement therapy in adrenocortical insufficiency.

Adverse reactions

Systemic corticosteroid therapy may suppress the hypothalamic-pituitary-adrenal (HPA) axis. Excessive use may cause cushingoid symptoms and various systemic disorders, such as diabetes and osteoporosis. Other effects may include euphoria, insomnia, edema, hypertension, peptic ulcer, increased appetite, fluid and electrolyte imbalances, dermatologic disorders, and immunosuppression.

Contraindications and precautions

• Contraindicated in patients with systemic fungal infection or hypersensitivity to drug or its components.
• Use with caution in patients with GI ulceration, renal disease, hypertension, osteoporosis, varicella, vaccinia, exanthema, diabetes mellitus, hypothyroidism, thromboembolic disorder, seizures, myasthenia gravis, heart failure, tuberculosis, ocular herpes simplex, hypoalbuminemia, emotional instability, or psychosis.
• **Geriatric use:** Elderly patients may be at increased risk for adverse reactions. Monitor closely.
• **Pediatric use:** Long-term use should be avoided, if possible; stunted growth may result.
• **Breast-feeding:** Corticosteroids are distributed in breast milk and could cause serious adverse effects in infants. Women should discontinue breast-feeding if corticosteroid therapy is required.

NURSING CONSIDERATIONS

Assessment
• Establish baseline blood pressure, fluid and electrolyte status, and weight; reassess regularly.
• Monitor patient closely for adverse reactions.
• Evaluate drug effectiveness at regular intervals.

Key nursing diagnoses
• Altered protection related to suppression of HPA axis with long-term therapy

• Risk for injury related to severe adverse reactions
• Risk for infection related to immunosuppression

⟩ Planning and implementation
• Administer drug early in the day to mimic circadian rhythm.
• Administer with food to prevent GI irritation.
• Take precautions to avoid exposing patient to infection.
• Do not discontinue drug abruptly.
• Notify doctor of severe or persistent adverse reactions.
Patient teaching
• Teach patient to take drug exactly as prescribed, and warn him never to discontinue drug suddenly.
• Tell patient to notify doctor if stress level increases; dosage may need to be temporarily increased.
• Instruct patient to take oral drug with food.
• Urge patient to report black tarry stools, bleeding, bruising, blurred vision, emotional changes, or other unusual effects.
• Encourage patient to carry medical identification at all times.

☑ Evaluation
• Patient does not exhibit signs and symptoms of adrenal insufficiency.
• Patient remains free from injury.
• Patient is free from infection.

Diuretics, loop
bumetanide
ethacrynate sodium
ethacrynic acid
furosemide
torsemide

Action

Loop diuretics inhibit sodium and chloride reabsorption in the ascending loop of Henle, thus increasing renal excretion of sodium, chloride, and water; like thiazide diuretics, loop diuretics increase excretion of potassium. Loop diuretics produce greater maximum diuresis and electrolyte loss than thiazide diuretics.

Indications

▶ Edema associated with heart failure, hepatic cirrhosis, or nephrotic syndrome; mild to moderate hypertension; adjunct treatment in acute pulmonary edema or hypertensive crisis.

Adverse reactions

Therapeutic doses commonly cause metabolic and electrolyte disturbances, particularly potassium depletion. They also may cause hypochloremic alkalosis, hyperglycemia, hyperuricemia, and hypomagnesemia. Rapid parenteral administration may cause hearing loss (including deafness) and tinnitus. High doses can produce profound diuresis, leading to hypovolemia and CV collapse.

Contraindications and precautions

• Contraindicated in patients with anuria, hepatic coma, severe electrolyte depletion, or known hypersensitivity to drug.
• Use with caution in pregnant women and in patients with severe renal disease.
• **Geriatric use:** Elderly patients are more susceptible to drug-induced diuresis. Reduced dosages may be indicated. Monitor closely.
• **Pediatric use:** Use with caution in neonates. The usual pediatric dose can be used, but dosage intervals should be extended.
• **Breast-feeding:** Loop diuretics should not be used in breast-feeding women.

NURSING CONSIDERATIONS

⟐ Assessment
• Monitor blood pressure and pulse rate (especially during rapid diuresis). Establish baseline values before therapy begins, and watch for significant changes.

• Establish baseline CBC, including white blood cell count; serum electrolyte, CO_2, magnesium, BUN, and creatinine levels; and liver function test results. Review periodically.
• Monitor for signs of excessive diuresis: hypotension, tachycardia, poor skin turgor, and excessive thirst.
• Monitor for edema and ascites. Observe lower extremities of ambulatory patients and sacral area of patients on bed rest.
• Weigh patient each morning immediately after voiding and before breakfast, in same type of clothing and on same scale. Weight provides a reliable indicator of patient's response to diuretic therapy.

🔲 **Key nursing diagnoses**
• Risk for fluid volume deficit related to excessive diuresis
• Altered urinary elimination related to change in diuresis pattern
• Altered protection related to electrolyte imbalance

▶ **Planning and implementation**
• Administer diuretics in morning to ensure that major diuresis occurs before bedtime. To prevent nocturia, do not administer diuretics after 6 p.m.
• If ordered, reduce dosage for patient with hepatic dysfunction, and increase dosage for patient with renal impairment, oliguria, or decreased diuresis (inadequate urine output may result in circulatory overload, causing water intoxication, pulmonary edema, and heart failure). If ordered, increase dosage of insulin or oral hypoglycemic in diabetic patient, and reduce dosage of other antihypertensive drugs.
• Take safety measures for all ambulatory patients until response to diuretic is known.
• Consult dietitian about need for potassium supplements.
• Have urinal or commode readily available to patient.
Patient teaching
• Explain rationale for therapy and importance of following the prescribed regimen.

• Review adverse effects, and urge patient to report symptoms promptly, especially chest, back, or leg pain; shortness of breath; dyspnea; increased edema or weight; or excess diuresis (weight loss of more than 0.9 kg [2 lb] daily).
• Advise patient to eat potassium-rich foods and to avoid high-sodium foods (lunch meat, smoked meats, processed cheeses). Caution him not to add table salt to foods.
• Encourage patient to keep follow-up appointments to monitor effectiveness of therapy.

☑ **Evaluation**
• Patient maintains adequate hydration.
• Patient states importance of taking diuretic early in day to prevent nocturia.
• Patient complies with therapy, as evidenced by improvement in underlying condition.

Diuretics, thiazide and thiazide-like
Thiazide
chlorothiazide
hydrochlorothiazide
Thiazide-like
indapamide
metolazone

Action

Thiazide and thiazide-like diuretics interfere with sodium transport across tubules of the nephron's cortical diluting segment, thereby increasing renal excretion of sodium, chloride, water, potassium, and calcium.

Thiazide diuretics also exert an antihypertensive effect; although the exact mechanism is unknown, direct arteriolar dilation may be partially responsible. In diabetes insipidus, thiazides cause a paradoxical decrease in urine volume and an increase in renal concentration of urine, possibly because of sodium depletion and decreased plasma volume; this increases water and sodium reabsorption in the kidneys.

Indications

► Edema associated with right-sided heart failure, mild to moderate left-sided heart failure, or nephrotic syndrome; edema and ascites secondary to hepatic cirrhosis; hypertension; diabetes insipidus, particularly nephrogenic diabetes insipidus.

Adverse reactions

Therapeutic doses cause electrolyte and metabolic disturbances, most commonly potassium depletion. Other abnormalities include hypochloremic alkalosis, hypomagnesemia, hyponatremia, hypercalcemia, hyperuricemia, hyperglycemia, and elevated cholesterol levels.

Contraindications and precautions

• Contraindicated in patients with anuria or known hypersensitivity to drug.
• Use with caution in pregnant women and in patients with severe renal disease, impaired hepatic function, or progressive liver disease.
• **Geriatric use:** Elderly patients are more susceptible to drug-induced diuresis. Reduced dosages may be indicated. Monitor closely.
• **Pediatric use:** Safety and efficacy have not been established in children.
• **Breast-feeding:** Thiazides are distributed in breast milk and are contraindicated in breast-feeding women.

NURSING CONSIDERATIONS

Assessment
• Monitor patient's intake and output and serum electrolyte levels regularly.
• Weigh patient each morning immediately after voiding and before breakfast, in same type of clothing and on same scale. Weight provides a reliable indicator of patient's response to diuretic therapy.
• Monitor blood glucose level in a diabetic patient. Diuretics may cause hyperglycemia.

• Monitor serum creatinine and BUN levels regularly. Drug is not as effective if these levels are more than twice normal. Also monitor blood uric acid levels.

Key nursing diagnoses
• Risk for fluid volume deficit related to excessive diuresis
• Altered urinary elimination related to change in diuresis pattern
• Altered protection related to electrolyte imbalance

Planning and implementation
• Administer drug in morning to prevent nocturia.
• Consult dietitian to provide high-potassium diet.
• Administer potassium supplements as prescribed to maintain acceptable serum potassium level.
• Have urinal or commode readily available to patient.

Patient teaching
• Explain rationale for therapy and importance of following the prescribed regimen.
• Tell patient to take drug at same time each day to prevent nighttime diuresis. Suggest taking drug with food to minimize gastric irritation.
• Urge patient to seek doctor's approval before taking any other drug, including OTC preparations.
• Advise patient to record weight each morning after voiding and before breakfast, in same type of clothing and on same scale.
• Review adverse effects, and urge patient to report symptoms promptly, especially chest, back, or leg pain; shortness of breath; dyspnea; increased edema or weight; or excess diuresis (weight loss of more than 0.9 kg [2 lb] daily). Warn him about photosensitivity reactions (these usually occur 10 to 14 days after initial sun exposure).
• Advise patient to eat potassium-rich foods and to avoid high-sodium foods (lunch meat, smoked meats, processed

cheeses). Caution him not to add table salt to foods.
• Encourage patient to keep follow-up appointments to monitor effectiveness of therapy.

☑ Evaluation
• Patient maintains adequate hydration.
• Patient states importance of taking diuretic early in day to prevent nocturia.
• Patient complies with therapy, as evidenced by improvement in underlying condition.

Estrogens
diethylstilbestrol
diethylstilbestrol diphosphate
esterified estrogens
estradiol
estradiol cypionate
estradiol valerate
estrogenic substances, conjugated
estrone
estropipate
ethinyl estradiol

Action

Conjugated estrogens and estrogenic substances are normally obtained from the urine of pregnant mares. Other estrogens are manufactured synthetically. Of the six naturally occurring estrogens in humans, three (estradiol, estrone, and estriol) are present in significant quantities.

Estrogens promote the development and maintenance of the female reproductive system and secondary sexual characteristics. They inhibit the release of pituitary gonadotropins and have various metabolic effects, including retention of fluid and electrolytes, retention and deposition in bone of calcium and phosphorus, and mild anabolic activity.

Estrogens and estrogenic substances administered as drugs have effects related to endogenous estrogen's mechanism of action. They can mimic the action of endogenous estrogen when used as replacement therapy and can inhibit ovulation or the growth of certain hormone-sensitive cancers.

Indications

▶ Prevention of vasomotor symptoms, such as hot flashes and dizziness; stimulation of vaginal tissue development, cornification, and secretory activity; inhibition of hormone-sensitive cancer growth; prevention of bone decalcification; ovulation control; prevention of conception.

Adverse reactions

Acute adverse reactions include changes in menstrual bleeding patterns (spotting, prolongation or absence of bleeding), abdominal cramps, swollen feet or ankles, bloated sensation (fluid and electrolyte retention), breast swelling and tenderness, weight gain, nausea, loss of appetite, headache, photosensitivity, loss of libido.

Chronic effects include elevated blood pressure (sometimes into hypertensive range), cholestatic jaundice, benign hepatomas, endometrial carcinoma (rare), and thromboembolic disease (risk increases markedly with cigarette smoking, especially in women over age 35).

Contraindications and precautions

• Contraindicated in pregnant women and in those with thrombophlebitis or thromboembolic disorders, undiagnosed abnormal genital bleeding, or estrogen-dependent neoplasia.
• Use with caution in patients with hypertension; metabolic bone disease; migraines; seizures; asthma; cardiac, renal, or hepatic impairment; blood dyscrasia; diabetes; family history of breast cancer; or fibrocystic disease.
• **Geriatric use:** Postmenopausal women with long-term estrogen use have an increased risk of endometrial cancer.
• **Pediatric use:** Because of their effects on epiphyseal closure, use estrogens with caution in adolescents whose bone growth is not complete.

Prototype drug

• **Breast-feeding:** Estrogens are contraindicated in breast-feeding women.

Assessment
• Monitor patient regularly to detect improvement or worsening of symptoms; observe for adverse reactions.
• Monitor patient with diabetes mellitus closely for loss of diabetes control.
• Monitor prothrombin time of patient receiving warfarin-type anticoagulant. If ordered, adjust dosage of anticoagulant.

Key nursing diagnoses
• Fluid volume excess related to drug-induced fluid retention
• Risk of injury related to adverse effects
• Noncompliance related to long-term therapy

Planning and implementation
• Notify pathologist of patient's estrogen therapy when sending specimens for evaluation.
• Keep in mind that estrogens are usually administered cyclically (once daily for 3 weeks, followed by 1 week without drugs; regimen is repeated as necessary).
Patient teaching
• Have patient read the package insert describing adverse reactions, and follow this with a verbal explanation. Tell her to keep the package insert for later reference.
• Instruct patient to notify doctor immediately if she experiences abdominal pain; pain, numbness, or stiffness in legs or buttocks; pressure or pain in chest; shortness of breath; severe headaches; visual disturbances, such as blind spots, flashing lights, or blurriness; vaginal bleeding or discharge; breast lumps; swelling of hands or feet; yellow skin and sclera; dark urine; or light-colored stools.
• Urge diabetic patient to report symptoms of hyperglycemia or glycosuria.
• Teach patient how to apply estrogen ointments or transdermal estrogen.

Review symptoms that accompany a systemic reaction to ointments.
• Advise patient to take drug with meals or at bedtime to relieve nausea. Reassure her that nausea usually disappears with continued therapy.
• If patient is on cyclic therapy for postmenopausal symptoms, explain that withdrawal bleeding may occur in week off drug but that fertility has not been restored and ovulation does not occur.
• Teach patient how to perform routine breast self-examination.
• Teach patient how to insert intravaginal estrogen suppository. Advise her to use sanitary pads instead of tampons when using suppository.
• Tell patient to stop taking drug immediately if she becomes pregnant; estrogens can harm fetus.
• Remind patient not to breast-feed during estrogen therapy.
• Explain that medical supervision is essential during prolonged therapy.
• Tell male patient on long-term therapy about possible gynecomastia and impotence, which will disappear when therapy is terminated.

Evaluation
• Patient experiences only minimal fluid retention.
• Serious complications associated with estrogen therapy do not develop.
• Patient complies with therapy, as evidenced by improvement in underlying condition or absence of pregnancy.

Hematinics, oral
ferrous fumarate
ferrous gluconate
ferrous sulfate

Action

Iron is an essential component of hemoglobin. It is needed in adequate amounts for erythropoiesis and for efficient oxygen transport in the blood. After absorption into the blood, iron is immediately bound to transferrin, a plasma protein that transports iron to bone marrow, where it is used during hemoglobin synthesis. Some iron is also used during synthesis of myoglobin and other nonhemoglobin heme units.

Indications

▶ Prevention and treatment of iron-deficiency anemia.

Adverse reactions

Because iron is corrosive, GI intolerance is common (5% to 20%); symptoms include nausea, vomiting, anorexia, constipation, and dark stools. Liquid preparations may stain teeth.

Contraindications and precautions

• Contraindicated in patients with hemochromatosis, hemolytic anemia, or hemosiderosis.
• Use with caution in patients with peptic ulcer disease, regional enteritis, ulcerative colitis, or sensitivity to sulfites or tartrazine (some products contain these ingredients).
• **Geriatric use:** Iron-induced constipation is common in elderly patients; stress proper diet to minimize this effect. Elderly patients also may need higher doses because reduced gastric secretions and achlorhydria may lower capacity for iron absorption.
• **Pediatric use:** Caution parents about the potentially lethal effects of iron overdose.
• **Breast-feeding:** Iron supplements are often recommended for breast-feeding women; no adverse effects have been documented.

NURSING CONSIDERATIONS

⚕ Assessment
• Monitor for adverse reactions, especially those related to bowel function.
• Monitor hemoglobin and reticulocyte counts during therapy.

⊕ Key nursing diagnoses
• Risk for fluid volume deficit related to GI upset
• Constipation related to adverse effect on bowel
• Noncompliance related to adverse effects or long-term use

▷ Planning and implementation
• Dilute liquid preparations in juice (preferably orange juice, which promotes iron absorption) or water, but not in milk or antacids. To avoid staining teeth, give liquid preparations through a straw. Administer antacids 1 hour before or 2 hours after iron product, if possible, to prevent interference with absorption.
• Don't crush tablets or capsules; if patient has trouble swallowing, use a liquid form.
Patient teaching
• Explain rationale for therapy, and urge him to follow his prescribed regimen.
• Tell patient to continue his regular dosage schedule if he misses a dose, and warn him not to take double doses.
• Advise patient to dilute liquid form in juice (preferably orange juice) or water, not milk or antacids. Suggest that he drink liquid through a straw to avoid staining teeth.
• Review possible adverse effects. Tell him that oral iron may turn stools black, and reassure him that this is harmless. Teach dietary measures to help prevent constipation.
• Explain iron's toxicity, and emphasize importance of keeping iron preparations away from children to prevent poisoning.
• Urge patient to report diarrhea or constipation because doctor may want to adjust dosage, modify diet, or order further tests.
• Explain that iron therapy may be required for 4 to 6 months after anemia resolves. Encourage compliance.

☑ Evaluation
• Patient maintains adequate hydration.
• Patient regains normal bowel pattern.

• Patient complies with therapy, as evidenced by return of normal hemoglobin levels and resolution of iron deficiency anemia.

Histamine$_2$-receptor antagonists
cimetidine
famotidine
nizatidine
ranitidine hydrochloride

Action

All H$_2$-receptor antagonists inhibit histamine's action at H$_2$ receptors in gastric parietal cells, reducing gastric acid output and concentration, regardless of the stimulatory drug (histamine, food, insulin, caffeine) or basal conditions.

Indications

▶ Acute duodenal or gastric ulcer, Zollinger-Ellison syndrome, gastroesophageal reflux.

Adverse reactions

H$_2$-receptor antagonists rarely cause adverse reactions. Mild and transient diarrhea, neutropenia, dizziness, fatigue, cardiac arrhythmias, and gynecomastia have been reported.

Contraindications and precautions

• Contraindicated in breast-feeding women and in patients with known hypersensitivity to drug.
• Use with caution in pregnant women and in patients with impaired renal or hepatic function.
• **Geriatric use:** Elderly patients have an increased risk of adverse reactions, particularly those affecting the CNS. Use with caution.
• **Pediatric use:** Safety and efficacy have not been established in children.
• **Breast-feeding:** H$_2$-receptor antagonists may be secreted in breast milk and

are contraindicated in breast-feeding women.

NURSING CONSIDERATIONS

☑ Assessment
• Monitor patient for adverse reactions, especially hypotension and arrhythmias.
• Periodically monitor laboratory tests, such as CBC and renal and hepatic studies, as ordered.

⊕ Key nursing diagnoses
• Risk for infection related to neutropenia
• Decreased cardiac output related to adverse CV effects (cimetidine)
• Fatigue related to drug's CNS effects

▷ Planning and implementation
• Administer once-daily dose at bedtime, twice-daily doses in morning and evening, and multiple doses with meals and at bedtime. Most clinicians prefer once-daily dose at bedtime to promote compliance.
• Do not exceed recommended infusion rates when administering drugs I.V.; doing so increases risk of adverse CV effects. Continuous I.V. infusion may suppress acid secretion more effectively.
• Administer antacids at least 1 hour before or after H$_2$-receptor antagonists. Antacids can decrease drug absorption.
• Anticipate dosage adjustment for patient with renal disease.
• Avoid discontinuing drug abruptly.
Patient teaching
• Teach patient how and when to take drug, and warn him not to stop drug suddenly.
• Review possible adverse reactions, and urge him to report unusual effects.
• Caution patient to avoid smoking during therapy; smoking stimulates gastric acid secretion and worsens the disease.

☑ Evaluation
• Patient is free from infection.
• Patient maintains a normal heart rhythm.

Prototype drug

• Patient states appropriate management plan for combating fatigue.

Hypoglycemics, oral

acarbose
acetohexamide
chlorpropamide
glimepiride
glipizide
glyburide
metformin hydrochloride
repaglinide
tolazamide
tolbutamide
troglitazone

Action

Except for metformin and troglitazone, all oral hypoglycemic drugs are sulfonylureas, sulfonamide derivatives that exert no antibacterial activity. They lower blood glucose levels by stimulating insulin release from the pancreas. These drugs work only in the presence of functioning beta cells in the islet tissue of the pancreas. After prolonged administration, they produce hypoglycemia through significant extrapancreatic effects, including reduction of hepatic glucose production and enhanced peripheral sensitivity to insulin. The latter may result from an increased number of insulin receptors or from changes in events after insulin binding. Sulfonylureas are divided into first-generation drugs (acetohexamide, chlorpropamide, tolbutamide, and tolazamide) and second-generation drugs (glyburide, glimepiride, and glipizide). Although their mechanisms of action are similar, the second-generation drugs carry a more lipophilic side chain, are more potent, and cause fewer adverse reactions. Clinically, their most important difference is their duration of action.

Metformin decreases hepatic glucose production, reduces intestinal glucose absorption, and improves insulin sensitivity (increases peripheral glucose uptake and utilization). With metformin therapy, insulin secretion remains unchanged, and fasting insulin levels and day-long plasma insulin response may actually decrease.

Troglitazone lowers glucose concentrations and decreases insulin secretion as pancreatic beta-cell production improves.

Indications

▶ Mild to moderately severe, stable, non-ketotic non-insulin-dependent diabetes mellitus (NIDDM) that cannot be controlled by diet alone.

Adverse reactions

Sulfonylureas cause dose-related reactions that usually respond to decreased dosage: headache, nausea, vomiting, anorexia, heartburn, weakness, and paresthesia. Hypoglycemia may follow excessive dosage, increased exercise, decreased food intake, or alcohol consumption.

The most serious reaction associated with metformin is lactic acidosis. Although rare, lactic acidosis is most likely to occur in patients with renal dysfunction. Other reactions to metformin include GI upset, megaloblastic anemia, rash, dermatitis, and unpleasant or metallic taste.

Contraindications and precautions

• Contraindicated in pregnant or breast-feeding women and in those with known hypersensitivity to drug or diabetic ketoacidosis with or without coma. In addition, metformin is contraindicated in patients with renal disease or metabolic acidosis and generally should be avoided in patients with hepatic disease.
• Use sulfonylureas with caution in patients with renal or hepatic disease. Use metformin with caution in patients with adrenal or pituitary insufficiency and in elderly, debilitated, or malnourished patients.
• **Geriatric use:** Elderly patients may be more sensitive to these drugs and usually require lower dosages. In addition, hypoglycemia may be more difficult to recognize, although it usually causes neurolog-

ic symptoms in such patients. Monitor
closely.
- **Pediatric use:** Oral hypoglycemics are
not effective in insulin-dependent (type 1,
juvenile-onset) diabetes mellitus.
- **Breast-feeding:** Oral hypoglycemics
are minimally excreted in breast milk and
may cause hypoglycemia in the breast-
feeding infant. They are contraindicated
for use in breast-feeding women.

NURSING CONSIDERATIONS

🔍 Assessment
- Monitor patient's blood glucose level
regularly. Increase monitoring during periods of increased stress (infection, fever,
surgery, or trauma).
- Monitor patient for adverse reactions.
- Assess patient's compliance with drug
therapy and other aspects of diabetic
treatment.

🔑 Key nursing diagnoses
- Risk for injury related to hypoglycemia
- Risk for fluid volume deficit related to
adverse GI effects
- Noncompliance related to long-term
therapy

➤ Planning and implementation
- Administer sulfonylureas 30 minutes
before morning meal (once-daily dosing)
or 30 minutes before morning and
evening meals (twice-daily dosing).
Administer metformin with morning and
evening meals.
- Keep in mind that patient transferring
from another oral hypoglycemic drug
(except chlorpropamide) usually needs
no transition period.
- Anticipate patient's need for insulin
during periods of increased stress.
Patient teaching
- Emphasize importance of following
prescribed regimen. Encourage patient to
adhere to diet, weight reduction, exercise,
and personal hygiene recommendations.
- Explain that therapy relieves symptoms
but does not cure the disease.

- Teach patient how to recognize and
treat hypoglycemia.

✅ Evaluation
- Patient remains free from injury.
- Patient maintains adequate hydration.
- Patient complies with therapy, as evi-
denced by normal or near-normal blood
glucose levels.

Laxatives

Bulk-forming
  calcium polycarbophil
  methylcellulose
  psyllium
Emollient
  docusate calcium
  docusate potassium
  docusate sodium
Hyperosmolar
  glycerin
  lactulose
  magnesium citrate
  magnesium hydroxide
  magnesium sulfate
  sodium phosphates
Lubricant
  mineral oil
Stimulant
  bisacodyl
  cascara sagrada
  castor oil
  senna

Action

Laxatives promote movement of intestinal materials from the colon and rectum.
Their classifications (bulk-forming,
emollient, hyperosmolar, lubricant, and
stimulant) indicate how they accomplish
this.

Indications

▶ Constipation, irritable bowel syndrome, diverticulosis.

Adverse reactions

All laxatives may cause flatulence, diarrhea, abdominal discomfort, weakness, and dependence. Bulk-forming laxatives may cause intestinal obstruction, impaction, or (rarely) esophageal obstruction. Emollient laxatives may cause a bitter taste or throat irritation. Hyperosmolar laxatives may cause fluid and electrolyte imbalances. Lubricant laxatives may cause impaired absorption of fat-soluble vitamins or anal irritation if given rectally. Stimulant laxatives may cause urine discoloration, malabsorption, and weight loss.

Contraindications and precautions

• Contraindicated in patients with GI obstruction or perforation, toxic colitis, megacolon, nausea and vomiting, or acute surgical abdomen.
• Use with caution in patients with rectal or anal conditions, such as rectal bleeding or large hemorrhoids.
• Additional contraindications and precautions exist. See individual drugs for complete listings.
• **Geriatric use:** Dependence is more likely to develop in elderly patients because of age-related changes in GI function. Monitor closely.
• **Pediatric use:** Infants and children are at increased risk for fluid and electrolyte disturbances. Use cautiously.
• **Breast-feeding:** Recommendations vary for use in breast-feeding women. See individual drugs for specific guidelines.

NURSING CONSIDERATIONS

⚜ Assessment
• Obtain baseline assessment of patient's bowel patterns and GI history before administering laxative.
• Monitor patient for adverse reactions.
• Monitor bowel pattern throughout therapy. Assess bowel sounds and color and consistency of stools.
• Monitor patient's fluid and electrolyte status during administration.

⬢ Key nursing diagnoses
• Diarrhea related to adverse GI effects
• Pain related to abdominal discomfort
• Altered health maintenance related to laxative dependence

⬢ Planning and implementation
• Don't crush enteric-coated tablets.
• Time administration so that bowel evacuation doesn't interfere with sleep.
• Make sure patient has easy access to bedpan or bathroom.
• Institute measures to prevent constipation.
Patient teaching
• Advise patient that therapy should be short-term. Point out that abuse or prolonged use can cause nutritional imbalances.
• Tell patient that stool softeners and bulk-forming laxatives may take several days to achieve results.
• Encourage patient to remain active and to drink plenty of fluids if he's taking a bulk-forming laxative.
• Explain that stimulant laxatives may cause harmless urine discoloration.

☑ Evaluation
• Patient regains normal bowel pattern.
• Patient states pain is relieved with stool evacuation.
• Patient discusses dangers of laxative abuse and importance of limiting laxative use.

Nonsteroidal anti-inflammatory drugs (NSAIDs)

diflunisal
etodolac
fenoprofen calcium
flurbiprofen
ibuprofen
indomethacin
indomethacin sodium trihydrate
ketoprofen
ketorolac tromethamine
meclofenamate

mefenamic acid
nabumetone
naproxen
naproxen sodium
oxaprozin
piroxicam
sulindac
tolmetin sodium

Action

The analgesic effect of NSAIDs may result from interference with the prostaglandins involved in pain. Prostaglandins appear to sensitize pain receptors to mechanical stimulation or to other chemical mediators. NSAIDs inhibit synthesis of prostaglandins peripherally and possibly centrally.

Like salicylates, NSAIDs exert an antiinflammatory effect that may result in part from inhibition of prostaglandin synthesis and release during inflammation. The exact mechanism has not been clearly established.

Indications

▶ Mild to moderate pain, inflammation, stiffness, swelling, or tenderness associated with headache, arthralgia, myalgia, neuralgia, dysmenorrhea, dental or surgical procedures, rheumatoid arthritis, juvenile arthritis, or osteoarthritis.

Adverse reactions

Adverse reactions chiefly involve the GI tract, particularly erosion of the gastric mucosa. Most common symptoms are dyspepsia, heartburn, epigastric distress, nausea, and abdominal pain. CNS reactions also may occur. Flank pain with other signs and symptoms of nephrotoxicity has occasionally been reported. Fluid retention may aggravate preexisting hypertension or heart failure.

Contraindications and precautions

• Contraindicated in patients with GI lesions or known hypersensitivity to drug.

• Use with caution in patients with cardiac decompensation, hypertension, fluid retention, or coagulation defects.
• **Geriatric use:** Patients older than age 60 may be more susceptible to toxic effects of NSAIDs because of decreased renal function.
• **Pediatric use:** Safety of long-term therapy in children under age 14 has not been established.
• **Breast-feeding:** NSAIDs are not recommended for use in breast-feeding women.

NURSING CONSIDERATIONS

⚗ Assessment
• Assess patient's level of pain and inflammation before therapy begins, and evaluate drug effectiveness after administration.
• Monitor for signs and symptoms of bleeding. Assess bleeding time if surgery is required.
• Monitor ophthalmic and auditory function before and periodically during therapy to detect toxicity.
• Monitor CBC, platelets, PT, and hepatic and renal function studies periodically to detect abnormalities.
• Monitor for bronchospasm in patients with known "triad" symptoms (aspirin hypersensitivity, rhinitis or nasal polyps, and asthma).

⊞ Key nursing diagnoses
• Risk for injury related to adverse reactions
• Fluid volume excess related to fluid retention
• Sensory-perceptual alterations (visual and auditory) related to toxicity

▷ Planning and implementation
• Administer oral NSAIDs with 8 oz (240 ml) of water to ensure adequate passage into stomach. Have patient sit up for 15 to 30 minutes after taking drug to prevent lodging in esophagus.
• Crush tablets or mix with food or fluid to aid swallowing. Administer with antacids to minimize gastric upset.

Patient teaching
• Encourage patient to take drug as directed to achieve desired effect. Explain that he may not notice benefits of drug for 2 to 4 weeks.
• Review methods to prevent or minimize gastric upset.
• Work with patient on chronic therapy to arrange for monitoring of laboratory parameters, especially BUN, serum creatinine, liver function tests, and CBC.
• Instruct patient to notify doctor of severe or persistent adverse reactions.

☑ **Evaluation**
• Patient remains free from injury.
• Patient does not exhibit signs of edema.
• Patient maintains normal visual and auditory function.

Opioids

alfentanil hydrochloride
codeine phosphate
codeine sulfate
difenoxin
diphenoxylate
fentanyl citrate
hydromorphone hydrochloride
meperidine hydrochloride
methadone hydrochloride
morphine sulfate
oxycodone hydrochloride
oxymorphone hydrochloride
propoxyphene hydrochloride
propoxyphene napsylate
sufentanil citrate

Action

Opioids act as agonists at specific opiate-receptor binding sites in the CNS and other tissues, altering the patient's perception of and emotional response to pain.

Indications

▶ Moderate to severe pain associated with acute and some chronic disorders; diarrhea; dry, nonproductive cough.

Prototype drug

Adverse reactions

Respiratory depression and circulatory depression (including orthostatic hypotension) are the major hazards of opioids. Other adverse CNS effects include dizziness, visual disturbances, mental clouding or depression, sedation, coma, euphoria, dysphoria, weakness, faintness, agitation, restlessness, nervousness, and seizures. Adverse GI effects include nausea, vomiting, constipation, and biliary colic. Urine retention or hypersensitivity also may occur. Tolerance or psychological or physical dependence may follow prolonged therapy.

Contraindications and precautions

• Contraindicated in patients with known hypersensitivity to drug or recent use of MAO inhibitors.
• Use with caution in pregnant women and in patients with head injury, increased intracranial or intraocular pressure, or hepatic or renal dysfunction.
• **Geriatric use:** Elderly patients may be more sensitive to opioids. Lower doses are usually indicated.
• **Pediatric use:** Safety and efficacy in children have not been established.
• **Breast-feeding:** Codeine, meperidine, methadone, morphine, and propoxyphene are excreted in breast milk and should be used with caution in breast-feeding women. Methadone has been shown to cause physical dependence in breast-feeding infants of women maintained on methadone.

NURSING CONSIDERATIONS

☑ **Assessment**
• Obtain baseline assessment of patient's pain, and reassess frequently to determine drug effectiveness.
• Evaluate patient's respiratory status before each dose; watch for respiratory rate below patient's baseline level and for restlessness, which may be a compensatory sign of hypoxia. Respiratory depression may last longer than analgesic effect.

• Monitor patient for other adverse reactions.
• Monitor for dependence. The first sign of tolerance to opioids is usually a shortened duration of effect.

🔅 Key nursing diagnoses
• Ineffective breathing pattern related to respiratory depression
• Risk for injury related to orthostatic hypotension
• Ineffective individual coping related to drug dependence

▶ Planning and implementation
• Keep resuscitative equipment and a narcotic antagonist (naloxone) available.
• Administer I.V. drug by slow injection, preferably in diluted solution. Rapid I.V. injection increases incidence of adverse effects.
• Give I.M. or S.C. injections cautiously to patients who have decreased platelet counts, are chilled, hypovolemic, or in shock; decreased perfusion may lead to drug accumulation and toxicity. Rotate injection sites to avoid induration.
• Carefully note strength of solution when measuring dose. Oral solutions of varying concentrations are available.
• Administer on regular dosage schedule rather than p.r.n. for maximum effectiveness.
• Institute safety precautions.
• Encourage postoperative patients to turn, cough, and deep-breathe every 2 hours to avoid atelectasis.
• Give oral products with food if gastric irritation occurs.
Patient teaching
• Teach patient to take drug exactly as prescribed. Urge him to call doctor if he is not experiencing desired effect or is experiencing significant adverse reactions.
• Warn patient to avoid hazardous activities that require alertness and coordination until drug's effects are known.
• Advise patient to avoid alcohol while taking opioids; it will cause additive CNS depression.

• Suggest measures to prevent constipation, such as increased fiber in diet and use of stool softener.
• Instruct patient to breathe deeply, cough, and change position every 2 hours to avoid respiratory complications.

☑ Evaluation
• Patient maintains adequate ventilation, as evidenced by normal respiratory rate and rhythm and pink color.
• Patient remains free from injury.
• Tolerance to therapy does not develop.

Penicillins
Natural penicillins
  penicillin G benzathine
  penicillin G potassium
  penicillin G procaine
  penicillin G sodium
  penicillin V potassium
Aminopenicillins
  amoxicillin/clavulanate potassium
  amoxicillin trihydrate
  ampicillin
  ampicillin sodium/sulbactam
    sodium
  ampicillin trihydrate
  bacampicillin hydrochloride
Penicillinase-resistant penicillins
  cloxacillin sodium
  dicloxacillin sodium
  nafcillin sodium
  oxacillin sodium
Extended-spectrum penicillins
  carbenicillin indanyl sodium
  mezlocillin sodium
  piperacillin sodium
  piperacillin sodium and tazobactam
    sodium
  ticarcillin disodium
  ticarcillin disodium/clavulanate
    potassium

Action

Penicillins are generally bactericidal. They inhibit synthesis of the bacterial cell wall, causing rapid cell lysis, and are most effective against fast-growing susceptible bacteria. Their sites of action are enzymes known as penicillin-binding proteins (PBPs). The affinity of certain penicillins for PBPs in various microorganisms helps explain differing spectra of activity in this class of antibiotics.

Susceptible aerobic gram-positive cocci include *Staphylococcus aureus;* nonenterococcal Group D streptococci, Groups A, B, D, G, H, K, L, and M streptococci; *S. viridans;* and enterococcus (usually in combination with an aminoglycoside). Susceptible aerobic gram-negative cocci include *Neisseria meningitidis* and non-penicillinase-producing *N. gonorrhoeae.*

Susceptible aerobic gram-positive bacilli include *Corynebacterium, Listeria*, and *Bacillus anthracis.* Susceptible anaerobes include *Peptococcus, Peptostreptococcus, Actinomyces, Clostridium, Fusobacterium, Veillonella,* and non-beta-lactamase-producing strains of *S. pneumoniae.* Susceptible spirochetes include *Treponema pallidum, T. pertenue, Leptospira, Borrelia recurrentis,* and, possibly, *Borrelia burgdorferi.*

Aminopenicillins offer a broader spectrum of activity, including many gram-negative organisms. Like natural penicillins, aminopenicillins are vulnerable to inactivation by penicillinase. Their activity spectrum includes *Escherichia coli, Proteus mirabilis, Shigella, Salmonella, S. pneumoniae, N. gonorrhoeae, Haemophilus influenzae, Staphylococcus aureus, Staphylococcus epidermidis* (non-penicillinase-producing *Staphylococcus*), and *Listeria monocytogenes.*

Penicillinase-resistant penicillins are semisynthetic penicillins designed to remain stable against hydrolysis by most staphylococcal penicillinases and thus are the drugs of choice against susceptible penicillinase-producing staphylococci. They also retain activity against most organisms susceptible to natural penicillins.

Extended-spectrum penicillins offer a wider range of bactericidal action than the other three classes and are usually given in combination with aminoglycosides. Susceptible strains include *Enterobacter, Klebsiella, Citrobacter, Serratia, Bacteroides fragilis, Pseudomonas aeruginosa; Proteus vulgaris, Providencia rettgeri,* and *Morganella morganii.* These penicillins are also vulnerable to beta-lactamase and penicillinases.

Indications

▶ Streptococcal pneumonia; enterococcal and nonenterococcal Group D endocarditis; diphtheria; anthrax; meningitis; tetanus; botulism; actinomycosis; syphilis; relapsing fever; Lyme disease; pneumococcal infections; rheumatic fever; bacterial endocarditis; neonatal Group B streptococcal disease; septicemia; gynecologic infections; infections of urinary, respiratory, and GI tracts; infections of skin, soft tissue, bones, and joints.

Adverse reactions

Hypersensitivity reactions occur with all penicillins; they range from mild rash, fever, and eosinophilia to fatal anaphylaxis. Hematologic reactions include hemolytic anemia, transient neutropenia, leukopenia, and thrombocytopenia.

Certain adverse reactions are more common with specific classes: For example, bleeding episodes are usually seen with high doses of extended-spectrum penicillins and GI adverse effects are most common with ampicillin. High doses, especially of penicillin G, irritate the CNS in patients with renal disease, causing confusion, twitching, lethargy, dysphagia, seizures, and coma. Hepatotoxicity is common with penicillinase-resistant penicillins; hyperkalemia and hypernatremia with extended-spectrum penicillins.

Local irritation from parenteral therapy may be severe enough to warrant administration by subclavian or centrally placed catheter or discontinuation of therapy.

Contraindications and precautions

• Contraindicated in patients with known hypersensitivity to drug.
• Use with caution in pregnant women and in patients with history of asthma or drug allergy, mononucleosis, hemorrhagic condition, or electrolyte imbalance.
• **Geriatric use:** Elderly patients are susceptible to superinfection and many have renal impairment, which decreases excretion of penicillins. Lower dosage is required. Use with caution.
• **Pediatric use:** Dosage recommendations have been established for most penicillins. See individual drugs for specific guidelines.
• **Breast-feeding:** Recommendations vary, depending on drug used. See individual drugs for specific guidelines.

NURSING CONSIDERATIONS

⚎ Assessment

• Assess patient's history of allergies. Try to ascertain whether previous reactions were true hypersensitivity reactions or adverse reactions (such as GI distress) that patient has interpreted as allergy.
• Keep in mind that a negative history for penicillin hypersensitivity does not preclude future allergic reactions; monitor patient continuously for possible allergic reactions or other untoward effects.
• Obtain results of culture and sensitivity tests before first dose; repeat tests periodically to assess drug's effectiveness.
• Monitor vital signs, electrolytes, and renal function studies.
• Assess level of consciousness and neurologic status when high doses are used; CNS toxicity can occur.
• Coagulation abnormalities, even frank bleeding, can follow high doses, especially of extended-spectrum penicillins; monitor PT, INR, and platelet counts; as-

sess patient for signs of occult or frank bleeding.
• Monitor patients on long-term therapy for possible superinfection, especially elderly and debilitated patients and others receiving immunosuppressants or radiation therapy.

⊞ Key nursing diagnoses

• Altered protection related to hypersensitivity
• Risk for infection related to superinfection
• Risk for fluid volume deficit related to adverse GI reactions

❭ Planning and implementation

• Administer penicillins at least 1 hour before bacteriostatic antibiotics (tetracyclines, erythromycins, and chloramphenicol); these drugs inhibit bacterial cell growth, decreasing rate of penicillin uptake by bacterial cell walls.
• Follow manufacturer's directions for reconstitution, dilution, and storage of drugs; check expiration dates.
• Give oral penicillin at least 1 hour before or 2 hours after meals to enhance gastric absorption.
• Refrigerate oral suspensions (stable for 14 days); shake well before administering to ensure correct dosage.
• Administer I.M. dose deep into large muscle mass (gluteal or midlateral thigh); rotate injection sites to minimize tissue injury; do not inject more than 2 g of drug per injection site. Apply ice to injection site to relieve pain.
• Do not add or mix other drugs with I.V. infusions, particularly aminoglycosides, which will be inactivated if mixed with penicillins. If other drugs must be given I.V., temporarily stop infusion of primary drug.
• Infuse I.V. drug continuously or intermittently (over 30 minutes); rotate infusion site every 48 hours; intermittent I.V. infusion may be diluted in 50 to 100 ml sterile water, 0.9% NaCl, dextrose 5% in

water, dextrose 5% in water and half normal saline, or lactated Ringer's solution.

Patient teaching
• Make sure patient understands how and when to take drug; urge him to complete prescribed regimen, to comply with instructions for around-the-clock dosage, and to keep follow-up appointments.
• Teach signs and symptoms of hypersensitivity and other adverse reactions. Urge him to report unusual reactions.
• Tell patient to check drug's expiration date and to discard unused drug. Warn him not to share drug with family or friends.

☑ **Evaluation**
• Patient exhibits no signs of hypersensitivity.
• Patient is free from infection.
• Patient maintains adequate hydration.

Phenothiazines

chlorpromazine hydrochloride
fluphenazine
mesoridazine besylate
perphenazine
prochlorperazine
promazine hydrochloride
promethazine
thioridazine hydrochloride
thiothixene
trifluoperazine hydrochloride

Action

Phenothiazines are believed to function as dopamine antagonists, blocking postsynaptic dopamine receptors in various parts of the CNS; their antiemetic effects result from blockage of the chemoreceptor trigger zone. They also produce varying degrees of anticholinergic and alpha-adrenergic receptor blocking actions.

Indications

▶ Agitated psychotic states, hallucinations, manic-depressive illness, excessive motor and autonomic activity, severe nausea and vomiting induced by CNS disturbances, moderate anxiety, behavioral problems associated with chronic organic mental syndrome, tetanus, acute intermittent porphyria, intractable hiccups, itching, symptomatic rhinitis.

Adverse reactions

Phenothiazines may produce extrapyramidal symptoms (dystonic movements, torticollis, oculogyric crises, parkinsonian symptoms) ranging from akathisia during early treatment to tardive dyskinesia after long-term use. A neuroleptic malignant syndrome resembling severe parkinsonism may occur (most often in young men taking fluphenazine). Other adverse reactions include orthostatic hypotension with reflex tachycardia, fainting, dizziness, arrhythmias, anorexia, nausea, vomiting, abdominal pain, local gastric irritation, seizures, endocrine effects, hematologic disorders, visual disturbances, skin eruptions, and photosensitivity. Allergic manifestations are usually marked by elevation of liver enzymes progressing to obstructive jaundice.

Contraindications and precautions

• Contraindicated in patients with CNS depression, bone marrow suppression, heart failure, circulatory collapse, coronary artery or cerebrovascular disorders, subcortical damage, or coma and with use of spinal or epidural anesthetics or adrenergic blockers.
• Use with caution in elderly or debilitated patients and in those with hepatic, renal, or CV disease; respiratory disorders; hypocalcemia; seizure disorders; suspected brain tumor or intestinal obstruction; glaucoma; or prostatic hyperplasia.
• **Geriatric use:** Elderly patients are more sensitive to therapeutic and adverse effects, especially cardiac toxicity, tardive dyskinesia, and other extrapyramidal effects. Lower doses are indicated. Titrate dosage to patient response.

• **Pediatric use:** Unless otherwise specified, phenothiazines are not recommended for children younger than age 12. Use with caution for nausea and vomiting; acutely ill children (chickenpox, measles, CNS infections, dehydration) are at greatly increased risk of dystonic reactions.

• **Breast-feeding:** Most phenothiazines are excreted in breast milk and have a direct effect on prolactin levels. If feasible, patient should not breast-feed during therapy.

NURSING CONSIDERATIONS

Assessment

• Check vital signs regularly for decreased blood pressure (especially before and after parenteral therapy) or tachycardia; observe patient carefully for other adverse reactions.

• Check intake and output for urine retention or constipation, which may require dosage reduction.

• Monitor bilirubin levels weekly for first 4 weeks; establish baseline CBC, ECG (for quinidine-like effects), liver and renal function studies, electrolyte levels (especially potassium), and eye examinations, and monitor periodically thereafter, especially in patients on long-term therapy.

• Observe patient for mood changes to monitor progress.

• Monitor for involuntary movements. Check patient receiving prolonged treatment at least once every 6 months.

Key nursing diagnoses

• Risk for injury related to adverse reactions

• Impaired mobility related to extrapyramidal symptoms

• Noncompliance related to long-term therapy

Planning and implementation

• Do not withdraw drug abruptly; although physical dependence does not occur with antipsychotic drugs, rebound exacerbation of psychotic symptoms may occur, and many drug effects persist.

• Follow manufacturer's guidelines for reconstitution, dilution, administration, and storage of drugs; slightly discolored liquids may or may not be acceptable for use. Check with pharmacist.

Patient teaching

• Teach patient how and when to take drug. Caution him not to increase his dosage or discontinue drug without his doctor's approval. Suggest taking full dose at bedtime if daytime sedation is troublesome.

• Explain that full therapeutic effect may not occur for several weeks.

• Teach signs and symptoms of adverse reactions, and urge him to report unusual effects, especially involuntary movements.

• Instruct patient to avoid beverages and drugs containing alcohol, and warn him not to take other drugs, including OTC products, without doctor's approval.

• Advise patient to avoid tasks requiring mental alertness and psychomotor coordination until drug's effects are established; emphasize that sedative effects will lessen after several weeks.

• Inform patient that excessive exposure to sunlight, heat lamps, or tanning beds may cause photosensitivity reactions. Advise him to avoid exposure to extremes of heat or cold.

• Explain that phenothiazines may cause pink to brown discoloration of urine.

Evaluation

• Patient remains free from injury.

• Extrapyramidal symptoms do not develop.

• Patient complies with therapy, as evidenced by improved thought processes.

Skeletal muscle relaxants
baclofen
carisoprodol
chlorzoxazone
cyclobenzaprine hydrochloride
methocarbamol
orphenadrine citrate

Action

All skeletal muscle relaxants except baclofen reduce impulse transmission from the spinal cord to skeletal muscle. Baclofen's mechanism of action is unclear.

Indications

▶ Painful musculoskeletal disorders, spasticity of multiple sclerosis.

Adverse reactions

Skeletal muscle relaxants may cause ataxia, confusion, depressed mood, dizziness, drowsiness, dry mouth, hallucinations, headache, hypotension, nervousness, tachycardia, tremor, and vertigo. Baclofen may cause seizures.

Contraindications and precautions

• Contraindicated in patients with known hypersensitivity to drug.
• Use with caution in patients with impaired renal or hepatic function.
• Additional contraindications and precautions exist. See individual drugs for complete listings.
• **Geriatric use:** Elderly patients are at greater risk for adverse reactions. Monitor carefully.
• **Pediatric use:** Recommendations vary for use in children. See individual drugs for specific guidelines.
• **Breast-feeding:** Recommendations vary for use in breast-feeding women. See individual drugs for specific guidelines.

NURSING CONSIDERATIONS

▨ Assessment
• Monitor patient for hypersensitivity reactions.
• Assess degree of relief obtained to help doctor determine when dosage can be reduced.
• Watch for increased seizures in epileptic patients receiving baclofen.
• Monitor CBC results closely.
• Monitor platelet counts in patients receiving cyclobenzaprine or orphenadrine.
• Observe for orthostatic hypotension in patient receiving methocarbamol.
• Monitor hepatic function and urinalysis results in patient receiving long-term orphenadrine therapy.
• Assess compliance in patient receiving long-term therapy.

▦ Key nursing diagnoses
• Risk for trauma related to baclofen-induced seizures
• Altered thought processes related to confusion
• Noncompliance related to long-term therapy

▶ Planning and implementation
• Do not stop baclofen or carisoprodol abruptly after long-term therapy unless required by severe adverse reactions.
• Institute safety precautions as needed.
• Give oral forms of drug with meals or milk to prevent GI distress.
• Obtain an order for a mild analgesic to relieve drug-induced headache.
Patient teaching
• Tell patient to take drug exactly as prescribed. Caution him not to stop baclofen or carisoprodol suddenly after long-term therapy.
• Instruct patient to avoid activities that require mental alertness until drug's CNS effects are known.
• Advise patient to avoid alcohol during therapy.
• Advise patient to follow his doctor's orders regarding rest and physical therapy.

Prototype drug

• Instruct patient receiving cyclobenzaprine or orphenadrine to report urinary hesitancy.

• Inform patient taking methocarbamol or chlorzoxazone that urine may be discolored.

☑ **Evaluation**

• Patient remains free from seizures.

• Patient exhibits normal thought processes.

• Patient complies with therapy, as evidenced by pain relief or improvement of spasticity.

Sulfonamides

co-trimoxazole (trimethoprim-
 sulfamethoxazole)
sulfadiazine
sulfamethoxazole
sulfasalazine
sulfisoxazole

Action

Sulfonamides are bacteriostatic. They inhibit biosynthesis of tetrahydrofolic acid, which is needed for bacterial cell growth. They are active against some strains of staphylococci, streptococci, *Nocardia asteroides* and *brasiliensis, Clostridium tetani* and *perfringens, Bacillus anthracis, Escherichia coli,* and *Neisseria gonorrhoeae* and *meningitidis.* They are also active against organisms causing urinary tract infections, such as *E. coli, Proteus mirabilis* and *vulgaris, Klebsiella, Enterobacter,* and *Staphylococcus aureus,* and genital lesions caused by *Haemophilus ducreyi* (chancroid).

Indications

▶ Bacterial infections, nocardiosis, toxoplasmosis, chloroquine-resistant *Plasmodium falciparum* malaria, inflammatory bowel disease.

Adverse reactions

Many adverse reactions are associated with hypersensitivity, including rash, fever, pruritus, erythema multiforme, erythema nodosum, Stevens-Johnson syndrome, Lyell's syndrome, exfoliative dermatitis, photosensitivity, joint pain, conjunctivitis, leukopenia, and bronchospasm. Hematologic reactions include granulocytopenia, thrombocytopenia, agranulocytosis, hypoprothrombinemia and, in G6PD deficiency, hemolytic anemia. Renal effects usually result from crystalluria (precipitation of sulfonamide in renal system). GI reactions include nausea, vomiting, anorexia, stomatitis, pancreatitis, diarrhea, and folic acid malabsorption.

Contraindications and precautions

• Contraindicated in pregnant women at term, in breast-feeding women, and in patients with known hypersensitivity to drug.

• Use with caution in patients with impaired renal or hepatic function, severe allergy, bronchial asthma, or G6PD.

• **Geriatric use:** Elderly patients are susceptible to bacterial and fungal superinfection and are at greater risk of folate deficiency anemia and adverse renal and hematologic effects.

• **Pediatric use:** Sulfonamides are contraindicated in infants younger than age 2 months, unless there is no therapeutic alternative. Use with caution in children with fragile X chromosome associated with mental retardation.

• **Breast-feeding:** Sulfonamides are secreted in breast milk and are contraindicated in breast-feeding women.

NURSING CONSIDERATIONS

☒ **Assessment**

• Assess patient's history of allergies, especially to sulfonamides or to any other drug containing sulfur (such as thiazides, furosemide, and oral sulfonylureas).

• Monitor patient for adverse reactions; patients with AIDS have a much higher incidence of adverse reactions.
• Obtain results of culture and sensitivity tests before first dose; check test results periodically to assess drug effectiveness.
• Monitor urine cultures, CBC, and urinalysis before and during therapy.
• Monitor patients on long-term therapy for possible superinfection.

🔲 **Key nursing diagnoses**
• Altered protection related to hypersensitivity
• Risk for infection related to superinfection
• Risk for fluid volume deficit related to adverse GI reactions

▶ **Planning and implementation**
• Give oral dose with 8 oz (240 ml) of water, and force fluids to 3,000 to 4,000 ml/day, depending on drug; patient's urine output should be at least 1,500 ml/day.
• Follow manufacturer's directions for reconstitution, dilution, and storage of drugs; check expiration dates.
• Shake oral suspensions well before administering to ensure correct dosage.
Patient teaching
• Urge patient to take drug exactly as prescribed, to complete the prescribed regimen, and to keep follow-up appointments.
• Advise patient to take oral drug with full glass of water and to drink plenty of fluids; explain that tablet may be crushed and swallowed with water to ensure maximal absorption.
• Teach signs and symptoms of hypersensitivity and other adverse reactions. Urge him to report bloody urine, difficult breathing, rash, fever, chills, or severe fatigue.
• Advise patient to avoid direct sun exposure and to use a sunscreen to help prevent photosensitivity reactions.
• Advise diabetic patient that sulfonamides may increase effects of oral hypo-glycemic. Tell him not to monitor urine glucose levels with Clinitest.
• Inform patient taking sulfasalazine that it may cause an orange-yellow discoloration of urine or skin and may permanently stain soft contact lenses yellow.

🔲 **Evaluation**
• Patient exhibits no signs of hypersensitivity.
• Patient is free from infection.
• Patient maintains adequate hydration.

Tetracyclines
demeclocycline hydrochloride
doxycycline
doxycycline hyclate
doxycycline hydrochloride
minocycline hydrochloride
oxytetracycline hydrochloride
tetracycline hydrochloride

Action

Tetracyclines are bacteriostatic but may be bactericidal against certain organisms. They bind reversibly to 30S and 50S ribosomal subunits, inhibiting bacterial protein synthesis.

Susceptible gram-positive organisms include *Bacillus anthracis, Actinomyces israelii, Clostridium perfringens, C. tetani, Listeria monocytogenes*, and *Nocardia*.

Susceptible gram-negative organisms include *Neisseria meningitidis, Pasteurella multocida, Legionella pneumophila, Brucella, Vibrio cholerae, Yersinia enterocolitica, Y. pestis, Bordetella pertussis, Haemophilus influenzae, H. ducreyi, Campylobacter fetus, Shigella*, and many other common pathogens.

Other susceptible organisms include *Rickettsia akari, R. typhi, R. prowazekii, R. tsutsugamushi, Coxiella burnetii, Chlamydia trachomatis, C. psittaci, Mycoplasma pneumoniae, M. hominis*,

Leptospira, Treponema pallidum, T. pertenue, and *Borrelia recurrentis.*

Indications

▶ Bacterial, antiprotozoal, rickettsial, and fungal infections.

Adverse reactions

The most common adverse effects involve the GI tract and are dose-related; they include anorexia; flatulence; nausea; vomiting; bulky, loose stools; epigastric burning; and abdominal discomfort. Superinfections also commonly occur. Photosensitivity reactions may be severe. Renal failure has been attributed to Fanconi's syndrome after use of outdated tetracycline. Permanent discoloration of teeth occurs when administered during tooth formation (in children younger than age 8).

Contraindications and precautions

• Contraindicated in pregnant or breast-feeding women, in children younger than age 8, and in patients with known hypersensitivity to tetracyclines.
• Use with caution in patients with impaired renal or hepatic function.
• **Geriatric use:** Some elderly patients have decreased esophageal motility; use with caution and monitor for local irritation from slowly passing oral forms. Elderly patients are also more susceptible to superinfection.
• **Pediatric use:** Children younger than age 8 should not receive tetracyclines. The drugs can cause permanent tooth discoloration, enamel hypoplasia, and a reversible decrease in bone calcification.
• **Breast-feeding:** Tetracyclines are excreted in breast milk and are contraindicated in breast-feeding women.

NURSING CONSIDERATIONS

⚕ Assessment
• Assess patient's allergic history.
• Monitor patient for adverse reactions.

• Obtain results of culture and sensitivity tests before first dose; check cultures periodically to assess drug effectiveness.
• Check expiration dates before administration. Outdated tetracyclines may cause nephrotoxicity.
• Monitor for bacterial and fungal superinfection, especially in elderly or debilitated patients or in those receiving immunosuppressants or radiation therapy; watch especially for oral candidiasis.

⊞ Key nursing diagnoses
• Altered protection related to hypersensitivity
• Risk for infection related to superinfection
• Risk for fluid volume deficit related to adverse GI reactions

⧐ Planning and implementation
• Give all oral tetracyclines except doxycycline and minocycline 1 hour before or 2 hours after meals for maximum absorption; do not give with food, milk or other dairy products, sodium bicarbonate, iron compounds, or antacids, which may impair absorption.
• Give water with and after oral drug to facilitate passage to stomach because incomplete swallowing can cause severe esophageal irritation; do not administer within 1 hour of bedtime to prevent esophageal reflux.
• Follow manufacturer's directions for reconstitution and storage; keep product refrigerated and away from light.
• Monitor I.V. injection sites and rotate routinely to minimize local irritation. I.V. administration may cause severe phlebitis.
Patient teaching
• Urge patient to take drug exactly as prescribed, to complete the prescribed regimen, and to keep follow-up appointments.
• Warn patient not to take drug with food, milk or other dairy products, sodium bicarbonate, or iron compounds because they may interfere with absorption.

Advise him to take antacids 3 hours after tetracycline.
• Instruct patient to check expiration dates and to discard any expired drug.
• Teach signs and symptoms of adverse reactions, and urge him to report these promptly.
• Advise patient to avoid direct exposure to sunlight and to use a sunscreen to help prevent photosensitivity reactions.

☑ **Evaluation**
• Patient exhibits no signs of hypersensitivity.
• Patient is free from infection.
• Patient maintains adequate hydration.

Thyroid hormones
levothyroxine sodium
liothyronine sodium
thyroid
thyrotropin

Action

Thyroid hormones have catabolic and anabolic effects and influence normal metabolism, growth, and development. Affecting every organ system, they are vital to normal CNS function. Thyrotropin (TSH) increases iodine uptake by the thyroid and increases formation and release of thyroid hormone. TSH is isolated from bovine anterior pituitary glands.

Indications

▶ Hypothyroidism, simple goiter, goitrogenesis.

Adverse reactions

Adverse reactions include nervousness, insomnia, tremor, tachycardia, palpitations, nausea, headache, fever, and sweating.

Contraindications and precautions
• Contraindicated in patients with MI, thyrotoxicosis, or uncorrected adrenal insufficiency.
• Use with extreme caution in patients with angina pectoris, hypertension or other CV disorders, renal insufficiency, or ischemia.
• Use with caution in patients with myxedema.
• **Geriatric use:** In patients older than age 60, initial hormone replacement dosage should be 25% less than the usual recommended starting dosage.
• **Pediatric use:** During first few months of therapy, children may suffer partial hair loss. Reassure child and parents that this is temporary.
• **Breast-feeding:** Minimal amounts of exogenous thyroid hormones are excreted in breast milk. However, problems have not been reported in breast-feeding infants.

NURSING CONSIDERATIONS

⚕ **Assessment**
• Assess patient's thyroid function studies regularly, as ordered.
• Monitor pulse rate and blood pressure.
• Monitor patient for signs of thyrotoxicosis or inadequate dosage therapy, including diarrhea, fever, irritability, listlessness, rapid heartbeat, vomiting, and weakness.
• Monitor PT and INR; patients taking anticoagulants usually require lower doses.

⚏ **Key nursing diagnoses**
• Risk for injury related to adverse CV reactions
• Sleep pattern disturbance related to insomnia
• Noncompliance related to long-term therapy

▶ **Planning and implementation**
• Keep in mind that thyroid hormone dosage varies widely among patients. As

ordered, begin treatment at lowest level, titrating to higher doses according to patient's symptoms and laboratory data, until euthyroid state is reached.

• Administer thyroid hormones at same time each day. Morning dosage is preferred to prevent insomnia.

Patient teaching

• Instruct patient to take drug exactly as prescribed. Suggest taking dose in morning to prevent insomnia.

• Advise patient to report signs and symptoms of overdose (chest pain, palpitations, sweating, nervousness) or aggravated CV disease (chest pain, dyspnea, tachycardia).

• Tell patient who has achieved a stable response not to change brands.

• Inform parents that child may lose hair during first months of therapy, but reassure them that this is temporary.

☑ Evaluation

• Patient does not experience injury from adverse reactions.

• Patient gets adequate sleep during the night.

• Patient complies with therapy, as evidenced by normal thyroid hormone levels and resolution of underlying disorder.

Xanthine derivatives
aminophylline
caffeine
theophylline

Action

Xanthine derivatives are structurally related; they directly relax smooth muscle, stimulate the CNS, induce diuresis, increase gastric acid secretion, inhibit uterine contractions, and exert weak inotropic and chronotropic effects on the heart. Of these drugs, theophylline exerts the greatest effect on smooth muscle.

The action of xanthine derivatives is not totally mediated by inhibition of phosphodiesterase. Current data suggest that inhibition of adenosine receptors or other as yet unidentified mechanisms may be responsible for therapeutic effects. By relaxing smooth muscle of the respiratory tract, they increase air flow and vital capacity. They also slow onset of diaphragmatic fatigue and stimulate the respiratory center in the CNS.

Indications

▶ Asthma and bronchospasm associated with emphysema and chronic bronchitis.

Adverse reactions

Adverse effects are dose-related, except for hypersensitivity, and can be controlled by dosage adjustment and monitored via serum levels. Common reactions include hypotension, palpitations, arrhythmias, restlessness, irritability, nausea, vomiting, urine retention, and headache.

Contraindications and precautions

• Contraindicated in patients with preexisting arrhythmias or known hypersensitivity to xanthines.

• Use with caution in patients with arrhythmias, cardiac or circulatory impairment, cor pulmonale, hepatic or renal disease, active peptic ulcers, hyperthyroidism, and diabetes mellitus.

• **Geriatric use:** Use with caution in elderly patients.

• **Pediatric use:** Small children may exhibit excessive CNS stimulation. Monitor closely.

• **Breast-feeding:** Xanthines are distributed in breast milk and should not be given to breast-feeding women; infants may experience serious adverse reactions.

NURSING CONSIDERATIONS

☉ Assessment

• Monitor theophylline blood levels closely; therapeutic levels range from 10 to 20 mcg/ml.

• Monitor patient closely for adverse reactions, especially toxicity.
• Monitor vital signs.

▦ Key nursing diagnoses
• Sleep pattern disturbance related to CNS effects
• Urine retention related to adverse effects on bladder
• Noncompliance related to long-term therapy

▷ Planning and implementation
• Do not crush or have patient chew timed-release preparations.
• Expect doctor to calculate dosage from lean body weight because theophylline does not distribute into fatty tissue.
• Anticipate adjustment of daily dosage in elderly patients and in those with heart failure or hepatic disease.
• Provide patient with sleep aids, such as a back rub or milk-based beverage.
Patient teaching
• Tell patient to take drug exactly as prescribed.
• Caution patient to check with doctor before using any other drug, including OTC products, or before switching brands.
• Inform patient who smokes that he may have decreased theophylline levels and to notify doctor if he quits because dose will need to be adjusted.

▨ Evaluation
• Patient sleeps usual number of hours without interruption.
• Patient does not experience change in voiding pattern.
• Patient complies with therapy, as evidenced by maintenance of therapeutic blood levels.

Alphabetical
Listing of Drugs

abciximab
(ab-SIKS-ih-mahb)
ReoPro

Pharmacologic class: fab fragment of chimeric human-murine monoclonal antibody 7E3
Therapeutic class: platelet aggregation inhibitor
Pregnancy risk category: C

How supplied

Injection: 2 mg/ml

Pharmacokinetics

Absorption: not applicable with I.V. administration.
Distribution: rapidly binds to platelet GPllb/llla receptors.
Metabolism: not reported.
Excretion: not reported. *Half-life:* initially, less than 10 minutes; second phase, about 30 minutes.

Route	Onset	Peak	Duration
I.V.	Almost immediate	Almost immediate	About 24 hr

Pharmacodynamics

Chemical effect: prevents binding of fibrinogen, von Willebrand factor, and other adhesive molecules to GPllb/llla receptor sites on activated platelets.
Therapeutic effect: inhibits platelet aggregation.

Indications and dosage

▶ **Adjunct to percutaneous transluminal coronary angioplasty (PTCA) or atherectomy for prevention of acute cardiac ischemic complications in patients at high risk for abrupt closure of treated coronary vessel.** *Adults:* 0.25 mg/kg as I.V. bolus 10 to 60 minutes before PTCA or atherectomy, followed by continuous I.V. infusion of 10 mcg/minute for 12 hours.

Adverse reactions

CNS: hypoesthesia, confusion.
CV: *hypotension,* bradycardia, peripheral edema.
EENT: abnormal vision.
GI: *nausea, vomiting.*
Hematologic: bleeding, *thrombocytopenia,* anemia, leukocytosis.
Respiratory: pleural effusion, pleurisy, pneumonia.
Other: pain.

Interactions

Drug-drug. *Antiplatelet agents, heparin, NSAIDs, other anticoagulants, thrombolytics:* increased risk of bleeding. Monitor patient closely.

Contraindications and precautions

• Contraindicated in patients with hypersensitivity to a drug component or to murine proteins; in those with active internal bleeding, GI or GU bleeding of clinical significance within 6 weeks, history of CVA within 2 years or with significant residual neurologic deficit, bleeding diathesis, thrombocytopenia (less than 100,000/mm³), major surgery or trauma within 6 weeks, intracranial neoplasm, intracranial arteriovenous malformation, intracranial aneurysm, severe uncontrolled hypertension, or history of vasculitis; when oral anticoagulants have been administered within 7 days unless PT is less than or equal to 1.2 times control; or with use of I.V. dextran before PTCA or intent to use it during PTCA.
• Use cautiously in patients at increased risk for bleeding (those who weigh under 75 kg, are older than age 65, have history of GI disease, or are receiving thrombolytic agents). Conditions that also increase risk of bleeding include PTCA within 12 hours of onset of symptoms for acute MI, prolonged PTCA (lasting more

than 70 minutes), failed PTCA, and concomitant use of heparin with abciximab.
• Use cautiously in pregnant or breast-feeding women.
• Safety of drug has not been established in children.

NURSING CONSIDERATIONS

⚕ Assessment
• Note patient's history. Patients at risk for abrupt closure (candidates for abciximab) include those undergoing PTCA with at least one of the following conditions: unstable angina or non-Q wave MI, acute Q wave MI within 12 hours of onset of symptoms, two type B lesions in artery to be dilated, one type B lesion in artery to be dilated in a woman older than age 65 or a patient with diabetes, one type C lesion in artery to be dilated, or angioplasty of infarct-related lesion within 7 days of MI.
• Assess vital signs and evaluate bleeding studies before therapy.
• Monitor patient closely for bleeding. Bleeding associated with therapy falls into two broad categories: that observed at arterial access site used for cardiac catheterization and internal bleeding involving GI or GU tract or retroperitoneal sites.
• Be alert for adverse reactions and drug interactions.
• Evaluate patient's and family's knowledge of drug therapy.

⬦ Nursing diagnoses
• Altered cerebral or cardiopulmonary tissue perfusion related to patient's underlying condition
• Risk of fluid volume deficit related to drug-induced bleeding
• Knowledge deficit related to drug therapy

⬥ Planning and implementation
• Inspect solution for particulate matter before administration. If opaque particles are found, discard solution and obtain new vial. Withdraw necessary amount of abciximab for I.V. bolus injection through sterile, nonpyrogenic, low-protein-binding 0.2- or 0.22-micron filter into syringe. I.V. bolus should be administered 10 to 60 minutes before procedure.
• Withdraw 4.5 ml of drug for continuous I.V. infusion through sterile, nonpyrogenic, low-protein-binding 0.2- or 0.22-micron filter into syringe. Inject into 250 ml of sterile 0.9% NaCl solution or 5% dextrose and infuse at 17 ml/hour for 12 hours via continuous infusion pump equipped with in-line filter. Discard unused portion.
• Administer drug in separate I.V. line; do not add other medication to infusion solution.
• Institute bleeding precautions. Maintain patient on bed rest for 6 to 8 hours after sheath removal or discontinuation of abciximab infusion, whichever is later.
• Keep epinephrine, dopamine, theophylline, antihistamines, and corticosteroids available in case anaphylaxis occurs.
• Know that drug is intended for use with aspirin and heparin.
Patient teaching
• Teach patient about his disease and therapy.
• Stress importance of reporting signs and symptoms.

☑ Evaluation
• Patient maintains adequate tissue perfusion.
• Patient maintains adequate hydration.
• Patient and family state understanding of drug therapy.

acarbose
(ay-KAR-bohs)
Precose

Pharmacologic class: alpha-glucosidase inhibitor
Therapeutic class: antidiabetic
Pregnancy risk category: B

How supplied
Tablets: 25 mg, 50 mg, 100 mg

Pharmacokinetics
Absorption: minimally absorbed.
Distribution: acts locally within GI tract.
Metabolism: metabolized exclusively within the GI tract, primarily by intestinal bacteria and to a lesser extent by digestive enzymes.
Excretion: almost completely excreted by the kidneys. *Half-life:* 2 hours.

Route	Onset	Peak	Duration
P.O.	Unknown	1 hr	2-4 hr

Pharmacodynamics
Chemical effect: an alpha-glucosidase inhibitor that delays digestion of carbohydrates.
Therapeutic effect: delayed glucose absorption and lower postprandial hyperglycemia.

Indications and dosages
▶ **Adjunct to diet to lower blood glucose in patients with type 2 (non-insulin-dependent) diabetes mellitus whose hyperglycemia cannot be managed by diet alone or by diet and a sulfonylurea.** *Adults:* Initially, 25 mg P.O. t.i.d. at start of each main meal. Subsequent dosage adjustment made q 4 to 8 weeks, based on 1-hour postprandial glucose level and tolerance. Maintenance dosage is 50 to 100 mg P.O. t.i.d.

Adverse reactions
GI: *abdominal pain, diarrhea, flatulence.*
Other: elevated serum transaminase levels.

Interactions
Drug-drug. *Calcium channel blockers, corticosteroids, estrogens, isoniazid, nicotinic acid, oral contraceptives, phenothiazines, phenytoin, sympathomimetics, thiazides and other diuretics, thyroid products:* may cause hyperglycemia during concomitant use or hypoglycemia when withdrawn. Monitor blood glucose level.
Digestive enzyme preparations containing carbohydrate-splitting enzymes (such as amylase, pancreatin), intestinal adsorbents (such as activated charcoal): may reduce effect of acarbose. Do not administer concomitantly.

Contraindications and precautions
• Contraindicated in patients with hypersensitivity to drug and in those with diabetic ketoacidosis, cirrhosis, inflammatory bowel disease, colonic ulceration, partial intestinal obstruction, predisposition to intestinal obstruction, chronic intestinal disease associated with marked disorder of digestion or absorption, or conditions that may deteriorate because of increased intestinal gas formation.
• Drug is not recommended in renally impaired patients or pregnant or breast-feeding women.
• Use cautiously in patients receiving a sulfonylurea or insulin. Acarbose may increase the hypoglycemic potential of the sulfonylurea.
• Safety and efficacy of drug have not been established in children.

NURSING CONSIDERATIONS

⚚ Assessment
• Monitor patient's plasma glucose level 1 hour after a meal to determine therapeutic effectiveness of acarbose and to identify appropriate dose. Report hyperglycemia to doctor.
• Monitor glycosylated hemoglobin every 3 months.
• Monitor serum transaminase level every 3 months in first year of therapy and periodically thereafter in patients receiving doses in excess of 50 mg t.i.d. Report abnormalities.
• Obtain baseline serum creatinine levels; drug is not recommended in patients with a serum creatinine greater than 2 mg/dl.
• Evaluate patient's and family's knowledge about drug therapy.

⊞ Nursing diagnoses
• Risk for fluid volume imbalance related to adverse GI effect
• Altered nutrition: Risk for less than body requirements related to patient's underlying condition
• Knowledge deficit related to drug therapy

⟫ Planning and implementation
• In patients weighing less than 60 kg (132 lb), do not exceed 50 mg P.O. t.i.d.
• Watch for elevations of serum transaminase and bilirubin levels and low serum calcium and plasma vitamin B$_6$ levels in doses exceeding 50 mg t.i.d.
• Know that acarbose may increase hypoglycemic potential of sulfonylureas. Monitor patient receiving both drugs closely. If hypoglycemia occurs, treat with oral glucose (dextrose), I.V. glucose infusion, or glucagon administration. Report hypoglycemia to doctor.
• Know that insulin therapy may be needed during increased stress (infection, fever, surgery, or trauma).
Patient teaching
• Tell patient to take drug daily with first bite of each of three main meals.
• Explain that therapy relieves symptoms but does not cure the disease.
• Stress importance of adhering to specific diet, weight reduction, exercise, and hygiene programs. Show patient how to monitor blood glucose level and to recognize and treat hyperglycemia.
• Teach patient to recognize hypoglycemia and to treat symptoms with a form of dextrose rather than with a product containing table sugar.
• Urge patient to carry medical identification at all times.

⊠ Evaluation
• Patient maintains adequate fluid volume balance.
• Patient does not experience hypoglycemic episodes.
• Patient and family state understanding of drug therapy.

acebutolol
(as-ih-BYOO-tuh-lol)
Monitan, Sectral

Pharmacologic class: beta blocker
Therapeutic class: antihypertensive, antiarrhythmic
Pregnancy risk category: B

How supplied
Capsules: 200 mg, 400 mg

Pharmacokinetics
Absorption: well absorbed after oral administration.
Distribution: about 25% protein–bound; minimal quantities detected in CSF.
Metabolism: undergoes extensive first-pass metabolism in liver.
Excretion: from 30% to 40% of dose is excreted in urine; remainder, in feces and bile. *Half-life:* 3 to 4 hours.

Route	Onset	Peak	Duration
P.O.	1-1.5 hr	2.5 hr	Up to 24 hr

Pharmacodynamics
Chemical effect: antihypertensive action unknown. Possible mechanisms include reduced cardiac output, decreased sympathetic outflow to peripheral vasculature, and inhibited renin release. Antiarrhythmic action decreases myocardial contractility and heart rate and has mild intrinsic sympathomimetic activity.
Therapeutic effect: lowers blood pressure and heart rate and restores normal sinus rhythm.

Indications and dosage
▶ **Hypertension.** *Adults:* 400 mg P.O. as single daily dose or in divided doses b.i.d. Patients may receive as much as 1,200 mg daily.
▶ **Suppression of PVCs.** *Adults:* 400 mg P.O. in divided doses b.i.d. Dosage increased to provide adequate clinical response. Usual dosage is 600 to 1,200 mg daily. In patients with impaired renal

---

Reactions may be *common*, uncommon, *life-threatening*, or COMMON AND LIFE-THREATENING.

function, dosage is reduced. Elderly patients may require lower dosage; dosage should not exceed 800 mg daily.

Adverse reactions

CNS: *fatigue,* headache, dizziness, insomnia.
CV: chest pain, edema, bradycardia, *heart failure, hypotension.*
GI: nausea, constipation, diarrhea, dyspepsia.
Respiratory: dyspnea, bronchospasm.
Skin: rash.
Other: fever, positive antinuclear antibody (ANA) test.

Interactions

Drug-drug. *Alpha-adrenergic agents stimulants:* increased hypertensive response. Use together cautiously.
Cardiac glycosides, diltiazem, verapamil: excessive bradycardia and increased depressant effect on myocardium. Use together cautiously.
Insulin, oral antidiabetic agents: can alter dosage requirements in previously stabilized diabetic patient. Observe patient carefully.
NSAIDs: decreased antihypertensive effect. Monitor blood pressure. Dosage may require adjustment.
Reserpine: additive effect. Monitor closely.

Contraindications and precautions

• Contraindicated in patients with persistently severe bradycardia, second- or third-degree heart block, overt heart failure, or cardiogenic shock and in breast-feeding women.
• Use cautiously in patients with heart failure, peripheral vascular disease, bronchospastic disease, or diabetes and in pregnant women.
• Safety of drug has not been established in children.

NURSING CONSIDERATIONS

✒ Assessment

• Assess patient's blood pressure and heart rate and rhythm before and during therapy.
• Monitor patient's energy level.
• Be alert for adverse reactions and drug interactions.
• Evaluate patient's and family's knowledge of drug therapy.

⊞ Nursing diagnoses

• Risk for injury related to patient's underlying condition
• Fatigue related to drug-induced CNS adverse reactions
• Knowledge deficit related to drug therapy

▶ Planning and implementation

• Be aware that dosage should be reduced in patients with decreased renal function and that elderly patients may require lower doses.
• Check apical pulse before giving drug; if slower than 60 beats/minute, withhold drug and call doctor.
• Do not discontinue abruptly; this can exacerbate angina and MI.
• Before surgery, notify anesthesiologist that patient is taking drug therapy.
Patient teaching
• Teach patient how to take his pulse, and instruct him to withhold dose and notify doctor if pulse rate is below 60 beats/minute.
• Warn patient that drug may cause dizziness. Instruct him to avoid sudden postural changes and to sit down immediately if dizziness occurs.
• Explain importance of taking drug as prescribed, even when feeling well.

☑ Evaluation

• Patient's blood pressure and heart rate and rhythm are normal.
• Patient effectively combats fatigue.
• Patient and family state understanding of drug therapy.

acetaminophen (APAP, paracetamol)

(as-ee-tuh-MIH-nuh-fin)

Abenol♦†; Aceta Elixir*†; Acetaminophen Uniserts†; Aceta Tablets†; Actamin†; Actimol♦†; Aminofen†; Anacin-3†; Anacin-3 Children's Elixir*†; Anacin-3 Children's Tablets†; Anacin-3 Extra Strength†; Anacin-3 Infants'†; Apacet Capsules†; Apacet Elixir*†; Apacet Extra Strength Caplets†; Apacet Infants'†; Apo-Acetaminophen♦†; Arthritis Pain Formula Aspirin Free†; Atasol Caplets♦†; Atasol Drops♦†; Atasol Elixir*♦†; Atasol Tablets♦†; Banesin†; Dapa†; Dapa XS†; Datril XS; Dolanex*†; Dorcol Children's Fever and Pain Reducer†; Dymadon◊†; Exdol♦†; Feverall, Children's◊; Feverall Junior Strength◊; Feverall Sprinkle Caps◊; Genapap Children's Elixir†; Genapap Children's Tablets†; Genapap Extra Strength Caplets†; Genapap, Infants'†; Genapap Regular Strength Tablets†; Genebs Extra Strength Caplets†; Genebs Regular Strength Tablets†; Genebs X-Tra†; Halenol Elixir*†; Liquiprin Infants' Drops†; Meda Cap†; Myapap Elixir*†; Myapap, Infants'†; Neopap†; Oraphen-PD†; Panadol†; Panadol, Children's†; Panadol Extra Strength†; Panadol, Infants'†; Panadol Maximum Strength Caplets†; Panamax◊†; Panex†; Panex-500†; Paralgin◊†; Paraspen◊†; Redutemp†; Ridenol Caplets†; Robigesic♦†; Rounox♦†; Setamol-500◊†; Snaplets-FR†; Stanback AF Extra Strength Powder; St. Joseph Aspirin-Free Fever Reducer for Children†; Suppap-120†; Suppap-325†; Suppap-650†; Tapanol Extra Strength Caplets†; Tapanol Extra Strength Tablets†; Tempra†; Tempra D.S.†; Tempra, Infants'†; Tempra Syrup†; Tenol†; Tylenol Children's Elixir†; Tylenol Children's Tablets†; Tylenol Extended Relief†; Tylenol Extra Strength Caplets†; Tylenol Infants'†; Tylenol Junior Strength Caplets†; Ty-Pap†; Ty-Pap, Infants'†; Ty-Pap Syrup†; Ty-Tab Caplets†; Ty-Tab Capsules†; Ty-Tab, Children's†; Ty-Tab Tablets†; Valorin†; Valorin Extra†

Pharmacologic class: para-aminophenol derivative
Therapeutic class: nonnarcotic analgesic, antipyretic
Pregnancy risk category: NR

How supplied

Tablets: 160 mg†, 325 mg†, 500 mg†, 650 mg†
Tablets (chewable): 80 mg†, 160 mg†
Caplets (extended-release): 650 mg
Capsules: 500 mg†
Oral solution: 48 mg/ml†, 100 mg/ml†
Oral suspension: 120 mg/5 ml◊, 100 mg/ml†, 160 mg/ml†
Oral liquid: 160 mg/5 ml†, 500 mg/15 ml†
Elixir: 120 mg/5 ml, 130 mg/5 ml*†, 160 mg/5 ml*†, 325 mg/5 ml*†
Granules: 80 mg/packet†, 325 mg/capful†
Powder for solution: 1 g/packet
Sprinkles: 80 mg/capsule, 160 mg/capsule
Tablets for solution: 325 mg
Suppositories: 120 mg†, 125 mg†, 300 mg†, 325 mg†, 650 mg†
Wafers: 120 mg†

Pharmacokinetics

Absorption: absorbed rapidly and completely via GI tract.
Distribution: 25% protein-bound. Plasma concentrations do not correlate well with analgesic effect but do correlate with toxicity.
Metabolism: from 90% to 95% metabolized in liver.
Excretion: excreted in urine. *Half-life:* 1 to 4 hours.

Route	Onset	Peak	Duration
P.O., P.R.	Unknown	1-3 hr	1-3 hr

Pharmacodynamics

Chemical effect: unknown. May produce analgesia by blocking pain impulses,

---

Reactions may be *common*, uncommon, *life-threatening*, or COMMON AND LIFE-THREATENING.

probably by inhibiting prostaglandin or other substances that sensitize pain receptors. May relieve fever by action in hypothalamic heat-regulating center.
Therapeutic effect: relieves pain and reduces fever.

Indications and dosage

▶ **Mild pain or fever.** *Adults and children over age 12:* 325 to 650 mg P.O. or P.R. q 4 hours, p.r.n.; or 1 g P.O. t.i.d. or q.i.d., p.r.n. Alternatively, 2 extended-release caplets P.O. q 8 hours. Maximum dosage should not exceed 4 g daily. Dosage for long-term therapy should not exceed 2.6 g daily. *Children ages 11 to 12:* 480 mg P.O. or P.R. q 4 to 6 hours. *Children ages 9 to 10:* 400 mg P.O. or P.R. q 4 to 6 hours. *Children ages 6 to 8:* 320 mg P.O. or P.R. q 4 to 6 hours. *Children ages 4 to 5:* 240 mg P.O. or P.R. q 4 to 6 hours. *Children ages 2 to 3:* 160 mg P.O. or P.R. q 4 to 6 hours. *Children ages 12 to 23 months:* 120 mg P.O. q 4 to 6 hours. *Children ages 4 to 11 months:* 80 mg P.O. q 4 to 6 hours. *Children up to age 3 months:* 40 mg P.O. q 4 to 6 hours.

Adverse reactions

Hematologic: hemolytic anemia, neutropenia, leukopenia, pancytopenia, thrombocytopenia (rare).
Hepatic: *severe liver damage* (with toxic doses), jaundice.
Skin: rash, urticaria.
Other: hypoglycemia.

Interactions

Drug-drug. *Barbiturates, carbamazepine, hydantoins, rifampin, sulfinpyrazone, isoniazid:* high doses or long-term use of these drugs may reduce therapeutic effects and enhance hepatotoxic effects of acetaminophen. Avoid concomitant use.
Warfarin: increased hypoprothrombinemic effects with long-term use with high doses of acetaminophen. Monitor PT and INR closely.
Zidovudine: may increase incidence of bone marrow suppression because of impaired zidovudine metabolism. Monitor patient closely.
Drug-food. *Caffeine:* may enhance analgesic effects of acetaminophen. Monitor for effect.
Drug-lifestyle. *Alcohol use:* increased risk of hepatic damage. Warn against concomitant use.

Contraindications and precautions

• No known contraindications.
• Use cautiously in patients with history of chronic alcohol abuse; hepatotoxicity has occurred after therapeutic doses.
• Use cautiously in pregnant or breast-feeding women.

NURSING CONSIDERATIONS

Assessment
• Assess patient's pain or temperature before and during therapy.
• Assess patient's medication history. Many OTC products contain acetaminophen; be aware of this when calculating total daily dosage.
• Be alert for adverse reactions and drug interactions.
• Evaluate patient's and family's knowledge of drug therapy.

Nursing diagnoses
• Pain related to patient's underlying condition
• Risk for injury related to drug-induced liver damage with toxic doses
• Knowledge deficit related to drug therapy

Planning and implementation
P.O. use: Administer liquid form to children and other patients who have difficulty swallowing.
P.R. use: Use this route in small children and other patients when oral administration is not feasible.
• Know that acetaminophen may interfere with laboratory tests for urinary 5-hydroxyindoleacetic acid and may pro-

---

duce false-positive decrease in blood glucose level in home monitoring system.
Patient teaching
• Tell parents to consult doctor before giving drug to children younger than 2 years.
• Tell patient that drug is for short-term use only. Doctor should be consulted if administering to children for more than 5 days or to adults for more than 10 days.
• Tell patient not to use drug for marked fever (over 103.1° F [39.5° C]), fever persisting longer than 3 days, or recurrent fever unless directed by doctor.
• Warn patient that high doses or unsupervised long-term use can cause hepatic damage. Excessive ingestion of alcoholic beverages may increase risk of hepatotoxicity.
• Tell breast-feeding patient that drug is found in breast milk in low concentrations (less than 1% of dose). Patient may use it safely if therapy is short-term and does not exceed recommended doses.

☑ **Evaluation**
• Patient reports pain relief with drug.
• Patient's liver function studies remain normal.
• Patient and family state understanding of drug therapy.

acetazolamide
(as-ee-tuh-ZOH-luh-mighd)
Acetazolam♦, Apo-Acetazolamide♦, Diamox, Diamox Sequels

acetazolamide sodium
Diamox Parenteral, Diamox Sodium

Pharmacologic class: carbonic anhydrase inhibitor
Therapeutic class: adjunct treatment of open-angle glaucoma and perioperative treatment for acute angle-closure glaucoma, anticonvulsant, management of edema, prevention and treatment of acute mountain sickness
Pregnancy risk category: C

How supplied
Tablets: 125 mg, 250 mg
Capsules (extended-release): 500 mg
Injection: 500 mg/vial

Pharmacokinetics
Absorption: well absorbed from GI tract after oral administration.
Distribution: distributed throughout body tissues.
Metabolism: none.
Excretion: excreted primarily in urine through tubular secretion and passive reabsorption. *Half-life:* 10 to 15 hours.

Route	Onset	Peak	Duration
P.O.			
Tablets	1-1.5 hr	2-4 hr	8-12 hr
Capsules	2 hr	8-12 hr	18-24 hr
I.V.	2 min	15 min	4-5 hr

Pharmacodynamics
Chemical effect: blocks action of carbonic anhydrase, promoting renal excretion of sodium, potassium, bicarbonate, and water, and decreases secretion of aqueous humor in eye. As anticonvulsant, may inhibit carbonic anhydrase in CNS and decrease abnormal paroxysmal or excessive neuronal discharge. In acute mountain sickness, carbonic anhydrase inhibitors produce respiratory and metabolic acidosis that may stimulate ventilation, increase cerebral blood flow, and promote release of oxygen from hemoglobin.
Therapeutic effect: lowers intraocular pressure, controls seizure activity, and may improve respiratory function.

Indications and dosage
▶ **Secondary glaucoma and preoperative management of acute angle-closure glaucoma.** *Adults:* 250 mg P.O. q 4 hours, or 250 mg P.O. or I.V. b.i.d. for short-term therapy. I.V. administration (100 to 500 mg/minute) is preferred.
▶ **Edema in heart failure.** *Adults:* 250 to 375 mg (5 mg/kg) P.O. daily in a.m.
▶ **Chronic open-angle glaucoma.** *Adults:* 250 mg to 1 g P.O. daily in divid-

ed doses q.i.d., or 500 mg (extended-release) P.O. b.i.d.

▶ **Prevention or amelioration of acute mountain sickness**. *Adults:* 500 mg to 1 g P.O. daily in divided doses q 8 to 12 hours, or 500 mg (extended-release) P.O. b.i.d. Treatment started 24 to 48 hours before ascent and continued for 48 hours while at high altitude.

▶ **Adjunct treatment of myoclonic, refractory generalized tonic-clonic, absence, or mixed seizures**. *Adults and children:* 8 to 30 mg/kg P.O. daily in divided doses. For adults, optimum dosage is 375 mg to 1 g daily. Usually given with other anticonvulsants.

Adverse reactions

CNS: drowsiness, paresthesia, confusion.
EENT: transient myopia.
GI: nausea, vomiting, anorexia, altered taste.
GU: crystalluria, renal calculi, hematuria.
Hematologic: *aplastic anemia,* hemolytic anemia, *leukopenia.*
Skin: rash.
Other: *pain at injection site,* sterile abscesses, hyperchloremic acidosis, hypokalemia, asymptomatic hyperuricemia.

Interactions

Drug-drug. *Amphetamines, anticholinergics, mecamylamine, quinidine, tricyclic antidepressants, procainamide:* decreased renal clearance of these agents, increasing toxicity. Monitor patient closely.
Lithium: increase lithium secretion. Monitor patient.
Methenamine: reduced effectiveness of acetazolamide. Avoid concomitant use.
Salicylates: possible accumulation and toxicity of acetazolamide, including CNS depression and metabolic acidosis. Monitor patient closely.

Contraindications and precautions

• Contraindicated in patients with hypersensitivity to drug; in those undergoing long-term therapy for chronic noncongestive angle-closure glaucoma; in those

with hyponatremia or hypokalemia, renal or hepatic disease or dysfunction, adrenal gland failure, or hyperchloremic acidosis; and in breast-feeding women.
• Use cautiously in patients with respiratory acidosis, emphysema, or chronic pulmonary disease; in patients receiving other diuretics; and in pregnant women.
• Safety of drug has not been established in children.

NURSING CONSIDERATIONS

⚗ Assessment
• Assess patient's underlying condition before and during therapy, including, as appropriate, eye discomfort and intraocular pressure in those with glaucoma; edema in those with heart failure; and neurologic status in those with seizures. Also monitor intake and output.
• Be alert for adverse reactions and drug interactions.
• Evaluate patient's and family's knowledge of drug therapy.

⊞ Nursing diagnoses
• Fluid volume excess related to patient's underlying condition
• Altered urinary elimination related to diuretic action of drug
• Knowledge deficit related to drug therapy

▷ Planning and implementation
P.O. use: Give oral preparations early in morning to avoid nocturia. Give second doses early in afternoon.
I.V. use: Reconstitute 500-mg vial with at least 5 ml of sterile water for injection. Use within 24 hours. Inject 100 to 500 mg/minute into large vein, using 21G or 23G needle. Intermittent or continuous infusion is not recommended.
• Check with pharmacist if patient cannot swallow oral forms. He may make suspension using crushed tablets in highly flavored syrup, such as cherry, raspberry, or chocolate. Although concentrations up to 500 mg/5 ml are feasible, concentra-

tions of 250 mg/5 ml are more palatable. Refrigeration improves palatability but doesn't improve stability. Suspensions are stable for 1 week.

• Diuretic effect decreases with acidosis but is reestablished by withdrawing drug for several days and then restarting it or by using intermittent administration.

• Withhold drug and notify doctor if hypersensitivity or adverse reactions occur.

• Be aware that drug may cause false-positive urine protein tests.

Patient teaching

• Advise patient to take drug early in day to avoid interruption of sleep caused by nocturia.

• Teach patient to monitor fluid volume by daily weight and intake and output.

• Encourage patient to avoid high-sodium foods and to choose high-potassium foods.

• Teach patient to recognize and report signs and symptoms of fluid and electrolyte imbalance.

☑ **Evaluation**

• Patient is free from edema.

• Patient adjusts lifestyle to accommodate altered patterns of urinary elimination.

• Patient and family state understanding of drug therapy.

---

acetohexamide
(ah-see-toh-HEKS-ah-mighd)
Dimelor♦, Dymelor

Pharmacologic class: sulfonylurea
Therapeutic class: antidiabetic
Pregnancy risk category: NR

How supplied
Tablets: 250 mg, 500 mg

Pharmacokinetics
Absorption: absorbed rapidly from GI tract.

Distribution: not fully understood, but probably similar to that of other sulfonylureas; drug is highly protein-bound.
Metabolism: metabolized in liver, primarily to potent active metabolite.
Excretion: about 80% excreted in urine.
Half-life: about 6 hours.

Route	Onset	Peak	Duration
P.O.	≤ 1 hr	≤ 2 hr	12-24 hr

Pharmacodynamics
Chemical effect: unknown. Probably stimulates insulin release from pancreatic beta cells and reduces glucose output by liver. Increases sensitivity to insulin at cellular level.
Therapeutic effect: lowers blood sugar.

Indications and dosage
▶ **Adjunct to diet to lower blood glucose level in patients with type 2 (non-insulin-dependent) diabetes mellitus.**
Adults: initially, 250 mg P.O. daily before breakfast; dosage increased q 5 to 7 days (by 250 to 500 mg) as needed to maximum of 1.5 g daily in divided doses b.i.d. or t.i.d. before meals.
▶ **Replacement of insulin therapy in patients with type 2 (non-insulin-dependent) diabetes mellitus.** *Adults:* if insulin dosage is less than 20 units daily, insulin is stopped and oral therapy started with 250 mg P.O. daily, before breakfast, and increased as above if needed. If insulin dosage is 20 to 40 units daily, oral therapy is started with 250 mg P.O. daily, before breakfast, while insulin dosage is reduced 25% to 30% daily or every other day, depending on response to oral therapy.

Adverse reactions
GI: nausea, heartburn, vomiting.
Hematologic: *thrombocytopenia, aplastic anemia, agranulocytosis, leukopenia.*
Skin: rash, pruritus, facial flushing.
Other: hypersensitivity reactions, sodium loss, hypoglycemia.

Reactions may be *common*, uncommon, *life-threatening*, or COMMON AND LIFE-THREATENING.

Interactions

Drug-drug. *Anabolic steroids, chloramphenicol, clofibrate, guanethidine, ketoconazole, MAO inhibitors, omeprazole, phenylbutazone, probenecid, salicylates, sulfonamides:* increased hypoglycemic activity. Monitor blood glucose level.
Beta blockers, clonidine: prolonged hypoglycemic effect and masked symptoms of hypoglycemia. Use together cautiously.
Corticosteroids, diazoxide, glucagon, hydantoins, rifampin, thiazide diuretics: decreased hypoglycemic response. Monitor blood glucose level.
Oral anticoagulants: increased hypoglycemic activity or enhanced anticoagulant effect. Monitor PT, INR, and blood glucose level.
Drug-lifestyle. *Alcohol use:* possible disulfiram-like reaction. Avoid concomitant use.

Contraindications and precautions

• Contraindicated in patients with type 1 diabetes or diabetes that can be adequately controlled by diet; type 2 diabetes complicated by ketosis, acidosis, or diabetic coma; hyperglycemia associated with primary renal disease; major surgery; severe infections or trauma; or hypersensitivity to sulfonylureas; and in pregnant or breast-feeding patients.
• Use cautiously in patients with history of porphyria or impaired hepatic or renal function and in debilitated, malnourished, or geriatric patients.
• Safety of drug has not been established in children.

NURSING CONSIDERATIONS

Assessment
• Assess patient's blood glucose level before and frequently during therapy.
• Monitor patient's glycosylated hemoglobin, as ordered.
• Be alert for adverse reactions and drug interactions.
• Evaluate patient's and family's knowledge of drug therapy.

Nursing diagnoses
• Altered health maintenance related to hyperglycemia
• Risk for injury related to drug-induced hypoglycemia
• Knowledge deficit related to drug therapy

Planning and implementation
• Consider that some patients taking drug may be controlled effectively on once-daily regimen, whereas others show better response with divided dosing.
• Administer once-daily doses with breakfast; divided doses, before morning and evening meals.
• Treat hypoglycemic reaction with oral form of rapid-acting glucose if patient is awake or with glucagon or I.V. glucose if patient cannot be aroused. Follow treatment with complex carbohydrate snack if mealtime is more than 1 hour away, and determine cause of reaction.
Patient teaching
• Emphasize importance of following prescribed diet, exercise, and medical regimens.
• Tell patient to take drug at same time each day; to take missed dose immediately, unless it's almost time for next dose; and to refrain from taking double doses.
• Advise patient to avoid alcohol during drug therapy. Remind him that many foods and OTC medications contain alcohol.
• Encourage patient to wear a medical identification bracelet or necklace.
• Tell patient to take drug with food (once-daily dosage with breakfast).
• Teach patient how to monitor blood glucose level.
• Teach patient how to recognize signs and symptoms of hyperglycemia and hypoglycemia and what to do if they occur.
• Stress importance of compliance with drug therapy.

Evaluation
• Patient's blood glucose level is normal.

• Patient recognizes hypoglycemia early and treats it effectively before injury occurs.
• Patient and family state understanding of drug therapy.

acetohydroxamic acid
(as-ee-toh-high-droks-AM-ik AS-id)
Lithostat

Pharmacologic class: urease inhibitor
Therapeutic class: antiurolithic, adjunct agent in treatment of urinary tract infection
Pregnancy risk category: X

How supplied
Tablets (scored): 250 mg

Pharmacokinetics
Absorption: absorbed rapidly, primarily in upper GI tract.
Distribution: distributed widely in body water. Drug crosses placenta; distribution in human breast milk unknown.
Metabolism: metabolized to non-urease-inhibiting compound, acetamide, through saturable or rate-limited process. Unchanged acetohydroxamic acid in urine is drug's active form.
Excretion: excreted primarily in urine.
Half-life: 3½ to 10 hours (increases with increasing dose). Not known if drug is dialyzable.

Route	Onset	Peak	Duration
P.O.	Unknown	15-60 min	Unknown

Pharmacodynamics
Chemical effect: prevents formation of renal stones by inhibiting bacterial urease activity.
Therapeutic effect: decreases ammonia in urine, which increases cure rate of urinary tract infection caused by kidney stones.

Indications and dosage
▶ **Adjunctive therapy in patients with chronic urinary tract infections caused by urease-producing bacteria.** *Adults:* 250 mg P.O. q 6 to 8 hours when stomach is empty. Maximum daily dosage is 1.5 g. *Children:* 10 mg/kg/day P.O. in two or three divided doses.

Adverse reactions
CNS: *mild headache, depression, anxiety, nervousness,* malaise.
CV: deep vein thrombosis, phlebitis, palpitations.
GI: *nausea, vomiting, diarrhea, constipation, anorexia.*
Hematologic: *hemolytic anemia.*
Skin: *nonpruritic, macular rash on arms and face.*
Other: alopecia.

Interactions
Drug-drug. *Methenamine:* may produce synergistic effects. Monitor closely.
Oral iron supplements: reduced absorption of iron. Check with doctor, who may prescribe I.M. administration of iron.
Drug-food. *Any food:* improved drug action if taken on empty stomach. Give 1 hour before or 2 hours after meals
Drug-lifestyle. *Alcohol use:* may cause flushing and rash. Avoid concomitant use.

Contraindications and precautions
• Contraindicated in patients whose physical status and disease are amenable to surgery and appropriate antibiotics, in those whose urine is infected by non-urease-producing organisms, in patients with poor renal function, and in pregnant or breast-feeding women.
• Safety of drug has not been established in children.

NURSING CONSIDERATIONS

🔍 **Assessment**
• Obtain patient's history of kidney stones and urinary tract infections.

• Determine whether female patient is pregnant or considering pregnancy or is breast-feeding.
• Be alert for adverse reactions and drug interactions.
• Monitor CBC, including reticulocyte count, after 2 weeks of therapy, then every 3 months during treatment, as ordered.
• Evaluate patient's and family's knowledge of drug therapy.

⊕ **Nursing diagnoses**
• Infection related to presence of urinary tract infection
• Risk for injury related to adverse effects of drug
• Knowledge deficit related to drug therapy

⊠ **Planning and implementation**
• Do not administer to women of child-bearing age until pregnancy has been ruled out and appropriate contraception is in effect.
• Anticipate using reduced dosage in patients with renal impairment.
• Administer 1 hour before or 2 hours after meals to improve drug action.
• Recognize that patient also may be given methenamine to enhance response to drug.
• Discontinue drug and notify doctor if laboratory findings indicate hemolytic anemia.
• Be aware that negative Coombs' test for hemolytic anemia has occurred in patients receiving drug.
• Know that iron should be administered parenterally; oral iron intake may interfere with drug absorption.
Patient teaching
• Advise patient to avoid alcohol during drug therapy.
• Warn patient to avoid pregnancy during treatment because drug is harmful to fetus.
• Warn patient to avoid oral iron supplements and all other oral preparations con-

taining iron because drug can chelate iron and decrease absorption.
• Stress importance of compliance with laboratory testing.
• Teach patient to recognize and report signs and symptoms of anemia.

☑ **Evaluation**
• Patient's urinary tract infection is eradicated.
• Patient does not experience injury from drug-induced adverse reactions.
• Patient and family state understanding of drug therapy.

acetylcysteine
(as-ee-til-SIS-teen)
Airbron♦, Mucomyst, Mucomyst 10, Mucosil-10, Mucosil-20, Parvolex♦ ◇

Pharmacologic class: amino acid (l-cysteine) derivative
Therapeutic class: mucolytic, antidote for acetaminophen overdose
Pregnancy risk category: NR

How supplied
Solution: 10%, 20%
Injection: 200 mg/ml♦ ◇

Pharmacokinetics
Absorption: most inhaled acetylcysteine acts directly on mucus in lungs; remainder is absorbed by pulmonary epithelium. After oral administration, drug is absorbed from GI tract.
Distribution: unknown.
Metabolism: metabolized in liver.
Excretion: unknown.

Route	Onset	Peak	Duration
P.O., I.V., inhalation	Unknown	Unknown	Unknown

Pharmacodynamics
Chemical effect: increases production of respiratory tract fluids to help liquefy and reduce viscosity of tenacious secretions.

---

*Liquid form contains alcohol   **May contain tartrazine   ♦ Canada   ◇ Australia   †OTC

Also restores glutathione in liver to treat acetaminophen toxicity.
Therapeutic effect: thins respiratory secretions and reverses toxic effects of acetaminophen.

Indications and dosage

▶ **Pneumonia, bronchitis, tuberculosis, cystic fibrosis, emphysema, atelectasis (adjunct), complications of thoracic and CV surgery.** *Adults and children:* 1 to 2 ml of 10% or 20% solution by direct instillation into trachea as often as hourly; or 3 to 5 ml of 20% solution or 6 to 10 ml of 10% solution by nebulization q 2 to 3 hours p.r.n. Alternatively, where available, 300 mg/kg by I.V. infusion in divided doses.

▶ **Acetaminophen toxicity.** *Adults and children:* initially, 140 mg/kg P.O., followed by 70 mg/kg P.O. q 4 hours for 17 doses; or, where available, 300 mg/kg by I.V. infusion.

Adverse reactions

EENT: *rhinorrhea, hemoptysis.*
GI: *stomatitis, nausea, vomiting.*
Respiratory: *bronchospasm* (especially in asthmatic patients).

Interactions

Drug-drug. *Activated charcoal:* limits acetylcysteine's effectiveness. Avoid concomitant use in treating drug toxicity.

Contraindications and precautions

• Contraindicated in patients with hypersensitivity to drug.
• Use cautiously in elderly or debilitated patients with severe respiratory insufficiency and in pregnant or breast-feeding women.

NURSING CONSIDERATIONS

🗓 Assessment
• Assess patient's respiratory secretions before and frequently during therapy.
• Be alert for adverse reactions and drug interactions.

• Evaluate patient's and family's knowledge of drug therapy.

🔲 Nursing diagnoses
• Ineffective airway clearance related to patient's underlying condition
• Altered oral mucous membrane related to drug-induced stomatitis
• Knowledge deficit related to drug therapy

▶ Planning and implementation
P.O. use: Dilute oral doses with cola, fruit juice, or water before administering to treat acetaminophen overdose. Dilute 20% solution to a concentration of 5% (add 3 ml of diluent to each ml of acetylcysteine). If patient vomits within 1 hour of loading or maintenance dose, repeat dose.
I.V. use: To prepare I.V. infusion, dilute calculated dose in D_5W. Dilute initial dose (150 mg/kg) in 200 ml of D_5W and infuse over 15 minutes. Dilute second dose (50 mg/kg) in 500 ml of D_5W and infuse over 4 hours. Dilute final dose (100 mg/kg) in 1,000 ml of D_5W and infuse over 16 hours.
Nebulization use: Use plastic, glass, stainless steel, or another nonreactive metal when administering by nebulization. Hand-bulb nebulizers are not recommended because output is too small and particle size too large.
– Before aerosol administration, have patient clear airway by coughing.
– After opening, store in refrigerator; use within 96 hours.
– Be aware that drug is physically or chemically incompatible with tetracyclines, erythromycin lactobionate, amphotericin B, and ampicillin sodium. If administered by aerosol inhalation, these drugs should be nebulized separately. Iodized oil, trypsin, and hydrogen peroxide are physically incompatible with acetylcysteine; don't add to nebulizer.
– Have suction equipment available in case patient cannot effectively clear his air passages.

• Be aware that acetylcysteine is administered to treat acetaminophen overdose within 24 hours after ingestion. Start treatment immediately as ordered; do not wait for results of drug blood levels.
• Alert doctor if patient's respiratory secretions thicken or become purulent or if bronchospasm occurs.
Patient teaching
• Instruct patient to follow directions on medication label exactly. Explain importance of not using more drug than directed.
• Tell patient to notify doctor if his condition does not improve within 10 days. Drug should not be used for prolonged period without direct medical supervision.
• Teach patient how to use and clean nebulizer.
• Inform patient that drug may have foul taste or smell.
• Instruct patient to clear his airway by coughing before aerosol administration to achieve maximum effect.
• Instruct patient to rinse mouth with water after nebulizer treatment because it may leave sticky coating on oral cavity.

☑ **Evaluation**
• Patient has clear lung sounds, decreased respiratory secretions, and reduced frequency and severity of cough.
• Patient's oral mucous membranes remain unchanged.
• Patient and family state understanding of drug therapy.

activated charcoal
(AK-tih-vay-ted CHAR-kohl)
Actidose-Aqua†, Charcoaid†, Charcocaps†, Liqui-Char†, Superchar†

Pharmacologic class: adsorbent.
Therapeutic class: antidote.
Pregnancy risk category: NR

How supplied
Tablets: 200 mg◊†, 300 mg◊†, 325 mg†, 650 mg†
Capsules: 260 mg†
Powder: 30 g†, 50 g†
Oral suspension: 0.625 g/5 ml†, 0.83 g/5 ml†, 1 g/5 ml†, 1.25 g/5 ml†

Pharmacokinetics
Absorption: none.
Distribution: none.
Metabolism: none.
Excretion: excreted in feces.

Route	Onset	Peak	Duration
P.O.	Immediate	Unknown	Unknown

Pharmacodynamics
Chemical effect: adheres to many drugs and chemicals, inhibiting their absorption from GI tract.
Therapeutic effect: used as antidote for selected poisons and overdoses.

Indications and dosage
▶ **Flatulence, dyspepsia.** *Adults:* 600 mg to 5 g P.O. t.i.d. after meals
▶ **Poisoning.** *Adults:* initially, 1 g/kg (30 to 100 g) P.O. or 5 to 10 times amount of poison ingested as suspension in 180 to 240 ml of water. *Children:* 5 to 10 times estimated weight of drug or chemical ingested, with minimum dose being 30 g P.O. in 240 ml of water to make a slurry, preferably within 30 minutes of poisoning. Larger dose is necessary if food is in stomach. Commonly used for treating poisoning or overdosage with acetaminophen, aspirin, atropine, barbiturates, cardiac glycosides, poisonous mushrooms, oxalic acid, parathion, phenol, phenylpropanolamine, phenytoin, propantheline, propoxyphene, strychnine, or tricyclic antidepressants. Check with poison control center for use in other types of poisonings or overdoses.

Adverse reactions
GI: black stools, nausea, constipation.

Interactions

Drug-drug. *Acetylcysteine, ipecac:* render charcoal ineffective. Don't administer together or lavage stomach until all charcoal is removed.

Contraindications and precautions

• No known contraindications.

NURSING CONSIDERATIONS

⚰ Assessment
• Obtain history of substance reportedly ingested, including time of ingestion, if possible. Drug is not effective for all drugs and toxic substances.
• Be alert for adverse reactions and drug interactions.
• Evaluate patient's and family's knowledge of drug therapy.

⊕ Nursing diagnoses
• Risk for injury related to ingestion of toxic substance or overdose
• Risk for fluid volume deficit related to drug-induced vomiting
• Knowledge deficit related to drug therapy

▶ Planning and implementation
• Give after emesis is complete because drug absorbs and inactivates syrup of ipecac.
• Do not give to semiconscious or unconscious persons unless airway is protected and nasogastric (NG) tube is in place for instillation.
• Mix powder form (most effective) with tap water to form consistency of thick syrup. Add small amount of fruit juice or flavoring to make mix more palatable.
• Give by NG tube after lavage if necessary.
• Don't give in ice cream, milk, or sherbet, which reduce absorptive capacity.
• Repeat dose if patient vomits shortly after administration.
• Keep airway, oxygen, and suction equipment nearby.

• Follow treatment with stool softener or laxative, as ordered, to prevent constipation.
Patient teaching
• Warn patient that feces will be black.
• Instruct patient to report respiratory difficulty immediately.

☑ Evaluation
• Patient does not experience injury because of ingestion of toxic substance or overdose.
• Patient exhibits no signs of fluid volume deficit.
• Patient or family state understanding of drug therapy.

acyclovir sodium
(ay-SIGH-kloh-veer SOH-dee-um)
Zovirax

Pharmacologic class: synthetic purine nucleoside
Therapeutic class: antiviral
Pregnancy risk category: C

How supplied

Capsules: 200 mg
Tablets: 400 mg, 800 mg
Suspension: 200 mg/5 ml
Injection: 500 mg/vial, 1 g/vial

Pharmacokinetics

Absorption: with oral administration, drug is absorbed slowly and incompletely (15% to 30%). Absorption is not affected by food.
Distribution: distributed widely to organ tissues and body fluids. CSF concentrations equal approximately 50% of serum concentrations. From 9% to 33% of dose binds to plasma proteins.
Metabolism: metabolized primarily inside viral cell to its active form. About 10% of dose is metabolized extracellularly.
Excretion: up to 92% of systemically absorbed acyclovir is excreted unchanged

by kidneys via glomerular filtration and tubular secretion. *Half-life:* 2 to 3½ hours with normal renal function; up to 19 hours with renal failure.

Route	Onset	Peak	Duration
P.O.	Unknown	Unknown	Unknown
I.V.	Immediate	Immediate	Unknown

Pharmacodynamics

Chemical effect: becomes incorporated into viral DNA and inhibits viral multiplication.
Therapeutic effect: kills susceptible viruses.

Indications and dosage

▶ **Initial and recurrent episodes of mucocutaneous herpes simplex virus (HSV-1 and HSV-2) infections in immunocompromised patients; severe initial episodes of herpes genitalis in nonimmunocompromised patients.**
Adults and children age 12 and over: 5 mg/kg I.V. at constant rate over 1 hour q 8 hours for 7 days (5 days for herpes genitalis). *Children under age 12:* 250 mg/m² I.V. at constant rate over 1 hour q 8 hours for 7 days (5 days for herpes genitalis).
▶ **Initial genital herpes.** *Adults:* 200 mg P.O. q 4 hours during waking hours (total of 5 capsules daily) for 10 days.
▶ **Intermittent therapy for recurrent genital herpes.** *Adults:* 200 mg P.O. q 4 hours during waking hours (total of 5 capsules daily) for 5 days. Start therapy at first sign of recurrence.
▶ **Chronic suppressive therapy for recurrent genital herpes.** *Adults:* 400 mg P.O. b.i.d. for up to 12 months.
▶ **Chickenpox.** *Adults and children age 2 and over weighing over 40 kg (88 lb):* 800 mg P.O. q.i.d. for 5 days.
▶ **Herpes zoster.** 800 mg P.O. q 4 hours, five times daily for 7 to 10 days.
▶ **Herpes simplex encephalitis.**
Adults: 10 mg/kg infused at a constant rate over 1 hour, q 8 hours for 10 days.
Children ages 6 months to 12 years:

500 mg/m² at a constant rate over at least 1 hour, q 8 hours for 10 days.
▶ **Varicella zoster in immunocompromised patients:** *Adults:* 10 mg/kg infused at a constant rate over 1 hour, q 8 hours for 7 days. *Children under age 12:* 500 mg/m² at a constant rate over at least 1 hour, q 8 hours for 7 days. Obese patients should be dosed at 10 mg/kg (ideal body weight). Maximum dose equivalent to 500 mg/m² q 8 hours should not be exceeded.

Adverse reactions

CNS: *encephalopathic changes (lethargy, obtundation, tremor, confusion, hallucinations, agitation, seizures, coma),* headache (associated with I.V. dosage).
CV: hypotension.
GI: *nausea, vomiting,* diarrhea.
GU: *transient elevations of serum creatinine level,* hematuria.
Skin: rash, itching.
Other: *inflammation, vesicular eruptions, phlebitis* (at injection site).

Interactions

Drug-drug. *Phenytoin:* possibly decreased phenytoin concentrations. Monitor patient closely.
Probenecid: increased acyclovir blood level. Monitor for possible toxicity.
Valproic acid: decreased valproic acid concentrations. Monitor patient closely.
Zidovudine: may cause drowsiness or lethargy. Use together cautiously.

Contraindications and precautions

● Contraindicated in patients with hypersensitivity to drug.
● Use cautiously in patients with underlying neurologic problems, renal disease, or dehydration and in those receiving other nephrotoxic drugs.
● Use cautiously in pregnant or breastfeeding women.
● Safety in children younger than age 2 has not been established.

NURSING CONSIDERATIONS

⚕ Assessment
• Assess infection before and regularly during therapy.
• Be alert for adverse reactions and drug interactions.
• Monitor patient for renal toxicity. Bolus injection, dehydration, preexisting renal disease, and concomitant use of other nephrotoxic drugs increase risk.
• Monitor patient's mental status when administering drug I.V. Encephalopathic changes are more likely in patients with neurologic disorders or in those who have had neurologic reactions to cytotoxic drugs.
• Monitor patient's hydration status if adverse GI reactions occur with oral administration.
• Evaluate patient's and family's knowledge of drug therapy.

⚙ Nursing diagnoses
• Infection related to presence of virus
• Risk for fluid volume deficit related to adverse GI reactions to oral drug
• Knowledge deficit related to drug therapy

▷ Planning and implementation
P.O. use: Follow normal protocol.
I.V. use: Administer I.V. infusion over at least 1 hour to prevent renal tubular damage.
– Don't give by bolus injection or administer I.M. or S.C.
– Be aware that concentrated solutions (10 mg/ml or more) may be associated with higher incidence of phlebitis.
• Know that patients with acute or chronic renal impairment require a dose adjustment.
• Keep in mind that Burroughs-Wellcome, the manufacturer, maintains an ongoing registry of women exposed to drug during pregnancy. Follow-up studies to date have not shown an increased risk for birth defects for infants born to patients exposed

during pregnancy. Health care providers are encouraged to report such exposures to registrar at (800) 722-9292.
Patient teaching
• Tell patient that drug effectively manages herpes infection but does not eliminate or cure it.
• Warn patient that drug will not prevent spread of infection to others.
• Urge patient to recognize early symptoms of herpes infection (tingling, itching, pain) so he can take acyclovir before infection fully develops.
• Tell patient to alert nurse if pain or discomfort occurs at I.V. injection site.

☑ Evaluation
• Patient's infection is eradicated.
• Patient maintains adequate hydration.
• Patient and family state understanding of drug therapy.

---

adenosine
(uh-DEN-oh-seen)
Adenocard

Pharmacologic class: nucleoside
Therapeutic class: antiarrhythmic
Pregnancy risk category: C

How supplied
Injection: 3 mg/ml in 2-ml vials

Pharmacokinetics
Absorption: not applicable with I.V. administration.
Distribution: rapidly taken up by erythrocytes and vascular endothelial cells.
Metabolism: metabolized within tissues to inosine and adenosine monophosphate.
Excretion: unknown. *Half-life:* less than 10 seconds.

Route	Onset	Peak	Duration
I.V.	Immediate	Immediate	Extremely short

Pharmacodynamics

Chemical effect: acts on AV node to slow conduction and inhibit reentry pathways. Adenosine also is useful in treating paroxysmal supraventricular tachycardia (PSVT) associated with accessory bypass tracts (Wolff-Parkinson-White syndrome).
Therapeutic effect: restores normal sinus rhythm.

Indications and dosage

▶ **Conversion of PSVT to sinus rhythm.** *Adults:* 6 mg I.V. by rapid bolus injection over 1 to 2 seconds. If PSVT is not eliminated in 1 to 2 minutes, 12 mg by rapid I.V. push may be given and repeated (if necessary). Single doses over 12 mg are not recommended.

Adverse reactions

CNS: apprehension, back pain, blurred vision, burning sensation, dizziness, heaviness in arms, light-headedness, neck pain, numbness, tingling in arms.
CV: chest pain, *facial flushing,* headache, hypotension, palpitations, diaphoresis.
GI: metallic taste, nausea.
Respiratory: *chest pressure, dyspnea, shortness of breath,* hyperventilation.
Other: *tightness in throat, groin pressure.*

Interactions

Drug-drug. *Carbamazepine:* higher degrees of heart block may occur. Monitor patient.
Digoxin, verapamil: combined use rarely associated with ventricular fibrillation. Use with caution.
Dipyridamole: may potentiate adenosine's effects. Smaller doses may be necessary.
Methylxanthines: antagonism of adenosine's effects. Patients receiving theophylline or caffeine may require higher doses or may not respond to adenosine therapy.

Drug-food. *Caffeine:* may antagonize adenosine's effects. May require higher doses

Contraindications and precautions

• Contraindicated in patients with hypersensitivity to drug and in those with second- or third-degree heart block or sick sinus syndrome unless artificial pacemaker is present. Adenosine decreases conduction through AV node and may produce transient first-, second-, or third-degree heart block. Patients in whom significant heart block develops should not receive additional doses.
• Use cautiously in patients with asthma because bronchoconstriction may occur.
• Safety of drug has not been established in pregnant or breast-feeding women or in children.

NURSING CONSIDERATIONS

⚞ Assessment
• Monitor patient's heart rate and rhythm before and during therapy.
• Be alert for adverse reactions and drug interactions.
• Evaluate patient's and family's knowledge of drug therapy.

⚙ Nursing diagnoses
• Decreased cardiac output related to arrhythmias
• Altered protection related to drug-induced proarrhythmias
• Knowledge deficit related to drug therapy

⚟ Planning and implementation
• Check solution for crystals, which may form if solution is cold. If crystals are visible, gently warm solution to room temperature. Do not use unclear solutions.
• Administer rapidly for effective drug action. Administer directly into vein if possible; if I.V. line is used, inject drug into most proximal port and follow with rapid saline flush to ensure that drug reaches systemic circulation quickly.

- Discard unused drug; it contains no preservatives.
- Withhold drug, obtain rhythm strip, and notify doctor immediately if ECG disturbances occur.
- Have emergency equipment and drugs on hand to treat new arrhythmias.

Patient teaching
- Teach patient about his disease and therapy.
- Stress importance of alerting nurse if chest pain or dyspnea occurs.
- Advise patient to avoid caffeine consumption.

☑ **Evaluation**
- Patient's arrhythmias are corrected.
- Patient does not experience proarrhythmias.
- Patient and family state understanding of drug therapy.

albumin 5%
(al-BYOO-min)
Albuminar 5%, Albutein 5%, Buminate 5%, Plasbumin 5%

albumin 25%
Albuminar 25%, Albumisol 25%, Albutein 25%, Buminate 25%, Plasbumin 25%

Pharmacologic class: blood derivative
Therapeutic class: plasma volume expander
Pregnancy risk category: C

How supplied
Injection: 50-ml, 250-ml, 500-ml, 1,000-ml vials (albumin 5%); 10-ml, 20-ml, 50-ml, 100-ml vials (albumin 25%)

Pharmacokinetics
Absorption: not applicable with I.V. administration.
Distribution: albumin accounts for about 50% of plasma proteins; it is distributed into intravascular space and extravascular sites, including skin, muscle, and lungs.

Metabolism: unknown.
Excretion: unknown, although liver, kidneys, or intestines may provide elimination mechanisms for albumin. *Half-life:* 15 to 20 days.

Route	Onset	Peak	Duration
I.V.	≤ 15 min for hydrated patient	≤ 15 min for hydrated patient	Up to several hr with reduced blood volume

Pharmacodynamics
Chemical effect: albumin 5% supplies colloid to blood and expands plasma volume. Albumin 25% provides intravascular oncotic pressure in 5:1 ratio, causing fluid shift from interstitial spaces to circulation and slightly increasing plasma protein concentration.
Therapeutic effect: relieves shock by increasing plasma volume and corrects plasma protein deficiency.

Indications and dosage
► **Hypovolemic shock.** *Adults:* initially, 500 ml 5% solution by I.V. infusion, repeated p.r.n. Dosage varies with patient's condition and response. Do not give more than 250 g in 48 hours. *Children:* 10 to 20 ml/kg 5% solution by I.V. infusion, repeated in 15 to 30 minutes if response is not adequate. Alternatively, 2.5 to 5 ml I.V. of 25% solution/kg, repeated after 10 to 30 minutes, if needed.
► **Hypoproteinemia.** *Adults:* 1,000 to 1,500 ml 5% solution by I.V. infusion daily, with maximum rate of 5 to 10 ml/minute; or 200 to 300 ml 25% solution by I.V. infusion daily, with maximum rate of 3 ml/minute. Dosage varies with patient's condition and response.
► **Hyperbilirubinemia.** *Infants:* 1 g albumin (4 ml 25%)/kg I.V. 1 to 2 hours before transfusion.

Adverse reactions
CV: *vascular overload* (after rapid infusion), hypotension, altered pulse rate.

Reactions may be *common*, uncommon, *life-threatening*, or COMMON AND LIFE-THREATENING.

GI: increased salivation, nausea, vomiting.
Respiratory: altered respiration.
Skin: urticaria, rash.
Other: chills, fever.

Interactions
None significant.

Contraindications and precautions
• Contraindicated in patients with hypersensitivity to drug.
• Use with extreme caution in patients with hypertension, cardiac disease, severe pulmonary infection, severe chronic anemia, or hypoalbuminemia with peripheral edema.
• Use with caution in pregnant women.

NURSING CONSIDERATIONS

☲ Assessment
• Assess patient's underlying condition.
• Be alert for adverse reactions.
• Monitor fluid intake and output, hemoglobin, hematocrit, and serum protein and electrolytes.
• Evaluate patient's and family's knowledge of drug therapy.

⛊ Nursing diagnoses
• Fluid volume deficit related to patient's underlying condition
• Fluid volume excess related to adverse effects of drug
• Knowledge deficit related to drug therapy

⏵ Planning and implementation
• Minimize waste when preparing and administering drug. This product is expensive, and random shortages occur often.
• Avoid rapid I.V. infusion. Specific rate is individualized according to patient's age, condition, and diagnosis. Dilute with 0.9% NaCl solution, or D₅W injection. Use solution promptly; it contains no preservatives. Discard unused solution. Don't use cloudy solutions or those con-

taining sediment. Solution should be clear amber.
• Do not give more than 250 g in 48 hours.
• Know that one volume of 25% albumin is equivalent to five volumes of 5% albumin in producing hemodilution and relative anemia.
• Follow storage instructions on bottle. Freezing may cause bottle to break.
• Withhold fluids in patient with cerebral edema for 8 hours after infusion to avoid fluid overload.
Patient teaching
• Explain how and why albumin is administered.
• Tell patient to report chills, fever, dyspnea, nausea, or rash immediately; normal serum albumin can cause allergic reaction.

☑ Evaluation
• Patient's fluid volume deficit is resolved.
• Patient does not experience fluid overload.
• Patient and family state understanding of drug therapy.

albuterol (salbutamol)
(al-BYOO-ter-ohl)
Asmol◊, Proventil, Respolin◊, Ventolin

albuterol sulfate (salbutamol sulfate)
Proventil, Proventil Repetabs, Respolin Autohaler Inhalation Device◊, Respolin Inhaler◊, Respolin Respirator Solution◊, Ventolin, Ventolin Obstetric Injection◊, Ventolin Rotacaps, Volmax

Pharmacologic class: adrenergic
Therapeutic class: bronchodilator
Pregnancy risk category: C

How supplied
Aerosol inhaler: 90 mcg/metered spray, 100 mcg/metered spray◊

Capsules for inhalation: 200 mcg
Tablets: 2 mg, 4 mg
Tablets (extended-release): 4 mg, 8 mg
Syrup: 2 mg/5 ml
Solution for inhalation: 0.083%, 0.5%
Injection: 1 mg/ml◊

Pharmacokinetics

Absorption: after oral inhalation, albuterol appears to be absorbed over several hours from respiratory tract; however, most of dose is swallowed and absorbed through GI tract. After oral administration, drug is well absorbed through GI tract.
Distribution: does not cross blood-brain barrier.
Metabolism: extensively metabolized in liver to inactive compounds.
Excretion: rapidly excreted in urine and feces. *Half-life:* about 4 hours.

Route	Onset	Peak	Duration
P.O.	15-30 min	2-3 hr	6-12 hr
I.V.	1-5 min	Unknown	Unknown
Inhalation	5-15 min	1-1.5 hr	3-6 hr

Pharmacodynamics

Chemical effect: relaxes bronchial and uterine smooth muscle by acting on $beta_2$-adrenergic receptors.
Therapeutic effect: improves ventilation.

Indications and dosage

▶ **Prevention or treatment of bronchospasm in patients with reversible obstructive airway disease.** *Adults and children ages 12 and over:* dosage and frequency vary with dosage form.
Aerosol inhalation—1 to 2 inhalations q 4 to 6 hours. More frequent administration or greater number of inhalations is not recommended. *Solution for inhalation*—2.5 mg t.i.d. or q.i.d. by nebulizer. To prepare solution, use 0.5 ml of 0.5% solution diluted with 2.5 ml of 0.9% NaCl. Alternatively, use 3 ml of 0.083% solution. *Capsules for inhalation*—200 mcg inhaled q 4 to 6 hours using Rotahaler inhalation device. Some pa-

tients may need 400 mcg q 4 to 6 hours. *Oral tablets*—2 to 4 mg P.O. t.i.d. or q.i.d. Maximum dosage is 8 mg q.i.d. *Extended-release tablets*—4 to 8 mg P.O. q 12 hours. Maximum dosage is 16 mg b.i.d. *Children ages 6 to 11:* 2 mg (1 teaspoonful) P.O. t.i.d. or q.i.d. *Children ages 2 to 5:* 0.1 mg/kg P.O. t.i.d., not to exceed 2 mg (1 teaspoonful) t.i.d. *Adults over age 65:* 2 mg P.O. t.i.d. or q.i.d.
▶ **Prevention of exercise-induced asthma.** *Adults:* 2 inhalations 15 minutes before exercise.

Adverse reactions

CNS: *tremor, nervousness,* dizziness, insomnia, headache.
CV: tachycardia, palpitations, hypertension.
EENT: drying and irritation of nose and throat (with inhaled form).
GI: heartburn, nausea, vomiting.
Respiratory: *bronchospasm.*
Other: muscle cramps, hypokalemia (with high doses).

Interactions

Drug-drug. *CNS stimulants:* increased CNS stimulation. Avoid concomitant use. *Levodopa:* risk of arrhythmias. Monitor patient closely.
MAO inhibitors, tricyclic antidepressants: increased adverse CV effects. Monitor patient closely.
Propranolol, other beta blockers: mutual antagonism. Monitor patient carefully.
Drug-food. *Caffeine-containing foods and beverages:* increased CNS stimulation. Avoid concomitant use.

Contraindications and precautions

● Contraindicated in patients with hypersensitivity to drug or its components and in breast-feeding women.
● Use cautiously in patients with CV disorders (including coronary insufficiency and hypertension), hyperthyroidism, or diabetes mellitus; in those unusually responsive to adrenergics; and during pregnancy.

Reactions may be *common,* uncommon, *life-threatening*, or **COMMON AND LIFE-THREATENING.**

• Use extended-release tablets cautiously in patients with preexisting GI narrowing.
• Safety of drug has not been established in children under age 12 for inhalation solution, aerosol, or Repetabs; in those under age 6 for tablets; and in those under age 2 for syrup.

NURSING CONSIDERATIONS

⚗ Assessment
• Obtain baseline assessment of patient's respiratory status, and monitor frequently throughout therapy.
• Be alert for adverse reactions and drug interactions.
• Evaluate patient's and family's knowledge of drug therapy.

🔁 Nursing diagnoses
• Impaired gas exchange related to underlying respiratory condition
• Risk for injury related to drug-induced adverse reactions
• Knowledge deficit related to drug therapy

➲ Planning and implementation
P.O. use: Remember that pleasant-tasting syrup may be taken by children as young as age 2. Syrup contains no alcohol or sugar.
• Recognize that patients may use tablets and aerosol concomitantly.
I.V. use: Be aware that I.V. form may be used, where available, to prepare infusion using NaCl injection, glucose injection, or NaCl and glucose injection. Do not administer drug without dilution, and do not mix with other medication. Discard unused diluted solution after 24 hours.
Inhalation use: Wait at least 2 minutes between doses if more than one dose is ordered. If steroid inhaler also is used, first have patient use bronchodilator, wait 5 minutes, and then have patient use steroid inhaler. This permits bronchodilator to open air passages for maximum effectiveness.

– Know that aerosol form may be prescribed for use 15 minutes before exercise to prevent exercise-induced bronchospasm.
Patient teaching
• Warn patient to discontinue drug immediately if paradoxical bronchospasm occurs.
• Give patient correct instructions for using metered-dose inhaler: Clear nasal passages and throat. Breathe out, expelling as much air from lungs as possible. Place mouthpiece well into mouth and, as dose is released, inhale deeply. Hold breath for several seconds, remove mouthpiece, and exhale slowly.
• Advise patient to wait at least 2 minutes before repeating procedure if more than one inhalation is ordered.
• Warn patient to avoid accidentally spraying inhalant form into eyes, which may blur vision temporarily.
• Tell patient to reduce intake of foods containing caffeine, such as coffee, colas, and chocolates, when taking bronchodilator.
• Show patient how to check pulse rate. Instruct him to check pulse before and after using bronchodilator and to call doctor if pulse rate increases more than 20 to 30 beats/minute.

☑ Evaluation
• Patient's respiratory signs and symptoms improve.
• Patient does not experience injury from adverse reactions associated with drug.
• Patient and family state understanding of drug therapy.

aldesleukin (interleukin-2, IL-2)
(al-des-LOO-kin)
Proleukin

Pharmacologic class: lymphokine
Therapeutic class: immunoregulatory agent
Pregnancy risk category: C

How supplied

Powder for injection: 22 million IU/vial

Pharmacokinetics

Absorption: not applicable with I.V. administration.

Distribution: about 30% of drug is rapidly distributed to plasma; balance is rapidly distributed to liver, kidneys, and lungs. Peak serum levels are proportional to dose.

Metabolism: metabolized by kidneys to amino acids within cells lining proximal convoluted tubules.

Excretion: excreted through kidneys by peritubular extraction and glomerular filtration. *Half-life:* 85 minutes.

Route	Onset	Peak	Duration
I.V.	Unknown	Unknown	Unknown

Pharmacodynamics

Chemical effect: unknown. May stimulate immunologic host reaction to tumor.
Therapeutic effect: eliminates or decreases kidney tumor size.

Indications and dosage

▶ **Metastatic renal cell carcinoma, metastatic melanoma.** *Adults:* 600,000 IU/kg (0.037 mg/kg) I.V. over 15 minutes q 8 hours for 5 days (total of 14 doses). After 9-day rest, sequence is repeated for another 14 doses. After rest period of at least 7 weeks, repeat courses may be administered.

Adverse reactions

CNS: headache, *mental status changes, dizziness, sensory dysfunction, special senses disorders, syncope, motor dysfunction,* **coma,** fatigue, weakness, malaise.

CV: *hypotension, sinus tachycardia, arrhythmias, bradycardia,* **PVCs,** *premature atrial contractions, myocardial ischemia,* **MI,** *heart failure,* **cardiac arrest,** myocarditis, endocarditis, *CVA,* pericardial effusion, thrombosis, *capillary leak syndrome (CLS).*

EENT: conjunctivitis.

GI: *nausea, vomiting, diarrhea, stomatitis, anorexia, bleeding, dyspepsia, constipation.*

GU: *oliguria,* **anuria,** *proteinuria, hematuria, dysuria,* urine retention, urinary frequency, urinary tract infection, *elevated BUN and serum creatinine levels.*

Hematologic: anemia, THROMBOCYTOPENIA, LEUKOPENIA, coagulation disorders, leukocytosis, eosinophilia.

Hepatic: *jaundice;* ascites; hepatomegaly; *elevated bilirubin, serum transaminase, alkaline phosphatase levels.*

Metabolic: *hypomagnesemia, acidosis, hypocalcemia, hypophosphatemia, hypokalemia, hyperuricemia, hypoalbuminemia, hypoproteinemia, hyponatremia, hyperkalemia.*

Musculoskeletal: abdominal, chest, or back pain; arthralgia; myalgia.

Respiratory: *pulmonary congestion, dyspnea,* **pulmonary edema, respiratory failure, pleural effusion, apnea, pneumothorax,** tachypnea.

Skin: *pruritus, erythema, rash, dryness,* **exfoliative dermatitis,** purpura, alopecia, petechiae.

Other: *fever, chills,* edema, infections of catheter tip or injection site, phlebitis, SEPSIS, weight gain or loss.

Interactions

Drug-drug. *Antihypertensives:* increased risk of hypotension. Monitor patient closely.

Cardiotoxic, hepatotoxic, myelotoxic, or nephrotoxic drugs: enhanced toxicity. Avoid concomitant use.

Corticosteroids: decreased antitumor effectiveness of aldesleukin. Avoid concomitant use.

Psychotropic agents: unpredictable interaction. Use together cautiously.

Contraindications and precautions

• Contraindicated in patients with hypersensitivity to drug or its components, in those with abnormal cardiac (thallium)

Reactions may be *common,* uncommon, *life-threatening*, or COMMON AND LIFE-THREATENING.

stress test or pulmonary function tests or organ allografts, and in breast-feeding women.
• Retreatment is contraindicated in patients who experience the following adverse effects: cardiac tamponade; disturbances in cardiac rhythm that were uncontrolled or unresponsive to intervention; sustained ventricular tachycardia (five beats or more); chest pain accompanied by ECG changes, indicating MI or angina pectoris; renal dysfunction requiring dialysis for 72 hours or more; coma or toxic psychosis lasting 48 hours or more; seizures that were repetitive or difficult to control; ischemia or perforation of bowel; or GI bleeding requiring surgery.
• Know that drug should not be used unless patient has had definitive tests documenting normal cardiac and pulmonary function. Use with extreme caution in patients with normal test results if they have a history of cardiac or pulmonary disease, in patients with a history of seizure disorders because drug may cause seizures, and during pregnancy.
• Use cautiously in patients who require large volumes of fluid (such as patients with hypercalcemia).
• Use cautiously and with close clinical monitoring in all patients because severe adverse effects usually accompany therapy at recommended dosage.
• Safety of drug has not been established in children.

NURSING CONSIDERATIONS

Assessment
• Obtain history of patient's renal carcinoma and underlying conditions.
• Assess status of patient's physical condition at onset of aldesleukin therapy and frequently throughout therapy.
• Obtain hematologic tests, serum electrolyte levels, renal and liver function tests, and chest X-ray before therapy and then daily during therapy, as ordered, and monitor results.

• Know that patient should be neurologically stable with negative computed tomography scan for CNS metastases before therapy is begun. Drug may exacerbate symptoms in patient with unrecognized or undiagnosed CNS metastases.
• Be alert for adverse reactions and drug interactions.
• Evaluate patient's and family's knowledge of drug therapy.

Nursing diagnoses
• Altered health maintenance related to neoplastic disease
• Altered protection related to drug-induced adverse reactions
• Knowledge deficit related to drug therapy

Planning and implementation
• Know that drug should be administered only in hospital under direction of doctor experienced in use of chemotherapeutic agents. Intensive care facility and intensive care or cardiopulmonary specialists must be readily available.
• Treat patient with bacterial infections before therapy is begun, as ordered.
• To avoid altering drug's pharmacologic properties, reconstitute and dilute carefully, and follow manufacturer's recommendations. Do not mix with other drugs or albumin.
• Reconstitute vial containing 22 million IU (1.3 mg) with 1.2 ml of sterile water for injection. Do not use bacteriostatic water or 0.9% NaCl injection; these diluents increase aggregation of drug. Direct stream of sterile water at sides of vial and gently swirl to reconstitute. Do not shake. Reconstituted solution will have concentration of 18 million IU (1.1 mg)/ml. It should be particle-free and colorless to slightly yellow.
• Add ordered dose of reconstituted drug to 50 ml of D_5W and infuse over 15 minutes. Do not use in-line filter. Plastic infusion bags are preferred because they provide consistent drug delivery.

• Discard unused portion. Vials are for single-dose use and contain no preservatives.
• Refrigerate powder for injection. Return drug to room temperature before administering to patient.
• Know that drug has been associated with CLS, a condition that results from loss of vascular tone, in which plasma proteins and fluids escape into extravascular space. Mean arterial blood pressure begins to drop within 2 to 12 hours of treatment; edema and effusions may be severe, and death can result from hypoperfusion of major organs. Other conditions that accompany CLS include arrhythmias, MI, angina, mental status changes, renal insufficiency, respiratory distress or failure, and GI bleeding or infarction.
• Be prepared to adjust dosage of other drugs, as ordered, to compensate for renal and hepatic impairment occurring during treatment. Modify dosage by withholding dose or interrupting therapy, as ordered, rather than by reducing dose.
• Withhold dose and notify doctor if moderate to severe lethargy or somnolence develops; continued administration can result in coma.
• Keep in mind that therapy is associated with impaired neutrophil function, which can lead to disseminated infection. Many studies used prophylactic antibiotic therapy with oxacillin, nafcillin, ciprofloxacin, or vancomycin; check protocol and administer antibiotics, as ordered.

Patient teaching
• Make sure patient understands that adverse effects are expected with normal doses and that serious toxicity may occur despite close clinical monitoring.
• Teach patient about specific adverse reactions associated with aldesleukin and how to manage them, including infection and bleeding precautions to take.
• Stress importance of compliance with extensive testing required during aldesleukin therapy.

• Advise patient to alert doctor when adverse reactions occur.

☑ Evaluation
• Patient's renal studies show positive response to drug.
• Patient exhibits positive response to measures used to limit severity of adverse reactions.
• Patient and family state understanding of drug therapy.

---

alendronate sodium
(ah-LEN-droh-nayt SOH-dee-um)
Fosamax

Pharmacologic class: inhibitor of osteoclast-mediated bone resorption
Therapeutic class: antiosteoporotic
Pregnancy risk category: C

How supplied
Tablets: 10 mg, 40 mg

Pharmacokinetics
Absorption: absorbed from GI tract; food or beverages can significantly decrease bioavailability.
Distribution: distributed to soft tissues but is then rapidly redistributed to bone or excreted in urine; about 78% protein–bound.
Metabolism: does not appear to be metabolized.
Excretion: excreted in urine.

Route	Onset	Peak	Duration
P.O.	1 mo	3-6 mo	3 wk

Pharmacodynamics
Chemical effect: suppresses osteoclast activity on newly formed resorption surfaces, reducing bone turnover.
Therapeutic effect: increases bone mass.

Indications and dosage
▶ **Treatment of osteoporosis in postmenopausal women.** *Adults:* 10 mg P.O. daily, at least 30 minutes before first

---

Reactions may be *common*, uncommon, *life-threatening*, or COMMON AND LIFE-THREATENING.

food, beverage, or medication of day, with plain water only.
▶ **Prevention of osteoporosis in post-menopausal women.** *Adults:* 5 mg P.O. daily, at least 30 minutes before first food, beverage, or medication of day, with plain water only.
▶ **Paget's disease of bone.** *Adults:* 40 mg P.O. daily for 6 months, at least 30 minutes before first food, beverage, or medication of day, with plain water only.

Adverse reactions

CNS: headache.
GI: abdominal pain, nausea, dyspepsia, constipation, diarrhea, flatulence, acid regurgitation, esophageal ulcer, vomiting, dysphagia, abdominal distention, gastritis.
Other: musculoskeletal pain, taste perversion.

Interactions

Drug-drug. *Antacids, calcium supplements:* interferes with alendronate absorption. Have patient wait 30 minutes after alendronate dose before taking other drugs.
Aspirin, NSAIDs: increased risk of upper GI reactions with alendronate doses over 10 mg/day. Monitor patient closely.
Hormone replacement therapy: not recommended when used with alendronate in treating osteoporosis; evidence of effectiveness is lacking.
Drug-food. *Any food:* decreased absorption of drug. Do not give drug with food.

Contraindications and precautions

• Contraindicated in patients with hypocalcemia, severe renal insufficiency, or hypersensitivity to drug or its component.
• Use cautiously in patients with dysphagia, esophageal diseases, gastritis, duodenitis, ulcers, or mild to moderate renal insufficiency.
• Safety of drug has not been established in breast-feeding women and in children.

NURSING CONSIDERATIONS

✍ Assessment
• Obtain history of patient's underlying disorder before therapy.
• Monitor serum calcium and phosphate levels throughout therapy, as ordered.
• Be alert for adverse reactions and drug interactions.
• Evaluate patient's and family's knowledge of drug therapy.

⊞ Nursing diagnoses
• Risk for injury related to decreased bone mass
• Risk for fluid volume deficit related to drug-induced GI upset
• Knowledge deficit related to drug therapy

▷ Planning and implementation
• Know that hypocalcemia and other disturbances of mineral metabolism (such as vitamin D deficiency) should be corrected before therapy begins.
• Administer drug in the morning at least 30 minutes before first meal, fluid, or other oral drug administration.
Patient teaching
• Warn patient not to lie down for at least 30 minutes after taking drug to facilitate delivery to stomach and reduce potential for esophageal irritation.
• Tell patient to take supplemental calcium and vitamin D, if daily dietary intake is inadequate.
• Show patient how to perform weight-bearing exercises, which help increase bone mass.
• Urge patient to limit or restrict smoking and alcohol use, if appropriate.

☑ Evaluation
• Patient remains free from bone fracture.
• Patient maintains adequate hydration.
• Patient and family state understanding of drug therapy.

---

alfentanil hydrochloride
(al-FEN-tah-nil high-droh-KLOR-ighd)
Alfenta

Pharmacologic class: opioid
Therapeutic class: analgesic, adjunct to anesthesia, anesthetic
Controlled substance schedule: II
Pregnancy risk category: C

How supplied
Injection: 500 mcg/ml

Pharmacokinetics
Absorption: not applicable with I.V. administration.
Distribution: over 90% is protein-bound.
Metabolism: metabolized in liver.
Excretion: excreted in urine. *Half-life:* about 1½ hours.

Route	Onset	Peak	Duration
I.V.	1 min	1.5-2 min	5-10 min

Pharmacodynamics
Chemical effect: binds with opiate receptors in CNS, altering perception of and emotional response to pain through unknown mechanism.
Therapeutic effect: enhances anesthetic effect and relieves pain.

Indications and dosage
▶ **Adjunct to general anesthetic.**
Adults: initially, 8 to 50 mcg/kg I.V.; then increments of 3 to 15 mcg/kg I.V. q 5 to 20 minutes. Reduced dosage needed for elderly and debilitated patients.
▶ **Primary anesthetic.** *Adults:* initially, 130 to 245 mcg/kg I.V.; then 0.5 to 1.5 mcg/kg/minute I.V. Reduced dosage needed for elderly and debilitated patients.

Adverse reactions
CNS: blurred vision, agitation, anxiety, headache, confusion.
CV: hypotension, hypertension, bradycardia, tachycardia, palpitations, orthostatic hypotension.
GI: nausea, vomiting.
Respiratory: *chest wall rigidity, bronchospasm, respiratory depression,* hypercapnia.
Skin: itching.
Other: intraoperative muscle movement.

Interactions
Drug-drug. *Cimetidine:* CNS toxicity. Monitor patient.
CNS depressants: additive effects. Use together cautiously.
Diazepam: CV depression and decreased blood pressure with high doses of alfentanil. Use cautiously together.
Drug-lifestyle. *Alcohol use:* additive effects. Use together cautiously.

Contraindications and precautions
• Contraindicated in patients with hypersensitivity to drug.
• Use cautiously in patients with head injury, pulmonary disease, decreased respiratory reserve, or hepatic or renal impairment and in pregnant or breast-feeding women.
• Safety of drug has not been established in children under age 12.

NURSING CONSIDERATIONS

Assessment
• Assess patient's CV and respiratory status before and during therapy.
• Know that drug decreases rate and depth of respirations. Monitoring arterial oxygen saturation may aid in assessing effects of respiratory depression.
• Be alert for adverse reactions and drug interactions.
• Evaluate patient's and family's knowledge of drug therapy.

Nursing diagnoses
• Altered health maintenance related to need for surgery

Reactions may be *common,* uncommon, *life-threatening*, or COMMON AND LIFE-THREATENING.

• Ineffective breathing pattern related to drug-induced respiratory depression
• Knowledge deficit related to drug therapy

⬧ Planning and implementation
• Be aware that drug should be administered only by those specifically trained in use of I.V. anesthetics.
• Know that drug is compatible with D_5W, D_5W in lactated Ringer's solution, and 0.9% NaCl. Most clinicians use infusions containing 25 to 80 mcg/ml.
• Discontinue infusion at least 10 to 15 minutes before end of surgery.
• Use tuberculin syringe to administer small volumes of alfentanil accurately.
• Keep narcotic antagonist (naloxone) and resuscitation equipment available.
• Notify doctor immediately if assessment findings deviate from expected norm. Patient who has developed tolerance to other opioids may become intolerant to alfentanil as well.
Patient teaching
• Explain anesthetic effect of drug.
• Inform patient that another analgesic will be available after effects of drug have worn off.
• Advise patient to avoid alcohol consumption during drug therapy.

☑ Evaluation
• Patient regains health maintenance after alfentanil administration and recovery from surgery.
• Patient's respiratory status returns to normal after effects of drug wear off.
• Patient and family state understanding of drug therapy.

---

allopurinol
(al-oh-PYOOR-ih-nol)
Alloremed◇, Capurate◇, Lopurin, Zyloprim

Pharmacologic class: xanthine oxidase inhibitor

Therapeutic class: antigout
Pregnancy risk category: C

How supplied
Tablets (scored): 100 mg, 300 mg
Capsules: 100 mg◇, 300 mg◇

Pharmacokinetics
Absorption: from 80% to 90% of dose is absorbed.
Distribution: distributed widely throughout body except brain, where concentrations are 50% of those found elsewhere. Allopurinol and oxypurinol are not bound to plasma proteins.
Metabolism: metabolized to oxypurinol by xanthine oxidase.
Excretion: excreted primarily in urine, with minute amount excreted in feces.
Half-life: allopurinol, 1 to 2 hours; oxypurinol, about 15 hours.

Route	Onset	Peak	Duration
P.O.	2-3 days	0.5-2 hr (allopurinol) 4.5-5 hr (oxypurinol)	1-2 wk

Pharmacodynamics
Chemical effect: reduces uric acid production by inhibiting biochemical reactions preceding its formation.
Therapeutic effect: alleviates gout symptoms.

Indications and dosage
▶ **Gout, primary or secondary to hyperuricemia; secondary to such diseases as acute or chronic leukemia, polycythemia vera, multiple myeloma, and psoriasis.** Dosage varies with severity of disease; can be given as single dose or in divided doses, but dosages larger than 300 mg should be divided. *Adults:* mild gout, 200 to 300 mg P.O. daily; severe gout with large tophi, 400 to 600 mg P.O. daily. Same dosage for maintenance in gout secondary to hyperuricemia.
▶ **Hyperuricemia secondary to malignancies.** *Children under age 6:* 50 mg

---

P.O. t.i.d. *Children ages 6 to 10:* 300 mg P.O. daily or divided t.i.d.
▶ **Prevention of acute gouty attacks.**
Adults: 100 mg P.O. daily; increase at weekly intervals by 100 mg without exceeding maximum dose (800 mg), until serum uric acid falls to 6 mg/100 ml or less.
▶ **Prevention of uric acid nephropathy during cancer chemotherapy.** *Adults:* 600 to 800 mg P.O. daily for 2 to 3 days, with high fluid intake.
▶ **Recurrent calcium oxalate calculi.** *Adults:* 200 to 300 mg P.O. daily in single or divided doses.
Note: *In adults with impaired renal function,* 100 mg q 3 days if creatinine clearance is up to 9 ml/minute; 100 mg q 2 days, 10 to 19 ml/minute; 100 mg daily, 20 to 39 ml/minute; 150 mg daily, 40 to 59 ml/minute; 200 mg daily, 60 to 79 ml/minute; 250 mg daily, 80 ml/minute.

Adverse reactions

CNS: drowsiness, headache.
EENT: cataracts, retinopathy.
GI: nausea, vomiting, diarrhea, abdominal pain.
GU: *renal failure,* uremia.
Hematologic: agranulocytosis, anemia, aplastic anemia, *thrombocytopenia.*
Hepatic: altered liver function studies, *hepatitis.*
Skin: *rash, usually maculopapular; exfoliative lesions;* urticarial and purpuric lesions; *erythema multiforme;* severe furunculosis of nose; ichthyosis; toxic epidermal necrolysis.

Interactions

Drug-drug. *ACE inhibitors:* higher risk of hyposensitivity reaction. Monitor closely.
Amoxicillin, ampicillin, bacampicillin: increased possibility of skin rash. Avoid concomitant use.
Anticoagulants, dicumarol: potentiation of anticoagulant effect. Dosage adjustments may be necessary.

Antineoplastic agents: increased potential for bone marrow suppression. Monitor patient carefully.
Azathioprine, mercaptopurine (purinethol): increased serum concentrations of these agents. Dosage adjustments may be necessary.
Chlorpropamide: possible increased hypoglycemic effect. Avoid concomitant use.
Diazoxide, diuretics, mecamylamine, pyrazinamide: increased serum acid concentration. Allopurinol dosage adjustment may be needed.
Ethacrynic acid, thiazide diuretics: increased risk of allopurinol toxicity. Reduce dosage of allopurinol and closely monitor renal function.
Uricosuric agents: additive effect. May be used to therapeutic advantage.
Urine-acidifying agents: may increase possibility of kidney stone formation. Monitor patient carefully.
Xanthines: increased serum theophylline level. Adjust dosage of theophylline.
Drug-lifestyle. *Alcohol use:* increased serum uric acid concentration. Avoid concomitant use.

Contraindications and precautions

• Contraindicated in patients with idiopathic hemochromatosis or hypersensitivity to drug.
• Use cautiously in pregnant and breast-feeding women.

NURSING CONSIDERATIONS

ᴿ Assessment

• Assess patient's uric acid results, joint stiffness, and pain before and during therapy. Optimal benefits may require 2 to 6 weeks of therapy.
• Monitor fluid intake and output. Daily urine output of at least 2 L and maintenance of neutral or slightly alkaline urine is desirable.
• Monitor CBC and hepatic and renal function at start of therapy and periodically during therapy, as ordered.

• Be alert for adverse reactions and drug interactions.
• Evaluate patient's and family's knowledge of drug therapy.

⊞ **Nursing diagnoses**
• Pain (joint) related to patient's underlying condition
• Risk for infection related to drug-induced agranulocytosis
• Knowledge deficit related to drug therapy

▶ **Planning and implementation**
• Administer drug with or immediately after meals to minimize adverse GI reactions.
• Have patient drink plenty of fluids while taking drug, unless contraindicated.
• Notify doctor if renal insufficiency occurs during treatment; this usually warrants dosage reduction.
• Administer colchicine with allopurinol, if ordered. This prophylactically treats acute gout attacks that may occur in first 6 weeks of therapy.
Patient teaching
• Advise patient to refrain from driving car or performing hazardous tasks requiring mental alertness until CNS effects of drug are known.
• Advise patient taking allopurinol for treatment of recurrent calcium oxalate stones to reduce intake of animal protein, sodium, refined sugars, oxalate-rich foods, and calcium.
• Tell patient to discontinue drug at first sign of rash, which may precede severe hypersensitivity or other adverse reaction. Rash is more common in patients taking diuretics and in those with renal disorders. Tell patient to report all adverse reactions immediately.
• Advise patient to avoid alcohol consumption during drug therapy.

☑ **Evaluation**
• Patient expresses relief of joint pain.
• Patient is free from infection.

• Patient and family state understanding of drug therapy.

---

alpha₁ proteinase inhibitor (human)
(AL-fah PROh-ten-ays in-HIB-ih-tor)
Prolastin

Pharmacologic class: enzyme inhibitor
Therapeutic class: orphan drug
Pregnancy risk category: C

How supplied
Injection: 500 mg, 1,000 mg

Pharmacokinetics
Absorption: not applicable with I.V. administration.
Distribution: may be distributed to lung tissues, but distribution is not well documented.
Metabolism: unknown.
Excretion: unknown.

Route	Onset	Peak	Duration
I.V.	≤ 3 wk	Immediate	Unknown

Pharmacodynamics
Chemical effect: replaces alpha₁ proteinase in patients with alpha₁ antitrypsin deficiency.
Therapeutic effect: replaces missing enzyme.

Indications and dosage
▶ **Chronic replacement therapy in patients with congenital alpha₁ antitrypsin deficiency and demonstrable panacinar emphysema.** *Adults:* 60 mg/kg I.V. once weekly.

Adverse reactions
Hematologic: possible viral transmission.

Interactions
Drug-lifestyle. *Smoking:* blocks drug's effects. Caution patient not to smoke.

Contraindications and precautions

- Contraindicated in patients with selective immunoglobulin A (IgA) deficiency who have known antibodies against IgA.
- Use cautiously in patients at risk for circulatory overload and in pregnant and breast-feeding women.
- Safety of drug has not been established in children.

NURSING CONSIDERATIONS

📝 Assessment

- Obtain baseline assessment of patient's condition.
- Be alert for viral infection.
- Determine whether patient smokes; cigarette smoke blocks drug's effects.
- Evaluate patient's and family's knowledge of drug therapy.

⊕ Nursing diagnoses

- Altered health maintenance related to underlying condition
- Risk for injury related to potential for viral transmission with use of drug
- Knowledge deficit related to drug therapy

⟩ Planning and implementation

- Carefully follow manufacturer's directions for use.
- Reconstitute drug using supplied diluent (sterile water for injection). After reconstitution, administer within 3 hours. Inject directly into vein; may give at rate of 0.08 ml/kg/minute or greater. Intermittent or continuous infusion is not recommended. Store powder for injection in refrigerator (36° to 46° F [2° to 8° C]).
- Know that prophylaxis against hepatitis B is recommended before drug is given.

Patient teaching
- Explain that product has been treated to minimize risk of transmission of hepatitis and AIDS but that hepatitis B vaccine is recommended before use.
- Advise patient who smokes to stop during therapy.

☑ Evaluation

- Patient shows positive response to therapy.
- Patient remains free from viral infection.
- Patient and family state understanding of drug therapy.

---

alprazolam
(al-PRAH-zoh-lam)
Apo-Alpraz♦, Novo-Alprazol♦, Nu-Alpraz♦, Xanax

Pharmacologic class: benzodiazepine
Therapeutic class: antianxiety
Controlled substance schedule: IV
Pregnancy risk category: D

How supplied

Tablets: 0.25 mg, 0.5 mg, 1 mg, 2 mg
Oral solution: 0.5 mg/5 ml, 1 mg/ml (concentrate)

Pharmacokinetics

Absorption: well absorbed.
Distribution: distributed widely throughout body; 80% to 90% of dose is bound to plasma protein.
Metabolism: metabolized in liver equally to alpha-hydroxyalprazolam and inactive metabolites.
Excretion: alpha-hydroxyalprazolam and other metabolites are excreted in urine.
Half-life: 12 to 15 hours.

Route	Onset	Peak	Duration
P.O.	Unknown	1-2 hr	Unknown

Pharmacodynamics

Chemical effect: unknown. Probably potentiates effects of gamma-aminobutyric acid, an inhibitory neurotransmitter, and depresses CNS at limbic and subcortical levels of brain.
Therapeutic effect: decreases anxiety.

Reactions may be *common*, uncommon, *life-threatening*, or COMMON AND LIFE-THREATENING.

Indications and dosage

▶ **Anxiety.** *Adults:* usual initial dose, 0.25 to 0.5 mg P.O. t.i.d. Maximum dosage is 4 mg daily in divided doses. *Elderly or debilitated patients or those with advanced liver disease:* usual initial dose, 0.25 mg P.O. b.i.d. or t.i.d. Maximum dosage is 4 mg daily in divided doses.
▶ **Panic disorders.** *Adults:* 0.5 mg P.O. t.i.d., increased q 3 to 4 days in increments of no more than 1 mg. Maximum dosage is 10 mg daily in divided doses.

Adverse reactions

CNS: *drowsiness, light-headedness,* headache, confusion, hostility, anterograde amnesia, restlessness, psychosis.
CV: transient hypotension, tachycardia.
EENT: vision disturbances.
GI: dry mouth, nausea, vomiting, constipation, discomfort.
GU: incontinence, urine retention, menstrual irregularities.

Interactions

Drug-drug. *Antihistamines, antipsychotics, CNS depressants:* increased CNS depression. Avoid concomitant use.
Cimetidine: increased sedation. Monitor patient carefully.
Digoxin: may increase serum level of digoxin, increasing toxicity. Monitor patient closely.
Fluoxetine, oral contraceptives: increase serum concentrations of alprazolam. Monitor for toxicity.
Tricyclic antidepressants: increased plasma level of tricyclic antidepressant. Monitor for toxicity.
Drug-lifestyle. *Alcohol use:* increased CNS depression. Avoid concomitant use.
Smoking: decreased effectiveness of benzodiazepine. Monitor patient closely.

Contraindications and precautions

• Contraindicated in patients with acute angle-closure glaucoma or hypersensitivity to drug or other benzodiazepines and in breast-feeding women.

• Use with extreme caution in pregnant women because infant could be at risk for withdrawal symptoms.
• Use cautiously in patients with hepatic, renal, or pulmonary disease.
• Safety of drug has not been established in children.

NURSING CONSIDERATIONS

☰ Assessment
• Assess patient's anxiety before and frequently after therapy.
• Monitor liver, renal, and hematopoietic function studies periodically, as ordered, in patient receiving repeated or prolonged therapy.
• Be alert for adverse reactions and drug interactions.
• Evaluate patient's and family's knowledge of drug therapy.

⊞ Nursing diagnoses
• Anxiety related to patient's underlying condition
• Risk for injury related to drug-induced CNS reactions
• Knowledge deficit related to drug therapy

⊵ Planning and implementation
• Know that drug should not be prescribed for everyday stress or for long-term use (more than 4 months).
• When administering drug, make sure patient has swallowed tablets before leaving bedside.
• Expect to administer lower doses at longer intervals in elderly or debilitated patients.
• Know that drug should not be withdrawn abruptly after long-term use; withdrawal symptoms may occur. Abuse or addiction is possible.
Patient teaching
• Warn patient to avoid hazardous activities that require alertness and psychomotor coordination until CNS effects of drug are known.

---

*Liquid form contains alcohol   **May contain tartrazine   ♦Canada   ◇Australia   †OTC

• Tell patient to avoid alcohol consumption and smoking while taking drug.
• Caution patient to take drug as prescribed and not to discontinue it without doctor's approval. Inform him of potential for dependence if taken longer than directed.
• Teach patient how to manage or avoid troublesome adverse reactions, such as constipation and drowsiness.

☑ **Evaluation**
• Patient is less anxious.
• Patient does not experience injury from adverse CNS reactions.
• Patient and family state understanding of drug therapy.

---

alprostadil
(al-PROS-tuh-dil)
Prostin VR Pediatric

Pharmacologic class: prostaglandin
Therapeutic class: ductus arteriosus patency adjunct
Pregnancy risk category: NR

How supplied
Injection: 500 mcg/ml

Pharmacokinetics
Absorption: not applicable with I.V. administration.
Distribution: distributed rapidly throughout body.
Metabolism: about 68% of dose is metabolized in one pass through lung, primarily by oxidation; 100% is metabolized within 24 hours.
Excretion: all metabolites are excreted in urine within 24 hours. *Half-life:* about 5 to 10 minutes.

Route	Onset	Peak	Duration
I.V.	5-10 min	≤ 20 min	1-3 hr

Pharmacodynamics
Chemical effect: relaxes smooth muscle of ductus arteriosus.
Therapeutic effect: improves cardiac circulation.

Indications and dosage
▶ **Palliative therapy for temporary maintenance of patent ductus arteriosus until surgery can be performed.**
Infants: 0.05 to 0.1 mcg/kg/minute by I.V. infusion. When therapeutic response is achieved, infusion rate reduced to lowest dosage that will maintain response. Maximum dosage is 0.4 mcg/kg/minute. Alternatively, drug can be administered through umbilical artery catheter placed at ductal opening.

Adverse reactions
CNS: *seizures.*
CV: bradycardia, *cardiac arrest,* hypotension, tachycardia.
GI: diarrhea.
Hematologic: *DIC.*
Other: APNEA, *flushing, fever, sepsis.*

Interactions
None significant.

Contraindications and precautions
• No known contraindications.
• Use cautiously in neonates with bleeding tendencies because drug inhibits platelet aggregation.

NURSING CONSIDERATIONS

☑ **Assessment**
• Obtain baseline assessment of infant's cardiopulmonary status before therapy.
• Measure drug's effectiveness by monitoring blood oxygenation of infants with restricted pulmonary blood flow and by monitoring systemic blood pressure and blood pH of infants with restricted systemic blood flow.
• Be alert for adverse reactions throughout therapy.

Reactions may be *common,* uncommon, *life-threatening,* or COMMON AND LIFE-THREATENING.

• Evaluate parent's knowledge of drug therapy.

🔲 **Nursing diagnoses**
• Altered cardiopulmonary tissue perfusion related to underlying condition
• Risk for injury related to drug-induced adverse reactions
• Knowledge deficit related to drug therapy

▶ **Planning and implementation**
• Know that a differential diagnosis should be made between respiratory distress syndrome and cyanotic heart disease before drug is administered. Do not use drug in neonates with respiratory distress syndrome.
• Dilute drug before administering. Prepare fresh solution daily; discard solution after 24 hours.
• Do not use diluents that contain benzyl alcohol. Fatal toxic syndrome may occur.
• Know that drug is not recommended for direct injection or intermittent infusion. Administer by continuous infusion using constant-rate pump. Infuse through large peripheral or central vein or through umbilical artery catheter placed at level of ductus arteriosus. If flushing occurs as a result of peripheral vasodilation, reposition catheter.
• Reduce infusion rate if fever or significant hypotension develops in infant.
• If apnea and bradycardia (may reflect drug overdose) develop, stop infusion immediately.
• Keep respiratory support available.
• Notify doctor if infant's cardiopulmonary status changes significantly.
Patient teaching
• Keep parents informed of infant's status.
• Explain that parents will be allowed as much time and physical contact with infant as feasible.

✔ **Evaluation**
• Patient demonstrates stable and effective cardiopulmonary status as indicated

by adequate cardiac and pulmonary parameters and peripheral systemic perfusion.
• Patient does not experience injury from adverse reactions associated with drug.
• Parents state understanding of drug therapy.

---

alteplase (tissue plasminogen activator, recombinant; tPA)
(AL-teh-plays)
Actilyse ◊, Activase

Pharmacologic class: enzyme
Therapeutic class: thrombolytic enzyme
Pregnancy risk category: C

How supplied
Injection: 20-mg (11.6 million-IU), 50-mg (29 million-IU), 100-mg (58 million-IU) vials

Pharmacokinetics
Absorption: not applicable with I.V. administration.
Distribution: rapidly cleared from plasma by liver (about 80% cleared within 10 minutes after infusion is discontinued).
Metabolism: primarily hepatic.
Excretion: over 85% excreted in urine, 5% in feces. *Half-life:* less than 10 minutes.

Route	Onset	Peak	Duration
I.V.	Immediate	About 45 min	About 4 hr

Pharmacodynamics
Chemical effect: binds to fibrin in thrombus and locally converts plasminogen to plasmin, which initiates local fibrinolysis.
Therapeutic effect: dissolves blood clots in coronary arteries and lungs.

Indications and dosage
▶ **Lysis of thrombi obstructing coronary arteries in acute MI.** *Adults:*
100 mg I.V. infusion over 3 hours as follows: 60 mg in first hour, of which 6 to 10 mg is given as bolus over first 1 to 2

---

minutes. Then 20 mg/hour infusion for 2 hours. Smaller adults (less than 65 kg) should receive 1.25 mg/kg in similar fashion (60% in first hour with 10% as bolus, then 20% of total dose per hour for 2 hours). Do not exceed 100-mg dose. Higher doses may increase risk of intracranial bleeding.

▶ **Management of acute massive pulmonary embolism.** *Adults:* 100 mg I.V. infusion over 2 hours. Heparin begun at end of infusion when PTT or PT returns to twice normal or less. Do not exceed 100-mg dose. Higher doses may increase risk of intracranial bleeding.

▶ **Management of acute ischemic strokes.** *Adults:* 0.9 mg/kg (maximum 90 mg) I.V. over 60 minutes with 10% of the total dose given as initial bolus over 1 minute.

Adverse reactions

CNS: *cerebral hemorrhage,* fever.
CV: hypotension, arrhythmias, edema.
GI: nausea, vomiting.
Hematologic: *severe, spontaneous bleeding (cerebral, retroperitoneal, GU, or GI).*
Other: bleeding at puncture sites, hypersensitivity reactions *(anaphylaxis),* urticaria, arthralgia.

Interactions

Drug-drug. *Aspirin, coumarin anticoagulants, dipyridamole, heparin:* increased risk of bleeding. Monitor patient carefully.

Contraindications and precautions

• Contraindicated in patients with active internal bleeding, intracranial neoplasm, arteriovenous malformation, aneurysm, severe uncontrolled hypertension, history of CVA, intraspinal or intracranial trauma or surgery within past 2 months, or known bleeding diathesis.
• Use cautiously in patients who had major surgery within past 10 days; in pregnancy and first 10 days postpartum; during lactation; in those with organ biopsy; trauma (including cardiopulmonary resus-

citation); GI or GU bleeding; cerebrovascular disease; hypertension; mitral stenosis, atrial fibrillation, or other condition that may lead to left-sided heart thrombus; acute pericarditis or subacute bacterial endocarditis; septic thrombophlebitis; or diabetic hemorrhagic retinopathy; in patients receiving anticoagulants; and in patients age 75 and older.
• Safety of drug has not been established in children.

NURSING CONSIDERATIONS

🔯 Assessment

• Assess patient's cardiopulmonary status (including ECG, vital signs, and coagulation studies) before and during therapy.
• Be alert for adverse reactions and drug interactions.
• Monitor patient for internal bleeding, and frequently check puncture sites.
• Evaluate patient's and family's knowledge of drug therapy.

🔯 Nursing diagnoses

• Altered cardiopulmonary tissue perfusion related to patient's underlying condition
• Risk for injury related to adverse effects of drug therapy
• Knowledge deficit related to drug therapy

▶ Planning and implementation

• Know that recanalization of occluded coronary arteries and improvement of heart function require initiation of alteplase as soon as possible after onset of symptoms.
• Reconstitute drug with sterile water for injection (without preservatives) only. Check manufacturer's label for specific information. Do not use vial if vacuum is not present. Reconstitute with large-bore (18G) needle, directing stream of sterile water at lyophilized cake. Do not shake. Slight foaming is common, and solution should be clear or pale yellow.

Reactions may be *common*, uncommon, *life-threatening*, or COMMON AND LIFE-THREATENING.

• Keep in mind that drug may be administered as reconstituted (1 mg/ml) or diluted with equal volume of 0.9% NaCl solution or D_5W to make 0.5 mg/ml solution. Adding other drugs to infusion is not recommended.

• Reconstitute alteplase solution immediately before use and administer within 8 hours because it contains no preservatives. Drug may be temporarily stored at 35° to 86° F (2° to 30° C), but it is only stable for 8 hours at room temperature. Discard unused solution.

• Be aware that heparin is frequently initiated after treatment with alteplase to reduce risk of rethrombosis.

• If arterial puncture is necessary, select site on an arm and apply pressure for 30 minutes afterward. Also use pressure dressings, sand bags, or ice packs on recent puncture sites to prevent bleeding.

• Notify doctor if severe bleeding occurs and doesn't stop with intervention; alteplase and heparin infusions will need to be discontinued.

• Have antiarrhythmic drugs available. Coronary thrombolysis is associated with arrhythmias induced by reperfusion of ischemic myocardium.

• Avoid invasive procedures during thrombolytic therapy.

Patient teaching

• Tell patient to report chest pain, dyspnea, changes in heart rate or rhythm, nausea, or bleeding immediately.

☑ **Evaluation**

• Patient's cardiopulmonary assessment findings demonstrate improved perfusion.

• Patient does not experience serious adverse reactions associated with drug.

• Patient and family state understanding of drug therapy.

altretamine
(hexamethylmelamine; HMM)
(al-TREH-tuh-meen)
Hexalen, Hexastat ♦

Pharmacologic class: alkylating-like agent
Therapeutic class: antineoplastic
Pregnancy risk category: D

How supplied

Capsules: 50 mg

Pharmacokinetics

Absorption: well absorbed from GI tract, but rapid and extensive demethylation causes variations in plasma levels.
Distribution: does not cross blood-brain barrier to significant extent; binds to plasma proteins.
Metabolism: rapid and extensive demethylation in liver.
Excretion: metabolites excreted primarily in urine; small amount eliminated through lungs in expired air; trace amount excreted in feces. *Half-life:* 5 to 10 hours.

Route	Onset	Peak	Duration
P.O.	Unknown	0.5-3 hr	Unknown

Pharmacodynamics

Chemical effect: unknown. Structurally similar to triethylenemelamine but is not an alkylating agent. Metabolism is important for antitumor activity; metabolites of drug are known alkylating agents.
Therapeutic effect: destroys rapidly replicating malignant cells.

Indications and dosage

▶ **Palliative treatment of patients with persistent or recurrent ovarian cancer after first-line therapy with cisplatin or alkylating agent-based combination therapy.** *Adults:* 260 mg/m² P.O. daily in four divided doses with meals and h.s. for 14 or 21 consecutive days in 28-day cycle.

Adverse reactions

CNS: *sensory neuropathy,* anorexia, ataxia, paresthesia, hyporeflexia, fatigue, *seizures.*
GI: *nausea, vomiting.*
Hematologic: *leukopenia, thrombocy-topenia, anemia.*
Skin: erythematous maculopapular eczema.
Other: increased serum creatinine and BUN levels, alopecia.

Interactions

Drug-drug. *Cimetidine:* may increase half-life and toxicity of altretamine. Monitor patient closely for toxicity.
MAO inhibitors: severe orthostatic hypotension. Avoid concomitant use.

Contraindications and precautions

• Contraindicated in patients with preexisting severe bone marrow suppression, severe neurologic toxicity, or hypersensitivity to drug. Use in pregnant or breast-feeding women is not recommended.
• Safety of drug has not been established in children.

NURSING CONSIDERATIONS

Assessment
• Assess patient's underlying condition before therapy.
• Obtain baseline CBC and platelet count before each course of therapy. Nadirs of WBC and platelet counts are reached by 3 to 4 weeks. Normal counts are regained by 6 weeks.
• Perform comprehensive neurologic assessment before each course of therapy and daily thereafter. Continuous high-dose daily treatment is associated with neurotoxicity, which appears to reverse when drug is discontinued.
• Be alert for adverse reactions and drug interactions.
• Evaluate patient's and family's knowledge of drug therapy.

Nursing diagnoses
• Altered health maintenance related to neoplastic disease
• Risk for fluid volume deficit related to drug-induced adverse reactions
• Knowledge deficit related to drug therapy

Planning and implementation
• If drug is given continuously, administer with antiemetics, as ordered. Anticipate altered dosage with severe nausea and vomiting.
• Be prepared to discontinue drug for at least 14 days if laboratory tests indicate platelet count below 75,000/mm^3, WBC count below 2,000 mm^3, or a granulocyte count below 1,000/mm^3.
• Anticipate temporary discontinuation of drug if severe GI distress unresponsive to symptomatic treatment or signs of progressive neuropathy develop. Drug should be discontinued if neurologic symptoms do not stabilize.
Patient teaching
• Instruct patient to report nausea, vomiting, or sensory neuropathy.
• Advise patient to take drug with meals to minimize nausea and vomiting.
• Advise patient to use contraception during treatment because drug can harm fetus.

Evaluation
• Patient shows positive response to therapy.
• Patient does not develop fluid volume deficit.
• Patient and family state understanding of drug therapy.

aluminum carbonate
(uh-LOO-mih-num KAR-buh-nayt)
Basaljel†

Pharmacologic class: inorganic aluminum salt

Therapeutic class: antacid, hypophos-
phatemic agent
Pregnancy risk category: B

How supplied

Tablets or capsules: equivalent to aluminum hydroxide 500 mg†
Oral suspension: equivalent to aluminum
hydroxide 400 mg/5 ml†

Pharmacokinetics

Absorption: small amounts absorbed sys-
temically.
Distribution: none.
Metabolism: none.
Excretion: excreted in feces.

Route	Onset	Peak	Duration
P.O.	20 min	Unknown	20-60 min if fasting; up to 3 hr if taken 1 hr after meal

Pharmacodynamics

Chemical effect: Reduces total acid load
in GI tract, elevates gastric pH to reduce
pepsin activity, strengthens gastric mucosal barrier, and increases esophageal
sphincter tone.
Therapeutic effect: relieves gastric discomfort and prevents phosphate stone
formation in urinary tract.

Indications and dosage

▶ **Antacid.** *Adults:* 10 ml of suspension
P.O. q 2 hours p.r.n.; or 1 to 2 tablets or
capsules P.O. q 2 hours p.r.n. Maximum
dosage is 24 capsules, tablets, or teaspoonfuls daily.
▶ **Prevention of urinary phosphate
stones (with low-phosphate diet).**
Adults: 1 g P.O. t.i.d. or q.i.d. Adjust to
lowest possible dosage after therapy is initiated, monitoring diet and serum levels.

Adverse reactions

GI: anorexia, *constipation,* intestinal obstruction.
Metabolic: hypophosphatemia.

Interactions

Drug-drug. *Allopurinol, antibiotics (including quinolones and tetracyclines),
corticosteroids, diflunisal, digoxin,
ethambutol, H_2 antagonists, iron, isoniazid, penicillamine, phenothiazines, thyroid hormones:* decreased pharmacologic
effect because of possible impaired absorption. Separate administration times.
Enteric-coated drugs: may release prematurely in stomach. Separate doses by
at least 1 hour.

Contraindications and precautions

• No known contraindications.
• Use cautiously in patients with chronic
renal disease.

NURSING CONSIDERATIONS

⚖ Assessment
• Assess patient's discomfort before therapy and regularly thereafter.
• Monitor long-term, high-dose use in patients on restricted sodium intake. Each
tablet, capsule, or 5 ml of suspension
contains about 3 mg of sodium.
• Be alert for adverse reactions and drug
interactions.
• Evaluate patient's and family's knowledge of drug therapy.

⊞ Nursing diagnoses
• Pain related to gastric hyperacidity
• Constipation related to drug's adverse
effects
• Knowledge deficit related to drug
therapy

▷ Planning and implementation
• Shake suspension well; give with small
amount of water or fruit juice to ease passage.
• When administering through nasogastric (NG) tube, make sure tube is patent
and placed correctly; after instilling,
flush tube with water to ensure passage to
stomach and to clear tube.
• Do not give other oral medications
within 2 hours of antacid administration.

This may cause premature release of enteric-coated drugs in stomach.

Patient teaching

• Caution patient to take aluminum carbonate only as directed, to shake suspension well, and to follow with sips of water or juice.

• Warn patient not to switch antacids without doctor's advice.

• Warn patient that drug may color stool white or cause white streaks.

• Teach patient how to prevent constipation.

☑ **Evaluation**

• Patient's pain is relieved.

• Patient maintains normal bowel function.

• Patient and family state understanding of drug therapy.

aluminum hydroxide
(uh-LOO-mih-num high-DROKS-ighd)
AlternaGEL†, Alu-Cap†, Alu-Tab†, Amphojel†, Dialume†, Nephrox†

Pharmacologic class: aluminum salt
Therapeutic class: antacid
Pregnancy risk category: C

How supplied

Tablets: 300 mg†, 500 mg†, 600 mg†
Capsules: 475 mg†, 500 mg†
Oral suspension: 320 mg/5 ml†, 600 mg/5 ml†

Pharmacokinetics

Absorption: small amounts absorbed systemically.
Distribution: none.
Metabolism: none.
Excretion: excreted in feces.

Route	Onset	Peak	Duration
P.O.	Varies: liquids more rapid-acting than tablets or capsules	Unknown	20-60 min if fasting; 3 hr if taken after meal

Pharmacodynamics

Chemical effect: reduces total acid load in GI tract, elevates gastric pH to reduce pepsin activity, strengthens gastric mucosal barrier, and increases esophageal sphincter tone.
Therapeutic effect: relieves gastric discomfort.

Indications and dosage

▶ **Antacid, hyperphosphatemia.**
Adults: 500 to 1,500 mg P.O. (tablet or capsule) 1 hour after meals and h.s.; or 5 to 30 ml (suspension) as needed 1 hour after meals and h.s.

Adverse reactions

GI: anorexia, *constipation,* intestinal obstruction.
Other: hypophosphatemia.

Interactions

Drug-drug. *Allopurinol, antibiotics (including quinolones and tetracyclines), corticosteroids, diflunisal, digoxin, ethambutol, H_2 antagonists, iron, isoniazid, penicillamine, phenothiazines, thyroid hormones:* decreased pharmacologic effect because of possible impaired absorption. Separate administration times.
Enteric-coated drugs: may release prematurely in stomach. Separate doses by at least 1 hour.

Contraindications and precautions

• No known contraindications.
• Use cautiously in patients with chronic renal disease.

NURSING CONSIDERATIONS

☒ **Assessment**

• Assess patient's discomfort before therapy and regularly thereafter.

• Monitor long-term, high-dose use in patient on restricted sodium intake. Each tablet, capsule, or 5 ml of suspension contains 2 to 3 mg of sodium.

• Be alert for adverse reactions and drug interactions.

Reactions may be *common,* uncommon, **life-threatening**, or COMMON AND LIFE-THREATENING.

• Evaluate patient's and family's knowledge of drug therapy.

⊞ Nursing diagnoses
• Pain related to gastric hyperacidity
• Constipation related to drug's adverse effects
• Knowledge deficit related to drug therapy

▶ Planning and implementation
• Shake suspension well; give with small amount of milk or water to ease passage.
• When administering through nasogastric (NG) tube, make sure tube is patent and placed correctly; after instilling, flush tube with water to ensure passage to stomach and to clear tube.
• Do not give other oral medications within 2 hours of antacid administration. This may cause premature release of enteric-coated drugs in stomach.
Patient teaching
• Advise patient not to take aluminum hydroxide indiscriminately or to switch antacids without doctor's advice.
• Instruct patient to shake suspension well and to follow with sips of water or juice.
• Warn patient that drug may color stool white or cause white streaks.
• Teach patient how to prevent constipation.

☑ Evaluation
• Patient's pain is relieved.
• Patient maintains normal bowel function.
• Patient and family state understanding of drug therapy.

---

aluminum phosphate
(uh-LOO-mih-num FOS-fayt)
Phosphaljel†

Pharmacologic class: aluminum salt
Therapeutic class: phosphate replacement
Pregnancy risk category: NR

How supplied
Oral suspension: 233 mg/5 ml†

Pharmacokinetics
Absorption: small amounts absorbed systemically.
Distribution: none.
Metabolism: none.
Excretion: excreted in feces.

Route	Onset	Peak	Duration
P.O.	About 20 min	Unknown	20-60 min if fasting; 3 hr if taken with meal

Pharmacodynamics
Chemical effect: reduces fecal excretion of phosphate.
Therapeutic effect: increases phosphate level in body.

Indications and dosage
▶ **To reduce fecal elimination of phosphate.** *Adults:* 15 to 30 ml undiluted P.O. q 2 hours between meals and h.s.

Adverse reactions
GI: *constipation,* intestinal obstruction.

Interactions
Drug-drug. *Allopurinol, antibiotics, corticosteroids, diflunisal, digoxin, ethambutol, H_2 antagonists, iron, isoniazid, penicillamine, phenothiazines, thyroid hormones:* decreased pharmacologic effect because of possible impaired absorption. Separate administration times.
Ciprofloxacin, other quinolones, tetracyclines: decreased antibiotic effect. Separate administration times.
Enteric-coated drugs: may release prematurely in stomach. Separate doses by at least 1 hour.

Contraindications and precautions
• No known contraindications.
• Use cautiously in patients with chronic renal disease.

NURSING CONSIDERATIONS

⟐ Assessment
• Assess patient's phosphate level before therapy and regularly thereafter.
• Monitor long-term, high-dose use in patient on restricted sodium intake.
• Be alert for adverse reactions and drug interactions.
• Evaluate patient's and family's knowledge of drug therapy.

⊕ Nursing diagnoses
• Altered protection related to reduced phosphate level
• Constipation related to drug's adverse effects
• Knowledge deficit related to drug therapy

⟩ Planning and implementation
• Shake suspension well; give with small amount of milk or water to ease passage.
• When administering through nasogastric (NG) tube, make sure tube is patent and placed correctly; after instilling, flush tube with water to ensure passage to stomach and to clear tube.
• Do not give other oral medications within 2 hours of administration.
Patient teaching
• Advise patient not to take drug indiscriminately or to switch antacids without doctor's advice.
• Instruct patient to shake suspension well and to follow with sips of water or juice.
• Warn patient that drug may color stool white or cause white streaks.
• Teach patient how to prevent constipation.

☑ Evaluation
• Patient's phosphate level is normal.
• Patient maintains normal bowel function.
• Patient and family state understanding of drug therapy.

amantadine hydrochloride
(uh-MAN-tah-deen high-droh-KLOR-ighd)
Antadine◇, Symadine, Symmetrel

Pharmacologic class: synthetic cyclic primary amine
Therapeutic class: antiviral, antiparkinsonian
Pregnancy risk category: C

How supplied
Capsules: 100 mg
Syrup: 50 mg/5 ml

Pharmacokinetics
Absorption: well absorbed from GI tract.
Distribution: distributed widely throughout body; crosses blood-brain barrier.
Metabolism: about 10% of drug is metabolized.
Excretion: about 90% is excreted unchanged in urine, primarily by tubular secretion. Portion of drug may be excreted in breast milk. Excretion rate depends on urine pH. *Half-life:* about 24 hours; with renal dysfunction, may be prolonged to 10 days.

Route	Onset	Peak	Duration
P.O.	48 hr (anti-dyskinetic)	2-4 hr	Unknown
	Unknown (antiviral)	Unknown	Unknown

Pharmacodynamics
Chemical effect: may interfere with influenza A virus penetration into susceptible cells. In parkinsonism, action unknown.
Therapeutic effect: protects against or reduces symptoms of influenza A viral infection and reduces extrapyramidal symptoms.

Indications and dosage
▶ **Prophylactic or symptomatic treatment of influenza type A virus; respi-**

Reactions may be *common*, uncommon, *life-threatening*, or COMMON AND LIFE-THREATENING.

ratory tract illnesses. *Adults up to age 64 and children ages 10 and over:* 200 mg P.O. daily in single dose or divided b.i.d. *Children ages 1 to 9:* 4.4 to 8.8 mg/kg P.O. daily in single dose or divided b.i.d. Maximum dose is 150 mg daily. *Adults over age 64:* 100 mg P.O. once daily. Treatment should continue for 24 to 48 hours after symptoms disappear. Prophylaxis should start as soon as possible after initial exposure and continue for at least 10 days. When inactivated influenza A vaccine unavailable, may continue prophylactic treatment for the duration of known influenza A in the community because of repeated or suspected exposures. If used with influenza vaccine, dose is continued for 2 to 4 weeks until protection from vaccine develops.
▶ **Drug-induced extrapyramidal reactions.** *Adults:* 100 mg P.O. b.i.d. Occasionally, patients whose responses are not optimal may benefit from an increase up to 300 mg P.O. daily in divided doses.
▶ **Idiopathic parkinsonism, parkinsonian syndrome.** *Adults:* 100 mg P.O. b.i.d.; in patients who are seriously ill or receiving other antiparkinsonian drugs, 100 mg daily for at least 1 week, then 100 mg b.i.d., p.r.n.

Adverse reactions

CNS: depression, fatigue, confusion, dizziness, psychosis, hallucinations, anxiety, *irritability,* ataxia, *insomnia,* weakness, headache, light-headedness, difficulty concentrating.
CV: peripheral edema, orthostatic hypotension, **heart failure.**
GI: anorexia, nausea, constipation, vomiting, dry mouth.
GU: urine retention.
Skin: *livedo reticularis* (with prolonged use).

Interactions

Drug-drug. *Anticholinergics:* increased adverse anticholinergic effects. Use together cautiously.

CNS stimulants: additive CNS stimulation. Use together cautiously.
Hydrochlorothiazide, triamterene: increased levels of amantadine. Use together cautiously.
Quinidine, quinine: reduced renal clearance of amantadine. Use together cautiously.
Sulfamethoxazole, trimethoprim: increased amantadine serum concentrations. Use together cautiously.
Thioridazine: worsened tremor in elderly patients. Monitor closely.

Contraindications and precautions

• Contraindicated in patients with hypersensitivity to drug.
• Use cautiously in patients with seizure disorders, heart failure, peripheral edema, hepatic disease, mental illness, eczematoid rash, renal impairment, orthostatic hypotension, or CV disease; in elderly patients; and in pregnant or breastfeeding women. Dosage may need adjustment in patients with renal failure.
• Safety of drug has not been established for children under age 1.

NURSING CONSIDERATIONS

Assessment
• Obtain baseline assessment of patient's exposure to influenza A virus or history of Parkinson's disease, as appropriate.
• Be alert for adverse reactions and drug interactions.
• Monitor patient's hydration status if adverse GI reactions occur.
• Evaluate patient's and family's knowledge of drug therapy.

Nursing diagnoses
• Altered health maintenance related to patient's underlying condition
• Risk for fluid volume deficit related to adverse GI reactions
• Knowledge deficit related to drug therapy

⧉ Planning and implementation
• Be aware that elderly patients are more susceptible to neurologic adverse effects. Giving drug in two daily doses rather than as single dose may reduce incidence of effects.
• Administer drug after meals for best absorption.
Patient teaching
• Advise patient to take drug several hours before bedtime to prevent insomnia.
• Advise patient not to stand or change positions too quickly to prevent orthostatic hypotension.
• Instruct patient to report adverse reactions, especially dizziness, depression, anxiety, nausea, and urine retention.
• Warn patient with parkinsonism not to discontinue drug abruptly; doing so could precipitate a parkinsonian crisis.

☑ Evaluation
• Patient exhibits improved health status.
• Patient maintains adequate hydration.
• Patient and family state understanding of drug therapy.

---

ambenonium chloride
(am-be-NOH-nee-um KLOR-ighd)
Mytelase

Pharmacologic class: cholinesterase inhibitor
Therapeutic class: antimyasthenic
Pregnancy risk category: NR

How supplied
Tablets: 10 mg

Pharmacokinetics
Absorption: poorly absorbed from GI tract.
Distribution: unknown.
Metabolism: unknown.
Excretion: unknown.

Route	Onset	Peak	Duration
P.O.	Unknown	Unknown	4-8 hr

Pharmacodynamics
Chemical effect: inhibits destruction of acetylcholine released from parasympathetic and somatic efferent nerves. Acetylcholine accumulates, promoting increased stimulation of receptor.
Therapeutic effect: relieves symptoms of myasthenia gravis.

Indications and dosage
▶ **Symptomatic treatment of myasthenia gravis in patients who cannot take neostigmine bromide or pyridostigmine bromide.** *Adults:* dosage individualized for each patient. Usual starting dose is 5 mg P.O. t.i.d. or q.i.d. Dosage increased and adjusted at 1- to 2-day intervals to avoid drug accumulation and overdosage. Usual dosage range is 5 to 25 mg P.O. t.i.d. or q.i.d., but some patients may require as much as 75 mg b.i.d. to q.i.d. *Children:* initially, 0.3 mg/kg/day or 10 mg/m^2/day P.O., up to 1.5 mg/kg/day or 50 mg/m^2/day respectively, in three or four doses.

Adverse reactions
CNS: headache, dizziness, weakness, incoordination, *seizures,* confusion, tremor, nervousness, sweating.
CV: bradycardia, hypotension.
EENT: miosis, lacrimation.
GI: *nausea, vomiting, diarrhea, abdominal cramps,* increased salivation.
GU: urinary frequency, incontinence.
Respiratory: bronchospasm, *bronchoconstriction,* increased bronchial secretions, *pulmonary edema, respiratory paralysis.*
Other: muscle cramps, sweating.

Interactions
Drug-drug. *Aminoglycosides, anesthetics, atropine, corticosteroids, magnesium, procainamide, quinidine:* prolonged or enhanced muscle weakness. Monitor closely.

Reactions may be *common*, uncommon, *life-threatening*, or COMMON AND LIFE-THREATENING.

Mecamylamine, other ganglionic blockers: increased toxicity. Avoid concomitant use.

Contraindications and precautions

• Contraindicated in patients with mechanical obstruction of intestine or urinary tract, in those receiving ganglionic blocking agents, and in breast-feeding women.
• Use with extreme caution in patients with bronchial asthma. Use cautiously in pregnant patients and in those with seizure disorder, bradycardia, recent coronary occlusion, vagotonia, hyperthyroidism, arrhythmias, postoperative atelectasis, or pneumonia.

NURSING CONSIDERATIONS

⬚ Assessment
• Obtain baseline assessment of patient's myasthenia gravis.
• Monitor patient's response to drug by regularly evaluating muscle strength.
• Be alert for adverse reactions (particularly if dosage exceeds 200 mg daily) and drug interactions.
• Evaluate patient's and family's knowledge of drug therapy.

⬚ Nursing diagnoses
• Ineffective breathing pattern related to myasthenia gravis
• Risk for injury related to drug's adverse reactions
• Knowledge deficit related to drug therapy

⬚ Planning and implementation
• Discontinue all other cholinergics, as ordered, before administering this drug.
• Know that large doses should be avoided in patients with decreased GI motility or megacolon.
• Administer each dose exactly as ordered, on time. Amount and frequency of dosing should vary with patient's activity level. Doctor probably will order larger

doses when patient is fatigued (for example, in afternoon and at mealtime).
• Give with milk or food to produce fewer adverse muscarinic reactions.
• Seek approval, when indicated, for hospitalized patients to have bedside supply of tablets. Patients with long-standing disease commonly insist on taking pills themselves.
• Check for weakness 30 to 60 minutes after administering dose (a warning sign of drug toxicity), and notify doctor immediately if it occurs. Doctor must determine whether severe muscle weakness is caused by toxicity or exacerbation of myasthenia gravis. Test dose of edrophonium I.V. will aggravate drug-induced weakness but will temporarily relieve weakness resulting from disease.
• Notify doctor of significant change in respiratory function. Always have atropine injection available, and be prepared to give 0.5 to 1 mg S.C. or slow I.V. push as ordered. Provide respiratory support as needed.
Patient teaching
• Teach patient to self-monitor for muscle weakness and to notify doctor of specific changes.
• Inform patient that drug will relieve symptoms of ptosis, double vision, difficulty in chewing and swallowing, and trunk and limb weakness. Stress importance of taking drug exactly as ordered.
• Explain to patient and family that drug is prescribed for chronic condition. Teach them about myasthenia gravis and drug's effect on symptoms.
• Advise patient to wear medical identification bracelet indicating his condition.

⬚ Evaluation
• Patient maintains effective breathing pattern.
• Patient does not experience injury from adverse reactions.
• Patient and family state understanding of drug therapy.

---

amifostine
(am-eh-FOS-teen)
Ethyol

Pharmacologic class: organic thiophosphate cytoprotective agent
Therapeutic class: antimetabolite
Pregnancy risk category: C

How supplied

Injection: 500 mg anhydrous base and 500 mg mannitol in 10-ml vial

Pharmacokinetics

Absorption: not applicable.
Distribution: less than 10% remains in plasma 6 minutes after administration.
Metabolism: metabolized to an active free thiol metabolite.
Excretion: renally excreted. *Half-life (elimination):* 8 minutes.

Route	Onset	Peak	Duration
I.V.	5-8 min	Unknown	Unknown

Pharmacodynamics

Chemical effect: dephosphoryated by alkaline phosphatase to pharmacologically active free thiol metabolite. Free thiol in normal tissues is available to bind to and detoxify reactive metabolites of cisplatin.
Therapeutic effect: reduction of toxic effects of cisplatin on renal tissue.

Indications and dosage

▶ **Reduction of cumulative renal toxicity associated with repeated administration of cisplatin in patients with advanced ovarian cancer or non-small-cell lung cancer.** *Adults:* 910 mg/m^2 daily as a 15-minute I.V. infusion, starting 30 minutes before chemotherapy. If hypotension occurs and blood pressure doesn't return to normal within 5 minutes after stopping treatment, subsequent cycles should use 740 mg/m^2.

Adverse reactions

CNS: dizziness, somnolence.

CV: *hypotension.*
GI: *nausea, vomiting.*
Other: flushing or feeling of warmth, chills or feeling of coldness, hiccups, sneezing, hypocalcemia, allergic reactions ranging from rash to rigors.

Interactions

Drug-drug. *Antihypertensive drugs, other drugs that could potentiate hypotension:* may potentiate hypotension. Give special consideration to administration of amifostine in patients receiving these agents.

Contraindications and precautions

• Contraindicated in patients hypersensitive to aminothiol compounds or mannitol. Do not use drug in patients receiving chemotherapy for potentially curable malignancies (including certain malignancies of germ cell origin), except for patients involved in clinical studies. Also contraindicated in hypotensive or dehydrated patients and in those receiving antihypertensive drugs that can't be stopped during the 24 hours preceding amifostine administration.
• Use cautiously in patients with ischemic heart disease, arrhythmias, heart failure, or history of stroke or transient ischemic attacks.
• Use cautiously in patients in whom the common adverse effects of nausea, vomiting, and hypotension are likely to have serious consequences.
• Use cautiously in elderly patients and in children; safety of drug use has not been established in these patients.

NURSING CONSIDERATIONS

☘ Assessment
• Be aware that patients receiving amifostine should be adequately hydrated before administration. Keep patient supine during infusion.
• Monitor blood pressure every 5 minutes during infusion. If hypotension occurs and requires interrupting therapy, notify

doctor and place patient in Trendelenburg's position. Then give an infusion of
0.9% NaCl solution, as ordered, using a
separate I.V. line. If blood pressure returns to normal within 5 minutes and patient is asymptomatic, restart infusion so
full dose of drug can be given. If full
dose can't be given, subsequent doses
should be limited to 740 mg/m².
• Know that antiemetic medication, including dexamethasone 20 mg I.V. and a
serotonin 5HT3 receptor antagonist,
should be administered before, and concurrent with, amifostine administration.
Additional antiemetics may be needed
based on chemotherapeutic drugs administered.
• Monitor patient's fluid balance when
drug is used with highly emetogenic
chemotherapy.
• Monitor serum calcium level in patients
at risk for hypocalcemia, such as those
with nephrotic syndrome. If necessary,
calcium supplements should be ordered
and administered.
• Evaluate patient's and family's knowledge of drug therapy.

⊕ Nursing diagnoses
• Altered health maintenance related to
neoplastic disease
• Knowledge deficit related to drug
therapy

▶ Planning and implementation
• Reconstitute each single-dose vial with
9.5 ml of sterile 0.9% NaCl injection. Do
not use other solutions to reconstitute
drug. Reconstituted solution (500 mg am-
ifostine/10 ml) is chemically stable for up
to 5 hours at room temperature (about
77° F [25° C]) or up to 24 hours under refrigeration (35° to 46° F [2° to 8° C]).
• Drug can be prepared in polyvinyl chloride bags in concentrations of 5 to 40 mg/
ml and has the same stability as when it
is reconstituted in single-use vial.
• Inspect vial for particulate matter and
discoloration before use, if possible.

Don't use if cloudiness or precipitate is
noted.
• If possible and if ordered, stop antihypertensive therapy 24 hours before drug
administration. If antihypertensive therapy can't be stopped, don't use amifostine
because severe hypotension may occur.
• Do not infuse for more than 15 minutes; a longer infusion has been associated with a higher incidence of adverse reactions.
Patient teaching
• Instruct patient to remain in a supine
position throughout infusion.
• Advise patient not to breast-feed; it is
unknown whether drug or its metabolites
are excreted in breast milk.

☑ Evaluation
• Patient shows positive response to drug.
• Patient and family state understanding
of drug therapy.

amikacin sulfate
(am-eh-KAY-sin SUL-fayt)
Amikin

Pharmacologic class: aminoglycoside
Therapeutic class: antibiotic
Pregnancy risk category: D

How supplied
Injection: 50 mg/ml, 250 mg/ml

Pharmacokinetics
Absorption: rapidly absorbed after I.M.
administration.
Distribution: distributed widely; protein
binding is minimal; drug crosses placenta.
Metabolism: none.
Excretion: excreted primarily in urine by
glomerular filtration. *Half-life:* 2 to 3
hours (adults); 30 to 86 hours (patients
with severe renal damage).

Route	Onset	Peak	Duration
I.V.	Immediate	Immediate	8-12 hr
I.M.	Unknown	1 hr	8-12 hr

Pharmacodynamics

Chemical effect: inhibits protein synthesis by binding directly to 30S ribosomal subunit. Generally bactericidal.
Therapeutic effect: kills susceptible bacteria. Its spectrum of activity includes many aerobic gram-negative organisms (including most strains of *Pseudomonas aeruginosa*) and some aerobic grampositive organisms. It is ineffective against anaerobes.

Indications and dosage

▶ **Serious infections caused by sensitive strains of** *Pseudomonas aeruginosa,* *Escherichia coli, Proteus, Klebsiella, Serratia, Enterobacter, Acinetobacter, Providencia, Citrobacter, Staphylococcus;* **meningitis.** *Adults and children:* 15 mg/kg/day divided q 8 to 12 hours I.M. or I.V. infusion. *Neonates:* initially, loading dose of 10 mg/kg I.V., followed by 7.5 mg/kg q 12 hours.
▶ **Uncomplicated urinary tract infections.** *Adults:* 250 mg I.M. or I.V. b.i.d.
▶ **Adults with impaired renal function.** *Adults:* initially, 7.5 mg/kg I.M. or I.V. Subsequent doses and frequency determined by amikacin blood level and renal function studies.

Adverse reactions

CNS: headache, lethargy, *neuromuscular blockade.*
EENT: *ototoxicity (tinnitus, vertigo, hearing loss).*
GU: *nephrotoxicity (cells or casts in urine, oliguria, proteinuria, decreased creatinine clearance, increased BUN and serum creatinine levels).*
Hepatic: *hepatic necrosis.*
Other: hypersensitivity reactions *(anaphylaxis).*

Interactions

Drug-drug. *Acyclovir, amphotericin B, cisplatin, methoxyflurane, other aminoglycosides, vancomycin:* increased nephrotoxicity. Use together cautiously.
Cephalothin: increased nephrotoxicity. Use together cautiously.
Dimenhydrinate: may mask symptoms of ototoxicity. Use with caution.
General anesthetics, neuromuscular blocking agents: may potentiate neuromuscular blockade. Monitor patient.
Indomethacin: may increase serum trough and peak levels of amikacin. Monitor serum amikacin level closely.
I.V. loop diuretics (such as furosemide): increased ototoxicity. Use together cautiously.
Parenteral penicillins (such as ticarcillin): amikacin inactivation in vitro. Don't mix.

Contraindications and precautions

• Contraindicated in patients with hypersensitivity to drug or other aminoglycosides and in breast-feeding women.
• Use with extreme caution in pregnant women and only if benefit outweighs risk to fetus.
• Use cautiously in patients with impaired renal function or neuromuscular disorders, in neonates and infants, and in elderly patients.

NURSING CONSIDERATIONS

Assessment
• Assess patient's infection, hearing, weight, and renal function studies before therapy and regularly thereafter.
• Monitor serum amikacin level. Obtain blood for peak amikacin level 1 hour after I.M. injection and 30 minutes to 1 hour after infusion ends; for trough level, draw blood just before next dose. Don't collect blood in heparinized tube because heparin is incompatible with aminoglycosides. Be aware that peak blood level above 35 mcg/ml and trough level above 10 mcg/ml may be associated with higher incidence of toxicity.
• Be alert for adverse reactions and drug interactions.
• Evaluate patient's and family's knowledge of drug therapy.

✦ Nursing diagnoses
- Infection related to bacteria
- Altered urinary elimination related to amikacin-induced nephrotoxicity
- Knowledge deficit related to drug therapy

▶ Planning and implementation
- Obtain specimen for culture and sensitivity tests before first dose. Therapy may begin pending results.

I.V. use: For adults, dilute in 100 to 200 ml of D_5W or 0.9% NaCl and infuse over 30 to 60 minutes. Volume for pediatric patients depends on dose of drug ordered. Infants should receive a 1- to 2-hour infusion. After I.V. infusion, flush line with 0.9% NaCl solution or D_5W.

I.M. use: Follow normal protocol.
- Know that therapy usually continues for 7 to 10 days.
- Be aware that drug potency is not affected if solution turns light yellow.
- Encourage adequate fluid intake; patient should be well hydrated while taking drug to minimize chemical irritation of renal tubules.
- Know that if no response occurs after 3 to 5 days, therapy may be stopped and new specimens obtained for culture and sensitivity testing.

Patient teaching
- Tell patient to immediately report changes in hearing or appearance or elimination pattern of urine. Teach patient how to measure intake and output.
- Emphasize importance of drinking 2,000 ml of fluid daily, if not contraindicated.
- Teach patient to watch for and promptly report signs of superinfection (continued fever and other signs of new infections, especially of upper respiratory tract).

☑ Evaluation
- Patient's infection is eradicated.
- Patient's renal function studies remain unchanged.
- Patient and family state understanding of drug therapy.

amiloride hydrochloride
(uh-MIL-uh-righd high-droh-KLOR-ighd)
Kaluril◇, Midamor

Pharmacologic class: potassium-sparing diuretic
Therapeutic class: diuretic, antihypertensive
Pregnancy risk category: B

How supplied
Tablets: 5 mg

Pharmacokinetics
Absorption: about 50% of dose is absorbed from GI tract; food decreases absorption to 30%.
Distribution: has wide extravascular distribution.
Metabolism: insignificant.
Excretion: excreted primarily in urine.
Half-life: 6 to 9 hours.

Route	Onset	Peak	Duration
P.O.	≤ 2 hr	6-10 hr	24 hr

Pharmacodynamics
Chemical effect: inhibits sodium reabsorption and potassium excretion in distal tubule.
Therapeutic effect: reduces blood pressure; promotes sodium and water excretion while blocking potassium excretion.

Indications and dosage
▶ **Hypertension; edema associated with heart failure, usually in patients also taking thiazide or other potassium-wasting diuretics.** *Adults:* usual dosage is 5 mg P.O. daily. Increased to 10 mg daily, if necessary. Maximum dosage is 20 mg daily.

Adverse reactions
CNS: *headache,* weakness, dizziness.
CV: orthostatic hypotension.
GI: *nausea, anorexia, diarrhea, vomiting,* abdominal pain, constipation.
GU: impotence.

Hematologic: *aplastic anemia.*
Metabolic: hyperkalemia.

Interactions

Drug-drug. *ACE inhibitors, potassium-containing salt substitutes, potassium-sparing diuretics, potassium supplements:* possible hyperkalemia. Avoid concomitant use.
Lithium: decreased lithium clearance, increasing risk of lithium toxicity. Monitor lithium level.
NSAIDs: decreased diuretic effectiveness. Avoid concomitant use.
Drug-food. *Foods high in potassium, potassium-containing salt substitutes:* possible hyperkalemia. Monitor serum potassium.

Contraindications and precautions

• Contraindicated in patients with elevated serum potassium level (over 5.5 mEq/L); in those receiving other potassium-sparing diuretics such as spironolactone; in those with anuria, acute or chronic renal insufficiency, diabetic nephropathy, or hypersensitivity to drug; and in breast-feeding women.
• Use with extreme caution, if at all, in patients with diabetes mellitus.
• Use cautiously in patients with severe hepatic insufficiency; in pregnant women; and in elderly or debilitated patients.
• Safety of drug has not been established in children.

NURSING CONSIDERATIONS

Assessment
• Assess patient's blood pressure, urine output, weight, serum electrolytes, and degree of edema before therapy and regularly thereafter.
• Be alert for adverse reactions and drug interactions.
• Evaluate patient's and family's knowledge of drug therapy.

Nursing diagnoses
• Fluid volume excess related to fluid retention
• Risk for injury related to potential for drug-induced hyperkalemia
• Knowledge deficit related to drug therapy

Planning and implementation
• Administer amiloride with meals to prevent nausea.
• Administer early in the day to prevent nocturia.
• Alert doctor immediately if potassium level exceeds 6.5 mEq/L, and expect drug to be discontinued.
• Choose diet with caution.
Patient teaching
• Advise patient to avoid sudden posture changes and to rise slowly to avoid orthostatic hypotension.
• Warn patient to limit potassium-rich foods (such as oranges and bananas), potassium-containing salt substitutes, and potassium supplements to prevent serious hyperkalemia.
• Teach patient and family to identify and report signs of hyperkalemia.
• Teach patient and family to monitor patient's fluid volume by recording daily weight and intake and output.

Evaluation
• Patient's fluid retention is relieved.
• Patient's serum potassium level remains normal.
• Patient and family state understanding of drug therapy.

amino acid infusions, crystalline
(uh-MEEN-oh AS-id in-FYOO-zhuns)
Aminosyn, Aminosyn II, Aminosyn-PF, FreAmine III, Novamine, Travasol, TrophAmine

amino acid infusions in dextrose
Aminosyn II with Dextrose

amino acid infusions with electrolytes

Aminosyn with Electrolytes, Aminosyn II with Electrolytes, FreAmine III with Electrolytes, ProcalAmine with Electrolytes, Travasol with Electrolytes

amino acid infusions with electrolytes in dextrose

Aminosyn II with Electrolytes in Dextrose

amino acid infusions for hepatic failure

HepatAmine

amino acid infusions for high metabolic stress

Aminosyn-HBC, BranchAmin, FreAmine HBC

amino acid infusions for renal failure

Aminess, Aminosyn-RF, Nephr-Amine, RenAmin

Pharmacologic class: protein substrate
Therapeutic class: parenteral nutritional therapy and caloric agent
Pregnancy risk category: C

How supplied

Injection: 250 ml, 500 ml, 1,000 ml, 2,000 ml containing amino acids in varying concentrations. *Crystalline:* Aminosyn, 3.5%, 5%, 7%, 8.5%, 10%. Aminosyn II, 3.5%, 5%, 7%, 8.5%, 10%. Aminosyn-PF, 7%, 10%. FreAmine III, 8.5%, 10%. Novamine, 11.4%, 15%. Travasol, 5.5%, 8.5%, 10%. TrophAmine, 6%, 10%. *In dextrose:* Aminosyn II, 3.5% in 5% dextrose, 3.5% in 25% dextrose, 4.25% in 10% dextrose, 4.25% in 20% dextrose, 4.25% in 25% dextrose, 5% in 25% dextrose. *With electrolytes:* Aminosyn, 3.5%, 7%, 8.5%. Aminosyn II, 3.5%, 7%, 8.5%, 10%. FreAmine III, 3%, 8.5%. ProcalAmine, 3%. Travasol, 3.5%, 5.5%, 8.5%. *With electrolytes in dextrose:* Aminosyn II,

3.5% with electrolytes in 5% dextrose, 4.25% with electrolytes in 10% dextrose. *For hepatic failure:* HepatAmine, 8%. *For high metabolic stress:* Aminosyn-HBC, 7%. BranchAmin, 4%. FreAmine HBC, 6.9%. *For renal failure:* Aminess, 5.2%. Aminosyn-RF, 5.2%. NephrAmine, 5.4%. RenAmin, 6.5%.

Pharmacokinetics

No information available.

Route	Onset	Peak	Duration
I.V.	Immediate	Immediate	Unknown

Pharmacodynamics

Chemical effect: provides substrate for protein synthesis or enhances conservation of existing body protein. Formulations for hepatic failure and high metabolic stress contain essential and nonessential amino acids, with high concentrations of branched chain amino acids isoleucine, leucine, and valine. Formulations for renal failure contain histidine and minimal amounts of essential amino acids; nonessential amino acids are synthesized from excess ammonia in blood of uremic patient, thus lowering azotemia.
Therapeutic effect: provides body with needed calories and protein.

Indications and dosage

▶ **Total parenteral nutrition in patients who cannot or will not eat.** *Adults:* 1 to 1.5 g/kg I.V. daily. *Children:* 2 to 3 g/kg I.V. daily.
▶ **Nutritional support in patients with cirrhosis, hepatitis, or hepatic encephalopathy.** *Adults:* 80 to 120 g of amino acids (12 to 18 g of nitrogen) I.V. daily using formulation for hepatic failure.
▶ **Nutritional support in patients with high metabolic stress.** *Adults:* 1.5 g/kg I.V. daily using formulation for high metabolic stress.

Adverse reactions

CNS: mental confusion, unconsciousness, headache, dizziness.
CV: hypervolemia, *heart failure* (in susceptible patients), *pulmonary edema,* exacerbation of hypertension (in predisposed patients), thrombophlebitis, thrombosis.
GI: nausea, vomiting.
GU: glycosuria, osmotic diuresis.
Hepatic: fatty liver.
Skin: chills, flushing, feeling of warmth.
Metabolic: *rebound hypoglycemia* (when long-term infusion is abruptly stopped), hyperglycemia, metabolic acidosis, alkalosis, hypophosphatemia, *hyperosmolar hyperglycemic nonketotic syndrome,* hyperammonemia, electrolyte imbalances.
Other: hypersensitivity reactions, tissue sloughing at infusion site caused by extravasation, *catheter sepsis,* dehydration (if hyperosmolar solutions are used).

Interactions

Drug-drug. *Tetracycline:* may reduce protein-sparing effects of infused amino acids because of its antianabolic activity. Monitor patient.

Contraindications and precautions

• Contraindicated in patients with anuria; inborn errors of amino acid metabolism, such as maple syrup urine disease and isovaleric acidemia; severe uncorrected electrolyte or acid-base imbalances; hyperammonemia; or decreased circulating blood volume.
• Use with extreme caution in pediatric patients and in neonates, especially those with low birth weight.
• Use cautiously in patients with renal insufficiency or failure, cardiac disease, or hepatic impairment.
• Use with caution in diabetic patients; insulin may be required to prevent hyperglycemia. Administer cautiously in cardiac insufficiency; may cause circulatory overload. Patients with fluid restriction may tolerate only 1 to 2 L.

NURSING CONSIDERATIONS

▨ Assessment

• Assess serum electrolyte, glucose, BUN, calcium, and phosphate levels before therapy, as ordered, and regularly thereafter.
• Be alert for adverse reactions and drug interactions.
• Check infusion site frequently for erythema, inflammation, irritation, tissue sloughing, necrosis, and phlebitis.
• Evaluate patient's and family's knowledge of drug therapy.

▣ Nursing diagnoses

• Altered nutrition (less than body requirements) related to patient's underlying condition
• Risk for fluid volume deficit related to adverse drug reactions
• Knowledge deficit related to drug therapy

▶ Planning and implementation

• Control infusion rate carefully with infusion pump. If infusion rate falls behind, notify doctor; do not increase rate to catch up.
• Know that peripheral infusions should be limited to 2.5% amino acids and dextrose 10%.
• Know that doctor will individualize dosage according to patient's metabolic and clinical response as determined by nitrogen balance and body weight corrected for fluid balance.
• Add vitamins, electrolytes, and trace elements, as ordered.
• If patient has chills, fever, or other signs of sepsis, replace I.V. tubing and bottle and send them to laboratory to be cultured.
Patient teaching
• Tell patient to report discomfort at injection site or unusual symptoms.

☑ Evaluation

• Patient's nutritional status improves.
• Patient maintains adequate hydration.

Reactions may be *common,* uncommon, *life-threatening*, or COMMON AND LIFE-THREATENING.

• Patient and family state understanding of drug therapy.

aminocaproic acid
(uh-mee-noh-kah-PROH-ik AS-id)
Amicar

Pharmacologic class: carboxylic acid derivative
Therapeutic class: fibrinolysis inhibitor
Pregnancy risk category: C

How supplied

Tablets: 500 mg
Syrup: 250 mg/ml
Injection: 5 g/20 ml for dilution, 24 g/96 ml for infusion

Pharmacokinetics

Absorption: rapidly and completely absorbed from GI tract when administered orally.
Distribution: readily permeates human blood cells and other body cells. It is not protein-bound.
Metabolism: insignificant.
Excretion: from 40% to 60% of single oral dose is excreted unchanged in urine in 12 hours.

Route	Onset	Peak	Duration
P.O.	≤ 1 hr	≤ 2 hr	Unknown
I.V.	≤ 1 hr	Unknown	< 3 hr

Pharmacodynamics

Chemical effect: inhibits plasminogen activator substances and blocks antiplasmin activity.
Therapeutic effect: promotes blood-clotting activity.

Indications and dosage

▶ **Excessive bleeding from hyperfibrinolysis.** *Adults:* 4 to 5 g I.V. or P.O. over first hour, followed with constant infusion of 1 g/hour for about 8 hours or until bleeding is controlled. Maximum dosage is 30 g/24 hours.

Adverse reactions

CNS: dizziness, headache, delirium, *seizures,* weakness, malaise.
CV: hypotension, bradycardia, *arrhythmias* (with rapid I.V. infusion).
EENT: tinnitus, nasal stuffiness, conjunctival suffusion.
GI: nausea, cramps, diarrhea.
Hematologic: generalized thrombosis.
Skin: rash.
Other: myopathy, *acute renal failure.*

Interactions

Drug-drug. *Estrogens, oral contraceptives:* increased probability of hypercoagulability. Use together cautiously.

Contraindications and precautions

• Contraindicated in patients with active intravascular clotting or DIC unless heparin is used concomitantly. Injectable form is contraindicated in newborns.
• Use cautiously in patients with cardiac, hepatic, or renal disease and in pregnant or breast-feeding women.
• Safety of drug has not been established in children.

NURSING CONSIDERATIONS

⚕ Assessment
• Assess history of blood loss, coagulation studies, blood pressure, and heart rhythm before therapy.
• Monitor coagulation studies throughout therapy, as ordered.
• Observe heart rhythm, especially when giving I.V. dose.
• Be alert for adverse reactions and drug interactions.
• Evaluate patient's and family's knowledge of drug therapy.

⚕ Nursing diagnoses
• Fluid volume deficit related to excessive bleeding
• Altered venous tissue perfusion related to drug-induced generalized thrombosis
• Knowledge deficit related to drug therapy

---

*Liquid form contains alcohol **May contain tartrazine ♦Canada ◊ Australia †OTC

⧉ Planning and implementation
P.O. use: Follow normal protocol.
I.V. use: Dilute solution with sterile water for injection, 0.9% NaCl injection, D₅W, or Ringer's injection. Infuse slowly. Don't give by direct or intermittent injection.
• Keep oxygen and resuscitation equipment nearby.
Patient teaching
• Explain all procedures to patient and family.
• Instruct patient and family to report respiratory difficulty, pain, or changes in mental status immediately.

☑ Evaluation
• Patient regains normal fluid volume status.
• Patient shows no signs of impaired venous tissue perfusion.
• Patient and family state understanding of drug therapy.

---

aminoglutethimide
(uh-mee-noh-gloo-TETH-ih-mighd)
Cytadren

Pharmacologic class: antiadrenal hormone
Therapeutic class: antineoplastic
Pregnancy risk category: D

How supplied
Tablets: 250 mg

Pharmacokinetics
Absorption: well absorbed through GI tract.
Distribution: distributed widely into body tissues.
Metabolism: metabolized extensively in liver.
Excretion: excreted primarily through kidneys, mostly as unchanged drug. *Half-life:* 12½ hours (7 hours with prolonged treatment).

Route	Onset	Peak	Duration
P.O.	Unknown	1.5 hr	1.5-3 days

Pharmacodynamics
Chemical effect: blocks conversion of cholesterol to delta-5-pregnenolone in adrenal cortex, inhibiting synthesis of adrenal steroids.
Therapeutic effect: decreases adrenocortical hormone levels.

Indications and dosage
▶ **Suppression of adrenal function in Cushing's syndrome and adrenal cancer.** *Adults:* 250 mg q.i.d. at 6-hour intervals. Dosage may be increased in increments of 250 mg daily q 1 to 2 weeks to maximum daily dosage of 2 g.

Adverse reactions
CNS: *drowsiness,* headache, dizziness.
CV: hypotension, tachycardia.
GI: nausea, anorexia.
Hematologic: transient leukopenia, *agranulocytosis, thrombocytopenia.*
Skin: *morbilliform rash,* pruritus, urticaria.
Other: fever, myalgia, adrenal insufficiency, masculinization, hirsutism, hypothyroidism.

Interactions
Drug-drug. *Dexamethasone, medroxyprogesterone:* increased hepatic metabolism of these agents. Monitor closely.
Digoxin: may increase drug clearance. Monitor patient closely.
Oral anticoagulants: decreased anticoagulant effect. Monitor PT.
Theophylline: reduced action of theophylline. Monitor patient closely.
Drug-lifestyle. *Alcohol use:* may potentiate effects of aminoglutethimide. Avoid concomitant use.

Contraindications and precautions
• Contraindicated in patients with hypersensitivity to drug or glutethimide and in breast-feeding women.

Reactions may be *common,* uncommon, *life-threatening*, or COMMON AND LIFE-THREATENING.

• Use with extreme caution in pregnancy because drug can harm fetus.
• Safety of drug has not been established in children.

NURSING CONSIDERATIONS

⚖ Assessment
• Assess patient's underlying condition before therapy and note improvement.
• Monitor for adrenal hypofunction, especially under stressful conditions, such as surgery, trauma, or acute illness.
• Be alert for adverse reactions and drug interactions.
• Evaluate patient's and family's knowledge of drug therapy.

🔁 Nursing diagnoses
• Altered health maintenance related to patient's underlying condition
• Altered protection related to drug-induced adrenal suppression
• Knowledge deficit related to drug therapy

⟫ Planning and implementation
• Administer on schedule and alert doctor if dose is delayed or missed.
• Know that patient may require more supplements during stress. For example, patient may need mineralocorticoid supplement to treat hyponatremia and orthostatic hypotension. Glucocorticoid replacement also may be necessary.
Patient teaching
• Instruct patient to notify doctor of stress; additional therapy may be required.
• Caution patient to watch for signs of infection (fever, sore throat, fatigue) and bleeding (easy bruising, nosebleeds, bleeding gums, melena). Tell patient to take temperature daily.
• Warn patient to avoid activities that require alertness and motor coordination until CNS effects of drug are known.
• Advise patient to stand up slowly to minimize orthostatic hypotension.

• Tell patient to report rash that persists for more than 8 days. Reassure patient that drowsiness, nausea, and loss of appetite usually diminish within 2 weeks after start of therapy, but advise him to notify doctor if symptoms persist.
• Advise patient to avoid alcohol consumption during drug therapy.

☑ Evaluation
• Patient's health is maintained.
• Patient does not exhibit hypoadrenalism.
• Patient and family state understanding of drug therapy.

aminophylline (theophylline and ethylenediamine)
(uh-mih-NOF-il-in)
Aminophyllin, Cardophyllin◇, Corophyllin♦, Phyllocontin, Phyllocontin-350, Somophyllin, Somophyllin-DF

Pharmacologic class: xanthine derivative
Therapeutic class: bronchodilator
Pregnancy risk category: C

How supplied
Tablets: 100 mg, 200 mg
Tablets (extended-release): 225 mg, 350 mg♦
Oral liquid: 105 mg/5 ml
Injection: 250 mg/10 ml, 500 mg/20 ml, 500 mg/2 ml, 100 mg/100 ml in 0.45% NaCl, 200 mg/100 ml in 0.45% NaCl
Rectal suppositories: 250 mg, 500 mg

Pharmacokinetics
Absorption: well absorbed except for suppository form, which is unreliable and slow. Food may alter rate but not extent of absorption of oral doses.
Distribution: distributed in all tissues and extracellular fluids except fatty tissue.
Metabolism: converted to theophylline, then metabolized to inactive compounds.

Excretion: excreted in urine as theophylline (10%). *Half-life:* depends on many variables, including smoking status, concurrent illness, age, and formulation used.

Route	Onset	Peak	Duration
P.O.			
Tablets	15-60 min	2 hr	Varies
Extended-release	Unknown	4-7 hr	Varies
Solution	15-60 min	≤ 1 hr	Varies
I.V.	15 min	Immediate	Varies
P.R.	Varies	Varies	Varies

Pharmacodynamics

Chemical effect: inhibits phosphodiesterase, the enzyme that degrades cAMP, thereby relaxing smooth muscle of bronchial airways and pulmonary blood vessels.
Therapeutic effect: eases breathing.

Indications and dosage

▶ **Symptomatic relief of bronchospasm.** *Patients not currently receiving theophylline products who require rapid relief of symptoms:* loading dose is 6 mg/kg (equivalent to 4.7 mg/kg anhydrous theophylline) I.V. (25 mg/minute or less), then maintenance infusion. *Adults (nonsmokers):* 0.7 mg/kg/hour I.V. for 12 hours; then 0.5 mg/kg/hour. *Otherwise healthy adult smokers:* 1 mg/kg/hour I.V. for 12 hours; then 0.8 mg/kg/hour. *Older patients and adults with cor pulmonale:* 0.6 mg/kg/hour I.V. for 12 hours; then 0.3 mg/kg/hour. *Adults with heart failure or liver disease:* 0.5 mg/kg/hour I.V. for 12 hours; then 0.1 to 0.2 mg/kg/hour. *Children ages 9 to 16:* 1 mg/kg/hour I.V. for 12 hours; then 0.8 mg/kg/hour. *Children ages 6 months to 9 years:* 1.2 mg/kg/hour for 12 hours; then 1 mg/kg/hour. *Patients currently receiving theophylline products:* aminophylline infusion of 0.63 mg/kg (0.5 mg/kg anhydrous theophylline) increases plasma level of theophylline by 1 mcg/ml. Some clinicians recommend dose of 3.1 mg/kg

(2.5 mg/kg anhydrous theophylline) with no obvious signs of theophylline toxicity.
▶ **Chronic bronchial asthma.** Dosage is highly individualized. Rectal dosage is same as that recommended for oral dosage. *Adults:* 600 to 1,600 mg P.O. daily in divided doses t.i.d. or q.i.d. *Children:* 12 mg/kg P.O. daily in divided doses t.i.d. or q.i.d.

Adverse reactions

CNS: *nervousness, restlessness, dizziness,* headache, *insomnia,* light-headedness, *seizures,* muscle twitching.
CV: *palpitations, sinus tachycardia,* extrasystole, flushing, marked hypotension, increased respiratory rate, *arrhythmias.*
GI: *nausea, vomiting, anorexia,* bitter aftertaste, dyspepsia, heavy feeling in stomach, diarrhea.
Respiratory: *respiratory arrest.*
Skin: urticaria.
Other: irritation (with rectal suppositories).

Interactions

Drug-drug. *Adenosine:* decreased antiarrhythmic effectiveness. Higher doses of adenosine may be necessary.
Alkali-sensitive drugs: reduced activity. Do not add to I.V. fluids containing aminophylline.
Allopurinol (high doses), cimetidine, influenza virus vaccine, macrolide antibiotics (such as erythromycin), oral contraceptives, quinolone antibiotics (such as ciprofloxacin): decreased hepatic clearance of theophylline; elevated theophylline blood level. Monitor for toxicity.
Amiodarone, ticlopidine, verapamil: increase theophylline levels. Use together cautiously.
Barbiturates, carbamazepine, nicotine, phenytoin, rifampin: enhanced metabolism and decreased theophylline blood level. Monitor for decreased aminophylline effect.
Beta blockers: antagonism. Propranolol and nadolol, especially, may cause bron-

chospasm in sensitive patients. Use together cautiously.
Ephedrine, other sympathomimetics:
theophylline may exhibit synergistic toxicity with these agents, predisposing patient to arrhythmias. Monitor closely.
Isoniazid, ketoconazole: decrease theophylline absorption.
Lithium: theophylline may increase lithium level. Monitor closely.
Drug-lifestyle. *Smoking:* may increase
clearance and decrease half-life of theophylline. Higher doses may be needed
to achieve desired effect.

Contraindications and precautions

• Contraindicated in patients with active
peptic ulcer disease, seizure disorders
(unless anticonvulsant therapy is given),
and hypersensitivity to xanthine compounds (caffeine, theobromine) or ethylenediamine.
• Use cautiously in neonates, infants,
young children, elderly patients, pregnant
or breast-feeding women, and patients
with heart failure or other cardiac or circulatory impairment, COPD, cor pulmonale, renal or hepatic disease, hyperthyroidism, diabetes mellitus, peptic ulcer, severe hypoxemia, or hypertension.

NURSING CONSIDERATIONS

Assessment
• Assess patient's underlying respiratory
condition.
• Monitor drug effectiveness by regularly
auscultating lungs and noting respiratory
rate and results of laboratory studies,
such as arterial blood gas analysis.
• Monitor patient's hydration status if adverse GI reactions occur.
• Be alert for adverse reactions and drug
interactions.
• Evaluate patient's and family's knowledge of drug therapy.

Nursing diagnoses
• Impaired gas exchange related to bronchospasm

• Risk for fluid volume deficit related to
drug-induced adverse GI reactions
• Knowledge deficit related to drug
therapy

Planning and implementation
• Ensure that patient has not had recent
theophylline therapy before giving loading dose.
P.O. use: Give oral drug with full glass
of water at meals. Food in stomach delays absorption. Enteric-coated tablets
may delay and impair absorption.
I.V. use: Because I.V. drug administration can cause burning, dilute with compatible I.V. solution and inject at rate no
faster than 25 mg/minute. Drug is compatible with most I.V. solutions except invert sugar, fructose, and fat emulsions.
P.R. use: Know that suppositories are
slowly and erratically absorbed.
Administer suppository if patient cannot
take drug orally, as ordered. Schedule after evacuation, if possible; may be retained better if given before meal. Have
patient remain recumbent 15 to 20 minutes after insertion.
• Know that aminophylline is a soluble
salt of theophylline and that dosage is adjusted by monitoring response, tolerance,
pulmonary function, and serum theophylline level. Theophylline concentration
should range from 10 to 20 mcg/ml; toxicity has been reported with level above
20 mcg/ml.
Patient teaching
• Supply instructions for home care and
dosage schedule. Some patients may require around-the-clock schedule.
• Warn elderly patients that dizziness is
a common adverse reaction at start of
therapy.
• Warn patient to check with doctor or
pharmacist before combining aminophylline with other drugs. OTC remedies
may contain ephedrine in combination
with theophylline salts; excessive CNS
stimulation may result.
• Advise patient to avoid switching brand
without consulting doctor.

• Tell patient to notify doctor if he has quit smoking. Dose may need to be reduced.

☑ Evaluation
• Patient's appearance, vital signs, and laboratory test results demonstrate improved gas exchange.
• Patient remains hydrated throughout therapy.
• Patient and family state understanding of drug therapy.

aminosalicylate sodium (para-amino salicylate, PAS)
(uh-MEE-noh-sal-ih-SIL-ate SOH-dee-um)
Nemasol Sodium♦, Sodium P.A.S., Tubasal

Pharmacologic class: structural analogue of aminobenzoic acid
Therapeutic class: antitubercular agent
Pregnancy risk category: NR

How supplied
Tablets: 500 mg

Pharmacokinetics
Absorption: absorbed rapidly from GI tract.
Distribution: widely distributed in various body fluids, especially in pleural and caseous tissue, but achieves low CSF concentration; only about 15% bound to protein.
Metabolism: metabolized in liver.
Excretion: over 80% excreted through kidneys as metabolites and free acid.
Half-life: about 1 hour (up to 23 hours in decreased renal function).

Route	Onset	Peak	Duration
P.O.	Unknown	1-2 hr	Unknown

Pharmacodynamics
Chemical effect: unknown. Believed to suppress growth and reproduction of *Mycobacterium tuberculosis* by inhibiting folic acid formation.

Therapeutic effect: thought to exert antitubercular effects.

Indications and dosage
▶ **Adjunct treatment of tuberculosis.**
Adults: 4 g P.O. q 8 hours. Maximum daily dosage is 12 g. Must be taken with other antitubercular agents. *Children:* 75 mg/kg P.O. q 12 hours. Maximum daily dosage is 12 g. Must be taken with other antitubercular agents.

Adverse reactions
GI: abdominal pain, nausea, vomiting, diarrhea, anorexia.
GU: crystalluria.
Hematologic: hemolytic anemia, *agranulocytosis, thrombocytopenia.*
Hepatic: *hepatitis.*
Skin: rash.
Other: hypersensitivity reactions (eosinophilia, joint pain, fever), mononucleosis-like syndrome, goiter or myxedema (with long-term therapy).

Interactions
Drug-drug. *Aminobenzoate derivatives:* decreased absorption of aminosalicylate sodium from GI tract. Avoid concomitant use.
Cyanocobalamin (vitamin B_{12}): decreased absorption of vitamin B_{12} from GI tract. Provide parenteral supplement as ordered.
Digoxin: may decrease digoxin absorption. Monitor patient closely.
Probenecid, sulfinpyrazone: decreased excretion of aminosalicylate sodium, resulting in toxicity. Monitor patient closely.
Rifampin: may impair rifampin absorption. Separate administration times by at least 6 hours.
Warfarin, other anticoagulants: enhanced anticoagulant effect. Monitor for bleeding.

Contraindications and precautions
• Contraindicated in patients with hypersensitivity to drug, other salicylates, or sulfonamides.

• Use cautiously in patients with peptic ulcer or other GI disease and in those with heart failure. Also use cautiously in patients who may become pregnant and in breast-feeding women.

NURSING CONSIDERATIONS

⚖ Assessment
• Assess patient's history of tuberculosis.
• Monitor patient's hydration status if adverse GI reactions occur.
• Be alert for adverse reactions and drug interactions.
• Evaluate patient's and family's knowledge of drug therapy.

🔅 Nursing diagnoses
• Altered health maintenance related to patient's underlying condition
• Risk for fluid volume deficit related to drug-induced adverse GI reactions
• Knowledge deficit related to drug therapy

⊠ Planning and implementation
• Be aware that therapy may last for 1 to 2 years (and sometimes indefinitely), although shorter treatment regimens have been effective in some patients.
• Administer with or after meals or with an antacid if gastric irritation occurs. If irritation persists, notify doctor, who may order temporary dosage reduction or rest period of up to 2 weeks. Drug may then be restarted in small daily doses and gradually increased to full therapeutic doses.
• Know that total daily dose may be given as single dose, if tolerated.
• Expect to administer other antitubercular agents concurrently.
• Be aware that urine glucose determinations may be false-positive with copper sulfate tests (Benedict's solution, Clinitest); glucose enzymatic tests (Diastix or Chemstrip uG) are not affected.
Patient teaching
• Advise patient to take drug with meals or antacids to minimize adverse GI ef-

fects. Children may tolerate drug better than adults.
• Tell patient to report back pain; pain during urination; unusual bruising or bleeding; fever or sore throat; yellow eyes, sclera, or skin; or severe joint pain.
• Encourage patient to comply with therapy, which may last several years.
• Instruct patient to store drug away from heat, humidity, and direct sunlight and not to take discolored tablets.

☑ Evaluation
• Patient's health is maintained.
• Patient remains hydrated throughout therapy.
• Patient and family state understanding of drug therapy.

---

amiodarone hydrochloride
(am-ee-OH-dah-rohn high-droh-KLOR-ighd)
Aratac◊, Cordarone, Cordarone X◊

Pharmacologic class: benzofuran derivative
Therapeutic class: ventricular antiarrhythmic
Pregnancy risk category: D

How supplied

Tablets: 100 mg♦ ◊, 200 mg
Injection: 50 mg/ml◊

Pharmacokinetics

Absorption: slow, variable absorption with oral administration.
Distribution: distributed widely, accumulating in adipose tissue and in organs with marked perfusion, such as lungs, liver, and spleen. It is highly protein–bound (96%).
Metabolism: metabolized extensively in liver to active metabolite, desethyl amiodarone.
Excretion: main excretory route is hepatic through biliary tree. *Half-life:* 25 to 110 days (usually, 40 to 50 days).

Route	Onset	Peak	Duration
P.O.	2-21 days	3-7 hr	Varies
I.V.	Unknown	Unknown	Unknown

Pharmacodynamics

Chemical effect: unknown; thought to prolong refractory period and action potential duration and decrease repolarization.
Therapeutic effect: abolishes ventricular arrhythmia.

Indications and dosage

▶ **Recurrent ventricular fibrillation and unstable ventricular tachycardia.**
Adults: loading dose of 800 to 1,600 mg P.O. daily for 1 to 3 weeks until initial therapeutic response occurs, then 650 to 800 mg P.O. daily for 1 month, then 200 to 600 mg P.O. daily as maintenance dosage. Or, for first 24 hours, 150 mg I.V. over 10 minutes (mixed in 100 ml D_5W); then 360 mg I.V. over 6 hours (mix 900 mg in 500 ml D_5W); then maintenance of 540 mg I.V. over 18 hours at a rate of 0.5 mg/minute. After first 24 hours, continue a maintenance infusion of 0.5 mg/minute in a 1 to 6 mg/ml concentration. For infusions greater than 1 hour, concentrations should not exceed 2 mg/ml unless a central venous catheter is used. Do not use for more than 3 weeks.

Adverse reactions

CNS: peripheral neuropathy, extrapyramidal symptoms, headache, muscle weakness, *malaise, fatigue.*
CV: bradycardia, hypotension, ***arrhythmias, heart failure, heart block, sinus arrest.***
EENT: *corneal microdeposits,* vision disturbances.
GI: *nausea, vomiting,* constipation.
Hepatic: *altered liver enzymes test results,* hepatic dysfunction.
Respiratory: SEVERE PULMONARY TOXICITY (PNEUMONITIS, ALVEOLITIS).
Skin: *photosensitivity,* blue-gray skin.

Other: hypothyroidism, hyperthyroidism, gynecomastia.

Interactions

Drug-drug. *Antiarrhythmics:* amiodarone may reduce hepatic or renal clearance of certain antiarrhythmics (especially flecainide, procainamide, or quinidine); concomitant use of amiodarone with other antiarrhythmics (especially mexiletine, propafenone, quinidine, disopyramide, or procainamide) may induce torsades de pointes. Monitor ECG closely.
Antihypertensives: increased hypotensive effect. Use together cautiously.
Beta blockers, calcium channel blockers: increased cardiac depressant effects; may potentiate slowing of sinus node and AV conduction. Use together cautiously.
Cardiac glycosides: increased serum digoxin level (average of 70% to 100%). Monitor digoxin level closely.
Cimetidine: interferes with action of amiodarone causing increased amiodarone levels. Avoid concomitant use.
Cholestyramine: decreased serum levels and half-life of amiodarone. Avoid concomitant use.
Cyclosporine: increased concentrations of cyclosporine. Monitor serum creatinine.
Phenytoin: may decrease phenytoin metabolism. Monitor serum phenytoin level.
Theophylline: increased theophylline level with toxicity may occur. Monitor serum theophylline level.
Warfarin: increased INR (average of 100% within 1 to 4 weeks of therapy). Warfarin dosage should be decreased 33% to 50% when amiodarone is initiated. Monitor patient closely.
Drug-lifestyle. *Sun exposure:* photosensitivity reaction may occur. Avoid prolonged or unprotected sun exposure.

Contraindications and precautions

• Contraindicated in patients with hypersensitive to drug; in those with severe sinus node disease resulting in preexisting

bradycardia; in those with second- or third-degree AV block unless artificial pacemaker is present; in those in whom bradycardia has caused syncope; and in breast-feeding women.
• Use with extreme caution in patients receiving other antiarrhythmics and in pregnant women.
• Use cautiously in patients with pulmonary or thyroid disease.
• Safety of drug has not been established in children.

NURSING CONSIDERATIONS

ℤ Assessment
• Assess CV status before therapy.
• Review pulmonary, liver, and thyroid function test results before and regularly during therapy.
• Continuously monitor cardiac status of patient receiving I.V. amiodarone to evaluate its effectiveness.
• Be alert for adverse reactions and drug interactions.
• Monitor carefully for pulmonary toxicity, which can be fatal. Incidence increases in patients receiving more than 400 mg/day.
• Monitor serum electrolytes, particularly potassium and magnesium levels.
• Evaluate patient's and family's knowledge of drug therapy.

Nursing diagnoses
• Decreased cardiac output related to ventricular arrhythmia
• Risk for injury related to drug-induced adverse reactions
• Knowledge deficit related to drug therapy

Planning and implementation
• Be aware that high incidence of adverse reactions limits drug's use.
• Administer loading doses in hospital setting with continuous ECG monitoring because of slow onset of antiarrhythmic effect and risk of life-threatening arrhythmias.

P.O. use: Divide oral loading dose into three equal doses and give with meals to decrease GI intolerance. Maintenance dosage may be given once daily or divided into two doses taken with meals if GI intolerance occurs.
I.V. use: Know that amiodarone may be given I.V. where facilities for close monitoring of cardiac function and resuscitation are available. Initial dosage of 5 mg/kg should be mixed in 250 ml of 5% dextrose solution. Repeat doses preferably should be administered through central venous catheter. Patient should receive maximum of 1.2 g in up to 500 ml of 5% dextrose solution daily.
• Maintain ECG monitoring during initiation and alteration of dosage. Notify doctor of any significant change.
• Recommend instillation of methylcellulose ophthalmic solution during amiodarone therapy to minimize corneal microdeposits.

Patient teaching
• Stress importance of taking medication exactly as prescribed.
• Emphasize importance of close follow-up and regular diagnostic studies to monitor drug action and assess for adverse reactions.
• Warn patient that drug may cause blue-gray skin pigmentation.
• Advise patient to use sunscreen to prevent photosensitivity reaction (burning or tingling skin followed by erythema and possible skin blistering).
• Inform patient that adverse effects are more prevalent at high doses but are generally reversible when therapy stops. Resolution of adverse reactions may take up to 4 months.

✓ Evaluation
• Patient's arrhythmia is corrected.
• Patient does not experience injury from adverse reactions.
• Patient and family state understanding of drug therapy.

---

amitriptyline hydrochloride
(am-ih-TRIP-tuh-leen high-droh-KLOR-ighd)
Apo-Amitriptyline♦, Elavil, Emitrip, Endep, Enovil, Levate♦, Novotriptyn♦, PMS-Amitriptyline, Tryptanol◊

amitriptyline pamoate
Elavil♦

Pharmacologic class: tricyclic antidepressant
Therapeutic class: antidepressant
Pregnancy risk category: NR

How supplied
Tablets: 10 mg, 25 mg, 50 mg, 75 mg, 100 mg, 150 mg
Injection: 10 mg/ml
Syrup: 10 mg/5 ml

Pharmacokinetics
Absorption: absorbed rapidly from GI tract after oral administration and from muscle tissue after I.M. administration.
Distribution: distributed widely into body, including CNS and breast milk. Drug is 96% protein–bound.
Metabolism: metabolized by liver to active metabolite nortriptyline; significant first-pass effect may account for variable serum concentrations in different patients taking same dosage.
Excretion: most of drug is excreted in urine.

Route	Onset	Peak	Duration
P.O., I.M.	Unknown	2-12 hr	Unknown

Pharmacodynamics
Chemical effect: unknown, but tricyclic antidepressant (TCA) increases norepinephrine, serotonin, or both in CNS by blocking their reuptake by presynaptic neurons.
Therapeutic effect: relieves depression.

Indications and dosage
▶ **Depression.** *Adults:* 50 to 100 mg P.O. h.s., increasing to 150 mg daily; maximum dosage is 300 mg daily, if needed. Or 20 to 30 mg I.M. q.i.d. *Elderly patients and adolescents:* 10 mg P.O. t.i.d. and 20 mg h.s. daily.

Adverse reactions
CNS: *drowsiness, dizziness,* excitation, tremors, weakness, confusion, headache, nervousness, EEG alterations, *seizures,* extrapyramidal reactions.
CV: *orthostatic hypotension, tachycardia, ECG changes,* hypertension, *MI, stroke, arrhythmias.*
EENT: *blurred vision,* tinnitus, mydriasis.
GI: *dry mouth, constipation,* nausea, vomiting, anorexia, paralytic ileus.
GU: *urine retention.*
Hematologic: *agranulocytosis, thrombocytopenia.*
Skin: rash, urticaria, photosensitivity.
Other: *diaphoresis,* hypersensitivity reactions.
After abrupt withdrawal of long-term therapy: nausea, headache, malaise (does not indicate addiction).

Interactions
Drug-drug. *Barbiturates, CNS depressants:* enhanced CNS depression. Avoid concomitant use.
Cimetidine, methylphenidate: increased TCA blood levels. Monitor for enhanced antidepressant effect.
Clonidine: hypertensive crises have occurred. Avoid concomitant use.
Epinephrine, norepinephrine: increased hypertensive effect. Use with caution.
Guanethidine: antagonize the antihypertensive action of guanethidine. Monitor patient.
MAO inhibitors: may cause severe excitation, hyperpyrexia, or seizures, usually with high dosage. Use with caution.
Drug-lifestyle. *Alcohol use:* enhanced CNS depression. Avoid concomitant use.

Reactions may be *common,* uncommon, *life-threatening,* or COMMON AND LIFE-THREATENING.

Smoking: may lower plasma concentrations of drug. Monitor for lack of effect.
Sun exposure: increased risk of photosensitivity reactions. Avoid prolonged or unprotected sun exposure.

Contraindications and precautions

• Contraindicated during acute recovery phase of MI, in patients with hypersensitivity to drug, in patients who have received an MAO inhibitor within past 14 days, and in breast-feeding women.
• Use cautiously in patients with history of seizures, urine retention, angle-closure glaucoma, or increased intraocular pressure; in those with hyperthyroidism, CV disease, diabetes, or impaired liver function; in those receiving thyroid medications; and during pregnancy.
• Don't use drug in children younger than age 12.

NURSING CONSIDERATIONS

⚚ Assessment
• Assess patient's depression before therapy.
• Be alert for adverse reactions and drug interactions.
• Evaluate patient's and family's knowledge of drug therapy.

⊕ Nursing diagnoses
• Ineffective individual coping related to depression
• Risk for injury related to adverse CNS reactions
• Knowledge deficit related to drug therapy

⊳ Planning and implementation
P.O. use: Oral therapy should replace injection as soon as possible.
I.M. use: Follow normal protocol. Effects may appear more rapidly than with oral administration.
• Administer full dose at bedtime when possible.
• Expect reduced dosage in elderly or debilitated patients and adolescents.

• Do not withdraw drug abruptly.
• Expect doctor to reduce dosage if signs of psychosis occur or increase. Allow patient only minimum supply of drug.
• Because hypertensive episodes have occurred during surgery in patients receiving TCAs, be aware that drug should be gradually discontinued several days before surgery.
Patient teaching
• Advise patient to take full dose at bedtime, but warn him of possible morning orthostatic hypotension.
• Tell patient to avoid alcohol and smoking while taking drug.
• Warn patient to avoid activities that require alertness and psychomotor coordination until CNS effects of drug are known. Drowsiness and dizziness usually subside after a few weeks.
• Advise patient to consult doctor before taking other prescription or OTC medications.
• Teach patient to relieve dry mouth with sugarless hard candy or gum. Saliva substitutes may be necessary.
• Advise patient to use sunblock, wear protective clothing, and avoid prolonged exposure to strong sunlight.
• Warn patient not to stop drug therapy abruptly.
• Tell patient to watch for urine retention and constipation. Instruct him to increase fluids and suggest stool softener or high-fiber diet as needed.

☑ Evaluation
• Patient behavior and communication indicate improvement of depression.
• Patient does not experience injury from CNS adverse reactions.
• Patient and family state understanding of drug therapy.

amlodipine besylate
(am-LOH-dih-peen BES-eh-layt)
Norvasc

Pharmacologic class: dihydropyridine calcium channel blocker
Therapeutic class: antianginal, antihypertensive
Pregnancy risk category: C

How supplied
Tablets: 2.5 mg, 5 mg, 10 mg

Pharmacokinetics
Absorption: absolute bioavailability from 64% to 90%.
Distribution: about 93% of circulating drug is bound to plasma proteins.
Metabolism: extensively metabolized in liver; about 90% of drug converted to inactive metabolites.
Excretion: excreted primarily in urine.
Half-life: 30 to 50 hours.

Route	Onset	Peak	Duration
P.O.	Unknown	6-9 hr	24 hr

Pharmacodynamics
Chemical effect: inhibits calcium ion influx across cardiac and smooth-muscle cells, thus decreasing myocardial contractility and oxygen demand. Also dilates coronary arteries and arterioles.
Therapeutic effect: reduces blood pressure and prevents anginal pain.

Indications and dosage
▶ **Chronic stable angina; vasospastic angina (Prinzmetal's [variant] angina).** *Adults:* initially, 10 mg P.O. daily. Small, frail, or elderly patients or patients with hepatic insufficiency should begin therapy at 5 mg daily. Most patients require 10 mg daily for adequate therapy.
▶ **Hypertension.** *Adults:* initially, 5 mg P.O. daily. Small, frail, or elderly patients; patients currently receiving other antihypertensives; or patients with hepatic insufficiency should begin therapy at 2.5 mg daily. Dosage adjusted based on patient response and tolerance. Maximum daily dosage is 10 mg.

Adverse reactions
CNS: *headache,* fatigue, somnolence.
CV: *edema,* dizziness, flushing, palpitation.
GI: nausea, abdominal pain.

Interactions
None reported.

Contraindications and precautions
• Contraindicated in patients with hypersensitivity to drug and in breast-feeding women.
• Use cautiously in patients receiving other peripheral vasodilators (especially those with severe aortic stenosis), in those with heart failure, and in pregnant women. Because drug is metabolized by liver, also use cautiously and in reduced dosage in patients with severe hepatic disease.
• Safety of drug has not been established in children.

NURSING CONSIDERATIONS

☒ Assessment
• Assess patient's blood pressure or anginal condition before therapy and regularly thereafter.
• Monitor patient carefully for pain. In some patients, especially those with severe obstructive coronary artery disease, increased frequency, duration, or severity of angina or even acute MI has developed after initiation of calcium channel blocker therapy or at time of dosage increase.
• Be alert for adverse reactions.
• Evaluate patient's and family's knowledge of drug therapy.

☒ Nursing diagnoses
• Pain related to increased oxygen demand in cardiac tissue
• Risk for injury related to hypertension

Reactions may be *common,* uncommon, *life-threatening,* or COMMON AND LIFE-THREATENING.

• Knowledge deficit related to drug therapy

≥ Planning and implementation
• Dosage should be adjusted by doctor based on patient response and tolerance.
• Administer S.L. nitroglycerin as needed for acute anginal symptoms.
Patient teaching
• Tell patient that S.L. nitroglycerin may be taken as needed for acute angina. If patient continues nitrate therapy during titration of amlodipine dosage, urge continued compliance.
• Caution patient to continue taking drug even when feeling better.

✓ Evaluation
• Patient's blood pressure is normal.
• Patient states anginal pain occurs with less frequency and severity.
• Patient and family state understanding of drug therapy.

---

ammonia, aromatic spirits†
(ah-MOH-nee-uh, ar-oh-MAT-ik SPIR-its)

Pharmacologic class: miscellaneous antagonist
Therapeutic class: antifainting agent
Pregnancy risk category: NR

How supplied
Solution: 30 ml†, 60 ml†, 120 ml†; pints†; gallons†
Inhalant: 0.33 ml†, 0.4 ml†

Pharmacokinetics
No information available.

Route	Onset	Peak	Duration
Inhalation	Immediate	Unknown	Unknown

Pharmacodynamics
Chemical effect: irritates sensory receptors in nasal membranes, producing reflex stimulation of respiratory centers.

Therapeutic effect: prevents fainting or awakens person from fainting.

Indications and dosage
▶ **Treatment or prevention of fainting.**
Adults and children: 1 broken capsule inhaled until awake or no longer faint; or 2 to 4 ml P.O. diluted in at least 30 ml of water.

Adverse reactions
EENT: irritation.

Interactions
None significant.

Contraindications and precautions
• No known contraindications or precautions.

NURSING CONSIDERATIONS

⚚ Assessment
• Determine that patient has palpable pulse and visible respirations.
• Evaluate patient's and family's knowledge of drug therapy.

⊕ Nursing diagnoses
• Knowledge deficit related to drug therapy

≥ Planning and implementation
• Avoid inhaling vapors when administering drug.
• Keep bottle tightly capped when not in use.
• Notify doctor if patient does not respond to drug.
Patient teaching
• Teach family when and how to administer drug.
• Instruct patient to notify doctor if drug is required so he can determine cause of fainting.

✓ Evaluation
• Patient and family state understanding of drug therapy.

ammonium chloride†
(ah-MOH-nee-um KLOR-ighd)

Pharmacologic class: acid-forming salt
Therapeutic class: acidifying agent,
expectorant
Pregnancy risk category: C

How supplied

Tablets: 500 mg†
Tablets (enteric-coated): 500 mg†,
1,000 mg†
Injection: 2.14% (0.4 mEq/ml), 26.75%
(5 mEq/ml)

Pharmacokinetics

Absorption: absorbed rapidly from GI
tract when administered orally.
Distribution: unknown.
Metabolism: metabolized in liver to urea
and hydrochloric acid.
Excretion: excreted in urine.

Route	Onset	Peak	Duration
P.O.	Unknown	Unknown	Unknown
I.V.	Immediate	Immediate	Unknown

Pharmacodynamics

Chemical effect: increases free hydrogen
ion concentration, resulting in acidosis.
Therapeutic effect: decreases pH; alleviates chloride deficiency.

Indications and dosage

▶ **Metabolic alkalosis (in the absence
of edema or hyponatremia)** *Adults:*
Dosage depends on the patient's condition and tolerance. I.V. dose (in mEq) is
equal to the serum chloride deficit (in
mEq/L) multiplied by the extracellular
fluid (estimated as 20% of the body
weight in kg). Half the calculated volume
should be given, then patient reassessed.
▶ **Acidification.** *Adults:* 4 to 12 g P.O.
daily in divided doses q 4 to 6 hours.
Children: 75 mg/kg P.O. daily in four divided doses.

Adverse reactions

CNS: headache, confusion, progressive
drowsiness, excitement alternating with
coma, hyperventilation, *calcium-
deficient tetany,* twitching, *tonic seizures,* hyperreflexia, EEG abnormalities.
CV: bradycardia.
GI: *gastric irritation, nausea, vomiting,*
thirst, anorexia, retching (with oral dose).
GU: glycosuria.
Metabolic: *metabolic acidosis, hyper-
chloremia, hypokalemia,* hyperglycemia.
Respiratory: irregular respirations with
periods of apnea.
Skin: rash, pallor.
Other: pain at injection site.

Interactions

Drug-drug. *Spironolactone:* increased
systemic acidosis. Use together cautiously.
Drug-food. *Dairy products:* decreased
effects. Do not give dairy products after
drug.

Contraindications and precautions

• Contraindicated in patients with primary respiratory acidosis and high total carbon dioxide (CO_2) and buffer base and in
those with severe hepatic or renal dysfunction (as self-medication).
• Use cautiously in patients with pulmonary insufficiency or cardiac edema,
in pregnant women, and in infants.
• Safety of drug has not been established
in breast-feeding women.

NURSING CONSIDERATIONS

☢ Assessment
• Obtain baseline assessment of patient's
acid-base imbalance.
• Monitor CO_2 combining power and
serum electrolytes during therapy to prevent acidosis. Each gram of ammonium
chloride reduces CO_2 combining power
by 1.1 volume percent.
• Monitor urine pH and output.
• Monitor rate and depth of respirations
frequently. Shortness of breath and increased ventilation indicate acidosis.

• Be alert for adverse reactions and drug interactions.
• Evaluate patient's and family's knowledge of drug therapy.

⚙ **Nursing diagnoses**
• Risk for injury related to acid-base imbalance
• Knowledge deficit related to drug therapy

▶ **Planning and implementation**
• Know that adverse reactions usually result from ammonia toxicity or too-rapid I.V. administration.
P.O. use: Give oral form after meals to decrease adverse GI reactions. Enteric-coated tablets also may minimize GI symptoms but are absorbed erratically.
I.V. use: Be aware that concentrated solutions of ammonium chloride crystallize when exposed to low temperatures; dissolve crystals by warming solution in water bath before use. Dilute concentrated form (26.75%) before administration. Add 100 to 200 mEq (20 to 40 ml of 26.75% solution) to 500 or 1,000 ml of 0.9% NaCl injection. Administer by infusion pump, not exceeding 5 ml/minute in adults.
• Lessen injection pain by decreasing infusion rate.
• Do not administer drug with milk or other alkaline solutions; they are not compatible.
Patient teaching
• Instruct patient to take oral drug after meals to decrease adverse GI reactions. Tell patient to notify doctor if GI reactions occur.
• Instruct patient not to consume dairy products after taking drug.
• Advise patient to take safety precautions because drug can adversely affect mental activity.
• Instruct patient receiving I.V. drug to report adverse reactions.

☑ **Evaluation**
• Patient regains normal acid-base balance.
• Patient and family state understanding of drug therapy.

amobarbital
(am-oh-BAR-bi-tahl)
Amytal

amobarbital sodium
Amytal Sodium

Pharmacologic class: barbiturate
Therapeutic class: sedative-hypnotic, anticonvulsant
Controlled substance schedule: II
Pregnancy risk category: D

How supplied

Tablets: 30 mg
Capsules: 200 mg
Powder for injection: 250 mg, 500 mg

Pharmacokinetics

Absorption: absorbed well after oral and I.M. administration.
Distribution: well distributed throughout body tissues and fluids.
Metabolism: metabolized in liver by oxidation to tertiary alcohol.
Excretion: less than 1% of dose is excreted unchanged in urine; remainder is excreted as metabolites. *Half-life:* 16 to 40 hours.

Route	Onset	Peak	Duration
P.O.	20-60 min	Unknown	6-8 hr
I.V.	Unknown	Unknown	6-8 hr
I.M.	Slightly faster than P.O.	Unknown	6-8 hr

Pharmacodynamics

Chemical effect: unknown. Probably interferes with transmission of impulses from thalamus to cortex of brain.

Therapeutic effect: promotes calmness and sleep, enhances anesthesia, and controls seizure activity.

Indications and dosage

▶ **Sedation.** *Adults:* usually 30 to 50 mg P.O. b.i.d. or t.i.d. *Children:* 2 mg/kg or 70 mg/m² P.O. daily in four equally divided doses.
▶ **Insomnia.** *Adults:* 65 to 200 mg P.O. or deep I.M. h.s. I.M. injection not to exceed 5 ml in any site. *Children:* 2 to 3 mg/kg I.M. h.s.
▶ **Preanesthetic sedation.** *Adults:* 200 mg P.O. 1 to 2 hours before surgery.
▶ **Labor.** *Adults:* 200 to 400 mg P.O. followed by 200 to 400 mg at 1- to 3-hour intervals, up to maximum dose of 1 g.
▶ **Manic reactions, adjunct in psychotherapy, anticonvulsant.** *Adults and children over age 6:* 65 to 500 mg slow I.V.; not to exceed 100 mg/minute. Maximum dosage is 1 g.

Adverse reactions

CNS: *drowsiness, lethargy, hangover,* paradoxical excitement.
CV: bradycardia, hypotension, syncope.
GI: nausea, vomiting.
Hematologic: exacerbation of porphyria.
Respiratory: respiratory depression.
Skin: rash; urticaria; *Stevens-Johnson syndrome;* pain, irritation, sterile abscess (at injection site).
Other: angioedema.

Interactions

Drug-drug. *Chloramphenicol, MAO inhibitors, valproic acid:* inhibit metabolism of barbiturates; may cause prolonged CNS depression. Reduced barbiturate dosage needed.
CNS depressants, including narcotic analgesics: excessive CNS and respiratory depression. Use together cautiously.
Corticosteroids, digitoxin, doxycycline, estrogens and oral contraceptives, oral anticoagulants, tricyclic antidepressants: amobarbital may enhance metabolism of these drugs. Monitor for decreased effect.

Griseofulvin: decreased absorption of griseofulvin. Monitor for decreased effect.
Rifampin: may decrease barbiturate level. Monitor for decreased effect.
Drug-lifestyle. *Alcohol use:* excessive CNS and respiratory depression. Use together cautiously.

Contraindications and precautions

• Contraindicated in patients with bronchopneumonia or other severe pulmonary insufficiency, porphyria, or hypersensitivity to barbiturates.
• Use with extreme caution in pregnant women only when absolutely necessary; fetal abnormalities may occur.
• Use cautiously in patients with acute or chronic pain, suicidal tendencies, depression, history of drug abuse, or hepatic or renal impairment and in breast-feeding women. Use parenteral form cautiously in patients with blood pressure alterations or pulmonary or CV disease.

NURSING CONSIDERATIONS

☒ Assessment
• Assess patient's sleep patterns and mental status before therapy and regularly thereafter.
• Be alert for adverse reactions and drug interactions.
• Monitor patient for skin changes. Skin eruptions may precede potentially fatal reactions to barbiturate therapy. Discontinue drug when skin reactions occur and notify doctor. In some patients, high fever, stomatitis, headache, or rhinitis may precede skin reactions.
• Monitor neonate's respiratory status closely if mother received drug during labor; excessive dosage may cause neonatal respiratory depression.
• After drug is discontinued, be alert for withdrawal symptoms.
• Evaluate patient's and family's knowledge of drug therapy.

Reactions may be *common*, uncommon, *life-threatening*, or COMMON AND LIFE-THREATENING.

⊕ Nursing diagnoses
• Sleep pattern disturbance related to underlying patient problem
• Risk for trauma related to adverse CNS reactions
• Knowledge deficit related to drug therapy

⊠ Planning and implementation
• To minimize deterioration, use injection solution within 30 minutes after opening container. Don't use cloudy or precipitated solution. Don't shake solution; mix with sterile water only.
P.O. use: Be aware that long-term use is not recommended; drug loses its efficacy in promoting sleep after 14 days of continued use.
I.V. use: Know that I.V. injection is reserved for emergency treatment. Close supervision required. Administer I.V. slowly; do not exceed 100 mg/minute.
– Have emergency resuscitation equipment available. I.V. administration of barbiturates may cause severe respiratory depression, laryngospasm, or hypotension.
– Assess patency of I.V. site before and during administration. Local tissue reactions and injection site pain have occurred with I.V. use.
I.M. use: Administer I.M. injection deeply. Superficial injection may cause pain, sterile abscess, and sloughing.
Patient teaching
• Inform patient that morning "hangover" is common after hypnotic dose, which also suppresses REM sleep. Patient may experience increased dreaming after drug is discontinued.
• Caution patient about performing activities that require mental alertness or physical coordination. For inpatient, supervise walking and raise bed rails, particularly for elderly patient.
• Warn patient that prolonged use may lead to physical dependence.
• Tell patient using oral contraceptives to consider alternate birth control methods; drug may enhance contraceptive hormone metabolism and decrease its effect.

☑ Evaluation
• Patient states drug effectively induced sleep.
• Patient's safety is maintained.
• Patient and family state understanding of drug therapy.

---

amoxapine
(uh-MOKS-uh-peen)
Asendin

Pharmacologic class: dibenzoxazepine, tricyclic antidepressant
Therapeutic class: antidepressant
Pregnancy risk category: C

How supplied
Tablets: 25 mg, 50 mg, 100 mg, 150 mg

Pharmacokinetics
Absorption: absorbed rapidly and completely from GI tract.
Distribution: distributed widely. Drug is 92% protein-bound.
Metabolism: metabolized by liver to active metabolite; significant first-pass effect may explain variable serum concentrations in different patients taking same dosage.
Excretion: excreted in urine and feces (7% to 18%); about 60% of dose is excreted as conjugated form within 6 days.
Half-life: 8 hours for amoxapine, 30 hours for its metabolite.

Route	Onset	Peak	Duration
P.O.	2-4 wk	About 90 min	Unknown

Pharmacodynamics
Chemical effect: increases amount of norepinephrine, serotonin, or both in CNS by blocking their reuptake by presynaptic neurons.
Therapeutic effect: relieves depression.

Indications and dosage

▶ **Depression.** *Adults:* initially, 50 mg
P.O. b.i.d. or t.i.d. Increased to 100 mg
b.i.d. or t.i.d. by the end of the first week.
Increases above 300 mg daily are made
only if 300 mg daily has been ineffective
during trial period of at least 2 weeks.
When effective dosage is established, entire dosage (not to exceed 300 mg) may
be given h.s.

Adverse reactions

CNS: *drowsiness, dizziness,* excitation,
tremors, weakness, confusion, headache,
nervousness, *tardive dyskinesia* (especially in elderly women); EEG changes,
seizures, extrapyramidal reactions (rare),
neuroleptic malignant syndrome (high
fever, tachycardia, tachypnea, profuse diaphoresis).
CV: *orthostatic hypotension, tachycardia, ECG changes,* hypertension.
EENT: *blurred vision,* tinnitus, mydriasis.
GI: *dry mouth, constipation,* nausea,
vomiting, anorexia, paralytic ileus.
GU: *urine retention, acute renal failure*
(with overdose).
Skin: rash, urticaria, photosensitivity.
Other: *diaphoresis,* weight gain and
craving for sweets, hypersensitivity reaction.
**After abrupt withdrawal of long-term
therapy:** nausea, headache, malaise
(does not indicate addiction).

Interactions

Drug-drug. *Barbiturates:* decreased tricyclic antidepressant blood level.
Monitor for decreased antidepressant effect.
*Cimetidine, methylphenidate, oral con-
traceptives:* may increase amoxapine
serum level. Monitor for increased adverse effects.
Clonidine, epinephrine, norepinephrine:
increased hypertensive effect. Use with
caution.
CNS depressants: enhanced CNS depression. Avoid concomitant use.

MAO inhibitors: may cause severe excitation, hyperpyrexia, or seizures, usually
with high dosage. Use with caution.
Drug-lifestyle. *Alcohol use:* enhanced
CNS depression. Avoid concomitant use.
Sun exposure: increased risk of photosensitivity. Avoid prolonged or unprotected
sun exposure.

Contraindications and precautions

• Contraindicated in patients with hypersensitivity to drug, during acute recovery
phase of MI, in patients who have received an MAO inhibitor within past 14
days, and in breast-feeding women.
• Use with extreme caution in patients
with history of seizure disorder or those
with overt or latent seizure disorders.
• Use cautiously in patients with history
of urine retention, angle-closure glaucoma, or increased intraocular pressure, as
well as patients with CV disease or during pregnancy.
• Don't use drug in children under age 12.

NURSING CONSIDERATIONS

⏏ Assessment
• Assess patient's depression before therapy and regularly thereafter.
• Be alert for adverse reactions and drug
interactions.
• Monitor for signs and symptoms of tardive dyskinesia, especially in elderly
women.
• Evaluate patient's and family's knowledge of drug therapy.

⊞ Nursing diagnoses
• Ineffective individual coping related to
patient's underlying condition
• Risk for injury related to drug-induced
adverse reactions
• Knowledge deficit related to drug
therapy

▶ Planning and implementation
• Administer full dose at bedtime when
possible. Expect delay of 2 weeks or

Reactions may be *common,* uncommon, *life-threatening,* or COMMON AND LIFE-THREATENING.

more before noticeable effect. Full effect may take 4 weeks or more.
• Be aware that dosage should be reduced in elderly or debilitated persons and adolescents.
• Do not withdraw drug abruptly.
• Because hypertensive episodes have occurred during surgery in patients receiving tricyclic antidepressants, be aware that drug should be gradually discontinued several days before surgery.
• If signs of psychosis occur or increase, expect doctor to reduce dosage. Allow patient only minimum supply of drug.
Patient teaching
• Warn patient not to stop therapy abruptly.
• Caution patient to avoid activities that require alertness and psychomotor coordination until CNS effects of drug are known. Drowsiness and dizziness usually subside after first few weeks.
• Tell patient to avoid alcohol consumption while on drug therapy.
• Advise patient to use sunblock, wear protective clothing, and avoid prolonged exposure to strong sunlight.

☑ **Evaluation**
• Patient behavior and communication indicate improvement of depression.
• Patient does not experience injury from adverse CNS reactions.
• Patient and family state understanding of drug therapy.

amoxicillin/clavulanate potassium
(uh-moks-uh-SIL-in/KLAV-yoo-lan-ayt poh-TAH-see-um)
Augmentin, Clavulin ♦

Pharmacologic class: aminopenicillin, beta-lactamase inhibitor
Therapeutic class: antibiotic
Pregnancy risk category: B

How supplied
Tablets (chewable): 125 mg amoxicillin trihydrate, 31.25 mg clavulanic acid; 250 mg amoxicillin trihydrate, 62.5 mg clavulanic acid
Tablets (film-coated): 250 mg amoxicillin trihydrate, 125 mg clavulanic acid; 500 mg amoxicillin trihydrate, 125 mg clavulanic acid; 875 mg amoxicillin trihydrate, 125 mg clavulanic acid
Oral suspension: 125 mg amoxicillin trihydrate and 31.25 mg clavulanic acid/ 5 ml (after reconstitution); 250 mg amoxicillin trihydrate and 62.5 mg clavulanic acid/5 ml (after reconstitution)

Pharmacokinetics
Absorption: well absorbed.
Distribution: both drugs distribute into pleural fluid, lungs, and peritoneal fluid; high urine concentrations are attained. Amoxicillin also distributes into synovial fluid, liver, prostate, muscle, and gallbladder and penetrates into middle ear effusions, maxillary sinus secretions, tonsils, sputum, and bronchial secretions. Both drugs have minimal protein binding.
Metabolism: amoxicillin is metabolized only partially; clavulanate potassium appears to undergo extensive metabolism.
Excretion: amoxicillin is excreted principally in urine by renal tubular secretion and glomerular filtration; clavulanate potassium is excreted by glomerular filtration. *Half-life:* amoxicillin, 1 to 1½ hours (7½ hours in severe renal impairment); clavulanate, about 1 to 1½ hours (4½ hours in severe renal impairment).

Route	Onset	Peak	Duration
P.O.	Unknown	1-2.5 hr	6-8 hr

Pharmacodynamics
Chemical effect: prevents bacterial cell-wall synthesis during replication. Clavulanic acid increases amoxicillin's effectiveness by inactivating beta lactamases, which destroy amoxicillin.
Therapeutic effect: kills susceptible bacteria. Active against penicillinase-

producing gram-positive bacteria, *Neisseria gonorrhoeae, N. meningitidis, Haemophilus influenzae, Escherichia coli, Proteus mirabilis, Citrobacter diversus, Klebsiella pneumoniae, P. vulgaris, Salmonella,* and *Shigella.*

Indications and dosage

▶ **Lower respiratory tract infections, otitis media, sinusitis, skin and skin structure infections, and urinary tract infections caused by susceptible strains of gram-positive and gram-negative organisms.** *Adults:* 250 mg (based on amoxicillin component) P.O. q 8 hours. For more severe infections, 500 mg q 8 hours, or 875 mg P.O. q 12 hours. *Children:* 20 to 40 mg/kg (based on amoxicillin component) P.O. daily in divided doses q 8 hours.

Adverse reactions

GI: *nausea,* vomiting, *diarrhea.*
Hematologic: anemia, ***thrombocytopenia,*** thrombocytopenic purpura, eosinophilia, ***leukopenia, agranulocytopenia.***
Other: hypersensitivity reactions (erythematous maculopapular rash, urticaria, ***anaphylaxis),*** overgrowth of nonsusceptible organisms.

Interactions

Drug-drug. *Allopurinol:* increased incidence of skin rash. Monitor patient. *Probenecid:* increased blood level of amoxicillin and other penicillins. Probenecid may be used for this purpose.

Contraindications and precautions

• Contraindicated in patients with hypersensitivity to drug or other penicillins and in those with history of amoxicillin-associated cholestatic jaundice or hepatic dysfunction.
• Use cautiously in patients with other drug allergies, especially to cephalosporins (possible cross-sensitivity); in those with mononucleosis (high inci-

dence of maculopapular rash); and in pregnant or breast-feeding women.

NURSING CONSIDERATIONS

⚷ Assessment
• Before therapy begins, assess patient's infection, ask him about allergic reactions to penicillin (negative history is no guarantee against allergic reaction), and obtain specimen for culture and sensitivity tests. Therapy may begin pending results.
• Be alert for adverse reactions and drug interactions.
• Monitor hydration status if adverse GI reactions occur.
• Evaluate patient's and family's knowledge of drug therapy.

⬣ Nursing diagnoses
• Infection related to susceptible bacteria
• Risk for fluid volume deficit related to drug-induced adverse GI reactions
• Knowledge deficit related to drug therapy

❯ Planning and implementation
• Give drug with food to prevent GI distress. Incidence of adverse effects, especially diarrhea, is greater than with amoxicillin alone.
• Give drug at least 1 hour before bacteriostatic antibiotics.
• Know that both 250-mg and 500-mg tablets contain same amount of clavulanic acid (125 mg). Therefore, two 250-mg tablets are not equal to one 500-mg tablet.
• Be aware that this drug combination is particularly useful with high prevalence of amoxicillin-resistant organisms.
• After reconstitution, refrigerate oral suspension and discard after 10 days.
• Know that urine glucose determinations may be false-positive with copper sulfate tests (Benedict's solution, Clinitest); glucose enzymatic tests (Diastix) are not affected.

Reactions may be *common,* uncommon, *life-threatening,* or COMMON AND LIFE-THREATENING.

Patient teaching
• Tell patient to take entire quantity of drug exactly as prescribed, even after he feels better.
• Tell patient to call doctor if rash develops (sign of allergic reaction).
• Instruct patient to take drug with food to prevent GI distress.

☑ **Evaluation**
• Patient is free from infection.
• Patient maintains adequate hydration.
• Patient and family state understanding of drug therapy.

---

amoxicillin trihydrate (amoxycillin trihydrate)
(uh-moks-uh-SIL-in trigh-HIGH-drayt)
Alphamox, Amoxil, Apo-Amoxi, Cilamox, Ibiamox, Larotid, Moxacin, Novamoxin, Nu-Amoxi, Polymox, Trimox, Wymox

Pharmacologic class: aminopenicillin
Therapeutic class: antibiotic
Pregnancy risk category: NR

How supplied
Tablets: 500 mg, 875 mg
Tablets (chewable): 125 mg, 250 mg
Capsules: 250 mg, 500 mg
Oral suspension: 50 mg/ml (pediatric drops), 125 mg/5 ml, 250 mg/5 ml (after reconstitution)

Pharmacokinetics
Absorption: about 80% absorbed after oral administration.
Distribution: distributed into pleural, peritoneal, and synovial fluids; lungs; prostate; muscle; liver; and gallbladder. Also penetrates middle ear, maxillary sinus and bronchial secretions, tonsils, and sputum. Amoxicillin readily crosses placenta and is 17% to 20% protein–bound.
Metabolism: only partially metabolized.
Excretion: excreted principally in urine by renal tubular secretion and glomerular filtration; also excreted in breast milk.

Half-life: 1 to 1½ hours (7½ hours in severe renal impairment).

Route	Onset	Peak	Duration
P.O.	Unknown	1-2 hr	6-8 hr

Pharmacodynamics
Chemical effect: inhibits cell-wall synthesis during bacterial multiplication.
Therapeutic effect: kills susceptible bacteria (*Streptococcus, Pneumococcus, Enterococcus, Haemophilus influenzae, Escherichia coli, Proteus mirabilis, Neisseria meningitidis, N. gonorrhoeae, Shigella, Salmonella, Borrelia burgdorferi*).

Indications and dosage
▶ **Systemic infections, acute and chronic urinary tract infections caused by susceptible strains of gram-positive and gram-negative organisms.** *Adults:* 250 mg P.O. q 8 hours. In adults and children over 20 kg who have severe infections or those caused by susceptible organisms, 500 mg P.O. q 8 hours or 875 mg P.O. q 12 hours may be needed. *Children:* 20 to 40 mg/kg P.O. daily, divided into doses given q 8 hours.
▶ **Uncomplicated gonorrhea.** *Adults:* 3 g P.O. as a single dose. *Children over age 2:* 50 mg/kg given with 25 mg/kg probenecid as a single dose.
▶ **Endocarditis prophylaxis for dental procedures.** *Adults:* initially, 3 g P.O. 1 hour before procedure; then 1.5 g 6 hours later. *Children:* initially, 50 mg/kg P.O. 1 hour before procedure; then half initial dose 6 hours later.
▶ *H. pylori* **eradication to reduce the risk of duodenal ulcer in combination with clarithromycin and/or lansoprazole. Triple therapy:** *Adults:* amoxicillin 1 g P.O., clarithromycin 500 mg P.O., lansoprazole 30 mg P.O.; each q 12 hours for 14 days. **Dual therapy:** *Adults:* amoxicillin 1 g P.O. and lansoprazole 30 mg P.O., each q 8 hours for 14 days.

Adverse reactions

CNS: *seizures.*
GI: *nausea,* vomiting, *diarrhea.*
Hematologic: anemia, *thrombocytopenia,* thrombocytopenic purpura, eosinophilia, *leukopenia, agranulocytosis.*
Other: hypersensitivity reactions (erythematous maculopapular rash, urticaria, *anaphylaxis),* overgrowth of nonsusceptible organisms.

Interactions

Drug-drug. *Allopurinol:* increased incidence of rash. Monitor patient.
Probenecid: increased blood level of amoxicillin and other penicillins. Probenecid may be used for this purpose.

Contraindications and precautions

• Contraindicated in patients hypersensitive to drug or other penicillins.
• Use cautiously in patients with other drug allergies, especially to cephalosporins (possible cross-sensitivity); in those with mononucleosis (high incidence of maculopapular rash); and in pregnant or breast-feeding women.

NURSING CONSIDERATIONS

⚗ Assessment

• Before therapy, assess patient's infection, ask him about allergic reactions to drug or other forms of penicillin (negative history does not guarantee future safety), and obtain specimen for culture and sensitivity tests. Therapy may begin pending test results.
• Be alert for adverse reactions and drug interactions.
• Monitor patient's hydration status if adverse GI reactions occur.
• Evaluate patient's and family's knowledge of drug therapy.

⬛ Nursing diagnoses

• Infection related to susceptible bacteria
• Risk for fluid volume deficit related to drug-induced adverse GI reactions

• Knowledge deficit related to drug therapy

⬢ Planning and implementation

• Give amoxicillin at least 1 hour before bacteriostatic antibiotics.
• Administer with food to prevent GI distress.
• Trimox oral suspension may be stored at room temperature for up to 2 weeks. Check individual product labels for storage information.
• Be aware that drug may cause false-positive urine glucose determinations with copper sulfate tests (Clinitest); drug does not affect glucose enzymatic tests (Diastix).
Patient teaching
• Advise patient in whom drug allergy has developed to wear medical identification bracelet or necklace stating this information.
• Tell patient to take entire quantity of drug exactly as ordered, even after he feels better.
• Tell patient to call doctor if rash (most common), fever, or chills develop.
• Instruct patient to take drug with food to prevent GI distress.
• Warn patient never to use leftover amoxicillin for a new illness or to share it with others.

✓ Evaluation

• Patient is free from infection.
• Patient maintains adequate hydration.
• Patient and family state understanding of drug therapy.

---

amphetamine sulfate
(am-FET-ah-meen SUL-fayt)

Pharmacologic class: amphetamine
Therapeutic class: CNS stimulant, short-term adjunct anorexigenic agent, sympathomimetic amine
Controlled substance schedule: II
Pregnancy risk category: C

How supplied

Tablets: 5 mg, 10 mg

Pharmacokinetics

Absorption: absorbed completely within 3 hours.
Distribution: distributed widely throughout body, with high concentrations in brain.
Metabolism: metabolized in liver.
Excretion: excreted in urine. *Half-life:* 10 to 30 hours.

Route	Onset	Peak	Duration
P.O.	Unknown	Unknown	Unknown

Pharmacodynamics

Chemical effect: unknown; probably promotes nerve impulse transmission by releasing stored norepinephrine from nerve terminals in brain. Main sites of activity appear to be cerebral cortex and reticular activating system.
Therapeutic effect: improves behavior in attention deficit disorder (ADD) with hyperactivity, helps prevent falling asleep, and aids in weight loss.

Indications and dosage

▶ **ADD with hyperactivity.** *Children ages 3 to 5:* 2.5 mg P.O. daily, with 2.5-mg increments weekly, p.r.n. *Children age 6 and older:* 5 mg P.O. daily, with 5-mg increments weekly, p.r.n. Give first dose on awakening; additional doses (one or two) at 4- to 6-hour intervals.
▶ **Narcolepsy.** *Adults:* 5 to 60 mg P.O. daily in divided doses.
▶ **Short-term adjunct in exogenous obesity.** *Adults:* 5 to 30 mg P.O. daily in divided doses 30 to 60 minutes before meals.

Adverse reactions

CNS: *restlessness,* tremors, *hyperactivity, talkativeness, insomnia,* irritability, dizziness, headache, chills, dysphoria.
CV: *tachycardia, palpitations,* hypertension, hypotension, *arrhythmias.*

GI: dry mouth, metallic taste, nausea, vomiting, cramps, diarrhea, constipation, anorexia, weight loss.
GU: impotence.
Skin: urticaria.
Other: altered libido.

Interactions

Drug-drug. *Acetazolamide, antacids, sodium bicarbonate:* increased renal reabsorption. Monitor for enhanced effect. *Ammonium chloride, ascorbic acid:* decreased serum levels and increased renal excretion of amphetamine. Monitor for decreased amphetamine effect.
Antihypertensives: reversal of antihypertensive action. Monitor blood pressure.
Haloperidol, phenothiazines, tricyclic antidepressants: increased CNS effect. Avoid concomitant use.
Insulin, oral antidiabetic agents: may decrease antidiabetic agent requirements. Monitor blood glucose level.
MAO inhibitors: severe hypertension; possibly hypertensive crisis. Don't use together or within 14 days after an MAO inhibitor has been discontinued.
Drug-food. *Caffeine:* may increase amphetamine and relate amine effects. Avoid concomitant use.

Contraindications and precautions

• Contraindicated in patients with hypersensitivity or idiosyncrasy to sympathomimetic amines, symptomatic CV disease, hyperthyroidism, moderate to severe hypertension, glaucoma, advanced arteriosclerosis, or history of drug abuse; within 14 days of MAO inhibitor therapy; and in agitated patients.
• Use cautiously in elderly, debilitated, or hyperexcitable patients and in those with psychopathic personalities or history of suicidal or homicidal tendencies; and in pregnant or breast-feeding women.
• Drug not recommended in children under age 12 for treatment of obesity and in children under age 3 for treatment of ADD with hyperactivity.

NURSING CONSIDERATIONS

⚕ Assessment
• Obtain history of patient's underlying condition.
• Be alert for adverse reactions and drug interactions.
• Monitor dietary intake when drug is used to treat obesity.
• Evaluate patient's and family's knowledge of drug therapy.

⚕ Nursing diagnoses
• Altered health maintenance related to underlying disorder
• Sleep pattern disturbance related to drug-induced insomnia
• Knowledge deficit related to drug therapy

⚕ Planning and implementation
• Know that drug is not recommended for first-line treatment of obesity or for treatment of obesity in children under age 12. Use as an anorexigenic agent is prohibited in some states.
• Be aware that drug should not be used to combat fatigue.
• Administer drug at least 6 hours before bedtime to avoid interference with sleep.
• When used for obesity, administer drug 30 to 60 minutes before meals.
• Know that drug should not be administered for a prolonged period because psychological dependence may occur. When used long term, reduce dosage gradually, as ordered, to prevent acute rebound depression.
• If tolerance to anorexigenic effect develops, know that drug should be discontinued. Notify doctor.
• Make sure obese patient is on a weight-reduction program.
Patient teaching
• Tell patient to take drug at least 6 hours before bedtime to avoid sleep pattern disturbance. If used to treat obesity, tell patient to take drug 30 to 60 minutes before meals.

• Warn patient to avoid activities that require alertness or good psychomotor coordination until CNS effects of drug are known.
• Tell patient to avoid drinks or foods containing caffeine, which increase effects of amphetamines and related amines.
• Tell patient to report signs of excess stimulation.
• Inform patient that fatigue may result as drug effects wear off. He will need more rest.
• Tell patient that when tolerance to anorexigenic effect develops, dosage should not be increased, but drug discontinued. He should report decreased effectiveness of drug. Warn patient against stopping drug abruptly.

⚕ Evaluation
• Patient's health is maintained during amphetamine sulfate therapy.
• Patient is able to sleep without difficulty.
• Patient and family state an understanding of drug therapy.

---

amphotericin B
(am-foh-TER-ah-sin bee)
Fungilin Oral◇, Fungizone Intravenous

Pharmacologic class: polyene macrolide
Therapeutic class: antifungal
Pregnancy risk category: B

How supplied

Tablets: 100 mg◇
Oral suspension: 100 mg/ml◇
Lozenges: 10 mg◇
Injection: 50-mg lyophilized cake

Pharmacokinetics

Absorption: absorbed poorly from GI tract.
Distribution: distributed well into pleural cavities and joints; less so into aqueous humor, bronchial secretions, pancreas,

---

bone, muscle, and parotid gland. Drug is 90% to 95% bound to plasma proteins. *Metabolism:* not well defined. *Excretion:* up to 5% excreted unchanged in urine. *Half-life:* initially, 24 hours; second phase, about 15 days.

Route	Onset	Peak	Duration
P.O.	Unknown	Unknown	Unknown
I.V.	Immediate	Immediate	Unknown

Pharmacodynamics

Chemical effect: may bind to sterol in fungal cell membrane and alter cell permeability, allowing leakage of intracellular components.
Therapeutic effect: decreases activity of or kills susceptible fungi, such as *Histoplasma capsulatum, Coccidioides immitis, Blastomyces dermatitidis, Cryptococcus neoformans, Candida, Aspergillus fumigatus, Mucor, Rhizopus, Absidia, Entomophthora, Basidiobolus, Paracoccidioides brasiliensis, Sporothrix schenckii,* and *Rhodotorula.*

Indications and dosage

▶ **Systemic fungal infections (histoplasmosis, coccidioidomycosis, blastomycosis, cryptococcosis, disseminated moniliasis, aspergillosis, mucormycosis); meningitis.** *Adults:* test dose of 1 mg I.V. in 20 ml of D_5W infused over 20 to 30 minutes may be recommended. If tolerated, daily dosage is then started as 0.25 to 0.3 mg/kg by slow I.V. infusion (0.1 mg/ml) over 2 to 6 hours. Dose is gradually increased, as patient tolerance develops, to maximum of 1 mg/kg daily. Therapy must not exceed 1.5 mg/kg daily. If drug is discontinued for 1 week or more, drug is resumed with initial dose and increased gradually.
▶ **Infections of GI tract caused by** *Candida albicans. Adults:* 100 mg P.O. q.i.d. for 2 weeks.
▶ **Oral and perioral candidal infections.** *Adults:* 1 lozenge q.i.d. for 7 to 14 days. Lozenge should be allowed to dissolve slowly.

Adverse reactions

CNS: headache, peripheral neuropathy, *seizures;* peripheral nerve pain, paresthesia (with I.V. use).
CV: hypotension, *arrhythmias, asystole.*
GI: *anorexia, weight loss, nausea,* vomiting, dyspepsia, diarrhea, epigastric cramps, *hemorrhagic gastroenteritis.*
GU: abnormal renal function with hypokalemia, azotemia, hyposthenuria, hypomagnesemia, renal tubular acidosis, nephrocalcinosis; *permanent renal impairment,* anuria, oliguria (with large doses).
Hematologic: normochromic normocytic anemia, *thrombocytopenia, agranulocytosis.*
Hepatic: *acute liver failure.*
Other: arthralgia, burning, stinging, irritation, tissue damage with extravasation, phlebitis, thrombophlebitis, pain at injection site, myalgia, muscle weakness from hypokalemia, *fever, chills,* malaise, generalized pain; *anaphylactoid reactions* (with topical use).

Interactions

Drug-drug. *Cardiac glycosides:* increased risk of digitalis toxicity in potassium-depleted patients. Monitor closely.
Corticosteroids: potassium depletion. Monitor potassium level.
Flucytosine: may increase flucytosine toxicity. Monitor closely.
Other nephrotoxic drugs (such as antibiotics, antineoplastic agents): may cause additive nephrotoxicity. Administer cautiously.

Contraindications and precautions

• Contraindicated in patients with hypersensitivity to drug and in breast-feeding women.
• Use cautiously in patients with impaired renal function and in pregnant women.
• Safety of drug has not been established in children.

NURSING CONSIDERATIONS

🔎 Assessment
• Obtain history of fungal infection and samples for culture and sensitivity tests before therapy. Reevaluate condition during therapy.
• Be alert for adverse reactions and drug interactions.
• Monitor patient's pulse, respiratory rate, temperature, and blood pressure every 30 minutes for at least 4 hours after administering drug I.V.; fever, shaking chills, and hypotension may appear 1 to 2 hours after start of I.V. infusion and should subside within 4 hours of discontinuation.
• Monitor BUN, serum creatinine (or creatinine clearance), and serum electrolyte levels; CBC; and liver function studies at least weekly, as ordered.
• Evaluate patient's and family's knowledge of drug therapy.

🔲 Nursing diagnoses
• Infection related to presence of susceptible fungal infection
• Risk for injury related to drug-induced adverse reactions
• Knowledge deficit related to drug therapy

🔳 Planning and implementation
P.O. use: Know that lozenge form of drug should be dissolved slowly.
I.V. use: Know that drug should be given parenterally only in hospitalized patients, under close supervision, when diagnosis of potentially fatal fungal infection has been confirmed. Be prepared to administer an initial test dose, as ordered; 1 mg is added to 20 ml of D_5W and infused over 20 to 30 minutes.
– Use an infusion pump and in-line filter with a mean pore diameter larger than 1 micron. Infuse over 6 hours; rapid infusion may cause CV collapse.
– Use I.V. sites in distal veins. If thrombosis occurs, alternate sites.

– Be aware that reconstituted solution is stable for 1 week in refrigerator or 24 hours at room temperature. It has 8-hour stability in room light.
– Give antibiotics separately; don't mix or piggyback with amphotericin B.
– Amphotericin B appears to be compatible with limited amounts of heparin sodium, hydrocortisone sodium succinate, and methylprednisolone sodium succinate.
– Store dry form at 35.6° to 46.4° F (2° to 8° C). Protect from light. Reconstitute with 10 ml of sterile water only. To avoid precipitation, do not mix with solutions containing NaCl, other electrolytes, or bacteriostatic agents (such as benzyl alcohol). Do not use if solution contains precipitate or foreign matter.
– If BUN level exceeds 40 mg/dl, or if serum creatinine level exceeds 3 mg/dl, doctor may reduce or stop drug until renal function improves. Drug may be stopped if alkaline phosphatase or bilirubin level increases.
– To reduce severe adverse reactions, be aware that patient may receive premedication with antipyretics, antihistamines, antiemetics, or small doses of corticosteroids; addition of phosphate buffer and heparin to solution; or an alternate-day schedule. For severe reactions, discontinue drug and notify doctor.
Patient teaching
• Teach patient signs and symptoms of hypersensitivity, and stress importance of reporting them immediately.
• Warn patient that therapy may take several months; teach personal hygiene and other measures to prevent spread and recurrence of lesions.
• Urge patient to comply with prescribed regimen and recommended follow-up.
• With oral form, instruct patient to let lozenges dissolve slowly.
• With I.V. therapy, warn patient that discomfort at injection site and adverse reactions may occur during therapy, which may last several months.

☑ Evaluation
• Patient is free from fungal infection.
• Patient does not experience injury as a result of drug-induced adverse reactions.
• Patient and family state understanding of drug therapy.

---

ampicillin
(am-pih-SIL-in)
Apo-Ampi♦, Novo-Ampicillin♦, Nu-Ampi♦, Omnipen, Principen

ampicillin sodium
Ampicin♦, Ampicyn Injection◇, Omnipen-N, Penbritin♦, Polycillin-N, Totacillin-N

ampicillin trihydrate
Ampicyn Oral◇, D-Amp, Omnipen, Penbritin◇, Polycillin, Principen-250, Principen-500, Totacillin

---

Pharmacologic class: aminopenicillin
Therapeutic class: antibiotic
Pregnancy risk category: B

How supplied

Capsules: 250 mg, 500 mg
Oral suspension: 100 mg/ml (pediatric drops), 125 mg/5 ml, 250 mg/5 ml, 500 mg/5 ml (after reconstitution)
Injection: 125 mg, 250 mg, 500 mg, 1 g, 2 g
Infusion: 500 mg, 1 g, 2 g

Pharmacokinetics

Absorption: about 42% is absorbed after an oral dose; unknown after I.M. administration.
Distribution: distributes into pleural, peritoneal and synovial fluids; lungs; prostate; liver; and gallbladder. Also penetrates middle ear effusions, maxillary sinus and bronchial secretions, tonsils, and sputum. Ampicillin is minimally protein-bound at 15% to 25%.
Metabolism: metabolized only partially.

Excretion: excreted in urine by renal tubular secretion and glomerular filtration. *Half-life:* about 1 to 1½ hours (10 to 24 hours in severe renal impairment).

Route	Onset	Peak	Duration
P.O.	Unknown	≤ 2 hr	6-8 hr
I.V.	Immediate	Immediate	Unknown
I.M.	Unknown	≤ 1 hr	Unknown

Pharmacodynamics

Chemical effect: inhibits cell-wall synthesis during microorganism multiplication.
Therapeutic effect: kills susceptible bacteria. Its spectrum of action includes non-penicillinase-producing gram-positive bacteria. It is also effective against many gram-negative organisms, including *Neisseria gonorrhoeae, N. meningitidis, Haemophilus influenzae, Escherichia coli, Proteus mirabilis, Salmonella,* and *Shigella.*

Indications and dosage

▶ **Systemic infections and acute and chronic urinary tract infections caused by susceptible strains of gram-positive and gram-negative organisms.** *Adults and children weighing 20 kg (44 lb) and over:* 250 to 500 mg P.O. q 6 hours; or 2 to 12 g I.M. or I.V. daily in divided doses q 4 to 6 hours. *Children weighing under 20 kg:* 50 to 100 mg/kg P.O. daily in divided doses q 6 hours; or 100 to 200 mg/kg I.M. or I.V. daily in divided doses q 6 hours.
▶ **Meningitis.** *Adults:* 8 to 14 g I.V. daily in divided doses q 3 to 4 hours. *Children age 2 months to 12 years:* up to 400 mg/kg I.V. daily for 3 days; then up to 300 mg/kg I.M. divided q 4 hours.
▶ **Uncomplicated gonorrhea.** *Adults and children weighing over 45 kg (99 lb):* 3.5 g P.O. with 1 g probenecid in a single dose.
▶ **Endocarditis prophylaxis for dental procedures.** *Adults:* 2 g I.V. or I.M. 30 minutes before procedure. *Children:*

---

50 mg/kg I.V. or I.M. 30 minutes before procedure.

Adverse reactions

CNS: *seizures*
CV: vein irritation, thrombophlebitis.
GI: *nausea,* vomiting, *diarrhea,* glossitis, stomatitis.
Hematologic: anemia, *thrombocytopenia,* thrombocytopenic purpura, eosinophilia, *leukopenia, agranulocytosis.*
Other: hypersensitivity reactions (maculopapular rash, urticaria, *anaphylaxis),* overgrowth of nonsusceptible organisms, pain at injection site.

Interactions

Drug-drug. *Allopurinol:* increased risk of rash.
Probenecid: increased blood level of ampicillin and other penicillins. Probenecid may be used for this purpose.

Contraindications and precautions

• Contraindicated in patients with hypersensitivity to drug or other penicillins.
• Use cautiously in patients with other drug allergies, especially to cephalosporins (possible cross-sensitivity); in those with mononucleosis (high incidence of maculopapular rash); and in pregnant or breast-feeding women.

NURSING CONSIDERATIONS

⬧ Assessment

• Obtain history of patient's infection before therapy and reassess for improvement regularly thereafter.
• Before giving drug, ask patient about previous allergic reaction to penicillin. Be aware that a negative history of penicillin allergy is no guarantee against a future reaction.
• Obtain specimen for culture and sensitivity tests before administering first dose.
• Be alert for adverse reactions and drug interactions.

• Monitor patient's hydration status if adverse GI reactions occur.
• Evaluate patient's and family's knowledge about drug therapy.

⬧ Nursing diagnoses

• Infection related to presence of susceptible bacterial infection
• Risk for fluid volume deficit related to drug-induced adverse GI reactions
• Knowledge deficit related to drug therapy

⬧ Planning and implementation

P.O. use: Give 1 hour before or 2 hours after meals. When given orally, drug may cause adverse GI reactions. Food may interfere with absorption.
I.V. use: Reconstitute with bacteriostatic water for injection. Use 5 ml for 125-mg, 250-mg, or 500-mg vials; 7.4 ml for 1-g vials; and 14.8 ml for 2-g vials. Give direct I.V. injections over 3 to 5 minutes for doses of 500 mg or less; over 10 to 15 minutes for larger doses. Don't exceed a rate of 100 mg/minute. Alternatively, dilute in 50 to 100 ml of 0.9% NaCl injection and give by intermittent infusion over 15 to 30 minutes. Don't mix with solutions containing dextrose or fructose because these solutions promote rapid breakdown of ampicillin.
– Use initial dilution within 1 hour. Follow manufacturer's directions for stability data when ampicillin is further diluted for I.V. infusion.
– Give intermittently to prevent vein irritation. Change site every 48 hours.
– Don't give I.V. unless prescribed and infection is severe or patient can't take oral dose.
I.M. use: Don't give I.M. unless prescribed and infection is severe or patient can't take oral dose.
• Know that dosage should be altered in patients with impaired renal function.
• Give ampicillin at least 1 hour before bacteriostatic antibiotics.
• Be aware that in pediatric meningitis, ampicillin may be given concurrently

---

Reactions may be *common,* uncommon, *life-threatening,* or COMMON AND LIFE-THREATENING.

with parenteral chloramphenicol for 24 hours pending culture results.

• Keep in mind that drug may cause false-positive urine glucose determinations with copper sulfate tests (Clinitest); drug does not affect glucose enzymatic tests (Diastix).

• Discontinue drug immediately if anaphylactic shock occurs. Notify doctor and prepare to administer immediate treatment (such as epinephrine, corticosteroids, antihistamines, and other resuscitative measures), as indicated.

Patient teaching

• Tell patient to take entire quantity of drug exactly as ordered, even after he feels better.

• Tell patient to call doctor if a rash (most common), fever, or chills develop.

• Warn patient never to use leftover ampicillin for a new illness or to share it with others.

• Tell patient to take oral ampicillin 1 hour before or 2 hours after meals for best absorption.

☑ **Evaluation**

• Patient is free from infection.

• Patient maintains adequate hydration.

• Patient and family state understanding of drug therapy.

---

ampicillin sodium/sulbactam sodium
(am-pih-SIL-in SOH-dee-um/ sul-BAC-tam SOH-dee-um)
Unasyn

Pharmacologic class: aminopenicillin/ beta-lactamase inhibitor combination
Therapeutic class: antibiotic
Pregnancy risk category: B

How supplied

Injection: vials and piggyback vials containing 1.5 g (1 g ampicillin sodium with 0.5 g sulbactam sodium) and 3 g (2 g

ampicillin sodium with 1 g sulbactam sodium)

Pharmacokinetics

Absorption: unknown.
Distribution: both drugs distribute into pleural, peritoneal, and synovial fluids; lungs; prostate; liver; and gallbladder. They also penetrate middle ear effusions, maxillary sinus and bronchial secretions, tonsils, and sputum. Ampicillin is minimally protein-bound at 15% to 25%; sulbactam is about 38% bound.
Metabolism: both drugs are metabolized only partially.
Excretion: both drugs excreted in urine by renal tubular secretion and glomerular filtration. *Half-life:* 1 to 1½ hours (10 to 24 hours in severe renal impairment).

Route	Onset	Peak	Duration
I.V.	Immediate	Immediate	Unknown
I.M.	Unknown	Unknown	Unknown

Pharmacodynamics

Chemical effect: ampicillin inhibits cell-wall synthesis during microorganism multiplication; sulbactam inactivates bacterial beta-lactamase, the enzyme that inactivates ampicillin and provides bacterial resistance to it.
Therapeutic effect: kills susceptible bacteria. Spectrum of activity includes beta-lactamase-producing strains of *Staphylococcus aureus, Escherichia coli, Klebsiella, Proteus mirabilis, Bacteroides, Enterobacter,* and *Acinetobacter calcoaceticus.*

Indications and dosage

▶ **Intra-abdominal, gynecologic, and skin structure infections caused by susceptible strains.** *Adults:* dosage expressed as total drug (each 1.5-g vial contains 1 g ampicillin sodium and 0.5 g sulbactam sodium)—1.5 to 3 g I.M. or I.V. q 6 hours. Maximum daily dosage is 4 g sulbactam (12 g of combined drugs).

Adverse reactions

CV: vein irritation, thrombophlebitis.
GI: *nausea,* vomiting, *diarrhea,* glossitis, stomatitis.
Hematologic: anemia, *thrombocytopenia,* thrombocytopenic purpura, eosinophilia, *leukopenia, agranulocytosis.*
Other: hypersensitivity reactions (erythematous maculopapular rash, urticaria, *anaphylaxis), overgrowth of nonsusceptible organisms,* pain at injection site.

Interactions

Drug-drug. *Allopurinol:* increased risk of rash. Monitor patient.
Probenecid: increased blood level of ampicillin. Probenecid may be used for this purpose.
Oral contraceptives: efficacy of oral contraceptives may be decreased.

Contraindications and precautions

• Contraindicated in patients with hypersensitivity to drug or other penicillins.
• Use cautiously in patients with other drug allergies, especially to cephalosporins (possible cross-sensitivity); in those with mononucleosis (high incidence of maculopapular rash); and in pregnant or breast-feeding women.
• Safety of drug has not been established in children younger than age 12.

NURSING CONSIDERATIONS

⚕ Assessment

• Obtain history of patient's infection before therapy, and observe for improvement in condition throughout therapy.
• Before giving drug, ask patient about previous allergic reaction to penicillin. Be aware that a negative history of penicillin allergy is no guarantee against a future reaction.
• Obtain specimen for culture and sensitivity tests before administering first dose.
• Be alert for adverse reactions and drug interactions.

• Monitor patient's hydration status if adverse GI reactions occur.
• Evaluate patient's and family's knowledge about drug therapy.

⚕ Nursing diagnoses

• Infection related to presence of susceptible bacterial infection
• Risk for fluid volume deficit related to drug-induced adverse GI reactions
• Knowledge deficit related to drug therapy

⚕ Planning and implementation

I.V. use: When preparing injection, reconstitute powder with any of the following diluents: 0.9% NaCl solution, D_5W, lactated Ringer's injection, 1/6 M sodium lactate, dextrose 5% and 0.45% NaCl injection, and 10% invert sugar. Stability varies with diluent, temperature, and concentration of solution.
– After reconstitution, allow vials to stand for a few minutes for foam to dissipate to permit visual inspection of contents for particles.
– Give dose by slow injection (over 10 to 15 minutes), or dilute in 50 to 100 ml of a compatible diluent and infuse over 15 to 30 minutes. If permitted, give intermittently to prevent vein irritation. Change site every 48 hours.
– Don't add or mix with other drugs because they might prove physically or chemically incompatible.
I.M. use: Reconstitute with sterile water for injection or 0.5% or 2% lidocaine hydrochloride injection. Add 3.2 ml to a 1.5-g vial (or 6.4 ml to a 3-g vial) to yield a concentration of 375 mg/ml. Administer deeply.
• Know that dosage should be altered in patients with impaired renal function.
• Give drug at least 1 hour before bacteriostatic antibiotics.
• Keep in mind that drug may cause false-positive urine glucose determinations with copper sulfate tests (Clinitest); drug does not affect glucose enzymatic tests (Diastix).

Reactions may be *common,* uncommon, *life-threatening,* or COMMON AND LIFE-THREATENING.

• Discontinue drug immediately if anaphylactic shock occurs. Notify doctor, and prepare to administer immediate treatment (such as epinephrine, corticosteroids, antihistamines, and other resuscitative measures), as indicated.
Patient teaching
• Tell patient to call doctor if rash (most common), fever, or chills develop.
• Advise female patient to use an additional form of contraception with oral contraceptives during drug therapy.

☑ Evaluation
• Patient is free from infection.
• Patient maintains adequate hydration.
• Patient and family state understanding of drug therapy.

amrinone lactate
(AM-rih-nohn LAK-tayt)
Inocor

Pharmacologic class: bipyridine derivative
Therapeutic class: inotropic, vasodilator
Pregnancy risk category: C

How supplied
Injection: 5 mg/ml

Pharmacokinetics
Absorption: not applicable with I.V. administration.
Distribution: sites unknown. Protein binding ranges from 10% to 49%.
Metabolism: metabolized in liver to several metabolites of unknown activity.
Excretion: excreted in urine. *Half-life:* about 4 hours (slightly longer in heart failure).

Route	Onset	Peak	Duration
I.V.	2-5 min	10 min	0.5-2 hr

Pharmacodynamics
Chemical effect: unknown; thought to produce inotropic action by increasing

cellular levels of cAMP. Produces vasodilation through a direct relaxant effect on vascular smooth muscle.
Therapeutic effect: increased cardiac output.

Indications and dosage
▶ **Short-term management of heart failure.** *Adults:* initially, 0.75 mg/kg I.V. bolus over 2 to 3 minutes. Then begin maintenance infusion of 5 to 10 mcg/kg/ minute. Additional bolus of 0.75 mg/kg may be given 30 minutes after start of therapy. Total daily dosage should not exceed 10 mg/kg.

Adverse reactions
CV: *arrhythmias,* hypotension, chest pain.
GI: nausea, vomiting, cramps, diarrhea, anorexia.
Hematologic: *thrombocytopenia* (depends on dose and duration of therapy).
Hepatic: elevated enzymes, hepatotoxicity (rare).
Other: burning at injection site, *hypersensitivity reactions* (pericarditis, ascites, myositis vasculitis, pleuritis), fever.

Interactions
Drug-drug. *Cardiac glycosides:* enhanced inotropic effect. Beneficial drug interaction. Give together.

Contraindications and precautions
• Contraindicated in patients with hypersensitivity to amrinone or bisulfites; in patients with severe aortic or pulmonic valvular disease in place of surgical correction of obstruction; or during acute phase of MI.
• Use cautiously in patients with hypertrophic cardiomyopathy and in pregnant or breast-feeding women.
• Safety of drug has not been established in children.

NURSING CONSIDERATIONS

⚕ Assessment
• Obtain history of patient's heart failure before therapy, and reassess regularly thereafter.
• Be alert for adverse reactions and drug interactions.
• Monitor ECG for arrhythmias.
• Evaluate patient's and family's knowledge of drug therapy.

⊞ Nursing diagnoses
• Fluid volume excess related to presence of heart failure.
• Risk for injury related to drug-induced arrhythmias
• Knowledge deficit related to drug therapy

⊠ Planning and implementation
• Administer amrinone with an infusion pump and use as supplied, or dilute in 0.45% or 0.9% NaCl to a concentration of 1 to 3 mg/ml. Use diluted solution within 24 hours.
• Don't dilute with solutions containing dextrose because a slow chemical reaction occurs over 24 hours. However, amrinone can be injected into free-flowing dextrose infusions through a Y-connector or directly into tubing.
• Don't administer furosemide and amrinone through same I.V. line because precipitation occurs.
• Patients with end-stage cardiac disease may receive home treatment with an amrinone drip while awaiting heart transplantation.
• If patient's blood pressure falls, slow or stop infusion and notify doctor.
• If platelet count falls below 150,000/mm^3, decrease dosage, as ordered.
• Be aware that amrinone is primarily prescribed for patients who have not responded to therapy with cardiac glycosides, diuretics, and vasodilators.
• Expect dosage to be based on clinical response, including assessment of pulmonary artery wedge pressure and cardiac output.

Patient teaching
• Warn patient that burning may occur at injection site.

☑ Evaluation
• Patient exhibits less fluid volume excess, such as improved lung sounds and decreased peripheral edema.
• Patient does not experience injury as a result of drug-induced arrhythmias.
• Patient and family state understanding of drug therapy.

anastrozole
(uh-NAS-truh-zohl)
Arimidex

Pharmacologic class: nonsteroidal aromatase inhibitor
Therapeutic class: antineoplastic
Pregnancy risk category: D

How supplied
Tablets: 1 mg

Pharmacokinetics
Absorption: absorbed from GI tract. Food affects extent of absorption.
Distribution: 40% bound to plasma proteins in therapeutic range.
Metabolism: metabolized in liver.
Excretion: about 11% excreted in urine as parent drug; about 60% excreted in urine as metabolites. *Half-life:* about 50 hours.

Route	Onset	Peak	Duration
P.O.	Unknown	Unknown	Unknown

Pharmacodynamics
Chemical effect: significantly lowers serum estradiol concentrations.
Therapeutic effect: hinders breast cancer cell growth.

Indications and dosage

▶ **Treatment of advanced breast cancer in postmenopausal women with disease progression after tamoxifen therapy.** *Adults:* 1 mg P.O. daily.

Adverse reactions

CNS: *asthenia, headache,* dizziness, depression, paresthesia.
CV: chest pain, edema.
GI: *nausea,* vomiting, diarrhea, constipation, dry mouth, abdominal pain, anorexia.
GU: pelvic pain, vaginal hemorrhage, vaginal dryness.
Musculoskeletal: *back pain,* bone pain.
Respiratory: dyspnea, increased cough, pharyngitis.
Skin: *hot flushes,* rash, sweating.
Other: *pain,* peripheral edema, weight gain, increased appetite, thromboembolic disease.

Interactions

None reported.

Contraindications and precautions

• Drug is not recommended for use in pregnant women.
• Use cautiously in breast-feeding women.
• Safety of drug has not been established in children.

NURSING CONSIDERATIONS

▨ **Assessment**
• Obtain history of patient's neoplastic disease before therapy.
• Be alert for adverse reactions.
• Evaluate patient's and family's knowledge of drug therapy.

✥ **Nursing diagnoses**
• Altered health maintenance related to neoplastic disease
• Risk for fluid volume deficit related to drug-induced adverse GI reactions
• Knowledge deficit related to drug therapy

▶ **Planning and implementation**
• Know that pregnancy must be ruled out before treatment can begin.
• Be aware that drug should be administered under supervision of a qualified doctor experienced in use of anticancer agents.
Patient teaching
• Instruct patient to report adverse reactions.
• Stress importance of follow-up care.

☑ **Evaluation**
• Patient exhibits positive response to therapy.
• Patient maintains adequate hydration.
• Patient and family state understanding of drug therapy.

---

anistreplase (anisoylated plasminogen-streptokinase activator complex; APSAC)
(uh-nIh-STREP-layz)
Eminase

Pharmacologic class: thrombolytic enzyme
Therapeutic class: thrombolytic enzyme
Pregnancy risk category: C

How supplied

Injection: 30 units/vial

Pharmacokinetics

Absorption: not applicable with I.V. administration.
Distribution: information not available.
Metabolism: immediately after injection, drug is deacylated by a nonenzymatic process to form active streptokinase-plasminogen complex.
Excretion: unknown. *Half-life:* 88 to 112 minutes.

Route	Onset	Peak	Duration
I.V.	Immediate	About 45 min	6 hr-2 days

Pharmacodynamics

Chemical effect: anistreplase, derived from Lys-plasminogen and streptokinase, is formulated into a fibrinolytic enzyme plus activator complex with activator temporarily blocked by an anisoyl group. Drug is activated in vivo by a nonenzymatic process that removes the anisoyl group. The active Lys-plasminogen—streptokinase activator complex is progressively formed in bloodstream or within thrombus.
Therapeutic effect: dissolves blood clots in coronary arteries.

Indications and dosage

▶ **Lysis of coronary artery thrombi after acute MI.** *Adults:* 30 units I.V. over 2 to 5 minutes by direct injection.

Adverse reactions

CNS: *intracranial hemorrhage.*
CV: ARRHYTHMIAS, conduction disorders, hypotension, edema.
EENT: hemoptysis, gum or mouth hemorrhage.
GI: *bleeding.*
GU: hematuria.
Hematologic: *bleeding tendency,* eosinophilia.
Skin: hematomas, urticaria, itching, flushing, delayed (2 weeks after therapy) purpuric rash.
Other: bleeding at puncture sites, *anaphylaxis or anaphylactoid reactions* (rare), arthralgias.

Interactions

Drug-drug. *Heparin, oral anticoagulants, drugs that alter platelet function (including aspirin, dipyridamole):* may increase risk of bleeding. Use together cautiously.

Contraindications and precautions

• Contraindicated in patients with history of severe allergic reaction to anistreplase or streptokinase and in those with active internal bleeding, CVA, recent (within past 2 months) intraspinal or intracranial surgery or trauma, aneurysm, arteriovenous malformation, intracranial neoplasm, uncontrolled hypertension, or known bleeding diathesis.
• Use cautiously in patients with recent (within 10 days) major surgery; trauma (including cardiopulmonary resuscitation); GI or GU bleeding; cerebrovascular disease; hypertension; mitral stenosis, atrial fibrillation, or other conditions that may lead to left-sided heart thrombus; acute pericarditis or subacute bacterial endocarditis; septic thrombophlebitis; diabetic hemorrhagic retinopathy; in pregnant women and during first 10 days postpartum; in breast-feeding women; in patients receiving anticoagulants; and in patients age 75 or older.
• Safety of drug has not been established in children.

NURSING CONSIDERATIONS

✍ Assessment
• Obtain history of patient's underlying cardiac condition before therapy.
• Monitor drug's effectiveness by carefully checking ECG and vital signs.
• Keep in mind that drug's efficacy may be limited if antistreptokinase antibodies are present. Antibody levels may be elevated if more than 5 days have elapsed since treatment with anistreplase or streptokinase or if patient has recently had a streptococcal infection.
• Be alert for adverse reactions and drug interactions.
• Evaluate patient's and family's knowledge about drug therapy.

⊞ Nursing diagnoses
• Altered tissue perfusion related to presence of coronary thrombosis
• Risk for injury related to drug-induced adverse reactions
• Knowledge deficit related to drug therapy

Reactions may be *common,* uncommon, *life-threatening,* or COMMON AND LIFE-THREATENING.

⧐ Planning and implementation

• Unlike other thrombolytics that must be infused, administer anistreplase by direct injection over 2 to 5 minutes.
• Reconstitute drug by slowly adding 5 ml of sterile water for injection. Direct stream against side of vial, not at drug itself. Gently roll vial to mix dry powder and water. To avoid excessive foaming, don't shake vial. The reconstituted solution should be colorless to pale yellow. Inspect for precipitate. If drug is not administered within 30 minutes of reconstituting, discard vial.
• Don't mix anistreplase with other drugs; don't dilute solution after reconstitution.
• Be prepared to treat bradycardia or ventricular irritability. Thrombolytic therapy is associated with reperfusion arrhythmias that may signify successful thrombolysis.
• Avoid I.M. injections and nonessential handling or moving of patient.
• If arterial puncture is necessary, select a compressible site (such as an arm), and apply pressure for 30 minutes afterward. Also, use pressure dressings, sandbags, or ice packs on recent puncture sites to prevent bleeding.
• Be aware that heparin therapy is frequently initiated after treatment with anistreplase to decrease risk of rethrombosis.
• Be aware that in vitro coagulation tests are affected by presence of anistreplase. This can be attenuated if blood samples are collected in presence of aprotinin (150 to 200 units/ml).
Patient teaching
• Teach patient to recognize signs of internal bleeding, and tell him to report them immediately. Advise patient about proper dental care to avoid excessive gum trauma.

✍ Evaluation

• Patient's ECG and vital signs reflect improvement in cardiopulmonary perfusion.

• Patient does not experience injury as a result of anistreplase therapy.
• Patient and family state understanding of drug therapy.

antihemophilic factor (AHF)
(an-tigh-hee-moh-FIL-ik FAK-tor)
Bioclate, Hemofil M, Helixate, Humate-P, Hyate:C, Koate-HP, Koate-HS, Kogenate, Monoclate, Monoclate-P, Profilate OSD, Recombinate

Pharmacologic class: blood derivative
Therapeutic class: antihemophilic
Pregnancy risk category: NR

How supplied

Injection: vials, with diluent. Units specified on label.

Pharmacokinetics

Absorption: not applicable with I.V. administration.
Distribution: equilibrates intravascular and extravascular compartments.
Metabolism: cleared rapidly from plasma.
Excretion: consumed during blood clotting. *Half-life:* 4 to 24 hours (averages 12 hours).

Route	Onset	Peak	Duration
I.V.	Immediate	1-2 hr	Unknown

Pharmacodynamics

Chemical effect: directly replaces deficient clotting factor that converts prothrombin to thrombin.
Therapeutic effect: causes blood clotting.

Indications and dosage

▶ **Hemophilia A (factor VIII deficiency).** *Adults and children:* dosage is highly individualized and depends on patient weight, severity of the deficiency, severity of the hemorrhage, presence of inhibitors, and level of factor VIII desired.

One AHF unit is equal to the activity present in 1 ml normal pooled human plasma less than 1 hour old. Do not confuse commercial product with blood bank-produced cryoprecipitated factor VIII from individual human donors. AHF is designed for I.V. use only; use plastic syringe, because solution adheres to glass surfaces.

Adverse reactions

CNS: headache, paresthesia, clouding or loss of consciousness, somnolence, lethargy.
CV: tachycardia, hypotension, tightness in chest.
EENT: visual disturbances.
GI: nausea, vomiting.
Hematologic: *hemolysis* (in patients with blood type A, B, or AB).
Respiratory: wheezing.
Skin: *erythema,* urticaria.
Other: *chills, fever, backache, flushing, hypersensitivity reactions,* rigor, stinging at injection site, risk of hepatitis B and HIV.

Interactions

None significant.

Contraindications and precautions

• Contraindicated in patients with hypersensitivity to murine (mouse) protein or to drug.
• Use cautiously in neonates, infants, pregnant women, and patients with hepatic disease because of susceptibility to hepatitis, which may be transmitted in AHF.
• Safety of drug has not been established in breast-feeding women.

NURSING CONSIDERATIONS

▨ Assessment
• Obtain thorough history of patient's underlying condition (including hematocrit, results of coagulation studies, and vital signs) before therapy begins and regularly throughout therapy.

• Be aware that inhibitors to factor VIII develop in some patients. This can eventually result in decreased response to drug.
• Assess the patient for adverse reactions to drug.
• Evaluate patient's and family's knowledge about drug therapy.

▨ Nursing diagnoses
• Altered health maintenance related to bleeding caused by underlying condition
• Risk for injury related to drug-induced adverse reactions
• Knowledge deficit related to drug therapy

▧ Planning and implementation
• As ordered, administer hepatitis B vaccine before administering drug.
• Take baseline pulse rate before administering. Use plastic syringe because drug may interact with glass syringe and bind to its surface. If pulse rate increases significantly, flow rate should be reduced or administration stopped.
• Refrigerate concentrate until ready to use. Warm concentrate and diluent bottles to room temperature before reconstituting. To mix drug, gently roll vial between hands.
• Use reconstituted solution within 3 hours. Store away from heat and do not refrigerate. Refrigeration after reconstitution may cause active ingredient to precipitate. Don't shake or mix with other I.V. solutions.
• Do not give S.C. or I.M.
• Keep in mind that a porcine product is available for patients with congenital hemophilia A who have antibodies to human factor VIII:C.
Patient teaching
• Educate patient about drug therapy.
• Inform patient about potential risks involved with drug therapy, such as risk of contracting hepatitis or HIV.
• Instruct patient to call doctor if adverse reactions develop.

Reactions may be *common,* uncommon, *life-threatening,* or COMMON AND LIFE-THREATENING.

☑ Evaluation
• Patient's vital signs and blood studies are within normal parameters with cessation of bleeding.
• Patient does not experience injury as a result of drug therapy.
• Patient and family state understanding of drug therapy.

anti-inhibitor coagulant complex
(an-tigh-in-HIB-eh-tor koh-AG-yoo-lant KOM-pleks)
Autoplex T, Feiba VH Immuno

Pharmacologic class: blood derivative
Therapeutic class: antihemophilic
Pregnancy risk category: C

How supplied
Injection: number of units of factor VIII correctional activity indicated on label of vial

Pharmacokinetics
Not fully evaluated.

Route	Onset	Peak	Duration
I.V.	10-30 min	Unknown	Unknown

Pharmacodynamics
Chemical effect: unknown. Efficacy may be related in part to presence of activated factors, which leads to more complete factor X activation in conjunction with tissue factor, phospholipid, and ionic calcium and allows coagulation process to proceed beyond those stages where factor VIII is needed.
Therapeutic effect: causes blood clotting.

Indications and dosage
▶ **Prevention and control of hemorrhagic episodes in certain patients with hemophilia A in whom inhibitor antibodies to antihemophilic factor have developed; management of bleeding in patients with acquired hemophilia who** have spontaneously acquired inhibitors to factor VIII. *Adults and children:* highly individualized and varies among manufacturers. For Autoplex T, 25 to 100 units/kg I.V., depending on severity of hemorrhage. If no hemostatic improvement occurs within 6 hours after administration, dosage repeated. For Feiba VH Immuno, 50 to 100 units/kg I.V. q 6 or 12 hours until clear signs of improvement.

Adverse reactions
CNS: dizziness, headache, lethargy, drowsiness.
CV: hypotension, transient chest discomfort, changes in pulse rate, *acute MI, thromboembolic events.*
GI: nausea, severe abdominal pain (rare).
Hematologic: *DIC.*
Respiratory: breathing difficulty.
Skin: flushing, rash, urticaria.
Other: fever, chills, hypersensitivity reactions (including *anaphylaxis), risk of hepatitis B and HIV.*

Interactions
Drug-drug. *Antifibrinolytic agents:* may alter effects of anti-inhibitor coagulant complex. Do not use together.

Contraindications and precautions
• Contraindicated in patients with signs of fibrinolysis, in those with DIC, and in those with a normal coagulation mechanism.
• Use with caution in patients with liver disease and in pregnant women.
• Safety of drug has not been established in breast-feeding women.

NURSING CONSIDERATIONS

☒ Assessment
• Obtain history of patient's underlying condition (including hematocrit, coagulation studies, and vital signs) before therapy and regularly throughout therapy.
• Be alert for adverse reactions and drug interactions.

• Evaluate patient's and family's knowledge about drug therapy.

⊞ **Nursing diagnoses**
• Altered health maintenance related to bleeding caused by underlying condition
• Risk for injury related to drug-induced adverse reactions
• Knowledge deficit related to drug therapy

▷ **Planning and implementation**
• As ordered, administer hepatitis B vaccine before administering drug.
• Warm drug and diluent to room temperature before reconstitution. Reconstitute according to manufacturer's directions. Use filter needle provided by manufacturer to withdraw reconstituted solution from vial into syringe; filter needle should then be replaced with a sterile injection needle for administration. Administer as soon as possible. Autoplex T infusions should be completed within 1 hour after reconstitution; Feiba VH Immuno infusions, within 3 hours.
• The rate of administration should be individualized according to patient's response. Autoplex T infusions may begin at a rate of 1 ml/minute; if well tolerated, infusion rate may be increased gradually to 10 ml/minute. Feiba VH Immuno infusion rate should not exceed 2 units/kg.
• Keep epinephrine readily available to treat anaphylaxis.
• If flushing, lethargy, headache, transient chest discomfort, or changes in blood pressure or pulse rate develop because of a rapid rate of infusion, stop drug and notify doctor. Know that these symptoms usually disappear with cessation of infusion. The infusion may then be resumed at a slower rate, as ordered.
Patient teaching
• Educate patient about anti-inhibitor coagulant complex therapy.
• Reassure patient that because of manufacturing process, risk of HIV transmission is extremely low.

☑ **Evaluation**
• Patient's vital signs and blood studies are within normal parameters with cessation of bleeding.
• Patient does not experience injury as a result of anti-inhibitor coagulant complex therapy.
• Patient and family state understanding of drug therapy.

antithrombin III, human (ATIII, heparin cofactor I)
(an-tigh-THROM-bin three, HYOO-mun)
ATnativ, Thrombate III

Pharmacologic class: glycoprotein
Therapeutic class: anticoagulant, antithrombotic
Pregnancy risk category: C

How supplied
Injection: 500 IU

Pharmacokinetics
Absorption: not applicable with I.V. administration.
Distribution: binding to epithelium and redistribution into extravascular compartment removes ATIII from blood. Special receptors on hepatocytes bind ATIII clotting factor complexes, rapidly removing them from circulation.
Metabolism: unknown.
Excretion: unknown. *Half-life:* 2 to 3 days.

Route	Onset	Peak	Duration
I.V.	Immediate	Unknown	About 4 days

Pharmacodynamics
Chemical effect: replaces deficient ATIII in patients with hereditary ATIII deficiency, normalizing coagulation inhibition and inhibiting thromboembolism. Also deactivates plasmin (to lesser extent than clotting factor).
Therapeutic effect: prevents or decreases blood clotting.

Reactions may be *common*, uncommon, *life-threatening*, or COMMON AND LIFE-THREATENING.

Indications and dosage

▶ **Thromboembolism associated with hereditary ATIII deficiency.** *Adults and children:* initial dose individualized to quantity required to increase ATIII activity to 120% of normal activity as determined 30 minutes after administration. Usual dose is 50 to 100 IU/minute I.V., not to exceed 100 IU/minute. Dose calculated based on anticipated 1% increase in plasma ATIII activity produced by 1 IU/kg of body weight using the formula: Dose (Units) is equal to desired activity (%) minus baseline activity (%) times weight (kg) divided by 1.4 (IU/kg). Maintenance dosage individualized to quantity required to increase ATIII activity to 80% of normal activity and is administered at 24-hour intervals. To calculate dosage, multiply desired ATIII activity (as % of normal) minus baseline ATIII activity (as % of normal) by body weight (in kg). Divide by actual increase in ATIII activity (in %) produced by 1 IU/kg as determined 30 minutes after administration of initial dose. Treatment is usually continued for 2 to 8 days but may be prolonged in pregnancy or when used with surgery or immobilization.

Adverse reactions

CV: vasodilation, lowered blood pressure. **GU:** diuresis.

Interactions

Drug-drug. *Heparin:* increased anticoagulant effect of both drugs. Heparin dose reduction may be necessary.

Contraindications and precautions

• No known contraindications.
• Use with extreme caution in children and neonates because safety and efficacy have not been established.

NURSING CONSIDERATIONS

Assessment

• Obtain history of patient's underlying condition before therapy, and reassess regularly throughout therapy.
• Because of risk of neonatal thromboembolism (sometimes fatal) in children of parents with hereditary ATIII deficiency, anticipate determination of ATIII levels immediately after birth.
• Obtain ATIII activity levels twice daily until dosage requirement has stabilized, then daily immediately before dose. Functional assays are preferred because quantitative immunologic test results may be normal despite decreased ATIII activity.
• Be alert for adverse reactions and drug interactions.
• Monitor for dyspnea and increased blood pressure, which may occur if administration rate is too rapid (1,500 IU in 5 minutes).
• Evaluate patient's and family's understanding of drug therapy.

Nursing diagnoses

• Altered tissue perfusion related to underlying condition
• Knowledge deficit related to drug therapy

Planning and implementation

• Reconstitute drug using 10 ml of sterile water (provided), 0.9% NaCl solution, or D₅W. Do not shake vial. Dilute further in same diluent solution, if desired.
• Keep in mind that 1 IU is equivalent to quantity of endogenous ATIII present in 1 ml of normal human plasma.
• Know that drug is not recommended for long-term prophylaxis of thrombotic episodes.
• Store drug at 36° to 46° F (2° to 8° C).
Patient teaching
• Tell patient to report difficulty breathing and any other sudden symptoms immediately while drug is being administered because a rate adjustment may be necessary.

• Inform patient that risk of hepatitis or HIV contraction is minimal.

☑ **Evaluation**
• Patient has adequate tissue perfusion.
• Patient and family state understanding of drug therapy.

---

aprobarbital
(ah-proh-BAR-bih-tahl)
Alurate*

Pharmacologic class: barbiturate
Therapeutic class: sedative-hypnotic
Controlled substance schedule: III
Pregnancy risk category: D

How supplied

Elixir: 40 mg/5 ml

Pharmacokinetics

Absorption: absorbed well.
Distribution: distributed widely throughout body tissues and fluids. Drug is 35% protein–bound.
Metabolism: metabolized in liver by oxidation to inactive metabolites.
Excretion: eliminated in urine; about 15% to 25% of dose is excreted as unchanged drug. **Half-life:** 14 to 34 hours.

Route	Onset	Peak	Duration
P.O.	45-60 min	≤ 3 hr	6-8 hr

Pharmacodynamics

Chemical effect: unknown; probably interferes with transmission of impulses from thalamus to cortex of brain.
Therapeutic effect: promotes sleep and calmness.

Indications and dosage

▶ **Sedation.** *Adults:* 40 mg P.O. t.i.d.
▶ **Insomnia.** *Adults:* 40 to 160 mg P.O. h.s.

Adverse reactions

CNS: *drowsiness, lethargy, hangover,* paradoxical excitement in elderly patients.
GI: nausea, vomiting.
Hematologic: exacerbation of porphyria.
Respiratory: respiratory depression.
Skin: *rash, urticaria, Stevens-Johnson syndrome.*
Other: *angioedema.*

Interactions

Drug-drug. *Chloramphenicol, MAO inhibitors, valproic acid:* inhibit metabolism of barbiturates; may cause prolonged CNS depression. Reduced barbiturate dosage needed.
CNS depressants, including narcotic analgesics: excessive CNS and respiratory depression. Use together cautiously.
Corticosteroids, digitoxin, doxycycline, estrogens and oral contraceptives, oral anticoagulants, tricyclic antidepressants: aprobarbital may enhance metabolism of these drugs. Monitor for decreased effectiveness.
Griseofulvin: decreased absorption of griseofulvin. Monitor for decreased effect.
Rifampin: may decrease barbiturate levels. Monitor for decreased effect.
Drug-lifestyle. *Alcohol use:* excessive CNS and respiratory depression. Use together cautiously.

Contraindications and precautions

• Contraindicated in patients with hypersensitivity to barbiturates, bronchopneumonia or other severe pulmonary insufficiency, or porphyria.
• Use with extreme caution in pregnant women only when absolutely necessary because fetal abnormality may occur.
• Use cautiously in patients with acute or chronic pain, suicidal tendencies, depression, history of drug abuse, or hepatic or renal impairment. Also use cautiously in breast-feeding women.

Reactions may be *common,* uncommon, *life-threatening*, or COMMON AND LIFE-THREATENING.

NURSING CONSIDERATIONS

⚖ Assessment
• Obtain history of patient's sleep patterns and mental status before therapy and reassess regularly thereafter.
• Be alert for adverse reactions and drug interactions.
• Assess patient's skin. Skin eruptions may precede potentially fatal reactions to barbiturate therapy. Discontinue drug when skin reactions occur. In some patients, high fever, stomatitis, headache, or rhinitis may precede skin reactions.
• Evaluate patient's and family's knowledge of drug therapy.

🖧 Nursing diagnoses
• Sleep pattern disturbance related to underlying problem
• Risk for trauma related to adverse CNS reactions caused by drug
• Knowledge deficit related to drug therapy

⫸ Planning and implementation
• Be aware that long-term use is not recommended; drug loses its efficacy in promoting sleep after 14 days of continued use.
Patient teaching
• Inform patient that morning "hangover" is common after hypnotic dose, which also suppresses REM sleep. Patients may experience increased dreaming after drug is discontinued.
• Caution patients about performing activities that require mental alertness or physical coordination. For inpatients, supervise walking and raise bed rails, particularly for elderly patients.
• Tell patient using oral contraceptives that she should consider alternate birth control methods because drug may enhance contraceptive hormone metabolism and decrease its effect.

🎶 Evaluation
• Patient states drug was effective in inducing sleep.

• Patient's safety is maintained throughout drug therapy.
• Patient and family state understanding of drug therapy.

---

aprotinin
(uh-proh-TIN-in)
Trasylol

Pharmacologic class: naturally occurring protease inhibitor
Therapeutic class: systemic hemostatic agent
Pregnancy risk category: B

How supplied
Injection: 10,000 KIU (kallikrein inactivator units)/ml (1.4 mg/ml) in 100-ml and 200-ml vials

Pharmacokinetics
Absorption: not applicable with I.V. administration.
Distribution: rapidly distributed into total extracellular space, leading to a rapid initial decrease in plasma concentrations.
Metabolism: unknown.
Excretion: 25% to 40% excreted in urine over 48 hours. *Half-life:* about 10 hours.

Route	Onset	Peak	Duration
I.V.	Unknown	Unknown	Unknown

Pharmacodynamics
Chemical effect: acts as systemic hemostatic agent, decreasing bleeding and turnover of coagulation factors. Aprotinin inhibits fibrinolysis by affecting kallikrein and plasmin, prevents triggering of contact phase of coagulation pathway, and increases resistance of platelets to damage from mechanical injury and high plasmin levels that occur during cardiopulmonary bypass.
Therapeutic effect: decreases bleeding.

Indications and dosage

▶ **To reduce blood loss or need for transfusion in patients undergoing coronary artery bypass grafts.** *Adults:* start with 10,000 KIU test dose at least 10 minutes before loading dose. If no allergic reaction is evident, anesthesia may be induced while loading dose of 2 million KIU is given slowly over 20 to 30 minutes. When loading dose is complete, sternotomy may be performed. Before bypass is initiated, cardiopulmonary bypass circuit is primed with 2 million KIU of drug by replacing an aliquot of priming fluid with drug. A continuous infusion at a rate of 500,000 KIU/hour is then given until patient leaves operating room. This is known as *regimen A.* A second regimen called *regimen B* may be given, which is half the dosage of *regimen A* (except for test dose).

Adverse reactions

CNS: *cerebral embolism, CVA.*
CV: *cardiac arrest, heart failure, MI, heart failure, ventricular tachycardia,* atrial fibrillation, atrial flutter, hypotension, supraventricular tachycardia.
GU: nephrotoxicity, *renal failure.*
Respiratory: pneumonia, respiratory disorder, *bronchospasm, pulmonary edema.*
Other: hypersensitivity reactions, *anaphylaxis,* fever.

Interactions

None significant.

Contraindications and precautions

• Contraindicated in patients hypersensitive to beef because drug is prepared from bovine lung.
• Use cautiously in pregnant women.
• Safety of drug has not been established in breast-feeding women and in children.

NURSING CONSIDERATIONS

☑ Assessment

• Obtain history of allergies. Patients with a history of allergic reactions to drugs or other substances may be at higher risk of development of an allergic reaction to aprotinin.
• Obtain history of patient's bleeding status before therapy and reassess regularly thereafter.
• Be alert for adverse reactions.
• Monitor laboratory studies, as ordered. Aprotinin prolongs activated clotting time and PTT. It may increase CK and transaminase levels and may falsely prolong whole blood clotting times when determined by surface activation methods.
• Evaluate patient's and family's understanding of drug therapy.

⊞ Nursing diagnoses

• Risk for fluid volume deficit related to potential bleeding during surgery
• Risk for injury related to drug-induced adverse reactions
• Knowledge deficit related to drug therapy

⊠ Planning and implementation

• Be prepared to administer a test dose. Test dose is particularly important in patients who have previously received drug because they have a higher risk of anaphylaxis. In such patients, pretreat with an antihistamine, as ordered.
• Keep in mind that aprotinin is incompatible with amino acids, corticosteroids, fat emulsions, heparin, and tetracyclines. Don't add any drugs to I.V. container and use a separate I.V.
• Administer all doses through a central line.
• To avoid hypotension, make sure patients are supine when loading dose is given.
• Store drug between 36° and 77° F (2° and 25° C). Protect from freezing.
• If symptoms of hypersensitivity occur (skin eruptions, itching, dyspnea, nausea, tachycardia), discontinue infusion immediately, call doctor, and provide supportive treatment.

Reactions may be *common,* uncommon, *life-threatening,* or COMMON AND LIFE-THREATENING.

Patient teaching
• Inform patient and family about aprotinin's use with cardiopulmonary bypass surgery and its potential adverse reactions.

☑ **Evaluation**
• Patient's bleeding during surgery is kept to a minimum as a result of aprotinin therapy.
• Patient does not experience injury as a result of aprotinin therapy.
• Patient and family state understanding of drug therapy.

---

asparaginase (L-asparaginase)
(as-PAR-ah-jin-ays)
Elspar, Kidrolase♦

Pharmacologic class: enzyme (L-asparagine amidohydrolase) (cell cycle-phase specific, G1 phase)
Therapeutic class: antineoplastic
Pregnancy risk category: C

How supplied
Injection: 10,000-unit vial

Pharmacokinetics
Absorption: unknown for I.M. administration.
Distribution: distributes primarily within intravascular space, with detectable concentrations in thoracic and cervical lymph. Minimal drug crosses blood-brain barrier.
Metabolism: hepatic sequestration by reticuloendothelial system may occur.
Excretion: unknown. *Half-life:* 8 to 30 hours.

Route	Onset	Peak	Duration
I.V.	Almost immediate	Almost immediate	23-33 days after stopping drug
I.M.	Almost immediate	4-24 hr	23-33 days after stopping drug

Pharmacodynamics
Chemical effect: destroys amino acid asparagine, which is needed for protein synthesis in acute lymphocytic leukemia. This leads to death of leukemic cell.
Therapeutic effect: kills leukemic cells.

Indications and dosage
► **Acute lymphocytic leukemia (in combination with other drugs).** *Adults and children:* 1,000 IU/kg I.V. daily for 10 days, injected over 30 minutes or by slow I.V. push; or 6,000 IU/m² I.M. at intervals specified in protocol.
► **Sole induction agent for acute lymphocytic leukemia.** *Adults:* 200 IU/kg I.V. daily for 28 days.

Adverse reactions
CNS: confusion, drowsiness, depression, hallucinations, nervousness, lethargy, somnolence.
GI: *vomiting* (may last up to 24 hours), *anorexia, nausea,* cramps, weight loss, HEMMORHAGIC PANCREATITIS.
GU: azotemia, *renal failure,* uric acid nephropathy, glycosuria, polyuria, *increased blood ammonia level.*
Hematologic: *anemia, hypofibrinogenemia,* depression of other clotting factors, *thrombocytopenia, leukopenia,* depressed serum albumin level.
Hepatic: elevated AST and ALT levels, *hepatotoxicity,* elevated bilirubin (direct and indirect) levels.
Metabolic: increase or decrease in total lipid level, *hyperuricemia, hyperglycemia.*
Skin: rash, urticaria.
Other: ANAPHYLAXIS, chills, fever, *death, fatal hyperthermia.*

Interactions
Drug-drug. *Methotrexate:* decreased methotrexate effectiveness. Monitor closely.
Prednisone, vincristine: increased toxicity. Monitor patient closely.

Contraindications and precautions
• Contraindicated in patients with pancreatitis or history of pancreatitis and previous hypersensitivity unless desensitized. Drug should also not be used in breast-feeding women.
• Use cautiously in patients with preexisting hepatic dysfunction and in pregnant women.

NURSING CONSIDERATIONS

⚖ Assessment
• Obtain history of patient's leukemic condition.
• Monitor effectiveness by evaluating CBC and bone marrow function tests, as ordered. Bone marrow regeneration may take 5 to 6 weeks.
• Be alert for adverse reactions and drug interactions.
• Evaluate patient's and family's knowledge of drug therapy.

⊕ Nursing diagnoses
• Altered health maintenance related to leukemic condition
• Altered protection related to drug-induced adverse reactions
• Knowledge deficit related to drug therapy

❯ Planning and implementation
• Know that drug should be administered in hospital setting with close supervision.
• Follow institutional policy to reduce risks. Preparation and administration of parenteral form is associated with carcinogenic, mutagenic, and teratogenic risks for personnel.
• Prevent occurrence of tumor lysis, which can result in uric acid nephropathy, by increasing fluid intake. Be aware that allopurinol should be started before therapy begins.
• Know that the risk of hypersensitivity reaction increases with repeated doses. An intradermal skin test should be performed before initial dose and when drug is given after an interval of a week or

more between doses. To perform skin test, give 2 IU of drug intradermally, as ordered. Observe site for at least 1 hour for erythema or a wheal, which indicates a positive response. An allergic reaction to the drug may still develop in a patient with a negative skin test.
• Know that a desensitization dose of 1 IU I.V. may be ordered. Dose is doubled q 10 minutes if no reaction occurs until total amount given equals patient's total dose for that day.
I.V. use: Give injection over 30 minutes through a running infusion of NaCl injection or 5% dextrose injection.
I.M. use: Limit dose at single injection site to 2 ml.
• Reconstitute with 2 to 5 ml of either sterile water for injection or NaCl injection. Don't shake vial. Don't use cloudy solutions.
• Know that drug should not be used as sole agent to induce remission unless combination therapy is inappropriate. Not recommended for maintenance therapy.
• Refrigerate unopened dry powder. Reconstituted solution is stable for 8 hours if refrigerated.
• If drug contacts skin or mucous membranes, wash with copious amounts of water for at least 15 minutes.
• Keep epinephrine, diphenhydramine, and I.V. corticosteroids available for treating anaphylaxis.
• Because of vomiting, administer parenteral fluids, as ordered, for 24 hours or until oral fluids are tolerated.
Patient teaching
• Tell patient to watch for signs of infection (fever, sore throat, fatigue) and bleeding (easy bruising, nosebleeds, bleeding gums, melena). Instruct patient to take temperature daily.
• Encourage patient to maintain an adequate fluid intake to increase urine output and facilitate excretion of uric acid.
• Tell patient that drowsiness may occur during therapy or for several weeks after treatment has ended. Warn patient to

---

Reactions may be *common,* uncommon, *life-threatening*, or COMMON AND LIFE-THREATENING.

avoid hazardous activities requiring mental alertness.

☑ Evaluation
• Patient is free of leukemic cells after asparaginase therapy.
• Patient does not experience injury as a result of drug-induced adverse reactions.
• Patient and family state understanding of drug therapy.

aspirin (acetylsalicylic acid)
(AS-prin)
Ancasal♦†, Arthrinol♦†, Artria S.R.†, ASA†, ASA Enseals†, Aspergum†, Aspro◊, Astrin♦†, Bayer Aspirin†, Bex◊, Coryphen♦†, Easprin†, Ecotrin†, Empirin†, Entrophen♦†, Halfprin, Measurin†, Norwich Aspirin Extra Strength†, Novasen♦†, Riphen-10♦†, Sal-Adult♦†, Sal-Infant♦†, Sloprin◊, Supasa♦†, Triaphen-10♦†, Vincent's Powders◊, Winsprin Capsules◊, ZORprin†

Pharmacologic class: salicylate
Therapeutic class: nonnarcotic analgesic, antipyretic, anti-inflammatory, antiplatelet
Pregnancy risk category: C (D in third trimester)

How supplied
Tablets†: 325 mg, 500 mg, 600 mg, 650 mg
Tablets (chewable): 81 mg†
Tablets (enteric-coated): 165 mg, 325 mg†, 500 mg†, 650 mg†, 975 mg
Tablets (extended-release): 800 mg
Tablets (timed-release): 650 mg†
Capsules: 325 mg†, 500 mg†
Powder: 500 mg
Chewing gum: 227.5 mg†
Suppositories: 60 mg, 65 mg, 120 mg, 125 mg, 130 mg, 195 mg, 200 mg, 300 mg, 325 mg, 600 mg, 650 mg, 1.2 g

Pharmacokinetics
Absorption: absorbed rapidly and completely from GI tract.
Distribution: distributed widely into most body tissues and fluids. Protein-binding to albumin is concentration-dependent; ranges from 75% to 90%, and decreases as serum concentration increases.
Metabolism: hydrolyzed partially in GI tract to salicylic acid with almost complete metabolism in liver.
Excretion: excreted in urine as salicylate and its metabolites. *Half-life:* 15 to 20 minutes.

Route	Onset	Peak	Duration
P.O.			
Solution	5-30 min	15-60 min	1-4 hr
Regular	5-30 min	25-40 min	1-4 hr
Buffered	5-30 min	1-2 hr	1-4 hr
Extended-release	5-30 min	1-2 hr	1-4 hr
Enteric-coated	5-30 min	4-8 hr	1-4 hr
P.R.	5-30 min	3-4 hr	1-4 hr

Pharmacodynamics
Chemical effect: produces analgesia by blocking prostaglandin synthesis (peripheral action). Aspirin and other salicylates may prevent lowering of pain threshold that occurs when prostaglandins sensitize pain receptors to mechanical and chemical stimulation. Exerts its anti-inflammatory effect by inhibiting prostaglandin synthesis; also may inhibit synthesis or action of other mediators of inflammatory response. Relieves fever by acting on hypothalamic heat-regulating center to cause peripheral vasodilation. This increases peripheral blood supply and promotes sweating, which leads to heat loss and to cooling by evaporation. In low doses, aspirin also appears to impede clotting by blocking prostaglandin synthesis, which prevents formation of platelet-aggregating substance thromboxane A_2.

Therapeutic effect: relieves pain, reduces fever and inflammation, and decreases incidence of transient ischemic attacks and MI.

Indications and dosage

▶ **Arthritis.** *Adults:* initially, 2.4 to 3.6 g P.O. daily in divided doses. Maintenance dosage is 3.6 to 5.4 g P.O. daily in divided doses. *Children:* 80 to 130 mg/kg P.O. daily in divided doses.
▶ **Mild pain or fever.** *Adults:* 325 to 650 mg P.O. or P.R. q 4 hours, p.r.n. *Children:* (for mild pain only) 65 mg/kg P.O. or P.R. daily in four to six divided doses.
▶ **Prevention of thrombosis.** *Adults:* 1.3 g P.O. daily in two to four divided doses.
▶ **Reduction of risk of heart attack in patients with previous MI or unstable angina.** *Adults:* 160 to 325 mg P.O. daily.
▶ **Kawasaki syndrome (mucocutaneous lymph node syndrome).** *Adults:* 80 to 100 mg/kg P.O. daily in four divided doses during febrile phase. Some patients may need up to 120 mg/kg. When fever subsides, decrease dosage to 3 to 8 mg/kg once daily, adjusted according to serum salicylate concentration.

Adverse reactions

EENT: *tinnitus, hearing loss.*
GI: *nausea, vomiting, GI distress, occult bleeding,* dyspepsia, *GI bleeding.*
Hematologic: *prolonged bleeding time, thrombocytopenia.*
Hepatic: altered liver function studies, *hepatitis.*
Skin: *rash,* bruising, urticaria, angioedema.
Other: hypersensitivity reactions, *(anaphylaxis,* asthma*), Reye's syndrome.*

Interactions

Drug-drug. *Ammonium chloride, other urine acidifiers:* increased blood levels of aspirin products. Monitor for aspirin toxicity.

Antacids in high doses (and other urine alkalinizers): decreased blood levels of aspirin products. Monitor for decreased aspirin effect.
Beta blockers: decreased antihypertensive effect. Avoid long-term aspirin use if patient is taking antihypertensives.
Corticosteroids: enhanced salicylate elimination. Monitor for decreased salicylate effect.
Heparin, oral anticoagulants: increased risk of bleeding. Avoid using together if possible.
Methotrexate: increased risk of methotrexate toxicity. Avoid concomitant use.
NSAIDs, steroids: increased risk of GI bleeding. Avoid concomitant use.
NSAIDs, including diflunisal, fenoprofen, ibuprofen, indomethacin, piroxicam, meclofenamate, naproxen: altered pharmacokinetics of these agents, leading to lowered serum levels and decreased effectiveness. Avoid concomitant use.
Oral antidiabetic agents: increased hypoglycemic effect. Monitor closely.
Probenecid, sulfinpyrazone: decreased uricosuric effect. Avoid aspirin during therapy with these agents.
Drug-food. *Caffeine:* may increase the absorption of aspirin. Monitor for increased effects.
Drug-lifestyle. *Alcohol use:* increased risk of GI bleeding. Avoid concomitant use.

Contraindications and precautions

• Contraindicated in patients with G6PD deficiency; bleeding disorders such as hemophilia, von Willebrand's disease, or telangiectasia; NSAID-induced sensitivity reactions; or hypersensitivity to drug.
• Use cautiously in patients with GI lesions, impaired renal function, hypoprothrombinemia, vitamin K deficiency, thrombocytopenia, thrombotic thrombocytopenic purpura, or severe hepatic impairment.
• Use cautiously in pregnant women. Safety has not been established in breast-feeding women.

Reactions may be *common,* uncommon, *life-threatening,* or COMMON AND LIFE-THREATENING.

• Because of epidemiologic association with Reye's syndrome, the Centers for Disease Control and Prevention recommends not giving salicylates to children or teenagers with chicken pox or influenza-like illness.

NURSING CONSIDERATIONS

⚗ Assessment
• Obtain history of patient's pain or fever before therapy and monitor throughout therapy.
• Be alert for adverse reactions and drug interactions.
• During chronic therapy, monitor serum salicylate level. Therapeutic level in arthritis is 10 to 30 mg/dl. With chronic therapy, mild toxicity may occur at plasma levels of 20 mg/dl. Tinnitus may occur at plasma levels of 30 mg/dl and above but does not reliably indicate toxicity, especially in very young patients and those older than age 60.
• Evaluate patient's and family's knowledge of drug therapy.

⊞ Nursing diagnoses
• Pain related to underlying condition.
• Risk for injury related to drug-induced adverse GI reactions
• Knowledge deficit related to drug therapy

⧉ Planning and implementation
P.O. use: Give aspirin with food, milk, antacid, or large glass of water to reduce adverse GI reactions. For patient who has difficulty swallowing, crush aspirin, combine it with soft food, or dissolve it in liquid. After mixing aspirin with a liquid, administer it immediately because drug doesn't stay in solution. Don't crush enteric-coated aspirin.
• Remember that enteric-coated products are slowly absorbed and not suitable for acute effects. They cause less GI bleeding and may be more suited for long-term therapy, for example, of arthritis.

P.R. use: Absorption following P.R. administration is slow and variable depending on how long suppository is retained. If retained for 2 to 4 hours, absorption of dose is 20% to 60%; if retained for at least 10 hours, absorption is 70% to 100%.
• Hold dose and notify doctor if bleeding, salicylism (tinnitus, hearing loss), or adverse GI reactions develop.
• Know that aspirin should be discontinued 5 to 7 days before elective surgery, as ordered.

Patient teaching
• Advise patient receiving high-dose prolonged treatment to watch for petechiae, bleeding gums, and signs of GI bleeding and to maintain adequate fluid intake. Encourage use of a soft toothbrush.
• Because of many possible drug interactions involving aspirin, warn patient taking prescription drugs to check with doctor or pharmacist before taking OTC combinations containing aspirin.
• Explain that various OTC preparations contain aspirin. Warn patient to read labels carefully to avoid overdose.
• Advise patient to avoid alcohol consumption during drug therapy.
• Advise patient to restrict intake of caffeine during drug therapy.
• Instruct patient to take aspirin with food or milk.
• Instruct patient not to chew enteric-coated products.
• Emphasize safe storage of medications in the home. Teach patient to keep aspirin and other drugs out of children's reach. Aspirin is a leading cause of poisoning in children. Encourage use of child-resistant containers in households that include children, even if only as occasional visitors.

☑ Evaluation
• Patient states aspirin has relieved pain.
• Patient remains free of adverse GI effects throughout drug therapy.
• Patient and family state understanding of drug therapy.

astemizole
(uh-STEH-mih-zohl)
Hismanal

Pharmacologic class: histamine$_1$-receptor antagonist
Therapeutic class: antiallergy
Pregnancy risk category: C

How supplied

Tablets: 10 mg
Oral suspension: 2 mg/ml* ◊

Pharmacokinetics

Absorption: rapidly absorbed from GI tract.
Distribution: about 90% bound to plasma proteins.
Metabolism: metabolized in liver.
Excretion: excreted primarily in feces.
Half-life: 1 to 2½ days.

Route	Onset	Peak	Duration
P.O.	≤ 24 hr	≤ 1 hr	Unknown

Pharmacodynamics

Chemical effect: blocks effects of histamine at H$_1$-receptor sites. Astemizole is a nonsedating antihistamine; its chemical structure prevents entry into CNS.
Therapeutic effect: relieves allergy symptoms.

Indications and dosage

▶ **Relief of symptoms associated with chronic idiopathic urticaria and seasonal allergic rhinitis.** *Adults and children over age 12:* 10 mg P.O. daily.

Adverse reactions

CNS: headache, nervousness, dizziness, drowsiness.
CV: *arrhythmias* (with high plasma levels).
EENT: dry mouth, pharyngitis, conjunctivitis.
GI: nausea, diarrhea, abdominal pain, increased appetite.

Other: arthralgia, weight gain, cholestatic jaundice.

Interactions

Drug-drug. *Fluconazole, HIV protease inhibitors, metronidazole, quinine, serotonin reuptake inhibitors, other potent CYP3A4 inhibitors:* may influence metabolism of astemizole, causing increased plasma concentrations. Avoid concomitant use.
Itraconazole, ketoconazole, macrolide antibiotics (such as clarithromycin, erythromycin, troleandomycin): risk of serious adverse cardiac reactions. Don't use together.
Drug-food. *Grapefruit juice:* can inhibit the hepatic metabolism of astemizole. Avoid grapefruit juice.

Contraindications and precautions

• Contraindicated in patients with hypersensitivity to astemizole and in those taking antifungal agents itraconazole or ketoconazole or macrolide antibiotics, including erythromycin.
• Use cautiously in patients with hepatic or renal disease and in pregnant or breast-feeding women.
• Also use cautiously in patients with lower respiratory tract diseases (including asthma); drying effects can increase risk of bronchial mucus plug formation.
• Safety of drug has not been established in children younger than age 12.

NURSING CONSIDERATIONS

 Assessment
• Obtain history of patient's allergic condition before therapy begins and reassess regularly thereafter.
• Be alert for adverse reactions and drug interactions.
• Monitor patient's fluid status if adverse GI reactions occur.
• Evaluate patient's and family's knowledge of drug therapy.

⊞ Nursing diagnoses
- Altered health maintenance related to underlying allergic condition
- Risk for fluid volume deficit related to drug-induced adverse GI reactions
- Knowledge deficit related to drug therapy

▷ Planning and implementation
- Administer astemizole to patient on an empty stomach at least 2 hours after a meal, and ensure that patient avoids eating for at least 1 hour after dosing.

Patient teaching
- Ensure that patient knows to take astemizole only once a day. If symptoms persist or worsen, warn patient not to increase dosage without consulting his doctor. High doses may increase risk of arrhythmias.
- Instruct patient to take drug on an empty stomach at least 2 hours after a meal and to avoid eating for at least 1 hour after dosing.
- Warn patient to stop taking drug 4 days before allergy skin tests to preserve accuracy of tests.
- Instruct patient not to drink grapefruit juice while on drug therapy, because the juice can inhibit the hepatic metabolism of astemizole.

☑ Evaluation
- Patient's allergic symptoms are relieved with drug.
- Patient maintains adequate hydration status during therapy.
- Patient and family state understanding of drug therapy.

---

atenolol
(uh-TEN-uh-lol)
Apo-Atenolol♦, Noten◇, Nu-Atenol♦, Tenormin

Pharmacologic class: beta blocker
Therapeutic class: antihypertensive, antianginal

Pregnancy risk category: D

How supplied
Tablets: 25 mg, 50 mg, 100 mg
Injection: 5 mg/10 ml

Pharmacokinetics
Absorption: about 50% to 60% of oral dose is absorbed.
Distribution: distributes into most tissues and fluids except brain and CSF. Approximately 5% to 15% protein-bound.
Metabolism: minimal.
Excretion: from 40% to 50% of dose is excreted unchanged in urine; remainder is excreted as unchanged drug and metabolites in feces. *Half-life:* 6 to 7 hours (increases as renal function decreases).

Route	Onset	Peak	Duration
P.O.	1 hr	2-4 hr	24 hr
I.V.	5 min	5 min	12 hr

Pharmacodynamics
Chemical effect: selectively blocks beta$_1$-adrenergic receptors; decreases cardiac output, peripheral resistance, and cardiac oxygen consumption; and depresses renin secretion.
Therapeutic effect: decreases blood pressure, relieves anginal symptoms, and reduces CV mortality rate and risk of reinfarction after acute MI.

Indications and dosage
▶ **Hypertension.** *Adults:* initially, 50 mg P.O. daily as a single dose. Dosage increased to 100 mg once daily after 7 to 14 days. Doses over 100 mg are unlikely to produce further benefit. Dosage adjustment required in patients with creatinine clearance below 35 ml/minute.
▶ **Angina pectoris.** *Adults:* 50 mg P.O. once daily. Increased as needed to 100 mg daily after 7 days for optimal effect. Maximum dosage is 200 mg daily.
▶ **Reduction of CV mortality rate and risk of reinfarction in patients with**

---

acute MI. *Adults:* 5 mg I.V. over 5 minutes, followed by another 5 mg 10 minutes later. After an additional 10 minutes, 50 mg P.O., followed by 50 mg P.O. in 12 hours. Thereafter, 100 mg P.O. daily (as a single dose or 50 mg b.i.d.) for at least 7 days. *In patients with renal insufficiency:* If creatinine clearance is 15 to 35 ml/minute, maximum dosage is 50 mg daily; if creatinine clearance is less than 15 ml/minute, maximum dosage is 25 mg daily. Hemodialysis patients require 25 mg or 50 mg after each dialysis session, but supervise closely because of risk of hypotension.

Adverse reactions

CNS: fatigue, lethargy.
CV: *bradycardia, hypotension,* **heart failure,** intermittent claudication.
GI: nausea, vomiting, diarrhea.
Respiratory: dyspnea, **bronchospasm.**
Skin: rash.
Other: fever.

Interactions

Drug-drug. *Antihypertensives:* enhanced hypotensive effect. Use together cautiously.
Cardiac glycosides, diltiazem, verapamil: excessive bradycardia and increased depressant effect on myocardium. Use together cautiously.
Insulin, oral antidiabetic agents: can alter dosage requirements in previously stabilized diabetic patients. Observe patient carefully.
Reserpine: may cause hypotension. Use with caution.

Contraindications and precautions

• Contraindicated in patients with sinus bradycardia, greater than first-degree heart block, overt cardiac failure, or cardiogenic shock.
• Don't use in pregnant women unless absolutely necessary because fetal harm can occur.
• Use cautiously in patients at risk for heart failure and in patients with bron-

chospastic disease, diabetes, and hyperthyroidism. Also use cautiously in breast-feeding women.
• Safety of drug has not been established in children.

NURSING CONSIDERATIONS

Assessment
• Obtain history of patient's underlying condition.
• Monitor effectiveness by frequently checking blood pressure if prescribed for hypertension, frequency and severity of anginal pain if prescribed for angina pectoris, and signs of reinfarction if prescribed to reduce CV mortality rate and risk of reinfarction after acute MI. Be aware that full antihypertensive effect may not appear for 1 to 2 weeks after initiating therapy.
• Be alert for adverse reactions and drug interactions.
• Evaluate patient's and family's understanding of drug therapy.

Nursing diagnoses
• Risk for injury related to underlying condition
• Decreased cardiac output related to drug-induced adverse CV reactions
• Knowledge deficit related to drug therapy

Planning and implementation
• Check patient's apical pulse before giving drug; if slower than 60 beats/minute, withhold drug and call doctor.
P.O. use: Administer as a single daily dose.
I.V. use: Give by slow injection, not to exceed 1 mg/minute. Doses may be mixed with D_5W, 0.9% NaCl, or dextrose and NaCl solutions. Solution is stable for 48 hours after mixing.
• Be prepared to treat shock or hypoglycemia because this drug masks common signs of these conditions.
• Notify doctor immediately if patient shows signs of decreased cardiac output.

Reactions may be *common,* uncommon, *life-threatening,* or COMMON AND LIFE-THREATENING.

Patient teaching
• Caution patient that abrupt discontinuation of drug can exacerbate angina and MI. Drug should be withdrawn gradually over a 2-week period.
• Counsel patient to take drug at same time every day.
• Tell female patient to notify doctor if pregnancy occurs. Drug will need to be discontinued.
• Teach patient how to take his pulse. Tell patient to withhold drug and call doctor if pulse rate is below 60 beats/minute.

☑ **Evaluation**
• Patient's underlying condition improves with drug therapy.
• Patient's cardiac output remains unchanged throughout drug therapy.
• Patient and family state understanding of drug therapy.

atorvastatin calcium
(uh-TOR-vah-stah-tin KAL-see-um)
Lipitor

Pharmacologic class: 3-hydroxy-3-methylglutaryl-coenzyme A (HMG-CoA) reductase inhibitor
Therapeutic class: antilipemic
Pregnancy risk category: X

How supplied
Tablets: 10 mg, 20 mg, 40 mg

Pharmacokinetics
Absorption: rapidly absorbed.
Distribution: 98% is bound to plasma proteins.
Metabolism: metabolized by liver.
Excretion: eliminated in bile.

Route	Onset	Peak	Duration
P.O.	Unknown	1-2 hr	Unknown

Pharmacodynamics
Chemical effect: selective inhibitor of HMG-CoA reductase, which converts HMG-CoA to mevalonate, a precursor of sterols.
Therapeutic effect: lowers plasma cholesterol and lipoprotein levels.

Indications and dosage
▶ **Adjunct to diet to reduce low-density lipoprotein (LDL), total cholesterol, apo B, and triglyceride levels in patients with primary hypercholesterolemia and mixed dyslipidemia.** *Adults:* initially, 10 mg P.O. once daily. Dosage increased p.r.n. to maximum of 80 mg daily as single dose. Dosage based on blood lipid levels drawn within 2 to 4 weeks after starting therapy.
▶ **Alone or as an adjunct to lipid-lowering treatments, such as LDL apheresis, in patients with homozygous familial hypercholesterolemia.** *Adults:* 10 to 80 mg P.O. once daily.

Adverse reactions
CNS: *headache,* asthenia.
GI: abdominal pain, constipation, diarrhea, dyspepsia, flatulence.
Musculoskeletal: back pain, arthralgia, myalgia.
Respiratory: sinusitis, pharyngitis.
Skin: rash.
Other: *infection,* accidental injury, flu-like syndrome, allergic reaction.

Interactions
Drug-drug. *Antacids:* decrease bioavailability. Administer separately.
Azole antifungals, cyclosporine, erythromycin, fibric acid derivatives, niacin: may cause rhabdomyolysis. Avoid use together.
Digoxin: may increase digoxin levels. Monitor serum digoxin levels.
Erythromycin: increases plasma drug levels. Monitor patient.
Oral contraceptives: increases hormone levels. Consider when selecting an oral contraceptive.

Contraindications and precautions

• Contraindicated in patients with active liver disease, conditions linked with unexplained persistent increases in serum transaminases, or hypersensitivity to drug; in pregnant or breast-feeding women; and in women of childbearing age (except those at no risk for becoming pregnant).

NURSING CONSIDERATIONS

⚐ Assessment
• Know that drug should be withheld or stopped in patients with serious, acute conditions that suggest myopathy or in those at risk for renal failure secondary to rhabdomyolysis due to trauma; major surgery; severe metabolic, endocrine, and electrolyte disorders; severe acute infection; hypotension; or uncontrolled seizures.
• Evaluate patient's and family's understanding of drug therapy.

⊞ Nursing diagnoses
• Risk for injury related to elevated cholesterol levels
• Knowledge deficit related to drug therapy

▷ Planning and implementation
• Use drug only after diet and other non-pharmacologic treatments prove ineffective. Know that patient should follow a standard low-cholesterol diet before and during therapy.
• Before initiating treatment, perform a baseline lipid profile to exclude secondary causes of hypercholesterolemia. Liver function tests and lipid levels should be done before therapy, after 6 and 12 weeks, or following an increase in dosage and periodically thereafter, as ordered.
Patient teaching
• Teach patient about proper dietary management, weight control, and exercise and explain their role in controlling elevated serum lipid levels.

• Warn patient to avoid alcohol.
• Tell patient to inform doctor of adverse reactions.
• Inform female patient to notify doctor if pregnancy is suspected.

☑ Evaluation
• Patient's blood cholesterol level is within normal limits.
• Patient and family state understanding of drug therapy.

---

atovaquone
(uh-TOH-vuh-kwohn)
Mepron

Pharmacologic class: ubiquinone analogue
Therapeutic class: antiprotozoal
Pregnancy risk category: C

How supplied
Tablets: 250 mg

Pharmacokinetics
Absorption: limited. Bioavailability is increased threefold when administered with meals. Fat has been shown to enhance absorption significantly.
Distribution: extensively bound (99.9%) to plasma proteins.
Metabolism: not metabolized.
Excretion: undergoes enterohepatic cycling and is primarily excreted in feces. Less than 0.6% is excreted in urine. *Half-life:* 2.2 to 2.9 days.

Route	Onset	Peak	Duration
P.O.	Unknown	1st peak 1-8 hr	Unknown
		2nd peak 1-4 days	

Pharmacodynamics
Chemical effect: unknown; appears to interfere with electron transport in protozoal mitochondria, inhibiting enzymes

---

Reactions may be *common*, uncommon, *life-threatening*, or COMMON AND LIFE-THREATENING.

needed for synthesis of nucleic acids and adenosine triphosphate. *Therapeutic effect:* kills *Pneumocystis carinii* protozoa.

Indications and dosage

▶ **Mild to moderate *P. carinii* in patients who cannot tolerate co-trimoxazole.**
Adults: 750 mg P.O. t.i.d. for 21 days.

Adverse reactions

CNS: *headache, insomnia,* asthenia, dizziness.
EENT: *cough.*
GI: *nausea, diarrhea, vomiting,* oral candidiasis, constipation, abdominal pain.
Skin: *rash,* pruritus.
Other: *fever.*

Interactions

Drug-drug. *Highly protein-bound drugs (phenytoin, coumadin):* may compete for receptor sites affecting drug concentrations. Use cautiously.
Rifampin, rifabutin: decreased atovaquone's steady-state concentrations. Avoid concurrent use.

Contraindications and precautions

• Contraindicated in patients with hypersensitivity to drug.
• Use cautiously in pregnant or breastfeeding women. Because drug is highly bound to plasma protein (greater than 99.9%), also use cautiously with other highly protein-bound drugs.
• Safety of drug has not been established in children.

NURSING CONSIDERATIONS

⚗ Assessment
• Obtain history of patient's protozoal respiratory infection and reassess regularly.
• Be alert for adverse reactions.
• Monitor patient's hydration status if adverse GI reactions occur.
• Evaluate patient's and family's knowledge of drug therapy.

⚗ Nursing diagnoses
• Infection related to presence of susceptible protozoal organisms
• Risk for fluid volume deficit related to drug-induced adverse GI reactions
• Knowledge deficit related to drug therapy

⚗ Planning and implementation
• Administer drug with food to improve bioavailability.
Patient teaching
• Instruct patient to take drug with meals because food enhances absorption significantly.
• Warn patient not to perform hazardous activities if dizziness occurs.
• Emphasize importance of taking drug for all 21 days, even if patient is feeling better.
• Tell patient to notify doctor if serious adverse reactions occur.

⚗ Evaluation
• Patient's infection is eradicated.
• Patient remains adequately hydrated throughout therapy.
• Patient and family state understanding of drug therapy.

atracurium besylate
(uh-trah-KYOO-ree-um BES-eh-layt)
Tracrium

Pharmacologic class: nondepolarizing neuromuscular blocker
Therapeutic class: skeletal muscle relaxant
Pregnancy risk category: C

How supplied

Injection: 10 mg/ml

Pharmacokinetics

Absorption: not applicable with I.V. administration.
Distribution: distributed into extracellular space. About 82% protein-bound.

Metabolism: rapidly metabolized by Hofmann elimination and by nonspecific enzymatic ester hydrolysis. The liver does not appear to play a major role. *Excretion:* atracurium and its metabolites are excreted in urine and feces. *Half-life:* 20 minutes.

Route	Onset	Peak	Duration
I.V.	≤ 2 min	3-5 min	35-70 min

Pharmacodynamics

Chemical effect: prevents acetylcholine from binding to receptors on muscle end plate, thus blocking depolarization and resulting in skeletal muscle paralysis. *Therapeutic effect:* relaxes skeletal muscles.

Indications and dosage

▶ **Adjunct to general anesthesia, to facilitate endotracheal intubation and to provide skeletal muscle relaxation during surgery or mechanical ventilation.** Dosage depends on anesthetic used, individual needs, and response. Dosages given here are representative and must be adjusted. *Adults and children over age 2:* 0.4 to 0.5 mg/kg by I.V. bolus. Maintenance dosage of 0.08 to 0.10 mg/kg within 20 to 45 minutes of initial dose should be administered during prolonged surgical procedures. Maintenance dosages may be administered q 15 to 25 minutes in patients receiving balanced anesthesia. For prolonged surgical procedures, a constant infusion of 5 to 9 mcg/kg/minute may be used after initial bolus. *Children ages 1 month to 2 years:* initial dose, 0.3 to 0.4 mg/kg. Frequent maintenance doses may be needed.

Adverse reactions

CV: increased heart rate, bradycardia, hypotension.
Respiratory: *prolonged dose-related apnea,* wheezing, increased bronchial secretions.

Skin: *flushing,* erythema, pruritus, urticaria.
Other: *anaphylaxis.*

Interactions

Drug-drug. *Aminoglycoside antibiotics (including amikacin, gentamicin, kanamycin, neomycin, streptomycin); polymyxin antibiotics (polymyxin B sulfate, colistin); clindamycin; quinidine; general anesthetics (such as enflurane, halothane, isoflurane):* potentiated neuromuscular blockade, leading to increased skeletal muscle relaxation and prolongation of effect. Use cautiously during surgical and postoperative periods. *Lithium, magnesium salts, opioid analgesics:* potentiated neuromuscular blockade, leading to increased skeletal muscle relaxation and, possibly, respiratory paralysis. Reduce dose of atracurium.

Contraindications and precautions

• Contraindicated in patients with hypersensitivity to drug.
• Use cautiously in patients with CV disease; severe electrolyte disorders; bronchogenic carcinoma; hepatic, renal, or pulmonary impairment; neuromuscular diseases; or myasthenia gravis.
• Also use cautiously in pregnant women, breast-feeding women, and elderly or debilitated patients.

NURSING CONSIDERATIONS

⚕ Assessment
• Obtain history of patient's neuromuscular status before therapy and reassess regularly.
• Be alert for adverse reactions and interactions.
• Monitor respirations closely until patient is fully recovered from neuromuscular blockade, as evidenced by tests of muscle strength (hand grip, head lift, and ability to cough).
• Be aware that a nerve stimulator and train-of-four monitoring are recommended to confirm antagonism of neuromus-

cular blockade and recovery of muscle strength. Before attempting pharmacologic reversal with neostigmine, some evidence of spontaneous recovery should be seen.
• Evaluate patient's and family's understanding of drug therapy.

⊕ **Nursing diagnoses**
• Risk for injury related to underlying condition
• Inability to sustain spontaneous ventilation related to drug-induced respiratory paralysis
• Knowledge deficit related to drug therapy

▶ **Planning and implementation**
• Administer sedatives or general anesthetics before neuromuscular blockers, as ordered. Neuromuscular blockers don't obtund consciousness or alter pain threshold.
• Use this drug only under direct medical supervision by personnel skilled in use of neuromuscular blockers and techniques for maintaining a patent airway. Don't use unless facilities and equipment for mechanical ventilation, oxygen therapy, and intubation as well as an antagonist are immediately available.
• Know that drug usually is administered by rapid I.V. bolus injection but may be given by intermittent infusion or continuous infusion. At concentrations of 0.2 mg/ml to 0.5 mg/ml, atracurium is compatible for 24 hours in D₅W, 0.9% NaCl injection, or dextrose 5% in 0.9% NaCl injection.
• Do not use lactated Ringer's solution. In lactated Ringer's injection, atracurium is stable for 8 hours at a concentration of 0.5 mg/ml. Because of an increased rate of drug degradation in this solution, it is not recommended.
• Do not administer by I.M. injection.
• Do not mix with acidic or alkaline solutions (precipitate may form).
• Know that prior administration of succinylcholine doesn't prolong duration of

action but quickens onset and may deepen neuromuscular blockade.
• Explain all events and happenings to patient because he can still hear.
• Administer analgesics, as ordered, for pain. Remember that patient can have pain but not be able to express it.
• Keep airway clear. Have emergency equipment and drugs immediately available.
• Once spontaneous recovery starts, be prepared to reverse atracurium-induced neuromuscular blockade with an anticholinesterase agent (such as neostigmine or edrophonium), as ordered. Such an agent usually is administered together with an anticholinergic (such as atropine).
Patient teaching
• Instruct patient and family about drug therapy.
• Reassure both patient and family that patient will be monitored at all times and that respiratory life-support will be used during paralysis.
• Reassure patient that pain medication will be given as needed.

☑ **Evaluation**
• Patient's underlying condition is resolved without causing injury.
• Patient is able to sustain spontaneous ventilation after effects of atracurium besylate wear off.
• Patient and family state understanding of drug therapy.

---

atropine sulfate
(AH-troh-peen SUL-fayt)

Pharmacologic class: anticholinergic, belladonna alkaloid
Therapeutic class: antiarrhythmic, vagolytic
Pregnancy risk category: C

How supplied
Tablets: 0.4 mg, 0.6 mg

Injection: 0.05 mg/ml, 0.1 mg/ml,
0.3 mg/ml, 0.4 mg/ml, 0.5 mg/ml,
0.6 mg/ml, 0.8 mg/ml, 1 mg/ml,
1.2 mg/ml

Pharmacokinetics

Absorption: well absorbed after P.O. and
I.M. administration; unknown for S.C.
administration.
Distribution: distributed throughout
body, including CNS. Only 18% binds
with plasma protein.
Metabolism: metabolized in liver to several metabolites.
Excretion: excreted primarily through
kidneys; small amount may be excreted
in feces and expired air. *Half-life:* initial,
2 hours; second phase, 12½ hours.

Route	Onset	Peak	Duration
P.O.	0.5-1 hr	2 hr	4 hr
I.V.	Immediate	2-4 min	4 hr
I.M.	30 min	1-1.6 hr	4 hr
S.C.	Unknown	Unknown	4 hr

Pharmacodynamics

Chemical effect: inhibits acetylcholine at
parasympathetic neuroeffector junction,
blocking vagal effects on SA node; this
enhances conduction through AV node
and speeds heart rate.
Therapeutic effect: increases heart rate;
antidote for anticholinesterase insecticide
poisoning; decreases secretions preoperatively; and slows GI motility.

Indications and dosage

▶ **Symptomatic bradycardia, bradyarrhythmia (junctional or escape
rhythm).** *Adults:* usually 0.5 to 1 mg I.V.
push; repeated q 3 to 5 minutes to maximum of 2 mg, p.r.n. Lower doses (less
than 0.5 mg) can cause bradycardia.
Children: 0.02 mg/kg I.V. up to maximum of 1 mg; or 0.3 mg/m²; may repeat
q 5 minutes.
▶ **Antidote for anticholinesterase insecticide poisoning.** *Adults and children:*
1 to 2 mg I.M. or I.V. repeated q 20 to 30
minutes until muscarinic symptoms dis-

appear or signs of atropine toxicity appear. Severe poisoning may require up to
6 mg q hour.
▶ **Preoperatively for decreasing secretions and blocking cardiac vagal reflexes.** *Adults and children weighing 20
kg or more:* 0.4 mg I.M. or S.C. 30 to 60
minutes before anesthesia. *Children
weighing less than 20 kg:* 0.1 mg I.M. for
3 kg, 0.2 mg I.M. for 4 to 9 kg, 0.3 mg
I.M. for 10 to 20 kg 30 to 60 minutes before anesthesia.
▶ **Adjunct treatment of peptic ulcer
disease; treatment of functional GI disorders such as irritable bowel syndrome.** *Adults:* 0.4 to 0.6 mg P.O. q 4 to
6 hours. *Children:* 0.01 mg/kg or
0.3 mg/m² (not to exceed 0.4 mg) q 4 to
6 hours.

Adverse reactions

CNS: *headache, restlessness,* ataxia, disorientation, hallucinations, delirium,
coma, *insomnia, dizziness;* excitement,
agitation, and confusion (especially in elderly patients).
CV: *tachycardia, palpitations* (with 1- to
2-mg doses); ***tachycardia, angina*** (with
doses over 2 mg).
EENT: *slight mydriasis,* photophobia
(with 1-mg dose); *blurred vision, mydriasis* (with 2-mg dose).
GI: *dry mouth (common even at low doses),* thirst, *constipation,* nausea, vomiting.
GU: urine retention.
Hematologic: leukocytosis.
Skin: flushing.
Other: severe allergic reactions, including ***anaphylaxis.***

Interactions

Drug-drug. *Antacids:* decreased absorption of anticholinergics. Separate administration times by at least 1 hour.
*Anticholinergics, drugs with anticholinergic effects (such as amantadine, glutethimide, meperidine, antiarrhythmics,
antiparkinsonian agents, phenothiazines,
tricyclic antidepressants):* additive anti-

---

cholinergic effects. Use together cautiously.
Ketoconazole, levodopa: decreased absorption. Avoid concomitant use.
Methotrimeprazine: may produce extrapyramidal symptoms. Monitor patient carefully.
Potassium chloride wax matrix tablets: increased risk of mucosal lesions. Use cautiously.

Contraindications and precautions

• Contraindicated in patients with acute angle-closure glaucoma, obstructive uropathy, obstructive disease of GI tract, paralytic ileus, toxic megacolon, intestinal atony, unstable CV status in acute hemorrhage, asthma, myasthenia gravis, or hypersensitivity to drug. Also not recommended for use in breast-feeding women.
• Use cautiously in patients with Down syndrome and in pregnant women.

NURSING CONSIDERATIONS

⚕ Assessment
• Obtain history of patient's underlying condition and reassess regularly.
• Be alert for adverse reactions and drug interactions.
• Monitor patients for paradoxical initial bradycardia, especially those receiving small doses (0.4 to 0.6 mg). This is caused by a drug effect in CNS and usually disappears within 2 minutes.
• Watch for tachycardia in cardiac patients because it may precipitate ventricular fibrillation.
• Evaluate patient's and family's knowledge of drug therapy.

☷ Nursing diagnoses
• Altered health maintenance related to underlying condition
• Risk for injury related to drug-induced adverse reactions
• Knowledge deficit related to drug therapy

⟩ Planning and implementation
P.O. use: Drug may be taken with or without food.
I.V. use: Administer by direct I.V. into a large vein or I.V. tubing over 1 to 2 minutes.
I.M. and S.C. use: Follow normal protocol.
• If ECG disturbances occur, withhold drug, obtain a rhythm strip, and notify doctor immediately.
• Have emergency equipment and drugs on hand to treat new arrhythmias. Be aware that other anticholinergic drugs may increase vagal blockage.
• Use physostigmine salicylate as antidote for atropine overdose.
Patient teaching
• Teach patient about atropine sulfate therapy.
• Instruct patient to ask for assistance with activities if adverse CNS reactions occur.
• Teach patient how to handle distressing anticholinergic effects.

✓ Evaluation
• Patient exhibits improvement of underlying condition.
• Patient does not experience injury as a result of therapy.
• Patient and family state understanding of drug therapy.

auranofin
(or-AN-uh-fin)
Ridaura

Pharmacologic class: gold salt
Therapeutic class: antiarthritic
Pregnancy risk category: C

How supplied
Capsules: 3 mg

Pharmacokinetics
Absorption: 25% absorbed through GI tract.

Distribution: distributed widely in body tissues. Synovial fluid levels are about 50% of blood concentrations. Drug is 60% protein-bound. *Metabolism:* unknown. *Excretion:* 60% of absorbed drug excreted in urine and remainder in feces. *Half-life:* 26 days.

Route	Onset	Peak	Duration
P.O.	1-3 mo	≤ 2 hr	Unknown

Pharmacodynamics

Chemical effect: unknown. Anti-inflammatory effects in rheumatoid arthritis are probably caused by inhibition of sulfhydryl systems, which alters cellular metabolism. Auranofin may also alter enzyme function and immune response and suppress phagocytic activity. *Therapeutic effect:* relieves symptoms of rheumatoid arthritis.

Indications and dosage

▶ **Rheumatoid arthritis.** *Adults:* 6 mg P.O. daily, either as 3 mg b.i.d. or 6 mg once daily. After 4 to 6 months, dosage may be increased to 9 mg daily.

Adverse reactions

CNS: confusion, *seizures.*
GI: *diarrhea, abdominal pain, nausea, vomiting,* stomatitis, enterocolitis, anorexia, metallic taste, dyspepsia, flatulence.
GU: proteinuria, hematuria, glomerulonephritis, *acute renal failure,* nephrotic syndrome.
Hematologic: *thrombocytopenia* (with or without purpura), *aplastic anemia, agranulocytosis, leukopenia,* eosinophilia.
Hepatic: jaundice, elevated liver enzyme levels.
Respiratory: interstitial pneumonitis.
Skin: *rash, pruritus, dermatitis, exfoliative dermatitis.*

Interactions

Drug-drug. *Phenytoin:* may raise phenytoin blood levels. Monitor for toxicity.

Contraindications and precautions

• Contraindicated in patients with history of severe gold toxicity, necrotizing enterocolitis, pulmonary fibrosis, exfoliative dermatitis, bone marrow aplasia, severe hematologic disorders, or history of severe toxicity resulting from previous exposure to other heavy metals. Also contraindicated in patients with urticaria, eczema, colitis, severe debilitation, hemorrhagic conditions, or systemic lupus erythematosus and in patients who have recently received radiation therapy.
• Use in breast-feeding women is not recommended.
• Use cautiously with other drugs that cause blood dyscrasia. Also use cautiously in patients who have preexisting renal, hepatic, or inflammatory bowel disease or rash or a history of bone marrow depression.
• Safety of drug has not been established in children.

NURSING CONSIDERATIONS

Assessment
• Obtain history of patient's joint pain and stiffness before therapy and reassess regularly thereafter.
• Be alert for adverse reactions and drug interactions.
• Monitor patient's hydration status if adverse GI reactions occur.
• Monitor patient's platelet count and CBC regularly, as ordered.
• Evaluate patient's and family's knowledge of drug therapy.

Nursing diagnoses
• Pain (arthritic) related to presence of rheumatoid arthritis
• Risk for fluid volume deficit related to drug-induced adverse GI reactions
• Knowledge deficit related to drug therapy

Reactions may be *common*, uncommon, *life-threatening*, or COMMON AND LIFE-THREATENING.

▶ Planning and implementation
• Store at controlled room temperature and in a light-resistant container.
• Administer concomitant drug therapy, such as NSAIDs, as ordered.
• Notify doctor and expect to discontinue drug if patient's platelet count falls below 100,000/mm³, if hemoglobin drops suddenly, if granulocytes are below 1,500/mm³, and if leukopenia (WBC count below 4,000/mm³) or eosinophilia (eosinophils greater than 75%) occurs.

Patient teaching
• Encourage patient to take drug as prescribed and not to alter dosage schedule.
• Tell patient to continue taking concomitant drug therapy, such as NSAIDs, if prescribed.
• Remind patient to see doctor monthly to monitor platelet counts. Know that auranofin should be discontinued if platelet count falls below 100,000/mm³, if hemoglobin drops suddenly, if granulocytes are below 1,500/mm³, or if leukopenia (WBC count below 4,000/mm³) or eosinophilia (eosinophils more than 75%) is present.
• Advise patient to have regular urinalysis. If proteinuria or hematuria is detected, discontinue drug because it can produce a nephrotic syndrome or glomerulonephritis, and notify doctor.
• Tell patient to continue taking drug if he experiences mild diarrhea and to contact doctor immediately if blood is noted in stool. Diarrhea is the most common adverse reaction.
• Advise patient to report any rashes or other skin problems immediately. Pruritus often precedes dermatitis; any pruritic skin eruption while patients are receiving auranofin should be considered a reaction to this drug until proven otherwise. Advise patient to stop therapy until reaction subsides and notify doctor.
• Advise patient that stomatitis is often preceded by a metallic taste, which should be reported to doctor immediately. Promote careful oral hygiene during therapy.

• Reassure patient that beneficial drug effect may be delayed as long as 3 months. If response is inadequate and maximum dosage has been reached, expect doctor to discontinue drug.
• Warn patient not to give drug to others. Auranofin, like injectable gold preparations, should be prescribed only for selected rheumatoid arthritis patients.

☑ Evaluation
• Patient expresses that his arthritic pain is relieved.
• Patient maintains fluid volume balance throughout therapy.
• Patient and family state understanding of drug therapy.

aurothioglucose
(or-oh-thigh-oh-GLOO-kohs)
Gold-50◇, Solganal

gold sodium thiomalate
(gohld SOH-dee-um thee-oh-MAH-layt)
Myochrysine

Pharmacologic class: gold salt
Therapeutic class: antiarthritic
Pregnancy risk category: C

How supplied
Injection (suspension): 50 mg/ml in sesame oil with aluminum monostearate 2% and propylparaben 0.1% in 10-ml container (aurothioglucose)
Injection: 25 mg/ml, 50 mg/ml with benzyl alcohol (gold sodium thiomalate)

Pharmacokinetics
Absorption: slow and erratic because drug is in oil suspension.
Distribution: distributed widely throughout body in lymph nodes, bone marrow, kidneys, liver, spleen, and tissues. About 85% to 90% is protein-bound.
Metabolism: not broken down into elemental form.

Excretion: about 70% excreted in urine; 30% in feces. *Half-life:* 14 to 40 days.

Route	Onset	Peak	Duration
I.M.	Unknown	3-6 hr	Unknown

Pharmacodynamics

Chemical effect: unknown. Anti-inflammatory effects in rheumatoid arthritis are probably caused by inhibition of sulfhydryl systems, which alters cellular metabolism. Gold salts may also alter enzyme function and immune response and suppress phagocytic activity.
Therapeutic effect: relieves signs and symptoms of rheumatoid arthritis.

Indications and dosage

▶ **Rheumatoid arthritis. Aurothioglucose.** *Adults:* initially, 10 mg I.M., followed by 25 mg for second and third doses at weekly intervals. Then, 50 mg weekly until 0.8 to 1 g has been given. If improvement occurs without toxicity, 50 mg is continued at 3- to 4-week intervals indefinitely as maintenance therapy. *Children ages 6 to 12:* one-fourth usual adult dosage, not to exceed 25 mg per dose. **Gold sodium thiomalate.** *Adults:* initially, 10 mg I.M., followed by 25 mg in 1 week. Then, 25 to 50 mg weekly until 14 to 20 doses have been given. If improvement occurs without toxicity, 25 to 50 mg is continued q 2 weeks for four doses; then, 25 to 50 mg q 3 weeks for four doses; then, 25 to 50 mg every month indefinitely as maintenance therapy. If relapse occurs during maintenance therapy, injections are resumed at weekly intervals. *Children:* 1 mg/kg I.M. weekly for 20 weeks. If response is good, may be given q 3 to 4 weeks indefinitely.

Adverse reactions

CNS: *dizziness,* syncope, *seizures.*
CV: bradycardia, hypotension.
EENT: corneal gold deposition, corneal ulcers.

GI: *metallic taste, stomatitis,* difficulty swallowing, nausea, vomiting.
GU: albuminuria, proteinuria, nephrotic syndrome, nephritis, acute tubular necrosis, *acute renal failure.*
Hematologic: *thrombocytopenia* (with or without purpura), *aplastic anemia, agranulocytosis, leukopenia,* eosinophilia.
Hepatic: hepatitis, jaundice.
Skin: photosensitivity; *rash and dermatitis* (occurs in 20% of patients; may lead to fatal *exfoliative dermatitis* if drug not stopped).
Other: *anaphylaxis, angioedema,* diaphoresis.

Interactions

None significant.

Contraindications and precautions

• Contraindicated in patients with hypersensitivity to drug; history of severe toxicity from exposure to gold or other heavy metals, hepatitis, or exfoliative dermatitis; severe uncontrollable diabetes; renal disease; hepatic dysfunction; uncontrolled heart failure; systemic lupus erythematosus; colitis; Sjögren's syndrome; urticaria; eczema; hemorrhagic conditions; severe hematologic disorders; or recent radiation therapy.
• Drug is not recommended in breast-feeding women.
• Use with extreme caution, if at all, in patients with rash, marked hypertension, compromised cerebral or CV circulation, or history of renal or hepatic disease, drug allergies, or blood dyscrasia.
• Use with caution in pregnant women.
• Safety of drug has not been established in children younger than age 6.

NURSING CONSIDERATIONS

⚗ Assessment
• Obtain history of patient's rheumatoid arthritis before therapy and reassess regularly thereafter.
• Be alert for adverse reactions.

• Analyze urine for protein and sediment changes before each injection.
• Monitor CBC, including platelet count, before every second injection, as ordered.
• Evaluate patient's and family's knowledge of drug therapy.

⊞ Nursing diagnoses
• Pain (joint) related to presence of rheumatoid arthritis
• Risk for injury related to drug-induced adverse reactions
• Knowledge deficit related to drug therapy

⧉ Planning and implementation
• Administer only under constant supervision of doctor who is thoroughly familiar with drug's toxicities and benefits.
• Know that gold compounds are typically used only in active rheumatoid arthritis that has not responded adequately to salicylates, rest, and physical therapy. Some clinicians advocate earlier use before disease progresses.
• Administer all gold salts I.M., as ordered, preferably intragluteally. Drug is pale yellow; don't use if it darkens.
• Immerse aurothioglucose (a suspension) vial in warm water, and shake vigorously before injecting.
• When giving gold sodium thiomalate, have patient lie down and remain recumbent for 10 to 20 minutes after injection to minimize hypotension.
• Observe patient for 30 minutes after administration because of possible anaphylactoid reaction.
• If adverse reactions develop and are mild, some rheumatologists resume gold therapy after 2 to 3 weeks' rest.
• Monitor platelet count if patient develops purpura or ecchymoses, as ordered.
• Keep dimercaprol on hand to treat acute toxicity.
Patient teaching
• Inform patient that benefits of therapy may not appear for 3 to 4 months or longer.

• Advise patient that increased joint pain may occur for 1 to 2 days after injection but usually subsides after a few injections.
• Advise patient to report any rashes or skin problems immediately. Pruritus often precedes dermatitis; pruritic skin eruptions that develop while patient is receiving gold salt therapy should be considered a reaction to therapy until proven otherwise. Advise patient to stop therapy until reaction subsides and to notify doctor.
• Advise patient that stomatitis is often preceded by metallic taste, which should be reported to doctor immediately. Promote careful oral hygiene during therapy.
• Tell patients to avoid sunlight and artificial ultraviolet light to minimize risk of photosensitivity.
• Stress need for close medical follow-ups and frequent blood and urine tests during therapy.

☑ Evaluation
• Patient expresses relief of joint stiffness and pain.
• Patient does not experience injury as result of drug-induced adverse reactions.
• Patient and family state understanding of drug therapy.

azatadine maleate
(uh-ZEH-tah-deen MAL-ee-ayt)
Optimine, Zadine◊

Pharmacologic class: piperidine antihistamine
Therapeutic class: antihistamine
Pregnancy risk category: B

How supplied

Tablets: 1 mg
Syrup: 0.5 mg/5 ml◊

Pharmacokinetics

Absorption: well absorbed from GI tract.

Distribution: not fully known; apparently crosses blood-brain barrier, resulting in CNS effects. It is minimally protein–bound.
Metabolism: 80% metabolized by liver.
Excretion: drug and metabolites excreted in urine; about 20% excreted unchanged.
Half-life: about 9 to 12 hours.

Route	Onset	Peak	Duration
P.O.	15-60 min	≤ 4 hr	12 hr

Pharmacodynamics

Chemical effect: competes with histamine for $histamine_1$-receptor sites on effector cells. Prevents but does not reverse histamine-mediated responses.
Therapeutic effect: relieves allergy symptoms.

Indications and dosage

▶ **Rhinitis, allergy symptoms, chronic urticaria.** *Adults and children age 12 and older:* 1 mg P.O. b.i.d.

Adverse reactions

CNS: (especially in elderly patients) *drowsiness, dizziness,* vertigo, disturbed coordination.
CV: hypotension, palpitations.
GI: anorexia, nausea, vomiting, *dry mouth and throat,* epigastric distress.
GU: urine retention.
Hematologic: *thrombocytopenia.*
Respiratory: thick bronchial secretions.
Skin: urticaria, rash.

Interactions

Drug-drug. *CNS depressants:* increased sedation. Use together cautiously.
MAO inhibitors: increased anticholinergic effects. Don't use together.

Contraindications and precautions

• Contraindicated in patients with acute asthmatic attacks and in breast-feeding women.
• Use cautiously in elderly patients, in pregnant women, and in patients with increased intraocular pressure, hyperthy-roidism, CV or renal disease, hypertension, bronchial asthma, urine retention, prostatic hyperplasia, bladder-neck obstruction, and stenosing peptic ulcerations.
• Safety of drug has not been established in children younger than age 12.

NURSING CONSIDERATIONS

Assessment
• Obtain history of patient's allergy condition before therapy and reassess regularly thereafter.
• Be alert for adverse reactions and drug interactions.
• Monitor CBC during long-term therapy, as ordered; watch for signs of blood dyscrasia.
• Evaluate patient's and family's understanding of drug therapy.

Nursing diagnoses
• Altered health maintenance related to underlying allergic condition
• Risk for injury related to drug-induced adverse CNS reactions
• Knowledge deficit related to drug therapy

Planning and implementation
• Administer with food or milk to reduce GI distress.
• If tolerance to drug develops, discuss this with doctor. It may be necessary to substitute another antihistamine.
Patient teaching
• Instruct patient to reduce GI distress by taking drug with food or milk.
• Tell patient to stop drug 4 days before allergy skin tests to preserve accuracy of tests.
• Warn patient to avoid alcohol and activities that require alertness until drug's CNS effects are known.
• Inform patient that coffee or tea may reduce drowsiness. Sugarless gum, sugarless hard candy, or ice chips may relieve dry mouth.

Reactions may be *common,* uncommon, *life-threatening,* or COMMON AND LIFE-THREATENING.

• Tell patient to notify doctor if tolerance develops; different antihistamine may need to be prescribed.

☑ **Evaluation**
• Patient's allergic signs and symptoms are relieved with drug therapy.
• Patient does not experience injury caused by drug-induced adverse reactions.
• Patient and family state understanding of drug therapy.

azathioprine
(ay-zuh-THIGH-oh-preen)
Imuran, Thioprine◊

Pharmacologic class: purine antagonist
Therapeutic class: immunosuppressive
Pregnancy risk category: D

How supplied
Tablets: 50 mg
Injection: 100 mg

Pharmacokinetics
Absorption: oral dose absorbed well from GI tract.
Distribution: azathioprine and its major metabolite, mercaptopurine, are distributed throughout body; both are 30% protein–bound.
Metabolism: metabolized primarily to mercaptopurine.
Excretion: small amounts of azathioprine and mercaptopurine are excreted in urine intact; most of given dose is excreted in urine as secondary metabolites. *Half-life:* about 5 hours.

Route	Onset	Peak	Duration
P.O., I.V.	4-8 wk	1-2 hr	Unknown

Pharmacodynamics
Chemical effect: unknown.
Therapeutic effect: suppresses immune system activity.

Indications and dosage
▶ **Immunosuppression in kidney transplantation.** *Adults and children:* initially, 3 to 5 mg/kg P.O. or I.V. daily, usually beginning on day of transplantation. Maintained at 1 to 3 mg/kg daily (dosage varies considerably according to patient response).
▶ **Severe, refractory rheumatoid arthritis.** *Adults:* initially, 1 mg/kg P.O. as single dose or as two doses. If patient response is not satisfactory after 6 to 8 weeks, dosage may be increased by 0.5 mg/kg daily (up to maximum of 2.5 mg/kg daily) at 4-week intervals.

Adverse reactions
GI: nausea, vomiting, anorexia, *pancreatitis,* steatorrhea, esophagitis, mouth ulceration.
Hematologic: LEUKOPENIA, *bone marrow suppression,* anemia, *pancytopenia,* THROMBOCYTOPENIA.
Hepatic: *hepatotoxicity,* jaundice.
Musculoskeletal: arthralgia, muscle wasting.
Skin: rash, alopecia, pruritus.
Other: *immunosuppression* (possibly profound), *infections,* increased risk of *neoplasia.*

Interactions
Drug-drug. *ACE inhibitors:* combination may cause severe leukopenia. Monitor closely.
Allopurinol: impaired inactivation of azathioprine. Decrease azathioprine dose to one-fourth or one-third normal dose.
Vaccines: decreased immune response. Postpone routine immunization.
Warfarin: may inhibit the anticoagulant effect of warfarin. Monitor PT/INR.

Contraindications and precautions
• Contraindicated in patients with hypersensitivity to drug.
• Drug is not recommended in breast-feeding women.
• Use cautiously in patients with hepatic or renal dysfunction.

• Don't use drug for treating rheumatoid arthritis in pregnant women.

NURSING CONSIDERATIONS

🔍 Assessment
• Obtain history of patient's immune status before therapy.
• Monitor effectiveness by observing for signs of organ rejection. Be aware that therapeutic response usually occurs within 8 weeks.
• Be alert for adverse reactions and drug interactions.
• Monitor hemoglobin, WBC, and platelet counts at least once monthly, as ordered—more often at beginning of treatment.
• Evaluate patient's and family's knowledge of drug therapy.

🔷 Nursing diagnoses
• Altered protection related to threat of organ rejection
• Risk for infection related to drug-induced immunosuppression
• Knowledge deficit related to drug therapy

▷ Planning and implementation
P.O. use: Administer drug in divided doses or after meals to minimize adverse GI effects.
I.V. use: Reconstitute 100-mg vial with 10 ml of sterile water for injection. Visually inspect for particles before giving. Drug may be administered by direct I.V. injection or further diluted in 0.9% NaCl injection or D_5W and infused over 30 to 60 minutes. Use only for patients unable to tolerate P.O. medications.
• Keep in mind that benefits must be weighed against risks with systemic viral infections, such as chickenpox and herpes zoster.
• Be aware that patients with rheumatoid arthritis previously treated with alkylating agents, such as cyclophosphamide, chlorambucil, and melphalan, may have prohibitive risk of neoplasia if treated with azathioprine.
• Know that drug should be stopped immediately when WBC count is less than 3,000/mm³ to prevent irreversible bone marrow suppression. Notify doctor.
• To prevent bleeding, avoid I.M. injections when platelet count is below 100,000/mm³.

Patient teaching
• Warn patient to report even mild infections (colds, fever, sore throat, and malaise) because drug is potent immunosuppressant.
• Instruct female patient to avoid conception during therapy and for 4 months after stopping therapy.
• Warn patient that some thinning of hair is possible.
• Tell patient taking this drug for refractory rheumatoid arthritis that it may take up to 12 weeks to be effective.

✅ Evaluation
• Patient exhibits no signs of organ rejection.
• Patient demonstrates no signs and symptoms of infection.
• Patient and family state understanding of drug therapy.

azelaic acid cream
(ah-zuh-LAY-ik AS-id KREEM)
Azelex 20%

Pharmacologic class: naturally occurring saturated dicarboxylic acid
Therapeutic class: antiacne agent
Pregnancy risk category: B

How supplied
Cream: 20%

Pharmacokinetics
Not applicable.

Route	Onset	Peak	Duration
Topical	Unknown	Unknown	Unknown

Pharmacodynamics

Chemical effect: unknown; antimicrobial action may be attributed to inhibition of microbial cellular protein synthesis. *Therapeutic effect:* resolves signs and symptoms of acne.

Indications and dosage

▶ **Mild to moderate inflammatory acne vulgaris.** *Adults:* Apply thin film and gently but thoroughly massage into affected areas b.i.d, in morning and evening.

Adverse reactions

Skin: pruritus, burning, stinging, tingling.

Interactions

None reported.

Contraindications and precautions

• Contraindicated in patients with hypersensitivity to drug or its components.
• Use cautiously in pregnant or breastfeeding women.
• Safety of drug has not been established in children under age 12.

NURSING CONSIDERATIONS

⚗ Assessment
• Obtain history of patient's skin condition before therapy.
• Be alert for adverse reactions.
• Monitor for early signs of hypopigmentation after use, especially in patient with dark complexion.
• Evaluate patient's and family's knowledge of drug therapy.

⚙ Nursing diagnoses
• Impaired skin integrity related to acne
• Knowledge deficit related to drug therapy

▷ Planning and implementation
• Thoroughly wash and pat dry affected areas before applying drug. Wash hands well after application.

• Notify doctor if sensitivity or severe irritation develops.
Patient teaching
• Tell patient to use drug for the prescribed period.
• Show him how to apply drug. Warn him not to apply occlusive dressings or wrappings to affected areas.
• Tell him to keep drug away from mouth, eyes, and other mucous membranes. If drug contacts his eyes, tell him to wash them with large amounts of water and to consult doctor if irritation persists.
• Advise patient with dark complexion to report abnormal changes in skin color to the doctor.
• Warn patient that temporary skin irritation may occur when drug is applied to broken or inflamed skin, usually at the start of therapy. Tell him to notify doctor if it persists.

☑ Evaluation
• Patient's acne is resolved.
• Patient and family state understanding of drug therapy.

azelastine hydrochloride
(ah-zuh-LAST-een high-droh-KLOR-ighd)
Astelin

Pharmacologic class: H₁-receptor agonist; antihistamine
Therapeutic class: anti-allergy
Pregnancy risk category: C

How supplied

Aerosol inhaler: 137 mcg/metered spray

Pharmacokinetics

Absorption: undefined.
Distribution: systemic bioavailability is 40%.
Metabolism: after dosing to a steady-state, plasma concentration ranges from 20% to 50%.

Excretion: oral dosage excreted in feces.
Half-life: 22 hours.

Route	Onset	Peak	Duration
Inhalation	1-3 hr	Plasma levels peak within 2-3 hr	12 hr

Pharmacodynamics

Chemical effect: exhibited histamine H_1-receptor agonist activity.
Therapeutic effect: relief of seasonal allergic rhinitis.

Indications and dosage

▶ **Seasonal allergic rhinitis.** *Adults and children age 12 and older:* two sprays per nostril b.i.d.

Adverse reactions

CNS: *headache, somnolence,* fatigue, dizziness.
EENT: *bitter taste,* nasal burning, dry mouth, epistaxis.
GI: nausea.
Musculoskeletal: myalgia.
Respiratory: pharyngitis, paroxysmal sneezing, rhinitis.
Other: weight increase.

Interactions

Drug-drug. *Cimetidine:* increased plasma levels of azelastine. Avoid concomitant use.
CNS depressants: increased sedation. Avoid concomitant use.
Drug-lifestyle. *Alcohol use*: increased sedation. Avoid concomitant use.

Contraindications and precautions

• Contraindicated in patients with known hypersensitivity to drug.

NURSING CONSIDERATIONS

🔍 **Assessment**
• Obtain history of patient's allergy condition before therapy begins and reassess regularly thereafter.

• Be alert for adverse reactions and drug interactions.
• Evaluate patient's and family's knowledge of drug therapy.

✣ **Nursing diagnoses**
• Altered health maintenance related to underlying allergic condition
• Knowledge deficit related to drug therapy

▶ **Planning and implementation**
• Know that drug should be used in pregnancy only if benefit justifies potential risk to fetus. Breast-feeding women should not take drug.
• Be aware that safety and effectiveness in patients under age 12 have not been established.
Patient teaching
• Warn patient not to drive or perform hazardous activities if somnolence occurs.
• Advise patient not to use alcohol, CNS depressants, or other antihistamines while taking drug.
• Teach patient proper usage of nasal spray. Instruct patient to replace child-resistant screw top on bottle with pump unit. Prime delivery system with four sprays or until a fine mist appears. Re-prime system with two sprays or until a fine mist appears if 3 or more days have elapsed since last use. Store bottle upright at room temperature with pump closed tightly. Keep unit away from children.
• Tell patient to avoid getting spray in eyes.

☑ **Evaluation**
• Patient's allergic symptoms are relieved with drug therapy.
• Patient and family state understanding of drug therapy.

azithromycin
(uh-zith-roh-MIGH-sin)
Zithromax

Pharmacologic class: azalide macrolide
Therapeutic class: antibiotic
Pregnancy risk category: B

How supplied

Tablets: 250 mg
Capsules: 250 mg
Injection: 500mg
Oral suspension: 100 mg/5 ml, 200 mg/
5 ml
Single dose powder for oral suspension: 1 g

Pharmacokinetics

Absorption: rapidly absorbed from GI
tract; food decreases both maximum
plasma concentrations and amount of
drug absorbed.
Distribution: rapidly distributed throughout body and readily penetrates cells; it
does not readily enter CNS. Drug concentrates in fibroblasts and phagocytes.
Significantly higher levels are reached in
tissues compared with plasma.
Metabolism: not metabolized.
Excretion: excreted mostly in feces after
excretion into bile. Less than 10% is excreted in urine. Terminal elimination
half-life: 68 hours.

Route	Onset	Peak	Duration
P.O.	Unknown	2.5-4.4 hr	Unknown
I.V.	Unknown	Unknown	Unknown

Pharmacodynamics

Chemical effect: binds to 50S subunit of
bacterial ribosomes, blocking protein
synthesis; bacteriostatic or bactericidal,
depending on concentration.
Therapeutic effect: hinders or kills susceptible bacteria. Spectrum of activity includes many gram-positive and gram-negative aerobic and anaerobic bacteria,
such as *Haemophilus influenzae, Moraxella (Branhamella) catarrhalis, Staph-*
ylococcus aureus, Streptococcus agalactiae, Streptococcus pneumoniae, Streptococcus pyogenes, and *Chlamydia trachomatis.*

Indications and dosage

▶ **Acute bacterial exacerbations of
COPD caused by** *Haemophilus influenzae, Moraxella (Branhamella) catarrhalis,* **or** *Streptococcus pneumoniae***;
uncomplicated skin and skin-structure
infections caused by** *Staphylococcus
aureus, Streptococcus pyogenes,* **or**
*Streptococcus agalactiae***; second-line
therapy of pharyngitis or tonsillitis
caused by** *S. pyogenes. Adults and adolescents age 16 and older:* 500 mg P.O.
as a single dose on day 1, followed by
250 mg P.O. daily on days 2 through 5.
Total dose is 1.5 g.
▶ **Community-acquired pneumonia
caused by** *Chlamydia pneumoniae, H.
influenzae, Mycoplasma pneumoniae, S.
pneumoniae***; I.V. form can also be used
for** *Legionella pneumophila, M. catarrhalis, and S. aureus. Adults and adolescents age 16 or older:* 500 mg P.O. as
a single dose on day 1, followed by
250 mg P.O. daily on days 2 through 5.
Total dose is 1.5 g. For patients requiring
initial I.V. therapy, 500 mg I.V. as a single daily dose for 2 days, followed by
500 mg P.O. as a single daily dose to
complete a 7-to 10-day course of therapy.
Switch from I.V. to P.O. therapy should
be done at doctor's discretion and based
on patient's clinical response.
▶ **Nongonococcal urethritis or cervicitis caused by** *Chlamydia trachomatis.*
Adults and adolescents age 16 and older:
1 g P.O. as a single dose.
▶ **Prevention of disseminated** *Mycobacterium avium* **complex disease in
patients with advanced HIV infection.**
Adults: 1,200 mg P.O. once weekly, as
indicated.
▶ **Urethritis and cervicitis due to**
Neisseria gonorrhoeae. Adults: 2 g P.O.
as a single dose.

▶ **Pelvic inflammatory disease caused by *C. trachomatis, N. gonorrhoeae, or Mycoplasma hominis* in patients who require initial I.V. therapy.** *Adults:* 500 mg I.V. as a single daily dose for 1 to 2 days, followed by 250 mg P.O. daily to complete a 7-day course of therapy. Switch from I.V. to P.O. therapy should be done at doctor's discretion and based on patient's clinical response.

▶ **Genital ulcer disease in men due to *Haemophilus ducreyi (chancroid).*** *Adults:* 1 g P.O. as a single dose.

▶ **Acute otitis media.** *Children over age 6 months:* 10 mg/kg (maximum 500 mg) P.O. on day 1, followed by 5 mg/kg (maximum 250 mg) on days 2 to 5.

▶ **Pharyngitis, tonsillitis.** *Children over age 2:* 12 mg/kg (maximum 500 mg) P.O. daily for 5 days.

Adverse reactions

CNS: dizziness, vertigo, headache, fatigue, somnolence.
CV: palpitations, chest pain.
GI: *nausea, vomiting, diarrhea, abdominal pain,* dyspepsia, flatulence, melena, cholestatic jaundice, pseudomembranous colitis.
GU: candidiasis, vaginitis, nephritis.
Skin: rash, photosensitivity.
Other: *angioedema.*

Interactions

Drug-drug. *Aluminum- and magnesium-containing antacids:* lowered peak plasma levels of azithromycin. Separate administration times by at least 2 hours.
Astemizole: potentially serious CV effects (prolongation of QT interval and ventricular tachycardia) have been associated with other macrolide antiinfectives. Monitor patient closely.
Digoxin: elevated digoxin levels. Monitor patient closely.
Dihydroergotamine, ergotamine: acute ergot toxicity. Avoid concomitant use.
Drugs metabolized by cytochrome P430 system: elevations of serum carbamaz-

epine, cyclosporine, hexobarbital, and phenytoin levels. Avoid concomitant use.
Theophylline: possibly increased plasma theophylline levels with other macrolides; effect of azithromycin is unknown. Monitor theophylline levels carefully.
Triazolam: increased pharmacologic effect of triazolam. Use with caution.
Warfarin: possibly increased PT with other macrolides; effect of azithromycin is unknown. Monitor PT and INR carefully.
Drug-food. *Any food:* decreased absorption. Give at least 1 hour before or 2 hours after a meal.
Drug-lifestyle. *Sun exposure:* photosensitivity reactions may occur. Avoid prolonged or unprotected sun exposure.

Contraindications and precautions

• Contraindicated in patients with hypersensitivity to erythromycin or other macrolides.
• Use cautiously in patients with impaired hepatic function and in pregnant or breast-feeding women.

NURSING CONSIDERATIONS

☢ Assessment
• Obtain history of patient's infection before therapy and reassess regularly thereafter.
• Obtain specimen for culture and sensitivity tests before first dose. Therapy may begin pending test results.
• Be alert for adverse reactions and drug interactions.
• Evaluate patient's and family's knowledge of drug therapy.

⊕ Nursing diagnoses
• Infection related to presence of susceptible bacteria
• Altered protection related to drug-induced superinfection
• Knowledge deficit related to drug therapy

⧁ Planning and implementation

P.O. use: Administer 1 hour before or 2 hours after meals; do not administer with antacids.

I.V. use: Reconstitute drug by adding 4.8 ml sterile water for injection to 500-mg vial and shake until all the drug is dissolved. Further dilute in 250 to 500 ml D₅W, 0.9 % NaCl, or other compatible solution. Infuse over 1 to 3 hours. Reconstituted solution is stable for 7 days if stored in refrigerator (41°F [5° C]).

Patient teaching
• Tell patient that drug should always be taken on an empty stomach because food or antacids decrease absorption.
• Tell patient to take all medication as prescribed, even after he feels better.
• Instruct patient to use sunblock and avoid prolonged exposure to the sun, to decrease risk of photosensitivity reactions.

☑ Evaluation
• Patient's infection is eradicated.
• Patient does not experience superinfection during therapy.
• Patient and family state understanding of drug therapy.

---

aztreonam
(az-TREE-oh-nam)
Azactam

Pharmacologic class: monobactam
Therapeutic class: antibiotic
Pregnancy risk category: B

How supplied

Injection: 500-mg, 1-g, 2-g vials

Pharmacokinetics

Absorption: absorbed rapidly and completely after I.M. administration.
Distribution: distributed rapidly and widely to all body fluids and tissues, including bile, breast milk, and CSF.

Metabolism: from 6% to 16% metabolized to inactive metabolites by nonspecific hydrolysis of beta-lactam ring; 56% to 60% protein-bound, less if renal impairment is present.
Excretion: excreted primarily unchanged in urine by glomerular filtration and tubular secretion; 1.5% to 3.5% excreted unchanged in feces. *Half-life:* averages 1.7 hours.

Route	Onset	Peak	Duration
I.V.	Immediate	Immediate	Unknown
I.M.	Unknown	0.6-1.3 hr	Unknown

Pharmacodynamics

Chemical effect: inhibits bacterial cell-wall synthesis, ultimately causing cell wall destruction; bactericidal.
Therapeutic effect: kills susceptible bacteria. Spectrum of activity is narrow and includes *Enterobacter, Escherichia coli, Klebsiella pneumoniae, Proteus mirabilis,* and *Pseudomonas aeruginosa.* It has limited activity against *Citrobacter, Haemophilus influenzae, Hafnia, Klebsiella oxytoca, Moraxella (Branhamella) catarrhalis, Neisseria gonorrhoeae, Providencia,* and *Serratia margaris.*

Indications and dosage

▶ **Urinary tract infections, lower respiratory tract infections, septicemia, skin and skin-structure infections, intra-abdominal infections, surgical infections, and gynecologic infections caused by various aerobic organisms.**
Adults: 500 mg to 2 g I.V. or I.M. q 8 to 12 hours. For severe systemic or life-threatening infections, 2 g q 6 to 8 hours may be given. Maximum dosage is 8 g daily.

Adverse reactions

CNS: *seizures,* headache, insomnia, confusion.
CV: hypotension.
EENT: halitosis, altered taste.
GI: diarrhea, nausea, vomiting.

Hematologic: *neutropenia,* anemia, *thrombocytopenia, pancytopenia.* **Hepatic:** transient elevation of ALT and AST levels. **Other:** hypersensitivity reactions (rash, *anaphylaxis*); rash, thrombophlebitis (at I.V. site); discomfort, swelling (at I.M. injection site).

Interactions

Drug-drug. *Aminoglycosides, beta-lactam antibiotics, other anti-infectives:* synergistic effect. Monitor closely. *Cefoxitin, imipenem:* possible antagonistic effect. Do not use together. *Furosemide, probenecid:* increased serum aztreonam levels. Avoid concomitant use.

Contraindications and precautions

• Contraindicated in patients with hypersensitivity to drug.
• Drug is not recommended in breast-feeding women.
• Use cautiously in elderly patients and in those with impaired renal function. Dosage adjustment may be necessary.
• Safety of drug has not been established in children.

NURSING CONSIDERATIONS

Assessment
• Obtain history of patient's infection before therapy and reassess regularly thereafter.
• Obtain urine specimen for culture and sensitivity tests before giving first dose. Therapy may begin pending test results.
• Be alert for adverse reactions and drug interactions.
• Be aware that patients allergic to penicillins or cephalosporins may not be allergic to aztreonam. However, closely monitor patients who have had an immediate hypersensitivity reaction to these antibiotics.
• Evaluate patient's and family's understanding of drug therapy.

Nursing diagnoses
• Infection related to presence of susceptible bacteria
• Altered protection related to drug-induced superinfection
• Knowledge deficit related to drug therapy

Planning and implementation
I.V. use: To administer bolus of aztreonam, inject drug slowly (over 3 to 5 minutes) directly into vein or I.V. tubing. Give infusions over 20 minutes to 1 hour.
I.M. use: Administer I.M. injection deep into large muscle mass, such as upper outer quadrant of gluteus maximus or lateral aspect of thigh. Give doses greater than 1 g I.V.
Patient teaching
• Warn patient receiving drug I.M. that pain and swelling may occur at injection site.
• Tell patient to report pain or discomfort at I.V. site.
• Instruct patient to report signs or symptoms that suggest superinfection is occurring.

Evaluation
• Patient is free of infection.
• Patient does not develop superinfection as result of therapy.
• Patient and family state understanding of drug therapy.

bacampicillin hydrochloride
(ba-cam-pi-SIL-in high-droh-KLOR-ighd)
Penglobe♦, Spectrobid

Pharmacologic class: aminopenicillin
Therapeutic class: antibiotic
Pregnancy risk category: B

How supplied

Tablets: 400 mg

Pharmacokinetics

Absorption: hydrolyzed rapidly to ampicillin both in GI tract and in plasma.
Distribution: no unchanged bacampicillin found in serum after P.O. administration. Ampicillin distributes into pleural, peritoneal, and synovial fluids; lungs; prostate; muscle; liver; and gallbladder; it also penetrates middle ear effusions, maxillary sinus and bronchial secretions, tonsils, and sputum. It is 15% to 25% protein-bound.
Metabolism: hydrolyzed to ampicillin; ampicillin is metabolized partially.
Excretion: excreted as ampicillin and metabolites in urine by renal tubular secretion and glomerular filtration. *Half-life:* 1 to 1½ hours (in adults); 7½ hours (in patients with renal impairment).

Route	Onset	Peak	Duration
P.O.	Unknown	30-90 min	6-8 hr

Pharmacodynamics

Chemical effect: inhibits cell-wall synthesis during microorganism multiplication.
Therapeutic effect: kills susceptible bacteria. Spectrum of activity includes non-penicillinase-producing gram-positive bacteria, such as *Enterococcus faecalis, Escherichia coli, Haemophilus influenzae, Neisseria gonorrhoeae, Neisseria meningitidis, Proteus mirabilis, Salmonella,* and *Shigella.*

Indications and dosage

▶ **Upper respiratory tract infections and otitis media caused by streptococci, pneumococci, staphylococci, and** *H. influenzae;* **urinary tract infections caused by** *E. coli, P. mirabilis,* **and** *Enterococcus faecalis;* **skin infections caused by streptococci and susceptible staphylococci.** *Adults and children weighing over 25 kg (55 lb):* 400 to 800 mg P.O. q 12 hours. *Children weighing 25 kg or less:* 25 mg/kg/day P.O. in divided doses q 12 hours.
▶ **Lower respiratory tract infections; other severe infections.** *Adults and children weighing over 25 kg:* 800 mg P.O. q 12 hours. *Children weighing 25 kg or less:* 50 mg/kg/day P.O. in divided doses q 12 hours.
▶ **Gonorrhea.** *Adults:* 1.6 g P.O. plus 1 g probenecid given as single dose.

Adverse reactions

GI: *nausea,* vomiting, *diarrhea,* glossitis, stomatitis.
Hematologic: anemia, thrombocytopenia, thrombocytopenic purpura, eosinophilia, leukopenia, **agranulocytosis.**
Other: hypersensitivity reactions (erythematous maculopapular rash, urticaria, **anaphylaxis**), overgrowth of nonsusceptible organisms.

Interactions

Drug-drug. *Allopurinol:* increased incidence of rash. Monitor patient.
Disulfiram: possible disulfiram-alcohol reaction. Do not give together.
Probenecid: increased blood levels of bacampicillin or other penicillins. Probenecid may be used for this purpose.

Contraindications and precautions

• Contraindicated in patients with hypersensitivity to drug or other penicillins.
• Use cautiously in patients with other drug allergies, especially to cephalosporins (possible cross-sensitivity), or in those with mononucleosis (high incidence of maculopapular rash).
• Also use cautiously in pregnant or breast-feeding women.

NURSING CONSIDERATIONS

Assessment
• Obtain history of infection before therapy and reassess regularly thereafter.

• Before giving drug, ask patient whether he has had an allergic reaction to penicillin. However, be aware that negative history of penicillin allergy is no guarantee against future reaction.
• Obtain specimen for culture and sensitivity tests before giving first dose. Therapy may begin pending test results.
• Be alert for adverse reactions and drug interactions.
• Monitor patient's hydration status if adverse GI reactions occur.
• Evaluate patient's and family's understanding of drug therapy.

⊞ **Nursing diagnoses**
• Infection related to presence of susceptible bacteria
• Risk for fluid volume deficit related to drug-induced reactions
• Knowledge deficit related to drug therapy

❱❱ **Planning and implementation**
• Administer bacampicillin, unlike ampicillin, with meals without fear of diminished drug absorption.
• Give drug at least 1 hour before bacteriostatic antibiotics.
• Know that tablets are indicated for children who weigh 25 kg or more.
• Be aware that bacampicillin is specially formulated to produce high blood levels of antibiotic when administered twice daily.
• Keep in mind that drug may cause false-positive urine glucose determinations with copper sulfate tests (Clinitest); drug does not affect glucose enzymatic tests (Diastix or Chemstrip uG).
• Notify doctor and anticipate discontinuing drug if patient develops rash.
Patient teaching
• Tell patient to take entire quantity of medication as prescribed, even after he feels better.
• Warn patient not to use leftover bacampicillin for new illness or to share it with others.

• Tell patient to call doctor if rash (most common), fever, or chills develop.

☑ **Evaluation**
• Patient is free from infection.
• Patient maintains adequate hydration throughout therapy.
• Patient and family state understanding of drug therapy.

bacillus Calmette-Guérin (BCG), live intravesical
(bah-SIL-us kal-MET geh-RAN, in-trah-VES-ih-kal)
ImmuCyst♦, TheraCys, TICE BCG

Pharmacologic class: bacterial agent
Therapeutic class: antineoplastic
Pregnancy risk category: C

How supplied
Suspension (freeze-dried) for bladder instillation: 2 ml vial containing 1 to 8×10^8 colony-forming units (CFU), equivalent to approximately 50 mg

Pharmacokinetics
No information available.

Route	Onset	Peak	Duration
Intravesical	Unknown	Unknown	Unknown

Pharmacodynamics
Chemical effect: unknown. Instillation of live bacterial suspension causes local inflammatory response. Local infiltration of histiocytes and leukocytes is followed by decrease in superficial tumors within bladder.
Therapeutic effect: decreases incidence of superficial bladder tumors.

Indications and dosage
▶ **In situ carcinoma of urinary bladder (primary and relapsed).** *Adults:* consult published protocols, specialized references, and manufacturer's recommendations.

Reactions may be *common*, uncommon, *life-threatening*, or COMMON AND LIFE-THREATENING.

Adverse reactions

GI: nausea, vomiting, anorexia, diarrhea, mild abdominal pain.
GU: *dysuria, urinary frequency, hematuria,* cystitis, urinary urgency, urinary incontinence, urinary tract infection, cramps, pain, decreased bladder capacity, tissue in urine, local infection, nephrotoxicity, genital pain.
Hematologic: anemia, *leukopenia, thrombocytopenia, DIC.*
Hepatic: elevated liver enzyme levels.
Musculoskeletal: myalgia, arthralgia.
Other: *hypersensitivity reaction,* malaise, *fever above 101°F (38.3° C),* chills.

Interactions

Drug-drug: *Antibiotics:* may attenuate response to BCG intravesical. Avoid concomitant use.
Bone marrow suppressants, immunosuppressants, radiation therapy: may impair response to BCG intravesical by decreasing immune response; also may increase risk of osteomyelitis or disseminated BCG infection. Avoid concomitant use.

Contraindications and precautions

• Contraindicated in immunocompromised patients, in those receiving immunosuppressive therapy (because of risk of bacterial infection), and in those with urinary tract infection (because of risk of increased bladder irritation or disseminated BCG infection).
• Also contraindicated in patients with fever of unknown origin. If fever is caused by an infection, withhold drug until patient has recovered.
• Use with caution in pregnant or breast-feeding women.
• Safety of drug has not been established in children.

NURSING CONSIDERATIONS

Assessment
• Determine patient's reactivity to tuberculin before therapy. Tuberculin sensitivity may be rendered positive by drug treatment.
• Obtain history of patient's bladder cancer.
• Monitor effectiveness by regularly checking tumor size and rate of growth through appropriate studies, as ordered, and by noting results of follow-up diagnostic tests and overall physical status.
• Be alert for adverse reactions and drug interactions.
• Closely monitor patient for evidence of systemic BCG infection. Such infections are seldom detected by positive cultures.
• Evaluate patient's and family's understanding of drug therapy.

Nursing diagnoses
• Risk for injury related to underlying condition
• Risk for trauma related to instillation procedure for drug therapy
• Knowledge deficit related to drug therapy

Planning and implementation
• Know that drug is not used as an immunizing agent for prevention of cancer or to prevent tuberculosis; drug should not be confused with BCG vaccine.
• Know that drug should not be handled or administered by caregiver with known immunologic deficiency.
• Be aware that BCG intravesical should not be administered within 7 to 14 days of transurethral resection or biopsy. Fatal disseminated BCG infection has occurred after traumatic catheterization.
• To administer TheraCys or ImmuCyst, reconstitute only with 1 ml of provided diluent per vial, just before use. Do not remove rubber stopper to prepare solution. Use immediately. Add contents of three reconstituted vials to 50 ml of sterile, preservative-free NaCl solution (final volume, 53 ml). Instill urethral catheter into bladder under aseptic conditions, drain bladder, and then infuse 53 ml of prepared solution by gravity feed.

Remove catheter and properly dispose of unused drug.
• To administer TICE BCG, use thermosetting plastic or sterile glass containers and syringes. Draw 1 ml of sterile, preservative-free NaCl solution into 3-ml syringe. Add to 1 ampule of drug; gently expel back into ampule three times to ensure thorough mixing. Use immediately. Dispense cloudy suspension into top end of catheter-tipped syringe that contains 49 ml of NaCl solution. Gently rotate syringe. Properly dispose of unused drug.
• Handle drug and all material used for instillation of drug as infectious material because it contains live attenuated mycobacteria. Dispose of all associated materials (syringes, catheters, and containers) as biohazardous waste.
• Use strict aseptic technique to administer drug in order to minimize trauma to GU tract and to prevent introduction of other contaminants to area.
• If there is evidence of traumatic catheterization, do not administer drug, and alert doctor. Subsequent treatment may resume after 1 week as if no interruption of schedule occurred.
• Know that therapy should be withheld if systemic infection is suspected (short-term high fever above 103° F [39.4° C], or persistent fever above 101° F [38.3° C] over 2 days, or with severe malaise). Doctor may contact an infectious disease specialist for initiation of fast-acting antituberculosis therapy.
• Be prepared to treat bladder irritation symptomatically with phenazopyridine, acetaminophen, and propantheline, as ordered. Systemic hypersensitivity can be treated with diphenhydramine. To minimize risk of systemic infection, some clinicians give isoniazid for 3 days starting on first day of treatment.
Patient teaching
• Tell patient to retain drug in bladder for 2 hours after instillation (if possible). For first hour, have patient lie prone for 15 minutes, supine for 15 minutes, and on each side for 15 minutes; second hour may be spent in sitting position.
• Instruct patient to sit when voiding.
• Instruct patient to disinfect urine for 6 hours after instillation of drug. To disinfect urine, add undiluted household bleach (5% sodium hypochlorite solution) in equal volume to voided urine in toilet; allow to stand for 15 minutes before flushing.
• Tell patient to call if symptoms worsen or if the following symptoms develop: blood in urine, frequent urge to urinate, painful urination, fever and chills, nausea, vomiting, joint pain, or rash.
• Caution patient that cough that develops after therapy could indicate life-threatening BCG infection and to notify doctor immediately.

☑ **Evaluation**
• Patient exhibits no further evidence of superficial bladder tumors.
• Patient does not experience trauma as result of drug use.
• Patient and family state understanding of drug therapy.

bacitracin
(bas-uh-TRAY-sin)

Pharmacologic class: polypeptide antibiotic
Therapeutic class: antibiotic
Pregnancy risk category: NR

How supplied

Injection: 10,000-unit, 50,000-unit vials

Pharmacokinetics

Absorption: absorbed rapidly and completely after I.M. injection.
Distribution: distributed widely throughout all body organs and fluids except CSF (unless meninges are inflamed). Drug binds to plasma proteins only minimally.
Metabolism: not significantly metabolized.

Excretion: 10% to 40% of dose excreted by kidneys.

Route	Onset	Peak	Duration
I.M.	Unknown	≤ 1 hr	Unknown

Pharmacodynamics

Chemical effect: hinders bacterial cell wall synthesis, damaging bacterial plasma membrane and making cell more vulnerable to osmotic pressure.
Therapeutic effect: hinders bacterial activity. Drug is effective against many gram-positive organisms, including *Clostridium difficile.* Drug is only minimally effective against gram-negative organisms.

Indications and dosage

▶ **Treatment of infants with pneumonia or empyema caused by susceptible staphylococci.** *Infants weighing over 2.5 kg (5.5 lb):* 1,000 units/kg I.M. daily in divided doses q 8 to 12 hours. *Infants weighing under 2.5 kg:* 900 units/kg I.M. daily in divided doses q 8 to 12 hours.

Adverse reactions

EENT: ototoxicity.
GI: nausea, vomiting, anorexia, diarrhea, rectal itching or burning.
GU: *nephrotoxicity (albuminuria,* cylindruria, oliguria, anuria, increased BUN, *tubular and glomerular necrosis).*
Hematologic: blood dyscrasia, eosinophilia.
Skin: urticaria, rash.
Other: superinfection, fever, *anaphylaxis, neuromuscular blockade,* pain at injection site.

Interactions

Drug-drug. *Inhalational anesthetics, neuromuscular blockers:* prolonged muscle weakness. Monitor patient for excessive muscle weakness or respiratory distress.
Nephrotoxic drugs (such as aminoglycosides): increased nephrotoxicity. Use together cautiously.

Contraindications and precautions

● Contraindicated in patients with impaired renal function or hypersensitivity to drug and in pregnant women.
● Use cautiously in patients with myasthenia gravis or neuromuscular disease.

NURSING CONSIDERATIONS

⚖ Assessment

● Obtain history of patient's infection before therapy and reassess regularly thereafter.
● Assess baseline renal function studies before starting therapy.
● Obtain urine specimen for culture and sensitivity tests before first dose. Therapy may begin pending test results.
● Be alert for adverse reactions and drug interactions.
● Evaluate patient's and family's understanding of drug therapy.

⚕ Nursing diagnoses

● Infection related to presence of susceptible bacteria
● Altered urinary elimination related to drug-induced nephrotoxicity
● Knowledge deficit related to drug therapy

▶ Planning and implementation

● Administer by deep I.M. injection only.
● Know that concentration of bacitracin should be between 5,000 and 10,000 units/ml. Store in refrigerator. Drug is inactivated if stored at room temperature.
● Provide measures to keep urine pH above 6 to reduce risk of nephrotoxicity, such as use of alkalinizing agents, as ordered, and adequate fluid intake.
Patient teaching
● Warn parent that injection may be painful.
● Instruct parents to report unusual signs or symptoms because drug causes many adverse reactions.

---

*Liquid form contains alcohol   **May contain tartrazine   ◆ Canada   ◇ Australia   †OTC

✓ Evaluation

- Patient is free of infection.
- Patient's kidney function remains normal throughout therapy.
- Patient and family state understanding of drug therapy.

---

baclofen
(BAH-kloh-fen)
Clofen◊, Lioresal, Lioresal Intrathecal

Pharmacologic class: chlorophenyl derivative
Therapeutic class: skeletal muscle relaxant
Pregnancy risk category: NR

How supplied

Tablets: 10 mg, 20 mg, 25 mg♦
Intrathecal injection: 500 mcg/ml, 2,000 mcg/ml

Pharmacokinetics

Absorption: rapidly and extensively absorbed from GI tract with P.O. administration but may vary.
Distribution: widely distributed throughout body, with small amounts crossing blood-brain barrier. It is about 30% plasma protein–bound.
Metabolism: about 15% metabolized in liver via deamination.
Excretion: 70% to 80% excreted in urine unchanged or as metabolites; remainder, in feces. *Half-life:* 2½ to 4 hours.

Route	Onset	Peak	Duration
P.O.	Hrs-wk	2-3 hr	Unknown
Intrathecal	0.5-1 hr	About 4 hr	4-8 hr

Pharmacodynamics

Chemical effect: unknown; appears to reduce transmission of impulses from spinal cord to skeletal muscle.
Therapeutic effect: relieves muscle spasms.

Indications and dosage

▶ **Spasticity in multiple sclerosis, spinal cord injury.** *Adults:* initially, 5 mg P.O. t.i.d. for 3 days. Dosage may be increased (based on response) at 3-day intervals by 15 mg (5 mg/dose) daily up to maximum of 80 mg daily (20 mg q.i.d.).
▶ **Management of severe spasticity in patients who do not respond to or cannot tolerate oral baclofen therapy.**
Adults (screening phase): after test dose to check responsiveness, drug is administered by an implantable infusion pump. The test dose is 1 ml of 50-mcg/ml dilution administered into intrathecal space by barbotage over 1 minute or more. Significantly decreased severity or frequency of muscle spasm or reduced muscle tone should be evident within 4 to 8 hours. If response is inadequate, second test dose of 75 mcg/1.5 ml is given 24 hours after the first. If response is still inadequate, final test dose of 100 mcg/2 ml is given 24 hours later. Patients unresponsive to 100-mcg dose shouldn't be considered candidates for implantable pump.
Adults (maintenance therapy): initial dose titrated based on screening dose that elicited an adequate response. This effective dose is doubled and administered over 24 hours. If screening dose efficacy is maintained for 8 hours or more, dose is not doubled. After first 24 hours, dose is increased slowly, as needed and tolerated, by 10% to 30% daily.

Adverse reactions

CNS: *drowsiness, dizziness,* headache, *weakness, fatigue,* hypotonia, confusion, insomnia, dysarthria, SEIZURES.
CV: hypotension.
EENT: nasal congestion, blurred vision.
GI: *nausea,* constipation, vomiting.
GU: urinary frequency.
Hepatic: increased AST and alkaline phosphatase levels.
Skin: rash, pruritus.
Other: ankle edema, excessive perspiration, hyperglycemia, weight gain, dyspnea.

Reactions may be *common,* uncommon, *life-threatening,* or COMMON AND LIFE-THREATENING.

Interactions

Drug-drug. *CNS depressants:* increased CNS depression. Avoid concomitant use. *MAO inhibitors, tricyclic antidepressants:* CNS and respiratory depression, hypotension. Avoid concomitant use. **Drug-lifestyle.** *Alcohol use:* increased CNS depression. Avoid concomitant use.

Contraindications and precautions

• Contraindicated in patients with hypersensitivity to drug.
• Use cautiously in patients with impaired renal function or seizure disorder or when spasticity is used to maintain motor function. Also use cautiously in pregnant or breast-feeding women.
• Safety of drug has not been established in children under age 12.

NURSING CONSIDERATIONS

Assessment
• Obtain history of patient's pain and muscle spasms related to underlying condition before therapy and reassess regularly thereafter.
• Be alert for adverse reactions and drug interactions.
• Watch for increased incidence of seizures in patient with seizure disorder.
• Evaluate patient's and family's understanding of drug therapy.

Nursing diagnoses
• Pain related to spasticity
• Risk for injury related to drug-induced adverse CNS reactions
• Knowledge deficit related to drug therapy

Planning and implementation
P.O. use: Give with meals or milk to prevent GI distress.
– Know that orally administered drug should not be used to treat muscle spasm caused by rheumatic disorders, cerebral palsy, Parkinson's disease, or CVA because efficacy hasn't been established.

Intrathecal use: Know that implantable pump or catheter failure can result in sudden loss of effectiveness of intrathecal baclofen.
• Do not administer intrathecal injection by I.V., I.M., S.C., or epidural route.
• Be aware that amount of relief determines if dose (and drowsiness) can be reduced.
• Do not withdraw drug abruptly after long-term use unless required by severe adverse reactions; abrupt withdrawal may precipitate hallucinations or rebound spasticity.
• Keep in mind that treatment for oral overdose is supportive only; emesis should not be induced nor respiratory stimulant used in obtunded patient.
• Know that experience with long-term intrathecal use suggests that about 10% of patients may develop tolerance to drug. In some cases, this may be treated by hospitalizing patient and slowly withdrawing drug over 2-week period.
• Institute safety precautions if patient develops adverse CNS reactions.
Patient teaching
• Tell patient to avoid activities that require alertness until drug's CNS effects are known. Drowsiness usually is transient.
• Tell patient to avoid alcohol while taking drug.
• Advise patient to follow doctor's orders about rest and physical therapy.
• Advise patient to take drug with food or milk to prevent GI distress.

Evaluation
• Patient reports pain and muscle spasms have ceased with drug therapy.
• Patient does not experience injury as a result of drug-induced drowsiness.
• Patient and family state understanding of drug therapy.

beclomethasone dipropionate
(bek-loh-METH-eh-sohn
digh-proh-PIGH-uh-nayt)
Aldecin Inhaler◇, Beclodisk◆, Becloforte Inhaler◇, Beclovent, Beclovent Rotacaps◆, Vanceril, Vanceril Double Strength Inhalation

Pharmacologic class: glucocorticoid
Therapeutic class: anti-inflammatory, antiasthmatic
Pregnancy risk category: NR

How supplied

Oral inhalation aerosol: 42 mcg/metered spray, 50 mcg /metered spray◇, 84 mcg/metered spray

Pharmacokinetics

Absorption: after oral inhalation, absorbed rapidly from lungs and GI tract.
Distribution: no evidence of tissue storage of beclomethasone or its metabolites. About 10% to 25% of an orally inhaled dose is deposited in respiratory tract. The remainder, deposited in mouth and oropharynx, is swallowed. When absorbed, it is 87% bound to plasma proteins.
Metabolism: most of drug metabolized in liver.
Excretion: unknown, although when drug is administered systemically, its metabolites are excreted mainly in feces and, to a lesser extent, in urine. *Half-life:* average 15 hours.

Route	Onset	Peak	Duration
Inhalation	1-4 wk	Unknown	Unknown

Pharmacodynamics

Chemical effect: decreases inflammation, mainly by stabilizing leukocyte lysosomal membranes.
Therapeutic effect: helps alleviate asthma symptoms.

Indications and dosage

▶ **Steroid-dependent asthma.** *Adults and children age 12 and over:* for regular strength, 2 inhalations t.i.d. or q.i.d or 4 inhalations b.i.d.; for double strength, 2 inhalations b.i.d. Maximum dosage is 840 mcg daily. *Children ages 6 to 12:* for regular strength, 1 to 2 inhalations t.i.d. or q.i.d. For double strength, 2 inhalations b.i.d. Maximum dosage is 420 mcg daily.

Adverse reactions

EENT: hoarseness, fungal infections of throat, throat irritation.
GI: dry mouth, fungal infections of mouth.
Other: *angioedema, bronchospasm, adrenal insufficiency.*

Interactions

None significant.

Contraindications and precautions

• Contraindicated in patients hypersensitive to drug or its components (fluorocarbons, oleic acid) and in those with status asthmaticus.
• Do not use in patients with asthma controlled by bronchodilators or other noncorticosteroids alone or in those with nonasthmatic bronchial diseases.
• Use with extreme caution, if at all, in patients with tuberculosis, fungal or bacterial infections, ocular herpes simplex, or systemic viral infections.
• Use with caution in patients receiving systemic corticosteroid therapy and in pregnant or breast-feeding women.
• Safety of drug has not been established in children under age 6.

NURSING CONSIDERATIONS

▨ **Assessment**
• Obtain history of patient's asthmatic condition before therapy and reassess regularly thereafter.
• Be alert for adverse reactions.
• Monitor patient closely during times of stress (trauma, surgery, or infection) because systemic corticosteroids may be

---

needed to prevent adrenal insufficiency in previously steroid-dependent patients.
• Know that periodic measurement of growth and development may be necessary during high-dose or prolonged therapy in children.
• Evaluate patient's and family's understanding of drug therapy.

⊞ **Nursing diagnoses**
• Impaired gas exchange related to asthmatic condition
• Altered oral mucous membranes related to drug-induced fungal infections
• Knowledge deficit related to drug therapy

⊠ **Planning and implementation**
• Never administer drug to relieve an emergency asthmatic attack because onset of action is too slow.
• Administer prescribed bronchodilators several minutes before beclomethasone.
• Have patient rest 1 minute between puffs and hold breath for a few seconds after each puff to enhance drug action.
• Be aware that spacer device may help ensure delivery of proper dose, although use of such a device with Becloforte Inhaler is not recommended.
• Taper oral glucocorticoid therapy slowly, as ordered. Acute adrenal insufficiency and death have occurred in asthmatics who changed abruptly from oral corticosteroids to beclomethasone.
• Notify doctor if decreased response is noted after administration of drug.
• Have patient drink glass of water after inhalations to help prevent oral fungal infections.
• Keep inhaler clean and unobstructed by washing it with warm water and drying it thoroughly after each use.
Patient teaching
• Inform patient that drug doesn't provide relief from acute asthma attacks.
• Tell patient requiring bronchodilator to use it several minutes before drug.
• Instruct patient to carry medical identification card indicating need for supple-

mental systemic glucocorticoids during stress.
• Advise patient to allow 1 minute to elapse before taking subsequent puffs of medication and to hold his breath for a few seconds after each puff to enhance action of drug.
• Instruct patient to contact doctor if response to therapy decreases or if symptoms don't improve within 3 weeks; dose may need to be adjusted. Tell patient not to exceed recommended dose on his own.
• Tell patient to keep inhaler clean and unobstructed by washing it with warm water and drying it thoroughly.
• Tell patient to prevent oral fungal infections by gargling or rinsing mouth with water after each use but not to swallow water.
• Tell patient to report symptoms associated with corticosteroid withdrawal, including fatigue, weakness, arthralgia, orthostatic hypotension, and dyspnea.
• Instruct patient to store drug between 36° and 86° F (2° and 30° C). Advise him to ensure delivery of proper dose by gently warming canister to room temperature before using. He may carry canister in pocket to keep it warm.

☑ **Evaluation**
• Patient's lungs are clear, and breathing and skin color are normal.
• Patient does not exhibit an oral fungal infection during therapy.
• Patient and family state understanding of drug therapy.

beclomethasone dipropionate monohydrate
(bek-loh-METH-eh-sohn digh-proh-PIGH-uh-nayt)
Beconase AQ Nasal Spray, Beconase Nasal Inhaler, Vancenase AQ Nasal Spray, Vancenase AQ 84 mcg, Vancenase Nasal Inhaler

Pharmacologic class: glucocorticoid

Therapeutic class: anti-inflammatory
Pregnancy risk category: C

How supplied

Nasal aerosol: 42 mcg/metered spray,
50 mcg/metered spray ◊
Nasal spray: 42 mcg/metered spray,
50 mcg/metered spray ◊, 84 mcg/metered
spray

Pharmacokinetics

Absorption: after nasal inhalation, drug
is absorbed primarily through nasal mucosa with minimal systemic absorption.
Distribution: unknown.
Metabolism: most of drug is metabolized
in liver.
Excretion: unknown, although when
drug is administered systemically, its
metabolites are excreted mainly in feces
and, to a lesser extent, in urine.
Biological half-life: average 15 hours.

Route	Onset	Peak	Duration
Inhalation	5-7 days	≤ 3 wk	Unknown

Pharmacodynamics

Chemical effect: decreases nasal inflammation, mainly by stabilizing leukocyte
lysosomal membranes.
Therapeutic effect: helps relieve nasal allergy symptoms.

Indications and dosage

▶ **Relief of symptoms of seasonal or
perennial rhinitis; prevention of recurrence of nasal polyps after surgical removal.** *Adults and children over age 6:*
for 42 mcg/metered spray, usual dosage is
1 or 2 sprays in each nostril, b.i.d. Maximum dosage is 168 to 336 mcg daily. For
84 mcg/metered spray, usual dosage is 1
to 2 inhalations daily. Maximum dosage
is 168 to 336 mcg daily.

Adverse reactions

CNS: headache.
EENT: *mild, transient nasal burning and
stinging;* nasal congestion; sneezing;
epistaxis; watery eyes; nasopharyngeal
fungal infections.
GI: nausea, vomiting.

Interactions

None significant.

Contraindications and precautions

• Contraindicated in patients hypersensitive to drug and in those experiencing
status asthmaticus or other acute episodes
of asthma.
• Use cautiously, if at all, in patients with
active or quiescent respiratory tract tubercular infections or untreated fungal, bacterial, systemic viral, or ocular herpes
simplex infections. Also use cautiously in
patients who have recently had nasal septal ulcers, nasal surgery, or trauma.
• Use cautiously in pregnant or breast-
feeding women.
• Safety of drug has not been established
in children under age 6.

NURSING CONSIDERATIONS

✍ Assessment
• Obtain history of patient's allergy
symptoms and nasal congestion before
therapy and reassess regularly thereafter.
• Be alert for adverse reactions.
• Monitor patient's hydration status if adverse GI reactions occur.
• Evaluate patient's and family's understanding of drug therapy.

❂ Nursing diagnoses
• Altered health maintenance related to
allergy-induced nasal congestion
• Risk for fluid volume deficit related to
drug-induced adverse GI reactions
• Knowledge deficit related to drug
therapy

❯ Planning and implementation
• Be aware that drug is not effective for
acute exacerbations of rhinitis. Decongestants or antihistamines may be needed.

Reactions may be *common,* uncommon, *life-threatening*, or COMMON AND LIFE-THREATENING.

• Shake container and invert. Have patient clear his nasal passages and then tilt his head back. Insert nozzle into nostril (pointed away from septum), holding other nostril closed. Deliver spray while patient inspires. Repeat in other nostril.
• Notify doctor if relief is not obtained or signs of infection appear.

Patient teaching
• Instruct patient to shake container before using, to blow nose to clear nasal passages, and to tilt head slightly forward and insert nozzle into nostril, pointing away from septum. Tell him to hold other nostril closed and then to inspire gently and spray. Next, have him shake container again and repeat in other nostril.
• Advise patient to pump new nasal spray three or four times before first use and then once or twice before first use each day thereafter. Also tell her to clean cap and nosepiece of activator in warm water every day, then to air-dry them.
• Advise patient to use drug regularly, as prescribed, because its effectiveness depends on regular use.
• Explain that drug's therapeutic effects, unlike those of decongestants, are not immediate. Most patients achieve benefit within a few days, but some may require 2 to 3 weeks.
• Warn patient not to exceed recommended doses because of risk of hypothalamic-pituitary-adrenal function suppression.
• Tell patient to notify doctor if symptoms don't improve within 3 weeks or if nasal irritation persists.
• Teach patient good nasal and oral hygiene.

☑ **Evaluation**
• Patient's nasal congestion subsides with therapy.
• Patient maintains adequate hydration throughout therapy.
• Patient and family state understanding of drug therapy.

belladonna leaf
(bel-ah-DON-ah LEEF)
Belladonna Tincture USP*

Pharmacologic class: belladonna alkaloid
Therapeutic class: antispasmodic
Pregnancy risk category: NR

How supplied
Oral solution: 27 to 33 mg belladonna alkaloids/dl in 67% alcohol solution

Pharmacokinetics
Absorption: well absorbed from GI tract.
Distribution: unknown.
Metabolism: hydrolyzed to tropine and tropic acid.
Excretion: 33% excreted unchanged by kidneys, while its derivatives are excreted in urine and, to a lesser extent, in feces.

Route	Onset	Peak	Duration
P.O.	Unknown	Unknown	Unknown

Pharmacodynamics
Chemical effect: blocks acetylcholine, which decreases GI motility and inhibits gastric acid secretion.
Therapeutic effect: decreases spasms in GI and GU tracts.

Indications and dosage
▶ **Adjunct therapy for peptic ulceration, irritable bowel syndrome, functional GI disorders, and neurogenic bowel disturbances.** *Adults:* 0.6 to 1 ml P.O. t.i.d. or q.i.d. *Children:* 0.1 ml/kg or 2.5 ml/m² tincture P.O. daily, given t.i.d. or q.i.d. Total dosage should not exceed 3.5 ml/day.

Adverse reactions
CNS: headache, insomnia, drowsiness, dizziness, nervousness, weakness; *confusion, excitement* (in elderly patients).
CV: *palpitations,* tachycardia.

EENT: *blurred vision,* mydriasis, increased intraocular pressure, cycloplegia, photophobia.
GI: *dry mouth,* dysphagia, heartburn, loss of taste, *constipation,* nausea, vomiting.
GU: *urinary hesitancy, urine retention,* impotence.
Skin: urticaria, decreased sweating or possibly anhidrosis, other dermal manifestations.
Other: fever, allergic reactions.
Note: Overdose may cause curare-like effects, such as respiratory paralysis.

Interactions

Drug-drug. *Amantadine, antihistamines, antiparkinsonian agents, disopyramide, glutethimide, meperidine, phenothiazines, procainamide, quinidine, tricyclic antidepressants:* additive adverse effects. Avoid concomitant use.
Antacids: decreased absorption of oral anticholinergics. Separate administration times by 2 to 3 hours.
Ketoconazole: anticholinergics may interfere with ketoconazole absorption. Avoid concomitant use.
Methotrimeprazine: anticholinergics may enhance risk of extrapyramidal reactions. Avoid concomitant use.

Contraindications and precautions

• Contraindicated in patients with angle-closure glaucoma, obstructive uropathy, obstructive disease of GI tract, severe ulcerative colitis, myasthenia gravis, paralytic ileus, intestinal atony, unstable CV status in acute hemorrhage, toxic megacolon, or hypersensitivity to anticholinergics.
• Drug is not recommended for use in breast-feeding women.
• Use cautiously in patients with autonomic neuropathy, hyperthyroidism, coronary artery disease, arrhythmias, heart failure, hypertension, hiatal hernia associated with reflux esophagitis, GI infections, hepatic or renal disease, partial obstructive uropathy, and ulcerative coli-

tis; in pregnant women; and in patients over age 40 because of increased incidence of glaucoma.
• Also use cautiously in hot or humid environments. Drug-induced heatstroke can develop.

NURSING CONSIDERATIONS

⚄ Assessment
• Obtain history of patient's underlying GI or GU condition before therapy and reassess regularly thereafter.
• Be alert for adverse reactions and drug interactions.
• Evaluate patient's and family's understanding of drug therapy.

⊕ Nursing diagnoses
• Pain related to spasms
• Risk for injury related to drug-induced adverse reactions
• Knowledge deficit related to drug therapy

⧁ Planning and implementation
• Give 30 minutes to 1 hour before meals and at bedtime. Bedtime dose can be larger; give at least 2 hours after last meal of day.
• Administer smaller doses to elderly patients, as ordered.
Patient teaching
• Instruct patient to avoid driving and other hazardous activities if he is drowsy or dizzy or has blurred vision; to drink plenty of fluids to help prevent constipation; and to report rash or local eruption.
• Tell patient to use sugarless gum or hard candy to relieve dry mouth.

▧ Evaluation
• Patient states spasms have been alleviated.
• Patient does not experience injury as result of drug-induced adverse reactions.
• Patient and family state understanding of drug therapy.

Reactions may be *common,* uncommon, *life-threatening,* or COMMON AND LIFE-THREATENING.

benazepril hydrochloride
(ben-AY-zuh-pril high-droh-KLOR-ighd)
Lotensin

Pharmacologic class: ACE inhibitor
Therapeutic class: antihypertensive
Pregnancy risk category: C (D in second and third trimesters)

How supplied
Tablets: 5 mg, 10 mg, 20 mg, 40 mg

Pharmacokinetics
Absorption: at least 37% is absorbed.
Distribution: serum protein binding of benazepril is about 96.7%; that of benazeprilat, 95.3%.
Metabolism: almost completely metabolized in liver to benazeprilat, which has much greater ACE inhibitory activity than benazepril, and to glucuronide conjugates of benazepril and benazeprilat.
Excretion: primarily in urine. *Half-life:* benazepril, 0.6 hours; benazeprilat, 10 to 12 hours.

Route	Onset	Peak	Duration
P.O.	≤ 1 hr	2-4 hr	24 hr

Pharmacodynamics
Chemical effect: inhibits ACE, preventing conversion of angiotensin I to angiotensin II, a potent vasoconstrictor. Reduced formation of angiotensin II decreases peripheral arterial resistance, thus decreasing aldosterone secretion. This reduces sodium and water retention and lowers blood pressure. Benazepril also has antihypertensive activity in patients with low-renin hypertension.
Therapeutic effect: lowers blood pressure.

Indications and dosage
▶ **Hypertension.** *Adults:* in patient not receiving diuretic, 10 mg P.O. daily (initially). Dose titrated, as needed and tolerated; most patients take 20 to 40 mg daily, divided into one or two doses.

Adverse reactions
CNS: asthenia, headache, dizziness, light-headedness, anxiety, amnesia, depression, insomnia, nervousness, neuralgia, neuropathy, paresthesia, somnolence.
CV: symptomatic hypotension, syncope, angina, *arrhythmias,* palpitations, *angioedema,* edema.
GI: nausea, vomiting, abdominal pain, constipation, dyspepsia, gastritis, dysphagia, increased salivation.
Metabolic: hyperkalemia.
Musculoskeletal: arthralgia, arthritis, myalgia.
Respiratory: dry, persistent, tickling, nonproductive cough; dyspnea.
Skin: hypersensitivity reactions, rash, dermatitis, pruritus, photosensitivity, purpura.
Other: impotence, increased diaphoresis, weight gain.

Interactions
Drug-drug. *Diuretics, other antihypertensives:* risk of excessive hypotension. Discontinue diuretic or lower dose of benazepril, as needed.
Lithium: increased serum lithium levels and lithium toxicity. Avoid concomitant use.
Potassium-sparing diuretics, potassium supplements: risk of hyperkalemia. Monitor patient closely.
Drug-food. *Food, especially high in fat:* can impair absorption. Instruct patient to take drug on an empty stomach.
Sodium substitutes containing potassium: risk of hyperkalemia. Monitor patient closely.

Contraindications and precautions
● Contraindicated in patients with hypersensitivity to ACE inhibitors.
● Use only if absolutely necessary in pregnant women, and then use with extreme caution. Drug is usually discontinued during pregnancy.
● Use cautiously in patients with impaired hepatic or renal function and in breast-feeding women.

• Safety of drug has not been established in children.

NURSING CONSIDERATIONS

☜ Assessment
• Obtain history of patient's blood pressure before therapy and reassess regularly thereafter. Measure blood pressure when drug levels are at peak (2 to 6 hours after dose) and at trough (just before dose) to verify adequate blood pressure control.
• Be alert for adverse reactions and drug interactions.
• Monitor patient's ECG.
• Monitor renal and hepatic function periodically, as ordered. Also monitor serum potassium levels.
• Monitor patient's CBC with differential every 2 weeks for first 3 months of therapy and periodically thereafter, as ordered. Other ACE inhibitors have been associated with agranulocytosis and neutropenia.
• Evaluate patient's and family's understanding of drug therapy.

☷ Nursing diagnoses
• Risk for injury related to hypertension
• Decreased cardiac output related to drug-induced arrhythmias
• Knowledge deficit related to drug therapy

☲ Planning and implementation
• Know that, if patient is receiving diuretic, dose should be lower than if patient is not receiving diuretic; excessive hypotension can occur when drug is given with diuretics.
• Dosage adjustment may be necessary in patients with renal impairment.
• Administer at about same time every day to maintain consistent effect on blood pressure.
• Administer drug when patient's stomach is empty.

Patient teaching
• Instruct patient to take this drug on an empty stomach; meals, particularly those high in fat, can impair absorption.
• Tell patient to avoid sodium substitutes; such products may contain potassium, which can cause hyperkalemia in patients taking drug.
• Tell patient to rise slowly to minimize risk of dizziness, which may occur during first few weeks of therapy. He should stop taking drug and call doctor immediately.
• Tell patient to use caution in hot weather and during exercise. Inadequate fluid intake, vomiting, diarrhea, and excessive perspiration can lead to light-headedness and syncope.
• Advise patient to report signs of infection, such as fever and sore throat. Also tell him to call doctor if the following signs or symptoms occur: easy bruising or bleeding; swelling of tongue, lips, face, eyes, mucous membranes, or extremities; difficulty swallowing or breathing; and hoarseness.
• Tell female patient to notify doctor if pregnancy occurs. Drug will need to be discontinued.

☑ Evaluation
• Patient's blood pressure is normal.
• Patient maintains adequate cardiac output during drug therapy.
• Patient and family state understanding of drug therapy.

benzonatate
(ben-ZOH-nuh-tayt)
Tessalon

Pharmacologic class: local anesthetic (ester)
Therapeutic class: nonnarcotic antitussive
Pregnancy risk category: C

How supplied
Capsules: 100 mg

Pharmacokinetics
Unknown.

Route	Onset	Peak	Duration
P.O.	15-20 min	Unknown	≤ 8 hr

Pharmacodynamics
Chemical effect: suppresses cough reflex by direct action on cough center in medulla. Also has local anesthetic action. *Therapeutic effect:* relieves cough.

Indications and dosage
▶ **Symptomatic relief of cough.** *Adults and children over age 10:* 100 mg P.O. t.i.d., increased as needed to maximum of 600 mg daily.

Adverse reactions
CNS: dizziness, drowsiness, headache, restlessness.
EENT: nasal congestion, burning sensation in eyes.
GI: nausea, constipation.
Skin: rash.
Other: chills.

Interactions
None significant.

Contraindications and precautions
● Contraindicated in patients hypersensitive to drug.
● Use cautiously in patients hypersensitive to para-aminobenzoic acid anesthetics (procaine, tetracaine) because cross-sensitivity reactions may occur and in pregnant women.
● Safety of drug has not been established in breast-feeding women and in children under age 10.

NURSING CONSIDERATIONS

🔍 Assessment
● Obtain history of patient's cough before therapy and reassess regularly thereafter.
● Be alert for adverse reactions.

● Evaluate patient's and family's understanding of drug therapy.

🔲 Nursing diagnoses
● Ineffective airway clearance related to underlying condition producing nonproductive cough
● Risk for injury related to drug-induced adverse CNS reactions
● Knowledge deficit related to drug therapy

🔆 Planning and implementation
● Don't use benzonatate when cough is valuable diagnostic sign or is beneficial (as after thoracic surgery).
● Make sure patient swallows capsules promptly; if capsules dissolve in mouth, CNS stimulation may cause restlessness.
● Use with percussion and chest vibration.
● Maintain fluid intake to help liquefy sputum.
Patient teaching
● Warn patient not to chew capsules or let them dissolve in his mouth because resulting local anesthesia may cause aspiration.
● Instruct patient not to take more of drug than directed.
● Tell patient to call doctor if cough persists more than 7 days.
● Advise patient to use humidifier to filter out dust, smoke, and air pollutants.
● Caution patient against performing hazardous activities that require alertness until CNS effects of drug are known.
● Explain importance of consuming 2,000 to 3,000 ml of fluid daily to liquefy sputum.

🔳 Evaluation
● Patient's cough is resolved.
● Patient does not experience injury as result of drug-induced adverse CNS reactions.
● Patient and family state understanding of drug therapy.

benzquinamide hydrochloride
(benz-KWIN-ah-mighd
high-droh-KLOR-ighd)
Emete-Con

Pharmacologic class: benzoquinolizine
derivative
Therapeutic class: antiemetic
Pregnancy risk category: NR

How supplied
Injection: 50 mg/vial

Pharmacokinetics
Absorption: not applicable for I.V. use;
unknown for I.M. use.
Distribution: distributed rapidly in body
tissues, with highest concentration in liver and kidneys. About 58% is plasma
protein–bound.
Metabolism: most of drug (90% to 95%)
metabolized in liver.
Excretion: 5% to 10% of drug excreted
unchanged in urine. Metabolites are excreted in urine, bile, and feces. *Plasma
half-life:* about 40 minutes.

Route	Onset	Peak	Duration
I.V.	≤ 15 min	Immediate	3-4 hr
I.M.	≤ 15 min	≤ 30 min	3-4 hr

Pharmacodynamics
Chemical effect: unknown; thought to
act on chemoreceptor trigger zone to inhibit nausea and vomiting.
Therapeutic effect: relieves nausea and
vomiting.

Indications and dosage
▶ **Nausea and vomiting associated with
anesthesia and surgery.** *Adults:* 25 mg
(0.2 to 0.4 mg/kg) I.V. as single dose, administered slowly (25 mg/minute), with
subsequent doses given I.M.; or 50 mg
I.M. (0.5 to 1 mg/kg), repeated in 1 hour
and, thereafter, q 3 to 4 hours, p.r.n.

Adverse reactions
CNS: *drowsiness,* fatigue, insomnia, restlessness, headache, excitation, tremors,
twitching, dizziness.
CV: sudden rise in blood pressure and
transient arrhythmias (premature atrial
and ventricular contractions, atrial fibrillation) after I.V. administration; hypertension; hypotension.
EENT: blurred vision.
GI: anorexia, nausea, salivation, dry
mouth.
Skin: urticaria, rash.
Other: muscle weakness, flushing, hiccups, sweating, chills, fever.

Interactions
Drug-drug. *CNS depressants:* enhanced
CNS depression. Avoid concomitant use.
Drug-lifestyle. *Alcohol use:* enhanced
CNS depression. Avoid concomitant use.

Contraindications and precautions
• I.V. use contraindicated in patients with
CV disease and within 15 minutes of administering preanesthetic or CV drugs.
Also contraindicated in patients with hypersensitivity to drug.
• Use in pregnant women is not recommended.
• Safety of drug has not been established
in children.

NURSING CONSIDERATIONS

⚕ Assessment
• Obtain history of patient's CV and GI
status before therapy and reassess regularly thereafter.
• Be alert for adverse reactions and drug
interactions.
• Evaluate patient's and family's understanding of drug therapy.

⚕ Nursing diagnoses
• Risk for aspiration related to nausea
and vomiting induced by anesthesia and
surgery

• Altered cardiopulmonary tissue perfusion related to drug-induced arrhythmias after I.V. administration
• Knowledge deficit related to drug therapy

>> **Planning and implementation**
I.V. use: Reconstitute drug with 2.2 ml of sterile water for injection or bacteriostatic water containing benzyl alcohol or propylparaben. Do not dilute further. Inject directly and slowly (25 mg/minute).
– Do not reconstitute with 0.9% NaCl injection.
I.M. use: Give injections in large muscle mass. Use deltoid area only if well developed.
• Store dry powder and reconstituted solution in light-resistant container. Reconstituted solution is stable for 14 days at room temperature.
• Position patient on side, if not contraindicated. Keep an airway and suction equipment nearby in case vomiting occurs.
Patient teaching
• Warn patient that drowsiness usually follows administration, and tell him to ask for assistance, as needed.

☑ **Evaluation**
• Patient does not experience nausea and vomiting and subsequent aspiration.
• Patient maintains adequate cardiopulmonary tissue perfusion throughout therapy.
• Patient and family state understanding of drug therapy.

---

benztropine mesylate
(BENZ-troh-peen MES-ih-layt)
Apo-Benztropine♦, Cogentin, PMS Benztropine♦

Pharmacologic class: anticholinergic
Therapeutic class: antiparkinsonian agent
Pregnancy risk category: NR

How supplied
Tablets: 0.5 mg, 1 mg, 2 mg
Injection: 1 mg/ml in 2-ml ampules

Pharmacokinetics
Absorption: absorbed from GI tract when administered P.O.
Distribution: largely unknown; however, drug crosses blood-brain barrier.
Metabolism: unknown.
Excretion: excreted in urine as unchanged drug and metabolites. After P.O. therapy, small amounts may be excreted in feces as unabsorbed drug.

Route	Onset	Peak	Duration
P.O.	1-2 hr	Unknown	24 hr
I.V., I.M.	≤ 15 min	Unknown	24 hr

Pharmacodynamics
Chemical effect: unknown; thought to block central cholinergic receptors, helping to balance cholinergic activity in basal ganglia.
Therapeutic effect: improves voluntary movement ability.

Indications and dosage
▶ **Drug-induced extrapyramidal disorders (except tardive dyskinesia).** *Adults:* 1 to 4 mg P.O. or I.V. once or twice daily.
▶ **Acute dystonic reaction.** *Adults:* 1 to 2 mg I.V. or I.M., followed by 1 to 2 mg P.O. b.i.d. to prevent recurrence.
▶ **Parkinsonism.** *Adults:* 0.5 to 6 mg P.O. daily. Initial dose is 0.5 mg to 1 mg. Increased by 0.5 mg q 5 to 6 days. Dose adjusted to meet individual requirements.

Adverse reactions
CNS: disorientation, restlessness, irritability, incoherence, hallucinations, headache, sedation, depression.
CV: palpitations, tachycardia, paradoxical bradycardia.
EENT: dilated pupils, blurred vision, photophobia, difficulty swallowing.
GI: dry mouth, *constipation,* nausea, vomiting, epigastric distress.

GU: urinary hesitancy, urine retention.
Musculoskeletal: muscle weakness.
Skin: flushing.
Note: Some adverse reactions may result from atropine-like toxicity and are dose-related.

Interactions

Drug-drug. *Amantadine, phenothiazines, tricyclic antidepressants:* additive anticholinergic adverse reactions, such as confusion and hallucinations. Reduce dose before administering.

Contraindications and precautions

• Contraindicated in patients with acute angle-closure glaucoma or hypersensitivity to drug or its components, in children under age 3, and in breast-feeding women.
• Use cautiously in patients exposed to hot weather, in those with mental disorders, in pregnant women, and in children age 3 and older.

NURSING CONSIDERATIONS

Assessment
• Obtain history of patient's dyskinetic movements and underlying condition before therapy.
• Monitor effectiveness by regularly checking body movements for signs of improvement; full effect of drug may take 2 to 3 days.
• Be alert for adverse reactions and drug interactions.
• Evaluate patient's and family's understanding of drug therapy.

Nursing diagnoses
• Impaired physical mobility related to dyskinetic movements
• Risk for injury related to drug-induced adverse CNS reactions
• Knowledge deficit related to drug therapy

Planning and implementation
P.O. use: Administer drug after meals to help prevent GI distress.
I.V. use: Be aware that drug is seldom used I.V. because of small difference in onset compared with I.M. route.
I.M. use: Know that I.M. route is preferred with parenteral administration.
• Give drug at bedtime if patient is to receive single daily dose.
• Never discontinue drug abruptly; reduce dose gradually.
Patient teaching
• Warn patient to avoid activities requiring alertness until CNS effects of drug are known.
• If patient is to receive single daily dose, tell him to take it at bedtime.
• If patient is to receive drug orally, tell him to take it after meals.
• Advise patient to report signs of urinary hesitancy or urine retention.
• Tell patient to relieve dry mouth with cool drinks, ice chips, sugarless gum, or hard candy.
• Advise patient to limit activities during hot weather because drug-induced anhidrosis may result in hyperthermia.

Evaluation
• Patient exhibits improved mobility with reduction in muscle rigidity, akinesia, and tremors.
• Patient does not experience injury as result of drug-induced adverse CNS reactions.
• Patient and family state understanding of drug therapy.

bepridil hydrochloride
(BEH-prih-dil high-droh-KLOR-ighd)
Vascor

Pharmacologic class: calcium channel blocker
Therapeutic class: antianginal
Pregnancy risk category: C

How supplied

Tablets: 200 mg, 300 mg, 400 mg

Pharmacokinetics

Absorption: rapidly and completely absorbed.
Distribution: more than 99% is plasma protein–bound.
Metabolism: metabolized in liver.
Excretion: over 10 days, 70% is excreted in urine, 22% in feces as metabolites.
Half-life: after multiple dosing, averages 42 hours.

Route	Onset	Peak	Duration
P.O.	Unknown	2-3 hr	24 hr

Pharmacodynamics

Chemical effect: inhibits calcium ion influx across cardiac and smooth-muscle cells. This action dilates coronary arteries, peripheral arteries, and arterioles; it may reduce heart rate, decrease myocardial contractility, and slow AV node conduction.
Therapeutic effect: prevents anginal pain.

Indications and dosage

► **Chronic stable angina in patients who cannot tolerate or who fail to respond to other agents.** *Adults:* initially, 200 mg P.O. daily. After 10 days, dosage increased based on response. Maintenance dosage in most patients is 300 mg/day. Maximum daily dosage is 400 mg.

Adverse reactions

CNS: dizziness.
CV: edema; flushing; palpitations; tachycardia; *ventricular arrhythmias, including torsades de pointes, ventricular tachycardia, ventricular fibrillation.*
GI: nausea, diarrhea.
Respiratory: dyspnea.
Skin: rash.

Interactions

Drug-drug. *Antiarrhythmic agents, tricyclic antidepressants:* could prolong QT interval. Use cautiously together.
Cardiac glycosides: could exaggerate AV nodal conduction. Use cautiously together.

Contraindications and precautions

• Contraindicated in patients with uncompensated cardiac insufficiency, sick sinus syndrome, or second- or third-degree AV block unless pacemaker is present; hypotension; congenital QT interval prolongation; hypersensitivity to drug; or history of serious ventricular arrhythmias. Also contraindicated in those receiving other drugs that prolong QT interval.
• Use cautiously in patients with left bundle branch block, sinus bradycardia (less than 50 beats/minute), impaired renal or hepatic function, or heart failure, and in pregnant women.
• Risk-benefit ratio must be assessed for use in breast-feeding women because of potential for serious adverse reactions in infants.
• Safe use of drug has not been established in children.

NURSING CONSIDERATIONS

🔳 **Assessment**
• Obtain history of patient's anginal status before therapy; reassess regularly thereafter.
• Be alert for adverse reactions and drug interactions.
• Monitor patient's ECG, heart rate, and rhythm regularly; use of bepridil may cause severe ventricular arrhythmias, including torsades de pointes.
• Monitor patient's CBC and differential; use of drug is associated with agranulocytosis.
• Evaluate patient's and family's understanding of drug therapy.

⊞ **Nursing diagnoses**
- Pain related to presence of angina
- Altered protection related to drug-induced ventricular arrhythmias
- Knowledge deficit related to drug therapy

▶ **Planning and implementation**
- Give drug following usual protocol for P.O. administration.
- Consult doctor if patient does not experience pain relief.

Patient teaching
- Tell patient to report unusual bruising or bleeding or signs of persistent infections promptly.
- Stress importance of taking drug exactly as prescribed, even when patient is feeling well.
- Tell patient to schedule activities to allow adequate rest.
- Encourage patient to restrict fluid and sodium intake to minimize edema.

☑ **Evaluation**
- Patient states anginal pain is relieved.
- Patient's ECG, heart rate, and rhythm are unchanged with therapy.
- Patient and family state understanding of drug therapy.

---

beractant
(natural lung surfactant)
(beh-RAK-tant)
Survanta

Pharmacologic class: bovine lung extract
Therapeutic class: lung surfactant
Pregnancy risk category: NR

How supplied

Suspension for intratracheal instillation: 25 mg/ml

Pharmacokinetics

Absorption: most of dose becomes lung-associated within hours.

Distribution: distributed across alveolar surface.
Metabolism: lipids enter endogenous surfactant pathway of recycling and reutilization.
Excretion: alveolar clearance of lipid components is rapid.

Route	Onset	Peak	Duration
Intratracheal	0.5-2 hr	Unknown	2-3 days

Pharmacodynamics

Chemical effect: lowers surface tension on alveolar surfaces during respiration and stabilizes alveoli against collapse. An extract of bovine lung containing neutral lipids, fatty acids, surfactant-associated proteins, and phospholipids that mimics naturally occurring surfactant; palmitic acid, tripalmitin, and colfosceril palmitate are added to standardize solution's composition.
Therapeutic effect: prevents respiratory distress syndrome in premature neonates with specific characteristics.

Indications and dosage

▶ **Prevention and rescue treatment of respiratory distress syndrome (RDS, or hyaline membrane disease), in premature infants weighing 1,250 g (2.75 lb) or less at birth or having symptoms of surfactant deficiency.**
Infants: 4 ml/kg administered by intratracheal instillation through a #5 French end-hole catheter inserted into the neonate's endotracheal tube with the tip of the catheter protruding just beyond the end of the tube above the carina. Length of catheter should be shortened before inserting it through the tube. Drug should not be instilled into a main-stem bronchus. Use the following dosing chart:

BERACTANT DOSING CHART

Weight (g)	Total dose (ml)
600 to 650	2.6
651 to 700	2.8
701 to 750	3
751 to 800	3.2
801 to 850	3.4
851 to 900	3.6
901 to 950	3.8
951 to 1000	4
1001 to 1050	4.2
1051 to 1100	4.4
1101 to 1150	4.6
1151 to 1200	4.8
1201 to 1250	5
1251 to 1300	5.2
1301 to 1350	5.4
1351 to 1400	5.6
1401 to 1450	5.8
1451 to 1500	6
1501 to 1550	6.2
1551 to 1600	6.4
1601 to 1650	6.6
1651 to 1700	6.8
1701 to 1750	7
1751 to 1800	7.2
1801 to 1850	7.4
1851 to 1900	7.6
1901 to 1950	7.8
1951 to 2000	8

Adverse reactions

CV: transient bradycardia, vasoconstriction, hypotension.
Hematologic: decreased oxygen saturation, hypocapnia, hypercapnia.
Respiratory: endotracheal tube reflux or blockage, *apnea*.
Other: pallor.

Interactions

None significant.

Contraindications and precautions

No known contraindications.

NURSING CONSIDERATIONS

Assessment
- Obtain history of neonate's respiratory status before therapy.
- Continuously monitor neonate before, during, and after beractant administration for effectiveness.
- Continuously monitor ECG and transcutaneous oxygen saturation; also, frequently monitor arterial blood pressure and sample arterial blood gas. Transient bradycardia and oxygen desaturation are common after dosing.
- Evaluate parent's understanding of drug therapy.

Nursing diagnoses
- Risk for injury related to potential for RDS
- Knowledge deficit related to drug therapy

Planning and implementation
- Know that beractant should be administered only by personnel experienced in care of clinically unstable premature neonates. Such personnel should have knowledge of neonatal intubation and airway management.
- Be aware that accurate determination of weight is essential to proper measurement of dose.
- Know that endotracheal tube may be suctioned before giving drug; allow neonate to stabilize before proceeding with administration.
- Refrigerate drug at 36° to 46° F (2° to 8° C). Warm before administration by allowing drug to stand at room temperature for at least 20 minutes or by holding in hand for at least 8 minutes. Do not use artificial warming methods. Unopened vials that have been warmed to room temperature may be returned to refrigerator within 8 hours; warm and return drug to refrigerator only once. Vials are for single use only; discard unused drug.
- Know that beractant does not require sonication or reconstitution before use.

---

*Liquid form contains alcohol   **May contain tartrazine   ◆ Canada   ◇ Australia   †OTC

Inspect contents before giving; ensure that color is off-white to light brown and contents are uniform. If settling occurs, swirl vial gently; do not shake. Some foaming is normal.
• Be aware that homogeneous distribution of drug is important. In clinical trials, each dose of drug was given in four quarter-doses, with patient positioned differently after each administration. Each quarter-dose was given over 2 to 3 seconds; catheter was removed and patient ventilated between quarter-doses. With head and body inclined slightly downward, first quarter-dose was given with head turned to right; second quarter-dose, with head turned to left. Then head and body were inclined slightly upward; third quarter-dose was given with head turned to right; fourth quarter-dose, with head turned to left.
• Know that moist breath sounds and crackles can occur immediately after administration. Do not suction neonate for 1 hour unless other signs of airway obstruction are evident.
• Know that audiovisual materials that describe dose and administration procedures are available from manufacturer.
• Know that beractant can rapidly affect oxygenation and lung compliance. Peak ventilator inspiratory pressures may need to be adjusted if chest expansion improves substantially after drug administration. Notify doctor and adjust immediately as directed because lung overdistention and fatal pulmonary air leakage may result.
Patient teaching
• Teach parents about beractant therapy.
• Reassure parents that neonate will be monitored at all times.

☑ **Evaluation**
• Patient does not develop RDS.
• Parents state understanding of drug therapy.

betamethasone
(bay-tuh-METH-uh-sohn)
Betnelan♦, Betnesol♦, Celestone*

betamethasone acetate and betamethasone sodium phosphate
Celestone Chronodose◇, Celestone Soluspan

betamethasone sodium phosphate
Celestone Phosphate, Selestoject

Pharmacologic class: glucocorticoid
Therapeutic class: anti-inflammatory
Pregnancy risk category: NR

How supplied

betamethasone
Tablets: 600 mcg
Tablets (extended-release): 1 mg
Tablets (effervescent): 500 mcg♦
Syrup: 600 mcg/5 ml
betamethasone acetate and betamethasone sodium phosphate
Injection (suspension): betamethasone acetate 3 mg and betamethasone sodium phosphate (equivalent to 3-mg base) per ml
betamethasone sodium phosphate
Tablets (effervescent): 500 mcg♦
Injection: 4 mg (equivalent to 3-mg base)/ml in 5-ml vials

Pharmacokinetics

Absorption: absorbed readily after P.O. administration. Systemic absorption occurs slowly after intra-articular injections.
Distribution: removed rapidly from blood and distributed to muscle, liver, skin, intestines, and kidneys. It is bound weakly to plasma proteins. Only unbound portion is active.
Metabolism: metabolized in liver to inactive glucuronide and sulfate metabolites.

Excretion: inactive metabolites and small amounts of unmetabolized drug are excreted in urine. Insignificant quantities of drug are also excreted in feces. *Half-life:* 36 to 54 hours.

Route	Onset	Peak	Duration
P.O.	Unknown	1-2 hr	3.25 days
I.V., I.M., intra-articular	Rapid	Unknown	7-14 days

Pharmacodynamics

Chemical effect: not completely defined. Decreases inflammation, mainly by stabilizing leukocyte lysosomal membranes; suppresses immune response; stimulates bone marrow; and influences protein, fat, and carbohydrate metabolism.
Therapeutic effect: causes immunosuppression.

Indications and dosage

▶ **Conditions with severe inflammation; conditions requiring immunosuppression.** *Adults:* 0.6 to 7.2 mg P.O. daily; or 0.5 to 9 mg I.V., I.M., or injected into joint or soft tissue daily; or 0.5 to 2 ml of sodium phosphate-acetate suspension injected into joint or soft tissue q 1 to 2 weeks, p.r.n.

Adverse reactions

Most adverse reactions are dose- or duration-dependent.
CNS: *euphoria, insomnia,* psychotic behavior, pseudotumor cerebri, *seizures.*
CV: *heart failure,* hypertension, edema, *thromboembolism.*
EENT: cataracts, glaucoma.
GI: *peptic ulceration,* GI irritation, increased appetite, pancreatitis.
Metabolic: hypokalemia, hyperglycemia, carbohydrate intolerance.
Musculoskeletal: muscle weakness, osteoporosis, growth suppression in children.
Skin: delayed wound healing, acne, various skin eruptions.

Other: hirsutism, susceptibility to infections, *acute adrenal insufficiency after stress (infection, surgery, or trauma) or abrupt withdrawal after long-term therapy.*
After abrupt withdrawal: rebound inflammation, fatigue, weakness, arthralgia, fever, dizziness, lethargy, depression, fainting, orthostatic hypotension, dyspnea, anorexia, hypoglycemia. *After prolonged use, sudden withdrawal may be fatal.*

Interactions

Drug-drug. *Aspirin, indomethacin, other NSAIDs:* increased risk of GI distress and bleeding. Give together cautiously.
Barbiturates, phenytoin, rifampin: decreased corticosteroid effect. Corticosteroid dosage may need to be increased.
Oral anticoagulants: altered dosage requirements. Monitor PT and INR closely.
Potassium-depleting drugs (such as thiazide diuretics): enhanced potassium-wasting effects of betamethasone. Monitor serum potassium levels.
Skin test antigens: decreased response. Defer skin testing until therapy is completed.
Toxoids, vaccines: decreased antibody response and increased risk of neurologic complications. Avoid concomitant use.

Contraindications and precautions

● Contraindicated in patients with viral or bacterial infections (except in life-threatening situations), systemic fungal infections, or hypersensitivity to drug.
● Use with extreme caution, and only in life-threatening situations, in patients with recent MI or peptic ulcer.
● Use cautiously in patients with renal disease, hypertension, osteoporosis, diabetes mellitus, hypothyroidism, cirrhosis, diverticulitis, nonspecific ulcerative colitis, recent intestinal anastomoses, thromboembolic disorders, seizures, myasthenia gravis, heart failure, tuberculosis, ocular herpes simplex, emotional

---

instability, or psychotic tendencies. Because some formulations contain sulfite preservatives, use cautiously in patients sensitive to sulfites. Also use cautiously in pregnant women.

• Breast-feeding should be discontinued if drug is given to breast-feeding women.

• Safety of drug has not been established in children under age 12.

NURSING CONSIDERATIONS

⊠ Assessment

• Obtain history of patient's underlying condition and current health status, including vital signs and weight.

• Be alert for adverse reactions and drug interactions.

• Monitor patient's weight, blood pressure, and blood glucose and serum potassium levels regularly, as ordered.

• Monitor for early signs of adrenal insufficiency or cushingoid symptoms. Adrenal suppression may last up to 1 year after drug is stopped.

• Monitor patient's stress level. Stress (fever, trauma, surgery, or emotional problems) may increase adrenal insufficiency.

• Evaluate patient's and family's understanding of drug therapy.

⊕ Nursing diagnoses

• Altered health maintenance related to underlying condition

• Risk for injury related to drug-induced adverse reactions

• Knowledge deficit related to drug therapy

⊠ Planning and implementation

P.O. use: Give drug with milk or food to reduce GI irritation.

I.V. use: Know that drug is compatible with 0.9% NaCl, D₅W, lactated Ringer's injection, dextrose 5% in lactated Ringer's injection, and dextrose 5% in Ringer's injection.

I.M. use: Give I.M. injection deeply to prevent muscle atrophy. Rotate injection sites.

Intra-articular use: Prepare drug for doctor to administer, as directed.

• Know that drug should not be used for alternate-day therapy.

• Give once-daily dose in the morning for best results and least toxicity.

• Be aware that drug should always be titrated to lowest effective dose.

• Gradually reduce drug dose after long-term therapy, as ordered.

• Expect to increase dose, as ordered, during times of physiologic stress (surgery, trauma, or infection).

• Know that potassium supplements may be necessary for patients receiving long-term therapy.

Patient teaching

• Tell patient not to stop drug abruptly or without doctor's consent.

• Tell patient using effervescent tablets to dissolve them in water immediately before ingestion.

• Teach patient about drug's effects. Warn patient on long-term therapy about cushingoid symptoms; instruct him to report sudden weight gain or swelling to doctor.

• Instruct patient to report symptoms associated with corticosteroid withdrawal, including fatigue, weakness, arthralgia, orthostatic hypotension, and dyspnea.

• Tell patient to contact doctor if symptoms worsen or drug is no longer effective. Also tell him not to increase dose without doctor's consent.

• Advise elderly patient receiving long-term therapy to consider exercise or physical therapy. Tell him to ask his doctor about vitamin D or calcium supplements.

• Advise patient receiving prolonged therapy to have periodic ophthalmic examinations.

• Tell patient to report slow healing.

• Instruct patient to carry medical identification card indicating his need for supplemental glucocorticoids during stress.

Reactions may be *common*, uncommon, *life-threatening*, or COMMON AND LIFE-THREATENING.

☑ **Evaluation**

• Patient's underlying condition is improved.
• Patient does not experience injury as a result of drug-induced adverse reactions.
• Patient and family state understanding of drug therapy.

betaxolol hydrochloride
(beh-TAKS-oh-lol high-droh-KLOR-ighd)
Kerlone

Pharmacologic class: beta blocker
Therapeutic class: antihypertensive
Pregnancy risk category: C

How supplied

Tablets: 10 mg, 20 mg

Pharmacokinetics

Absorption: absorbed completely. Small first-pass effect reduces bioavailability by about 10%.
Distribution: about 50% bound to plasma proteins.
Metabolism: metabolized in liver.
Excretion: excreted primarily in urine (about 80%) as metabolites. *Half-life:* 14 to 22 hours.

Route	Onset	Peak	Duration
P.O.	≤ 3 hr	2-4 hr (anti-hypertensive effects peak in 7-14 days)	24-48 hr

Pharmacodynamics

Chemical effect: unknown.
Therapeutic effect: reduces blood pressure.

Indications and dosage

▶ **Hypertension.** *Adults:* initially, 10 mg P.O. once daily. If necessary, 20 mg P.O. once daily if desired response not achieved in 7 to 14 days.

Adverse reactions

CNS: dizziness, fatigue, headache, lethargy, anxiety.
CV: bradycardia, chest pain, hypotension, worsening of angina, peripheral vascular insufficiency, *heart failure,* edema, syncope, postural hypotension, conduction disturbances.
GI: flatulence, constipation, nausea, diarrhea, vomiting, anorexia, dry mouth.
Respiratory: dyspnea, wheezing, *bronchospasm.*
Skin: rash.

Interactions

Drug-drug. *Calcium channel blockers:* increased risk of hypotension, left ventricular failure, and AV conduction disturbances. Use I.V. calcium channel blockers with caution.
Catecholamine-depleting drugs, reserpine: may have an additive effect. Monitor patient closely.
General anesthetics: increased hypotensive effects. Observe carefully for excessive hypotension, bradycardia, and orthostatic hypotension.
Lidocaine: may increase the effects of lidocaine. Monitor patient closely.

Contraindications and precautions

• Contraindicated in patients with severe bradycardia, greater than first-degree heart block, cardiogenic shock, uncontrolled heart failure, or hypersensitivity to drug.
• Use cautiously in patients with heart failure controlled by cardiac glycosides and diuretics because they may exhibit signs of cardiac decompensation with beta blocker therapy.
• Also use with caution in pregnant or breast-feeding women.
• Safety of drug has not been established in children.

NURSING CONSIDERATIONS

⚕ Assessment
• Obtain history of patient's blood pressure before therapy and reassess regularly thereafter.
• Be alert for adverse reactions and drug interactions.
• Monitor blood glucose levels regularly in diabetic patients. Beta blockade may inhibit glycogenolysis and signs and symptoms of hypoglycemia (such as tachycardia and blood pressure changes).
• Evaluate patient's and family's understanding of drug therapy.

Nursing diagnoses
• Risk for injury related to presence of hypertension
• Decreased cardiac output related to drug-induced adverse CV reactions
• Knowledge deficit related to drug therapy

Planning and implementation
• Never discontinue drug abruptly because angina pectoris may occur in patients with unrecognized coronary artery disease. Obtain guidelines from doctor as to how dose should be tapered before discontinuing drug.
• Advise anesthesiologist when surgical patient is receiving beta blocker so that isoproterenol or dobutamine is made readily available for reversal of drug's cardiac effects.
• Know that beta blockers may mask tachycardia associated with hyperthyroidism. In patients with suspected thyrotoxicosis, withdraw beta blocker gradually, as ordered, to avoid thyroid storm.
Patient teaching
• Explain importance of taking drug as prescribed, even when feeling well. Tell patient not to discontinue drug suddenly but to call doctor if unpleasant adverse reactions occur.
• Teach patient signs of heart failure, including shortness of breath or difficulty breathing, unusually fast heartbeat, cough, or fatigue with exertion, and tell patient to report such signs immediately.

✓ Evaluation
• Patient's blood pressure is within normal limits.
• Patient's cardiac output remains unchanged throughout therapy.
• Patient and family state understanding of drug therapy.

---

bethanechol chloride
(beh-THAN-eh-kol KLOR-ighd)
Duvoid, Urabeth, Urocarb Liquid◇, Urocarb Tablets◇

Pharmacologic class: cholinergic agonist
Therapeutic class: urinary tract stimulant
Pregnancy risk category: C

How supplied
Tablets: 5 mg, 10 mg, 25 mg, 50 mg
Injection: 5 mg/ml

Pharmacokinetics
Absorption: poorly absorbed from GI tract after P.O. administration; unknown after S.C. administration.
Distribution: unknown.
Metabolism: unknown.
Excretion: unknown.

Route	Onset	Peak	Duration
P.O.	30-90 min	About 1 hr	≤ 6 hr
S.C.	5-15 min	5-30 min	About 2 hr

Pharmacodynamics
Chemical effect: directly stimulates cholinergic receptors, mimicking action of acetylcholine.
Therapeutic effect: relieves urine retention.

Indications and dosage
▶ **Acute postoperative and postpartum nonobstructive (functional) urine retention, neurogenic atony of urinary bladder with urine retention.** *Adults:*

Reactions may be *common*, uncommon, *life-threatening*, or COMMON AND LIFE-THREATENING.

10 to 50 mg P.O. b.i.d. to q.i.d; or 2.5 to 5 mg S.C. Never give I.V. or I.M. When used for urine retention, some patients may require 50 to 100 mg P.O. per dose. Use such doses with extreme caution.

Test dose is 2.5 mg S.C. repeated at 15- to 30-minute intervals to total of four doses to determine minimal effective dose; then minimal effective dose used q 6 to 8 hours. All doses must be adjusted individually.

Adverse reactions

CNS: headache, malaise.
CV: bradycardia, hypotension, reflex tachycardia.
EENT: lacrimation, miosis.
GI: *abdominal cramps, diarrhea,* excessive salivation, nausea, vomiting, belching, borborygmus, esophageal spasms.
GU: urinary urgency.
Respiratory: *bronchoconstriction,* increased bronchial secretions.
Skin: flushing, sweating.

Interactions

Drug-drug. *Anticholinergic agents, atropine, procainamide, quinidine:* may reverse cholinergic effects. Observe for lack of drug effect.
Anticholinesterase agents, cholinergic agonists, may cause additive effects or increase toxicity. Avoid concomitant use.
Ganglionic blockers: may cause hypotension. Avoid concomitant use.

Contraindications and precautions

• Contraindicated for I.V. or I.M. use; in patients hypersensitive to drug or its components; in those with hyperthyroidism, peptic ulceration, latent or active bronchial asthma, pronounced bradycardia or hypotension, vasomotor instability, cardiac or coronary artery disease, seizure disorder, Parkinson's disease, spastic GI disturbances, acute inflammatory lesions of GI tract, peritonitis, mechanical obstruction of GI or urinary tract, marked vagotonia, or uncertain strength or integrity of bladder wall and when in-

creased muscle activity of GI or urinary tract is harmful.
• Use cautiously in pregnant women.
• Breast feeding should be discontinued if drug must be administered to breast-feeding women.
• Safety of drug has not been established in children.

NURSING CONSIDERATIONS

Assessment
• Obtain history of patient's bladder condition before therapy and reassess regularly throughout therapy.
• Be alert for adverse reactions and drug interactions.
• Evaluate patient's and family's understanding of drug therapy.

Nursing diagnoses
• Altered urinary elimination related to underlying bladder condition
• Ineffective breathing pattern related to drug-induced bronchoconstriction
• Knowledge deficit related to drug therapy

Planning and implementation
P.O. use: Give drug on empty stomach to prevent nausea and vomiting.
S.C. use: Know that onset of action is more rapid but duration is shorter than with P.O. use. Also know that P.O. and S.C. doses are not interchangeable.
• Never give I.V. or I.M.; could cause circulatory collapse, hypotension, severe abdominal cramping, bloody diarrhea, shock, or cardiac arrest.
• Always have atropine injection readily available, and be prepared to give 0.5 mg S.C. or slow I.V. push, as ordered. Provide respiratory support, as necessary.
Patient teaching
• Advise patient to take P.O. dose on an empty stomach.
• Tell patient to report breathing difficulty immediately.

☑ Evaluation

• Patient is able to void without urine retention.
• Patient's respiratory function remains normal during therapy.
• Patient and family state understanding of drug therapy.

---

bicalutamide
(bigh-kah-LOO-tuh-mighd)
Casodex

Pharmacologic class: nonsteroidal antiandrogen
Therapeutic class: antineoplastic
Pregnancy risk category: X

How supplied

Tablets: 50 mg

Pharmacokinetics

Absorption: well absorbed from GI tract.
Distribution: 96% protein-bound.
Metabolism: undergoes stereo-specific metabolism. The S (inactive) isomer is metabolized primarily by glucuronidation. The R (active) isomer also undergoes glucuronidation but is predominantly oxidized to an inactive metabolite.
Excretion: excreted in urine and feces.

Route	Onset	Peak	Duration
P.O.	Unknown	Unknown	Unknown

Pharmacodynamics

Chemical effect: competitively inhibits action of androgens by binding to cytosol androgen receptors in target tissue.
Therapeutic effect: counteracts the effect of androgen or removes its source.

Indications and dosage

► **Adjunct therapy for treatment of advanced prostate cancer.** *Adults:* 50 mg P.O. once daily in morning or evening.

Adverse reactions

CNS: *asthenia,* headache, dizziness, paresthesia, insomnia.
CV: *hot flashes,* hypertension, chest pain, peripheral edema.
GI: *constipation, nausea, diarrhea,* abdominal pain, flatulence, increased liver enzymes, vomiting, weight loss.
GU: nocturia, hematuria, urinary tract infection, impotence, gynecomastia, urinary incontinence.
Hematologic: hypochromic anemia, iron deficiency anemia.
Musculoskeletal: *back, pelvic,* and bone pain.
Respiratory: dyspnea.
Skin: rash, diaphoresis.
Other: *general pain infection,* flu syndrome, hyperglycemia.

Interactions

Drug-drug. *Coumarin anticoagulants:* displacement of these drugs from protein-binding sites. Monitor PT and INR closely; adjust anticoagulant dosage, as necessary.

Contraindications and precautions

• Contraindicated in patients with hypersensitivity to drug or its components.
• Use cautiously in patients with moderate-to-severe hepatic impairment; drug is extensively metabolized by liver.
• Safety of drug has not been established in children.

NURSING CONSIDERATIONS

☑ Assessment
• Obtain history of patient's neoplastic disease before therapy.
• Regularly monitor serum prostate specific antigen (PSA) levels, as ordered.
• Monitor liver function studies, as ordered.
• Be alert for adverse reactions and drug interactions.
• Evaluate patient's and family's understanding of drug therapy.

Reactions may be *common,* uncommon, *life-threatening*, or COMMON AND LIFE-THREATENING.

✥ Nursing diagnoses
• Altered health maintenance related to neoplastic disease
• Pain related to drug-induced adverse reactions
• Knowledge deficit related to drug therapy

⫸ Planning and implementation
• Be aware that bicalutamide is used with a luteinizing hormone–releasing hormone analogue. Treatment should be started at the same time for both.
• Administer drug at the same time each day.
• Report elevated PSA levels to doctor, who should evaluate patient to determine disease progression.
• Know that bicalutamide should be discontinued if patient develops jaundice or exhibits laboratory evidence of liver injury in absence of liver metastases. Abnormalities are usually reversible by discontinuing drug.
Patient teaching
• Inform patient that drug may be taken without regard to meals.
• Advise patient to take drug at same time each day.
• Tell patient not to interrupt or stop drug without consulting doctor.

▨ Evaluation
• Patient shows positive response to drug.
• Patient states that he is pain free.
• Patient and family state understanding of drug therapy.

biperiden hydrochloride
(bih-PEH-rih-den high-droh-KLOR-ighd)
Akineton

biperiden lactate
Akineton Lactate

Pharmacologic class: anticholinergic
Therapeutic class: antiparkinsonian agent
Pregnancy risk category: C

How supplied
biperiden hydrochloride
Tablets: 2 mg
biperiden lactate
Injection: 5 mg/ml in 1-ml ampules

Pharmacokinetics
Absorption: well absorbed from GI tract.
Distribution: well distributed throughout body.
Metabolism: unknown.
Excretion: excreted in urine as unchanged drug and metabolites.

Route	Onset	Peak	Duration
P.O.	≤ 1 hr	Unknown	6-12 hr
I.V.	≤ 30 min	Unknown	1-8 hr
I.M.	Unknown	Unknown	Unknown

Pharmacodynamics
Chemical effect: blocks central cholinergic receptors, helping to balance cholinergic activity in basal ganglia.
Therapeutic effect: improves voluntary movement.

Indications and dosage
▶ **Drug-induced extrapyramidal disorders.** *Adults:* 2 mg P.O. once daily, b.i.d., or t.i.d., depending on severity. Usual dosage is 2 mg P.O. daily or 2 mg I.V. or I.M. q 30 minutes, not to exceed four doses or 8 mg daily.
▶ **Parkinsonism.** *Adults:* 2 mg P.O. t.i.d. or q.i.d., not to exceed 16 mg/day.

Adverse reactions
Adverse reactions are dose-related and may resemble those of atropine toxicity.
CNS: disorientation, euphoria, restlessness, irritability, incoherence, dizziness, increased tremors.
CV: transient postural hypotension (with parenteral use).
EENT: blurred vision.
GI: dry mouth, *constipation,* nausea, vomiting, epigastric distress.
GU: urinary hesitancy, urine retention.
Skin: rash, urticaria.

Interactions

Drug-drug. *Amantadine, phenothiazines, tricyclic antidepressants:* excessive CNS anticholinergic effects. Avoid concomitant use.
Drug-lifestyle. *Alcohol use:* increased sedative affect. Don't use together.

Contraindications and precautions

• Contraindicated in patients with angle-closure glaucoma, bowel obstruction, megacolon, or hypersensitivity to drug.
• Use cautiously in patients with prostatic hyperplasia, arrhythmias, manifest glaucoma, and seizure disorder.
• Also use cautiously in pregnant or breast-feeding women.
• Safety of drug has not been established in children.

NURSING CONSIDERATIONS

Assessment
• Obtain history of patient's underlying condition.
• Monitor effectiveness by regularly checking body movements for signs of improvement. However, in severe parkinsonism, tremors may increase as spasticity is relieved.
• Be alert for adverse reactions and drug interactions.
• Evaluate patient's and family's understanding of drug therapy.

Nursing diagnoses
• Impaired physical mobility related to underlying parkinsonism or other extrapyramidal disorders
• Risk for injury related to drug-induced adverse CNS reactions
• Knowledge deficit related to drug therapy

Planning and implementation
P.O. use: Give oral doses with or after meals to decrease adverse GI effects.
I.V. use: Administer drug very slowly.
– When giving parenterally, keep patient in supine position. Parenteral administra-

tion may cause transient postural hypotension and coordination disturbances.
I.M. use: Follow normal protocol. No local tissue reactions have been reported with I.M. use.
• Notify doctor if tolerance to drug develops; dose will need to be increased.
• Notify doctor if patient develops serious adverse reactions that may require dose reduction.
Patient teaching
• Warn patient to avoid activities that require alertness until CNS effects of drug are known.
• Tell patient to report urinary hesitancy or urine retention.
• Advise patient to relieve dry mouth with cool drinks, ice chips, sugarless gum, or hard candy.

Evaluation
• Patient exhibits improved mobility with reduction in muscle rigidity and tremors.
• Patient does not experience injury as result of drug-induced adverse CNS reactions.
• Patient and family state understanding of drug therapy.

bisacodyl

(bigh-suh-KOH-dil)
Bisac-Evac†, Bisacolax♦†, Bisalax◇, Bisco-Lax**†, Carter's Little Pills†, Dacodyl†, Deficol†, Dulcolax†, Durolax◇, Fleet Bisacodyl†, Fleet Bisacodyl Prep†, Fleet Laxative†, Laxit♦†, Theralax†

Pharmacologic class: diphenylmethane derivative
Therapeutic class: stimulant laxative
Pregnancy risk category: B

How supplied

Tablets (enteric-coated): 5 mg†
Enema: 0.33 mg/dl†, 10 mg/5 ml (microenema)◇

Powder for rectal solution (bisacodyl tannex): 1.5 mg bisacodyl and 2.5 g tannic acid
Suppositories: 5 mg†, 10 mg◊

Pharmacokinetics

Absorption: minimal.
Distribution: distributed locally.
Metabolism: up to 15% of P.O. dose may enter enterohepatic circulation.
Excretion: excreted primarily in feces; some excreted in urine.

Route	Onset	Peak	Duration
P.O.	6-12 hr	Variable	Variable
P.R.	15-60 min	Variable	Variable

Pharmacodynamics

Chemical effect: increases peristalsis, probably by acting directly on smooth muscle of intestine. Thought to irritate musculature or stimulate colonic intramural plexus. Also promotes fluid accumulation in colon and small intestine.
Therapeutic effect: relieves constipation.

Indications and dosage

▶ **Chronic constipation; preparation for delivery, surgery, or rectal or bowel examination.** *Adults and children age 12 and over:* 10 to 15 mg P.O. in evening or before breakfast. Up to 30 mg P.O., as needed and ordered, or 10 mg P.R. for evacuation before examination or surgery. *Children ages 6 to 12:* 5 mg P.O. or P.R. h.s. or before breakfast.

Adverse reactions

GI: *nausea, vomiting, abdominal cramps,* diarrhea (with high doses), *burning sensation in rectum* (with suppositories), laxative dependence (with long-term or excessive use).
Metabolic: alkalosis, hypokalemia, fluid and electrolyte imbalance.
Other: tetany, protein-losing enteropathy (with excessive use), muscle weakness (with excessive use).

Interactions

Drug-drug. *Antacids:* gastric irritation or dyspepsia from premature dissolution of enteric coating. Avoid concurrent use.
Drug-food. *Milk:* gastric irritation or dyspepsia from premature dissolution of enteric coating. Avoid concurrent use.

Contraindications and precautions

• Contraindicated in patients with rectal bleeding, gastroenteritis, intestinal obstruction, or hypersensitivity to drug and in those with abdominal pain, nausea, vomiting, or other symptoms of appendicitis or acute surgical abdomen.
• Use cautiously in pregnant women.

NURSING CONSIDERATIONS

Assessment
• Obtain history of bowel disorder, GI status, fluid intake, nutritional status, exercise habits, and normal patterns of elimination.
• Monitor effectiveness by checking frequency and characteristics of stools.
• Be alert for adverse reactions and drug interactions.
• Auscultate bowel sounds at least once a shift. Assess for presence of pain and cramping.
• Evaluate patient's and family's understanding of drug therapy.

Nursing diagnoses
• Constipation related to interruption of normal pattern of elimination
• Pain related to drug-induced abdominal cramps
• Knowledge deficit related to drug therapy

Planning and implementation
P.O. use: Do not give tablets within 30 minutes of milk or antacid intake.
P.R. use: Insert suppository as high as possible into rectum and try to position suppository against rectal wall. Avoid embedding within fecal material because this may delay onset of action.

• Time administration of drug so as not to interfere with scheduled activities or sleep. Soft, formed stool usually produced 15 to 60 minutes after P.R. administration.
• Know that tablets and suppositories are used together to clean colon before and after surgery and before barium enema.
• Store tablets and suppositories at temperature below 86° F (30° C).

Patient teaching
• Advise patient to swallow enteric-coated tablet whole to avoid GI irritation. Tell him not to take tablet within 1 hour of milk or antacid intake.
• Advise patient to report adverse effects to doctor.
• Teach patient about dietary sources of bulk, including bran and other cereals, fresh fruit, and vegetables.
• Caution patient against excessive use of drug.

☑ Evaluation
• Patient reports return of normal bowel pattern of elimination.
• Patient is free from abdominal pain and cramping.
• Patient and family state understanding of drug therapy.

bismuth subgallate
(BIS-muth sub-GAL-ayt)
Devrom†

bismuth subsalicylate
Maximum Strength Pepto-Bismol Liquid†, Pepto-Bismol†

Pharmacologic class: adsorbent
Therapeutic class: antidiarrheal
Pregnancy risk category: NR

How supplied
bismuth subgallate
Tablets (chewable): 200 mg†
bismuth subsalicylate
Tablets (chewable): 262.5 mg†

Oral suspension: 262.5 mg/15 ml†, 525 mg/15 ml†

Pharmacokinetics
Absorption: absorbed poorly; significant salicylate absorption may occur after using bismuth subsalicylate.
Distribution: distributed locally in gut.
Metabolism: metabolized minimally.
Excretion: bismuth subsalicylate is excreted in urine.

Route	Onset	Peak	Duration
P.O.	≤ 1 hr	Unknown	Unknown

Pharmacodynamics
Chemical effect: unknown; has mild water-binding capacity. Also may adsorb toxins and provide protective coating for mucosa.
Therapeutic effect: relieves diarrhea.

Indications and dosage
▶ **Mild, nonspecific diarrhea.** *Adults:* 1 to 2 tablets (subgallate) P.O., chewed or swallowed whole t.i.d.; or 30 ml or 2 tablets (subsalicylate) P.O. q 30 to 60 minutes up to maximum of eight doses and for no longer than 2 days. *Children ages 3 to 6:* 5 ml or ⅓ tablet P.O. *Children ages 6 to 9:* 10 ml or ⅔ tablet P.O. *Children ages 9 to 12:* 15 ml or 1 tablet P.O.

Adverse reactions
GI: temporary darkening of tongue and stools.
Other: salicylism (with high doses).

Interactions
Drug-drug. *Aspirin, other salicylates:* risk of salicylate toxicity. Monitor patient closely.
Oral anticoagulants, oral antidiabetic agents: theoretical risk of increased effects of these agents after high doses of bismuth subsalicylate. Monitor patient closely.

Reactions may be *common*, uncommon, *life-threatening*, or COMMON AND LIFE-THREATENING.

Probenecid: theoretical risk of decreased uricosuric effects after high doses of bismuth subsalicylate. Monitor patient closely.
Tetracycline: decreased tetracycline absorption. Separate administration times by at least 2 hours.

Contraindications and precautions

• Contraindicated in patients hypersensitive to salicylates.
• Use cautiously in patients already taking aspirin and in pregnant or breast-feeding women.

NURSING CONSIDERATIONS

⚖ Assessment
• Obtain history of patient's bowel disorder, GI status, and frequency of loose stools before therapy.
• Monitor effectiveness by checking frequency and characteristics of stools.
• Be alert for adverse reactions and drug interactions.
• Check hearing if patient is taking drug in large doses.
• Evaluate patient's and family's understanding of drug therapy.

⊞ Nursing diagnoses
• Diarrhea related to underlying GI condition
• Sensory or perceptual alteration (auditory) related to drug-induced salicylism
• Knowledge deficit related to drug therapy

❯ Planning and implementation
• Avoid use before GI radiologic procedures because bismuth is radiopaque and may interfere with X-rays.
• Read label carefully because dosage varies with form of drug.
• Discontinue therapy and notify doctor if tinnitus occurs.
Patient teaching
• Advise patient that drug contains large amount of salicylate. (Each tablet pro-

vides 102 mg salicylate; regular-strength liquid provides 130 mg/15 ml, and extra-strength liquid provides 230 mg/15 ml.)
• Instruct patient to chew tablets well or to shake liquid before measuring dose.
• Tell patient to report diarrhea that persists for more than 2 days or is accompanied by high fever.
• Tell patient to consult with doctor before giving bismuth subsalicylate to children or teenagers during or after recovery from flu or chickenpox.
• Inform patient that both liquid and tablet forms of Pepto-Bismol are effective against traveler's diarrhea. Tablets may be more convenient to carry.

☑ Evaluation
• Patient reports decrease or absence of loose stools.
• Patient remains free from signs and symptoms of salicylism.
• Patient and family state understanding of drug therapy.

bisoprolol fumarate
(bis-OP-roh-lol FYOO-muh-ayt)
Zebeta

Pharmacologic class: beta blocker
Therapeutic class: antihypertensive
Pregnancy risk category: C

How supplied

Tablets: 5 mg, 10 mg

Pharmacokinetics

Absorption: bioavailability after 10-mg dose is about 80%.
Distribution: about 30% of drug binds to serum proteins.
Metabolism: first-pass metabolism of drug is about 20%.
Excretion: excreted equally by renal and nonrenal pathways, with about 50% of dose appearing unchanged in urine and

remainder appearing as inactive metabolites. Less than 2% of dose is excreted in feces. *Half-life:* 9 to 12 hours.

Route	Onset	Peak	Duration
P.O.	Unknown	2-4 hr	About 24 hr

Pharmacodynamics

Chemical effect: not completely defined. Bisoprolol is a beta$_1$-selective blocker that decreases myocardial contractility, heart rate, and cardiac output; lowers blood pressure; and reduces myocardial oxygen consumption.
Therapeutic effect: decreases blood pressure.

Indications and dosage

▶ **Hypertension.** *Adults:* initially, 5 mg P.O. once daily. If response is inadequate, increased to 10 mg once daily or to 20 mg P.O. daily, if needed. Maximum recommended dosage is 20 mg daily. For patients with renal or hepatic impairment, 2.5 mg P.O. daily initially. Subsequent dosage titration is done cautiously.

Adverse reactions

CNS: asthenia, fatigue, dizziness, headache, hypoesthesia, vivid dreams, depression, insomnia.
CV: bradycardia, peripheral edema, chest pain, *heart failure*.
EENT: pharyngitis, rhinitis, sinusitis.
GI: nausea, vomiting, diarrhea, dry mouth.
Respiratory: cough, dyspnea.
Other: sweating, arthralgia.

Interactions

Drug-drug. *Beta blockers:* can cause extreme hypotension. Don't use together. *Calcium channel blockers:* can cause myocardial depression and AV conductive inhibition. Monitor closely. *Guanethidine, reserpine:* can cause hypotension. Monitor closely. *NSAIDs:* decreased antihypertensive effect. Monitor blood pressure and adjust dosage.

Rifampin: increased metabolic clearance of bisoprolol. Monitor patient.

Contraindications and precautions

• Contraindicated in patients with cardiogenic shock, overt cardiac failure, marked sinus bradycardia, second- or third-degree AV block, or hypersensitivity to drug.
• Use cautiously in patients with bronchospastic disease. In general, these patients should avoid beta blockers because blockade of beta$_1$ receptors is not absolute and blockage of pulmonary beta$_2$ receptors may result in worsening of symptoms. A bronchodilator should be made available.
• Also use cautiously in patients with diabetes, peripheral vascular disease, or thyroid disease; in those with history of heart failure; and in pregnant and breast-feeding women.
• Safety of drug has not been established in children.

NURSING CONSIDERATIONS

⚛ Assessment
• Obtain history of patient's hypertensive status before therapy, and check blood pressure regularly throughout therapy.
• Be alert for adverse reactions and drug interactions.
• Monitor patient's hydration status if adverse GI reactions occur.
• Closely monitor blood glucose levels in diabetic patients. Beta blockers may mask some manifestations of hypoglycemia, such as tachycardia.
• Evaluate patient's and family's understanding of drug therapy.

⚛ Nursing diagnoses
• Risk for injury related to presence of hypertension
• Risk for fluid volume deficit related to drug-induced adverse GI reactions
• Knowledge deficit related to drug therapy

Reactions may be *common*, uncommon, *life-threatening*, or COMMON AND LIFE-THREATENING.

⟩ Planning and implementation

• Be sure that a beta$_2$ agonist (bronchodilator) is available for patients with bronchospastic disease.
• Do not discontinue drug abruptly because angina may occur in patients with unrecognized coronary artery disease.
Patient teaching
• Tell patient to take drug as prescribed, even when he's feeling well. Warn him that abruptly discontinuing drug can exacerbate angina and precipitate MI and that drug must be withdrawn gradually over 1 to 2 weeks.
• Instruct patient to call doctor if unpleasant adverse reactions occur.
• Tell diabetic patient to closely monitor blood glucose levels.
• Tell patient to check with doctor or pharmacist before taking OTC medications.

☑ Evaluation

• Patient's blood pressure is normal.
• Patient maintains adequate fluid balance throughout therapy.
• Patient and family state understanding of drug therapy.

bitolterol mesylate
(bigh-TOL-ter-ol MES-i-layt)
Tornalate

Pharmacologic class: adrenergic, beta$_2$ agonist
Therapeutic class: bronchodilator
Pregnancy risk category: C

How supplied

Aerosol inhaler: 370 mcg/metered spray
Solution for inhalation (0.2%): 10 ml, 30 ml, 60 ml

Pharmacokinetics

Absorption: after oral inhalation, bronchodilation results from local action on bronchial tree, with most of inhaled dose being swallowed.

Distribution: widely distributed throughout body.
Metabolism: hydrolyzed by esterases to active metabolites.
Excretion: bitolterol and its metabolites excreted primarily in urine.

Route	Onset	Peak	Duration
Inhalation	3-4 min	0.5-1 hr	5-8 hr

Pharmacodynamics

Chemical effect: relaxes bronchial smooth muscle by acting on beta$_2$-adrenergic receptors.
Therapeutic effect: relieves bronchospasm.

Indications and dosage

▶ **To prevent or treat bronchial asthma and bronchospasm.** *Adults and children over age 12:* **Inhaler:** to treat bronchospasm, two inhalations with an interval of at least 1 minute, followed by a third inhalation, if needed. To prevent bronchospasm, usual dosage is two inhalations q 8 hours. In either case, dosage should never exceed three inhalations q 6 hours or two inhalations q 4 hours.
Nebulizer: dosage varies based on patient's requirements. Usual frequency of treatments is t.i.d. May be increased up to q.i.d.; however, interval between treatments should not be less than 4 hours. Maximum daily dose should not exceed 8 mg with intermittent flow nebulization system or 14 mg with continuous flow nebulization system.

Adverse reactions

CNS: *tremors,* nervousness, headache, dizziness, light-headedness.
CV: palpitations, chest discomfort, tachycardia.
EENT: throat irritation.
GI: nausea.
Respiratory: cough, dyspnea.
Other: *hypersensitivity.*

Interactions

None significant.

Contraindications and precautions

• Contraindicated in patients with hypersensitivity to drug.

• Use cautiously in patients with ischemic heart disease, hypertension, hyperthyroidism, diabetes mellitus, arrhythmias, seizure disorders, or history of unusual responsiveness to beta-adrenergic agonists.

• Also use cautiously in pregnant and breast-feeding women.

• Safety of drug has not been established in children age 12 and younger.

NURSING CONSIDERATIONS

Assessment

• Obtain history of patient's respiratory status and underlying condition.

• Monitor effectiveness by regularly auscultating lungs, taking respiratory rate, and noting results of laboratory studies, such as arterial blood gases.

• Be alert for adverse reactions.

• Evaluate patient's and family's understanding of drug therapy.

Nursing diagnoses

• Impaired gas exchange related to presence of bronchospasm

• Risk of injury related to drug-induced adverse reactions

• Knowledge deficit related to drug therapy

Planning and implementation

• If more than one inhalation is ordered, have patient wait at least 1 minute before repeating procedure for second dose. If patient is also to use steroid inhaler, be sure he uses bronchodilator first and then waits about 5 minutes before using steroid inhaler to allow bronchodilator to open air passages for maximum effectiveness.

• Know that solution for inhalation should be added to nebulizer just prior to use and not left in nebulizer.

• Do not mix other drugs in nebulizer, such as cromolyn sodium or acetylcys-teine, due to chemical or physical incompatibilities.

Patient teaching

• Advise patient not to exceed recommended dosages. Too frequent use may cause tachycardia.

• Remind patient that beneficial effects last for up to 8 hours, longer than most other, similar bronchodilators.

• Teach patient to perform oral inhalation correctly. Give following instructions for using metered-dose inhaler: Clear nasal passages and throat. Breathe out, expelling as much air from lungs as possible. Place mouthpiece well into mouth as dose from inhaler is released, and inhale deeply and slowly for about 10 seconds. Hold breath for several seconds, remove mouthpiece, and exhale slowly.

• If more than one inhalation is ordered, tell patient to wait at least 1 minute before repeating procedure for second inhalation.

• Tell patient who also is using steroid inhaler to use bronchodilator first, then wait about 5 minutes before using steroid to allow bronchodilator to open air passages for maximum effectiveness.

• Inform patient that manufacturer recommends rinsing plastic mouthpiece daily with warm tap water, then drying it, to ensure proper delivery of drug.

• Instruct patient to report an unusual smell or taste associated with use of inhalation solution.

Evaluation

• Patient exhibits adequate gas exchange.

• Patient does not experience injury related to drug-induced adverse reactions.

• Patient and family state understanding of drug therapy.

Reactions may be *common*, uncommon, *life-threatening*, or COMMON AND LIFE-THREATENING.

bleomycin sulfate
(blee-oh-MIGH-sin SUL-fayt)
Blenoxane

Pharmacologic class: antibiotic, antineoplastic (cell cycle–phase specific, G2 and M phase)
Therapeutic class: antineoplastic
Pregnancy risk category: NR

How supplied

Injection: 15- and 30-unit vials (1 unit = 1 mg)

Pharmacokinetics

Absorption: I.M. administration results in lower serum levels than those that occur after equivalent I.V. doses.
Distribution: distributes widely into total body water, mainly in skin, lungs, kidneys, peritoneum, and lymphatic tissue.
Metabolism: metabolic fate of drug is undetermined; however, extensive tissue inactivation occurs in liver and kidneys and much less in skin and lungs.
Excretion: drug and its metabolites excreted primarily in urine. *Half-life:* 2 hours.

Route	Onset	Peak	Duration
I.V., I.M., S.C.	Unknown	Unknown	Unknown

Pharmacodynamics

Chemical effect: unknown; thought to inhibit DNA synthesis and cause scission of single- and double-stranded DNA.
Therapeutic effect: kills selected types of cancer cells.

Indications and dosage

Indications and dosage may vary. Check treatment protocol with doctor.
▶ **Hodgkin's lymphoma, squamous cell carcinoma, non-Hodgkin's lymphoma, testicular cancer.** *Adults:* 10 to 20 units/ m² (0.25 to 0.5 units/kg) I.V., I.M., or S.C. once or twice weekly. After 50% response in patients with Hodgkin's dis-

ease, maintenance dosage is 1 unit I.V. or I.M. daily or 5 units I.V. or I.M. weekly.

Adverse reactions

CNS: hyperesthesia of scalp and fingers, headache.
GI: *stomatitis, prolonged anorexia, nausea, vomiting,* diarrhea.
Hematologic: leukocytosis.
Respiratory: PNEUMONITIS, *pulmonary fibrosis, pulmonary adverse reactions (fine crackles, dyspnea), nonproductive cough.*
Skin: *erythema, vesiculation, hardening and discoloration of palmar and plantar skin;* desquamation of hands, feet, and pressure areas; *hyperpigmentation; acne.*
Other: *reversible alopecia,* swelling of interphalangeal joints, hypersensitivity reaction *(fever up to 106° F [41.1° C] with chills up to 5 hours after injection; anaphylaxis),* fever.

Interactions

Drug-drug. *Cardiac glycosides:* decreased serum digoxin levels. Monitor patient closely.
Phenytoin: decreased serum phenytoin levels. Monitor patient closely.

Contraindications and precautions

• Contraindicated in patients with hypersensitivity to drug.
• Use cautiously in patients with renal or pulmonary impairment.
• Safety of drug has not been established in pregnant or breast-feeding women or in children.

NURSING CONSIDERATIONS

✎ Assessment
• Obtain history of patient's overall physical status, especially respiratory status, CBC, and pulmonary and renal function tests, before therapy and reassess regularly thereafter.
• Be alert for adverse reactions and drug interactions.

• Be aware that adverse pulmonary reactions are common in patients over age 70. Fatal pulmonary fibrosis occurs in 1% of patients, especially when cumulative dose exceeds 400 units.
• Monitor for bleomycin-induced fever, which is common and usually occurs within 3 to 6 hours after administering drug.
• Watch for hypersensitivity reactions, which may be delayed for several hours, especially in patients with lymphoma.
• Evaluate patient's and family's understanding of drug therapy.

⊕ Nursing diagnoses
• Risk for injury related to underlying neoplastic condition
• Impaired gas exchange related to drug-induced adverse pulmonary reactions
• Knowledge deficit related to drug therapy

▶ Planning and implementation
• Follow institutional policy for administration of drug to reduce risks. Preparation and administration of parenteral form of this drug are associated with carcinogenic, mutagenic, and teratogenic risks for personnel.
I.V. use: Reconstitute drug with 5 ml or more of D_5W or 0.9% NaCl injection. For I.V. infusion, dilute with 50 to 100 ml of D_5W or 0.9% NaCl injection. Bleomycin may adsorb to plastic I.V. bags. For prolonged stability, use glass containers.
I.M. use: Dilute drug in 1 to 5 ml of sterile water for injection, bacteriostatic water for injection, 0.9% NaCl injection, or D_5W.
S.C. use: Follow manufacturer's guidelines for administering bleomycin S.C.
• Refrigerate unopened vials containing dry powder.
• Know that refrigerated, reconstituted solution is stable for 4 weeks; at room temperature, it is stable for 2 weeks.

• Know that drug should be stopped if pulmonary function test shows a marked decline.
• To prevent linear streaking from drug concentrating in keratin of squamous epithelium, don't use adhesive dressings on skin.
• In patients prone to post-treatment fever, give acetaminophen, as ordered, before treatment and for 24 hours after treatment.
• If ordered after treatment, give supplemental oxygen at an FIO_2 no higher than 25% to avoid potential lung damage.
Patient teaching
• Explain risks associated with drug therapy, especially potential for serious pulmonary reactions in high-risk patients.
• Explain necessity for monitoring and type of monitoring to be done.
• Tell patient that alopecia may occur, but that it is usually reversible.

☑ Evaluation
• Patient exhibits positive response to therapy with follow-up diagnostic test results.
• Patient's gas exchange remains normal throughout therapy.
• Patient and family state understanding of drug therapy.

bretylium tosylate
(breh-TIL-ee-um TOH-si-layt)
Bretylate♦ ◊, Bretylol

Pharmacologic class: adrenergic blocker
Therapeutic class: ventricular antiarrhythmic
Pregnancy risk category: C

How supplied
Injection: 50 mg/ml

Pharmacokinetics
Absorption: not applicable with I.V. administration.

Reactions may be *common,* uncommon, *life-threatening,* or COMMON AND LIFE-THREATENING.

Distribution: distributed widely throughout body. Only about 1% to 10% is plasma protein–bound.
Metabolism: no metabolites have been identified.
Excretion: excreted in urine. *Half-life:* 5 to 10 hours (longer in patients with renal impairment).

Route	Onset	Peak	Duration
I.V.	3 min-2 hr	6-9 hr	6-24 hr

Pharmacodynamics
Chemical effect: unknown; considered a class III antiarrhythmic that initially exerts transient adrenergic stimulation through release of norepinephrine. Subsequent depletion of norepinephrine causes adrenergic blocking actions to predominate, prolonging repolarization and increasing duration of action potential and effective refractory period.
Therapeutic effect: abolishes ventricular arrhythmias.

Indications and dosage
▶ **Ventricular fibrillation or hemodynamically unstable ventricular tachycardia unresponsive to other antiarrhythmics.** *Adults:* 5 mg/kg by I.V. push over 1 minute. If necessary, dose increased to 10 mg/kg and repeated q 15 to 30 minutes until 35 to 40 mg/kg have been given. For continuous suppression, diluted solution administered at 1 to 2 mg/minute continuously, or 5 to 10 mg/kg diluted and given over more than 8 minutes q 6 hours.

Adverse reactions
CNS: *vertigo, dizziness, light-headedness, syncope* (usually secondary to hypotension).
CV: SEVERE HYPOTENSION (especially orthostatic), bradycardia, anginal pain, *transient arrhythmias,* transient hypertension.
GI: severe nausea, vomiting (with rapid infusion).

Other: muscle atrophy, tissue necrosis (with repeated injections).

Interactions
Drug-drug. *Antihypertensives:* may potentiate hypotension. Monitor blood pressure.
Other antiarrhythmics: additive or antagonistic antiarrhythmic effects. Monitor for additive toxicity.
Sympathomimetics: bretylium may potentiate effects of drugs given to correct hypotension. Monitor blood pressure.

Contraindications and precautions
• Contraindicated in patients taking a cardiac glycoside unless arrhythmia is life-threatening, not caused by digitalis, and unresponsive to other antiarrhythmics.
• Use with extreme caution in patients with fixed cardiac output (aortic stenosis and pulmonary hypertension). Drug may cause severe and sudden drop in blood pressure.
• Use with caution in pregnant or breast-feeding women.
• Safety of drug has not been established in children.

NURSING CONSIDERATIONS
Assessment
• Obtain history of patient's heart rate and rhythm before therapy.
• Monitor effectiveness by evaluating continuous ECG recordings, blood pressure, and heart rate. Initial release of norepinephrine caused by drug may induce transient hypertension and arrhythmias.
• Be alert for adverse reactions and drug interactions.
• Evaluate patient's and family's understanding of drug therapy.

Nursing diagnoses
• Decreased cardiac output related to presence of ventricular arrhythmia
• Altered cerebral tissue perfusion related to drug-induced severe hypotension

• Knowledge deficit related to drug therapy

> **Planning and implementation**
• When used in maintenance therapy, dilute using dextrose or NaCl injection before administering. Follow manufacturer's guidelines for specific dilution (varies according to dosage). When administering as direct I.V. injection, use 20G to 22G needle and inject over 1 minute into vein or I.V. line containing free-flowing compatible solution.
• Know that drug is used with other cardiac life-support measures, such as cardiopulmonary resuscitation, countershock, epinephrine, sodium bicarbonate, and lidocaine.
• To prevent nausea and vomiting, follow dosage directions carefully.
• Keep patient in supine position until tolerance to hypotension develops. Have patient avoid sudden position changes.
• If supine systolic blood pressure falls below 75 mm Hg, expect that doctor may order norepinephrine, dopamine, or volume expanders to raise blood pressure.
Patient teaching
• Tell patient to report chest pain or dyspnea immediately.
• Tell patient to avoid sudden position changes.

☑ **Evaluation**
• Patient's ECG reveals that arrhythmia has been corrected.
• Patient's blood pressure remains normal throughout therapy.
• Patient and family state understanding of drug therapy.

bromocriptine mesylate
(broh-moh-KRIP-teen MES-ih-layt)
Parlodel

Pharmacologic class: dopamine receptor agonist

Therapeutic class: semisynthetic ergot alkaloid, dopaminergic agonist, antiparkinsonian agent, inhibitor of prolactin and growth hormone release
Pregnancy risk category: NR

How supplied
Tablets: 2.5 mg
Capsules: 5 mg

Pharmacokinetics
Absorption: 28% absorbed.
Distribution: 90% to 96% bound to serum albumin.
Metabolism: first-pass metabolism occurs with more than 90% of absorbed dose. Drug is metabolized completely in liver.
Excretion: major route of excretion is through bile. Only 2.5% to 5.5% of dose excreted in urine. *Half-life:* 15 hours.

Route	Onset	Peak	Duration
P.O.	0.5-2 hr	1-3 hr	12-24 hr

Pharmacodynamics
Chemical effect: inhibits secretion of prolactin and acts as dopamine-receptor agonist by activating postsynaptic dopamine receptors.
Therapeutic effect: reverses amenorrhea and galactorrhea associated with hyperprolactinemia, increases female fertility, improves voluntary movement, and inhibits prolactin and growth hormone release.

Indications and dosage
▶ **Amenorrhea and galactorrhea associated with hyperprolactinemia; female infertility or hypogonadism.**
Adults: 1.25 to 2.5 mg P.O. daily. Increased by 2.5 mg daily at 3- to 7-day intervals until desired effect is achieved. Maintenance dosage is usually 5 to 7.5 mg/day, but may be 2.5 to 15 mg/day.
▶ **Parkinson's disease.** *Adults:* 1.25 to 2.5 mg P.O. b.i.d. with meals. Dosage increased q 14 to 28 days, up to 100 mg daily, as needed.

▶ **Acromegaly.** *Adults:* 1.25 to 2.5 mg P.O. with h.s. snack for 3 days. An additional 1.25 to 2.5 mg may be added q 3 to 7 days until patient receives therapeutic benefit. Maximum dosage is 100 mg/day.

Adverse reactions

CNS: confusion, hallucinations, uncontrolled body movements, *dizziness, headache,* fatigue, mania, delusions, nervousness, insomnia, depression, *seizures.*
CV: *hypotension,* orthostatic hypotension, hypertension, *CVA,* syncope, *acute MI.*
EENT: nasal congestion, tinnitus, blurred vision.
GI: *nausea,* vomiting, *abdominal cramps,* constipation, diarrhea.
GU: urine retention, urinary frequency.
Skin: coolness and pallor of fingers and toes.

Interactions

Drug-drug. *Antihypertensives:* increased hypotensive effects. Adjust dosage of antihypertensive, as necessary.
Ergot alkaloids, estrogens, oral contraceptives, progestins: interfere with effects of bromocriptine. Don't use concomitantly.
Erythromycin: increased serum bromocriptine levels. Adjust bromocriptine dosage, as necessary.
Haloperidol, loxapine, methyldopa, metoclopramide, MAO inhibitors, phenothiazines, reserpine: interferes with effects of bromocriptine. Increase bromocriptine dosage, as necessary.
Levodopa: additive effects. Adjusted levodopa dosage, as necessary.
Drug-lifestyle. *Alcohol use:* disulfiram-like reaction. Don't use together.

Contraindications and precautions

• Contraindicated in patients with uncontrolled hypertension, toxemia of pregnancy, or hypersensitivity to ergot derivatives.
• Use cautiously in patients with impaired renal or hepatic function or history of MI with residual arrhythmias.

• Because drug inhibits lactation, it should not be used in women who intend to breast-feed.
• Safety of drug has not been established in children under age 15.

NURSING CONSIDERATIONS

☑ **Assessment**
• Obtain history of patient's underlying condition before therapy and reassess regularly thereafter.
• Perform baseline and periodic evaluations of cardiac, hepatic, renal, and hematopoietic function during prolonged therapy.
• Be alert for adverse reactions and drug interactions. Incidence of adverse reactions is high (about 68%), particularly at beginning of therapy; most are mild to moderate, with nausea being most common. Adverse reactions are more frequent when drug is used for Parkinson's disease.
• Evaluate patient's and family's understanding of drug therapy.

🔲 **Nursing diagnoses**
• Altered health maintenance related to underlying condition
• Risk for injury related to drug-induced adverse CNS or CV reactions
• Knowledge deficit related to drug therapy

▶ **Planning and implementation**
• Be aware that patients with impaired renal function may require dosage adjustments.
• Give drug with meals.
• Gradually titrate doses to effective levels, as ordered, to minimize adverse reactions.
• Know that, for Parkinson's disease, bromocriptine usually is given in addition to either levodopa or carbidopa-levodopa.
Patient teaching
• Advise patient to use contraceptive methods other than oral contraceptives or subdermal implants during treatment.

• Advise patient to avoid dizziness and fainting by rising slowly to an upright position and avoiding sudden position changes.

• Advise patient that resumption of menses and suppression of galactorrhea may take 6 weeks or longer.

• Warn patient to avoid hazardous activities that require alertness until CNS and CV effects of drug are known.

• Tell patient to take drug with meals to minimize GI distress.

☑ **Evaluation**

• Patient exhibits improvement in underlying condition.

• Patient does not experience injury as a result of drug-induced adverse reactions.

• Patient and family state understanding of drug therapy.

---

brompheniramine maleate
(brom-fen-IR-ah-meen MAL-ee-ayt)
Bromphen*†, Codimal-A, Cophene-B, Dehist, Diamine T.D., Dimetane*†, Dimetane Extentabs†, Histaject, Nasahist B, ND-Stat, Oraminic II, Veltane

Pharmacologic class: alkylamine antihistamine
Therapeutic class: antihistamine (H₁-receptor antagonist)
Pregnancy risk category: C

How supplied

Tablets: 4 mg†
Tablets (extended-release): 8 mg†, 12 mg†
Elixir: 2 mg/5 ml*†
Injection: 10 mg/ml

Pharmacokinetics

Absorption: absorbed readily from GI tract; unknown for parenteral administration.
Distribution: distributed widely throughout body.
Metabolism: about 90% to 95% metabolized by liver.

Excretion: drug and its metabolites excreted primarily in urine; small amount excreted in feces. *Half-life:* 12 to 34½ hours.

Route	Onset	Peak	Duration
P.O.	15-60 min	2-5 hr	4-8 hr (longer for extended-release)
I.V., I.M., S.C.	15-60 min	2-5 hr	4-8 hr

Pharmacodynamics

Chemical effect: competes with histamine for H₁-receptor sites on effector cells. Prevents but does not reverse histamine-mediated responses.
Therapeutic effect: relieves allergy symptoms.

Indications and dosage

▶ **Rhinitis, allergy symptoms.** *Adults:* 4 to 8 mg P.O. t.i.d. or q.i.d.; or 8 to 12 mg extended-release P.O. b.i.d. or t.i.d.; or 5 to 20 mg q 6 to 12 hours I.V., I.M., or S.C. Maximum dosage is 40 mg daily. *Children age 6 and over:* 2 to 4 mg P.O. t.i.d. or q.i.d.; or 8 to 12 mg extended-release P.O. q 12 hours; or 0.5 mg/kg I.V., I.M., or S.C. daily in divided doses t.i.d. or q.i.d. *Children under age 6:* 0.5 mg/kg P.O., I.V., I.M., or S.C. daily in divided doses t.i.d. or q.i.d. *Note:* Children under age 12 should use only as directed by doctor.

Adverse reactions

CNS: dizziness, tremors, irritability, insomnia, *drowsiness, stimulation* (especially in elderly patients).
CV: hypotension, palpitations.
GI: anorexia, nausea, vomiting, *dry mouth and throat.*
GU: urine retention.
Hematologic: *thrombocytopenia, agranulocytosis.*
Skin: urticaria, rash.
Other: local stinging, diaphoresis, syncope (after parenteral administration).

Reactions may be *common,* uncommon, *life-threatening*, or COMMON AND LIFE-THREATENING.

Interactions
Drug-drug. *CNS depressants:* increased sedation. Use together cautiously.
MAO inhibitors: increased anticholinergic effects. Don't use together.

Contraindications and precautions
• Contraindicated in patients with acute asthmatic attacks, severe hypertension, coronary artery disease, angle-closure glaucoma, urine retention, peptic ulcer, or hypersensitivity to drug's ingredients; in breast-feeding women; and within 14 days of MAO inhibitor therapy.
• Use cautiously during pregnancy, in elderly patients, and in those with increased intraocular pressure, diabetes, ischemic heart disease, hyperthyroidism, hypertension, bronchial asthma, or prostatic hyperplasia.
• Drug is not recommended for use in neonates; children, especially those under age 6, may experience paradoxical hyperexcitability. Timed-release tablets are not recommended for children age 11 and under.

NURSING CONSIDERATIONS

Assessment
• Assess patient's allergy symptoms before therapy and regularly thereafter.
• Be alert for adverse reactions and drug interactions.
• Monitor CBC during long-term therapy, as ordered; observe for signs of blood dyscrasias.
• Monitor patient's hydration status if adverse GI reactions occur.
• Evaluate patient's and family's understanding of drug therapy.

Nursing diagnoses
• Altered health maintenance related to allergy symptoms
• Risk for fluid volume deficit related to drug-induced adverse GI reactions
• Knowledge deficit related to drug therapy

Planning and implementation
P.O. use: Give drug with food or milk to reduce GI distress.
I.V. use: Injectable form containing 10 mg/ml can be given diluted or undiluted very slowly I.V. Do not give 100 mg/ml injection I.V.
I.M. and S.C. use: Follow normal protocol.
• Alert doctor if patient appears to be developing tolerance for drug. A different antihistamine may need to be substituted.
Patient teaching
• Instruct patient to reduce GI distress by taking drug with food or milk.
• Warn patient to avoid alcohol and activities that require alertness until drug's CNS effects are known.
• Tell patient that coffee or tea may reduce drug-induced drowsiness; although drug causes less drowsiness than some other antihistamines.
• Tell patient to relieve dry mouth with ice chips, sugarless gum, or sour hard candy.
• Instruct patient to notify doctor if tolerance develops because different antihistamine may need to be ordered.
• Instruct patient to stop drug 4 days before skin tests to preserve accuracy of tests.

Evaluation
• Patient's allergy symptoms are relieved.
• Patient maintains adequate hydration throughout therapy.
• Patient and family state understanding of drug therapy.

buclizine hydrochloride
(BYOO-kli-zeen high-droh-KLOR-ighd)
Bucladin-S Softabs**

Pharmacologic class: piperazine derivative antihistamine
Therapeutic class: antiemetic, antivertigo
Pregnancy risk category: NR

How supplied
Tablets (chewable): 50 mg

Pharmacokinetics

Route	Onset	Peak	Duration
P.O.	Unknown	Unknown	4-6 hr

Pharmacodynamics
Chemical effect: may affect neural pathways originating in labyrinth to inhibit nausea and vomiting, but exact mechanism of action is unknown.
Therapeutic effect: prevents motion sickness and vertigo.

Indications and dosage
▶ **Prevention of motion sickness.** *Adults:* 50 mg P.O. at least 30 minutes before beginning travel. If needed, repeat after 4 to 6 hours.
▶ **Vertigo.** *Adults:* 50 mg P.O. once to three times daily. Maintenance dosage is 50 mg b.i.d.

Adverse reactions
CNS: *drowsiness,* headache, dizziness, jitters.
EENT: blurred vision.
GI: dry mouth.
GU: urine retention.

Interactions
Drug-drug. *CNS depressants:* additive CNS depression. Avoid concomitant use.
Drug-lifestyle. *Alcohol use:* additive CNS depression. Don't use together.

Contraindications and precautions
• Contraindicated in patients hypersensitive to drug. Drug contains tartrazine, which may precipitate allergic reactions in certain people, including those allergic to aspirin. Also contraindicated in pregnant or breast-feeding women.
• Safety of drug has not been established in children.

NURSING CONSIDERATIONS

☑ **Assessment**
• Obtain history of patient's underlying condition.
• Monitor effectiveness by observing patient for nausea and vomiting or determining if vertigo is still present.
• Be alert for adverse reactions and drug interactions.
• Evaluate patient's and family's understanding of drug therapy.

⊞ **Nursing diagnoses**
• Risk for fluid volume deficit related to motion sickness–induced nausea and vomiting
• Sensory or perceptual alteration (visual) related to drug-induced blurred vision
• Knowledge deficit related to drug therapy

▷ **Planning and implementation**
• Know that tablets may be placed in mouth and allowed to dissolve without water or may be chewed or swallowed whole.
Patient teaching
• Instruct patient to place tablets in mouth and allow them to dissolve without water or to chew them or swallow them whole.
• Tell patient to take drug at least 30 minutes before beginning travel.
• Advise patient to refrain from driving or performing other activities that require alertness until CNS effects of drug are known.

☑ **Evaluation**
• Patient demonstrates no sign of fluid volume deficit.
• Patient states that vision is normal.
• Patient and family state understanding of drug therapy.

Reactions may be *common,* uncommon, *life-threatening,* or COMMON AND LIFE-THREATENING.

budesonide
(byoo-DES-oh-nighd)
Rhinocort◊

Pharmacologic class: nonhalozenated glucocorticoid
Therapeutic class: anti-inflammatory
Pregnancy risk category: C

How supplied
Nasal spray: 32 mcg/metered spray (7-g canister)

Pharmacokinetics
Absorption: amount of intranasal dose that reaches systemic circulation is generally low (approximately 20%).
Distribution: 88% protein-bound in plasma.
Metabolism: rapidly and extensively metabolized in liver.
Excretion: excreted in urine (about 67%) and feces (about 33%). *Half-life:* about 2 hours.

Route	Onset	Peak	Duration
Inhalation	Unknown	Unknown	Unknown

Pharmacodynamics
Chemical effect: unknown; probably decreases nasal inflammation, mainly by inhibiting activities of specific cells and mediators involved in allergic response.
Therapeutic effect: decreases nasal congestion.

Indications and dosage
▶ **Symptoms of seasonal or perennial allergic rhinitis and non-allergic perennial rhinitis.** *Adults:* two sprays (64 mcg) in each nostril in morning and evening or four sprays (128 mcg) in each nostril in morning. Maintenance dosage should be fewest number of sprays needed to control symptoms.
▶ **Symptoms of seasonal or perennial allergic rhinitis.** *Children age 6 and older:* two sprays (64 mcg) in each nostril in morning and evening or four sprays (128 mcg) in each nostril in morning. Maintenance dosage should be fewest number of sprays needed to control symptoms.

Adverse reactions
CNS: nervousness.
EENT: *nasal irritation, epistaxis, pharyngitis,* reduced sense of smell, nasal pain, hoarseness.
GI: bad taste, dry mouth, dyspepsia, nausea.
Respiratory: *cough,* candidiasis, wheezing, dyspnea.
Skin: facial edema, rash, pruritus, contact dermatitis.
Other: myalgia, *hypersensitivity reactions*.

Interactions
None significant.

Contraindications and precautions
● Contraindicated in patients hypersensitive to drug or its components and in those who have had recent septal ulcers, nasal surgery, or nasal trauma, until total healing has occurred.
● Use cautiously in patients with tuberculous infections; untreated fungal, bacterial, or systemic viral infections; or ocular herpes simplex and in pregnant or breast-feeding women.
● Safety of drug has not been established in children under age 6.

NURSING CONSIDERATIONS

Assessment
● Obtain history of patient's allergy symptoms and nasal congestion before therapy and reassess regularly thereafter.
● Be alert for adverse reactions.
● Evaluate patient's and family's understanding of drug therapy.

Nursing diagnoses
● Altered health maintenance related to allergy-induced nasal congestion

---

*Liquid form contains alcohol   **May contain tartrazine   ◆Canada   ◊Australia   †OTC

• Impaired gas exchange related to drug-induced wheezing
• Knowledge deficit related to drug therapy

⟩ **Planning and implementation**
• Before giving drug, shake container and invert. Have patient clear his nasal passages, then tilt his head back. Insert nozzle into nostril (pointed away from septum), holding other nostril closed. Deliver spray while patient inspires. Repeat in other nostril.
• Notify doctor if relief is not obtained or signs of infection appear.
• Obtain specimen for culture, as ordered, if signs of nasal infection occur.
Patient teaching
• Instruct patient to shake container before using, blow nose to clear nasal passages, and insert nozzle into nostril, pointing away from septum. Tell him to hold other nostril closed, inspire gently, and spray; then shake container again and repeat in other nostril.
• Tell patient that product should be used by one person only to prevent spread of infection.
• Advise patient not to break, incinerate, or store canister in extreme heat; contents are under pressure.
• Warn patient not to exceed prescribed dose or use for long periods because of risk of hypothalamic-pituitary-adrenal axis suppression.
• Tell patient to report worsened condition or symptoms that do not improve in 3 weeks.
• Teach patient good nasal and oral hygiene.

☑ **Evaluation**
• Patient's nasal congestion subsides.
• Patient has adequate gas exchange.
• Patient and family state understanding of drug therapy.

bumetanide
(byoo-MEH-tuh-nighd)
Bumex, Burinex◇

Pharmacologic class: loop diuretic
Therapeutic class: diuretic
Pregnancy risk category: C

How supplied

Tablets: 0.5 mg, 1 mg, 2 mg
Injection: 0.25 mg/ml

Pharmacokinetics

Absorption: after P.O. administration, 85% to 95% absorbed; food delays absorption of P.O. dose. I.M. bumetanide is completely absorbed.
Distribution: about 92% to 96% protein bound; unknown if drug enters CSF.
Metabolism: metabolized by liver to at least five metabolites.
Excretion: excreted in urine (80%) and feces (10% to 20%). *Half-life:* 1 to 1½ hours.

Route	Onset	Peak	Duration
P.O.	30-60 min	1-2 hr	4-6 hr
I.V.	≤ 3 min	15-30 min	3.5-4 hr
I.M.	40 min	Unknown	Unknown

Pharmacodynamics

Chemical effect: inhibits sodium and chloride reabsorption at ascending portion of loop of Henle.
Therapeutic effect: promotes sodium and water excretion.

Indications and dosage

▶ **Edema in heart failure or hepatic or renal disease.** *Adults:* 0.5 to 2 mg P.O. once daily. If diuretic response is not adequate, second or third dose may be given at 4- to 5-hour intervals. Maximum dosage is 10 mg/day. May be administered parenterally if P.O. not feasible. Usual initial dose is 0.5 to 1 mg given I.V. over 1 to 2 minutes or I.M. If response is not adequate, second or third dose may be given at 2- to 3-hour intervals. Maximum dosage is 10 mg/day.

Adverse reactions

CNS: dizziness, headache.
CV: volume depletion and dehydration, orthostatic hypotension, ECG changes.
EENT: transient deafness.
GI: nausea.
GU: *renal failure,* nocturia, polyuria, frequent urination, oliguria.
Hematologic: azotemia, *thrombocytopenia.*
Metabolic: hypokalemia; hypochloremic alkalosis; asymptomatic hyperuricemia; fluid and electrolyte imbalances, including dilutional hyponatremia, hypocalcemia, hypomagnesemia; hyperglycemia and glucose intolerance impairment.
Musculoskeletal: muscle pain and tenderness.
Skin: rash.

Interactions

Drug-drug. *Aminoglycoside antibiotics:* potentiated ototoxicity. Use together cautiously.
Antihypertensives: increased risk of hypotension. Use together cautiously.
Cardiac glycosides: increased risk of digitalis toxicity from bumetanide-induced hypokalemia. Monitor potassium and digitalis levels.
Indomethacin, NSAIDs, probenecid: inhibited diuretic response. Use together cautiously.
Lithium: decreased lithium clearance, increasing risk of lithium toxicity. Monitor lithium level.
Metolazone: profound diuresis and potential electrolyte loss. Monitor patient for fluid and electrolyte imbalances.
Other potassium-wasting drugs: increased risk of hypokalemia. Use together cautiously.

Contraindications and precautions

• Contraindicated in patients with hypersensitivity to drug or to sulfonamides (possible cross-sensitivity), in those with anuria or hepatic coma, in patients in states of severe electrolyte depletion, and in breast-feeding women.
• Use cautiously in patients with hepatic cirrhosis and ascites or depressed renal function and in pregnant women.
• Safety of drug has not been established in children.

NURSING CONSIDERATIONS

⚚ Assessment

• Obtain history of patient's urine output, vital signs, serum electrolyte levels, breath sounds, peripheral edema, and weight before therapy and reassess regularly thereafter.
• Be alert for adverse reactions and drug interactions.
• Evaluate patient's and family's understanding of drug therapy.

⚚ Nursing diagnoses

• Fluid volume excess related to underlying condition
• Altered urinary elimination related to therapeutic effect of drug therapy
• Knowledge deficit related to drug therapy

⚚ Planning and implementation

P.O. and I.M. use: Follow normal protocol.
I.V. use: Give I.V. doses directly using 21G or 23G needle over 1 to 2 minutes. For intermittent infusion, give diluted drug through an intermittent infusion device, or piggyback into an I.V. line containing free-flowing compatible solution. Infuse at ordered rate. Continuous infusion not recommended.
• To prevent nocturia, give in morning. If second dose is necessary, give in early afternoon.
• Be aware that safest and most effective dosage schedule for control of edema is intermittent dosage given on alternate days or given for 3 to 4 days with 1- or 2-day rest periods.

• Keep in mind that drug can be safely used in patients allergic to furosemide; 1 mg of bumetanide equals 40 mg of furosemide. Bumetanide may be less ototoxic than furosemide, but clinical relevance has not been determined.

• If oliguria or azotemia develops or increases, anticipate that doctor may stop drug.

• Notify doctor if drug-related hearing changes occur.

Patient teaching

• Advise patient to stand up slowly to prevent dizziness and to limit alcohol intake and strenuous exercise in hot weather to avoid exacerbating orthostatic hypotension.

• Teach patient to monitor fluid volume by measuring weight and fluid intake and output daily.

• Encourage patient to avoid high-sodium foods and to choose high-potassium foods.

• Advise patient to take drug early in day to avoid sleep interruption caused by nocturia.

• Tell diabetic patient receiving bumetanide to monitor blood glucose levels closely.

☑ **Evaluation**

• Patient is free from edema.

• Patient demonstrates adjustment of lifestyle to deal with altered patterns of urinary elimination.

• Patient and family state understanding of drug therapy.

---

buprenorphine hydrochloride
(byoo-preh-NOR-feen high-droh-KLOR-ighd)
Buprenex, Temgesic Injection◊

Pharmacologic class: narcotic agonist-antagonist, opioid partial agonist
Therapeutic class: analgesic
Controlled substance schedule: V
Pregnancy risk category: C

How supplied
Injection: 0.324 mg (equivalent to 0.3 mg base/ml).

Pharmacokinetics
Absorption: absorbed rapidly after I.M. administration.
Distribution: about 96% protein-bound.
Metabolism: metabolized in liver.
Excretion: excreted primarily in feces as unchanged drug; about 30% excreted in urine. *Half-life:* 1.2 to 7.2 hours.

Route	Onset	Peak	Duration
I.V., I.M.	≤ 15 min	≤ 1 hr	About 6 hr

Pharmacodynamics
Chemical effect: binds with opiate receptors in CNS, altering both perception of and emotional response to pain through an unknown mechanism.
Therapeutic effect: relieves pain.

Indications and dosage
▶ **Moderate to severe pain.** *Adults and children age 13 and over:* 0.3 mg I.M. or slow I.V. q 6 hours, p.r.n., or around clock; may repeat 0.3 mg or increase to 0.6 mg, if needed, 30 to 60 minutes after initial dose. *Children ages 2 to 12:* 2 to 6 mcg/kg I.V. or I.M. q 4 to 6 hours.

Adverse reactions
CNS: *dizziness, sedation, headache,* confusion, nervousness, euphoria, *increased intracranial pressure.*
CV: *hypotension,* bradycardia, tachycardia, hypertension.
EENT: *miosis,* blurred vision.
GI: *nausea,* vomiting, constipation.
GU: urine retention.
Respiratory: *respiratory depression,* hypoventilation.
Skin: pruritus, *sweating.*

Interactions
Drug-drug. *CNS depressants, MAO inhibitors:* additive effects. Use together cautiously.

Reactions may be *common,* uncommon, *life-threatening,* or COMMON AND LIFE-THREATENING.

Narcotic analgesics: possibly decreased analgesic effect. Avoid concomitant use. **Drug-lifestyle.** *Alcohol use:* additive effects. Use together cautiously

Contraindications and precautions

• Contraindicated in patients with hypersensitivity to drug.
• Use cautiously in elderly or debilitated patients and in pregnant or breast-feeding women. Also use cautiously in patients with head injury; intracranial lesions; increased intracranial pressure; severe respiratory, liver, or kidney impairment; CNS depression or coma; thyroid irregularities; adrenal insufficiency; prostatic hyperplasia; urethral stricture; acute alcoholism; alcohol withdrawal syndrome; or kyphoscoliosis.

NURSING CONSIDERATIONS

Assessment
• Obtain history of patient's pain before and after drug use.
• Be alert for adverse reactions and drug interactions.
• Monitor respiratory status frequently for at least 1 hour after administration, and notify doctor of evidence of respiratory depression.
• Evaluate patient's and family's understanding drug therapy.

Nursing diagnoses
• Pain related to underlying condition
• Ineffective breathing pattern related to drug-induced respiratory depression
• Knowledge deficit related to drug therapy

Planning and implementation
I.V. use: Give by direct I.V. injection slowly into vein or through tubing of free-flowing compatible I.V. solution over not less than 2 minutes.
I.M. use: Follow normal protocol.
• S.C. administration not recommended.
• Be aware that analgesic potency of 0.3 mg of buprenorphine is equal to that of 10 mg of morphine and 75 mg of meperidine and that buprenorphine has longer duration of action than morphine or meperidine.
• Notify doctor and discuss increasing dose or frequency of drug if pain is not relieved.
• If patient's respiratory rate falls below 8 breaths/minute, withhold dose, arouse patient to stimulate breathing, and notify doctor.
• Know that naloxone will not completely reverse respiratory depression caused by buprenorphine overdose; mechanical ventilation may be necessary. Larger-than-usual doses of naloxone (more than 0.4 mg) and doxapram also may be ordered.
• Be aware that drug's narcotic antagonist properties may precipitate withdrawal syndrome in narcotic-dependent patients.
• Know that if dependence occurs, withdrawal symptoms may appear up to 14 days after drug is stopped.
Patient teaching
• Caution ambulatory patient about getting out of bed or walking due to dizziness or hypotensive adverse effects.
• When drug is used postoperatively, encourage patient to turn, cough, and deep-breathe to prevent atelectasis.

Evaluation
• Patient reports pain relief.
• Patient's respiratory status is within normal limits.
• Patient and family state understanding of drug therapy.

---

bupropion hydrochloride
(byoo-PROH-pee-on high-droh-KLOR-ighd)
Wellbutrin, Wellbutrin SR

Pharmacologic class: aminoketone
Therapeutic class: antidepressant
Pregnancy risk category: B

How supplied

Tablets: 75 mg, 100 mg
Tablets (sustained-release): 100 mg, 150 mg

Pharmacokinetics

Absorption: unknown.
Distribution: at plasma concentrations up to 200 mcg/ml, drug appears to be about 80% bound to plasma proteins.
Metabolism: probably metabolized in liver; several active metabolites have been identified.
Excretion: primarily excreted in urine.
Half-life: 8 to 24 hours.

Route	Onset	Peak	Duration
P.O.	1-3 wk	≤ 2 hr	Unknown

Pharmacodynamics

Chemical effect: unknown. Drug is not a tricyclic antidepressant, does not inhibit MAO, and is a weak inhibitor of norepinephrine, dopamine, and serotonin reuptake.
Therapeutic effect: relieves depression.

Indications and dosage

▶ **Depression**. *Adults:* initially, 100 mg P.O. b.i.d. Dosage increased after 3 days to 100 mg P.O. t.i.d., if needed. If no response occurs after several weeks of therapy, dosage increased to 150 mg t.i.d. For sustained-release tablets, 150 mg P.O. q morning; increased to target dose of 150 mg P.O. b.i.d., as tolerated, as early as day 4 of dosing. The usual adult dose is 300 mg/day.

Adverse reactions

CNS: *headache*, akathisia, *seizures,* agitation, anxiety, *confusion,* delusions, euphoria, hostility, impaired sleep quality, insomnia, sedation, sensory disturbance, tremors.
CV: *arrhythmias,* hypertension, hypotension, palpitations, syncope, tachycardia.
EENT: auditory disturbance, blurred vision.
GI: dry mouth, taste disturbance, increased appetite, constipation, dyspepsia, nausea, vomiting.
GU: impotence, menstrual complaints, urinary frequency, decreased libido.
Skin: pruritus, rash, cutaneous temperature disturbance, diaphoresis.
Other: arthritis, fever, chills.

Interactions

Drug-drug. *Levodopa, MAO inhibitors, phenothiazines, tricyclic antidepressants; recent and rapid withdrawal of benzodiazepines:* increased risk of adverse reactions, including seizures. Monitor closely.
Drug-lifestyle. *Alcohol use:* increased risk of adverse reactions, including seizures. Monitor closely.

Contraindications and precautions

• Contraindicated in patients with seizure disorders, hypersensitivity to drug, or history of bulimia or anorexia nervosa and in those who have taken MAO inhibitors within previous 14 days.
• Use cautiously in pregnant women and in patients with renal or hepatic impairment or recent history of MI or unstable heart disease.
• Breast-feeding should be discontinued if drug must be administered to breast-feeding women.
• Safety of drug has not been established in children.

NURSING CONSIDERATIONS

⚄ Assessment
• Obtain history of patient's depression before therapy and reassess regularly thereafter.
• Be alert for adverse reactions and drug interactions.
• Monitor patient with history of bipolar disorder closely. Antidepressants can cause manic episodes during depressed phase of bipolar disorder.
• Evaluate patient's and family's understanding of drug therapy.

⊕ **Nursing diagnoses**
• Ineffective individual coping related to underlying condition
• Risk for injury related to drug-induced adverse CNS reactions
• Knowledge deficit related to drug therapy

▶ **Planning and implementation**
• Know that risk of seizures may be minimized by not exceeding 450 mg/day and by administering daily dosage in three to four equally divided doses. Be aware that many patients who experience seizures have predisposing factors, including history of head trauma, seizures, or CNS tumors, or they may be taking drug that lowers seizure threshold.
• Make sure patient has swallowed dose before leaving bedside.
• Know that patient may experience period of increased restlessness, agitation, insomnia, and anxiety, especially at beginning of therapy.
• Don't confuse drug with Zyban which is used to aid smoking cessation.
Patient teaching
• Advise patient to take drug as scheduled and to take each day's dosage in three divided doses to minimize risk of seizures.
• Tell patient to avoid alcohol while taking drug because alcohol use may contribute to development of seizures.
• Advise patient to avoid hazardous activities that require alertness and good psychomotor coordination until CNS effects of drug are known.
• Advise patient not to take Zyban in combination with Wellbutrin and to seek medical advice before taking other prescription or OTC medications.
• Tell patient not to crush, chew, or divide sustained-release tablets.

✂ **Evaluation**
• Patient's behavior and communication indicate improvement of depression.
• Patient does not experience injury from drug-induced adverse CNS reactions.

• Patient and family state understanding of drug therapy.

---

buspirone hydrochloride
(byoo-SPEER-ohn high-droh-KLOR-ighd)
BuSpar

Pharmacologic class: azaspirodecane-dione derivative
Therapeutic class: antianxiety agent
Pregnancy risk category: B

How supplied
Tablets: 5 mg, 10 mg, 15 mg

Pharmacokinetics
Absorption: absorbed rapidly and completely, but extensive first-pass metabolism limits absolute bioavailability to between 1% and 13% of P.O. dose. Food slows absorption but increases amount of unchanged drug in systemic circulation.
Distribution: 95% protein-bound; does not displace other highly protein-bound medications.
Metabolism: metabolized in liver, resulting in at least one active metabolite.
Excretion: 29% to 63% excreted in urine in 24 hours, primarily as metabolites; 18% to 38% excreted in feces. *Half-life:* 2 to 3 hours.

Route	Onset	Peak	Duration
P.O.	Unknown	40-90 min	Unknown

Pharmacodynamics
Chemical effect: unknown; may inhibit neuronal firing and reduce serotonin turnover in cortical, amygdaloid, and septohippocampal tissue.
Therapeutic effect: relieves anxiety.

Indications and dosage
▶ **Anxiety disorders, short-term relief of anxiety.** *Adults:* initially, 7.5 mg P.O. b.i.d. Dosage increased at 2- to 3-day intervals in 5-mg/day increments. Usual maintenance dosage is 20 to 30 mg daily

---

in divided doses. Do not exceed 60 mg daily.

Adverse reactions

CNS: *dizziness, drowsiness,* nervousness, excitement, insomnia, headache.
GI: dry mouth, nausea, diarrhea.
Other: fatigue.

Interactions

Drug-drug. *CNS depressants:* increased CNS depression. Avoid concomitant use.
MAO inhibitors: may elevate blood pressure. Avoid concomitant use.
Drug-lifestyle. *Alcohol use:* increased CNS depression. Don't use together.

Contraindications and precautions

• Contraindicated in patients hypersensitive to drug or within 14 days of taking MAO inhibitors.
• Avoid use in breast-feeding women, if possible.
• Use cautiously in patients with hepatic or renal failure and in pregnant women.
• Safety of drug has not been established in children.

NURSING CONSIDERATIONS

🔎 **Assessment**
• Obtain history of patient's anxiety before therapy and reassess regularly thereafter. Signs of improvement are usually evident within 7 to 10 days; optimal results are achieved after 3 to 4 weeks of therapy.
• Be alert for adverse reactions and drug interactions.
• Evaluate patient's and family's understanding of drug therapy.

🔲 **Nursing diagnoses**
• Anxiety related to underlying condition
• Fatigue related to drug-induced adverse reactions
• Knowledge deficit related to drug therapy

▶ **Planning and implementation**
• Be aware that, although drug has shown no potential for abuse and has not been classified as controlled substance, it is not recommended for relief of everyday stress.
• Before initiating therapy in patient already being treated with a benzodiazepine, make sure he does not stop benzodiazepine abruptly; withdrawal reaction may occur.
• Administer drug with food or milk.
• Know that dosage may be increased, as ordered, in 2- to 3-day intervals.
Patient teaching
• Tell patient to take drug with food.
• Warn patient to avoid performing hazardous activities that require alertness and good psychomotor coordination until CNS effects of drug are known.
• Review energy-saving measures with patient and family.
• If patient is already being treated with benzodiazepine, warn him not to abruptly discontinue drug because withdrawal reaction can occur. Teach him how and when benzodiazepine can be withdrawn safely.

☑ **Evaluation**
• Patient's anxiety is reduced.
• Patient states that energy-saving measures help combat fatigue caused by therapy.
• Patient and family state understanding of drug therapy.

busulfan
(byoo-SUL-fan)
Myleran

Pharmacologic class: alkylating agent (cell cycle–phase nonspecific)
Therapeutic class: antineoplastic
Pregnancy risk category: D

How supplied

Tablets: 2 mg

Pharmacokinetics

Absorption: well absorbed from GI tract.
Distribution: unknown.
Metabolism: metabolized in liver.
Excretion: cleared rapidly from plasma
and excreted in urine. *Half-life:* about 2½
hours.

Route	Onset	Peak	Duration
P.O.	1-2 wk	Unknown	Unknown

Pharmacodynamics

Chemical effect: unknown; thought to
cross-link strands of cellular DNA and
interfere with RNA transcription, causing
an imbalance of growth that leads to cell
death. Cell cycle–phase nonspecific.
Therapeutic effect: kills selected type of
cancer cell.

Indications and dosage

Dosage and indications may vary. Check
current literature for recommended protocol.
▶ **Chronic myelocytic (granulocytic)
leukemia.** *Adults:* for remission induction, 4 to 8 mg P.O. daily (0.06 mg/kg or
1.8 mg/m^2). For maintenance therapy, 1
to 3 mg P.O. daily. *Children:* 0.06 mg/kg
or 1.8 mg/m^2 P.O. daily.

Adverse reactions

CNS: *seizures,* unusual tiredness or
weakness.
GI: nausea, vomiting, diarrhea, cheilosis,
glossitis.
GU: amenorrhea, testicular atrophy, impotence.
Hematologic: WBC count falling after
about 10 days and continuing to fall for 2
weeks after stopping drug, *thrombocytopenia, anemia, severe pancytopenia.*
Respiratory: persistent cough; dyspnea;
*irreversible pulmonary fibrosis, com-
monly termed "busulfan lung."*
Skin: transient hyperpigmentation, rash,
urticaria, anhidrosis, alopecia.
Other: gynecomastia, Addison-like wasting syndrome, profound hyperuricemia
caused by increased cell lysis.

Interactions

Drug-drug. *Anticoagulants, aspirin:* increased risk of bleeding. Avoid concomitant use.
Thioguanine: may cause hepatotoxicity,
esophageal varices, or portal hypertension. Use together cautiously.

Contraindications and precautions

• Contraindicated in patients with chronic
myelogenous leukemia, which is known
to be resistant to drug, and in breast-
feeding women.
• Use with extreme caution, if at all, in
pregnant women.
• Use cautiously in patients recently giv-
en other myelosuppressive drugs or radiation therapy and in those with depressed
neutrophil or platelet count. Because
high-dose therapy has been associated
with seizures, use such therapy cautiously in patients with history of head trauma
or seizures and in patients receiving other
drugs that lower seizure threshold.

NURSING CONSIDERATIONS

◪ Assessment
• Obtain history of patient's underlying
neoplastic disease.
• Monitor effectiveness by noting results
of follow-up diagnostic tests and overall
physical status. Note patient response (increased appetite and sense of well-being,
decreased total WBC count, reduced size
of spleen), which usually begins within 1
to 2 weeks.
• Monitor WBC and platelet counts
weekly while patient is receiving drug.
• Monitor serum uric acid level.
• Be alert for adverse reactions and drug
interactions. Pulmonary fibrosis may occur as late as 4 to 6 months after treatment.
• Evaluate patient's and family's understanding of drug therapy.

⊞ Nursing diagnoses
• Altered health maintenance related to
presence of neoplastic disease

---

*Liquid form contains alcohol **May contain tartrazine ◆Canada ◇Australia †OTC

• Risk for infection related to drug-induced immunosuppression
• Knowledge deficit related to drug therapy

≫ **Planning and implementation**
• Follow institutional policy regarding preparation and handling of drug. Label as hazardous drug.
• Administer drug at same time each day.
• Ensure that patient is adequately hydrated.
• Remember that dosage is adjusted based on patient's weekly WBC counts and that doctor may temporarily stop drug therapy if severe leukocytopenia develops.
• Know that drug is often administered with allopurinol to prevent symptoms of gout.
Patient teaching
• Warn patient to watch for signs of infection (fever, sore throat, fatigue) and bleeding (easy bruising, nosebleeds, bleeding gums, melena) and to take temperature daily.
• Instruct patient to report symptoms of toxicity so that dosage adjustments can be made. Such symptoms include persistent cough and progressive dyspnea with alveolar exudate, suggestive of pneumonia.
• Instruct patient to avoid OTC products containing aspirin.
• Advise women of childbearing age to avoid becoming pregnant during therapy. Recommend that patient consult with doctor before becoming pregnant.
• Advise breast-feeding women to discontinue breast-feeding because of possibility of toxicity in infant.

☑ **Evaluation**
• Patient exhibits positive response to drug therapy.
• Patient remains free from infection.
• Patient and family state understanding of drug therapy.

butabarbital sodium (butabarbitone sodium)
(byoo-tah-BAR-bih-tal SOH-dee-um)
Butalan*, Butisol* **, Sarisol No. 2* **

Pharmacologic class: barbiturate
Therapeutic class: sedative-hypnotic agent
Controlled substance schedule: III
Pregnancy risk category: D

How supplied
Tablets: 15 mg, 30 mg, 50 mg, 100 mg
Elixir: 30 mg/5 ml, 33.3 mg/5 ml

Pharmacokinetics
Absorption: well absorbed after P.O. administration.
Distribution: well distributed throughout body tissues and fluids.
Metabolism: metabolized extensively in liver by oxidation.
Excretion: inactive metabolites excreted in urine. Only 1% to 2% of dose excreted unchanged in urine. *Half-life:* 30 to 40 hours.

Route	Onset	Peak	Duration
P.O.	45-60 min	≤ 3 hr	6-8 hr

Pharmacodynamics
Chemical effect: unknown; probably interferes with transmission of impulses from thalamus to cortex of brain.
Therapeutic effect: promotes sleep and calmness.

Indications and dosage
▶ **Sedation.** *Adults:* 15 to 30 mg P.O. t.i.d. or q.i.d. *Children:* 2 mg/kg or 60 mg/m² P.O. t.i.d. Dosage range is 7.5 to 30 mg P.O. t.i.d.
▶ **Preoperative sedation.** *Adults:* 50 to 100 mg P.O. 60 to 90 minutes before surgery. *Children:* 2 to 6 mg/kg P.O. (not to exceed 100 mg) 60 to 90 minutes before surgery.
▶ **Insomnia.** *Adults:* 50 to 100 mg P.O. h.s.

Reactions may be *common*, uncommon, *life-threatening*, or COMMON AND LIFE-THREATENING.

Adverse reactions

CNS: *drowsiness, lethargy, hangover;* paradoxical excitement (in elderly patients).
CV: *angioedema.*
GI: nausea, vomiting.
Hematologic: exacerbation of porphyria.
Respiratory: *respiratory depression.*
Skin: rash, urticaria, *Stevens-Johnson syndrome.*

Interactions

Drug-drug. *Chloramphenicol, MAO inhibitors, valproic acid:* inhibited metabolism of barbiturates; may cause prolonged CNS depression. Reduce barbiturate dosage, as necessary.
CNS depressants, including narcotic analgesics: excessive CNS and respiratory depression. Use together cautiously.
Corticosteroids, digitoxin, doxycycline, estrogens and oral contraceptives, oral anticoagulants, tricyclic antidepressants: barbiturates may enhance metabolism of these drugs. Monitor for decreased effectiveness.
Griseofulvin: decreased absorption of griseofulvin. Monitor for decreased effect.
Rifampin: may decrease barbiturate levels. Monitor for decreased effect.
Drug-lifestyle. *Alcohol use:* excessive CNS and respiratory depression. Don't use together.

Contraindications and precautions

• Contraindicated in patients with bronchopneumonia or other severe pulmonary insufficiency, porphyria, or hypersensitivity to barbiturates and in breast-feeding women.
• Use cautiously in patients with acute or chronic pain, depression, suicidal tendencies, history of drug abuse, or hepatic or renal impairment.
• Also use cautiously in pregnant women and in children.

NURSING CONSIDERATIONS

Assessment
• Obtain history of patient's sleeping patterns and CNS status before therapy and reassess regularly thereafter.
• Be alert for adverse reactions and drug interactions.
• Evaluate patient's and family's understanding of drug therapy.

Nursing diagnoses
• Sleep pattern disturbance related to underlying condition
• Risk for injury related to drug-induced adverse CNS reactions
• Knowledge deficit related to drug therapy

Planning and implementation
• Before leaving bedside, make sure patient has swallowed drug.
• Be aware that long-term use is not recommended; drug loses its efficacy in promoting sleep after 14 days. A drug-free interval of at least 1 week is advised if continued treatment is appropriate. Long-term high dosage may cause drug dependence, and patient may experience withdrawal symptoms if drug is suddenly stopped. Withdraw barbiturates gradually.
• Discontinue drug when skin reactions occur because skin eruptions may precede potentially fatal reaction to barbiturate therapy. In some patients, high fever, stomatitis, headache, or rhinitis may precede skin reactions.
Patient teaching
• Inform patient that morning hangover is common after hypnotic dose and that hypnotic doses suppress REM sleep; patient may experience increased dreaming after drug is discontinued.
• Caution patient about performing activities that require mental alertness or physical coordination. For inpatients, particularly those who are elderly, supervise walking and raise bed rails.
• Tell patient using oral contraceptive that she should consider alternative birth

control methods because drug may enhance contraceptive hormone metabolism and decrease its effect.
• Warn patient that drug may cause physical dependence.

☑ **Evaluation**
• Patient states that drug effectively induces sleep.
• Patient does not experience injury as a result of drug-induced adverse reactions.
• Patient and family state understanding of drug therapy.

---

butoconazole nitrate
(byoo-tah-KON-ah-zohl NIGH-trayt)
Femstat

Pharmacologic class: synthetic imidazole derivative
Therapeutic class: topical fungistat
Pregnancy risk category: C

How supplied

Vaginal cream: 2% supplied with applicators

Pharmacokinetics

Absorption: about 5.5% absorbed through vaginal walls.
Distribution: unknown.
Metabolism: appears to be metabolized in liver.
Excretion: appears to be excreted in urine and feces.

Route	Onset	Peak	Duration
Topical (vaginal)	Unknown	Unknown	Unknown

Pharmacodynamics

Chemical effect: unknown; thought to control or destroy fungus by disrupting cell membrane permeability, causing osmotic instability.
Therapeutic effect: controls or eliminates vaginal *Candida* infections.

Indications and dosage

▶ **Vulvovaginal mycotic infections caused by *Candida*.** *Adults:* for nonpregnant women, 1 applicator intravaginally h.s. for 3 days. If necessary, treatment can be extended for another 3 days. For pregnant women during second or third trimester, 1 applicator intravaginally h.s. for 6 days.

Adverse reactions

GU: vulvovaginal itching, soreness, swelling.
Skin: finger itching.

Interactions

None significant.

Contraindications and precautions

• Contraindicated in patients hypersensitive to drug.
• Use cautiously in pregnant or breast-feeding women.
• Safety of drug has not been established in female children.

NURSING CONSIDERATIONS

☒ **Assessment**
• Obtain history of patient's vaginal infection before therapy and monitor for response throughout therapy.
• Be alert for adverse reactions.
• Evaluate patient's and family's understanding of drug therapy.

✪ **Nursing diagnoses**
• Infection related to presence of vaginal fungal infection
• Knowledge deficit related to drug therapy

▷ **Planning and implementation**
• Confirm diagnosis of *Candida* vulvovaginal infection by smears or cultures, as ordered.
• Be aware that butoconazole may be used with oral contraceptive and antibiotic therapy.

Patient teaching
• Teach patient how to apply drug, and tell her not to use tampons during treatment.
• Advise patient to keep affected area cool and dry, wear loose-fitting cotton clothing, avoid feminine hygiene sprays, wash daily with unscented soap, dry thoroughly with clean towel, and maintain proper hygiene by wiping perineum from front to back to prevent reinfection.
• Tell patient's sexual partner to wear condom during intercourse until treatment is complete and to consult doctor if he experiences penile itching, redness, or discomfort.

☑ **Evaluation**
• Patient's vaginal infection is resolved.
• Patient and family state understanding of drug therapy.

butorphanol tartrate
(byoo-TOR-fah-nohl TAR-trayt)
Stadol, Stadol NS

Pharmacologic class: narcotic agonist-antagonist; opioid partial agonist
Therapeutic class: analgesic, adjunct to anesthesia
Pregnancy risk category: C

How supplied
Injection: 1 mg/ml, 2 mg/ml
Nasal spray: 10 mg/ml

Pharmacokinetics
Absorption: well absorbed after I.M. administration; unknown after nasal administration.
Distribution: about 80% bound to plasma proteins. After I.V. administration, mean volume of distribution is about 500 L. Drug rapidly crosses placenta and neonatal serum levels are 0.4 to 1.4 times maternal levels.
Metabolism: extensively metabolized in liver to inactive metabolites.

Excretion: excreted in inactive form, mainly by kidneys. About 11% to 14% of parenteral dose excreted in feces.

Route	Onset	Peak	Duration
I.V.	2-3 min	0.5-1 hr	2-4 hr
I.M.	10-30 min	0.5-1 hr	3-4 hr
Intranasal	≤ 15 min	1-2 hr	4-5 hr

Pharmacodynamics
Chemical effect: binds with opiate receptors in CNS, altering both perception of and emotional response to pain through unknown mechanism.
Therapeutic effect: relieves pain and enhances anesthesia.

Indications and dosage
▶ **Moderate to severe pain.** *Adults:* 0.5 to 2 mg I.V. q 3 to 4 hours, p.r.n. or around the clock; or 1 to 4 mg I.M. q 3 to 4 hours, p.r.n. or around the clock. Not to exceed 4 mg per dose. Alternatively, 1 mg by nasal spray q 3 to 4 hours (1 spray in one nostril); repeated in 60 to 90 minutes if pain relief is inadequate.
▶ **Labor for patients at full term and in early labor.** *Adults:* 1 to 2 mg I.V. or I.M., repeated after 4 hours, p.r.n.
▶ **Preoperative anesthesia or preanesthesia.** *Adults:* 2 mg I.M. 60 to 90 minutes before surgery.
▶ **Adjunct to balanced anesthesia.** *Adults:* 2 mg I.V. shortly before induction or 0.5 to 1 mg I.V. in increments during anesthesia.

Adverse reactions
CNS: *sedation, headache, vertigo, floating sensation,* lethargy, *confusion,* nervousness, unusual dreams, agitation, euphoria, hallucinations, flushing, increased intracranial pressure.
CV: palpitations, fluctuation in blood pressure.
EENT: diplopia, blurred vision, *nasal congestion* (with nasal spray).
GI: nausea, vomiting, constipation, *dry mouth.*
Respiratory: *respiratory depression.*

---

*Liquid form contains alcohol   **May contain tartrazine   ◆ Canada   ◇ Australia   †OTC

Skin: rash, urticaria, *clamminess, excessive sweating.*

Interactions

Drug-drug. *CNS depressants:* additive effects. Use together cautiously. *Narcotic analgesics:* possibly decreased analgesic effect. Avoid concomitant use. **Drug-lifestyle.** *Alcohol use:* additive effects. Use together cautiously.

Contraindications and precautions

• Contraindicated in patients with narcotic addiction; may precipitate withdrawal syndrome. Also contraindicated in patients with hypersensitivity to drug or to preservative (benzethonium chloride) and in breast-feeding women.
• Use with extreme caution, if at all, in pregnant women.
• Use cautiously in patients with head injury, increased intracranial pressure, acute MI, ventricular dysfunction, coronary insufficiency, respiratory disease or depression, or renal or hepatic dysfunction. Also use cautiously in patients who have recently received repeated doses of narcotic analgesic.
• Use cautiously in children; drug may cause paradoxical excitement.

NURSING CONSIDERATIONS

⚐ **Assessment**
• Obtain history of patient's pain before and after drug administration.
• Be alert for adverse reactions and drug interactions.
• Periodically monitor postoperative vital signs and bladder function. Because drug decreases both rate and depth of respirations, monitoring arterial oxygen saturation may aid in assessing respiratory depression.
• Evaluate patient's and family's understanding of drug therapy.

⊞ **Nursing diagnoses**
• Pain related to underlying condition

• Risk for injury related to drug-induced adverse CNS reactions
• Knowledge deficit related to drug therapy

≽ **Planning and implementation**
I.V. use: Give drug by direct I.V. injection into vein or into I.V. line containing free-flowing compatible solution.
I.M. use: Follow normal protocol.
Intranasal use: Have patient clear nasal passages before administering drug. Shake container. Tilt patient's head slightly backward; insert nozzle into nostril, pointing away from septum. Have patient hold other nostril closed, and spray while patient is inspiring gently.
• S.C. route not recommended.
• Be aware that psychological and physical addiction may occur.
• Notify doctor and discuss increasing dose or frequency if pain persists.
• Keep narcotic antagonist (naloxone) and resuscitative equipment readily available.
Patient teaching
• Caution ambulatory patient about getting out of bed or walking. Warn outpatient to refrain from driving and performing other potentially hazardous activities that require mental alertness until drug's CNS effects are known.
• Warn patient that drug can cause physical and psychological dependence. Tell him that he should use drug only as directed and that abrupt withdrawal after chronic use produces intense withdrawal symptoms.

☑ **Evaluation**
• Patient reports relief of pain.
• Patient does not experience injury as a result of therapy.
• Patient and family state understanding of drug therapy.

caffeine
(ka-FEEN)
Caffedrine Caplets†, NoDoz†, Quick Pep†,
Vivarin†

Pharmacologic class: methylxanthine
Therapeutic class: CNS stimulant
Pregnancy risk category: B

How supplied
Tablets: 100 mg†, 150 mg†, 200 mg†
Capsules (timed-release): 200 mg†

Pharmacokinetics
Absorption: well absorbed from GI tract.
Distribution: distributed rapidly through-
out body; crosses blood-brain barrier;
about 17% protein-bound.
Metabolism: metabolized by liver.
Excretion: excreted in urine. *Half-life:* 3
to 7 hours.

Route	Onset	Peak	Duration
P.O.	Unknown	50-75 min	Unknown

Pharmacodynamics
Chemical effect: inhibits phosphodi-
esterase, enzyme that degrades cAMP.
Therapeutic effect: stimulates CNS.

Indications and dosage
▶ **CNS stimulant.** *Adults:* 100 to
200 mg P.O. q 4 hours, p.r.n

Adverse reactions
CNS: *stimulation, insomnia,* restlessness,
nervousness, mild delirium, headache,
excitement, agitation, muscle tremors,
twitches.
CV: *tachycardia, palpitations.*
GI: nausea, vomiting.
GU: *diuresis.*
Skin: hyperesthesia.

Other: dehydration, fever, hyperglycemia, abrupt withdrawal symptoms
(headache, irritability).

Interactions
Drug-drug. *Beta-adrenergic agonists,
cimetidine, fluoroquinolones, oral contraceptives, phenylpropanolamine, theophylline:* excessive CNS stimulation.
Avoid concomitant use.
Drug-food. *Caffeine-containing foods
and beverages:* excessive CNS stimulation. Limit concomitant use.

Contraindications and precautions
• Contraindicated in patients with hypersensitivity to drug.
• Use cautiously in patients with history
of peptic ulcer, symptomatic arrhythmias,
or palpitations; during first several days
to weeks after acute MI; and in pregnant
women.
• Avoid use of caffeine tablets or capsules in breast-feeding women.
• Safety of drug has not been established
in children.

NURSING CONSIDERATIONS

Assessment
• Assess patient's CNS depression before
therapy and regularly thereafter.
• Be alert for adverse reactions and drug
interactions.
• Monitor patient for tolerance or psychological dependence.
• Evaluate patient's and family's knowledge of drug therapy.

Nursing diagnoses
• Altered health maintenance related to
patient's underlying condition
• Fatigue related to caffeine-induced
CNS stimulation
• Knowledge deficit related to drug
therapy

Planning and implementation
• Be aware that single dose should not
exceed 1 g.

• Recognize that sudden discontinuation may cause headache and irritability.
• Know that caffeine does not reverse alcohol intoxication or CNS depressant effects of alcohol.
• Restrict caffeine-containing beverages in patients who experience palpitations. Caffeine content per 180 ml: cola, 17 to 55 mg; tea, 40 to 100 mg; instant coffee, 60 to 180 mg; brewed coffee, 100 to 150 mg; decaffeinated coffee, 1 to 6 mg.

Patient teaching
• Caution patient not to use drug excessively; tolerance or psychological dependence may occur.
• Tell patient to restrict caffeine-containing beverages.
• Instruct patient to stop using drug and notify doctor if palpitations occur.

☑ Evaluation
• Patient exhibits CNS stimulation.
• Patient does not develop fatigue.
• Patient and family state understanding of drug therapy.

calcifediol
(kal-sih-fih-DIGH-al)
Calderol

Pharmacologic class: vitamin D analogue
Therapeutic class: antihypocalcemic
Pregnancy risk category: C

How supplied
Capsules: 20 mcg, 50 mcg

Pharmacokinetics
Absorption: absorbed readily from small intestine.
Distribution: distributed widely; highly protein-bound.
Metabolism: metabolized in liver and kidney.
Excretion: excreted in urine and bile.
Half-life: 16 days.

Route	Onset	Peak	Duration
P.O.	Unknown	4 hr	15-20 days

Pharmacodynamics
Chemical effect: stimulates calcium absorption from GI tract; promotes calcium secretion from bone to blood.
Therapeutic effect: raises blood calcium level.

Indications and dosage
▶ **Metabolic bone disease associated with chronic renal failure.** *Adults:* initially, 300 to 350 mcg/week P.O. daily or every other day. Dosage increased at 4-week intervals if necessary.

Adverse reactions
Vitamin D intoxication associated with hypercalcemia:
CNS: headache, somnolence.
EENT: conjunctivitis, photosensitivity reactions, rhinorrhea.
GI: nausea, vomiting, constipation, metallic taste, dry mouth, anorexia, diarrhea.
GU: polyuria.
Other: weakness, bone and muscle pain.

Interactions
Drug-drug. *Cholestyramine, colestipol:* decreased absorption of orally administered vitamin D analogues. Avoid concomitant use.
Corticosteroids: counteracts vitamin D analogue effects. Don't use together.
Cardiac glycosides: increased risk of arrhythmias. Avoid concomitant use.
Magnesium-containing antacids: possible hypermagnesemia, especially in patients with chronic renal failure. Avoid concomitant use.
Other vitamin D analogues: increased toxicity. Avoid concomitant use.

Contraindications and precautions
• Contraindicated in patients with hypercalcemia or vitamin D toxicity.
• Use cautiously in pregnant or breast-feeding women.

• Safety of drug has not been established in children.

NURSING CONSIDERATIONS

⚖ **Assessment**
• Assess patient's metabolic bone disease before therapy and regularly thereafter.
• Monitor drug effectiveness by regularly checking serum calcium level, as ordered: serum calcium times serum phosphate should not exceed 70. During titration, determine serum calcium level at least weekly.
• Be alert for adverse reactions and drug interactions.
• Evaluate patient's and family's knowledge of drug therapy.

⊞ **Nursing diagnoses**
• Risk for injury related to patient's underlying bone condition
• Altered protection related to potential for drug-induced vitamin D intoxication
• Knowledge deficit related to drug therapy

❱ **Planning and implementation**
• Be aware that optimal dosage is highly individualized.
• Notify doctor if hypercalcemia occurs; drug should be discontinued until serum calcium level returns to normal.
• Ensure that patient's daily calcium intake is adequate.
Patient teaching
• Advise patient to adhere to diet and calcium supplementation and to avoid OTC drugs.
• Teach patient to report signs and symptoms of hypercalcemia.

☑ **Evaluation**
• Patient's underlying condition improves and serum calcium level rises.
• Patient does not experience drug-induced vitamin D intoxication.
• Patient and family state understanding of drug therapy.

calcitonin (human)
(kal-sih-TOH-nin)
Cibacalcin

calcitonin (salmon)
Calcimar, Miacalcin, Osteocalcin, Salmonine

Pharmacologic class: thyroid hormone
Therapeutic class: hypocalcemic
Pregnancy risk category: C

How supplied
calcitonin (human)
Injection: 0.5 mg/vial
calcitonin (salmon)
Injection: 100 IU/ml, 1-ml ampules; 200 IU/ml, 2-ml ampules
Nasal spray: 200 IU/activation in 2-ml bottle

Pharmacokinetics
Absorption: unknown.
Distribution: unknown.
Metabolism: rapidly metabolized in kidneys; additional activity in blood and peripheral tissues.
Excretion: excreted in urine as inactive metabolites. *Half-life:* of calcitonin human, 60 minutes; of calcitonin salmon, 70 to 90 minutes.

Route	Onset	Peak	Duration
I.M., S.C.	≤ 15 min	≤ 4 hr	8-24 hr
Intranasal	Rapid	30 min	1 hr

Pharmacodynamics
Chemical effect: decreases osteoclastic activity by inhibiting osteocytic osteolysis; decreases mineral release and matrix or collagen breakdown in bone.
Therapeutic effect: prohibits bone and kidney (tubular) resorption of calcium.

Indications and dosage
▶ **Paget's disease of bone (osteitis deformans).** *Adults:* initially, 100 IU of calcitonin (salmon) daily I.M. or S.C.; maintenance dosage is 50 to 100 IU daily or

every other day. Alternatively, calcitonin (human) 0.5 mg S.C. daily. If patient improves sufficiently, dosage reduced to 0.25 mg daily two or three times weekly. Some patients may need as much as 1 mg daily.

▶ **Hypercalcemia.** *Adults:* 4 IU/kg of calcitonin (salmon) q 12 hours I.M. or S.C. If response is inadequate after 1 or 2 days, dose increased to 8 IU/kg I.M. q 12 hours. If response remains unsatisfactory after 2 more days, dosage increased to maximum of 8 IU/kg q 6 hours.

▶ **Postmenopausal osteoporosis.** *Adults:* 100 IU of calcitonin (salmon) daily I.M. or S.C. Alternatively, 200 IU (one activation) of calcitonin (salmon) daily intranasally, alternating nostrils daily. Patients should receive adequate vitamin D and calcium supplements.

Adverse reactions

CNS: headache.
GI: transient nausea, unusual taste, diarrhea, anorexia.
GU: transient diuresis.
Other: inflammation at injection site, rash, *facial flushing;* hypocalcemia; hyperglycemia; hand swelling, tingling, and tenderness; hypersensitivity reactions, *anaphylaxis.*

Interactions

None significant.

Contraindications and precautions

• Calcitonin may inhibit lactation and thus should not be used in breast-feeding women. Additionally, calcitonin salmon is contraindicated in patients with hypersensitivity to drug.
• Use cautiously in pregnant women.
• Safety of drug has not been established in children.

NURSING CONSIDERATIONS

 Assessment
• Assess patient's serum calcium level before therapy and regularly thereafter.

• Monitor serum alkaline phosphatase and 24-hour urine hydroxyproline levels to evaluate drug effectiveness, as ordered.
• Know that periodic examinations of urine sediment are advisable.
• Be alert for adverse reactions.
• Evaluate patient's and family's knowledge of drug therapy.

 Nursing diagnoses
• Risk for trauma related to patient's underlying bone condition
• Altered protection related to potential for drug-induced anaphylaxis
• Knowledge deficit related to drug therapy

 Planning and implementation
• Be aware that skin test is usually performed before therapy.
• Know that calcitonin human is especially indicated in patients who have developed resistance to calcitonin salmon. Calcitonin human is associated with risk of diminishing efficacy caused by antibody formation or hypersensitivity reactions.
• Administer drug at bedtime when possible to minimize nausea and vomiting.
I.M. use: I.M. route is preferred if volume of dose to be administered exceeds 2 ml. Follow normal protocol.
S.C. use: Follow normal protocol.
Intranasal use: Alternate nostrils daily.
• Use freshly reconstituted solution within 2 hours.
• Keep parenteral calcium available during first doses in case hypocalcemic tetany occurs.
• Store calcitonin human at room temperature (77° F [25° C]); refrigerate calcitonin salmon at 36° to 46° F (2° to 8° C). Store open nasal spray at room temperature.
• In patients with positive initial response who then suffer relapse, expect to evaluate for antibody response to hormone protein.

Reactions may be *common,* uncommon, *life-threatening*, or COMMON AND LIFE-THREATENING.

• Keep epinephrine handy: systemic allergic reactions are possible because hormone is protein.
• If symptoms have been relieved after 6 months, know that treatment may be discontinued until symptoms or radiologic signs recur.

Patient teaching
• Teach patient how to self-administer drug.
• Teach patient to activate nasal spray before first use. He should hold bottle upright and depress side arms six times until a faint mist occurs. This signifies that pump is ready for use.
• Instruct patient to report signs of nasal irritation with nasal spray.
• Tell patient to handle missed doses as follows: With daily dosing, take as soon as possible, but do not take double dose. With every-other-day dosing, take as soon as possible, then restart alternate days from this dose.
• Reassure patient that facial flushing and warmth (which occur in 20% to 30% of patients within minutes of injection) usually subside in about 1 hour.
• Remind patient with postmenopausal osteoporosis to take adequate calcium and vitamin D supplements.
• Tell patient in whom drug loses its hypocalcemic activity that further drug or increased dosages will be of no value.

☑ **Evaluation**
• Patient's serum calcium levels are normal.
• Patient does not experience anaphylaxis.
• Patient and family state understanding of drug therapy.

calcitriol
(1,25-dihydroxycholecalciferol)
(kal-SIH-tree-ohl)
Rocaltrol, Calcijex

Pharmacologic class: vitamin D analogue
Therapeutic class: antihypocalcemic
Pregnancy risk category: C

How supplied
Capsules: 0.25 mcg, 0.5 mcg
Injection: 1 mcg/ml, 2 mcg/ml

Pharmacokinetics
Absorption: absorbed readily.
Distributed: distributed widely; protein-bound.
Metabolism: metabolized in liver and kidney.
Excretion: excreted primarily in feces.
Half-life: 3 to 6 hours.

Route	Onset	Peak	Duration
P.O.	2-6 hr	3-6 hr	3-5 days
I.V.	Immediate	Unknown	3-5 days

Pharmacodynamics
Chemical effect: stimulates calcium absorption from GI tract; promotes calcium secretion from bone to blood.
Therapeutic effect: raises blood calcium levels.

Indications and dosage
▶ **Hypocalcemia in patients undergoing chronic dialysis.** *Adults:* initially, 0.25 mcg P.O. daily. Dosage may be increased by 0.25 mcg daily at 4- to 8-week intervals. Maintenance dosage is 0.25 mcg every other day up to 1.25 mcg daily. Or, 0.5 mcg I.V. three times weekly approximately every other day. If response is inadequate to initial dose, may increase by 0.5 to 1 mcg at 2- to 4-week intervals. Maintenance dose is 0.5 to 3 mcg I.V. three times weekly.
▶ **Hypoparathyroidism and pseudohypoparathyroidism.** *Adults and children*

age 1 and older: initially, 0.25 mcg P.O. daily. Dosage may be increased at 2- to 4-week intervals. Maintenance dosage is 0.25 to 2 mcg daily.

Adverse reactions

Vitamin D intoxication associated with hypercalcemia:
CNS: headache, somnolence.
EENT: conjunctivitis, photophobia, rhinorrhea.
GI: nausea, vomiting, constipation, metallic taste, dry mouth, anorexia.
GU: polyuria.
Musculoskeletal: weakness, bone and muscle pain.

Interactions

Drug-drug. *Cardiac glycosides:* increased risk of arrhythmias. Avoid concomitant use.
Cholestyramine, colestipol, excessive use of mineral oil: decreased absorption of orally administered vitamin D analogues. Avoid concomitant use.
Corticosteroids: counteracts vitamin D analogue effects. Don't use together.
Magnesium-containing antacids: may induce hypermagnesemia, especially in patients with chronic renal failure. Avoid concomitant use.

Contraindications and precautions

• Contraindicated in patients with hypercalcemia or vitamin D toxicity.
• Use cautiously in pregnant or breast-feeding women.

NURSING CONSIDERATIONS

🏵 Assessment
• Assess patient's serum calcium level before therapy, and reassess regularly thereafter to monitor drug effectiveness; serum calcium level times serum phosphate level should not exceed 70. During titration, determine serum calcium level twice weekly.
• Be alert for adverse reactions and drug interactions.

• Evaluate patient's and family's knowledge of drug therapy.

🏵 Nursing diagnoses
• Risk for injury related to patient's underlying condition
• Altered protection related to potential for drug-induced vitamin D intoxication
• Knowledge deficit related to drug therapy

🔊 Planning and implementation
P.O. use: Follow normal protocol.
I.V. use: Administer I.V. dose by rapid injection via dialysis catheter at end of hemodialysis treatment.
• Protect drug from heat and light.
• Administer drug at same time daily or every other day as ordered.
• Discontinue drug and notify doctor if hypercalcemia occurs; resume after serum calcium level returns to normal. The patient should receive 1,000 mg of calcium daily.
Patient teaching
• Tell patient to immediately report early symptoms of vitamin D intoxication: weakness, nausea, vomiting, dry mouth, constipation, muscle or bone pain, or metallic taste.
• Instruct patient to adhere to diet and calcium supplements and to avoid unapproved OTC drugs and magnesium-containing antacids.
• Warn patient that calcitriol is most potent form of vitamin D available and must not be taken by anyone for whom it was not prescribed because it can cause severe toxicity.

🗹 Evaluation
• Patient's serum calcium level is normal.
• Patient does not experience injury from drug-induced vitamin D toxicity.
• Patient and family state understanding of drug therapy.

calcium acetate
(KAL-see-um AS-ih-tayt)
Phos-Ex†, Phos-Lo

calcium carbonate
Apo-Cal◆†, Cal-Carb-HD†, Calci-Chew†, Calciday 667†, Calci-Mix†, Calcite 500◆†, Calcium 500◆†, Calcium 600†, Cal-Plus†, Calsan◆†, Caltrate 600◆†, Chooz†, Gencalc 600†, Mallamint†, Nephro-Calci†, Nu-Cal◆†, Os-Cal◆†, Os-Cal 500†, Os-Cal Chewable◆†, Oysco†, Oysco 500 Chewable◆†, Oyst-Cal 500†, Oystercal 500†, Oyster Shell Calcium-500†, Rolaids Calcium Rich†, Super Calcium 1200†, Titralac†, Tums†, Tums E-X†

calcium chloride†
Calciject◆

calcium citrate†
Citrical†, Citrical Liquitabs◆†

calcium glubionate†
Calcium-Sandoz◆, Neo-Calglucon

calcium gluceptate†

calcium gluconate

calcium lactate†

calcium phosphate, dibasic†

calcium phosphate, tribasic
Posture†

Pharmacologic class: calcium supplement
Therapeutic class: therapeutic agent for electrolyte balance, cardiotonic
Pregnancy risk category: C

How supplied

calcium acetate
Contains 253 mg or 12.7 mEq of elemental calcium/g
Tablets: 250 mg†, 500 mg†, 667 mg, 668 mg†, 1,000 mg†
Injection: 0.5 mEq Ca^{++} per ml

calcium carbonate
Contains 400 mg or 20 mEq of elemental calcium/g
Tablets: 650 mg†, 667 mg†, 750 mg†, 1.25 g†, 1.5 g†
Tablets (chewable): 350 mg†, 420 mg†, 500 mg†, 625 mg†, 750 mg†, 850 mg†, 1.25 g†
Capsules: 364 mg†, 1.25 g†
Oral suspension: 1.25 g/5 ml†
Powder packets: 6.5 g (2,400 mg calcium) per packet†
calcium chloride
Contains 270 mg or 13.5 mEq of elemental calcium/g
Injection: 10% solution in 10-ml ampules, vials, and syringes
calcium citrate
Contains 211 mg or 10.6 mEq of elemental calcium/g
Tablets: 950 mg†
Effervescent tablets: 2,376 mg†
calcium glubionate
Contains 64 mg or 3.2 mEq of elemental calcium/g
Syrup: 1.8 g/5 ml
calcium gluceptate
Contains 82 mg or 4.1 mEq of elemental calcium/g
Injection: 1.1 g/5 ml in 5-ml ampules or 10-ml vials
calcium gluconate
Contains 90 mg or 4.5 mEq of elemental calcium/g
Tablets: 500 mg†, 650 mg†, 975 mg†, 1 g†
Injection: 10% solution in 10-ml ampules and vials, 10-ml or 50-ml vials
Pharmacy bulk vials: 100 ml, 200 ml
calcium lactate
Contains 130 mg or 6.5 mEq of elemental calcium/g
Tablets: 325 mg, 650 mg
calcium phosphate, dibasic
Contains 230 mg or 11.5 mEq of elemental calcium/g
Tablets: 468 mg†
calcium phosphate, tribasic
Contains 400 mg or 20 mEq of elemental calcium/g
Tablets: 600 mg†

Pharmacokinetics

Absorption: absorbed actively in duodenum and proximal jejunum and, to lesser extent, in distal part of small intestine after oral administration. Pregnancy and reduced calcium intake may enhance absorption. Vitamin D in active form is required for absorption.

Distribution: enters extracellular fluid and is incorporated rapidly into skeletal tissue. Bone contains 99% of total calcium; 1% is distributed equally between intracellular and extracellular fluids. CSF concentrations are about 50% of serum calcium concentrations.

Metabolism: insignificant.

Excretion: excreted mainly in feces, minimally in urine.

Route	Onset	Peak	Duration
P.O.	Unknown	Unknown	Unknown
I.V.	Immediate	Immediate	0.5-2 hr
I.M.	Unknown	Unknown	Unknown

Pharmacodynamics

Chemical effect: replaces and maintains calcium.

Therapeutic effect: raises blood calcium level.

Indications and dosage

▶ **Hypocalcemic emergency.** *Adults:* 7 to 14 mEq calcium I.V. May be given as 10% calcium gluconate solution, 2% to 10% calcium chloride solution, or 22% calcium gluceptate solution (calcium gluceptate sodium may be given I.M. in emergent situations only). *Children:* 1 to 7 mEq calcium I.V. *Infants:* up to 1 mEq calcium I.V.

▶ **Hypocalcemic tetany.** *Adults:* 4.5 to 16 mEq calcium I.V. Repeated until tetany is controlled. *Children:* 0.5 to 0.7 mEq calcium I.V. t.i.d. or q.i.d. until tetany is controlled. *Neonates:* 2.4 mEq I.V. daily in divided doses.

▶ **Adjunct treatment of cardiac arrest.** *Adults:* 0.027 to 0.054 mEq calcium chloride I.V., 4.5 to 6.3 mEq calcium gluceptate I.V., or 2.3 to 3.7 mEq calcium

gluconate I.V. *Children:* 0.27 mEq/kg calcium chloride I.V. Repeated in 10 minutes if necessary; determine serum calcium levels before administering further doses.

▶ **Adjunct treatment of magnesium intoxication.** *Adults:* initially, 7 mEq I.V. Subsequent doses based on patient's response.

▶ **During exchange transfusions.** *Adults:* 1.35 mEq concurrently with each 100 ml citrated blood. *Neonates:* 0.45 mEq after each 100 ml citrated blood.

▶ **Hyperphosphatemia in end-stage renal failure.** *Adults:* 2 to 4 tablets calcium acetate P.O. with each meal.

▶ **Dietary supplement.** *Adults:* 800 mg to 1.2 g P.O. daily.

Adverse reactions

CNS: tingling sensations, sense of oppression or heat waves (with I.V. use); syncope (with rapid I.V. injection).

CV: mild decrease in blood pressure; vasodilation, bradycardia, *arrhythmias, cardiac arrest* (with rapid I.V. injection).

GI: irritation, hemorrhage, *constipation* (with oral use); chalky taste (with I.V. use); hemorrhage, nausea, vomiting, thirst, abdominal pain (with oral calcium chloride).

GU: hypercalcemia, polyuria, renal calculi.

Skin: local reactions including burning, necrosis, tissue sloughing, cellulitis, soft-tissue calcification (with I.M. use).

Other: pain, irritation (with S.C. injection); *vein irritation* (with I.V. use).

Interactions

Drug-drug. *Atenolol, tetracyclines, fluoroquinolones:* decreased bioavailability of these agents and calcium when oral preparations are taken together. Separate administration times.

Calcium channel blockers: decreased calcium effectiveness. Avoid concomitant use.

Reactions may be *common*, uncommon, *life-threatening*, or COMMON AND LIFE-THREATENING.

Cardiac glycosides: increased digitalis toxicity; administer calcium cautiously (if at all) to digitalized patients.
Sodium polystyrene sulfonate: risk of metabolic acidosis in patients with renal disease. Avoid concomitant use.
Thiazide diuretics: risk of hypercalcemia. Avoid concomitant use.
Drug-food. *Foods containing oxalic acid (rhubarb, spinach), phytic acid (bran, whole cereals), and phosphorus (milk, dairy products):* may interfere with calcium absorption. Tell patient to avoid these foods.

Contraindications and precautions

• Contraindicated in patients with ventricular fibrillation, hypercalcemia, hypophosphatemia, or renal calculi.
• Use all calcium products with extreme caution in patients with sarcoidosis and renal or cardiac disease and in digitalized patients. Use calcium chloride cautiously in patients with cor pulmonale, respiratory acidosis, and respiratory failure.
• Use I.V. route cautiously in children.

NURSING CONSIDERATIONS

Assessment
• Assess patient's serum calcium level before therapy, and reassess frequently thereafter to monitor drug effectiveness. Hypercalcemia may result after large doses in chronic renal failure.
• Be alert for adverse reactions and drug interactions.
• Evaluate patient's and family's knowledge of drug therapy.

Nursing diagnoses
• Altered protection related to calcium deficiency
• Risk for injury related to drug-induced adverse reactions
• Knowledge deficit related to drug therapy

Planning and implementation
• Warm solutions to body temperature before administration.
P.O. use: If GI upset occurs, give oral calcium products 1 to 1½ hours after meals.
• Ensure that doctor specifies calcium form to administer because crash carts usually contain both calcium gluconate and calcium chloride.
• Withhold drug and notify doctor if hypercalcemia occurs. Be prepared to provide emergency supportive care as needed until calcium level returns to normal.
I.V. use: Administer direct injection slowly through small needle into large vein or through I.V. line containing freeflowing, compatible solution at rate not exceeding 1 ml/minute (1.5 mEq/minute) for calcium chloride, 1.5 to 5 ml/minute for calcium gluconate, and 2 ml/minute for calcium gluceptate. Do not use scalp veins in children.
– When administering intermittent infusion, infuse diluted solution through I.V. line containing compatible solution. Maximum rate of 200 mg/minute suggested for calcium gluceptate and calcium gluconate.
– Give calcium chloride I.V. only. When adding to parenteral solutions that contain other additives (especially phosphorus or phosphate), observe closely for precipitate. Use in-line filter.
– After injection, ensure that patient remains recumbent for 15 minutes.
– Monitor ECG when giving calcium I.V. Stop if patient complains of discomfort, and notify doctor.
– Stop drug immediately if extravasation occurs (severe necrosis and tissue sloughing), and change I.V. site before continuing drug.
I.M. use: Give injection in gluteal region in adults; lateral thigh in infants. Only calcium gluceptate can be given via the I.M. route in emergencies when no I.V. route available.

Patient teaching
• Tell patient to take oral calcium 1 to 1½ hours after meals if GI upset occurs.
• Warn patient to avoid oxalic acid (found in rhubarb and spinach), phytic acid (in bran and whole cereals), and phosphorus (in milk and dairy products) because these substances may interfere with calcium absorption.
• Teach patient to recognize and report signs and symptoms of hypercalcemia.
• Stress importance of follow-up care and regular blood samples to monitor calcium level.

☑ **Evaluation**
• Patient's calcium level is normal.
• Patient does not experience injury from calcium-induced adverse reactions.
• Patient and family state understanding of drug therapy.

---

calcium carbonate
(KAL-see-um KAR-buh-nayt)
Alka-Mints†, Amitone†, Calcimax◇, Cal-Sup◇, Chooz†, Effercal-600◇, Equilet†, Mallamint†, Rolaids Calcium Rich†, Titralac†,Titralac Extra Strength†, Titralac Plus†, Tums†, Tums E-X†, Tums Liquid Extra Strength†

Pharmacologic class: calcium supplement
Therapeutic class: therapeutic agent for electrolyte balance, antacid
Pregnancy risk category: NR

How supplied
Calcium carbonate contains 40% calcium; 20 mEq calcium/g.
Tablets (chewable): 350 mg†, 420 mg†, 500 mg†, 750 mg, 850 mg, 1,000 mg, 1,250 mg◇
Tablets: 500 mg†, 600 mg†, 650 mg†, 1,000 mg†, 1,250 mg†
Chewing gum: 500 mg/piece
Oral suspension: 1 g/5 ml†, 250 mg/5 ml
Lozenges: 600 mg†

Pharmacokinetics
Absorption: absorbed actively in small intestine. Pregnancy and reduced calcium intake may enhance absorption. Vitamin D in its active form is required for absorption.
Distribution: enters extracellular fluid and is incorporated rapidly into skeletal tissue. Bone contains 99% of total calcium; 1% is distributed equally between intracellular and extracellular fluids. CSF concentrations are about 50% of serum calcium concentrations.
Metabolism: insignificant.
Excretion: excreted mainly in feces, minimally in urine.

Route	Onset	Peak	Duration
P.O.	≤ 20 min	Unknown	20-60 min (fasting) 3 hr (nonfasting)

Pharmacodynamics
Chemical effect: reduces total acid load in GI tract, elevates gastric pH to reduce pepsin activity, strengthens gastric mucosal barrier, and increases esophageal sphincter tone.
Therapeutic effect: raises blood calcium level and relieves mild gastric discomfort.

Indications and dosage
▶ **Antacid, calcium supplement.**
Adults: 350 mg to 1.5 g P.O. or two pieces of chewing gum 1 hour after meals and h.s. p.r.n.

Adverse reactions
GI: *constipation,* gastric distention, flatulence, rebound hyperacidity, *nausea.*

Interactions
Drug-drug. *Antibiotics (including quinolones and tetracyclines), hydantoins, iron, isoniazid, salicylates:* decreased pharmacologic effect because of possible impaired absorption. Separate administration times.

Reactions may be *common,* uncommon, *life-threatening,* or COMMON AND LIFE-THREATENING.

Enteric-coated drugs: may release prematurely in stomach. Separate doses by at least 1 hour.
Drug-food. *Milk, other foods high in vitamin D:* possible milk-alkali syndrome (headache, confusion, distaste for food, nausea, vomiting, hypercalcemia, hypercalciuria, calcinosis, and hypophosphatemia). Avoid concomitant use.

Contraindications and precautions
• Contraindicated in patients with ventricular fibrillation or hypercalcemia.
• Use cautiously, if at all, in patients with sarcoidosis or renal or cardiac disease and in patients receiving cardiac glycosides.

NURSING CONSIDERATIONS

Assessment
• Assess patient's underlying condition before therapy and regularly thereafter.
• Monitor serum calcium level, especially in patient with mild renal impairment.
• Be alert for adverse reactions and drug interactions.
• Evaluate patient's and family's knowledge of drug therapy.

Nursing diagnoses
• Altered nutrition: less than body requirements related to insufficient calcium intake
• Risk for injury related to calcium-induced hypercalcemia
• Knowledge deficit related to drug therapy

Planning and implementation
• Administer 1 hour after meals as needed.
• Ensure that patient with calcium deficiency is receiving adequate calcium in diet.
Patient teaching
• Advise patient not to take calcium carbonate indiscriminately or to switch antacids without consulting doctor.
• Tell patient to take drug 1 hour after meals and at bedtime, as needed.

Evaluation
• Patient's symptoms are alleviated.
• Patient's blood calcium level is normal.
• Patient and family state understanding of drug therapy.

---

calcium polycarbophil
(KAL-see-um pah-lee-KAR-boh-fil)
Equalactin†, Fiberall†, FiberCon†, Fiber-Lax†, FiberNorm†, Mitrolan†

Pharmacologic class: hydrophilic agent
Therapeutic class: bulk laxative, antidiarrheal
Pregnancy risk category: NR

How supplied
Tablets: 500 mg†, 625 mg†, 1,250 mg†
Tablets (chewable): 500 mg†

Pharmacokinetics
Absorption: none.
Distribution: none.
Metabolism: none.
Excretion: excreted in feces.

Route	Onset	Peak	Duration
P.O.	12-24 hr	≤ 3 days	Varies

Pharmacodynamics
Chemical effect: as laxative, absorbs water and expands to increase bulk and moisture content of stool, which encourages peristalsis and bowel movement. As antidiarrheal, absorbs free fecal water, thereby producing formed stools.
Therapeutic effect: relieves constipation; relieves diarrhea caused by irritable bowel syndrome.

Indications and dosage
▶ **Constipation.** *Adults and children age 12 and over:* 1 g P.O. q.i.d. as required. Maximum dosage is 6 g daily. *Children ages 6 to 12:* 500 mg P.O. one to three times daily as required. Maximum dosage is 3 g daily. *Children ages 2 to 6:* 500 mg P.O. b.i.d. as required. Maximum

---

dosage is 1.5 g daily. Use must be directed by doctor.

▶ **Diarrhea associated with irritable bowel syndrome; acute nonspecific diarrhea.** *Adults and children age 12 and over:* 1 g P.O. q.i.d. as required. Maximum dosage is 6 g daily. *Children ages 6 to 12:* 500 mg P.O. t.i.d. as required. Maximum dosage is 3 g daily. *Children ages 2 to 6:* 500 mg P.O. b.i.d. as required. Maximum dosage is 1.5 g daily. Use must be directed by doctor.

Adverse reactions

GI: abdominal fullness, increased flatus, intestinal obstruction.
Other: laxative dependence (with long-term or excessive use).

Interactions

Drug-drug. *Tetracyclines:* impaired absorption of tetracyclines. Avoid use together.

Contraindications and precautions

• Contraindicated in patients with signs of GI obstruction.

NURSING CONSIDERATIONS

▨ Assessment
• Assess patient's bowel condition.
• Before administering drug for constipation, determine if patient has adequate fluid intake, exercise, and diet.
• Monitor drug effectiveness by evaluating frequency and characteristics of patient's stools.
• Be alert for adverse reactions and drug interactions.
• Evaluate patient's and family's knowledge of drug therapy.

▣ Nursing diagnoses
• Constipation related to underlying condition
• Diarrhea related to irritable bowel syndrome
• Knowledge deficit related to drug therapy

▧ Planning and implementation
• Give drug with full glass of water when used to treat constipation. Do not give drug with water when used for diarrhea.
• Know that dose may be repeated every 30 minutes, if ordered, for severe diarrhea, but maximum daily dosage should not be exceeded.
• Do not give to patient with signs of GI obstruction.
Patient teaching
• Advise patient to chew Equalactin or Mitrolan tablets thoroughly before swallowing and to drink a full glass of water with each dose. Tell patient *not* to drink with water when used as antidiarrheal.
• Teach patient about dietary sources of bulk, including bran and other cereals, fresh fruit, and vegetables.
• For severe diarrhea, advise patient to repeat dose every 30 minutes, but tell him not to exceed maximum daily dosage.

▨ Evaluation
• Patient's elimination pattern returns to normal.
• Patient and family state understanding of drug therapy.

candesartan cilexetil
(kan-dih-SAR-ten se-LEKS-ih-til)
Atacand

Pharmacologic class: angiotensin II receptor antagonist
Therapeutic class: antihypertensive
Pregnancy risk category: C (D in second and third trimesters)

How supplied

Tablets: 4 mg, 8 mg, 16 mg, 32 mg

Pharmacokinetics:

Absorption: absolute bioavailability is approximately 15%.
Distribution: greater than 99% bound to plasma protein and does not penetrate RBCs.

Metabolism: rapidly and completely bioactivated by ester hydrolysis to candesartan.
Excretion: approximately 33% is recovered in the urine (26% unchanged) and 67% in the feces. *Half-life:* 9 hours.

Route	Onset	Peak	Duration
P.O.	Unknown	3-4 hr	24 hr

Pharmacodynamics

Chemical effect: inhibits the vasoconstrictive action of angiotensin II by blocking the angiotensin II receptor on the surface of vascular smooth muscle and other tissue cells.
Therapeutic effect: vasodilates blood vessels to decrease blood pressure.

Indications & dosages

▶ **Treatment of hypertension (used alone or in combination with other antihypertensive agents):** *Adults:* initially16 mg P.O. once daily when used as monotherapy; usual dosage range is 8 to 32 mg P.O. daily as a single dose or divided b.i.d.

Adverse reactions

CNS: dizziness, fatigue, headache.
CV: chest pain, peripheral edema.
EENT: pharyngitis, rhinitis, sinusitis.
GI: abdominal pain, diarrhea, nausea, vomiting.
GU: albuminuria.
Musculoskeletal: arthralgia, back pain.
Respiratory: coughing, bronchitis, upper respiratory tract infection.

Interactions

None reported.

Contraindications and precautions

• Contraindicated in those with hypersensitivity to drug or its components.
• Use cautiously in patients whose renal function depends on the renin-angiotensin-aldosterone system (such as patients with heart failure) due to risk of oliguria and progressive azotemia with acute renal failure or death.
• Use cautiously in patients who are volume- or salt-depleted due to risk of symptomatic hypotension.
• Know that drugs that act directly on the renin-angiotension system (such as candesartan) can cause fetal and neonatal morbidity and death when given to pregnant women. These problems have not been detected when exposure has been limited to first trimester. If pregnancy is suspected, notify doctor because drug should be discontinued.

NURSING CONSIDERATIONS

⚕ Assessment

• Monitor patient's electrolytes and assess patient for volume or salt depletion (vigorous diuretic use) prior to initiation of drug therapy.
• Carefully monitor therapeutic response and the occurrence of adverse reactions especially in elderly patients and patients with renal impairment.
• Evaluate patient's and family's knowledge of drug therapy.

🔧 Nursing diagnoses

• Decreased cardiac output related to risk for symptomatic hypotension in volume- or salt-depleted patients
• Risk for fluid volume imbalance in patients with impaired renal function related to drug-induced oliguria
• Knowledge deficit related to drug therapy

▷ Planning and implementation

• Be certain patient is adequately hydrated before starting therapy.
• Observe patient for hypotension. If it occurs after a dose of candesartan, place patient in supine position and, if necessary, give an I.V. infusion of normal saline, as ordered.
• Know that most of antihypertensive effect is present within 2 weeks. Maximal antihypertensive effect is obtained within

4 to 6 weeks. Diuretic may be added if blood pressure is not controlled by drug alone.

• Be aware that drug cannot be removed by hemodialysis.

Patient teaching

• Advise female patient of childbearing age of risk of second and third trimester exposure to drug. If pregnancy is suspected, tell her to notify doctor immediately.

• Advise breast-feeding patient about risk for adverse drug effects on infant and need to either stop breast-feeding or discontinue drug.

• Instruct patient to store drug at room temperature and to keep container tightly sealed.

• Inform patient to promptly report adverse reactions.

• Instruct patient to take drug exactly as directed.

• Tell patient that drug may be taken without regard to meals.

☑ **Evaluation**

• Patient's volume or salt depletion is corrected so that symptomatic hypotension does not occur.

• Patient maintains fluid balance.

• Patient and family state understanding of drug therapy.

---

capreomycin sulfate
(kap-ree-oh-MIGH-sin SUL-fayt)
Capastat

Pharmacologic class: polypeptide antibiotic
Therapeutic class: antitubercular agent
Pregnancy risk category: C

How supplied
Injection: 1 g/vial

Pharmacokinetics
Absorption: unknown.
Distribution: unknown.
Metabolism: unknown.

Excretion: excreted primarily unchanged in urine. *Half-life:* 4 to 6 hours.

Route	Onset	Peak	Duration
I.M.	Unknown	1-2 hr	Unknown

Pharmacodynamics
Chemical effect: unknown.
Therapeutic effect: helps eradicate tuberculosis.

Indications and dosage
▶ **Adjunct treatment of tuberculosis.**
Adults: 15 mg/kg/day up to 1 g I.M. daily injected deeply into large muscle mass for 60 to 120 days; then 1 g two to three times weekly for 18 to 24 months. Maximum dosage should not exceed 20 mg/kg/day. Must be given with another antitubercular drug. Dose must be reduced in renal function impairment.

Adverse reactions
CNS: headache, *neuromuscular blockade.*
EENT: ototoxicity (tinnitus, vertigo, hearing loss).
GU: *nephrotoxicity* (elevated BUN and nonprotein nitrogen levels, casts, RBC counts, leukocytes; tubular necrosis; proteinuria; decreased creatinine clearance).
Hematologic: eosinophilia, leukocytosis, leukopenia, *thrombocytopenia.*
Hepatic: hepatotoxicity.
Metabolic: hypokalemia, alkalosis.
Other: *hypersensitivity reactions;* pain, induration, excessive bleeding, sterile abscesses (at injection site).

Interactions
Drug-drug. *Nephrotoxic or ototoxic drugs (such as aminoglycosides, colistin, polymyxin B, vancomycin):* increased risk of additive toxicity. Avoid concomitant use.

Contraindications and precautions
• Contraindicated in patients with hypersensitivity to drug.

Reactions may be *common,* uncommon, *life-threatening*, or COMMON AND LIFE-THREATENING.

• Use with extreme caution in patients receiving other ototoxic or nephrotoxic drugs.
• Use cautiously in patients with impaired renal function, hearing impairment, or history of allergies and in pregnant or breast-feeding women.
• Safety of drug has not been established in children.

NURSING CONSIDERATIONS

⚕ Assessment
• Assess patient's respiratory status before therapy.
• Assess patient's renal function and hearing before therapy and regularly thereafter.
• Monitor drug effectiveness by regularly assessing for improved pulmonary status and by evaluating results of culture and sensitivity tests.
• Be alert for adverse reactions and drug interactions.
• Evaluate patient's and family's knowledge of drug therapy.

🔀 Nursing diagnoses
• Infection related to pulmonary tuberculosis
• Sensory/perceptual alterations (auditory) related to drug-induced ototoxicity
• Knowledge deficit related to drug therapy

🔀 Planning and implementation
• Give deep I.M. injection to minimize local reactions. Apply ice to injection site as needed for pain. Never give drug I.V. because this may cause neuromuscular blockade.
• Be aware that straw- or dark-colored solution after reconstitution does not indicate loss in potency. Do not administer solutions that contain precipitate.
• Notify doctor if patient complains of tinnitus, vertigo, or hearing impairment or if renal function decreases. Dosage must be reduced in renal impairment.

• Be aware that capreomycin is considered a "second-line" drug in treatment of tuberculosis and should always be administered with other antitubercular agents to prevent development of resistant organisms.

Patient teaching
• Teach family member or friend how to administer I.M. injection.
• Tell patient to notify doctor promptly of tinnitus, vertigo, or hearing impairment.
• Warn patient that injection may be painful. Suggest applying ice to injection site as needed for pain.

☑ Evaluation
• Patient is free from pulmonary tuberculosis.
• Patient's auditory function does not diminish.
• Patient and family state understanding of drug therapy.

captopril
(KAP-toh-pril)
Apo-Capto♦, Capoten, Novo-Captopril♦

Pharmacologic class: ACE inhibitor
Therapeutic class: antihypertensive, adjunct treatment of heart failure and diabetic nephropathy
Pregnancy risk category: C (D in second and third trimesters)

How supplied
Tablets: 12.5 mg, 25 mg, 50 mg, 100 mg

Pharmacokinetics
Absorption: absorbed through GI tract; food may reduce absorption by up to 40%.
Distribution: distributed into most body tissues except CNS; 25% to 30% protein-bound.
Metabolism: about 50% metabolized in liver.

Excretion: excreted primarily in urine, minimally in feces. *Half-life:* less than 2 hours.

Route	Onset	Peak	Duration
P.O.	15-60 min	30-90 min	6-12 hr

Pharmacodynamics

Chemical effect: thought to inhibit ACE, preventing conversion of angiotensin I to angiotensin II. Reduced formation of angiotensin II decreases peripheral arterial resistance, thus decreasing aldosterone secretion.
Therapeutic effect: reduces sodium and water retention, lowers blood pressure, and helps improve renal function adversely affected by diabetes.

Indications and dosage

▶ **Hypertension.** *Adults:* initially, 25 mg P.O. b.i.d. or t.i.d. If blood pressure isn't controlled in 1 to 2 weeks, dosage increased to 50 mg b.i.d. or t.i.d. If not controlled after another 1 to 2 weeks, expect a thiazide diuretic to be added to regimen. If further blood pressure reduction is necessary, dosage may be raised to as high as 150 mg t.i.d. while continuing diuretic. Maximum dosage is 450 mg daily.
▶ **Heart failure; to reduce risk of death and to slow development of heart failure after MI.** *Adults:* 6.25 to 12.5 mg P.O. t.i.d. initially. Gradually increased to 50 to 100 mg t.i.d. as needed. Maximum daily dosage is 450 mg.
▶ **Diabetic nephropathy.** *Adults:* 25 mg P.O. t.i.d.

Adverse reactions

CNS: dizziness, fainting.
CV: *tachycardia, hypotension,* angina pectoris, *heart failure,* pericarditis.
GI: anorexia, *dysgeusia.*
GU: *proteinuria, nephrotic syndrome, membranous glomerulopathy, renal failure* (in patients with preexisting renal disease or those receiving high dosages), urinary frequency.

Hematologic: *leukopenia, agranulocytosis, pancytopenia, thrombocytopenia.*
Hepatic: transient increase in hepatic enzymes.
Respiratory: dry, persistent, tickling, nonproductive cough.
Skin: urticarial rash, maculopapular rash, pruritus.
Other: fever, *angioedema of face and extremities,* hyperkalemia.

Interactions

Drug-drug. *Antacids:* decreased captopril effect. Separate administration times.
Cardiac glycosides: may increase serum digoxin concentration by 15% to 30%.
Diuretics, other antihypertensives: risk of excessive hypotension. Diuretic may need to be discontinued or captopril dosage lowered.
Insulin, oral antidiabetic agents: risk of hypoglycemia when captopril therapy is initiated. Monitor closely.
Lithium: increased lithium levels and symptoms of toxicity may occur. Monitor patient closely.
NSAIDs: may reduce antihypertensive effect. Monitor blood pressure.
Potassium supplements, potassium-sparing diuretics: increased risk of hyperkalemia. Avoid these agents unless hypokalemic blood levels are confirmed.
Drug-food. *Any food:* may reduce absorption. Administer drug 1 hour before meals.

Contraindications and precautions

• Contraindicated in patients with hypersensitivity to drug or other ACE inhibitors.
• Use with extreme caution, if at all, in pregnant women. Drug usually is discontinued if pregnancy occurs.
• Use cautiously in patients with impaired renal function or serious autoimmune disease (particularly systemic lupus erythematosus); in patients exposed to other drugs known to affect WBC counts or immune response; and in breast-feeding women.

Reactions may be *common*, uncommon, **life-threatening**, or COMMON AND LIFE-THREATENING.

• Safety of drug has not been established in children.

NURSING CONSIDERATIONS

℞ Assessment
• Assess patient's underlying condition before therapy and regularly thereafter.
• Monitor blood pressure and pulse rate frequently.
• Monitor WBC and differential counts before therapy, every 2 weeks for first 3 months of therapy, and periodically thereafter, as ordered.
• Monitor serum potassium level and renal function (BUN and creatinine clearance levels, urinalysis), as ordered.
• Be alert for adverse reactions and drug interactions.
• Evaluate patient's and family's knowledge of drug therapy.

⊡ Nursing diagnoses
• Risk for injury related to patient's underlying condition
• Altered protection related to drug-induced blood disorder
• Knowledge deficit related to drug therapy

⊵ Planning and implementation
• Administer 1 hour before meals because food may reduce absorption.
• Because antacids decrease drug's effect, separate administration times.
• Withhold dose and notify doctor if patient develops fever, sore throat, leukopenia, hypotension, or tachycardia.
• Notify doctor of abnormal laboratory studies.
Patient teaching
• Instruct patient to take drug 1 hour before meals; food in GI tract may reduce absorption.
• Inform patient that light-headedness can occur, especially during first few days of therapy. Tell patient to rise slowly to minimize this effect and to report symptoms to doctor. Tell patient who ex-

periences syncope to stop taking drug and call doctor immediately.
• Tell patient to use caution in hot weather and during exercise. Inadequate fluid intake, vomiting, diarrhea, and excessive perspiration can lead to light-headedness and syncope.
• Advise patient to report signs of infection, such as fever and sore throat.
• Tell female patient to notify doctor if pregnancy occurs. Drug will be discontinued.

☑ Evaluation
• Patient's underlying condition improves.
• Patient's WBC and differential counts are normal.
• Patient and family state understanding of drug therapy.

carbamazepine
(kar-buh-MEH-zuh-peen)
Apo-Carbamazepine♦, Atretol, Carbamazepine Chewable Tablets, Carbatrol, Epitol, Novocarbamaz♦, Tegretol, Tegretol CR♦, Tegretol-XR

Pharmacologic class: iminostilbene derivative
Therapeutic class: anticonvulsant, analgesic
Pregnancy risk category: D

How supplied
Tablets: 200 mg
Tablets (chewable): 100 mg
Tablets (extended-release): 100 mg, 200 mg, 400 mg
Capsules (extended-release): 200 mg, 300 mg
Oral suspension: 100 mg/5 ml

Pharmacokinetics
Absorption: absorbed slowly from GI tract.
Distribution: distributed widely throughout body; about 75% protein-bound.

Metabolism: metabolized by liver to active metabolite; may also induce its own metabolism.
Excretion: excreted in urine (70%) and feces (30%). *Half-life:* 25 to 65 hours with single dosing; 8 to 29 hours with chronic dosing.

Route	Onset	Peak	Duration
P.O.	Hrs-days (suspension) 4-12 hr (tablets)	1.5 hr	Unknown

Pharmacodynamics

Chemical effect: may stabilize neuronal membranes and limit seizure activity by increasing efflux or decreasing influx of sodium ions across cell membranes in motor cortex during generation of nerve impulses.
Therapeutic effect: prevents seizure activity; eliminates pain caused by trigeminal neuralgia.

Indications and dosage

▶ **Generalized tonic-clonic and complex partial seizures, mixed seizure patterns.** *Adults and children over age 12:* initially, 200 mg P.O. b.i.d. for tablets or 1 teaspoon of suspension P.O. q.i.d. May be increased at weekly intervals by 200 mg P.O. daily, in divided doses at 6- to 8-hour intervals. Adjusted to minimum effective level when control is achieved. Maximum daily dosage is 1 g in children ages 12 to 15, or 1.2 g in patients over age 15. *Children ages 6 to 12:* initially, 100 mg P.O. b.i.d. or ½ teaspoon of suspension P.O. q.i.d. Increased at weekly intervals by 100 mg P.O. daily. Maximum daily dosage is 1 g.
▶ **Trigeminal neuralgia.** *Adults:* initially, 100 mg P.O. b.i.d. or ½ teaspoon of suspension P.O. q.i.d. with meals. Increased by 100 mg q 12 hours for tablets or ½ teaspoon of suspension q.i.d. until pain is relieved. Maximum daily dosage is 1.2 g. Maintenance dosage is 200 to 1,200 mg P.O. daily. Decrease dose to minimum effective level or discontinue drug at least once q 3 months.

Adverse reactions

CNS: *dizziness, vertigo, drowsiness,* fatigue, *ataxia,* **worsening of seizures** (usually in patients with mixed seizure disorders, including atypical absence seizures).
CV: *heart failure,* hypertension, hypotension, aggravation of coronary artery disease.
EENT: conjunctivitis, dry mouth and pharynx, blurred vision, diplopia, nystagmus.
GI: *nausea, vomiting,* abdominal pain, diarrhea, anorexia, stomatitis, glossitis.
GU: urinary frequency, urine retention, impotence, albuminuria, glycosuria, elevated BUN.
Hematologic: *aplastic anemia, agranulocytosis,* eosinophilia, leukocytosis, *thrombocytopenia.*
Hepatic: abnormal liver function test results, *hepatitis.*
Respiratory: pulmonary hypersensitivity.
Skin: rash, urticaria, erythema multiforme, *Stevens-Johnson syndrome.*
Other: excessive sweating, fever, chills, water intoxication.

Interactions

Drug-drug. *Cimetidine, danazol, diltiazem, macrolides (such as erythromycin), isoniazid, propoxyphene, valproic acid, verapamil:* may increase carbamazepine blood levels. Use cautiously.
Doxycycline, haloperidol, oral contraceptives, phenytoin, theophylline, warfarin: carbamazepine may decrease blood levels of these drugs. Monitor for decreased effect.
Lithium: increased CNS toxicity of lithium. Avoid concomitant use.
MAO inhibitors: increased depressant and anticholinergic effects. Don't use together.

Reactions may be *common,* uncommon, *life-threatening,* or COMMON AND LIFE-THREATENING.

Phenobarbital, phenytoin, primidone: may decrease carbamazepine levels. Monitor for decreased effect.

Contraindications and precautions

• Contraindicated in patients with previous bone marrow suppression or hypersensitivity to drug or tricyclic antidepressants and in those who have taken an MAO inhibitor within 14 days of therapy.
• Breast-feeding should be discontinued if drug must be used in breast-feeding women.
• Use cautiously in patients with mixed seizure disorders (they may experience increased incidence of seizures, usually atypical absence or generalized) and in pregnant women.
• Safety of drug has not been established in children under age 6.

NURSING CONSIDERATIONS

⚖ Assessment

• Assess patient's seizure disorder or trigeminal neuralgia before therapy and regularly thereafter.
• Obtain baseline determinations of urinalysis, BUN level, liver function, CBC, platelet and reticulocyte counts, and serum iron level. Reassess regularly, as ordered.
• Monitor blood levels and effects closely (therapeutic carbamazepine blood level is 4 to 12 mcg/ml).
• Be alert for adverse reactions and drug interactions.
• Evaluate patient's and family's knowledge of drug therapy.

⊞ Nursing diagnoses

• Risk for injury related to seizure disorder
• Pain related to trigeminal neuralgia
• Knowledge deficit related to drug therapy

⊠ Planning and implementation

• Administer drug in divided doses, when possible, to maintain consistent blood levels.
• Administer drug with food to minimize GI distress.
• Shake oral suspension well before measuring dose.
• When administering by nasogastric tube, mix dose with equal volume of water, 0.9% NaCl, or D_5W. Flush tube with 100 ml of diluent after administering dose.
• Never discontinue suddenly when treating seizures or status epilepticus. Notify doctor immediately if adverse reactions occur. Expect him to increase dosage gradually to minimize adverse reactions.

Patient teaching

• Tell patient to take drug with food to minimize GI distress.
• Tell patient to keep tablets in original container, tightly closed, and away from moisture. Some formulations may harden when exposed to excess moisture, resulting in decreased bioavailability and loss of seizure control.
• Inform patient with trigeminal neuralgia that doctor may attempt to decrease dosage or withdraw drug every 3 months.
• Tell patient to notify doctor immediately of fever, sore throat, mouth ulcers, or easy bruising or bleeding.
• Warn patient that drug may cause mild to moderate dizziness and drowsiness when first taken. Advise patient to avoid hazardous activities until effects disappear (usually within 3 to 4 days).
• Advise patient to have periodic ophthalmic examinations.

▨ Evaluation

• Patient remains free from seizure activity.
• Patient reports pain relief.
• Patient and family state understanding of drug therapy.

carbenicillin indanyl sodium
(kar-ben-ih-SIL-in in-DAN-il SOH-dee-um)
Geocillin, Geopen Oral♦

Pharmacologic class: extended-spectrum penicillin, alpha-carboxy-penicillin
Therapeutic class: antibiotic
Pregnancy risk category: B

How supplied
Tablets: 382 mg

Pharmacokinetics
Absorption: absorbed partially (30% to 40%) from GI tract.
Distribution: distributed widely, but concentrations insufficient to treat systemic infections; 30% to 60% protein-bound.
Metabolism: hydrolyzed rapidly in plasma to carbenicillin, which is partially metabolized.
Excretion: excreted primarily (79% to 99%) in urine by renal tubular secretion and glomerular filtration. *Half-life:* about 1 hour.

Route	Onset	Peak	Duration
P.O.	Unknown	≤ 30 min	≤ 6 hr

Pharmacodynamics
Chemical effect: inhibits cell-wall synthesis during microorganism multiplication; bacteria resist carbenicillin by producing penicillinases—enzymes that hydrolyze its active form.
Therapeutic effect: kills susceptible bacteria (many gram-negative aerobic and anaerobic bacilli; some gram-positive aerobic and anaerobic bacilli; and many gram-positive and gram-negative aerobic cocci).

Indications and dosage
▶ **Urinary tract infection and prostatitis caused by susceptible strains of gram-negative organisms.** *Adults:* 382 to 764 mg P.O. q.i.d.

Adverse reactions
GI: *nausea,* vomiting, *diarrhea, flatulence, abdominal cramps, unpleasant taste.*
Hematologic: leukopenia, neutropenia, eosinophilia, *hemolytic anemia,* thrombocytopenia.
Other: hypersensitivity reactions (rash, chills, fever, urticaria, pruritus, *anaphylaxis*), overgrowth of nonsusceptible organisms.

Interactions
Drug-food. *Any food:* may interfere with absorption. Give drug 1 to 2 hours before or 2 to 3 hours after meals.

Contraindications and precautions
• Contraindicated in patients with hypersensitivity to drug or other penicillins.
• Use cautiously in patients with other drug allergies, especially to cephalosporins (possible cross-sensitivity), and in pregnant or breast-feeding women.
• Safety of drug has not been established in children.

NURSING CONSIDERATIONS

⚄ Assessment
• Assess patient's infection before and during therapy.
• Be alert for adverse reactions.
• Monitor patient's hydration status if adverse GI reactions occur.
• Evaluate patient's and family's knowledge of drug therapy.

⚄ Nursing diagnoses
• Infection related to bacteria
• Risk for fluid volume deficit related to drug-induced GI adverse reactions
• Knowledge deficit related to drug therapy

⚄ Planning and implementation
• Ask patient about allergic reactions to penicillin before administering drug, (negative history is no guarantee against future allergic reaction).

• Obtain specimen for culture and sensitivity tests before first dose. Therapy may begin pending results.

• Know that drug is used only when patient's creatinine clearance is at least 10 ml/minute.

• Give 1 to 2 hours before or 2 to 3 hours after meals because food may interfere with absorption.

• Know that urine glucose determinations may be false-positive with copper sulfate tests (Benedict's solution, Clinitest); glucose enzymatic tests (Diastix or Chemstrip uG) are not affected.

• Be aware that drug also may interfere with direct results of Coombs' test and certain tests for serum uric acid.

Patient teaching

• Tell patient to take drug exactly as prescribed, even after he feels better.

• Tell patient to notify doctor of rash, fever, or chills. A rash is most common allergic reaction.

• Warn patient never to use leftover drug for a new illness or to share it with anyone.

• Advise patient to take drug 1 to 2 hours before or 2 to 3 hours after meals.

☑ **Evaluation**

• Patient is free from infection.

• Patient maintains adequate hydration.

• Patient and family state understanding of drug therapy.

---

carbidopa-levodopa
(kar-bih-DOH-puh LEE-vuh-doh-puh)
Sinemet, Sinemet CR

Pharmacologic class: decarboxylase inhibitor-dopamine precursor combination
Therapeutic class: antiparkinsonian agent
Pregnancy risk category: NR

How supplied

Tablets: carbidopa 10 mg with levodopa 100 mg (Sinemet 10-100), carbidopa 25 mg with levodopa 100 mg (Sinemet 25-100), carbidopa 25 mg with levodopa 250 mg (Sinemet 25-250)
Tablets (extended-release): carbidopa 25 mg with levodopa 100 mg, carbidopa 50 mg with levodopa 200 mg, (Sinemet CR)

Pharmacokinetics

Absorption: 40% to 70% of dose absorbed.
Distribution: distributed widely in body tissues except CNS.
Metabolism: carbidopa is not metabolized extensively. It inhibits metabolism of levodopa in GI tract, thus increasing its absorption from GI tract and its concentration in plasma.
Excretion: 30% of dose excreted unchanged in urine within 24 hours. When given with carbidopa, amount of levodopa excreted unchanged in urine is increased by about 6%. *Half-life:* 1 to 2 hours.

Route	Onset	Peak	Duration
P.O.	Unknown (regular-release)	40 min	Unknown
	2.5 hr (extended-release)		

Pharmacodynamics

Chemical effect: unknown for levodopa. Thought to be decarboxylated to dopamine, countering depletion of striatal dopamine in extrapyramidal centers. Carbidopa inhibits peripheral decarboxylation of levodopa without affecting levodopa's metabolism within CNS. Therefore, more levodopa is available to be decarboxylated to dopamine in brain.
Therapeutic effect: improves voluntary movement.

Indications and dosage

▶ **Idiopathic Parkinson's disease, postencephalitic parkinsonism, and symptomatic parkinsonism resulting from carbon monoxide or manganese intoxi-**

---

cation. *Adults:* 1 tablet of 25 mg carbidopa/100 mg levodopa or carbidopa 10 mg/levodopa 100 mg P.O. daily t.i.d. followed by increase of 1 tablet daily or every other day as necessary to maximum daily dosage of 8 tablets. 25 mg carbidopa/250 mg levodopa or 10 mg carbidopa/100 mg levodopa tablets are substituted as required to obtain maximum response. Optimum daily dosage must be determined by careful titration for each patient. Patients treated with conventional tablets may receive extended-release tablets; dosage is calculated on current levodopa intake. Initially, extended-release tablets given equal to 10% more levodopa per day; increased as needed and tolerated to 30% more levodopa per day. Administered in divided doses at intervals of 4 to 8 hours.

Adverse reactions

CNS: *choreiform, dystonic, dyskinetic movements; involuntary grimacing, head movements, myoclonic body jerks, ataxia,* tremors, muscle twitching; bradykinetic episodes; psychiatric disturbances, memory loss, nervousness, anxiety, disturbing dreams, euphoria, malaise, fatigue; severe depression, suicidal tendencies, dementia, delirium, hallucinations (may necessitate reduction or withdrawal of drug).
CV: *orthostatic hypotension,* **cardiac irregularities,** flushing, hypertension, phlebitis.
EENT: blepharospasm, blurred vision, diplopia, mydriasis or miosis, widening of palpebral fissures, activation of latent Horner's syndrome, oculogyric crises, nasal discharge, excessive salivation.
GI: dry mouth, bitter taste, nausea, vomiting, anorexia, weight loss at start of therapy; constipation; flatulence; diarrhea; epigastric pain; bleeding (rare).
GU: urinary frequency, urine retention, urinary incontinence, darkened urine, excessive and inappropriate sexual behavior, priapism.
Hematologic: *hemolytic anemia.*
Hepatic: hepatotoxicity.

Other: dark perspiration, hyperventilation, hiccups.

Interactions

Drug-drug. *Antihypertensives:* additive hypotensive effects. Use together cautiously.
MAO inhibitors: risk of severe hypertension. Avoid concomitant use.
Papaverine, phenytoin: antagonism of antiparkinsonian actions. Don't use together.
Phenothiazines, other antipsychotics: may antagonize antiparkinsonian actions. Use together cautiously.
Drug-food. *Foods high in protein:* decreased absorption of levodopa. Don't give levodopa with high-protein foods.

Contraindications and precautions

• Contraindicated in patients with acute angle-closure glaucoma, melanoma, undiagnosed skin lesions, or hypersensitivity to drug; within 14 days of MAO inhibitor therapy; and in breast-feeding women.
• Use with extreme caution, if at all, in pregnant women.
• Use cautiously in patients with severe CV, renal, hepatic, endocrine, or pulmonary disorders; history of peptic ulcer; psychiatric illness; MI with residual arrhythmias; bronchial asthma; emphysema; or well-controlled, chronic open-angle glaucoma.
• Safety of drug has not been established in children.

NURSING CONSIDERATIONS

Assessment
• Assess patient's underlying condition before therapy and regularly thereafter; therapeutic response usually follows each dose and disappears within 5 hours but varies considerably.
• Be alert for adverse reactions and drug interactions.
• Immediately report muscle twitching and blepharospasm (twitching of eye-

lids), which may be early signs of drug overdose.

• Know that patients receiving long-term therapy should be tested regularly for diabetes and acromegaly and should have periodic tests of liver, renal, and hematopoietic function, as ordered.

• Evaluate patient's and family's knowledge of drug therapy.

🕮 Nursing diagnoses
• Impaired physical mobility related to underlying parkinsonian syndrome
• Altered thought processes related to drug-induced CNS adverse reactions
• Knowledge deficit related to drug therapy

⧉ Planning and implementation
• Know that if patient is being treated with levodopa, drug should be discontinued at least 8 hours before starting carbidopa-levodopa.
• Administer drug with food to minimize adverse GI reactions.
• Be aware that dosage will be adjusted according to patient's response and tolerance.
• Withhold dose and notify doctor if significant changes in vital signs or mental status occur. Reduced dosage or discontinuation may be necessary.
• Depending on reagent and test method used, expect possible false-positive increases in levels of uric acid, urine ketones, urine catecholamines, and urine vanillylmandelic acid.
• False-positive tests for urine glucose can occur if reagents using copper sulfate are used; false-negative results can occur with tests that use glucose enzymatic methods. An accurate measure can be obtained if paper strip is only partially immersed in urine sample. Urine will migrate up strip, as with an ascending chromatographic system. Read only top of strip.
Patient teaching
• Tell patient to take drug with food to minimize GI upset.

• Caution patient and family not to increase dosage without doctor's orders.
• Warn patient of possible dizziness and orthostatic hypotension, especially at start of therapy. Tell patient to change position slowly and dangle legs before getting out of bed. Elastic stockings may control this adverse reaction in some patients.
• Instruct patient to report adverse reactions and therapeutic effects.
• Inform patient that pyridoxine (vitamin B_6) does not reverse beneficial effects of carbidopa-levodopa. Multivitamins can be taken without losing control of symptoms.

☑ Evaluation
• Patient exhibits improved mobility with reduction of muscular rigidity and tremor.
• Patient remains mentally alert.
• Patient and family state understanding of drug therapy.

---

carboplatin
(KAR-boh-plat-in)
Paraplatin, Paraplatin-AQ♦

Pharmacologic class: alkylating agent (cell cycle–phase nonspecific)
Therapeutic class: antineoplastic
Pregnancy risk category: D

How supplied
Injection: 50-mg, 150-mg, 450-mg vials

Pharmacokinetics
Absorption: not applicable with I.V. administration.
Distribution: volume distributed is approximately equal to that of total body water; no significant protein binding occurs.
Metabolism: hydrolyzed to form hydroxylated and aquated species.

Excretion: 65% excreted by kidneys within 12 hours, 71% within 24 hours.
Half-life: 5 hours.

Route	Onset	Peak	Duration
I.V.	Unknown	Unknown	Unknown

Pharmacodynamics

Chemical effect: probably produces cross-linking of DNA strands. Cell cycle–phase nonspecific.
Therapeutic effect: impairs ovarian cancer cells.

Indications and dosage

▶ **Palliative treatment of ovarian cancer.** *Adults:* 360 mg/m^2 I.V. on day 1 q 4 weeks; doses should not be repeated until platelet count exceeds 100,000/mm^3 and neutrophil count exceeds 2,000/mm^3. Subsequent doses are based on blood counts.
For patients with renal dysfunction: starting dose is 250 mg/m^2 in patients with creatinine clearance of 41 to 59 ml/minute or 200 mg/m^2 in those with creatinine clearance of 16 to 40 ml/minute. Recommended dosage adjustments are not available for patients with creatinine clearance of 15 ml/minute or less.

Adverse reactions

CNS: dizziness, confusion, peripheral neuropathy, ototoxicity, central neurotoxicity, *CVA.*
CV: *cardiac failure, embolism.*
GI: constipation, diarrhea, *nausea, vomiting.*
GU: increased BUN and creatinine levels.
Hematologic: THROMBOCYTOPENIA, *leukopenia,* NEUTROPENIA, *anemia,* BONE MARROW SUPPRESSION.
Hepatic: hepatotoxicity, increased AST or alkaline phosphatase levels.
Other: alopecia; *hypersensitivity reactions.*

Interactions

Drug-drug. *Bone marrow depressants, including radiation therapy:* increased

hematologic toxicity. Monitor patient closely.
Nephrotoxic agents: enhanced nephrotoxicity of carboplatin. Monitor patient closely.

Contraindications and precautions

• Contraindicated in patients with hypersensitivity to cisplatin, platinum-containing compounds, or mannitol or with severe bone marrow suppression or bleeding.
• Drug should not be used during pregnancy if at all possible because fetal harm may occur.
• Safety of drug has not been established in breast-feeding women and children.

NURSING CONSIDERATIONS

Assessment
• Assess patient's condition before therapy and regularly thereafter.
• Determine serum electrolyte, creatinine, and BUN levels; creatinine clearance; CBC; and platelet count before first infusion and before each course of treatment. WBC and platelet count nadirs usually occur by day 21. Levels usually return to baseline by day 28.
• Be alert for adverse reactions and drug interactions.
• Be aware that patients over age 65 are at greater risk for neurotoxicity.
• Evaluate patient's and family's knowledge of drug therapy.

Nursing diagnoses
• Altered health maintenance related to ovarian cancer
• Altered protection related to drug-induced adverse reactions
• Knowledge deficit related to drug therapy

Planning and implementation
• Follow institutional policy to reduce risks because preparation and administration of parenteral form is associated with

mutagenic, teratogenic, and carcinogenic risks for personnel.
• Check ordered dose against laboratory test results carefully. Only one increase in dosage is recommended. Subsequent doses should not exceed 125% of starting dose.
• Reconstitute with D$_5$W, 0.9% NaCl solution, or sterile water for injection to make concentration of 10 mg/ml. Add 5 ml of diluent to 50-mg vial, 15 ml of diluent to 150-mg vial, or 45 ml of diluent to 450-mg vial. It can then be further diluted for infusion with 0.9% NaCl solution or D$_5$W. Concentration as low as 0.5 mg/ml can be prepared. Give drug by continuous or intermittent infusion over at least 15 minutes.
• Do not use needles or I.V. administration sets containing aluminum to administer carboplatin; precipitation and loss of drug's potency may occur.
• Keep in mind that bone marrow suppression may be more severe in patients with creatinine clearance below 60 ml/minute; dosage adjustments are recommended for such patients.
• Know that dose should not be repeated unless platelet count exceeds 100,000/mm^3.
• Store unopened vials at room temperature. Once reconstituted and diluted as directed, drug is stable at room temperature for 8 hours. Because drug does not contain antibacterial preservatives, discard unused drug after 8 hours.
• Have epinephrine, corticosteroids, and antihistamines available when administering carboplatin because anaphylactoid reactions may occur within minutes of administration.
• Administer antiemetic therapy as ordered. Carboplatin can produce severe vomiting.
Patient teaching
• Warn patient to watch for signs of infection (fever, sore throat, fatigue) and bleeding (easy bruising, nose bleeds, bleeding gums, melena). Take temperature daily.

• Instruct patient to avoid OTC products containing aspirin.
• Advise woman of childbearing age to avoid pregnancy during therapy and to consult doctor before becoming pregnant.
• Advise breast-feeding patient to discontinue breast-feeding because of risk of infant toxicity.

☑ Evaluation
• Patient exhibits positive response to carboplatin as evidenced by follow-up diagnostic tests.
• Patient does not experience injury from drug therapy.
• Patient and family state understanding of drug therapy.

carboprost tromethamine
(KAR-boh-prost troh-METH-ah-meen)
Hemabate

Pharmacologic class: prostaglandin
Therapeutic class: oxytocic
Pregnancy risk category: C

How supplied
Injection: 250 mcg/ml

Pharmacokinetics
Absorption: unknown.
Distribution: unknown.
Metabolism: enzymatic deactivation occurs in maternal tissues.
Excretion: excreted primarily in urine.

Route	Onset	Peak	Duration
I.M.	Unknown	15-60 min	16-24 hr

Pharmacodynamics
Chemical effect: produces strong, prompt contractions of uterine smooth muscle, possibly mediated by calcium and cAMP.
Therapeutic effect: aborts fetus and stops postpartum hemorrhage.

Indications and dosage

▶ **Abortion between 13th and 20th weeks of gestation.** *Adults:* initially, 250 mcg deep I.M. Subsequent doses of 250 mcg administered at intervals of 1½ to 3½ hours, depending on uterine response. Dosage may be increased in increments to 500 mcg if contractility is inadequate after several 250-mcg doses. Total dosage should not exceed 12 mg.

▶ **Postpartum hemorrhage caused by uterine atony not managed by conventional methods.** *Adults:* 250 mcg by deep I.M. injection. Repeat doses administered at 15- to 90-minute intervals, p.r.n. Maximum total dosage is 2 mg.

Adverse reactions

CV: *arrhythmias.*
GI: *vomiting, diarrhea,* nausea.
Other: *fever,* chills, flushing, *uterine rupture.*

Interactions

Drug-drug. *Other oxytocics:* may potentiate action. Avoid concomitant use.

Contraindications and precautions

• Contraindicated in patients hypersensitive to drug and in those with acute pelvic inflammatory disease or active cardiac, pulmonary, renal, or hepatic disease.
• Use cautiously in patients with history of asthma; hypotension; hypertension; CV, adrenal, renal, or hepatic disease; anemia; jaundice; diabetes; seizure disorders; or previous uterine surgery.

NURSING CONSIDERATIONS

⚗ Assessment
• Assess patient's pregnancy status before therapy.
• Monitor drug effectiveness by evaluating uterine contractions, expulsion of products of conception, or cessation of postpartum hemorrhage.
• Be alert for adverse reactions.
• Evaluate patient's and family's knowledge of drug therapy.

⊞ Nursing diagnoses
• Impaired adjustment related to pregnancy
• Risk for altered body temperature related to drug-induced fever
• Knowledge deficit related to drug therapy

▷ Planning and implementation
• Know that, unlike other prostaglandin abortifacients, carboprost is administered by I.M. injection. Injectable form avoids risk of expelling vaginal suppositories, which may occur with profuse vaginal bleeding.
• Know that drug should be used only by trained personnel in hospital setting.
• Consult doctor if uterine contractions are ineffective or postpartum bleeding persists.
Patient teaching
• Explain importance of follow-up care.
• Tell patient to report adverse reactions immediately.

☑ Evaluation
• Patient aborts successfully.
• Patient's temperature remains normal.
• Patient and family state understanding of drug therapy.

---

carisoprodol
(kar-ih-soh-PROH-dol)
Soma

Pharmacologic class: caramate derivative
Therapeutic class: skeletal muscle relaxant
Pregnancy risk category: NR

How supplied

Tablets: 350 mg

Pharmacokinetics

Absorption: unknown.
Distribution: widely distributed throughout body.
Metabolism: metabolized in liver.

Reactions may be *common,* uncommon, *life-threatening,* or COMMON AND LIFE-THREATENING.

Excretion: excreted in urine mainly as metabolites; less than 1% of dose excreted unchanged. *Half-life:* 8 hours.

Route	Onset	Peak	Duration
P.O.	≤ 30 min	≤ 4 hr	4-6 hr

Pharmacodynamics

Chemical effect: appears to modify central perception of pain without modifying pain reflexes. Blocks interneuronal activity in descending reticular activating system and in spinal cord.
Therapeutic effect: relieves musculoskeletal pain.

Indications and dosage

▶ **Adjunct in acute, painful musculoskeletal conditions.** *Adults:* 350 mg P.O. t.i.d. and h.s.

Adverse reactions

CNS: *drowsiness, dizziness,* vertigo, ataxia, tremor, agitation, irritability, headache, depressive reactions, insomnia.
CV: orthostatic hypotension, tachycardia, facial flushing.
GI: nausea, vomiting, hiccups, increased bowel activity, epigastric distress.
Hematologic: eosinophilia.
Respiratory: asthmatic episodes.
Skin: rash, erythema multiforme, pruritus.
Other: fever, angioedema, *anaphylaxis.*

Interactions

Drug-drug. *CNS depressants:* increased CNS depression. Avoid concomitant use.
Drug-lifestyle. *Alcohol use:* increased CNS depression. Don't use together.

Contraindications and precautions

• Contraindicated in patients with intermittent porphyria or hypersensitivity to related compounds (such as meprobamate, tybamate).
• Use cautiously in patients with impaired hepatic or renal function.

NURSING CONSIDERATIONS

✍ Assessment
• Assess patient's pain before and after drug administration.
• Monitor drug effectiveness by regularly assessing severity and frequency of muscle spasms.
• Be alert for adverse reactions and drug interactions.
• Watch for idiosyncratic reactions after first to fourth dose (weakness, ataxia, visual and speech difficulties, fever, skin eruptions, and mental changes) and for severe reactions (bronchospasm, hypotension, and anaphylactic shock).
• Evaluate patient's and family's knowledge of drug therapy.

⊕ Nursing diagnoses
• Pain related to patient's underlying condition
• Risk for injury related to drug-induced drowsiness
• Knowledge deficit related to drug therapy

▷ Planning and implementation
• Give drug with meals or milk to prevent GI distress.
• Know that amount of pain relief obtained determines if dosage can be reduced.
• Withhold dose and notify doctor immediately if unusual reactions occur.
• Do not stop drug abruptly; mild withdrawal effects (such as insomnia, headache, nausea, and abdominal cramps) may result.
Patient teaching
• Warn patient to avoid activities that require alertness until drug's CNS effects are known. Drowsiness is transient.
• Advise patient to avoid combining drug with alcohol or other CNS depressants.
• Advise patient to follow doctor's orders about rest and physical therapy.
• Tell patient to take drug with meals or milk to prevent GI distress.

☑ Evaluation

• Patient reports pain has ceased.
• Patient does not experience injury from drug-induced CNS adverse reactions.
• Patient and family state understanding of drug.

carmustine (BCNU)
(kar-MUHS-teen)
BiCNU, Gliadel

Pharmacologic class: alkylating agent; nitrosourea (cell cycle–phase nonspecific)
Therapeutic class: antineoplastic
Pregnancy risk category: D

How supplied

Injection: 100-mg vial (lyophilized), with 3-ml vial of absolute alcohol supplied as diluent
Wafer: 7.7 mg

Pharmacokinetics

Absorption: not applicable with I.V. administration
Distribution: distributed rapidly into CSF.
Metabolism: metabolized extensively in liver.
Excretion: from 60% to 70% excreted in urine within 96 hours, 6% to 10% excreted as carbon dioxide by lungs, and 1% excreted in feces. *Half-life:* 15 to 30 minutes.

Route	Onset	Peak	Duration
I.V., wafer	Unknown	Unknown	Unknown

Pharmacodynamics

Chemical effect: inhibits enzymatic reactions involved with DNA synthesis, cross-links strands of cellular DNA, and interferes with RNA transcription, causing growth imbalance that leads to cell death. Cell cycle–phase nonspecific.
Therapeutic effect: kills selected cancer cells.

Indications and dosage

▶ **Brain tumors, Hodgkin's disease, non-Hodgkin's lymphoma, and multiple myeloma.** *Adults:* 75 to 100 mg/m^2 I.V. by slow infusion daily for 2 days; repeated q 6 weeks if platelet count is above 100,000/mm^3 and WBC count is above 4,000/mm^3. Dosage is reduced by 30% when WBC count is 2,000 to 3,000/mm^3 and platelet count is 25,000 to 75,000/mm^3. Dosage is reduced by 50% when WBC count is below 2,000/mm^3 and platelet count is below 25,000/mm^3. *Alternative therapy:* 150 to 200 mg/m^2 I.V. by slow infusion as single dose, repeated q 6 weeks.
▶ **Recurrent glioblastoma and metastatic brain tumors (adjunct to surgery to prolong survival):** *Adults:* implant 8 wafers into resection cavity as size of cavity allows.

Adverse reactions

CNS: ataxia, drowsiness.
GI: *nausea beginning in 2 to 6 hours (can be severe), vomiting, anorexia, dysphagia, esophagitis, diarrhea.*
GU: *nephrotoxicity, renal failure.*
Hematologic: *cumulative bone marrow suppression* (delayed 4 to 6 weeks, lasting 1 to 2 weeks); *leukopenia; thrombocytopenia; acute leukemia or bone marrow dysplasia* (may occur after long-term use).
Hepatic: *hepatotoxicity.*
Respiratory: *pulmonary fibrosis.*
Skin: facial flushing, hyperpigmentation (if drug contacts skin).
Other: *intense pain* (at infusion site from venous spasm); possible hyperuricemia (in lymphoma patients when rapid cell lysis occurs).

Interactions

Drug-drug. *Anticoagulants, aspirin:* increased risk of bleeding. Avoid concomitant use.
Cimetidine: may increase carmustine's bone marrow toxicity. Avoid combination if possible.

Reactions may be *common*, uncommon, *life-threatening*, or COMMON AND LIFE-THREATENING.

Digoxin, phenytoin: Serum levels of these drugs may be reduced. Use together cautiously.

Contraindications and precautions

• Contraindicated in patients with hypersensitivity to drug and in pregnant or breast-feeding women.
• Safety of drug has not been established in children.

NURSING CONSIDERATIONS

Assessment
• Assess patient's neoplastic disorder before therapy and regularly thereafter.
• Obtain baseline pulmonary function tests as ordered before therapy because pulmonary toxicity appears to be dose-related. Then evaluate results of liver, renal, and pulmonary function tests periodically thereafter.
• Monitor CBC and serum uric acid level, as ordered.
• Be alert for adverse reactions and drug interactions.
• Evaluate patient's and family's knowledge of drug therapy.

Nursing diagnoses
• Altered health maintenance related to neoplastic disease
• Risk for injury related to drug-induced adverse reactions
• Knowledge deficit related to drug therapy

Planning and implementation
• Follow institutional policy to reduce risks because preparation and administration of parenteral form is associated with carcinogenic, mutagenic, and teratogenic risks for personnel.
• To reduce nausea, give antiemetic before administering drug, as ordered.
I.V. use: To reconstitute, dissolve 100 mg of carmustine in 3 ml of absolute alcohol provided by manufacturer. Dilute solution with 27 ml of sterile water for injection. Resultant solution contains 3.3 mg

of carmustine/ml in 10% alcohol. Dilute in 0.9% NaCl solution or D_5W for I.V. infusion. Give at least 250 ml over 1 to 2 hours. To reduce pain on infusion, dilute further or slow infusion rate.
• Discard drug if powder liquefies or appears oily (decomposition has occurred).
• Administer only in glass containers. Solution is unstable in plastic I.V. bags.
• Don't mix with other drugs during administration.
• Store reconstituted solution in refrigerator for 48 hours. May decompose at temperatures above 80° F (26.6° C).
• Avoid contact with skin because carmustine will cause brown stain. If drug contacts skin, wash off thoroughly.
Wafer use: Unopen foil packs are stable at room temperature for 6 hours. Store below –4° F. Use double gloves if handling wafer in operating room.
• Know that allopurinol may be used with adequate hydration to prevent hyperuricemia and uric acid nephropathy.
Patient teaching
• Warn patient to watch for signs of infection (fever, sore throat, fatigue) and bleeding (easy bruising, nosebleeds, bleeding gums, melena). Take temperature daily.
• Instruct patient to avoid OTC products containing aspirin.
• Advise breast-feeding women to discontinue breast-feeding during therapy because of possible infant toxicity.
• Advise female patient of childbearing age to avoid pregnancy during therapy and to consult doctor before becoming pregnant.

Evaluation
• Patient exhibits positive response to drug therapy as evidenced by follow-up diagnostic studies.
• Patient does not experience injury from drug-induced adverse reactions.
• Patient and family state understanding of drug therapy.

---

carteolol hydrochloride
(KAR-tee-oh-lol)
Cartrol

Pharmacologic class: beta blocker
Therapeutic class: antihypertensive
Pregnancy risk category: C

How supplied
Tablets: 2.5 mg, 5 mg

Pharmacokinetics
Absorption: bioavailability is about 85%.
Distribution: 20% to 30% bound to plasma proteins.
Metabolism: 30% to 50% metabolized in liver to active and inactive metabolites.
Excretion: excreted primarily by kidneys. *Half-life:* about 6 hours.

Route	Onset	Peak	Duration
P.O.	Unknown	1-3 hr	Unknown

Pharmacodynamics
Chemical effect: unknown. Nonselective beta-adrenergic blocker with intrinsic sympathomimetic activity. Antihypertensive effects probably caused by decreased sympathetic outflow from brain and decreased cardiac output. Carteolol does not have consistent effect on renin output.
Therapeutic effect: lowers blood pressure.

Indications and dosage
▶ **Hypertension.** *Adults:* initially, 2.5 mg P.O. as single daily dose. Gradually increased to 5 or 10 mg as single daily dose, as needed. Dosages exceeding 10 mg daily do not produce greater response and may decrease response. *In patients with substantial renal failure:* if creatinine clearance is over 60 ml/minute, administer drug at 24-hour intervals; 20 to 60 ml/minute, at 48-hour intervals; below 20 ml/minute, at 72-hour intervals.

Adverse reactions
CNS: lassitude, tiredness, fatigue, somnolence, *asthenia.*
CV: conduction disturbances.
Other: *muscle cramps.*

Interactions
Drug-drug. *Calcium channel blockers:* increased risk of hypotension, left ventricular failure, and AV conduction disturbances. Use I.V. calcium antagonists with caution.
Cardiac glycosides: may produce additive effects on slowing AV node conduction. Avoid concomitant use.
Catecholamine-depleting drugs, reserpine: may have additive effect. Monitor patient.
General anesthetics: increased hypotensive effects. Observe carefully for excessive hypotension or bradycardia or orthostatic hypotension.
Insulin, oral antidiabetic agents: may alter hypoglycemic response. Adjust dosage as necessary.

Contraindications and precautions
• Contraindicated in patients with bronchial asthma, severe bradycardia, greater than first-degree heart block, cardiogenic shock, or uncontrolled heart failure.
• Use cautiously in patients with heart failure controlled by cardiac glycosides and diuretics (patients may exhibit signs of cardiac decompensation with beta-blocker therapy) and in pregnant or breast-feeding women.
• Safety of drug has not been established in children.

NURSING CONSIDERATIONS

⚕ Assessment
• Assess patient's blood pressure before therapy and regularly thereafter.
• Be alert for adverse reactions and drug interactions.
• Be aware that patients with unrecognized coronary artery disease may exhibit

signs of angina pectoris on withdrawal of drug. Monitor closely.
• Evaluate patient's and family's knowledge of drug therapy.

⊞ **Nursing diagnoses**
• Risk for injury related to hypertension
• Pain related to drug-induced muscle cramps
• Knowledge deficit related to drug therapy

❯ **Planning and implementation**
• Be aware that patients with significant renal failure should receive usual dose of carteolol at longer intervals.
• Know that withdrawal of beta-blocker therapy before surgery is controversial. Advise anesthesiologist that patient is receiving a beta blocker so that isoproterenol or dobutamine is made readily available for reversal of drug's cardiac effects.
• Gradually withdraw beta-blocker therapy, as ordered, to avoid thyroid storm in patients with suspected thyrotoxicosis.
Patient teaching
• Explain importance of taking drug as prescribed, even when feeling well. Tell patient not to discontinue drug suddenly, but to notify doctor of distressing reactions, such as muscle cramps.
• Emphasize importance of reporting signs of heart failure, including shortness of breath, difficulty breathing, unusually fast heartbeat, cough, and fatigue with exertion.

☑ **Evaluation**
• Patient's blood pressure is normal.
• Patient does not experience muscle cramps.
• Patient and family state understanding of drug therapy.

carvedilol
(kar-VAY-deh-lol)
Coreg

Pharmacologic class: alpha$_1$-, beta-adrenergic blocker
Therapeutic class: antihypertensive, adjunct treatment for heart failure
Pregnancy risk category: C

How supplied

Tablets: 3.125 mg, 6.25 mg, 12.5 mg, 25 mg

Pharmacokinetics

Absorption: rapidly and extensively absorbed with absolute bioavailability of 25% to 35% because of significant first-pass metabolism.
Distribution: extensively distributed into extravascular tissues; about 98% bound to plasma proteins.
Metabolism: primarily metabolized by aromatic ring oxidation and glucuronidation.
Excretion: metabolites are primarily excreted via bile in the feces. Less than 2% is excreted unchanged in urine. *Half-life:* 7 to 10 hours.

Route	Onset	Peak	Duration
P.O.	Unknown	1-2 hr	7-10 hr

Pharmacodynamics

Chemical effect: nonselective beta-adrenergic blocker with alpha$_1$-blocking activity causes significant reductions in systemic blood pressure, pulmonary arterial pressure, pulmonary capillary wedge pressure and heart rate.
Therapeutic effect: lowers blood pressure and heart rate

Indications and dosage

▶ **Hypertension.** *Adults:* dosage highly individualized. Initially, 6.25 mg P.O. b.i.d. with food. Obtain a standing blood pressure 1 hour after initial dose. If tolerated, continue dosage for 7 to 14 days.

---

*Liquid form contains alcohol   **May contain tartrazine   ◆Canada   ◇Australia   †OTC

May increase to 12.5 mg P.O. b.i.d. for 7 to 14 days, following blood pressure monitoring protocol noted above. Maximum dosage is 25 mg P.O. b.i.d. as tolerated.

▶ **Heart failure.** *Adults:* dosage highly individualized and titrated carefully. Initially, 3.125 mg P.O. b.i.d. with food for 2 weeks; if tolerated, can increase to 6.25 mg P.O. b.i.d. Dosage may be doubled q 2 weeks as tolerated. At initiation of new dose, observe patient for dizziness or light-headedness for 1 hour. Maximum dosage for patients weighing less than 85 kg (187 lb) is 25 mg P.O. b.i.d.; for those weighing over 85 kg, dosage is 50 mg P.O. b.i.d.

Adverse reactions

CNS: *dizziness, fatigue,* headache, hypesthesia, insomnia, pain, paresthesia, somnolence, vertigo, malaise.
CV: aggravated angina pectoris, *AV block, bradycardia, chest pain,* fluid overload, hypertension, hypotension, postural hypotension, syncope.
EENT: abnormal vision, rhinitis, pharyngitis, sinusitis..
GI: abdominal pain, *diarrhea,* melena, nausea, periodontitis, vomiting.
GU: abnormal renal function, albuminuria, hematuria, impotence, urinary tract infection.
Hematologic: decreased PT, purpura, *thrombocytopenia.*
Hepatic: increased ALT, AST.
Metabolic: dehydration, glycosuria, gout, hypercholesterolemia, *hyperglycemia,* hypertriglyceridemia, hypervolemia, hypovolemia, hyperuricemia, hypoglycemia, hyponatremia, weight gain.
Musculoskeletal: arthralgia, back pain.
Respiratory: bronchitis, dyspnea, *upper respiratory tract infection.*
Other: allergy, edema, fever, increased sweating, myalgia, peripheral edema, *sudden death,* viral infection.

Interactions

Drug-drug. *Calcium channel blockers:* can cause isolated conduction disturbances. Monitor patient's heart rhythm and blood pressure.
Catecholamine-depleting agents (such as reserpine, MAO inhibitors): may cause bradycardia or severe hypotension. Monitor patient closely.
Cimetidine: increased bioavailability of carvedilol. Monitor vital signs carefully.
Clonidine: may potentiate blood pressure and heart rate lowering effects. Monitor vital signs closely
Digoxin: increased concentrations of digoxin by about 15% while on concurrent therapy. Monitor digoxin levels and vital signs carefully.
Insulin, oral antidiabetic agents: concomitant use may enhance hypoglycemic properties. Monitor blood glucose levels.
Rifampin: reduced plasma concentrations of carvedilol by 70%. Monitor vital signs closely.
Drug-food. *Any food:* delayed rate of absorption of carvedilol but does not alter extent of bioavailability. Advise patient to take drug with food to minimize orthostatic effects.

Contraindications and precautions

• Contraindicated in patients with New York Heart Association class IV decompensated cardiac failure requiring I.V. inotropic therapy, bronchial asthma or related bronchospastic conditions, second- or third- degree AV block, sick sinus syndrome (unless a permanent pacemaker is in place), cardiogenic shock, severe bradycardia, or hypersensitivity to drug. Drug is not recommended in patients with symptomatic hepatic impairment.
• Use cautiously in hypertensive patients with left ventricular failure, perioperative patients who receive anesthetics that depress myocardial function, or diabetic patients receiving insulin or oral antidiabetic agents and in those subject to spontaneous hypoglycemia. Also use with caution in patients with thyroid disease, pheochromocytoma, Prinzmetal's variant angina, bronchospastic disease, or peripheral vascular disease.

Reactions may be *common,* uncommon, *life-threatening,* or COMMON AND LIFE-THREATENING.

• Safety and efficacy in patients under age 18 have not been established.

NURSING CONSIDERATIONS

⚖ Assessment
• Monitor patient for decreased PT and increased serum alkaline phosphatase, BUN, ALT, and AST.
• Assess patient with heart failure for worsened condition, renal dysfunction, or fluid retention; diuretics may need to be increased, as ordered.
• Monitor diabetic patient closely; drug may mask signs of hypoglycemia, or hyperglycemia may be worsened.
• Observe patient for dizziness or lightheadedness for 1 hour after administration of each dose.
• Evaluate patient's and family's knowledge of drug therapy.

⊞ Nursing diagnoses
• Altered health maintenance related to underlying disorder
• Altered cerebral tissue perfusion secondary to therapeutic action of drug
• Knowledge deficit related to drug therapy

⊠ Planning and implementation
• Notify doctor if pulse is below 55 beats/minute because dose of drug may need to be reduced.
• Be aware that before drug can be started, dosages of digoxin, diuretics, or ACE inhibitors should be stabilized.
• Monitor elderly patients carefully; plasma levels are about 50% higher in elderly patients.
• Give drug with food to reduce risk of orthostatic hypotension.
Patient teaching
• Tell patient not to interrupt or discontinue drug without medical approval. Drug should be withdrawn gradually over 1 to 2 weeks.
• Advise heart failure patient to call doctor if weight gain or shortness of breath occurs.

• Inform patient that he may experience low blood pressure when standing. If dizziness or fainting (rare) occurs, advise him to sit or lie down.
• Caution patient against driving or performing hazardous tasks until CNS effects of are known.
• Tell patient to notify doctor if dizziness or faintness occurs; dose may need to be adjusted.
• Inform breast feeding patient that effects on the infant are unknown. Breastfeeding should be discontinued during drug therapy.
• Advise diabetic patient to report changes in blood glucose promptly.
• Inform patient who wears contact lenses that decreased lacrimation may occur.

☑ Evaluation
• Patient responds well to therapy.
• Patient does not experience dizziness or light-headedness.
• Patient and family state understanding of drug therapy.

---

cascara sagrada†
(kas-KAR-uh suh-GRAH-duh)

cascara sagrada aromatic fluidextract†

cascara sagrada fluidextract†

Pharmacologic class: anthraquinone glycoside mixture
Therapeutic class: laxative
Pregnancy risk category: C

How supplied
Tablets: 325 mg†
Aromatic fluidextract: 1 g/ml†
Fluidextract: 1 g/ml†

Pharmacokinetics
Absorption: minimally absorbed in small intestine.

Distribution: distributed in bile, saliva, colonic mucosa, and breast milk.
Metabolism: hydrolyzed by colonic flora enzymes to active free anthraquinones, which are metabolized in liver.
Excretion: excreted in feces via biliary elimination, in urine, or both.

Route	Onset	Peak	Duration
P.O.	6-10 hr	Varies	Varies

Pharmacodynamics

Chemical effect: increases peristalsis, probably by direct effect on smooth muscle of intestine. Thought to irritate musculature or stimulate colonic intramural plexus. Also promotes fluid accumulation in colon and small intestine.
Therapeutic effect: relieves constipation.

Indications and dosage

▶ **Acute constipation; preparation for bowel or rectal examination.** *Adults and children over age 12:* 1 tablet P.O. h.s.; 0.5 to 1 ml fluidextract P.O. daily; or 5 ml aromatic fluid extract P.O. daily. *Children ages 2 to 12:* one-half adult dosage. *Children under age 2:* one-quarter adult dosage.

Adverse reactions

GI: *nausea;* vomiting; diarrhea; loss of normal bowel function (with excessive use); *abdominal cramps,* especially in severe constipation; malabsorption of nutrients; "cathartic colon" (syndrome resembling ulcerative colitis radiologically and pathologically) in chronic misuse; discoloration of rectal mucosa (after long-term use).
Other: hypokalemia, protein enteropathy, electrolyte imbalance (with excessive use), laxative dependence (with long-term or excessive use).

Interactions

None significant.

Contraindications and precautions

• Contraindicated in patients with abdominal pain, nausea, vomiting, or other symptoms of appendicitis or acute surgical abdomen; acute surgical delirium; fecal impaction; or intestinal obstruction or perforation.
• Use cautiously in patients with rectal bleeding, in pregnant or breast-feeding women, and in children.

NURSING CONSIDERATIONS

℞ Assessment
• Assess patient's constipation before therapy, and evaluate drug effectiveness after administration.
• Determine if patient has adequate fluid intake, exercise, and diet before giving for constipation.
• Monitor patient for adverse reactions.
• Monitor serum electrolytes during prolonged use.
• Evaluate patient's and family's knowledge of drug therapy.

Nursing diagnoses
• Constipation related to patient's underlying condition
• Pain related to drug-induced abdominal cramps
• Knowledge deficit related to drug therapy

Planning and implementation
• Check doctor's orders and read drug label carefully to ensure administration of correct drug form.
• Be aware that cascara sagrada aromatic fluid extract is less active and less bitter than nonaromatic fluid extract.
• Know that liquid preparations are more reliable than solid dosage forms.
Patient teaching
• Discourage excessive use of laxatives.
• Warn patient that drug may turn alkaline urine red-pink and acidic urine yellow-brown.

• Teach patient about dietary sources of bulk, including bran and other cereals, fresh fruit, and vegetables.
• Warn patient that abdominal cramping may occur because cascara works by increasing intestinal peristalsis.

☑ **Evaluation**
• Patient's elimination pattern returns to normal.
• Patient remains free from pain.
• Patient and family state understanding of drug therapy.

castor oil
(KAS-tir oyl)
Emulsoil†, Fleet Flavored Castor Oil†, Neoloid†, Purge†

Pharmacologic class: glyceride, *Ricinus communis* derivative
Therapeutic class: stimulant laxative
Pregnancy risk category: NR

How supplied
Oral liquid: 36.4% (Neoloid†), 67% (Fleet†), 95% (Emulsoil†, Purge†)

Pharmacokinetics
Absorption: unknown.
Distribution: distributed locally, primarily in small intestine.
Metabolism: metabolized by intestinal enzymes into its active form, ricinoleic acid.
Excretion: excreted in feces.

Route	Onset	Peak	Duration
P.O.	2-6 hr	Varies	Varies

Pharmacodynamics
Chemical effect: increases peristalsis, probably by direct effect on smooth muscle of intestine. Thought to irritate musculature or stimulate colonic intramural plexus. Also promotes fluid accumulation in colon and small intestine.
Therapeutic effect: cleanses bowel.

Indications and dosage
▶ **Preparation for rectal or bowel examination or for surgery.** For all patients, administered as single dose about 16 hours before surgery or procedure.
Adults and children age 12 and older: 15 to 60 ml P.O. *Children ages 2 to 12:* 5 to 15 ml P.O. *Children under age 2:* 2.5 to 7.5 ml P.O. Increased dose produces no greater effect.

Adverse reactions
GI: *nausea;* vomiting; diarrhea; loss of normal bowel function (with excessive use); *abdominal cramps,* especially in severe constipation; malabsorption of nutrients; "cathartic colon" (syndrome resembling ulcerative colitis radiologically and pathologically; with chronic misuse); laxative dependence (with long-term or excessive use). May cause constipation after catharsis.
GU: pelvic congestion (in menstruating women).
Other: hypokalemia, protein-losing enteropathy, other electrolyte imbalances (with excessive use).

Interactions
None significant.

Contraindications and precautions
• Contraindicated in patients with ulcerative bowel lesions; abdominal pain, nausea, vomiting, or other symptoms of appendicitis or acute surgical abdomen; or anal or rectal fissures, fecal impaction, or intestinal obstruction or perforation; and during menstruation or pregnancy.
• Use cautiously in patients with rectal bleeding.
• Breast-feeding women should seek medical approval before using castor oil.

NURSING CONSIDERATIONS

☑ **Assessment**
• Assess patient's underlying condition.

• Monitor drug effectiveness by noting if diagnostic testing provides accurate results.
• Be aware that failure to respond to drug may indicate acute condition requiring surgery.
• Be alert for adverse reactions and drug interactions.
• Evaluate patient's and family's knowledge of drug therapy.

⊕ **Nursing diagnoses**
• Health-seeking behavior (seeking diagnostic testing) related to underlying condition
• Pain related to drug-induced abdominal cramps
• Knowledge deficit related to drug therapy

❱ **Planning and implementation**
• Have patient suck on ice before drug administration and give drug with juice or carbonated beverage to mask oily taste. Stir mixture and have patient drink it promptly.
• Shake emulsion well before measuring dose. Emulsion is better tolerated but more expensive. Store below 40° F (4.4° C). Don't freeze.
• Time drug administration so that it doesn't interfere with scheduled activities or sleep.
• Give drug on empty stomach for best results.
• Know that increased intestinal motility lessens absorption of concomitantly administered oral drugs. Separate administration times.
Patient teaching
• Tell patient not to expect another bowel movement for 1 to 2 days after castor oil has emptied bowel.

✓ **Evaluation**
• Patient obtains accurate results of diagnostic testing.
• Patient does not experience pain from therapy.

• Patient and family state understanding of drug therapy.

cefaclor
(SEH-fuh-klor)
Ceclor, Ceclor CD

Pharmacologic class: second-generation cephalosporin
Therapeutic class: antibiotic
Pregnancy risk category: B

How supplied
Tablets: (extended-release): 375 mg, 500 mg
Capsules: 250 mg, 500 mg
Oral suspension: 125 mg/5 ml, 250 mg/5 ml, 187 mg/5 ml, 375 mg/5 ml

Pharmacokinetics
Absorption: well absorbed from GI tract. Food will delay but not prevent complete GI tract absorption.
Distribution: distributed widely into most body tissues and fluids; CSF penetration is poor. Drug is 25% protein-bound.
Metabolism: none.
Excretion: excreted primarily in urine by renal tubular secretion and glomerular filtration. *Half-life:* 0.5 to 1 hour.

Route	Onset	Peak	Duration
P.O.	Unknown	30-60 min	Unknown

Pharmacodynamics
Chemical effect: inhibits cell-wall synthesis, promoting osmotic instability; usually bactericidal.
Therapeutic effect: hinders or kills susceptible bacteria: many gram-positive cocci, including penicillinase-producing *Staphylococcus aureus* and *Staphylococcus epidermidis, Streptococcus pneumoniae,* group B streptococci, and group A beta-hemolytic streptococci; gram-negative organisms, including *Klebsiella pneumoniae, Escherichia coli, Proteus*

---

mirabilis, and *Shigella;* and other organisms, such as *Moraxella (Branhamella) catarrhalis, Haemophilus influenzae, Enterobacter, Citrobacter, Providencia, Acinetobacter, Serratia,* and *Neisseria.*

Indications and dosage

▶ **Respiratory or urinary tract, skin, and soft-tissue infections and otitis media caused by** *H. influenzae, S. pneumoniae, S. pyogenes, E. coli, P. mirabilis, Klebsiella* **species, and staphylococci.** *Adults:* 250 to 500 mg P.O. q 8 hours. Total daily dosage should not exceed 4 g. For extended-release forms, 500 mg P.O. q 12 hours for 7 days for bronchitis; for pharyngitis or skin and skin-structure infections, 375 mg P.O. q 12 hours for 10 days and 7 to 10 days respectively. *Children:* 20 mg/kg P.O. daily in divided doses q 8 hours. For more serious infections, 40 mg/kg daily are recommended, not to exceed 1 g daily.

Adverse reactions

CNS: dizziness, headache, somnolence, malaise.
GI: *nausea,* vomiting, *diarrhea,* anorexia, dyspepsia, abdominal cramps, pseudomembranous colitis, oral candidiasis.
GU: red and white cells in urine, vaginal candidiasis, vaginitis.
Hematologic: *transient leukopenia,* lymphocytosis, anemia, eosinophilia, *thrombocytopenia.*
Hepatic: transient increases in liver enzymes.
Skin: *maculopapular rash,* dermatitis.
Other: hypersensitivity reactions (serum sickness, *anaphylaxis*), fever.

Interactions

Drug-drug. *Chloramphenicol:* antagonistic effect. Do not use together.
Probenecid: may inhibit excretion and increase blood levels of cefaclor. Monitor patient.

Contraindications and precautions

• Contraindicated in patients with hypersensitivity to other cephalosporins.
• Use cautiously in patients with impaired renal function or history of sensitivity to penicillin and in pregnant or breast-feeding women.

NURSING CONSIDERATIONS

▣ Assessment

• Assess patient's infection before therapy and regularly thereafter.
• Obtain specimen for culture and sensitivity tests before first dose. Therapy may begin pending test results.
• Ask patient about previous reactions to cephalosporin or penicillin before administering first dose.
• Be alert for adverse reactions and drug interactions.
• Monitor patient's hydration status if adverse GI reactions occur.
• Evaluate patient's and family's knowledge of drug therapy.

▣ Nursing diagnoses

• Infection related to bacteria susceptible to drug
• Risk for fluid volume deficit related to drug-induced adverse GI reactions
• Knowledge deficit related to drug therapy

▣ Planning and implementation

• Administer drug with food to prevent or minimize GI upset.
• Store reconstituted suspension in refrigerator (stable for 14 days). Keep tightly closed and shake well before using.
• Be aware that urine glucose determinations may be false-positive with copper sulfate tests (Clinitest); glucose enzymatic tests (Diastix or Chemstrip uG) are not affected.
Patient teaching
• Tell patient that drug may be taken with meals.
• Advise patient to take drug exactly as prescribed, even after he feels better.

---

*Liquid form contains alcohol   **May contain tartrazine   ♦Canada   ◊ Australia   †OTC

• Instruct patient to call doctor if rash develops.
• Teach patient how to store drug.

☑ **Evaluation**
• Patient is free from infection.
• Patient maintains adequate hydration.
• Patient and family state understanding of drug therapy.

---

cefadroxil monohydrate
(seh-fuh-DROKS-il MON-oh-HIGH-drayt)
Duricef

Pharmacologic class: first-generation cephalosporin
Therapeutic class: antibiotic
Pregnancy risk category: B

How supplied
Tablets: 1 g
Capsules: 500 mg
Oral suspension: 125 mg/5 ml, 250 mg/ 5 ml, 500 mg/5 ml

Pharmacokinetics
Absorption: absorbed rapidly and completely from GI tract.
Distribution: distributed widely into most body tissues and fluids; CSF penetration is poor. Drug is 20% protein-bound.
Metabolism: none.
Excretion: excreted primarily unchanged in urine. *Half-life:* about 1 to 2 hours.

Route	Onset	Peak	Duration
P.O.	Unknown	1-2 hr	Unknown

Pharmacodynamics
Chemical effect: inhibits cell-wall synthesis, promoting osmotic instability; usually bactericidal.
Therapeutic effect: hinders or kills susceptible bacteria: many gram-positive cocci, including penicillinase-producing *Staphylococcus aureus* and *Staphylo-*

coccus epidermidis, Streptococcus pneumoniae, group B streptococci, and group A beta-hemolytic streptococci; and gram-negative organisms, including *Klebsiella pneumoniae, Escherichia coli, Proteus mirabilis,* and *Shigella.*

Indications and dosage
▶ **Urinary tract infections caused by *E. coli, P. mirabilis,* and *Klebsiella* species; skin and soft-tissue infections; and streptococcal pharyngitis.** *Adults:* 1 to 2 g P.O. daily, depending on infection treated, usually once or twice daily.
Children: 30 mg/kg P.O. daily in two divided doses. Course of treatment is usually at least 10 days.

Adverse reactions
CNS: dizziness, headache, malaise, paresthesia.
GI: pseudomembranous colitis, *nausea,* anorexia, vomiting, *diarrhea,* glossitis, *dyspepsia,* abdominal cramps, anal pruritus, tenesmus, oral candidiasis.
GU: genital pruritus, candidiasis.
Hematologic: *transient neutropenia,* eosinophilia, *leukopenia,* anemia, *agranulocytosis, thrombocytopenia.*
Hepatic: transient increases in liver enzymes.
Respiratory: dyspnea.
Skin: *maculopapular and erythematous rashes.*
Other: hypersensitivity reactions (serum sickness, *anaphylaxis*).

Interactions
Drug-drug. *Probenecid:* may inhibit excretion and increase blood levels of cefadroxil. Monitor patient.

Contraindications and precautions
• Contraindicated in patients with hypersensitivity to drug or other cephalosporins.
• Use cautiously in patients with impaired renal function (dosage adjustments may be necessary) or history of sensitivi-

---

ty to penicillin and in pregnant or breast-feeding women.

NURSING CONSIDERATIONS

⚕ Assessment
• Assess patient's infection before therapy and regularly thereafter.
• Obtain specimen for culture and sensitivity tests before first dose. Therapy may begin pending test results.
• Be alert for adverse reactions and drug interactions.
• Monitor patient's hydration status if adverse GI reactions occur.
• Evaluate patient's and family's knowledge of drug therapy.

⚕ Nursing diagnoses
• Infection related to bacteria susceptible to drug
• Risk for fluid volume deficit related to drug-induced adverse GI reactions
• Knowledge deficit related to drug therapy

⚕ Planning and implementation
• Know that drug's half-life permits once- or twice-daily dosing.
• Expect doctor to lengthen dosage interval to prevent drug accumulation if creatinine clearance is below 50 ml/minute.
• Store reconstituted suspension in refrigerator. Keep container tightly closed and shake well before using.
• Keep in mind that 40% to 75% of patients receiving cephalosporins show false-positive direct Coombs' test.
• Be aware that urine glucose determinations may be false-positive with copper sulfate tests (Clinitest); glucose enzymatic tests (Diastix or Chemstrip uG) are not affected.
Patient teaching
• Tell patient to take drug exactly as prescribed, even after he feels better.
• Advise patient to take drug with food or milk to lessen GI discomfort.
• Tell patient to call doctor if rash develops.

• Inform patient using oral suspension to shake it well before using and to refrigerate mixture in tightly closed container.

✓ Evaluation
• Patient is free from infection.
• Patient maintains adequate hydration.
• Patient and family state understanding of drug therapy.

---

cefazolin sodium
(sef-EH-zoh-lin SOH-dee-um)
Ancef, Kefzol, Zolicef

Pharmacologic class: first-generation cephalosporin
Therapeutic class: antibiotic
Pregnancy risk category: B

How supplied
Injection (parenteral): 250 mg, 500 mg, 1 g
Infusion: 500 mg/50 ml or 100 ml vial, 1 g/50 ml or 100 ml vial, 500 mg or 1 g RediVials, Faspaks, or ADD-Vantage vials

Pharmacokinetics
Absorption: unknown after I.M. administration.
Distribution: distributed widely into most body tissues and fluids; CSF penetration is poor; 74% to 86% protein-bound.
Metabolism: none.
Excretion: excreted primarily in urine.
Half-life: about 1 to 2 hours.

Route	Onset	Peak	Duration
I.V.	Immediate	Immediate	Unknown
I.M.	Unknown	1-2 hr	Unknown

Pharmacodynamics
Chemical effect: inhibits cell-wall synthesis, promoting osmotic instability; usually bactericidal.
Therapeutic effect: hinders or kills susceptible bacteria: many gram-positive

---

cocci, including penicillinase-producing *Staphylococcus aureus, Streptococcus pneumoniae,* group A beta-hemolytic streptococci, *Klebsiella, Escherichia coli, Enterobacteriaceae,* gonococci, *Proteus mirabilis,* and *Haemophilus influenzae.*

Indications and dosage

▶ **Serious infections of respiratory, biliary, and GU tracts; skin, soft-tissue, bone, and joint infections; septicemia; and endocarditis caused by** *E. coli,* **Enterobacteriaceae, gonococci,** *H. influenzae, Klebsiella, P. mirabilis, S. aureus, S. pneumoniae,* **and group A beta-hemolytic streptococci.** *Adults:* 250 mg I.V. or I.M. q 8 hours to 1 g q 6 hours. Maximum 12 g/day in life-threatening situations. *Children over age 1 month:* 50 to 100 mg/kg or 1.25 g/m^2 daily I.V. or I.M. in three or four divided doses.

▶ **Perioperative prophylaxis in contaminated surgery.** *Adults:* 1 g I.V. or I.M. 30 to 60 minutes before surgery; then 0.5 to 1 g I.V. or I.M. q 6 to 8 hours for 24 hours. In operations lasting over 2 hours, another 0.5 to 1 g dose may be administered intraoperatively. *Note:* In cases where infection would be devastating, prophylaxis may be continued for 3 to 5 days.

Adverse reactions

CNS: dizziness, headache, malaise, paresthesia.
GI: pseudomembranous colitis, nausea, anorexia, vomiting, *diarrhea,* glossitis, dyspepsia, abdominal cramps, anal pruritus, tenesmus, oral candidiasis.
GU: genital pruritus and candidiasis, vaginitis.
Hematologic: *transient neutropenia, leukopenia,* eosinophilia, anemia, *thrombocytopenia.*
Hepatic: transient increases in liver enzymes.
Respiratory: dyspnea.
Skin: *maculopapular and erythematous rashes, urticaria.*

Other: hypersensitivity reactions (serum sickness, *anaphylaxis*); *Stevens-Johnson syndrome: pain, induration, sterile abscesses, tissue sloughing* (at injection site); *phlebitis, thrombophlebitis* (with I.V. injection).

Interactions

Drug-drug. *Probenecid:* may inhibit excretion and increase blood levels of cefazolin. Monitor patient.

Contraindications and precautions

● Contraindicated in patients with hypersensitivity to other cephalosporins.
● Use cautiously in patients with history of sensitivity to penicillin, in pregnant or breast-feeding women, and with dosage adjustments in patients with renal failure.

NURSING CONSIDERATIONS

▨ Assessment
● Assess patient's infection before therapy and regularly thereafter.
● Obtain specimen for culture and sensitivity tests. Therapy may begin pending test results.
● Ask patient about previous reactions to cephalosporin or penicillin before administering first dose.
● Be alert for adverse reactions and drug interactions.
● Monitor patient's hydration status if adverse GI reactions occur.
● Evaluate patient's and family's knowledge of drug therapy.

▦ Nursing diagnoses
● Infection related to bacteria susceptible to drug
● Risk for fluid volume deficit related to drug-induced adverse GI reactions
● Knowledge deficit related to drug therapy

▶ Planning and implementation
I.V. use: Reconstitute with sterile water, bacteriostatic water, or 0.9% NaCl solution as follows: 2 ml to 500-mg vial;

Reactions may be *common,* uncommon, *life-threatening,* or COMMON AND LIFE-THREATENING.

2.5 ml to 1-g vial. Shake well until dissolved. Resultant concentration: 225 mg/ml or 330 mg/ml, respectively.
– For direct injection, further dilute Ancef with 5 ml of sterile water (Kefzol with 10 ml). Inject into large vein or into tubing of free-flowing I.V. solution over 3 to 5 minutes. For intermittent infusion, add reconstituted drug to 50 to 100 ml of compatible solution or use premixed solution. Commercially available frozen solutions of cefazolin in D_5W should be given only by intermittent or continuous I.V. infusion.
– Alternate injection sites if I.V. therapy lasts longer than 3 days. Use of small I.V. needles in larger available veins may be preferable.
I.M. use: After reconstitution, inject I.M. drug without further dilution (not as painful as other cephalosporins). Inject deeply into large muscle mass, such as gluteus maximus or lateral aspect of thigh.
• Know that reconstituted drug is stable for 24 hours at room temperature and 96 hours if refrigerated.
• Be aware that dose and dosing interval will be adjusted if creatinine clearance is below 55 ml/minute.
• Know that because of long duration of effect, most infections can be treated with dose every 8 hours.
• Be aware that urine glucose determinations may be false-positive with copper sulfate tests (Clinitest); glucose enzymatic tests (Diastix or Chemstrip uG) are not affected.
Patient teaching
• Tell patient to report if adverse reactions occur.

☑ **Evaluation**
• Patient is free from infection.
• Patient maintains adequate hydration.
• Patient and family state understanding of drug therapy.

cefdinir
(SEF-dih-neer)
Omnicef

Pharmacologic class: third-generation cephalosporin
Therapeutic class: antibiotic
Pregnancy risk category: B

How supplied
Capsules: 300 mg
Suspension: 125 mg/5 ml

Pharmacokinetics
Absorption: bioavailability of drug is approximately 21% after 300-mg capsule dose, 16% after 600-mg capsule dose, and 25% for suspension.
Distribution: 60% to 70% bound to plasma proteins.
Metabolism: not appreciably metabolized; activity is due mainly to parent drug.
Excretion: eliminated primarily by renal excretion. *Half-life:* 1.7 hours,

Route	Onset	Peak	Duration
P.O.	Unknown	2-4 hr	Unknown

Pharmacodynamics
Chemical effect: bactericidal activity results from inhibition of cell-wall synthesis.
Therapeutic effect: is stable in the presence of some beta-lactamase enzymes, causing some microorganisms resistant to penicillins and cephalosporins to be susceptible to cefdinir. Excluding *Pseudomonas, Enterobacter, Enterococcus,* and methicillin-resistant *Staphylococcus* species, cefdinir's spectrum of activity includes a broad range of gram-positive and gram-negative aerobic microorganisms.

Indications and dosages
▶ **Treatment of mild to moderate infections caused by susceptible strains of microorganisms for conditions of community-acquired pneumonia,**

acute exacerbations of chronic bronchitis, acute maxillary sinusitis, acute bacterial otitis media, and uncomplicated skin and skin-structure infection. *Adults and children age 13 and older:* 300 mg P.O. q 12 hours or 600 mg P.O. q 24 hours for 10 days. (Use q-12-hour dosages for pneumonia and skin infections.) *Children ages 6 months to 12 years:* 7 mg/kg P.O. q 12 hours or 14 mg/kg P.O. q 24 hours for 10 days, up to maximum dose of 600 mg daily. (Use q-12-hour dosages for skin infections.) Dosage is adjusted for patients with impaired renal function and is based on creatinine clearance.

▶ **Treatment of pharyngitis and tonsillitis.** *Adults and children age 13 and older:* 300 mg P.O. q 12 hours for 5 to 10 days or 600 mg P.O. q 24 hours for 10 days. *Children ages 6 months to 12 years:* 7 mg/kg P.O. q 12 hours for 5 to 10 days or 14 mg/kg P.O. q 24 hours for 10 days, up to a maximum dose of 600 mg daily.

Adverse reactions

CNS: headache.
GI: abdominal pain, *diarrhea*, nausea, vomiting.
GU: vaginal candidiasis, vaginitis, increased urine proteins and RBCs.
Skin: rash.

Interactions

Drug-drug. *Antacids (magnesium- and aluminum-containing), iron supplements, multivitamins containing iron:* decrease cefdinir's rate of absorption and bioavailability. Administer such preparations 2 hours before or after cefdinir dose.
Probenecid: inhibits the renal excretion of cefdinir. Monitor patient.

Contraindications and precautions

• Contraindicated in patients with known allergy to cephalosporins.
• Use cautiously in patients with known hypersensitivity to penicillin because of risk of cross-sensitivity with other beta-lactam antibiotics. Also, use with caution in patients with history of colitis and renal insufficiency.

NURSING CONSIDERATIONS

⚨ Assessment
• Ask patient about previous reactions to cephalosporins or penicillins before administering first dose.
• Obtain specimen for culture and sensitivity tests as ordered before giving first dose.
• Monitor patient for symptoms of superinfection.
• Assess patients with diarrhea carefully; pseudomembranous colitis has been reported with drug.
• Evaluate patient's and family's knowledge of drug therapy.

⚙ Nursing diagnoses
• Infection related to susceptible bacteria
• Risk for fluid volume deficit related to drug-induced adverse GI reactions
• Knowledge deficit related to drug therapy

⬗ Planning and implementation
• Begin therapy pending culture and sensitivity test results.
• Know that patients with renal insufficiency require reduced dosage.
• Notify doctor if allergic reaction is suspected; drug should be discontinued and emergency treatment may be required.
Patient teaching
• Instruct patient to take antacids and iron supplements 2 hours before or after dose of cefdinir.
• Inform diabetic patient that each teaspoon of suspension contains 2.86 g of sucrose.
• Tell patient that drug may be taken without regard to meals.
• Advise patient to report severe diarrhea or diarrhea accompanied by abdominal pain.
• Tell patient to report adverse reactions or symptoms of superinfection promptly.

Reactions may be *common*, uncommon, *life-threatening*, or COMMON AND LIFE-THREATENING.

☑ Evaluation
• Patient is free from infection.
• Patient maintains adequate hydration.
• Patient and family state understanding of drug therapy.

cefixime
(sef-IKS-eem)
Suprax

Pharmacologic class: third-generation cephalosporin
Therapeutic class: antibiotic
Pregnancy risk category: B

How supplied

Tablets: 200 mg, 400 mg
Oral suspension: 100 mg/5 ml (after re-constitution)

Pharmacokinetics

Absorption: well absorbed from GI tract.
Distribution: widely distributed; enters CSF in patients with inflamed meninges; about 65% bound to plasma proteins.
Metabolism: about 50% of drug is me-tabolized.
Excretion: excreted primarily in urine.
Half-life: 3 to 4 hours.

Route	Onset	Peak	Duration
P.O.	Unknown	3.1-4.4 hr	Unknown

Pharmacodynamics

Chemical effect: inhibits cell-wall syn-thesis, promoting osmotic instability; usually bactericidal.
Therapeutic effect: hinders or kills bac-teria: *Haemophilus influenzae, Moraxella (Branhamella) catarrhalis, Streptococcus pyogenes, Streptococcus pneumoniae, Escherichia coli,* and *Proteus mirabilis.*

Indications and dosage

▶ **Uncomplicated urinary tract infec-tions caused by** *E. coli* **and** *P. mirabilis;* **otitis media caused by** *H. influenzae* **(beta-lactamase positive and negative**

strains), *M. catarrhalis,* **and** *S. pyo-genes***; pharyngitis and tonsillitis caused by** *S. pyogenes;* **acute bronchitis and acute exacerbations of chronic bronchitis caused by** *S. pneumoniae* **and** *H. influenzae* **(beta-lactamase pos-itive and negative strains).** *Adults and children over age 12 or weighing over 50 kg (110 lb):* 400 mg/day P.O. as single 400-mg tablet or 200 mg q 12 hours. *Children age 12 and younger or weigh-ing 50 kg or less:* 8 mg/kg P.O. daily dose in one or two divided doses. For oti-tis media, use suspension only.
▶ **Uncomplicated gonorrhea caused by** *Neisseria gonorrhoeae. Adults:* 400 mg P.O. as single dose.

Adverse reactions

CNS: headaches, dizziness, nervousness, malaise, fatigue, somnolence, insomnia.
GI: *diarrhea,* loose stools, abdominal pain, nausea, vomiting, dyspepsia, flatu-lence, pseudomembranous colitis.
GU: genital pruritus, vaginitis, genital candidiasis, transient increases in BUN and serum creatinine levels.
Hematologic: *thrombocytopenia, leuko-penia,* eosinophilia.
Skin: pruritus, rash, urticaria, *Stevens-Johnson syndrome.*
Other: drug fever, transient increases in liver enzymes, hypersensitivity reactions (serum sickness, *anaphylaxis*).

Interactions

Drug-drug. *Probenecid:* may inhibit ex-cretion and increase blood levels of ce-fixime. Monitor patient.
Salicylates: may displace cefixime from plasma protein–binding sites. Clinical significance is unknown.

Contraindications and precautions

• Contraindicated in patients with hyper-sensitivity to drug or other cephalosporins.
• Use cautiously in patients with renal dysfunction (reduced dosage necessary with creatinine clearance below 60 ml/minute) or history of sensitivity to peni-

cillin and in pregnant or breast-feeding women.

NURSING CONSIDERATIONS

⚕ Assessment
• Assess patient's infection before therapy and regularly thereafter.
• Obtain specimen for culture and sensitivity tests before first dose. Therapy may begin pending test results.
• Ask patient about previous reactions to cephalosporin or penicillin before administering first dose.
• Be alert for adverse reactions and drug interactions.
• Monitor patient's hydration status if adverse GI reactions occur.
• Evaluate patient's and family's knowledge of drug therapy.

⊞ Nursing diagnoses
• Infection related to bacteria susceptible to drug
• Risk for fluid volume deficit related to drug-induced adverse GI reactions
• Knowledge deficit related to drug therapy

⊠ Planning and implementation
• To prepare oral suspension: add required amount of water to powder in two portions. Shake well after each addition. After mixing, suspension is stable for 14 days (no need to refrigerate). Keep tightly closed. Shake well before using.
• Be aware that urine glucose determinations may be false-positive with copper sulfate tests (Clinitest); glucose enzymatic tests (Diastix or Chemstrip uG) are not affected.
Patient teaching
• Tell patient to take drug exactly as prescribed, even after he feels better.
• Tell patient to call doctor if rash develops.
• Teach patient how to store drug.

☑ Evaluation
• Patient is free from infection.

• Patient maintains adequate hydration.
• Patient and family state understanding of drug therapy.

cefmetazole sodium (cefmetazone)
(sef-MET-ah-zohl SOH-dee-um)
Zefazone

Pharmacologic class: second-generation cephalosporin
Therapeutic class: antibiotic
Pregnancy risk category: B

How supplied
Injection: 1 g, 2 g

Pharmacokinetics
Absorption: not applicable with I.V. administration.
Distribution: distributed widely into most body tissues and fluids; CSF penetration is P.O.; 65% protein-bound.
Metabolism: about 15% of dose is metabolized, probably in liver.
Excretion: excreted primarily in urine.
Half-life: about 1.5 hours.

Route	Onset	Peak	Duration
I.V.	Unknown	Immediate	Unknown

Pharmacodynamics
Chemical effect: inhibits cell-wall synthesis, promoting osmotic instability; usually bactericidal.
Therapeutic effect: hinders or kills susceptible bacteria: many gram-positive organisms and enteric gram-negative bacilli, including *Staphylococcus aureus, Staphylococcus epidermidis,* streptococci, *Klebsiella, Escherichia coli* and other coliform bacteria, *Haemophilus influenzae,* and *Bacteroides* species.

Indications and dosage
▶ **Lower respiratory tract infections caused by *Streptococcus pneumoniae,* *S. aureus* (penicillinase- and non-**

penicillinase–producing strains), *E. coli,* and *H. influenzae* (non-penicillinase–producing strains); intra-abdominal infections caused by *E. coli* or *Bacteroides fragilis;* skin and skin-structure infections caused by *S. aureus* (penicillinase- and non-penicillinase–producing strains), *S. epidermidis, Streptococcus pyogenes, Strep. agalactiae, E. coli, Proteus mirabilis, Klebsiella pneumoniae,* and *B. fragilis. Adults:* 2 g I.V. q 6 to 12 hours for 5 to 14 days.

▶ **Urinary tract infections caused by *E. coli.*** *Adults:* 2 g I.V. q 12 hours.

▶ **Prophylaxis in patients undergoing vaginal hysterectomy.** *Adults:* 2 g I.V. 30 to 90 minutes before surgery as single dose; or 1 g I.V. 30 to 90 minutes before surgery, repeated in 8 and 16 hours.

▶ **Prophylaxis in patients undergoing abdominal hysterectomy.** *Adults:* 1 g I.V. 30 to 90 minutes before surgery, repeated in 8 and 16 hours.

▶ **Prophylaxis in patients undergoing cesarean section.** *Adults:* 2 g I.V. as single dose after clamping cord; or 1 g I.V. after clamping cord, repeated in 8 and 16 hours.

▶ **Prophylaxis in patients undergoing colorectal surgery.** *Adults:* 2 g I.V. as single dose 30 to 90 minutes before surgery. Some clinicians follow with additional 2-g doses in 8 and 16 hours.

▶ **Prophylaxis in patients undergoing cholecystectomy (high risk).** *Adults:* 1 g I.V. 30 to 90 minutes before surgery, repeated in 8 and 16 hours.

Adverse reactions

CNS: headache.
CV: *shock,* hypotension.
EENT: epistaxis.
GI: nausea, vomiting, *diarrhea,* epigastric pain, pseudomembranous colitis.
GU: vaginitis.
Respiratory: pleural effusion, dyspnea, respiratory distress.
Skin: rash, pruritus, generalized erythema.

Other: fever, bacterial or fungal superinfection, hypersensitivity reactions (serum sickness, *anaphylaxis*), altered color perception, pain at injection site, phlebitis.

Interactions

Drug-drug. *Aminoglycosides:* potential for increased risk of nephrotoxicity. Monitor closely.
Probenecid: may inhibit excretion and increase blood levels of cefmetazole. Sometimes used for this effect.
Drug-lifestyle. *Alcohol use:* possible disulfiram-like reaction. Avoid alcohol consumption for 24 hours before and after administration of cefmetazole.

Contraindications and precautions

• Contraindicated in patients with hypersensitivity to drug or other cephalosporins.
• Use cautiously in patients with history of sensitivity to penicillin and in pregnant women.
• Know that traces of drug have been detected in breast milk. Breast-feeding should be discontinued temporarily during therapy.
• Safety of drug has not been established in children.

NURSING CONSIDERATIONS

☑ **Assessment**
• Assess patient's infection before therapy and regularly thereafter.
• Obtain specimen for culture and sensitivity tests before first dose. Therapy may begin pending test results.
• Ask patient about previous reactions to cephalosporin or penicillin before administering first dose.
• Be alert for adverse reactions and drug interactions.
• Monitor patient's hydration status if adverse GI reactions.
• Evaluate patient's and family's knowledge of drug therapy.

---

*Liquid form contains alcohol   **May contain tartrazine   ◆Canada   ◇Australia   †OTC

🔢 Nursing diagnoses
• Infection related to bacteria susceptible to drug
• Risk for fluid volume deficit related to drug-induced adverse GI reactions
• Knowledge deficit related to drug therapy

❯ Planning and implementation
• Reconstitute with bacteriostatic water for injection, sterile water for injection, or 0.9% NaCl injection. After reconstitution, drug may be further diluted to concentrations ranging from 1 to 20 mg/ml by adding it to 0.9% NaCl injection, D₅W, or lactated Ringer's injection. Reconstituted or dilute solutions are stable for 24 hours at room temperature (77° F [25° C]) or 1 week if refrigerated at 46° F (8° C).
• Be aware that urine glucose determinations may be false-positive with copper sulfate tests (Clinitest); glucose enzymatic tests (Diastix or Chemstrip uG) are not affected.
Patient teaching
• Instruct patient to report if adverse reactions occur.

☑ Evaluation
• Patient is free from infection.
• Patient maintains adequate hydration.
• Patient and family state understanding of drug therapy.

---

cefonicid sodium
(sef-ON-eh-sid SOH-dee-um)
Monocid

Pharmacologic class: second-generation cephalosporin
Therapeutic class: antibiotic
Pregnancy risk category: B

How supplied
Injection: 1 g
Infusion: 1 g/100 ml

Pharmacokinetics
Absorption: unknown after I.M. administration.
Distribution: distributed widely into most body tissues and fluids; CSF penetration is P.O.; 90% to 98% protein-bound.
Metabolism: none.
Excretion: excreted primarily in urine.
Half-life: about 3.5 to 6 hours.

Route	Onset	Peak	Duration
I.V.	Immediate	Immediate	Unknown
I.M.	Unknown	1-2 hr	Unknown

Pharmacodynamics
Chemical effect: inhibits cell-wall synthesis, promoting osmotic instability; usually bactericidal.
Therapeutic effect: hinders or kills susceptible bacteria: many gram-positive organisms and enteric gram-negative bacilli, such as *Staphylococcus aureus, Staphylococcus epidermidis, Streptococcus pyogenes, Streptococcus pneumoniae, Klebsiella pneumoniae, Escherichia coli, Proteus mirabilis,* and *Haemophilus influenzae.*

Indications and dosage
▶ **Perioperative prophylaxis in contaminated surgery.** *Adults:* 1 g I.V. or I.V. 60 minutes before surgery.
▶ **Serious infections of lower respiratory and urinary tracts, skin and skin-structure infections, septicemia, bone and joint infections, and perioperative prophylaxis. Susceptible microorganisms include S. pneumoniae, K. pneumoniae, E. coli, H. influenzae, P. mirabilis, S. aureus, S. epidermidis, and S. pyogenes.** *Adults:* usual dosage is 1 g I.V. or I.M. q 24 hours. In life-threatening infections, 2 g q 24 hours.

Adverse reactions
CNS: dizziness, headache, malaise, paresthesia.
GI: pseudomembranous colitis, nausea, anorexia, vomiting, diarrhea, glossitis,

---

dyspepsia, abdominal cramps, anal pruritus, tenesmus, oral candidiasis.
GU: genital pruritus and candidiasis, vaginitis, *acute renal failure.*
Hematologic: *transient neutropenia, leukopenia,* eosinophilia, anemia, *thrombocytopenia.*
Skin: *maculopapular and erythematous rashes, urticaria.*
Other: dyspnea; hypersensitivity reactions (serum sickness, *anaphylaxis*); *pain, induration, sterile abscesses, tissue sloughing* (at injection site); *phlebitis, thrombophlebitis* (with I.V. injection).

Interactions

Drug-drug. *Aminoglycosides:* potential increased risk of nephrotoxicity. Monitor closely.
Probenecid: may inhibit excretion and increase blood levels of cefonicid. Monitor patient.

Contraindications and precautions

• Contraindicated in patients with hypersensitivity to drug or other cephalosporins.
• Use cautiously in patients with history of sensitivity to penicillin, in pregnant or breast-feeding women, and with dosage adjustments in patients with renal failure.
• Safety of drug has not been established in children.

NURSING CONSIDERATIONS

Assessment
• Assess patient's infection before therapy and regularly thereafter.
• Obtain specimen for culture and sensitivity tests before first dose. Therapy may begin pending test results.
• Ask patient about previous reactions to cephalosporin or penicillin before administering first dose.
• Be alert for adverse reactions and drug interactions.
• Monitor patient's hydration status if adverse GI reactions occur.

• Evaluate patient's and family's knowledge of drug therapy.

Nursing diagnoses
• Infection related to bacteria susceptible to drug
• Risk for fluid volume deficit related to drug-induced adverse GI reactions
• Knowledge deficit related to drug therapy

Planning and implementation
I.V. use: Reconstitute 500-mg vial with 2 ml of sterile water for injection (yields concentration of 225 mg/ml) and 1-g vial with 2.5 ml of sterile water for injection (yields concentration of 325 mg/ml). Shake well. Reconstitute piggyback vials with 50 to 100 ml of 5% dextrose in water or 0.9% NaCl.
I.M. use: When administering 2-g I.M. doses once daily, divide dose equally and inject deeply into large muscle masses, such as gluteus maximus or lateral aspect of thigh.
• Be aware that dosing interval will be adjusted for patients with renal impairment.
• Be aware that urine glucose determinations may be false-positive with copper sulfate tests (Clinitest); glucose enzymatic tests (Diastix or Chemstrip uG) are not affected.
Patient teaching
• Tell patient to report adverse reactions.

Evaluation
• Patient is free from infection.
• Patient maintains adequate hydration.
• Patient and family state understanding of drug therapy.

cefoperazone sodium
(sef-oh-PER-ah-zohn SOH-dee-um)
Cefobid

Pharmacologic class: third-generation cephalosporin

Therapeutic class: antibiotic
Pregnancy risk category: B

How supplied

Infusion: 1 g, 2 g piggyback
Parenteral: 1 g, 2 g
Pharmacy bulk package: 10-g vial

Pharmacokinetics

Absorption: unknown after I.M. administration.
Distribution: distributed widely into most body tissues and fluids; CSF penetration in patients with inflamed meninges; 82% to 93% protein-bound.
Metabolism: insubstantial.
Excretion: excreted primarily in urine.
Half-life: about 1.5 to 2.5 hours.

Route	Onset	Peak	Duration
I.V.	Immediate	Immediate	Unknown
I.M.	Unknown	1-2 hr	Unknown

Pharmacodynamics

Chemical effect: inhibits cell-wall synthesis, promoting osmotic instability; usually bactericidal.
Therapeutic effect: hinders or kills susceptible bacteria: some gram-positive organisms and many enteric gram-negative bacilli, including *Streptococcus pneumoniae* and *Streptococcus pyogenes, Staphylococcus aureus, Staphylococcus epidermidis,* enterococcus, *Escherichia coli, Klebsiella, Haemophilus influenzae, Enterobacter, Citrobacter, Proteus,* some *Pseudomonas* species (including *Pseudomonas aeruginosa*), and *Bacteroides fragilis.*

Indications and dosage

▶ **Serious infections of respiratory tract; intra-abdominal, gynecologic, and skin infections; bacteremia; and septicemia. Susceptible microorganisms include S. pneumoniae and S. pyogenes; S. aureus (penicillinase- and non-penicillinase–producing) and S. epidermidis; enterococci; E. coli; Klebsiella; H. influenzae; Enterobacter; Citrobacter;** *Proteus;* some *Pseudomonas,* including *P. aeruginosa;* and *B. fragilis. Adults:* usual dosage is 1 to 2 g q 12 hours I.V. or I.M. In severe infections or those caused by less sensitive organisms, total daily dosage may be increased to 16 g/day.

Adverse reactions

CNS: headache, malaise, paresthesia, dizziness.
GI: pseudomembranous colitis, nausea, anorexia, vomiting, *diarrhea,* glossitis, dyspepsia, abdominal cramps, tenesmus, anal pruritus, oral candidiasis.
GU: genital pruritus and candidiasis.
Hematologic: *transient neutropenia,* eosinophilia, hemolytic anemia, hypoprothrombinemia, bleeding.
Skin: *maculopapular and erythematous rashes, urticaria.*
Other: dyspnea; mildly elevated liver enzymes; hypersensitivity reactions (serum sickness, *anaphylaxis*); *pain, induration, sterile abscesses, temperature elevation, tissue sloughing* (at injection site) *phlebitis, thrombophlebitis* (with I.V. injection).

Interactions

Drug-drug. *Anticoagulant:* effects of anticoagulant may be increased. Use with caution.
Probenecid: may inhibit excretion and increase blood levels of cefoperazone. Monitor patient.
Drug-lifestyle. *Alcohol use:* possible disulfiram-like reaction. Caution patients to avoid alcohol consumption for several days after discontinuing cefoperazone.

Contraindications and precautions

• Contraindicated in patients with hypersensitivity to drug or other cephalosporins.
• Use cautiously in patients with impaired renal function or history of sensitivity to penicillin and in pregnant or breast-feeding patients.
• Safety of drug has not been established in children under age 12.

Reactions may be *common,* uncommon, *life-threatening,* or COMMON AND LIFE-THREATENING.

NURSING CONSIDERATIONS

⚕ Assessment
• Assess patient's infection before therapy and regularly thereafter.
• Obtain specimen for culture and sensitivity tests before first dose. Therapy may begin pending test results.
• Ask patient about previous reactions to cephalosporin or penicillin before administering first dose.
• Be alert for adverse reactions and drug interactions.
• Monitor hydration status if patient develops adverse GI reactions. Be aware that cefoperazone may increase risk of diarrhea over other cephalosporins.
• Evaluate patient's and family's knowledge of drug therapy.

⊕ Nursing diagnoses
• Infection related to bacteria susceptible to drug
• Risk for fluid volume deficit related to drug-induced adverse GI reactions
• Knowledge deficit related to drug therapy

⟩ Planning and implementation
• Administer doses of 4 g/day cautiously to patients with hepatic disease or biliary obstruction. Higher dosages require monitoring of serum levels.
I.V. use: Reconstitute 1- or 2-g vial with minimum of 2.8 ml of compatible I.V. solution; manufacturer recommends using 5 ml/g. Give by direct injection into large vein or into tubing of free-flowing I.V. solution over 3 to 5 minutes. When giving by intermittent infusion, add reconstituted drug to 20 to 40 ml of compatible I.V. solution and infuse over 15 to 30 minutes.
I.M. use: To prepare drug for I.M. injection: using 1-g vial, dissolve drug with 2 ml of sterile water for injection; then add 0.6 ml of 2% lidocaine hydrochloride for final concentration of 333 mg/ml. Alternatively, dissolve drug with 2.8 ml of sterile water for injection; then add

1 ml of 2% lidocaine hydrochloride for final concentration of 250 mg/ml. When using 2-g vial, dissolve drug with 3.8 ml of sterile water for injection; then add 1.2 ml of 2% lidocaine hydrochloride for final concentration of 333 mg/ml. Alternatively, dissolve drug with 5.4 ml of sterile water for injection; then add 1.8 ml of 2% lidocaine hydrochloride for final concentration of 250 mg/ml.
– Inject deeply into large muscle mass, such as gluteus maximus or lateral aspect of thigh.
– Be aware that urine glucose determinations may be false-positive with copper sulfate tests (Clinitest); glucose enzymatic tests (Diastix or Chemstrip uG) are not affected.
Patient teaching
• Tell patient to report adverse reactions.

☑ Evaluation
• Patient is free from infection.
• Patient maintains adequate hydration.
• Patient and family state understanding of drug therapy.

cefotaxime sodium
(sef-oh-TAKS-eem SOH-dee-um)
Claforan

Pharmacologic class: third-generation cephalosporin
Therapeutic class: antibiotic
Pregnancy risk category: B

How supplied
Injection: 500 mg, 1 g, 2 g
Infusion: 1 g, 2 g
Pharmacy bulk package: 10-g vial

Pharmacokinetics
Absorption: unknown after I.M. administration.
Distribution: distributed widely into most body tissues and fluids; adequate CSF penetration when meninges are inflamed; 13% to 38% protein-bound.

Metabolism: partially metabolized to active metabolite, desacetylcefotaxime.
Excretion: excreted primarily in urine.
Half-life: 1 to 2 hours.

Route	Onset	Peak	Duration
I.V.	Immediate	Immediate	Unknown
I.M.	Unknown	30 min	Unknown

Pharmacodynamics

Chemical effect: inhibits cell-wall synthesis, promoting osmotic instability; usually bactericidal.
Therapeutic effect: hinders or kills susceptible bacteria: some gram-positive organisms and many enteric gram-negative bacilli, including streptococci (*Streptococcus pneumoniae* and *pyogenes*), *Staphylococcus aureus, Staphylococcus epidermidis, Escherichia coli, Klebsiella* species, *Haemophilus influenzae, Enterobacter* species, *Proteus* species, and *Peptostreptococcus* species, and some strains of *Pseudomonas aeruginosa.*

Indications and dosage

▶ **Perioperative prophylaxis in contaminated surgery.** *Adults:* 1 g I.V. or I.M. 30 to 60 minutes before surgery. Patients undergoing cesarean section should receive 1 g I.V. or I.M. as soon as umbilical cord is clamped, followed by 1 g I.V. or I.M. 6 and 12 hours later.
▶ **Serious infections of lower respiratory and urinary tracts, CNS, skin, bone, and joints; gynecologic and intra-abdominal infections; bacteremia; and septicemia. Susceptible microorganisms include streptococci, including *S. pneumoniae* and *S. pyogenes; S. aureus* (penicillinase- and non-penicillinase–producing) and *S. epidermidis; E. coli; Klebsiella; H. influenzae; Enterobacter; Proteus*; and *Peptostreptococcus*.** *Adults:* usual dose is 1 g I.V. or I.M. q 6 to 12 hours. Up to 12 g daily can be administered in life-threatening infections. *Children weighing at least 50 kg (110 lb):* usual adult dose but dosage should not exceed 12 g daily. *Children*

ages 1 month to 12 years weighing under 50 kg: 50 to 180 mg/kg/day I.V. or I.M. in four to six divided doses. *Neonates ages 1 to 4 weeks:* 50 mg/kg I.V. q 8 hours. *Neonates up to age 1 week:* 50 mg/kg I.V. q 12 hours.

Adverse reactions

CNS: headache, malaise, paresthesia, dizziness.
GI: pseudomembranous colitis, nausea, anorexia, vomiting, *diarrhea,* glossitis, dyspepsia, abdominal cramps, tenesmus, anal pruritus, oral candidiasis.
GU: genital pruritus and candidiasis.
Hematologic: *transient neutropenia,* eosinophilia, hemolytic anemia, *thrombocytopenia, agranulocytosis.*
Hepatic: transient increases in liver enzymes.
Respiratory: dyspnea.
Skin: *maculopapular and erythematous rashes, urticaria.*
Other: hypersensitivity reactions (serum sickness, *anaphylaxis*); elevated temperature; *pain, induration, sterile abscesses, temperature elevation, tissue sloughing* (at injection site); *phlebitis, thrombophlebitis* (with I.V. injection).

Interactions

Drug-drug. *Aminoglycosides:* may increase risk of nephrotoxicity. Monitor closely.
Probenecid: may inhibit excretion and increase blood levels of cefotaxime. Use together cautiously.

Contraindications and precautions

• Contraindicated in patients with hypersensitivity to drug or other cephalosporins.
• Use cautiously in patients with history of sensitivity to penicillin, in pregnant or breast-feeding patients, and with dosage adjustments in patients with renal failure.

NURSING CONSIDERATIONS

⚕ Assessment
- Assess patient's infection before therapy and regularly thereafter.
- Obtain specimen for culture and sensitivity tests. Therapy may begin before test results are known.
- Ask patient about previous reactions to cephalosporin or penicillin before administering first dose.
- Be alert for adverse reactions and drug interactions.
- Monitor patient's hydration status if adverse GI reactions occur.
- Evaluate patient's and family's knowledge of drug therapy.

⊞ Nursing diagnoses
- Infection related to bacteria susceptible to drug
- Risk for fluid volume deficit related to drug-induced adverse GI reactions
- Knowledge deficit related to drug therapy

❯ Planning and implementation
I.V. use: For direct injection, reconstitute 500-mg, 1-g, or 2-g vials with 10 ml of sterile water for injection. Solutions containing 1 g/14 ml are isotonic. Inject drug into large vein or into tubing of free-flowing I.V. solution over 3 to 5 minutes.
– For I.V. infusion, reconstitute infusion vials with 50 to 100 ml of D₅W or 0.9% NaCl solution. Infuse drug over 20 to 30 minutes. Interrupt flow of primary I.V. solution during infusion.
I.M. use: Inject deeply into large muscle mass, such as gluteus maximus or lateral aspect of thigh.
- Be aware that urine glucose determinations may be false-positive with copper sulfate tests (Clinitest); glucose enzymatic tests (Diastix or Chemstrip uG) are not affected.
Patient teaching
- Tell patient to report adverse reactions.

✓ Evaluation
- Patient is free from infection.
- Patient maintains adequate hydration.
- Patient and family state understanding of drug therapy.

---

cefotetan disodium
(SEF-oh-teh-tan die-SOH-dee-um)
Cefotan

Pharmacologic class: second-generation cephalosporin
Therapeutic class: antibiotic
Pregnancy risk category: B

How supplied
Injection: 1 g, 2 g
Infusion: 1 g, 2 g piggyback
Pharmacy bulk package: 10-g vial

Pharmacokinetics
Absorption: unknown after I.M. administration.
Distribution: distributed widely into most body tissues and fluids; CSF penetration is poor; 75% to 90% protein-bound.
Metabolism: none.
Excretion: excreted primarily in urine.
Half-life: about 3 to 4.5 hours.

Route	Onset	Peak	Duration
I.V.	Immediate	Immediate	Unknown
I.M.	Unknown	1.5-2 hr	Unknown

Pharmacodynamics
Chemical effect: inhibits cell-wall synthesis, promoting osmotic instability; usually bactericidal.
Therapeutic effect: hinders or kills susceptible bacteria: many gram-positive organisms and enteric gram-negative bacilli, such as streptococci, *Staphylococcus aureus* and *Staphylococcus epidermidis*, *Escherichia coli, Klebsiella* species, *Enterobacter* species, *Proteus* species, *Haemophilus influenzae, Neisseria gonorrhoeae*, and *Bacteroides* species.

Indications and dosage

▶ **Serious urinary tract and lower respiratory tract infections and gynecologic, skin and skin-structure, intra-abdominal, and bone and joint infections caused by susceptible streptococci,** *S. aureus* **and** *S. epidermidis, Escherichia coli, Klebsiella, Enterobacter, Proteus, H. influenzae, N. gonorrhoeae,* **and** *Bacteroides,* **including** *B. fragilis;* **and perioperative prophylaxis.** *Adults:* 500 mg to 3 g I.V. or I.M. q 12 hours for 5 to 10 days. In life-threatening infections, up to 6 g daily.

Adverse reactions

CNS: headache, malaise, paresthesia, dizziness.
GI: pseudomembranous colitis, nausea, anorexia, vomiting, *diarrhea,* glossitis, dyspepsia, abdominal cramps, tenesmus, anal pruritus.
GU: genital pruritus and candidiasis, *nephrotoxicity.*
Hematologic: *transient neutropenia,* eosinophilia, hemolytic anemia, hypoprothrombinemia, bleeding, *agranulocytosis, thrombocytopenia.*
Hepatic: transient increases in liver enzymes.
Respiratory: dyspnea.
Skin: *maculopapular and erythematous rashes, urticaria.*
Other: hypersensitivity reactions (serum sickness, *anaphylaxis*); elevated temperature; *pain, induration, sterile abscesses, tissue sloughing* (at injection site); *phlebitis, thrombophlebitis* (with I.V. injection).

Interactions

Drug-drug. *Aminoglycosides:* possible synergistic effect and possible increased risk of nephrotoxicity. Use with caution.
Anticoagulants: effects of anticoagulants may be increased. Use with caution.
Probenecid: may inhibit excretion and increase blood levels of cefotetan. Sometimes used for this effect.

Drug-lifestyle. *Alcohol use:* possible disulfiram-like reaction. Caution patient to avoid alcohol consumption for several days after discontinuing cefotetan.

Contraindications and precautions

• Contraindicated in patients with hypersensitivity to drug or other cephalosporins.
• Use cautiously in patients with history of sensitivity to penicillin, in pregnant or breast-feeding women, and with dosage adjustments in patients with renal failure.
• Safety of drug has not been established in children.

NURSING CONSIDERATIONS

⚗ Assessment
• Assess patient's infection before therapy and regularly thereafter.
• Obtain specimen for culture and sensitivity tests before first dose. Therapy may begin pending test results.
• Ask patient about previous reactions to cephalosporin or penicillin before administering first dose.
• Be alert for adverse reactions and drug interactions.
• Monitor patient's hydration status if adverse GI reactions occur.
• Evaluate patient's and family's knowledge of drug therapy.

⚕ Nursing diagnoses
• Infection related to bacteria susceptible to drug
• Risk for fluid volume deficit related to drug-induced adverse GI reactions
• Knowledge deficit related to drug therapy

⧐ Planning and implementation
I.V. use: Reconstitute drug with sterile water for injection. Then may be mixed with 50 to 100 ml of D_5W or 0.9% NaCl solution. Interrupt flow of primary I.V. solution during drug infusion. For direct injection, give solutions containing 1 or 2 g of solution over 3 to 5 minutes.

Reactions may be *common,* uncommon, *life-threatening,* or COMMON AND LIFE-THREATENING.

I.M. use: Reconstitute I.M. injection with sterile water or bacteriostatic water for injection, 0.9% NaCl for injection, or 0.5% or 1% lidocaine hydrochloride. Shake to dissolve and let stand until clear.
• Know that reconstituted solution remains stable for 24 hours at room temperature or 96 hours if refrigerated.
• Be aware that urine glucose determinations may be false-positive with copper sulfate tests (Clinitest); glucose enzymatic tests (Diastix or Chemstrip uG) are not affected.
Patient teaching
• Tell patient to report adverse reactions.

☑ **Evaluation**
• Patient is free from infection.
• Patient maintains adequate hydration.
• Patient and family state understanding of drug therapy.

cefoxitin sodium
(sef-OKS-ih-tin SOH-dee-um)
Mefoxin

Pharmacologic class: second-generation cephalosporin
Therapeutic class: antibiotic
Pregnancy risk category: B

How supplied

Injection: 1 g, 2 g
Infusion: 1 g, 2 g in 50-ml or 100-ml container

Pharmacokinetics

Absorption: unknown after I.M. administration.
Distribution: distributed widely into most body tissues and fluids; CSF penetration is poor; 50% to 80% protein-bound.
Metabolism: insignificant (about 2%).
Excretion: excreted primarily in urine.
Half-life: about 0.5 to 1 hours.

Route	Onset	Peak	Duration
I.V.	Immediate	Immediate	Unknown

Pharmacodynamics

Chemical effect: inhibits cell-wall synthesis, promoting osmotic instability; usually bactericidal.
Therapeutic effect: hinders or kills susceptible bacteria: many gram-positive organisms and enteric gram-negative bacilli, such as *Escherichia coli* and other coliform bacteria, streptococci, *Staphylococcus aureus, Staphylococcus epidermidis, Klebsiella, Haemophilus influenzae,* and *Bacteroides* species.

Indications and dosage

▶ **Serious infections of respiratory and GU tracts, skin, soft-tissue, bone, and joint infections, and bloodstream and intra-abdominal infections caused by susceptible E. coli and other coliform bacteria, S. aureus (penicillinase- and non-penicillinase–producing) and S. epidermidis, streptococci, Klebsiella, H. influenzae, and Bacteroides, including B. fragilis; and perioperative prophylaxis.** *Adults:* 1 to 2 g I.V. q 6 to 8 hours for uncomplicated forms of infection. In life-threatening infections, up to 12 g daily. *Children over age 3 months:* 80 to 160 mg/kg I.V. daily given in four to six equally divided doses. Maximum daily dose is 12 g.
▶ **Prophylactic use in surgery.** *Adults:* 2 g I.V. 30 to 60 minutes before surgery, then 2 g I.V. q 6 hours for 24 hours. *Children age 3 months or older:* 30 to 40 mg/kg I.V. 30 to 60 minutes before surgery, then 30 mg/kg q 6 hours for 24 hours.

Adverse reactions

CNS: headache, malaise, paresthesia, dizziness.
GI: pseudomembranous colitis, nausea, anorexia, vomiting, *diarrhea,* glossitis, dyspepsia, abdominal cramps, tenesmus, anal pruritus, oral candidiasis.
GU: genital pruritus and candidiasis, *acute renal failure.*

Hematologic: transient neutropenia, eosinophilia, *hemolytic anemia, thrombocytopenia.*
Hepatic: transient increases in liver enzymes.
Respiratory: dyspnea.
Skin: *maculopapular and erythematous rashes, urticaria.*
Other: hypersensitivity reactions (serum sickness, *anaphylaxis*), elevated temperature, *phlebitis, thrombophlebitis* (with I.V. injection).

Interactions

Drug-drug. *Nephrotoxic agents:* possible increased risk of nephrotoxicity. Monitor closely.
Probenecid: may inhibit excretion and increase blood levels of cefoxitin. Sometimes used for this effect.

Contraindications and precautions

• Contraindicated in patients with hypersensitivity to drug or other cephalosporins.
• Use cautiously in patients with history of sensitivity to penicillin, in pregnant or breast-feeding patients, and with dosage adjustments in patients with renal failure.

NURSING CONSIDERATIONS

Assessment
• Assess patient's infection before therapy and regularly thereafter.
• Obtain specimen for culture and sensitivity tests before first dose. Therapy may begin pending test results.
• Ask patient about previous reactions to cephalosporin or penicillin before administering first dose.
• Be alert for adverse reactions and drug interactions.
• Assess I.V. site frequently for thrombophlebitis.
• Monitor patient's hydration status if adverse GI reactions occur.
• Evaluate patient's and family's knowledge of drug therapy.

Nursing diagnoses
• Infection related to bacteria susceptible to drug
• Risk for fluid volume deficit related to drug-induced adverse GI reactions
• Knowledge deficit related to drug therapy

Planning and implementation
• Reconstitute 1 g with at least 10 ml of sterile water for injection and 2 g with 10 to 20 ml of sterile water for injection. Solutions of dextrose 5% and 0.9% NaCl for injection can also be used. For direct injection, inject drug into large vein or into tubing of free-flowing I.V. solution over 3 to 5 minutes. For intermittent infusion, add reconstituted drug to 50 or 100 ml of dextrose 5% or 10% in water or 0.9% NaCl injection. Interrupt flow of primary I.V. solution during infusion.
• After reconstitution, store for 24 hours at room temperature or refrigerate for 1 week.
• Be aware that urine glucose determinations may be false-positive with copper sulfate tests (Clinitest); glucose enzymatic tests (Diastix or Chemstrip uG) are not affected.
• Know that patients with renal dysfunction require dosage adjustment.
Patient teaching
• Tell patient to report adverse reactions.

Evaluation
• Patient is free from infection.
• Patient maintains adequate hydration.
• Patient and family state understanding of drug therapy.

cefpodoxime proxetil
(sef-poh-DOKS-eem PROKS-eh-til)
Vantin

Pharmacologic class: third-generation cephalosporin
Therapeutic class: antibiotic
Pregnancy risk category: B

Reactions may be *common*, uncommon, **life-threatening**, or COMMON AND LIFE-THREATENING.

How supplied

Tablets (film-coated): 100 mg, 200 mg
Oral suspension: 50 mg/5 ml,
100 mg/5 ml in 100-ml bottles

Pharmacokinetics

Absorption: absorbed from GI tract.
Distribution: distributed widely into
most body tissues and fluids except CSF;
22% to 33% protein-bound in serum and
21% to 29% protein-bound in plasma.
Metabolism: drug is de-esterified to its
active metabolite, cefpodoxime.
Excretion: excreted primarily in urine.
Half-life: 2.1 to 2.8 hours.

Route	Onset	Peak	Duration
P.O.	Unknown	2-3 hr	Unknown

Pharmacodynamics

Chemical effect: inhibits cell-wall synthesis, promoting osmotic instability;
usually bactericidal.
Therapeutic effect: hinders or kills susceptible bacteria: many gram-positive aerobes, such as *Staphylococcus aureus,*
Staphylococcus saprophyticus, Streptococ-
cus pneumoniae, and *Streptococcus pyo-*
genes; and gram-negative aerobes, including *Klebsiella pneumoniae, Escherichia*
coli, Proteus mirabilis, Moraxella (Bran-
hamella) catarrhalis, Haemophilus in-
fluenzae, and *Neisseria gonorrhoeae.*

Indications and dosage

▶ **Acute, community-acquired pneu-**
monia caused by non-beta-lactamase–
producing strains of *H. influenzae* or *S.*
pneumoniae. *Adults and children age 13*
and older: 200 mg P.O. q 12 hours for 14
days.
▶ **Acute bacterial exacerbation of**
chronic bronchitis caused by *S. pneu-*
***moniae, H. influenzae* (non-beta-**
lactamase–producing strains only), or
M. catarrhalis. *Adults and children age*
13 and older: 200 mg P.O. q 12 hours for
10 days.
▶ **Uncomplicated gonorrhea in men**
and women; rectal gonococcal infec-

tions in women. *Adults and children age*
13 and older: 200 mg P.O. as single dose.
Follow with doxycycline 100 mg P.O.
b.i.d. for 7 days.
▶ **Uncomplicated skin and skin-**
structure infections caused by *S.*
aureus* or *S. pyogenes. *Adults and chil-*
dren age 13 and older: 400 mg P.O. q 12
hours for 7 to 14 days.
▶ **Acute otitis media caused by *S.***
pneumoniae, H. influenzae,* or *M.
catarrhalis. *Children age 5 months and*
over: 5 mg/kg (not to exceed 200 mg)
P.O. q 12 hours or 10 mg/kg (not to exceed 400 mg) P.O. q.d. for 10 days.
▶ **Pharyngitis or tonsillitis caused by**
S. pyogenes. *Adults and children age 13*
and older: 100 mg P.O. q 12 hours for 7
to 10 days. *Children age 5 months to 12*
years: 5 mg/kg (not to exceed 100 mg)
P.O. q 12 hours for 10 days.
▶ **Uncomplicated urinary tract infec-**
tions caused by *E. coli, Klebsiella pneu-*
moniae, P. mirabilis,* or *S. saprophyticus.
Adults: 100 mg P.O. q 12 hours for 7 days.
In patients with renal failure: if creatinine
clearance is below 30 ml/minute, dosage
interval should be increased to q 24 hours.
Patients receiving dialysis should get drug
three times weekly, after dialysis.

Adverse reactions

CNS: headache.
GI: *diarrhea,* nausea, vomiting, abdomi-
nal pain.
GU: vaginal fungal infections.
Skin: rash.
Other: hypersensitivity reactions (*ana-*
phylaxis).

Interactions

Drug-drug. *Antacids, H_2 antagonists:*
decreased absorption of cefpodoxime.
Avoid concomitant use.
Probenecid: decreased excretion of cefpodoxime. Monitor for toxicity.
Drug-food. *Any food:* increases absorption. Give drug with food.

Contraindications and precautions

• Contraindicated in patients with hypersensitivity to drug or other cephalosporins.
• Use cautiously in patients with history of hypersensitivity to penicillin (risk of cross-sensitivity), in patients receiving nephrotoxic drugs (other cephalosporins have had nephrotoxic potential), and in pregnant or breast-feeding women.
• Safety of drug has not been established in children under age 6 months.

NURSING CONSIDERATIONS

☞ Assessment
• Assess patient's infection before therapy and regularly thereafter.
• Obtain specimen for culture and sensitivity tests before first dose. Therapy may begin pending test results.
• Ask patient about previous reactions to cephalosporin or penicillin before administering first dose.
• Be alert for adverse reactions and drug interactions.
• Monitor patient's hydration status if adverse GI reactions occur.
• Evaluate patient's and family's knowledge of drug therapy.

⊕ Nursing diagnoses
• Infection related to bacteria susceptible to drug
• Risk for fluid volume deficit related to drug-induced adverse GI reactions
• Knowledge deficit related to drug therapy

⊠ Planning and implementation
• Administer drug with food to minimize adverse GI reactions. Shake well before using.
• Store suspension in refrigerator (36° to 46° F [2° to 8° C]). Discard unused portion after 14 days.
• Be aware that urine glucose determinations may be false-positive with copper sulfate tests (Clinitest); glucose enzymatic tests (Diastix or Chemstrip uG) are not affected.

Patient teaching
• Advise patient to take drug with meals to minimize adverse GI reactions.
• Tell patient to take drug exactly as prescribed, even after he feels better.
• Instruct patient to notify doctor if rash develops.
• Teach patient how to store drug.

☑ Evaluation
• Patient is free from infection.
• Patient maintains adequate hydration.
• Patient and family state understanding of drug therapy.

cefprozil
(SEF-pruh-zil)
Cefzil

Pharmacologic class: second-generation cephalosporin
Therapeutic class: antibiotic
Pregnancy risk category: B

How supplied

Tablets: 250 mg, 500 mg
Oral suspension: 125 mg/5 ml, 250 mg/5 ml

Pharmacokinetics

Absorption: about 95% absorbed from GI tract.
Distribution: about 35% protein-bound; distributed into various body tissues and fluids.
Metabolism: probably metabolized by the liver.
Excretion: excreted primarily in urine. *Half-life:* 1.3 hours in patients with normal renal function; 2 hours in patients with impaired hepatic function; and 5.2 to 5.9 hours in patients with end-stage renal disease.

Route	Onset	Peak	Duration
P.O.	Unknown	Unknown	Unknown

Pharmacodynamics

Chemical effect: inhibits cell-wall synthesis, promoting osmotic instability; usually bactericidal.

Therapeutic effect: hinders or kills susceptible bacteria: *Staphylococcus aureus, Streptococcus pyogenes, Streptococcus pneumoniae, Moraxella (Branhamella) catarrhalis,* and *Haemophilus influenzae.*

Indications and dosage

▶ **Pharyngitis or tonsillitis caused by** *S. pyogenes. Adults and children age 13 and older:* 500 mg P.O. daily for at least 10 days.

▶ **Otitis media caused by** *S. pneumoniae, H. influenzae,* **and** *M. catarrhalis. Infants and children age 6 months to 12 years:* 15 mg/kg P.O. q 12 hours for 10 days.

▶ **Secondary bacterial infections of acute bronchitis and acute bacterial exacerbation of chronic bronchitis caused by** *S. pneumoniae, H. influenzae,* **and** *M. catarrhalis. Adults and children age 13 and older:* 500 mg P.O. q 12 hours for 10 days.

▶ **Uncomplicated skin and skin-structure infections caused by** *S. aureus* **and** *S. pyogenes. Adults and children age 13 and older:* 250 mg P.O. b.i.d., or 500 mg daily to b.i.d. for 10 days.

Adverse reactions

CNS: dizziness, hyperactivity, headache, nervousness, insomnia.
GI: *diarrhea, nausea,* vomiting, abdominal pain.
GU: elevated BUN level, elevated serum creatinine level, genital pruritus, vaginitis.
Hematologic: decreased leukocyte count, eosinophilia.
Hepatic: elevated liver enzymes, cholestatic jaundice (rare).
Skin: rash, urticaria, diaper rash.
Other: superinfection, hypersensitivity reactions (serum sickness, *anaphylaxis*).

Interactions

Drug-drug. *Aminoglycosides:* increased risk of nephrotoxicity. Monitor closely.
Probenecid: may inhibit excretion and increase blood levels of cefprozil. Monitor patient.

Contraindications and precautions

• Contraindicated in patients with hypersensitivity to drug or other cephalosporins.
• Use cautiously in patients with history of sensitivity to penicillin, in pregnant or breast-feeding women, and in those with impaired hepatic or renal function.

NURSING CONSIDERATIONS

⚗ Assessment
• Assess patient's infection before therapy and regularly thereafter.
• Obtain specimen for culture and sensitivity tests before first dose. Therapy may begin pending test results.
• Ask patient about previous reactions to cephalosporin or penicillin before administering first dose.
• Be alert for adverse reactions and drug interactions.
• Monitor patient's hydration status if adverse GI reactions occur.
• Evaluate patient's and family's knowledge of drug therapy.

⊞ Nursing diagnoses
• Infection related to bacteria susceptible to drug
• Risk for fluid volume deficit related to drug-induced adverse GI reactions
• Knowledge deficit related to drug therapy

▷ Planning and implementation
• Know that patients with creatinine clearance less than 30 ml/minute should receive 50% of usual dose.
• Administer drug after hemodialysis treatment is completed; drug is removed by hemodialysis.

• Refrigerate reconstituted suspension (stable for 14 days). Keep tightly closed and shake well before using.

• Be aware that urine glucose determinations may be false-positive with copper sulfate tests (Clinitest); glucose enzymatic tests (Diastix or Chemstrip uG) are not affected.

Patient teaching

• Tell patient to shake suspension well before measuring dose.

• Advise patient to take drug as prescribed, even after he feels better.

• Inform patient that oral suspensions contain drug in bubble-gum-flavored form to improve palatability and promote compliance in children. Tell him to refrigerate reconstituted suspension and to discard unused portion after 14 days.

☑ Evaluation

• Patient is free from infection.
• Patient maintains adequate hydration.
• Patient and family state understanding of drug therapy.

ceftazidime
(SEF-TAZ-ih-deem)
Ceptaz, Fortaz, Tazicef, Tazidime

Pharmacologic class: third-generation cephalosporin
Therapeutic class: antibiotic
Pregnancy risk category: B

How supplied

Injection (with sodium carbonate): 500 mg, 1 g, 2 g;
Injection (with arginine): 1 g, 2 g;
Infusion: 1 g, 2 g in 50-ml and 100-ml vials (premixed)

Pharmacokinetics

Absorption: unknown after I.M. administration.
Distribution: distributed widely into most body tissues and fluids, including

CSF (unlike most other cephalosporins); 5% to 24% protein-bound.
Metabolism: none.
Excretion: excreted primarily in urine.
Half-life: about 1.5 to 2 hours.

Route	Onset	Peak	Duration
I.V.	Immediate	Immediate	Unknown
I.M.	Unknown	≤ 1 hr	Unknown

Pharmacodynamics

Chemical effect: inhibits cell-wall synthesis, promoting osmotic instability; usually bactericidal.
Therapeutic effect: hinders or kills susceptible bacteria: some gram-positive organisms and many enteric gram-negative bacilli, as well as streptococci (*Streptococcus pneumoniae* and *S. pyogenes*); *Staphylococcus aureus; Escherichia coli; Klebsiella* species; *Proteus* species; *Enterobacter* species; *Haemophilus influenzae; Pseudomonas* species; and some strains of *Bacteroides*.

Indications and dosage

▶ **Serious infections of lower respiratory and urinary tracts; gynecologic, intra-abdominal, CNS, and skin infections; bacteremia; and septicemia. Among susceptible microorganisms are streptococci, including *S. pneumoniae* and *S. pyogenes; S. aureus; E. coli; Klebsiella; Proteus; Enterobacter; H. influenzae; Pseudomonas;* and some strains of *Bacteroides*.** *Adults and children age 12 and older:* 1 g I.V. or I.M. q 8 to 12 hours; up to 6 g daily in life-threatening infections. *Children age 1 month to 12 years:* 30 to 50 mg/kg I.V. q 8 hours. *Neonates up to 4 weeks:* 30 mg/kg I.V. q 12 hours.

Adverse reactions

CNS: headache, dizziness, *seizures*.
GI: pseudomembranous colitis, nausea, vomiting, diarrhea, dysgeusia, abdominal cramps.
GU: genital pruritus and candidiasis.

Hematologic: eosinophilia, thrombocytosis, leukopenia, *agranulocytosis.*
Skin: *maculopapular and erythematous rashes, urticaria.*
Other: hypersensitivity reactions (serum sickness, *anaphylaxis*); transient elevation in liver enzymes; dyspnea; elevated temperature; *pain, induration, sterile abscesses, tissue sloughing* (at injection site); *phlebitis, thrombophlebitis* (with I.V. injection).

Interactions
Drug-drug. *Chloramphenicol:* antagonistic effect. Avoid concomitant use.

Contraindications and precautions
• Contraindicated in patients with hypersensitivity to drug or other cephalosporins.
• Use cautiously in patients with history of sensitivity to penicillin, in pregnant or breast-feeding women, and with dosage adjustments in patients with renal failure.
• Know that commercially available preparations contain either sodium carbonate (Fortaz, Tazicef, Tazidime) or arginine (Ceptaz) to facilitate dissolution of drug. Safety and efficacy of arginine-containing solutions in children age 12 and younger have not been established.

NURSING CONSIDERATIONS

Assessment
• Assess patient's infection before therapy and regularly thereafter.
• Obtain specimen for culture and sensitivity tests before first dose. Therapy may begin pending test results.
• Ask patient about previous reactions to cephalosporin or penicillin before administering first dose.
• Be alert for adverse reactions and drug interactions.
• Monitor patient's hydration status if adverse GI reactions occur.
• Evaluate patient's and family's knowledge of drug therapy.

Nursing diagnoses
• Infection related to bacteria susceptible to drug
• Risk for fluid volume deficit related to drug-induced adverse GI reactions
• Knowledge deficit related to drug therapy

Planning and implementation
I.V. use: Reconstitute sodium carbonate-containing solutions with sterile water for injection. Add 5 ml to 500-mg vial; 10 ml to 1-g or 2-g vial. Shake well to dissolve drug. Carbon dioxide is released during dissolution, and positive pressure will develop in vial. Reconstitute arginine-containing solutions with 10 ml of sterile water for injection. This formulation won't release gas bubbles. Each brand of ceftazidime includes specific instructions for reconstitution. Read and follow these instructions carefully.
I.M. use: Inject deeply into large muscle mass, such as gluteus maximus or lateral aspect of thigh.
• Know that ceftazidime is removed by hemodialysis; supplemental dose of drug is indicated after each dialysis period, as ordered.
• Be aware that urine glucose determinations may be false-positive with copper sulfate tests (Clinitest); glucose enzymatic tests (Diastix or Chemstrip uG) are not affected.
Patient teaching
• Tell patient to report adverse reactions.

Evaluation
• Patient is free from infection.
• Patient maintains adequate hydration.
• Patient and family state understanding of drug therapy.

---

ceftibuten
(sef-tih-BY00-tin)
Cedax

Pharmacologic class: third-generation cephalosporin
Therapeutic class: antibiotic
Pregnancy risk category: B

How supplied

Capsules: 400 mg
Oral suspension: 90 mg/5 ml, 180 mg/5 ml

Pharmacokinetics

Absorption: rapidly absorbed.
Distribution: 65% bound to plasma proteins.
Metabolism: by kidneys.
Excretion: mainly in urine.

Route	Onset	Peak	Duration
P.O.	Unknown	2-4 hr	Unknown

Pharmacodynamics

Chemical effect: exerts its bacterial action by binding to essential target proteins of the bacterial cell wall, thus inhibiting cell-wall synthesis.
Therapeutic effect: hinders or kills susceptible bacteria.

Indications and dosage

▶ **Acute bacterial exacerbation of chronic bronchitis due to** *Haemophilus influenzae, Moraxella (Branhamella) catarrhalis,* **or penicillin-susceptible strains of** *Streptococcus pneumoniae. Adults and children age 12 and over:* 400 mg P.O. daily for 10 days.
▶ **Pharyngitis and tonsillitis due to** *Streptococcus pyogenes,* **acute bacterial otitis media due to** *H. influenzae, M. catarrhalis,* **or** *S. pyogenes. Adults and children age 12 and over:* 400 mg P.O. daily for 10 days. *Children under age 12:* 9 mg/kg P.O. daily for 10 days. *Children weighing over 45 kg (99 lb):* should re-ceive maximum dose of 400 mg P.O. daily for 10 days.
In patients with renal impairment: if creatinine clearance is 30 to 49 ml/minute, 4.5 mg/kg or 200 mg P.O. q 24 hours; if it is 5 to 29 ml/minute, 2.25 mg/kg or 100 mg P.O. q 24 hours.

Adverse reactions

CNS: headache, dizziness, aphasia, psychosis.
GI: nausea, vomiting, diarrhea, dyspepsia, abdominal pain, loose stools, pseudomembranous colitis.
GU: elevated levels of BUN, toxic nephropathy, renal dysfunction.
Hematologic: elevated levels of eosinophils, decreased hemoglobin levels, altered platelet count, aplastic anemia, hemolytic anemia, *hemorrhage, neutropenia, agranulocytosis, pancytopenia.*
Hepatic: hepatic cholestasis, elevated liver enzymes and bilirubin.
Skin: *Stevens-Johnson syndrome.*
Other: allergic reaction, *anaphylaxis,* drug fever.

Interactions

Drug-food. *Any food:* decreases bioavailability of drug. Administer drug 2 hours before or 1 hour after a meal.

Contraindications and precautions

• Contraindicated in patients with hypersensitivity to cephalosporins.
• Use cautiously in patients with history of hypersensitivity to penicillin, GI disease, or impaired renal function and in the elderly.

NURSING CONSIDERATIONS

📋 Assessment
• Obtain specimen for *Clostridium difficile,* as ordered, in patient who develops diarrhea after therapy.
• Obtain specimen for culture and sensitivity tests before starting drug.
• Evaluate patient's and family's knowledge of drug therapy.

Reactions may be *common,* uncommon, *life-threatening,* or COMMON AND LIFE-THREATENING.

⊞ Nursing diagnoses
• Infection related to bacteria susceptible to drug
• Knowledge deficit related to drug therapy

⧉ Planning and implementation
• To prepare oral suspension, tap bottle to loosen powder. Follow chart supplied by manufacturer for mixing instructions. Suspension is stable for 14 days if refrigerated.
• Shake suspension well before use.
• Stop drug if allergic reaction occurs.
• Monitor patient for superinfection.
Patient teaching
• Instruct patient to take drug as prescribed, even after he feels better.
• Instruct patient using oral suspension to shake bottle before use and to take it at least 2 hours before or 1 hour after a meal.
• Instruct patient to store oral suspension in the refrigerator, with lid tightly closed, and to discard unused drug after 14 days.
• Warn breast-feeding patient that it is unclear if drug occurs in breast milk.
• Tell diabetic patient that suspension has 1 g sucrose per teaspoon.

☑ Evaluation
• Patient is free from infection.
• Patient and family state understanding of drug therapy.

---

ceftizoxime sodium
(sef-tih-ZOKS-eem SOH-dee-um)
Cefizox

Pharmacologic class: third-generation cephalosporin
Therapeutic class: antibiotic
Pregnancy risk category: B

How supplied

Injection: 500 mg, 1 g, 2 g
Infusion: 1 g, 2 g in 100-mg vials or in 50 ml of D₅W
Pharmacy bulk package: 10 g

Pharmacokinetics
Absorption: unknown after I.M. administration.
Distribution: distributed widely into most body tissues and fluids; unlike many other cephalosporins, ceftizoxime has good CSF penetration and achieves adequate concentration in inflamed meninges. Drug is 28% to 31% protein-bound.
Metabolism: none.
Excretion: excreted primarily in urine.
Half-life: about 1.5 to 2 hours.

Route	Onset	Peak	Duration
I.V.	Immediate	Immediate	Unknown
I.M.	Unknown	0.5-1.5 hr	Unknown

Pharmacodynamics
Chemical effect: inhibits cell-wall synthesis, promoting osmotic instability; usually bactericidal.
Therapeutic effect: hinders or kills susceptible bacteria: some gram-positive organisms and many enteric gram-negative bacilli, as well as streptococci (*Streptococcus pneumoniae* and *S. pyogenes*); *Staphylococcus aureus; Escherichia coli; Klebsiella* species; *Proteus* species; *Enterobacter* species; *Haemophilus influenzae; Pseudomonas* species; and some strains of *Bacteroides*.

Indications and dosage

▶ **Serious infections of lower respiratory and urinary tracts, gynecologic infections, bacteremia, septicemia, meningitis, intra-abdominal infections, bone and joint infections, and skin infections. Among susceptible microorganisms are streptococci, including *S. pneumoniae* and *S. pyogenes; S. aureus* (penicillinase- and non-penicillinase–producing) and *S. epidermidis; E. coli; Klebsiella; H. influenzae; Enterobacter; Proteus;* some *Pseudomonas;* and *Peptostreptococcus.* Adults:** usual dosage is 500 mg to 2 g I.V. or I.M. q 8 to 12 hours. In life-threatening infections, 3 to 4 g I.V. q 8 hours. *Children over age 6 months:* 50 mg/kg I.V. q 6 to 8 hours. For

---

serious infections, up to 200 mg/kg/day in divided doses may be used. Don't exceed 12 g/day.

Adverse reactions

CNS: headache, malaise, paresthesia, dizziness.
GI: pseudomembranous colitis, nausea, anorexia, vomiting, *diarrhea,* glossitis, dyspepsia, abdominal cramps, tenesmus, anal pruritus.
GU: genital pruritus and candidiasis.
Hematologic: *transient neutropenia,* eosinophilia, hemolytic anemia, *thrombocytopenia.*
Skin: *maculopapular and erythematous rashes, urticaria.*
Other: hypersensitivity reactions (serum sickness, *anaphylaxis*); dyspnea; elevated temperature; *pain, induration, sterile abscesses, tissue sloughing* (at injection site); *phlebitis, thrombophlebitis* (with I.V. injection).

Interactions

Drug-drug. *Probenecid:* may inhibit excretion and increase blood levels of ceftizoxime. Sometimes used for this effect.

Contraindications and precautions

• Contraindicated in patients with hypersensitivity to drug or other cephalosporins.
• Use cautiously in patients with history of sensitivity to penicillin, in pregnant or breast-feeding women, and with dosage adjustments in patients with renal failure.
• Safety of drug has not been established in infants under age 6 months.

NURSING CONSIDERATIONS

Assessment
• Assess patient's infection before therapy and regularly thereafter.
• Obtain specimen for culture and sensitivity tests before giving first dose. Therapy may begin pending test results.
• Ask patient about previous reactions to cephalosporin or penicillin before administering first dose.

• Be alert for adverse reactions and drug interactions.
• Monitor patient's hydration status if adverse GI reactions occur.
• Evaluate patient's and family's knowledge of drug therapy.

Nursing diagnoses
• Infection related to bacteria susceptible to drug
• Risk for fluid volume deficit related to drug-induced adverse GI reactions
• Knowledge deficit related to drug therapy

Planning and implementation
I.V. use: To reconstitute powder, add 5 ml of sterile water to 500-mg vial, 10 ml to 1-g vial, or 20 ml to 2-g vial. Reconstitute piggyback vials with 50 to 100 ml of 0.9% NaCl solution or D_5W. Shake vial well.
I.M. use: Inject deeply into large muscle mass, such as gluteus maximus or lateral aspect of thigh. Larger doses (2 g) should be divided and administered at two separate sites.
• Be aware that urine glucose determinations may be false-positive with copper sulfate tests (Clinitest); glucose enzymatic tests (Diastix or Chemstrip uG) are not affected.
Patient teaching
• Tell patient to report adverse reactions.

Evaluation
• Patient is free from infection.
• Patient maintains adequate hydration.
• Patient and family state understanding of drug therapy.

ceftriaxone sodium
(**sef-trigh-AKS-ohn SOH-dee-um**)
Rocephin

Pharmacologic class: third-generation cephalosporin
Therapeutic class: antibiotic

Reactions may be *common*, uncommon, *life-threatening*, or COMMON AND LIFE-THREATENING.

Pregnancy risk category: B

How supplied

Injection: 250 mg, 500 mg, 1 g, 2 g
Infusion: 1 g, 2 g
Pharmacy bulk package: 10 g

Pharmacokinetics

Absorption: unknown after I.M. administration.
Distribution: distributed widely into most body tissues and fluids; unlike many other cephalosporins, ceftriaxone has good CSF penetration. Drug is 58% to 96% protein-bound.
Metabolism: partially metabolized.
Excretion: excreted primarily in urine, minimally in bile. *Half-life:* about 5.5 to 11 hours.

Route	Onset	Peak	Duration
I.V.	Immediate	Immediate	Unknown
I.M.	Unknown	1.5-4 hr	Unknown

Pharmacodynamics

Chemical effect: inhibits cell-wall synthesis, promoting osmotic instability; usually bactericidal.
Therapeutic effect: hinders or kills susceptible bacteria: some gram-positive organisms and many enteric gram-negative bacilli, as well as streptococci; *Staphylococcus epidermidis; Escherichia coli; Klebsiella* species; *Proteus* species; *Enterobacter* species; *Haemophilus influenzae; Pseudomonas* species; and some strains of *Pseudomonas* species and *Peptostreptococcus* and spirochetes such as *Borrelia burgdorferi.*

Indications and dosage

▶ **Uncomplicated gonococcal vulvovaginitis, urethritis, or proctitis.** *Adults:* 125 to 250 mg I.M. as single dose, followed with 100 mg of doxycycline P.O. q 12 hours for 7 days.
Children: 125 mg I.M. as single dose.
▶ **Serious infections of lower respiratory and urinary tracts; gynecologic, bone and joint, intra-abdominal, and**

skin infections; bacteremia; septicemia; and Lyme disease caused by such susceptible microorganisms as streptococci, including *Streptococcus pneumoniae* and *S. pyogenes; Staphylococcus aureus* and *S. epidermidis; Escherichia coli; Klebsiella; H. influenzae; Neisseria meningitidis; Neisseria gonorrhoeae; Enterobacter; Proteus; Pseudomonas; Peptostreptococcus,* and *Serratia marcescens. Adults and children over age 12:* 1 to 2 g I.V. or I.M. daily or in equally divided doses b.i.d. Total daily dosage should not exceed 4 g. *Children age 12 and under:* 50 to 75 mg/kg, not to exceed 2 g/day, given in divided doses q 12 hours.
▶ **Gonococcal meningitis and endocarditis.** *Adults:* 1 to 2 g I.V. q 12 hours for 10 to 14 days (meningitis) or 3 to 4 weeks (endocarditis). *Children:* 100 mg/kg as a single dose or divided q 12 hours for 10 to 14 days (meningitis) or 28 days (endocarditis). Maximum daily dose is 4 g.
▶ **Preoperative prophylaxis.** *Adults:* 1 g I.V. as single dose ½ to 2 hours before surgery.

Adverse reactions

CNS: headache, dizziness.
GI: pseudomembranous colitis, nausea, vomiting, diarrhea, dysgeusia.
GU: genital pruritus and candidiasis.
Hematologic: eosinophilia, thrombocytosis, leukopenia.
Skin: pain, induration, tenderness (at injection site); phlebitis; *rash.*
Other: hypersensitivity reactions (serum sickness, *anaphylaxis*), elevated temperature.

Interactions

Drug-drug. *Probenecid:* high doses may shorten ceftriaxone's half-life. Avoid concomitant use.

Contraindications and precautions

• Contraindicated in patients with hypersensitivity to drug or other cephalosporins.

• Use cautiously in patients with history of sensitivity to penicillin and in pregnant or breast-feeding women.

NURSING CONSIDERATIONS

🗐 Assessment

• Assess patient's infection before therapy and regularly thereafter.

• Obtain specimen for culture and sensitivity tests. Therapy may begin before test results are known.

• Ask patient about previous reactions to cephalosporin or penicillin before administering first dose.

• Be alert for adverse reactions and drug interactions.

• Monitor patient's hydration status if adverse GI reactions occur.

• Evaluate patient's and family's knowledge of drug therapy.

🗐 Nursing diagnoses

• Infection related to bacteria susceptible to drug

• Risk for fluid volume deficit related to drug-induced adverse GI reactions

• Knowledge deficit related to drug therapy

🗐 Planning and implementation

I.V. use: Reconstitute with sterile water for injection, 0.9% NaCl injection, dextrose 5% or 10% injection, or combination of NaCl and dextrose injection and other compatible solutions. Reconstitute by adding 2.4 ml of diluent to 250-mg vial, 4.8 ml to 500-mg vial, 9.6 ml to 1-g vial, and 19.2 ml to 2-g vial. All reconstituted solutions yield concentration that averages 100 mg/ml. After reconstitution, dilute further for intermittent infusion to desired concentration. I.V. dilutions are stable for 24 hours at room temperature.

I.M. use: Inject deeply into large muscle mass, such as gluteus maximus or lateral aspect of thigh. May use lidocaine 1% without epinephrine to dilute for I.M. use if ordered by the physician.

• Be aware that urine glucose determinations may be false-positive with copper sulfate tests (Clinitest); glucose enzymatic tests (Diastix or Chemstrip uG) are not affected.

Patient teaching

• Tell patient to report adverse reactions.

🗹 Evaluation

• Patient is free from infection.

• Patient maintains adequate hydration.

• Patient and family state understanding of drug therapy.

cefuroxime axetil
(sef-yoor-OKS-eem AKS-eh-til)
Ceftin

cefuroxime sodium
Kefurox, Zinacef

Pharmacologic class: second-generation cephalosporin
Therapeutic class: antibiotic
Pregnancy risk category: B

How supplied

cefuroxime axetil
Tablets: 125 mg, 250 mg, 500 mg
Suspension: 125 mg/5 ml, 250 mg/5 ml
cefuroxime sodium
Injection: 750 mg, 1.5 g
Infusion: 750 mg, 1.5 g premixed, frozen solution

Pharmacokinetics

Absorption: cefuroxime axetil is absorbed from GI tract with 37% to 52% of oral dose reaching systemic circulation. Food appears to enhance absorption. Cefuroxime sodium is not well absorbed from GI tract; absorption from I.M. administration is unknown.

Distribution: distributed widely into most body tissues and fluids; CSF penetration is greater than that of most first- and second-generation cephalosporins and achieves adequate therapeutic levels in inflamed meninges. It is 33% to 50% protein-bound.
Metabolism: none.
Excretion: excreted primarily in urine.
Half-life: 1 to 2 hours.

Route	Onset	Peak	Duration
P.O.	Unknown	≤ 2 hr	Unknown
I.V.	Unknown	Immediate	Unknown
I.M.	Unknown	15-60 min	Unknown

Pharmacodynamics

Chemical effect: inhibits cell-wall synthesis, promoting osmotic instability; usually bactericidal.
Therapeutic effect: hinders or kills susceptible bacteria: many gram-positive organisms and enteric gram-negative bacilli.

Indications and dosage

▶ **Injectable form is for serious infections of lower respiratory and urinary tracts; skin and skin-structure infections; bone and joint infections; septicemia; meningitis; and gonorrhea; and for perioperative prophylaxis; oral form is used to treat otitis media, pharyngitis, tonsillitis, infections of urinary and lower respiratory tracts, and skin and skin-structure infections. Among susceptible organisms are *Streptococcus pneumoniae* and S. *pyogenes, Haemophilus influenzae, Klebsiella, Staphylococcus aureus, Escherichia coli, Enterobacter,* and *Neisseria gonorrhoeae. Adults and children age 12 and older:* usual dosage of cefuroxime sodium is 750 mg to 1.5 g I.V. or I.M. q 8 hours for 5 to 10 days. For life-threatening infections and infections caused by less susceptible organisms, 1.5 g I.V. or I.M. q 6 hours; for bacterial meningitis, up to 3 g I.V. q 8 hours. Alternatively,**

250 mg cefuroxime axetil P.O. q 12 hours for 10 days. For severe infections, dosage may be increased to 500 mg q 12 hours. *Children and infants over age 3 months:* 50 to 100 mg/kg/day cefuroxime sodium I.V. or I.M. in equally divided doses q 6 to 8 hours. Higher doses are administered when treating meningitis. Alternatively, 125 to 250 mg cefuroxime axetil P.O. q 12 hours; for bacterial meningitis, 200 to 240 mg/kg I.V. in divided doses q 6 to 8 hours, reduced to 100 mg/kg daily when clinical improvement occurs.
▶ **Uncomplicated urinary tract infections.** *Adults:* 125 to 250 mg P.O. q 12 hours for 10 days.
▶ **Otitis media.** *Children age 3 months to 12 years:* 30 mg/kg/day oral suspension P.O. divided in two doses (maximum dose, 1 g), or 250-mg tablet P.O. b.i.d. for 10 days.
▶ **Perioperative prophylaxis.** *Adults:* 1.5 g I.V. 30 to 60 minutes before surgery; in lengthy operations, 750 mg I.V. or I.M. q 8 hours. For open-heart surgery, 1.5 g I.V. at induction of anesthesia and then q 12 hours for total dosage of 6 g.

Adverse reactions

CNS: headache, malaise, paresthesia, dizziness.
GI: pseudomembranous colitis, nausea, anorexia, vomiting, *diarrhea,* glossitis, dyspepsia, abdominal cramps, tenesmus, anal pruritus.
GU: genital pruritus and candidiasis.
Hematologic: *transient neutropenia,* eosinophilia, *hemolytic anemia,* decrease in hemoglobin and hematocrit, *thrombocytopenia.*
Hepatic: transient increases in liver enzymes.
Respiratory: dyspnea.
Skin: *maculopapular and erythematous rashes, urticaria.*
Other: hypersensitivity reactions (serum sickness, *anaphylaxis*); *pain, induration, sterile abscesses, temperature elevation, tissue sloughing* (at injection site);

---

phlebitis, thrombophlebitis (with I.V. injection).

Interactions

Drug-drug. *Diuretics:* increased risk of adverse renal reactions. Monitor closely. *Probenecid:* may inhibit excretion and increase blood levels of cefuroxime. Sometimes used for this effect.
Drug-food. *Any food:* increased absorption. Give drug with food.

Contraindications and precautions

• Contraindicated in patients with hypersensitivity to drug or other cephalosporins.
• Use cautiously in patients with history of sensitivity to penicillin, in pregnant or breast-feeding women, and with reduced dosage in patients with impaired renal function.
• Safety of drug has not been established in infants under age 3 months.

NURSING CONSIDERATIONS

Assessment
• Assess patient's infection before therapy and regularly thereafter.
• Obtain specimen for culture and sensitivity tests before first dose. Therapy may begin pending test results.
• Ask patient about previous reactions to cephalosporin or penicillin before administering first dose.
• Be alert for adverse reactions and drug interactions.
• Monitor patient's hydration status if adverse GI reactions occur.
• Evaluate patient's and family's knowledge of drug therapy.

Nursing diagnoses
• Infection related to bacteria susceptible to drug
• Risk for fluid volume deficit related to drug-induced adverse GI reactions
• Knowledge deficit related to drug therapy

Planning and implementation
P.O. use: Know that food enhances absorption of cefuroxime axetil.
– Keep in mind that cefuroxime axetil is available only in tablet form, which may be crushed for patients who cannot swallow tablets. Tablets may be allowed to dissolve in small amounts of apple, orange, or grape juice or chocolate milk. However, drug has bitter taste that is difficult to mask, even with food.
I.V. use: For each 750-mg vial of Kefurox, reconstitute with 9 ml of sterile water for injection. Withdraw 8 ml from vial for proper dose. For each 1.5-g vial of Kefurox, reconstitute with 14 ml of sterile water for injection; withdraw entire contents of vial for dose. For each 750-mg vial of Zinacef, reconstitute with 8 ml of sterile water for injection; for each 1.5-g vial, reconstitute with 16 ml. In each case, withdraw entire contents of vial for dose.
– To give by direct injection, inject into large vein or into tubing of free-flowing I.V. solution over 3 to 5 minutes.
– For intermittent infusion, add reconstituted drug to 100 ml D_5W, 0.9% NaCl injection, or other compatible I.V. solution. Infuse over 15 to 60 minutes.
I.M. use: Inject deeply into large muscle mass, such as gluteus maximus or lateral aspect of thigh.
• Be aware that urine glucose determinations may be false-positive with copper sulfate tests (Clinitest); glucose enzymatic tests (Diastix or Chemstrip uG) are not affected.
Patient teaching
• Instruct patient to take drug exactly as prescribed, even after he feels better.
• Advise patient to take oral drug with food to enhance absorption. Explain that tablets may be crushed, but drug has bitter taste that is difficult to mask, even with food.
• Tell patient to report adverse reactions.

☑ **Evaluation**
• Patient is free from infection.
• Patient maintains adequate hydration.
• Patient and family state understanding of drug therapy.

cephalexin hydrochloride
(sef-uh-LEK-sin high-droh-KLOR-ighd)
Keftab

cephalexin monohydrate
Apo-Cephalex♦, Cefanex, Keflex, Novo-Lexin♦, Nu-Cephalex◇

Pharmacologic class: first-generation cephalosporin
Therapeutic class: antibiotic
Pregnancy risk category: B

How supplied
cephalexin hydrochloride
Tablets: 500 mg
cephalexin monohydrate
Tablets: 250 mg, 500 mg, 1 g
Capsules: 250 mg, 500 mg
Oral suspension: 125 mg/5 ml, 250 mg/5 ml

Pharmacokinetics
Absorption: absorbed rapidly and completely from GI tract. Food delays but does not prevent complete absorption.
Distribution: distributed widely into most body tissues and fluids; CSF penetration is poor. Drug is 6% to 15% protein-bound.
Metabolism: none.
Excretion: excreted primarily unchanged in urine. *Half-life:* about 0.5 to 1 hour.

Route	Onset	Peak	Duration
P.O.	Unknown	≤ 1 hr	Unknown

Pharmacodynamics
Chemical effect: inhibits cell-wall synthesis, promoting osmotic instability; usually bactericidal.

Therapeutic effect: hinders or kills susceptible bacteria: many gram-positive cocci, including penicillinase-producing *Staphylococcus aureus* and *Staphylococcus epidermidis, Streptococcus pneumoniae,* group B streptococci, and group A beta-hemolytic streptococci; and gram-negative organisms, including *Klebsiella pneumoniae, Escherichia coli, Proteus mirabilis,* and *Shigella.*

Indications and dosage
▶ **Respiratory tract, GI tract, skin, soft-tissue, bone, and joint infections and otitis media caused by *E. coli* and other coliform bacteria, group A beta-hemolytic streptococci, *Haemophilus influenzae, Klebsiella, Moraxella (Branhamella) catarrhalis, P. mirabilis, S. pneumoniae,* and staphylococci.** *Adults:* 250 mg to 1 g P.O. q 6 hours. *Children:* 25 to 50 mg/kg P.O. daily, divided into four doses.

Adverse reactions
CNS: dizziness, headache, malaise, paresthesia.
GI: pseudomembranous colitis, *nausea, anorexia,* vomiting, *diarrhea,* glossitis, dyspepsia, abdominal cramps, anal pruritus, tenesmus, oral candidiasis.
GU: genital pruritus and candidiasis, vaginitis.
Hematologic: transient neutropenia, eosinophilia, anemia, **thrombocytopenia.**
Skin: *maculopapular and erythematous rashes, urticaria.*
Other: transient increases in liver enzymes, hypersensitivity reactions (serum sickness, *anaphylaxis*), dyspnea.

Interactions
Drug-drug. *Probenecid:* may increase blood levels of cephalosporins. Sometimes used for this effect.

Contraindications and precautions
• Contraindicated in patients with hypersensitivity to cephalosporins.

• Use cautiously in patients with impaired renal function, in those with history of hypersensitivity to penicillin, and in pregnant or breast-feeding women.

NURSING CONSIDERATIONS

⚕ Assessment
• Assess patient's infection before therapy and regularly thereafter.
• Obtain specimen for culture and sensitivity tests before giving first dose. Therapy may begin pending test results.
• Ask patient about previous reactions to cephalosporin or penicillin before administering first dose.
• Be alert for adverse reactions and drug interactions.
• Monitor patient's hydration status if adverse GI reactions occur.
• Evaluate patient's and family's knowledge of drug therapy.

⊞ Nursing diagnoses
• Infection related to bacteria susceptible to drug
• Risk for fluid volume deficit related to drug-induced adverse GI reactions
• Knowledge deficit related to drug therapy

⧁ Planning and implementation
• To prepare oral suspension: Add required amount of water to powder in two portions. Shake well after each addition. After mixing, store in refrigerator (will remain stable for 14 days without significant loss of potency). Keep tightly closed, and shake well before using.
• Administer drug with food or milk to minimize adverse GI reactions.
• Know that group A beta-hemolytic streptococcal infections should be treated for minimum of 10 days.
• Be aware that urine glucose determinations may be false-positive with copper sulfate tests (Clinitest); glucose enzymatic tests (Diastix or Chemstrip uG) are not affected.

Patient teaching
• Inform patient that drug may be taken with meals.
• Instruct patient to take drug exactly as prescribed, even after he feels better.
• Tell patient to call doctor if rash develops.
• Teach patient how to store drug.

☑ Evaluation
• Patient is free from infection.
• Patient maintains adequate hydration.
• Patient and family state understanding of drug therapy.

cephradine
(SEF-ruh-deen)
Velosef**

Pharmacologic class: first-generation cephalosporin
Therapeutic class: antibiotic
Pregnancy risk category: B

How supplied
Capsules: 250 mg, 500 mg
Oral suspension: 125 mg/5 ml, 250 mg/5 ml

Pharmacokinetics
Absorption: absorbed rapidly and completely from GI tract.
Distribution: distributed widely into most body tissues and fluids; CSF penetration is poor. Drug is 6% to 20% protein-bound.
Metabolism: none.
Excretion: excreted primarily in urine.
Half-life: about 0.5 to 2 hours.

Route	Onset	Peak	Duration
P.O.	Unknown	≤ 1 hr	Unknown

Pharmacodynamics
Chemical effect: inhibits cell-wall synthesis, promoting osmotic instability; usually bactericidal.

Therapeutic effect: hinders or kills susceptible bacteria: many gram-positive organisms and some gram-negative organisms, such as *Escherichia coli* and other coliform bacteria, group A beta-hemolytic streptococci, *Haemophilus influenzae, Klebsiella, Proteus mirabilis, Staphylococcus aureus, Streptococcus pneumoniae,* staphylococci, and *Streptococcus viridans.*

Indications and dosage

▶ **Serious infections of respiratory, GU, or GI tract; skin and soft-tissue infections; bone and joint infections; septicemia; endocarditis; and otitis media caused by such susceptible organisms as *E. coli* and other coliform bacteria, group A beta-hemolytic streptococci, *H. influenzae, Klebsiella, P. mirabilis, S. aureus, S. pneumoniae, S. viridans,* and staphylococci; and perioperative prophylaxis.** *Adults:* 250 to 500 mg P.O. q 6 hours or 500 mg to 1 g q 12 hours. For severe or chronic infections, larger doses may be needed but dosage should not exceed 4 g/day. *Children over age 9 months:* 25 to 50 mg/kg/day P.O. given in equally divided doses q 6 to 12 hours. For otitis media, usual dosage is 75 to 100 mg/kg/day P.O. in equally divided doses q 6 to 12 hours. Dose should not exceed 4g/day.

Adverse reactions

CNS: dizziness, headache, malaise, paresthesia.
GI: pseudomembranous colitis, *nausea, anorexia,* vomiting, heartburn, glossitis, dyspepsia, abdominal cramping, *diarrhea,* tenesmus, anal pruritus, oral candidiasis.
GU: genital pruritus and candidiasis, vaginitis.
Hematologic: *transient neutropenia,* eosinophilia, *thrombocytopenia.*
Hepatic: transient increases in liver enzymes.
Skin: *maculopapular and erythematous rashes, urticaria.*

Other: hypersensitivity reactions (serum sickness, *anaphylaxis*), dyspnea.

Interactions

Drug-drug. *Probenecid:* may increase blood levels of cephalosporins. Sometimes used for this effect.

Contraindications and precautions

• Contraindicated in patients with hypersensitivity to drug and other cephalosporins.
• Use cautiously in patients with impaired renal function, in those with history of sensitivity to penicillin, and in pregnant or breast-feeding patients.

NURSING CONSIDERATIONS

Ⅶ Assessment
• Assess patient's infection before therapy and regularly thereafter.
• Obtain specimen for culture and sensitivity tests before first dose. Therapy may begin pending test results.
• Ask patient about previous reactions to cephalosporin or penicillin before administering first dose.
• Be alert for adverse reactions and drug interactions.
• Monitor patient's hydration status if adverse GI reactions occur.
• Evaluate patient's and family's knowledge of drug therapy.

⊕ Nursing diagnoses
• Infection related to bacteria susceptible to drug
• Risk for fluid volume deficit related to drug-induced adverse GI reactions
• Knowledge deficit related to drug therapy

⊠ Planning and implementation
• Administer drug with food to prevent or minimize GI upset.
• Know that group A beta-hemolytic streptococcal infections should be treated for minimum of 10 days.

---

*Liquid form contains alcohol   **May contain tartrazine   ♦Canada   ◇ Australia   †OTC

• Store reconstituted suspension for 7 days at room temperature or 14 days if refrigerated. Keep tightly closed, and shake well before using.

• Be aware that urine glucose determinations may be false-positive with copper sulfate tests (Clinitest); glucose enzymatic tests (Diastix or Chemstrip uG) are not affected.

Patient teaching

• Inform patient that drug may be taken with meals.

• Instruct patient to take drug exactly as prescribed, even after he feels better.

• Tell patient to call doctor if rash develops.

• Teach patient how to store drug.

☑ **Evaluation**

• Patient is free from infection.

• Patient maintains adequate hydration.

• Patient and family state understanding of drug therapy.

---

cerivastatin sodium
(seh-rih-vah-STAH-tin SOH-dee-um)
Baycol

Pharmacologic class:3-hydroxy-3-methylglutaryl-coenzyme A (HMG-CoA) reductase inhibitor
Therapeutic class: antilipemic
Pregnancy risk category: X

How supplied

Tablets: 0.2 mg, 0.3 mg

Pharmacokinetics

Absorption: mean absolute bioavailability is 60% following administration of 0.2-mg dose.
Distribution: more than 99% is bound to plasma protein, primarily albumin.
Metabolism: converted to two active metabolites, M1 and M23, with relative potencies of 50% and 80% of parent compound, respectively. Cholesterol-lowering effect is primarily due to parent drug.
Excretion: M1 and M23 metabolites are excreted by about 24% in urine and 70% in feces; none of parent compound is excreted in urine or feces. *Half-life:* 2 to 3 hours.

Route	Onset	Peak	Duration
P.O.	Unknown	2.5 hr	Unknown

Pharmacodynamics

Chemical effect: competitive inhibitor of HMG-CoA reductase that is responsible for converting HMG-CoA to mevalonate, a precursor of sterols including cholesterol.
Therapeutic effect: reduction in plasma cholesterol level.

Indications and dosages

▶ **Adjunct to diet, to reduce total and low-density lipoprotein (LDL) cholesterol levels in patients with primary hypercholesterolemia and mixed dyslipidemia when diet and other nonpharmacologic measures have been inadequate.** *Adults:* 0.3 mg P.O. daily in the evening. Recommended starting dose in patients with significant renal impairment is 0.2 mg P.O. daily in the evening.

Adverse reactions

CNS: asthenia, dizziness, *headache*.
CV: chest pain, peripheral edema.
EENT: *pharyngitis, rhinitis,* sinusitis.
GI: abdominal pain, constipation, diarrhea, dyspepsia, flatulence, nausea.
GU: urinary tract infection.
Musculoskeletal: arthralgia, back or leg pain, myalgia.
Respiratory: increased cough.
Skin: rash.
Other: flu syndrome.

Interactions

Drug-drug. *Azole antifungals, cyclosporine, erythromycin, fibric acid derivatives, niacin:* may increase the incidence of myopathy. Use cautiously together.

Reactions may be *common*, uncommon, **life-threatening**, or COMMON AND LIFE-THREATENING.

Cholestyramine: when given within 4 hours of drug, results in decreased absorption and decreased peak plasma levels of cerivastatin. Use cautiously together. *Erythromycin:* may decrease hepatic metabolism of drug; has resulted in increases of cerivastatin of up to 50%. Monitor closely.

Contraindications and precautions

• Contraindicated in patients with hypersensitivity to drug, active liver disease, or unexplained persistent elevations of serum transaminases and during pregnancy or breast-feeding.
• Use cautiously in patients with history of liver disease or chronic alcohol use.
• Safety and efficacy in children have not been established.
• Drug should be given to women of childbearing age only if conception is highly unlikely and they have been warned of potential risks to fetus.

NURSING CONSIDERATIONS

⚗ Assessment

• Monitor lipid levels and liver function tests prior to initiation of treatment and at scheduled intervals thereafter as ordered.
• Assess if female patient of childbearing age is using effective birth control methods. Drug is contraindicated in pregnancy because of risk of fetal harm.
• Evaluate patient's and family's knowledge of drug therapy.

🔳 Nursing diagnoses

• Altered nutrition: less than body requirements related to drug-induced adverse GI reactions
• Risk for injury related to underlying condition
• Knowledge deficit related to drug therapy

▷ Planning and implementation

• Council patient regarding appropriate diet, exercise, and weight reduction before starting therapy.

• Know that patients with moderate or severe renal dysfunction require a reduced dosage.
• Withhold drug temporarily in patients experiencing an acute or serious condition predisposing them to renal failure secondary to rhabdomyolysis.

Patient teaching

• Tell patient to take drug in the evening with or without food.
• Inform patient that it may take up to 4 weeks for full therapeutic effect to occur.
• Caution female patient to stop drug and notify doctor if pregnancy occurs or is suspected.
• Advise breast-feeding patient to discontinue breast feeding during drug therapy.
• Tell patient to notify doctor if an unexplained muscle pain, tenderness, or weakness (particularly if accompanied by fever or malaise) occurs.

☑ Evaluation

• Patient maintains adequate nutritional intake.
• Patient remains free from injury and improvement of underlying condition.
• Patient and family state understanding of drug therapy.

chloral hydrate
(KLOR-ul HIGH-drayt)
Aquachloral Supprettes, Noctec
Novo-Chlorhydrate◆

Pharmacologic class: general CNS depressant
Therapeutic class: sedative-hypnotic
Controlled substance schedule: IV
Pregnancy risk category: C

How supplied

Capsules: 250 mg, 500 mg
Syrup: 250 mg/5 ml, 500 mg/5 ml
Suppositories: 324 mg, 500 mg, 648 mg

Pharmacokinetics

Absorption: absorbed well after oral and rectal administration.
Distribution: distributed throughout body tissue and fluids; active metabolite trichloroethanol is 35% to 41% protein-bound.
Metabolism: metabolized rapidly and nearly completely in liver and erythrocytes to active metabolite trichloroethanol; further metabolized in liver and kidneys to trichloroacetic acid and other inactive metabolites.
Excretion: inactive metabolites are excreted primarily in urine, minimally in bile. *Half-life:* 8 to 10 hours for trichloroethanol.

Route	Onset	Peak	Duration
P.O.	≤ 30 min	Unknown	4-8 hr
P.R.	Unknown	Unknown	4-8 hr

Pharmacodynamics

Chemical effect: unknown; sedative effects may be caused by trichloroethanol.
Therapeutic effect: promotes sleep and calmness.

Indications and dosage

▶ **Sedation.** *Adults:* 250 mg P.O. or P.R. t.i.d. after meals. *Children:* 8 mg/kg P.O. or P.R. t.i.d. Maximum daily dosage is 500 mg t.i.d.
▶ **Insomnia.** *Adults:* 500 mg to 1 g P.O. or P.R. 15 to 30 minutes before bedtime. *Children:* 50 mg/kg P.O. or P.R. 15 to 30 minutes before bedtime. Maximum single dose is 1 g.
▶ **Preoperatively.** *Adults:* 500 mg to 1 g P.O. or P.R. 30 minutes before surgery.
▶ **Premedication for EEG.** *Children:* 20 to 25 mg/kg P.O. or P.R.
▶ **Management of alcohol withdrawal symptoms.** *Adults:* 500 mg to 1 g P.O. or P.R. q 6 hours, p.r.n. Generally, single doses or daily dosage for adults should not exceed 2 g.

Adverse reactions

CNS: hangover, drowsiness, nightmares, dizziness, ataxia, paradoxical excitement.
GI: *nausea, vomiting, diarrhea,* flatulence.
Hematologic: eosinophilia, leukopenia.
Skin: hypersensitivity reactions.

Interactions

Drug-drug. *Alkaline solutions:* incompatible with aqueous solutions of chloral hydrate. Don't mix together.
CNS depressants, including narcotic analgesics: excessive CNS depression or vasodilation reaction. Use together cautiously.
Furosemide I.V.: sweating, flushes, variable blood pressure, and uneasiness. Use together cautiously or use different hypnotic drug.
Oral anticoagulants: increased risk of bleeding. Monitor patient closely.
Phenytoin: decreased phenytoin levels. Monitor closely.
Drug-lifestyle. *Alcohol use:* excessive CNS depression or vasodilation reaction. Use together cautiously.

Contraindications and precautions

• Contraindicated in patients hypersensitive to chloral hydrate and in those with hepatic or renal impairment. Oral administration contraindicated in patients with gastric disorders.
• Avoid use in breast-feeding women because small amounts of drug pass into breast milk and may cause drowsiness in infants.
• Use with extreme caution in patients with severe cardiac disease.
• Use cautiously in patients with mental depression, suicidal tendencies, or history of drug abuse.

NURSING CONSIDERATIONS

⚕ Assessment
• Assess patient's underlying condition.
• Evaluate drug effectiveness after administration.

• Monitor BUN levels as ordered. Large dosage may raise BUN levels.
• Be alert for adverse reactions and drug interactions.
• Evaluate patient's and family's knowledge of drug therapy.

🖲 **Nursing diagnoses**
• Sleep pattern disturbance related to patient's underlying condition
• Risk for trauma related to adverse CNS reactions
• Knowledge deficit related to drug therapy

⧊ **Planning and implementation**
P.O. use: Note two strengths of oral liquid form. Double-check dose, especially when administering to children. Fatal overdoses have occurred.
– To minimize unpleasant taste and stomach irritation, dilute or administer drug with liquid. Drug should be taken after meals.
P.R. use: Store rectal suppositories in refrigerator.
• Be aware that long-term use is not recommended; drug loses its efficacy in promoting sleep after 14 days of continued use. Long-term use may cause drug dependence, and patient may experience withdrawal symptoms if drug is suddenly stopped.
• Know that drug may interfere with fluorometric tests for urine catecholamines and Reddy-Jenkins-Thorn test for urine 17-hydroxycorticosteroids. Do not administer drug for 48 hours before fluorometric test as ordered. May also cause false-positive tests for urine glucose when using copper sulfate tests (Clinitest). Use glucose enzymatic tests (Diastix or Chemstrip uG) instead.
Patient teaching
• Caution patient about performing activities that require mental alertness or physical coordination. For inpatients, supervise walking and raise bed rails, particularly for elderly patients.

• Tell patient to store capsules or syrup in dark container; store suppositories in refrigerator.
• Explain that drug may cause morning "hangover." Encourage patient to report severe hangover or feelings of oversedation so doctor can be consulted to adjust dosage or change drug.

☑ **Evaluation**
• Patient states drug effectively induced sleep.
• Patient's safety is maintained.
• Patient and family state understanding of drug therapy.

chlorambucil
(klor-AM-byoo-sil)
Leukeran

Pharmacologic class: alkylating agent (cell cycle–phase nonspecific)
Therapeutic class: antineoplastic
Pregnancy risk category: D

How supplied
Tablets: 2 mg

Pharmacokinetics
Absorption: well absorbed from GI tract.
Distribution: not well understood; drug and its metabolites are highly bound to plasma and tissue proteins.
Metabolism: metabolized in liver; primary metabolite, phenylacetic acid mustard, also possesses cytotoxic activity.
Excretion: metabolites are excreted in urine. *Half-life:* 2 hours for parent compound; 2.5 hours for phenylacetic acid metabolite.

Route	Onset	Peak	Duration
P.O.	3-4 wk	1 hr	Unknown

Pharmacodynamics
Chemical effect: cross-links strands of cellular DNA and interferes with RNA transcription, causing growth imbalance

that leads to cell death. Cell cycle–phase nonspecific. *Therapeutic effect:* kills selected cancer cells.

Indications and dosage

▶ **Chronic lymphocytic leukemia; malignant lymphomas including lymphosarcoma, giant follicular lymphoma, and Hodgkin's disease.** *Adults:* 0.1 to 0.2 mg/kg P.O. daily for 3 to 6 weeks; then adjusted for maintenance (usually 4 to 10 mg daily).

Adverse reactions

CNS: seizures (with overdose).
GI: *nausea, vomiting, stomatitis.*
GU: *azoospermia, infertility.*
Hematologic: *neutropenia* (delayed up to 3 weeks, lasting up to 10 days after last dose); *thrombocytopenia; anemia; myelosuppression* (usually moderate, gradual, and rapidly reversible).
Hepatic: *hepatotoxicity* (rare).
Respiratory: interstitial pneumonitis, *pulmonary fibrosis* (rare).
Skin: exfoliative dermatitis, rash, *Stevens-Johnson syndrome.*
Other: allergic febrile reaction, hyperuricemia.

Interactions

Drug-drug. *Anticoagulants, aspirin:* increased risk of bleeding. Avoid concomitant use.

Contraindications and precautions

• Contraindicated in patients with hypersensitivity or resistance to previous therapy (those hypersensitive to other alkylating agents also may be hypersensitive to chlorambucil) and in breast-feeding women.
• Use with extreme caution, if at all, in pregnant women because fetal harm may occur.
• Use cautiously in patients with history of head trauma or seizures and in patients receiving other drugs that lower seizure threshold.

• Safety of drug has not been established in children.

NURSING CONSIDERATIONS

⚕ Assessment
• Assess patient's underlying neoplastic disorder before therapy and reassess regularly throughout therapy.
• Monitor CBC and serum uric acid level, as ordered.
• Be alert for adverse reactions and drug interactions.
• Evaluate patient's and family's knowledge about drug therapy.

⊞ Nursing diagnoses
• Altered health maintenance related to presence of neoplastic disease
• Altered protection related to drug-induced hematologic adverse reactions
• Knowledge deficit related to drug therapy

⊠ Planning and implementation
• Dose is individualized according to patient's response.
• Give drug 1 hour before breakfast and at least 2 hours after evening meal.
• Know that nausea and vomiting associated with drug use can usually be controlled with antiemetics.
• Know that allopurinol may be used with adequate hydration to prevent hyperuricemia with resulting uric acid nephropathy.
• Follow institutional policy for infection control in immunocompromised patients if WBC count falls below 2,000/mm³ or granulocyte count falls below 1,000/mm³. Severe neutropenia is reversible up to cumulative dosage of 6.5 mg/kg in single course.
Patient teaching
• Warn patient to watch for signs of infection (fever, sore throat, fatigue) and bleeding (easy bruising, nosebleeds, bleeding gums, melena). Tell him to take temperature daily.

Reactions may be *common,* uncommon, *life-threatening*, or COMMON AND LIFE-THREATENING.

• Instruct patient to avoid OTC products containing aspirin.
• Tell patient to take drug 1 hour before breakfast and 2 hours after evening meal if bothered by nausea and vomiting.
• Instruct patient to maintain fluid intake of 2,400 to 3,000 ml/day, if not contraindicated.

☑ Evaluation
• Patient exhibits improvement in underlying neoplastic condition on follow-up diagnostic tests.
• Patient remains infection free and does not bleed abnormally.
• Patient and family state understanding of drug therapy.

chloramphenicol sodium succinate
(klor-am-FEN-eh-kol SOH-dee-um SUK-seh-nayt)
Chloromycetin Sodium Succinate, Pentamycetin ◆

Pharmacologic class: dichloroacetic acid derivative
Therapeutic class: antibiotic
Pregnancy risk category: NR

How supplied
Injection: 1 g

Pharmacokinetics
Absorption: well absorbed from GI tract after oral administration.
Distribution: distributed widely to most body tissues and fluids. Approximately 50% to 60% bound to plasma protein.
Metabolism: parent drug is metabolized primarily by hepatic glucuronyl transferase to inactive metabolites.
Excretion: 8% to 12% of dose is excreted by kidneys as unchanged drug; remainder is excreted as inactive metabolites. *Half-life:* about 1.5 to 4.5 hours.

Route	Onset	Peak	Duration
P.O.	Unknown	1-3 hr	Unknown
I.V.	Immediate	Immediate	Unknown

Pharmacodynamics
Chemical effect: inhibits bacterial protein synthesis by binding to 50S subunit of ribosome; bacteriostatic.
Therapeutic effect: inhibits growth of susceptible bacteria. Spectrum of activity includes *Rickettsia, Chlamydia,* and *Mycoplasma* and certain *Salmonella* strains, as well as most gram-positive and gram-negative organisms.

Indications and dosage
▶ **Haemophilus influenzae meningitis, acute *Salmonella typhi* infection, and meningitis, bacteremia, or other severe infections caused by sensitive *Salmonella* species, *Rickettsia,* lymphogranuloma, psittacosis, or various sensitive gram-negative organisms.** *Adults and children:* 50 to 100 mg/kg P.O. or I.V. daily, divided q 6 hours. Maximum dosage is 100 mg/kg daily. *Full-term infants over age 2 weeks with normal metabolic processes:* up to 50 mg/kg I.V. daily, divided q 6 hours. *Premature infants, neonates age 2 weeks or younger, and children and infants with immature metabolic processes:* 25 mg/kg I.V. once daily. I.V. route must be used to treat meningitis.

Adverse reactions
CNS: headache, mild depression, confusion, delirium; peripheral neuropathy (with prolonged therapy).
EENT: optic neuritis (in patients with cystic fibrosis), glossitis, decreased visual acuity.
GI: nausea, vomiting, stomatitis, diarrhea, enterocolitis.
Hematologic: *aplastic anemia, hypoplastic anemia, thrombocytopenia, agranulocytosis.*
Other: infections from nonsusceptible organisms, hypersensitivity reactions (fever, rash, urticaria, *anaphylaxis*), jaun-

---

dice, *gray syndrome in neonates, (abdominal distention, gray cyanosis, vasomotor collapse, respiratory distress, death within few hours of onset of symptoms).*

Interactions

Drug-drug. *Chlorpropamide, dicumarol, phenobarbital, phenytoin, tolbutamide:* increased blood levels possible. Monitor for toxicity.
Folic acid, iron supplements, vitamin B_{12}: possible delayed response in patients with anemia. Monitor closely.

Contraindications and precautions

• Contraindicated in patients with hypersensitivity to drug.
• Breast-feeding women should temporarily stop breast-feeding during therapy because drug is excreted in breast milk, posing risk of bone marrow depression and slight risk of gray syndrome.
• Use cautiously in patients with impaired hepatic or renal function, acute intermittent porphyria, or G6PD deficiency; in those taking other drugs that cause bone marrow suppression or blood disorders; and in pregnant women.

NURSING CONSIDERATIONS

⚕ Assessment
• Assess patient's infection before therapy and reassess regularly throughout therapy.
• Obtain specimen for culture and sensitivity tests before first dose. Therapy may begin pending results.
• Monitor plasma concentration levels. Therapeutic plasma concentrations are 5 to 25 mcg/ml.
• Monitor CBC, platelets, serum iron, and reticulocytes before and every 2 days during therapy, as ordered.
• Be alert for adverse reactions and drug interactions.
• Evaluate patient's and family's knowledge about drug therapy.

⚕ Nursing diagnoses
• Infection related to presence of bacteria susceptible to drug
• Altered protection related to drug-induced aplastic anemia
• Knowledge deficit related to drug therapy

⚕ Planning and implementation
P.O. use: Administer oral drug forms on empty stomach 1 hour before or 2 hours after meals. (If patient develops adverse GI effects, however, administer with food).
I.V. use: Give I.V. slowly over at least 1 minute. Check injection site daily for phlebitis and irritation.
– Reconstitute 1-g vial of powder for injection with 10 ml of sterile water for injection. Concentration will be 100 mg/ml. Stable for 30 days at room temperature, but refrigeration recommended. Do not use cloudy solutions.
• Stop drug immediately and notify doctor if anemia, reticulocytopenia, leukopenia, or thrombocytopenia develops.
• If patient's serum drug level exceeds 25 mcg/ml, take bleeding precautions and infection-control measures because bone marrow suppression can occur.
Patient teaching
• Instruct patient to report adverse reactions to doctor, especially nausea, vomiting, diarrhea, fever, confusion, sore throat, or mouth sores.
• Stress importance of having frequent blood tests to monitor therapeutic effectiveness and adverse reactions.

⚕ Evaluation
• Patient is free from infection after drug therapy.
• Patient's hematologic status remains unchanged with drug therapy.
• Patient and family state understanding of drug therapy.

---

chlordiazepoxide
(klor-digh-eh-zuh-POKS-ighd)
Libritabs

chlordiazepoxide hydrochloride
Apo-Chlordiazepoxide♦, Librium,
Novopoxide♦

Pharmacologic class: benzodiazepine
Therapeutic class: antianxiety agent,
sedative-hypnotic agent
Controlled substance schedule: IV
Pregnancy risk category: NR

How supplied
chlordiazepoxide
Tablets: 5 mg, 10 mg, 25 mg
chlordiazepoxide hydrochloride
Capsules: 5 mg, 10 mg, 25 mg
Powder for injection: 100 mg/ampule

Pharmacokinetics
Absorption: when given orally, drug is
absorbed well through GI tract; unknown
after I.M. administration.
Distribution: distributed widely throughout body. Drug is 80% to 90% protein-
bound.
Metabolism: metabolized in liver to several active metabolites.
Excretion: most metabolites of drug are
excreted in urine. *Half-life:* 5 to 30 hours.

Route	Onset	Peak	Duration
P.O., I.V., I.M.	Unknown	0.5-4 hr	Unknown

Pharmacodynamics
Chemical effect: unknown. Thought to
depress CNS at limbic and subcortical
levels of brain.
Therapeutic effect: relieves anxiety and
promotes sleep and calmness.

Indications and dosage
▶ **Mild to moderate anxiety.** *Adults:* 5
to 10 mg P.O. t.i.d. or q.i.d. *Children over
age 6:* 5 mg P.O. b.i.d. to q.i.d. Maximum
dosage is 10 mg P.O. b.i.d. or t.i.d.

▶ **Severe anxiety.** *Adults:* 20 to 25 mg
P.O. t.i.d. or q.i.d.
▶ **Withdrawal symptoms of acute alcoholism.** *Adults:* 50 to 100 mg P.O., I.V.,
or I.M. Repeated in 2 to 4 hours, p.r.n.
Maximum dosage is 300 mg daily.
▶ **Preoperative apprehension and anxiety.** *Adults:* 5 to 10 mg P.O. t.i.d. or
q.i.d. on day preceding surgery; or 50 to
100 mg I.M. 1 hour before surgery.

Adverse reactions
CNS: *drowsiness, lethargy, hangover,*
fainting, restlessness, psychosis, *suicidal
tendencies.*
CV: *thrombophlebitis,* transient hypoten-
sion.
EENT: visual disturbances.
GI: nausea, vomiting, abdominal dis-
comfort.
GU: incontinence, urine retention, men-
strual irregularities.
Hematologic: *agranulocytosis.*
Skin: *swelling, pain at injection site.*

Interactions
Drug-drug. *Cimetidine:* increased seda-
tion. Monitor carefully.
Digoxin: increased serum digoxin levels
and risk of toxicity. Monitor closely.
CNS depressants: increased CNS depres-
sion. Avoid concomitant use.
Drug-lifestyle. *Alcohol use:* increased
CNS depression. Don't use together.
Smoking: increased clearance of benzodi-
azepines. Monitor for lack of effect.

Contraindications and precautions
• Contraindicated in patients hypersensitive to drug and during pregnancy.
• Drug should not be administered to
breast-feeding women because of potential for adverse effects to infant.
• Use cautiously in patients with mental
depression, porphyria, or hepatic or renal
disease.
• Safety of drug has not been established
in children under age 6; safety of parenteral use has not been established in
children under age 12.

---

*Liquid form contains alcohol   **May contain tartrazine   ♦ Canada   ◊ Australia   †OTC

NURSING CONSIDERATIONS

⚥ Assessment
• Assess patient's underlying condition before therapy and reassess regularly thereafter.
• Monitor respirations every 5 to 15 minutes after I.V. administration and before each repeated I.V. dose.
• Monitor liver, renal, and hematopoietic function studies periodically in patients receiving repeated or prolonged therapy as ordered.
• Monitor for abuse and addiction.
• Be alert for adverse reactions and drug interactions.
• Evaluate patient's and family's knowledge about drug therapy.

⊕ Nursing diagnoses
• Anxiety related to patient's underlying condition
• Risk for injury related to drug-induced CNS reactions
• Knowledge deficit related to drug therapy

⧁ Planning and implementation
• Know that dosage should be reduced in elderly or debilitated patients.
• Also know that drug should not be prescribed regularly for everyday stress.
P.O. use: Make sure patient has swallowed tablets before leaving bedside.
• Injectable form (as hydrochloride) comes in two types of ampules—as diluent and as powdered drug. Read directions carefully.
• Do not mix injectable form with any other parenteral drug.
I.V. use: Use 5 ml of 0.9% NaCl solution or sterile water for injection as diluent; do not give packaged diluent I.V. Administer over 1 minute.
– Be sure equipment and personnel needed for emergency airway management are available.
I.M. use: Add 2 ml of diluent to powder and agitate gently until clear. Use imme-
diately. I.M. form may be erratically absorbed.
• Recommended for I.M. use only, but may be given I.V.
• Refrigerate powder and keep away from light; mix just before use and discard remainder.
• Drug should not be withdrawn abruptly after long-term administration; withdrawal symptoms may occur.
• May cause false-positive reaction in Gravindex pregnancy test. May also interfere with certain tests for urine 17-ketosteroids.
Patient teaching
• Warn patient to avoid hazardous activities that require alertness and good psychomotor coordination until CNS effects of drug are known.
• Tell patient to avoid alcohol while taking drug.
• Warn patient to take this drug only as directed and not to discontinue it without doctor's approval. Inform patient of drug's potential for dependence if taken longer than directed.

☑ Evaluation
• Patient states he is less anxious.
• Patient's safety is maintained.
• Patient and family state understanding of drug therapy.

chloroquine hydrochloride
(KLOR-uh-qwin high-droh-KLOR-ighd)
Aralen HCl

chloroquine phosphate
Aralen Phosphate, Chlorquin◊

Pharmacologic class: 4-amino-quinoline
Therapeutic class: antimalarial, amebicide
Pregnancy risk category: C

How supplied

chloroquine hydrochloride
Injection: 50 mg/ml (40-mg/ml base)

chloroquine phosphate
Tablets: 250 mg (150-mg base), 500 mg
(300-mg base)

Pharmacokinetics

Absorption: absorbed readily and almost
completely.
Distribution: concentrates in liver,
spleen, kidneys, heart, and brain and is
strongly bound in melanin-containing
cells.
Metabolism: about 30% of dose is metabolized by liver to monodesethyl-
chloroquine and bidesethylchloroquine.
Excretion: about 70% of administered
dose is excreted unchanged in urine; unabsorbed drug is excreted in feces. Small
amounts of drug may be present in urine
for months after drug is discontinued.
Renal excretion is enhanced by urinary
acidification. *Half-life:* 1 to 2 months.

Route	Onset	Peak	Duration
P.O.	Unknown	1-3 hr	Unknown
I.M.	Unknown	30 min	Unknown

Pharmacodynamics

Chemical effect: unknown. As antimalarial, chloroquine may bind to and alter
properties of DNA in susceptible parasites.
Therapeutic effect: prevents or eradicates malarial infections; eradicates amebiasis.

Indications and dosage

▶ **Acute malarial attacks caused by**
Plasmodium vivax, P. malariae, P. ovale,
and susceptible strains of ***P. falci-***
parum. *Adults:* 1 g (600-mg base) P.O.
followed by 500 mg (300-mg base) P.O.
after 6 to 8 hours; then a single dose of
500 (300-mg base) P.O. for next 2 days
or 4 to 5 ml (160- to 200-mg base) I.M.
and repeated in 6 hours, if needed,
changing to P.O. as soon as possible.
Children: initially, 10 mg (base)/kg P.O.,
then 5 mg (base)/kg at 6, 24, and 48
hours (do not exceed adult dose). Or

5 mg (base)/kg I.M. initially; repeated in
6 hours p.r.n. Do not exceed 10 mg
(base)/kg/24 hours. Patient should be
switched to oral therapy as soon as possible.
▶ **Malaria prophylaxis.** *Adults:* 500 mg
(300-mg base) P.O. on same day once
weekly, beginning 2 weeks before exposure. Continue for 4 weeks after leaving
endemic area. *Children:* 5 mg (base)/kg
P.O. on the same day once weekly (not to
exceed adult dosage), beginning 2 weeks
before exposure.
▶ **Extraintestinal amebiasis.** *Adults:* 1 g
(600-mg base) chloroquine phosphate
P.O. daily for 2 days; then 500 mg
(300-mg base) daily for at least 2 to 3
weeks. Treatment is usually combined
with intestinal amebicide.

Adverse reactions

CNS: mild and transient headache, neu-
romyopathy, psychic stimulation, fatigue,
irritability, nightmares, *seizures,* dizziness.
CV: hypotension, ECG changes.
EENT: *visual disturbances* (blurred vision; difficulty in focusing; reversible
corneal changes; typically irreversible,
sometimes progressive or delayed retinal
changes, such as narrowing of arterioles;
macular lesions; pallor of optic disk; optic atrophy; patchy retinal pigmentation,
typically leading to blindness); ototoxicity (nerve deafness, vertigo, tinnitus).
GI: anorexia, abdominal cramps, diarrhea, nausea, vomiting, stomatitis.
Hematologic: *agranulocytosis, aplastic*
anemia, hemolytic anemia, *thrombocy-*
topenia.
Skin: pruritus, lichen planus eruptions,
skin and mucosal pigmentary changes,
pleomorphic skin eruptions.

Interactions

Drug-drug. *Cimetidine:* decreased hepatic metabolism of chloroquine. Monitor for toxicity.

Kaolin, magnesium and aluminum salts: decreased GI absorption. Separate administration times.
Drug-lifestyle. *Sun exposure:* may exacerbate drug-induced dermatomes. Tell patient to avoid excessive sun exposure.

Contraindications and precautions

• Contraindicated in patients with retinal or visual field changes, porphyria, or hypersensitivity to drug. Use during pregnancy is not recommended except for suppression or treatment of malaria (since malaria poses greater potential danger to mother and fetus than prophylactic administration) or hepatic amebiasis.
• Use with extreme caution in patients with severe GI, neurologic, or blood disorders.
• Use cautiously in patients with hepatic disease or alcoholism (drug concentrates in liver), in those with G6PD deficiency or psoriasis (drug may exacerbate these conditions), and in breast-feeding women.

NURSING CONSIDERATIONS

☒ Assessment
• Assess patient's infection before therapy and reassess regularly throughout therapy.
• Ensure that baseline and periodic ophthalmic examinations are performed. Check periodically for ocular muscle weakness after long-term use.
• Assist patient with obtaining audiometric examinations before, during, and after therapy, especially if long-term.
• Monitor CBC and liver function studies periodically during long-term therapy, as ordered.
• Be alert for adverse reactions and drug interactions.
• Assess patient for possible overdose, which can quickly lead to toxic symptoms: headache, drowsiness, visual disturbances, cardiovascular collapse, and seizures, followed by cardiopulmonary arrest. Children are extremely susceptible to toxicity.

• Evaluate patient's and family's knowledge about drug therapy.

⊞ Nursing diagnoses
• Infection related to presence of organisms susceptible to drug
• Sensory or perceptual alterations (visual or auditory) related to adverse reactions to drug
• Knowledge deficit related to drug therapy

▷ Planning and implementation
• Administer drug at same time of same day each week.
• Missed doses should be given as soon as possible. To avoid doubling doses in regimens requiring more than one dose per day, administer missed dose within 1 hour of scheduled time or omit dose.
P.O. use: Administer drug with milk or meals to minimize GI distress. Tablets may be crushed and mixed with food or chocolate syrup for patients with difficulty swallowing; however drug has bitter taste and patients may find mixture unpleasant. Crushed tablets may be placed inside empty gelatin capsules, which are easier to swallow.
I.M. use: Substitute with oral administration as soon as possible.
• Store drug in amber-colored containers to protect from light.
• Be aware that prophylactic antimalarial therapy should begin 2 weeks before exposure and should continue for 4 weeks after patient leaves endemic area.
• Monitor patient's weight for significant changes because dosage is calculated by patient's weight.
• Notify doctor if patient develops severe blood disorder not attributable to disease; drug may need to be discontinued.
Patient teaching
• Tell patient to take drug with food at same time on same day each week.
• Instruct patient to avoid excessive sun exposure to prevent exacerbation of drug-induced dermatoses.

Reactions may be *common,* uncommon, *life-threatening,* or COMMON AND LIFE-THREATENING.

• Tell patient to report blurred vision, increased sensitivity to light, or muscle weakness.
• Warn patient to avoid alcohol while taking drug.
• Teach patient how to take missed doses.

☑ **Evaluation**
• Patient is free from infection.
• Patient maintains normal visual and auditory function.
• Patient and family state understanding of drug therapy.

---

chlorothiazide
(klor-oh-THIGH-uh-zighd)
Chlotride◇, Diurigen, Diuril

chlorothiazide sodium
Sodium Diuril

Pharmacologic class: thiazide diuretic
Therapeutic class: diuretic, antihypertensive
Pregnancy risk category: D

How supplied
Tablets: 250 mg, 500 mg
Oral suspension: 250 mg/5 ml
Injection: 500-mg vial

Pharmacokinetics
Absorption: absorbed incompletely and variably from GI tract.
Distribution: unknown.
Metabolism: none.
Excretion: excreted unchanged in urine.
Half-life: 1 to 2 hours.

Route	Onset	Peak	Duration
P.O.	≤ 2 hr	About 4 hr	6-12 hr
I.V.	≤ 15 min	30 min	6-12 hr

Pharmacodynamics
Chemical effect: increases sodium and water excretion by inhibiting sodium reabsorption in nephron's cortical diluting site.

Therapeutic effect: promotes sodium and water excretion.

Indications and dosage
▶ **Edema, hypertension.** *Adults:* 500 mg to 2 g P.O. or I.V. daily or in divided doses.
▶ **Diuresis, hypertension.** *Children age 6 months and over:* 20 mg/kg P.O. or I.V. daily in divided doses. *Children under age 6 months:* May require 30 mg/kg P.O. or I.V. daily in two divided doses.

Adverse reactions
CV: volume depletion and dehydration, orthostatic hypotension.
GI: anorexia, nausea, pancreatitis.
GU: nocturia, polyuria, frequent urination, *renal failure.*
Hematologic: *aplastic anemia, agranulocytosis,* leukopenia, thrombocytopenia.
Hepatic: hepatic encephalopathy.
Skin: dermatitis, photosensitivity, rash.
Other: impotence, hypersensitivity reactions, such as pneumonitis and vasculitis; hypokalemia; asymptomatic hyperuricemia; hyperglycemia and impairment of glucose tolerance; fluid and electrolyte imbalances, including dilutional hyponatremia and hypochloremia, metabolic alkalosis, hypercalcemia; gout.

Interactions
Drug-drug. *Barbiturates, opiates:* increased orthostatic hypotensive effect. Monitor closely.
Cardiac glycosides: increased risk of digitalis toxicity from chlorothiazide-induced hypokalemia. Monitor potassium and digitalis levels.
Cholestyramine, colestipol: decreased intestinal absorption of thiazides. Separate doses.
Diazoxide: increased antihypertensive, hyperglycemic, and hyperuricemic effects. Use together cautiously.
Lithium: decreased lithium clearance, increasing risk of lithium toxicity. Monitor lithium level.

NSAIDs: increased risk of NSAID-induced renal failure. Monitor patient for renal failure.

Drug-lifestyle. *Alcohol use:* increased orthostatic hypotensive effect. Monitor closely.

Contraindications and precautions

• Contraindicated in patients with anuria or hypersensitivity to other thiazides or other sulfonamide-derived drugs.
• Use cautiously in patients with severe renal disease and impaired hepatic function.
• Safety of drug has not been established in pregnant or breast-feeding women.

NURSING CONSIDERATIONS

Assessment
• Assess patient's underlying condition.
• Monitor effectiveness by regularly checking blood pressure, fluid intake and urine output, blood pressure, and weight.
• Be aware that therapeutic response may be delayed several days in patients with hypertension
• Monitor serum electrolyte and blood glucose levels.
• Monitor serum creatinine and BUN regularly. Drug not as effective if these levels are more than twice normal.
• Monitor blood uric acid level, especially in patients with history of gout.
• Be alert for adverse reactions and drug interactions.
• Evaluate patient's and family's knowledge about drug therapy.

Nursing diagnoses
• Fluid volume excess related to patient's underlying condition
• Altered urinary elimination related to drug therapy
• Knowledge deficit related to drug therapy

Planning and implementation
• To prevent nocturia, give drug in the morning.

P.O. use: Don't give more than 250 mg P.O. at any one time. Bioavailability studies show that 250 mg P.O. every 6 hours is better absorbed than single dose of 1 g.
I.V. use: Reconstitute 500 mg with 18 ml of sterile water for injection. Inject reconstituted drug directly into vein, through I.V. line containing free-flowing, compatible solution, or through intermittent infusion device. Store reconstituted solutions at room temperature up to 24 hours. Compatible with I.V. dextrose or NaCl solutions.
– Avoid I.V. infiltration; can be very painful.
• Never inject I.M. or S.C.
• Avoid simultaneous administration with whole blood and its derivatives.
• Hold drug and notify doctor if hypersensitivity reactions occur.
• Know that drug may be used with potassium-sparing diuretic to prevent potassium loss.
• As ordered, discontinue thiazides and thiazide-like diuretics before parathyroid function tests are performed.
Patient teaching
• Teach patient and family to identify and report signs of hypersensitivity and hypokalemia.
• Teach patient to monitor fluid intake and output and daily weight.
• Instruct patient to avoid high-sodium foods and to choose high-potassium foods.
• Tell patient to take drug early in day to avoid interruptions of sleep due to nocturia.
• Advise patient to avoid sudden posture changes and to rise slowly to avoid orthostatic hypotension.
• Advise patient to use sunblock to prevent photosensitivity reactions.

Evaluation
• Patient is free from edema.
• Patient adjusts lifestyle to deal with altered patterns of urinary elimination
• Patient and family state understanding of drug therapy.

Reactions may be *common*, uncommon, *life-threatening*, or COMMON AND LIFE-THREATENING.

chlorpheniramine maleate
(klor-fen-EER-uh-meen MAL-ee-ayt)
Aller-Chlor*†, Chlo-Amine†, Chlor-100†, Chlorate†, Chlor-Niramine†, Chlor-Pro, Chlor-Pro 10, Chlor-Trimeton*†, Chlor-Trimeton Allergy 12 Hour†, Chlor-Tripolon♦†, Gen-Allerate†, Novopheniram◊†, Pfeiffer's Allergy†, Phenetron*, Teldrin†

Pharmacologic class: propylamine-derivative antihistamine
Therapeutic class: antihistamine (H₁-receptor antagonist)
Pregnancy risk category: B

How supplied
Tablets: 4 mg†
Tablets (chewable): 2 mg†
Tablets (timed-release): 8 mg†, 12 mg†
Capsules (timed-release): 8 mg†, 12 mg†
Syrup: 2 mg/5 ml.*†
Injection: 10 mg/ml, 100 mg/ml

Pharmacokinetics
Absorption: well absorbed from GI tract after oral administration. Food delays absorption but does not affect bioavailability. Unknown for I.M. or S.C. administration.
Distribution: distributed extensively into body; drug is about 72% protein-bound.
Metabolism: metabolized largely in GI mucosal cells and liver (first-pass effect).
Excretion: drug and metabolites are excreted in urine. *Half-life:* 12 to 43 hours in adults; 10 to 13 hours in children.

Route	Onset	Peak	Duration
P.O.	15-60 min	2-6 hr	< 24 hr
I.V.	15-60 min	Immediate	24 hr
I.M., S.C.	15-60 min	Unknown	< 24 hr

Pharmacodynamics
Chemical effect: competes with histamine for H₁-receptor sites on effector cells. Prevents, but does not reverse, histamine-mediated responses.
Therapeutic effect: relieves allergy symptoms.

Indications and dosage
▶ **Rhinitis, allergy symptoms.** *Adults and children age 12 and older:* 4 mg P.O. q 4 to 6 hours or 8 to 12 mg timed-release P.O. q 8 to 12 hours, not to exceed 24 mg/day; or 10 to 20 mg I.M., or S.C. as single dose. *Children ages 6 to 11:* 2 mg P.O. q 4 to 6 hours, not to exceed 12 mg/day. Alternatively, may give 8 mg timed-release P.O. h.s. *Children ages 2 to 5:* 1 mg P.O. q 4 to 6 hours.
▶ **Anaphylaxis.** *Adults:* 10 to 20 mg P.O. as a single dose.

Adverse reactions
CNS: *stimulation,* sedation, *drowsiness* (especially in elderly patients), excitability (in children).
CV: hypotension, palpitations.
GI: epigastric distress, *dry mouth.*
GU: urine retention.
Respiratory: thick bronchial secretions.
Skin: rash, urticaria.
Other: local stinging, burning sensation, pallor, weak pulse, transient hypotension (after parenteral administration).

Interactions
Drug-drug. *CNS depressants:* increased sedation. Use together cautiously.
MAO inhibitors: increased anticholinergic effects. Don't use together.
Drug-lifestyle. *Alcohol use:* increased sedation. Use together cautiously.

Contraindications and precautions
• Contraindicated in patients with acute asthmatic attacks.
• Antihistamines are not recommended for breast-feeding patients because small amounts of drug are excreted in breast milk nor for use in premature or newborn infants.
• Use cautiously in elderly patients and in those with increased intraocular pressure, hyperthyroidism, CV or renal disease, hypertension, bronchial asthma, urine retention, prostatic hyperplasia, bladder-neck obstruction, and stenosing peptic ulcerations.

---

*Liquid form contains alcohol   **May contain tartrazine   ♦Canada   ◊ Australia   †OTC

• Safety of drug has not been established for use in pregnant women.

NURSING CONSIDERATIONS

🔬 Assessment
• Assess patient's underlying allergy condition and reassess regularly thereafter.
• Be alert for adverse reactions and drug interactions.
• Evaluate patient's and family's knowledge about drug therapy.

🔆 Nursing diagnoses
• Altered health maintenance related to underlying allergy condition
• Risk for injury related to drug-induced CNS adverse reactions
• Knowledge deficit related to drug therapy

⏩ Planning and implementation
P.O. use: Give drug with food or milk to reduce GI distress.
I.V. use: Drug is available in 10 mg/ml ampules for I.V.,I.M., or S.C. administration; do not give the 100 mg/ml strength I.V. Drug is compatible with most I.V. solutions. Check with pharmacist before mixing with other I.V. solutions to verify specific compatibilities. Give injection over 1 minute.
I.M. and S.C. use: Follow normal protocol.
• Notify doctor if patient develops tolerance. Doctor may substitute another antihistamine.
• If symptoms occur during or after parenteral dose, discontinue drug. Notify doctor.
Patient teaching
• Instruct patient to take oral drug with food or milk.
• Warn patients to avoid alcohol and other CNS depressants and driving or other activities that require alertness until drug's CNS effects are known.
• Tell patient that coffee or tea may reduce drowsiness. Also, recommend sugarless gum, sugarless sour hard candy, or ice chips to relieve dry mouth.

• Advise patients to stop drug 4 days before allergy skin tests to preserve accuracy of tests.
• Tell patient to notify doctor if tolerance develops because different antihistamine may need to be prescribed.
• Tell parents that drug, including extended-release products, should not be used in children under age 12 unless directed by doctor.

☑ Evaluation
• Patient's allergic symptoms are relieved with drug therapy.
• Patient does not experience injury as a result of drug-induced adverse reactions.
• Patient and family state understanding of drug therapy.

---

chlorpromazine hydrochloride
(klor-PROH-meh-zeen high-droh-KLOR-ighd)
Chlorpromanyl-5♦, Chlorpromanyl-20♦, Chlorpromanyl-40♦, Largactil♦◇, Novo-Chlorpromazine♦, Thorazine

Pharmacologic class: aliphatic phenothiazine
Therapeutic class: antipsychotic, antiemetic
Pregnancy risk category: C

How supplied
Tablets: 10 mg, 25 mg, 50 mg, 100 mg, 200 mg
Capsules (controlled-release): 30 mg, 75 mg, 150 mg, 200 mg, 300 mg
Oral concentrate: 30 mg/ml, 100 mg/ml
Syrup: 10 mg/5 ml
Injection: 25 mg/ml
Suppositories: 25 mg, 100 mg

Pharmacokinetics
Absorption: absorption of oral administration is erratic and variable. Absorption of I.M. administration is rapid.
Distribution: distributed widely into body; concentration is usually higher in

---

CNS than plasma. Drug is 91% to 99% protein-bound.
Metabolism: metabolized extensively by liver and forms 10 to 12 metabolites; some are pharmacologically active.
Excretion: most of drug is excreted as metabolites in urine; some is excreted in feces. Chlorpromazine may undergo enterohepatic circulation.

Route	Onset	Peak	Duration
All	Varies	Varies	Varies

Pharmacodynamics

Chemical effect: unknown. An aliphatic phenothiazine that probably blocks postsynaptic dopamine receptors in brain and inhibits medullary chemoreceptor trigger zone.
Therapeutic effect: relieves nausea and vomiting; hiccups; signs and symptoms of psychosis, acute intermittent porphyria, and tetanus; and produces calmness and sleep preoperatively.

Indications and dosage

▶ **Psychosis.** *Adults:* initially, 30 to 75 mg P.O. daily in two to four divided doses. Dosage increased by 20 to 50 mg twice weekly until symptoms are controlled. Up to 800 mg daily may be required in some patients. Should be switched to oral therapy as soon as possible. *Children age 6 months and older:* 0.55 mg/kg P.O. or I.M. q 4 to 6 hours; or 1.1 mg/kg P.R. q 6 to 8 hours. Maximum I.M. dose in children under age 5 or weighing under 22.7 kg (50 lb) is 40 mg. Maximum I.M. dose in children ages 5 to 12 or weighing 22.7 to 45.5 kg (100 lb) is 75 mg.
▶ **Nausea and vomiting.** *Adults:* 10 to 25 mg P.O. q 4 to 6 hours, p.r.n.; or 50 to 100 mg P.R. q 6 to 8 hours, p.r.n. or 25 mg I.M. If no hypotension occurs, may give 25 to 50 mg I.M. q 3 to 4 hours p.r.n. until vomiting stops. *Children age 6 months and older:* 0.55 mg/kg P.O. or I.M. q 4 to 6 hours; or 1.1 mg/kg P.R. q 6 to 8 hours. Maximum I.M. dose in children under age 5 or weighing under

22.7 kg is 40 mg. Maximum I.M. dose in children ages 5 to 12 or weighing 22.7 to 45.5 kg is 75 mg.
▶ **Intractable hiccups, acute intermittent porphyria.** *Adults:* 25 to 50 mg P.O. t.i.d. or q.i.d. If symptoms persist for 2 to 3 days, 25 to 50 mg I.M. If symptoms still persist, 25 to 50 mg diluted in 500 to 1,000 ml of saline and infused slowly.
▶ **Tetanus.** *Adults:* 25 to 50 mg I.V. or I.M. t.i.d. or q.i.d. *Children age 6 months or older:* 0.55 mg/kg I.M. or I.V. q 6 to 8 hours. Maximum parenteral dosage in children weighing under 22.7 kg is 40 mg daily; for children weighing 22.7 to 45.5 kg is 75 mg daily, except in severe cases.
▶ **Surgery.** *Adults:* preoperatively, 25 to 50 mg P.O. 2 to 3 hours before surgery or 12.5 to 25 mg I.M. 1 to 2 hours before surgery; during surgery, 12.5 mg I.M. repeated in 30 minutes if needed or fractional 2 mg doses I.V. at 2 minute intervals up to maximum dose of 25 mg; postoperatively, 10 to 25 mg P.O. q 4 to 6 hours or 12.5 mg to 25 mg I .M. repeated in 1 hour if needed. *Children age 6 months and older:* preoperatively, 0.55 mg/kg P.O. 2 to 3 hours before surgery or I.M. 1 to 2 hours before surgery; during surgery, 0.275 mg/kg I.M. repeated in 30 minutes if needed or fractional 1 mg doses I.V. at 2 minute intervals up to total of 0.275 mg/kg, may repeat fractional I.V. regimen in 30 minutes if needed; postoperatively, 0.55 mg/kg P.O. q 4 to 6 hours or I.M. 1 hour if needed and hypotension does not occur.

Adverse reactions

CNS: *extrapyramidal reactions* (moderate incidence), *sedation* (high incidence), *seizures, tardive dyskinesia,* pseudoparkinsonism, dizziness.
CV: *orthostatic hypotension,* tachycardia, ECG changes.
EENT: ocular changes, blurred vision.
GI: *dry mouth, constipation.*
GU: *urine retention,* menstrual irregularities, gynecomastia, inhibited ejaculation.

Hematologic: transient leukopenia, *agranulocytosis*, hyperprolactinemia, *aplastic anemia, thrombocytopenia.*
Hepatic: cholestatic jaundice, abnormal liver function test results.
Skin: *mild photosensitivity,* allergic reactions, *I.M. injection site pain,* sterile abscess.
Other: *neuroleptic malignant syndrome.*
After abrupt withdrawal of long-term therapy: gastritis, nausea, vomiting, dizziness, tremors.

Interactions

Drug-drug. *Antacids:* inhibited absorption of oral phenothiazines. Separate antacid and phenothiazine doses by at least 2 hours.
Anticholinergics, including antidepressants and antiparkinsonian agents: increased anticholinergic activity, aggravated parkinsonian symptoms. Use with caution.
Barbiturates, lithium: may decrease phenothiazine effect. Observe patient.
Centrally acting antihypertensives: decreased antihypertensive effect. Monitor patient.
CNS depressants: increased CNS depression. Avoid concomitant use.
Propranolol: increased levels of both propranolol and chlorpromazine. Monitor patient.
Warfarin: decreased effect of oral anticoagulants. Monitor PT and INR.
Drug-lifestyle. *Alcohol use:* increased CNS depression. Avoid concomitant use.
Sun exposure: increased risk of photosensitivity. Avoid prolonged or unprotected exposure to sun. Wear protective sunglasses.

Contraindications and precautions

• Contraindicated in patients with hypersensitivity to drug or in patients experiencing CNS depression, bone marrow suppression, subcortical damage, and coma. Also not recommended for use in pregnant or breast-feeding women.

• Use cautiously in elderly or debilitated patients and in those with hepatic or renal disease; severe CV disease (may cause sudden drop in blood pressure); exposure to extreme heat or cold (including antipyretic therapy), to organophosphate insecticides; respiratory disorders; hypocalcemia; seizure disorders (may lower seizure threshold); severe reactions to insulin or electroconvulsive therapy; glaucoma; or prostatic hyperplasia.
• Use cautiously in acutely ill or dehydrated children.

NURSING CONSIDERATIONS

⚖ Assessment
• Assess patient's underlying condition and reassess regularly thereafter.
• Be alert for adverse reactions and drug interactions.
• Monitor blood pressure regularly. Watch for orthostatic hypotension, especially with parenteral administration. Monitor blood pressure before and after I.M. administration.
• Monitor patient for tardive dyskinesia. Be aware that tardive dyskinesia may occur after prolonged use. It may not appear until months or years later and may disappear spontaneously or persist for life despite discontinuation of drug.
• Watch for symptoms of neuroleptic malignant syndrome. It is rare, but frequently fatal. It is not necessarily related to length of drug use or type of neuroleptic, but over 60% of affected patients are men.
• Monitor therapy with weekly bilirubin tests during first month; periodic blood tests (CBC and liver function); and ophthalmic tests (long-term use), as ordered.
• Evaluate patient's and family's knowledge about drug therapy.

⊞ Nursing diagnoses
• Altered health maintenance related to patient's underlying condition
• Impaired physical mobility related to drug-induced extrapyramidal reactions

---

Reactions may be *common*, uncommon, *life-threatening*, or COMMON AND LIFE-THREATENING.

• Knowledge deficit related to drug therapy

▶ **Planning and implementation**
P.O. use: Protect liquid concentrate from light. Dilute with fruit juice, milk, or semisolid food just before administration.
– Sustained-release preparations should not be crushed but administered whole.
– Shake syrup before administration.
I.V. use: For direct injection, drug may be diluted with 0.9% NaCl injection and administered into large vein or through tubing of free-flowing I.V. solution. Do not exceed 1 mg/minute for adults or 0.5 mg/minute for children. Drug also may be given as I.V. infusion; dilute with 500 or 1000 ml of 0.9% NaCl and administer slowly. Chlorpromazine is compatible with most common I.V. solutions, including D_5W, Ringer's injection, lactated Ringer's injection, and 0.9% NaCl injection.
• Slight yellowing of injection or concentrate is common; does not affect potency. Discard markedly discolored solutions.
I.M. use: Give deep I.M. only in upper outer quadrant of buttocks. Massage slowly afterward to prevent sterile abscess. Injection stings.
• Wear gloves when preparing solutions, and prevent any contact with skin and clothing. Oral liquid and parenteral forms can cause contact dermatitis.
P.R. use: Follow normal protocol for administering suppository.
– Store suppositories in cool place.
• Keep patient supine for 1 hour after parenteral administration and advise him to get up slowly.
• Do not withdraw drug abruptly unless required by severe adverse reactions.
• Withhold dose and notify doctor if patient develops jaundice, symptoms of blood dyscrasia (fever, sore throat, infection, cellulitis, weakness), persistent extrapyramidal reactions (longer than a few hours), or any such reaction in pregnancy or in children.

• Know that acute dystonic reactions may be treated with diphenhydramine.
Patient teaching
• Warn patients to avoid activities that require alertness or good psychomotor coordination until CNS effects of drug are known. Drowsiness and dizziness usually subside after first few weeks.
• Instruct patient to avoid alcohol while taking drug.
• Tell patient to notify doctor if urine retention or constipation occurs.
• Tell patient to use sunblock and to wear protective clothing to avoid photosensitivity reactions. Chlorpromazine causes higher incidence of photosensitivity than other drugs in its class.
• Tell patient to take sugarless gum or hard candy to relieve dry mouth.
• Tell patient not to stop taking drug suddenly but to take it exactly as prescribed and not to take double doses to compensate for missed ones.
• Instruct patient about which fluids are appropriate for diluting concentrate and show dropper technique for measuring dose. Warn patient to avoid spilling liquid preparation on skin because it may cause rash and irritation.
• Advise patient that injection stings.

✓ **Evaluation**
• Patient's health improves as result of diminished signs and symptoms of underlying condition with drug.
• Patient maintains physical mobility throughout drug therapy.
• Patient and family state understanding of drug therapy.

chlorpropamide
(klor-PROH-puh-mighd)
Apo-Chlorpropamide♦, Diabinese,
Novo-Propamide♦

Pharmacologic class: sulfonylurea
Therapeutic class: antidiabetic
Pregnancy risk category: C

How supplied

Tablets: 100 mg, 250 mg

Pharmacokinetics

Absorption: absorbed readily from GI tract.
Distribution: unknown although it is highly protein-bound.
Metabolism: approximately 80% of drug is metabolized by liver.
Excretion: excreted in urine. Rate of excretion depends on urinary pH; it increases in alkaline urine and decreases in acidic urine. *Half-life:* 36 hours.

Route	Onset	Peak	Duration
P.O.	≤ 1 hr	3-6 hr	< 60 hr

Pharmacodynamics

Chemical effect: unknown. A sulfonylurea that may stimulate insulin release from pancreatic beta cells, reduce glucose output by liver, and increase peripheral sensitivity to insulin. Also exerts antidiuretic effect in patients with diabetes insipidus.
Therapeutic effect: lowers blood sugar; also promotes water excretion in patients with diabetes insipidus.

Indications and dosage

▶ **Adjunct to diet to lower blood glucose level in patients with type 2 (non-insulin-dependent) diabetes mellitus.**
Adults: 250 mg P.O. daily with breakfast or in divided doses if GI disturbances occur. First dosage increased after 5 to 7 days because of extended duration of action; then increased q 3 to 5 days by 50 to 125 mg, if needed, to maximum of 750 mg daily. Some patients with mild diabetes respond well to dosages of 100 mg or less daily. *Adults over age 65:* initially, 100 to 125 mg P.O. daily.
▶ **To change from insulin to oral therapy.** *Adults:* if insulin dosage is less than 40 units daily, insulin stopped and oral therapy started as above. If insulin dosage is 40 units or more daily, oral therapy started as above with insulin re-

duced 50%. Insulin dosage reduced further based on patient response.

Adverse reactions

GI: nausea, heartburn, vomiting.
GU: tea-colored urine.
Hematologic: *thrombocytopenia, aplastic anemia, agranulocytosis.*
Skin: rash, pruritus, facial flushing.
Other: *hypersensitivity reactions, prolonged hypoglycemia, dilutional hyponatremia.*

Interactions

Drug-drug. *Anabolic steroids, chloramphenicol, clofibrate, guanethidine, MAO inhibitors, phenylbutazone, salicylates, sulfonamides:* increased hypoglycemic activity. Monitor blood glucose level.
Beta blockers, clonidine: prolonged hypoglycemic effect and masked symptoms of hypoglycemia. Use together cautiously.
Corticosteroids, glucagon, rifampin, thiazide diuretics: decreased hypoglycemic response. Monitor blood glucose level.
Hydantoins: increased blood levels of hydantoins. Monitor closely.
Oral anticoagulants: increased hypoglycemic activity or enhanced anticoagulant effect. Monitor blood glucose level and PT and INR.
Drug-lifestyle. *Alcohol use:* possible disulfiram-like reaction. Don't use together.

Contraindications and precautions

• Contraindicated for treating patients with type 1 (insulin-dependent) diabetes mellitus or diabetes that can be adequately controlled by diet. Also contraindicated in patients with type 2 diabetes complicated by ketosis, acidosis, diabetic coma, major surgery, severe infections, or severe trauma; during pregnancy or breast-feeding; and in patients with hypersensitivity to drug.
• Use cautiously in patients with porphyria, impaired hepatic or renal function and in debilitated, malnourished, or elderly patients.

Reactions may be *common*, uncommon, *life-threatening*, or COMMON AND LIFE-THREATENING.

• Safety of drug has not been established in children.

NURSING CONSIDERATIONS

🔊 Assessment
• Assess patient's diabetes mellitus before therapy.
• Monitor effectiveness by checking patient's blood glucose level regularly and monitoring patient for signs and symptoms of hyperglycemia which may indicate drug is ineffective.
• Monitor patient's hemoglobin A_{1C} regularly as ordered.
• Monitor serum alkaline phosphatase levels routinely, as ordered. Progressive increases may indicate need to discontinue drug.
• Be alert for adverse reactions and drug interactions. Be aware adverse effects of chlorpropamide, especially hypoglycemia, may be more frequent or severe than with some other sulfonylureas because of its long duration of action.
• If hypoglycemia occurs, monitor patients closely for minimum of 3 to 5 days.
• Evaluate patient's and family's knowledge about drug therapy.

🔲 Nursing diagnoses
• Altered health maintenance related to hyperglycemia
• Risk for injury related to drug-induced hypoglycemia
• Knowledge deficit related to drug therapy

⟩ Planning and implementation
• Administer once-daily doses with breakfast; divided doses are usually given before morning and evening meals.
• Notify doctor if blood glucose levels remain elevated or frequent episodes of hypoglycemia occur.
• Treat hypoglycemic reaction with oral form of rapid-acting glucose if patient is able to swallow or with glucagon or I.V. glucose if patient cannot swallow. Follow up treatment with complex carbohydrate snack when patient is awake and determine cause of reaction.

Patient teaching
• Instruct patient about nature of disease, importance of following therapeutic regimen, adhering to specific diet, weight reduction, exercise, and personal hygiene programs, and about avoiding infection. Explain how and when to perform self-monitoring of blood glucose level, and teach recognition of and intervention for hypoglycemia and hyperglycemia.
• Make sure patient understands that therapy relieves symptoms but doesn't cure disease.
• Tell patient not to change drug dosage without doctor's consent, and to report abnormal blood or urine glucose test results.
• Instruct patient to carry candy or other simple sugars to treat mild hypoglycemic episodes. Severe episodes may require hospital treatment.
• Advise patient not to take other medications, including OTC drugs, without first checking with doctor.
• Advise patient to avoid intake of alcohol. Chlorpropamide-alcohol flush is characterized by facial flushing, lightheadedness, headache, and occasional breathlessness. Even very small amounts of alcohol can produce this reaction.
• Advise patient to carry medical identification identifying him as a diabetic patient.

🗹 Evaluation
• Patient's blood glucose level is normal with drug therapy.
• Patient does not experience injury as a result of drug-induced hypoglycemia.
• Patient and family state understanding of drug therapy.

---

chlorzoxazone
(klor-ZOKS-uh-zohn)
Paraflex, Parafon Forte DSC, Remular-S

Pharmacologic class: benzoxazole derivative

Therapeutic class: skeletal muscle relaxant
Pregnancy risk category: NR

How supplied

Tablets: 250 mg
Caplets: 500 mg

Pharmacokinetics

Absorption: rapidly and completely absorbed from GI tract.
Distribution: widely distributed in body.
Metabolism: metabolized in liver to inactive metabolites.
Excretion: excreted in urine as glucuronide metabolite. *Half-life:* 1 to 2 hours.

Route	Onset	Peak	Duration
P.O.	1 hr	1-2 hr	3-4 hr

Pharmacodynamics

Chemical effect: unknown. Appears to modify central perception of pain without modifying pain reflexes. Blocks interneuronal activity in descending reticular activating system and in spinal cord.
Therapeutic effect: relaxes skeletal muscles.

Indications and dosage

▶ **As adjunct in acute, painful musculoskeletal conditions.** *Adults:* 250 to 750 mg P.O. t.i.d. or q.i.d.

Adverse reactions

CNS: *drowsiness, dizziness, lightheadedness,* malaise, headache, overstimulation, tremor.
GI: anorexia, nausea, vomiting, heartburn, abdominal distress, constipation, diarrhea.
GU: urine discoloration (orange or purple-red).
Hematologic: anemia, *agranulocytosis.*
Hepatic: hepatic dysfunction.
Skin: urticaria, redness, itching, petechiae, bruising.
Other: *anaphylaxis.*

Interactions

Drug-drug. *CNS depressants:* increased CNS depression. Avoid concomitant use.
Drug-lifestyle. *Alcohol use:* increased CNS depression. Don't use together.

Contraindications and precautions

● Contraindicated in patients with impaired hepatic function or hypersensitivity to drug.
● Use cautiously in patients with history of drug allergies and in pregnant or breast-feeding women.

NURSING CONSIDERATIONS

ᴶᴱ Assessment
● Assess patient's underlying condition before therapy.
● Monitor effectiveness by regularly assessing severity and frequency of muscle spasms.
● Know that amount of relief determines if dosage (and drowsiness) can be reduced.
● Be alert for adverse reactions and drug interactions.
● Evaluate patient's and family's knowledge about drug therapy.

Nursing diagnoses
● Pain related to patient's underlying condition
● Risk for injury related to drug-induced adverse CNS reactions
● Knowledge deficit related to drug therapy

Planning and implementation
● Administer drug with meals or milk to prevent GI distress.
● Withhold dose and notify doctor of unusual reactions.
Patient teaching
● Tell patient to avoid activities that require mental alertness, such as driving, until drug's adverse CNS effects are known.
● Advise patient to avoid combining drug with alcohol or other CNS depressants.

Reactions may be *common*, uncommon, **life-threatening**, or COMMON AND LIFE-THREATENING.

• Instruct patient to take drug with food or milk to prevent GI distress.
• Tell patient that drug may discolor urine orange or purple-red.
• Advise patient to follow doctor's orders regarding physical activity.

☑ Evaluation
• Patient reports pain has decreased or ceased as result of chlorzoxazone therapy.
• Patient does not experience injury as result of drug-induced adverse CNS reactions.
• Patient and family state understanding of drug therapy.

cholestyramine
(koh-leh-STIGH-ruh-meen)
Questran**, Questran Light, Questran Lite◊

Pharmacologic class: anion exchange resin
Therapeutic class: antilipemic, bile acid sequestrant
Pregnancy risk category: NR

How supplied

Powder: 78-g cans, 9-g single-dose packets. Each scoop of powder or single-dose packet contains 4 g of cholestyramine resin.

Pharmacokinetics

Absorption: drug is not absorbed.
Distribution: none.
Metabolism: none.
Excretion: insoluble cholestyramine with bile acid complex is excreted in feces.

Route	Onset	Peak	Duration
P.O.	1-2 wk	Unknown	2-4 wk

Pharmacodynamics

Chemical effect: a bile-acid sequestrant that combines with bile acid to form insoluble compound that is excreted. The liver must synthesize new bile acid from cholesterol, which reduces low-density-lipoprotein cholesterol levels.
Therapeutic effect: lowers blood cholesterol levels and relieves itching caused by partial bile obstruction.

Indications and dosage

▶ **Primary hyperlipidemia or pruritus caused by partial bile obstruction; adjunct for reduction of elevated serum cholesterol in patients with primary hypercholesterolemia.** *Adults:* 4 g P.O. once or twice daily. Maintenance dosage is 8 to 16 g P.O. daily. Maximum daily dosage is 24 g P.O.

Adverse reactions

GI: *constipation,* fecal impaction, hemorrhoids, *abdominal discomfort,* flatulence, *nausea,* vomiting, steatorrhea.
Skin: *rash;* irritation of skin, tongue, and perianal area.
Other: *vitamin A, D, and K deficiency;* hyperchloremic acidosis (with long-term use or very high dosage).

Interactions

Drug-drug. *Acetaminophen, beta blockers, cardiac glycosides, corticosteroids, fat-soluble vitamins (A, D, E, and K), iron preparations, thiazide diuretics, thyroid hormones, warfarin and other coumarin derivatives:* absorption may be substantially decreased by cholestyramine. Administer at least 2 hours apart.

Contraindications and precautions

• Contraindicated in patients with complete biliary obstruction or hypersensitivity to bile-acid sequestering resins.
• Use cautiously in patients at risk for constipation and those with conditions aggravated by constipation, such as severe, symptomatic coronary artery disease.
• Use cautiously in pregnant or breast-feeding women because of potential for interference of fat-soluble vitamin absorption.
• Safety of drug has not been established for children.

NURSING CONSIDERATIONS

⚐ Assessment

• Assess patient's blood cholesterol level or pruritus before therapy.

• Monitor effectiveness by checking serum cholesterol and triglyceride levels every 4 weeks, as ordered, or asking patient if pruritus has diminished or abated.

• Be alert for adverse reactions and drug interactions.

• Monitor for fat-soluble vitamin deficiency as long-term use may be associated with deficiency of vitamins A, D, E, and K and folic acid.

• Evaluate patient's and family's knowledge about drug therapy.

⊞ Nursing diagnoses

• Risk for injury related to elevated cholesterol levels

• Constipation related to drug-induced adverse GI reactions

• Knowledge deficit related to drug therapy

❱ Planning and implementation

• To mix powder, sprinkle on surface of preferred beverage or wet food (like soup, applesauce or crushed pineapple). Let stand a few minutes, then stir to obtain uniform suspension. Mixing with carbonated beverages may result in excess foaming. Use large glass and mix slowly.

• Administer drug before meals and at bedtime.

• If drug therapy is discontinued, adjust dosage of cardiac glycosides, as ordered and applicable, to avoid toxicity.

• If severe constipation develops, decrease dosage, add stool softener, or discontinue drug, as ordered.

• Administer all other drugs at least 1 hour before or 4 to 6 hours after cholestyramine to avoid blocking their absorption.

Patient teaching

• Instruct patient never to take drug in its dry form; esophageal irritation or severe constipation may result. Using large glass, patient should sprinkle powder on surface of preferred beverage; let mixture stand a few minutes; then stir thoroughly. The best diluents are water, milk, and juice (especially pulpy fruit juice). Mixing with carbonated beverages may result in excess foaming. After drinking this preparation, patient should swirl small additional amount of liquid in same glass and then drink it to ensure ingestion of entire dose.

• Advise patient to take all other drugs at least 1 hour before or 4 to 6 hours after cholestyramine to avoid blocking their absorption.

• Teach patient about proper dietary management of serum lipids (restricting total fat and cholesterol intake), as well as measures to control other cardiac disease risk factors. When appropriate, recommend weight control, exercise, and smoking cessation programs.

☑ Evaluation

• Patient's blood cholesterol level is normal with drug therapy.

• Patient maintains normal bowel patterns throughout drug therapy.

• Patient and family state understanding of drug therapy.

---

cidofovir
(sigh-doh-FOH-veer)
Vistide

Pharmacologic class: inhibitor of viral DNA synthesis
Therapeutic class: antiviral
Pregnancy risk category: C

How supplied

Injection: 75 mg/ml in 5-ml ampule

Pharmacokinetics

Absorption: not applicable with I.V. administration.
Distribution: less than 6% plasma protein-bound.

Reactions may be *common,* uncommon, *life-threatening*, or COMMON AND LIFE-THREATENING.

Metabolism: mainly by kidneys.
Excretion: by renal tubular secretion.

Route	Onset	Peak	Duration
I.V.	Unknown	Unknown	Unknown

Pharmacodynamics

Chemical effect: selective inhibition of CMV DNA polymerase; inhibits DNA viral synthesis.
Therapeutic effect: reduces rate of CMV replication.

Indications and dosage

▶ **CMV retinitis in patients with AIDS.**
Adults: 5 mg/kg I.V. infused over 1 hour once weekly for 2 consecutive weeks, followed by a maintenance dose of 5 mg/kg I.V. infused over 1 hour once q 2 weeks. Probenecid and prehydration with 0.9% NaCl I.V. must be given concomitantly and may reduce risk of nephrotoxicity. Dosage may need adjustment in patients with renal impairment.

Adverse reactions

CNS: *asthenia, headache,* amnesia, anxiety, confusion, *seizures,* depression, dizziness, malaise, abnormal gait, hallucinations, insomnia, neuropathy, paresthesia, somnolence.
CV: hypotension, postural hypotension, pallor, syncope, tachycardia, vasodilation.
EENT: amblyopia, conjunctivitis, eye disorders, *ocular hypotony,* iritis, retinal detachment, uveitis, abnormal vision, taste perversion.
GI: *nausea, vomiting, diarrhea, anorexia, abdominal pain,* dry mouth, colitis, constipation, tongue discoloration, dyspepsia, dysphagia, flatulence, gastritis, melena, oral candidiasis, rectal disorders, stomatitis, aphthous stomatitis, mouth ulcerations.
GU: *elevated creatinine levels, nephrotoxicity, proteinuria,* decreased creatinine clearance levels, glycosuria, hematuria, urinary incontinence, urinary tract infection.

Hematologic: *neutropenia, thrombocytopenia, anemia.*
Hepatic: hepatomegaly, abnormal liver function tests, increased alkaline phosphatase levels.
Respiratory: asthma, bronchitis, coughing, *dyspnea,* hiccups, increased sputum, lung disorders, pharyngitis, pneumonia, rhinitis, sinusitis.
Metabolic: fluid imbalance, hyperglycemia, hyperlipemia, hypocalcemia, hypokalemia, weight loss, decreased serum bicarbonate level.
Musculoskeletal: arthralgia, myasthenia, myalgia.
Skin: *rash, alopecia,* acne, skin discoloration, dry skin, herpes simplex, pruritus, sweating, urticaria.
Other: *fever, infections, chills,* allergic reactions, facial edema, *sarcoma, sepsis,* pain in back, chest, or neck.

Interactions

Drug-drug. *Nephrotoxic agents (such as aminoglycosides, amphotericin B, foscarnet, I.V. pentamidine):* may increase nephrotoxicity. Avoid concomitant use.
Probenecid: interacts with metabolism or renal tubular excretion of many drugs. Monitor closely.

Contraindications and precautions

● Contraindicated in patients with hypersensitivity to drug or history of clinically severe hypersensitivity to probenecid or other sulfur-containing drug. Don't give to breast-feeding women or as intraocular injection.
● Use cautiously in patients with impaired renal function.

NURSING CONSIDERATIONS

⚕ Assessment

● Monitor WBC counts with differential and renal function before each dose.
● Monitor intraocular pressure, visual acuity, and ocular symptoms periodically.
● Do not use drug in patients with baseline serum creatinine above 1.5 mg/dl or

---

calculated creatinine clearance of 55 ml/minute or below unless potential benefits outweigh potential risks.
• Evaluate patient's and family's knowledge about drug therapy.

⊕ **Nursing diagnoses**
• Infection related to presence of virus
• Altered protection related to adverse renal reactions
• Knowledge deficit related to drug therapy

❯ **Planning and implementation**
• Use I.V. prehydration with 0.9% NaCl solution and administer probenecid with each cidofovir infusion, as ordered.
• Administer 1 L of 0.9% NaCl solution, as ordered, usually over 1- to 2-hour period immediately before each cidofovir infusion.
• To prepare drug for infusion, remove appropriate amount of drug from vial using syringe, and transfer dose to an infusion bag containing 100 ml of 0.9% NaCl solution. Infuse entire volume I.V. at constant rate over 1 hour. Use a standard infusion pump.
• Prepare drug in a class II laminar flow biological safety cabinet.
• Know that cidofovir infusion admixtures should be given within 24 hours of preparation. Let drug reach room temperature before use.
Patient teaching
• Inform patient that drug is not a cure for CMV retinitis and that regular ophthalmologic follow-up examinations are necessary.
• Explain that close monitoring of renal function is critical.
• Tell patient to take probenecid with food to reduce drug-associated nausea and vomiting.
• Advise male patient to practice barrier contraception during and for 3 months after drug treatment.

☑ **Evaluation**
• Patient's infection is eradicated.

• Patient does not experience serious renal reactions.
• Patient and family state understanding of drug therapy.

cimetidine
(sih-MEH-tih-deen)
Tagamet

Pharmacologic class: H_2-receptor antagonist
Therapeutic class: antiulcer agent
Pregnancy risk category: B

How supplied

Tablets: 100 mg, 200 mg, 300 mg, 400 mg, 800 mg
Tablets (effervescent): 800 mg◊
Oral liquid: 300 mg/5 ml
Injection: 100 mg/ml◊, 150 mg/ml; 300 mg in 50 ml 0.9% NaCl solution injection

Pharmacokinetics

Absorption: 60% to 75% of oral dose is absorbed. Absorption rate but not extent may be affected by food. Degree of absorption unknown after I.M. administration.
Distribution: distributed to many body tissues. About 15% to 20% of drug is protein-bound.
Metabolism: 30% to 40% of dose is metabolized in liver.
Excretion: excreted primarily in urine (48% of oral dose, 75% of parenteral dose); 10% of oral dose excreted in feces.
Half-life: 2 hours.

Route	Onset	Peak	Duration
P.O.	Unknown	45-90 min	4-5 hr
I.V.	Unknown	Immediate	Unknown
I.M.	Unknown	Unknown	Unknown

Pharmacodynamics

Chemical effect: competitively inhibits action of H_2 at receptor sites of parietal cells, decreasing gastric acid secretion.

Reactions may be *common*, uncommon, *life-threatening*, or COMMON AND LIFE-THREATENING.

Therapeutic effect: lessens upper GI irritation caused by increased gastric acid secretion.

Indications and dosage

▶ **Duodenal ulcer (short-term treatment).** *Adults and children age 16 and over:* 800 mg P.O. h.s. Alternatively, 400 mg P.O. b.i.d. or 300 mg q.i.d. (with meals and h.s.). Treatment continued for 4 to 6 weeks unless endoscopy shows healing. For maintenance therapy, 400 mg h.s. For parenteral therapy, 300 mg diluted to 20 ml with 0.9% NaCl solution or other compatible I.V. solution by I.V. push over 1 to 2 minutes q 6 hours; or 300 mg diluted in 100 ml D₅W or other compatible I.V. solution by I.V. infusion over 15 to 20 minutes q 6 hours; or 300 mg I.M. q 6 hours (no dilution necessary). Parenteral dosage increased by giving 300-mg doses more frequently to maximum daily dosage of 2,400 mg as needed. Alternatively, 900 mg/day (37.5 mg/hour) I.V. diluted in 100 to 1,000 ml of compatible solution by continuous I.V. infusion.

▶ **Active benign gastric ulceration.** *Adults:* 800 mg P.O. h.s., or 300 mg P.O. q.i.d., with meals and h.s., for up to 8 weeks.

▶ **Pathologic hypersecretory conditions (such as Zollinger-Ellison syndrome, systemic mastocytosis, and multiple endocrine adenomas).** *Adults and children age 16 and over:* 300 mg P.O. q.i.d. with meals and h.s.; adjusted to patient needs. Maximum oral daily dosage is 2,400 mg. For parenteral therapy, 300 mg diluted to 20 ml with 0.9% NaCl solution or other compatible I.V. solution by I.V. push over 1 to 2 minutes q 6 hours; or 300 mg diluted in 100 ml D₅W or other compatible I.V. solution by I.V. infusion over 15 to 20 minutes q 6 hours. Parenteral dosage increased by giving 300-mg doses more frequently to maximum daily dosage of 2,400 mg as needed.

▶ **Gastroesophageal reflux disease.** *Adults:* 800 mg P.O. b.i.d. or 400 mg q.i.d. before meals and h.s.

▶ **Prevention of upper GI bleeding in critically ill patients.** *Adults:* 50 mg/ hour by continuous I.V. infusion for up to 7 days; 25 mg/hour to patients with creatinine clearance below 30 ml/minute/ 1.73 m².

Adverse reactions

CNS: confusion, dizziness, headaches, peripheral neuropathy.
CV: bradycardia.
GI: *mild and transient diarrhea.*
GU: transient elevations in serum creatinine levels.
Hematologic: *agranulocytosis, neutropenia, thrombocytopenia, aplastic anemia* (rare).
Hepatic: jaundice (rare).
Skin: acnelike rash, urticaria.
Other: hypersensitivity reactions, muscle pain, mild gynecomastia (if used longer than 1 month).

Interactions

Drug-drug. *Antacids:* interference with cimetidine absorption. Separate administration by at least 1 hour if possible.
Lidocaine, phenytoin, propranolol, some benzodiazepines, warfarin: inhibited hepatic microsomal enzyme metabolism of these drugs. Monitor serum levels of these drugs.

Contraindications and precautions

• Contraindicated in patients hypersensitive to drug and in breast-feeding women.
• Use cautiously in elderly or debilitated patients because they may be more susceptible to drug-induced confusion and in pregnant women.
• Safety of drug has not been established in children under age 16.

NURSING CONSIDERATIONS

☒ Assessment
• Assess patient's underlying upper GI condition before therapy and reassess regularly throughout therapy.

• Be alert for adverse reactions and drug interactions.
• Identify tablet strength when obtaining drug history.
• Monitor patient's CV status during I.V. administration; drug can cause profound bradycardia and other cardiotoxic effects when given too rapidly I.V.
• Evaluate patient's and family's knowledge about drug therapy.

⊞ **Nursing diagnoses**
• Impaired tissue integrity related to patient's underlying condition
• Diarrhea related to drug-induced adverse reaction
• Knowledge deficit related to drug therapy

▷ **Planning and implementation**
P.O. use: Give tablets with meals to ensure more consistent therapeutic effect.
I.V. use: Dilute I.V. solutions with 0.9% NaCl solution, D_5W and dextrose 10% in water (and combinations of these), lactated Ringer's solution, or 5% sodium bicarbonate injection. Do not dilute with sterile water for injection.
– Don't infuse I.V. too rapidly; may cause bradycardia. When administering cimetidine I.V. in 100 ml of diluent solution, do not infuse so rapidly that circulatory overload is produced. Some authorities recommend infusing drug over at least 30 minutes, to minimize risk of adverse cardiac effects. Sometimes administered as continuous I.V. infusion. Use infusion pump if given in total volume of 250 ml over 24 hours or less.
I.M. use: Be aware that I.M. administration may be painful.
• Schedule cimetidine dose at end of hemodialysis treatment. Hemodialysis reduces blood levels of cimetidine. Adjust dosage as ordered in patients with renal failure.
Patient teaching
• Remind patient taking drug once daily to take it at bedtime for best results.

• Warn patient to take drug as directed and to continue taking it even after pain subsides, to allow for adequate healing.
• Remind patient not to take antacid within 1 hour of taking drug.
• Urge patient to avoid cigarette smoking because it may increase gastric acid secretion and worsen disease.
• Instruct patient to report immediately signs of black tarry stools; diarrhea; confusion; or rash.

☑ **Evaluation**
• Patient has experienced decrease in or relief of upper GI symptomatology with drug therapy.
• Patient maintains normal bowel habits throughout drug therapy.
• Patient and family state understanding of drug therapy.

cinoxacin
(sin-OKS-uh-sin)
Cinobac

Pharmacologic class: fluoroquinolone antibiotic
Therapeutic class: urinary tract antiseptic
Pregnancy risk category: B

How supplied
Capsules: 250 mg, 500 mg

Pharmacokinetics
Absorption: well absorbed from GI tract. Food decreases peak concentrations but not total absorption.
Distribution: drug concentrates in renal tissue; it is 60% to 80% protein-bound and has only fair prostatic penetration (30% to 60% of plasma levels).
Metabolism: 30% to 40% of drug is metabolized in liver to inactive compounds.
Excretion: inactive metabolites and unchanged drug are excreted in urine. *Half-life:* 1 to 1.5 hours.

Reactions may be *common*, uncommon, *life-threatening*, or COMMON AND LIFE-THREATENING.

Route	Onset	Peak	Duration
P.O.	Unknown	≤ 2 hr (plasma) 2-4 hr (urine)	≤ 12 hr

Pharmacodynamics

Chemical effect: inhibits microbial DNA synthesis.
Therapeutic effect: hinders or kills susceptible bacteria in urine. Spectrum of activity includes most strains of *Escherichia coli, Klebsiella, Enterobacter, Proteus mirabilis*, and *P. vulgaris.*

Indications and dosage

▶ **Initial and recurrent urinary tract infections caused by susceptible strains of *E. coli, Klebsiella, Enterobacter, P. mirabilis, P. vulgaris,* and *Citrobacter.*** *Adults and children over age 12:* 1 g P.O. daily, in two to four divided doses for 7 to 14 days. Note: Not recommended for children under age 12.

Adverse reactions

CNS: *dizziness, headache,* drowsiness, insomnia, *seizures.*
EENT: tinnitus.
GI: *nausea, vomiting, abdominal pain,* diarrhea, distorted taste.
Skin: rash, urticaria, pruritus, photosensitivity.
Other: elevated liver enzymes, *Stevens-Johnson syndrome, thrombocytopenia, anaphylaxis.*

Interactions

Drug-drug. *Oral anticoagulants:* increased anticoagulant effect. Monitor for bleeding.
Probenecid: may decrease urine levels of cinoxacin by inhibiting renal tubular secretion. Monitor for increased toxicity and reduced antibacterial effectiveness.
Theophylline: increased effects of these drugs. Monitor closely.
Drug-lifestyle. *Caffeine:* increased effects of these drugs. Monitor closely

Contraindications and precautions

• Contraindicated in patients with hypersensitivity to drug or other fluoroquinolones and in breast-feeding women.
• Use cautiously in patients with impaired renal and hepatic function and in pregnant women.
• Safety of drug has not been established in children under age 12.

NURSING CONSIDERATIONS

☑ Assessment
• Assess patient's urinary tract infection before therapy and reassess regularly throughout therapy.
• Obtain clean-catch urine specimen for culture and sensitivity tests before starting therapy and repeat as needed. Therapy may begin pending results.
• Be alert for adverse reactions and drug interactions.
• Monitor patient's hydration status if adverse GI reactions occur.
• Evaluate patient's and family's knowledge about drug therapy.

⊞ Nursing diagnoses
• Infection related to presence of bacteria susceptible to drug therapy
• Risk for fluid volume deficit related to drug-induced adverse GI reactions
• Knowledge deficit related to drug therapy

❯ Planning and implementation
• Give cinoxacin with meals to help decrease adverse GI reactions.
• Know that high urine levels permit twice-daily dosing.
• Report adverse CNS reactions immediately. They indicate toxicity and usually mean that patient should stop taking drug.
Patient teaching
• Remind patient to take entire amount of this drug as prescribed, even when he feels better.
• Warn patient about photosensitizing effects of drug, and advise him to avoid bright sunlight and to wear sunblock.

• Warn patient to avoid driving and other hazardous tasks that require alertness until CNS effects of drug are known or if they occur until effects abate. Tell patient to notify doctor if CNS reactions occur as drug may need to be discontinued.

☑ **Evaluation**
• Patient is free from infection after drug therapy.
• Patient maintains adequate hydration throughout drug therapy.
• Patient and family state understanding of drug therapy.

---

ciprofloxacin
(sih-proh-FLOKS-uh-sin)
Cipro, Cipro I.V., Ciproxin◇

Pharmacologic class: fluoroquinolone antibiotic
Therapeutic class: antibiotic
Pregnancy risk category: C

How supplied

Tablets: 250 mg, 500 mg, 750 mg
Infusion (premixed): 200 mg in 100 ml D_5W, 400 mg in 200 ml D_5W
Injection: 200 mg, 400 mg

Pharmacokinetics

Absorption: about 70% of drug absorbed after oral administration. Food delays rate of absorption but not extent.
Distribution: drug is 20% to 40% protein-bound. Cerebrospinal fluid levels are only about 10% of plasma levels.
Metabolism: unknown but probably hepatic. Four metabolites have been identified; each has less antimicrobial activity than parent compound.
Excretion: primarily renal. *Half-life:* about 4 hours.

Route	Onset	Peak	Duration
P.O.	Unknown	0.5-2.3 hr	Unknown
I.V.	Immediate	Immediate	Unknown

Pharmacodynamics

Chemical effect: unknown. Bactericidal effects may result from drug's inhibiting bacterial DNA gyrase and preventing replication in susceptible bacteria.
Therapeutic effect: kills susceptible bacteria. Spectrum of activity includes *Campylobacter jejuni, Citrobacter diversus, Citrobacter freundii, Enterobacter cloacae, Escherichia coli, Haemophilus parainfluenzae, Klebsiella pneumoniae, Morganella organii, Proteus mirabilis, Proteus vulgaris, Providencia stuartii, Providencia rettgeri, Pseudomonas aeruginosa, Serratia marcescens, Shigella flexneri, Shigella sonnei, Staphylococcus aureus, Staphylococcus epidermidis, Streptococcus faecalis,* and *Streptococcus pyogenes.*

Indications and dosage

▶ **Mild to moderate urinary tract infections.** *Adults:* 250 mg P.O. or 200 mg I.V. q 12 hours.
▶ **Severe or complicated urinary tract infections; mild to moderate bone and joint infections; mild to moderate respiratory tract infections; mild to moderate skin and skin-structure infections; infectious diarrhea.** *Adults:* 500 mg P.O. or 400 mg I.V. q 12 hours.
▶ **Severe or complicated bone or joint infections; severe respiratory tract infections; severe skin and skin-structure infections.** *Adults:* 750 mg P.O. q 12 hours.

Adverse reactions

CNS: headache, restlessness, tremor, light-headedness, confusion, hallucinations, **seizures,** paresthesia.
GI: *nausea, diarrhea,* vomiting, abdominal pain or discomfort, oral candidiasis.
GU: crystalluria, increased serum creatinine and BUN levels, interstitial nephritis.
Hematologic: eosinophilia, *leukopenia, neutropenia, thrombocytopenia.*
Hepatic: elevated liver enzymes.

Musculoskeletal: arthralgia, joint or back pain, joint inflammation, joint stiffness, achiness, neck or chest pain.
Skin: *rash,* photosensitivity, *Stevens-Johnson syndrome.*
Other: thrombophlebitis, burning, pruritus, erythema, swelling (with I.V. administration).

Interactions

Drug-drug. *Antacids containing magnesium hydroxide or aluminum hydroxide, sucralfate, iron supplements:* decreased ciprofloxacin absorption. Separate administration by at least 2 hours.
Probenecid: may elevate serum level of ciprofloxacin. Monitor for toxicity.
Theophylline: increased plasma theophylline concentrations and prolonged theophylline half-life. Monitor blood levels of theophylline and observe for adverse effects.
Drug-lifestyle. *Caffeine:* increased effect of caffeine. Monitor closely.

Contraindications and precautions

• Contraindicated in patients sensitive to fluoroquinolone antibiotics and in breast-feeding women.
• Use cautiously in patients with CNS disorders, such as severe cerebral arteriosclerosis or seizure disorders, and in those at increased risk for seizures. May cause CNS stimulation. Also use cautiously in pregnant women.
• Safety of drug has not been established in children under age 18.

NURSING CONSIDERATIONS

Assessment
• Assess patient's infection before therapy and reassess regularly throughout therapy.
• Obtain specimen for culture and sensitivity tests before first dose. Therapy may begin pending results.
• Be alert for adverse reactions and drug interactions.

• Monitor patient's hydration status if adverse GI reactions occur.
• Evaluate patient's and family's knowledge of drug therapy.

Nursing diagnoses
• Infection related to presence of bacteria susceptible to drug
• Risk for fluid volume deficit related to drug-induced adverse GI reactions
• Knowledge deficit related to drug therapy

Planning and implementation
P.O. use: Administer oral form 2 hours after meal or 2 hours before or after taking antacids, sucralfate, or products that contain iron (such as vitamins with mineral supplements). Food does not affect absorption but may delay peak serum levels.
I.V. use: Dilute drug using D_5W or 0.9% NaCl injection to final concentration of 1 to 2 mg/ml before use. Infuse slowly (over 1 hour) into large vein.
• Be aware that dosage adjustments are necessary in patients with renal dysfunction.
• Have patient drink plenty of fluids to reduce risk of crystalluria.
Patient teaching
• Tell patient to take drug 2 hours after meal and to take prescribed antacids at least 2 hours after taking drug.
• Advise patient to drink plenty of fluids to reduce risk of crystalluria.
• Warn patient to avoid hazardous tasks that require alertness, such as driving, until CNS effects of drug are known.
• Advise patient to avoid caffeine while taking drug because of potential for cumulative caffeine effects.
• Advise patient that hypersensitivity reactions may occur even after first dose. If he notices rash or other allergic reactions, tell him to stop drug immediately and notify doctor.
• Instruct patient to discontinue breast-feeding during treatment or be treated

---

with another drug. Drug is excreted in breast milk.

☑ Evaluation
• Patient is free from infection after drug therapy.
• Patient maintains adequate hydration throughout drug therapy.
• Patient and family state understanding of drug therapy.

---

cisapride
(SIS-uh-prighd)
Propulsid

Pharmacologic class: serotonin-4 receptor agonist
Therapeutic class: GI prokinetic agent
Pregnancy risk category: C

How supplied
Tablets: 10 mg, 20 mg
Suspension: 1 mg/ml

Pharmacokinetics
Absorption: rapidly absorbed.
Distribution: extensively distributed; 97.5% to 98% binds to plasma proteins, mainly albumin.
Metabolism: extensively metabolized in liver.
Excretion: excreted in urine and feces. Unchanged drug accounts for less than 10% of urinary and fecal recovery. *Half-life:* 6 to 12 hours.

Route	Onset	Peak	Duration
P.O.	30-60 min	1-2 hr	Unknown

Pharmacodynamics
Chemical effect: stimulates serotonin-4 (5-HT$_4$) receptors, enhancing release of acetylcholine at myenteric plexus and increasing GI motility.
Therapeutic effect: relieves nocturnal heartburn caused by gastroesophageal reflux disease.

Indications and dosage
▶ **Symptoms of nocturnal heartburn caused by gastroesophageal reflux disease.** *Adults:* initially, 10 mg P.O. q.i.d. at least 15 minutes before meals and h.s. If response is inadequate, increased to 20 mg q.i.d.

Adverse reactions
CNS: *headache.*
CV: tachycardia.
GI: *diarrhea, abdominal pain,* nausea, constipation, flatulence, dyspepsia.
GU: frequency, urgency, vaginitis.
Respiratory: rhinitis, sinusitis, cough.
Skin: rash, pruritus.
Other: flulike symptoms, pain, fever.

Interactions
Drug-drug. *Anticholinergics:* decreased effectiveness of cisapride. Avoid concomitant use.
Anticoagulants: may increase clotting times. Monitor closely.
Benzodiazepines: enhanced sedation. Avoid concomitant use.
Drugs known to prolong the QT interval (quinidine, procainamide, amitriptyline, maprotiline, astemizole): increased risk of arrhythmias. Avoid concomitant use.
Cimetidine, ranitidine: increased absorption of these agents; cimetidine increases cisapride levels. Use together cautiously.
Clarithromycin, erythromycin, fluconazole, indinavir, itraconazole, ketoconazole, I.V. miconazole, nefazodone, ritonavir, troleandomycin: increased cisapride levels which may cause ventricular arrhythmias. Avoid concomitant use.
Drug-lifestyle. *Alcohol use:* enhanced sedation. Avoid concomitant use.

Contraindications and precautions
• Contraindicated in patients hypersensitive to drug. Also contraindicated in patients who have history of prolonged QT intervals, renal failure, ventricular arrhythmias, ischemic heart disease, heart failure, uncorrected electrolyte disorders, respiratory failure and concomitant drugs

---

known to prolong the QT interval and in whom increased GI motility may be harmful, such as those with mechanical obstruction, hemorrhage, or perforation of GI tract.
• Use cautiously in pregnant and breast-feeding women.
• Safety has not been established in children.

NURSING CONSIDERATIONS

⚠ Assessment
• Assess patient's gastroesophageal reflux disease before therapy and reassess regularly thereafter.
• Be alert for adverse reactions and drug interactions.
• Monitor patient's hydration status if adverse GI reactions occur.
• Evaluate patient's and family's knowledge about drug therapy.

⊞ Nursing diagnoses
• Pain related to nocturnal heartburn
• Risk of fluid volume deficit related to drug-induced adverse GI reactions
• Knowledge deficit related to drug therapy

❯ Planning and implementation
• Administer at least 15 minutes before meals and at bedtime.
• Use suspension formula if patient has difficulty swallowing tablets.
Patient teaching
• Remind patient to avoid alcohol and sedatives while using drug.
• Advise patient to report adverse effects to doctor immediately.
• Tell patient to take drug at least 15 minutes before meals and at bedtime.

✓ Evaluation
• Patient states nocturnal heartburn is relieved with drug therapy.
• Patient maintains adequate hydration throughout drug therapy.
• Patient and family state understanding of drug therapy.

cisplatin (cis-platinum)
(sis-PLAH-tin)
Platinol AQ

Pharmacologic class: alkylating agent (cell cycle–phase nonspecific).
Therapeutic class: antineoplastic.
Pregnancy risk category: D

How supplied
Injection: 0.5 mg/ml♦, 1 mg/ml

Pharmacokinetics
Absorption: not applicable as drug is given I.V.
Distribution: distributes widely into tissues, with highest concentrations found in kidneys, liver, and prostate. Drug does not readily cross blood-brain barrier. Drug is extensively and irreversibly bound to plasma proteins and tissue proteins.
Metabolism: unknown.
Excretion: excreted primarily unchanged in urine. *Half-life:* initial phase, 25 to 79 minutes; terminal phase, 58 to 78 hours.

Route	Onset	Peak	Duration
I.V.	Unknown	Unknown	Several days

Pharmacodynamics
Chemical effect: unknown. Probably cross-links strands of cellular DNA and interferes with RNA transcription, causing imbalance of growth that leads to cell death. Cell cycle–phase nonspecific.
Therapeutic effect: kills selected cancer cells.

Indications and dosage
▶ **Adjunct therapy in metastatic testicular cancer.** *Adults:* 20 mg/m² I.V. daily for 5 days. Repeated q 3 weeks for three cycles or longer.
▶ **Adjunct therapy in metastatic ovarian cancer.** *Adults:* 100 mg/m² I.V.; repeated q 4 weeks. Or, 75 to 100 mg/m² I.V. once q 4 weeks in combination with cyclophosphamide.

▶ **Advanced bladder cancer.** *Adults:* 50 to 70 mg/m² I.V. q 3 to 4 weeks. Patients who have received other antineoplastic agents or radiation therapy should receive 50 mg/m² q 4 weeks. *Note:* Prehydration and mannitol diuresis may reduce renal toxicity and ototoxicity significantly.

Adverse reactions

CNS: *peripheral neuritis,* loss of taste, *seizures.*
EENT: *tinnitus, hearing loss.*
GI: *nausea, vomiting, beginning 1 to 4 hours after dose and lasting 24 hours;* diarrhea; metallic taste.
GU: *more prolonged and* SEVERE RENAL TOXICITY *with repeated courses of therapy.*
Hematologic: MILD MYELOSUPPRESSION, *leukopenia, thrombocytopenia, anemia;* nadirs in circulating platelet and WBC counts on days 18 to 23, with recovery by day 39.
Other: *anaphylactoid reaction,* hypomagnesemia, hypokalemia, hypocalcemia.

Interactions

Drug-drug. *Aminoglycoside antibiotics:* additive nephrotoxicity. Monitor renal function studies very carefully.
Bumetanide, ethacrynic acid, furosemide: additive ototoxicity. Avoid concomitant use.
Phenytoin: decreased serum phenytoin levels. Monitor serum levels.

Contraindications and precautions

• Contraindicated in patients with hypersensitivity to drug or to other platinum-containing compounds and in those with severe renal disease, hearing impairment, or myelosuppression. Also not recommended for use in breast-feeding patients.
• Use with extreme caution and only when absolutely necessary in pregnant women because fetal harm may occur.
• Safety of drug has not been established in children.

NURSING CONSIDERATIONS

✐ Assessment

• Assess patient's underlying neoplastic disease before therapy and reassess regularly throughout therapy.
• Monitor CBC, electrolyte levels (especially potassium and magnesium), platelet count, and renal function studies before initial and subsequent dosages, as ordered.
• To detect permanent hearing loss, perform audiometry before initial dosage and subsequent courses, as ordered.
• Be alert for adverse reactions and drug interactions.
• Evaluate patient's and family's knowledge about drug therapy.

🔲 Nursing diagnoses

• Altered health maintenance related to presence of neoplastic disease
• Altered protection related to drug-induced adverse reactions
• Knowledge deficit related to drug therapy

▷ Planning and implementation

• Administer mannitol as 12.5-g I.V. bolus before starting cisplatin infusion, as ordered. Follow, if ordered, by infusion of mannitol at rate of up to 10 g/hour p.r.n. to maintain urine output during and 6 to 24 hours after drug infusion.
• Hydrate patient with 0.9% NaCl solution before giving drug, as ordered. Maintain urine output of 100 ml/hour for 4 consecutive hours before therapy and for 24 hours after therapy.
• Follow institutional policy to reduce risks because preparation and administration of parenteral form of drug is associated with carcinogenic, mutagenic, and teratogenic risks for personnel.
• Dilute with dextrose 5% in 0.3% NaCl injection or dextrose 5% in 0.45% NaCl injection. Solutions are stable for 20 hours at room temperature. Don't refrigerate.
• Keep in mind that infusions are most stable in chloride-containing solutions

---

Reactions may be *common*, uncommon, *life-threatening*, or COMMON AND LIFE-THREATENING.

(such as 0.9% NaCl, 0.45% NaCl, and 0.22% NaCl).
• Be aware that manufacturer recommends administering drug as I.V. infusion in 2 L of 0.9% NaCl solution with 37.5 g of mannitol over 6 to 8 hours.
• Do not use needles or I.V. administration sets that contain aluminum because it will displace platinum, causing loss of potency and formation of black precipitate.
• Know that renal toxicity is cumulative. Renal function must return to normal before next dose can be given.
• Know that dosage should not be repeated unless platelet count is over 100,000/ mm^3, WBC count is over 4,000/mm^3, creatinine level is under 1.5 mg/dl, or BUN level is under 25 mg/dl.
• Check current protocol. Some clinicians use I.V. sodium thiosulfate to minimize toxicity.
• Administer antiemetics as ordered. Nausea and vomiting may be severe and protracted (up to 24 hours). Provide I.V. hydration as ordered until patient can tolerate adequate oral intake.
• Keep in mind that ondansetron, granisetron, or high-dose metoclopramide has been used very effectively to treat and prevent nausea and vomiting. Some clinicians combine metoclopramide with dexamethasone and antihistamines, or ondansetron or granisetron with dexamethasone.
• Be alert that delayed-onset vomiting (3 to 5 days after treatment) has been reported. Patients may need prolonged antiemetic treatment.
• To prevent hypokalemia, know that potassium chloride (10 to 20 mEq/L) is frequently added to I.V. fluids before and after cisplatin therapy.
• Immediately administer epinephrine, corticosteroids, or antihistamines for anaphylactoid reactions, as ordered.
Patient teaching
• Warn patient to watch for signs of infection (fever, sore throat, fatigue) and bleeding (easy bruising, nosebleeds, bleeding gums, melena). Take temperature daily.

• Tell patient to report tinnitus immediately.
• Instruct patient to avoid OTC products containing aspirin.
• Teach patient to record intake and output on daily basis; and to report edema or decrease in urine output.
• Encourage patient to notify doctor if any concerns arise during drug therapy.

☑ **Evaluation**
• Patient exhibits positive response to cisplatin therapy according to follow-up diagnostic studies.
• Patient does not experience permanent injury as a result of drug-induced adverse reactions.
• Patient and family state understanding of drug therapy.

citalopram hydrobromide
(sih-TAL-oh-pram high-droh-BROH-mighd)
Celexa

Pharmacologic class: selective serotonin reuptake inhibitor (SSRI)
Therapeutic class: antidepressant
Pregnancy risk category: C

How supplied
Tablets: 20 mg, 40 mg

Pharmacokinetics
Absorption: absolute bioavailability is 80%.
Distribution: about 80% bound to plasma proteins.
Metabolism: metabolized primarily by the liver.
Excretion: about 10% of drug is recovered in urine. *Half-life:* 35 hours.

Route	Onset	Peak	Duration
P.O.	Unknown	4 hr	Unknown

Pharmacodynamics

Chemical effect: probably enhances serotonergic activity in CNS resulting from its inhibition of CNS neuronal reuptake of serotonin.
Therapeutic effect: relieves depression.

Indications and dosages

▶ **Depression.** *Adults:* initially, 20 mg, P.O. once daily, increasing to 40 mg daily after no less than 1 week. Maximum recommended dose is 40 mg daily. *Elderly:* 20 mg P.O. daily with titration to 40 mg daily only for nonresponding patients.

Adverse reactions

CNS: tremor, *somnolence, insomnia,* anxiety, agitation, dizziness, paresthesia, migraine, impaired concentration, amnesia, depression, apathy, *suicide attempt,* confusion, decreased libido, fatigue.
CV: tachycardia, postural hypotension, hypotension.
EENT: *dry mouth,* rhinitis, sinusitis, abnormal accommodation, taste perversion.
GI: *nausea,* diarrhea, anorexia, dyspepsia, vomiting, abdominal pain, increased saliva, flatulence, decreased and increased weight, increased appetite.
GU: dysmenorrhea, amenorrhea, ejaculation disorder, impotence, polyuria.
Respiratory: upper respiratory tract infection, coughing.
Skin: rash, pruritus.
Other: *increased sweating,* fever, arthralgia, myalgia, yawning.

Interactions

Drug-drug. *Carbamazepine:* may increase citalopram clearance. Monitor for effects.
CNS drugs: Increased CNS effects. Use caution when taken with citalopram.
Drugs that inhibit cytochrome P-450 isoenzymes 3A4 (such as ketoconazole, erythromycin, fluconazole, itraconazole) and 2C19 (such as omeprazole): decreased clearance of citalopram. Monitor closely.

Imipramine, other tricyclic antidepressants: concentration of imipramine metabolite desipramine increased by approximately 50%. Use together cautiously.
MAO inhibitors: serious, sometimes fatal, reactions may occur. Do not use drug with MAO inhibitors or within 14 days of stopping MAO inhibitor use.
Lithium: may enhance serotonergic effect of citalopram. Use with caution, and monitor lithium levels.
Warfarin: prothrombin time increased by 5%. Monitor closely.
Drug-lifestyle. *Alcohol use:* increased CNS effects. Don't use together.

Contraindications and precautions

● Contraindicated in patients taking MAO inhibitors or within 14 days of stopping MAO inhibitor therapy and in those with hypersensitivity to drug or its inactive ingredients.
● Use cautiously in patients with history of mania, seizures, suicidal ideation, or hepatic or renal impairment.
● Safety and effectiveness have not been established in children.

NURSING CONSIDERATIONS

� Assessment
● Assess patient's underlying condition before therapy and reassess regularly thereafter.
● Check vital signs regularly for decreased blood pressure or tachycardia.
● Closely supervise high-risk patients at start of drug therapy.
● Evaluate patient's and family's knowledge of drug therapy.

� Nursing diagnoses
● Risk for injury related to patient's underlying condition
● Ineffective individual coping related to patient's underlying condition
● Knowledge deficit related to drug therapy

Reactions may be *common,* uncommon, *life-threatening,* or COMMON AND LIFE-THREATENING.

⟫ Planning and implementation

• Be aware that a reduced dosage is indicated for elderly patients and in those with hepatic impairment.
• Do not give until at least 14 days have elapsed between stopping MAO inhibitor therapy and starting citalopram therapy.
Patient teaching
• Inform patient that although improvement may occur within 1 to 4 weeks, he should continue therapy as prescribed.
• Instruct patient to exercise caution when operating hazardous machinery, including automobiles, because psychoactive drugs can impair judgment, thinking, and motor skills.
• Advise patient to consult doctor before taking other prescriptions or OTC drugs or breast feeding an infant..
• Warn patient not to use alcohol.
• Instruct female patient of childbearing age to use birth control during drug therapy and to notify doctor immediately if pregnancy is suspected.
• Tell patient that drug may be taken without regard to meals.

☑ Evaluation

• Patient's safety is maintained.
• Patient's condition is improved with drug.
• Patient and family state understanding of drug therapy.

---

cladribine
(2-chlorodeoxyadenosine)
(klah-DRIGH-been)
Leustatin

Pharmacologic class: purine nucleoside analogue
Therapeutic class: antineoplastic
Pregnancy risk category: D

How supplied

Injection: 1 mg/ml

Pharmacokinetics

Absorption: not applicable as drug is given I.V.
Distribution: about 20% of drug is bound to plasma proteins.
Metabolism: unknown.
Excretion: unknown. *Half-life:* 5.4 hours.

Route	Onset	Peak	Duration
I.V.	4 mo	Unknown	> 8 mo

Pharmacodynamics

Chemical effect: unknown. A purine nucleoside analogue that enters tumor cells, is phosphorylated by deoxycytidine kinase, and is subsequently converted into active triphosphate deoxynucleotide. This metabolite probably impairs synthesis of new DNA, inhibits repair of existing DNA, and disrupts cellular metabolism.
Therapeutic effect: kills selected cancer cells.

Indications and dosage

▶ **Active hairy cell leukemia.** *Adults;* 0.09 mg/kg daily by continuous I.V. infusion for 7 days.

Adverse reactions

CNS: headache, fatigue, dizziness, insomnia, asthenia.
CV: tachycardia, edema.
EENT: epistaxis.
GI: nausea, decreased appetite, vomiting, diarrhea, constipation, abdominal pain.
GU: acute renal insufficiency.
Hematologic: NEUTROPENIA, *anemia, thrombocytopenia.*
Respiratory: abnormal breath or chest sounds, cough, shortness of breath.
Skin: *rash, pruritus, erythema,* purpura, petechiae.
Other: fever, INFECTION, local reactions at the injection site, chills, diaphoresis, malaise, trunk pain, myalgia, arthralgia, hyperuricemia.

Interactions

None significant.

Contraindications and precautions

• Contraindicated in patients hypersensitive to drug and in breast-feeding women.
• Use with extreme caution and only if absolutely necessary in pregnant women because fetal harm may occur.
• Use cautiously in patients with renal or hepatic impairment.
• Safety of drug has not been established in children.

NURSING CONSIDERATIONS

🕮 Assessment

• Assess patient's underlying neoplastic disease before therapy and reassess regularly throughout therapy.
• Monitor hematologic function closely as ordered, especially during first 4 to 8 weeks of therapy.
• Be alert for adverse reactions and drug interactions.
• Evaluate patient's and family's knowledge about drug therapy.

🕮 Nursing diagnoses

• Altered health maintenance related to presence of neoplastic disease
• Altered protection related to drug-induced hematologic adverse reactions
• Knowledge deficit related to drug therapy

🕮 Planning and implementation

• For 24-hour infusion, add calculated dose to 500-ml infusion bag of 0.9% NaCl injection. Once diluted, administer promptly or begin administration within 8 hours. Don't use solutions that contain dextrose because studies have shown increased degradation of drug. Because drug product doesn't contain any bacteriostatic agents, use strict aseptic technique to prepare admixture. Repeat daily for 7 consecutive days.
• Alternatively, prepare 7-day infusion solution, using bacteriostatic NaCl injection, which contains 0.9% benzyl alcohol. Studies have shown acceptable physical and chemical stability using Pharmacia

Deltec medication cassettes. First, pass calculated amount of drug through disposable 0.22-micron hydrophilic syringe filter into sterile infusion reservoir. Next, add sufficient bacteriostatic NaCl injection to bring total volume to 100 ml. Clamp off line; then disconnect and discard filter. If necessary, aseptically aspirate air bubbles from reservoir using new filter or sterile vent filter assembly.
• Be aware that because calculated dose dilutes benzyl alcohol preservative, 7-day infusion solutions prepared for patients weighing more than 85 kg (187 lb) may have reduced preservative effectiveness.
• Refrigerate unopened vials at 36° to 46° F (2° to 8° C) and protect from light. Although freezing doesn't adversely affect drug, precipitate may form; this will disappear if drug is allowed to warm to room temperature gradually and vial is vigorously shaken. Don't heat or microwave; don't refreeze.
• Because of risk of hyperuricemia from tumor lysis, administer allopurinol as ordered during therapy.
• Keep in mind that fever is commonly observed during first month of therapy. In clinical trials, virtually all patients received parenteral antibiotics.

Patient teaching
• Warn patient to watch for signs of infection (fever, sore throat, fatigue) and bleeding (easy bruising, nosebleeds, bleeding gums, melena). Take temperature daily.
• Instruct patient on infection control and bleeding precautions.
• Instruct patient to notify doctor if other adverse reactions occur.

🕮 Evaluation

• Patient exhibits positive response to drug therapy according to follow-up diagnostic studies.
• Patient does not experience injury as a result of drug-induced hematologic adverse reactions.
• Patient and family state understanding of drug therapy.

Reactions may be *common*, uncommon, *life-threatening*, or COMMON AND LIFE-THREATENING.

clarithromycin
(klah-rith-roh-MIGH-sin)
Biaxin

Pharmacologic class: macrolide
Therapeutic class: antibiotic
Pregnancy risk category: C

How supplied

Tablets: 250 mg, 500 mg
Suspension: 125 mg/5 ml, 250 mg/5 ml

Pharmacokinetics

Absorption: rapidly absorbed from GI tract.
Distribution: widely distributed; because it readily penetrates cells, tissue concentrations are higher than plasma levels.
Metabolism: drug's major metabolite, 14-hydroxy clarithromycin, has significant antimicrobial activity; it is about twice as active against *Haemophilus influenzae* as parent drug.
Excretion: 20% to 30% excreted in urine unchanged. The major metabolite accounts for about 15% of drug in urine.
Half-life: 5 to 6 hours with 250 mg q 12 hours; 7 hours with 500 mg q 12 hours.

Route	Onset	Peak	Duration
P.O.	Unknown	2-3 hr	Unknown

Pharmacodynamics

Chemical effect: binds to 50S subunit of bacterial ribosomes, blocking protein synthesis; bacteriostatic or bactericidal, depending on concentration.
Therapeutic effect: hinders or kills susceptible bacteria. Spectrum of activity includes *Streptococcus pyogenes, Streptococcus pneumoniae, Moraxella (Branhamella) catarrhalis, Mycoplasma pneumoniae, H. influenzae,* and *Staphylococcus aureus.*

Indications and dosage

▶ **Pharyngitis or tonsillitis caused by** *S. pyogenes. Adults:* 250 mg P.O. q 12 hours for 10 days. *Children:*
15 mg/kg/day P.O. in divided doses q 12 hours for 10 days.
▶ **Acute maxillary sinusitis caused by** *S. pneumoniae. Adults:* 500 mg P.O. q 12 hours for 14 days. *Children:* 15 mg/kg/day P.O. in divided doses q 12 hours for 10 days.
▶ **Acute exacerbations of chronic bronchitis caused** *by M. catarrhalis* or *S. pneumoniae*; pneumonia caused by *S. pneumoniae* or *M. pneumoniae. Adults:* 250 mg P.O. q 12 hours for 7 to 14 days.
▶ **Acute exacerbations of chronic bronchitis caused by** *H. influenzae. Adults:* 500 mg P.O. q 12 hours for 7 to 14 days.
▶ **Uncomplicated skin and skin-structure infections caused by** *S. aureus* or *S. pyogenes. Adults:* 250 mg P.O. q 12 hours for 7 to 14 days. *Children:* 15 mg/kg/day P.O. in divided doses q 12 hours for 10 days.
▶ **Acute otitis media.** *Children:* 15 mg/kg/day P.O. in divided doses q 12 hours for 10 days.
▶ **Active duodenal ulcer associated with** *Helicobacter pylori* **infection.** *Adults:* 500 mg P.O. t.i.d. for 14 days with omeprazole 40 mg P.O. each morning. Omeprazole therapy should continue at a dose of 20 mg P.O. each morning for days 15-28. Or, 500 mg P.O. t.i.d. for 14 days with ranitidine bismuth citrate 400 mg P.O. b.i.d. Ranitidine bismuth citrate therapy continues for days 15-28.
▶ **Eradication of** *H. pylori* **infection in patients with duodenal ulcer disease** *Adults:* 500 mg P.O. plus lansoprazole 30 mg P.O. and amoxicillin 1 g P.O. each q 12 hours for 14 days.

Adverse reactions

CNS: headache.
CV: *ventricular arrhythmias.*
Hematologic: *leukopenia, thrombocytopenia.*
GI: *diarrhea, nausea, abnormal taste,* dyspepsia, abdominal pain or discomfort.
Skin: *Stevens-Johnson syndrome.*

Interactions

Drug-drug. *Carbamazepine:* may increase serum levels of carbamazepine. Monitor blood levels.
Theophylline: increased plasma theophylline levels possible with other macrolides; effect of clarithromycin is unknown. Monitor theophylline levels carefully.
Warfarin: increased PT and INR possible with other macrolides; effect of clarithromycin is unknown. Monitor PT and INR carefully.

Contraindications and precautions

• Contraindicated in patients with hypersensitivity to erythromycin or other macrolides.
• Use cautiously in patients with hepatic or renal impairment and in pregnant or breast-feeding women.
• Safety of drug has not been established in children under age 6 months.

NURSING CONSIDERATIONS

⚖ Assessment
• Assess patient's infection before therapy and reassess regularly throughout therapy.
• Obtain urine specimen for culture and sensitivity tests before first dose. Therapy may begin pending results.
• Be alert for adverse reactions and drug interactions.
• Monitor patient's hydration status if adverse GI reactions occur.
• Evaluate patient's and family's knowledge about drug therapy.

⊞ Nursing diagnoses
• Infection related to presence of bacteria susceptible to drug
• Risk for fluid volume deficit related to drug-induced adverse GI reactions
• Knowledge deficit related to drug therapy

❯ Planning and implementation
• Administer drug without regard to meals.

Patient teaching
• Tell patient to take all of drug as prescribed, even after he feels better.
• Tell patient to notify doctor if adverse reactions occur.

☑ Evaluation
• Patient is free from infection after drug therapy.
• Patient maintains adequate hydration throughout drug therapy.
• Patient and family state understanding of drug therapy.

---

clemastine fumarate
(KLEM-eh-steen FOO-muh-rayt)
Tavist, Tavist-1†

Pharmacologic class: ethanolamine-derivative antihistamine
Therapeutic class: antihistamine (H-receptor antagonist)
Pregnancy risk category: B

How supplied

Tablets: 1.34 mg†, 2.68 mg
Syrup: 0.67 mg per 5 ml

Pharmacokinetics

Absorption: absorbed readily from GI tract.
Distribution: unknown.
Metabolism: drug is extensively metabolized, probably in liver.
Excretion: excreted in urine.

Route	Onset	Peak	Duration
P.O.	15-60 min	2-4 hr	12 hr

Pharmacodynamics

Chemical effect: competes with histamine for H-receptor sites on effector cells. Prevents, but does not reverse, histamine-mediated responses.
Therapeutic effect: relieves allergy symptoms.

Reactions may be *common,* uncommon, *life-threatening*, or COMMON AND LIFE-THREATENING.

Indications and dosage

▶ **Rhinitis, allergy symptoms.** *Adults and children age 12 and over:* 1.34 mg P.O. q 12 hours, or 2.68 mg P.O. once daily to t.i.d. as needed. *Children ages 6 to 12:* 0.67 to 1.34 mg P.O. b.i.d.

Adverse reactions

CNS: (especially in elderly patients) *sedation, drowsiness, seizures.*
CV: hypotension, palpitations, tachycardia.
GI: epigastric distress, anorexia, nausea, vomiting, constipation, *dry mouth.*
GU: urine retention.
Hematologic: hemolytic anemia, *thrombocytopenia, agranulocytosis.*
Respiratory: thick bronchial secretions.
Skin: rash, urticaria.
Other: *anaphylactic shock.*

Interactions

Drug-drug. *CNS depressants:* increased sedation. Use together cautiously.
MAO inhibitors: increased anticholinergic effects. Don't use together.
Drug-lifestyle. *Sun exposure:* photosensitivity may occur. Use protection.

Contraindications and precautions

• Contraindicated in patients with acute asthmatic attacks or hypersensitivity to drug or other antihistamines of similar chemical structure; in neonates or premature infants; and in breast-feeding patients.
• Use cautiously in elderly patients and in those with angle-closure glaucoma, increased intraocular pressure, hyperthyroidism, CV disease, hypertension, bronchial asthma, prostatic hyperplasia, bladder-neck obstruction, pyloroduodenal obstruction, and stenosing peptic ulcerations. Also use cautiously in pregnant women.

NURSING CONSIDERATIONS

Assessment
• Assess patient's allergy condition before therapy and reassess regularly thereafter.

• Monitor blood counts during long-term therapy, as ordered; observe for signs of blood dyscrasias.
• Be alert for adverse reactions and drug interactions.
• Evaluate patient's and family's knowledge about drug therapy.

Nursing diagnoses
• Altered health maintenance related to patient's underlying allergy condition
• Ineffective airway clearance related to drug-induced thickened bronchial secretions
• Knowledge deficit related to drug therapy

Planning and implementation
• Know that children under age 12 should use only as directed by doctor.
• Administer drug with food or milk to minimize GI distress.
• Notify doctor if tolerance occurs because another antihistamine may need to be substituted for clemastine.
Patient teaching
• Warn patient to avoid driving or other activities that require alertness until drug's CNS effects are known.
• Warn patient to avoid alcohol while taking drug; it will increase drowsiness.
• Tell patient that coffee or tea may reduce drowsiness and that sugarless gum, sugarless sour hard candy, or ice chips may relieve dry mouth.
• Advise patient to stop drug 4 days before allergy skin tests to preserve accuracy of tests.
• Tell patient to notify doctor if tolerance develops because different antihistamine may need to be prescribed.
• Advise patient to increase fluid intake, if not contraindicated, to help keep bronchial secretions thin.

Evaluation
• Patient's allergy symptoms are relieved with drug therapy.
• Patient maintains adequate air exchange throughout drug therapy.

• Patient and family state understanding of drug therapy.

---

clindamycin hydrochloride
(klin-duh-MIGH-sin high-droh-KLOR-ighd)
Cleocin HCl, Dalacin C♦◊

clindamycin palmitate hydrochloride
Cleocin Pediatric, Dalacin C♦◊

clindamycin phosphate
Cleocin Phosphate, Dalacin C♦◊, Dalacin C Phosphate

Pharmacologic class: lincomycin derivative
Therapeutic class: antibiotic
Pregnancy risk category: B

How supplied
clindamycin hydrochloride
Capsules: 75 mg, 150 mg, 300 mg
clindamycin palmitate hydrochloride
Oral solution: 75 mg/5 ml
clindamycin phosphate
Injection: 150 mg/ml

Pharmacokinetics
Absorption: when administered orally, drug is absorbed rapidly and almost completely from GI tract. Drug is absorbed well after I.M. administration.
Distribution: distributed widely to most body tissues and fluids (except CSF). Drug is approximately 93% bound to plasma proteins.
Metabolism: metabolized partially to inactive metabolites.
Excretion: about 10% of clindamycin dose is excreted unchanged in urine; rest is excreted as inactive metabolites. *Half-life:* 2.5 to 3 hours.

Route	Onset	Peak	Duration
P.O.	Unknown	0.75-1 hr	Unknown
I.V.	Immediate	Immediate	Unknown
I.M.	Unknown	3 hr	Unknown

Pharmacodynamics
Chemical effect: inhibits bacterial protein synthesis by binding to 50S subunit of ribosome.
Therapeutic effect: hinders or kills susceptible bacteria. Spectrum of activity includes most aerobic gram-positive cocci and anaerobic gram-negative and gram-positive organisms. It is considered first-line drug in treatment of *Bacteroides fragilis* and most other gram-positive and gram-negative anaerobes. It is also effective against *Mycoplasma pneumoniae, Leptotrichia buccalis*, and some gram-positive cocci and bacilli.

Indications and dosage
▶ **Infections caused by sensitive staphylococci, streptococci, pneumococci, Bacteroides, Fusobacterium, Clostridium perfringens, and other sensitive aerobic and anaerobic organisms.** *Adults:* 150 to 450 mg P.O. q 6 hours; or 600 to 2,700 mg I.V. or I.M. daily divided into two to four equal doses. *Children over age 1 month:* 8 to 20 mg/kg P.O. daily, in divided doses q 6 to 8 hours; or 15 to 40 mg/kg I.M. or I.V. daily, in divided doses q 6 hours.
▶ **Endocarditis prophylaxis for dental procedures in patients allergic to penicillin.** *Adults:* initially, 300 mg P.O. 1 hour before procedure; then 150 mg 6 hours later. *Children:* initially, 10 mg/kg P.O. 1 hour before procedure; then half initial dose 6 hours later.

Adverse reactions
GI: *nausea,* vomiting, abdominal pain, *diarrhea, pseudomembranous colitis,* esophagitis, flatulence, anorexia, *bloody or tarry stools, dysphagia.*
Hematologic: *transient leukopenia,* eosinophilia, *thrombocytopenia.*
Skin: maculopapular rash, urticaria.
Other: unpleasant or bitter taste; *anaphylaxis;* elevated alkaline phosphatase, AST, bilirubin; *pain,* induration, *sterile abscess* (with I.M. injection); thrombophlebitis, erythema, pain (after I.V. administration).

Reactions may be *common,* uncommon, *life-threatening,* or COMMON AND LIFE-THREATENING.

Interactions

Drug-drug. *Erythromycin:* may block clindamycin site of action. Don't use together.
Kaolin: decreased absorption of oral clindamycin. Separate administration times.
Neuromuscular blockers: potentiated neuromuscular blockade possible. Monitor closely.
Drug-food. *Diet foods with sodium cyclamate:* decreased serum drug concentration. Do not use together.

Contraindications and precautions

• Contraindicated in patients with hypersensitivity to antibiotic congener lincomycin.
• Know that breast-feeding women should use alternative feeding method during drug therapy.
• Use cautiously in neonates and patients with renal or hepatic disease, asthma, history of GI disease, or significant allergies.

NURSING CONSIDERATIONS

Assessment

• Assess patient's infection before therapy and reassess regularly throughout therapy.
• Obtain urine specimen for culture and sensitivity tests before first dose. Therapy may begin pending results.
• Monitor renal, hepatic, and hematopoietic functions during prolonged therapy, as ordered.
• Be alert for adverse reactions and drug interactions.
• Monitor patient's hydration status if adverse GI reactions occur.
• Evaluate patient's and family's knowledge about drug therapy.

Nursing diagnoses

• Infection related to presence of bacteria susceptible to drug
• Risk for fluid volume deficit related to drug-induced adverse GI reactions

• Knowledge deficit related to drug therapy

Planning and implementation

P.O. use: Don't refrigerate reconstituted oral solution, because it will thicken. Drug is stable for 2 weeks at room temperature.
– Administer capsule form with full glass of water to prevent dysphagia.
I.V. use: When giving I.V., check site daily for phlebitis and irritation. For I.V. infusion, dilute each 300 mg in 50 ml solution, and give no faster than 30 mg/minute (over 10 to 60 minutes). Never give undiluted as bolus.
I.M. use: Inject drug deeply. Rotate sites. Warn patient that I.M. injection may be painful. Doses over 600 mg per injection are not recommended.
– Be aware that I.M. injection may raise CK in response to muscle irritation.
Patient teaching
• Advise patient taking capsule form to take with full glass of water to prevent dysphagia.
• Inform patient how to store oral solution.
• Instruct patient to take drug for as long as prescribed, exactly as directed.
• Tell patient to take entire amount prescribed even after he feels better.
• Warn patient that I.M. injection may be painful.
• Instruct patient to report diarrhea and to avoid self-treatment.
• Tell patient receiving drug I.V. to tell nurse of discomfort at infusion site.

Evaluation

• Patient is free from infection after drug therapy.
• Patient maintains adequate hydration during drug therapy.
• Patient and family state understanding of drug therapy.

clofazimine
(kloh-FAH-zih-meen)
Lamprene

Pharmacologic class: substituted iminophenazine dye
Therapeutic class: leprostatic
Pregnancy risk category: C

How supplied
Capsules: 50 mg, 100 mg

Pharmacokinetics
Absorption: absorption is variable (45% to 62%) after oral administration.
Distribution: highly lipophilic, drug is distributed widely into fatty tissues and is taken up by macrophages into reticuloendothelial system. Little, if any, crosses blood-brain barrier or enters CNS.
Metabolism: not totally known; some evidence exists of enterohepatic cycling.
Excretion: most is excreted in feces; some in sputum, sebum, and sweat; very little in urine. *Half-life:* up to 70 days.

Route	Onset	Peak	Duration
P.O.	Unknown	1-6 hr	Unknown

Pharmacodynamics
Chemical effect: unknown. Thought to inhibit mycobacterial growth by binding preferentially to mycobacterial DNA. Also has anti-inflammatory effects that suppress skin reactions of erythema nodosum leprosum.
Therapeutic effect: adjunct leprosy therapy. Relieves inflammation of erythema nodosum leprosum.

Indications and dosage
▶ **Dapsone-resistant leprosy (Hansen's disease).** *Adults:* 100 mg P.O. daily in combination with other antileprotics for 3 years. Then, clofazimine *alone,* 100 mg daily.
▶ **Erythema nodosum leprosum.** *Adults:* 100 to 200 mg P.O. daily for up to 3 months. Dosage is tapered to 100 mg daily as soon as possible. Dosages above 200 mg daily are not recommended.

Adverse reactions
EENT: conjunctival and corneal pigmentation.
GI: *epigastric pain, diarrhea, nausea, vomiting, GI intolerance, bowel obstruction, GI bleeding.*
Skin: *pink to brownish black pigmentation, ichthyosis and dryness,* rash, itching.
Other: *splenic infarction,* discolored body fluids and excrement.

Interactions
Drug-drug. *Dapsone:* impaired anti-inflammatory effects of clofazimine. No intervention appears necessary.
Isoniazid: may decrease skin levels and increase serum and urine levels of clofazimine. Monitor for decreased effectiveness.
Rifampin: decreased rifampin bioavailability. Monitor for decreased effectiveness.

Contraindications and precautions
• No known contraindications although drug should not be administered to breast-feeding women unless potential benefit to mother exceeds risk to infant.
• Use cautiously in patients with GI dysfunction, such as abdominal pain and diarrhea and in pregnant women.
• Safety of drug has not been established in children.

NURSING CONSIDERATIONS

⁊ Assessment
• Assess patient's leprosy or erythema nodosum leprosum before therapy and reassess regularly thereafter.
• Be alert for adverse reactions and drug interactions.
• Monitor patient's hydration status if adverse GI reactions occur.
• Evaluate patient's and family's knowledge about drug therapy.

Reactions may be *common,* uncommon, *life-threatening,* or COMMON AND LIFE-THREATENING.

🔟 Nursing diagnoses
• Altered health maintenance related to patient's underlying condition
• Risk for fluid volume deficit related to drug-induced adverse GI reactions
• Knowledge deficit related to drug therapy

▶ Planning and implementation
• Administer drug with food or milk.
• Be aware that doses that exceed 100 mg daily should be given for as short a period as possible and only under close medical supervision.
• If patient complains of colic, burning abdominal pain, or other GI symptoms, notify doctor, who may reduce dose or increase interval between doses.
Patient teaching
• Advise patient to take drug with meals or milk.
• Warn patient that drug may discolor skin, body fluids, and excrement. The color ranges from red to brownish black. Reassure patient that unsightly skin discoloration is reversible but may not disappear until several months or years after drug treatment ends.
• Recommend application of skin oil or cream to help reverse skin dryness or ichthyosis.

☑ Evaluation
• Patient exhibits improvement of underlying condition with drug therapy.
• Patient maintains adequate hydration throughout drug therapy.
• Patient and family state understanding of drug therapy.

---

clofibrate
(kloh-FIGH-brayt)
Atromid-S, Claripex♦, Novofibrate♦

Pharmacologic class: fibric acid derivative
Therapeutic class: antilipemic
Pregnancy risk category: C

How supplied
Capsules: 500 mg

Pharmacokinetics
Absorption: absorbed slowly but completely from GI tract.
Distribution: distributed into extracellular space as its active form, clofibric acid, which is up to 98% protein-bound.
Metabolism: drug is hydrolyzed by serum enzymes to clofibric acid, which is metabolized by liver.
Excretion: 20% of clofibric acid is excreted unchanged in urine; 70% is eliminated in urine as conjugated metabolite.
Half-life: 6 to 25 hours.

Route	Onset	Peak	Duration
P.O.	2-5 days	3 wk	≤ 3 wk

Pharmacodynamics
Chemical effect: unknown. Seems to inhibit biosynthesis of cholesterol at early stage.
Therapeutic effect: lowers blood cholesterol levels.

Indications and dosage
▶ **Hyperlipidemia.** *Adults:* 2 g P.O. daily in divided doses. Some patients may respond to lower doses as assessed by serum lipid monitoring.

Adverse reactions
CNS: fatigue, weakness.
CV: *arrhythmias.*
GI: *nausea, diarrhea, vomiting,* stomatitis, *dyspepsia,* flatulence.
GU: impotence and decreased libido, *acute renal failure.*
Hematologic: leukopenia, anemia.
Hepatic: gallstones, *transient and reversible elevations of liver function tests.*
Skin: rash, urticaria, pruritus, dry skin and hair.
Other: myalgia and arthralgia, resembling flulike syndrome; *weight gain; polyphagia;* fever.

Interactions

Drug-drug. *Furosemide, sulfonylureas:* clofibrate may potentiate clinical effects of these agents. Monitor patient closely.
Lovastatin, pravastatin, simvastatin: risk of myositis, rhabdomyolysis, and renal failure. Avoid concomitant use.
Oral anticoagulants: clofibrate may potentiate anticoagulant effects of warfarin or dicumarol. Decrease anticoagulant dosage.
Oral contraceptives, rifampin: may antagonize clofibrate's lipid-lowering effect. Monitor serum lipids.
Probenecid: increased clofibrate effect. Monitor for toxicity.

Contraindications and precautions

• Contraindicated in patients with significant hepatic or renal dysfunction, primary biliary cirrhosis, or hypersensitivity to drug and in pregnant or breast-feeding women.
• Use cautiously in patients with peptic ulcer.
• Safety of drug has not been established in children.

NURSING CONSIDERATIONS

⚖ Assessment
• Assess patient's blood cholesterol level before therapy.
• Monitor effectiveness by evaluating serum cholesterol and triglyceride levels regularly during therapy.
• Monitor renal and hepatic function, blood counts, and serum electrolyte and blood glucose levels.
• Be alert for adverse reactions and drug interactions.
• Evaluate patient's and family's knowledge about drug therapy.

⊞ Nursing diagnoses
• Risk for injury related to elevated blood cholesterol
• Altered urinary elimination related to drug-induced acute renal failure

• Knowledge deficit related to drug therapy

❱ Planning and implementation
• If liver function tests show steady rise, drug may be discontinued.
• Know that drug typically is discontinued if significant lipid lowering is not achieved within 3 months.
Patient teaching
• Teach patient about proper dietary management of serum lipids (restricting total fat and cholesterol intake) as well as measures to control other cardiac disease risk factors. When appropriate, recommend weight control, exercise, and smoking cessation programs.
• Advise patients to report flulike symptoms immediately because their occurrence may indicate rhabdomyolysis-induced renal failure.

☑ Evaluation
• Patient's blood cholesterol level is normal with drug therapy.
• Patient maintains normal urinary elimination pattern throughout drug therapy.
• Patient and family state understanding of drug therapy.

clomiphene citrate
(KLOH-meh-feen SIGH-trayt)
Clomid, Serophene

Pharmacologic class: chlorotrianisene derivative
Therapeutic class: ovulation stimulant
Pregnancy risk category: X

How supplied

Tablets: 50 mg

Pharmacokinetics

Absorption: absorbed readily from GI tract.
Distribution: may undergo enterohepatic recirculation or may be stored in body fat.
Metabolism: metabolized by liver.

Excretion: excreted principally in feces via biliary elimination. *Half-life:* about 5 days.

Route	Onset	Peak	Duration
P.O.	Unknown	Unknown	Unknown

Pharmacodynamics
Chemical effect: unknown. Appears to stimulate release of pituitary gonadotropins, follicle-stimulating hormone, and luteinizing hormone. This results in maturation of ovarian follicle, ovulation, and development of corpus luteum.
Therapeutic effect: causes female patient to ovulate.

Indications and dosage
▶ **Induction of ovulation.** *Adults:* 50 to 100 mg P.O. daily for 5 days, starting any time; or 50 to 100 mg P.O. daily starting on day 5 of menstrual cycle (first day of menstrual flow is day 1). Repeated until conception occurs or until three courses of therapy are completed.

Adverse reactions
CNS: headache, restlessness, insomnia, dizziness, light-headedness, depression, fatigue, tension.
CV: hypertension.
EENT: blurred vision, diplopia, scotoma, photophobia.
GI: nausea, vomiting, bloating, distention, increased appetite, weight gain.
GU: urinary frequency and polyuria; ovarian enlargement and cyst formation, which regress spontaneously when drug is stopped.
Skin: urticaria, rash, dermatitis.
Other: *hot flashes,* reversible alopecia, *breast discomfort, hyperglycemia.*

Interactions
None significant.

Contraindications and precautions
• Contraindicated during pregnancy and in patients with undiagnosed abnormal genital bleeding, ovarian cyst not due to polycystic ovarian syndrome, hepatic disease or dysfunction, uncontrolled thyroid or adrenal dysfunction, or presence of organic intracranial lesion (such as pituitary tumor).

NURSING CONSIDERATIONS

☙ Assessment
• Assess patient's underlying condition before therapy.
• Monitor effectiveness by assessing ovulation through biphasic body temperature measurement, postovulatory urinary levels of pregnanediol, estrogen excretion, and changes in endometrial tissues.
• Be alert for adverse reactions.
• Evaluate patient's and family's knowledge about drug therapy.

☙ Nursing diagnoses
• Fluid volume excess related to drug-induced fluid retention.
• Sexual dysfunction related to underlying condition
• Knowledge deficit related to drug therapy

☙ Planning and implementation
• Prepare administration instructions for patient: Begin daily dosage on fifth day of menstrual flow for 5 consecutive days.
• Know that no more than three courses of therapy should be given in attempt for conception to occur.
Patient teaching
• Tell patient about risk of multiple births with drug use; risk increases with higher doses.
• Teach patient how to take and chart basal body temperature and to ascertain whether ovulation has occurred.
• Reassure patient that ovulation generally occurs after first course of therapy. If pregnancy does not occur, course of therapy may be repeated twice.
• Advise patient to stop drug and contact doctor immediately if pregnancy is suspected because drug may have teratogenic effect.

• Advise patient to stop drug and contact doctor immediately if abdominal symptoms or pain occurs because these may indicate ovarian enlargement or ovarian cyst.

• Tell patient to immediately report signs of impending visual toxicity, such as blurred vision, diplopia, scotoma, or photophobia.

• Warn patient to avoid hazardous activities, such as driving or operating machinery, until CNS effects are known. Drug may cause dizziness or visual disturbances.

☑ **Evaluation**

• Patient is free from fluid retention at cessation of drug therapy.

• Patient ovulates with drug therapy.

• Patient and family state understanding of drug therapy.

---

clomipramine hydrochloride
(kloh-MIH-pruh-meen
high-droh-KLOR-ighd)
Anafranil

Pharmacologic class: tricyclic antidepressant (TCA)
Therapeutic class: antiobsessional agent
Pregnancy risk category: C

How supplied

Capsules: 25 mg, 50 mg, 75 mg

Pharmacokinetics

Absorption: well absorbed from the GI tract, but extensive first-pass metabolism limits bioavailability to about 50%.
Distribution: distributes well into lipophilic tissues; it is about 98% bound to plasma proteins.
Metabolism: primarily hepatic. Several metabolites have been identified; desmethylclomipramine is primary active metabolite.
Excretion: about 66% is excreted in urine; remainder in feces. *Half-life:* par-

ent compound, about 36 hours; desmethylclomipramine, 4.4 to 233 days.

Route	Onset	Peak	Duration
P.O.	≥ 2 wk	Unknown	Unknown

Pharmacodynamics

Chemical effect: unknown but a TCA that selectively inhibits reuptake of serotonin.
Therapeutic effect: relieves obsessive-compulsive behaviors.

Indications and dosage

▶ **Obsessive-compulsive disorder.**
Adults: initially, 25 mg P.O. daily in divided doses with meals, gradually increased to 100 mg daily during first 2 weeks. Thereafter, increased to maximum dosage of 250 mg daily in divided doses with meals as needed. After titration, total daily dosage may be given h.s.
Children and adolescents: initially, 25 mg P.O. daily in divided doses with meals, gradually increased to daily maximum of 3 mg/kg or 100 mg P.O., whichever is smaller. Maximum daily dosage is 3 mg/kg or 200 mg, whichever is smaller; may be given h.s. after titration. Periodic reassessment and adjustment necessary.

Adverse reactions

CNS: *somnolence, tremors, dizziness,* headache, insomnia, *nervousness, myoclonus, fatigue, EEG changes, seizures,* extrapyramidal reactions, asthenia, aggressiveness.
CV: orthostatic hypotension, palpitations, tachycardia.
EENT: otitis media (in children), abnormal vision, laryngitis, pharyngitis, rhinitis.
GI: dry mouth, constipation, nausea, dyspepsia, increased appetite, diarrhea, anorexia, abdominal pain, eructation, *nausea.*
GU: *urinary hesitancy,* urinary tract infection, dysmenorrhea, *ejaculation failure,* impotence.
Hematologic: anemia, bone marrow suppression.

Reactions may be *common,* uncommon, *life-threatening,* or COMMON AND LIFE-THREATENING.

Skin: *diaphoresis,* rash, pruritus, photosensitivity, dry skin.
Other: myalgia, weight gain, *altered libido.*

Interactions

Drug-drug. *Barbiturates:* decreased TCA blood levels. Monitor for decreased antidepressant effect.
Cimetidine, methylphenidate: increased TCA blood levels. Monitor for enhanced antidepressant effect.
Clonidine, epinephrine, norepinephrine: increased hypertensive effect. Use with caution.
CNS depressants: enhanced CNS depression. Avoid concomitant use.
MAO inhibitors: may cause hyperpyretic crisis, seizures, coma, or death. Don't use together.
Drug-lifestyle. *Alcohol use:* enhanced CNS depression. Don't use together.
Sun exposure: photosensitivity may occur. Use precautions.

Contraindications and precautions

• Contraindicated in patients hypersensitive to drug or other TCAs, in those who have taken MAO inhibitors within the previous 14 days, and in patients during acute recovery period after MI.
• Use cautiously in patients with history of seizure disorders or with brain damage of varying etiology; in those receiving other seizure threshold-lowering drugs; in patients at risk for suicide; in patients with history of urine retention or angle-closure glaucoma, increased intraocular pressure, CV disease, impaired hepatic or renal function, or hyperthyroidism; in patients with tumors of the adrenal medulla; in patients receiving thyroid drug or electroconvulsive therapy; and in those undergoing elective surgery.
• Also use cautiously in pregnant or breast-feeding women.

NURSING CONSIDERATIONS

⚕ Assessment
• Assess patient's underlying condition before therapy and reassess regularly throughout therapy.
• Evaluate patient's and family's knowledge about drug therapy.

✚ Nursing diagnoses
• Ineffective individual coping related to patient's underlying condition
• Risk for injury related to drug-induced adverse reactions
• Knowledge deficit related to drug therapy

▶ Planning and implementation
• Know that total daily dose may be taken at bedtime after titration. During titration, dosage may be divided and given with meals to minimize GI effects.
• Do not withdraw drug abruptly.
• Because hypertensive episodes have occurred during surgery in patients receiving TCAs, know that drug should be gradually discontinued several days before surgery.
Patient teaching
• Warn patient to avoid hazardous activities requiring alertness and good psychomotor coordination, especially during titration. Daytime sedation and dizziness may occur.
• Tell patient to avoid alcohol while taking drug.
• Warn patient not to withdraw drug suddenly.
• Advise patient to use sunblock, wear protective clothing, and avoid prolonged exposure to strong sunlight to prevent photosensitivity reactions.

☑ Evaluation
• Patient's behavior and communication indicate improvement of obsessive-compulsive pattern.
• Patient does not experience injury from drug-induced adverse CNS reactions.
• Patient and family state understanding of drug therapy.

---

clonazepam
(kloh-NEH-zuh-pam)
Klonopin, Rivotril◊ ♦

Pharmacologic class: benzodiazepine
Therapeutic class: anticonvulsant
Controlled substance schedule: IV
Pregnancy risk category: C

How supplied
Tablets: 0.5 mg, 1 mg, 2 mg
Injection: 1mg/ml◊

Pharmacokinetics
Absorption: well absorbed from GI tract.
Distribution: distributed widely throughout body; it is about 47% protein-bound.
Metabolism: metabolized by liver to several metabolites.
Excretion: excreted in urine. *Half-life:* 18 to 50 hours.

Route	Onset	Peak	Duration
P.O.	Unknown	1-2 hr	Unknown
I.V.	Unknown	Unknown	Unknown

Pharmacodynamics
Chemical effect: unknown. A benzodiazepine that probably acts by facilitating effects of inhibitory neurotransmitter gamma-aminobutyric acid (GABA).
Therapeutic effect: prevents or stops seizure activity.

Indications and dosage
▶ **Lennox-Gastaut syndrome; atypical absence seizures; akinetic and myoclonic seizures.** *Adults:* initially, not to exceed 1.5 mg P.O. daily in three divided doses. May be increased by 0.5 to 1 mg q 3 days until seizures are controlled. If given in unequal doses, largest dose given h.s. Maximum recommended daily dosage is 20 mg. *Children up to age 10 or 30 kg:* initially, 0.01 to 0.03 mg/kg' P.O. daily (not to exceed 0.05 mg/kg daily), in two or three divided doses. Increased by 0.25 to 0.5 mg q third day

to maximum maintenance dosage of 0.1 to 0.2 mg/kg daily as needed.
▶ **Status epilepticus (where parenteral form is available).** *Adults:* 1 mg by slow I.V. infusion. *Children:* 0.5 mg by slow I.V. infusion.

Adverse reactions
CNS: *drowsiness, ataxia, behavioral disturbances* (especially in children), slurred speech, tremor, confusion, psychosis, agitation.
EENT: *increased salivation,* diplopia, nystagmus, abnormal eye movements, sore gums.
GI: constipation, gastritis, change in appetite, nausea, abnormal thirst.
GU: dysuria, enuresis, nocturia, urine retention.
Hematologic: *leukopenia, thrombocytopenia,* eosinophilia.
Respiratory: *respiratory depression.*
Skin: rash.

Interactions
Drug-drug. *CNS depressants:* increased CNS depression. Monitor closely.
Drug-lifestyle. *Alcohol use:* increased CNS depression. Don't use together.

Contraindications and precautions
• Contraindicated in patients with acute angle-closure glaucoma, significant hepatic disease, or sensitivity to benzodiazepines.
• Use cautiously in patients with mixed type of seizure because drug may precipitate generalized tonic-clonic seizures. Also use cautiously in children and in patients with chronic respiratory disease or open-angle glaucoma.
• Safety of drug has not been established in breast-feeding women.

NURSING CONSIDERATIONS

🎗 **Assessment**
• Assess patient's seizure condition before therapy and reassess regularly thereafter.

Reactions may be *common,* uncommon, *life-threatening,* or COMMON AND LIFE-THREATENING.

• Monitor blood levels. Therapeutic blood level is 20 to 80 ng/ml.
• Monitor CBCs and liver function tests, as ordered.
• Be alert for adverse reactions and drug interactions.
• Evaluate patient's and family's knowledge about drug therapy.

⊞ Nursing diagnoses
• Risk for injury related to potential for seizure activity
• Activity intolerance related to drug-induced sedation
• Knowledge deficit related to drug therapy

❯ Planning and implementation
P.O. use: Know that dosage should be increased gradually, as ordered.
I.V. use: Give slowly by direct injection or by slow I.V. infusion. Drug may be diluted with D₅W, dextrose 2.5% in water, 0.9% NaCl, or 0.45% NaCl.
– Mix solutions in glass bottles because drug binds to polyvinyl chloride plastics. If polyvinyl chloride infusion bags are used, administer immediately and infuse at rate of 60 ml/hour or greater.
• Never withdraw suddenly because seizures may worsen. Call doctor at once if adverse reactions develop.
• Know that withdrawal symptoms are similar to those of barbiturates.
• Maintain seizure precautions.
Patient teaching
• Advise patient to avoid driving or other potentially hazardous activities that require mental alertness until drug's CNS effects are known.
• Instruct parents to monitor child's school performance because drug may interfere with attentiveness in school.
• Instruct patient and family never to stop drug abruptly because seizures may occur.
• Instruct patient or family to notify doctor if oversedation or other adverse reactions develop or questions arise about drug therapy.

☑ Evaluation
• Patient is free from seizure activity with drug therapy.
• Patient is able to meet daily activity needs.
• Patient and family state understanding of drug therapy.

clonidine hydrochloride
(KLON-uh-deen high-droh-KLOR-ighd)
Catapres, Catapres-TTS, Dixarit♦◇

Pharmacologic class: centrally acting antiadrenergic
Therapeutic class: antihypertensive
Pregnancy risk category: C

How supplied
Tablets: 0.025 mg♦◇, 0.1 mg, 0.2 mg, 0.3 mg
Transdermal: TTS-1 (releases 0.1 mg/24 hours), TTS-2 (releases 0.2 mg/24 hours), TTS-3 (releases 0.3 mg/24 hours)

Pharmacokinetics
Absorption: absorbed well from GI tract when administered orally. Also absorbed well percutaneously after transdermal topical administration.
Distribution: distributed widely into body.
Metabolism: metabolized in liver, where nearly 50% is transformed to inactive metabolites.
Excretion: approximately 65% of drug is excreted in urine; 20% in feces. *Half-life:* 6 to 20 hours.

Route	Onset	Peak	Duration
P.O.	15-30 min	1.5-2.5 hr	6-8 hr
Transdermal	2-3 days	2-3 days	Several days

Pharmacodynamics
Chemical effect: unknown. Thought to inhibit central vasomotor centers, thereby decreasing sympathetic outflow to heart,

kidneys, and peripheral vasculature; this results in decreased peripheral vascular resistance, decreased systolic and diastolic blood pressure, and decreased heart rate.
Therapeutic effect: lowers blood pressure.

Indications and dosage

▶ **Essential, renal, and malignant hypertension.** *Adults:* initially, 0.1 mg P.O. b.i.d. Then increased by 0.1 to 0.2 mg daily on weekly basis. Usual dosage range is 0.2 to 0.6 mg daily in divided doses; infrequently, dosages as high as 2.4 mg daily are used. Or, transdermal patch is applied to nonhairy area of intact skin on upper arm or torso, once q 7 days. Start with 0.1-mg system and titrate after 1 to 2 weeks with another 0.1-mg system or larger system if increases are needed to maintain normal pressure.

Adverse reactions

CNS: *drowsiness, dizziness,* fatigue, sedation, nervousness, headache, vivid dreams.
CV: orthostatic hypotension, bradycardia, *severe rebound hypertension.*
GI: *constipation, dry mouth,* nausea, vomiting.
GU: urine retention, impotence.
Skin: *pruritus, dermatitis* (with transdermal patch).
Other: transient glucose intolerance (with large doses).

Interactions

Drug-drug. *CNS depressants:* enhanced CNS depression. Use together cautiously. *MAO inhibitors, tricyclic antidepressants:* may decrease antihypertensive effect. Use together cautiously. *Propranolol, other beta blockers:* severe rebound hypertension. Monitor carefully.

Contraindications and precautions

● Contraindicated in patients with hypersensitivity to drug. Transdermal form is contraindicated in patients with hypersensitivity to any component of adhesive layer of transdermal system.
● Use cautiously in patients with severe coronary insufficiency, recent MI, cerebrovascular disease, chronic renal failure, or impaired liver function. Also use cautiously in breast-feeding women.
● Safety of drug has not been established in children or pregnant women.

NURSING CONSIDERATIONS

Assessment
● Assess patient's blood pressure before therapy and reassess regularly thereafter.
● Know that antihypertensive effects of transdermal clonidine may take 2 to 3 days to become apparent. Oral antihypertensive therapy may have to be continued in interim.
● Be alert for adverse reactions and drug interactions.
● Observe for patient tolerance to drug's therapeutic effects, which may require increased dosage.
● Be aware that periodic eye examinations are recommended.
● Monitor site of transdermal patch for dermatitis. Ask patient about pruritus.
● Evaluate patient's and family's knowledge about drug therapy.

Nursing diagnoses
● Risk for injury related to presence of hypertension
● Altered protection related to severe rebound hypertension caused by abrupt cessation of drug
● Knowledge deficit related to drug therapy

Planning and implementation
● Know that drug may be given to rapidly lower blood pressure in some hypertensive emergency situations.
● Dosage is usually adjusted to patient's blood pressure and tolerance.
● Administer last dose of day at bedtime.
P.O. use: Follow normal protocol.

Reactions may be *common*, uncommon, *life-threatening*, or COMMON AND LIFE-THREATENING.

Transdermal use: To provide additional adherence of patch, apply adhesive "overlay." Place patch at different site each week.
– Remove transdermal patch before defibrillation to prevent arcing.
• When stopping therapy in patients receiving both clonidine and beta blocker, gradually withdraw beta blocker first to minimize adverse reactions, as ordered.
• Be aware that discontinuation of clonidine for surgery is not recommended.
Patient teaching
• Advise patient that abrupt discontinuation of drug may cause severe rebound hypertension. Reduce dosage gradually over 2 to 4 days, as ordered.
• Tell patient to take last dose of day immediately before bedtime.
• Reassure patient that transdermal patch usually adheres despite showering and other routine daily activities. Instruct him on use of adhesive "overlay" to provide additional skin adherence if necessary. Also tell patient to place patch at different site each week.
• Caution patient that drug can cause drowsiness, but that tolerance to this adverse effect will develop.
• Inform patient that orthostatic hypotension can be minimized by rising slowly and avoiding sudden position changes.

☑ **Evaluation**
• Patient's blood pressure is normal with drug therapy.
• Patient states understanding of not abruptly stopping drug therapy.
• Patient and family state understanding of drug therapy.

clopidogrel bisulfate
(kloh-PIH-doh-grel bigh-SUL-fayt)
Plavix

Pharmacologic class: inhibitor of adenosine diphosphate (ADP) induced platelet aggregation

Therapeutic class: antiplatelet
Pregnancy risk category: B

How supplied
Tablets: 75 mg

Pharmacokinetics
Absorption: rapidly absorbed following oral administration.
Distribution: highly bound to plasma protein.
Metabolism: extensively metabolized by the liver.
Excretion: about 50% is excreted in urine and 46% in feces. *Half-life:* 8 hours

Route	Onset	Peak	Duration
P.O.	2 hr	Unknown	5 days

Pharmacodynamics
Chemical effect: inhibits platelet aggregation by inhibiting binding of ADP to its platelet receptor inhibiting ADP-mediated activation and subsequent platelet aggregation. Because clopidogrel acts by irreversibly modifying the platelet ADP receptor, platelets exposed to drug are affected for their life span.
Therapeutic effect: prevent clot formation.

Indications and dosage
▶ **To reduce atherosclerotic events in patients with atherosclerosis documented by recent CVA, MI, or peripheral arterial disease.** *Adults:* 75 mg P.O. daily.

Adverse reactions
CNS: headache, dizziness, fatigue, depression.
CV: chest pain, edema, hypertension.
EENT: rhinitis.
GI: *hemorrhage,* abdominal pain, dyspepsia, gastritis, constipation, diarrhea, ulcers.
GU: urinary tract infection.
Hematologic: purpura, epistaxis.
Respiratory: bronchitis, coughing, dyspnea, upper respiratory infection.

Skin: *rash,* pruritus.
Other: arthralgia, back pain, flu symptoms, pain.

Interactions

Drug-drug. *Aspirin, NSAIDs:* may increase risk for GI bleeding. Use together cautiously.
Heparin, warfarin: safety has not been established. Use together cautiously.

Contraindications and precautions

• Contraindicated in patients with pathologic bleeding, such as peptic ulcer or intracranial hemorrhage, and in those hypersensitive to drug or its components.
• Use with caution in patients at risk for increased bleeding from trauma, surgery or other pathologic conditions and in those with hepatic impairment.

NURSING CONSIDERATIONS

⚙ Assessment
• Assess concurrent use of OTC drugs such as aspirin or NSAIDs.
• Assess patient for increased bleeding or bruising tendencies before initiating drug therapy and after therapy begins.
• Evaluate patient's and family's knowledge of drug therapy.

⊞ Nursing diagnoses
• Risk for injury related to potential for atherosclerotic events from underlying condition
• Altered protection related to increased risk of bleeding
• Knowledge deficit related to drug therapy

▷ Planning and implementation
• Know that platelet aggregation will return to normal 5 days after drug has been discontinued.
• Withhold drug from patients with hepatic impairment and those at increased risk for bleeding from trauma, surgery, or other pathologic conditions.

Patient teaching
• Inform patient it may take longer than usual to stop bleeding. Tell him to refrain from activities in which trauma and bleeding may occur; encourage use of seat belt when in a car.
• Instruct patient to notify doctor if unusual bleeding or bruising occurs.
• Tell patient to inform doctor or dentist that he is taking drug before having surgery or starting new drug therapy.
• Inform patient that drug may be taken without regard to meals.

▣ Evaluation
• Patient has reduced risk of CVA, MI, and vascular death.
• Patient states appropriate bleeding precautions to take.
• Patient and family state understanding of drug therapy.

clorazepate dipotassium
(klor-AYZ-eh-payt digh-po-TAH-see-um)
Apo-Clorazepate♦, Gen-XENE,
Novoclopate♦, Tranxene, Tranxene-SD,
Tranxene-T-Tab

Pharmacologic class: benzodiazepine
Therapeutic class: antianxiety, anticonvulsant, sedative-hypnotic agent
Controlled substance schedule: IV
Pregnancy risk category: D

How supplied

Tablets: 3.75 mg, 7.5 mg, 11.25 mg, 15 mg, 22.5 mg
Capsules: 3.75 mg, 7.5 mg, 15 mg

Pharmacokinetics

Absorption: absorbed completely and rapidly after being hydrolyzed in stomach to desmethyldiazepam.
Distribution: distributed widely throughout body. About 80% to 95% of drug is bound to plasma protein.
Metabolism: metabolized in liver to oxazepam.

Excretion: inactive glucuronide metabo-lites are excreted in urine. *Half-life:* 30 to 200 hours.

Route	Onset	Peak	Duration
P.O.	Unknown	0.5-2 hr	Unknown

Pharmacodynamics

Chemical effect: unknown. A benzodi-azepine that probably facilitates action of inhibitory neurotransmitter gamma-aminobutyric acid. Depresses CNS at limbic and subcortical levels of brain and suppresses spread of seizure activity pro-duced by epileptogenic foci in cortex, thalamus, and limbic structures.
Therapeutic effect: relieves anxiety, pre-vents seizure activity, and promotes sleep and calmness.

Indications and dosage

► **Acute alcohol withdrawal.** *Adults:* day 1—30 mg P.O. initially, followed by 30 to 60 mg P.O. in divided doses; day 2—5 to 90 mg P.O. in divided doses; day 3—22.5 to 45 mg P.O. in divided doses; day 4—5 to 30 mg P.O. in divided doses; then grad-ually reduce dosage to 7.5 to 15 mg daily. Maximum daily dose is 90 mg.
► **Anxiety.** *Adults:* 15 to 60 mg P.O. daily.
► **Adjunct in partial seizure disorder.** *Adults and children over age 12:* maxi-mum recommended initial dosage is 7.5 mg P.O. t.i.d. Dosage increases should not exceed 7.5 mg/week; maxi-mum dosage should not exceed 90 mg daily. *Children ages 9 to 12:* maximum recommended initial dosage is 7.5 mg P.O. b.i.d. Dosage increases should not exceed 7.5 mg/week; maximum dosage should not exceed 60 mg daily.

Adverse reactions

CNS: *drowsiness, lethargy, hangover,* fainting, restlessness, psychosis.
CV: transient hypotension.
EENT: visual disturbances.
GI: nausea, vomiting, abdominal dis-comfort, dry mouth
GU: urine retention, incontinence.

Interactions

Drug-drug. *Cimetidine:* increased seda-tion. Monitor carefully.
CNS depressants: increased CNS depres-sion. Avoid concomitant use.
Digoxin: may increase serum levels of digoxin, increasing toxicity. Monitor closely.
Drug-lifestyle. *Alcohol use:* increased CNS depression. Don't use together.
Smoking: increased clearance of benzodi-azepines. Monitor for lack of effect.

Contraindications and precautions

• Contraindicated in patients with acute angle-closure glaucoma or hypersensitiv-ity to drug.
• Know that drug should be avoided dur-ing pregnancy, especially first trimester.
• Use cautiously in patients with suicidal tendencies, renal or hepatic impairment, or history of drug abuse.
• Safety of drug has not been established for children under age 9.

NURSING CONSIDERATIONS

Assessment
• Assess patient's underlying condition before therapy and reassess regularly thereafter.
• Monitor liver, renal, and hematopoietic function studies periodically in patients receiving repeated or prolonged therapy as ordered.
• Be alert for adverse reactions and drug interactions.
• Evaluate patient's and family's knowl-edge about drug therapy.

Nursing diagnoses
• Anxiety related to patient's underlying condition
• Risk of injury related to drug-induced adverse CNS reactions
• Knowledge deficit related to drug therapy

⋙ Planning and implementation

• Know that dosage should be reduced in elderly or debilitated patients.

• Know that possibility of abuse and addiction exists. Do not withdraw drug abruptly after prolonged use; withdrawal symptoms may occur.

Patient teaching

• Warn patient to avoid activities that require alertness and good psychomotor coordination until CNS effects of drug are known.

• Tell patient to avoid alcohol while taking drug.

• Suggest taking sugarless chewing gum or hard candy to relieve dry mouth.

• Warn patient to take drug only as directed and not to discontinue taking it without doctor's approval. Inform patient of drug's potential for dependence if taken longer than directed.

✔ Evaluation

• Patient states he is less anxious after taking drug therapy.

• Patient does not experience injury as a result of drug-induced adverse CNS reactions.

• Patient and family state understanding of drug therapy.

cloxacillin sodium

(kloks-uh-SIL-in SOH-dee-um)
Alclox◇, Apo-Cloxi◆, Cloxapen,
Novocloxin◆, Nu-Cloxi◆, Orbenin◆

Pharmacologic class: penicillinase-resistant penicillin
Therapeutic class: antibiotic
Pregnancy risk category: B

How supplied

Capsules: 250 mg, 500 mg
Oral solution: 125 mg/5 ml (after reconstitution)

Pharmacokinetics

Absorption: absorbed rapidly but incompletely (37% to 60%) from GI tract. Food may decrease both rate and extent of absorption.
Distribution: distributed widely. CSF penetration is poor but enhanced in meningeal inflammation. Drug is 90% to 96% protein-bound.
Metabolism: only partially metabolized.
Excretion: drug and metabolites are excreted in urine. *Half-life:* 0.5 to 1 hour.

Route	Onset	Peak	Duration
P.O.	Unknown	0.5-2 hr	About 6 hr

Pharmacodynamics

Chemical effect: a penicillinase-resistant penicillin that inhibits cell-wall synthesis during microorganism multiplication; bacteria resist penicillins by producing penicillinases—enzymes that convert penicillins to inactive penicilloic acid. Cloxacillin resists these enzymes.
Therapeutic effect: hinders bacterial activity. Spectrum of activity include many strains of penicillinase-producing bacteria of which most pronounced activity occurs against penicillinase-producing staphylococci. It is also active against gram-positive aerobic and anaerobic bacilli.

Indications and dosage

▶ **Systemic infections caused by penicillinase-producing staphylococci.** *Adults and children weighing over 20 kg (44 lb):* 250 to 500 mg P.O. q 6 hours. *Children weighing 20 kg or less:* 50 to 100 mg/kg P.O. daily, in divided doses q 6 hours.

Adverse reactions

CNS: *seizures.*
GI: *nausea,* vomiting, *epigastric distress, diarrhea.*
Hematologic: eosinophilia, *thrombocytopenia, agranulocytosis, leukopenia.*
Other: hypersensitivity reactions (rash, urticaria, chills, fever, sneezing, wheezing, *anaphylaxis),* intrahepatic cholesta-

sis, overgrowth of nonsusceptible organisms.

Interactions

Drug-drug. *Probenecid:* increased blood levels of cloxacillin. Probenecid may be used for this purpose.
Drug-food. *Any food:* may interfere with absorption. Give 1 to 2 hours before or 2 to 3 hours after meals.
Carbonated beverages, fruit juice: will inactivate drug. Don't give together.

Contraindications and precautions

• Contraindicated in patients with hypersensitivity to drug or other penicillins.
• Use cautiously in patients with mononucleosis (high risk of maculopapular rash) or other drug allergies, especially to cephalosporins (possible cross-sensitivity).
• Also use cautiously in pregnant or breast-feeding women.

NURSING CONSIDERATIONS

Assessment
• Assess patient's infection before therapy and reassess regularly throughout therapy.
• Before giving, ask patient about any allergic reactions to penicillin. However, negative history of penicillin allergy is no guarantee against future allergic reaction.
• Obtain specimen for culture and sensitivity tests before first dose. Therapy may begin pending results.
• Periodically assess renal, hepatic, and hematopoietic function in patients receiving long-term therapy, as ordered.
• Be alert for adverse reactions and drug interactions.
• Monitor patient's hydration status if adverse GI reactions occur.
• Evaluate patient's and family's knowledge about drug therapy.

Nursing diagnoses
• Infection related to presence of bacteria susceptible to drug

• Risk for fluid volume deficit related to drug-induced adverse GI reactions
• Knowledge deficit related to drug therapy

Planning and implementation
• Give drug 1 to 2 hours before or 2 to 3 hours after meals to avoid GI disturbances. Food may interfere with its absorption. Give each dose with full glass of water, not fruit juice or carbonated beverage because acid will inactivate drug.
• Give drug at least 1 hour before bacteriostatic antibiotics.
• Know that drug may falsely elevate or cause false-positive results with certain tests for urine or serum proteins.
Patient teaching
• Tell patient to take entire quantity of drug exactly as prescribed, even after he feels better. Also tell him to take drug on empty stomach.
• Tell patient to call doctor if rash, fever, or chills develop. A rash is most common allergic reaction.
• Instruct patient to take each dose with full glass of water, not with fruit juice or carbonated beverage, because their acid will inactivate drug.
• Warn patient never to use leftover drug for new illness or to share it with family and friends.

Evaluation
• Patient is free from infection after drug.
• Patient maintains adequate hydration throughout drug therapy.
• Patient and family state understanding of drug therapy.

---

clozapine
(KLOH-zuh-peen)
Clozaril

Pharmacologic class: tricyclic dibenzodiazepine derivative
Therapeutic class: antipsychotic

Pregnancy risk category: B

How supplied

Tablets: 25 mg, 100 mg

Pharmacokinetics

Absorption: thought to be absorbed from GI tract.
Distribution: about 95% bound to serum proteins.
Metabolism: metabolism is nearly complete.
Excretion: about 50% of drug appears in urine and 30% in feces, mostly as metabolites. *Half-life:* appears proportional to dose and may range from 8 to 12 hours.

Route	Onset	Peak	Duration
P.O.	Unknown	2.5 hr	4-12 hr

Pharmacodynamics

Chemical effect: unknown. Binds to dopaminergic receptors (both D-1 and D-2) within limbic system of CNS and may interfere with adrenergic, cholinergic, histaminergic, and serotoninergic receptors.
Therapeutic effect: relieves psychotic signs and symptoms.

Indications and dosage

▶ **Schizophrenia in severely ill patients unresponsive to other therapies.**
Adults: initially, 25 mg P.O. once daily or b.i.d., titrated upward at 25 to 50 mg daily (if tolerated) to 300 to 450 mg daily by end of 2 weeks. Because potentially adverse effects have been reported at initiation of therapy, some clinicians advise an initial dose of 12.5 mg P.O. once or twice daily. Individual dosage based on clinical response, patient tolerance, and adverse reactions. Subsequent dosage should not be increased more than once or twice weekly, and should not exceed 100 mg. Many patients respond to dosages of 300 to 600 mg daily, but some may require as much as 900 mg daily. Do not exceed 900 mg daily.

Adverse reactions

CNS: *drowsiness, sedation, seizures,* dizziness, syncope, vertigo, headache, tremor, disturbed sleep or nightmares, restlessness, hypokinesia or akinesia, agitation, rigidity, akathisia, confusion, fatigue, insomnia, hyperkinesia, weakness, lethargy, ataxia, slurred speech, depression, myoclonus, anxiety.
CV: tachycardia, hypotension, hypertension, chest pain, ECG changes, orthostatic hypotension.
GI: dry mouth, constipation, nausea, vomiting, *excessive salivation,* heartburn, constipation.
GU: urinary abnormalities (urinary frequency or urgency, urine retention), incontinence, abnormal ejaculation.
Hematologic: *leukopenia, agranulocytosis.*
Musculoskeletal: muscle pain or spasm, muscle weakness.
Skin: rash.
Other: fever, weight gain.
After abrupt withdrawal of long-term therapy: possible abrupt recurrence of psychotic symptoms. Monitor closely.

Interactions

Drug-drug. *Anticholinergics:* may potentiate anticholinergic effects of clozapine. Avoid concomitant use.
Antihypertensives: may potentiate hypotensive effects. Monitor blood pressure.
Bone marrow suppressants: may increase bone marrow toxicity. Don't use together.
Digoxin, warfarin, other highly proteinbound drugs: may increase serum levels of these drugs. Monitor closely for adverse reactions.
Psychoactive drugs: may produce additive effects. Use together cautiously.
Drug-food. *Caffeine-containing beverages:* may inhibit antipsychotic effects of clozapine. Monitor closely.
Drug-lifestyle. *Alcohol use:* increased CNS depression. Don't use together.

Contraindications and precautions

• Contraindicated in patients with uncontrolled epilepsy, history of drug-induced agranulocytosis, myelosuppressive disorders, severe CNS depression or coma, or WBC count below 3,500/mm³; in those taking other drugs that suppress bone marrow function; and in breast-feeding women.

• Use cautiously in patients with prostatic hyperplasia or angle-closure glaucoma because clozapine has potent anticholinergic effects and in those with hepatic, renal, or cardiac disease or receiving general anesthesia. Also use cautiously in pregnant women.

• Safety of drug has not been established in children under age 16.

NURSING CONSIDERATIONS

⚅ Assessment

• Assess patient's psychotic condition before therapy and reassess regularly thereafter.

• Know that baseline WBC and differential counts are required before therapy and weekly thereafter.

• Be alert for adverse reactions and drug interactions.

• Monitor WBC counts weekly for at least 4 weeks after drug therapy is discontinued, as ordered, and also monitor closely for recurrence of psychotic symptoms.

• Evaluate patient's and family's knowledge about drug therapy.

⊞ Nursing diagnoses

• Altered thought processes related to patient's underlying condition

• Risk of infection related to potential for drug-induced agranulocytosis

• Knowledge deficit related to drug therapy

❯ Planning and implementation

• Know that drug carries significant risk of agranulocytosis. If possible, patients should receive at least two trials of stan-dard antipsychotic drug therapy before clozapine therapy is initiated.

• Give drug with meals if patient develops GI distress.

• Ensure that no more than 1-week supply of drug is distributed.

• Know that WBC count is used to help determine safety of therapy. If WBC count drops below 3,500/mm³ after therapy is initiated or it exhibits substantial drop from baseline, monitor patient closely for signs of infection. If WBC count is 3,000 to 3,500/mm³ and granulocyte count is above 1,500/mm³, perform WBC and differential count twice weekly. If WBC count drops below 3,000/mm³ and granulocyte count drops below 1,500/mm³, interrupt therapy, notify doctor, and monitor patient for signs of infection. Be aware that therapy may be restarted cautiously if WBC count returns to above 3,000/mm³ and granulocyte count returns above 1,500/mm³. Continue monitoring of WBC and differential counts twice weekly until WBC count exceeds 3,500/mm³, as ordered.

• Follow usual guidelines for dosage increase if therapy is reinstated in patients withdrawn from drug. However, reexposure of patient to drug may increase severity and risk of adverse reactions. If therapy was withdrawn for WBC counts below 2,000/mm³ or granulocyte counts below 1,000/mm³, don't expect drug to be continued.

• Monitor patient for seizures because seizures may occur, especially in those receiving high doses.

• Be aware that some patients experience transient fevers (temperature over 100.4° F [38° C]), especially in first 3 weeks of therapy. Monitor patient closely.

• Know that if WBC count drops below 2,000/mm³ and granulocyte count drops below 1,000/mm³, patient may require protective isolation. If patient develops infection, prepare cultures according to institutional policy and administer antibiotics as ordered. Some clinicians may perform bone marrow aspiration to assess

bone marrow function. Future clozapine therapy is contraindicated in such patients.
• Be aware that drug usually is withdrawn gradually (over 1- to 2-week period) if it must be discontinued. However, changes in patient's medical condition (including development of leukopenia) may require abrupt discontinuation of drug.

Patient teaching
• Warn patient about risk of agranulocytosis. Tell him drug is available only through special monitoring program that requires weekly blood tests to monitor for agranulocytosis. Advise patient to report flulike symptoms, fever, sore throat, lethargy, malaise, or other signs of infection.
• Warn patient to avoid hazardous activities that require alertness and good psychomotor coordination while taking drug.
• Tell patient to rise slowly to avoid orthostatic hypotension.
• Advise patient to check with doctor before taking OTC drugs or alcohol.
• Recommend ice chips or sugarless candy or gum to help relieve dry mouth.

☑ **Evaluation**
• Patient demonstrates reduction in psychotic symptoms with drug therapy.
• Patient does not develop infection throughout drug therapy.
• Patient and family state understanding of drug therapy.

---

codeine phosphate
(KOH-deen FOS-fayt)
Paveral ♦

codeine sulfate

Pharmacologic class: opioid
Therapeutic class: analgesic, antitussive
Controlled substance schedule: II
Pregnancy risk category: C

How supplied

codeine phosphate
Oral solution: 15 mg/5 ml, 10 mg/ml ♦

Injection: 30 mg/ml, 60 mg/ml
Soluble tablets: 30 mg, 60 mg
codeine sulfate
Tablets: 15 mg, 30 mg, 60 mg

Pharmacokinetics

Absorption: well absorbed after oral or parenteral administration. It is about two thirds as potent orally as parenterally.
Distribution: distributed widely throughout body.
Metabolism: metabolized mainly in liver.
Excretion: excreted mainly in urine.
Half-life: 2.5 to 4 hours.

Route	Onset	Peak	Duration
P.O.	30-45 min	1-2 hr	4-6 hr
I.V.	Immediate	Immediate	4-6 hr
I.M.	10-30 min	0.5-1 hr	4-6 hr
S.C.	10-30 min	Unknown	4-6 hr

Pharmacodynamics

Chemical effect: binds with opiate receptors in CNS, altering both perception of and emotional response to pain through unknown mechanism. Also suppresses cough reflex by direct action on cough center in medulla.
Therapeutic effect: relieves pain and cough.

Indications and dosage

▶ **Mild to moderate pain.** *Adults:* 15 to 60 mg P.O. or 15 to 60 mg (phosphate) S.C., I.M., or I.V. q 4 to 6 hours, p.r.n. *Children over age 1:* 0.5 mg/kg P.O., I.M., or S.C. q 4 hours, p.r.n.
▶ **Nonproductive cough.** *Adults:* 10 to 20 mg P.O. q 4 to 6 hours. Maximum dosage is 120 mg/24 hours. *Children ages 6 to 12:* 5 to 10 mg P.O. q 4 to 6 hours. Maximum dosage is 60 mg/24 hours. *Children ages 2 to 6:* 2.5 to 5 mg P.O. q 6 hours. Do not exceed 30 mg in 24 hours.

Adverse reactions

CNS: *sedation, clouded sensorium, euphoria,* dizziness, **seizures** (with large doses).

CV: *hypotension,* bradycardia.
GI: *nausea, vomiting, constipation, dry mouth,* ileus.
GU: *urine retention.*
Respiratory: *respiratory depression.*
Skin: pruritus, flushing.
Other: physical dependence.

Interactions

Drug-drug. *CNS depressants, general anesthetics, hypnotics, MAO inhibitors, other narcotic analgesics, sedatives, tranquilizers, tricyclic antidepressants:* additive effects. Use together with extreme caution. Monitor patient response.
Drug-lifestyle. *Alcohol use:* additive effects. Use together with extreme caution. Monitor patient response.

Contraindications and precautions

• Contraindicated in patients with hypersensitivity to drug.
• Use with extreme caution in patients with head injury, increased intracranial pressure, increased CSF pressure, hepatic or renal disease, hypothyroidism, Addison's disease, acute alcoholism, seizures, severe CNS depression, bronchial asthma, COPD, respiratory depression, and shock. Also use with extreme caution in elderly or debilitated patients.
• Use cautiously in pregnant or breast-feeding women and in children.

NURSING CONSIDERATIONS

Assessment

• Assess patient's pain or cough before and after drug administration.
• Be alert for adverse reactions and drug interactions.
• Evaluate patient's and family's knowledge about drug therapy.

Nursing diagnoses

• Pain related to patient's underlying condition
• Fatigue related to presence of cough

• Knowledge deficit related to drug therapy

Planning and implementation

• Administer drug before patient has intense pain for full analgesic effect.
• Be aware that drug is an antitussive and should not be used when cough is valuable diagnostic sign or is beneficial (as after thoracic surgery).
P.O. use: Administer drug with food or milk to minimize adverse GI reactions.
I.V. use: Give drug by direct injection into large vein. Administer very slowly. Don't mix with other solutions because codeine phosphate is incompatible with many drugs.
I.M. and S.C. use: Follow normal protocol.
• Don't administer discolored injection solution.
• Know that codeine and aspirin or acetaminophen are often prescribed together to provide enhanced pain relief.
• Be aware that codeine's abuse potential is much lower than morphine's.
• Notify doctor if patient does not experience pain or cough relief after codeine administration.
• Keep narcotic antagonist (naloxone) and resuscitative equipment available, if administering drug intravenously.
Patient teaching
• Advise patient to take drug with milk or meals to minimize GI distress caused by oral administration.
• Advise patient to ask for or take drug (if at home) before pain becomes severe.
• Caution ambulatory patient about getting out of bed or walking. Warn outpatient to avoid driving and other potentially hazardous activities that require mental alertness until drug's CNS effects are known.
• Tell patient to report adverse drug reactions.

Evaluation

• Patient is free of pain after drug administration.

• Patient's cough is suppressed after drug administration.
• Patient and family state understanding of drug therapy.

colchicine
(KOHL-chih-seen)
Colchicine MR◇, Colgout◇

Pharmacologic class: Colchicum autumnate alkaloid
Therapeutic class: antigout agent
Pregnancy risk category: D

How supplied
Tablets: 0.5 mg (1/120 grain), 0.6 mg (¹⁄₁₀₀ grain) as sugar-coated granules
Injection: 0.5 mg/ml

Pharmacokinetics
Absorption: rapidly absorbed from GI tract when orally administered. Unchanged drug may be reabsorbed from intestine by biliary processes.
Distribution: distributed rapidly into various tissues. It is concentrated in leukocytes and distributed into kidneys, liver, spleen, and intestinal tract, but is absent in heart, skeletal muscle, and brain.
Metabolism: metabolized partially in liver and also slowly metabolized in other tissues.
Excretion: drug and its metabolites are excreted primarily in feces, with lesser amounts excreted in urine. *Half-life:* 1 to 10.5 hours.

Route	Onset	Peak	Duration
P.O.	≤ 12 hr	0.5-2 hr	Unknown
I.V.	6-12 hr	0.5-2 hr	Unknown

Pharmacodynamics
Chemical effect: unknown. As antigout agent, apparently decreases WBC motility, phagocytosis, and lactic acid production, decreasing urate crystal deposits and reducing inflammation. As antiosteolytic agent, apparently inhibits mitosis of os-

teoprogenitor cells and decreases osteoclast activity.
Therapeutic effect: relieves gout signs and symptoms.

Indications and dosage
▶ **Prevention of acute gout attacks as prophylactic or maintenance therapy.** *Adults:* 0.5 or 0.6 mg P.O. daily. Patients who normally have one attack per year or less should receive drug only 1 to 4 days per week; patients who have more than one attack per year should receive drug daily. In severe cases, 1 to 1.8 mg daily.
▶ **Prevention of gout attacks in patients undergoing surgery.** *Adults:* 0.5 to 0.6 mg P.O. t.i.d. 3 days before and 3 days after surgery.
▶ **Acute gout, acute gouty arthritis.** *Adults:* initially, 0.5 to 1.2 mg P.O., then 0.5 or 0.6 mg q 1 to 2 hours until pain is relieved; nausea, vomiting, or diarrhea ensues. Usual range in a course of oral therapy is 4 to 8 mg. Alternatively, 2 mg I.V. followed by 0.5mg I.V. q 6 hours if necessary. (Note that some clinicians prefer to give a single injection of 3 mg I.V.) Total I.V. dosage over 24 hours (one course of treatment) should not exceed 4 mg.

Adverse reactions
CNS: peripheral neuritis.
GI: *nausea, vomiting, abdominal pain, diarrhea.*
Hematologic: *aplastic anemia, thrombocytopenia, agranulocytosis* (with prolonged use); nonthrombocytopenic purpura.
Hepatic: *hepatic necrosis.*
Skin: alopecia, urticaria, dermatitis.
Other: severe local irritation (if extravasation occurs), *hypersensitivity, anaphylaxis.*

Interactions
Drug-drug. *Loop diuretics:* may decrease efficacy of colchicine prophylaxis. Avoid concomitant use.

Phenylbutazone: may increase risk of leukopenia or thrombocytopenia. Avoid concomitant use.

Vitamin B$_{12}$: impaired absorption of vitamin B$_{12}$. Avoid concomitant use.

Drug-lifestyle. *Alcohol use:* may impair efficacy of colchicine prophylaxis. Don't use together.

Contraindications and precautions

• Contraindicated in patients with serious cardiac disease, renal disease, or GI disorders, and in elderly or debilitated patients.
• Use with extreme caution, if at all, in pregnant women because fetal harm may occur.
• Use cautiously in elderly or debilitated patients or in patients with early manifestations of cardiac, renal, or GI disease.
• Safety of drug has not been established in children or breast-feeding women.

NURSING CONSIDERATIONS

Assessment
• Assess patient's underlying condition before therapy and reassess regularly thereafter.
• Obtain baseline laboratory studies, including CBC and uric acid levels, prior to therapy and repeat regularly, as ordered.
• Be alert for adverse reactions and drug interactions.
• Evaluate patient's and family's knowledge about drug therapy.

Nursing diagnoses
• Pain related to presence of gout
• Altered protection related to drug-induced hematologic adverse reactions
• Knowledge deficit related to drug therapy

Planning and implementation
P.O. use: Give drug with meals to reduce GI effects as maintenance therapy. May be used with uricosuric agents.
I.V. use: Give drug by slow I.V. push over 2 to 5 minutes. Be sure to avoid ex-

travasation because colchicine is very irritating to tissues. Don't dilute colchicine injection with dextrose 5% injection or other fluids that might change pH of colchicine solution. If lower concentration of colchicine injection is needed, dilute with 0.9% NaCl solution or sterile water for injection and administer over 2 to 5 minutes by direct injection. Preferably, inject into tubing of free-flowing I.V. solution. However, don't inject if diluted solution becomes turbid.
• Know that after full course of I.V. colchicine (4 mg), no more colchicine should be given by any other route for at least 7 days. Colchicine is toxic and death can result from overdose.
• Do not administer I.M. or S.C.; severe local irritation occurs.
• Store drug in tightly closed, light-resistant container.
• Discontinue drug as soon as gout pain is relieved or at first sign of GI symptoms, as ordered.
• Force fluids to maintain output at 2,000 ml daily.
Patient teaching
• Instruct patient how to take drug.
• Advise patient to report rash, sore throat, fever, unusual bleeding, bruising, fatigue, weakness, numbness, or tingling.
• Instruct patient on when drug should be discontinued.
• Tell patient to avoid alcohol during drug therapy because it may inhibit drug action.
• Advise patient to avoid all drugs containing aspirin as these may precipitate gout.

Evaluation
• Patient becomes pain free after drug therapy.
• Patient's CBC and platelet counts remain normal throughout drug therapy.
• Patient and family state understanding of drug therapy.

colestipol hydrochloride
(koh-LEH-stih-pohl
high-droh-KLOR-ighd)
Colestid

Pharmacologic class: anion exchange
resin
Therapeutic class: antilipemic
Pregnancy risk category: B

How supplied
Granules: 300-g and 500-g bottles, 5-g
packets
Tablets: 1 g

Pharmacokinetics
Absorption: not absorbed.
Distribution: distributed locally in
intestines.
Metabolism: none.
Excretion: excreted in feces.

Route	Onset	Peak	Duration
P.O.	1-2 days	1 mo	≤ 1 mo

Pharmacodynamics
Chemical effect: combines with bile acid
to form insoluble compound that is excreted. The liver must synthesize new
bile acid from cholesterol; this leads to
reduced low-density-lipoprotein cholesterol levels.
Therapeutic effect: lowers low-density-
lipoprotein blood cholesterol levels.

Indications and dosage
▶ **Primary hypercholesterolemia.**
Adults: 5 to 30 g P.O. once daily or in
divided doses.

Adverse reactions
CNS: headache, dizziness.
GI: constipation, fecal impaction, hemorrhoids, abdominal discomfort, flatulence,
nausea, vomiting, steatorrhea.
Skin: rash; irritation of tongue and perianal area.
Other: vitamin A, D, E, and K deficiency (from decreased absorption); hyper-

chloremic acidosis (with long-term use or
high dosage).

Interactions
Drug-drug. *Orally administered drugs:*
colestipol may decrease absorption. Separate administration times; give other
drugs at least 1 hour before or 4 hours after colestipol.
Oral antidiabetic agents: may antagonize
response to colestipol. Monitor serum
lipids.

Contraindications and precautions
• Contraindicated in patients with hypersensitivity reactions to bile-acid sequestering resins.
• Use cautiously in patients predisposed
to constipation and in those with conditions aggravated by constipation, such as
severe, symptomatic coronary artery disease. Also use cautiously in pregnant
women.
• Safety of drug has not been established
in children or breast-feeding women.

NURSING CONSIDERATIONS

⚕ Assessment
• Assess patient's blood cholesterol level
before therapy.
• Monitor effectiveness by evaluating
serum cholesterol and triglyceride levels
regularly during therapy.
• Be alert for adverse reactions and drug
interactions.
• Monitor patient for signs of fat-soluble
vitamin deficiencies.
• Evaluate patient's and family's knowledge about drug therapy.

⚙ Nursing diagnoses
• Risk for injury related to elevated blood
cholesterol
• Constipation related to drug-induced
adverse GI reactions
• Knowledge deficit related to drug
therapy

≥ Planning and implementation
• To prepare, use large glass containing water, milk, or juice (especially pulpy fruit juice). Sprinkle powder on surface of preferred beverage; let mixture stand few minutes; then stir thoroughly to obtain uniform suspension. After patient drinks this preparation, swirl small additional amount of liquid in same glass and then have him drink it to ensure ingestion of entire dose.
• If severe constipation develops, decrease dosage or add stool softener as ordered. Encourage diet high in fiber and fluids.
• Administer all other drugs at least 1 hour before or 4 to 6 hours after colestipol to avoid blocking their absorption.
Patient teaching
• Instruct patient never to take drug in its dry form; esophageal irritation or severe constipation may result.
• Teach patient how to mix and take drug. To enhance palatability, tell him to mix and refrigerate the next daily dose the previous evening.
• Advise patient to take all other drugs at least 1 hour before or 4 to 6 hours after colestipol to avoid blocking their absorption.
• Teach patient about proper dietary management of serum lipids (restricting total fat and cholesterol intake) as well as measures to control other cardiac disease risk factors. When appropriate, recommend weight control, exercise, and smoking cessation programs.
• Inform patient that long-term use may be associated with deficiency of vitamins A, D, E, and K and folic acid. Instruct patient to report unusual signs and symptoms and to ask doctor about taking multivitamins.

☑ Evaluation
• Patient's blood cholesterol level is normal.
• Patient's constipation is relieved.
• Patient and family state understanding of drug therapy.

corticotropin
(adrenocorticotropic hormone, ACTH)
(kor-teh-koh-TROH-pin)
ACTH, Acthar

repository corticotropin
Acthar Gel (H.P.)♦, ACTH Gel, Acthar Gel

Pharmacologic class: anterior pituitary hormone
Therapeutic class: diagnostic aid, replacement hormone
Pregnancy risk category: C

How supplied
Aqueous injection: 25 units/vial, 40 units/vial
Repository injection: 40 units/ml, 80 units/ml

Pharmacokinetics
Absorption: absorbed rapidly after I.M. administration; unknown for S.C. administration.
Distribution: unknown.
Metabolism: unknown.
Excretion: excreted by kidneys. *Half-life:* about 15 minutes.

Route	Onset	Peak	Duration
I.V.	Rapid	Varies	2 hr for zinc form; ≤ 3 days for repository form
I.M.	Varies	Varies	2 hr for zinc form; ≤ 3 days for repository form
S.C.	Varies	Varies	2 hr for zinc form; ≤ 3 days for repository form

Pharmacodynamics
Chemical effect: by replacing body's own tropic hormone, stimulates secretion of adrenal cortex hormones.
Therapeutic effect: diagnoses or treats adrenocortical hormonal deficiency.

---

*Liquid form contains alcohol   **May contain tartrazine   ♦Canada   ◊ Australia   †OTC

Indications and dosage

► **Diagnostic test of adrenocortical function.** *Adults:* up to 80 units repository form I.M. or S.C. in divided doses or as single dose; or 10 to 25 units aqueous form in 500 ml of D_5W I.V. over 8 hours, between blood samplings. Individual dosages generally vary with adrenal glands' sensitivity to stimulation as well as with specific disease. Infants and younger children require larger doses per kilogram than older children and adults.
► **For therapeutic use.** *Adults:* 20 units aqueous form S.C. or I.M. in four divided doses; or 40 to 80 units q 24 to 72 hours (repository form).

Adverse reactions

CNS: *seizures, dizziness, papilledema,* headache, *euphoria, insomnia,* mood swings, personality changes, depression, psychosis, *increased intracranial pressure.*
CV: *shock.*
EENT: cataracts, glaucoma.
GI: peptic ulceration (with perforation and hemorrhage), pancreatitis, abdominal distention, ulcerative esophagitis, nausea, vomiting.
Skin: impaired wound healing, thin fragile skin, petechiae, ecchymoses, facial erythema, diaphoresis, acne, hyperpigmentation, allergic skin reactions, hirsutism.
Other: muscle weakness, steroid myopathy, loss of muscle mass, osteoporosis, vertebral compression fractures, cushingoid symptoms, suppression of growth in children, activation of latent diabetes mellitus, progressive increase in antibodies, loss of corticotropin stimulatory effect, hypersensitivity reactions (rash, *bronchospasm*), *sodium and fluid retention,* calcium and potassium loss, hypokalemic alkalosis, negative nitrogen balance, menstrual irregularities.

Interactions

Drug-drug. *Anticonvulsants, barbiturates, rifampin:* increased metabolism of corticotropin and decreased effectiveness. Monitor for lack of effect.
Estrogens: may potentiate effects of cortisol. Dosage adjustments may be necessary.
NSAIDs, salicylates: increased risk of GI bleeding. Avoid concomitant use.
Oral anticoagulants: altered PT. Monitor PT and INR. Dosage adjustments may be necessary.
Potassium-wasting diuretics: increased risk of hypokalemia. Monitor serum potassium levels.

Contraindications and precautions

• Contraindicated in patients with peptic ulcer, scleroderma, osteoporosis, systemic fungal infections, ocular herpes simplex, peptic ulceration, heart failure, hypertension, adrenocortical hyperfunction or primary insufficiency, Cushing's syndrome, or hypersensitivity to pork and pork products. Also contraindicated in those who have had recent surgery.
• Use cautiously in pregnant women and in women of childbearing age. Also use cautiously in patients being immunized and in those with latent tuberculosis or tuberculin reactivity, hypothyroidism, cirrhosis, acute gouty arthritis, psychotic tendencies, renal insufficiency, diverticulitis, nonspecific ulcerative colitis, thromboembolic disorders, seizures, uncontrolled hypertension, or myasthenia gravis.
• Also use cautiously in children because prolonged use of drug will inhibit skeletal growth. Intermittent administration is recommended.
• Safety of drug has not been established in breast-feeding women.

NURSING CONSIDERATIONS

⚕ Assessment
• Assess patient's underlying condition before therapy and reassess regularly during therapy.
• Know that corticotropin treatment should be preceded by verification of adrenal responsiveness and test for hypersensitivity and allergic reactions.

Reactions may be *common,* uncommon, *life-threatening,* or COMMON AND LIFE-THREATENING.

• Be alert for adverse reactions and drug interactions.

• Note and record weight changes, fluid exchange, and resting blood pressures until minimal effective dosage is achieved.

• Watch neonates of corticotropin-treated mothers for signs of hypoadrenalism.

• Monitor patient for stress.

• Evaluate patient's and family's knowledge about drug test or therapy.

🔁 **Nursing diagnoses**
• Altered protection related to underlying condition
• Risk for injury related to drug-induced adverse reactions
• Knowledge deficit related to drug test or therapy

▷ **Planning and implementation**
• Be aware that corticotropin should be adjunct, not sole, therapy. Oral agents are preferred for long-term therapy.
I.V. use: Use only aqueous form for I.V. administration. Dilute in 500 ml of D₅W and infuse over 8 hours.
I.M. use: If administering gel, warm it to room temperature, draw into large needle, and give slowly as deep I.M. injection with 21G or 22G needle. Warn patient that injection is painful.
• Refrigerate reconstituted solution and use within 24 hours.
• Counteract edema by low-sodium, high-potassium intake; nitrogen loss by high-protein diet; and psychotic changes by reducing corticotropin dosage or administering sedatives as ordered.
• Unusual stress may require additional use of rapidly acting corticosteroids. When possible, gradually reduce corticotropin dosage to smallest effective dose as ordered to minimize induced adrenocortical insufficiency. Know that therapy can be reinstituted if stressful situation (trauma, surgery, severe illness) occurs shortly after stopping drug.
Patient teaching
• Stress importance of informing health care team members about corticotropin

use because unusual stress may need additional use of rapidly acting corticosteroids. If corticotropin was recently stopped, therapy may have to be reinstituted.
• Tell patient to restrict sodium intake and consume high-protein, high-potassium diet.
• Advise patient to have close follow-up care.
• Warn patient that injections, especially I.M. injections, are painful.

☑ **Evaluation**
• Patient's underlying condition improves with drug therapy.
• Patient does not experience injury as result of drug-induced adverse reactions.
• Patient and family state understanding of drug test or therapy.

cortisone acetate
(KOR-tih-sohn AS-ih-tayt)
Cortate◇, Cortone Acetate

Pharmacologic class: glucocorticoid, mineralocorticoid
Therapeutic class: anti-inflammatory, replacement therapy
Pregnancy risk category: NR

How supplied
Tablets: 5 mg, 10 mg, 25 mg
Injection (suspension): 50 mg/ml

Pharmacokinetics
Absorption: absorbed readily after oral administration; unknown for I.M. administration.
Distribution: distributed rapidly to muscle. liver, skin, intestines, and kidneys. Cortisone is extensively bound to plasma proteins. Only unbound portion is active.
Metabolism: metabolized in liver to active metabolite hydrocortisone, which is metabolized to inactive glucuronide and sulfate metabolites.
Excretion: inactive metabolites and small amounts of unmetabolized drug are

---

excreted by kidneys. Insignificant quantities of drug also excreted in feces. *Half-life:* 8 to 12 hours.

Route	Onset	Peak	Duration
P.O.	Rapid	2 hr	1.25-1.5 days
I.M.	Slow	20-48 hr	Varies

Pharmacodynamics

Chemical effect: not completely defined. Decreases inflammation, mainly by stabilizing leukocyte lysosomal membranes; suppresses immune response; stimulates bone marrow; and influences protein, fat, and carbohydrate metabolism. *Therapeutic effect:* reduces inflammation; raises corticosteroid therapy.

Indications and dosage

▶ **Adrenal insufficiency, allergy, inflammation.** *Adults:* 25 to 300 mg P.O. or 20 to 300 mg I.M. daily or on alternate days. Dosages are highly individualized, depending on severity of disease.

Adverse reactions

Most adverse reactions are dose- or duration-dependent.
CNS: *euphoria, insomnia,* psychotic behavior, pseudotumor cerebri, *seizures.*
CV: *arrhythmias, heart failure, thromboembolism,* hypertension, edema.
EENT: cataracts, glaucoma.
GI: *peptic ulceration,* GI irritation, increased appetite, pancreatitis.
Metabolic: possible hypokalemia, hyperglycemia, and carbohydrate intolerance.
Musculoskeletal: muscle weakness, osteoporosis, growth suppression in children.
Skin: delayed wound healing, acne, various skin eruptions; atrophy (at I.M. injection site).
Other: hirsutism, susceptibility to infections; *acute adrenal insufficiency may follow increased stress (infection, surgery, or trauma) or abrupt withdrawal after long-term therapy.*
After abrupt withdrawal: rebound inflammation, fatigue, weakness, arthralgia, fever, dizziness, lethargy, depression, fainting, orthostatic hypotension, dyspnea, anorexia, hypoglycemia. *After prolonged use, sudden withdrawal may be fatal.*

Interactions

Drug-drug. *Aspirin, indomethacin, other NSAIDs:* increased risk of GI distress and bleeding. Give together cautiously.
Barbiturates, phenytoin, rifampin: decreased corticosteroid effect. Increase corticosteroid dosage, as ordered.
Live-attenuated virus vaccines, other toxoids and vaccines: decreased antibody response and increased risk of neurologic complications. Avoid concomitant use.
Oral anticoagulants: altered dosage requirements. Monitor PT closely.
Potassium-depleting drugs (such as thiazide diuretics): enhanced potassium-wasting effects of cortisone. Monitor serum potassium levels.
Skin-test antigens: decreased response. Defer skin testing until therapy is completed.
Drug-lifestyle. *Alcohol use:* increase risk of gastric irritation. Avoid use.

Contraindications and precautions

● Contraindicated in patients with systemic fungal infections or hypersensitivity to drug or its ingredients.
● Use with extreme caution in patient with recent MI.
● Use cautiously in patients with GI ulcer, renal disease, hypertension, osteoporosis, diabetes mellitus, hypothyroidism, cirrhosis, diverticulitis, nonspecific ulcerative colitis, recent intestinal anastomoses, thromboembolic disorders, seizures, myasthenia gravis, heart failure, tuberculosis, ocular herpes simplex, emotional instability, and psychotic tendencies.
● Use cautiously in pregnant or breast-feeding women.
● Know that chronic use of drug in children is not recommended because delayed growth and maturation may occur.

Reactions may be *common,* uncommon, *life-threatening,* or COMMON AND LIFE-THREATENING.

NURSING CONSIDERATIONS

▣ Assessment
• Assess patient's underlying condition before therapy and reassess regularly thereafter.
• Monitor serum electrolyte and blood glucose levels as ordered. Check patient's weight and vital signs regularly.
• Monitor patient's stress level.
• Be alert for adverse reactions and drug interactions.
• Evaluate patient's and family's knowledge about drug therapy.

▣ Nursing diagnoses
• Altered protection related to underlying condition
• Risk for injury related to drug-induced adverse reactions
• Knowledge deficit related to drug therapy

▣ Planning and implementation
P.O. use: Give drug with milk or food to reduce GI irritation.
– Give once-daily dose in morning for best results and least toxicity.
I.M. use: I.M. route causes slow onset of action. Should not be used in acute conditions where rapid effect is required. May be used on twice-daily schedule matching diurnal variation. Rotate injection sites to prevent muscle atrophy.
• Mixing or diluting parenteral suspension may alter absorption rate and decrease drug's effectiveness.
• Know that drug is not for I.V. use.
• Know that drug should always be titrated to lowest effective dose.
• Gradually reduce drug dosage after long-term therapy, as ordered.
• Notify doctor if signs of adrenal insufficiency increase. Unusual stress may require additional use of rapidly acting corticosteroids.
Patient teaching
• Tell patient not to discontinue drug abruptly or without doctor's consent.

• Advise patient receiving long-term therapy to consider exercise or physical therapy. Also tell him to ask doctor about vitamin D or calcium supplements.
• Tell patient to restrict sodium intake and consume high-protein, high-potassium diet.
• Tell patient to report slow healing.
• Warn patient on long-term therapy about cushingoid symptoms and to report sudden weight gain or swelling to doctor.
• Instruct patient to carry card indicating their need for supplemental glucocorticoids during stress.

▣ Evaluation
• Patient exhibits improvement in underlying condition with drug therapy.
• Patient does not experience injury as result of drug-induced adverse reactions.
• Patient and family state understanding of drug therapy.

---

cosyntropin
(koh-sin-TROH-pin)
Cortrosyn

Pharmacologic class: anterior pituitary hormone
Therapeutic class: diagnostic agent
Pregnancy risk category: C

How supplied
Injection: 0.25 mg/vial

Pharmacokinetics
Absorption: absorbed rapidly after I.M. administration.
Distribution: unknown.
Metabolism: unknown.
Excretion: thought to be excreted by kidneys.

Route	Onset	Peak	Duration
I.V.	≤ 5 min	1 hr	Unknown
I.M.	Unknown	1 hr	Unknown

Pharmacodynamics
Chemical effect: by replacing body's own tropic hormone, stimulates secretion of adrenal cortex hormones. *Therapeutic effect:* aid in diagnosing adrenocortical dysfunction.

Indications and dosage
▶ **Diagnostic test of adrenocortical function.** *Adults and children age 2 and older:* 0.25 to 1 mg I.V. or I.M. (unless label prohibits I.V. administration) between blood samplings. *Children under age 2:* 0.125 mg I.V. or I.M.

Adverse reactions
CNS: *seizures, increased intracranial pressure with papilledema.*
Skin: pruritus.
Other: flushing, hypersensitivity reactions (*anaphylaxis* [rare]).

Interactions
Drug-drug. *Blood and plasma products:* inactivates cosyntropin. Avoid concomitant administration.
Cortisone, hydrocortisone: may interfere with test results of cortisol levels if administered on test day.
Spironolactone: may interfere with fluorometric analysis of cortisol levels. Avoid concomitant use.

Contraindications and precautions
• Contraindicated in patients with hypersensitivity to drug.
• Use cautiously in patients hypersensitive to natural corticotropin.
• Safety of drug has not been established in pregnant or breast-feeding women and children under age 2.

NURSING CONSIDERATIONS

☒ Assessment
• Assess patient's reason for test before administration. Evaluate test results.
• Be alert for adverse reactions and drug interactions.

• Monitor patients for allergic reactions, rashes, dyspnea, wheezing, or evidence of anaphylaxis.
• Evaluate patient's and family's knowledge about drug test.

☒ Nursing diagnoses
• Risk for injury related to potential for cosyntropin to cause hypersensitivity reactions
• Knowledge deficit related to drug test

☒ Planning and implementation
I.V. use: Reconstitute drug with 1 ml of supplied diluent. For direct injection, administer over at least 2 minutes. May be further diluted with D_5W or 0.9% NaCl and infused at a rate of 0.04 mg/hr over 6 hours. Solution is stable for 12 hours at room temperature.
I.M. use: Follow normal protocol.
• Notify doctor if hypersensitivity occurs, and be prepared to administer emergency care.
Patient teaching
• Instruct patient to notify doctor immediately if pruritus or other signs of hypersensitivity occur.
• Explain how drug test is performed.

☒ Evaluation
• Patient does not exhibit hypersensitivity reaction to drug administration.
• Patient and family state understanding of drug test.

---

co-trimoxazole (sulfamethoxazole-trimethoprim)
(koh-trigh-MOX-uh-zohl)
Apo-Sulfatrim♦, Apo-Sulfatrim DS♦, Bactrim*, Bactrim DS, Bactrim I.V. Infusion, Cotrim, Cotrim D.S., Novotrimel♦, Novotrimel DS♦, Resprim◇, Roubac♦, Septra*, Septra DS, Septra I.V. Infusion, Septrin◇, SMZ-TMP

Pharmacologic class: sulfonamide and folate antagonist

Therapeutic class: antibiotic
Pregnancy risk category: C (contraindicated at term)

How supplied

Tablets: trimethoprim 80 mg and sulfamethoxazole 400 mg; trimethoprim 160 mg and sulfamethoxazole 800 mg
Oral suspension: trimethoprim 40 mg and sulfamethoxazole 200 mg/5 ml
Injection: trimethoprim 16 mg and sulfamethoxazole 80 mg/ml (5 ml/ampule)

Pharmacokinetics

Absorption: well absorbed from GI tract after oral administration.
Distribution: distributed widely into body tissues and fluids, including middle ear fluid, prostatic fluid, bile, aqueous humor, and CSF. Protein binding is 44% for trimethoprim, 70% for sulfamethoxazole.
Metabolism: both components of drug are metabolized by liver.
Excretion: both components of drug are excreted primarily in urine. *Half-life:* trimethoprim, 8 to 11 hours; sulfamethoxazole, 10 to 13 hours.

Route	Onset	Peak	Duration
P.O.	Unknown	1-4 hr	Unknown
I.V.	Immediate	Immediate	Unknown

Pharmacodynamics

Chemical effect: sulfamethoxazole component inhibits formation of dihydrofolic acid from PABA; trimethoprim component inhibits dihydrofolate reductase. Both decrease bacterial folic acid synthesis.
Therapeutic effect: inhibits susceptible bacterial activity. Spectrum of activity include *Escherichia coli, Klebsiella, Enterobacter, Proteus mirabilis, Haemophilus influenzae, Streptococcus pneumoniae, Staphylococcus aureus, Acinetobacter, Salmonella, Shigella,* and *Pneumocystis carinii.*

Indications and dosage

▶ **Urinary tract infections and shigellosis.** *Adults:* 160 mg trimethoprim/

800 mg sulfamethoxazole (double strength tablet) P.O. q 12 hours for 10 to 14 days in urinary tract infections and for 5 days in shigellosis. For simple cystitis or acute urethral syndrome, one to three double-strength tablets may be given as single dose. If indicated, I.V. infusion is given: 8 to 10 mg/kg/day (based on trimethoprim component) in two to four divided doses q 6, 8, or 12 hours for up to 14 days. Maximum daily dose is 960 mg trimethoprim. *Children age 2 months and over:* 8 mg/kg trimethoprim/40 mg/kg sulfamethoxazole P.O. per 24 hours, in two divided doses q 12 hours (10 days for urinary tract infections; 5 days, for shigellosis). If indicated, I.V. infusion is given: 8 to 10 mg/kg/day (based on trimethoprim component) in two to four divided doses q 6, 8, or 12 hours. Adult dose should not be exceeded.
▶ **Otitis media in patients with penicillin allergy or penicillin-resistant infections.** *Children age 2 months and over:* 8 mg/kg trimethoprim/40 mg/kg sulfamethoxazole P.O. per 24 hours, in two divided doses q 12 hours for 10 days.
▶ *Pneumocystis carinii* **pneumonia.** *Adults and children age 2 months and over:* 20 mg/kg trimethoprim/100 mg/kg sulfamethoxazole P.O. per 24 hours, in equally divided doses q 6 hours for 14 days. If indicated, I.V. infusion may be given 15 to 20 mg/kg/day (based on trimethoprim component) in three or four divided doses q 6 to 8 hours for up to 14 days.
▶ **Chronic bronchitis.** *Adults:* 160 mg trimethoprim/800 mg sulfamethoxazole P.O. q 12 hours for 10 to 14 days.
▶ **Traveler's diarrhea.** *Adults:* 160 mg trimethoprim/800 mg sulfamethoxazole P.O. b.i.d. for 3 to 5 days. Some patients may require 2 days of therapy or less.
▶ **Urinary tract infections in males with prostatitis.** *Adults:* 160 mg trimethoprim/800 mg sulfamethoxazole P.O. b.i.d. for 3 to 6 months.

▶ **Chronic urinary tract infections.**
Adults: 40 mg trimethoprim/200 mg sulfamethoxazole (½ tablet) or 80 mg trimetoprim/400 mg sulfamethoxazole P.O. daily or three times week for 3 to 6 months.

Adverse reactions

CNS: headache, mental depression, *seizures,* hallucinations, ataxia, nervousness, fatigue, muscle weakness, vertigo, insomnia.
GI: *nausea, vomiting, diarrhea,* abdominal pain, anorexia, stomatitis.
GU: *toxic nephrosis with oliguria and anuria,* crystalluria, hematuria.
Hematologic: *agranulocytosis, aplastic anemia,* megaloblastic anemia, *thrombocytopenia, leukopenia, hemolytic anemia.*
Hepatic: jaundice, *hepatic necrosis.*
Skin: *erythema multiforme (Stevens-Johnson syndrome), generalized skin eruption, epidermal necrolysis, exfoliative dermatitis,* photosensitivity, urticaria, pruritus.
Other: hypersensitivity reactions (serum sickness, drug fever, *anaphylaxis*), thrombophlebitis.

Interactions

Drug-drug. *Oral anticoagulants:* increased anticoagulant effect. Monitor for bleeding.
Oral antidiabetic agents: increased hypoglycemic effect. Monitor blood glucose levels.
Oral contraceptives: decreased contraceptive effectiveness and increased risk of breakthrough bleeding. Suggest nonhormonal form of contraception.
Phenytoin: may inhibit hepatic metabolism of phenytoin. Monitor closely.
Drug-lifestyle. *Sun exposure:* Photosensitivity reactions may occur. Take precautions.

Contraindications and precautions

• Contraindicated in patients with megaloblastic anemia caused by folate deficiency, porphyria, severe renal impairment (creatinine clearance less than 15 ml/minute), or hypersensitivity to trimethoprim or sulfonamides; in pregnant women at term; and in breast-feeding women.
• Use cautiously and in reduced dosages in patients with impaired hepatic or renal function (creatinine clearance of 15 to 30 ml/minute), severe allergy or bronchial asthma, G6PD deficiency, and blood dyscrasia.
• Safety of drug has not been established in infants under age 2 months.

NURSING CONSIDERATIONS

Assessment
• Assess patient's infection before therapy and reassess regularly thereafter.
• Obtain specimen for culture and sensitivity tests before first dose. Therapy may begin pending results.
• Be alert for adverse reactions and drug interactions.
• Monitor patient's hydration status if adverse GI reactions occur.
• Monitor intake and output. Urine output should be at least 1,500 ml/day to ensure proper hydration. Inadequate urine output can lead to crystalluria or tubular deposits of drug.
• Evaluate patient's and family's knowledge about drug therapy.

Nursing diagnoses
• Infection related to presence of bacteria susceptible to drug
• Risk for fluid volume deficit related to drug induced adverse GI reactions
• Knowledge deficit related to drug therapy

Planning and implementation
P.O. use: Administer drug with full glass of water at least 1 hour before or 2 hours after meals for maximum absorption. Shake oral suspension thoroughly before administering.
I.V. use: Dilute contents of 5-ml ampule of drug in 125 ml of D_5W before admin-

istration. If patient is on a fluid restriction, dilute 5 ml of drug in 75 ml D₅W. Don't mix with other drugs or solutions. Infuse slowly over 60 to 90 minutes. Don't give by rapid infusion or bolus injection. Don't refrigerate.
• Never administer I.M.
• Note that "DS" or "F" product means "double strength."

Patient teaching
• Tell patient to take entire amount of medication exactly as prescribed, even if he feels better.
• Tell patient to take drug with full glass of water and to drink at least 3,000 to 4,000 ml/day of water.
• Advise patient to avoid exposure to direct sunlight because of risk of photosensitivity reaction.
• Tell patient to report signs of rash, sore throat, fever, or mouth sores as drug may need to be discontinued.

☑ **Evaluation**
• Patient is free from infection after drug therapy.
• Patient maintains adequate hydration after drug therapy.
• Patient and family state understanding of drug therapy.

cromolyn sodium (sodium cromoglycate)
(KROH-moh-lin SOH-dee-um)
Crolom, Gastrocrom, Intal, Intal Aerosol Spray, Intal Nebulizer Solution, Nasalcrom, Rynacrom♦

Pharmacologic class: chromone derivative
Therapeutic class: mast cell stabilizer, antiasthmatic
Pregnancy risk category: B

How supplied

Capsules (for oral solution): 100 mg
Aerosol: 800 mcg/metered spray

Nasal solution: 5.2 mg/metered spray (40 mg/ml)
Solution (for nebulization): 20 mg/2 ml
Ophthalmic solution: 4% (with benzalkonium chloride 0.01%, EDTA 0.01%, and phenylethyl ethanol 0.4%)

Pharmacokinetics

Absorption: only 0.5% to 2% of oral dose, 7% of intranasal dose, and 0.03% of ophthalmic dose is absorbed.
Distribution: drug does not cross most biological membranes.
Metabolism: none significant.
Excretion: excreted unchanged in urine (50%) and bile (about 50%). Small amounts may be excreted in feces or exhaled. *Half-life:* 81 minutes.

Route	Onset	Peak	Duration
All routes	Unknown	Unknown	Unknown

Pharmacodynamics

Chemical effect: inhibits degranulation of sensitized mast cells that occurs after patient's exposure to specific antigens. Also inhibits release of histamine and slow-reacting substance of anaphylaxis. *Therapeutic effect:* adjunct to preventing bronchospasms and allergy symptoms.

Indications and dosage

▶ **Adjunct in severe perennial bronchial asthma.** *Adults and children age 5 and over:* 2 metered sprays using inhaler q.i.d. at regular intervals. Alternatively, 20 mg via nebulization q.i.d. at regular intervals.
▶ **Prevention and treatment of allergic rhinitis.** *Adults and children over age 5:* 1 spray in each nostril t.i.d or q.i.d. Maximal administration is six times daily.
▶ **Prevention of exercise-induced bronchospasm.** *Adults and children age 5 and over:* 2 metered sprays inhaled no more than 1 hour before anticipated exercise.
▶ **Allergic ocular disorders.** *Adults and children age 4 and older:* 1 to 2 drops in

each eye four to six times daily at regular intervals.

▶ **Systemic mastocytosis.** *Adults and children over age 12:* 200 mg P.O. q.i.d. before meals and h.s. *Children ages 2 to 12:* 100 mg P.O. q.i.d. 30 minutes before meals or h.s.

Adverse reactions

CNS: dizziness, headache.
EENT: *irritation of throat and trachea,* nasal congestion, pharyngeal irritation, lacrimation.
GI: nausea, esophagitis.
GU: dysuria, urinary frequency.
Respiratory: *bronchospasm* (after inhalation of dry powder); *cough,* wheezing, *eosinophilic pneumonia.*
Skin: rash, urticaria.
Other: joint swelling and pain, swollen parotid gland, *angioedema.*

Interactions

None significant.

Contraindications and precautions

• Contraindicated in patients experiencing acute asthma attacks and status asthmaticus and in those with hypersensitivity to drug.
• Use with caution in pregnant or breast-feeding women.
• Administer drug with caution in children. Use of cromolyn oral inhalation solution is *not* recommended in children under age 2; cromolyn powder or aerosol for oral inhalation, not recommended in children under age 5; and cromolyn nasal solution, not recommended in children under age 6.
• Use inhalation form cautiously in patients with coronary artery disease or history of arrhythmias.

NURSING CONSIDERATIONS

☑ Assessment

• Assess patient's underlying condition before therapy and reassess regularly thereafter.

• Monitor pulmonary function tests to demonstrate bronchodilator-reversible component of airway obstruction.
• Monitor patient for eosinophilic pneumonia.
• Watch for recurrence of asthmatic symptoms when dosage is decreased, especially when corticosteroids are also used.
• Be alert for adverse reactions.
• Evaluate patient's and family's knowledge about drug therapy.

☑ Nursing diagnoses

• Impaired gas exchange related to patient's underlying condition
• Impaired tissue integrity related to drug-induced adverse EENT reactions
• Knowledge deficit related to drug therapy

☑ Planning and implementation

• Know that drug should be used only when acute episode of asthma has been controlled, airway is cleared, and patient can inhale independently.
• Be aware that oral cromolyn sodium should be used in full-term neonates and infants *only* for severe, incapacitating disease when benefits clearly outweigh risks.
P.O. use: Dissolve powder in capsules for oral dose in hot water and further dilute with cold water before ingestion. Do not mix with fruit juice, milk, or food.
Inhalation use: Insert inhalation capsule into inhalation device as described in manufacturer's directions. Have patient exhale completely. Then place mouthpiece between patient's lips; have him inhale deeply and rapidly with steady, even breath; remove inhaler from mouth, have patient hold his breath for few seconds, and then exhale. Repeat until all powder has been inhaled.
Intranasal and ophthalmic use: Follow normal protocol.
• Discontinue drug if patient develops eosinophilic pneumonia, indicated by

---

Reactions may be *common*, uncommon, *life-threatening*, or COMMON AND LIFE-THREATENING.

eosinophilia and infiltrates on chest X-ray film.
• Aid in relief of esophagitis by use of antacids, as ordered, or milk.
Patient teaching
• Instruct patient on how to administer form of drug prescribed. Warn him to avoid excessive handling of capsules for inhalation.
• Tell patient that esophagitis may be relieved by antacids or glass of milk.
• Instruct patient to notify doctor if adverse reactions occur with frequency or become troublesome or severe.

☑ **Evaluation**
• Patient exhibits adequate air exchange with drug therapy.
• Patient demonstrates management of adverse EENT reactions appropriately.
• Patient and family state understanding of drug therapy.

cyanocobalamin (vitamin B₁₂)
(sigh-an-oh-koh-BAH-luh-meen)
Anacobin♦, Bedoz♦, Crystamine, Crysti 1000, Cyanocobalamin, Cyanoject, Cyomin

hydroxocobalamin (vitamin B₁₂)
Hydro-Cobex, LA-12

Pharmacologic class: water-soluble vitamin
Therapeutic class: vitamin, nutrition supplement
Pregnancy risk category: A (C if used in doses above RDA)

How supplied
cyanocobalamin
Tablets: 25 mcg†, 50 mcg†, 100 mcg†, 250 mcg†, 500 mcg†, 1,000 mcg†
Injection: 1,000 mcg/ml
hydroxocobalamin
Injection: 1,000 mcg/ml

Pharmacokinetics
Absorption: after oral administration, vitamin B₁₂ is absorbed irregularly from distal small intestine. Vitamin B₁₂ is protein-bound. Absorption depends on sufficient intrinsic factor and calcium. Vitamin B₁₂ is absorbed rapidly from I.M. and S.C. administration sites.
Distribution: distributed into liver, bone marrow, and other tissues.
Metabolism: metabolized in liver.
Excretion: amount of vitamin B₁₂ needed by body is reabsorbed; excess is excreted in urine. *Half-life:* about 6 days.

Route	Onset	Peak	Duration
P.O.	Unknown	8-12 hr	Unknown
I.M.	Unknown	60 min	Unknown
S.C.	Unknown	Unknown	Unknown

Pharmacodynamics
Chemical effect: coenzyme that stimulates metabolic functions. Necessary for cell replication, hematopoiesis, and nucleoprotein and myelin synthesis.
Therapeutic effect: increases vitamin B₁₂ level.

Indications and dosage
▶ **RDA for cyanocobalamin.** *Neonates and infants to age 6 months:* 0.3 mcg. *Infants ages 6 months to 1 year:* 0.5 mcg. *Children over age 1 to age 3:* 0.7 mcg. *Children ages 4 to 6:* 1 mcg. *Children ages 7 to 10:* 1.4 mcg. *Adults and children age 11 and over:* 2 mcg. *Pregnant women:* 2.2 mcg. *Breast-feeding women:* 2.6 mcg.
▶ **Vitamin B₁₂ deficiency caused by inadequate diet, subtotal gastrectomy, or any other condition, disorder, or disease except malabsorption related to pernicious anemia or other GI disease.** *Adults:* 30 mcg hydroxocobalamin I.M. daily for 5 to 10 days, depending on severity of deficiency. Maintenance dosage is 100 to 200 mcg I.M. once monthly. For subsequent prophylaxis, advise adequate nutrition and daily RDA vitamin B₁₂ supplements. *Children:* 1 to 5 mg hydroxo-

cobalamin spread over 2 or more weeks in doses of 100 mcg I.M., depending on severity of deficiency. Maintenance dosage is 30 to 50 mcg/month I.M. For subsequent prophylaxis, advise adequate nutrition and daily RDA vitamin B_{12} supplements.

▶ **Pernicious anemia or vitamin B_{12} malabsorption.** *Adults:* initially, 100 mcg cyanocobalamin I.M. or S.C. daily for 6 to 7 days, then 100 mcg I.M. or S.C. once monthly. *Children:* 30 to 50 mcg I.M. or S.C. daily over 2 or more weeks; then 100 mcg I.M. or S.C. monthly for life.

▶ **Methylmalonic aciduria.** *Neonates:* 1,000 mcg cyanocobalamin I.M. daily.

▶ **Schilling test flushing dose.** *Adults and children:* 1,000 mcg hydroxocobalamin I.M. in single dose.

Adverse reactions

CV: peripheral vascular thrombosis, pulmonary edema, heart failure.
GI: transient diarrhea.
Skin: itching, transitory exanthema, urticaria.
Other: *anaphylaxis, anaphylactoid reactions* (with parenteral administration); pain, burning (at S.C. or I.M. injection sites).

Interactions

Drug-drug. *Aminoglycosides, chloramphenicol, colchicine, para-aminosalicylic acid and salts:* malabsorption of vitamin B_{12}. Don't use concomitantly.
Drug-lifestyle. *Alcohol use:* malabsorption of vitamin B_{12}. Don't use together.

Contraindications and precautions

• Contraindicated in patients with early Leber's disease or hypersensitivity to vitamin B_{12} or cobalt.
• Use cautiously in anemic patients with coexisting cardiac, pulmonary, or hypertensive disease and in those with severe vitamin B_{12}-dependent deficiencies.

• Use cautiously in premature infants. Some products contain benzyl alcohol which may cause "gasping syndrome."

NURSING CONSIDERATIONS

⧖ Assessment
• Assess patient's vitamin B_{12} deficiency before therapy.
• Determine reticulocyte count, hematocrit, B_{12}, iron, and folate levels before beginning therapy, as ordered.
• Monitor effectiveness by assessing patient for improvement in signs and symptoms of vitamin B_{12} deficiency. Also monitor reticulocyte count, hematocrit, B_{12}, iron, and folate levels between fifth and seventh day of therapy and periodically thereafter, as ordered.
• Be aware that infection, tumors, or renal, hepatic, and other debilitating diseases may reduce therapeutic response.
• Closely monitor serum potassium levels for first 48 hours. Be alert for adverse reactions and drug interactions.
• Evaluate patient's and family's knowledge about drug therapy.

⊕ Nursing diagnoses
• Altered health maintenance related to underlying vitamin B_{12} deficiency
• Risk for injury related to parenteral administration of drug-induced hypersensitivity reactions
• Knowledge deficit related to drug therapy

▷ Planning and implementation
• Don't mix parenteral liquids in same syringe with other medications.
• Keep in mind that drug is physically incompatible with dextrose solutions, alkaline or strongly acidic solutions, oxidizing or reducing agents, heavy metals, chlorpromazine, phytonadione, prochlorperazine, and many other drugs.
P.O. use: Do not administer large oral doses of vitamin B_{12} routinely as drug is lost through excretion.

I.M. use: Follow normal protocol. Know
that hydroxocobalamin is approved for
I.M. use only.
S.C. use: Follow normal protocol.
• Protect vitamin from light. Do not re-
frigerate or freeze.
• Give potassium supplement if neces-
sary, as ordered.
• Be aware that drug may cause false-
positive intrinsic factor antibody test.
Patient teaching
• Stress need for patients with pernicious
anemia to return for monthly injections.
Although total body stores may last 3 to
6 years, anemia will recur if not treated
monthly.
• Emphasize importance of well-
balanced diet.
• Tell patient to store oral tablets in tightly closed container at room temperature.

☑ **Evaluation**
• Patient's vitamin B$_{12}$ deficiency is
resolved with drug therapy.
• Patient does not experience hypersensitivity reactions following parenteral
administration of drug.
• Patient and family state understanding
of drug therapy.

---

cyclizine hydrochloride
(SIGH-klih-zeen high-droh-KLOR-ighd)
Marezine†

cyclizine lactate
Marezine, Marzine♦

Pharmacologic class: piperazine-
derivative antihistamine
Therapeutic class: antiemetic, antivertigo agent
Pregnancy risk category: B

How supplied
cyclizine hydrochloride
Tablets: 50 mg†
cyclizine lactate
Injection: 50 mg/ml♦

Pharmacokinetics
Absorption: unknown after oral adminis-
tration.
Distribution: well distributed throughout
body.
Metabolism: metabolized in liver.
Excretion: unknown.

Route	Onset	Peak	Duration
P.O., I.M.	0.5-1 hr	Unknown	4-6 hr

Pharmacodynamics
Chemical effect: unknown. An antihistamine that may affect neural pathways
originating in labyrinth to inhibit nausea
and vomiting, but exact mechanism of
action is unknown.
Therapeutic effect: prevents or relieves
motion sickness.

Indications and dosage
▶ **Prevention or treatment of motion
sickness.** *Adults and children age 12 and
older:* 50 mg P.O. (hydrochloride) 30
minutes before travel, then q 4 to 6 hours,
p.r.n., to maximum of 200 mg daily; or
50 mg I.M. (lactate) q 4 to 6 hours, p.r.n.
Children ages 6 to 12: 25 mg (hydrochloride) P.O. q 4 to 6 hours, p.r.n., to maximum of 75 mg daily.

Adverse reactions
CNS: *drowsiness,* dizziness, auditory and
visual hallucinations.
CV: hypotension.
EENT: blurred vision.
GI: constipation, dry mouth.
GU: urine retention.

Interactions
Drug-drug. *CNS depressants:* additive
CNS depression. Avoid concomitant use.
Drug-lifestyle. *Alcohol use:* additive
CNS depression. Don't use together.

Contraindications and precautions
• Contraindicated in patients hypersensitive to drug and in breast-feeding women.

• Use cautiously in patients with severe heart failure and after surgery and in pregnant women.
• Safety of drug has not been established in children under age 6.

NURSING CONSIDERATIONS

⚚ Assessment
• Assess patient's motion sickness before and after drug administration.
• Be alert for adverse reactions and drug interactions.
• Evaluate patient's and family's knowledge about drug therapy.

⊞ Nursing diagnoses
• Altered health maintenance related to motion sickness
• Risk for injury related to drug-induced adverse CNS reactions
• Knowledge deficit related to drug therapy

⧉ Planning and implementation
P.O. and I.M. use: Follow normal protocol.
• Know that drug should be administered 30 minutes before anticipated motion sickness.
• Store drug in cool place. When stored at room temperature, injection may turn slightly yellow; this change does not indicate loss of potency.
Patient teaching
• Advise patient to avoid driving and other activities that require alertness until CNS effects of drug are known.
• Tell patient to take oral drug at least 30 minutes before beginning travel.
• Advise patient that repeat doses may be necessary in 4 to 6 hours.

☑ Evaluation
• Patient's motion sickness is relieved or prevented with drug therapy.
• Patient does not experience injury as result of drug-induced adverse CNS reactions.

• Patient and family state understanding of drug therapy.

cyclobenzaprine hydrochloride
(sigh-kloh-BEN-zah-preen high-droh-KLOR-ighd)
Flexeril

Pharmacologic class: tricyclic antidepressant derivative
Therapeutic class: skeletal muscle relaxant
Pregnancy risk category: B

How supplied
Tablets: 10 mg

Pharmacokinetics
Absorption: almost completely absorbed during first pass through GI tract.
Distribution: 93% plasma protein-bound.
Metabolism: during first pass through GI tract and liver, drug and metabolites undergo enterohepatic recycling.
Excretion: excreted primarily in urine as conjugated metabolites; also in feces via bile as unchanged drug. *Half-life:* 1 to 3 days.

Route	Onset	Peak	Duration
P.O.	≤ 1 hr	3-8 hr	12-24 hr

Pharmacodynamics
Chemical effect: unknown.
Therapeutic effect: relieves muscle spasms.

Indications and dosage
▶ **Short-term treatment of muscle spasm.** *Adults:* 10 mg P.O. t.i.d. for 7 days. Maximum dosage is 60 mg daily; maximum duration of treatment is 2 to 3 weeks.

Adverse reactions
CNS: *drowsiness,* euphoria, weakness, headache, insomnia, nightmares, pares-

---

Reactions may be *common,* uncommon, *life-threatening,* or COMMON AND LIFE-THREATENING.

thesia, dizziness, depression, visual disturbances, *seizures*.
CV: tachycardia, *arrhythmias*.
EENT: blurred vision, dry mouth.
GI: abdominal pain, dyspepsia, abnormal taste, constipation.
GU: urine retention.
Skin: rash, urticaria, pruritus.

Interactions

Drug-drug. *Anticholinergics:* additive anticholinergic effects. Avoid concomitant use.
CNS depressants: may cause additive CNS depression. Avoid concomitant use.
MAO inhibitors: may exacerbate CNS depression or anticholinergic effects. Don't give within 14 days after discontinuing MAO inhibitors.
Drug-lifestyle. *Alcohol use:* may cause additive CNS depression. Don't use together.

Contraindications and precautions

• Contraindicated in patients who have received MAO inhibitors within 14 days; during acute recovery phase of MI; and in patients with hyperthyroidism, heart block, arrhythmias, conduction disturbances, heart failure, hypersensitivity to drug.
• Use cautiously in patients with history of urine retention, acute angle-closure glaucoma, and increased intraocular pressure and in elderly or debilitated patients.
• Safety of drug has not been established in pregnant or breast-feeding women or children.

NURSING CONSIDERATIONS

Assessment
• Assess patient's underlying condition before therapy.
• Monitor effectiveness by assessing severity and frequency of patient's muscle spasms.
• Be alert for adverse reactions and drug interactions.

• Be alert for nausea, headache, and malaise, which may occur if drug is stopped abruptly after long-term use.
• Evaluate patient's and family's knowledge about drug therapy.

Nursing diagnoses
• Pain related to presence of muscle spasms
• Risk for injury related to potential for drug-induced CNS adverse reactions
• Knowledge deficit related to drug therapy

Planning and implementation
• Do not administer drug with other CNS depressants.
• With high doses, watch for adverse reactions similar to those of other TCAs.
• Notify doctor immediately if toxicity is suspected and have physostigmine available.
Patient teaching
• Advise patient to report urinary hesitancy or urine retention. If constipation occurs, tell him to increase fluid intake and suggest use of a stool softener.
• Warn patient to avoid activities that require alertness until drug's CNS effects are known.
• Warn patient to avoid combining drug with alcohol or other CNS depressants.
• Tell patient that dry mouth may be relieved with sugarless candy or gum.

Evaluation
• Patient is free from pain with drug therapy.
• Patient does not experience injury as a result of drug-induced adverse CNS reactions.
• Patient and family state understanding of drug therapy.

---

*Liquid form contains alcohol   **May contain tartrazine   ◆Canada   ◇Australia   †OTC

cyclophosphamide
(sigh-kloh-FOS-fuh-mighd)
Cycloblastin◇, Cytoxan**, Cytoxan
Lyophilized, Endoxan-Asta◇, Neosar,
Procytox◆

Pharmacologic class: alkylating agent
(cell cycle–phase nonspecific)
Therapeutic class: antineoplastic
Pregnancy risk category: D

How supplied
Tablets: 25 mg, 50 mg
Injection: 100-mg, 200-mg, 500-mg, 1-g,
2-g vials

Pharmacokinetics
Absorption: almost completely absorbed
from GI tract at oral doses of 100 mg or
less. Higher doses (300 mg) are about
75% absorbed.
Distribution: distributed throughout
body, although only minimal amounts
have been found in saliva, sweat, and
synovial fluid. Active metabolites are
about 50% bound to plasma proteins.
Metabolism: metabolized to its active
form by hepatic microsomal enzymes.
Activity of these metabolites is terminated by metabolism to inactive forms.
Excretion: drug and its metabolites are
eliminated primarily in urine, with 15%
to 30% excreted as unchanged drug.
Half-life: 4 to 6.5 hours.

Route	Onset	Peak	Duration
P.O., I.V.	Unknown	Unknown	Unknown

Pharmacodynamics
Chemical effect: cross-links strands of
cellular DNA and interferes with RNA
transcription, causing imbalance of
growth that leads to cell death. Cell
cycle–phase nonspecific.
Therapeutic effect: kills specific types of
cancer cells; improves renal function in
mild nephrotic syndrome in children.

Indications and dosage
▶ **Breast, head, neck, prostate, lung,
and ovarian cancers; Hodgkin's disease; chronic lymphocytic leukemia;
chronic myelocytic leukemia; acute
lymphoblastic leukemia; acute myelocytic leukemia; neuroblastoma; retino-
blastoma; non-Hodgkin's lymphoma;
multiple myeloma; mycosis fungoides;
sarcoma.** *Adults and children:* initially,
40 to 50 mg/kg I.V. in divided doses over
2 to 5 days. Alternatively, 10 to 15 mg/kg
I.V. q 7 to 10 days, 3 to 5 mg/kg I.V.
twice weekly, or 1 to 5 mg/kg P.O. daily,
based on patient tolerance. Subsequent
dosages adjusted according to evidence
of antitumor activity or leukopenia.
Children: same dosage as adults.
▶ **"Minimal change" nephrotic syndrome in children.** *Children:* 2.5 to
3 mg/kg P.O. daily for 60 to 90 days.

Adverse reactions
CV: *cardiotoxicity* (with very high doses
and in combination with doxorubicin).
GI: anorexia, *nausea and vomiting beginning within 6 hours,* stomatitis, mucositis.
GU: gonadal suppression (may be irreversible), HEMORRHAGIC CYSTITIS,
bladder fibrosis.
Hematologic: *leukopenia,* nadir between
days 8 and 15, recovery in 17 to 28 days;
thrombocytopenia; anemia.
Respiratory: *pulmonary fibrosis* (with
high doses).
Other: *reversible alopecia in 50% of patients, especially with high doses; secondary malignancies; anaphylaxis;* hyperuricemia; SIADH (with high doses).

Interactions
Drug-drug. *Barbiturates:* increased
pharmacologic effect and enhanced cyclophosphamide toxicity due to induction
of hepatic enzymes. Monitor patient
closely.
Cardiotoxic drugs: additive adverse cardiac effects. Monitor patient closely.

Chloramphenicol, corticosteroids: reduced activity of cyclophosphamide. Use cautiously.
Digoxin: may decrease serum digoxin levels. Monitor levels closely.
Succinylcholine: prolonged neuromuscular blockade. Don't use together.

Contraindications and precautions

• Contraindicated in patients with severe bone marrow depression or hypersensitivity to drug and in breast-feeding women.
• Use with extreme caution, if at all, in pregnant women because fetal harm may occur.
• Use cautiously in patients with leukopenia, thrombocytopenia, malignant cell infiltration of bone marrow, or hepatic or renal disease and in those who have recently undergone radiation therapy or chemotherapy.

NURSING CONSIDERATIONS

Assessment

• Assess patient's underlying condition before therapy and reassess regularly during therapy.
• Monitor CBC, serum uric acid levels, and renal and liver function tests, as ordered.
• Monitor for cyclophosphamide toxicity if patient's corticosteroid therapy is discontinued.
• Be alert for adverse reactions and drug interactions.
• Evaluate patient's and family's knowledge about drug therapy.

Nursing diagnoses

• Altered health maintenance related to underlying condition
• Risk for injury related to drug-induced adverse reactions
• Knowledge deficit related to drug therapy

Planning and implementation

• Follow institutional policy to reduce risks. Preparation and administration of parenteral form of this drug is associated with carcinogenic, mutagenic, and teratogenic risks for personnel.
P.O. use: Know that tablets are used for children with minimal change nephrotic syndrome and not to treat neoplastic disease.
I.V. use: Reconstitute powder using sterile water for injection or bacteriostatic water for injection containing only parabens. For nonlyophilized product, add 5 ml to 100-mg vial, 10 ml to 200-mg vial, 25 ml to 500-mg vial, 50 ml to 1-g vial, or 100 ml to 2-g vial to produce solution containing 20 mg/ml. Shake to dissolve; this may take up to 6 minutes and it may be difficult to completely dissolve drug. Lyophilized preparation is much easier to reconstitute; check package insert for quantity of diluent needed to reconstitute drug.
– After reconstitution, administer as ordered by direct I.V. injection or infusion. For I.V. infusion, further dilute with D_5W, dextrose 5% in 0.9% NaCl injection, dextrose 5% in Ringer's injection, lactated Ringer's injection, sodium lactate injection, or 0.45% NaCl injection.
– Check reconstituted solution for small particles. Filter solution if necessary.
– Know that reconstituted solution is stable for 6 days refrigerated or 24 hours at room temperature. However, use stored solutions cautiously because drug contains no preservatives.
• To prevent hyperuricemia with resulting uric acid nephropathy, know that allopurinol may be used with adequate hydration.
Patient teaching
• Warn patient that alopecia is likely to occur, but that it is reversible.
• Warn patient to watch for signs of infection (fever, sore throat, fatigue) and bleeding (easy bruising, nosebleeds, bleeding gums, melena),and to take temperature daily.

• Instruct patient to avoid OTC products containing aspirin.

• Encourage patient to void every 1 to 2 hours while awake and to drink at least 3 L of fluid daily to minimize risk of hemorrhagic cystitis. Tell patient not to take drug at bedtime; infrequent urination during night may increase possibility of cystitis. If cystitis occurs, tell him to discontinue drug and notify doctor. Cystitis can occur months after therapy ceases. Mesna may be given to lower incidence and severity of bladder toxicity.

• Advise male and female patients to practice contraception while taking drug and for 4 months after; drug is potentially teratogenic.

• Advise female patient of childbearing age to avoid becoming pregnant during therapy. Also recommend consulting with doctor before becoming pregnant.

☑ **Evaluation**

• Patient exhibits positive response to drug therapy.

• Patient does not experience injury as a result of drug-induced adverse reactions.

• Patient and family state understanding of drug therapy.

cycloserine
(sigh-kloh-SER-een)
Seromycin

Pharmacologic class: isoxizolidone, d-alanine analogue
Therapeutic class: antitubercular agent
Pregnancy risk category: C

How supplied

Capsules: 250 mg

Pharmacokinetics

Absorption: about 80% is absorbed from GI tract.
Distribution: distributed widely into body tissues and fluids, including CSF. It does not bind to plasma proteins.

Metabolism: may be metabolized partially.
Excretion: excreted primarily in urine.
Half-life: 10 hours.

Route	Onset	Peak	Duration
P.O.	Unknown	3-4 hr	Unknown

Pharmacodynamics

Chemical effect: inhibits cell-wall biosynthesis by interfering with bacterial use of amino acids (bacteriostatic).
Therapeutic effect: aids in eradicating tuberculosis.

Indications and dosage

▶ **Adjunct treatment in pulmonary or extrapulmonary tuberculosis**. *Adults:* initially, 250 mg P.O. q 12 hours for 2 weeks; then, if blood levels are below 25 to 30 mcg/ml and no toxicity has developed, 250 mg q 8 hours for 2 weeks. If optimum blood levels are not achieved, and no toxicity has developed, dose is increased to 250 mg q 6 hours. Maximum dosage is 1 g/day. If CNS toxicity occurs, drug is discontinued for 1 week, then resumed at 250 mg daily for 2 weeks. If no serious toxic effects occur, dosage is increased by 250-mg increments q 10 days until the blood level is 25 to 30 mcg/ml.

Adverse reactions

CNS: *seizures,* drowsiness, headache, tremor, dysarthria, vertigo, confusion, loss of memory, *possible suicidal tendencies* and other psychotic symptoms, *nervousness, hallucinations, depression,* hyperirritability, paresthesia, paresis, hyperreflexia, *coma.*
Other: hypersensitivity reactions (allergic dermatitis).

Interactions

Drug-drug. *Ethionamide, isoniazid:* increased risk of CNS toxicity (seizures, dizziness, or drowsiness). Monitor closely.
Drug-lifestyle. *Alcohol use:* increased risk of CNS toxicity. Advise patient to refrain from alcohol consumption during therapy.

Contraindications and precautions

• Contraindicated in patients with seizure disorders, depression or severe anxiety, psychosis, severe renal insufficiency, or hypersensitivity to drug and in those who concurrently consume excessive amounts of alcohol.
• Use cautiously in patients with impaired renal function; reduced dosage is required. Also use cautiously in pregnant or breast-feeding women.
• Safety of drug has not been established in children.

NURSING CONSIDERATIONS

Assessment
• Assess patient's underlying condition before therapy.
• Obtain specimen for culture and sensitivity tests before therapy begins and periodically thereafter to detect possible resistance.
• Monitor effectiveness by evaluating culture and sensitivity results and for improvement in patient's underlying condition.
• Monitor serum cycloserine levels periodically as ordered, especially in patients receiving high doses (more than 500 mg daily) because toxic reactions may occur with blood levels above 30 mcg/ml.
• Monitor results of hematologic tests and renal and liver function studies.
• Be alert for adverse reactions and drug interactions.
• Evaluate patient's and family's knowledge about drug therapy.

Nursing diagnoses
• Altered health maintenance related to presence of tuberculosis
• Risk for injury related to drug-induced CNS adverse reactions
• Knowledge deficit related to drug therapy

Planning and implementation
• Know that cycloserine is considered "second-line" drug in treatment of tuber-

culosis and should always be administered with other antitubercular agents to prevent development of resistant organisms.
• Expect to adjust dose according to blood levels, clinical toxicity, or ineffectiveness, as ordered.
• Administer pyridoxine, anticonvulsants, tranquilizers, or sedatives, as ordered, to relieve adverse reactions.
Patient teaching
• Warn patient to avoid alcohol, which may cause serious neurologic reactions.
• Instruct patient to take drug exactly as prescribed; warn against discontinuing drug without doctor's approval.
• Stress importance of having laboratory studies done as ordered to monitor drug effectiveness and toxicity.

Evaluation
• Patient is able to maintain health after drug therapy.
• Patient does not experience injury as a result of drug-induced adverse reactions.
• Patient and family state understanding of drug therapy.

cyclosporine (cyclosporin)
(sigh-kloh-SPOOR-een)
Neoral, Sandimmun◊, Sandimmune

Pharmacologic class: polypeptide antibiotic
Therapeutic class: immunosuppressant
Pregnancy risk category: C

How supplied

Oral solution: 100 mg/ml
Injection: 50 mg/ml
Capsules: 25 mg, 50 mg, 100 mg
Capsules for microemulsion: 25 mg, 100 mg

Pharmacokinetics

Absorption: absorption varies widely after oral administration between patients and in same patient. Only 30% of

Sandimmune oral dose reaches systemic circulation while 60% of Neoral reaches the systemic circulation.
Distribution: distributed widely outside blood volume. In plasma, about 90% is bound to proteins.
Metabolism: metabolized extensively in liver.
Excretion: excreted primarily in feces with only 6% of drug found in urine.
Half-life: 10 to 27 hours.

Route	Onset	Peak	Duration
P.O. (Sandimmune)	Unknown	3.5 hr	Unknown
(Neoral)	Unknown	1.5-2 hr	Unknown
I.V.	Unknown	Unknown	Unknown

Pharmacodynamics

Chemical effect: inhibits proliferation of T lymphocytes.
Therapeutic effect: prevents organ rejection.

Indications and dosage

▶ **Prophylaxis of organ rejection in kidney, liver, or heart transplantation.** *Adults and children:* 15 mg/kg P.O. 4 to 12 hours before transplantation and continued daily postoperatively for 1 to 2 weeks. Then dosage reduced by 5% each week to maintenance level of 5 to 10 mg/kg/day. Alternatively, 5 to 6 mg/kg I.V. concentrate 4 to 12 hours before transplantation. Postoperatively, dosage repeated daily until patients can tolerate P.O. forms. For microemulsion, oral doses are the same and dosage adjustments are made according to a predefined cyclosporine blood level.
▶ **Severe, active rheumatoid arthritis that has not adequately responded to methotrexate (Neoral only).** *Adults:* 2.5 mg/kg/day P.O., taken b.i.d. as divided dose.
▶ **Recalcitrant, plaque psoriasis that is not adequately responsive to at least one systemic therapy or in patients for whom other systemic therapy is con-**traindicated or cannot be tolerated (Neoral only). *Adults:* initially 2.5 mg/kg/day P.O. divided b.i.d. Initially dose should be maintained for 4 weeks. If dosage increase is necessary increase at 2 week intervals, 0.5 mg/kg/day to a maximum of 4 mg/kg/day

Adverse reactions

CNS: *tremor,* headache, *seizures.*
CV: hypertension.
EENT: *gum hyperplasia,* oral thrush.
GI: nausea, vomiting, diarrhea.
GU: NEPHROTOXICITY.
Hematologic: anemia, *leukopenia, thrombocytopenia.*
Hepatic: *hepatotoxicity.*
Skin: acne.
Other: sinusitis, flushing, increased low-density lipoprotein levels, *infections,* hirsutism, *anaphylaxis.*

Interactions

Drug-drug. *Aminoglycosides, amphotericin B, co-trimoxazole, NSAIDs:* increased risk of nephrotoxicity. Monitor for toxicity.
Amphotericin B, cimetidine, diltiazem, erythromycin, imipenem, cilastatin, ketoconazole, metoclopramide, prednisolone: may increase blood levels of cyclosporine. Monitor for increased toxicity.
Azathioprine, corticosteroids, cyclophosphamide, verapamil: increased immunosuppression. Monitor patient closely.
Carbamazepine, isoniazid, phenobarbital, phenytoin, rifampin: possible decreased immunosuppressant effect. May need to increase cyclosporine dosage.
Vaccines: decreased immune response. postpone routine immunization.
Drug-food. *Grapefruit juice:* slows metabolism of drug. Avoid concomitant use.

Contraindications and precautions

• Contraindicated in patients hypersensitive to drug or to polyoxyethylated castor oil (found in injectable form). Neoral contraindicated in patients with psoriasis or rheumatoid arthritis who also have ab-

---

Reactions may be *common,* uncommon, *life-threatening,* or COMMON AND LIFE-THREATENING.

normal renal function, uncontrolled hypertension, or malignancies.
• Use cautiously in pregnant women.
• Safety of drug has not been established in breast-feeding women.

NURSING CONSIDERATIONS

✎ Assessment
• Assess patient's organ transplant before therapy.
• Monitor effectiveness by evaluating patient for signs and symptoms of organ rejection.
• Monitor cyclosporine blood levels at regular intervals.
• Monitor BUN and serum creatinine levels as nephrotoxicity may develop 2 to 3 months after transplant surgery, possibly requiring dosage reduction.
• Monitor liver function tests, as ordered, for hepatotoxicity, which usually occurs during first month after transplant.
• Monitor CBC and platelet counts regularly.
• Be alert for adverse reactions and drug interactions.
• Evaluate patient's and family's knowledge about drug therapy.

🏥 Nursing diagnoses
• Risk for injury related to potential for organ rejection
• Altered protection related to drug-induced immunosuppression
• Knowledge deficit related to drug therapy

❱ Planning and implementation
P.O. use: Measure oral doses carefully in oral syringe. To increase palatability, mix with whole milk, chocolate milk, or fruit juice (except grapefruit juice). Oral cyclosporine solution for emulsion is less palatable when mixed with milk. Use glass container to minimize adherence to container walls.
• Administer drug with meals to minimize GI distress.

I.V. use: Administer cyclosporine I.V. concentrate at one-third oral dose and dilute before use. Dilute each milliliter of concentrate in 20 to 100 ml of D_5W or 0.9% NaCl injection. Dilute immediately before administration; infuse over 2 to 6 hours. Usually reserved for patients who cannot tolerate oral drugs.
• Know that Sandimmune and Neoral are not bioequivalent and cannot be used interchangeably without physician supervision. Conversion from Neoral to Sandimmune should be made with increased monitoring as ordered to avoid the potential of underdosing.
• Be aware that psoriasis patients who are treated with Neoral should not receive concomitant PUVA or UVB therapy, methotrexate or other immunosuppressive agents, coal tar or radiation therapy.
• Always give drug concomitantly with adrenal corticosteroids, as ordered.
Patient teaching
• Encourage patient to take drug at same times each day.
• Advise patient to take Neoral on an empty stomach. Don't mix with grapefruit juice.
• Advise patient to take with meals if drug causes nausea. Anorexia, nausea, and vomiting are usually transient and most frequently occur at start of therapy.
• Stress that therapy should not be stopped without doctor's approval.
• Instruct patient to swish and swallow nystatin four times daily to prevent thrush.
• Instruct patient on infection control and bleeding precaution measures, as indicated by CBC and platelet count results.

☑ Evaluation
• Patient does not experience organ rejection while taking drug.
• Patient is free from infection and serious bleeding episodes throughout drug therapy.
• Patient and family state understanding of drug therapy.

---

cyproheptadine hydrochloride
(sigh-proh-HEP-tah-deen
high-droh-KLOR-ighd)
Periactin

Pharmacologic class: piperidine-derivative antihistamine
Therapeutic class: antihistamine
(H_1-receptor antagonist), antipruritic
Pregnancy risk category: B

How supplied

Tablets: 4 mg
Syrup: 2 mg/5 ml

Pharmacokinetics

Absorption: well absorbed from GI tract.
Distribution: unknown.
Metabolism: appears to be almost completely metabolized in liver.
Excretion: drug's metabolites are excreted primarily in urine; unchanged drug is not excreted in urine but small amounts of unchanged cyproheptadine and metabolites are excreted in feces.

Route	Onset	Peak	Duration
P.O.	15-60 min	6-9 hr	8 hr

Pharmacodynamics

Chemical effect: competes with histamine for H_1-receptor sites on effector cells. Prevents, but does not reverse, histamine-mediated responses.
Therapeutic effect: relieves allergy symptoms and itching.

Indications and dosage

▶ **Allergy symptoms, pruritus.** *Adults:*
4 to 20 mg P.O. daily in divided doses.
Maximum dosage is 0.5 mg/kg daily.
Children ages 7 to 14: 4 mg P.O. b.i.d. or t.i.d. Maximum dosage is 16 mg daily.
Children ages 2 to 6: 2 mg P.O. b.i.d. or t.i.d. Maximum dosage is 12 mg daily.

Adverse reactions

CNS: *drowsiness,* dizziness, headache, fatigue, *seizures* (especially in elderly patients).
GI: nausea, vomiting, epigastric distress, *dry mouth.*
GU: urine retention.
Hematologic: *agranulocytosis, thrombocytopenia.*
Skin: rash.
Other: weight gain, *anaphylactic shock.*

Interactions

Drug-drug. *CNS depressants:* increased sedation. Use together cautiously.
MAO inhibitors: increased anticholinergic effects. Don't use together.
Drug-lifestyle. *Sun exposure:* photosensitivity reactions may occur. Use protection.

Contraindications and precautions

• Contraindicated in patients with hypersensitivity to drug or other drugs of similar chemical structure; in those with acute asthmatic attacks, angle-closure glaucoma, stenosing peptic ulcer, symptomatic prostatic hypertrophy, bladder-neck obstruction, and pyloroduodenal obstruction; in therapy with MAO inhibitors; in neonates or premature infants; in elderly or debilitated patients, and in breast-feeding patients.
• Use cautiously in patients with increased intraocular pressure, hyperthyroidism, CV disease, hypertension, or bronchial asthma and in pregnant women.

NURSING CONSIDERATIONS

Assessment
• Assess patient's underlying condition before therapy and reassess regularly during therapy.
• Be alert for adverse reactions and drug interactions.
• Evaluate patient's and family's knowledge about drug therapy.

Nursing diagnoses
- Altered health maintenance related to underlying condition
- Risk for injury related to potential for drug-induced adverse CNS reactions
- Knowledge deficit related to drug therapy

Planning and implementation
- Reduce GI distress by giving drug with food or milk.
- Notify doctor if tolerance is suspected; another antihistamine may need to be used.

Patient teaching
- Instruct patient to take drug with food or milk to reduce GI distress.
- Warn patient to avoid alcohol and driving or other activities that require alertness until drug's CNS effects are known.
- Tell patient that coffee or tea may reduce drowsiness. Sugarless gum, sugarless sour hard candy, or ice chips may relieve dry mouth.
- Advise patient to stop drug 4 days before allergy skin tests to preserve accuracy of tests.
- Instruct patient to notify doctor if tolerance develops; different antihistamine may need to be prescribed.

Evaluation
- Patient is free from allergy symptoms or pruritus with drug therapy.
- Patient does not experience injury as result of drug-induced CNS adverse reactions.
- Patient and family state understanding of drug therapy.

---

cysteamine bitartrate
(sis-TEE-uh-meen bigh-TAR-trayt)
Cystagon

Pharmacologic class: aminothiol derivative
Therapeutic class: cystine reduction agent
Pregnancy risk category: C

How supplied
Capsules: 50 mg, 150 mg

Pharmacokinetics
Not available.

Route	Onset	Peak	Duration
P.O.	Unknown	Unknown	Unknown

Pharmacodynamics
Chemical effect: reacts with cystine, thereby decreasing cystine level in cells. *Therapeutic effect:* relieves signs and symptoms of nephropathic cystinosis.

Indications and dosage
▶ **Management of nephropathic cystinosis.** *Adults and children over age 12 and weighing over 50 kg (110 lb):* initially, one-fourth to one-sixth of maintenance dosage, then increased gradually over 4 to 6 weeks to achieve maintenance dosage. Maintenance dosage is 2 g (free base) P.O. in four divided doses. *Children age 12 and under:* initially, one-fourth to one-sixth of maintenance dosage, then increased gradually over 4 to 6 weeks to achieve maintenance dosage. Maintenance dosage is 1.3 g/m² (free base) P.O. daily in four divided doses.

Adverse reactions
CNS: *lethargy,* somnolence, *encephalopathy,* headache, *seizures,* ataxia, confusion, tremor, hyperkinesis, decreasing hearing, dizziness, jitteriness, nervousness, abnormal thinking, depression, emotional lability, hallucinations, nightmares.
CV: hypertension.
GI: *vomiting, anorexia, diarrhea,* nausea, abdominal pain, dyspepsia, constipation, gastroenteritis, duodenitis, duodenal ulcer.
Hematologic: anemia, *leukopenia.*
Hepatic: abnormal liver function.
Skin: *rash,* urticaria.
Other: *fever,* dehydration, bad breath.

Interactions

None reported.

Contraindications and precautions

• Contraindicated in patients with hypersensitivity to drug, cysteamine, or penicillamine.

• Safety of drug has not been established in pregnant or breast-feeding women.

NURSING CONSIDERATIONS

⚡ Assessment

• Assess patient's underlying condition before therapy. Know that drug therapy should begin as soon as diagnosis of nephropathic cystinosis has been confirmed by increased level of cystine in increased WBCs.

• Monitor effectiveness by measuring leukocyte cystine levels because they are useful in determining adequate dosage and compliance. When drug is well tolerated, goal of therapy is to keep leukocyte cystine levels below 1 mmol/½ cystine/mg protein 5 to 6 hours after administration of drug. Measurements should be done at least every 3 months.

• Monitor patient's CBC and liver function studies, as ordered, to detect adverse hematologic reactions.

• Be alert for adverse reactions.

• Evaluate patient's and family's knowledge about drug therapy.

⊕ Nursing diagnoses

• Altered health maintenance related to underlying condition

• Risk of injury related to drug-induced adverse GI reactions

• Knowledge deficit related to drug therapy

⊠ Planning and implementation

• If rash develops, notify doctor because drug will need to be withheld until rash clears. Doctor may restart drug at lower dosage and slowly titrate dosage to achieve therapeutic effect. However, if severe rash (such as erythema multiforme

bullosa or toxic epidermal necrolysis) develops, drug should not be restarted.

• Notify doctor if adverse CNS or GI reactions develop; dosage will need to be adjusted or drug temporarily withheld.

• Know that patients with cystinosis taking cysteamine hydrochloride or phosphocysteamine solutions may be transferred to equimolar doses of drug.

Patient teaching

• Inform the patient and parents that dosage of cysteamine is based on patient's weight and that doctor's directions should be followed exactly.

• Instruct patient and parents that if dose of drug is missed, it should be taken as soon as possible. However, if it is within 2 hours of next dose, patient should skip missed dose and go back to regular dosing schedule. Tell patient not to double dose.

• Tell parents of child under age 6 not to give child capsule to swallow because he may choke or aspirate it. Instead, capsule may be opened and contents sprinkled on food or mixed in formula.

• Inform patient or parent that supplements also will be given to replace electrolytes lost through kidneys and that periodic blood tests will need to be performed to help determine correct dosage of drug. Compliance with these measures is extremely important for maximal effectiveness of drug.

• Instruct patient not to engage in hazardous activities (such as driving) until drug's CNS effects are known.

• Advise patient and parents to store the drug in dry place, away from light.

☑ Evaluation

• Patient's health is restored with drug therapy.

• Patient maintains adequate hydration throughout drug therapy.

• Patient and family state understanding of drug therapy.

Reactions may be *common,* uncommon, *life-threatening*, or COMMON AND LIFE-THREATENING.

cytarabine
(ara-C, cytosine arabinoside)
(sigh-TAR-uh-been)
Cytosar♦, Cytosar-U

Pharmacologic class: antimetabolite
(cell cycle–phase specific, S phase)
Therapeutic class: antineoplastic
Pregnancy risk category: D

How supplied
Injection: 100-mg, 500-mg, 1-g, 2-g
vials

Pharmacokinetics
Absorption: unknown after S.C. administration.
Distribution: rapidly distributes widely throughout body. About 13% of drug is bound to plasma proteins. Drug penetrates the blood-brain barrier only slightly after rapid I.V. dose; however, when drug is administered by continuous I.V. infusion, CSF levels achieve concentration 40% to 60% of that of plasma levels.
Metabolism: metabolized primarily in liver but also in kidneys, GI mucosa, and granulocytes.
Excretion: drug and its metabolites are excreted in urine. Less than 10% of dose is excreted as unchanged drug in urine.
Half-life: elimination of cytarabine is biphasic, with initial half-life of 8 minutes and terminal phase half-life of 1 to 3 hours.

Route	Onset	Peak	Duration
I.V.	Unknown	Unknown	Unknown
S.C.	Unknown	20-60 min	Unknown
Intrathecal	Unknown	Unknown	Unknown

Pharmacodynamics
Chemical effect: inhibits DNA synthesis.
Therapeutic effect: kills selected cancer cells.

Indications and dosage
▶ **Acute nonlymphocytic leukemia, acute lymphocytic leukemia, blast phase of chronic myelocytic leukemia.** *Adults and children:* 100 mg/m² daily by continuous I.V. infusion or 100 mg/m² I.V. q 12 hours. Given for 5 days and repeated q 2 weeks. For maintenance, 1 mg/kg S.C. once or twice weekly.
▶ **Meningeal leukemia.** *Adults and children:* highly variable from 5 to 75 mg/m² intrathecally. Frequency also varies from once a day for 4 days to once q 4 days. Most common dosage is 30 mg/m², q 4 days until CSF is normal, followed by one more dose.

Adverse reactions
CNS: neurotoxicity, including ataxia and cerebellar dysfunction (with high doses).
EENT: keratitis, nystagmus.
GI: nausea, vomiting, diarrhea, dysphagia; reddened area at juncture of lips, followed by sore mouth, oral ulcers in 5 to 10 days; high dose given rapid I.V. may cause projectile vomiting.
Hematologic: *leukopenia,* with initial WBC count nadir 7 to 9 days after drug is stopped and second (more severe) nadir 15 to 24 days after drug is stopped; anemia; reticulocytopenia; *thrombocytopenia,* with platelet count nadir occurring on day 10; *megaloblastosis.*
Hepatic: hepatotoxicity (usually mild and reversible).
Skin: rash.
Other: flulike syndrome, hyperuricemia, urate nephropathy, *anaphylaxis.*

Interactions
Drug-drug. *Digoxin:* may decrease serum digoxin levels. Monitor closely.
Flucytosine: decreased flucytosine activity. Monitor closely.
Gentamicin: decreased activity against *Klebsiella pneumoniae.* Don't use.

Contraindications and precautions
• Contraindicated in patients hypersensitive to drug and in breast-feeding women.
• Know that drug is not recommended for use in pregnant women because fetal harm may occur.

• Use cautiously in patients with hepatic disease.

NURSING CONSIDERATIONS

☢ Assessment

• Assess patient's underlying condition before therapy and reassess regularly throughout therapy.
• Monitor serum uric acid level, hepatic and renal function studies and CBC, as ordered.
• Be alert for adverse reactions and drug interactions.
• Assess patient receiving high doses for neurotoxicity, which may first appear as nystagmus, but can progress to ataxia and cerebellar dysfunction.
• Evaluate patient's and family's knowledge about drug therapy.

⊕ Nursing diagnoses

• Altered health maintenance related to underlying condition
• Risk for injury related to drug-induced adverse hematologic reactions
• Knowledge deficit related to drug therapy

⊠ Planning and implementation

• Follow institutional policy to reduce risks. Preparation and administration of parenteral form of this drug is associated with carcinogenic, mutagenic, and teratogenic risks for personnel.
• To reduce nausea, give antiemetic before administering, as ordered. Nausea and vomiting are more frequent when large doses are administered rapidly by I.V. push. These reactions are less frequent when given by infusion.
I.V. use: Reconstitute drug using provided diluent, which is bacteriostatic water for injection containing benzyl alcohol. Avoid this diluent when preparing drug for neonates or for intrathecal use. Reconstitute 100-mg vial with 5 ml of diluent or 500-mg vial with 10 ml of diluent. Reconstituted solution is stable

for 48 hours. Discard cloudy reconstituted solution.
– For I.V. infusion, further dilute using 0.9% NaCl injection, D_5W, or sterile water for injection.
S.C. use: Follow manufacturer guidelines.
Intrathecal use: Use preservative-free 0.9% NaCl. Add 5 ml to 100-mg vial or 10 ml to 500-mg vial. Use immediately after reconstitution. Discard unused drug.
• Maintain high fluid intake and give allopurinol, if ordered, to avoid urate nephropathy in leukemia induction therapy.
• Know that therapy may be modified or stopped if granulocyte count is below 1,000/mm³ or if platelet count is below 50,000/mm³.
• Know that corticosteroid eye drops are prescribed to prevent drug-induced keratitis.

Patient teaching

• Warn patient to watch for signs of infection (fever, sore throat, fatigue) and bleeding (easy bruising, nosebleeds, bleeding gums, melena). Tell patient to take temperature daily.
• Instruct patient on infection control and bleeding precautions.
• Advise female patient of childbearing age to avoid becoming pregnant during therapy. Also recommend consulting with doctor before becoming pregnant.
• Encourage patient to drink at least 3 L of fluids daily.
• Instruct patient about need for frequent oral hygiene.

☑ Evaluation

• Patient demonstrates positive response to drug therapy.
• Patient does not experience injury as result of drug therapy.
• Patient and family state understanding of drug therapy.

Reactions may be *common*, uncommon, *life-threatening*, or COMMON AND LIFE-THREATENING.

cytomegalovirus immune globulin, intravenous (CMV-IGIV)
(sigh-toh-meh-GEH-loh VIGH-rus
ih MYOON GLOH-byoo-lin)
CytoGam

Pharmacologic class: immune globulin
Therapeutic class: immune serum
Pregnancy risk category: C

How supplied
Solution for injection: ± 10 mg/ml in
20 ml and 50 ml vials.

Pharmacokinetics
Unknown.

Route	Onset	Peak	Duration
I.V.	Unknown	Unknown	Unknown

Pharmacodynamics
Chemical effect: supplies relatively high
concentration of immunoglobulin g (IgG)
antibodies against CMV. Increasing these
antibody levels in CMV-exposed patients
may attenuate or reduce incidence of serious CMV disease.
Therapeutic effect: provides passive immunity against CMV.

Indications and dosage
► **To attenuate primary CMV disease
in seronegative kidney transplant recipients who receive kidney from a
CMV seropositive donor.** *Adults:* administered I.V. according to following
schedule:
– within 72 hours of transplantation:
150 mg/kg
– 2 weeks after transplantation:
100 mg/kg
– 4 weeks after transplantation:
100 mg/kg
– 6 weeks after transplantation:
100 mg/kg
– 8 weeks after transplantation:
100 mg/kg
– 12 weeks after transplantation:
50 mg/kg

– 16 weeks after transplantation:
50 mg/kg.
  Initial dose administered at 15 mg/kg/
hour. Increased to 30 mg/kg/hour after 30
minutes if no untoward reactions occur,
then increased to 60 mg/kg/hour after another 30 minutes if no untoward reactions
occur. Volume should not exceed 75 ml/
hour. Subsequent doses may be administered at 15 mg/kg/hour for 15 minutes,
increasing at 15-minute intervals in stepwise fashion to 60 mg/kg/hour.

Adverse reactions
CVS: hypotension.
GI: nausea, vomiting.
Other: wheezing, *anaphylaxis,* flushing,
chills, muscle cramps, back pain, fever.

Interactions
Drug-drug. *Live-virus vaccines:* may interfere with immune response to live-
virus vaccines. Defer vaccination for at
least 3 months.

Contraindications and precautions
• Contraindicated in patients with selective IgA deficiency or history of sensitivity to other human immunoglobulin
preparations.
• Use with caution in pregnant women.
• Safety of drug has not been established
for breast-feeding women or children.

NURSING CONSIDERATIONS

☑ Assessment
• Assess patient's kidney transplant before therapy.
• Take vital signs prior to beginning therapy, then in midinfusion, postinfusion,
and before any increase in infusion rate.
• Monitor effectiveness by evaluating
kidney function.
• Be alert for adverse reactions and drug
interactions.
• Evaluate patient's and family's knowledge about drug therapy.

⊕ Nursing diagnoses
• Risk for injury related to potential for organ rejection
• Decreased cardiac output related to drug-induced hypotension
• Knowledge deficit related to drug therapy

⧉ Planning and implementation
• Remove tab portion of vial cap and clean rubber stopper with 70% alcohol or equivalent. *Do not shake vial; avoid foaming.* Infuse solution only if it is colorless, free of particulate matter and not turbid. Pre-dilution before infusion is not recommended.
• If possible, administer through separate I.V. line using constant infusion pump. Filters are unnecessary. If unable to administer through separate line, piggyback into preexisting line of NaCl injection or one of following dextrose solutions with or without NaCl: dextrose 2.5% in water, D_5W, dextrose 10% in water, or dextrose 20% in water. Do not dilute more than 1:2 with any of above solutions.
• Refrigerate drug at 36° to 46° F (2° to 8° C).
• If anaphylaxis or drop in blood pressure occurs, discontinue infusion, notify doctor, and be prepared to administer CPR and such drugs as diphenhydramine and epinephrine.
Patient teaching
• Teach patient about drug therapy.
• Instruct patient to notify doctors immediately if adverse reactions develop.

✔ Evaluation
• Patient does not reject transplanted kidney with drug therapy.
• Patient maintains normal cardiac output throughout drug therapy.
• Patient and family state understanding of drug therapy.

dacarbazine (DTIC)
(deh-KAR-buh-zeen)
DTIC♦, DTIC-Dome

Pharmacologic class: alkylating agent (cell cycle–phase nonspecific)
Therapeutic class: antineoplastic
Pregnancy risk category: C

How supplied
Injection: 100-mg, 200-mg vials

Pharmacokinetics
Absorption: not applicable with I.V. administration.
Distribution: thought to localize in body tissues, especially the liver; minimally bound to plasma proteins.
Metabolism: rapidly metabolized in liver to several compounds, some of which may be active.
Excretion: about 30% to 45% of dose excreted in urine. *Half-life:* initial, 19 minutes; terminal, 5 hours.

Route	Onset	Peak	Duration
I.V.	Unknown	Unknown	Unknown

Pharmacodynamics
Chemical effect: unknown; probably cross-links strands of cellular DNA and interferes with RNA transcription, causing imbalance of growth that leads to cell death.
Therapeutic effect: kills selected cancer cells.

Indications and dosage
▶ **Metastatic malignant melanoma.**
Adults: 2 to 4.5 mg/kg I.V. daily for 10 days; then repeated q 4 weeks as tolerated. Or 250 mg/m² I.V. daily for 5 days, repeated at 3-week intervals.

Reactions may be *common*, uncommon, *life-threatening*, or COMMON AND LIFE-THREATENING.

► **Hodgkin's disease.** *Adults:* 150 mg/m²
I.V. daily (in combination with other
agents) for 5 days, repeated q 4 weeks; or
375 mg/m² on first day of combination
regimen, repeated q 15 days.

Adverse reactions

GI: *severe nausea and vomiting, anorexia.*
Hematologic: *leukopenia, thrombocytopenia* (nadir between 3 and 4 weeks).
Hepatic: transient increase in liver enzyme levels, *hepatotoxicity* (rare).
Skin: phototoxicity.
Other: *flulike syndrome* (fever, malaise,
myalgia beginning 7 days after treatment
has stopped and possibly lasting 7 to 21
days), alopecia, *anaphylaxis;* severe pain
(if I.V. solution infiltrates or if solution is
too concentrated), tissue damage, hyperuricemia.

Interactions

Drug-drug. *Allopurinol:* additive hypo-
uricemic effects. Monitor patient closely.
Anticoagulants, aspirin: increased risk of
bleeding. Avoid concomitant use.
Bone marrow suppressants: additive toxicity. Monitor patient closely.
*Phenobarbital, phenytoin, other drugs
that induce hepatic metabolism:* enhanced dacarbazine activation and risk of
toxicity. Monitor patient closely.
Drug-lifestyle. *Sun exposure:* photosensitivity reactions may occur, especially
during the first 2 days of therapy. Take
precautions.

Contraindications and precautions

• Contraindicated in patients hypersensitive to drug and in breast-feeding women.
• Use with extreme caution and only
when absolutely necessary in pregnant
women because fetal harm may occur.
• Use cautiously if bone marrow function
is impaired.
• Safety of drug has not been established
in children.

NURSING CONSIDERATIONS

▨ Assessment
• Obtain history of patient's underlying
neoplastic disease before therapy, and reassess regularly throughout therapy.
• Monitor CBC, platelet count, and liver
enzyme levels, as ordered.
• Be alert for adverse reactions and drug
interactions.
• Evaluate patient's and family's knowledge of drug therapy.

▨ Nursing diagnoses
• Altered health maintenance related to
presence of neoplastic disease
• Risk for injury related to potential of
drug-induced adverse reactions
• Knowledge deficit related to drug
therapy

▶ Planning and implementation
• Follow institutional policy to reduce
risks. Preparation and administration of
parenteral form are associated with carcinogenic, mutagenic, and teratogenic
risks for personnel.
• Administer antiemetics, as ordered, before giving dacarbazine to help decrease
nausea. Nausea and vomiting may subside after several doses.
• Reconstitute drug, using sterile water
for injection. Add 9.9 ml to 100-mg vial
or 19.7 ml to 200-mg vial. The resulting
solution is colorless to clear yellow. For
infusion, further dilute, using up to
250 ml of 0.9% NaCl injection or D₅W;
infuse over 30 minutes.
• During infusion, protect bag from direct
sunlight to avoid possible drug breakdown. Solution may be diluted further or
infusion slowed to decrease pain at infusion site.
• Keep in mind that reconstituted solutions are stable for 8 hours at room temperature and normal lighting conditions,
or up to 3 days if refrigerated. Diluted solutions are stable for 8 hours at room
temperature and normal light, or up to 24
hours if refrigerated. If solutions turn

---

pink, decomposition has occurred; discard drug.
• Discard refrigerated solution after 72 hours, and room temperature solution after 8 hours.
• Take care not to allow extravasation during infusion. If I.V. solution infiltrates, discontinue immediately, apply ice to area for 24 to 48 hours, and notify doctor.
• For Hodgkin's disease, be aware that drug is usually given with bleomycin, vinblastine, and doxorubicin.
Patient teaching
• Warn patient to watch for signs of infection (fever, sore throat, fatigue) and bleeding (easy bruising, nosebleeds, bleeding gums, melena). Tell patient to take temperature daily.
• Instruct patient to avoid OTC products containing aspirin.
• Advise patient to avoid sunlight and sunlamps for first 2 days after treatment.
• Reassure patient that flulike syndrome may be treated with mild antipyretics, such as acetaminophen.

☑ **Evaluation**
• Patient exhibits positive response to therapy, as evidenced on follow-up diagnostic studies and overall physical status.
• Patient does not experience injury as result of drug-induced adverse reactions.
• Patient and family state understanding of drug therapy.

---

dactinomycin (actinomycin-D)
(dak-tih-noh-MIGH-sin)
Cosmegen

Pharmacologic class: antibiotic antineoplastic (cell cycle–phase nonspecific)
Therapeutic class: antineoplastic
Pregnancy risk category: C

How supplied

Injection: 500 mcg/vial

Pharmacokinetics

Absorption: not applicable with I.V. administration.
Distribution: widely distributed in body tissues, with highest levels found in bone marrow and nucleated cells.
Metabolism: only minimally metabolized in liver.
Excretion: drug and its metabolites excreted in urine and bile. *Half-life:* 36 hours.

Route	Onset	Peak	Duration
I.V.	Unknown	Unknown	Unknown

Pharmacodynamics

Chemical effect: unknown; thought to interfere with DNA-dependent RNA synthesis by intercalation.
Therapeutic effect: kills selected cancer cells.

Indications and dosage

Indications and dosage may vary. Check treatment protocol with doctor.
► **Sarcoma, trophoblastic tumors in women, testicular cancer.** *Adults:* 500 mcg (0.5 mg) I.V. daily for 5 days. Maximum dosage is 15 mcg/kg/day or 400 to 600 mcg/m^2/day for 5 days. After bone marrow recovery, course may be repeated.
► **Wilms' tumor, rhabdomyosarcoma, Ewing's sarcoma.** *Children:* 10 to 15 mcg/kg or 450 mcg/m^2/day I.V. for 5 days. Maximum dosage is 500 mcg/day or 2.5 mg/m^2 I.V. in equally divided daily doses over 7-day period. After bone marrow recovery, course may be repeated.

Adverse reactions

GI: *anorexia, nausea, vomiting,* abdominal pain, diarrhea, *stomatitis,* ulceration, proctitis.
Hematologic: *anemia, leukopenia, thrombocytopenia, pancytopenia, aplastic anemia, agranulocytosis.*
Hepatic: *hepatotoxicity.*
Skin: *erythema;* desquamation; *hyperpigmentation of skin, especially in previ-*

ously irradiated areas; acnelike eruptions (reversible).
Other: phlebitis and severe damage to soft tissue at injection site; reversible alopecia, malaise, fatigue, lethargy, fever, myalgia, hypocalcemia, *anaphylactoid reaction, death.*

Interactions

Drug-drug. *Bone marrow suppressants:* additive toxicity. Monitor patient closely. *Vitamin K derivatives:* decreased effectiveness. Monitor patient closely.

Contraindications and precautions

• Contraindicated in patients with chickenpox or herpes zoster and in breast-feeding women.
• Use with extreme caution and only when absolutely necessary in pregnant women because fetal harm may occur.

NURSING CONSIDERATIONS

▧ Assessment
• Obtain history of patient's underlying neoplastic disease before therapy, and reassess regularly throughout therapy.
• Monitor CBC, platelet count, and kidney and liver function tests, as ordered.
• Be alert for adverse reactions and drug interactions.
• Evaluate patient's and family's knowledge of drug therapy.

✛ Nursing diagnoses
• Altered health maintenance related to presence of neoplastic disease
• Risk for injury related to potential of drug-induced adverse reactions
• Knowledge deficit related to drug therapy

▷ Planning and implementation
• Follow institutional policy to reduce risks. Preparation and administration of parenteral form are associated with carcinogenic, mutagenic, and teratogenic risks for personnel.

• Administer antiemetics, as ordered, before giving drug to help decrease nausea.
• Use only sterile water (without preservatives) as diluent for reconstitution. Add 1.1 ml to vial to yield gold-colored solution containing 0.5 mg/ml. Give by direct injection into vein or through I.V. line of free-flowing compatible I.V. solution of 0.9% NaCl injection or D₅W.
• For I.V. infusion, dilute with up to 50 ml of D₅W or 0.9% NaCl injection, and infuse over 15 minutes.
• Administer drug through running I.V. line with good blood return.
• If accidental skin contact occurs, irrigate area with copious amounts of water for at least 15 minutes.
• Be aware that dosage must be reduced in patient who has recently been treated with or who will receive concomitant treatment with radiation therapy or other chemotherapeutic drugs.
• In event of spill, keep in mind that manufacturer recommends using solution of trisodium phosphate 5% to inactivate drug.
• Discard unused portions of solutions because they do not contain preservative.
• Know that stomatitis, diarrhea, leukopenia, and thrombocytopenia may require that dosage and schedule be modified.
• Be aware that dactinomycin is a vesicant. If infiltration occurs, apply cold compresses to area and notify doctor.
Patient teaching
• Warn patient to watch for signs of infection (fever, sore throat, fatigue) and bleeding (easy bruising, nosebleeds, bleeding gums, melena). Tell patient to take temperature daily.
• Instruct patient to avoid OTC products containing aspirin.
• Tell patient that alopecia may occur but that it's usually reversible.

☑ Evaluation
• Patient exhibits positive response to therapy, as evidenced on follow-up diagnostic studies and overall physical status.

• Patient does not experience injury as result of drug-induced adverse reactions.
• Patient and family state understanding of drug therapy.

dalteparin sodium
(dal-TEH-puh-rin SOH-dee-um)
Fragmin

Pharmacologic class: low-molecular-weight heparin
Therapeutic class: anticoagulant
Pregnancy risk category: B

How supplied

Syringe: 2,500 anti-factor Xa IU/0.2 ml; 5,000 anti-factor Xa IU/0.2 ml

Pharmacokinetics

Absorption: unknown.
Distribution: unknown.
Metabolism: unknown.
Excretion: excreted in urine. *Half-life:* 3 to 5 hours after S.C. administration.

Route	Onset	Peak	Duration
S.C.	Unknown	About 4 hr	Unknown

Pharmacodynamics

Chemical effect: enhances inhibition of factor Xa and thrombin by antithrombin.
Therapeutic effect: prevents deep vein thrombosis (DVT) in selected patients.

Indications and dosage

▶ **Prophylaxis against DVT in patients undergoing abdominal surgery who are at risk for thromboembolic complications.** *Adults:* 2,500 IU S.C. daily, starting 1 to 2 hours before surgery and repeated once daily for 5 to 10 days postoperatively.

Adverse reactions

Hematologic: *thrombocytopenia.*
Skin: pruritus, rash.
Local: *hematoma at injection site,* pain or skin necrosis (rare) at injection site.

Other: *hemorrhage,* ecchymosis, bleeding complications, fever, *anaphylactoid reactions* (rare).

Interactions

Drug-drug. *Antiplatelet agents, oral anticoagulants:* may increase risk of bleeding. Use together cautiously.

Contraindications and precautions

• Contraindicated in patients with hypersensitivity to drug, heparin, or pork products; active major bleeding; or thrombocytopenia associated with positive in vitro tests for antiplatelet antibody in presence of drug.
• Use with extreme caution in patients with history of heparin-induced thrombocytopenia; in patients with increased risk of hemorrhage, such as those with severe uncontrolled hypertension, bacterial endocarditis, congenital or acquired bleeding disorders, active ulceration and angiodysplastic GI disease, or hemorrhagic stroke; or in those who recently have undergone brain, spinal, or ophthalmologic surgery.
• Use with caution in patients with bleeding diathesis, thrombocytopenia, platelet defects, severe liver or kidney insufficiency, hypertensive or diabetic retinopathy, or recent GI bleeding. Also use cautiously in pregnant or breast-feeding women.
• Safety of drug has not been established in children.

NURSING CONSIDERATIONS

⚶ Assessment
• Obtain history of patient's underlying condition before therapy.
• Monitor effectiveness by assessing patient for evidence of DVT.
• Know that periodic, routine CBCs (including platelet count) and fecal occult blood tests are recommended during course of treatment. Patient does not require regular monitoring of PT or activated partial thromboplastin time.

• Be alert for adverse reactions and drug interactions.
• Evaluate patient's and family's knowledge of drug therapy.

⊕ **Nursing diagnoses**
• Risk for injury related to potential development of DVT as result of underlying condition
• Altered protection related to drug-induced adverse hematologic reactions
• Knowledge deficit related to drug therapy

▶ **Planning and implementation**
• Know that candidates for dalteparin therapy are at risk for DVT. Patients at risk include those who are over age 40, obese, or undergoing surgery under general anesthesia lasting longer than 30 minutes and those who have additional risk factors (such as cancer or a history of DVT or pulmonary embolism).
• Have patient assume sitting or supine position when administering drug. Administer S.C. injection deeply. Injection sites include U-shaped area around navel, upper outer side of thigh, and upper outer quadrangle of buttock. Rotate sites daily. When area around navel or thigh is used, use thumb and forefinger to lift up fold of skin while giving injection. The entire length of needle should be inserted at a 45- to 90-degree angle.
• Never administer drug I.M.
• Do not mix with other injections or infusions unless specific compatibility data are available that support such mixing.
• Be aware that drug is not interchangeable (unit for unit) with unfractionated heparin or other low-molecular-weight heparin derivatives.
• Be aware that drug should be discontinued if thromboembolic event occurs despite dalteparin prophylaxis.
Patient teaching
• Instruct patient and family to watch for signs of bleeding and notify doctor immediately.

• Tell patient to avoid OTC medications containing aspirin or other salicylates.

☑ **Evaluation**
• Patient does not develop DVT.
• Patient maintains hematologic function.
• Patient and family state understanding of drug therapy.

---

danaparoid sodium
(deh-neh-PEH-royd SOH-dee-um)
Orgaran

Pharmacologic class: heparinoid derivative
Therapeutic class: antithrombotic
Pregnancy risk category: B

How supplied
Ampule: 750 anti-Xa units/0.6 ml
Syringe: 750 anti-Xa units/0.6 ml

Pharmacokinetics
Absorption: 100% bioavailability.
Distribution: nonspecific.
Metabolism: unknown.
Excretion: excreted in urine.

Route	Onset	Peak	Duration
S.C.	Unknown	2-5 hr	Unknown

Pharmacodynamics
Chemical effect: prevents fibrin formation in the coagulation pathway via thrombin generation inhibition by anti-Xa and anti-IIa effects.
Therapeutic effect: prevents deep vein thrombosis (DVT).

Indications and dosage
▶ **Prophylaxis for postoperative DVT in patients undergoing elective hip replacement surgery.** *Adults:* 750 units S.C. b.i.d. starting 1 to 4 hours preoperatively, then no sooner than 2 hours after surgery. Continue treatment for 7 to 10 days postoperatively, or until risk of DVT has diminished.

Adverse reactions

CNS: insomnia, headache, asthenia, dizziness.
CV: peripheral edema, *hemorrhage*.
GI: *nausea, constipation,* vomiting.
GU: urinary tract infection, urine retention.
Hematologic: anemia.
Musculoskeletal: joint disorder.
Skin: rash, pruritus.
Other: fever, injection site pain, infection.

Interactions

Drug-drug. *Oral anticoagulants, platelet inhibitors:* may increase risk of bleeding. Use together cautiously.

Contraindications and precautions

• Contraindicated in patients with hypersensitivity to drug or to pork products, severe hemorrhagic diathesis, active major bleeding, or thrombocytopenia associated with positive in vitro test for antiplatelet antibody in the presence of drug.
• Use cautiously in patients with impaired renal function or increased risk of bleeding and in breast-feeding patients.

NURSING CONSIDERATIONS

⚕ Assessment
• Know that drug contains sodium sulfite, which can cause allergic reactions in some patients.
• Monitor periodically CBCs (including platelet count) and fecal occult blood tests during therapy; PT and PTT not required.
• Monitor patient's hematocrit and blood pressure closely.
• Evaluate patient's and family's knowledge of drug therapy.

✤ Nursing diagnoses
• Risk for injury related to potential for blood clot formation
• Altered protection related to increased risk of bleeding
• Knowledge deficit related to drug therapy

➤ Planning and implementation
• Alternate abdominal wall injection sites; do not rub.
• Be aware that drug is not interchangeable (unit for unit) with heparin or low-molecular-weight heparin.
• Store ampules at room temperature, away from light; refrigerate syringes at 35.6° to 46.4° F (2° to 8° C).
Patient teaching
• Instruct patient and family to watch for and report signs of bleeding.
• Tell patient to avoid OTC drugs containing aspirin or other salicylates.

☑ Evaluation
• Patient does not develop blood clots.
• Patient states appropriate bleeding precautions to take.
• Patient and family state understanding of drug therapy.

danazol
(DAN-eh-zol)
Cyclomen♦, Danocrine

Pharmacologic class: androgen
Therapeutic class: antiestrogen, androgen
Pregnancy risk category: X

How supplied

Capsules: 50 mg, 100 mg, 200 mg

Pharmacokinetics

Absorption: amount absorbed by body is not proportional to administered dose.
Distribution: unknown.
Metabolism: metabolized to 2-hydroxymethylethisterone.
Excretion: unknown. *Half-life:* about 4½ hours.

Route	Onset	Peak	Duration
P.O.	≤ 1 mo	1.5-3 mo	Unknown

Pharmacodynamics

Chemical effect: not clearly defined; gonadotropin inhibitor that suppresses

pituitary-ovarian axis and inhibits estrogenic effects.
Therapeutic effect: relieves symptoms of endometriosis and fibrocystic breast disease; prevents hereditary angioedema occurrence.

Indications and dosage

▶ **Mild endometriosis.** *Women:* initially, 100 to 200 mg P.O. b.i.d. Subsequent dosage based on patient response.
▶ **Moderate to severe endometriosis.** *Women:* 400 mg P.O. b.i.d. uninterrupted for 3 to 6 months; may be continued for 9 months.
▶ **Fibrocystic breast disease.** *Women:* 100 to 400 mg P.O. daily in two divided doses uninterrupted for 2 to 6 months.
▶ **Prevention of hereditary angioedema.** *Adults:* 200 mg P.O. b.i.d to t.i.d., continued until favorable response is achieved. Then dosage decreased 50% at 1- to 3-month intervals.

Adverse reactions

CNS: dizziness, headache, sleep disorders, fatigue, tremors, irritability, excitation, lethargy, depression, paresthesia.
CV: elevated blood pressure.
EENT: visual disturbances.
GI: gastric irritation, nausea, vomiting, diarrhea, constipation, change in appetite.
GU: hematuria.
Hematologic: *thrombocytopenia,* elevated serum lipid levels.
Hepatic: reversible jaundice, peliosis hepatis, elevated liver enzyme levels, *liver cell tumors.*
Other: muscle cramps or spasms; androgenic effects in women *(weight gain, hirsutism,* hoarseness, clitoral enlargement, *decrease in breast size,* changes in libido, *oily skin or hair,* voice deepening); *hypoestrogenic effects (flushing, diaphoresis, vaginitis [including itching, dryness, and burning]; vaginal bleeding, nervousness, emotional lability, menstrual irregularities),* chills, *allergic reactions.*

Interactions

Drug-drug. *Carbamazepine:* may increase carbamazepine levels. Monitor closely.
Cyclosporine: can increase cyclosporine levels and increase chance of nephrotoxicity. Monitor closely.
Warfarin: may prolong PT in patients stabilized on warfarin. Monitor PT and INR.

Contraindications and precautions

• Contraindicated in patients with undiagnosed abnormal genital bleeding, porphyria, or impaired renal, cardiac, or hepatic function and in pregnant or breast-feeding women. Avoid use in women of childbearing age until pregnancy is ruled out.
• Use cautiously in patients with seizure disorder or migraine headache.
• Safety of drug has not been established in children.

NURSING CONSIDERATIONS

🔍 Assessment
• Obtain history of patient's underlying condition before therapy.
• Monitor effectiveness by assessing severity of pain and other signs and symptoms of underlying condition.
• Periodically evaluate liver function, as ordered. Semen evaluation is performed routinely every 3 to 4 months, especially in adolescent boys.
• Be alert for adverse reactions.
• Monitor patient closely for signs of virilization. Some androgenic effects, such as deepening of voice, may not be reversible on discontinuation of drug.
• Evaluate patient's and family's knowledge of drug therapy.

🔟 Nursing diagnoses
• Pain related to underlying condition
• Body image disturbance related to drug-induced adverse androgenic reactions
• Knowledge deficit related to drug therapy

⊠ Planning and implementation

• Be aware that long-term therapy may be required.

• Know that periodic dosage decreases or gradual drug withdrawal is best.

• Notify doctor of signs of virilization in women.

• Have patient seek counseling if body image disturbance is serious.

Patient teaching

• Make sure patient understands the importance of using effective nonhormonal contraceptive during therapy.

• Tell patient that ovulation and cyclic menstrual bleeding usually return in 2 to 3 months after withdrawal of treatment; fibrocystic disease symptoms return within 1 year in 50% of patients.

• Advise patient who is taking danazol for fibrocystic breast disease to examine breasts regularly and to call doctor immediately if breast nodule enlarges during treatment.

• Instruct patient to wash after intercourse to decrease risk of vaginitis. Tell patient to wear only cotton underwear.

• Prepare female patient for possible changes in appearance as a result of virilization, and instruct her to report any changes immediately to doctor.

✓ Evaluation

• Patient is free from pain.

• Patient states acceptance of body image throughout therapy.

• Patient and family state understanding of drug therapy.

---

dantrolene sodium
(DAN-troh-leen SOH-dee-um)
Dantrium, Dantrium Intravenous

Pharmacologic class: hydantoin derivative
Therapeutic class: skeletal muscle relaxant
Pregnancy risk category: C

How supplied

Capsules: 25 mg, 50 mg, 100 mg
Injection: 20 mg/vial

Pharmacokinetics

Absorption: 35% of P.O. dose absorbed through GI tract.
Distribution: substantially plasma protein–bound, mainly to albumin.
Metabolism: metabolized in liver to its less active 5-hydroxy derivatives and to its amino derivative by reductive pathways.
Excretion: excreted in urine as metabolites. *Half-life:* P.O., 8.7 hours; I.V., 4 to 8 hours.

Route	Onset	Peak	Duration
P.O.	≤ 1 wk	5 hr	Unknown
I.V.	Unknown	Unknown	Unknown

Pharmacodynamics

Chemical effect: acts directly on skeletal muscle to interfere with intracellular calcium movement.
Therapeutic effect: relieves muscle spasms.

Indications and dosage

▶ **Spasticity and sequelae secondary to severe chronic disorders (such as multiple sclerosis, cerebral palsy, spinal cord injury, CVA).** *Adults:* 25 mg P.O. daily. Increased gradually in increments of 25 mg, up to 100 mg b.i.d. to q.i.d., to maximum of 400 mg daily. *Children:* initially, 0.5 mg/kg P.O. b.i.d.; increased to t.i.d., and then q.i.d. Dosage increased as needed by 0.5 mg/kg daily to 3 mg/kg b.i.d. to q.i.d. Maximum dosage is 100 mg q.i.d.

▶ **Management of malignant hyperthermia crisis.** *Adults and children:* 1 mg/kg I.V. initially; repeated as needed up to cumulative dose of 10 mg/kg.

▶ **Prevention or attenuation of malignant hyperthermia crisis in susceptible patients who require surgery.** *Adults:* 4 to 8 mg/kg P.O. daily in three or four divided doses for 1 or 2 days before proce-

dure. Final dose administered 3 to 4 hours before procedure, or 2.5 mg/kg I.V. infused over 1 hour approximately 1 hour prior to anesthesia. Additional doses, which must be individualized, may be given intraoperatively if necessary.
► **Prevention of recurrence of malignant hyperthermia crisis.** *Adults:* 4 to 8 mg/kg/day P.O. in four divided doses for up to 3 days after hyperthermic crisis.

Adverse reactions

CNS: *muscle weakness, drowsiness, dizziness,* light-headedness, *malaise,* headache, confusion, nervousness, insomnia, hallucinations, *seizures.*
CV: tachycardia, blood pressure changes.
EENT: excessive lacrimation, auditory or visual disturbances.
GI: anorexia, constipation, cramping, dysphagia, metallic taste, severe diarrhea, bleeding.
GU: urinary frequency, hematuria, incontinence, nocturia, dysuria, crystalluria, difficulty achieving erection.
Hepatic: *hepatitis.*
Respiratory: pleural effusion.
Skin: eczematous eruption, pruritus, urticaria, photosensitivity.
Other: abnormal hair growth, drooling, diaphoresis, myalgia, chills, fever.

Interactions

Drug-drug. *CNS depressants:* increased CNS depression. Avoid concomitant use. *Estrogens:* may increase risk of hepatotoxicity. Use together cautiously. *I.V. verapamil:* may result in CV collapse. Stop verapamil before administering I.V. dantrolene.
Drug-lifestyle. *Alcohol use:* increased CNS depression. Avoid concomitant use.

Contraindications and precautions

• Contraindicated in patients when spasticity is used to maintain motor function, in those with upper motor neuron disorders, for spasms in rheumatic disorders, in patients with active hepatic disease, and in breast-feeding women.

• Use cautiously in patients with severely impaired cardiac or pulmonary function or preexisting hepatic disease, in women (including pregnant women), and in patients over age 35.

NURSING CONSIDERATIONS

⚞ Assessment
• Obtain history of patient's spasticity disorder before therapy.
• Obtain liver function tests at beginning of therapy.
• Monitor effectiveness by evaluating severity of spasticity.
• Be alert for adverse reactions and drug interactions.
• Evaluate patient's and family's knowledge of drug therapy.

⊞ Nursing diagnoses
• Pain related to presence of spasticity disorder
• Risk for injury related to drug-induced adverse reactions
• Knowledge deficit related to drug therapy

❯ Planning and implementation
• For optimum drug effect, give daily dosage in four divided doses.
P.O. use: Give drug with meals or milk to prevent GI distress.
– Prepare oral suspension for single dose by dissolving capsule contents in juice or other suitable liquid. For multiple doses, use acid vehicle, such as citric acid in USP syrup; refrigerate. Use within several days.
I.V. use: Administer as soon as malignant hyperthermia reaction is recognized, as ordered. Reconstitute each vial by adding 60 ml of sterile water for injection and shaking vial until clear. Don't use diluent that contains bacteriostatic agent. Protect contents from light, and use within 6 hours. Be careful to avoid extravasation.
• Know that amount of relief in patient determines if dosage (and drowsiness) can be reduced.

• If hepatitis, severe diarrhea or weakness, or sensitivity reactions occur, withhold dose and notify doctor.
Patient teaching
• Tell patient to use caution when eating to avoid choking. Some patients may experience difficulty swallowing during therapy.
• Warn patient to refrain from driving and performing other hazardous activities until drug's CNS effects are known.
• Advise patient to avoid combining dantrolene with alcohol or other CNS depressants.
• Tell patient to avoid photosensitivity reactions by using sunblock and wearing protective clothing, to report GI problems immediately, and to follow doctor's orders regarding rest and physical therapy.

☑ Evaluation
• Patient states that pain from muscle spasticity has lessened.
• Patient does not experience injury as result of drug-induced adverse reactions.
• Patient and family state understanding of drug therapy.

dapsone
(DAP-sohn)
Avlosulfon♦, Dapsone◊

Pharmacologic class: synthetic sulfone
Therapeutic class: antileprotic, antimalarial
Pregnancy risk category: C

How supplied
Tablets: 25 mg, 100 mg

Pharmacokinetics
Absorption: absorbed completely but rather slowly from GI tract.
Distribution: distributed widely in most body tissues and fluids; 50% to 80% protein-bound.
Metabolism: undergoes acetylation by liver enzymes; rate varies and is genetically determined. Almost 50% of blacks and whites are slow acetylators, whereas more than 80% of Chinese, Japanese, and Eskimos are fast acetylators. Dosage adjustment may be required.
Excretion: dapsone and metabolites excreted primarily in urine; small amounts excreted in feces. *Half-life:* 10 to 50 hours.

Route	Onset	Peak	Duration
P.O.	Unknown	4-8 hr	Unknown

Pharmacodynamics
Chemical effect: unknown; may inhibit folic acid biosynthesis in susceptible organisms (bacteriostatic).
Therapeutic effect: hinders or kills selected bacteria. Spectrum of activity includes *Mycobacterium leprae* and *Mycobacterium tuberculosis.* Drug has some activity against *Pneumocystis carinii* and *Plasmodium.*

Indications and dosage
▶ **All forms of leprosy (Hansen's disease).** *Adults:* 100 mg P.O. daily indefinitely; give with rifampin 600 mg daily for 6 months. *Children:* 1 to 2 mg/kg/day P.O. once daily; maximum of 100 mg/day.
▶ **Dermatitis herpetiformis.** *Adults:* 50 mg P.O. daily; increased to 300 mg daily, p.r.n.

Adverse reactions
CNS: insomnia, psychosis, headache, dizziness, lethargy, severe malaise, paresthesia, peripheral neuropathy (with loss of motor function), vertigo.
CV: tachycardia.
EENT: tinnitus, blurred vision, allergic rhinitis.
GI: anorexia, abdominal pain, *pancreatitis,* nausea, vomiting.
GU: albuminuria, nephrotic syndrome, renal papillary necrosis, male infertility.
Hematologic: *aplastic anemia, agranulocytosis, hemolytic anemia, methemoglobinemia,* possibly *leukopenia.*

Reactions may be *common*, uncommon, **life-threatening**, or COMMON AND LIFE-THREATENING.

Hepatic: *hepatitis,* cholestatic jaundice.
Skin: allergic dermatitis (generalized or fixed maculopapular rash), lupus erythematosus, phototoxicity, *exfoliative dermatitis, toxic erythema, erythema multiforme, toxic epidermal necrolysis,* morbilliform and scarlatiniform reactions, urticaria, *erythema nodosum.*
Other: fever, pulmonary eosinophilia, infectious mononucleosis–like syndrome, *sulfone syndrome* (fever, malaise, jaundice [with hepatic necrosis]), lymphadenopathy.

Interactions

Drug-drug. *Folic acid antagonists (such as methotrexate):* increased risk of adverse hematologic reactions. Avoid concomitant use.
Rifampin: increased hepatic metabolism of dapsone. Monitor for lack of efficacy.

Contraindications and precautions

• Contraindicated in patients with hypersensitivity to drug and in breast-feeding women.
• Use cautiously in patients with chronic renal, hepatic, or CV disease; refractory types of anemia; or G6PD deficiency.
• Also use cautiously in pregnant women.

NURSING CONSIDERATIONS

Assessment
• Obtain history of patient's underlying infection and CBC before therapy.
• Monitor effectiveness by assessing for improvement of infection and evaluating culture and sensitivity test results, as ordered.
• Monitor CBC weekly for first month, monthly for 6 months, and semiannually thereafter.
• Be alert for adverse reactions and drug interactions.
• Evaluate patient's and family's knowledge of drug therapy.

Nursing diagnoses
• Infection related to presence of susceptible bacteria
• Risk of impaired skin integrity related to drug-induced adverse dermatologic reactions
• Knowledge deficit related to drug therapy

Planning and implementation
• Be prepared to reduce dosage or temporarily discontinue drug if hemoglobin falls below 9 g/dl; if WBC count falls below 5,000/mm^3; or if RBC count falls below 2.5 million/mm^3 or remains low.
• If generalized, diffuse dermatitis occurs, notify doctor and prepare to interrupt therapy regimen.
• Administer antihistamines, as ordered, to combat drug-induced allergic dermatitis.
• In severe cases of erythema nodosum, know that therapy should be stopped and glucocorticoids given cautiously.
Patient teaching
• Inform patient of need for periodic laboratory studies.
• Teach patient to watch for and promptly report adverse dermatologic changes because such reactions may require discontinuation of drug.
• Warn patient not to perform hazardous activities that require alertness if adverse CNS reactions occur.

Evaluation
• Patient is free from infection.
• Patient maintains normal skin integrity throughout therapy.
• Patient and family state understanding of drug therapy.

daunorubicin hydrochloride
(daw-noh-ROO-buh-sin high-droh-KLOR-ighd)
Cerubidine

Pharmacologic class: antibiotic antineoplastic (cell cycle–phase nonspecific)

Therapeutic class: antineoplastic
Pregnancy risk category: D

How supplied
Injection: 20 mg/vial

Pharmacokinetics
Absorption: not applicable with I.V. administration.
Distribution: widely distributed in body tissues; drug does not cross blood-brain barrier.
Metabolism: extensively metabolized in liver. One of metabolites has cytotoxic activity.
Excretion: daunorubicin and its metabolites primarily excreted in bile, with small portion excreted in urine. *Half-life:* initial, 45 minutes; terminal, 18½ hours.

Route	Onset	Peak	Duration
I.V.	Unknown	Unknown	Unknown

Pharmacodynamics
Chemical effect: unknown; thought to interfere with DNA-dependent RNA synthesis by intercalation.
Therapeutic effect: kills selected cancer cells.

Indications and dosage
Indications and dosage may vary. Check treatment protocol with doctor.
▶ **Remission induction in acute non-lymphocytic (myelogenous, monocytic, erythroid) leukemia.** *Adults:* in combination, 30 to 45 mg/m²/day I.V. on days 1, 2, and 3 of first course and on days 1 and 2 of subsequent courses with cytarabine infusions.
▶ **Remission induction in acute lymphocytic leukemia.** *Adults:* 45 mg/m²/day I.V. on days 1, 2, and 3. *Children age 2 and older:* 25 mg/m² I.V. on day 1 every week for up to 6 weeks, if needed. *Children under age 2 or with body surface area of less than 0.5 mg/m²:* dose should be calculated based on body weight (1 mg/kg) rather than body surface area.

Adverse reactions
CV: *irreversible cardiomyopathy* (dose-related), ECG changes, *arrhythmias,* pericarditis, myocarditis.
GI: *nausea, vomiting, stomatitis, esophagitis,* anorexia, diarrhea.
GU: red urine (transient).
Hematologic: *bone marrow suppression* (lowest blood counts 10 to 14 days after administration).
Hepatic: *hepatotoxicity.*
Skin: rash, pigmentation of fingernails and toenails.
Other: *severe cellulitis, tissue sloughing* (if drug extravasates); *generalized alopecia,* fever, chills, hyperuricemia, *anaphylactoid reaction.*

Interactions
Drug-drug. *Doxorubicin:* additive cardiotoxicity. Monitor patient closely.
Hepatotoxic drugs: increased risk of additive hepatotoxicity. Monitor patient closely.

Contraindications and precautions
• No known contraindications. However, breast-feeding is not recommended during therapy.
• Use with extreme caution, if at all, in pregnant women.
• Use cautiously in patients with myelosuppression and in those with impaired cardiac, renal, or hepatic function.

NURSING CONSIDERATIONS

☒ Assessment
• Obtain history of patient's underlying neoplastic disease before therapy and reassess regularly throughout therapy.
• Check ECG before treatment.
• Monitor CBC and liver function tests, as ordered; monitor ECG every month during therapy.
• Monitor pulse rate closely. Light resting pulse rate is a sign of adverse cardiac reactions.
• Be alert for adverse reactions and drug interactions.

• Monitor for nausea and vomiting, which may be severe and last for 24 to 48 hours. Monitor patient's hydration status during episodes of nausea and vomiting.
• Evaluate patient's and family's knowledge of drug therapy.

🔟 **Nursing diagnoses**
• Risk for injury related to presence of neoplastic disease
• Risk for fluid volume deficit related to drug-induced nausea and vomiting
• Knowledge deficit related to drug therapy

▶ **Planning and implementation**
• Follow institutional policy to reduce risks. Preparation and administration of parenteral form are associated with carcinogenic, mutagenic, and teratogenic risks for personnel.
• Reconstitute drug using 4 ml of sterile water for injection to produce 5-mg/ml solution.
• Withdraw desired dose into syringe containing 10 to 15 ml of 0.9% NaCl injection. Inject into I.V. line containing free-flowing compatible solution of D_5W or 0.9% NaCl injection over 2 to 3 minutes. Alternatively, dilute in 50 ml of 0.9% NaCl injection and infuse over 10 to 15 minutes, or dilute in 100 ml and infuse over 30 to 45 minutes.
• Avoid extravasation. If extravasation occurs, discontinue I.V. infusion immediately, apply ice to area for 24 to 48 hours, and notify doctor.
• Don't infuse with dexamethasone or heparin; a precipitate may form.
• Never give drug I.M. or S.C.
• Be aware that cumulative dosage is limited to 500 to 600 mg/m² (450 mg/m² when patients also are receiving or have received cyclophosphamide or radiation therapy to cardiac area).
• Know that color is similar to that of doxorubicin. Take care to avoid confusing these two drugs.
• Optimally, use within 8 hours of preparation. Reconstituted solution is stable for 24 hours at room temperature, or 48 hours if refrigerated.
• Notify doctor if adverse cardiac reactions occur. Stop drug immediately if signs of heart failure or cardiomyopathy develop and notify doctor.
• Give antiemetics to help control nausea and vomiting.
Patient teaching
• Warn patient to watch for signs of infection and bleeding.
• Advise patient that red urine for 1 to 2 days is normal and does not indicate presence of blood in urine.
• Inform patient that alopecia may occur but that it's usually reversible.
• Advise female patient of childbearing age to avoid becoming pregnant during therapy. Also recommend that she consult with doctor before becoming pregnant.
• Instruct patient about need for protective measures, including conservation of energy, balanced diet, adequate rest, personal cleanliness, clean environment, and avoidance of exposure to people with infections.

☑ **Evaluation**
• Patient shows positive response to therapy as evidenced by reports of follow-up diagnostic tests and improved physical status.
• Patient maintains adequate hydration throughout therapy.
• Patient and family state understanding of drug therapy.

deferoxamine mesylate
(deh-fer-OKS-uh-meen MES-ih-layt)
Desferal

Pharmacologic class: chelating agent
Therapeutic class: heavy metal antagonist
Pregnancy risk category: C

How supplied
Powder for injection: 500 mg

Pharmacokinetics

Absorption: unknown after S.C. or I.M. administration.
Distribution: distributed widely in body after parenteral administration.
Metabolism: small amounts of drug metabolized by plasma enzymes.
Excretion: excreted in urine as unchanged drug or as ferrioxamine, deferoxamine-iron complex. *Half-life:* about 6 hours.

Route	Onset	Peak	Duration
All routes	Unknown	Unknown	Unknown

Pharmacodynamics

Chemical effect: chelates iron by binding ferric ions.
Therapeutic effect: abolishes acute iron intoxication.

Indications and dosage

▶ **Adjunct treatment of acute iron intoxication.** *Adults and children:* 1 g I.M. or I.V. followed by 500 mg I.M. or I.V. for two doses q 4 hours; then 500 mg I.M. or I.V. q 4 to 12 hours. Maximum dosage is 6 g in 24 hours.
▶ **Chronic iron overload from multiple transfusions.** *Adults and children:* 500 mg to 1 g I.M. daily, and 2 g slow I.V. infusion in separate solution along with each unit of blood transfused. Maximum dosage is 6 g daily. Alternatively, 20 to 40 mg/kg by S.C. infusion pump daily.

Adverse reactions

CV: tachycardia (with long-term use).
EENT: blurred vision, cataracts, hearing loss.
GI: diarrhea, abdominal discomfort (with long-term use).
GU: dysuria (with long-term use).
Other: *hypersensitivity reactions* (cutaneous wheal formation, pruritus, rash, *anaphylaxis*); pain, induration (at injection site); leg cramps, fever; *erythema, urticaria, hypotension, shock* (after rapid I.V. administration).

Interactions

Drug-drug. *Ascorbic acid:* may enhance effects of deferoxamine and increase tissue toxicity of iron. Use together with extreme caution and close monitoring.

Contraindications and precautions

• Contraindicated in patients with severe renal disease or anuria.
• Use cautiously in patients with impaired kidney function and in pregnant women.
• Safety of drug has not been established in breast-feeding women.

NURSING CONSIDERATIONS

⚕ Assessment
• Obtain history of patient's iron intoxication before therapy.
• Monitor effectiveness by monitoring serum iron levels and assessing patient for decreased signs of iron intoxication.
• Observe for signs of anaphylactic reaction immediately after injection.
• Check respiratory status and vital signs frequently until stable.
• Be alert for adverse reactions and drug interactions.
• Evaluate patient's and family's knowledge of drug therapy.

⊞ Nursing diagnoses
• Risk for poisoning related to iron intoxication
• Risk for injury related to drug-induced hypersensitivity reactions
• Knowledge deficit related to drug therapy

⊠ Planning and implementation
• To reconstitute, add 2 ml of sterile water for injection to each ampule. Make sure drug is dissolved completely. Reconstituted solution is good for 1 week at room temperature. Protect from light.
I.V. use: After reconstitution, add to 0.9% NaCl solution, D_5W, or lactated Ringer's solution, and infuse at rate not exceeding

15 mg/kg hourly. Change to I.M. route as soon as possible, as ordered.
I.M. use: Preferred method of administration is I.M. injection. Follow normal protocol.
S.C. use: Follow normal protocol.
• Have epinephrine 1:1,000 readily available to treat hypersensitivity reaction.
• Apply ice or cold compresses to injection site to alleviate local discomfort.
Patient teaching
• Instruct patient to report respiratory difficulty or decreased urine output immediately.
• Warn patient that urine may be red.
• Advise patient to have eye examinations regularly during long-term therapy.
• Warn patient that pain and induration may occur at injection site.

☑ Evaluation
• Patient's iron intoxication is resolved.
• Patient does not exhibit hypersensitivity to therapy.
• Patient and family state understanding of drug therapy.

---

delavirdine mesylate
(deh-luh-VEER-deen MES-ih-layt)
Rescriptor

Pharmacologic class: nonnucleoside reverse transcriptase inhibitor
Therapeutic class: antiviral
Pregnancy risk category: C

How supplied
Tablets: 100 mg

Pharmacokinetics
Absorption: rapidly absorbed after oral administration.
Distribution: 98% bound to plasma protein.
Metabolism: extensively converted to inactive metabolites. Primarily metabolized in liver by cytochrome enzyme systems.

Excretion: 51% excreted in the urine (less than 5% unchanged), 44% excreted in the feces. *Half-life:* 5.8 hours.

Route	Onset	Peak	Duration
P.O.	Unknown	1 hr	Unknown

Pharmacodynamics
Chemical effect: drug binds directly to reverse transcriptase and blocks RNA- and DNA-dependent DNA polymerase activities, inhibiting viral replication.
Therapeutic effect: inhibits HIV replication.

Indications and dosage
▶ **Treatment of HIV-1 infection.**
Adults: 400 mg P.O. t.i.d. in combination with other appropriate antiretroviral agents.

Adverse reactions
CNS: abnormal coordination, agitation, amnesia, anxiety, change in dreams, cognitive impairment, confusion, depression, disorientation, dizziness, emotional lability, fatigue, hallucinations, headache, hyperesthesia, hyperreflexia, hypesthesia, impaired concentration, insomnia, lethargy, malaise, manic symptoms, migraine, nervousness, neuropathy, nightmares, pallor, paralysis, paranoid symptoms, paresthesia, restlessness, somnolence, tingling, tremor, vertigo, weakness.
CV: *bradycardia,* edema (generalized or localized), palpitation, orthostatic hypotension, syncope, tachycardia, vasodilation, chest pain.
EENT: blepharitis, conjunctivitis, diplopia, dry eyes, ear pain, epistaxis, nystagmus, pharyngitis, photophobia, rhinitis, sinusitis, taste perversion, tinnitus.
GI: abdominal cramps, distention, pain (generalized or localized), anorexia, aphthous stomatitis, bloody stools, colitis, constipation, decreased appetite, diarrhea, diverticulitis, duodenitis, dry mouth, dyspepsia, dysphagia, enteritis, esophagitis, fecal incontinence, flatulence, gagging, gastritis, gastroesopha-

geal reflux, GI bleeding, gingivitis, gum hemorrhage, increased thirst and appetite, increased saliva, mouth ulcer, *nausea*, nonspecific hepatitis, pancreatitis, rectal disorder, sialadenitis, stomatitis, tongue edema or ulceration, vomiting.
GU: epididymitis, hematuria, hemospermia, impotence, renal calculi, renal pain, metrorrhagia, nocturia, polyuria, proteinuria, vaginal candidiasis.
Hematologic: anemia, ecchymosis, eosinophilia, granulocytosis, *neutropenia, pancytopenia,* petechiae, prolonged PTT, purpura, spleen disorder, *thrombocytopenia.*
Hepatic: increased ALT and AST levels.
Metabolic: alcohol intolerance; bilirubinemia; hyperkalemia; hyperuricemia; hypocalcemia; hyponatremia; hypophosphatemia; increased gamma glutamyl transpeptidase, lipase, serum alkaline phosphatase, serum amylase, serum CK, and serum creatinine levels; peripheral edema; weight gain or loss.
Musculoskeletal: arthralgia or arthritis of single and multiple joints, asthenia, back pain, bone disorder, bone pain, leg cramps, muscle cramps, muscular weakness, myalgia, neck rigidity, tendon disorder, tenosynovitis, tetany.
Respiratory: bronchitis, chest congestion, cough, dyspnea, laryngismus, upper respiratory infection.
Skin: alopecia, angioedema, dermal leukocytoblastic vasculitis, dermatitis, desquamation, diaphoresis, dry skin, epidermal cyst, erythema, erythema multiforme, folliculitis, fungal dermatitis, maculopapular rash, nail disorder, petechial rash, pruritus, *rash,* sebaceous cyst, seborrhea, skin nodule, *Stevens-Johnson syndrome,* urticaria, vesiculobullous rash.
Other: allergic reaction, breast enlargement, chills, decreased libido, fever, flank pain, flu syndrome, lip edema, pain (generalized or localized), trauma.

Interactions

Drug-drug. *Amphetamines, astemizole, benzodiazepines, calcium channel blockers, cisapride, ergot alkaloid preparations, quinidine:* may result in potentially serious or life-threatening adverse events. Avoid concomitant use.
Antacids: reduced absorption of delavirdine. Separate doses by at least 1 hour.
Carbamazepine, phenobarbital, phenytoin, rifampin: substantially decreased plasma delavirdine levels. Avoid coadministration.
Clarithromycin: increased concentrations of both drugs. Monitor carefully.
Dapsone, warfarin: delavirdine increases plasma concentrations of these drugs. Monitor carefully.
Didanosine: coadministration with delavirdine results in a 20% decrease in absorption of both drugs. Separate administration by at least 1 hour.
Fluoxetine, ketoconazole: increased delavirdine trough levels. Monitor patient.
H₂-receptor antagonists: may reduce absorption of delavirdine. Long-term use of these drugs with delavirdine is not recommended.
Indinavir: increased plasma concentrations of indinavir. May require lower dose of indinavir.
Rifabutin: decreased delavirdine levels and increased rifabutin levels. Monitor closely.
Saquinavir: fivefold increase in systemic levels of saquinavir. Monitor AST and ALT levels frequently when used together.

Contraindications and precautions

• Contraindicated in patients with hypersensitivity to drug's formulation.
• Use cautiously in patients with impaired hepatic function.

NURSING CONSIDERATIONS

Assessment
• Assess patient's underlying condition, before therapy and regularly thereafter.

• Be alert for potential adverse reactions and drug interactions.
• Monitor patient for drug-induced rash.
• Evaluate patient's and family's knowledge of drug therapy.

🔁 Nursing diagnoses
• Risk for impaired skin integrity related to potential side effects of medication
• Risk for infection related to patient's underlying condition
• Knowledge deficit related to drug therapy

⊠ Planning and implementation
• Administer diphenhydramine, hydroxyzine, or topical corticosteroids as ordered to relieve symptoms if rash develops.
• Know that resistance develops rapidly when drug is used as monotherapy. Always give in combination with appropriate antiretroviral therapy.
• Know that drug may be dispersed in water before ingestion. Add tablets to at least 3 oz (90 ml) of water, allow to stand for a few minutes; then stir well. Have patient drink promptly, rinse glass, and swallow the rinse to ensure that entire dose is consumed.
Patient teaching
• Tell patient to discontinue drug and call doctor if severe rash or rash accompanied by such symptoms as fever, blistering, oral lesions, conjunctivitis, swelling, or muscle or joint aches occurs.
• Tell patient that drug is not a cure for HIV-1 infection and that he may continue to acquire illnesses associated with HIV-1 infection.
• Advise patient to remain under medical supervision when taking drug because long-term effects are not known.
• Tell patient to take drug as prescribed and not to alter doses without doctor's approval. If a dose is missed, take next dose as soon as possible; do not double next dose.
• Inform patient that drug may be taken without regard for food.

• Tell patient with achlorhydria to take drug with an acidic beverage, such as orange or cranberry juice.
• Advise patient to report use of other prescription or OTC drugs.

☑ Evaluation
• Patient's skin integrity is maintained.
• Patient is free from opportunistic infections.
• Patient and family state understanding of drug therapy.

---

demeclocycline hydrochloride
(dee-meh-kloh-SIGH-kleen high-droh-KLOR-ighd)
Declomycin

Pharmacologic class: tetracycline antibiotic
Therapeutic class: antibiotic
Pregnancy risk category: D

How supplied
Tablets: 150 mg, 300 mg
Capsules: 150 mg

Pharmacokinetics
Absorption: 60% to 80% absorbed from GI tract. Food or milk reduces absorption by 50%.
Distribution: distributed widely in body tissues and fluids; however, CSF penetration is poor. Drug is 36% to 91% protein-bound.
Metabolism: not metabolized.
Excretion: excreted primarily unchanged in urine. *Half-life:* 10 to 17 hours.

Route	Onset	Peak	Duration
P.O.	Unknown	3-4 hr	Unknown

Pharmacodynamics
Chemical effect: unknown; thought to exert bacteriostatic effect by binding to 30S ribosomal subunit of microorganisms, thus inhibiting protein synthesis.

Therapeutic effect: inhibits bacterial activity. Spectrum of activity includes many gram-negative and gram-positive organisms, *Mycoplasma, Rickettsia, Chlamydia,* and spirochetes.

Indications and dosage

▶ **Infections caused by susceptible gram-negative and gram-positive organisms, including** *Campylobacter fetus,* **Haemophilus ducreyi, rickettsiae,** *Mycoplasma pneumoniae, Yersinia pestis.* **Also indicated for organism causing psittacosis, lymphogranuloma venereum, granuloma inguinale, relapsing fever, and trachoma.** *Adults:* 150 mg P.O. q 6 hours or 300 mg P.O. q 12 hours. *Children over age 8:* 6 to 12 mg/kg P.O. daily in divided doses q 6 to 12 hours.
▶ **Gonorrhea.** *Adults:* initially, 600 mg P.O., then 300 mg P.O. q 12 hours for 4 days (total 3 g).

Adverse reactions

CNS: *intracranial hypertension (pseudotumor cerebri),* dizziness.
CV: pericarditis.
EENT: dysphagia, glossitis, tinnitus, visual disturbances.
GI: anorexia, *nausea, vomiting, diarrhea,* enterocolitis, anogenital inflammation, dysphagia, glossitis, *pancreatitis.*
Hematologic: *neutropenia,* eosinophilia, *thrombocytopenia, hemolytic anemia.*
Skin: *maculopapular and erythematous rashes, photosensitivity, increased pigmentation, urticaria.*
Other: hypersensitivity reactions (*anaphylaxis*), elevated liver enzyme levels, *increased BUN level,* diabetes insipidus syndrome (polyuria, polydipsia, weakness), permanent tooth discoloration or bone growth retardation if used in children under age 8.

Interactions

Drug-drug. *Antacids (including sodium bicarbonate) and laxatives containing aluminum, magnesium, or calcium; an-*

tidiarrheals: decreased antibiotic absorption. Give antibiotic 1 hour before or 2 hours after any of above.
Ferrous sulfate and other iron products, zinc: decreased antibiotic absorption. Give antibiotic 3 hours after or 2 hours before iron administration.
Methoxyflurane: may cause nephrotoxicity with tetracyclines. Monitor patient carefully.
Oral anticoagulants: increased anticoagulant effect. Monitor PT and INR and adjust dosage, as ordered.
Oral contraceptives: decreased contraceptive effectiveness and increased risk of breakthrough bleeding. Use nonhormonal birth control method.
Penicillins: may interfere with bactericidal action of penicillins. Avoid using together.
Drug-food. *Food, milk, other dairy products:* decreased antibiotic absorption. Give antibiotic 1 hour before or 2 hours after any of above.
Drug-lifestyle. *Sun exposure:* photosensitivity reactions may occur. Take precautions.

Contraindications and precautions

• Contraindicated in patients with hypersensitivity to drug or other tetracyclines and in breast-feeding women.
• Use cautiously in patients with impaired kidney or liver function. Use of these drugs during last half of pregnancy and in children under age 8 may cause permanent discoloration of teeth, enamel defects, and bone growth retardation.

NURSING CONSIDERATIONS

⚕ Assessment
• Obtain history of patient's infection before therapy, and reassess regularly throughout therapy.
• Obtain specimen for culture and sensitivity tests before giving first dose. Therapy may begin, pending test results.
• Be alert for adverse reactions and drug interactions.

• Monitor patient's hydration status if adverse GI reactions occur.
• Evaluate patient's and family's knowledge of drug therapy.

⊞ **Nursing diagnoses**
• Infection related to presence of susceptible organism
• Risk of fluid volume deficit related to drug-induced adverse GI reactions
• Knowledge deficit related to drug therapy

▷ **Planning and implementation**
• Check expiration date. Outdated or deteriorated tetracyclines have been associated with reversible nephrotoxicity (Fanconi's syndrome).
• Don't expose these drugs to light or heat; store in tight container.
• Do not administer with milk or other dairy products, food, antacids, or iron products because they reduce effectiveness. Administer with full glass of water at least 1 hour before meals or 2 hours afterward. Give at least 1 hour before bedtime to prevent esophagitis.
• Be aware that demeclocycline may cause a false-negative reading in urine tests using glucose oxidase reagent (Diastix, Chemstrip uG).
• Notify doctor if patient develops superinfection. Drug may need to be discontinued and another antibiotic substituted.
Patient teaching
• Explain that drug's effectiveness is reduced when taken with milk or other dairy products, food, antacids, or iron products. Tell patient to take each dose with full glass of water at least 1 hour before or 2 hours after meals and to remain standing for 90 seconds after ingestion. Tell patient to take drug at least 1 hour before bedtime to prevent esophagitis.
• Instruct patient to take entire amount of medication, exactly as prescribed, even after he feels better.
• Stress good oral hygiene.
• Warn patient to avoid direct sunlight and ultraviolet light. A sunscreen may help prevent photosensitivity reactions. Photosensitivity persists for some time after discontinuation of drug.
• Tell patient to check expiration date and discard outdated demeclocycline because it may become toxic.
• Advise female patient taking oral contraceptive to use alternative means of contraception during drug therapy and for 1 week after it is discontinued.

☑ **Evaluation**
• Patient is free from infection.
• Patient maintains adequate hydration throughout therapy.
• Patient and family state understanding of drug therapy.

---

desipramine hydrochloride
(deh-SIP-rah-meen high-droh-KLOR-ighd)
Norpramin**, Pertofran♦◊

Pharmacologic class: dibenzazepine tricyclic antidepressant (TCA)
Therapeutic class: antidepressant
Pregnancy risk category: C

How supplied
Tablets: 10 mg, 25 mg, 50 mg, 75 mg, 100 mg, 150 mg
Capsules: 25 mg, 50 mg

Pharmacokinetics
Absorption: absorbed rapidly from GI tract.
Distribution: distributed widely throughout body, including CNS; 90% protein-bound.
Metabolism: metabolized by liver; significant first-pass effect may explain variability of serum concentrations in different patients taking same dosage.
Excretion: excreted primarily in urine.

Route	Onset	Peak	Duration
P.O.	2-4 wk	4-6 hr	Unknown

Pharmacodynamics

Chemical effect: unknown; increases amount of norepinephrine, serotonin, or both in CNS by blocking their reuptake by neurons.
Therapeutic effect: relieves depression.

Indications and dosage

▶ **Depression.** *Adults:* initially, 100 to 200 mg P.O. daily in divided doses; increased to maximum of 300 mg daily. Or entire dosage can be given h.s. *Elderly patients and adolescents:* 25 to 100 mg P.O. daily in divided doses; increased gradually to maximum of 150 mg daily, if needed.

Adverse reactions

CNS: *drowsiness, dizziness,* excitation, tremors, weakness, confusion, headache, nervousness, EEG changes, *seizures,* extrapyramidal reactions.
CV: orthostatic hypotension, *tachycardia, ECG changes,* hypertension (especially during surgery).
EENT: *blurred vision,* tinnitus, mydriasis.
GI: *dry mouth, constipation,* nausea, vomiting, anorexia, paralytic ileus.
GU: *urine retention.*
Skin: rash, urticaria, photosensitivity.
Other: *diaphoresis, hypersensitivity reaction, sudden death* (children).
After abrupt withdrawal of long-term therapy: nausea, headache, malaise (does not indicate addiction).

Interactions

Drug-drug. *Barbiturates, CNS depressants:* enhanced CNS depression. Avoid concomitant use.
Cimetidine, methylphenidate: may increase desipramine serum levels. Monitor for adverse reactions.
Clonidine, epinephrine, norepinephrine: increased hypertensive effect. Use with caution.
MAO inhibitors: may cause severe excitation, hyperpyrexia, or seizures, usually with high dosage. Use with caution.

Drug-lifestyle. *Alcohol use:* enhanced CNS depression. Avoid concomitant use.
Smoking: may lower plasma concentrations of desipramine. Monitor for lack of effect.
Sun exposure: increased risk of photosensitivity. Avoid unprotected or prolonged sun exposure.

Contraindications and precautions

• Contraindicated in patients with hypersensitivity to drug, in those who have taken MAO inhibitors within previous 14 days, and in patients during acute recovery phase of MI.
• Use with extreme caution in patients with CV disease, seizure disorder, glaucoma, thyroid disorder, or history of urine retention and in those taking thyroid medication.
• Use cautiously in pregnant or breast-feeding women.
• Safety of drug has not been established in children under age 12.

NURSING CONSIDERATIONS

Assessment
• Obtain history of patient's depression before therapy, and reassess regularly thereafter.
• Be alert for adverse reactions and drug interactions.
• Evaluate patient's and family's knowledge of drug therapy.

Nursing diagnoses
• Ineffective individual coping related to depression
• Risk for injury related to drug-induced adverse reactions
• Knowledge deficit related to drug therapy

Planning and implementation
• Do not withdraw drug abruptly.
• Know that because desipramine produces fewer anticholinergic effects than other TCAs, it is prescribed often for patients with cardiac problems.

Reactions may be *common*, uncommon, *life-threatening*, or COMMON AND LIFE-THREATENING.

• Because hypertensive episodes have occurred during surgery in patients receiving TCAs, know that this drug should be discontinued gradually several days before surgery.
• If signs of psychosis occur or increase, expect doctor to reduce dosage.
Patient teaching
• Warn patient not to perform hazardous activities that require alertness and good psychomotor coordination until CNS effects of drug are known. Drowsiness and dizziness usually subside after a few weeks.
• Tell patient to avoid alcohol while taking this drug because it may antagonize effects of desipramine.
• Warn patient not to stop drug therapy suddenly.
• Advise patient to consult doctor before taking other prescription or OTC drugs.
• Instruct patient to use sunblock, wear protective clothing, and avoid prolonged exposure to strong sunlight.

☑ **Evaluation**
• Patient behavior and communication indicate improvement of depression.
• Patient does not experience injury as a result of drug-induced adverse reactions.
• Patient and family state understanding of drug therapy.

---

desmopressin acetate
(dez-moh-PREH-sin AS-ih-tayt)
DDAVP, Stimate

Pharmacologic class: posterior pituitary hormone
Therapeutic class: antidiuretic; hemostatic agent
Pregnancy risk category: B

How supplied
Nasal solution: 0.1 mg/ml, 1.5 mg/ml
Injection: 4 mcg/ml
Tablets: 0.1 mg, 0.2 mg

Pharmacokinetics
Absorption: after intranasal administration, 10% to 20% of dose absorbed through nasal mucosa. Absorption after S.C. administration is unknown. Following oral administration, drug is minimally absorbed from the GI tract.
Distribution: unknown.
Metabolism: unknown.
Excretion: unknown. *Half-life:* fast phase, about 8 minutes; slow phase, 75½ minutes.

Route	Onset	Peak	Duration
P.O.	1 hr	4-7 hr	Unknown
I.V.	15-30 min	1.5-2 hr	4-12 hr
S.C.	Unknown	Unknown	Unknown
Intranasal	≤ 1 hr	1-5 hr	8-12 hr

Pharmacodynamics
Chemical effect: increases permeability of renal tubular epithelium to adenosine monophosphate and water; epithelium promotes reabsorption of water and produces concentrated urine (ADH effect). Desmopressin also increases factor VIII activity by releasing endogenous factor VIII from plasma storage sites.
Therapeutic effect: decreases diuresis and promotes clotting.

Indications and dosage
▶ **Nonnephrogenic diabetes insipidus, temporary polyuria and polydipsia associated with pituitary trauma.** *Adults:* 0.1 to 0.4 ml intranasally in one to three divided doses daily. Morning and evening doses adjusted separately for adequate diurnal rhythm of water turnover. Alternately, 0.05 mg P.O. b.i.d. Each dose should be adjusted separately for an adequate diurnal rhythm of water turnover. Total oral daily dosage should be increased or decreased in range of 0.1 to 1.2 mg divided into two or three daily doses. Oral therapy should be initiated 12 hours after last intranasal dose. Alternatively, injectable form administered in dosage of 0.5 to 1 ml I.V. or S.C. daily, usually in two equally divided doses.

Children ages 3 months to 12 years (nasal spray): 0.05 to 0.3 ml intranasally daily in one or two doses. *Children age 4 and older (oral form):* begin with 0.05 mg P.O. b.i.d. Each dose should be adjusted separately for an adequate diurnal rhythm of water turnover. Total oral daily dosage should be increased or decreased in range of 0.1 to 1.2 mg divided into two or three daily doses. Oral therapy should be initiated 12 hours after the last intranasal dose. *Children under age 4 (oral form):* dosage must be individually adjusted in order to prevent an excessive decrease in plasma osmolality.

► **Hemophilia A and von Willebrand's disease.** *Adults and children:* 0.3 mcg/kg diluted in 0.9% NaCl and infused I.V. over 15 to 30 minutes. Dose repeated if necessary based on laboratory response and patient's clinical condition. Intranasal dose is 1 spray (of solution containing 1.5 mg/ml) into each nostril to provide total of 300 mcg. In patients weighing under 50 kg (110 lb), use 1 spray into a single nostril (150 mcg).

► **Primary nocturnal enuresis.** *Children age 6 and over:* initially, 20 mcg intranasally h.s. Dosage adjusted according to response. Maximum recommended dosage is 40 mcg daily. Alternately, 0.2 mg P.O. h.s. Dose may be titrated up to 0.6 mg P.O. to achieve desired response. Oral therapy may be initiated 24 hours after last intranasal dose.

Adverse reactions

CNS: headache.
CV: slight rise in blood pressure (with high dosage).
EENT: nasal congestion, rhinitis, epistaxis, sore throat, cough.
GI: nausea, abdominal cramps.
GU: vulval pain.
Other: flushing, local erythema, swelling or burning after injection.

Interactions

Drug-drug. *Clofibrate:* enhanced and prolonged effects of desmopressin. Monitor patient carefully.
Demeclocycline, epinephrine, heparin, lithium: increased risk of adverse effects. Monitor patient closely.
Drug-lifestyle. *Alcohol use:* increased risk of adverse effects. Monitor patient closely.

Contraindications and precautions

• Contraindicated in patients with type IIB von Willebrand's disease or hypersensitivity to drug.
• Use cautiously in patients with coronary artery insufficiency or hypertensive CV disease and in those with conditions associated with fluid and electrolyte imbalance, such as cystic fibrosis, because these patients are prone to hyponatremia. Also use cautiously in pregnant or breast-feeding women.
• Use of drug in infants under age 3 months is not recommended because of infants' increased tendency to develop fluid imbalance; safety of parenteral form of drug has not been established for management of diabetes insipidus in children under age 12.

NURSING CONSIDERATIONS

Assessment
• Obtain history of patient's underlying condition before therapy.
• Monitor effectiveness by checking patient's fluid intake and output, serum and urine osmolality, and urine specific gravity for treatment of diabetes insipidus or relief of symptoms of other disorders.
• Be alert for adverse reactions and drug interactions.
• Monitor patient carefully for hypertension during high-dose treatment.
• Evaluate patient's and family's knowledge of drug therapy.

◉ Nursing diagnoses
• Fluid volume deficit related to underlying condition
• Pain related to drug-induced headache
• Knowledge deficit related to drug therapy

❯ Planning and implementation
P.O. use: Follow normal protocol.
I.V. use: Dilute drug with 0.9% NaCl according to doctor's instructions when administering I.V. for treatment of hemophilia A and von Willebrand's disease.
S.C. use: Follow normal protocol. Rotate injection sites.
Intranasal use: Follow manufacturer's instructions exactly for administration.
• Know that desmopressin injection should not be used to treat hemophilia A with factor VIII levels of 0% to 5%, or severe cases of von Willebrand's disease.
• Know that when drug is used to treat diabetes insipidus, dosage or frequency of administration may be adjusted according to patient's fluid output. Morning and evening doses are adjusted separately for adequate diurnal rhythm of water turnover.
• Intranasal use can cause changes in nasal mucosa, resulting in erratic, unreliable absorption. Report worsening condition to doctor, who may prescribe injectable DDAVP.
Patient teaching
• Instruct patient to clear nasal passages before administering drug intranasally.
• Patient may have difficulty measuring and inhaling drug into nostrils. Teach patient and caregiver correct method of administration.
• Advise patient to report conditions such as nasal congestion, allergic rhinitis, or upper respiratory tract infection; dosage adjustment may be required.
• Teach patient using S.C. desmopressin to rotate injection sites to avoid tissue damage.
• Warn patient to drink only enough water to satisfy thirst.
• Inform patient that when treating hemophilia A and von Willebrand's disease,

giving desmopressin may avoid hazards of using blood products.
• Advise patient to wear medical identification indicating use of drug.

☑ Evaluation
• Patient achieves normal fluid and electrolyte balance.
• Patient states that headache is relieved with mild analgesic.
• Patient and family state understanding of drug therapy.

dexamethasone
(deks-ah-METH-uh-sohn)
Decadron*, Dexamethasone Intensol*, Dexasone♦, Dexone 0.5, Dexone 0.75, Dexone 1.5, Dexone 4, Hexadrol*, Mymethasone*

dexamethasone acetate
Dalalone D.P., Dalalone L.A., Decadron-LA, Decaject-L.A., Dexacen LA-8, Dexasone-L.A., Dexone L.A., Solurex-LA

dexamethasone sodium phosphate
Ak-Dex, Dalalone, Decadrol, Decadron Phosphate, Decaject, Dexacen-4, Dexone, Hexadrol Phosphate, Solurex

Pharmacologic class: glucocorticoid
Therapeutic class: anti-inflammatory, immunosuppressant
Pregnancy risk category: NR

How supplied
dexamethasone
Tablets: 0.25 mg, 0.5 mg, 0.75 mg, 1 mg, 1.5 mg, 2 mg, 4 mg, 6 mg
Oral solution: 0.5 mg/5 ml, 1 mg/ml
Elixir: 0.5 mg/5 ml*
dexamethasone acetate
Injection: 8 mg/ml, 16 mg/ml suspension

dexamethasone sodium phosphate

Injection: 4 mg/ml, 10 mg/ml, 20 mg/ml, 24 mg/ml

Pharmacokinetics

Absorption: absorbed readily after P.O. administration. Absorption of suspension for injection depends on whether it is injected into an intra-articular space, a muscle, or blood supply to a muscle.
Distribution: distributed to muscle, liver, skin, intestines, and kidneys. Drug is bound weakly to plasma proteins (transcortin and albumin). Only unbound portion is active.
Metabolism: metabolized in liver to inactive glucuronide and sulfate metabolites.
Excretion: inactive metabolites and small amounts of unmetabolized drug excreted by kidneys. Insignificant quantities of drug also are excreted in feces. *Half-life:* 36 to 54 hours.

Route	Onset	Peak	Duration
P.O.	1-2 hr	1-2 hr	2.5 days
I.V., I.M.	≤ 1 hr	1 hr	2 days-3 wk

Pharmacodynamics

Chemical effect: not clearly defined; decreases inflammation, mainly by stabilizing leukocyte lysosomal membranes; suppresses immune response; stimulates bone marrow; and influences protein, fat, and carbohydrate metabolism.
Therapeutic effect: relieves cerebral edema, reduces inflammation and immune response, and reverses shock.

Indications and dosage

▶ **Cerebral edema. Phosphate.** *Adults:* initially, 10 mg I.V.; then 4 to 6 mg I.M. q 6 hours until symptoms subside (usually 2 to 4 days); then tapered over 5 to 7 days.
▶ **Inflammatory conditions, allergic reactions, neoplasias. Phosphate.** *Adults:* 0.75 to 9 mg/day P.O. or 0.5 to 9 mg/day I.M. **Acetate.** *Adults:* 4 to 16 mg I.M. into joint or soft tissue q 1 to 3 weeks, or 0.8 to 1.6 mg into lesions q 1 to 3 weeks.

▶ **Shock. Phosphate.** *Adults:* 1 to 6 mg/ kg I.V. as single dose; or 40 mg I.V. q 2 to 6 hours, p.r.n.
▶ **Dexamethasone suppression test for Cushing's syndrome.** *Adults:* after determining baseline 24-hour urine levels of 17-hydroxycorticosteroids, 0.5 mg P.O. q 6 hours for 48 hours; 24-hour urine collection made for determination of 17-hydroxycorticosteroid excretion again during second 24 hours of dexamethasone administration.

Adverse reactions

Most adverse reactions to corticosteroids are dose- or duration-dependent.
CNS: *euphoria, insomnia,* psychotic behavior, pseudotumor cerebri, *seizures.*
CV: *heart failure,* hypertension, edema, *arrhythmias, thromboembolism.*
EENT: cataracts, glaucoma.
Endocrine: menstrual irregularities, cushingoid state (moonface, buffalo hump, central obesity).
GI: *peptic ulceration,* GI irritation, increased appetite, *pancreatitis.*
Metabolic: hypokalemia, hyperglycemia, carbohydrate intolerance,
Musculoskeletal: muscle weakness, osteoporosis, growth suppression in children.
Skin: hirsutism, delayed wound healing, acne, various skin eruptions; atrophy (at I.M. injection sites).
Other: susceptibility to infections, *acute adrenal insufficiency may follow increased stress (infection, surgery, or trauma) or abrupt withdrawal after long-term therapy.*
After abrupt withdrawal: rebound inflammation, fatigue, weakness, arthralgia, fever, dizziness, lethargy, depression, fainting, orthostatic hypotension, dyspnea, anorexia, hypoglycemia. *After prolonged use, sudden withdrawal may be fatal.*

Interactions

Drug-drug. *Antidiabetic agents, including insulin:* decreased response. May need dose adjustment.

Aspirin, indomethacin, other NSAIDs: increased risk of GI distress and bleeding. Give together cautiously.
Barbiturates, phenytoin, rifampin: decreased corticosteroid effect. Increase corticosteroid dosage, as ordered.
Cardiac glycosides: increased possibility of arrhythmia due to hypokalemia. May warrant dosage adjustment.
Oral anticoagulants: altered dosage requirements. Monitor PT and INR closely.
Potassium-depleting drugs (such as thiazide diuretics): enhanced potassium-wasting effects of dexamethasone. Monitor serum potassium levels.
Salicylates: decreased serum salicylate levels.
Skin-test antigens: decreased response. Defer skin testing until therapy is completed.
Toxoids, vaccines: decreased antibody response and increased risk of neurologic complications. Avoid concomitant use.
Drug-lifestyle. *Alcohol use:* increased risk of gastric irritation and GI ulceration.

Contraindications and precautions

• Contraindicated in patients with systemic fungal infections or hypersensitivity to drug or its components.
• Drug is not recommended for use in breast-feeding women.
• Use with extreme caution in patient with recent MI.
• Use cautiously in pregnant women and in patients with GI ulcer, renal disease, hypertension, osteoporosis, diabetes mellitus, hypothyroidism, cirrhosis, diverticulitis, nonspecific ulcerative colitis, recent intestinal anastomoses, thromboembolic disorders, seizures, myasthenia gravis, heart failure, tuberculosis, ocular herpes simplex, emotional instability, or psychotic tendencies. Because some formulations contain sulfite preservatives, also use cautiously in patients sensitive to sulfites.
• Long-term use of drug in children and adolescents may delay growth and maturation.

NURSING CONSIDERATIONS

Assessment
• Obtain history of patient's underlying condition before therapy.
• Monitor patient's weight, blood pressure, blood glucose level, and serum electrolyte levels.
• Be alert for adverse reactions and drug interactions.
• Watch for depression or psychotic episodes, especially in high-dose therapy.
• Evaluate patient's and family's knowledge of drug therapy.

Nursing diagnoses
• Altered health maintenance related to underlying condition
• Risk for injury related to drug-induced adverse reactions
• Knowledge deficit related to drug therapy

Planning and implementation
• For better results and less toxicity, give once-daily dose in morning.
P.O. use: Give oral dose with food when possible.
I.V. use: When administering as direct injection, inject undiluted over at least 1 minute. When administering as intermittent or continuous infusion, dilute solution according to manufacturer's instructions and give over prescribed duration. If used for continuous infusion, change solution every 24 hours.
I.M. use: Give I.M. injection deeply into gluteal muscle. Rotate injection sites to prevent muscle atrophy.
• Avoid S.C. injection because atrophy and sterile abscesses may occur.
• Always titrate to lowest effective dose, as ordered.
• Gradually reduce drug dosage after long-term therapy, as ordered.
• Unless contraindicated, give patient low-sodium diet high in potassium and protein. Know that doctor may also prescribe potassium supplements, as needed.

• Notify doctor if patient is experiencing increased stress (physical or psychological) because dosage may need to be increased.

• Also notify doctor if patient develops adverse reactions, and be prepared to provide supportive and symptomatic treatment, as prescribed.

Patient teaching

• Tell patient not to discontinue drug abruptly or without doctor's consent.

• Teach patient signs of early adrenal insufficiency: fatigue, muscle weakness, joint pain, fever, anorexia, nausea, dyspnea, dizziness, and fainting.

• Instruct patient to carry medical identification card indicating need for supplemental systemic glucocorticoids during stress, especially as dosage is decreased.

• Warn patient on long-term therapy about cushingoid symptoms and to report sudden weight gain or swelling to doctor.

• Warn patient about easy bruising.

• Advise patient receiving long-term therapy to consider exercise or physical therapy. Give vitamin D or calcium supplements, as ordered.

• Advise patient receiving long-term therapy to have periodic ophthalmologic examinations.

☑ Evaluation

• Patient's condition being treated with drug therapy shows improvement.

• Patient does not experience injury as a result of drug therapy.

• Patient and family state understanding of drug therapy.

---

dexrazoxane
(deks-rah-ZOKS-ayn)
Zinecard

Pharmacologic class: intracellular chelating agent
Therapeutic class: cardioprotective agent
Pregnancy risk category: C

How supplied
Injection: 250 mg, 500 mg

Pharmacokinetics
Absorption: not applicable with I.V. administration.
Distribution: not bound to plasma proteins.
Metabolism: not thought to be metabolized.
Excretion: excreted primarily in urine.

Route	Onset	Peak	Duration
I.V.	Unknown	15 min	Unknown

Pharmacodynamics
Chemical effect: unknown; cyclic derivative of ethylenediamine tetra-acetic acid that readily penetrates cell membranes and may be converted to ring-opened chelating agent that interferes with iron-mediated free radical generation.
Therapeutic effect: prevents doxorubicin-induced cardiomyopathy or reduces its severity.

Indications and dosage
▶ **Reduction of incidence and severity of doxorubicin-induced cardiomyopathy in women with metastatic breast cancer who have received a cumulative doxorubicin dose of 300 mg/m² but would benefit from continued therapy with doxorubicin.** *Adults:* dosage ratio of dexrazoxane to doxorubicin must be 10:1, such as 500 mg/m² of dexrazoxane to 50 mg/m² of doxorubicin. After reconstitution, dexrazoxane should be given by slow I.V. push or rapid drip I.V. infusion. After completion of dexrazoxane administration (and less than 30 minutes from the beginning of this administration), I.V. injection of doxorubicin should be given.

Adverse reactions
CNS: *fatigue, malaise,* **neurotoxicity.**
GI: *nausea, vomiting, anorexia, stomatitis, diarrhea,* esophagitis, dysphagia.
Hematologic: **immunosuppression, hemorrhage.**

Reactions may be *common*, uncommon, *life-threatening*, or COMMON AND LIFE-THREATENING.

Skin: erythema, urticaria, skin reaction.
Other: *alopecia, fever, infection, pain on injection, sepsis,* streaking at I.V. insertion site, phlebitis, extravasation.
Note: The adverse reactions listed above, with the exception of pain on injection, may be attributed to the FAC regimen (fluorouracil, doxorubicin, cyclophosphamide) given shortly after dexrazoxane.

Interactions
None reported.

Contraindications and precautions
• Contraindicated in patients who are not receiving chemotherapy regimens that contain an anthracycline.
• Drug is not recommended for use in pregnant or breast-feeding women.
• Use cautiously in all patients. Additive effects of immunosuppression may result from required concomitant administration of cytotoxic drugs.
• Safety of drug has not been established in children.

NURSING CONSIDERATIONS

⚖ Assessment
• Obtain history of patient's underlying condition before drug administration.
• Monitor CBC closely, as ordered. Dexrazoxane is always used with other cytotoxic drugs, and it may add to their myelosuppressive effects.
• Be alert for adverse reactions.
• Evaluate patient's and family's knowledge of drug therapy.

⊞ Nursing diagnoses
• Risk for injury related to doxorubicin-induced cardiomyopathy
• Altered protection related to immunosuppression induced by dexrazoxane and concomitant cardiotoxic drug therapy
• Knowledge deficit related to drug therapy

▣ Planning and implementation
• Be aware that dexrazoxane is recommended for use only when patient has already received an accumulated doxorubicin dose of 300 mg/m^2 and continuation of doxorubicin is desired.
• Know that drug must be diluted with the diluent supplied with drug (0.167 molar sodium lactate injection) to give a concentration of 10 mg dexrazoxane for each milliliter of sodium lactate. The reconstituted solution should be given by slow I.V. push or rapid drip I.V. infusion from a bag.
• Reconstituted solution, when transferred to an empty infusion bag, is stable for 6 hours from the time of reconstitution when stored at controlled room temperature (36° to 46° F [2° to 8°C]) or under refrigeration. Discard unused solution.
• Reconstituted drug may be diluted with either normal saline solution or 5% dextrose injection to a concentration range of 1.3 to 5.0 mg/ml in I.V. infusion bags. The resultant solution is also stable for 6 hours under the same storage conditions as the diluted drug.
• Dexrazoxane should not be mixed with other drugs because of possible incompatibility.
• When handling and preparing reconstituted solution, use the same precautions as those for handling antineoplastic agents. Use of gloves is recommended.
• If drug powder or solution contacts skin or mucosa, immediately wash thoroughly with soap and water.
• Institute infection-control and bleeding precautions, as indicated by CBC results.
Patient teaching
• Inform patient of the need for drug during continued doxorubicin therapy.
• Warn patient to watch for signs of infection (fever, sore throat, fatigue) and bleeding (easy bruising, nosebleeds, bleeding gums, melena). Emphasize importance of infection-control and bleeding precautions. Tell patient to take her temperature daily.

• Warn patient that alopecia may occur but that it's usually reversible.

☑ **Evaluation**
• Patient does not exhibit signs and symptoms of cardiomyopathy (or, if present before dexrazoxane therapy, does not develop worsening signs and symptoms).
• Patient does not develop serious complications from drug-induced immunosuppression.
• Patient and family state understanding of drug therapy.

dextran, high-molecular-weight (dextran 70, dextran 75)
(DEKS-tran, high moh-LEH-kyoo-ler wayt)
Dextran 75, Gentran 70, Gentran 75, Macrodex

Pharmacologic class: glucose polymer
Therapeutic class: plasma volume expander
Pregnancy risk category: C

How supplied
Injection: dextran 70 in 0.9% NaCl solution or dextrose 5%; 6% dextran 75 in 0.9% NaCl solution or dextrose 5%

Pharmacokinetics
Absorption: not applicable with I.V. administration.
Distribution: distributed throughout vascular system.
Metabolism: dextran molecules with molecular weights above 50,000 are enzymatically degraded by dextranase to glucose at rate of about 70 to 90 mg/kg/day. This process is variable.
Excretion: dextran molecules with molecular weights below 50,000 are eliminated by renal excretion.

Route	Onset	Peak	Duration
I.V.	Immediate	Immediate	Unknown

Pharmacodynamics
Chemical effect: expands plasma volume by way of colloidal osmotic effect, drawing fluid from interstitial to intravascular space, providing fluid replacement.
Therapeutic effect: expands plasma volume.

Indications and dosage
▶ **Plasma expander.** *Adults:* 30 g (500 ml of 6% solution) I.V. In emergencies, may be administered at rate of 1.2 to 2.4 g (20 to 40 ml)/minute. In normovolemic or nearly normovolemic patients, rate of infusion should not exceed 240 mg (4 ml)/minute. Total dosage during first 24 hours not to exceed 1.2 g/kg; actual dosage depends on amount of fluid loss and resultant hemoconcentration and must be determined for each patient.

Adverse reactions
GI: nausea, vomiting.
GU: increased specific gravity and viscosity of urine, tubular stasis and blocking, oliguria, anuria.
Hematologic: decreased level of hemoglobin and hematocrit; with doses of 15 ml/kg, prolonged bleeding time and significant suppression of platelet function.
Hepatic: increased AST and ALT levels.
Skin: *hypersensitivity reactions,* urticaria.
Other: fever, arthralgia, nasal congestion, fluid overload, thrombophlebitis, *anaphylaxis.*

Interactions
Drug-drug. *Abciximab, aspirin, heparin, thrombolytics, warfarin:* increased bleeding if given in combination. Use together with extreme caution.

Contraindications and precautions
• Contraindicated in patients with hypersensitivity to dextran and in those with marked hemostatic defects, marked cardiac decompensation, renal disease with

---

Reactions may be *common,* uncommon, *life-threatening,* or COMMON AND LIFE-THREATENING.

severe oliguria or anuria, hypervolemic
conditions, or severe bleeding disorders.
• It is recommended that breast-feeding
women discontinue breast-feeding or that
drug should not be used.
• Use cautiously in patients with active
hemorrhage, thrombocytopenia, impaired
renal clearance, chronic liver disease, or
abdominal conditions and in patients undergoing bowel surgery. Also use cautiously in pregnant women.
• Safety of drug has not been established
in children.

NURSING CONSIDERATIONS

⚕ Assessment
• Obtain history of patient's underlying
condition and hydration status before
therapy, and reassess regularly throughout therapy; frequently assess vital signs
and fluid intake and output as well as
urine or serum osmolarity levels, as ordered.
• Be alert for adverse reactions.
• Observe patient closely during early
phase of infusion, when most anaphylactic reactions occur.
• Watch for circulatory overload and rise
in central venous pressure. Plasma expansion is slightly greater than volume
infused.
• Check hemoglobin and hematocrit levels, as ordered.
• Evaluate patient's and family's knowledge of drug therapy.

⊞ Nursing diagnoses
• Decreased cardiac output related to underlying condition
• Risk for injury related to potential for
drug-induced hypersensitivity reaction
• Knowledge deficit related to drug
therapy

▷ Planning and implementation
• As ordered, use D_5W solution instead
of 0.9% NaCl solution because drug is
hazardous for patients with heart failure,

especially when given in 0.9% NaCl solution.
• Be aware that doctor may order dextran
1 to protect against drug-induced anaphylaxis. Administer 20 ml of dextran 1
(containing 150 mg/ml) I.V. over 60 seconds 1 to 2 minutes before I.V. infusion
of dextran.
• Store drug at constant 77° F (25° C).
Dextran may precipitate in storage, but it
can be heated to dissolve, if necessary.
• If oliguria or anuria occurs or is not relieved by infusion, stop dextran and give
loop diuretic, as ordered.
• If hematocrit values fall below 30% by
volume, notify doctor.
• Be aware that drug may interfere with
analyses of blood grouping, crossmatching, and bilirubin, blood glucose, and
protein levels.
Patient teaching
• Inform patient, if alert, and family
about dextran therapy.
• Instruct patient to notify doctor if adverse reactions, such as itching, occur.

☑ Evaluation
• Patient's vital signs and urine output return to normal.
• Patient does not develop hypersensitivity reaction to drug.
• Patient and family state understanding
of drug therapy.

dextran, low-molecular-weight (dextran 40)
(DEKS-tran, loh moh-LEH-kyoo-ler wayt)
Dextran 40, Gentran 40, 10% LMD,
Rheomacrodex

Pharmacologic class: glucose polymer
Therapeutic class: plasma volume
expander
Pregnancy risk category: C

How supplied

Injection: 10% dextran 40 in D_5W or
0.9% NaCl solution

Pharmacokinetics

Absorption: not applicable with I.V. administration.
Distribution: distributed throughout vascular system.
Metabolism: dextran molecules with molecular weights above 50,000 are enzymatically degraded by dextranase to glucose at a rate of about 70 to 90 mg/kg/day. This is a variable process.
Excretion: drug molecules with molecular weights below 50,000 are excreted by kidneys.

Route	Onset	Peak	Duration
I.V.	Immediate	Immediate	≤ 3 hr

Pharmacodynamics

Chemical effect: expands plasma volume by way of colloidal osmotic effect, drawing fluid from interstitial to intravascular space, providing fluid replacement.
Therapeutic effect: expands plasma volume.

Indications and dosage

▶ **Plasma volume expansion.** *Adults:* dosage by I.V. infusion depends on amount of fluid loss. Initially, 10 ml/kg of dextran infused rapidly with central venous pressure monitoring; remainder of dose administered slowly. Total dosage not to exceed 20 ml/kg daily. If therapy is continued longer than 24 hours, do not exceed 10 ml/kg daily. Continued for no longer than 5 days.
▶ **Prophylaxis of venous thrombosis.** *Adults:* 10 ml/kg (500 to 1,000 ml) I.V. on day of procedure; 500 ml on days 2 and 3.
▶ **Hemodiluent in extracorporeal circulation.** *Adults:* 10 to 20 ml/kg added to perfusion circuit. Total dosage not to exceed 20 ml/kg.

Adverse reactions

GI: nausea, vomiting.
GU: tubular stasis and blocking, increased urine viscosity.

Hematologic: *decreased hemoglobin and hematocrit levels;* increased bleeding time (with higher doses).
Hepatic: increased AST and ALT levels.
Skin: *hypersensitivity reactions,* urticaria.
Other: *anaphylaxis,* thrombophlebitis.

Interactions

None significant.

Contraindications and precautions

• Contraindicated in patients with marked hemostatic defects, marked cardiac decompensation, renal disease with severe oliguria or anuria, and hypersensitivity to drug.
• It is recommended that breast-feeding women discontinue breast-feeding or that drug should not be used.
• Use cautiously in patients with active hemorrhage, thrombocytopenia, or diabetes mellitus. Also use cautiously in pregnant women.
• Safety of drug has not been established in children.

NURSING CONSIDERATIONS

🔎 **Assessment**
• Obtain history of patient's underlying condition and hydration status before therapy, and reassess regularly throughout therapy; frequently assess vital signs and fluid intake and output as well as urine or serum osmolarity levels, as ordered.
• Be alert for adverse reactions.
• Observe patient closely during early phase of infusion, when most anaphylactic reactions occur.
• Watch for circulatory overload and rise in central venous pressure. Plasma expansion is slightly greater than volume infused.
• Check hemoglobin and hematocrit levels, as ordered.
• Evaluate patient's and family's knowledge of drug therapy.

Reactions may be *common,* uncommon, *life-threatening,* or COMMON AND LIFE-THREATENING.

❂ Nursing diagnoses
• Decreased cardiac output related to underlying condition
• Risk for injury related to potential for drug-induced hypersensitivity reaction
• Knowledge deficit related to drug therapy

❯ Planning and implementation
• As ordered, use D₅W solution instead of 0.9% NaCl solution because drug is hazardous for patients with heart failure, especially when given in 0.9% NaCl solution.
• Be aware that doctor may order dextran 1 to protect against drug-induced anaphylaxis. Administer 20 ml of dextran 1 (containing 150 mg/ml) I.V. over 60 seconds 1 to 2 minutes before I.V. infusion of dextran.
• Store at constant 77° F (25° C). Dextran may precipitate in storage, but it can be heated to dissolve, if necessary.
• If oliguria or anuria occurs or is not relieved by infusion, stop dextran and give loop diuretic, as ordered.
• If hematocrit values fall below 30% by volume, notify doctor.
• Be aware that drug may interfere with analyses of blood grouping, crossmatching, and bilirubin, blood glucose, and protein levels.
Patient teaching
• Inform patient, if alert, and family about dextran therapy.
• Instruct patient to notify doctor if adverse reactions, such as itching, occur.

☑ Evaluation
• Patient's vital signs and urine output return to normal.
• Patient does not develop hypersensitivity reaction to drug.
• Patient and family state understanding of drug therapy.

dextroamphetamine sulfate
(deks-troh-am-FET-uh-meen SUL-fayt)
Dexedrine* **, Dexedrine Spansule, Ferndex, Oxydess II, Spancap #1

Pharmacologic class: amphetamine
Therapeutic class: CNS stimulant, sympathomimetic amine
Controlled substance schedule: II
Pregnancy risk category: C

How supplied
Tablets: 5 mg, 10 mg
Capsules (sustained-release): 5 mg, 10 mg, 15 mg
Elixir: 5 mg/5 ml

Pharmacokinetics
Absorption: rapidly absorbed from GI tract; longer-acting capsules are absorbed more slowly.
Distribution: distributed widely throughout body.
Metabolism: unknown.
Excretion: excreted in urine. *Half-life:* 10 to 12 hours.

Route	Onset	Peak	Duration
P.O.	Unknown	Unknown	Unknown

Pharmacodynamics
Chemical effect: unknown; probably promotes nerve impulse transmission by releasing stored norepinephrine from nerve terminals in brain. Main sites of activity appear to be the cerebral cortex and reticular activating system. In children with hyperkinesis, amphetamines have paradoxical calming effect.
Therapeutic effect: helps prevent sleep and calms hyperactive children.

Indications and dosage
▶ **Narcolepsy.** *Adults:* 5 to 60 mg P.O. daily in divided doses. *Children age 12 and older:* 10 mg P.O. daily, with 10-mg increments weekly, p.r.n. *Children ages 6 to 12:* 5 mg P.O. daily, with 5-mg increments weekly, p.r.n. Give first dose on

*Liquid form contains alcohol   **May contain tartrazine   ♦Canada   ◊Australia   †OTC

awakening, additional doses (one or two) at intervals of 4 to 6 hours.

► **Attention deficit disorder with hyperactivity.** *Children age 6 and older:* 5 mg P.O. once daily or b.i.d., with 5-mg increments weekly, p.r.n. *Children ages 3 to 5:* 2.5 mg P.O. daily, with 2.5-mg increments weekly, p.r.n. Only in rare cases is it necessary to exceed total of 40 mg/day.

Adverse reactions

CNS: *restlessness,* tremors, *insomnia,* dizziness, headache, overstimulation, dysphoria.
CV: *tachycardia, palpitations,* hypertension, *arrhythmias.*
GI: dry mouth, unpleasant taste, diarrhea, constipation, anorexia, weight loss, and other GI disturbances.
GU: impotence.
Skin: urticaria.
Other: altered libido, chills.

Interactions

Drug-drug. *Acetazolamide, alkalizing agents, antacids, sodium bicarbonate:* increased renal reabsorption. Monitor for enhanced amphetamine effects.
Acidifying agents, ammonium chloride, ascorbic acid: decreased blood levels and increased renal clearance of dextroamphetamine. Monitor for decreased amphetamine effects.
Adrenergic blockers: adrenergic blockers inhibited by amphetamines. Avoid concomitant use.
Antihistamines: amphetamines may counteract sedative effects of antihistamines.
Chlorpromazine: inhibits central stimulant effects of amphetamines; may be used to treat amphetamine poisoning.
Haloperidol, phenothiazines, tricyclic antidepressants: increased CNS effects. Avoid concomitant use.
Insulin, oral antidiabetic agents: may decrease antidiabetic agent requirements. Monitor blood glucose levels.
Lithium carbonate: may inhibit antiobesity and stimulating effects of amphetamines.
MAO inhibitors: severe hypertension; possibly hypertensive crisis. Don't use together or within 14 days after MAO inhibitor has been discontinued.
Meperidine: amphetamines potentiate analgesic effect. Use together cautiously.
Methenamine: increased urinary excretion of amphetamines and efficacy reduced. Monitor effects.
Norepinephrine: amphetamines enhance adrenergic effect of norepinephrine.
Phenobarbital, phenytoin: amphetamines may delay absorption. Monitor patient closely.
Propoxyphene: in cases of propoxyphene overdose, amphetamine CNS stimulation is potentiated and fatal seizures can occur.
Veratrum alkaloids: amphetamines inhibit hypotensive effect of *Veratrum* alkaloids. Monitor blood pressure closely.
Drug-food. *Caffeine:* may increase amphetamine and related amine effects. Monitor patient closely.

Contraindications and precautions

• Contraindicated in patients with hypersensitivity or idiosyncratic reaction to sympathomimetic amines; within 14 days of MAO inhibitor therapy; and in those with hyperthyroidism, moderate to severe hypertension, symptomatic CV disease, glaucoma, advanced arteriosclerosis, or history of drug abuse.
• Use cautiously in patients with motor and phonic tics or Tourette syndrome and in those in agitated states. Also use cautiously in pregnant women.
• Safety of drug has not been established in breast-feeding women.

NURSING CONSIDERATIONS

Assessment
• Obtain history of patient's underlying condition before therapy, and reassess regularly throughout therapy.

• Be alert for adverse reactions and drug interactions.
• Monitor sleeping pattern, and observe for signs of excessive stimulation.
• Evaluate patient's and family's knowledge of drug therapy.

🔶 **Nursing diagnoses**
• Altered health maintenance related to underlying condition
• Sleep pattern disturbance related to drug-induced insomnia
• Knowledge deficit related to drug therapy

▶ **Planning and implementation**
• Give at least 6 hours before bedtime to avoid sleep interference.
• Know that prolonged administration may cause psychological dependence or habituation, especially in patients with history of drug addiction. After prolonged use, reduce dosage gradually to prevent acute rebound depression, as ordered.
Patient teaching
• Warn patient to avoid activities that require alertness or good psychomotor coordination until CNS effects of drug are known.
• Tell patient to avoid drinks containing caffeine, which increases effects of amphetamines and related amines.
• Inform patient that fatigue may result as drug effects wear off. He will need more rest.
• Instruct patient to report signs of excessive stimulation.
• Inform patient that when tolerance to anorexigenic effect develops, dosage should not be increased, but drug discontinued. Tell him to report decreased effectiveness of drug. Warn patient against stopping drug abruptly.

☑ **Evaluation**
• Patient demonstrates clinical improvement in underlying condition.
• Patient is able to sleep without difficulty.

• Patient and family state understanding of drug therapy.

---

dextromethorphan hydrobromide
(deks-troh-meth-OR-fan
high-droh-BROH-mighd)
Balminil D.M.†, Benylin DM†, Broncho-Grippol-DM♦, Children's Hold†, DM Syrup†, Hold†, Koffex♦, Mediquell†, Neo-DM♦, Ornex-DM 15†, Ornex-DM 30†, Pertussin Cough Suppressant†, Pertussin CS†, Pertussin ES†, Robidex♦, Robitussin Pediatric†, Sedatuss♦, St. Joseph Cough Suppressant for Children†, Sucrets Cough Control Formula†, Trocal†, Vicks Formula 44 Pediatric Formula†

More commonly available in combination products such as: Anti-Tuss DM Expectorant†, Cheracol D Cough†, Extra Action Cough†, Glycotuss dm†, Guiamid D.M. Liquid†, Guiatuss-DM†, Halotussin-DM Expectorant†, Kolephrin GG/DM†, Mytussin DM†, Naldecon Senior DX†, Pertussin All-Night CS†, Rhinosyn-DMX Expectorant†, Robitussin-DM†, Silexin Cough†, Tolu-Sed DM†, Tuss-DM†, Unproco†, Vicks Children's Cough Syrup†

Pharmacologic class: levorphanol derivative (dextrorotatory methyl ether)
Therapeutic class: antitussive (nonnarcotic)
Pregnancy risk category: C

How supplied
Liquid (extended-release): 30 mg/5 ml†
Lozenges: 5 mg†, 7.5 mg†, 15 mg
Solution: 3.5 mg/5 ml, 5 mg/5 ml*†, 7.5 mg/5 ml*†, 10 mg/5 ml*†, 15 mg/5 ml*†

Pharmacokinetics
Absorption: absorbed readily from GI tract.
Distribution: unknown.
Metabolism: metabolized extensively by liver.

Excretion: small amount excreted unchanged. Metabolites excreted primarily in urine; about 7% to 10% excreted in feces. *Half-life:* about 11 hours.

Route	Onset	Peak	Duration
P.O.	≤ 30 min	Unknown	3-12 hr

Pharmacodynamics

Chemical effect: suppresses cough reflex by direct action on cough center in medulla.
Therapeutic effect: prevents cough.

Indications and dosage

▶ **Nonproductive cough.** *Adults and children age 12 and over:* 10 to 20 mg P.O. q 4 hours, or 30 mg q 6 to 8 hours. Or, 60 mg extended-release liquid b.i.d. Maximum dosage is 120 mg daily.
Children ages 6 to 12: 5 to 10 mg P.O. q 4 hours, or 15 mg q 6 to 8 hours. Or, 30 mg extended-release liquid b.i.d. Maximum dosage is 60 mg daily.
Children ages 2 to 6: 2.5 to 5 mg P.O. q 4 hours, or 7.5 mg q 6 to 8 hours. Or, 15 mg extended-release liquid b.i.d. Maximum dosage is 30 mg daily.
   Dosages for children under age 2 must be individualized.

Adverse reactions

CNS: drowsiness, dizziness.
GI: nausea, vomiting, stomach pain.

Interactions

Drug-drug. *MAO inhibitors:* risk of hypotension, coma, hyperpyrexia, and death. Avoid concomitant use.
Selegiline: risk of confusion, coma, hyperpyrexia. Avoid concurrent use.

Contraindications and precautions

• Contraindicated in patients taking MAO inhibitors or within 2 weeks of discontinuing MAO inhibitors.
• Use with caution in atopic children, sedated or debilitated patients, and patients confined to supine position. Also, use cautiously in patients with aspirin sensitivity and in pregnant women.
• Safety of drug has not been established in breast-feeding women.

NURSING CONSIDERATIONS

⚕ Assessment
• Obtain history of patient's cough before and after drug administration.
• Be alert for adverse reactions and drug interactions.
• Evaluate patient's and family's knowledge of drug therapy.

⊕ Nursing diagnoses
• Fatigue related to presence of nonproductive cough
• Risk for injury related to drug-induced adverse CNS reactions
• Knowledge deficit related to drug therapy

❯ Planning and implementation
• Don't use drug when cough is valuable diagnostic sign or is beneficial (as after thoracic surgery).
• Know that 15 to 30 mg of dextromethorphan is equivalent to 8 to 15 mg of codeine as an antitussive.
• Use drug with chest percussion and vibration.
• Notify doctor if cough is unrelieved with drug.
Patient teaching
• Instruct patient to follow directions on medication bottle exactly; stress importance of not taking more of drug than directed.
• Tell patient to call doctor if cough persists more than 7 days.
• Suggest sugarless throat lozenges to decrease throat irritation and resulting cough.
• Advise patient to use humidifier to filter out dust, smoke, and air pollutants.

☑ Evaluation
• Patient's cough is relieved.

Reactions may be *common*, uncommon, *life-threatening*, or COMMON AND LIFE-THREATENING.

• Patient does not experience injury as result of therapy.
• Patient and family state understanding of drug therapy.

dextrose (d-glucose)
(DEKS-tros)

Pharmacologic class: carbohydrate
Therapeutic class: total parenteral nutrition (TPN) component, caloric agent, fluid volume replacement
Pregnancy risk category: C

How supplied

Injection: 3-ml ampule (10%); 5-ml ampule (10%); 10 ml (25%); 50 ml (5% and 50% available in vial, ampule, and Bristoject); 70-ml pin-top vial (70% for additive use only); 100 ml (5%); 250 ml (5%, 10%); 400 ml (5%); 500 ml (5%, 10%, 20%, 30%, 40%, 50%, 60%, 70%); 650 ml (38.5%); 1,000 ml (2.5%, 5%, 10%, 20%, 30%, 40%, 50%, 60%, 70%)

Pharmacokinetics

Absorption: not applicable with I.V. administration.
Distribution: distributed throughout plasma volume.
Metabolism: metabolized to carbon dioxide and water.
Excretion: excess excreted in urine.

Route	Onset	Peak	Duration
I.V.	Immediate	Immediate	Unknown

Pharmacodynamics

Chemical effect: simple water-soluble sugar that minimizes glyconeogenesis and promotes anabolism in patient who can't receive sufficient oral caloric intake.
Therapeutic effect: provides supplemental calories and fluid.

Indications and dosage

▶ **Fluid replacement and caloric supplementation in patients who can't maintain adequate oral intake or who are restricted from doing so.** *Adults and children:* dosage depends on fluid and caloric requirements. Peripheral I.V. infusion of 2.5%, 5%, or 10% solution or central I.V. infusion of 20% solution is used for minimal fluid needs; 25% solution is used to treat acute hypoglycemia in neonate or older infant; 50% solution is used to treat insulin-induced hypoglycemia; 10%, 20%, 30%, 40%, 50%, 60%, and 70% solutions diluted in admixtures, normally amino acid solutions, for TPN are given through the central vein.

Adverse reactions

CNS: confusion, *unconsciousness in hyperosmolar hyperglycemic nonketotic syndrome.*
CV: *pulmonary edema, exacerbated hypertension, heart failure* (with fluid overload in susceptible patients); *phlebitis, venous sclerosis,* tissue necrosis (with prolonged or concentrated infusions, especially with peripheral administration).
GU: glycosuria, osmotic diuresis.
Metabolic: hyperglycemia, hypervolemia, hyperosmolarity (with rapid infusion of concentrated solution or prolonged infusion); hypoglycemia from rebound hyperinsulinemia (rapid termination of long-term infusions).
Skin: sloughing, tissue necrosis (if extravasation occurs with concentrated solutions).

Interactions

Drug-drug. *Corticosteroids:* may cause salt and water retention and increased potassium excretion. Monitor glucose, sodium, and potassium.

Contraindications and precautions

• Contraindicated in patients in diabetic coma, while blood glucose level remains

excessively high. Use of concentrated solutions is contraindicated in patients with intracranial or intraspinal hemorrhage, in dehydrated patients with delirium tremens, and in patients with severe dehydration, anuria, hepatic coma, or glucose-galactose malabsorption syndrome.
• Use cautiously in patients with cardiac or pulmonary disease, hypertension, renal insufficiency, urinary obstruction, or hypovolemia.

NURSING CONSIDERATIONS

⚕ Assessment
• Obtain history of patient's underlying condition before therapy, and reassess regularly throughout therapy.
• Be alert for adverse reactions.
• Evaluate patient's and family's knowledge of drug therapy.

⊞ Nursing diagnoses
• Altered nutrition: less than body requirements related to underlying condition
• Altered health maintenance related to drug-induced hyperglycemia
• Knowledge deficit related to drug therapy

⊠ Planning and implementation
• Control infusion rate carefully; maximal rate is 0.5 g/kg/hour. Use infusion pump when infusing with amino acids for TPN. Never infuse concentrated solutions rapidly; this may cause hyperglycemia and fluid shift.
• Don't give dextrose solutions without NaCl solution in blood transfusions; this may cause clumping of RBCs. Use central veins to infuse dextrose solutions with concentrations greater than 10%.
• Take care to prevent extravasation.
• Never stop hypertonic solutions abruptly. If necessary, have dextrose 10% in water solution available to treat hypoglycemia if rebound hyperinsulinemia occurs.

Patient teaching
• Inform patient of need for dextrose therapy, how it will be administered, and what adverse reactions to report.

⚕ Evaluation
• Patient exhibits improvement of underlying condition.
• Patient maintains normal blood glucose level throughout therapy.
• Patient and family state understanding of drug therapy.

dezocine
(DEZ-oh-seen)
Dalgan

Pharmacologic class: opioid (narcotic) agonist-antagonist
Therapeutic class: analgesic
Pregnancy risk category: C

How supplied
Injection: 5 mg/ml, 10 mg/ml, 15 mg/ml

Pharmacokinetics
Absorption: rapidly and completely absorbed after I.M. administration.
Distribution: unknown.
Metabolism: unknown, although thought to be hepatic.
Excretion: excreted primarily in urine.
Half-life: about 2.4 hours.

Route	Onset	Peak	Duration
I.V.	≤ 15 min	0.5-2.5 hr	Unknown
I.M.	≤ 30 min	0.5-2.5 hr	Unknown

Pharmacodynamics
Chemical effect: unknown; produces postoperative analgesia qualitatively similar to that produced by morphine.
Therapeutic effect: relieves pain.

Indications and dosage
▶ **Management of moderate to severe pain.** *Adults:* 5 to 20 mg I.M. q 3 to 6 hours or 2.5 to 10.0 mg I.V. q 2 to 4

hours. Maximum recommended single I.M. dose is 20 mg, with maximum daily dosage of 120 mg. Maximum dosage for I.V. use has not been determined.

Adverse reactions

CNS: *sedation, dizziness, vertigo,* anxiety, mood disorders, sleep disturbances, headache, slurred speech.
CV: edema, hypotension, irregular heartbeat, hypertension, chest pain, thrombophlebitis.
GI: *nausea, vomiting,* constipation, diarrhea, abdominal distress, dry mouth.
Hematologic: low hemoglobin level.
Respiratory: *respiratory depression.*
Skin: rash, pruritus, *irritation at injection site.*
Other: sweating, chills, flushing, pallor.

Interactions

Drug-drug. *CNS depressants:* may increase risk of CNS depression. Monitor patient closely.
Opioids: opioid-dependent patients may experience withdrawal symptoms after receiving dezocine; may increase risk of CNS depression. Avoid concomitant use.
Drug-lifestyle. *Alcohol use:* may increase risk of CNS depression. Avoid concomitant use.

Contraindications and precautions

• Contraindicated in patients with hypersensitivity to drug and in those physically dependent on narcotics.
• Because it is not known if dezocine is excreted in breast milk, breast-feeding is not recommended.
• Drug is not recommended for patients with chronic pain because of limited clinical experience and because drug can precipitate withdrawal syndrome in patients with substantial tolerance to opioids.
• Use with extreme caution in patients with head injury because drug's CNS depressant effects may obscure clinical signs.
• Use cautiously and in lower doses in patients with chronic respiratory disease

and in patients undergoing biliary surgery.
• Administer with caution to elderly patients, those who have recently received substantial amounts of narcotic medication, and pregnant women.
• Use cautiously in patients with renal or hepatic failure.

NURSING CONSIDERATIONS

⚗ Assessment
• Obtain history of patient's pain before therapy, and reassess regularly thereafter.
• Be alert for adverse reactions and drug interactions.
• Monitor patient for allergic reactions. The injection contains sulfite preservatives, which may cause allergic reactions in certain sensitive patients.
• Be aware that plasma concentrations higher than 45 ng/ml are associated with increased incidence of adverse reactions.
• Evaluate patient's and family's knowledge of drug therapy.

⊞ Nursing diagnoses
• Pain related to underlying condition
• Ineffective breathing pattern related to drug-induced respiratory depression
• Knowledge deficit related to drug therapy

⊠ Planning and implementation
• Dezocine produces dose-dependent respiratory depression similar to that produced by morphine. Use only in clinical settings where adequate respiratory support and opioid antagonist (naloxone) are available to reverse respiratory depression.
I.V. use: Give drug by direct injection into large vein. Avoid mixing with other drugs because there is little information regarding drug and solution compatibility. Infuse over at least 5 minutes.
I.M. use: Follow normal protocol.
• Notify doctor and discuss increase of dosage or frequency if pain is not relieved.

• Hold dose and notify doctor if patient's respirations are below 12 breaths/minute.
Patient teaching
• Caution ambulatory patient about getting out of bed or walking. Warn outpatient to refrain from driving and performing other potentially hazardous activities that require mental alertness until drug's CNS effects are known.

☑ **Evaluation**
• Patient is free from pain.
• Patient maintains effective respiratory pattern throughout therapy.
• Patient and family state understanding of drug therapy.

diazepam
(digh-AZ-uh-pam)
Apo-Diazepam♦, Diazemuls♦◇, Diazepam Intensol, Novo-Dipam♦, PMS-Diazepam♦, Valium, Valrelease, Vivol♦, Zetran

Pharmacologic class: benzodiazepine
Therapeutic class: antianxiety, skeletal muscle relaxant, anticonvulsant, sedative-hypnotic agent
Controlled substance schedule: IV
Pregnancy risk category: D

How supplied
Tablets: 2 mg, 5 mg, 10 mg
Capsules (extended-release): 15 mg
Oral solution: 5 mg/ml, 5 mg/5 ml
Injection: 5 mg/ml
Sterile emulsion for injection: 5 mg/ml♦

Pharmacokinetics
Absorption: when administered P.O., absorbed through GI tract. I.M. administration results in erratic absorption.
Distribution: distributed widely throughout body; about 85% to 95% bound to plasma protein.
Metabolism: metabolized in liver to active metabolite, desmethyldiazepam.

Excretion: most metabolites of diazepam excreted in urine, with only small amount excreted in feces. *Half-life:* 30 to 200 hours.

Route	Onset	Peak	Duration
P.O.	30 min	0.5-2 hr	3-8 hr
I.V.	1-5 min	≤ 15 min	15-60 min
I.M.	Unknown	2 hr	Unknown

Pharmacodynamics
Chemical effect: unknown; probably depresses CNS at limbic and subcortical levels of brain; suppresses spread of seizure activity produced by epileptogenic foci in cortex, thalamus, and limbic structures.
Therapeutic effect: relieves anxiety, muscle spasms, and seizures (parenteral form); promotes calmness and sleep.

Indications and dosage
▶ **Anxiety.** *Adults:* depending on severity, 2 to 10 mg P.O. b.i.d. to q.i.d. or 15 to 30 mg extended-release capsules once daily. Alternatively, 2 to 10 mg I.M. or I.V. q 3 to 4 hours, if needed. *Children age 6 months and older:* 1.0 to 2.5 mg P.O. t.i.d or q.i.d., increased gradually as needed and tolerated.
▶ **Acute alcohol withdrawal.** *Adults:* 10 mg P.O. t.i.d. or q.i.d. first 24 hours, reduced to 5 mg P.O. t.i.d. or q.i.d., p.r.n. Alternatively, initially, 10 mg I.M. or I.V., then 5 to 10 mg I.M. or I.V. in 3 to 4 hours, if necessary.
▶ **Before endoscopic procedures.** *Adults:* I.V. dose titrated to desired sedative response (up to 20 mg). Alternatively, 5 to 10 mg I.M. 30 minutes before procedure.
▶ **Muscle spasm.** *Adults:* 2 to 10 mg P.O. b.i.d. to q.i.d. daily or 15 to 30 mg extended-release capsules once daily. Alternatively, 5 to 10 mg I.M. or I.V. initially, then 5 to 10 mg I.M. or I.V. in 3 to 4 hours, p.r.n. For tetanus, larger doses may be required. *Children age 5 or older:* 5 to 10 mg I.M. or I.V. q 3 to 4 hours, p.r.n. *Children over age 30 days to 5*

years: 1 to 2 mg I.M. or I.V. slowly repeated q 3 to 4 hours, p.r.n.
▶ **Preoperative sedation.** *Adults:* 10 mg I.M. (preferred) or I.V. before surgery.
▶ **Cardioversion.** *Adults:* 5 to 15 mg I.V. within 5 to 10 minutes before procedure.
▶ **Adjunct in seizure disorders.** *Adults:* 2 to 10 mg P.O. b.i.d. to q.i.d.. *Children age 6 months and older:* 1.0 to 2.5 mg P.O. t.i.d. or q.i.d initially; increased as tolerated and needed.
▶ **Status epilepticus and severe recurrent seizures.** *Adults:* 5 to 10 mg I.V. (preferred) or I.M. initially. Repeated q 10 to 15 minutes, p.r.n., up to maximum dose of 30 mg. Repeated in 2 to 4 hours, p.r.n. *Children age 5 and older:* 1 mg I.V. q 2 to 5 minutes up to maximum of 10 mg. Repeated in 2 to 4 hours, p.r.n. *Children over age 30 days to 5 years:* 0.2 to 0.5 mg I.V. slowly q 2 to 5 minutes up to maximum of 5 mg. Repeated in 2 to 4 hours, p.r.n.

Adverse reactions

CNS: *drowsiness, lethargy, hangover,* *ataxia,* fainting, depression, restlessness, anterograde amnesia, psychosis, slurred speech, tremors, headache, insomnia.
CV: transient hypotension, *bradycardia, CV collapse.*
EENT: diplopia, blurred vision, nystagmus.
GI: nausea, vomiting, abdominal discomfort, constipation.
GU: incontinence, urine retention.
Respiratory: *respiratory depression.*
Skin: rash, urticaria, desquamation.
Other: physical or psychological dependence, *acute withdrawal syndrome* after sudden discontinuation in physically dependent people, *pain, phlebitis at injection site.*

Interactions

Drug-drug. *Cimetidine:* increased sedation. Monitor patient carefully.
CNS depressants: increased CNS depression. Avoid concomitant use.

Digoxin: may increase serum levels of digoxin, increasing toxicity. Monitor patient closely.
Phenobarbital: increased effects of both drugs. Use together cautiously.
Drug-lifestyle. *Alcohol use:* increased CNS depression. Avoid concomitant use.
Smoking: increased clearance of benzodiazepines. Monitor for lack of effect.

Contraindications and precautions

● Contraindicated in patients with angle-closure glaucoma or hypersensitivity to drug; in those experiencing shock, coma, or acute alcohol intoxication (parenteral form); and in children under age 6 months (oral form).
● Avoid use of drug in pregnant women, especially during the first trimester, and in breast-feeding women.
● Use cautiously in patients with hepatic or renal impairment, depression, or chronic open-angle glaucoma and in elderly and debilitated patients.
● Dosage should be reduced in elderly or debilitated patients because they may be more susceptible to adverse CNS effects of drug.

NURSING CONSIDERATIONS

🌡 Assessment
● Obtain history of patient's underlying condition before therapy, and reassess regularly thereafter.
● Monitor respirations every 5 to 15 minutes and before each repeated I.V. dose.
● Periodically monitor liver, kidney, and hematopoietic function studies in patient receiving repeated or prolonged therapy, as ordered.
● Be alert for adverse reactions and drug interactions.
● Evaluate patient's and family's knowledge of drug therapy.

🔲 Nursing diagnoses
● Altered health maintenance related to underlying condition

• Risk for injury related to drug-induced adverse CNS reactions
• Knowledge deficit related to drug therapy

▶ **Planning and implementation**
P.O. use: When oral concentrate solution is used, dilute dose just before administering. Use water, juice, or carbonated beverages, or mix with semisolid food, such as applesauce or pudding.
I.V. use: Give drug at rate not exceeding 5 mg/minute. When injecting, administer directly into vein. If this is impossible, inject slowly through infusion tubing as near to vein insertion site as possible. Watch daily for phlebitis at injection site.
• Avoid extravasation. Do not inject into small veins.
• Have emergency resuscitation equipment and oxygen at bedside when administering drug I.V.
I.M. use: I.M. administration is not recommended because absorption is variable and injection is painful. Used only when I.V. route and P.O. route are not applicable.
• Do not mix injectable form with other drugs because diazepam is incompatible with most drugs.
• Do not store parenteral solution in plastic syringes.
• Parenteral emulsion—a stabilized oil-in-water emulsion—should appear milky white and uniform. Avoid mixing with any other drugs or solutions, and avoid infusion sets or containers made from polyvinyl chloride. If dilution is necessary, drug may be mixed with I.V. fat emulsion. Use admixture within 6 hours.
• Possibility of abuse and addiction exists. Do not withdraw drug abruptly after long-term use; withdrawal symptoms may occur.
• Institute safety measures.
Patient teaching
• Warn patient to avoid activities that require alertness and good psychomotor coordination until CNS effects of drug are known.

• Tell patient to avoid alcohol during drug therapy.
• Warn patient to take this drug only as directed and not to discontinue it without doctor's approval. Inform patient of drug's potential for causing dependence if taken longer than directed.

☑ **Evaluation**
• Patient exhibits improvement in underlying condition.
• Patient does not experience injury as result of drug-induced adverse CNS reactions.
• Patient and family state understanding of drug therapy.

diazoxide
(digh-uz-OKS-ighd)
Hyperstat IV

Pharmacologic class: peripheral vasodilator
Therapeutic class: antihypertensive
Pregnancy risk category: C

How supplied
Injection: 15 mg/ml, 300 mg/20 ml

Pharmacokinetics
Absorption: not applicable with I.V. administration.
Distribution: distributed throughout body; about 90% protein-bound.
Metabolism: metabolized partially in liver.
Excretion: diazoxide and its metabolites excreted slowly by kidneys. *Half-life:* 21 to 36 hours.

Route	Onset	Peak	Duration
I.V.	≤ 1 min	2-5 min	2-12 hr

Pharmacodynamics
Chemical effect: unknown; directly relaxes arteriolar smooth muscle and decreases peripheral vascular resistance.

Therapeutic effect: lowers blood pressure.

Indications and dosage

▶ **Hypertensive crisis.** *Adults and children:* 1 to 3 mg/kg by I.V. bolus (up to maximum of 150 mg) q 5 to 15 minutes until adequate response is seen. Repeat at 4- to 24-hour intervals, p.r.n.

Adverse reactions

CNS: *headache,* dizziness, light-headedness, euphoria, *cerebral ischemia, seizures, paralysis.*
CV: *sodium and water retention, orthostatic hypotension,* diaphoresis, flushing, warmth, angina, myocardial ischemia, *arrhythmias,* ECG changes, *shock, MI.*
GI: *nausea, vomiting,* abdominal discomfort, dry mouth, constipation, diarrhea.
Hematologic: *thrombocytopenia.*
Metabolic: *hyperglycemia,* hyperuricemia.
Other: inflammation, pain (resulting from extravasation).

Interactions

Drug-drug. *Antihypertensives:* may cause severe hypotension. Use together cautiously.
Hydantoins: may decrease levels of hydantoins, resulting in decreased anticonvulsant action. Monitor closely.
Sulfonylureas: may cause hyperglycemia. Monitor serum glucose levels.
Thiazide diuretics: may increase diazoxide's effects. Use together cautiously.

Contraindications and precautions

• Contraindicated in patients with hypersensitivity to drug, other thiazides, or other sulfonamide-derived drugs. Also contraindicated in treatment of compensatory hypertension (such as in coarctation of the aorta or arteriovenous shunt).
• Use of drug not recommended in breast-feeding women.
• Use cautiously in patients with impaired cerebral or cardiac function or uremia and in pregnant women.

NURSING CONSIDERATIONS

⚖ Assessment
• Obtain history of patient's blood pressure before therapy.
• Monitor effectiveness by monitoring blood pressure and ECG continuously during drug administration.
• Weigh patient daily.
• Monitor blood glucose level daily; watch closely for signs of severe hyperglycemia or hyperosmolar nonketotic syndrome.
• Check patient's uric acid levels frequently, as ordered.
• Be alert for adverse reactions and drug interactions.
• Evaluate patient's and family's knowledge of drug therapy.

⊕ Nursing diagnoses
• Risk for injury related to presence of hypertension
• Fluid volume excess related to drug-induced fluid retention
• Knowledge deficit related to drug therapy

❯ Planning and implementation
• Place patient in supine position or in Trendelenburg's position during and for 1 hour after infusion.
• Protect I.V. solutions from light. Darkened I.V. solutions of diazoxide are subpotent and should not be used.
• Take care to avoid extravasation.
• Check patient's standing blood pressure before discontinuing drug.
• Notify doctor immediately if severe hypotension develops and keep norepinephrine available.
• Know that if fluid or sodium retention develops, doctor may order diuretics.
Patient teaching
• Inform patient that orthostatic hypotension can be minimized by rising slowly and avoiding sudden position changes. Instruct patient to remain in supine position for 30 minutes after injection.

☑ **Evaluation**
• Patient's blood pressure returns to normal.
• Patient maintains normal fluid and electrolyte balance during therapy.
• Patient and family state understanding of drug therapy.

diclofenac potassium
(digh-KLOH-fen-ek poh-TAH-see-um)
Cataflam

diclofenac sodium
Voltaren, Voltaren SR♦, Voltaren-XR

Pharmacologic class: NSAID
Therapeutic class: antiarthritic, anti-inflammatory
Pregnancy risk category: B

How supplied
diclofenac potassium
Tablets: 50 mg
diclofenac sodium
Tablets (delayed-release/enteric-coated): 25 mg, 50 mg, 75 mg
Tablets (extended-release): 100 mg♦
Suppositories: 50 mg♦, 100 mg♦

Pharmacokinetics
Absorption: after P.O. or P.R. administration, rapidly and almost completely absorbed. Absorption is delayed by food.
Distribution: highly (nearly 100%) protein-bound.
Metabolism: undergoes first-pass metabolism, with 60% of unchanged drug reaching systemic circulation.
Excretion: about 40% to 60% excreted in urine; balance is excreted in bile. *Half-life:* 1.2 to 1.8 hours after P.O. dose.

Route	Onset	Peak	Duration
P.O., P.R.	30 min	Unknown	8 hr
P.O. (enteric-coated)	30 min	2-3 hr	8 hr

Pharmacodynamics
Chemical effect: unknown; produces anti-inflammatory, analgesic, and antipyretic effects, possibly by inhibiting prostaglandin synthesis.
Therapeutic effect: relieves inflammation, pain, and fever.

Indications and dosage
▶ **Ankylosing spondylitis.** *Adults:* 25 mg P.O. q.i.d. (and h.s., p.r.n.).
▶ **Osteoarthritis.** Diclofenac sodium. *Adults:* 50 mg P.O. b.i.d. or t.i.d., or 75 mg P.O. b.i.d.
▶ **Rheumatoid arthritis.** *Adults:* 50 mg P.O. t.i.d. or q.i.d. Alternatively, 75 mg P.O. b.i.d. (diclofenac sodium only) or 50 to 100 mg P.R. (where available) h.s. as substitute for last P.O. dose of day. Not to exceed 225 mg daily.
▶ **Analgesia and primary dysmenorrhea.** Diclofenac potassium. *Adults:* 50 mg P.O. t.i.d.

Adverse reactions
CNS: anxiety, depression, dizziness, drowsiness, insomnia, irritability, myoclonus, migraine, *headache.*
CV: *heart failure,* hypertension, edema, fluid retention.
EENT: *tinnitus, laryngeal edema,* swelling of lips and tongue, blurred vision, eye pain, night blindness, epistaxis, taste disorder, reversible hearing loss.
GI: *abdominal pain or cramps, constipation, diarrhea, indigestion, nausea,* abdominal distention, flatulence, peptic ulceration, *bleeding,* melena, bloody diarrhea, appetite change, colitis.
GU: azotemia, proteinuria, *acute renal failure,* oliguria, interstitial nephritis, papillary necrosis, *nephrotic syndrome, fluid retention.*
Hepatic: elevated liver enzyme levels, jaundice, *hepatitis, hepatotoxicity.*
Metabolic: hypoglycemia; hyperglycemia.
Musculoskeletal: back, leg, or joint pain.
Respiratory: asthma.

Reactions may be *common,* uncommon, *life-threatening,* or COMMON AND LIFE-THREATENING.

Skin: rash, pruritus, urticaria, eczema, dermatitis, alopecia, photosensitivity, bullous eruption, *Stevens-Johnson syndrome* (rare), allergic purpura.
Other: *anaphylaxis; anaphylactoid reactions,* angioedema.

Interactions

Drug-drug. *Anticoagulants, including warfarin:* possibly increased incidence of bleeding. Monitor patient closely.
Aspirin: may increase risk of bleeding. Concomitant use not recommended by manufacturer.
Beta blockers: antihypertensive effect may be blunted. Monitor closely.
Cyclosporine, digoxin, lithium, methotrexate: diclofenac may reduce renal clearance of these drugs and increase risk of toxicity. Monitor patient closely.
Diuretics: decreased effectiveness of diuretics. Monitor patient closely.
Insulin, oral antidiabetic agents: diclofenac may alter requirements for antidiabetic agents. Monitor patient closely.
Phenytoin: increased serum levels. Monitor for toxicity.
Potassium-sparing diuretics: enhanced potassium retention and increased serum potassium levels. Monitor for hyperkalemia.
Drug-lifestyle. *Sun exposure:* may cause photosensitivity reactions; take precautions.

Contraindications and precautions

• Contraindicated in patients with history of asthma, urticaria, or other allergic reactions after taking aspirin or other NSAIDs; hypersensitivity to drug; or hepatic porphyria. Drug is not recommended for use during late pregnancy or breast-feeding.
• Use cautiously in patients with history of peptic ulcer disease, hepatic dysfunction, cardiac disease, hypertension, conditions associated with fluid retention, or impaired kidney function.
• Safety of drug has not been established in children.

NURSING CONSIDERATIONS

⚖ Assessment
• Obtain history of patient's underlying condition before therapy.
• Monitor effectiveness by assessing patient for pain relief.
• Know that liver test results may become elevated during therapy. Monitor serum transaminase levels, especially ALT levels, periodically in patients undergoing long-term therapy, as ordered. First serum transaminase measurement should be no later than 8 weeks after initiation of therapy.
• Be alert for adverse reactions and drug interactions.
• Evaluate patient's and family's knowledge of drug therapy.

❖ Nursing diagnoses
• Pain related to underlying condition
• Risk for injury related to drug-induced adverse reactions
• Knowledge deficit related to drug therapy

❱ Planning and implementation
P.O. use: Administer drug with milk or food if GI distress occurs.
• Notify doctor immediately if patient develops signs of GI bleeding or hepatotoxicity or other adverse reactions.
P.R. use: Not commercially available in the United States. May be substituted for the last oral dose of the day.
Patient teaching
• Tell patient to take drug with milk or food to minimize GI distress.
• Instruct patient not to crush, break, or chew enteric-coated tablets.
• Teach patient signs and symptoms of GI bleeding, and tell him to contact doctor immediately if they occur.
• Teach patient signs and symptoms of hepatotoxicity, including nausea, fatigue, lethargy, pruritus, jaundice, right upper quadrant tenderness, and flulike symptoms. Tell him to contact doctor immediately if these symptoms appear.

• Tell pregnant patient to avoid use of drug during last trimester.

☑ **Evaluation**
• Patient is free from pain.
• Patient does not experience injury as result of drug-induced adverse reactions.
• Patient and family state understanding of drug therapy.

dicloxacillin sodium
(digh-kloks-uh-SIL-in SOH-dee-um)
Dycill, Dynapen, Pathocil

Pharmacologic class: penicillinase-resistant penicillin
Therapeutic class: antibiotic
Pregnancy risk category: B

How supplied
Capsules: 125 mg, 250 mg, 500 mg
Oral suspension: 62.5 mg/5 ml (after reconstitution)

Pharmacokinetics
Absorption: absorbed rapidly but incompletely (35% to 76%) from GI tract; food may decrease both rate and extent of absorption.
Distribution: distributed widely in bone, bile, and pleural and synovial fluids. CSF penetration is poor but is enhanced by meningeal inflammation. Drug is 95% to 99% protein-bound.
Metabolism: metabolized only partially.
Excretion: dicloxacillin and metabolites excreted in urine. *Half-life:* 30 to 60 minutes.

Route	Onset	Peak	Duration
P.O.	Unknown	0.5-2 hr	About 6 hr

Pharmacodynamics
Chemical effect: inhibits cell wall synthesis during microorganism multiplication. Bacteria resist penicillins by producing penicillinases—enzymes that convert penicillins to inactive penicilloic acid. Dicloxacillin resists these enzymes. *Therapeutic effect:* kills susceptible bacteria. Spectrum of activity includes many strains of penicillinase-producing bacteria. This activity is most important against penicillinase-producing staphylococci; some strains may remain resistant. Dicloxacillin is also active against few gram-positive aerobic and anaerobic bacilli but has no significant effect on gram-negative bacilli.

Indications and dosage
▶ **Systemic infections caused by penicillinase-producing staphylococci.**
Adults and children weighing over 40 kg (88 lb): 125 to 250 mg P.O. q 6 hours. *Children weighing 40 kg or less:* 25 to 50 mg/kg P.O. daily in divided doses q 6 hours.

Adverse reactions
CNS: neuromuscular irritability, *seizures*, lethargy, hallucinations, anxiety, confusion, agitation, depression, dizziness, fatigue.
GI: *nausea,* vomiting, *epigastric distress,* flatulence, *diarrhea,* enterocolitis, pseudomembranous colitis, black "hairy" tongue, abdominal pain.
Hematologic: eosinophilia, anemia, *thrombocytopenia, agranulocytosis, leukopenia,* hemolytic anemia.
Other: *hypersensitivity reactions* (pruritus, urticaria, rash, *anaphylaxis*), overgrowth of nonsusceptible organisms.

Interactions
Drug-drug. *Oral contraceptives:* efficacy of oral contraceptives may be decreased. Additional form of contraception recommended during penicillin therapy. *Probenecid:* increased blood levels of dicloxacillin and other penicillins. Probenecid may be used for this purpose.

Contraindications and precautions
• Contraindicated in patients with hypersensitivity to drug or other penicillins.

Reactions may be *common,* uncommon, *life-threatening*, or COMMON AND LIFE-THREATENING.

• Use cautiously in patients with other drug allergies, especially to cephalosporins (possible cross-sensitivity), and in those with mononucleosis (high incidence of maculopapular rash).
• Also use cautiously in pregnant or breast-feeding women.

NURSING CONSIDERATIONS

⚕ Assessment
• Obtain history of patient's infection before therapy, and reassess regularly thereafter.
• Before giving drug, ask patient about any allergic reactions to penicillin. Negative history of penicillin allergy is no guarantee against future allergic reactions.
• Obtain specimen for culture and sensitivity tests before first dose. Therapy may begin, pending test results.
• As ordered, periodically assess renal, hepatic, and hematopoietic function in patients receiving long-term therapy.
• Be alert for adverse reactions and drug interactions.
• Monitor patient's hydration status if adverse GI reactions occur.
• Evaluate patient's and family's knowledge of drug therapy.

🔷 Nursing diagnoses
• Infection related to presence of susceptible bacteria
• Risk for fluid volume deficit related to drug-induced adverse GI reactions
• Knowledge deficit related to drug therapy

⊵ Planning and implementation
• Give drug 1 to 2 hours before or 2 to 3 hours after meals. It may cause GI disturbances. Food may interfere with absorption.
• Give drug at least 1 hour before bacteriostatic antibiotics.
• Notify doctor if adverse reactions occur, especially rash, because dicloxacillin

may need to be discontinued and another antibiotic substituted.
Patient teaching
• Tell patient to take entire quantity of medication exactly as prescribed, even after he feels better.
• Tell patient to call doctor if rash develops.
• Warn patient not to use leftover drug for new illness or share it with others.

☑ Evaluation
• Patient is free from infection.
• Patient maintains adequate hydration throughout therapy.
• Patient and family state understanding of drug therapy.

dicyclomine hydrochloride
(digh-SIGH-kloh-meen high-droh-KLOR-ighd)
Antispas, Bemote, Bentyl, Bentylol◆, Byclomine, Dibent, Dilomine, Di-Spaz, Formulex◆, Lomine◆, Neoquess, Or-Tyl, Spasmoban◆, Spasmoject

Pharmacologic class: anticholinergic
Therapeutic class: antimuscarinic, GI antispasmodic
Pregnancy risk category: B

How supplied
Tablets: 10 mg◇, 20 mg
Capsules: 10 mg, 20 mg
Syrup: 5 mg/5 ml◇, 10 mg/5 ml
Injection: 10 mg/ml

Pharmacokinetics
Absorption: about 67% of P.O. dose absorbed from GI tract; unknown after I.M. administration.
Distribution: unknown.
Metabolism: unknown.
Excretion: after P.O. administration, 80% excreted in urine and 10% in feces; unknown after I.M. administration. *Half-life:* initial, 1.8 hours; secondary, 9 to 10 hours.

Route	Onset	Peak	Duration
P.O.	Unknown	1-1.5 hr	Unknown
I.M.	Unknown	Unknown	Unknown

Pharmacodynamics

Chemical effect: unknown; appears to exert nonspecific, nondirect spasmolytic action on smooth muscle. Dicyclomine also possesses local anesthetic properties that may be partly responsible for spasmolysis.
Therapeutic effect: relieves GI spasms.

Indications and dosage

▶ **Irritable bowel syndrome and other functional GI disorders.** *Adults:* initially, 20 mg P.O. q.i.d., increased to 40 mg q.i.d.; or 20 mg I.M. q 4 to 6 hours. *Children age 2 and older:* 10 mg P.O. t.i.d. or q.i.d. *Children ages 6 months to 2 years:* 5 to 10 mg P.O. t.i.d. or q.i.d.

Adverse reactions

CNS: *headache, dizziness,* insomnia, drowsiness; nervousness, confusion, excitement (in elderly patients).
CV: *palpitations,* tachycardia.
EENT: blurred vision, increased intraocular pressure, mydriasis.
GI: nausea, vomiting, *constipation, dry mouth,* abdominal distention, heartburn, paralytic ileus.
GU: *urinary hesitancy, urine retention,* impotence.
Skin: urticaria, decreased sweating or possibly anhidrosis, other dermal manifestations.
Other: fever, allergic reactions.
Note: Drug is synthetic tertiary derivative that may have atropine-like adverse reactions. Overdose may cause curare-like effects, such as respiratory paralysis.

Interactions

Drug-drug. *Amantadine, antihistamines, antiparkinsonian agents, disopyramide, glutethimide, meperidine, phenothiazines, procainamide, quinidine, tricyclic antidepressants:* additive adverse effects. Avoid concomitant use.

Antacids: decreased absorption of oral anticholinergics. Separate administration times by 2 to 3 hours.
Ketoconazole: anticholinergics may interfere with ketoconazole absorption. Avoid concomitant use.
Methotrimeprazine: anticholinergics may enhance risk of extrapyramidal reactions. Avoid concomitant use.

Contraindications and precautions

• Contraindicated in patients with obstructive uropathy, obstructive disease of GI tract, reflux esophagitis, severe ulcerative colitis, myasthenia gravis, unstable CV status in acute hemorrhage, glaucoma, or hypersensitivity to anticholinergics. Also contraindicated in breastfeeding women and in children under age 6 months.
• Use cautiously in patients with autonomic neuropathy, hyperthyroidism, coronary artery disease, arrhythmias, heart failure, hypertension, hiatal hernia, hepatic or renal disease, prostatic hypertrophy, ulcerative colitis, and during pregnancy.

NURSING CONSIDERATIONS

⚗ Assessment
• Obtain history of patient's underlying condition before therapy.
• Monitor effectiveness by regularly evaluating for pain relief and improvement of underlying condition.
• Be alert for adverse reactions and drug interactions.
• Evaluate patient's and family's knowledge of drug therapy.

⚙ Nursing diagnoses
• Pain related to underlying condition
• Risk for injury related to drug-induced adverse CNS reactions
• Knowledge deficit related to drug therapy

Reactions may be *common*, uncommon, *life-threatening*, or COMMON AND LIFE-THREATENING.

⯈ Planning and implementation

P.O. use: Give 30 to 60 minutes before meals and at bedtime. Bedtime dose can be larger; give at least 2 hours after last meal of day.

I.M. use: Follow normal protocol.

• Do not use S.C. or I.V.

• Be prepared to adjust dosage according to patient's needs and response, as ordered. Doses up to 40 mg P.O. q.i.d. have been used in adults, but safety and efficacy for more than 2 weeks have not been established.

Patient teaching

• Instruct patient to refrain from driving and performing other hazardous activities if he is drowsy or dizzy or has blurred vision; to drink plenty of fluids to help prevent constipation; and to report rash or skin eruption.

• Tell patient to use sugarless gum or hard candy to relieve dry mouth.

☑ Evaluation

• Patient is free from pain.

• Patient does not experience injury as a result of drug-induced adverse CNS reactions.

• Patient and family state understanding of drug therapy.

---

didanosine (ddI)
(digh-DAN-uh-zeen)
Videx

Pharmacologic class: purine analogue
Therapeutic class: antiviral
Pregnancy risk category: B

How supplied

Tablets (chewable): 25 mg, 50 mg, 100 mg, 150 mg
Powder for oral solution (buffered): 100 mg/packet, 167 mg/packet, 250 mg/packet, 375 mg/packet
Powder for oral solution (pediatric): 10 mg/ml in 2- and 4-g bottles

Pharmacokinetics

Absorption: degrades rapidly in gastric acid. Commercially available preparations contain buffers to raise stomach pH. Bioavailability averages about 33%; tablets may exhibit better bioavailability than buffered powder for oral solution. Food can decrease absorption by 50%.

Distribution: widely distributed; drug penetration into CNS varies, but CSF levels average 46% of concurrent plasma levels.

Metabolism: not fully understood; probably similar to that of endogenous purines.

Excretion: excreted in urine. *Half-life:* 0.8 hours.

Route	Onset	Peak	Duration
P.O.	Unknown	0.5-1 hr	Unknown

Pharmacodynamics

Chemical effect: unknown; appears to inhibit replication of HIV by preventing DNA replication.

Therapeutic effect: inhibits replication of HIV.

Indications and dosage

⯈ **Treatment of HIV infection when antiretroviral therapy is warranted.**
Adults weighing 60 kg (132 lb) and over: 200 mg (tablets) P.O. q 12 hours; or 250 mg buffered powder q 12 hours.
Adults weighing below 60 kg: 125 mg (one 100-mg tablet and one 25-mg tablet) P.O. q 12 hours; or 167 mg buffered powder q 12 hours. *Children:* 120 mg/m^2 P.O. q 12 hours.

Adverse reactions

CNS: *headache,* insomnia, *dizziness, seizures,* confusion, anxiety, nervousness, hypertonia, abnormal thinking, twitching, depression, asthenia, pain, *peripheral neuropathy.*
CV: hypertension, edema, hyperlipemia, *heart failure.*
GI: *diarrhea, nausea, vomiting, abdominal pain, pancreatitis,* dry mouth, dyspepsia, flatulence.

Hematologic: *thrombocytopenia,*
leukopenia, granulocytosis, anemia.
Hepatic: liver abnormalities, *hepatic*
failure.
Musculoskeletal: myalgia, arthritis, myopathy.
Respiratory: cough, dyspnea, pneumonia.
Skin: rash, pruritus, alopecia.
Other: infection, sarcoma, *allergic reac-*
tion, increased serum uric acid levels,
chills, fever.

Interactions

Drug-drug. *Antacids containing magne-*
sium or aluminum hydroxides: enhanced
adverse effects of antacid component (including diarrhea or constipation) when
administered with didanosine tablets or
pediatric suspension. Avoid concomitant
use.
Dapsone, ketoconazole, drugs that re-
quire gastric acid for adequate absorp-
tion: decreased absorption from buffering
action. Administer these drugs 2 hours
before didanosine.
Fluoroquinolones, tetracyclines: decreased absorption from buffering agents
in didanosine tablets or antacids in pediatric suspension. Monitor for decreased
effectiveness.
Itraconazole: decreased serum concentrations of itraconazole. Avoid concomitant use.
Drug-food. *Any food:* increased rate of
absorption. Give drug on an empty stomach.

Contraindications and precautions

• Contraindicated in patients with hypersensitivity to drug or its components.
• Use of drug is not recommended in
breast-feeding women.
• Use cautiously in patients with history
of pancreatitis. Also use cautiously in patients with peripheral neuropathy, renal
or hepatic impairment, or hyperuricemia
and in pregnant women.

NURSING CONSIDERATIONS

☒ Assessment
• Obtain history of patient's underlying
condition before therapy, and reassess
regularly thereafter.
• Be alert for adverse reactions and drug
interactions.
• Evaluate patient's and family's knowledge of drug therapy.

⊞ Nursing diagnoses
• Infection related to presence of HIV infection
• Diarrhea related to drug-induced adverse effect on bowel
• Knowledge deficit related to drug
therapy

⊠ Planning and implementation
• Administer drug on empty stomach, regardless of dosage form used; administering drug with meals can decrease absorption by 50%.
• Know that most patients should receive
two tablets per dose.
• To administer single-dose packets containing buffered powder for oral solution,
pour contents into 4 oz of water. Do not
use fruit juice or other beverages that
may be acidic. Stir for 2 to 3 minutes until powder dissolves completely.
Administer immediately.
• Use care when preparing powder or
crushing tablets to avoid excessive dis-
persal of powder into air.
• Know that pediatric powder for oral solution must be prepared by pharmacist
before dispensing. It must be constituted
with Purified Water, USP, then diluted
with antacid (either Mylanta Double
Strength Liquid or Maalox TC
Suspension) to final concentration of
10 mg/ml. The admixture is stable for 30
days if refrigerated (at 36° to 46° F [2° to
8° C]). Shake solution well before measuring dose.
• Notify doctor if patient taking powder
form develops diarrhea; in early clinical
trials, powder for oral solution was asso-

ciated with high incidence of diarrhea. The manufacturer suggests switching to tablet formulation if diarrhea is a problem, although no evidence suggests that other formulations may be associated with lower incidence of diarrhea.

Patient teaching
• Instruct patient to chew tablets thoroughly before swallowing and to drink at least 1 oz of water with each dose because tablets contain buffers that raise stomach pH to levels that prevent degradation of active drug. If tablets are manually crushed, stir them thoroughly in 1 oz of water to disperse particles uniformly, then have patient drink mixture immediately.
• Inform patient on sodium-restricted diet that each 2-tablet dose of didanosine contains 529 mg of sodium; each single packet of buffered powder for oral solution contains 1.38 g of sodium.
• Warn patient about adverse CNS reactions and tell patient to take safety precautions.
• Tell patient to notify doctor if adverse GI reactions occur.

☑ **Evaluation**
• Patient exhibits improvement with therapy.
• Patient regains normal bowel pattern.
• Patient and family state understanding of drug therapy.

diethylstilbestrol (stilbestrol)
(digh-eh-thil-stil-BES-trohl)
DES

diethylstilbestrol diphosphate
DES, Honvol♦, Stilphostrol

Pharmacologic class: estrogen
Therapeutic class: estrogen replacement, antineoplastic
Pregnancy risk category: X

How supplied
diethylstilbestrol
Tablets: 1 mg, 5 mg
diethylstilbestrol diphosphate
Tablets: 50 mg, 83 mg♦
Injection: 50 mg/ml♦

Pharmacokinetics
Absorption: well absorbed from GI tract with P.O. administration.
Distribution: distributed to most body tissue.
Metabolism: undergoes conjugation with glucuronic acid in liver.
Excretion: excreted in urine and feces.

Route	Onset	Peak	Duration
P.O., I.V.	Unknown	Unknown	Unknown

Pharmacodynamics
Chemical effect: increases synthesis of DNA, RNA, and protein in responsive tissues; also reduces release of follicle-stimulating hormone and luteinizing hormone from pituitary gland.
Therapeutic effect: inhibits growth of hormone-sensitive tissue.

Indications and dosage
▶ **Prostate cancer.** *Men:* initially, 1 to 3 mg P.O. daily, may be reduced to 1 mg daily; or 50 mg P.O. diphosphate t.i.d., then increased up to 200 mg or more t.i.d., p.r.n.; or 0.5 g I.V. followed by 1 g daily for 5 or more days, p.r.n. Maintenance dosage is 0.25 to 0.5 g I.V. once or twice weekly.
▶ **Metastatic, advanced breast cancer.** *Men and postmenopausal women:* 15 mg P.O. daily.

Adverse reactions
CNS: headache, dizziness, chorea, depression, lethargy, *seizures.*
CV: thrombophlebitis; *thromboembolism;* hypertension; edema; *increased risk of CVA, pulmonary embolism, and MI.*
EENT: worsening of myopia or astigmatism, intolerance of contact lenses.

GI: *nausea,* vomiting, abdominal cramps, bloating, diarrhea, constipation, anorexia, increased appetite, excessive thirst, weight changes, *pancreatitis.*
GU: breakthrough bleeding, altered menstrual flow, dysmenorrhea, amenorrhea, cervical erosion, *increased risk of endometrial cancer, possibility of increased risk of breast cancer,* altered cervical secretions, enlargement of uterine fibromas, vaginal candidiasis, loss of libido (in women); gynecomastia, testicular atrophy, impotence.
Hepatic: cholestatic jaundice, *hepatic adenoma* (in men).
Metabolic: hyperglycemia, hypercalcemia, folic acid deficiency.
Skin: melasma, urticaria, acne, seborrhea, oily skin, hirsutism or hair loss, erythema nodosum, dermatitis.
Other: leg cramps, breast tenderness or enlargement, gallbladder disease.

Interactions

Drug-drug. *Bromocriptine:* may cause amenorrhea, interfering with bromocriptine's effects. Avoid concomitant use.
Carbamazepine, phenobarbital, rifampin: decreased effectiveness of estrogen therapy. Monitor closely.
Corticosteroids: possibly enhanced effects. Monitor patient closely.
Cyclosporine: increased risk of toxicity. Use together with caution and frequently monitor cyclosporine levels.
Dantrolene, other hepatotoxic drugs: increased risk of hepatotoxicity. Monitor patient closely.
Oral anticoagulants: dosage adjustments may be necessary. Monitor PT and INR.
Tamoxifen: estrogens may interfere with effectiveness of tamoxifen. Avoid concomitant use.
Drug-food. *Caffeine:* may increase serum caffeine concentrations. Monitor effects.
Drug-lifestyle. *Smoking:* increased risk of adverse CV effects. If smoking continues, may need alternative therapy.

Contraindications and precautions

• Contraindicated in men with known or suspected breast cancer except in selected patients being treated for metastatic disease; in patients with active thrombophlebitis or thromboembolic disorders, estrogen-dependent neoplasia, undiagnosed abnormal genital bleeding, or history of thrombophlebitis, thrombosis, or thromboembolic disorders associated with estrogen use; and in pregnant women.
• Drug is not recommended for use in breast-feeding women.
• Use cautiously in patients with hypertension; depression; bone disease; migraine; seizures; diabetes mellitus; cardiac, hepatic, or renal dysfunction; and cerebrovascular or coronary artery disease.

NURSING CONSIDERATIONS

Assessment
• Obtain history of patient's underlying condition before therapy, and reassess regularly thereafter.
• Ensure that patient has a thorough physical examination before initiating estrogen therapy. Patient receiving long-term therapy should have yearly examinations.
• Periodically monitor patient's body weight, blood pressure, liver function, and serum lipid levels.
• Be alert for adverse reactions and drug interactions.
• Evaluate patient's and family's knowledge of drug therapy.

Nursing diagnoses
• Altered health maintenance related to underlying condition
• Risk for injury related to drug-induced adverse reactions
• Knowledge deficit related to drug therapy

Reactions may be *common,* uncommon, *life-threatening,* or COMMON AND LIFE-THREATENING.

>> Planning and implementation

P.O. use: Give drug with or immediately after meals if patient experiences GI upset.

I.V. use: Mix ordered dose in 250 to 500 ml of D₅W or 0.9% NaCl. Infuse at 1 to 2 ml/minute for first 15 minutes; if no adverse reactions occur, increase infusion rate to administer entire dose within 1 hour.

• Notify pathologist about patient receiving estrogen therapy.

• Because of risk of thromboembolism, know that therapy should be discontinued at least 1 month before procedures associated with prolonged immobilization or thromboembolism, such as knee or hip surgery.

Patient teaching
• Tell diabetic patient to report elevated blood glucose test results so antidiabetic medication dosage can be adjusted.

• Instruct patient not to crush, break, or chew enteric-coated tablets.

• Tell patient that package insert describing estrogen's adverse effects is available; also provide verbal explanation.

• Warn patient to immediately report abdominal pain; pain, numbness, or stiffness in legs or buttocks; pressure or pain in chest; shortness of breath; severe headache; visual disturbances, such as blind spots, flashing lights, or blurriness; vaginal bleeding or discharge; breast lumps; sudden weight gain; swelling of hands or feet; yellow sclera or skin; dark urine; and light-colored stools.

• Teach female patient how to perform breast self-examination.

☑ Evaluation

• Patient exhibits improved health.
• Patient does not experience injury as a result of therapy.
• Patient and family state understanding of drug therapy.

diflunisal
(digh-FLOO-neh-sol)
Dolobid

Pharmacologic class: NSAID, salicylic acid derivative
Therapeutic class: nonnarcotic analgesic, antipyretic, anti-inflammatory
Pregnancy risk category: C

How supplied

Tablets: 250 mg, 500 mg

Pharmacokinetics

Absorption: absorbed rapidly and completely by way of GI tract.
Distribution: highly protein-bound.
Metabolism: metabolized in liver.
Excretion: excreted in urine. *Half-life:* 8 to 12 hours.

Route	Onset	Peak	Duration
P.O.	1 hr	2-3 hr	8-12 hr

Pharmacodynamics

Chemical effect: unknown; probably related to inhibition of prostaglandin synthesis.
Therapeutic effect: relieves inflammation and pain; reduces body temperature.

Indications and dosage

▶ **Mild to moderate pain, osteoarthritis, rheumatoid arthritis.** *Adults:* 500 to 1,000 mg P.O. daily in two divided doses, usually q 12 hours. Maximum dosage is 1,500 mg daily. *Adults over age 65:* one-half usual adult dose.

Adverse reactions

CNS: *dizziness,* somnolence, insomnia, *headache,* fatigue.
EENT: *tinnitus,* visual disturbances (rare).
GI: *nausea, dyspepsia, GI pain, diarrhea,* vomiting, constipation, flatulence.
GU: renal impairment, hematuria, *interstitial nephritis.*

Skin: rash, pruritus, sweating, stomatitis, *erythema multiforme, Stevens-Johnson syndrome.*
Other: dry mucous membranes.

Interactions

Drug-drug. *Acetaminophen, hydrochlorothiazide, indomethacin:* diflunisal may substantially increase blood levels, increasing risk of toxicity. Avoid concomitant use.
Antacids, aspirin: decreased diflunisal blood levels. Monitor for possible decreased therapeutic effect.
Cyclosporine: diflunisal may enhance nephrotoxicity of cyclosporine. Avoid concomitant use.
Methotrexate: diflunisal may enhance toxicity of methotrexate. Avoid concomitant use.
Oral anticoagulants, thrombolytic agents: diflunisal may enhance pharmacologic effects of these agents. Use together cautiously.
Sulindac: diflunisal decreases blood levels of sulindac's active metabolite. Monitor for decreased pharmacologic effect.

Contraindications and precautions

• Contraindicated in patients with hypersensitivity to drug and in those whose acute asthmatic attacks, urticaria, or rhinitis is precipitated by aspirin or other NSAIDs.
• Use of drug is not recommended in breast-feeding women.
• Because of epidemiologic association with Reye's syndrome, Centers for Disease Control and Prevention recommends not giving salicylates to children and teenagers with chickenpox or influenza-like illness.
• Use cautiously in patients with GI bleeding, history of peptic ulcer disease, renal impairment, or compromised cardiac function, hypertension, or other conditions predisposing patient to fluid retention.

NURSING CONSIDERATIONS

⚕ Assessment
• Obtain history of patient's underlying condition before therapy, and reassess regularly thereafter.
• Be alert for adverse reactions and drug interactions.
• Evaluate patient's and family's knowledge of drug therapy.

⊕ Nursing diagnoses
• Pain related to underlying condition
• Risk for fluid volume deficit related to drug-induced adverse reactions
• Knowledge deficit related to drug therapy

▷ Planning and implementation
• Administer with milk or food to minimize adverse GI reactions.
Patient teaching
• Advise patient to take with water, milk, or meals.
• Warn patient to check with doctor or pharmacist before taking OTC medications to avoid possible interactions with drugs, such as those containing aspirin.

☑ Evaluation
• Patient is free from pain.
• Patient maintains adequate hydration throughout therapy.
• Patient and family state understanding of drug therapy.

digoxin
(dih-JOKS-in)
Digoxin, Lanoxicaps, Lanoxin*, Novodigoxin♦

Pharmacologic class: cardiac glycoside
Therapeutic class: antiarrhythmic, inotropic
Pregnancy risk category: C

How supplied
Tablets: 0.125 mg, 0.25 mg, 0.5 mg

Capsules: 0.05 mg, 0.1 mg, 0.2 mg
Elixir: 0.05 mg/ml
Injection: 0.05 mg/ml♦, 0.1 mg/ml
(pediatric), 0.25 mg/ml

Pharmacokinetics

Absorption: with tablet or elixir administration, 60% to 85% of dose is absorbed. With capsule form, bioavailability increases, with about 90% to 100% of dose absorbed.
Distribution: distributed widely in body tissues; about 20% to 30% bound to plasma proteins.
Metabolism: small amount of digoxin is thought to be metabolized in liver and gut by bacteria. This metabolism varies and may be substantial in some patients. Drug undergoes some enterohepatic recirculation (also variable). Metabolites have minimal cardiac activity.
Excretion: most of dose excreted by kidneys as unchanged drug, although some patients excrete a substantial amount of metabolized or reduced drug. In patients with renal failure, biliary excretion is more important excretion route. *Half-life:* 30 to 40 hours.

Route	Onset	Peak	Duration
P.O.	0.5-2 hr	2-6 hr	3-4 days
I.V.	5-30 min	1-4 hr	3-4 days

Pharmacodynamics

Chemical effect: inhibits sodium–potassium–activated adenosine triphosphatase, thereby promoting movement of calcium from extracellular to intracellular cytoplasm and strengthening myocardial contraction. Digoxin also acts on CNS to enhance vagal tone, slowing conduction through SA and AV nodes and providing antiarrhythmic effect.
Therapeutic effect: strengthens myocardial contractions and slows conduction through SA and AV nodes.

Indications and dosage

▶ **Heart failure, paroxysmal supraventricular tachycardia, atrial fibrillation**

and flutter. *Adults:* loading dose is 0.5 to 1 mg I.V. or P.O. in divided doses over 24 hours; maintenance dosage is 0.125 to 0.5 mg I.V. or P.O. daily (average is 0.25 mg). Depending on patient response, larger doses may be needed for treatment of arrhythmias. Smaller loading and maintenance doses are given to patients with impaired kidney function. *Adults over age 65:* 0.125 mg P.O. daily as maintenance dose. Frail or underweight elderly patients may require only 0.0625 mg daily or 0.125 mg every other day. *Children over age 2:* loading dose is 0.02 to 0.04 mg/kg P.O. daily divided q 8 hours over 24 hours; I.V. loading dose is 0.015 to 0.035 mg/kg; maintenance dosage is 0.012 mg/kg P.O. daily divided q 12 hours. *Children ages 1 month to 2 years:* loading dose is 0.035 to 0.06 mg/kg P.O. in three divided doses over 24 hours; I.V. loading dose is 0.03 to 0.05 mg/kg; maintenance dosage is 0.01 to 0.02 mg/kg P.O. daily divided q 12 hours. *Neonates:* loading dose is 0.035 mg/kg P.O. divided q 8 hours over 24 hours; I.V. loading dose is 0.02 to 0.03 mg/kg; maintenance dosage is 0.01 mg/kg P.O. daily divided q 12 hours. *Premature neonates:* loading dose is 0.025 mg/kg I.V. in three divided doses over 24 hours; maintenance dosage is 0.01 mg/kg daily divided q 12 hours.

Adverse reactions

The following signs of toxicity may occur with all cardiac glycosides.
CNS: *fatigue, generalized muscle weakness, agitation, hallucinations,* headache, malaise, dizziness, vertigo, stupor, paresthesia.
CV: *arrhythmias* (most commonly, conduction disturbances with or without AV block, PVCs, and supraventricular arrhythmias); arrhythmias may lead to increased severity of *heart failure* and hypotension. *Toxic effects on heart may be life-threatening and require immediate attention.*

EENT: yellow-green halos around visual images, blurred vision, light flashes, photophobia, diplopia.
GI: *anorexia, nausea,* vomiting, diarrhea.

Interactions

Drug-drug. *Amiloride:* inhibited digoxin effect and increased digoxin excretion. Monitor for altered digoxin effect.
Amiodarone, diltiazem, nifedipine, quinidine, verapamil: increased digoxin blood levels. Monitor for toxicity.
Amphotericin B, carbenicillin, corticosteroids, diuretics (including loop diuretics, chlorthalidone, metolazone, and thiazides), ticarcillin: hypokalemia, predisposing patient to digitalis toxicity. Monitor serum potassium levels.
Antacids, kaolin-pectin: decreased absorption of oral digoxin. Schedule doses as far as possible from P.O. digoxin administration.
Anticholinergics: may increase absorption of digoxin tablets. Monitor blood levels and observe for toxicity.
Cholestyramine, colestipol, metoclopramide: decreased absorption of P.O. digoxin. Monitor for decreased effect and low blood levels. Increase dosage, if necessary and as ordered.
Parenteral calcium, thiazides: hypercalcemia and hypomagnesemia, predisposing patient to digitalis toxicity. Monitor serum calcium and magnesium levels.

Contraindications and precautions

• Contraindicated in patients with hypersensitivity to drug; digitalis-induced toxicity; ventricular fibrillation; or ventricular tachycardia unless caused by heart failure.
• Use with extreme caution in elderly patients and in those with acute MI, incomplete AV block, sinus bradycardia, PVCs, chronic constrictive pericarditis, hypertrophic cardiomyopathy, renal insufficiency, severe pulmonary disease, or hypothyroidism. Reduce dosage in patients with renal impairment.

• Use cautiously in pregnant or breast-feeding women.

NURSING CONSIDERATIONS

Assessment
• Obtain history of patient's underlying condition before therapy.
• Monitor effectiveness by taking apical-radial pulse for 1 full minute before each dose. Evaluate ECG when ordered, and regularly assess patient's cardiopulmonary status for signs of improvement.
• Monitor serum digoxin levels. Therapeutic blood levels of digoxin range from 0.5 to 2.0 ng/ml. Obtain blood for digoxin levels 8 hours after last P.O. dose.
• Monitor serum potassium level carefully.
• Be alert for adverse reactions and drug interactions.
• Evaluate patient's and family's knowledge of drug therapy.

Nursing diagnoses
• Decreased cardiac output related to underlying condition
• Altered protection related to digitalis toxicity caused by drug
• Knowledge deficit related to drug therapy

Planning and implementation
• Be aware that hypothyroid patients are extremely sensitive to glycosides; hyperthyroid patients may need larger doses.
• Before administering loading dose, obtain baseline data (heart rate and rhythm, blood pressure, and electrolyte levels), and question patient about recent use of cardiac glycosides (within previous 2 to 3 weeks).
• Be aware that loading dose is always divided over first 24 hours unless clinical situation indicates otherwise.
• Before giving, take apical-radial pulse for 1 full minute. Record and report to doctor significant changes (sudden increase or decrease in pulse rate, pulse deficit, irregular beats and, particularly,

regularization of previously irregular rhythm). If these changes occur, check blood pressure and obtain 12-lead ECG.
P.O. use: Because absorption of digoxin from parenteral route and from liquid-filled capsules is superior to absorption from tablets or elixir, expect dosage reduction of 20% to 25% when changing from tablets or elixir to liquid-filled capsules or parenteral therapy.
I.V. use: Infuse drug slowly over at least 5 minutes.
• Withhold drug and notify doctor if pulse rate slows to 60 beats/minute or less.
• For digitalis toxicity, administer agents that bind drug in intestine (for example, colestipol or cholestyramine). Treat arrhythmias with phenytoin I.V. or lidocaine I.V. and potentially life-threatening toxicity with specific antigen-binding fragments (such as digoxin immune Fab), as ordered.
• Withhold drug for 1 to 2 days before elective cardioversion, as ordered. Adjust dose after cardioversion, as ordered.
Patient teaching
• Instruct patient and responsible family member about drug action, dosage regimen, pulse taking, reportable signs, and follow-up plans.
• Instruct patient not to substitute one brand of digoxin for another.
• Tell patient to eat potassium-rich foods.

☑ **Evaluation**
• Patient exhibits adequate cardiac output.
• Patient does not experience digitalis toxicity.
• Patient and family state understanding of drug therapy.

---

digoxin immune Fab (ovine)
(dih-JOKS-in ih-MYOON Fab)
Digibind

Pharmacologic class: antibody fragment

Therapeutic class: cardiac glycoside antidote
Pregnancy risk category: C

How supplied
Injection: 38-mg vial

Pharmacokinetics
Absorption: not applicable with I.V. administration.
Distribution: unknown.
Metabolism: unknown.
Excretion: excreted in urine. *Half-life:* 15 to 20 hours.

Route	Onset	Peak	Duration
I.V.	Varies	On completion of I.V.	2-6 hr

Pharmacodynamics
Chemical effect: binds molecules of digoxin and digitoxin, making them unavailable for binding at site of action on cells.
Therapeutic effect: reverses digitalis intoxication.

Indications and dosage
▶ **Potentially life-threatening digoxin or digitoxin intoxication.** *Adults and children:* I.V. dosage varies according to amount of digoxin or digitoxin to be neutralized. Each vial binds about 0.5 mg of digoxin or digitoxin. Average dosage is 6 vials (228 mg). If toxicity resulted from acute digoxin ingestion and neither serum digoxin level nor estimated ingestion amount is known, 20 vials (760 mg) may be required. See package insert for complete, specific dosage instructions.

Adverse reactions
CV: *heart failure,* rapid ventricular rate (both caused by reversal of cardiac glycoside's therapeutic effects).
Other: *hypersensitivity reactions* (*anaphylaxis*), hypokalemia.

Interactions
None reported.

Contraindications and precautions

• No known contraindications.
• Use cautiously in patients known to be allergic to ovine proteins. In these high-risk patients, skin testing is recommended because drug is derived from digoxin-specific antibody fragments obtained from immunized sheep. Also use cautiously in pregnant or breast-feeding women.

NURSING CONSIDERATIONS

⚄ Assessment
• Obtain history of patient's digitalis intoxication before therapy.
• Monitor effectiveness by observing for decreased signs and symptoms of digitalis toxicity; know that in most patients, signs of digitalis toxicity disappear within a few hours.
• Be aware that because drug interferes with digitalis immunoassay measurements, standard serum digoxin levels are misleading until drug is cleared from body (about 2 days).
• Be alert for adverse reactions.
• Evaluate patient's and family's knowledge of drug therapy.

⊞ Nursing diagnoses
• Altered health maintenance related to digitalis intoxication
• Decreased cardiac output related to drug-induced heart failure
• Knowledge deficit related to drug therapy

⊠ Planning and implementation
• Refrigerate powder for injection. Reconstitute drug immediately before use. Reconstituted solutions may be refrigerated for 4 hours.
• Reconstitute 38-mg vial with 4 ml of sterile water for injection. Gently roll vial to dissolve powder. Reconstituted solution contains 9.5 mg/ml. Drug may be given by direct injection if cardiac arrest seems imminent. Alternatively, dilute

with 0.9% NaCl injection to appropriate volume and give by intermittent infusion.
• Infuse drug through 0.22-micron membrane filter.
• Know that drug is used only for life-threatening overdose in patients in shock or cardiac arrest; with ventricular arrhythmias, such as ventricular tachycardia or fibrillation; with progressive bradycardia, such as severe sinus bradycardia; or with second- or third-degree AV block not responsive to atropine.
• Administer oxygen, as ordered. Keep resuscitation equipment nearby.
Patient teaching
• Instruct patient to report respiratory difficulty, chest pain, or dizziness immediately.

☑ Evaluation
• Patient exhibits improved health with alleviation of digitalis toxicity.
• Patient demonstrates adequate cardiac output through normal vital signs and urine output and clear mental status.
• Patient and family state understanding of drug therapy.

dihydroergotamine mesylate
(digh-high-droh-er-GAH-tuh-meen MES-ih-layt)
D.H.E. 45, Dihydroergotamine-Sandoz♦, Migranal

Pharmacologic class: ergot alkaloid
Therapeutic class: vasoconstrictor
Pregnancy risk category: X

How supplied

Injection: 1 mg/ml
Intranasal solution: 0.5 mg/metered spray (4 mg/ml)

Pharmacokinetics

Absorption: unknown for S.C. and I.M. administration.
Distribution: 90% plasma protein–bound.

Metabolism: extensively metabolized, probably in liver (extensive first-pass metabolism).
Excretion: 10% excreted in urine as metabolites; rest in feces by biliary elimination.

Route	Onset	Peak	Duration
I.V.	≤ 5 min	≤ 15 min	8 hr
I.M.	15-30 min	≤ 30 min	8 hr
S.C.	Unknown	15-45 min	8 hr
Intranasal	Rapid	0.5-1 hr	Unknown

Pharmacodynamics

Chemical effect: causes peripheral vasoconstriction primarily by stimulating alpha-adrenergic receptors; may abort vascular headaches by direct vasoconstriction of dilated carotid artery bed with decline in amplitude of pulsations. *Therapeutic effect:* prevents or relieves vascular or migraine headache.

Indications and dosage

▶ **To prevent or abort vascular or migraine headache.** *Adults:* 1 mg I.M. or I.V. Repeated q 1 to 2 hours, p.r.n., up to total of 2 mg I.V. or 3 mg I.M. per attack. Maximum weekly dosage is 6 mg.
Adults: 1 spray into each nostril; repeat in 15 minutes for total of 4 sprays (2 mg).

Adverse reactions

CNS: dizziness.
CV: numbness and tingling in fingers and toes, transient tachycardia or bradycardia, precordial distress and pain, increased arterial pressure.
EENT: rhinitis, taste perversion, application site reaction, pharyngitis, sinusitis, dry mouth.
GI: *nausea, vomiting.*
Musculoskeletal: weakness in legs, muscle pain in extremities, localized edema, uterine contractions.
Skin: itching.

Interactions

Drug-drug. *Erythromycin, other macrolides:* may cause symptoms of ergot toxi-
city. Vasodilators (nitroprusside, nifedipine, or prazosin) may be ordered to treat such an attack. Monitor patient closely. *Propranolol, other beta blockers:* blocked natural pathway for vasodilation in patients receiving ergot alkaloids; may result in excessive vasoconstriction and cold extremities. Watch closely if drugs are used together.
Drug-lifestyle. *Smoking:* nicotine may promote vasoconstriction, predisposing patient to a greater ischemic response. Avoid concomitant use.

Contraindications and precautions

• Contraindicated in patients with peripheral and occlusive vascular disease, coronary artery disease, uncontrolled hypertension, severe hepatic or renal dysfunction, sepsis, or hypersensitivity to drug and in pregnant or breast-feeding women.
• Do not use drug in patients with hemiplegic or basilar migraines.
• Safety of drug has not been established in children.

NURSING CONSIDERATIONS

⚏ Assessment
• Obtain history of patient's vascular or migraine headache before therapy, and reassess regularly thereafter.
• Be alert for adverse reactions and drug interactions.
• Be alert for ergotamine rebound or increase in frequency and duration of headache, which may occur when drug is stopped.
• Evaluate patient's and family's knowledge of drug therapy.

⚏ Nursing diagnoses
• Pain related to vascular or migraine headache
• Sensory or perceptual alteration (tactile) related to drug-induced adverse reactions
• Knowledge deficit related to drug therapy

⟩ **Planning and implementation**
• Know that drug is most effective when used at first sign of migraine or soon after onset.
I.V. use: Directly inject solution into vein over 3 minutes. Continuous or intermittent infusion is not recommended.
I.M. and S.C. use: Follow normal protocol.
Intranasal use: Pump spray four times before using to prepare unit for administration. Discard spray ampule 8 hours after opening.
• Do not give drug within 24 hours of a 5-HT agonist (sumatriptan), ergotamine-containing or ergot-type medication, or methysergide.
• Avoid prolonged administration; don't exceed recommended dosage, as ordered. Adjust to most effective minimal dosage, as ordered, for best results.
• Protect ampules from heat and light. Discard if solution is discolored.
• Protect extremities, fingers, and toes from injury if tactile adverse reactions occur.
Patient teaching
• Tell patient when using intranasal spray, do not tilt head back or sniff while spraying drug.
• Instruct patient to lie down and relax in quiet, low-light environment after administration of drug.
• Tell patient to report coldness in extremities or tingling in fingers and toes. Severe vasoconstriction may result in tissue damage. Keep extremities warm and administer vasodilators, as ordered.
• Help patient to evaluate underlying causes of stress, which may precipitate attacks.

☑ **Evaluation**
• Patient's pain is relieved.
• Patient does not experience injury as result of drug-induced adverse tactile reactions.
• Patient and family state understanding of drug therapy.

dihydrotachysterol
(digh-high-droh-tak-ES-ster-ol)
DHT Intensol*, Hytakerol

Pharmacologic class: vitamin D analogue
Therapeutic class: antihypocalcemic
Pregnancy risk category: C

How supplied
Tablets: 0.125 mg, 0.2 mg, 0.4 mg
Capsules: 0.125 mg
Oral solution: 0.2 mg/5 ml, 0.2 mg/ml* (DHT Intensol*), 0.25 mg/ml (in sesame oil)
Note: 1 mg of dihydrotachysterol is equal to 120,000 units of ergocalciferol (vitamin D_2).

Pharmacokinetics
Absorption: absorbed readily from small intestine.
Distribution: distributed widely; largely protein-bound.
Metabolism: metabolized in liver.
Excretion: excreted in urine and bile.

Route	Onset	Peak	Duration
P.O.	Several hr	1-2 wk	< 9 wk

Pharmacodynamics
Chemical effect: stimulates calcium absorption from GI tract and promotes secretion of calcium from bone to blood.
Therapeutic effect: raises blood calcium level.

Indications and dosage
▶ **Hypocalcemia associated with hypoparathyroidism and pseudohypoparathyroidism.** *Adults:* initially, 0.75 to 2.5 mg P.O. daily for several days. Maintenance dosage is 0.2 to 1 mg daily.
Children: initially, 1 to 5 mg P.O. for 4 days. Dosage is then continued or reduced to one-fourth the initial amount. Maintenance dosage is 0.5 to 1.5 mg daily.

Reactions may be *common*, uncommon, *life-threatening*, or COMMON AND LIFE-THREATENING.

▶ **Prophylaxis of hypocalcemic tetany after thyroid surgery.** *Adults:* 0.25 mg P.O. daily (with calcium supplements).

Adverse reactions

Vitamin D intoxication associated with hypercalcemia.
CNS: headache, somnolence, vertigo, irritability, psychosis (rare).
CV: hypertension, *arrhythmias*.
EENT: conjunctivitis, photophobia, rhinorrhea, tinnitus.
GI: nausea, vomiting, constipation, metallic taste, dry mouth, anorexia, diarrhea, *pancreatitis*.
GU: polyuria, nocturia.
Other: weakness, bone and muscle pain, thirst, weight loss, hyperthermia, decreased libido, nephrocalcinosis.

Interactions

Drug-drug. *Cholestyramine, colestipol, excessive use of mineral oil:* decreased absorption of orally administered vitamin D analogues. Avoid concomitant use.
Corticosteroids: counteracts vitamin D analogue effects. Don't use together.
Cardiac glycosides: increased risk of arrhythmias. Avoid concomitant use.
Magnesium-containing antacids: possibly hypermagnesemia, especially in patients with chronic renal failure. Avoid concomitant use.
Other vitamin D analogues: increased toxicity. Avoid concomitant use.
Thiazide diuretics: may cause hypercalcemia.

Contraindications and precautions

• Contraindicated in patients with hypercalcemia or vitamin D toxicity.
• Use of drug is not recommended in breast-feeding women.
• Use cautiously in pregnant women.

NURSING CONSIDERATIONS

Assessment
• Obtain history of patient's blood calcium level before therapy.

• Monitor effectiveness by checking serum and urine calcium levels, as ordered; serum calcium level multiplied by serum phosphate level should not exceed 70. During titration, determine serum calcium level twice weekly.
• Be alert for adverse reactions and drug interactions.
• Evaluate patient's and family's knowledge of drug therapy.

Nursing diagnoses
• Altered health maintenance related to hypocalcemia
• Altered protection related to potential for vitamin D intoxication caused by drug therapy
• Knowledge deficit related to drug therapy

Planning and implementation
• Be aware that optimal dosage is highly individualized.
• Store in tightly closed, light-resistant container. Don't refrigerate.
• Discontinue if hypercalcemia occurs, and notify doctor. Know that drug can be resumed after serum calcium level returns to normal.
• Ensure that patient is consuming adequate daily intake of calcium (1,000 mg).
Patient teaching
• Advise patient to adhere to diet and calcium supplementation and to avoid OTC drugs.
• Teach patient the signs and symptoms of hypercalcemia, and instruct him to report them if they occur.
• Tell patient how to store drug properly.

Evaluation
• Patient's serum and urine calcium levels are within normal range.
• Patient does not experience drug-induced adverse reactions.
• Patient and family state understanding of drug therapy.

---

diltiazem hydrochloride
(dil-TIGH-uh-zem high-droh-KLOR-ighd)
Cardizem, Cardizem CD, Cardizem SR,
Dilacor XR, Tiazac

Pharmacologic class: calcium channel
blocker
Therapeutic class: antianginal
Pregnancy risk category: C

How supplied

Tablets: 30 mg, 60 mg, 90 mg, 120 mg
*Capsules (extended-release; Cardizem
CD, Dilacor XR, Tiazac):* 120 mg,
180 mg, 240 mg, 300 mg (Cardizem CD
only), 360 mg (Tiazac only)
*Capsules (sustained-release; Cardizem
SR):* 60 mg, 90 mg, 120 mg
Injection: 5 mg/ml

Pharmacokinetics

Absorption: about 80% of dose is absorbed rapidly from GI tract. Only about
40% of drug enters systemic circulation
because of significant first-pass effect in
liver.
Distribution: about 70% to 85% of circulating diltiazem is bound to plasma proteins.
Metabolism: metabolized in liver.
Excretion: about 35% excreted in urine
and about 65% in bile as unchanged drug
and inactive and active metabolites. *Half-
life:* 3 to 9 hours.

Route	Onset	Peak	Duration
P.O.	0.5-3 hr	2-14 hr	6-24 hr
I.V.	3 min	Immediate	1-3 hr (bolus); < 10 hr (infusion)

Pharmacodynamics

Chemical effect: inhibits calcium ion influx across cardiac and smooth-muscle
cells, decreasing myocardial contractility
and oxygen demand; also dilates coronary arteries and arterioles.

Therapeutic effect: relieves anginal pain,
lowers blood pressure, and restores normal sinus rhythm.

Indications and dosage

► **Vasospastic angina (Prinzmetal's
[variant] angina), classic chronic stable
angina pectoris.** *Adults:* 30 mg P.O. t.i.d.
or q.i.d. before meals and h.s. Dosage increased gradually to maximum of
360 mg/day in divided doses. Alternatively, 120 to 180 mg (extended-release)
P.O. once daily. Dosage may be titrated
up to 480 mg once daily, if necessary.
► **Hypertension.** *Adults:* 60 to 120 mg
P.O. b.i.d. (sustained-release capsule).
Titrated to effect. Maximum recommended dosage is 360 mg/day. Alternatively,
180 to 240 mg daily (extended-release
capsule) initially. Dosage adjusted as
necessary.
► **Atrial fibrillation or flutter; paroxysmal supraventricular tachycardia.**
Adults: 0.25 mg/kg as I.V. bolus injection
over 2 minutes. If response is inadequate,
0.35 mg/kg I.V. after 15 minutes, followed with continuous infusion of
10 mg/hour. Some patients respond well
to infusion rates of 5 mg/hour; maximum
dosage is 15 mg/hour.

Adverse reactions

CNS: *headache,* somnolence, dizziness,
insomnia, asthenia.
CV: *edema, arrhythmias,* flushing,
bradycardia, hypotension, conduction
abnormalities, *heart failure, AV block,*
abnormal ECG.
GI: *nausea, constipation,* vomiting, diarrhea, abdominal discomfort.
GU: nocturia, polyuria.
Hepatic: transient elevation of liver enzyme levels.
Skin: rash, pruritus, photosensitivity.

Interactions

Drug-drug. *Anesthetics:* effects may be
potentiated.
Cimetidine: may inhibit diltiazem metabolism. Monitor for toxicity.

Cyclosporine: diltiazem may increase serum cyclosporine levels, possibly by decreasing its metabolism, leading to increased risk of cyclosporine toxicity. Avoid concomitant use.
Digoxin: diltiazem may increase serum levels of digoxin. Monitor for toxicity.
Propranolol, other beta blockers: may precipitate heart failure or prolong cardiac conduction time. Use together cautiously.

Contraindications and precautions

• Contraindicated in patients with sick sinus syndrome or second- or third-degree AV block in absence of artificial pacemaker, hypotension (systolic blood pressure below 90 mm Hg), acute MI, pulmonary congestion (documented by X-ray), or hypersensitivity to drug.
• Breast-feeding should be discontinued during drug use.
• Use cautiously in elderly patients, in patients with heart failure, and in those with impaired liver or kidney function. Also use cautiously in pregnant women.
• Safety of drug has not been established in children.

NURSING CONSIDERATIONS

Assessment
• Obtain history of patient's underlying condition before therapy, and reassess regularly thereafter.
• Monitor blood pressure during initiation of therapy and dosage adjustments.
• Monitor patient's ECG and heart rate and rhythm regularly.
• Be alert for adverse reactions and drug interactions.
• Evaluate patient's and family's knowledge of drug therapy.

Nursing diagnoses
• Altered health maintenance related to underlying condition
• Decreased cardiac output related to drug-induced adverse reactions

• Knowledge deficit related to drug therapy

Planning and implementation
P.O. use: Administer tablets before meals and at bedtime.
I.V. use: Know that infusions lasting longer than 24 hours are not recommended.
– Know that furosemide forms a precipitate when mixed with diltiazem injection. Administer through separate I.V. lines.
• If systolic blood pressure is below 90 mm Hg or heart rate is below 60 beats/minute, withhold dose and notify doctor.
• Assist patient with ambulation during initiation of drug therapy because dizziness may occur.
• Restrict patient's fluid and sodium intake to minimize edema.
Patient teaching
• If nitrate therapy is prescribed during titration of diltiazem dosage, urge patient compliance. Tell patient that sublingual nitroglycerin, especially, may be taken concomitantly as needed and ordered when anginal symptoms are acute.
• Tell patient to swallow extended- and sustained-release capsules whole. Do not open, crush, or chew.
• Instruct patient to take drug exactly as prescribed, even when feeling well.
• Advise patient to minimize exposure to direct sunlight and to take precautions when in sun because of drug-induced photosensitivity.
• Instruct patient to limit fluid and sodium intake to minimize edema.

Evaluation
• Patient exhibits improvement in underlying condition.
• Patient maintains adequate cardiac output throughout therapy.
• Patient and family state understanding of drug therapy.

dimenhydrinate
(digh-men-HIGH-drih-nayt)
Apo-Dimenhydrinate♦, Calm X†,
Children's Dramamine†, Dimetabs, Dinate,
Dommanate, Dramamine†*, Dramamine
Chewable†**, Dramamine Liquid†*,
Dramanate, Dramocen, Dramoject,
Dymenate, Gravol♦, Gravol L/A♦,
Hydrate, Marmine†, Nico-Vert†, PMS-
Dimenhydrinate♦, Tega-Vert†, Triptone
Caplets†, Wehamine

Pharmacologic class: ethanolamine
derivative antihistamine
Therapeutic class: antihistamine
(H_1-receptor antagonist), antiemetic,
antivertigo
Pregnancy risk category: B

How supplied

Tablets: 50 mg†
Tablets (chewable): 50 mg†
Capsules: 50 mg†
Elixir: 15 mg/5 ml♦
Syrup: 12.5 mg/4 ml*†, 15.62 mg/5 ml
Injection: 50 mg/ml

Pharmacokinetics

Absorption: well absorbed after P.O. and
I.M. administration.
Distribution: well distributed throughout
body.
Metabolism: metabolized in liver.
Excretion: excreted in urine. *Half-life:* 1
to 4 hours.

Route	Onset	Peak	Duration
P.O.	20-30 min	Unknown	3-6 hr
I.V.	Immediate	Unknown	3-6 hr
I.M.	15-20 min	Unknown	3-6 hr

Pharmacodynamics

Chemical effect: unknown; may affect
neural pathways originating in labyrinth
to inhibit nausea and vomiting.
Therapeutic effect: prevents and relieves
motion sickness.

Indications and dosage

▶ **Prevention and treatment of motion
sickness.** *Adults and children age 12 and
over:* 50 to 100 mg P.O. q 4 to 6 hours;
50 mg I.M., p.r.n.; or 50 mg I.V. diluted
in 10 ml NaCl injection, injected over 2
minutes. Maximum dosage is 400 mg
daily. *Children ages 6 to 12:* 25 to 50 mg
P.O. q 6 to 8 hours, not to exceed 150 mg
in 24 hours. *Children ages 2 to 6:* 12.5 to
25.0 mg P.O. q 6 to 8 hours, not to exceed 75 mg in 24 hours.

Adverse reactions

CNS: *drowsiness,* headache, confusion,
nervousness, insomnia (especially in
children), vertigo, tingling and weakness
of hands, lassitude, excitation, incoordination, dizziness.
CV: palpitations, hypotension, tachycardia.
EENT: blurred vision, diplopia, nasal
congestion, tinnitus, dry respiratory passages.
GI: dry mouth, nausea, vomiting, diarrhea, epigastric distress, constipation,
anorexia.
Respiratory: wheezing, thickened
bronchial secretions.
Skin: photosensitivity, urticaria, rash.
Other: *anaphylaxis,* tightness of chest.

Interactions

Drug-drug. *CNS depressants:* additive
CNS depression. Avoid concomitant use.
Drug-lifestyle. *Alcohol use:* additive
CNS depression. Avoid concomitant use.

Contraindications and precautions

• No known contraindications, although
drug is not recommended for use in
breast-feeding women.
• Use cautiously in patients with seizures,
acute angle-closure glaucoma, or enlarged prostate gland or in patients receiving ototoxic drugs. Also use cautiously in pregnant women.

NURSING CONSIDERATIONS

☆ Assessment
• Obtain history of patient's underlying condition before therapy.
• Monitor effectiveness by evaluating patient for nausea and vomiting.
• Be alert for adverse reactions and drug interactions.
• Evaluate patient's and family's knowledge of drug therapy.

⊕ Nursing diagnoses
• Risk for fluid volume deficit related to nausea and vomiting induced by motion sickness
• Risk for injury related to drug-induced adverse CNS reactions
• Knowledge deficit related to drug therapy

❯ Planning and implementation
P.O. use: Administer drug at least 30 minutes before patient is to travel to prevent motion sickness.
I.V. use: Before administration, dilute each milliliter of drug with 10 ml of sterile water for injection, D_5W, or 0.9% NaCl injection. Give by direct injection over not less than 2 minutes.
– Know that undiluted solution is irritating to veins and may cause sclerosis.
I.M. use: Follow normal protocol.
• Because incompatibilities are common, avoid mixing parenteral preparation with other drugs.
Patient teaching
• Advise patient to refrain from driving and performing other activities that require alertness until CNS effects of drug are known.
• Tell patient to take drug at least 30 minutes before beginning travel.

☑ Evaluation
• Patient maintains adequate hydration.
• Patient does not experience injury as result of drug-induced adverse CNS reactions.

• Patient and family state understanding of drug therapy.

dimercaprol
(digh-mer-KAP-rohl)
BAL in Oil

Pharmacologic class: chelating agent
Therapeutic class: heavy metal antagonist
Pregnancy risk category: NR

How supplied
Injection: 100 mg/ml

Pharmacokinetics
Absorption: unknown.
Distribution: distributed to all tissues, mainly intracellular space.
Metabolism: uncomplexed dimercaprol is metabolized rapidly to inactive products.
Excretion: most dimercaprol metal complexes and inactive metabolites are excreted in urine and feces.

Route	Onset	Peak	Duration
I.M.	Unknown	30-60 min	4 hr

Pharmacodynamics
Chemical effect: forms complexes with heavy metals.
Therapeutic effect: treats heavy metal intoxication.

Indications and dosage
❯ **Severe arsenic or gold poisoning.**
Adults and children: 3 mg/kg deep I.M. q 4 hours for 2 days, then q.i.d. on third day, then b.i.d. for 10 days.
❯ **Mild arsenic or gold poisoning.**
Adults and children: 2.5 mg/kg deep I.M. q.i.d. for 2 days, then b.i.d. on third day, then once daily for 10 days.
❯ **Mercury poisoning.** *Adults and children:* initially, 5 mg/kg deep I.M., then 2.5 mg/kg daily or b.i.d. for 10 days.

▶ **Acute lead encephalopathy or lead level exceeding 100 mcg/dl.** *Adults and children:* 4 mg/kg deep I.M., then q 4 hours with edetate calcium disodium (250 mg/m² I.M.). Use separate sites. Maximum dosage is 5 mg/kg per dose.

Adverse reactions

CNS: headache; paresthesia; muscle pain or weakness.
CV: *transient increase in blood pressure* (returns to normal in 2 hours), *tachycardia.*
EENT: blepharospasm, conjunctivitis, lacrimation, rhinorrhea, excessive salivation.
GI: *halitosis; nausea; vomiting; burning sensation in lips, mouth, and throat; abdominal pain.*
GU: *dysuria;* renal damage (if alkaline urine not maintained).
Other: *fever* (especially in children), pain or tightness in throat, chest, or hands; diaphoresis, pain in teeth, sterile abscess, pain at injection site, decreased iodine uptake.

Interactions

Drug-drug. *Iron:* toxic metal complex formed; concurrent therapy contraindicated. Wait 24 hours after last dimercaprol dose.
131I uptake thyroid tests: decreased. Don't schedule patient for this test during course of dimercaprol therapy.

Contraindications and precautions

• Contraindicated in patients with hepatic dysfunction (except postarsenical jaundice).
• Use cautiously in patients with hypertension or oliguria.
• Safety of drug has not been established in pregnant or breast-feeding women.

NURSING CONSIDERATIONS

Assessment
• Obtain history of patient's toxicity before therapy.

• Monitor effectiveness by monitoring serum level of substance ingested and for improvement in patient's condition.
• Be alert for adverse reactions and drug interactions.
• Monitor patient's hydration status if adverse GI reactions occur.
• Observe injection site for local reaction.
• Evaluate patient's and family's knowledge of drug therapy.

Nursing diagnoses
• Risk for poisoning related to exposure to toxic substance
• Risk for fluid volume deficit related to drug-induced nausea and vomiting
• Knowledge deficit related to drug therapy

Planning and implementation
• Don't give I.V.; give by deep I.M. route only. Massage injection site after administration.
• Be careful not to let drug come in contact with skin because it may cause skin reaction.
• Know that solution with slight sediment is usable.
• Know that drug is ineffective in arsine gas poisoning.
• Do not use for iron, cadmium, or selenium toxicity. Complex formed is highly toxic, even fatal.
• Use ephedrine or antihistamine, as ordered, to prevent or relieve mild adverse reactions.
• Keep urine alkaline to prevent renal damage. Oral sodium bicarbonate may be ordered.
• Apply ice or cold compresses to injection site to alleviate local discomfort.
Patient teaching
• Warn patient that drug has unpleasant garlic-like odor.
• Advise patient that drug may cause pain at injection site.
• Instruct patient to report changes in urine output, fever, pain, nausea, or vomiting immediately.

Reactions may be *common,* uncommon, *life-threatening*, or COMMON AND LIFE-THREATENING.

☑ **Evaluation**
• Patient's toxicity is eliminated.
• Patient maintains adequate hydration throughout therapy.
• Patient and family state understanding of drug therapy.

---

dinoprostone
(digh-noh-PROS-tohn)
Cervidil, Prepidil, Prostin E$_2$

Pharmacologic class: prostaglandin
Therapeutic class: oxytocic
Pregnancy risk category: C

How supplied

Vaginal suppositories: 20 mg
Vaginal insert: 10 mg
Endocervical gel: 0.5 mg/application (2.5-ml syringe)

Pharmacokinetics

Absorption: after vaginal insertion, drug is diffused slowly into maternal blood. There is also some local absorption into uterus through cervix or local vascular and lymphatic channels, but this accounts for only small portion of dose.
Distribution: distributed widely in mother.
Metabolism: metabolized in lungs, liver, kidneys, spleen, and other maternal tissues.
Excretion: drug and metabolites are excreted primarily in urine, with small amounts in feces. *Half-life:* less than 1 minute.

Route	Onset	Peak	Duration
Intra-vaginal	10-60 min	Unknown	About 17 hr (suppositories); unknown (gel); 12 hr (vaginal insert)

Pharmacodynamics

Chemical effect: produces strong, prompt contractions of uterine smooth muscle, possibly mediated by calcium and cAMP.
Therapeutic effect: causes abortion to occur.

Indications and dosage

▶ **To abort second-trimester pregnancy; to evacuate uterus in missed abortion, intrauterine fetal deaths up to 28 weeks of gestation, or benign hydatidiform mole (suppository only).** *Adults:* 20-mg suppository inserted high into posterior vaginal fornix. Repeated q 3 to 5 hours until abortion is complete.
▶ **Ripening of unfavorable cervix in pregnant patients at or near term (gel only).** *Adults:* contents of one syringe administered intravaginally; if cervix remains unfavorable after 6 hours, dosage repeated. No more than 1.5 mg (three applications) should be given per 24 hours. Place one insert with retrieval system intravaginally. Remove the insert upon onset of active labor or 12 hours after insertion.

Adverse reactions

CNS: *headache, dizziness,* anxiety, hot flashes, paresthesia, weakness, syncope.
CV: chest pain, *arrhythmias,* hypotension (in large doses).
EENT: blurred vision, eye pain.
GI: *nausea, vomiting, diarrhea.*
GU: vaginal pain, vaginitis, endometritis.
Musculoskeletal: *nocturnal leg cramps,* backache, muscle cramps.
Respiratory: coughing, dyspnea, *bronchospasm.*
Skin: rash
Other: *fever, shivering, chills,* breast tenderness, diaphoresis.

Interactions

Drug-drug. *Other oxytocics:* may potentiate action. Avoid concomitant use.
Drug-lifestyle. *Alcohol use:* inhibited effectiveness of dinoprostone with high doses. Avoid concomitant use.

Contraindications and precautions

• Gel form contraindicated when prolonged contractions of uterus are considered inappropriate and in patients with hypersensitivity to prostaglandins or constituents of gel. Drug also contraindicated in patients with placenta previa or unexplained vaginal bleeding during this pregnancy and in whom vaginal delivery is not indicated (that is, because of vasa previa or active herpes genitalia).

• Suppository form contraindicated in patients with hypersensitivity to drug, acute pelvic inflammatory disease, or active cardiac, pulmonary, renal, or hepatic disease.

• Use suppository form cautiously in patients with asthma; seizure disorders; anemia; diabetes; hypertension or hypotension; jaundice; CV, renal, or hepatic disease; scarred uterus; cervicitis; or acute vaginitis.

• Use gel form cautiously in patients with asthma or history of asthma, glaucoma or raised intraocular pressure, or renal or hepatic dysfunction, and in patients with ruptured membranes.

NURSING CONSIDERATIONS

Assessment
• Obtain history of patient's pregnancy status before therapy.
• Monitor effectiveness by observing patient for desired response to drug. Keep in mind that abortion should be complete within 30 hours when suppository form is used.
• Be alert for adverse reactions and drug interactions.
• Monitor patient's hydration status if adverse GI reactions occur.
• Evaluate patient's and family's knowledge of drug therapy.

Nursing diagnoses
• Risk for fluid volume deficit related to potential drug-induced adverse GI reactions

• Risk for altered body temperature related to possible drug-induced fever
• Knowledge deficit related to drug therapy

Planning and implementation
• Administer only when critical care facilities are readily available.
• Just before use, warm dinoprostone suppositories in their wrapping to room temperature. After administration, patient should remain supine for 10 minutes.
• When used for cervical ripening, have patient lying on her back, with cervix visualized using speculum. Assist with insertion: using aseptic technique, catheter provided with drug is used to administer gel into cervical canal just below level of internal os.
• Be aware that when gel form is used, contents of syringe are used for one patient only. Discard syringe, catheter, and unused drug after administration; do not attempt to administer small amount of drug remaining in catheter.
• Freeze suppositories at –4° F (–20° C).
• When used as abortifacient, be prepared to pretreat patient with antiemetic and antidiarrheal agents.
• Treat dinoprostone-induced fever (self-limiting and transient and occurs in approximately 50% of all patients) with water or alcohol sponging and increased fluid intake, not with aspirin.
• A dosing interval of at least 30 minutes is recommended for sequential use of oxytocin following the removal of a vaginal insert.

Patient teaching
• Instruct patient to remain supine for 10 minutes after administration.

Evaluation
• Patient maintains adequate hydration throughout therapy.
• Patient's body temperature returns to normal.
• Patient and family state understanding of drug therapy.

Reactions may be *common*, uncommon, *life-threatening*, or COMMON AND LIFE-THREATENING.

diphenhydramine hydrochloride

(digh-fen-HIGH-drah-meen
high-droh-KLOR-ighd)

Allerdryl ♦ †, AllerMax Caplets†,
Allermed†, Banophen†, Banophen
Caplets†, Beldin†, Belix†, Benadryl†,
Benadryl 25†, Benadryl Kapseals†,
Benylin Cough†, Bydramine Cough†,
Compoz†, Diphenadryl†, Diphen Cough†,
Diphenhist†, Diphenhist Captabs†,
Genahist†, Hyrexin-50, Nytol Maximum
Strength†, Nytol with DPH†, Sleep-Eze 3†,
Sominex Formula 2†, Tusstat†, Twilite
Caplets†, Uni-Bent Cough†

Pharmacologic class: ethanolamine
derivative antihistamine
Therapeutic class: antihistamine
(H_1-receptor antagonist), antiemetic,
antivertigo, antitussive, sedative-
hypnotic, antidyskinetic (anticholinergic)
Pregnancy risk category: B

How supplied

Tablets: 25 mg†, 50 mg†
Chewable tablets: 12.5 mg
Capsules: 25 mg†, 50 mg†
Elixir: 12.5 mg/5 ml (14% alcohol)*†
Syrup: 12.5 mg/5 ml†, 13.3 mg/5 ml (5%
alcohol)†
Injection: 10 mg/ml, 50 mg/ml

Pharmacokinetics

Absorption: well absorbed from GI tract
after P.O. administration; unknown after
I.M. administration.
Distribution: distributed widely throughout body, including CNS; about 82%
protein-bound.
Metabolism: metabolized in liver.
Excretion: drug and metabolites excreted
primarily in urine. *Half-life:* about 3½
hours.

Route	Onset	Peak	Duration
P.O.	≤ 15 min	1-4 hr	6-8 hr
I.V.	Immediate	1-4 hr	6-8 hr
I.M.	Unknown	1-4 hr	6-8 hr

Pharmacodynamics

Chemical effect: competes with histamine for H_1-receptor sites on effector
cells. Diphenhydramine prevents but does
not reverse histamine-mediated responses,
particularly histamine's effects on smooth
muscle of bronchial tubes, GI tract,
uterus, and blood vessels. Structurally related to local anesthetics, diphenhydramine provides local anesthesia by preventing initiation and transmission of
nerve impulses. It also suppresses cough
reflex by direct effect in medulla of brain.
Therapeutic effect: relieves allergy
symptoms, motion sickness, and cough;
improves voluntary movement; and promotes sleep and calmness.

Indications and dosage

▶ **Rhinitis, allergy symptoms, motion
sickness, Parkinson's disease.** *Adults
and children age 12 and over:* 25 to
50 mg P.O. t.i.d. or q.i.d.; or 10 to 50 mg
deep I.M. or I.V. Maximum I.M. or I.V.
dosage is 400 mg daily. *Children under
age 12:* 5 mg/kg daily P.O., deep I.M., or
I.V. in divided doses q.i.d. Maximum
dosage is 300 mg daily.
▶ **Sedation.** *Adults:* 25 to 50 mg P.O. or
deep I.M., p.r.n.
▶ **Nighttime sleep aid.** *Adults:* 50 mg
P.O. h.s.
▶ **Nonproductive cough.** *Adults:* 25 mg
P.O. q 4 to 6 hours (up to 150 mg daily).
Children ages 6 to 12: 12.5 mg P.O. q 4
to 6 hours (up to 75 mg daily). *Children
ages 2 to 6:* 6.25 mg P.O. q 4 to 6 hours
(up to 25 mg daily).

Adverse reactions

CNS: *drowsiness,* confusion, insomnia,
headache, vertigo, *sedation, sleepiness,
dizziness,* incoordination, fatigue, restlessness, tremor, nervousness, *seizures.*
CV: palpitations, hypotension, tachycardia.
EENT: diplopia, blurred vision, nasal
congestion, tinnitus.

GI: *nausea,* vomiting, diarrhea, *dry mouth,* constipation, *epigastric distress,* anorexia.
GU: dysuria, urine retention, urinary frequency.
Hematologic: *hemolytic anemia, thrombocytopenia, agranulocytosis.*
Respiratory: thickening of bronchial secretions, nasal congestion.
Skin: urticaria, photosensitivity, rash.
Other: *anaphylactic shock.*

Interactions

Drug-drug. *CNS depressants:* increased sedation. Use together cautiously.
MAO inhibitors: increased anticholinergic effects. Don't use together.
Drug-lifestyle. *Sun exposure:* photosensitivity reactions may occur.

Contraindications and precautions

• Contraindicated in patients with hypersensitivity to drug, during acute asthmatic attacks, and in newborns or premature neonates and breast-feeding women.
• Use with extreme caution in patients with angle-closure glaucoma, prostatic hyperplasia, pyloroduodenal and bladder-neck obstruction, asthma or COPD, increased intraocular pressure, hyperthyroidism, CV disease, hypertension, or stenosing peptic ulcer.
• Use cautiously in pregnant women.
• Children under age 12 should use only as directed by doctor.

NURSING CONSIDERATIONS

⚕ Assessment
• Obtain history of patient's underlying condition before therapy, and reassess regularly thereafter.
• Be alert for adverse reactions and drug interactions.
• Evaluate patient's and family's knowledge of drug therapy.

⊞ Nursing diagnoses
• Altered health maintenance related to underlying condition

• Risk for injury related to drug-induced adverse CNS reactions
• Knowledge deficit related to drug therapy

⊠ Planning and implementation
P.O. use: Reduce GI distress by giving drug with food or milk.
I.V. use: Follow manufacturer's guidelines.
I.M. use: Alternate injection sites to prevent irritation. Administer I.M. injection deeply into large muscle.
• Notify doctor if tolerance is observed because another antihistamine may need to be substituted.
Patient teaching
• Instruct patient to take drug 30 minutes before travel to prevent motion sickness.
• Warn patient to avoid alcohol and to refrain from driving or performing other hazardous activities that require alertness until drug's CNS effects are known.
• Tell patient that coffee or tea may reduce drowsiness.
• Inform patient that ice chips or sugarless gum or sour hard candy may relieve dry mouth.
• Advise patient to stop drug 4 days before allergy skin tests to preserve accuracy of tests.
• Tell patient to notify doctor if tolerance develops because different antihistamine may need to be prescribed.
• Warn patient of possible photosensitivity. Advise use of sunblock.

☑ Evaluation
• Patient exhibits improvement in underlying condition.
• Patient does not experience injury as result of therapy.
• Patient and family state understanding of drug therapy.

diphenoxylate hydrochloride and atropine sulfate
(digh-fen-OKS-ul-ayt high-droh-KLOR-ighd and AH-troh-peen SUL-fayt)
Lomanate, Lomotil*, Lonox

Pharmacologic class: opioid
Therapeutic class: antidiarrheal
Controlled substance schedule: V
Pregnancy risk category: C

How supplied

Tablets: 2.5 mg (with atropine sulfate 0.025 mg)
Liquid: 2.5 mg/5 ml (with atropine sulfate 0.025 mg/5 ml)*

Pharmacokinetics

Absorption: about 90% absorbed.
Distribution: unknown.
Metabolism: metabolized extensively by liver.
Excretion: metabolites excreted mainly in feces with lesser amounts excreted in urine. *Half-life:* diphenoxylate, 2½ hours; its major metabolite, diphenoxylic acid, 4½ hours; atropine, 2½ hours.

Route	Onset	Peak	Duration
P.O.	45-60 min	About 3 hr	3-4 hr

Pharmacodynamics

Chemical effect: unknown; probably increases smooth-muscle tone in GI tract, inhibits motility and propulsion, and diminishes secretions.
Therapeutic effect: relieves diarrhea.

Indications and dosage

▶ **Acute, nonspecific diarrhea.** *Adults:* initially, 5 mg P.O. q.i.d., then dosage adjusted as needed. *Children ages 2 to 12:* 0.3 to 0.4 mg/kg liquid form P.O. daily in four divided doses. Maintenance dosage can be 1/4 of original dose.

Adverse reactions

CNS: *sedation, dizziness,* headache, drowsiness, lethargy, restlessness, depression, euphoria, malaise, confusion, numbness in the extremities.
CV: tachycardia.
EENT: mydriasis.
GI: *dry mouth,* nausea, vomiting, abdominal discomfort or distention, *paralytic ileus,* anorexia, fluid retention in bowel (may mask depletion of extracellular fluid and electrolytes, especially in young children treated for acute gastroenteritis), possibly physical dependence with long-term use, *pancreatitis.*
GU: urine retention.
Respiratory: *respiratory depression.*
Skin: pruritus, rash.
Other: *angioedema, anaphylaxis.*

Interactions

Drug-drug. *Barbiturates, CNS depressants, narcotic agents, tranquilizers:* enhanced CNS depression. Closely monitor patient.
MAO inhibitors: possibly hypertensive crisis. Avoid concomitant use.
Drug-lifestyle. *Alcohol use:* enhanced CNS depression. Do not use concomitantly.

Contraindications and precautions

● Contraindicated in patients with hypersensitivity to diphenoxylate or atropine, acute diarrhea resulting from poison until toxic material is eliminated from GI tract, acute diarrhea caused by organisms that penetrate intestinal mucosa, or diarrhea resulting from antibiotic-induced pseudomembranous enterocolitis. Also contraindicated in jaundiced patients and in children under age 2.
● Drug is not recommended for use in breast-feeding women.
● Use cautiously in children age 2 and over; in patients with hepatic disease, narcotic dependence, or acute ulcerative colitis; and in pregnant women. Stop therapy immediately if abdominal disten-

tion or other signs of toxic megacolon develop, and notify doctor.

NURSING CONSIDERATIONS

◪ Assessment
• Assess patient's diarrhea before and regularly during therapy.
• Be alert for adverse reactions and drug interactions.
• Evaluate patient's and family's knowledge of drug therapy.

⊞ Nursing diagnoses
• Diarrhea related to underlying condition
• Ineffective breathing pattern related to drug-induced respiratory depression
• Knowledge deficit related to drug therapy

⊠ Planning and implementation
• Correct fluid and electrolyte disturbances before starting drug. Dehydration, especially in young children, may increase risk of delayed toxicity.
• Keep in mind that dose of 2.5 mg is as effective as 5 ml of camphorated opium tincture.
• Know that drug is not indicated for treating antibiotic-induced diarrhea.
• Be aware that drug is unlikely to be effective if no response occurs within 48 hours.
• Know that risk of physical dependence increases with high dosage and long-term use. Atropine sulfate helps discourage abuse.
• Use naloxone, as ordered, to treat respiratory depression caused by overdose.
Patient teaching
• Tell patient not to exceed recommended dosage.
• Warn patient not to use drug to treat acute diarrhea for longer than 2 days. Encourage him to seek medical attention if diarrhea continues.
• Advise patient to avoid hazardous activities, such as driving, until CNS effects of drug are known.

☑ Evaluation
• Patient regains normal bowel pattern.
• Patient maintains normal breathing pattern throughout therapy.
• Patient and family state understanding of drug therapy.

---

dipyridamole
(digh-peer-IH-duh-mohl)
Apo-Dipyridamole♦, Dipridacot, I.V. Persantine, Novodipiradol♦, Persantin◇, Persantin 100◇, Persantine**

Pharmacologic class: pyrimidine analogue
Therapeutic class: coronary vasodilator, platelet aggregation inhibitor
Pregnancy risk category: B

How supplied
Tablets: 25 mg, 50 mg, 75 mg
Injection: 10 mg/2 ml

Pharmacokinetics
Absorption: variable and slow; bioavailability ranges from 27% to 59%.
Distribution: wide distribution in body tissues. Protein binding ranges from 91% to 97%.
Metabolism: metabolized by liver.
Excretion: elimination occurs by way of biliary excretion of glucuronide conjugates. Some dipyridamole and conjugates may undergo enterohepatic circulation and fecal excretion; small amount is excreted in urine. *Half-life:* 1 to 12 hours.

Route	Onset	Peak	Duration
P.O.	Unknown	45-150 min	Unknown
I.V.	Unknown	2 min after infusion completed	Unknown
I.M.	Unknown	Unknown	Unknown

Pharmacodynamics
Chemical effect: unknown; may involve its ability to increase adenosine, which is

---

a coronary vasodilator and platelet aggregation inhibitor.
Therapeutic effect: dilates coronary arteries and helps prevent clotting.

Indications and dosage

▶ **Inhibition of platelet adhesion in prosthetic heart valves (in combination with warfarin or aspirin).** *Adults:* 75 to 100 mg P.O. q.i.d.
▶ **Alternative to exercise in evaluation of coronary artery disease during thallium-201 myocardial perfusion scintigraphy.** *Adults:* 0.57 mg/kg as I.V. infusion at constant rate over 4 minutes (0.142 mg/kg/minute).
▶ **Acute coronary insufficiency.** *Adults:* 10 mg I.V. or I.M.

Adverse reactions

CNS: *headache, dizziness,* weakness.
CV: flushing, fainting, hypotension, chest pain, ECG abnormalities, blood pressure lability, hypertension (with I.V. infusion).
GI: *nausea,* vomiting, diarrhea, abdominal distress.
Skin: rash, irritation (with undiluted injection), pruritus.

Interactions

Drug-drug. *Heparin:* may cause increased bleeding. Monitor patient closely.
Theophylline: may prevent the coronary vasodilation by I.V. dipyridamole. Avoid concomitant use.

Contraindications and precautions

• No known contraindications.
• Use cautiously in patients with hypotension and in pregnant women.
• Safety of drug has not been established in breast-feeding women or in children.

NURSING CONSIDERATIONS

⚕ Assessment
• Obtain history of patient's underlying condition before therapy, and reassess regularly thereafter.

• Be alert for adverse reactions and drug interactions.
• Evaluate patient's and family's knowledge of drug therapy.

⊞ Nursing diagnoses
• Altered cardiopulmonary tissue perfusion related to underlying condition
• Pain related to drug-induced headache
• Knowledge deficit related to drug therapy

⧉ Planning and implementation
P.O. use: Administer drug 1 hour before meals. If patient develops adverse GI reactions, administer drug with meals.
I.V. use: If administering drug as diagnostic agent, dilute in 0.45% or 0.9% NaCl or D_5W in at least a 1:2 ratio for total volume of 20 to 50 ml. Inject thallium-201 within 5 minutes after completing 4-minute dipyridamole infusion.
I.M. use: Follow normal protocol.
Patient teaching
• Instruct patient when to take drug.
• Tell patient to have his blood pressure checked frequently.
• Advise patient to take mild analgesic if headache occurs.
• Instruct patient to notify doctor if chest pain occurs.

☑ Evaluation
• Patient maintains adequate tissue perfusion and cellular oxygenation.
• Patient obtains relief from drug-induced headache with use of mild analgesic.
• Patient and family state understanding of drug therapy.

dirithromycin
(digh-rith-roh-MIGH-sin)
Dynabac

Pharmacologic class: macrolide
Therapeutic class: antibiotic
Pregnancy risk category: C

How supplied

Tablets (enteric-coated): 250 mg

Pharmacokinetics

Absorption: rapidly absorbed from GI tract and converted by nonenzymatic hydrolysis to the microbiologically active compound erythromycyclamine. Food slightly increases bioavailability.
Distribution: widely distributed throughout body; protein binding ranges from 15% to 30%.
Metabolism: undergoes little to no hepatic metabolism.
Excretion: eliminated primarily in bile; small amount excreted in urine. *Half-life:* about 8 hours.

Route	Onset	Peak	Duration
P.O.	Unknown	About 4 hr	Unknown

Pharmacodynamics

Chemical effect: inhibits bacterial RNA-dependent protein synthesis by binding to 5OS subunit of ribosome.
Therapeutic effect: hinders susceptible bacterial activity. Spectrum of activity includes gram-positive aerobes, such as *Staphylococcus aureus* (methicillin-susceptible strains only), *Streptococcus pneumoniae,* and *Streptococcus pyogenes;* gram-negative aerobes, such as *Legionella pneumophila* and *Moraxella (Branhamella) catarrhalis;* and other bacteria, such as *Mycoplasma pneumoniae.*

Indications and dosage

▶ **Acute bacterial exacerbations of chronic bronchitis due to *M. (Bran-hamella) catarrhalis* or *S. pneumoniae;* secondary bacterial infection of acute bronchitis due to *M. (Branhamella) catarrhalis* or *S. pneumoniae;* uncomplicated skin and skin structure infections due to *S. aureus* (methicillin-susceptible strains only).** *Adults and children age 12 and older:* 500 mg P.O. daily with food for 7 days.

▶ **Community-acquired pneumonia due to *L. pneumophila, M. pneumoniae,* or *S. pneumoniae.*** *Adults and children age 12 and older:* 500 mg P.O. daily with food for 14 days.

▶ **Pharyngitis or tonsillitis due to *S. pyogenes.*** *Adults and children age 12 and older:* 500 mg P.O. daily with food for 10 days.

Adverse reactions

CNS: asthenia, headache, dizziness, vertigo, insomnia.
GI: abdominal pain, nausea, diarrhea, vomiting, dyspepsia, GI disorder, flatulence.
Hematologic: increased platelet, eosinophil, and neutrophil counts.
Metabolic: hyperkalemia, decreased bicarbonate levels.
Respiratory: increased cough, dyspnea.
Skin: rash, pruritus, urticaria.
Other: pain (nonspecific), increased CK and liver enzyme levels.

Interactions

Drug-drug. *Antacids, H_2 antagonists:* absorption slightly enhanced when dirithromycin is administered immediately after these drugs.
Theophylline: may alter steady-state plasma concentration of theophylline. Monitor theophylline plasma concentrations. Dosage adjustments may be needed.
Note: Alfentanil, oral anticoagulants, astemizole, bromocriptine, carbamazepine, cyclosporine, digoxin, disopyramide, ergotamine, hexobarbital, lovastatin, phenytoin, triazolam, and valproate have been reported to interact with erythromycin products. It is not known whether these same drug interactions occur with dirithromycin. Until further data are available, caution should be used during coadministration.
Drug-food. *Any food:* increased absorption. Administer drug with food.

Contraindications and precautions

• Contraindicated in patients with hypersensitivity to drug, erythromycin, or other macrolide antibiotics.
• Use cautiously in patients with hepatic insufficiency and in pregnant or breast-feeding women.
• Safety of drug has not been established in children under age 12.

NURSING CONSIDERATIONS

Assessment
• Obtain history of patient's infection before therapy.
• Obtain culture and sensitivity tests before first dose. Therapy may begin, pending test results.
• Be alert for adverse reactions and drug interactions.
• Evaluate patient's and family's knowledge of drug therapy.

Nursing diagnoses
• Infection related to susceptible bacteria
• Risk of fluid volume deficit related to adverse GI reactions
• Knowledge deficit related to drug therapy

Planning and implementation
• Be aware that drug should not be used in patient with known, suspected, or potential bacteremia; serum levels are inadequate to provide antibacterial coverage of the bloodstream.
• Administer drug with food or within 1 hour of food intake.
Patient teaching
• Tell patient to take all of drug, as ordered, even if he feels better.
• Advise him to take drug with food or within 1 hour of having eaten. Tell him not to cut, chew, or crush the tablet.

Evaluation
• Patient is free from infection.
• Patient maintains adequate hydration.
• Patient and family state understanding of drug therapy.

disopyramide
(digh-so-PEER-uh-mighd)
Rythmodan♦◊

disopyramide phosphate
Norpace, Norpace CR, Rythmodan LA♦

Pharmacologic class: pyridine derivative
Therapeutic class: antiarrhythmic
Pregnancy risk category: C

How supplied

disopyramide
Capsules: 100 mg♦, 150 mg♦
disopyramide phosphate
Tablets (sustained-release): 250 mg♦
Capsules: 100 mg, 150 mg
Capsules (controlled-release): 100 mg, 150 mg
Injection: 10 mg/ml♦◊

Pharmacokinetics

Absorption: rapidly and well absorbed from GI tract with P.O. administration.
Distribution: well distributed throughout extracellular fluid but not extensively bound to tissues. Plasma protein binding varies but generally ranges from about 50% to 65%.
Metabolism: metabolized in liver.
Excretion: excreted in urine. *Half-life:* about 7 hours.

Route	Onset	Peak	Duration
P.O.	0.5-3.5 hr	2-2.5 hr	1.5-8.5 hr
I.V.	Unknown	Unknown	Unknown

Pharmacodynamics

Chemical effect: unknown; considered class Ia antiarrhythmic that depresses phase O and prolongs action potential. All class I drugs have membrane-stabilizing effects.
Therapeutic effect: restores normal sinus rhythm.

Indications and dosage

▶ **Symptomatic PVCs (unifocal, multifocal, or coupled); ventricular tachycardia not severe enough to require cardioversion.** *Adults weighing over 50 kg (110 lb):* 150 mg q 6 hours with conventional capsules or 300 mg q 12 hours with controlled-release preparations. *Adults weighing 50 kg or less:* highly individualized. *Children ages 12 to 18:* 6 to 15 mg/kg P.O. daily. *Children ages 4 to 12:* 10 to 15 mg/kg P.O. daily. *Children ages 1 to 4:* 10 to 20 mg/kg P.O. daily. *Children under age 1:* 10 to 30 mg/kg P.O. daily. For pediatric dosages, divide into equal amounts and give q 6 hours.

Recommended dosages in advanced renal insufficiency: if creatinine clearance is 30 to 40 ml/minute, 100 mg q 8 hours; if creatinine clearance is 15 to 30 ml/minute, 100 mg q 12 hours; if creatinine clearance is less than 15 ml/minute, 100 mg q 24 hours. *For parenteral use in adults:* 2 mg/kg I.V. slowly (over not less than 15 minutes). Administer until arrhythmia is eliminated or patient has received 150 mg. Repeat dosage if conversion is successful but arrhythmia returns. Total I.V. dosage should not exceed 300 mg in first hour. Follow with I.V. infusion of 0.4 mg/kg/hour (usually 20 to 30 mg/hour) to maximum of 800 mg/day.

Adverse reactions

CNS: dizziness, agitation, depression, fatigue, headache, acute psychosis.
CV: *hypotension,* syncope, *heart failure, heart block,* edema, weight gain, *arrhythmias,* shortness of breath, chest pain.
EENT: blurred vision, dry eyes, dry nose.
GI: nausea, vomiting, anorexia, bloating, abdominal pain, constipation, dry mouth, diarrhea.
GU: urine retention, urinary hesitancy.
Hepatic: cholestatic jaundice.
Metabolic: hypoglycemia (rare).

Musculoskeletal: aches, pain, muscle weakness.
Skin: rash, pruritus, dermatosis.

Interactions

Drug-drug. Antiarrhythmics: possibly additive or antagonized antiarrhythmic effects. Monitor patient closely.
Erythromycin: increased disopyramide levels may occur, causing arrhythmias and prolonged QT_c. Monitor closely.
Phenytoin: increased metabolism of disopyramide. Monitor for decreased antiarrhythmic effect.
Rifampin: disopyramide levels may be decreased. Monitor for decreased effectiveness.

Contraindications and precautions

• Contraindicated in patients with second- or third-degree heart block in absence of artificial pacemaker, cardiogenic shock, or hypersensitivity to drug.
• Drug is not recommended for use in breast-feeding women.
• Use with extreme caution and avoid, if possible, in patients with heart failure. Use cautiously in patients with underlying conduction abnormalities, urinary tract diseases (especially prostatic hypertrophy), hepatic or renal impairment, myasthenia gravis, or acute angle-closure glaucoma.
• Also use cautiously in pregnant women.

NURSING CONSIDERATIONS

⚗ Assessment
• Obtain history of patient's arrhythmia before therapy.
• Monitor effectiveness by assessing patient's ECG pattern and apical pulse rate.
• Be alert for adverse reactions and drug interactions.
• Evaluate patient's and family's knowledge of drug therapy.

⚙ Nursing diagnoses
• Decreased cardiac output related to underlying arrhythmia

Reactions may be *common,* uncommon, *life-threatening,* or COMMON AND LIFE-THREATENING.

• Altered protection related to drug-induced proarrhythmias
• Knowledge deficit related to drug therapy

≫ **Planning and implementation**
• Correct any underlying electrolyte abnormalities before therapy begins, as ordered.
• Check apical pulse before administering drug. Notify doctor if pulse rate is slower than 60 beats/minute or faster than 120 beats/minute.
P.O. use: Know that sustained-release and controlled-release preparations should not be used for rapid control of ventricular arrhythmias; when therapeutic blood levels must be rapidly attained; in patients with cardiomyopathy or possible cardiac decompensation; or in those with severe renal impairment.
• Know that for administration to young children, pharmacist may prepare disopyramide suspension from 100-mg capsules, using cherry syrup. Suspension should be dispensed in amber glass bottles and protected from light.
I.V. use: Add 200 mg to 500 ml of compatible solution, such as 0.9% NaCl or D₅W. Use an infusion pump to administer drug. Do not mix with other drugs; switch to P.O. therapy as soon as possible.
• Discontinue drug if heart block develops, if QRS complex widens by more than 25%, or if QT interval lengthens by more than 25% above baseline; also notify doctor.
Patient teaching
• When transferring patient from immediate-release to sustained-release capsules, advise him to take sustained-release capsule 6 hours after last immediate-release capsule was taken.
• Teach patient importance of taking drug on time and exactly as prescribed. This may require use of alarm clock for night doses.
• Advise patient to chew gum or hard candy to relieve dry mouth.

☑ **Evaluation**
• Patient's ECG reveals that arrhythmia has been corrected.
• Patient does not develop a new arrhythmia as result of therapy.
• Patient and family state understanding of drug therapy.

disulfiram
(digh-SUL-fih-ram)
Antabuse

Pharmacologic class: aldehyde dehydrogenase inhibitor
Therapeutic class: alcoholic deterrent
Pregnancy risk category: NR

How supplied
Tablets: 250 mg, 500 mg

Pharmacokinetics
Absorption: absorbed completely from GI tract.
Distribution: drug is highly lipid-soluble and initially localized in adipose tissue.
Metabolism: mostly oxidized in liver.
Excretion: primarily excreted in urine; 5% to 20% eliminated in feces.

Route	Onset	Peak	Duration
P.O.	1-2 hr	Unknown	< 14 days

Pharmacodynamics
Chemical effect: blocks oxidation of ethanol at acetaldehyde stage. Excess acetaldehyde produces highly unpleasant reaction in presence of even small amounts of ethanol.
Therapeutic effect: deters alcohol consumption.

Indications and dosage
▶ **Adjunct in management of chronic alcoholism.** *Adults:* 250 to 500 mg P.O. as single dose in morning for 1 to 2 weeks. Can be taken in evening if drowsiness occurs. Maintenance dosage is 125 to 500 mg P.O. daily (average

dosage 250 mg) until permanent self-control is established. Treatment may continue for months or years.

Adverse reactions

CNS: drowsiness, headache, fatigue, delirium, depression, neuritis, peripheral neuritis, polyneuritis, restlessness, and psychotic reactions.
EENT: optic neuritis.
GI: metallic or garlic aftertaste.
GU: impotence.
Skin: acneiform or allergic dermatitis.
Other: disulfiram reaction (precipitated by ethanol use), which may include flushing, throbbing headache, dyspnea, nausea, copious vomiting, diaphoresis, thirst, chest pain, palpitations, hyperventilation, hypotension, syncope, anxiety, weakness, blurred vision, confusion. *In severe reactions—respiratory depression, CV collapse, arrhythmias, MI, acute heart failure, seizures, unconsciousness, or death.*

Interactions

Drug-drug. *Alfentanil:* prolonged duration of effect. Closely monitor patient.
Anticoagulants: increased anticoagulant effect. Adjust dosage of anticoagulant.
Bacampicillin: lowered concentrations of ethanol and acetaldehyde. Monitor patient closely.
CNS depressants: increased CNS depression. Use together cautiously.
Isoniazid: ataxia or marked change in behavior. Don't use concomitantly.
Metronidazole: psychotic reaction. Don't use concomitantly.
Midazolam: increased plasma levels of midazolam. Use together cautiously.
Paraldehyde: toxic levels of acetaldehyde. Don't use concomitantly.
Phenytoin: increased blood levels of phenytoin. Monitor phenytoin blood levels, and expect doctor to adjust phenytoin dosages.
Tricyclic antidepressants, especially amitriptyline: transient delirium. Closely monitor patient.

Drug-lifestyle. *Alcohol use (all sources, including cough syrups, liniments, shaving lotion, back-rub preparations):* may precipitate disulfiram reaction. Don't use concomitantly. Alcohol reaction may occur as long as 2 weeks after single disulfiram dose; the longer patient remains on drug, the more sensitive he is to alcohol.

Contraindications and precautions

• Contraindicated during alcohol intoxication and within 12 hours of alcohol ingestion; in patients with hypersensitivity to disulfiram or to other thiram derivatives used in pesticides and rubber vulcanization; in patients with psychoses, myocardial disease, or coronary occlusion; and in patients receiving metronidazole, paraldehyde, alcohol, or alcohol-containing preparations.
• Drug should not be administered to pregnant women.
• Use with extreme caution in patients with diabetes mellitus, hypothyroidism, seizure disorder, cerebral damage, or nephritis or hepatic cirrhosis or insufficiency and with concurrent phenytoin therapy.
• Use cautiously in breast-feeding women.
• Safety of drug has not been established in children.

NURSING CONSIDERATIONS

⏳ Assessment
• Obtain history of patient's alcoholism before therapy.
• Know that complete physical examination and laboratory studies, including CBC, chemistry panel, and transaminase determination, should precede therapy. Repeat physical examination and laboratory studies regularly, as ordered.
• Monitor effectiveness by assessing patient's abstinence from alcohol.
• Obtain measurement of serum alcohol level on weekly basis.
• Be alert for adverse reactions and drug interactions.

Reactions may be *common,* uncommon, *life-threatening,* or COMMON AND LIFE-THREATENING.

• Evaluate patient's and family's knowledge of drug therapy.

🔁 **Nursing diagnoses**
• Altered health maintenance related to alcoholism
• Pain related to drug-induced headache
• Knowledge deficit related to drug therapy

❯ **Planning and implementation**
• Use only under close medical and nursing supervision. Never administer until patient has abstained from alcohol for at least 12 hours. Patients should clearly understand consequences of disulfiram therapy and give permission for its use. Use drug only in patients who are cooperative, well motivated, and receiving supportive psychiatric therapy.
• Know that administration is usually during the day, although drug may be given at night if drowsiness occurs. Establish lowered maintenance dose until permanent self-control is practiced. Keep in mind that treatment may continue for months or years.
Patient teaching
• Caution patient's family that disulfiram should never be given to the patient without his knowledge; severe reaction or death could result if the patient ingests alcohol.
• Warn patient to avoid all sources of alcohol (for example, sauces and cough syrups). Even external application of liniments, shaving lotion, and back-rub preparations may precipitate disulfiram reaction. Tell patient that alcohol reaction may occur as long as 2 weeks after single dose of disulfiram; the longer patient remains on drug, the more sensitive he becomes to alcohol.
• Tell patient to wear a medical identification bracelet or carry a card supplied by drug manufacturer identifying him as a disulfiram user. *Note:* Mild reactions may occur in sensitive patients with blood alcohol levels of 5 to 10 mg/dl; symptoms are fully developed at

50 mg/dl; unconsciousness typically occurs at 125- to 150-mg/dl level. Reaction may last from 30 minutes to several hours or as long as alcohol remains in blood.
• Reassure patient that drug-induced adverse reactions (unrelated to concomitant alcohol use), such as drowsiness, fatigue, impotence, headache, peripheral neuritis, and metallic or garlic taste, subside after about 2 weeks of therapy.

☑ **Evaluation**
• Patient abstains from alcohol consumption.
• Patient's headache is relieved with mild analgesic therapy.
• Patient and family state understanding of drug therapy.

---

dobutamine hydrochloride
(doh-BYOO-tuh-meen high-droh-KLOR-ighd)
Dobutrex

Pharmacologic class: adrenergic, beta$_1$ agonist
Therapeutic class: inotropic agent
Pregnancy risk category: B

How supplied

Injection: 12.5 mg/ml in 20-ml vials (parenteral)

Pharmacokinetics

Absorption: not applicable with I.V. administration.
Distribution: widely distributed throughout body.
Metabolism: metabolized by liver.
Excretion: excreted mainly in urine with minor amounts in feces. *Half-life:* about 2 minutes.

Route	Onset	Peak	Duration
I.V.	1-2 min	≤ 10 min	< 5 min after drug stopped

Pharmacodynamics

Chemical effect: directly stimulates beta₁ receptors to increase myocardial contractility and stroke volume. At therapeutic dosages, drug decreases peripheral vascular resistance (afterload), reduces ventricular filling pressure (preload), and may facilitate AV node conduction.
Therapeutic effect: increases cardiac output.

Indications and dosage

► **To increase cardiac output in short-term treatment of cardiac decompensation caused by depressed contractility, such as during refractory heart failure, and as adjunct in cardiac surgery.** *Adults:* 2.5 to 10.0 mcg/kg/minute I.V. infusion. Rates up to 40 mcg/kg/minute may be needed (rare).

Adverse reactions

CNS: headache.
CV: *increased heart rate, hypertension,* PVCs, angina, nonspecific chest pain, hypotension.
GI: nausea, vomiting.
Respiratory: shortness of breath, *asthmatic episodes.*
Other: mild leg cramps or tingling sensation, phlebitis, *anaphylaxis.*

Interactions

Drug-drug. *Beta blockers:* may antagonize dobutamine effects. Do not use together.
Bretylium: may potentiate action of vasopressors on adrenergic receptors; arrhythmias may result.
General anesthetics: greater incidence of ventricular arrhythmias. Monitor patient closely.
Tricyclic antidepressants: may potentiate pressor response. Monitor patient closely.

Contraindications and precautions

• Contraindicated in patients with idiopathic hypertrophic subaortic stenosis or hypersensitivity to drug or its components.

• Use cautiously in patients with history of hypertension. Drug may precipitate exaggerated pressor response.
• Safety of drug has not been established in pregnant or breast-feeding women and in children.

NURSING CONSIDERATIONS

⚕ Assessment
• Assess patient's condition before therapy and regularly thereafter.
• Continuously monitor ECG, blood pressure, pulmonary capillary wedge pressure, cardiac condition, and urine output.
• Monitor serum electrolyte levels, as ordered. Drug may lower serum potassium level.
• Be alert for adverse reactions and drug interactions.
• Evaluate patient's and family's knowledge of drug therapy.

⊕ Nursing diagnoses
• Decreased cardiac output related to underlying condition
• Pain related to headache
• Knowledge deficit related to drug therapy

⊠ Planning and implementation
• Before initiating therapy with dobutamine, correct hypovolemia with plasma volume expanders, as ordered.
• Administer cardiac glycoside before dobutamine, as ordered. Because drug increases AV node conduction, patients with atrial fibrillation may develop rapid ventricular rate.
• Administer using central venous catheter or large peripheral vein. Titrate infusion according to doctor's orders and patient's condition. Use infusion pump.
• Dilute concentrate for injection before administration. Compatible solutions include D_5W, 0.45% NaCl injection, 0.9% NaCl injection, and lactated Ringer's injection. The contents of one vial (250 mg) diluted with 1,000 ml of solution yields

concentration of 250 mcg/ml; diluted with 500 ml, concentration of 500 mcg/ml; diluted with 250 ml, concentration of 1,000 mcg/ml. Maximum concentration should not exceed 5 mg/ml.
• Avoid extravasation; it may cause inflammatory response.
• Do not administer through same I.V. line with other drugs. Drug is incompatible with heparin, hydrocortisone sodium succinate, cefazolin, cefamandole, neutral cephalothin, penicillin, and ethacrynate sodium.
• Do not mix with sodium bicarbonate injection because drug is incompatible with alkaline solutions.
• Keep in mind that I.V. solutions remain stable for 24 hours.
• Be aware that oxidation of drug may slightly discolor admixtures containing dobutamine. This does not indicate significant loss of potency, provided drug is used within 24 hours of reconstitution.
• Change I.V. sites regularly to avoid phlebitis.
Patient teaching
• Tell patient to report shortness of breath and headache.

☑ **Evaluation**
• Patient regains adequate cardiac output exhibited by stable vital signs, normal urine output, and clear mental status.
• Patient's headache is relieved with analgesic administration.
• Patient and family state understanding of drug therapy.

docetaxel
(doks-uh-TAKX-ul)
Taxotere

Pharmacologic class: taxoid antineoplastic
Therapeutic class: antineoplastic
Pregnancy risk category: D

How supplied
Injection: 20 mg, 80 mg

Pharmacokinetics
Absorption: not applicable with I.V. administration.
Distribution: 94% is protein-bound.
Metabolism: partly by liver.
Excretion: mainly in feces.

Route	Onset	Peak	Duration
I.V.	Immediate	Unknown	Unknown

Pharmacodynamics
Chemical effect: disrupts the microtubular network essential for mitotic and interphase cellular functions.
Therapeutic effect: inhibits mitosis, producing antineoplastic effect.

Indications and dosage
▶ **Treatment of patients with locally advanced or metastatic breast cancer who have progressed during anthracycline-based therapy or have relapsed during anthracycline-based adjuvant therapy.** *Adults:* 60 to 100 mg/m^2 I.V. over 1 hour q 3 weeks.

Adverse reactions
CNS: *asthenia,* paresthesia, dysesthesia, pain (including burning sensation), weakness.
CV: *fluid retention,* hypotension.
GI: *stomatitis, nausea, vomiting, diarrhea.*
Hematologic: *anemia,* NEUTROPENIA, FEBRILE NEUTROPENIA, MYELOSUPPRESSION (DOSE LIMITING), LEUKOPENIA, THROMBOCYTOPENIA, *septic and nonseptic death.*
Hepatic: increased liver function tests.
Musculoskeletal: back pain, *myalgia,* arthralgia.
Respiratory: dyspnea.
Skin: *alopecia,* skin eruptions, desquamation, nail pigmentation alterations, nail pain, flushing, rash.

Other: HYPERSENSITIVITY REACTIONS, infection, chest tightness, drug fever, chills.

Interactions

Drug-drug. *Agents that are induced, inhibited, or metabolized by cytochrome P-450 3A4 (cyclosporin, terfenadine, ketoconazole, erythromycin, troleandomycin):* may modify docetaxel metabolism when given together. Use cautiously.

Contraindications and precautions

• Contraindicated in patients with history of hypersensitivity to drug or to other polysorbate 80–containing drugs and in those with neutrophil counts below 1,500 cells/mm³.

NURSING CONSIDERATIONS

Assessment
• Premedicate patient with oral corticosteroids.
• Monitor blood count frequently during therapy.
• Evaluate patient's and family's knowledge of drug therapy.

Nursing diagnoses
• Altered health maintenance related to neoplastic disease
• Knowledge deficit related to drug therapy

Planning and implementation
• Dilute drug with diluent supplied before administration. Allow drug and diluent to stand at room temperature for 5 minutes before mixing. After adding diluent contents to vial, rotate vial gently for 15 seconds. Let solution stand for few minutes for foam to dissipate.
• To prepare solution for infusion, withdraw required amount of premixed solution from vial and inject it into 250 ml 0.9% NaCl solution or D₅W to produce a final concentration of 0.3 to 0.9 mg/ml.
• Wear gloves during drug preparation and administration.

Patient teaching
• Warn patient that alopecia occurs in almost 80% of all patients.
• Tell patient to promptly report sore throat, fever, or unusual bruising or bleeding and signs of fluid retention.

Evaluation
• Patient shows positive response to drug.
• Patient and family state understanding of drug therapy.

---

docusate calcium (dioctyl calcium sulfosuccinate)
(DOK-yoo-sayt KAL-see-um)
Pro-Cal-Soft†, Surfak†

docusate potassium (dioctyl potassium sulfosuccinate)
Diocto-K†, Kasof†

docusate sodium (dioctyl sodium sulfosuccinate)
Colace†, Coloxyl◇, Coloxyl Enema Concentrate◇, Dialose†, Diocto†, Dioeze†, Disonate†, DOK†, DOS Softgels†, Doxinate†, D-S-S†, Modane Soft†, Pro-Sof†, Regulax SS†, Regulex♦†, Regutol†, Therevac Plus†, Therevac-SB†

Pharmacologic class: surfactant
Therapeutic class: emollient laxative
Pregnancy risk category: C

How supplied

docusate calcium
Capsules: 50 mg†, 240 mg†
docusate potassium
Capsules: 100 mg†, 240 mg†
docusate sodium
Tablets: 100 mg†
Capsules: 50 mg†, 60 mg†, 100 mg†, 240 mg†, 250 mg†
Oral liquid: 150 mg/15 ml†
Oral solution: 50 mg/ml†
Syrup: 50 mg/15 ml†, 60 mg/15 ml†

Reactions may be *common*, uncommon, *life-threatening*, or COMMON AND LIFE-THREATENING.

Enema concentrate: 18 g/100 ml (must be diluted)◊

Pharmacokinetics

Absorption: absorbed minimally in duodenum and jejunum.
Distribution: distributed primarily locally, in gut.
Metabolism: none.
Excretion: excreted in feces.

Route	Onset	Peak	Duration
P.O.	Varies	Varies	24-72 hr
P.R.	Unknown	Unknown	Unknown

Pharmacodynamics

Chemical effect: reduces surface tension of interfacing liquid contents of bowel. This detergent activity promotes incorporation of additional liquid into stool, thus forming softer mass.
Therapeutic effect: softens stool.

Indications and dosage

▶ **Stool softener.** *Adults and children over age 12:* 50 to 360 mg P.O. daily until bowel movements are normal. Alternatively, give enema (where available). Dilute 1:24 with sterile water before administration, and give 100 to 150 ml (retention enema), 300 to 500 ml (evacuation enema), or 0.5 to 1.5 liters (flushing enema). *Children ages 6 to 12:* 40 to 120 mg docusate sodium P.O. daily. *Children ages 3 to 6:* 20 to 60 mg docusate sodium P.O. daily. *Children under age 3:* 10 to 40 mg docusate sodium P.O. daily.

Higher dosages used for initial therapy. Dosage adjusted to individual response. Usual dosage in children and adults with minimal needs is 50 to 150 mg (docusate calcium) P.O. daily.

Adverse reactions

EENT: throat irritation.
GI: bitter taste, mild abdominal cramping, diarrhea, laxative dependence (with long-term or excessive use).

Interactions

Drug-drug. *Mineral oil:* may increase mineral oil absorption and cause toxicity and lipoid pneumonia. Separate administration times.

Contraindications and precautions

• Contraindicated in patients with intestinal obstruction, undiagnosed abdominal pain, vomiting or other signs of appendicitis, fecal impaction, acute surgical abdomen, or hypersensitivity to drug.
• Use cautiously in pregnant women.

NURSING CONSIDERATIONS

🛂 Assessment
• Obtain history of patient's bowel patterns before therapy, and reassess regularly thereafter.
• Before giving for constipation, determine if patient has adequate fluid intake, exercise, and diet.
• Be alert for adverse reactions and drug interactions.
• Evaluate patient's and family's knowledge of drug therapy.

🔁 Nursing diagnoses
• Constipation related to underlying condition
• Diarrhea related to prolonged or excessive use of drug
• Knowledge deficit related to drug therapy

❯ Planning and implementation
P.O. use: Give liquid in milk, fruit juice, or infant formula to mask bitter taste.
P.R. use: Follow manufacturer's directions.
• Be aware that drug is laxative of choice for patients who should not strain during defecation, including patients recovering from MI or rectal surgery; for those with rectal or anal disease that makes passage of firm stool difficult; and for those with postpartum constipation.
• Store drug at 59° to 86° F (15° to 30° C), and protect liquid from light.

• Discontinue if abdominal cramping occurs and notify doctor; docusate does not stimulate intestinal peristaltic movements.

Patient teaching

• Teach patient about dietary sources of bulk, which include bran and other cereals, fresh fruit, and vegetables.

• Instruct patient to use only occasionally and not to use for more than 1 week without doctor's knowledge.

• Tell patient to discontinue if severe cramping occurs and notify doctor.

☑ **Evaluation**

• Patient's constipation is relieved.

• Patient remains free from diarrhea during therapy.

• Patient and family state understanding of drug therapy.

---

dolasetron mesylate
(doh-LEH-seh-trohn MES-ih layt)
Anzemet

Pharmacologic class: selective serotonin 5-HT$_3$ receptor antagonist
Therapeutic class: antiemetic
Pregnancy risk category: B

How supplied

Tablets: 50 mg, 100 mg
Injection: 20 mg/ml as 12.5 mg/0.625 ml ampule or 100 mg/5 ml vials

Pharmacokinetics

Absorption: rapid for hydrodolasetron, an active metabolite that has an absolute bioavailability of 75%. Absorption of the parent compound is rarely seen.
Distribution: widely distributed with 69% to 77% bound to plasma protein.
Metabolism: dolasetron is metabolized to an active metabolite; hydrodolasetron by carbonyl reductase. Rarely detected in plasma due to rapid and complete metabolism.

Excretion: about two-thirds of hydrodolasetron is recovered in urine; one-third in feces. *Half-life:* 8.1 hours.

Route	Onset	Peak	Duration
P.O.	Rapid	1 hr	8 hr
I.V.	Rapid	36 min	7 hr

Pharmacodynamics

Chemical effect: selective serotonin 5-HT$_3$ receptor antagonist that blocks the action of serotonin, thereby preventing serotonin from stimulating the vomiting reflex.
Therapeutic effect: prevents nausea and vomiting.

Indications and dosage

▶ **Prevention of nausea and vomiting associated with cancer chemotherapy.** *Adults:* 100 mg P.O. given as a single dose 1 hour before chemotherapy; or 1.8 mg/kg (or a fixed dose of 100 mg) as a single I.V. dose given 30 minutes before chemotherapy.
Children ages 2 to 16: 1.8 mg/kg P.O. 1 hour before chemotherapy, or 1.8 mg/kg as single I.V. dose 30 minutes before chemotherapy. Injectable formulation can be mixed with apple juice and administered P.O. Maximum dose is 100 mg.
▶ **Prevention of postoperative nausea and vomiting.** *Adults:* 100 mg P.O. within 2 hours before surgery; or 12.5 mg as single I.V. dose about 15 minutes before cessation of anesthesia. *Children ages 2 to 16:* 1.2 mg/kg P.O. given within 2 hours before surgery, up to maximum of 100 mg; or 0.35 mg/ kg (up to 12.5 mg) as single I.V. dose about 15 minutes before cessation of anesthesia. Injectable formulation can be mixed with apple juice and administered P.O.
▶ **Treatment of postoperative nausea and vomiting (I.V. form only).** *Adults:* 12.5 mg as a single I.V. dose as soon as nausea or vomiting presents. *Children ages 2 to 16:* 0.35 mg/kg, up to maximum dose of 12.5 mg, as a single I.V. dose as soon as nausea or vomiting presents.

Adverse reactions

CNS: *headache*, dizziness, drowsiness, fatigue.
CV: *arrhythmias, bradycardia,* ECG changes, hypotension, hypertension, tachycardia.
GI: *diarrhea,* dyspepsia, abdominal pain, constipation, anorexia.
GU: oliguria, urine retention.
Skin: pruritus, rash.
Other: fever, elevation of liver function tests, chills, pain at injection site.

Interactions

Drug-drug. *Drugs that prolong ECG intervals (such as antiarrhythmic drugs):* increased risk of arrhythmia. Monitor patient closely.
Drugs that inhibit P-450 enzymes (such as cimetidine): increased hydrodolasetron levels. Monitor patient for adverse effects
Drugs that induce P-450 enzymes (such as rifampin): decreased hydrodolasetron levels. Monitor patient for decreased efficacy of drug.

Contraindications and precautions

• Contraindicated in patients hypersensitive to drug.
• Administer with caution in patients who have or may develop prolonged cardiac conduction intervals, such as those with electrolyte abnormalities, history of arrhythmias, and cumulative high-dose anthracycline therapy.
• Drug is not recommended for use in children under age 2. Use cautiously in breast-feeding women.

NURSING CONSIDERATIONS

☝ Assessment
• Assess patient for history of nausea and vomiting associated with chemotherapy or postoperatively.
• Be alert for potential adverse reactions and drug interactions.

• Monitor ECG carefully in patients who have or may develop prolonged cardiac conduction intervals.
• Evaluate patient's and family's knowledge of drug therapy.

☒ Nursing diagnoses
• Altered nutrition: less than body requirements related to nausea and vomiting
• Risk for injury related to drug-induced adverse CNS reaction
• Knowledge deficit related to drug therapy

❯ Planning and implementation
P.O. use: Injection for oral administration is stable in apple juice for 2 hours at room temperature.
I.V. use: Injection can be infused as rapidly as 100 mg/30 seconds or diluted in 50 ml compatible solution and infused over 15 minutes.
• Discontinue drug and notify doctor immediately if arrhythmia occurs.
Patient teaching
• Tell patient about potential adverse effects.
• Instruct patient not to mix injection in juice for oral administration until just before dosing.
• Tell patient to report nausea or vomiting.

☑ Evaluation
• Patient does not experience nausea and vomiting.
• Patient is free from injury.
• Patient and family state understanding of drug therapy

donepezil hydrochloride
(doh-NEH-peh-zil high-droh-KLOR-ighd)
Aricept

Pharmacologic class: reversible inhibitor of acetylcholinesterase

---

Therapeutic class: psychotherapeutic agent for Alzheimer's disease
Pregnancy risk category: C

How supplied

Tablets: 5 mg, 10 mg

Pharmacokinetics

Absorption: well absorbed.
Distribution: 96% plasma protein–bound, mainly to albumin.
Metabolism: extensively metabolized.
Excretion: in urine and feces.

Route	Onset	Peak	Duration
P.O.	Unknown	3-4 hr	Unknown

Pharmacodynamics

Chemical effect: reversibly inhibits acetylcholinesterase in the CNS, thereby increasing the concentration of acetylcholine.
Therapeutic effect: temporarily improves the cognitive function in patients with Alzheimer's disease.

Indications and dosage

▶ **Mild to moderate dementia of the Alzheimer's type.** *Adults:* initially, 5 mg P.O. daily h.s. After 4 to 6 weeks, may increase dosage to 10 mg daily.

Adverse reactions

CNS: *headache, insomnia,* dizziness, depression, abnormal dreams, somnolence, *seizures,* tremor, irritability, paresthesia, aggression, vertigo, ataxia, increased libido, restlessness, abnormal crying, fatigue, nervousness, aphasia.
CV: syncope, chest pain, hypertension, vasodilation, atrial fibrillation, hot flashes, hypotension.
EENT: cataract, blurred vision, eye irritation.
GI: *nausea, diarrhea,* vomiting, anorexia, fecal incontinence, GI bleeding, bloating, epigastric pain.
GU: frequent urination.
Hematologic: ecchymosis.

Musculoskeletal: muscle cramps, arthritis, toothache, bone fracture.
Respiratory: *dyspnea, sore throat, bronchitis.*
Skin: pruritus, urticaria, diaphoresis.
Other: pain, accident, weight decrease, influenza, dehydration.

Interactions

Drug-drug. *Anticholinergics:* may interfere with anticholinergic activity. Monitor patient.
Bethanechol, succinylcholine: additive effects. Monitor patient closely.
Carbamazepine, dexamethasone, rifampin, phenytoin, phenobarbital: may increase rate of elimination of donepezil. Monitor patient.
Cholinomimetics, cholinesterase inhibitors: synergistic effect. Monitor patient closely.

Contraindications and precautions

• Contraindicated in patients with known hypersensitivity to drug or to piperidine derivatives.
• Use cautiously in patients with history of ulcer disease, CV disease, asthma or obstructive pulmonary disease, or urinary outflow impairment and in those currently taking NSAIDs.

NURSING CONSIDERATIONS

Assessment
• Monitor for symptoms of active or occult GI bleeding.
• Evaluate patient's and family's knowledge of drug therapy.

Nursing diagnoses
• Risk for injury related to adverse effects of drug
• Knowledge deficit related to drug therapy

Planning and implementation
• Use only in pregnancy if benefit justifies risk to fetus. Tell patient to avoid breast-feeding during therapy.

• Know that safety and effectiveness in children have not been established.
Patient teaching
• Explain that drug does not alter underlying degenerative disease but can alleviate symptoms.
• Tell caregiver to give drug in the evening, just before bedtime.
• Advise patient and caregiver to immediately report significant adverse effects or changes in overall health status. Also tell them to inform health-care team that patient is taking drug before anesthesia is given.

☑ **Evaluation**
• Patient remains free from injury.
• Patient and family state understanding of drug therapy.

dopamine hydrochloride
(DOH-puh-meen high-droh-KLOR-ighd)
Intropin, Revimine◆

Pharmacologic class: adrenergic
Therapeutic class: inotropic, vasopressor
Pregnancy risk category: C

How supplied
Injection: 40 mg/ml, 80 mg/ml, 160 mg/ml concentrate for injection for I.V. infusion; 0.8 mg/ml (200 or 400 mg) in dextrose 5%; 1.6 mg/ml (400 or 800 mg) in dextrose 5%, 3.2 mg/ml (800 mg) in dextrose 5% parenteral injection for I.V. infusion.

Pharmacokinetics
Absorption: not applicable with I.V. administration.
Distribution: widely distributed throughout body; does not cross blood-brain barrier.
Metabolism: metabolized to inactive compounds in liver, kidneys, and plasma.
Excretion: excreted in urine, mainly as its metabolites. *Half-life:* about 9 minutes.

Route	Onset	Peak	Duration
I.V.	≤ 5 min	Unknown	≤ 10 min after drug stopped

Pharmacodynamics
Chemical effect: stimulates dopaminergic, beta-adrenergic, and alpha-adrenergic receptors of sympathetic nervous system.
Therapeutic effect: increases cardiac output and blood pressure.

Indications and dosage
▶ **To treat shock and correct hemodynamic imbalances; to improve perfusion to vital organs; to increase cardiac output; to correct hypotension.** *Adults:* initially, 1 to 5 mcg/kg/minute by I.V. infusion, up to 50 mcg/kg/minute. Dosage titrated to desired hemodynamic or renal response, and increased by 1 to 4 mcg/kg/minute at 10- to 30-minute intervals.

Adverse reactions
CNS: headache.
CV: *arrhythmias,* ectopic beats, tachycardia, anginal pain, palpitations, *hypotension; bradycardia,* widening of QRS complex, conduction disturbances, vasoconstriction, hypertension (less common).
GI: nausea, vomiting.
Other: necrosis, tissue sloughing (with extravasation); piloerection, dyspnea, *anaphylaxis, asthmatic episodes,* azotemia.

Interactions
Drug-drug. *Alpha blockers, beta blockers:* may antagonize dopamine's effects. Monitor patient closely.
Ergot alkaloids: extreme elevations in blood pressure. Don't use together.
Inhalation anesthetics: increased risk of arrhythmias or hypertension. Monitor patient closely.
MAO inhibitors: may cause hypertensive crisis. Avoid if possible.

Oxytocic drugs: potentiation of pressor effect resulting in severe hypertension. Avoid if possible.

Phenytoin: may lower blood pressure of dopamine-stabilized patients. Monitor patient carefully.

Tricyclic antidepressants: potentiate adverse sympathomimetic effects of dopamine. Monitor closely.

Contraindications and precautions

• Contraindicated in patients with uncorrected tachyarrhythmias, pheochromocytoma, or ventricular fibrillation.

• Use cautiously in patients with occlusive vascular disease, cold injuries, diabetic endarteritis, and arterial embolism; in pregnant women; and in those taking MAO inhibitors.

• Safety of drug has not been established in breast-feeding women and in children.

NURSING CONSIDERATIONS

Assessment

• Obtain history of patient's underlying condition before therapy.

• During infusion, frequently monitor ECG, blood pressure, cardiac output, central venous pressure, pulmonary capillary wedge pressure, pulse rate, urine output, and color and temperature of extremities.

• Be alert for adverse reactions and drug interactions.

• Be aware that acidosis decreases effectiveness of dopamine.

• After drug is stopped, watch closely for sudden drop in blood pressure.

• Evaluate patient's and family's knowledge of drug therapy.

Nursing diagnoses

• Altered tissue perfusion (cerebral, cardiopulmonary, and renal) related to underlying condition

• Risk for injury related to drug-induced adverse reactions

• Knowledge deficit related to drug therapy

Planning and implementation

• Remember that drug is not used to treat blood or fluid volume deficit. If deficit exists, replace fluid before administering vasopressors, as ordered.

• Use central line or large vein, such as in antecubital fossa, to minimize risk of extravasation.

• Don't mix with alkaline solutions. Use D_5W, 0.9% NaCl solution, or combination of D_5W and 0.9% NaCl solution. Mix just before use.

• Do not mix other drugs in I.V. container with dopamine. Do not give alkaline drugs (for example, sodium bicarbonate or phenytoin sodium) through I.V. line containing dopamine.

• Use continuous infusion pump to regulate flow rate.

• Keep in mind that patient response depends on dosage and pharmacologic effect. Dosages of 0.5 to 2.0 mcg/kg/minute predominantly stimulate dopamine receptors and produce vasodilation of renal vasculature. Dosages of 2 to 10 mcg/kg/minute stimulate beta-adrenergic receptors for positive inotropic effect. Higher dosages also stimulate alpha-adrenergic receptors, causing vasoconstriction and increased blood pressure.

• Know that most patients are satisfactorily maintained on dosages less than 20 mcg/kg/minute.

• Taper dosage slowly to evaluate stability of blood pressure, as ordered.

• Discard after 24 hours or earlier if solution is discolored.

• If disproportionate rise in diastolic pressure (a marked decrease in pulse pressure) is observed in patient receiving dopamine, decrease infusion rate, as ordered, and observe carefully for further evidence of predominant vasoconstrictor activity, unless such effect is desired.

• If extravasation occurs, stop infusion immediately and call doctor. Extravasation may require treatment by infiltration of area with 5 to 10 mg of phentolamine and 10 to 15 ml of 0.9% NaCl solution.

Reactions may be *common*, uncommon, *life-threatening*, or COMMON AND LIFE-THREATENING.

• If adverse reactions develop, notify doctor, who will adjust or discontinue dosage. Also, if urine flow decreases without hypotension, notify doctor because dosage may need to be reduced.
Patient teaching
• Emphasize importance of reporting discomfort at I.V. site immediately.

☑ **Evaluation**
• Patient regains adequate cerebral, cardiopulmonary, and renal tissue perfusion.
• Patient does not experience injury as result of drug-induced adverse reactions.
• Patient and family state understanding of drug therapy.

doxacurium chloride
(doks-uh-KYOO-ree-um KLOR-ighd)
Nuromax

Pharmacologic class: nondepolarizing neuromuscular blocker
Therapeutic class: skeletal muscle relaxant
Pregnancy risk category: C

How supplied
Injection: 1 mg/ml

Pharmacokinetics
Absorption: not applicable with I.V. administration.
Distribution: plasma protein binding is about 30% in human plasma.
Metabolism: thought not to be metabolized.
Excretion: eliminated primarily unchanged in urine and bile. *Half-life:* 86 to 123 minutes.

Route	Onset	Peak	Duration
I.V.	≤ 5 min	3-9 min	1-4 hr

Pharmacodynamics
Chemical effect: competes with acetylcholine for receptor sites at motor end plate. Because this action may be antago-nized by cholinesterase inhibitors, doxacurium is considered a competitive antagonist.
Therapeutic effect: relaxes skeletal muscles.

Indications and dosage
► **To provide skeletal muscle relaxation during surgery as adjunct to general anesthesia.** Dosage is highly individualized. Note that all times of onset and duration of neuromuscular blockade are averages and considerable individual variation is normal. *Adults:* 0.05 mg/kg rapid I.V. produces adequate conditions for endotracheal intubation in 5 minutes in about 90% of patients when used as part of thiopental-narcotic induction technique. Lower doses may require longer delay before intubation is possible. Neuromuscular blockade at this dose lasts for average of 100 minutes.
Children over age 2: initial dose of 0.03 mg/kg I.V. administered during halothane anesthesia produces effective blockade in 7 minutes with duration of 30 minutes. Under same conditions, 0.05 mg/kg produces blockade in 4 minutes with duration of 45 minutes.
► **Maintenance of neuromuscular blockade during long procedures.**
Adults and children: after initial dose of 0.05 mg/kg I.V., maintenance doses of 0.005 to 0.01 mg/kg prolong neuromuscular blockade for an average of 30 minutes. Children usually require more frequent administration of maintenance doses.

Adverse reactions
Respiratory: dyspnea, *respiratory depression, respiratory insufficiency or apnea.*
Musculoskeletal: prolonged muscle weakness.

Interactions
Drug-drug. *Alkaline solutions (such as barbiturate solutions):* physically incompatible; precipitate may form. Do not administer through same I.V. line.

Aminoglycosides (gentamicin, kanamycin, neomycin, streptomycin), bacitracin, colistimethate, colistin, polymyxin B, tetracyclines: potentiated neuromuscular blockade leading to increased skeletal muscle relaxation and prolongation of effect. Use together cautiously.
Carbamazepine, phenytoin: may prolong time to maximal block or shorten duration of block with neuromuscular blocking agents.
Inhalation anesthetics, quinidine: may enhance activity (or prolonged action) of nondepolarizing neuromuscular blockers. *Magnesium salts:* may enhance neuromuscular blockade. Monitor for excessive weakness.

Contraindications and precautions

• Contraindicated in patients with hypersensitivity to drug and in neonates. Drug contains benzyl ethanol, which has been associated with fatalities in neonates.
• Use cautiously, possibly at reduced dosage, in debilitated patients; in patients with metastatic cancer, severe electrolyte disturbances, or neuromuscular diseases; and in those in whom potentiation or difficulty in reversal of neuromuscular blockade is anticipated. Patients with myasthenia gravis or myasthenic syndrome (Eaton-Lambert syndrome) are particularly sensitive to effects of nondepolarizing relaxants. Shorter-acting agents are recommended for use in such patients.
• Also use cautiously in breast-feeding women.
• Because of lack of data supporting safety, be aware that this drug is not recommended for use in patients requiring prolonged mechanical ventilation in intensive care unit, before or after administration of nondepolarizing neuromuscular blocking agents, or during cesarean delivery.
• Safety of drug has not been established in children under age 2.

NURSING CONSIDERATIONS

✐ Assessment
• Obtain history of patient's underlying condition before therapy.
• Monitor patient continuously throughout drug administration.
• Be alert for adverse reactions and drug interactions.
• Because drug has minimal vagolytic action, monitor for bradycardia, which may occur during anesthesia.
• Monitor respirations closely until patient is fully recovered from neuromuscular blockade, as evidenced by tests of muscle strength (hand grip, head lift, and ability to cough).
• Evaluate patient's and family's knowledge of drug therapy.

✿ Nursing diagnoses
• Altered health maintenance related to underlying condition
• Inability to sustain spontaneous ventilation related to drug's effects on respiratory muscles
• Knowledge deficit related to drug therapy

▷ Planning and implementation
• To avoid distress to patient, do not administer drug until patient's consciousness is obtunded by general anesthetic. Doxacurium has no effect on consciousness or pain threshold.
• Keep in mind that dosage should be adjusted to ideal body weight in obese patients (patients 30% or more above their ideal weight) to avoid prolonged neuromuscular blockade.
• Use drug only under direct medical supervision by personnel skilled in use of neuromuscular blocking agents and techniques for maintaining patent airway. Do not use unless facilities and equipment for intubation, mechanical ventilation, oxygen therapy, and drug antagonist are within reach.
• Know that higher initial doses may be required in patients with severe burns and

in some patients with severe liver disease. Higher doses (0.8 mg/kg) produce intubating conditions more rapidly (4 minutes), with neuromuscular blockade for 160 minutes or more. Consequently, higher doses should be reserved for long procedures. Administration during steady-state anesthesia with enflurane, halothane, or isoflurane may allow 33% reduction of dose.
• Prepare drug for I.V. use with D_5W, 0.9% NaCl injection, dextrose 5% in 0.9% NaCl injection, lactated Ringer's injection, or dextrose 5% in lactated Ringer's injection.
• When diluted as directed, keep in mind that doxacurium is compatible with alfentanil, fentanyl, and sufentanil.
• Recommend that product be administered immediately after reconstitution. Diluted solutions are stable for 24 hours at room temperature; however, because reconstitution dilutes preservative, risk of contamination increases. Unused solutions should be discarded after 8 hours.
• Know that experimental evidence suggests that acid-base and electrolyte balance may influence actions of nondepolarizing neuromuscular blockers. Alkalosis may counteract paralysis, and acidosis may enhance it.
• Be aware that nerve stimulator and train-of-four monitoring are recommended to document antagonism of neuromuscular blockade and recovery of muscle strength. Before attempting pharmacologic reversal with neostigmine, some evidence of spontaneous recovery should be evident.
• Provide respiratory support as required.
• Administer pain medication regularly if pain is thought to be present; patient may experience pain but not be able to demonstrate that pain is present.
Patient teaching
• If patient is not under influence of anesthesia, talk to patient and keep him informed of surroundings because drug does not affect consciousness. Reassure him that all his vital needs are being met and that he is being monitored constantly.

☑ **Evaluation**
• Patient exhibits improvement of underlying condition.
• Patient regains ability to maintain spontaneous ventilation after effects of drug have subsided.
• Patient and family state understanding of drug therapy.

doxapram hydrochloride
(DOKS-uh-prahm high-droh-KLOR-ighd)
Dopram

Pharmacologic class: analeptic
Therapeutic class: CNS and respiratory stimulant
Pregnancy risk category: B

How supplied

Injection: 20 mg/ml (benzyl alcohol 0.9%)

Pharmacokinetics

Absorption: not applicable with I.V. administration.
Distribution: distributed throughout body.
Metabolism: 99% metabolized by liver.
Excretion: metabolites excreted in urine.

Route	Onset	Peak	Duration
I.V.	20-40 sec	1-2 min	5-12 min

Pharmacodynamics

Chemical effect: not clearly defined; acts either directly on central respiratory centers in medulla or indirectly on chemoreceptors.
Therapeutic effect: stimulates respirations.

Indications and dosage

▶ **Postanesthesia respiratory stimulation, drug-induced CNS depression, chronic pulmonary disease associated with acute hypercapnia.** *Adults:* 0.5 to 1 mg/kg of body weight (up to 2 mg/kg in CNS depression) by I.V. injection or

infusion. Repeated q 5 minutes, if needed. Maximum dosage is 4 mg/kg, up to 3 g in 1 day.
▶ **COPD.** *Adults:* 1 to 2 mg/minute by I.V. infusion. Maximum dosage is 3 mg/minute for maximum duration of 2 hours.

Adverse reactions

CNS: *seizures,* *headache,* dizziness, apprehension, disorientation, pupillary dilation, bilateral Babinski's signs, paresthesia.
CV: *chest pain and tightness, variations in heart rate, hypertension,* lowered T waves, *arrhythmias.*
EENT: sneezing, *laryngospasm.*
GI: nausea, vomiting, diarrhea.
GU: urine retention, bladder stimulation with incontinence.
Respiratory: cough, *bronchospasm, dyspnea.*
Skin: pruritus.
Other: hiccups, rebound hypoventilation, fever, muscle spasms, diaphoresis, flushing.

Interactions

Drug-drug. *MAO inhibitors, sympathomimetics:* potentiate adverse CV effects. Use together cautiously.

Contraindications and precautions

• Contraindicated in patients with seizure disorders; head injury; CV disorders; frank uncompensated heart failure; severe hypertension; CVA; respiratory failure or incompetence secondary to neuromuscular disorders, muscle paresis, flail chest, obstructed airway, pulmonary embolism, pneumothorax, restrictive respiratory disease, acute bronchial asthma, or extreme dyspnea; or hypoxia not associated with hypercapnia.
• Use cautiously in patients with bronchial asthma, severe tachycardia or arrhythmias, cerebral edema or increased CSF pressure, hyperthyroidism, pheochromocytoma, or metabolic disorders. Also use cautiously in pregnant women.

• Safety of drug has not been established in breast-feeding women and in children.

NURSING CONSIDERATIONS

Assessment
• Obtain history of patient's underlying condition before therapy.
• Assess blood pressure, heart rate, deep tendon reflexes, and arterial blood gases before giving drug and closely throughout therapy.
• Monitor effectiveness by observing patient for improvement in CNS and respiratory function.
• Be alert for adverse reactions and drug interactions.
• Evaluate patient's (if appropriate) and family's knowledge of drug therapy.

Nursing diagnoses
• Ineffective breathing pattern related to underlying condition
• Risk for trauma related to potential for drug-induced seizure activity
• Knowledge deficit related to drug therapy

Planning and implementation
• Establish adequate airway before administering drug. Prevent patient from aspirating vomitus by placing him on his side.
• Administer drug slowly; rapid infusion may cause hemolysis. Doxapram is physically incompatible with strongly alkaline drugs such as thiopental sodium, aminophylline, and sodium bicarbonate.
• Avoid extravasation, which may lead to thrombophlebitis and local skin irritation.
• Be aware that drug is used only in surgical or emergency department situations.
• Keep airway patent and patient on side to prevent aspiration. Have suction equipment nearby.
• Discontinue drug and notify doctor if patient shows signs of increased arterial carbon dioxide or oxygen tension or if mechanical ventilation is started.

Reactions may be *common,* uncommon, *life-threatening,* or COMMON AND LIFE-THREATENING.

Patient teaching
• If patient is alert, instruct him to report chest pain or tightness immediately.

☑ **Evaluation**
• Patient regains normal respiratory pattern.
• Patient does not experience seizures as result of therapy.
• Patient and family state understanding of drug therapy.

doxazosin mesylate
(doks-AY-zoh-sin MES-ih-layt)
Cardura

Pharmacologic class: alpha-adrenergic blocker
Therapeutic class: antihypertensive
Pregnancy risk category: C

How supplied

Tablets: 1 mg, 2 mg, 4 mg, 8 mg

Pharmacokinetics

Absorption: readily absorbed from GI tract.
Distribution: 98% protein-bound.
Metabolism: extensively metabolized in liver.
Excretion: 63% excreted in bile and feces; 9% excreted in urine. *Half-life:* 19 to 22 hours.

Route	Onset	Peak	Duration
P.O.	1-2 hr	5-6 hr	24 hr

Pharmacodynamics

Chemical effect: acts on peripheral vasculature to produce vasodilation.
Therapeutic effect: lowers blood pressure.

Indications and dosage

▶ **Essential hypertension.** *Adults:* initially, 1 mg P.O. daily. If necessary, dose is increased to 2 mg daily. To minimize adverse reactions, dosage is titrated slowly (dosage typically increased only q 2 weeks). If necessary, dose is increased to 4 mg daily, then 8 mg. Maximum daily dosage is 16 mg, but dosage that exceeds 4 mg daily is associated with greater incidence of adverse reactions.
▶ **BPH.** *Adults:* initially, 1 mg P.O. once daily in the morning or evening; may be increased to 2 mg and, thereafter, 4 mg and 8 mg once daily p.r.n. Recommended titration interval is 1 to 2 weeks.

Adverse reactions

CNS: *dizziness,* vertigo, *asthenia, headache,* somnolence, drowsiness.
CV: *orthostatic hypotension,* hypotension, edema, palpitations, *arrhythmias,* tachycardia.
EENT: rhinitis, pharyngitis, abnormal vision.
GI: nausea, vomiting, diarrhea, constipation.
Musculoskeletal: arthralgia, myalgia.
Respiratory: dyspnea.
Skin: rash, pruritus.
Other: pain.

Interactions

None significant.

Contraindications and precautions

• Contraindicated in patients with hypersensitivity to drug and quinazoline derivatives (including prazosin and terazosin).
• Drug is not recommended for breast-feeding women because it accumulates in breast milk in levels about 20 times greater than those in maternal plasma.
• Use cautiously in patients with impaired liver function and in pregnant women.
• Safety in children has not been established.

NURSING CONSIDERATIONS

☷ **Assessment**
• Obtain history of patient's blood pressure before therapy, and reassess regularly thereafter.

• Determine effect on standing and supine blood pressure at 2 to 6 hours and 24 hours after administration.
• Be alert for adverse reactions.
• Monitor patient's ECG for arrhythmias.
• Evaluate patient's and family's knowledge of drug therapy

🔟 **Nursing diagnoses**
• Risk for injury related to presence of hypertension
• Decreased cardiac output related to drug-induced adverse CV reactions
• Knowledge deficit related to drug therapy

⟩ **Planning and implementation**
• Know that dosage increases must be titrated gradually, with adjustments every 2 weeks.
• If syncope occurs, place patient in recumbent position and treat supportively. A transient hypotensive response is not considered a contraindication to continued therapy.
Patient teaching
• Advise patient taking doxazosin that he is susceptible to "first-dose" effect similar to that produced by other alpha-adrenergic blockers—marked orthostatic hypotension accompanied by dizziness or syncope. Orthostatic hypotension is most common after first dose, but it also can occur when therapy is interrupted or during dosage adjustments.
• Warn patient that dizziness or fainting may occur. Advise patient to refrain from driving and performing other hazardous activities until drug's adverse CNS effects are known.
• Stress importance of regular follow-up visits.

☑ **Evaluation**
• Patient's blood pressure becomes normal.
• Patient maintains adequate cardiac output throughout therapy.
• Patient and family state understanding of drug therapy.

doxepin hydrochloride
(DOKS-eh-pin high-droh-KLOR-ighd)
Adapin, Deptran◇, Novo-Doxepin♦, Sinequan, Triadapin♦

Pharmacologic class: tricyclic antidepressant
Therapeutic class: antidepressant
Pregnancy risk category: NR

How supplied
Capsules: 10 mg, 25 mg, 50 mg, 75 mg, 100 mg, 150 mg
Oral concentrate: 10 mg/ml

Pharmacokinetics
Absorption: absorbed rapidly from GI tract.
Distribution: distributed widely in body, including CNS; 90% protein-bound.
Metabolism: metabolized by liver. A significant first-pass effect may explain variability of serum concentrations in different patients taking same dosage.
Excretion: most of drug excreted in urine.

Route	Onset	Peak	Duration
P.O.	Unknown	≤ 2 hr	Unknown

Pharmacodynamics
Chemical effect: unknown; increases amount of norepinephrine, serotonin, or both in CNS by blocking their reuptake by presynaptic neurons.
Therapeutic effect: relieves depression and anxiety.

Indications and dosage
▶ **Depression, anxiety.** *Adults:* initially, 25 to 75 mg P.O. daily in divided doses to maximum of 300 mg daily. Alternatively, entire maintenance dosage may be given once daily with maximum dose of 150 mg P.O.

Adverse reactions
CNS: *drowsiness, dizziness,* excitation, tremors, weakness, confusion, headache,

---

Reactions may be *common*, uncommon, *life-threatening*, or COMMON AND LIFE-THREATENING.

nervousness, EEG changes, *seizures*, extrapyramidal reactions, ataxia, paresthesia, hallucinations.
CV: *orthostatic hypotension, tachycardia, ECG changes,* hypertension.
EENT: *blurred vision,* tinnitus, mydriasis.
GI: *dry mouth, glossitis, constipation,* nausea, vomiting, anorexia.
GU: *urine retention.*
Hematologic: eosinophilia, *bone marrow depression.*
Skin: rash, urticaria, photosensitivity.
Other: *diaphoresis,* *hypersensitivity reaction.*
After abrupt withdrawal of long-term therapy: nausea, headache, malaise (does not indicate addiction).

Interactions

Drug-drug. *Barbiturates, CNS depressants:* enhanced CNS depression. Avoid concomitant use.
Cimetidine, fluoxetine, sertraline, methylphenidate: may increase doxepin serum levels. Monitor for increased adverse reactions.
Clonidine, epinephrine, norepinephrine: increased hypertensive effect. Use with caution.
MAO inhibitors: may cause severe excitation, hyperpyrexia, or seizures, usually with high dosage. Avoid concomitant use.
Drug-food. *Carbonated beverages, grape juice:* drug is physically incompatible with these beverages. Do not give together.
Drug-lifestyle. *Alcohol use:* enhanced CNS depression. Avoid concomitant use.
Sun exposure: increased risk of photosensitivity reactions. Avoid unprotected or prolonged exposure to the sun.

Contraindications and precautions

• Contraindicated in patients with glaucoma, hypersensitivity to drug, or tendency to experience urine retention.
• Breast-feeding not recommended during use of drug.

• Safety of drug has not been established in pregnant women or in children under age 12.

NURSING CONSIDERATIONS

⊠ Assessment
• Assess patient's depression or anxiety before and during therapy.
• Be alert for adverse reactions and drug interactions.
• Evaluate patient's and family's knowledge of drug therapy.

⊞ Nursing diagnoses
• Ineffective individual coping related to underlying condition
• Risk for injury related to drug-induced adverse CNS reactions
• Knowledge deficit related to drug therapy

⊠ Planning and implementation
• Be aware that dosage should be reduced in elderly or debilitated patients, adolescents, and those receiving other medications (especially anticholinergics).
• Dilute oral concentrate with 120 ml of water, milk, or juice. Do not mix with carbonated beverages because of incompatibility.
• Do not withdraw drug abruptly.
• Because hypertensive episodes have occurred during surgery in patients receiving tricyclic antidepressants, be aware that drug should be discontinued gradually several days before surgery.
• If signs of psychosis occur or increase, notify doctor and expect dosage to be reduced.
Patient teaching
• Tell patient to dilute oral concentrate with 120 ml of water, milk, or juice (orange, grapefruit, tomato, prune, or pineapple). Drug is incompatible with carbonated beverages.
• Advise patient to take full dose at bedtime, but warn of possible morning orthostatic hypotension.

---

*Liquid form contains alcohol   **May contain tartrazine   ♦ Canada   ◊ Australia   †OTC

• Warn patient to avoid hazardous activities that require alertness and good psychomotor coordination until CNS effects of drug are known. Drowsiness and dizziness usually subside after a few weeks.
• Tell patient to avoid alcohol during drug therapy.
• Warn patient not to stop drug therapy suddenly.
• Advise patient to consult the doctor before taking other prescription or OTC medications.
• Advise patient to use sunblock, wear protective clothing, and avoid prolonged exposure to strong sunlight.

☑ **Evaluation**
• Patient behavior and communication indicate improvement of depression or anxiety.
• Patient does not experience injury as result of drug-induced adverse CNS reactions.
• Patient and family state understanding of drug therapy.

doxorubicin hydrochloride
(doks-oh-ROO-bih-sin high-droh-KLOR-ighd)
Adriamycin◇, Adriamycin PFS, Adriamycin RDF, Rubex

Pharmacologic class: antineoplastic antibiotic (cell cycle–phase nonspecific)
Therapeutic class: antineoplastic
Pregnancy risk category: D

How supplied

Injection (preservative-free): 2 mg/ml
Powder for injection: 10-mg, 20-mg, 50-mg, 100-mg, 150-mg vials

Pharmacokinetics

Absorption: not applicable with I.V. administration.
Distribution: distributed widely in body tissues; does not cross blood-brain barrier.

Metabolism: extensively metabolized by hepatic microsomal enzymes to several metabolites, one of which possesses cytotoxic activity.
Excretion: excreted primarily in bile, minimally in urine. *Half-life:* initial, 30 minutes; terminal, 16½ hours.

Route	Onset	Peak	Duration
I.V.	Unknown	Unknown	Unknown

Pharmacodynamics

Chemical effect: unknown; thought to interfere with DNA-dependent RNA synthesis by intercalation.
Therapeutic effect: hinders or kills selected cancer cells.

Indications and dosage

Dosage and indications may vary. Check treatment protocol with doctor.
▶ **Bladder, breast, lung, ovarian, stomach, testicular, and thyroid cancers; Hodgkin's disease; acute lymphoblastic and myeloblastic leukemia; Wilms' tumor; neuroblastoma; lymphoma; sarcoma.** *Adults:* 60 to 75 mg/m² I.V. as single dose q 3 weeks; or 30 mg/m² I.V. in single daily dose on days 1 through 3 of 4-week cycle. Alternatively, 20 mg/m² I.V. once weekly. Maximum cumulative dosage is 550 mg/m².

Adverse reactions

CV: cardiac depression, seen in such ECG changes as sinus tachycardia, T-wave flattening, ST-segment depression, voltage reduction; *arrhythmias; irreversible cardiomyopathy.*
EENT: conjunctivitis.
GI: *nausea, vomiting, diarrhea, stomatitis,* esophagitis, anorexia.
GU: red urine (transient).
Hematologic: *leukopenia* during days 10 through 15, with recovery by day 21; *thrombocytopenia,* MYELOSUPPRESSION.
Skin: urticaria, facial flushing, *hyperpigmentation of nails, dermal creases, or*

Reactions may be *common*, uncommon, *life-threatening*, or COMMON AND LIFE-THREATENING.

skin (especially in previously irradiated areas).
Other: *severe cellulitis or tissue sloughing if drug extravasates;* hyperuricemia; *complete alopecia within 3 to 4 weeks* (hair may regrow 2 to 5 months after drug is stopped); *anaphylaxis.*

Interactions

Drug-drug. *Calcium channel blockers:* may potentiate cardiotoxic effects. Monitor closely.
Digoxin: may decrease serum digoxin levels. Monitor patient closely.
Phenytoin: decreased serum levels of phenytoin. Check levels.
Streptozocin: increased and prolonged blood levels. Dosage may have to be adjusted.

Contraindications and precautions

• Contraindicated in patients with marked myelosuppression induced by previous treatment with other antitumor agents or by radiotherapy and in those who have received lifetime cumulative dosage of 550 mg/m².
• Drug is not recommended for use in pregnant or breast-feeding women.
• Safety of drug has not been established in children.

NURSING CONSIDERATIONS

Assessment
• Obtain history of patient's neoplastic disorder before therapy, and reassess regularly thereafter.
• Assess ECG before treatment.
• Monitor CBC and liver function tests, as ordered; monitor ECG monthly during therapy.
• Be alert for adverse reactions and drug interactions.
• Evaluate patient's and family's knowledge of drug therapy.

Nursing diagnoses
• Altered health maintenance related to presence of neoplastic disease

• Decreased cardiac output related to drug-induced cardiotoxicity
• Knowledge deficit related to drug therapy

Planning and implementation
• Premedicate with antiemetic, as ordered, to reduce nausea.
• Follow institutional policy to reduce risks. Preparation and administration of parenteral form are associated with carcinogenic, mutagenic, and teratogenic risks for personnel.
• Know that dosage modification may be required in patients with myelosuppression or impaired cardiac or hepatic function and in elderly patients.
• Never give this drug I.M. or S.C.
• Know that red color of doxorubicin is similar to that of daunorubicin. Take care to avoid confusing these two drugs.
• Reconstitute using preservative-free 0.9% NaCl injection. Add 5 ml to 10-mg vial, 10 ml to 20-mg vial, or 25 ml to 50-mg vial. Shake vial and allow drug to dissolve; final concentration is 2 mg/ml. Give by direct injection into I.V. line of free-flowing compatible I.V. solution containing D₅W or 0.9% NaCl injection.
• Avoid extravasation; don't place I.V. line over joints or in extremities with poor venous or lymphatic drainage.
• If extravasation occurs, discontinue I.V. infusion immediately, apply ice to area for 24 to 48 hours, and notify doctor. Monitor area closely because extravasation reaction may be progressive. Early consultation with plastic surgeon may be advisable.
• Know that a precipitate may form if drug is mixed with aminophylline, cephalothin, dexamethasone, fluorouracil, heparin, or hydrocortisone.
• If skin or mucosal contact occurs, immediately wash area with soap and water.
• In the event of a leak or spill, inactivate drug with 5% sodium hypochlorite solution (household bleach).

• Be prepared to stop drug or slow rate of infusion if tachycardia develops, and notify doctor.
• Stop drug immediately if signs of heart failure develop, and notify doctor. Know that in many instances, heart failure can be prevented by limiting cumulative dosage to 550 mg/m^2 (400 mg/m^2 when patients are also receiving or have received cyclophosphamide or radiation therapy to cardiac area).
• Be aware that alternative dosage schedule (once-weekly dosing) causes a lower incidence of cardiomyopathy.
• If vein streaking occurs, slow administration rate. If welts occur, stop administration and report this to doctor.
• Be prepared to decrease dosage if serum bilirubin level is increased: 50% dosage when bilirubin level is 1.2 to 3 mg/dl; 25% dosage when bilirubin level is greater than 3 mg/dl.
• Keep in mind that refrigerated, reconstituted solution is stable for 48 hours; at room temperature, it's stable for 24 hours.
• Provide adequate hydration; alkalinizing urine or administering allopurinol may prevent or minimize uric acid nephropathy.
• Report adverse reactions to doctor, and be prepared to provide supportive care to treat such reactions.
Patient teaching
• Warn patient to watch for signs of infection (fever, sore throat, fatigue) and bleeding (easy bruising, nosebleeds, bleeding gums, melena). Have patient take temperature daily.
• Advise patient that orange to red urine for 1 to 2 days is normal and does not indicate presence of blood in urine.
• Tell patient that alopecia may occur but is usually reversible.
• Instruct patient to report symptoms of heart failure and other cardiac signs and symptoms promptly to doctor.
• Tell patient to use safety precautions to prevent injury.

☑ **Evaluation**
• Patient exhibits positive response to therapy, as noted on improvement of follow-up studies.
• Patient maintains adequate cardiac output throughout therapy.
• Patient and family state understanding of drug therapy.

doxycycline
(doks-ee-SIGH-kleen)
Doxylin◇, Vibramycin

doxycycline hyclate
Apo-Doxy♦, Doryx, DoxyCaps, Doxycin♦, Doxy-Tabs, Monodox, Novo-Doxylin♦, Vibramycin, Vibra-Tabs

doxycycline hydrochloride
Doryx◇, Vibramycin◇, Vibramycin IV, Vibra-Tabs 50◇

Pharmacologic class: tetracycline
Therapeutic class: antibiotic
Pregnancy risk category: D

How supplied

doxycycline
Tablets: 50 mg◇, 100 mg◇
Oral suspension: 25 mg/5 ml
Syrup: 50 mg/5 ml
doxycycline hyclate
Tablets: 50 mg, 100 mg
Capsules: 50 mg, 100 mg
Capsules (coated pellets): 100 mg
Injection: 100 mg, 200 mg
doxycycline hydrochloride
Tablets: 50 mg◇, 100 mg◇
Capsules: 50 mg◇, 100 mg◇, 250 mg◇
Injection: 100 mg◇
Powder for injection: 200 mg

Pharmacokinetics

Absorption: 90% to 100% absorbed after P.O. administration; absorption is insignificantly altered by milk or other dairy products.

Distribution: distributed widely in body tissues and fluids. CSF penetration is poor. Drug is 25% to 93% protein-bound.
Metabolism: insignificantly metabolized; some hepatic degradation occurs.
Excretion: excreted primarily unchanged in urine; some drug is excreted in feces.
Half-life: 22 to 24 hours after multiple dosing.

Route	Onset	Peak	Duration
P.O.	Unknown	1.5-4 hr	Unknown
I.V.	Immediate	Unknown	Unknown

Pharmacodynamics

Chemical effect: unknown; thought to exert bacteriostatic effect by binding to 30S ribosomal subunit of microorganisms, thus inhibiting protein synthesis.
Therapeutic effect: hinders bacterial growth. Spectrum of activity includes many gram-negative and gram-positive organisms, *Chlamydia, Mycoplasma, Rickettsia,* and spirochetes.

Indications and dosage

▶ **Infections caused by sensitive gram-negative and gram-positive organisms, Chlamydia, Mycoplasma, Rickettsia, and organisms that cause trachoma and Lyme disease.** *Adults and children weighing over 45 kg (99 lb):* 100 mg P.O. q 12 hours on first day, then 100 mg P.O. daily; or 200 mg I.V. on first day in one or two infusions, then 100 to 200 mg I.V. daily. *Children over age 8 and weighing under 45 kg:* 4.4 mg/kg P.O. or I.V. daily in divided doses q 12 hours on first day, then 2.2 to 4.4 mg/kg daily.

Give I.V. infusion slowly (minimum 1 hour). Infusion must be completed within 12 hours (within 6 hours in lactated Ringer's solution or dextrose 5% in lactated Ringer's solution).
▶ **Gonorrhea in patients allergic to penicillin.** *Adults:* 100 mg P.O. b.i.d. for 7 days, or 300 mg P.O. initially and repeat dose in 1 hour.
▶ **Primary or secondary syphilis in patients allergic to penicillin.** *Adults:*

100 mg P.O. b.i.d. for 2 weeks (early detection) or 4 weeks (if more than 1 year's duration).
▶ **Uncomplicated urethral, endocervical, or rectal infection caused by** *Chlamydia trachomatis* **or** *Ureaplasma urealyticum.* *Adults:* 100 mg P.O. b.i.d. for at least 7 days.
▶ **Prophylaxis of malaria.** *Adults:* 100 mg P.O. daily. *Children over age 8:* 2 mg/kg P.O. once daily. Dosage should not exceed adult dose. *Note:* Prophylaxis should begin 1 to 2 days before travel to malarious area and be continued throughout travel and for 4 weeks thereafter.

Adverse reactions

CNS: *intracranial hypertension (pseudotumor cerebri).*
CV: pericarditis, thrombophlebitis.
EENT: glossitis, dysphagia.
GI: anorexia, *epigastric distress, nausea,* vomiting, *diarrhea,* oral candidiasis, enterocolitis, anogenital inflammation.
Hematologic: *neutropenia,* eosinophilia, *thrombocytopenia,* hemolytic anemia.
Skin: *maculopapular and erythematous rash, photosensitivity, increased pigmentation, urticaria.*
Other: *hypersensitivity reactions (anaphylaxis);* elevated liver enzyme levels; permanent discoloration of teeth, enamel defects, bone growth retardation if used in children under age 9; superinfection.

Interactions

Drug-drug. *Antacids (including sodium bicarbonate) and laxatives containing aluminum, magnesium, or calcium; antidiarrheals:* decreased antibiotic absorption. Give antibiotic 1 hour before or 2 hours after any of above.
Ferrous sulfate and other iron products, zinc: decreased antibiotic absorption. Give drug 3 hours after or 2 hours before iron administration.
Methoxyflurane: may cause nephrotoxicity with tetracyclines. Monitor patient carefully.

Oral anticoagulants: increased anticoagulant effect. Monitor PT and INR and adjust dosage, as ordered.
Oral contraceptives: decreased contraceptive effectiveness and increased risk of breakthrough bleeding. Use nonhormonal form of birth control.
Penicillins: may interfere with bactericidal action of penicillins. Avoid using together.
Carbamazepine, phenobarbital: decreased antibiotic effect. Avoid if possible.
Drug-lifestyle. *Alcohol use:* decreased antibiotic effect. Avoid concomitant use.
Sun exposure: photosensitivity reactions may occur. Take precautions.

Contraindications and precautions

• Contraindicated in patients with hypersensitivity to drug or other tetracyclines.
• Avoid use of drug in breast-feeding women.
• Use cautiously in patients with impaired kidney or liver function. Use of these drugs during last half of pregnancy and in children under age 8 may cause permanent discoloration of teeth, enamel defects, and bone growth retardation.

NURSING CONSIDERATIONS

Assessment

• Obtain history of patient's infection before therapy, and reassess regularly thereafter.
• Obtain specimen for culture and sensitivity tests before first dose. Therapy may begin, pending test results.
• Be alert for adverse reactions and drug interactions.
• Monitor I.V. infusion site for signs of thrombophlebitis, which may occur with I.V. administration.
• Monitor patient's hydration status if adverse GI reactions occur.
• Evaluate patient's and family's knowledge of drug therapy.

Nursing diagnoses

• Infection related to presence of susceptible bacteria
• Risk for fluid volume deficit related to drug-induced adverse GI reactions
• Knowledge deficit related to drug therapy

Planning and implementation

• Check expiration date. Outdated or deteriorated tetracyclines have been associated with reversible nephrotoxicity (Fanconi's syndrome).
P.O. use: Administer drug with milk or food if adverse GI reactions develop.
• Be alert that parenteral form may cause false-positive reading of copper sulfate tests (Clinitest). All forms may cause false-negative reading of glucose oxidase reagent (Diastix or Chemstrip uG).
I.V. use: Reconstitute powder for injection with sterile water for injection. Use 10 ml in 100-mg vial and 20 ml in 200-mg vial. Dilute solution to 100 to 1,000 ml for I.V. infusion. Avoid extravasation. Don't infuse solutions that are more concentrated than 1 mg/ml.
• Don't expose drug to light or heat. Protect it from sunlight during infusion.
• Know that reconstituted injectable solution is stable for 72 hours if refrigerated.
• Notify doctor of adverse reactions. Some adverse reactions, such as superinfection, may necessitate substitution of another antibiotic.
Patient teaching
• Tell patient to take entire amount of medication exactly as prescribed, even after he feels better.
• Instruct patient to take oral doxycycline with milk or food but not antacids if adverse GI reactions develop and not less than 1 hour before bedtime (to prevent irritation from esophageal reflux).
• Tell patient to use sunscreen and avoid strong sunlight during therapy to prevent photosensitivity reactions.
• Stress good oral hygiene.

Reactions may be *common,* uncommon, *life-threatening*, or COMMON AND LIFE-THREATENING.

• Tell patient to check expiration dates and to discard outdated doxycycline because it may become toxic.

• Advise patient taking oral contraceptive to use alternative means of contraception during doxycycline therapy and for 1 week after therapy is discontinued.

☑ **Evaluation**
• Patient is free from infection.
• Patient maintains adequate hydration throughout therapy.
• Patient and family state understanding of drug therapy.

dronabinol
(delta-9-tetrahydrocannabinol)
(droh-NAB-eh-nohl)
Marinol

Pharmacologic class: cannabinoid
Therapeutic class: antiemetic or appetite stimulant
Controlled substance schedule: II
Pregnancy risk category: C

How supplied
Capsules: 2.5 mg, 5 mg, 10 mg

Pharmacokinetics
Absorption: almost 90% to 95% absorbed.
Distribution: distributed rapidly in many tissue sites; 97% to 99% protein-bound.
Metabolism: undergoes extensive metabolism in liver. Metabolite activity is unknown.
Excretion: excreted primarily in feces.
Half-life: 25 to 35 hours.

Route	Onset	Peak	Duration
P.O.	Unknown	2-4 hr	4-6 hr

Pharmacodynamics
Chemical effect: unknown.
Therapeutic effect: relieves nausea and vomiting caused by chemotherapy and stimulates appetite.

Indications and dosage
▶ **Nausea and vomiting associated with chemotherapy.** *Adults:* 5 mg/m² P.O. 1 to 3 hours before administration of chemotherapy. Then same dose q 2 to 4 hours after chemotherapy for total of four to six doses per day. If needed, dosage increased in increments of 2.5 mg/m² to maximum of 15 mg/m² per dose.
▶ **Anorexia and weight loss in patients with AIDS.** *Adults:* 2.5 mg P.O. b.i.d. before lunch and dinner, increased p.r.n. to maximum of 20 mg daily.

Adverse reactions
CNS: *dizziness, drowsiness, euphoria, ataxia,* depersonalization, disorientation, hallucinations, somnolence, headache, muddled thinking, asthenia, amnesia, confusion, *paranoia.*
CV: tachycardia, orthostatic hypotension, palpitations, vasodilation.
EENT: visual disturbances.
GI: *dry mouth, nausea, vomiting, abdominal pain,* diarrhea.

Interactions
Drug-drug. *CNS depressants, psychotomimetic substances, sedatives:* additive effects. Avoid concomitant use.
Drug-lifestyle. *Alcohol use:* additive effects. Avoid concomitant use.

Contraindications and precautions
• Contraindicated in patients who are hypersensitive to sesame oil or cannabinoids.
• Drug is not recommended for use in breast-feeding women.
• Use cautiously in elderly patients and in those with heart disease, psychiatric illness, or history of drug abuse.
• Safety of drug has not been established in children.

NURSING CONSIDERATIONS

☒ **Assessment**
• Obtain history of patient's underlying condition before therapy.

• Monitor effectiveness by assessing for nausea and vomiting or weight gain. Drug's effects may persist for days after treatment ends.
• Be alert for adverse reactions and drug interactions.
• Monitor patient for dependence. Know that dronabinol is principal active substance present in *Cannabis sativa* (marijuana). This substance can produce both physical and psychological dependence and has high potential for abuse.
• Monitor patient's hydration status, weight, and nutritional status regularly.
• Evaluate patient's and family's knowledge of drug therapy.

⊞ **Nursing diagnoses**
• Risk for fluid volume deficit related to nausea and vomiting associated with chemotherapy
• Altered thought processes related to drug-induced adverse CNS reactions
• Knowledge deficit related to drug therapy

▷ **Planning and implementation**
• Expect this drug to be prescribed only for patients who have not responded satisfactorily to other antiemetics.
• Give 1 to 3 hours before beginning chemotherapy and again 2 to 4 hours after chemotherapy is administered.
Patient teaching
• Inform patient that drug may induce unusual changes in mood or other adverse behavioral effects.
• Advise patient to avoid hazardous activities that require alertness until CNS effects of drug are known.
• Warn family members to ensure that patient is supervised by responsible person during and immediately after treatment.

☑ **Evaluation**
• Patient maintains adequate hydration.
• Patient regains normal thought processes after effects of drug therapy have dissipated.

• Patient and family state understanding of drug therapy.

edetate calcium disodium
(ED-eh-tayt KAL-see-um digh-SOH-dee-um)
Calcium Disodium Versenate, Calcium EDTA

Pharmacologic class: chelating agent
Therapeutic class: heavy metal antagonist
Pregnancy risk category: NR

How supplied
Injection: 200 mg/ml

Pharmacokinetics
Absorption: well absorbed after I.M. administration.
Distribution: distributed primarily in extracellular fluid.
Metabolism: none.
Excretion: excreted in urine. *Half-life:* 20 minutes to 1½ hours.

Route	Onset	Peak	Duration
I.V., I.M.	1 hr	24-48 hr	Unknown

Pharmacodynamics
Chemical effect: forms stable, soluble complexes with metals, particularly lead.
Therapeutic effect: abolishes effects of lead poisoning.

Indications and dosage
▶ **Acute lead encephalopathy or blood lead levels above 70 mcg/dl.** *Adults and children:* 1.5 g/m² I.V. or I.M. daily in divided doses at 12-hour intervals for 3 to 5 days, usually in conjunction with dimercaprol. A second course may be administered in 5 to 7 days.

Reactions may be *common,* uncommon, *life-threatening*, or COMMON AND LIFE-THREATENING.

► **Lead poisoning without encephalopathy or asymptomatic with blood levels below 70 mcg/dl.** *Children:* 1 g/m² I.V. or I.M. daily in divided doses.

Adverse reactions

CNS: headache, paresthesia, numbness, fatigue.
CV: *arrhythmias,* hypotension.
EENT: sneezing and nasal congestion.
GI: anorexia, nausea, vomiting.
GU: proteinuria, hematuria; *nephrotoxicity with renal tubular necrosis leading to fatal nephrosis.*
Other: arthralgia, myalgia, hypercalcemia; sudden fever, chills, excessive thirst.

Interactions

Drug-drug. *Zinc insulin:* interferes with action of insulin by binding with zinc. Monitor closely.

Contraindications and precautions

• Contraindicated in patients with anuria, hepatitis, or acute renal disease.
• Use with extreme caution in patients with mild renal disease. Expect dosages to be reduced.
• Use cautiously in pregnant women.

NURSING CONSIDERATIONS

Assessment
• Obtain history of patient's underlying condition before therapy.
• Monitor effectiveness by checking serum lead level and observing for decreasing signs and symptoms of lead poisoning.
• Monitor fluid intake and output, urinalysis, BUN, and ECG daily, as ordered.
• Be alert for adverse reactions.
• Observe injection site for local reaction.
• Evaluate patient's and family's knowledge of drug therapy.

Nursing diagnoses
• Risk for injury related to lead poisoning

• Altered renal tissue perfusion related to drug-induced fatal nephrosis
• Knowledge deficit related to drug therapy

Planning and implementation
I.V. use: Dilute drug with D₅W or 0.9% NaCl injection to concentration of 2 to 4 mg/ml. Infuse one-half of daily dose over 1 hour in asymptomatic patients or 2 hours in symptomatic patients. Give rest of infusion at least 6 hours later. Alternatively, give by slow infusion over at least 8 hours.
I.M. use: Add procaine hydrochloride, as ordered, to I.M. solution to minimize pain. Watch for local reactions.
• Because I.V. use may increase intracranial pressure, do not administer by that route to treat lead encephalopathy. Give by I.M. route instead.
• Know that I.M. route is preferred, especially for children and patients with lead encephalopathy.
• Do not confuse with edetate disodium, which is used to treat hypercalcemia.
• Force fluids to facilitate lead excretion, except in patients with lead encephalopathy.
• To avoid toxicity, use with dimercaprol, as ordered.
• Apply ice or cold compresses to injection site to ease local reaction.
Patient teaching
• Warn patient that some adverse reactions like fever, chills, thirst, and nasal congestion may occur 4 to 8 hours after administration.
• Encourage patient and family to identify and remove source of lead in home.

Evaluation
• Patient does not experience injury as result of lead poisoning.
• Patient does not exhibit signs of altered renal tissue perfusion.
• Patient and family state understanding of drug therapy.

edetate disodium
(ED-eh-tayt digh-SOH-dee-um)
EDTA, Disotate, Endrate

Pharmacologic class: chelating agent
Therapeutic class: heavy metal antagonist
Pregnancy risk category: NR

How supplied
*Injection:*150 mg/ml

Pharmacokinetics
Absorption: not applicable with I.V. administration.
Distribution: distributed widely throughout body but does not enter CSF in significant amounts.
Metabolism: none.
Excretion: excreted in urine.

Route	Onset	Peak	Duration
I.V.	Unknown	Unknown	Unknown

Pharmacodynamics
Chemical effect: chelates with metals, such as calcium, to form stable, soluble complex.
Therapeutic effect: lowers blood calcium level.

Indications and dosage
▶ **Hypercalcemic crisis.** *Adults:*
50 mg/kg by slow I.V. infusion added to 500 ml of D_5W or 0.9% NaCl solution administered over 3 or more hours. Maximum dosage is 3 g/day. *Children:*
40 to 70 mg/kg by slow I.V. infusion, diluted to maximum concentration of 30 mg/ml in D_5W or 0.9% NaCl solution administered over 3 or more hours. Maximum dosage is 70 mg/kg/day.
▶ **Cardiac glycoside–induced arrhythmias.** *Adults and children:*
15 mg/kg/hour I.V. with maximum daily dosage of 60 mg/kg.

Adverse reactions
CNS: circumoral paresthesia, numbness, headache.
CV: hypertension, thrombophlebitis, orthostatic hypotension.
EENT: erythema.
GI: nausea, vomiting, diarrhea, anorexia, abdominal cramps.
GU: nephrotoxicity with urinary urgency, nocturia, dysuria, polyuria, proteinuria, renal insufficiency, *renal failure, tubular necrosis* (in excessive doses).
Skin: dermatitis.
Other: *severe hypocalcemia,* decreased magnesium level, pain at site of infusion.

Interactions
None significant.

Contraindications and precautions
• Contraindicated in patients with anuria, known or suspected hypocalcemia, significant renal disease, active or healed tubercular lesions, history of seizures or intracranial lesions, or hypersensitivity to drug.
• Use cautiously in patients with limited cardiac reserve, heart failure, or hypokalemia. Also use cautiously in pregnant or breast-feeding women.

NURSING CONSIDERATIONS

☼ Assessment
• Obtain history of patient's calcium level before therapy.
• Monitor effectiveness by obtaining serum calcium level after each dose, as ordered. If used to treat cardiac glycoside–induced arrhythmias, evaluate patient's ECG frequently.
• Monitor kidney function tests frequently, as ordered.
• Be alert for adverse reactions.
• Evaluate patient's and family's knowledge of drug therapy.

⊞ Nursing diagnoses
• Risk for injury related to hypercalcemia

• Altered protection related to drug-induced hypocalcemia
• Knowledge deficit related to drug therapy

❯ Planning and implementation
• Read label carefully; do not confuse with edetate calcium disodium, which is used for lead toxicity.
• Dilute before use. Avoid rapid I.V. infusion; profound hypocalcemia may occur, leading to tetany, seizures, arrhythmias, and respiratory arrest. Drug is not recommended for direct or intermittent injection. Avoid extravasation.
• Record I.V. site used, and avoid repeated use of same site, which increases likelihood of thrombophlebitis.
• Keep I.V. calcium available to treat hypocalcemia.
• Keep patient in bed for 15 minutes after infusion to avoid orthostatic hypotension.
• If generalized systemic reactions—fever, chills, back pain, emesis, muscle cramps, urinary urgency—occur 4 to 8 hours after infusion, report them to doctor. Treatment is usually supportive. Symptoms generally subside within 12 hours.
• Don't use to treat lead toxicity; know that edetate calcium disodium should be used instead.
• Know that other drug treatments for hypercalcemia are safer and more effective than edetate disodium.
Patient teaching
• Instruct patient to report respiratory difficulty, dizziness, and muscle cramping immediately.
• Advise patient to move from sitting or lying position slowly to avoid dizziness.
• Reassure patient that generalized systemic reaction usually subsides within 12 hours.

☑ Evaluation
• Patient does not experience injury as result of hypercalcemia.

• Patient's blood calcium level does not fall below normal after edetate disodium therapy.
• Patient and family state understanding of drug therapy.

---

edrophonium chloride
(ed-roh-FOH-nee-um KLOR-ighd)
Enlon, Reversol, Tensilon

Pharmacologic class: cholinesterase inhibitor
Therapeutic class: cholinergic agonist, diagnostic agent
Pregnancy risk category: NR

How supplied
Injection: 10 mg/ml in 1-ml ampules or in 10-ml or 15-ml vials

Pharmacokinetics
Unknown.

Route	Onset	Peak	Duration
I.V.	30-60 sec	Unknown	5-10 min
I.M.	2-10 min	Unknown	5-30 min

Pharmacodynamics
Chemical effect: inhibits destruction of acetylcholine released from parasympathetic and somatic efferent nerves. Acetylcholine accumulates, promoting increased stimulation of receptor.
Therapeutic effect: reverses nondepolarizing neuromuscular blocker.

Indications and dosage
▶ **As curare antagonist (to reverse nondepolarizing neuromuscular blocking action).** *Adults:* 10 mg I.V. given over 30 to 45 seconds. Dose may be repeated as necessary to 40 mg maximum dosage. Larger dosages may potentiate effect of curare.
▶ **Diagnostic aid in myasthenia gravis (Tensilon test).** *Adults:* 1 to 2 mg I.V. over 15 to 30 seconds, then 8 mg if no response (increase in muscle strength) oc-

---

*Liquid form contains alcohol   **May contain tartrazine   ◆Canada   ◊Australia   †OTC

curs. Alternatively, 10 mg I.M. If cholinergic reaction occurs, 2 mg I.M. is given 30 minutes later to rule out false-negative response. *Children weighing over 34 kg (75 lb):* 2 mg I.V. If no response within 45 seconds, 1 mg q 45 seconds to maximum of 10 mg. Alternatively, 5 mg I.M. *Children weighing under 34 kg:* 1 mg I.V. If no response within 45 seconds, 1 mg q 45 seconds to maximum of 5 mg. Alternatively, 2 mg I.M. (I.M. route may be used in children because of difficulty with I.V. route.) Expect same reactions as with I.V. test, but they appear after 2- to 10-minute delay. *Infants:* 0.5 mg to 1 mg I.M. or S.C.

▶ **To differentiate myasthenic crisis from cholinergic crisis.** *Adults:* 1 mg I.V. If no response in 1 minute, dose is repeated once. Increased muscle strength confirms myasthenic crisis; no increase or exaggerated weakness confirms cholinergic crisis.

Adverse reactions

CNS: *seizures,* weakness, dysarthria.
CV: hypotension, *bradycardia, AV block, cardiac arrest.*
EENT: excessive lacrimation, diplopia, miosis, conjunctival hyperemia, dysphagia.
GI: nausea, vomiting, *diarrhea, abdominal cramps,* excessive salivation.
GU: urinary frequency, incontinence.
Musculoskeletal: muscle cramps, muscle fasciculation.
Respiratory: *respiratory paralysis, bronchospasm, laryngospasm,* increased bronchial secretions.
Other: diaphoresis.

Interactions

Drug-drug. *Aminoglycosides, anesthetics:* prolonged or enhanced muscle weakness. Monitor patient closely.
Cardiac glycosides: may increase heart's sensitivity to edrophonium. Use together cautiously.

Cholinergics: increased effects. Stop all other cholinergics before giving drug, as ordered.
Corticosteroids, magnesium, procainamide, quinidine: may antagonize cholinergic effects. Observe for lack of drug effect.

Contraindications and precautions

● Contraindicated in patients with mechanical obstruction of intestine or urinary tract and hypersensitivity to anticholinesterase agents.
● Use cautiously in patients with bronchial asthma or arrhythmias.
● Safety of drug has not been established in pregnant or breast-feeding women.

NURSING CONSIDERATIONS

⚕ Assessment
● Obtain history of patient's underlying condition before therapy.
● Monitor effectiveness by evaluating reduction of symptoms of underlying condition. When giving drug to differentiate myasthenic crisis from cholinergic crisis, observe patient's muscle strength closely.
● Be alert for adverse reactions and drug interactions.
● Evaluate patient's and family's knowledge of drug therapy.

⊞ Nursing diagnoses
● Altered health maintenance related to underlying condition
● Impaired gas exchange related to drug-induced bronchospasm
● Knowledge deficit related to drug therapy

▶ Planning and implementation
● Stop all other cholinergics before giving this drug, as ordered.
I.V. use: For easier parenteral administration, use tuberculin syringe with I.V. needle.
I.M. use: Use I.M. route, as ordered, for administration of drug to children be-

cause of difficulty with I.V. insertion in children.
• Always have atropine injection readily available, and be prepared to give 0.5 to 1 mg S.C. or slow I.V. push, as ordered. Provide respiratory support, as needed.
Patient teaching
• Tell patient to report adverse reactions immediately, especially difficulty breathing.

☑ **Evaluation**
• Patient exhibits improvement in underlying condition.
• Patient maintains adequate gas exchange throughout therapy.
• Patient and family state understanding of drug therapy.

efavirenz
(eh-fah-VEER-enz)
Sustiva

Pharmacologic class: nonnucleoside, reverse transcriptase inhibitor
Therapeutic class: antiviral
Pregnancy risk category: C

How supplied
Capsules: 50 mg, 100 mg, 200 mg

Pharmacokinetics
Absorption: oral absorption produces peak concentrations in 3 to 5 hours with steady-state concentrations in 6 to 10 days.
Distribution: highly bound to human plasma proteins, predominantly albumin.
Metabolism: primarily metabolized by cytochrome P-450 system to metabolites that are inactive against HIV-1.
Excretion: excreted primarily in feces with a small number of metabolites excreted in urine.

Route	Onset	Peak	Duration
P.O.	Unknown	3-5 hr	Unknown

Pharmacodynamics
Chemical effect: a nonnucleoside, reverse transcriptase inhibitor (NNRTI) that inhibits the transcription of HIV-1 RNA to DNA, a critical step in the viral replication process.
Therapeutic effect: lowers amount of HIV in the blood (viral load) and increases CD4 lymphocytes.

Indications and dosage
▶ **Treatment of HIV-1 infection.**
Adults: 600 mg P.O. once daily in combination with a protease inhibitor or nucleoside analogue reverse transcriptase inhibitors. *Children age 3 and older weighing 40 kg (88 lb) or more:* 600 mg P.O. once daily in combination with a protease inhibitor or nucleoside analogue reverse transcriptase inhibitors. *Children age 3 and older weighing 10 to under 15 kg (22 to under 33 lb):* 200 mg P.O. once daily; weighing 15 to under 20 kg (33 to under 44 lb): 250 mg P.O. once daily; weighing 20 to under 25 kg (44 to under 55 lb): 300 mg P.O. once daily; weighing 25 to under 32.5 kg (55 to under 72 lb): 350 mg P.O. once daily; weighing 32.5 to under 40 kg (72 to under 88 lb): 400 mg P.O. once daily.*
Give above doses in combination with a protease inhibitor or nucleoside analogue reverse transcriptase inhibitors.

Adverse reactions
CNS: abnormal dreams or thinking, agitation, amnesia, confusion, depersonalization, depression, *dizziness*, euphoria, fatigue, hallucinations, headache, hypesthesia, impaired concentration, insomnia, somnolence, nervousness.
GI: abdominal pain, anorexia, *diarrhea,* dyspepsia, flatulence, *nausea*, vomiting.
GU: hematuria, kidney stones.
Hepatic: increase in AST, ALT, and total cholesterol levels.
Skin: increased sweating, *erythema multiforme, Stevens-Johnson syndrome, toxic epidermal necrolysis, rash,* pruritus.
Other: fever.

---

*Liquid form contains alcohol   **May contain tartrazine   ◆Canada   ◇ Australia   †OTC

Interactions

Drug-drug. *Astemizole, cisapride, ergot derivatives, midazolam, triazolam:* competition for cytochrome P-450 enzyme system may result in inhibition of the metabolism of these drugs and cause serious or life-threatening adverse events (such as arrhythmias, prolonged sedation, or respiratory depression). Avoid concomitant use.

Clarithromycin, indinavir: decreased plasma concentrations. Alternate therapy or dosage adjustment may be indicated.

Drugs that induce cytochrome P-450 enzyme system (such as phenobarbital, rifampin, rifabutin): increased clearance of efavirenz resulting in lowered plasma concentrations. Avoid concomitant use.

Estrogens, ritonavir: increased plasma concentrations. Monitor patient.

Oral contraceptives: potential interaction of efavirenz with oral contraceptive has not been determined. Advise use of a reliable method of barrier contraception in addition to oral contraceptives.

Psychoactive drugs: additive CNS effects. Avoid concomitant use.

Saquinavir: plasma concentrations of saquinavir decreased significantly. Do not use with saquinavir as sole protease inhibitor.

Warfarin: plasma concentrations and effects potentially increased or decreased. Monitor INR.

Drug-food. *High-fat meals:* increased absorption of drug. Instruct patient to maintain a proper low-fat diet.

Drug-lifestyle. *Alcohol use:* enhanced CNS effects. Avoid concomitant use.

Contraindications and precautions

• Contraindicated in patients with hypersensitivity to drug or its components.
• Use cautiously in patients with hepatic impairment or in those concurrently receiving hepatotoxic drugs.

NURSING CONSIDERATIONS

⚖ Assessment

• Monitor liver function test results in patients with prior history of hepatitis B or C and in those also taking ritonavir.
• Monitor cholesterol levels.
• Know that children may be more prone to adverse reactions, especially diarrhea, nausea, vomiting, and rash.
• Evaluate patient's and family's knowledge of drug therapy.

✛ Nursing diagnoses

• Risk for infection related to patient's underlying condition
• Risk for impaired skin integrity related to potential adverse effects of drug
• Knowledge deficit related to drug therapy

❯ Planning and implementation

• Drug should be used in combination with other antiretroviral agents because resistant viruses emerge rapidly when used alone. Drug should not be used as monotherapy, or added on as a single agent to a failing regimen.
• Combination with ritonavir is associated with a higher frequency of adverse effects (such as dizziness, nausea, paresthesia) and laboratory abnormalities (elevated liver enzymes).
• Be aware that pregnancy must be ruled out before starting therapy in female patients of childbearing age.
• Administer drug at bedtime to decrease noticeable CNS adverse effects.

Patient teaching

• Instruct patient to take drug with water, juice, milk, or soda. It may be taken without regard to meals.
• Inform patient about need for scheduled blood tests to monitor liver function and cholesterol levels.
• Tell patient to use reliable method of barrier contraception in addition to oral contraceptives and to notify doctor immediately if pregnancy is suspected.

Reactions may be *common,* uncommon, *life-threatening*, or COMMON AND LIFE-THREATENING.

• Inform patient that drug is not a cure for HIV infection and that it will not affect the development of opportunistic infections and other complications associated with HIV disease or transmission of HIV to others through sexual contact or blood contamination.

• Instruct patient to take drug at same time daily and always in combination with other antiretroviral drugs.

• Tell patient to take drug exactly as prescribed and not to discontinue without medical approval. Also instruct patient to report any adverse reactions.

• Inform patient that rash is most common adverse effect. If it occurs, tell patient to report it immediately because it may be serious in rare cases.

• Instruct patient to report use of other medications.

• Advise patient that dizziness, difficulty sleeping or concentrating, drowsiness, or unusual dreams may occur the first few days of therapy. Reassure patient that these symptoms generally resolve after 2 to 4 weeks and may be less problematic if drug is taken at bedtime.

• Tell patient to avoid alcoholic beverages, driving, or operating machinery until drug's effects are known.

🗹 **Evaluation**
• Patient is free from opportunistic infections.
• Patient's skin integrity is maintained.
• Patient and family state understanding of drug therapy.

---

enalaprilat
(eh-NAH-leh-prel-at)
Vasotec I.V.

enalapril maleate
Amprace◊, Renitec◊, Vasotec

Pharmacologic class: ACE inhibitor
Therapeutic class: antihypertensive

Pregnancy risk category: C (D in second and third trimesters)

How supplied
Tablets: 2.5 mg, 5 mg, 10 mg, 20 mg
Injection: 1.25 mg/ml

Pharmacokinetics
Absorption: about 60% of P.O. dose absorbed from GI tract.
Distribution: unknown.
Metabolism: metabolized extensively to active metabolite enalaprilat.
Excretion: about 94% excreted in urine and feces as enalaprilat and enalapril.
Half-life: 12 hours.

Route	Onset	Peak	Duration
P.O.	1 hr	4-6 hr	24 hr
I.V.	15 min	1-4 hr	6 hr

Pharmacodynamics
Chemical effect: unknown, but does inhibit ACE, preventing conversion of angiotensin I to angiotensin II, a potent vasoconstrictor. Reduced formation of angiotensin II decreases peripheral arterial resistance, thus decreasing aldosterone secretion.
Therapeutic effect: lowers blood pressure.

Indications and dosage
▶ **Hypertension.** *Adults:* for patient not receiving diuretics, initially 5 mg P.O. once daily, then adjusted according to response. Usual dosage range is 10 to 40 mg daily as single dose or two divided doses. Alternatively, 1.25 mg I.V. over 5 minutes q 6 hours. For patient on diuretics, initially 2.5 mg P.O. once daily. Alternatively, 0.625 mg I.V. over 5 minutes, repeated in 1 hour if needed, then followed by 1.25 mg I.V. q 6 hours.
▶ **To convert from I.V. to P.O. therapy.** *Adults:* initially, 5 mg P.O. once daily; if patient was receiving 0.625 mg I.V., then 2.5 mg P.O. once daily. Dosage is adjusted to response.

► **To convert from P.O. to I.V. therapy.**
Adults: 1.25 mg I.V. over 5 minutes q 6 hours. Higher doses have not demonstrated greater efficacy.
► **Renal impairment or hyponatremia.** If serum creatinine level is above 1.6 mg/dl or serum sodium level is below 130 mEq/L, dosage is initiated at 2.5 mg P.O. daily and titrated slowly.

Adverse reactions

CNS: *headache, dizziness, fatigue,* vertigo, asthenia, syncope.
CV: *hypotension,* chest pain.
GI: diarrhea, nausea, abdominal pain, vomiting.
GU: decreased renal function (in patients with bilateral renal artery stenosis or heart failure).
Hematologic: *neutropenia, thrombocytopenia, agranulocytosis.*
Respiratory: *dry, persistent, tickling, nonproductive cough,* dyspnea.
Skin: rash.
Other: *angioedema.*

Interactions

Drug-drug. *Diuretics:* excessive reduction of blood pressure. Monitor patient.
Insulin, oral antidiabetic agents: risk of hypoglycemia, especially at initiation of enalapril therapy. Monitor patient closely.
Lithium: lithium toxicity can occur. Monitor lithium levels.
NSAIDs: may reduce antihypertensive effect. Monitor blood pressure.
Potassium supplements, potassium-sparing diuretics: increased risk of hyperkalemia. Avoid these drugs unless hypokalemic blood levels are confirmed.

Contraindications and precautions

• Contraindicated in patients with hypersensitivity to drug or history of angioedema related to previous treatment with ACE inhibitor.
• Use with extreme caution and only when absolutely necessary in pregnant women because fetal harm may occur.

• Use cautiously in patients with renal impairment.
• Safety of drug has not been established in breast-feeding women and in children.

NURSING CONSIDERATIONS

◪ Assessment
• Obtain history of patient's blood pressure before therapy, and reassess regularly thereafter.
• Monitor CBC with differential counts before therapy, every 2 weeks for first 3 months of therapy, and periodically thereafter.
• Monitor potassium intake and serum potassium level.
• Be alert for adverse reactions and drug interactions.
• Evaluate patient's and family's knowledge of drug therapy.

⊞ Nursing diagnoses
• Risk for injury related to presence of hypertension
• Risk for infection related to drug-induced adverse hematologic reactions
• Knowledge deficit related to drug therapy

◪ Planning and implementation
P.O. use: Follow normal protocol.
I.V. use: Inject drug slowly over at least 5 minutes, or dilute in 50 ml of compatible solution and infuse over 15 minutes. Compatible solutions include D_5W, 0.9% NaCl injection, dextrose 5% in lactated Ringer's injection, and dextrose 5% in 0.9% NaCl injection.
• Notify doctor immediately if CBC becomes abnormal or if signs and symptoms of infection occur.
• If angioedema occurs, notify doctor and discontinue treatment immediately. Institute appropriate therapy (epinephrine solution 1:1,000 [0.3 to 0.5 ml] S.C.), and take measures to ensure patent airway.

Patient teaching
• Advise patient to report signs or symptoms of angioedema, such as swelling of face, eyes, lips, or tongue or breathing difficulty. Angioedema (including laryngeal edema) may occur, especially after first dose.
• Instruct patient to report signs of infection, such as fever and sore throat.
• Advise patient that light-headedness can occur, especially during first few days of therapy. Tell patient to rise slowly to minimize this effect and to report symptoms to doctor. If patient experiences syncope, he should stop taking drug and call doctor immediately.
• Tell patient to use caution in hot weather and during exercise. Inadequate fluid intake, vomiting, diarrhea, and excessive perspiration can lead to light-headedness and syncope.
• Advise patient to avoid sodium substitutes; these products may contain potassium, which can cause hyperkalemia in patients taking drug.
• Tell female patient to notify doctor if pregnancy occurs. Drug will need to be discontinued.

☑ Evaluation
• Patient's blood pressure becomes normal.
• Patient's CBC remains normal throughout therapy.
• Patient and family state understanding of drug therapy.

enoxacin
(eh-NOKS-uh-sin)
Penetrex

Pharmacologic class: fluoroquinolone antibacterial
Therapeutic class: antibiotic
Pregnancy risk category: C

How supplied
Tablets: 200 mg, 400 mg

Pharmacokinetics
Absorption: absolute oral bioavailability is about 90% after absorption.
Distribution: about 40% bound to plasma proteins.
Metabolism: five metabolites of drug have been identified; they account for 15% to 20% of administered dose.
Excretion: excreted primarily in urine.
Half-life: 3 to 6 hours.

Route	Onset	Peak	Duration
P.O.	Unknown	1-3 hr	Unknown

Pharmacodynamics
Chemical effect: inhibits bacterial DNA synthesis, mainly by blocking DNA gyrase; bactericidal.
Therapeutic effect: kills susceptible bacteria. Spectrum of activity includes most strains of gram-positive aerobes, such as *Staphylococcus epidermidis* and *Staphylococcus saprophyticus,* and many gram-negative aerobes, such as *Enterobacter cloacae, Escherichia coli, Klebsiella pneumoniae, Neisseria gonorrhoeae, Proteus mirabilis,* and *Pseudomonas aeruginosa.*

Indications and dosage
▶ **Uncomplicated urinary tract infections.** *Adults:* 200 mg P.O. q 12 hours for 7 days.
▶ **Severe or complicated urinary tract infections.** *Adults:* 400 mg P.O. q 12 hours for 14 days.
▶ **Uncomplicated urethral or endocervical gonorrhea.** *Adults:* 400 mg P.O. as single dose. Doxycycline therapy may follow to treat possible coexisting chlamydial infection.
Note: In patients with renal failure with creatinine clearance of 30 ml/minute or less, therapy started with usual initial dose. Subsequent doses are decreased by 50%.

Adverse reactions

CNS: headache, restlessness, tremors, light-headedness, confusion, hallucinations, *seizures.*
GI: *nausea, diarrhea,* vomiting, abdominal pain or discomfort, oral candidiasis.
GU: crystalluria.
Other: *rash,* photosensitivity, eosinophilia, dyspnea, cough, elevated liver enzyme levels, pruritus, hypersensitivity.

Interactions

Drug-drug. *Aminophylline, cyclosporine, theophylline:* increased levels of these drugs because of decreased metabolism. Use together cautiously.
Antacids containing magnesium hydroxide or aluminum hydroxide, oral iron supplements, sucralfate: decreased enoxacin absorption. Separate administration times by at least 2 hours.
Bismuth subsalicylate: bioavailability of enoxacin is decreased when given within 60 minutes of bismuth subsalicylate. Separate administration times.
Digoxin: may increase digoxin serum levels. Monitor closely for toxicity.
Oral anticoagulants: increased anticoagulant effect. Use together cautiously.
Drug-food. *Any food:* affects absorption. Give drug on an empty stomach.
Caffeine: increased effect of caffeine. Monitor closely.

Contraindications and precautions

• Contraindicated in patients with hypersensitivity to drug or other fluoroquinolone antibiotics.
• Use cautiously in patients with CNS disorders, such as severe cerebral arteriosclerosis or seizure disorders, and in those at increased risk for seizures. Drug may cause CNS stimulation.
• Use cautiously and with dosage adjustments in patients with impaired kidney or liver function. Also use cautiously in pregnant women.
• Safety of drug has not been established in breast-feeding women and in children.

NURSING CONSIDERATIONS

⚗ Assessment
• Obtain history of patient's infection before therapy, and reassess regularly thereafter.
• Obtain specimen for culture and sensitivity tests before first dose. Therapy may begin, pending test results.
• Have patient being treated for gonorrhea obtain initial serologic test for syphilis before therapy starts. Drug is not effective in treating syphilis and may mask signs and symptoms of infection. Have patient repeat serologic test in 1 to 3 months.
• Be alert for adverse reactions and drug interactions.
• Monitor patient's hydration status if adverse GI reactions occur.
• Evaluate patient's and family's knowledge of drug therapy.

🔑 Nursing diagnoses
• Infection related to presence of susceptible bacteria
• Risk for fluid volume deficit related to drug-induced adverse GI reactions
• Knowledge deficit related to drug therapy

❯ Planning and implementation
• Administer 2 hours after a meal or 2 hours before or after antacids containing magnesium hydroxide or aluminum hydroxide, sucralfate, or products that contain iron (such as vitamins with mineral supplements).
Patient teaching
• Advise patient to avoid overexposure to direct sunlight while taking drug and to use sunblock and wear protective clothing when outdoors.
• Warn patient not to drink beverages containing caffeine while taking enoxacin. Drug inhibits metabolism of caffeine and can result in toxicity.
• Advise patient to liberally increase fluid intake while taking drug because simi-

---

lar drugs have caused urine microcrystal formation.

• Warn patient to refrain from driving and performing other hazardous activities until adverse CNS effects of drug are known.

☑ **Evaluation**

• Patient is free from infection.
• Patient maintains adequate hydration throughout therapy.
• Patient and family state understanding of drug therapy.

enoxaparin sodium
(eh-NOKS-uh-pah-rin SOH-dee-um)
Lovenox

Pharmacologic class: low-molecular-weight heparin derivative
Therapeutic class: anticoagulant
Pregnancy risk category: B

How supplied

Injection: 30 mg/0.3 ml; 40 mg/0.4 ml; 60 mg/0.6 ml; 80 mg/0.8 ml; 100 mg/ml

Pharmacokinetics

Absorption: unknown.
Distribution: unknown.
Metabolism: unknown.
Excretion: unknown. *Half-life:* about 4½ hours after S.C. administration.

Route	Onset	Peak	Duration
S.C.	Unknown	3-5 hr	< 24 hr

Pharmacodynamics

Chemical effect: accelerates formation of antithrombin IIIB–thrombin complex and deactivates thrombin, preventing conversion of fibrinogen to fibrin. Enoxaparin has higher antifactor Xa–antifactor IIa activity ratio.
Therapeutic effect: prevents pulmonary embolism and deep vein thrombosis (DVT).

Indications and dosage

► **Prevention of pulmonary embolism and DVT after hip or knee replacement surgery.** *Adults:* 30 mg S.C. q 12 hours for 7 to 10 days. Initial dose given 12 to 24 hours after surgery, provided hemostasis has been established.
Alternatively, for hip replacement surgery, 40 mg S.C. once daily given initially 12 hours before surgery. May continue with 40 mg S.C. once daily or 30 mg S.C. q 12 hours for 3 weeks.
► **Prevention of pulmonary embolism and DVT in patients after abdominal surgery.** *Adults:* 40 mg S.C. once daily for 7 to 10 days with initial dose given 2 hours prior to surgery.
► **Prevention of ischemic complications of unstable angina and non–Q-wave MI, when concurrently administered with aspirin.** *Adults:* 1 mg/kg S.C. q 12 hours for 2 to 8 days together with oral aspirin therapy (100 to 325 mg/day).

Adverse reactions

CNS: confusion, *neurologic injury* (when used with spinal or epidural puncture).
CV: edema, peripheral edema, *CV toxicity* (chest pain, dizziness, irregular heartbeat).
GI: nausea.
Hematologic: hypochromic anemia, *thrombocytopenia, hemorrhage,* bleeding complications.
Other: irritation, pain, hematoma, or erythema at injection site; fever; pain; ecchymosis, *angioedema, rash, hives.*

Interactions

Drug-drug. *Anticoagulants, antiplatelet agents, NSAIDs:* increased risk of bleeding. Don't use together.
Plicamycin, valproic acid: may cause hypoprothrombinemia and inhibit platelet aggregation. Monitor closely.

Contraindications and precautions

• Contraindicated in patients with hypersensitivity to drug or to heparin or pork products; in those with active major

---

bleeding or thrombocytopenia; and in those who demonstrate antiplatelet antibodies in presence of drug.

• Use with extreme caution, if at all, in patients with postoperative indwelling epidural catheters or patients who have had epidural or spinal anesthesia. Epidural and spinal hematomas have been reported, resulting in long-term or permanent paralysis.

• Use with extreme caution in patients with history of heparin-induced thrombocytopenia.

• Use cautiously in patients with conditions that put them at increased risk for hemorrhage, such as bacterial endocarditis, and in patients with congenital or acquired bleeding disorders, ulcer disease, angiodysplastic GI disease, hemorrhagic stroke, or recent spinal, eye, or brain surgery.

• Use cautiously in pregnant or breast-feeding women.

• Safe use in children has not been established.

NURSING CONSIDERATIONS

◆ Assessment

• Obtain history of patient's coagulation parameters before therapy.

• Monitor effectiveness by evaluating patient for signs and symptoms of pulmonary embolism or DVT.

• Monitor platelet counts regularly. Patient with normal coagulation does not require regular monitoring of PT, INR, and PTT.

• Frequently monitor neurological status in patients who have had spinal or epidural anesthesia. Alert the doctor immediately if neurological compromise is noted.

• Be alert for adverse reactions and drug interactions.

• Evaluate patient's and family's knowledge of drug therapy.

◆ Nursing diagnoses

• Risk for injury related to potential for pulmonary embolism or DVT development after knee or hip replacement surgery

• Altered protection related to drug-induced bleeding complications

• Knowledge deficit related to drug therapy

◆ Planning and implementation

• Never administer drug I.M.

• Don't massage after S.C. injection. Rotate sites and keep accurate record.

• Know that enoxaparin cannot be used interchangeably (unit for unit) with unfractionated heparin or other low-molecular-weight heparins.

• Don't mix enoxaparin with other injections or infusions.

• Avoid excessive I.M. injections of other drugs to prevent or minimize hematomas. If possible, don't give I.M. injections.

• To treat severe overdose, give protamine sulfate (a heparin antagonist) by slow I.V. infusion at concentration of 1% to equal dosage of enoxaparin injected, as ordered.

Patient teaching

• Instruct patient and family to watch for signs of bleeding and notify doctor immediately.

• Tell patient to avoid OTC medications containing aspirin or other salicylates.

◆ Evaluation

• Patient does not develop pulmonary embolism or DVT.

• Patient does not experience bleeding complications during therapy.

• Patient and family state understanding of drug therapy.

---

ephedrine sulfate
(eh-FED-rin SUL-fayt)
Vicks Vatronol Nose Drops

Pharmacologic class: adrenergic
Therapeutic class: bronchodilator, vasopressor (parenteral form), nasal decongestant.
Pregnancy risk category: C

Reactions may be *common,* uncommon, *life-threatening,* or COMMON AND LIFE-THREATENING.

How supplied

Tablets: 30 mg◊
Capsules: 25 mg, 50 mg
Injection: 25 mg/ml, 50 mg/ml
Nasal solution: 0.5%

Pharmacokinetics

Absorption: rapidly and completely absorbed after P.O., I.M., or S.C. administration; unknown after nasal administration.
Distribution: widely distributed throughout body.
Metabolism: slowly metabolized in liver.
Excretion: excreted unchanged in urine. Rate of excretion depends on urine pH.
Half-life: 3 to 6 hours.

Route	Onset	Peak	Duration
P.O.	15-60 min	Unknown	3-5 hr
I.V.	≤ 5 min	Unknown	Unknown
I.M.	10-20 min	Unknown	0.5-1 hr
S.C.	Unknown	Unknown	0.5-1 hr
Intranasal	Unknown	Unknown	Unknown

Pharmacodynamics

Chemical effect: stimulates alpha- and beta-adrenergic receptors; direct- and indirect-acting sympathomimetic.
Therapeutic effect: raises blood pressure, causes bronchodilation, and relieves nasal decongestion.

Indications and dosage

▶ **To correct hypotension.** *Adults:* 25 to 50 mg I.M. or S.C., or 10 to 25 mg I.V., p.r.n., to maximum of 150 mg/24 hours. *Children:* 3 mg/kg or 100 mg/m² S.C. or I.V. daily in four to six divided doses.
▶ **Bronchodilation, nasal decongestion.** *Adults and children age 12 and over:* 12.5 to 50.0 mg P.O. b.i.d., t.i.d., or q.i.d. Maximum dosage is 400 mg daily in six to eight divided doses. As nasal decongestant, 0.5% solution applied topically to nasal mucosa as drops or on nasal pack. Instill no more often than q 4 hours. *Children ages 2 to 12:* 2 to 3 mg/ kg P.O. daily in four to six divided doses.

Adverse reactions

CNS: *insomnia, nervousness,* dizziness, headache, muscle weakness, diaphoresis, euphoria, confusion, delirium.
CV: *palpitations,* tachycardia, hypertension, precordial pain.
EENT: dryness of nose and throat.
GI: nausea, vomiting, anorexia.
GU: urine retention, painful urination due to visceral sphincter spasm.

Interactions

Drug-drug. *Acetazolamide:* increased serum ephedrine levels. Monitor for toxicity.
Alpha-adrenergic blockers: unopposed beta-adrenergic effects, resulting in hypotension. Monitor blood pressure.
Antihypertensives: decreased effects. Monitor blood pressure.
Beta blockers: unopposed alpha-adrenergic effects, resulting in hypertension. Monitor blood pressure.
Cardiac glycosides, general anesthetics (halogenated hydrocarbons): increased risk of ventricular arrhythmias. Monitor patient closely.
Ergot alkaloids: enhanced vasoconstrictor activity. Monitor patient closely.
Guanadrel, guanethidine: enhanced pressor effects of ephedrine. Monitor patient closely.
Levodopa: enhanced risk of ventricular arrhythmias. Monitor patient closely.
MAO inhibitors, tricyclic antidepressants: when given with sympathomimetics, may cause severe hypertension (hypertensive crisis). Avoid concomitant use.
Methyldopa, reserpine: may inhibit effects of ephedrine. Use together cautiously.

Contraindications and precautions

• Contraindicated in patients with hypersensitivity to ephedrine and other sympathomimetic drugs; in those with porphyria, severe coronary artery disease, arrhythmias, angle-closure glaucoma, psychoneurosis, angina pectoris, substan-

tial organic heart disease, or CV disease; and in those taking MAO inhibitors.
• Breast-feeding should be avoided during treatment with ephedrine.
• Use with extreme caution in elderly men and in those with hypertension, hyperthyroidism, nervous or excitable states, diabetes, or prostatic hyperplasia.
• Use cautiously in pregnant women and in children.

NURSING CONSIDERATIONS

⚖ Assessment
• Obtain history of patient's underlying condition before therapy, and reassess regularly thereafter.
• Be alert for adverse reactions and drug interactions.
• Evaluate patient's and family's knowledge of drug therapy.

🔲 Nursing diagnoses
• Altered health maintenance related to underlying condition
• Risk for fluid volume deficit related to drug-induced adverse GI reactions
• Knowledge deficit related to drug therapy

❯ Planning and implementation
• Know that hypoxia, hypercapnia, and acidosis, which may reduce effectiveness or increase incidence of adverse reactions, must be identified and corrected before or during ephedrine administration.
• Know that volume deficit must be corrected before administering vasopressors. This drug is not a substitute for blood or fluid volume replenishment.
• To prevent insomnia, avoid giving within 2 hours before bedtime.
P.O. use: Follow normal protocol.
I.V. use: Give 10 to 25 mg by I.V. injection slowly; repeat in 5 to 10 minutes, if necessary. Compatible with most common I.V. solutions.
I.M., S.C., and intranasal use: Follow normal protocol.

• Notify doctor if effectiveness decreases. Effectiveness decreases after 2 to 3 weeks, as tolerance develops. Doctor may need to increase dosage. Drug is not addictive.
Patient teaching
• Warn patient not to take OTC drugs that contain ephedrine without informing doctor.
• Teach patient how to instill nose drops and caution him not to exceed recommended dosage.
• Advise patient to notify doctor if effectiveness decreases because dosage may need to be adjusted.
• Instruct patient to notify doctor if adverse reactions occur.
• Caution patient not to perform hazardous activities if adverse CNS reactions occur.

✔ Evaluation
• Patient exhibits improvement in underlying condition.
• Patient maintains adequate hydration throughout therapy.
• Patient and family state understanding of drug therapy.

epinephrine (adrenaline)
(eh-pih-NEF-rin)
Adrenalin†, Bronkaid Mist†, Bronkaid Mistometer♦, Primatene Mist†

epinephrine bitartrate
AsthmaHaler Mist†, Bronitin Mist†, Bronkaid Mist Suspension†, Medihaler-Epi†, Primatene Mist Suspension†

epinephrine hydrochloride
Adrenalin Chloride†, EpiPen Auto-Injector, EpiPen Jr. Auto-Injector, Sus-Phrine

Pharmacologic class: adrenergic
Therapeutic class: bronchodilator, vasopressor, cardiac stimulant, local anesthetic, topical antihemorrhagic
Pregnancy risk category: C

Reactions may be *common*, uncommon, *life-threatening*, or COMMON AND LIFE-THREATENING.

How supplied

Aerosol inhaler: 160 mcg†, 200 mcg†, 220 mcg†, 250 mcg/metered spray†
Nebulizer inhaler: 1% (1:100)♦†, 1.25%♦†, 2.25%♦†
Injection: 0.01 mg/ml (1:100,000), 0.1 mg/ml (1:10,000), 0.5 mg/ml (1:2,000), 1 mg/ml (1:1,000) parenteral; 5 mg/ml (1:200) parenteral suspension

Pharmacokinetics

Absorption: well absorbed after S.C. or I.M. injection. Rapidly absorbed after inhalation administration.
Distribution: distributed widely throughout body.
Metabolism: metabolized at sympathetic nerve endings, liver, and other tissues to inactive metabolites.
Excretion: excreted in urine, mainly as its metabolites and conjugates.

Route	Onset	Peak	Duration
I.V.	Immediate	≤ 5 min	1-4 hr
I.M.	Varies	Unknown	1-4 hr
S.C.	6-15 min	≤ 30 min	1-4 hr
Inhalation	3-5 min	Unknown	1-3 hr

Pharmacodynamics

Chemical effect: stimulates alpha- and beta-adrenergic receptors within sympathetic nervous system.
Therapeutic effect: relaxes bronchial smooth muscle, causes cardiac stimulation, relieves allergic signs and symptoms, stops local bleeding, and decreases pain sensation.

Indications and dosage

► **Bronchospasm, hypersensitivity reactions, anaphylaxis.** *Adults:* 0.1 to 0.5 ml of 1:1,000 S.C. or I.M.; repeated q 10 to 15 minutes, p.r.n. Or, 0.1 to 0.25 ml of 1:1,000 (1.0 to 2.5 ml of commercially available 1:10,000 injection or of 1:10,000 dilution prepared by diluting 1 ml of commercially available 1:1,000 injection with 10 ml of water for injection or 0.9% NaCl injection) I.V. slowly over 5 to 10 minutes. *Children:* 0.01 ml (10 mcg) of 1:1,000/kg S.C.; repeated q 20 minutes to 4 hours, p.r.n. Or 0.005 ml/ kg of 1:200 (Sus-Phrine) S.C.; repeated q 8 to 12 hours, p.r.n.

► **Hemostasis.** *Adults:* 1:50,000 to 1:1,000 applied topically.

► **Acute asthmatic attacks.** *Adults and children age 4 and over:* 160 to 250 mcg (metered aerosol), which is equivalent to one inhalation, repeated once if necessary after at least 1 minute; subsequent doses should not be administered for at least 3 hours. Alternatively, 1% (1:100) solution of epinephrine or 2.25% solution of racepinephrine administered by hand-bulb nebulizer as one to three deep inhalations, repeated q 3 hours, p.r.n.

► **Prolongation of local anesthetic effect.** *Adults and children:* 1:500,000 to 1:50,000 mixed with local anesthetic.

► **Restoration of cardiac rhythm in cardiac arrest.** *Adults:* 0.5 to 1.0 mg I.V. or into endotracheal tube. Drug may be given intracardiac if no I.V. route or intratracheal route is available. Some clinicians advocate higher dose (up to 5 mg), especially in patients who don't respond to usual I.V. dose. After initial I.V. administration, drug may be infused I.V. at rate of 1 to 4 mcg/minute. *Children:* 10 mcg/kg I.V., or 5 to 10 mcg (0.05 to 0.1 ml of 1:10,000)/kg intracardiac.
Note: 1 mg = 1 ml of 1:1,000 or 10 ml of 1:10,000.

Adverse reactions

CNS: *nervousness, tremors*, euphoria, anxiety, coldness of extremities, vertigo, *headache, drowsiness*, diaphoresis, disorientation, agitation, fear, weakness, *cerebral hemorrhage, CVA;* increased rigidity and tremors (in patients with Parkinson's disease).
CV: *palpitations;* widened pulse pressure; *hypertension; tachycardia; ventricular fibrillation; shock;* anginal pain; ECG changes, including decreased T-wave amplitude.
GI: *nausea,* vomiting.
Respiratory: dyspnea.

Skin: urticaria, pain, hemorrhage (at injection site).
Other: pallor, hyperglycemia, glycosuria.

Interactions

Drug-drug. *Alpha-adrenergic blockers:* hypotension due to unopposed beta-adrenergic effects. Monitor blood pressure.
Antihistamines, thyroid hormones, tricyclic antidepressants: when given with sympathomimetics, may cause severe adverse cardiac effects. Avoid giving together.
Beta blockers (such as propranolol): vasoconstriction and reflex bradycardia. Monitor patient carefully.
Cardiac glycosides, general anesthetics (halogenated hydrocarbons): increased risk of ventricular arrhythmias. Monitor patient closely.
Doxapram, mazindol, methylphenidate: enhanced CNS stimulation or pressor effects. Monitor patient closely.
Ergot alkaloids: enhanced vasoconstrictor activity. Monitor patient closely.
Guanadrel, guanethidine: enhanced pressor effects of epinephrine. Monitor patient closely.
Levodopa: enhanced risk of cardiac arrhythmias. Monitor patient closely.
MAO inhibitors: increased risk of hypertensive crisis. Avoid concomitant use.

Contraindications and precautions

• Contraindicated in patients with angle-closure glaucoma, shock (other than anaphylactic shock), organic brain damage, cardiac dilation, arrhythmias, coronary insufficiency, or cerebral arteriosclerosis. Also contraindicated in patients during general anesthesia with halogenated hydrocarbons or cyclopropane and in patients in labor (may delay second stage).
• Some commercial products contain sulfites: contraindicated in patients with sulfite allergies except when epinephrine is being used for treatment of serious allergic reactions or in other emergency situations.

• In conjunction with local anesthetics, epinephrine is contraindicated for use in fingers, toes, ears, nose, or genitalia.
• Breast-feeding should be avoided during drug use.
• Use with extreme caution in patients with long-standing bronchial asthma or emphysema who have developed degenerative heart disease. Also use cautiously in elderly patients and in those with hyperthyroidism, CV disease, hypertension, psychoneurosis, or diabetes, as well as in pregnant women not in labor and in children.

NURSING CONSIDERATIONS

⚕ Assessment
• Obtain history of patient's underlying condition before therapy, and reassess regularly thereafter.
• When administering I.V., monitor blood pressure, heart rate, and ECG when therapy is initiated and frequently thereafter.
• Be alert for adverse reactions and drug interactions.
• Evaluate patient's and family's knowledge of drug therapy.

⬛ Nursing diagnoses
• Altered health maintenance related to underlying condition
• Decreased cardiac output related to drug-induced adverse CV effects
• Knowledge deficit related to drug therapy

▶ Planning and implementation
• Be aware that epinephrine is drug of choice in emergency treatment of acute anaphylactic reactions.
• Discard epinephrine solution after 24 hours or if solution is discolored or contains precipitate. Keep solution in light-resistant container, and don't remove before use.
I.V. use: Don't mix with alkaline solutions. Use D_5W, 0.9% NaCl injection, lactated Ringer's injection, or combinations of dextrose in NaCl. Mix just before use.

Reactions may be *common*, uncommon, *life-threatening*, or COMMON AND LIFE-THREATENING.

I.M. use: Avoid I.M. administration of parenteral suspension into buttocks. Gas gangrene may occur because epinephrine reduces oxygen tension of tissues, encouraging growth of contaminating organisms.
– Massage site after I.M. injection to counteract possible vasoconstriction. Repeated local injection can cause necrosis, resulting from vasoconstriction at injection site.

S.C. use: Follow normal protocol.

Inhalation use: Always wait 2 minutes between inhalations, if bronchodilator is administered by way of inhalant and more than one inhalation is ordered. Always administer bronchodilator first and wait 5 minutes before administering the other, if more than one type of inhalant is ordered. Remember that patient should not receive more than 12 bronchodilator inhalations in 24 hours.

• Giving medication on time is extremely important.

• Notify doctor if adverse reactions develop; he may adjust dosage or discontinue drug. Also notify doctor if patient's pulse increases by 20% or more when epinephrine is administered.

• Know that if blood pressure rises sharply, rapid-acting vasodilators, such as nitrites or alpha-adrenergic blockers, can be given to counteract marked pressor effect of large doses of epinephrine.

• Know that epinephrine is destroyed rapidly by oxidizing agents, such as iodine, chromates, nitrates, nitrites, oxygen, and salts of easily reducible metals (such as iron).

Patient teaching
• Tell patient to take medication exactly as prescribed and to take it around the clock.
• Teach patient to perform oral inhalation correctly. Give following instructions for using metered-dose inhaler:
– Clear nasal passages and throat.
– Breathe out, expelling as much air from lungs as possible.
– Place mouthpiece well into mouth as dose from inhaler is released, and inhale deeply.

– Hold breath for several seconds, remove mouthpiece, and exhale slowly.
• If more than one inhalation is ordered, tell patient to wait at least 2 minutes before repeating procedure.
• Tell patient who also is using steroid inhaler to use bronchodilator first, then wait about 5 minutes before using steroid. This allows bronchodilator to open air passages for maximum effectiveness.
• Instruct patient who has acute hypersensitivity reactions, such as to bee stings, to self-inject epinephrine at home.
• Tell patient to reduce intake of foods containing caffeine, such as coffee, colas, and chocolates, when taking bronchodilator.
• Instruct patient to contact doctor immediately if he experiences fluttering of heart, rapid beating of heart, shortness of breath, or chest pain.
• Tell patient not to self-medicate with any OTC drugs without medical approval while taking this drug.
• Show patient how to check pulse. Instruct him to check pulse before and after using bronchodilator and to call doctor if pulse rate increases more than 20 beats/minute.

☑ Evaluation
• Patient exhibits improvement in underlying condition.
• Patient maintains adequate cardiac output throughout therapy.
• Patient and family state understanding of drug therapy.

epinephrine hydrochloride
(eh-pih-NEF-rin high-droh-KLOR-ighd)
Adrenalin Chloride

Pharmacologic class: adrenergic
Therapeutic class: decongestant, topical antihemorrhagic
Pregnancy risk category: NR

How supplied

Nasal solution: 0.1%

Pharmacokinetics

Unknown.

Route	Onset	Peak	Duration
Nasal	≤ 1 min	Unknown	Unknown

Pharmacodynamics

Chemical effect: causes local vasoconstriction of dilated arterioles, reducing blood flow and nasal congestion.
Therapeutic effect: relieves nasal decongestion and stops local bleeding.

Indications and dosage

▶ **Nasal congestion, local superficial bleeding.** *Adults and children:* instill 1 or 2 drops of solution.

Adverse reactions

CNS: nervousness, excitation.
CV: *tachycardia.*
EENT: rebound nasal congestion, slight sting on application.

Interactions

None significant.

Contraindications and precautions

• Contraindicated in patients with hypersensitivity to drug.
• Breast-feeding should be avoided during drug therapy.
• Use cautiously in patients with hyperthyroidism, coronary artery disease, hypertension, or diabetes mellitus.
• Also use cautiously in pregnant women and in children.

NURSING CONSIDERATIONS

Assessment
• Obtain history of patient's underlying condition before therapy, and reassess regularly thereafter.
• Monitor effectiveness by noting if patient experiences decreased nasal congestion or cessation of bleeding.

• Be alert for adverse reactions.
• Evaluate patient's and family's knowledge of drug therapy.

Nursing diagnoses
• Altered health maintenance related to underlying condition
• Knowledge deficit related to drug therapy

Planning and implementation
• Follow normal protocol for instilling nose drops.
Patient teaching
• Teach patient how to instill nose drops.
• Instruct patient that product should be used by only one person to prevent spread of infection.
• Tell patient not to exceed recommended dosage and to use only when needed.

Evaluation
• Patient exhibits improvement of underlying condition.
• Patient and family state understanding of drug therapy.

epoetin alfa (erythropoietin)
(ee-POH-eh-tin AL-fah)
Epogen, Procrit

Pharmacologic class: glycoprotein
Therapeutic class: antianemic
Pregnancy risk category: C

How supplied

Injection: 2,000 units/ml, 3,000 units/ml, 4,000 units/ml, 10,000 units/ml, 20,000 units/ml

Pharmacokinetics

Unknown.

Route	Onset	Peak	Duration
I.V.	1-6 wk	Immediate	Unknown
S.C.	1-6 wk	4-24 hr	Unknown

Reactions may be *common,* uncommon, *life-threatening*, or COMMON AND LIFE-THREATENING.

Pharmacodynamics

Chemical effect: mimics effects of erythropoietin, a naturally occurring hormone produced by the kidneys. Epoetin alfa is one of factors controlling rate of RBC production. It acts on erythroid tissues in bone marrow, stimulating mitotic activity of erythroid progenitor cells and early precursor cells. It functions as a growth factor and as a differentiating factor, enhancing rate of RBC production. **Therapeutic effect:** eliminates anemia.

Indications and dosage

► **Anemia due to reduced production of endogenous erythropoietin caused by end-stage renal disease.** *Adults:* dosage is individualized. Starting dose is 50 to 100 units/kg I.V. three times weekly. (Nondialysis patients with chronic renal failure or patients receiving continuous peritoneal dialysis may receive drug by S.C. injection or I.V.) Dosage reduced when target hematocrit is reached or if hematocrit rises more than 4 points in any 2-week period. Dosage increased if hematocrit does not increase by 5 to 6 points after 8 weeks of therapy. Maintenance dosage is individualized.

► **Adjunct treatment of HIV-infected patients with anemia secondary to zidovudine therapy.** *Adults:* 100 units/kg I.V. or S.C. three times weekly for 8 weeks or until target hemoglobin is reached.

► **Anemia secondary to chemotherapy.** *Adults:* 150 units/kg S.C. three times weekly for 8 weeks or until target hemoglobin is reached. Dosage then increased up to 300 units/kg S.C. three times weekly, if needed.

Adverse reactions

CNS: *headache,* **seizures,** *paresthesia, fatigue,* dizziness, *asthenia.*
CV: *hypertension, edema.*
GI: *nausea, vomiting, diarrhea.*
Hematologic: iron deficiency, elevated platelet count.
Respiratory: *cough, shortness of breath.*

Skin: *rash, injection site reactions, urticaria.*
Other: increased clotting of arteriovenous grafts, *pyrexia, arthralgia.*

Interactions

None significant.

Contraindications and precautions

• Contraindicated in patients with uncontrolled hypertension, hypersensitivity to mammalian cell–derived products or albumin (human).
• Use cautiously in pregnant or breast-feeding women.
• Safety of drug has not been established in children.

NURSING CONSIDERATIONS

⚗ Assessment
• Assess patient's blood count and blood pressure before therapy.
• Monitor effectiveness by monitoring blood count results, as ordered. Know that hematocrit may rise and cause excessive clotting. Watch for signs and symptoms of blood clot formation.
• Know that patient's response to epoetin alfa depends on amount of endogenous erythropoietin in plasma. Patients with levels of 500 units/L or more usually have transfusion-dependent anemia and will probably not respond to drug. Those with levels below 500 units/L usually respond well.
• Be alert for adverse reactions.
• Monitor blood pressure closely. Up to 80% of patients with chronic renal failure have hypertension. Blood pressure may rise, especially when hematocrit is increasing in early part of therapy.
• After injection (usually within 2 hours), know that some patients complain of pain or discomfort in their limbs (long bones) and pelvis and of coldness and sweating. Symptoms may persist for up to 12 hours and then disappear.
• Monitor patient's hydration status if adverse GI reactions occur.

• Evaluate patient's and family's knowledge of drug therapy.

✚ **Nursing diagnoses**
• Altered protection related to reduced production of endogenous erythropoietin
• Risk for fluid volume deficit related to drug-induced adverse GI reactions
• Knowledge deficit related to drug therapy

▶ **Planning and implementation**
I.V. use: Give drug by direct injection without dilution. Solution contains no preservatives. Discard unused portion. Do not mix with other drugs.
S.C. use: Follow normal protocol.
• When used in HIV-infected patient, be prepared to individualize dosage based on response, as ordered. Dosage recommendations are for patients with endogenous erythropoietin levels of 500 units/liter or less and cumulative zidovudine doses of 4.2 g/week or less.
• Be aware that patient treated with epoetin alfa may require additional heparin to prevent clotting during dialysis treatments.
• Institute diet restrictions or drug therapy to control blood pressure. Reduce dosage in patient who exhibits rapid rise in hematocrit (more than 4 points in a 2-week period), as ordered, because of risk of hypertension.
Patient teaching
• Advise patient that blood specimens will be drawn weekly for blood counts and that dosage adjustments may be made based on results.
• Warn patient to avoid hazardous activities, such as driving or operating heavy machinery, during initiation of therapy. A relation between excessively rapid hematocrit rise and seizures may exist.
• Tell patient to notify doctor if adverse reactions occur.

☑ **Evaluation**
• Patient's blood count is normal.
• Patient maintains adequate hydration throughout therapy.

• Patient and family state understanding of drug therapy.

ergotamine tartrate
(er-GAH-tuh-meen TAR-trayt)
Ergodryl Mono◇, Ergomar, Ergostat, Gynergen♦

Pharmacologic class: ergot alkaloid
Therapeutic class: vasoconstrictor
Pregnancy risk category: X

How supplied
Capsules: 1 mg◇
Tablets: 1 mg♦
Tablets (sublingual): 2 mg
Aerosol inhaler: 360 mcg/metered spray♦
Suppositories: 2 mg

Pharmacokinetics
Absorption: rapidly absorbed after inhalation and variably absorbed after P.O. or P.R. administration.
Distribution: widely distributed throughout body.
Metabolism: extensively metabolized in liver.
Excretion: thought to be primarily excreted in feces; 4% excreted in urine.

Route	Onset	Peak	Duration
P.O.	Varies	0.5-3 hr	Varies
P.R., S.L., inhalation	Varies	Unknown	Varies

Pharmacodynamics
Chemical effect: stimulates alpha-adrenergic receptors, causing peripheral vasoconstriction. Drug also inhibits reuptake of norepinephrine, increasing vasoconstrictor activity.
Therapeutic effect: relieves vascular or migraine headache.

Indications and dosage
▶ **Vascular or migraine headache.**
Adults: initially, 2 mg P.O. or S.L., then 1

Reactions may be *common,* uncommon, *life-threatening*, or COMMON AND LIFE-THREATENING.

to 2 mg P.O. or S.L. q ½ hour to maximum of 6 mg per attack and 10 mg weekly. Alternatively, use of aerosol inhaler: 1 spray (360 mcg) initially, repeated q 5 minutes, p.r.n., to maximum of 6 sprays (2.16 mg) per 24 hours or 15 sprays (5.4 mg) weekly.

Patient also may use suppositories. Initially, 2 mg P.R. at onset of attack, repeated in 1 hour, p.r.n. Maximum dosage is two suppositories per attack or five suppositories weekly.

Adverse reactions

CV: numbness and tingling in fingers and toes, transient tachycardia or *bradycardia,* precordial distress and pain, increased arterial pressure, angina pectoris, peripheral vasoconstriction.
GI: nausea, *vomiting.*
Skin: itching, localized edema.
Other: weakness in legs, muscle pain in extremities, uterine contractions.

Interactions

Drug-drug. *Erythromycin, other macrolides:* may cause symptoms of ergot toxicity. Vasodilators (nitroprusside, nifedipine, or prazosin) may be ordered to treat such an attack. Monitor patient closely. *Propranolol, other beta blockers:* blocked natural pathway for vasodilation in patients receiving ergot alkaloids; may result in excessive vasoconstriction. Watch closely if drugs are used together.

Contraindications and precautions

• Contraindicated in pregnant women and in those with peripheral or occlusive vascular diseases, coronary artery disease, hypertension, hepatic or renal dysfunction, severe pruritus, sepsis, or hypersensitivity to ergot alkaloids.
• Use cautiously in breast-feeding women. Excessive dosage or prolonged administration of drug may inhibit lactation.
• Safety of drug has not been established in children.

NURSING CONSIDERATIONS

⚗ Assessment
• Obtain history of patient's headache before therapy, and reassess regularly thereafter.
• Be alert for adverse reactions and drug interactions.
• Be alert for ergotamine rebound or increase in frequency and duration of headache, which may occur if drug is discontinued suddenly.
• Evaluate patient's and family's knowledge of drug therapy.

⊕ Nursing diagnoses
• Pain related to presence of vascular or migraine headache
• Decreased peripheral tissue perfusion related to vasoconstriction
• Knowledge deficit related to drug therapy

⧽ Planning and implementation
• Be aware that drug is most effective when used during prodromal stage of headache or as soon as possible after onset.
• Avoid prolonged administration; don't exceed recommended dosage.
• Know that S.L. tablets are preferred for use during early stage of attack because of their rapid absorption.
• Store drug in light-resistant container.
P.O. and inhalation use: Follow normal protocol.
P.R. use: Chill suppository in ice-cold water while still in wrapper, if it has become softened.
S.L. use: Do not give drug with food or drink while tablets are dissolving.
Patient teaching
• Tell patient not to eat, drink, or smoke while tablet is dissolving. S.L. tablets are preferred during early stage of attack because of their rapid absorption.
• Warn patient not to increase dosage without first consulting doctor.
• Advise patient to avoid prolonged exposure to cold weather whenever possi-

ble. Cold may increase adverse reactions to drug.
• Instruct patient who is on long-term therapy to check for and report coldness in extremities or tingling in fingers and toes. Severe vasoconstriction may result in tissue damage.
• Instruct patient on correct use of inhaler.
• Help patient evaluate underlying causes of stress, which may precipitate attacks.

☑ Evaluation
• Patient is free from pain.
• Patient maintains adequate tissue perfusion to extremities throughout therapy.
• Patient and family state understanding of drug therapy.

erythromycin base

(eh-rith-roh-MIGH-sin bays)
Apo-Erythro♦, EMU-V◇, E-Mycin, Erybid♦, ERYC, ERYC-125♦, ERYC-250♦, Ery-Tab, Erythromid♦, Erythromycin Base Filmtab, Novo-Rythro♦, PCE Dispertab

erythromycin estolate

Ilosone, Novo-rythro♦

erythromycin ethylsuccinate

Apo-Erythro-ES♦, E.E.S., EES-400◇, EES granules◇, EryPed, Erythrocin

erythromycin gluceptate

Ilotycin Gluceptate

erythromycin lactobionate

Erythrocin

erythromycin stearate

Apo-Erythro-S♦, Erythrocin, My-E, Novo-Rythro♦

Pharmacologic class: erythromycin
Therapeutic class: antibiotic
Pregnancy risk category: B

How supplied

erythromycin base
Tablets (enteric-coated): 250 mg, 333 mg, 500 mg
Tablets (filmtabs): 250 mg, 500 mg
Capsules (enteric-coated pellets): 250 mg
erythromycin estolate
Tablets: 500 mg
Capsules: 250 mg
Oral suspension: 125 mg/5 ml, 250 mg/5 ml
erythromycin ethylsuccinate
Tablets: 400 mg
Tablets (chewable): 200 mg
Oral suspension: 200 mg/5 ml, 400 mg/5 ml, 100 mg/2.5 ml
erythromycin gluceptate
Injection: 1-g vial
erythromycin lactobionate
Injection: 500-mg, 1-g vials
erythromycin stearate
Tablets (film-coated): 250 mg, 500 mg

Pharmacokinetics

Absorption: most erythromycin salts are absorbed in duodenum. Because erythromycin base is acid-sensitive, it must be buffered or have enteric coating to prevent destruction by gastric acid. Acid salts and esters (estolate, ethylsuccinate, and stearate) are not affected by gastric acidity and, therefore, are well absorbed; they are unaffected or possibly even enhanced by presence of food. Base and stearate preparations should be given on empty stomach.
Distribution: widely distributed in most body tissues and fluids except CSF, where it appears in low concentrations. About 80% of erythromycin base and 96% of erythromycin estolate are protein-bound.
Metabolism: partially metabolized in liver to inactive metabolites.
Excretion: mainly excreted unchanged in bile; small amount (less than 5%) excreted in urine. *Half-life:* about 1½ hours.

Route	Onset	Peak	Duration
P.O.	Unknown	1-4 hr	Unknown
I.V.	Immediate	Immediate	Unknown

Pharmacodynamics

Chemical effect: inhibits bacterial protein synthesis by binding to 50S subunit of ribosome.
Therapeutic effect: inhibits bacterial growth. Spectrum of activity includes *Bordetella pertussis, Corynebacterium diphtheriae, Corynebacterium minutissimum, Entamoeba histolytica, Haemophilus influenzae, Legionella pneumophila,* and *Mycoplasma pneumoniae*. It also may be used to treat infections caused by *Chlamydia trachomatis, Listeria monocytogenes, Neisseria gonorrhoeae, Staphylococcus aureus, Streptococcus pneumoniae, Streptococcus viridans,* and *Treponema pallidum*.

Indications and dosage

▶ **Acute pelvic inflammatory disease caused by *N. gonorrhoeae*.** *Adults:* 500 mg I.V. (erythromycin gluceptate, lactobionate) q 6 hours for 3 days, then 250 mg (erythromycin base, estolate, stearate) or 400 mg (erythromycin ethylsuccinate) P.O. q 6 hours for 7 days.
▶ **Endocarditis prophylaxis for dental procedures in patients allergic to penicillin.** *Adults:* initially, 800 mg (ethylsuccinate) or 1 g (stearate) P.O. 2 hours before procedure; then 400 mg (ethylsuccinate) or 500 mg (stearate) P.O. 6 hours later. *Children:* initially, 20 mg/kg (ethylsuccinate or stearate) P.O. 2 hours before procedure; then one-half initial dose 6 hours later.
▶ **Intestinal amebiasis.** *Adults:* 250 mg (base, estolate, stearate) or 400 mg (ethylsuccinate) P.O. q 6 hours for 10 to 14 days. *Children:* 30 to 50 mg/kg (base, estolate, ethylsuccinate, stearate) P.O. daily in divided doses q 6 hours for 10 to 14 days.
▶ **Mild to moderately severe respiratory tract, skin, and soft-tissue infections caused by sensitive group A beta-**hemolytic streptococci, *B. pertussis, C. diphtheriae, Diplococcus pneumoniae, L. monocytogenes, M. pneumoniae.* *Adults:* 250 to 500 mg (erythromycin base, estolate, stearate) P.O. q 6 hours; or 400 to 800 mg (erythromycin ethylsuccinate) P.O. q 6 hours; or 15 to 20 mg/kg I.V. daily as continuous infusion or in divided doses q 6 hours. *Children:* 30 to 50 mg/kg (oral erythromycin salts) P.O. daily in divided doses q 6 hours; or 15 to 20 mg/kg I.V. daily in divided doses q 4 to 6 hours.
▶ **Syphilis.** *Adults:* 500 mg (erythromycin base, estolate, stearate) P.O. q.i.d. for 15 days.
▶ **Legionnaires' disease.** *Adults:* 1 to 4 g P.O. or I.V. daily in divided doses for 10 to 21 days.
▶ **Uncomplicated urethral, endocervical, or rectal infections when tetracyclines are contraindicated.** *Adults:* 500 mg (base, estolate, stearate) or 800 mg (ethylsuccinate) P.O. q.i.d. for at least 7 days.
▶ **Urogenital *C. trachomatis* infections during pregnancy.** *Adults:* 500 mg (base, estolate, stearate) P.O. q.i.d. for at least 7 days, or 250 mg (base, estolate, stearate) or 400 mg (ethylsuccinate) P.O. q.i.d. for at least 14 days.
▶ **Conjunctivitis caused by *C. trachomatis* in neonates.** *Neonates:* 50 mg/kg P.O. daily in four divided doses for at least 2 weeks.
▶ **Pneumonia of infancy caused by *C. trachomatis*.** *Infants:* 50 mg/kg daily in four divided doses for at least 3 weeks.

Adverse reactions

CV: *ventricular arrhythmias; venous irritation, thrombophlebitis* (after I.V. injection).
EENT: hearing loss (with high I.V. doses).
GI: *abdominal pain and cramping, nausea, vomiting, diarrhea.*
Hepatic: cholestatic jaundice (with erythromycin estolate).
Skin: urticaria, rash, eczema.

---

*Liquid form contains alcohol   **May contain tartrazine   ◆Canada   ◇Australia   †OTC

Other: overgrowth of nonsusceptible bacteria or fungi, *anaphylaxis,* fever.

Interactions

Drug-drug. *Astemizole:* decreased metabolism, leading to increased levels of antihistamines and cardiotoxicity. Avoid concomitant use.
Carbamazepine: increased carbamazepine blood levels and increased risk of toxicity. Monitor patient closely.
Cisapride: may increase cisapride concentrations, leading to toxicity including arrhythmias.
Clindamycin, lincomycin: may be antagonistic. Don't use together.
Cyclosporine: increased concentrations of cyclosporine. Monitor patient closely.
Digoxin: increased serum digoxin levels. Monitor for digoxin toxicity.
Disopyramide: increased disopyramide plasma levels, resulting, in some cases, in arrhythmias and increased QT intervals. Monitor ECG.
Midazolam, triazolam: increased effects of these drugs. Monitor patient closely.
Oral anticoagulants: increased anticoagulant effects. Monitor PT and INR closely.
Theophylline: decreased erythromycin blood level and increased theophylline toxicity. Use together cautiously.

Contraindications and precautions

• Contraindicated in patients with hypersensitivity to drug or other macrolides. Erythromycin estolate is contraindicated in patients with hepatic disease.
• Use other erythromycin salts cautiously in patients with impaired liver function. Also use cautiously in pregnant or breast-feeding women.

NURSING CONSIDERATIONS

⚖ Assessment
• Obtain history of patient's infection before therapy, and reassess regularly thereafter.

• Obtain urine specimen for culture and sensitivity tests before first dose. Therapy may begin, pending test results.
• Be alert for adverse reactions and drug interactions.
• Monitor patient's hydration status if adverse GI reactions occur.
• Monitor liver function (increased serum levels of alkaline phosphatase, ALT, AST, and bilirubin may occur). Erythromycin estolate may cause serious hepatotoxicity in adults (reversible cholestatic jaundice). Other erythromycin salts cause hepatotoxicity to lesser degree. Patients who develop hepatotoxicity from estolate may react similarly to treatment with other erythromycin preparations.
• Evaluate patient's and family's knowledge of drug therapy.

✥ Nursing diagnoses
• Infection related to presence of susceptible bacteria
• Risk for fluid volume deficit related to potential for drug-induced adverse GI reactions
• Knowledge deficit related to drug therapy

❯ Planning and implementation
P.O. use: When administering suspension, be sure to note concentration.
– For best absorption, give oral form of drug with full glass of water 1 hour before or 2 hours after meals. Coated tablets may be taken with meals. Tell patient not to drink fruit juice with drug. Chewable erythromycin tablets should not be swallowed whole.
I.V. use: Reconstitute drug according to manufacturer's directions, and dilute each 250 mg in at least 100 ml of 0.9% NaCl solution. Infuse over 1 hour.
– Do not administer erythromycin lactobionate with other drugs.
• Keep in mind that drug may falsely elevate concentrations of urinary catecholamines, 17-hydroxycorticosterone, and 17-ketosteroids.

Reactions may be *common*, uncommon, *life-threatening*, or COMMON AND LIFE-THREATENING.

• Be aware that drug may interfere with colorimetric assays, resulting in falsely elevated AST and ALT concentrations.

• Keep in mind that coated tablets or encapsulated pellets have caused fewer instances of GI upset; they may be more tolerable in patients who cannot tolerate erythromycin.

Patient teaching

• Instruct patient how to take oral drug.

• Tell patient to take entire amount of drug exactly as prescribed, even after he feels better.

• Instruct patient to notify doctor if adverse reactions occur, especially nausea, abdominal pain, and fever.

☑ Evaluation

• Patient is free from infection.

• Patient maintains adequate hydration with therapy.

• Patient and family state understanding of drug therapy.

---

esmolol hydrochloride
(EZ-moh-lohl high-droh-KLOR-ighd)
Brevibloc

Pharmacologic class: beta blocker
Therapeutic class: antiarrhythmic
Pregnancy risk category: C

How supplied

Injection: 10 mg/ml, 250 mg/ml

Pharmacokinetics

Absorption: not applicable with I.V. administration.
Distribution: distributed rapidly throughout plasma; 55% protein-bound.
Metabolism: hydrolyzed rapidly by plasma esterase.
Excretion: excreted by kidneys as metabolites. *Half-life:* about 9 minutes.

Route	Onset	Peak	Duration
I.V.	Almost immediate	About 30 min	< 30 min

Pharmacodynamics

Chemical effect: a class II antiarrhythmic, esmolol is ultrashort-acting selective beta$_1$-adrenergic blocker that decreases heart rate, myocardial contractility, and blood pressure.
Therapeutic effect: restores normal sinus rhythm.

Indications and dosage

▶ **Supraventricular tachycardia; control of ventricular rate in patients with atrial fibrillation or flutter in perioperative, postoperative, or other emergent circumstances; noncompensatory sinus tachycardia when heart rate requires specific interventions.** *Adults:* loading dose is 500 mcg/kg/minute by I.V. infusion over 1 minute, followed by 4-minute maintenance infusion of 50 mcg/kg/minute. If adequate response does not occur within 5 minutes, loading dose is repeated and followed by maintenance infusion of 100 mcg/kg/minute for 4 minutes. Loading dose is repeated and maintenance infusion is increased in stepwise manner, p.r.n. Maximum maintenance infusion for tachycardia is 200 mcg/kg/minute.

▶ **Management of perioperative and postoperative tachycardia or hypertension.** *Adults:* for perioperative treatment, 80 mg (about 1 mg/kg) I.V. bolus over 30 seconds, followed by 150 mcg/kg/minute I.V., if needed. Adjust infusion rate, p.r.n., up to maximum of 300 mcg/kg/minute; for postoperative treatment, same as for supraventricular tachycardia.

Adverse reactions

CNS: dizziness, somnolence, headache, agitation, fatigue, confusion.
CV: HYPOTENSION (sometimes with diaphoresis), peripheral ischemia.
GI: *nausea,* vomiting.
Respiratory: *bronchospasm,* wheezing, dyspnea, nasal congestion.
Other: inflammation, induration (at infusion site).

---

*Liquid form contains alcohol   **May contain tartrazine   ♦ Canada   ◇ Australia   †OTC

Interactions

Drug-drug. *Digoxin:* esmolol may increase serum digoxin levels by 10% to 20%. Monitor serum digoxin levels.
Morphine: may increase esmolol blood levels. Titrate esmolol carefully.
Reserpine, other catecholamine-depleting drugs: may cause additive bradycardia and hypotension. Titrate esmolol carefully.
Succinylcholine: esmolol may prolong neuromuscular blockade. Monitor patient.

Contraindications and precautions

• Contraindicated in patients with sinus bradycardia, heart block greater than first-degree, cardiogenic shock, or overt heart failure.
• Use cautiously in patients with impaired kidney function, diabetes, or bronchospasm. Also use cautiously in pregnant or breast-feeding women.
• Safety of drug has not been established in children.

NURSING CONSIDERATIONS

Assessment
• Obtain history of patient's arrhythmias before therapy.
• Monitor ECG and blood pressure continuously during infusion. Up to 50% of all patients treated with esmolol develop hypotension. Monitor closely, especially if patient's pretreatment blood pressure was low.
• Be alert for adverse reactions and drug interactions.
• Evaluate patient's and family's knowledge of drug therapy.

Nursing diagnoses
• Decreased cardiac output related to presence of arrhythmias
• Altered cerebral tissue perfusion related to drug-induced hypotension
• Knowledge deficit related to drug therapy

Planning and implementation
• Don't give by I.V. push; use infusion-control device. The 10-mg/ml single-dose vial may be used without diluting, but injection concentrate (250 mg/ml) must be diluted to maximum concentration of 10 mg/ml before infusion. Remove 20 ml from 500 ml of D_5W, lactated Ringer's solution, or 0.45% or 0.9% NaCl solution and add two ampules of esmolol (final concentration 10 mg/ml).
• Be aware that hypotension can usually be reversed within 30 minutes by decreasing dose or, if necessary, stopping infusion. Notify doctor if this becomes necessary.
• Remember that esmolol solutions are incompatible with diazepam, furosemide, sodium bicarbonate, and thiopental sodium.
• Know that when patient's heart rate becomes stable, esmolol will be replaced by alternative (longer-acting) antiarrhythmic, such as propranolol, digoxin, or verapamil. A half-hour after first dose of alternative agent is administered, reduce infusion rate by 50%. Monitor patient response, and if heart rate is controlled for 1 hour after administration of second dose of alternative drug, discontinue esmolol infusion.
• If local reaction develops at infusion site, change to another site. Avoid using butterfly needles.
Patient teaching
• Inform patient of need for continuous ECG, blood pressure, and heart rate monitoring to assess effectiveness of drug and detect adverse reactions.

Evaluation
• Patient regains normal cardiac output with correction of arrhythmias.
• Patient's blood pressure remains normal throughout therapy.
• Patient and family state understanding of drug therapy.

---

estazolam
(eh-STAZ-uh-lam)
ProSom

Pharmacologic class: benzodiazepine
Therapeutic class: hypnotic
Controlled substance schedule: IV
Pregnancy risk category: X

How supplied
Tablets: 1 mg, 2 mg

Pharmacokinetics
Absorption: rapidly and completely absorbed through GI tract.
Distribution: 93% protein-bound.
Metabolism: extensively metabolized in liver.
Excretion: metabolites excreted primarily in urine. Less than 5% excreted in urine as unchanged drug; 4% of 2-mg dose excreted in feces. *Half-life:* 10 to 24 hours.

Route	Onset	Peak	Duration
P.O.	Unknown	1-3 hr	Unknown

Pharmacodynamics
Chemical effect: unknown; thought to act on limbic system and thalamus of CNS by binding to specific benzodiazepine receptors.
Therapeutic effect: promotes sleep.

Indications and dosage
▶ **Insomnia.** *Adults:* 1 mg P.O. h.s. Some patients may require 2 mg.
Elderly: 1 mg P.O. h.s. Use higher doses with extreme care. Frail elderly or debilitated patients may take 0.5 mg, but this low dose may be only marginally effective.

Adverse reactions
CNS: fatigue, dizziness, *daytime drowsiness, somnolence, asthenia, hypokinesia,* headache, abnormal thinking.
GI: dyspepsia, abdominal pain.
Musculoskeletal: back pain, stiffness.

Interactions
Drug-drug. *Cimetidine, disulfiram, isoniazid, oral contraceptives:* may impair metabolism and clearance of benzodiazepines and prolong their plasma half-life. Monitor for increased CNS depression.
CNS depressants, including antihistamines, opioid analgesics, and other benzodiazepines: increased CNS depression. Avoid concomitant use.
Digoxin, phenytoin: increased serum levels of these drugs, resulting in toxicity. Monitor closely.
Rifampin: may increase metabolism and clearance and decrease plasma half-life. Monitor for decreased effectiveness.
Theophylline: pharmacologic antagonism. Monitor for decreased effectiveness.
Drug-lifestyle. *Alcohol use:* increased CNS and respiratory depression. Avoid concomitant use.
Smoking: may increase metabolism and clearance and decrease plasma half-life. Monitor for decreased effectiveness.

Contraindications and precautions
● Contraindicated during pregnancy and in patients with hypersensitivity to drug.
● Drug is not recommended for use in breast-feeding women.
● Use cautiously in patients with hepatic, renal, or pulmonary disease; depression; or suicidal tendencies.
● Safety of drug has not been established in children.

NURSING CONSIDERATIONS

Assessment
● Obtain history of patient's sleep pattern before therapy, and reassess regularly thereafter.
● Monitor liver and kidney function and CBC periodically during long-term therapy, as ordered.
● Be alert for adverse reactions and drug interactions.

• Monitor for possible withdrawal symptoms. Be aware that patients who receive prolonged treatment with benzodiazepines may experience withdrawal symptoms if drug is discontinued suddenly (possibly after 6 weeks of continuous therapy).
• Evaluate patient's and family's knowledge of drug therapy.

⊞ **Nursing diagnoses**
• Sleep pattern disturbance related to underlying condition
• Risk for trauma related to drug-induced adverse CNS reactions
• Knowledge deficit related to drug therapy

▶ **Planning and implementation**
• Before leaving bedside, make sure patient has swallowed medication.
• Take precautions to prevent hoarding by depressed, suicidal, or drug-dependent patient or patient who has history of drug abuse.
Patient teaching
• Tell patient not to increase dosage of drug but to inform doctor if he thinks that drug is no longer effective.
• Caution patient about performing activities that require mental alertness or physical coordination. For inpatient, supervise walking and raise bed rails, particularly for elderly patient.
• Warn patient that additive depressant effects can occur if alcohol is consumed while taking drug or within 24 hours after its use.
• Tell patient using oral contraceptives that she should consider alternate birth control methods when taking this drug because drug may enhance contraceptive hormone metabolism and decrease its effect.

☑ **Evaluation**
• Patient is able to sleep.
• Patient's safety is maintained.
• Patient and family state understanding of drug therapy.

estradiol (oestradiol)
(eh-struh-DIGH-ol)
Climara, Estrace**, Estrace Vaginal Cream, Estraderm, Vivelle

estradiol cypionate
depGynogen, Depo-Estradiol, Dura-Estrin, E-Cypionate, Estro-Cyp, Estrofem, Estroject-L.A.

estradiol valerate (oestradiol valerate)
Delestrogen, Dioval, Duragen-10, Duragen-20, Duragen-40, Estradiol L.A., Estra-L 20, Estra-L 40, Femogex, Gynogen L.A., Menaval, Primogyn Depot◇, Valergen-10, Valergen-20, Valergen-40

Pharmacologic class: estrogen
Therapeutic class: estrogen replacement, antineoplastic
Pregnancy risk category: X

How supplied
estradiol
Tablets (micronized): 0.5 mg, 1 mg, 2 mg
Transdermal: 0.0375 mg/24 hours, 0.05 mg/24 hours, 0.075 mg/24 hours, 0.1 mg/24 hours; 4 mg/10 cm^2 (delivers 0.05 mg/24 hours); 8 mg/20 cm^2 (delivers 0.1 mg/24 hours).
Vaginal cream (in nonliquefying base): 0.1 mg/g
estradiol cypionate
Injection (in oil): 1 mg/ml, 5 mg/ml
estradiol valerate
Injection (in oil): 10 mg/ml, 20 mg/ml, 40 mg/ml

Pharmacokinetics
Absorption: after P.O. administration, estradiol and other natural unconjugated estrogens are well absorbed but substantially inactivated by liver. After I.M. administration, absorption begins rapidly and continues for days. Topically applied estradiol is absorbed readily into systemic circulation.

Reactions may be *common,* uncommon, *life-threatening*, or COMMON AND LIFE-THREATENING.

Distribution: distributed throughout body with highest concentrations appearing in fat. Estradiol and other natural estrogens are about 50% to 80% plasma protein–bound.
Metabolism: metabolized primarily in liver.
Excretion: excreted primarily through kidneys.

Route	Onset	Peak	Duration
All routes	Unknown	Unknown	Unknown

Pharmacodynamics

Chemical effect: increases synthesis of DNA, RNA, and protein in responsive tissues; also reduces release of follicle-stimulating hormone and luteinizing hormone from pituitary gland.
Therapeutic effect: relieves vasomotor menopausal symptoms, provides estrogen replacement, relieves vaginal dryness, and provides palliative action for advanced prostate or breast cancer.

Indications and dosage

▶ **Vasomotor menopausal symptoms, female hypogonadism, female castration, primary ovarian failure.**
Estradiol. *Adults:* 1 to 2 mg P.O. daily in cycles of 21 days on and 7 days off or cycles of 5 days on and 2 days off; or 1 transdermal system (Estraderm) delivering 0.05 mg/24 hours applied twice weekly; or as a system (Vivelle) delivering either 0.05 mg/24 hours or 0.0375 mg/24 hours applied twice weekly; or as a system (Climara) delivering 0.05 mg/24 hours or 0.1 mg/24 hours applied once weekly in cycles of 3 weeks on and 1 week off. **Cypionate.** *Adults:* 1 to 5 mg I.M. q 3 to 4 weeks. **Valerate.** *Adults:* 10 to 20 mg I.M. q 4 weeks, p.r.n.
▶ **Atrophic vaginitis, kraurosis vulvae.**
Estradiol. *Adults:* 2 to 4 g intravaginal applications of cream daily for 1 to 2 weeks. When vaginal mucosa is restored, maintenance dosage of 1 g one to three times weekly in cyclic regimen.
Climara. *Adults:* 0.05 mg/24 hours applied weekly in a cyclic regimen.
Estraderm. *Adults:* 0.05 mg/24 hours applied twice weekly in a cyclic regimen.
Valerate. *Adults:* 10 to 20 mg I.M. q 4 weeks, p.r.n.
▶ **Palliative treatment of advanced, inoperable breast cancer. Estradiol.** *Men and postmenopausal women:* 10 mg P.O. t.i.d. for 3 months.
▶ **Palliative treatment of advanced inoperable prostate cancer. Estradiol.** *Men:* 1 to 2 mg P.O. t.i.d. **Valerate.** *Men:* 30 mg I.M. q 1 to 2 weeks.

Adverse reactions

CNS: headache, dizziness, chorea, depression, *seizures*.
CV: thrombophlebitis, *thromboembolism,* hypertension, edema.
EENT: worsening of myopia or astigmatism, intolerance of contact lenses.
GI: *nausea,* vomiting, abdominal cramps, bloating, diarrhea, constipation, increased appetite, weight changes, *pancreatitis.*
GU: breakthrough bleeding, altered menstrual flow, dysmenorrhea, amenorrhea, *increased risk of endometrial cancer, possibility of increased risk of breast cancer,* cervical erosion, altered cervical secretions, enlargement of uterine fibromas, vaginal candidiasis (in women); gynecomastia, testicular atrophy, impotence (in men).
Hepatic: cholestatic jaundice, gallbladder disease, *hepatic adenoma.*
Metabolic: hyperglycemia, hypercalcemia.
Skin: melasma, urticaria, erythema nodosum, dermatitis, hair loss.
Other: breast changes (tenderness, enlargement, secretion).

Interactions

Drug-drug. *Bromocriptine:* may cause amenorrhea, interfering with bromocriptine's effects. Avoid concomitant use. *Carbamazepine, phenobarbital, rifampin:* decreased effectiveness of estrogen therapy. Monitor patient closely.

Corticosteroids: possibly enhanced effects. Monitor patient closely.
Cyclosporine: increased risk of toxicity. Use together with caution, and frequently monitor cyclosporine levels.
Dantrolene, other hepatotoxic drugs: increased risk of hepatotoxicity. Monitor patient closely.
Oral anticoagulants: dosage adjustments may be necessary. Monitor PT and INR.
Tamoxifen: estrogens may interfere with effectiveness of tamoxifen. Avoid concomitant use.
Drug-food. *Caffeine:* may increase serum caffeine concentrations. Monitor effects.
Drug-lifestyle. *Smoking:* increased risk of CV effects. If smoking continues, may need alternative therapy.

Contraindications and precautions

• Contraindicated in patients with thrombophlebitis or thromboembolic disorders, estrogen-dependent neoplasia, breast or reproductive organ cancer (except for palliative treatment), or undiagnosed abnormal genital bleeding and in pregnant or breast-feeding women. Also contraindicated in patients with history of thrombophlebitis or thromboembolic disorders linked to estrogen use (except for palliative treatment of breast and prostate cancer).
• Use cautiously in patients with cerebrovascular or coronary artery disease, asthma, bone diseases, migraine, seizures, or cardiac, hepatic, or renal dysfunction and in women with strong family history of breast cancer or who have breast nodules, fibrocystic disease, or abnormal mammographic findings.
• Drug should not be used in children.

NURSING CONSIDERATIONS

☜ Assessment
• Obtain history of patient's underlying condition before therapy, and reassess regularly thereafter.

• Ensure that patient has thorough physical examination before initiating estrogen therapy.
• Ask patient about allergies, especially to foods or plants. Estradiol is available as aqueous solution or as solution in peanut oil; estradiol cypionate, as solution in cottonseed oil or vegetable oil; estradiol valerate, as solution in castor oil, sesame oil, or vegetable oil.
• Patient receiving long-term therapy should have repeat examinations yearly. Periodically monitor serum lipid levels, blood pressure, body weight, and liver function, as ordered.
• Evaluate patient's and family's knowledge of drug therapy.

⊕ Nursing diagnoses
• Altered health maintenance related to underlying condition
• Altered tissue perfusion (cerebral, peripheral, pulmonary, or myocardial) related to drug-induced thromboembolism
• Knowledge deficit related to drug therapy

❯ Planning and implementation
P.O. use: Administer oral preparations at mealtimes or bedtime (if only one daily dose is required) to minimize nausea.
I.M. use: To administer as I.M. injection, make sure drug is well dispersed in solution by rolling vial between palms. Inject deep I.M. into large muscle. Rotate injection sites to prevent muscle atrophy. Never give drug I.V.
Intravaginal use: Follow normal protocol.
Transdermal use: Apply transdermal patch to clean, dry, hairless, intact skin on abdomen or buttocks. Do not apply to breasts, waistline, or other areas where clothing can loosen patch. When applying, ensure good contact with skin, especially around edges, and hold in place with palm for about 10 seconds. Rotate application sites.
• Know that in women who are currently taking oral estrogen, treatment with

---

Reactions may be *common*, uncommon, *life-threatening*, or COMMON AND LIFE-THREATENING.

Estraderm transdermal patch can begin 1 week after withdrawal of oral therapy, or sooner if menopausal symptoms appear before end of week.
• Because of risk of thromboembolism, know that therapy should be discontinued at least 1 month before procedures associated with prolonged immobilization or thromboembolism, such as knee or hip surgery. Also withhold drug and notify doctor if thromboembolic event is suspected; be prepared to provide supportive care as indicated.
• Notify pathologist of patient receiving estrogen therapy.

Patient teaching
• Inform patient that package insert that describes estrogen's adverse effects is available; also provide verbal explanation.
• Emphasize importance of regular physical examinations. Studies suggest that postmenopausal women who use estrogen replacement for more than 5 years to treat menopausal symptoms may be at increased risk for endometrial carcinoma. This risk is reduced by using cyclic rather than continuous therapy and lowest possible dosages of estrogen. Adding progestins to regimen decreases incidence of endometrial hyperplasia; it isn't known if progestins affect incidence of endometrial carcinoma. Most studies show no increased risk of breast cancer.
• Teach patient how to use vaginal cream. Patient should wash vaginal area with soap and water before applying. Tell her to apply drug at bedtime or to lie flat for 30 minutes after application to minimize drug loss.
• Warn patient to immediately report abdominal pain; pain, numbness, or stiffness in legs or buttocks; pressure or pain in chest; shortness of breath; severe headaches; visual disturbances, such as blind spots, flashing lights, or blurriness; vaginal bleeding or discharge; breast lumps; swelling of hands or feet; yellow skin or sclera; dark urine; and light-colored stools.

• Explain to patient on cyclic therapy for postmenopausal symptoms that although withdrawal bleeding may occur during week off drug, fertility has not been restored. Pregnancy cannot occur because patient has not ovulated.
• Tell diabetic patient to report elevated blood glucose test results so antidiabetic medication dosage can be adjusted.
• Teach female patient how to perform routine breast self-examination.

☑ **Evaluation**
• Patient exhibits improvement in underlying condition.
• Patient does not experience thromboembolic event during therapy.
• Patient and family state understanding of drug therapy.

estramustine phosphate sodium
(es-truh-MUS-teen FOS-fayt SOE-dee-um)
Emcyt, Estracyt ◊

Pharmacologic class: estrogen, alkylating agent
Therapeutic class: antineoplastic
Pregnancy risk category: NR

How supplied
Capsules: 140 mg

Pharmacokinetics
Absorption: about 75% absorbed in GI tract.
Distribution: distributed widely in body tissues.
Metabolism: extensively metabolized in liver.
Excretion: excreted primarily in feces, with small amount excreted in urine.
Half-life: 20 hours.

Route	Onset	Peak	Duration
P.O.	Unknown	Unknown	Unknown

Pharmacodynamics

Chemical effect: unknown; probably acts by its ability to bind selectively to protein present in human prostate.
Therapeutic effect: hinders prostatic cancer growth.

Indications and dosage

▶ **Palliative treatment of metastatic or progressive prostate cancer.** *Adults:* 10 to 16 mg/kg P.O. in three to four divided doses. Usual dosage is 14 mg/kg daily. Therapy continued for up to 3 months and, if successful, maintained as long as patient responds.

Adverse reactions

CNS: lethargy, insomnia, headache, anxiety.
CV: *MI,* sodium and fluid retention, thrombophlebitis, *heart failure, stroke,* hypertension.
GI: *nausea, vomiting,* diarrhea, anorexia, flatulence, GI bleeding, thirst.
GU: loss of libido.
Hematologic: *leukopenia, thrombocytopenia.*
Respiratory: dyspnea, *pulmonary embolism.*
Skin: rash, pruritus, dry skin, thinning of hair, flushing.
Other: *edema, painful gynecomastia and breast tenderness.*

Interactions

Drug-drug. *Calcium-containing drugs (such as antacids):* impaired absorption of estramustine. Do not administer together.
Drug-food. *Calcium-rich foods (milk, dairy products):* impaired absorption of estramustine. Do not administer together.

Contraindications and precautions

• Contraindicated in patients hypersensitive to estradiol or nitrogen mustard and in those with active thrombophlebitis or thromboembolic disorders, except when actual tumor mass is cause of thromboembolic phenomenon.

• Use cautiously in patients with history of thrombophlebitis or thromboembolic disorders and cerebrovascular or coronary artery disease. Monitor weight regularly in these patients. Estramustine may exaggerate preexisting peripheral edema or heart failure.

NURSING CONSIDERATIONS

☷ Assessment

• Obtain history of patient's neoplastic disease before therapy, and reassess regularly thereafter.
• Monitor blood pressure and glucose tolerance periodically throughout therapy. Also monitor CBC and ECG periodically during therapy.
• Be alert for adverse reactions and drug interactions.
• Evaluate patient's and family's knowledge of drug therapy.

☷ Nursing diagnoses

• Altered health maintenance related to neoplastic disease
• Risk for injury related to drug-induced adverse reactions
• Knowledge deficit related to drug therapy

☷ Planning and implementation

• Administer drug on empty stomach.
• Be aware that patient may continue therapy as long as response is favorable. Some patients have taken drug for more than 3 years.
• Store capsules in refrigerator.
• Be aware that each 140-mg capsule contains 12.5 mg of sodium. Limit patient's sodium intake if not contraindicated to minimize sodium and fluid retention.
Patient teaching
• Tell patient to take drug on empty stomach (2 hours before or 1 hour after meals) and to avoid taking with milk or dairy products.
• Advise patient and partner to use contraception if woman is of childbearing age.

Reactions may be *common,* uncommon, *life-threatening*, or COMMON AND LIFE-THREATENING.

☑ **Evaluation**
• Patient exhibits improvement in health.
• Patient does not experience injury as result of therapy.
• Patient and family state understanding of drug therapy.

---

estrogens, conjugated
(estrogenic substances, conjugated; oestrogens, conjugated)
(ES-troh-jenz, KAHN-jih-gayt-ed)
C.E.S.◆, Premarin, Premarin Intravenous

Pharmacologic class: estrogen
Therapeutic class: estrogen replacement, antineoplastic, antiosteoporotic
Pregnancy risk category: X

How supplied
Tablets: 0.3 mg, 0.625 mg, 0.9 mg, 1.25 mg, 2.5 mg
Injection: 25 mg/5 ml
Vaginal cream: 0.625 mg/g

Pharmacokinetics
Absorption: not well characterized after P.O. or intravaginal administration. After I.M. administration, absorption begins rapidly and continues for days.
Distribution: distributed throughout body with highest concentrations appearing in fat; about 50% to 80% plasma protein–bound.
Metabolism: metabolized primarily in liver.
Excretion: majority of estrogen elimination occurs through kidneys.

Route	Onset	Peak	Duration
All routes	Unknown	Unknown	Unknown

Pharmacodynamics
Chemical effect: increases synthesis of DNA, RNA, and protein in responsive tissues; also reduces release of follicle-stimulating hormone and luteinizing hormone from pituitary gland.
Therapeutic effect: provides estrogen replacement, relieves vasomotor menopausal symptoms and vaginal dryness, helps prevent severity of osteoporosis, and provides palliative action for prostate and breast cancer.

Indications and dosage
▶ **Abnormal uterine bleeding (hormonal imbalance).** *Women:* 25 mg I.V. or I.M. Repeated in 6 to 12 hours, p.r.n.
▶ **Palliative treatment of breast cancer (at least 5 years after menopause).** *Men and postmenopausal women:* 10 mg P.O. t.i.d. for 3 months or more.
▶ **Female castration, primary ovarian failure.** *Women:* 1.25 mg P.O. daily in cycles of 3 weeks on and 1 week off.
▶ **Osteoporosis.** *Postmenopausal women:* 0.625 mg P.O. daily in cyclic regimen (3 weeks on, 1 week off).
▶ **Hypogonadism.** *Women:* 2.5 to 7.5 mg P.O. daily in divided doses for 20 consecutive days each month.
▶ **Vasomotor menopausal symptoms.** *Women:* 0.3 to 1.25 mg P.O. daily in cycles of 3 weeks on and 1 week off.
▶ **Atrophic vaginitis, kraurosis vulvae.** *Women:* 2 to 4 g intravaginally once daily on cyclic basis (3 weeks on and 1 week off).
▶ **Palliative treatment of inoperable prostate cancer.** *Men:* 1.25 to 2.5 mg P.O. t.i.d.

Adverse reactions
CNS: headache, dizziness, chorea, depression, lethargy, *seizures*.
CV: thrombophlebitis; *thromboembolism;* hypertension; edema; *increased risk of CVA, pulmonary embolism, and MI.*
EENT: worsening of myopia or astigmatism, intolerance of contact lenses.
GI: *nausea,* vomiting, abdominal cramps, bloating, diarrhea, constipation, anorexia, increased appetite, weight changes, *pancreatitis.*

GU: breakthrough bleeding, altered menstrual flow, dysmenorrhea, amenorrhea, *increased risk of endometrial cancer, possibility of increased risk of breast cancer,* cervical erosion, altered cervical secretions, enlargement of uterine fibromas, vaginal candidiasis (in women); gynecomastia, testicular atrophy, impotence (in men).

Hepatic: gallbladder disease, cholestatic jaundice, *hepatic adenoma.*

Metabolic: hyperglycemia, hypercalcemia.

Skin: melasma, urticaria, erythema nodosum, dermatitis, flushing (with rapid I.V. administration), hirsutism, hair loss.

Other: breast changes (tenderness, enlargement, secretion).

Interactions

Drug-drug. *Bromocriptine:* may cause amenorrhea, interfering with bromocriptine's effects. Avoid concomitant use.
Carbamazepine, phenobarbital, rifampin: decreased estrogen effectiveness. Monitor patient closely.
Corticosteroids: possibly enhanced effects. Monitor patient closely.
Cyclosporine: increased risk of toxicity. Use together with caution and frequently monitor cyclosporine levels.
Dantrolene, other hepatotoxic drugs: increased risk of hepatotoxicity. Monitor patient closely.
Oral anticoagulants: dosage adjustments may be necessary. Monitor PT and INR.
Tamoxifen: estrogens may interfere with effectiveness of tamoxifen. Avoid concomitant use.

Drug-food. *Caffeine:* may increase serum caffeine concentrations. Monitor effects.

Drug-lifestyle. *Smoking:* increased risk of CV effects. If smoking continues, patient may need an alternative therapy.

Contraindications and precautions

• Contraindicated in patients with thrombophlebitis or thromboembolic disorders, estrogen-dependent neoplasia, breast or reproductive organ cancer (except for palliative treatment), or undiagnosed abnormal genital bleeding and in pregnant or breast-feeding women.

• Use cautiously in patients with cerebrovascular or coronary artery disease, asthma, bone disease, migraine, seizures, or cardiac, hepatic, or renal dysfunction and in women with family history (mother, grandmother, sister) of breast or genital tract cancer or who have breast nodules, fibrocystic disease, or abnormal mammographic findings.

• Drug should not be used in children.

NURSING CONSIDERATIONS

Assessment

• Obtain history of patient's underlying condition before therapy, and reassess regularly thereafter.

• Ensure that patient has thorough physical examination before initiating estrogen therapy.

• Patient receiving long-term therapy should have repeat examinations yearly. Periodically monitor serum lipid levels, blood pressure, body weight, and liver function, as ordered.

• Be alert for adverse reactions and drug interactions.

• Evaluate patient's and family's knowledge of drug therapy.

Nursing diagnoses

• Altered health maintenance related to underlying condition

• Altered tissue perfusion (cerebral, peripheral, pulmonary, or myocardial) related to drug-induced thromboembolism

• Knowledge deficit related to drug therapy

Planning and implementation

• Know that I.M. or I.V. use is preferred for rapid treatment of dysfunctional uterine bleeding or reduction of surgical bleeding.

• Refrigerate before reconstituting. Agitate gently after adding diluent.

P.O. use: Administer oral preparations at mealtimes or h.s. (if only one daily dose is required) to minimize nausea.

I.V. use: When giving by direct I.V. injection, administer slowly to avoid flushing reaction. Reconstitute powder for injection with diluent provided (sterile water for injection with benzyl alcohol). To facilitate introduction of diluent, withdraw 5 ml of air from vial before adding diluent. Gently agitate to mix drug. Avoid shaking container. Avoid mixing with solutions of acidic pH to prevent incompatibility.

I.M. use: When administering by I.M. injection, inject deeply into large muscle. Rotate injection sites to prevent muscle atrophy.

Intravaginal use: Follow normal protocol.

• Because of risk of thromboembolism, know that therapy should be discontinued at least 1 month before procedures associated with prolonged immobilization or thromboembolism, such as knee or hip surgery.

• Withhold drug and notify doctor if thromboembolic event is suspected; be prepared to provide supportive care as indicated.

• Notify pathologist of patient receiving estrogen therapy.

Patient teaching

• Inform patient that package insert that describes estrogen's adverse effects is available; also provide verbal explanation.

• Emphasize importance of regular physical examinations. Studies suggest that postmenopausal women who use estrogen replacement for more than 5 years to treat menopausal symptoms may be at increased risk for endometrial carcinoma. This risk is reduced by using cyclic rather than continuous therapy and lowest possible dosages of estrogen. Adding progestins to regimen decreases incidence of endometrial hyperplasia; it isn't known if progestins affect incidence of endometrial carcinoma. Most studies show no increased risk of breast cancer.

• Teach patient how to use vaginal cream. Patient should wash vaginal area with soap and water before applying. Tell her to apply drug at bedtime or to lie flat for 30 minutes after application to minimize drug loss.

• Explain to patient on cyclic therapy for postmenopausal symptoms that although withdrawal bleeding may occur during week off drug, fertility has not been restored. Pregnancy cannot occur because she has not ovulated.

• Warn patient to immediately report abdominal pain; pain, numbness, or stiffness in legs or buttocks; pressure or pain in chest; shortness of breath; severe headaches; visual disturbances, such as blind spots, flashing lights, or blurriness; vaginal bleeding or discharge; breast lumps; swelling of hands or feet; yellow skin or sclera; dark urine; and light-colored stools.

• Tell diabetic patient to report elevated blood glucose test results so antidiabetic medication dosage can be adjusted.

• Teach female patient how to perform routine breast self-examination.

☑ **Evaluation**

• Patient exhibits improvement in underlying condition.

• Patient does not experience thromboembolic event during therapy.

• Patient and family state understanding of drug therapy.

---

estrogens, esterified
(ES-troh-jenz, ES-ter-eh-fighd)
Estratab, Menest, Neo-Estrone♦

Pharmacologic class: estrogen
Therapeutic class: antineoplastic
Pregnancy risk category: X

How supplied

Tablets: 0.3 mg, 0.625 mg, 1.25 mg, 2.5 mg
Tablets (film-coated): 0.3 mg, 0.625 mg, 1.25 mg, 2.5 mg

Pharmacokinetics

Absorption: well absorbed but substantially inactivated by liver.
Distribution: distributed throughout body with highest concentrations appearing in fat; about 50% to 80% plasma protein–bound.
Metabolism: metabolized primarily in liver.
Excretion: excreted primarily by kidneys.

Route	Onset	Peak	Duration
P.O.	Unknown	Unknown	Unknown

Pharmacodynamics

Chemical effect: increases synthesis of DNA, RNA, and protein in responsive tissues; also reduces release of follicle-stimulating hormone and luteinizing hormone from pituitary gland.
Therapeutic effect: provides estrogen replacement, hinders prostate and breast cancer cell growth, and relieves vasomotor menopausal symptoms and vaginal dryness.

Indications and dosage

▶ **Inoperable prostate cancer.** *Men:* 1.25 to 2.5 mg P.O. t.i.d.
▶ **Breast cancer.** *Men and postmenopausal women:* 10 mg P.O. t.i.d. for 3 or more months.
▶ **Female hypogonadism.** *Women:* 2.5 to 7.5 mg P.O. daily in divided doses in cycles of 20 days on, 10 days off.
▶ **Castration, primary ovarian failure.** *Women:* 2.5 mg P.O. daily to t.i.d. in cycles of 3 weeks on, 1 week off.
▶ **Vasomotor menopausal symptoms.** *Women:* average dosage is 1.25 mg P.O. daily in cycles of 3 weeks on, 1 week off.
▶ **Atrophic vaginitis or urethritis.** *Women:* 0.3 to 1.25 mg P.O. daily in cycles of 3 weeks on, 1 week off.

Adverse reactions

CNS: headache, dizziness, chorea, depression, lethargy, *seizures.*
CV: thrombophlebitis; *thromboembolism;* hypertension; edema; *increased risk of CVA, pulmonary embolism, and MI.*
EENT: worsening of myopia or astigmatism, intolerance of contact lenses.
GI: *nausea,* vomiting, abdominal cramps, bloating, diarrhea, constipation, anorexia, increased appetite, weight changes, *pancreatitis.*
GU: breakthrough bleeding, altered menstrual flow, dysmenorrhea, amenorrhea, *increased risk of endometrial cancer, possibility of increased risk of breast cancer,* cervical erosion, altered cervical secretions, enlargement of uterine fibromas, vaginal candidiasis (in women); gynecomastia, testicular atrophy, impotence (in men).
Hepatic: cholestatic jaundice, *hepatic adenoma.*
Skin: melasma, rash, erythema nodosum, dermatitis, hirsutism, hair loss.
Other: breast changes (tenderness, enlargement, secretion), hypercalcemia, gallbladder disease.

Interactions

Drug-drug. *Bromocriptine:* may cause amenorrhea, interfering with bromocriptine's effects. Avoid concomitant use.
Carbamazepine, phenobarbital, rifampin: decreased effectiveness of estrogen therapy. Monitor patient closely.
Corticosteroids: possibly enhanced effects. Monitor patient closely.
Cyclosporine: increased risk of toxicity. Use together with caution and frequently monitor cyclosporine levels.
Dantrolene, other hepatotoxic drugs: increased risk of hepatotoxicity. Monitor patient closely.
Oral anticoagulants: dosage adjustments may be necessary. Monitor PT and INR.
Tamoxifen: estrogens may interfere with effectiveness of tamoxifen. Avoid concomitant use.
Drug-food. *Caffeine:* may increase serum caffeine concentrations. Monitor effects.
Drug-lifestyle. *Smoking:* increased risk of CV effects. If smoking continues, patient may need an alternative therapy.

Reactions may be *common,* uncommon, *life-threatening,* or COMMON AND LIFE-THREATENING.

Contraindications and precautions

• Contraindicated in patients with breast cancer (except metastatic disease), estrogen-dependent neoplasia, active thrombophlebitis or thromboembolic disorders, undiagnosed abnormal genital bleeding, hypersensitivity to drug, or history of thromboembolic disease and in pregnant or breast-feeding women.

• Use cautiously in patients with history of hypertension, depression, cardiac or renal dysfunction, liver impairment, bone diseases, migraine, seizures, or diabetes mellitus.

• Drug should not be used in children.

NURSING CONSIDERATIONS

Assessment

• Obtain history of patient's underlying condition before therapy, and reassess regularly thereafter.

• Ensure that patient has thorough physical examination before initiating esterified estrogens therapy.

• Patient receiving long-term therapy should have repeat examinations yearly. Periodically monitor serum lipid levels, blood pressure, body weight, and liver function, as ordered.

• Be alert for adverse reactions and drug interactions.

• Evaluate patient's and family's knowledge of drug therapy.

Nursing diagnoses

• Altered health maintenance related to underlying condition

• Altered tissue perfusion (cerebral, peripheral, pulmonary, or myocardial) related to drug-induced thromboembolism

• Knowledge deficit related to drug therapy

Planning and implementation

• Administer oral preparations at mealtimes or bedtime (if only one daily dose is required) to minimize nausea.

• Because of risk of thromboembolism, know that therapy should be discontinued at least 1 month before procedures associated with prolonged immobilization or thromboembolism, such as knee or hip surgery.

• Withhold drug and notify doctor if thromboembolic event is suspected; be prepared to provide supportive care as indicated.

• Notify pathologist of patient receiving estrogen therapy.

Patient teaching

• Inform patient that package insert that describes estrogen's adverse effects is available; also provide verbal explanation.

• Emphasize importance of regular physical examinations. Studies suggest that postmenopausal women who use estrogen replacement for more than 5 years to treat menopausal symptoms may be at increased risk for endometrial carcinoma. This risk is reduced by using cyclic rather than continuous therapy and lowest possible dosages of estrogen. Adding progestins to regimen decreases incidence of endometrial hyperplasia; it isn't known if progestins affect incidence of endometrial carcinoma. Most studies show no increased risk of breast cancer.

• Explain to patient on cyclic therapy for postmenopausal symptoms that although withdrawal bleeding may occur during week off drug, fertility has not been restored. Pregnancy cannot occur because she has not ovulated.

• Warn patient to immediately report abdominal pain; pain, numbness, or stiffness in legs or buttocks; pressure or pain in chest; shortness of breath; severe headaches; visual disturbances, such as blind spots, flashing lights, or blurriness; vaginal bleeding or discharge; breast lumps; swelling of hands or feet; yellow skin or sclera; dark urine; and light-colored stools.

• Tell diabetic patient to report elevated blood glucose test results so antidiabetic medication dosage can be adjusted.

• Teach female patient how to perform routine breast self-examination.

☑ **Evaluation**
• Patient exhibits improvement in underlying condition.
• Patient does not experience thromboembolic event during therapy.
• Patient and family state understanding of drug therapy.

---

estrone (oestrone)
(ES-trohn)
Estro-A, Estrone 5, Gynogen, Kestrone-5

Pharmacologic class: estrogen
Therapeutic class: estrogen replacement
Pregnancy risk category: X

How supplied
Injection (aqueous suspension):
5 mg/ml

Pharmacokinetics
Absorption: after I.M. administration, absorption begins rapidly and continues for days.
Distribution: distributed throughout body with highest concentrations appearing in fat; about 50% to 80% plasma protein–bound.
Metabolism: metabolized primarily in liver.
Excretion: majority of estrogen elimination occurs through kidneys.

Route	Onset	Peak	Duration
I.M.	Unknown	Unknown	Unknown

Pharmacodynamics
Chemical effect: increases synthesis of DNA, RNA, and protein in responsive tissues; also reduces release of follicle-stimulating hormone and luteinizing hormone from pituitary.
Therapeutic effect: provides estrogen replacement, relieves vasomotor menopausal symptoms and vaginal dryness, and provides palliative action for prostate cancer.

Indications and dosage
▶ **Atrophic vaginitis, kraurosis vulvae, vasomotor menopausal symptoms.** *Women:* 0.1 to 0.5 mg I.M. two or three times weekly.
▶ **Female hypogonadism or castration, primary ovarian failure.** *Women:* 0.1 to 1.0 mg I.M. weekly as single dose or in divided doses.
▶ **Palliative treatment of inoperable prostate cancer.** *Men:* 2 to 4 mg I.M. two or three times weekly.

Adverse reactions
CNS: headache, dizziness, chorea, depression, lethargy, *seizures.*
CV: thrombophlebitis *thromboembolism;* hypertension; edema; *increased risk of CVA, pulmonary embolism, and MI.*
EENT: worsening of myopia or astigmatism, intolerance of contact lenses.
GI: *nausea,* vomiting, abdominal cramps, bloating, diarrhea, constipation, anorexia, increased appetite, weight changes, *pancreatitis.*
GU: breakthrough bleeding, altered menstrual flow, dysmenorrhea, amenorrhea, *increased risk of endometrial cancer, possibility of increased risk of breast cancer,* cervical erosion, altered cervical secretions, enlargement of uterine fibromas, vaginal candidiasis (in women); gynecomastia, testicular atrophy, impotence (in men).
Hepatic: cholestatic jaundice, *hepatic adenoma.*
Skin: melasma, rash, erythema nodosum, dermatitis, hirsutism, hair loss.
Other: breast changes (tenderness, enlargement, secretion), hypercalcemia, gallbladder disease.

Interactions
Drug-drug. *Bromocriptine:* may cause amenorrhea, interfering with bromocriptine's effects. Avoid concomitant use.
Carbamazepine, phenobarbital, rifampin: decreased effectiveness of estrogen therapy. Monitor patient closely.

Reactions may be *common*, uncommon, *life-threatening*, or COMMON AND LIFE-THREATENING.

Corticosteroids: possibly enhanced effects. Monitor patient closely.
Cyclosporine: increased risk of toxicity. Use together with caution and frequently monitor cyclosporine levels.
Dantrolene, other hepatotoxic drugs: increased risk of hepatotoxicity. Monitor patient closely.
Oral anticoagulants: dosage adjustments may be necessary. Monitor PT and INR.
Tamoxifen: estrogens may interfere with effectiveness of tamoxifen. Avoid concomitant use.
Drug-food. *Caffeine:* may increase serum caffeine concentrations. Monitor effects.
Drug-lifestyle. *Smoking:* increased risk of CV effects. If smoking continues, may need an alternate therapy.

Contraindications and precautions

• Contraindicated in patients with thrombophlebitis or thromboembolic disorders, estrogen-dependent neoplasia, breast or reproductive organ cancer (except for palliative treatment), or undiagnosed abnormal genital bleeding and in pregnant or breast-feeding women.
• Use cautiously in patients with cerebrovascular or coronary artery disease, asthma, bone diseases, depression, migraine, seizures, or cardiac, hepatic, or renal dysfunction and in women with family history (mother, grandmother, sister) of breast or genital tract cancer or who have breast nodules, fibrocystic disease, or abnormal mammographic findings.
• Drug should not be used in children.

NURSING CONSIDERATIONS

Assessment
• Obtain history of patient's underlying condition before therapy, and reassess regularly thereafter.
• Ensure that patient has thorough physical examination before initiating estrone therapy.
• Patient receiving long-term therapy should have repeat examinations yearly. Periodically monitor serum lipid levels,

blood pressure, body weight, and liver function, as ordered.
• Be alert for adverse reactions and drug interactions.
• Evaluate patient's and family's knowledge of drug therapy.

Nursing diagnoses
• Altered health maintenance related to underlying condition
• Altered tissue perfusion (cerebral, peripheral, pulmonary, or myocardial) related to drug-induced thromboembolism
• Knowledge deficit related to drug therapy

Planning and implementation
• Administer estrone I.M. Rotate injection sites to prevent muscle atrophy.
• Because of risk of thromboembolism, know that therapy should be discontinued at least 1 month before procedures associated with prolonged immobilization or thromboembolism, such as knee or hip surgery.
• Withhold drug and notify doctor if thromboembolic event is suspected; be prepared to provide supportive care as indicated.
• Notify pathologist of patient receiving estrone therapy.
Patient teaching
• Inform patient that package insert that describes estrone's adverse effects is available; also provide verbal explanation.
• Emphasize importance of regular physical examinations. Studies suggest that postmenopausal women who use estrone replacement for more than 5 years to treat menopausal symptoms may be at increased risk for endometrial carcinoma. This risk is reduced by using cyclic rather than continuous therapy and lowest possible dosages of estrogen. Adding progestins to regimen decreases incidence of endometrial hyperplasia; it isn't known if progestins affect incidence of endometrial carcinoma. Most studies show no increased risk of breast cancer.

• Explain to patient on cyclic therapy for postmenopausal symptoms that although withdrawal bleeding may occur during week off drug, fertility has not been restored. Pregnancy cannot occur because she has not ovulated.

• Warn patient to immediately report abdominal pain; pain, numbness, or stiffness in legs or buttocks; pressure or pain in chest; shortness of breath; severe headaches; visual disturbances, such as blind spots, flashing lights, or blurriness; vaginal bleeding or discharge; breast lumps; swelling of hands or feet; yellow skin or sclera; dark urine; and light-colored stools.

• Tell diabetic patient to report elevated blood glucose test results so antidiabetic medication dosage can be adjusted.

• Teach female patient how to perform routine breast self-examination.

☑ **Evaluation**
• Patient exhibits improvement in underlying condition.
• Patient does not experience thromboembolic event during therapy.
• Patient and family state understanding of drug therapy.

estropipate (piperazine estrone sulfate)
(ES-troh-pih-payt)
Ogen, Ortho-Est

Pharmacologic class: estrogen
Therapeutic class: estrogen replacement
Pregnancy risk category: X

How supplied
Tablets: 0.75 mg, 1.5 mg, 3 mg, 6 mg
Vaginal cream: 1.5 mg/g

Pharmacokinetics
Absorption: not well characterized after P.O. or intravaginal administration.
Distribution: distributed throughout body with highest concentrations appearing in

fat; about 50% to 80% plasma protein–bound.
Metabolism: metabolized primarily in liver.
Excretion: eliminated primarily by kidneys.

Route	Onset	Peak	Duration
P.O., intravaginal	Unknown	Unknown	Unknown

Pharmacodynamics
Chemical effect: increases synthesis of DNA, RNA, and protein in responsive tissues. Also reduces release of follicle-stimulating hormone and luteinizing hormone from pituitary gland.
Therapeutic effect: provides estrogen replacement, relieves vasomotor menopausal symptoms, and helps reduce severity of osteoporosis.

Indications and dosage
▶ **Vulval and vaginal atrophy.** *Women:* 0.625 to 5.0 mg P.O. daily 3 weeks on, 1 week off, or 2 to 4 g of vaginal cream daily. Typically, dosage given on cyclic, short-term basis.
▶ **Primary ovarian failure, female castration, female hypogonadism.** *Women:* administered on cyclic basis—1.25 to 7.5 mg P.O. daily for first 3 weeks, followed by rest period of 8 to 10 days. If bleeding does not occur by end of rest period, cycle repeated.
▶ **Vasomotor menopausal symptoms.** *Women:* 0.625 to 5.0 mg P.O. daily in cyclic method of 3 weeks on, 1 week off.
▶ **Prevention of osteoporosis.** *Women:* 0.625 mg P.O. daily for 25 days of 31-day cycle.

Adverse reactions
CNS: depression, headache, dizziness, migraine, *seizures.*
CV: edema; thrombophlebitis; *increased risk of CVA, pulmonary embolism, thromboembolism, and MI.*
GI: nausea, vomiting, abdominal cramps, bloating, weight changes.

Reactions may be *common,* uncommon, *life-threatening,* or COMMON AND LIFE-THREATENING.

GU: increased size of uterine fibromas, *increased risk of endometrial cancer, possibility of increased risk of breast cancer,* vaginal candidiasis, cystitis-like syndrome, dysmenorrhea, amenorrhea, breakthrough bleeding, condition resembling premenstrual syndrome.
Hepatic: cholestatic jaundice.
Skin: hemorrhagic eruption, erythema nodosum, *erythema multiforme,* hirsutism, melasma, hair loss.
Other: breast engorgement or enlargement, hypercalcemia, aggravation of porphyria, libido changes.

Interactions

Drug-drug. *Bromocriptine:* may cause amenorrhea, interfering with bromocriptine's effects. Avoid concomitant use.
Carbamazepine, phenobarbital, rifampin: decreased effectiveness of estrogen therapy. Monitor patient closely.
Corticosteroids: possibly enhanced effects. Monitor patient closely.
Cyclosporine: increased risk of toxicity. Use together with caution and frequently monitor cyclosporine levels.
Dantrolene, other hepatotoxic drugs: increased risk of hepatotoxicity. Monitor patient closely.
Oral anticoagulants: dosage adjustments may be necessary. Monitor PT and INR.
Tamoxifen: estrogens may interfere with effectiveness of tamoxifen. Avoid concomitant use.
Drug-food. *Caffeine:* may increase serum caffeine concentrations. Monitor effects.
Drug-lifestyle. *Smoking:* increased risk of CV effects. If smoking continues, may need an alternate therapy.

Contraindications and precautions

• Contraindicated in patients with active thrombophlebitis or thromboembolic disorders, estrogen-dependent neoplasia, undiagnosed genital bleeding, or breast, reproductive organ, or genital cancer and in pregnant or breast-feeding women.

• Use cautiously in patients with cerebrovascular or coronary artery disease, asthma, depression, bone disease, migraine, seizures, or cardiac, hepatic, or renal dysfunction and in women with family history (mother, grandmother, sister) of breast or genital tract cancer or who have breast nodules, fibrocystic disease, or abnormal mammographic findings.
• Drug should not be used in children.

NURSING CONSIDERATIONS

✍ Assessment
• Obtain history of patient's underlying condition before therapy, and reassess regularly thereafter.
• Ensure that patient has thorough physical examination before initiating estropipate therapy.
• Patient receiving long-term therapy should have repeat examinations yearly. Periodically monitor serum lipid levels, blood pressure, body weight, and liver function, as ordered.
• Be alert for adverse reactions and drug interactions.
• Evaluate patient's and family's knowledge of drug therapy.

🔷 Nursing diagnoses
• Altered health maintenance related to underlying condition
• Altered tissue perfusion (cerebral, peripheral, pulmonary, or myocardial) related to drug-induced thromboembolism
• Knowledge deficit related to drug therapy

❯ Planning and implementation
P.O. use: Administer oral preparations with meals or at bedtime (if only one daily dose is required) to minimize nausea.
Intravaginal use: Follow normal protocol.
• Because of risk of thromboembolism, know that therapy should be discontinued at least 1 month before procedures associated with prolonged immobilization or

thromboembolism, such as knee or hip surgery.
• Withhold drug and notify doctor if thromboembolic event is suspected; be prepared to provide supportive care as indicated.
• Notify pathologist about patient receiving this drug.

Patient teaching
• Inform patient that package insert that describes estrogen's adverse effects is available; also provide verbal explanation.
• Emphasize importance of regular physical examinations. Studies suggest that postmenopausal women who use estrogen replacement for more than 5 years to treat menopausal symptoms may be at increased risk for endometrial carcinoma. This risk is reduced by using cyclic rather than continuous therapy and lowest possible dosages of estrogen. Adding progestins to regimen decreases incidence of endometrial hyperplasia; it isn't known if progestins affect incidence of endometrial carcinoma. Most studies show no increased risk of breast cancer.
• Teach patient how to use vaginal cream. Patient should wash vaginal area with soap and water before applying. Tell her to use drug at bedtime or to lie flat for 30 minutes after application to minimize drug loss.
• Explain to patient on cyclic therapy for postmenopausal symptoms that although withdrawal bleeding may occur during week off drug, fertility has not been restored. Pregnancy cannot occur because she has not ovulated.
• Explain to patient being treated for hypogonadism that duration of therapy necessary to produce withdrawal bleeding depends on patient's endometrial response to drug. If satisfactory withdrawal bleeding does not occur, oral progestin is added to regimen. Explain to patient that despite return of withdrawal bleeding, pregnancy cannot occur because she is not ovulating.
• Warn patient to immediately report abdominal pain; pain, numbness, or stiffness in legs or buttocks; pressure or pain in

chest; shortness of breath; severe headaches; visual disturbances, such as blind spots, flashing lights, or blurriness; vaginal bleeding or discharge; breast lumps; swelling of hands or feet; yellow skin or sclera; dark urine; and light-colored stools.
• Tell diabetic patient to report elevated blood glucose test results so antidiabetic medication dosage can be adjusted.
• Teach female patient how to perform routine breast self-examination.

☑ Evaluation
• Patient exhibits improvement in underlying condition.
• Patient does not experience thromboembolic event during therapy.
• Patient and family state understanding of drug therapy.

ethacrynate sodium
(eth-uh-KRIH-nayt SOH-dee-um)
Sodium Edecrin

ethacrynic acid
Edecril◊, Edecrin

Pharmacologic class: loop diuretic
Therapeutic class: diuretic
Pregnancy risk category: B

How supplied
Tablets: 25 mg, 50 mg
Injection: 50 mg (with 62.5 mg of mannitol and 0.1 mg of thimerosal)

Pharmacokinetics
Absorption: ethacrynic acid is absorbed rapidly from GI tract. Ethacrynate sodium is administered I.V. and does not require absorption.
Distribution: unknown.
Metabolism: unknown.
Excretion: unknown.

Route	Onset	Peak	Duration
P.O.	30 min	2 hr	6-8 hr
I.V.	5 min	15-30 min	2 hr

Reactions may be *common*, uncommon, *life-threatening*, or COMMON AND LIFE-THREATENING.

Pharmacodynamics

Chemical effect: inhibits sodium and chloride reabsorption at renal tubules and ascending loop of Henle.
Therapeutic effect: promotes sodium and water excretion.

Indications and dosage

▶ **Acute pulmonary edema.** *Adults:* 50 mg or 0.5 to 1 mg/kg I.V. to maximum dose of 100 mg. Usually only one dose is needed; occasionally, second dose may be required.
▶ **Edema.** *Adults:* 50 to 200 mg P.O. daily. Refractory cases may require up to 200 mg b.i.d. *Children:* initial dose is 25 mg P.O., increased cautiously in 25-mg increments daily until desired effect is achieved.

Adverse reactions

CNS: confusion, fatigue, vertigo, headache, nervousness.
CV: volume depletion and dehydration, orthostatic hypotension.
EENT: transient deafness (with too-rapid I.V. injection), blurred vision, tinnitus, hearing loss.
GI: cramping, diarrhea, anorexia, nausea, vomiting, *GI bleeding, pancreatitis.*
GU: nocturia, polyuria, frequent urination, oliguria, hematuria.
Hematologic: *agranulocytosis,* neutropenia, *thrombocytopenia,* azotemia.
Skin: dermatitis.
Other: hypokalemia; hypochloremic alkalosis; asymptomatic hyperuricemia; rash; fever, chills; malaise; fluid and electrolyte imbalances, including dilutional hyponatremia, hypocalcemia, hypomagnesemia; hyperglycemia and impairment of glucose tolerance.

Interactions

Drug-drug. *Aminoglycoside antibiotics:* potentiated ototoxic adverse reactions of both drugs. Use together cautiously.
Antihypertensives: increased risk of hypotension. Use together cautiously.

Cardiac glycosides: increased risk of digoxin toxicity from ethacrynate-induced hypokalemia. Monitor potassium and digoxin levels.
Cisplatin: increased risk of ototoxicity. Avoid concomitant use.
Lithium: decreased lithium clearance, increasing risk of lithium toxicity. Monitor lithium level.
Metolazone: profound diuresis and enhanced electrolyte loss. Use together cautiously.
NSAIDs: decreased diuretic effectiveness. Use together cautiously.
Warfarin: potentiated anticoagulant effect. Use together cautiously.

Contraindications and precautions

● Contraindicated in patients with hypersensitivity to drug, in those with anuria, and in infants.
● Ethacrynic acid is not recommended for use in breast-feeding women.
● Use cautiously in patients with electrolyte abnormalities or hepatic impairment. Also use cautiously in pregnant women.

NURSING CONSIDERATIONS

⁂ Assessment
● Obtain history of patient's underlying condition before therapy.
● Monitor effectiveness by regularly checking urine output, weight, peripheral edema, and breath sounds.
● Monitor fluid intake, blood pressure, and serum electrolyte levels.
● Monitor blood uric acid levels, especially in patients with history of gout.
● Be alert for adverse reactions and drug interactions.
● Evaluate patient's and family's knowledge of drug therapy.

⊞ Nursing diagnoses
● Fluid volume excess related to underlying condition
● Altered urinary elimination related to diuretic therapy

• Knowledge deficit related to drug therapy

⊠ **Planning and implementation**
P.O. use: Give drug with food or milk.
P.O. use may cause GI upset.
– To prevent nocturia, give P.O. doses in morning.
I.V. use: Reconstitute vacuum vial with 50 ml of D_5W or 0.9% NaCl solution. Give slowly through I.V. line of running infusion over several minutes. Discard unused solution after 24 hours. Don't use cloudy or opalescent solutions.
– If more than one I.V. dose is necessary, use new injection site to avoid thrombophlebitis.
– Don't mix with whole blood or its derivatives.
• Don't give S.C. or I.M. because of local pain and irritation.
• Know that potassium chloride and sodium supplements may be needed.
• Notify doctor if diarrhea occurs because severe diarrhea may necessitate discontinuing drug.
Patient teaching
• Advise patient to avoid sudden posture changes and to rise slowly to avoid orthostatic hypotension.
• Advise diabetic patient to closely monitor blood glucose levels.
• Teach patient and family to identify and report signs of hypersensitivity or fluid and electrolyte disturbances.
• Teach patient to monitor fluid volume by daily weight and intake and output.
• Tell patient to take oral drug early in day to avoid interruption of sleep by nocturia.

☑ **Evaluation**
• Patient is free from edema.
• Patient demonstrates adjustment of lifestyle to deal with altered patterns of urinary elimination.
• Patient and family state understanding of drug therapy.

ethambutol hydrochloride
(ee-THAM-byoo-tol
high-droh-KLOR-ighd)
Etibi♦, Myambutol

Pharmacologic class: semisynthetic antitubercular
Therapeutic class: antitubercular agent
Pregnancy risk category: NR

How supplied
Tablets: 100 mg, 400 mg

Pharmacokinetics
Absorption: absorbed rapidly from GI tract.
Distribution: distributed widely in body tissues and fluids; 8% to 22% protein-bound.
Metabolism: undergoes partial hepatic metabolism.
Excretion: after 24 hours, about 50% of unchanged drug and 8% to 15% of its metabolites are excreted in urine; 20% to 25% is excreted in feces. *Half-life:* about 3½ hours.

Route	Onset	Peak	Duration
P.O.	Unknown	2-4 hr	Unknown

Pharmacodynamics
Chemical effect: unknown; appears to interfere with synthesis of one or more metabolites of susceptible bacteria, altering cellular metabolism during cell division (bacteriostatic).
Therapeutic effect: hinders bacterial growth. Spectrum of activity includes *Mycobacterium bovis, Mycobacterium marinum, Mycobacterium tuberculosis,* and some strains of *Mycobacterium avium, Mycobacterium fortuitum, Mycobacterium intracellulare,* and *Mycobacterium kansasii.*

Indications and dosage
▶ **Adjunct treatment in pulmonary tuberculosis.** *Adults and children over age 13:* for patients who have not received

previous antitubercular therapy, 15 mg/kg P.O. daily in single dose. *Retreatment:* 25 mg/kg P.O. daily as single dose for 60 days with at least one other antitubercular drug; then decreased to 15 mg/kg/day as single dose.

Adverse reactions

CNS: headache, dizziness, confusion, possibly hallucinations, peripheral neuritis (numbness and tingling of extremities).
EENT: optic neuritis (related to dose—vision loss and loss of color discrimination, especially red and green).
GI: anorexia, nausea, vomiting, abdominal pain.
Hematologic: *thrombocytopenia.*
Skin: dermatitis, pruritus, *toxic epidermal necrolysis.*
Other: *anaphylactoid reactions,* fever, malaise, bloody sputum, elevated uric acid level, precipitation of gout, abnormal liver function tests.

Interactions

Drug-drug. *Aluminum salts:* may delay and reduce absorption of ethambutol. Separate administrations by several hours.

Contraindications and precautions

• Contraindicated in patients with optic neuritis or hypersensitivity to drug and in children under age 13.
• Use cautiously in patients with impaired kidney function, cataracts, recurrent eye inflammations, gout, and diabetic retinopathy. Also use cautiously in pregnant or breast-feeding women.

NURSING CONSIDERATIONS

🔍 Assessment
• Obtain history of patient's infection before therapy.
• Perform visual acuity and color discrimination tests and obtain AST and ALT levels, as ordered, before therapy.

• Monitor effectiveness by regularly assessing for improvement in patient's condition and evaluating culture and sensitivity test results.
• Monitor AST and ALT levels every 2 to 4 weeks, as ordered, and perform visual acuity and color discrimination tests during treatment.
• Monitor serum uric acid level, as ordered; observe patient for symptoms of gout.
• Be alert for adverse reactions and drug interactions.
• Evaluate patient's and family's knowledge of drug therapy.

🔧 Nursing diagnoses
• Infection related to presence of susceptible bacteria
• Sensory or perceptual alterations (visual) related to drug-induced adverse reactions
• Knowledge deficit related to drug therapy

▶ Planning and implementation
• Anticipate dosage reduction in patient with impaired kidney function.
• Know that ethambutol should always be administered with other antitubercular agents to prevent development of resistant organisms.
Patient teaching
• Reassure patient that visual disturbances will disappear several weeks to months after drug is stopped. Caution patient not to perform hazardous activities if visual disturbances or adverse CNS reactions occur.
• Emphasize need for regular follow-up care.

☑ Evaluation
• Patient is free from infection.
• Patient regains pretreatment visual ability after therapy has stopped.
• Patient and family state understanding of drug therapy.

ethinyl estradiol
(ethinyloestradiol)
(ETH-uh-nil es-truh-DIGH-ol)
Estinyl**

Pharmacologic class: estrogen
Therapeutic class: estrogen replacement, antineoplastic
Pregnancy risk category: X

How supplied

Tablets: 0.02 mg, 0.05 mg, 0.5 mg

Pharmacokinetics

Absorption: well absorbed but substantially inactivated by liver.
Distribution: distributed throughout body with highest concentrations appearing in fat; about 50% to 80% plasma protein–bound.
Metabolism: metabolized primarily in liver.
Excretion: excreted primarily by kidneys.

Route	Onset	Peak	Duration
P.O.	Unknown	Unknown	Unknown

Pharmacodynamics

Chemical effect: increases synthesis of DNA, RNA, and protein in responsive tissues; also reduces release of follicle-stimulating hormone and luteinizing hormone from pituitary gland.
Therapeutic effect: replaces estrogen, hinders prostate and breast cancer cell growth, and relieves vasomotor menopausal symptoms.

Indications and dosage

▶ **Palliative treatment of metastatic breast cancer (at least 5 years after menopause).** *Women:* 1 mg P.O. t.i.d. for at least 3 months.
▶ **Female hypogonadism.** *Women:* 0.05 mg P.O. once daily to t.i.d. 2 weeks a month, followed by 2 weeks of progesterone therapy; continued for three to six monthly dosing cycles, followed by 2 months off.
▶ **Vasomotor menopausal symptoms.** *Women:* 0.02 to 0.05 mg P.O. daily for cycles of 3 weeks on and 1 week off.
▶ **Palliative treatment of metastatic inoperable prostate cancer.** *Men:* 0.15 to 2 mg P.O. daily.

Adverse reactions

CNS: headache, dizziness, chorea, depression, lethargy, *seizures.*
CV: thrombophlebitis, *thromboembolism,* hypertension, edema, *increased risk of CVA, pulmonary embolism, MI.*
EENT: worsening of myopia or astigmatism, intolerance to contact lenses.
GI: *nausea,* vomiting, abdominal cramps, bloating, diarrhea, constipation, anorexia, increased appetite, weight changes.
GU: breakthrough bleeding, altered menstrual flow, dysmenorrhea, amenorrhea, cervical erosion, increased risk of endometrial cancer, *possibility of increased risk of breast cancer,* altered cervical secretions, enlarged uterine fibromas, vaginal candidiasis (in women); gynecomastia, testicular atrophy, impotence (in men).
Hepatic: cholestatic jaundice, *hepatic adenoma.*
Skin: melasma, urticaria, acne, seborrhea, oily skin, hirsutism or hair loss, erythema nodosum, dermatitis.
Other: breast changes (tenderness, enlargement, secretion), hyperglycemia, hypercalcemia, gallbladder disease.

Interactions

Drug-drug. *Bromocriptine:* may cause amenorrhea, interfering with bromocriptine's effects. Avoid concomitant use.
Carbamazepine, phenobarbital, rifampin: decreased effectiveness of estrogen therapy. Monitor patient closely.
Corticosteroids: possibly enhanced effects. Monitor patient closely.

Reactions may be *common,* uncommon, *life-threatening,* or COMMON AND LIFE-THREATENING.

Cyclosporine: increased risk of toxicity. Use together with caution and frequently monitor cyclosporine levels.
Dantrolene, other hepatotoxic drugs: increased risk of hepatotoxicity. Monitor patient closely.
Oral anticoagulants: dosage adjustments may be necessary. Monitor PT and INR.
Tamoxifen: estrogens may interfere with effectiveness of tamoxifen. Avoid concomitant use.
Drug-food. *Caffeine:* may increase serum caffeine concentrations. Monitor effects.
Drug-lifestyle. *Smoking:* increased risk of CV effects. If smoking continues, may need an alternate therapy.

Contraindications and precautions

• Contraindicated in patients with thrombophlebitis or thromboembolic disorders, estrogen-dependent neoplasia, breast or reproductive organ cancer (except for palliative treatment), or undiagnosed abnormal genital bleeding and in pregnant or breast-feeding women.
• Use cautiously in patients with cerebrovascular or coronary artery disease, asthma, depression, bone disease, or cardiac, hepatic, or renal dysfunction and in women with family history (mother, grandmother, sister) of breast or genital tract cancer or who have breast nodules, fibrocystic disease, or abnormal mammographic findings.
• Drug should not be used in children.

NURSING CONSIDERATIONS

Assessment
• Obtain history of patient's underlying condition before therapy, and reassess regularly thereafter.
• Ensure that patient has thorough physical examination before initiating ethinyl estradiol therapy.
• Patient receiving long-term therapy should have repeat examinations yearly. Periodically monitor serum lipid levels,

blood pressure, body weight, and liver function, as ordered.
• Be alert for adverse reactions and drug interactions.
• Evaluate patient's and family's knowledge of drug therapy.

Nursing diagnoses
• Altered health maintenance related to underlying condition
• Altered tissue perfusion (cerebral, peripheral, pulmonary, or myocardial) related to drug-induced thromboembolism
• Knowledge deficit related to drug therapy

Planning and implementation
• Administer oral preparations with meals or at bedtime (if only one daily dose is required) to minimize nausea.
• Because of risk of thromboembolism, know that therapy should be discontinued at least 1 month before procedures associated with prolonged immobilization or thromboembolism, such as knee or hip surgery.
• Withhold drug and notify doctor if thromboembolic event is suspected; be prepared to provide supportive care as indicated.
• Notify pathologist of patient receiving this drug.
Patient teaching
• Inform patient that package insert that describes estrogen's adverse effects is available; also provide verbal explanation.
• Emphasize importance of regular physical examinations. Studies suggest that postmenopausal women who use estrogen replacement for more than 5 years to treat menopausal symptoms may be at increased risk for endometrial carcinoma. This risk is reduced by using cyclic rather than continuous therapy and lowest possible dosages of estrogen. Adding progestins to regimen decreases incidence of endometrial hyperplasia; it isn't known if progestins affect incidence of

endometrial carcinoma. Most studies show no increased risk of breast cancer.
• Explain to patient on cyclic therapy for postmenopausal symptoms that although withdrawal bleeding may occur during week off drug, fertility has not been restored. Pregnancy cannot occur because patient has not ovulated.
• Warn patient to immediately report abdominal pain; pain, numbness, or stiffness in legs or buttocks; pressure or pain in chest; shortness of breath; severe headaches; visual disturbances, such as blind spots, flashing lights, or blurriness; vaginal bleeding or discharge; breast lumps; swelling of hands or feet; yellow skin or sclera; dark urine; and light-colored stools.
• Tell diabetic patient to report elevated blood glucose test results so antidiabetic medication dosage can be adjusted.
• Teach female patient how to perform routine breast self-examination.

☑ Evaluation
• Patient exhibits improvement in underlying condition.
• Patient does not experience thromboembolic event during therapy.
• Patient and family state understanding of drug therapy.

ethinyl estradiol and desogestrel
(ETH-uh-nil es-truh-DIGH-ol and DAY-so-jest-rul)
monophasic: Desogen, Ortho-Cept

ethinyl estradiol and ethynodiol diacetate
monophasic: Demulen 1/35, Demulen 1/50

ethinyl estradiol and levonorgestrel
monophasic: Levlen, Nordette
triphasic: Tri-Levlen, Triphasil

ethinyl estradiol and norethindrone
monophasic: Brevicon, Genora 0.5/35, Genora 1/35, ModiCon, N.E.E. 1/35, Nelova 0.5/35E, Nelova 1/35E, Norcept-E 1/35, Norethin 1/35E, Norinyl 1+35, Ortho-Novum 1/35, Ovcon-35, Ovcon-50
biphasic: Nelova 10/11, Ortho-Novum 10/11
triphasic: Ortho-Novum 7/7/7, Tri-Norinyl

ethinyl estradiol and norethindrone acetate
monophasic: Loestrin 21 1/20, Loestrin 21 1.5/30, Norlestrin 21 1/50, Norlestrin 21 2.5/50

ethinyl estradiol and norgestimate
monophasic: Ortho-Cyclen
triphasic: Ortho Tri-Cyclen

ethinyl estradiol and norgestrel
monophasic: Lo/Ovral, Ovral

ethinyl estradiol, norethindrone acetate, and ferrous fumarate
monophasic: Loestrin Fe 1/20, Loestrin Fe 1.5/30, Norlestrin Fe 1/50, Norlestrin Fe 2.5/50

mestranol and norethindrone
monophasic: Genora 1/50, Nelova 1/50 M, Norethin 1/50 M, Norinyl 1+50, Ortho-Novum 1/50

mestranol and norethynodrel
monophasic: Enovid 5 mg, Enovid 10 mg

Pharmacologic class: estrogen with progestin
Therapeutic class: oral contraceptive
Pregnancy risk category: X

How supplied

Monophasic oral contraceptives
ethinyl estradiol and desogestrel
Tablets: ethinyl estradiol 30 mcg and desogestrel 0.15 mg (Desogen, Ortho-Cept)

ethinyl estradiol and ethynodiol diacetate
Tablets: ethinyl estradiol 35 mcg and ethynodiol diacetate 1 mg (Demulen 1/35); ethinyl estradiol 50 mcg and ethynodiol diacetate 1 mg (Demulen 1/50)
ethinyl estradiol and levonorgestrel
Tablets: ethinyl estradiol 30 mcg and levonorgestrel 0.15 mg (Levlen, Nordette)
ethinyl estradiol and norethindrone
Tablets: ethinyl estradiol 35 mcg and norethindrone 0.4 mg (Ovcon-35); ethinyl estradiol 35 mcg and norethindrone 0.5 mg (Brevicon, Genora 0.5/35, ModiCon, Nelova 0.5/35E); ethinyl estradiol 35 mcg and norethindrone 1 mg (Genora 1/35, N.E.E. 1/35, Nelova 1/35E, Norcept-E 1/35, Norethin 1/35E, Norinyl 1+35, Ortho-Novum 1/35); ethinyl estradiol 50 mcg and norethindrone 1 mg (Ovcon-50)
ethinyl estradiol and norethindrone acetate
Tablets: ethinyl estradiol 20 mcg and norethindrone acetate 1 mg (Loestrin 21 1/20); ethinyl estradiol 30 mcg and norethindrone acetate 1.5 mg (Loestrin 21 1.5/30); ethinyl estradiol 50 mcg and norethindrone acetate 1 mg (Norlestrin 21 1/50); ethinyl estradiol 50 mcg and norethindrone acetate 2.5 mg (Norlestrin 21 2.5/50)
ethinyl estradiol and norgestimate
Tablets: ethinyl estradiol 35 mcg and norgestimate 0.25 mg (Ortho Cyclen)
ethinyl estradiol and norgestrel
Tablets: ethinyl estradiol 30 mcg and norgestrel 0.3 mg (Lo/Ovral); ethinyl estradiol 50 mcg and norgestrel 0.5 mg (Ovral)
ethinyl estradiol, norethindrone acetate, and ferrous fumarate
Tablets: ethinyl estradiol 20 mcg, norethindrone acetate 1 mg, and ferrous fumarate 75 mg (Loestrin Fe 1/20); ethinyl estradiol 30 mcg, norethindrone acetate 1.5 mg, and ferrous fumarate 75 mg (Loestrin Fe 1.5/30); ethinyl estradiol 50 mcg, norethindrone acetate 1 mg,

and ferrous fumarate 75 mg (Norlestrin Fe 1/50); ethinyl estradiol 50 mcg, norethindrone acetate 2.5 mg, and ferrous fumarate 75 mg (Norlestrin Fe 2.5/50)
mestranol and norethindrone
Tablets: mestranol 50 mcg and norethindrone 1 mg (Genora 1/50, Nelova 1/50 M, Norethin 1/50 M, Norinyl 1+50, Ortho-Novum 1/50)
mestranol and norethynodrel
Tablets: mestranol 75 mg and norethynodrel 5 mg (Enovid 5 mg); mestranol 150 mg and norethynodrel 9.85 mg (Enovid 10 mg).
Biphasic oral contraceptives
ethinyl estradiol and norethindrone
Tablets: ethinyl estradiol 35 mcg and norethindrone 0.5 mg during phase 1 [10 days]; ethinyl estradiol 35 mcg and norethindrone 1 mg during phase 2 [11 days] (Nelova 10/11, Ortho-Novum 10/11)
Triphasic oral contraceptives
ethinyl estradiol and levonorgestrel
Tablets: (Tri-Levlen, Triphasil) ethinyl estradiol 35 mcg and levonorgestrel 0.05 mg during phase 1 [6 days]; ethinyl estradiol 35 mcg and levonorgestrel 0.075 mg during phase 2 [5 days]; ethinyl estradiol 35 mcg and levonorgestrel 0.125 mg during phase 3 [10 days]
ethinyl estradiol and norethindrone
Tablets: (Tri-Norinyl) ethinyl estradiol 35 mcg and norethindrone 0.5 mg during phase 1 [7 days]; ethinyl estradiol 35 mcg and norethindrone 1 mg during phase 2 [9 days]; ethinyl estradiol 35 mcg and norethindrone 0.5 mg during phase 3 [5 days]; (Ortho-Novum 7/7/7) ethinyl estradiol 35 mcg and norethindrone 0.5 mg during phase 1 [7 days]; ethinyl estradiol 35 mcg and norethindrone 0.75 mg during phase 2 [7 days]; ethinyl estradiol 35 mcg and norethindrone 1 mg during phase 3 [7 days]
ethinyl estradiol and norgestimate
Tablets: (Ortho Tri-Cyclen) ethinyl estradiol 35 mcg and norgestimate 0.18 mg during phase 1 (7 days); ethinyl estradiol 35 mcg and norgestimate 0.215 mg dur-

---

ing phase 2 (7 days); ethinyl estradiol 35 mcg and norgestimate 0.25 mg during phase 3 (7 days).

Pharmacokinetics
Absorption: mostly well absorbed.
Distribution: widely distributed and extensively bound to plasma proteins.
Metabolism: metabolized mainly in liver.
Excretion: excreted in urine and feces.

Route	Onset	Peak	Duration
P.O.	Unknown	Varies	Unknown

Pharmacodynamics
Chemical effect: inhibit ovulation through negative feedback mechanism directed at hypothalamus; also may prevent transport of ovum through fallopian tubes.

Estrogen suppresses secretion of follicle-stimulating hormone, blocking follicular development and ovulation.

Progestin suppresses secretion of luteinizing hormone so ovulation cannot occur even if follicle develops. Progestin thickens cervical mucus, which interferes with sperm migration, and causes endometrial changes that prevent implantation of fertilized ovum.
Therapeutic effect: prevent pregnancy and relieve signs and symptoms of endometriosis.

Indications and dosage
▶ **Contraception. Monophasic oral contraceptives.** *Adults:* 1 tablet P.O. daily, beginning on day 5 of menstrual cycle (first day of menstrual flow is day 1). With 20- and 21-tablet packages, new dosing cycle begins 7 days after last tablet taken. With 28-tablet packages, dosage is 1 tablet daily without interruption; extra tablets are placebos or contain iron. **Biphasic oral contraceptives.** *Adults:* 1 color tablet P.O. daily for 10 days; then next color tablet for 11 days. **Triphasic oral contraceptives.** *Adults:* 1 tablet P.O. daily in sequence specified by brand.

▶ **Endometriosis.** *Adults:* 1 tablet Enovid 5 mg or 10 mg P.O. daily for 2 weeks starting on day 5 of menstrual cycle. Continued without interruption for 6 to 9 months, increasing dosage by 5 to 10 mg q 2 weeks, up to 20 mg daily; up to 40 mg daily as needed and ordered if breakthrough bleeding occurs.

Adverse reactions
CNS: *headache, dizziness,* depression, lethargy, migraine.
CV: *thromboembolism,* hypertension, edema, *pulmonary embolism, CVA.*
EENT: worsening of myopia or astigmatism, intolerance of contact lenses, exophthalmos, diplopia.
GI: *nausea,* vomiting, abdominal cramps, bloating, diarrhea, constipation, anorexia, changes in appetite, weight gain, *pancreatitis.*
GU: *breakthrough bleeding,* granulomatous colitis, dysmenorrhea, amenorrhea, cervical erosion or abnormal secretions, enlargement of uterine fibromas, vaginal candidiasis.
Hepatic: gallbladder disease, cholestatic jaundice, *liver tumors.*
Metabolic: hyperglycemia, hypercalcemia.
Skin: rash, acne, *erythema multiforme.*
Other: breast changes (*tenderness,* enlargement, secretion).

Interactions
Drug-drug. *Bromocriptine:* may cause amenorrhea, interfering with bromocriptine's effects. Avoid concomitant use.
Carbamazepine, phenobarbital, phenytoin, rifampin: decreased effectiveness of estrogen therapy. Monitor patient closely.
Corticosteroids: possibly enhanced effects. Monitor patient closely.
Dantrolene, other hepatotoxic drugs: increased risk of hepatotoxicity. Monitor patient closely.
Griseofulvin, penicillins, sulfonamides, tetracyclines: may decrease effectiveness of oral contraceptives. Avoid concomitant use, if possible.

Reactions may be *common*, uncommon, **life-threatening**, or COMMON AND LIFE-THREATENING.

Oral anticoagulants: dosage adjustments may be necessary. Monitor PT and INR.
Tamoxifen: estrogens may interfere with effectiveness of tamoxifen. Avoid concomitant use.
Drug-food. *Caffeine:* may increase serum caffeine concentrations. Monitor effects.
Drug-lifestyle. *Smoking:* increased risk of CV effects. If smoking continues, may need an alternate therapy.

Contraindications and precautions

• Contraindicated in patients with thromboembolic disorders, cerebrovascular or coronary artery disease, diplopia or ocular lesion arising from ophthalmic vascular disease, classic migraine, MI, known or suspected breast cancer, known or suspected estrogen-dependent neoplasia, benign or malignant liver tumors, active liver disease or history of cholestatic jaundice with pregnancy or prior use of oral contraceptives, or undiagnosed abnormal vaginal bleeding; in known or suspected pregnancy; and in breast-feeding women.
• Use cautiously in patients with cardiac, renal, or hepatic insufficiency; hyperlipidemia; hypertension; migraine; seizure disorders; or asthma.
• To avoid later fertility and menstrual problems, hormonal contraception is not advised for adolescent until after at least 2 years of well-established menstrual cycles and completion of physiologic maturation.

NURSING CONSIDERATIONS

▨ Assessment
• Obtain history of patient's pregnancy status or underlying endometriosis before therapy.
• Monitor effectiveness by determining if pregnancy test is negative or if patient with endometriosis has diminished signs and symptoms.
• Periodically monitor serum lipid levels, blood pressure, body weight, and liver function, as ordered.

• Be alert for adverse reactions and drug interactions.
• Evaluate patient's and family's knowledge of drug therapy.

▨ Nursing diagnoses
• Health-seeking behavior (prevention of pregnancy) related to family planning
• Pain related to drug-induced headache
• Knowledge deficit related to drug therapy

▨ Planning and implementation
• Ensure that patient has been properly instructed about prescribed oral contraceptive before she takes first dose.
• Ensure that negative pregnancy test has been obtained before drug therapy is initiated.
• Know that many laboratory tests are affected by oral contraceptives.
• Discontinue if patient develops granulomatous colitis while on oral contraceptives, and notify doctor.
• Know that drug should be discontinued at least 1 week before surgery to decrease risk of thromboembolism. Tell patient to use alternative method of birth control.
Patient teaching
• Tell patient to take tablets at same time each day; nighttime dosing may reduce nausea and headaches.
• Advise patient to use additional method of birth control, such as condoms or diaphragm with spermicide, for first week of administration in initial cycle.
• Tell patient that missed doses in midcycle greatly increase likelihood of pregnancy.
• If one tablet is missed, tell patient to take it as soon as remembered or to take two tablets the next day and continue regular schedule. If patient misses 2 consecutive days, instruct her to take two tablets daily for 2 days and then resume normal schedule. Also advise her to use additional method of birth control for 7 days after two missed doses. If three or more doses are missed, tell patient to discard remaining tablets in monthly package and to

substitute another contraceptive method. If next menstrual period doesn't begin on schedule, warn patient to rule out pregnancy before starting new dosing cycle. If menstrual period begins, have patient start new dosing cycle 7 days after last tablet was taken.

• Warn patient that headache, nausea, dizziness, breast tenderness, spotting, and breakthrough bleeding are common at first. These effects should diminish after three to six dosing cycles (months).

• Instruct patient to weigh herself at least twice weekly and to report sudden weight gain or edema to doctor.

• Warn patient to avoid exposure to ultraviolet light or prolonged exposure to sunlight.

• Warn patient to immediately report abdominal pain; numbness, stiffness, or pain in legs or buttocks; pressure or pain in chest; shortness of breath; severe headache; visual disturbances, such as blind spots, blurriness, or flashing lights; undiagnosed vaginal bleeding or discharge; two consecutive missed menstrual periods; lumps in breast; swelling of hands or feet; or severe pain in abdomen (tumor rupture in liver).

• Advise patient of increased risks associated with simultaneous use of cigarettes and oral contraceptives.

• Teach patient how to perform routine breast self-examination.

• If one menstrual period is missed and tablets have been taken on schedule, tell patient to continue taking them. If two consecutive menstrual periods are missed, tell patient to stop drug and have pregnancy test. Progestins may cause birth defects if taken early in pregnancy.

• Advise patient not to take same drug for longer than 12 months without consulting doctor. Stress importance of Papanicolaou test and annual gynecologic examination.

• Advise patient to check with doctor about how soon pregnancy may be attempted after hormonal therapy is stopped. Many doctors recommend that women not become pregnant within 2 months after stopping drug.

• Warn patient of possible delay in achieving pregnancy when drug is discontinued.

• Tell patient that many doctors advise women on prolonged therapy (5 years or longer) to stop drug and use other birth control methods. Periodically reassess patient while off hormone therapy.

☑ Evaluation
• Patient does not become pregnant.
• Patient obtains relief from drug-induced headache with administration of mild analgesic.
• Patient and family state understanding of drug therapy.

---

ethosuximide
(eth-oh-SUKS-ih-mighd)
Zarontin

Pharmacologic class: succinimide derivative
Therapeutic class: anticonvulsant
Pregnancy risk category: NR

How supplied

Capsules: 250 mg
Syrup: 250 mg/5 ml

Pharmacokinetics

Absorption: absorbed from GI tract.
Distribution: distributed widely throughout body; protein binding is minimal.
Metabolism: metabolized extensively in liver.
Excretion: excreted in urine with small amounts excreted in bile and feces. *Half-life:* about 60 hours.

Route	Onset	Peak	Duration
P.O.	Unknown	3-7 hr	Unknown

Pharmacodynamics

Chemical effect: not well defined; may increase seizure threshold. Reduces

---

paroxysmal spike-and-wave pattern of absence seizures by depressing nerve transmission in motor cortex.
Therapeutic effect: prevents seizures.

Indications and dosage

▶ **Absence seizures.** *Adults and children age 6 and older:* 500 mg P.O. daily. Optimal dose is 20 mg/kg/day. *Children ages 3 to 6:* 250 mg P.O. daily. Optimal dose is 20 mg/kg/day.

Adverse reactions

CNS: *drowsiness, headache, fatigue, dizziness, ataxia, irritability, hiccups, euphoria, lethargy, depression, psychosis.*
EENT: myopia, tongue swelling, gingival hyperplasia.
GI: *nausea, vomiting, diarrhea, weight loss, cramps, anorexia, epigastric and abdominal pain.*
GU: vaginal bleeding, urinary frequency.
Hematologic: *leukopenia,* eosinophilia, *agranulocytosis, pancytopenia.*
Skin: urticaria, pruritic and erythematous rashes, hirsutism.

Interactions

Drug-drug. *Phenytoin:* serum phenytoin levels may be increased. Monitor levels closely.
Drug-lifestyle. *Alcohol use:* increased CNS depression. Avoid concomitant use.

Contraindications and precautions

• Contraindicated in patients with hypersensitivity to succinimide derivatives.
• Use with extreme caution in patients with hepatic or renal disease.
• Safety of drug has not been established in pregnant or breast-feeding women.

NURSING CONSIDERATIONS

❄ Assessment
• Obtain history of patient's seizure disorder before therapy.
• Monitor effectiveness by assessing patient for absence of seizure activity.
Know that drug may increase frequency of generalized tonic-clonic seizures when used alone in patients who have mixed types of seizures.
• Monitor blood levels. Therapeutic blood levels are 40 to 80 mcg/ml.
• Obtain CBC every 3 to 6 months, as ordered.
• Be alert for adverse reactions.
• Evaluate patient's and family's knowledge of drug therapy.

❄ Nursing diagnoses
• Risk for injury related to seizure disorder
• Altered protection related to drug-induced blood disorders
• Knowledge deficit related to drug therapy

❄ Planning and implementation
• Be aware that ethosuximide is drug of choice for treating absence seizures.
• Administer with food to minimize GI distress.
• Never withdraw drug suddenly. Abrupt withdrawal may precipitate absence seizures. Call doctor immediately if adverse reactions develop.
• Know that drug may cause positive direct Coombs' test.
Patient teaching
• Advise patient to take drug with food to minimize GI distress.
• Caution patient to refrain from driving or performing other potentially hazardous activities that require mental alertness until drug's CNS effects are known.
• Warn patient and parents not to stop drug abruptly but to call doctor if adverse reactions occur.

❄ Evaluation
• Patient is free from seizure activity.
• Patient maintains normal CBC throughout therapy.
• Patient and family state understanding of drug therapy.

etidronate disodium

(eh-tih-DROH-nayt digh-SOH-dee-um)
Didronel

Pharmacologic class: pyrophosphate analogue
Therapeutic class: antihypercalcemic
Pregnancy risk category: C

How supplied

Tablets: 200 mg, 400 mg
Injection: 50 mg/ml

Pharmacokinetics

Absorption: absorption after P.O. dose is variable and decreased in presence of food. Absorption may also be dose-related.
Distribution: about half of dose is distributed to bone.
Metabolism: not metabolized.
Excretion: about 50% excreted within 24 hours in urine. *Half-life:* 5 to 7 hours.

Route	Onset	Peak	Duration
P.O., I.V.	Variable	Variable	Variable

Pharmacodynamics

Chemical effect: decreases osteoclastic activity by inhibiting osteocytic osteolysis and decreases mineral release and matrix or collagen breakdown in bone.
Therapeutic effect: slows excessive remodeling of pagetic or heterotropic bone and lowers blood calcium levels in malignant disease.

Indications and dosage

▶ **Symptomatic Paget's disease of bone (osteitis deformans).** *Adults:* 5 to 10 mg/kg P.O. daily in single dose 2 hours before meal with water or juice. Maximum dosage is 20 mg/kg P.O. daily.
▶ **Heterotopic ossification in spinal cord injuries.** *Adults:* 20 mg/kg P.O. daily for 2 weeks, then 10 mg/kg daily for 10 weeks. Total treatment period is 12 weeks.

▶ **Heterotopic ossification after total hip replacement.** *Adults:* 20 mg/kg P.O. daily for 1 month before total hip replacement and for 3 months afterward.
▶ **Malignancy-associated hypercalcemia.** *Adults:* 7.5 mg/kg I.V. daily for 3 consecutive days. Maintenance dosage is 20 mg/kg P.O. daily for 30 days. May be used for maximum of 90 days.

Adverse reactions

GI: diarrhea, increased frequency of bowel movements, nausea, constipation, stomatitis (with dosage of 20 mg/kg/day).
Other: increased or recurrent bone pain, pain at previously asymptomatic sites, increased risk of fracture, *elevated serum phosphate level,* fever, fluid overload, dyspnea, *seizures,* abnormal hepatic function, **hypersensitivity reactions.**

Interactions

Drug-drug. *Antacids containing calcium, magnesium, or aluminum; mineral supplements containing calcium, iron, magnesium, or aluminum:* can inhibit absorption. Avoid use within 2 hours of dose.
Drug-food. *Foods containing large amounts of calcium (such as milk, dairy products):* can prevent oral absorption. Avoid use within 2 hours of dose.

Contraindications and precautions

• No known contraindications.
• Use cautiously in patients with impaired kidney function. Also use cautiously in pregnant or breast-feeding women.
• Safety of drug has not been established in children.

NURSING CONSIDERATIONS

Assessment
• Obtain history of patient's underlying condition before therapy.
• Assess kidney function before therapy and then during therapy, as ordered.

• Monitor effectiveness by evaluating serum alkaline phosphatase level and urinary hydroxyproline excretion; both decrease if therapy is effective.
• Evaluate patient's and family's knowledge of drug therapy.

🖐 **Nursing diagnoses**
• Risk for injury related to underlying bone condition
• Diarrhea related to drug-induced adverse GI reactions
• Knowledge deficit related to drug therapy

▶ **Planning and implementation**
• Know that drug should not be given longer than 3 months at doses above 10 mg/kg daily. Therapy can be resumed after 3 months, if needed, but should not exceed 6 months.
• Know that some patients may receive I.V. etidronate for up to 7 days. However, risk of hypokalemia increases after 3 days of treatment.
P.O. use: Don't give drug with food, milk, or antacids; they may reduce absorption.
I.V. use: Dilute daily dose in at least 250 ml of 0.9% NaCl solution or D_5W, and infuse over at least 2 hours.
• Notify doctor if elevated serum phosphate level occurs, especially in patients receiving higher doses. However, serum phosphate level usually returns to normal 2 to 4 weeks after drug is discontinued.
Patient teaching
• Stress importance of diet high in calcium and vitamin D.
• Tell patient not to eat for 2 hours after daily dose.
• Tell patient that improvement may not occur for up to 3 months but may continue for months after drug is stopped.

✔ **Evaluation**
• Patient exhibits improvement of underlying condition.
• Patient does not experience severe diarrhea throughout therapy.

• Patient and family state understanding of drug therapy.

etodolac (ultradol)
(eh-toh-DOH-lak)
Lodine, Lodine XL

Pharmacologic class: NSAID
Therapeutic class: antiarthritic
Pregnancy risk category: C

How supplied
Capsules: 200 mg, 300 mg
Tablets (extended-release): 400 mg, 500 mg, 600 mg

Pharmacokinetics
Absorption: well absorbed from GI tract.
Distribution: distributed to liver, lungs, heart, and kidneys.
Metabolism: extensively metabolized in liver.
Excretion: excreted in urine primarily as metabolites; 16% is excreted in feces.

Route	Onset	Peak	Duration
P.O.	≤ 30 min	1-2 hr	4-12 hr

Pharmacodynamics
Chemical effect: unknown; may inhibit prostaglandin synthesis.
Therapeutic effect: relieves inflammation and pain.

Indications and dosage
▶ **Short- and long-term management of osteoarthritis and pain.** *Adults:* Lodine 200 to 400 mg P.O. q 6 to 8 hours, p.r.n., not to exceed 1,200 mg daily or Lodine XL 400 to 1,000 mg P.O. once daily. For patients weighing 60 kg (132 lb) or less, total daily dose should not exceed 20 mg/kg.

Adverse reactions
CNS: *asthenia, malaise, dizziness,* depression, drowsiness, nervousness, insomnia, headache.

CV: hypertension, *heart failure*, syncope, flushing, palpitations, edema, fluid retention.
EENT: blurred vision, tinnitus, photophobia, dry mouth.
GI: *dyspepsia,* flatulence, abdominal pain, diarrhea, nausea, constipation, gastritis, melena, vomiting, anorexia, peptic ulceration with or without *GI bleeding* or *perforation,* ulcerative stomatitis, thirst.
GU: dysuria, urinary frequency, *renal failure.*
Hematologic: anemia (rare), hemolytic anemia, *leukopenia, thrombocytopenia, agranulocytosis.*
Hepatic: *hepatitis.*
Respiratory: asthma.
Skin: pruritus, rash, photosensitivity, *Stevens-Johnson syndrome.*
Other: chills, fever, weight gain.

Interactions

Drug-drug. *Antacids:* may decrease peak levels of drug. Monitor for decreased effect of etodolac.
Aspirin: reduced protein-binding of etodolac without altering its clearance. Clinical significance unknown. Recommend avoiding concomitant use.
Beta blockers, diuretics: effects may be blunted. Monitor closely.
Cyclosporine: impaired elimination and increased risk of nephrotoxicity. Avoid concomitant use.
Digoxin, lithium, methotrexate: etodolac may impair elimination of these drugs, resulting in increased levels and risk of toxicity. Monitor blood levels.
Phenytoin: increased serum levels of phenytoin. Monitor for toxicity.
Warfarin: etodolac decreases protein-binding of warfarin but does not change its clearance. Although no dosage adjustment is necessary, monitor PT and INR closely and watch for bleeding.
Drug-lifestyle. *Alcohol use:* increased chance of adverse effects. Avoid use.
Sun exposure: photosensitivity reactions may occur; take precautions.

Contraindications and precautions

• Contraindicated in patients with hypersensitivity to drug and in those with history of aspirin- or NSAID-induced asthma, rhinitis, urticaria, or other allergic reactions.
• Use of drug during third trimester of pregnancy is not recommended.
• Use cautiously in patients with history of GI bleeding, ulceration, and perforation and renal or hepatic impairment. Also use cautiously in pregnant women during first and second trimesters and breast-feeding women.
• Safety of drug has not been established in children under age 18.

NURSING CONSIDERATIONS

⚖ Assessment
• Obtain history of patient's underlying condition before therapy.
• Monitor effectiveness by evaluating patient for decreased inflammation and pain.
• Be alert for adverse reactions and drug interactions.
• Evaluate patient's and family's knowledge of drug therapy.

Nursing diagnoses
• Pain related to underlying condition
• Risk for injury related to drug-induced adverse reactions
• Knowledge deficit related to drug therapy

Planning and implementation
• Give drug with milk or meals to minimize GI discomfort.
• Know that metabolites of etodolac may cause false-positive test for urinary bilirubin, decreased serum uric acid levels, and borderline elevations of one or more liver function tests.
Patient teaching
• Advise patient that serious GI toxicity, including peptic ulceration and bleeding, can occur as a result of taking NSAIDs, despite absence of GI symptoms. Teach patient signs and symptoms of GI bleed-

---

Reactions may be *common,* uncommon, *life-threatening*, or COMMON AND LIFE-THREATENING.

ing, and tell him to contact doctor immediately if they occur. Also tell patient to take drug with milk or food.

• Instruct patient to notify doctor if other adverse reactions occur or pain relief is not obtained with drug administration.

• Advise patient to use sunblock, wear protective clothing, and avoid prolonged exposure to sunlight to prevent photosensitivity reactions.

• Tell patient that use during last trimester of pregnancy should be avoided.

☑ **Evaluation**
• Patient is free from pain.
• Patient does not experience injury as result of drug-induced adverse reactions.
• Patient and family state understanding of drug therapy.

etoposide (VP-16)
(eh-toh-POH-sighd)
VePesid

Pharmacologic class: podophyllotoxin (cell cycle–phase specific, G2 and late S phases)
Therapeutic class: antineoplastic
Pregnancy risk category: D

How supplied

Capsules: 50 mg
Injection: 100 mg/5 ml

Pharmacokinetics

Absorption: only moderately absorbed across GI tract after P.O. administration. Bioavailability ranges from 25% to 75%, with average of 50% of dose being absorbed.
Distribution: distributed widely in body tissues; crosses blood-brain barrier to limited and variable extent. Etoposide is about 94% protein-bound.
Metabolism: only small portion of dose is metabolized in liver.
Excretion: excreted primarily in urine as unchanged drug; smaller portion excreted

in feces. *Half-life:* initial, 30 minutes to 2 hours; terminal, 5½ to 11 hours.

Route	Onset	Peak	Duration
P.O., I.V.	Unknown	Unknown	Unknown

Pharmacodynamics

Chemical effect: unknown.
Therapeutic effect: inhibits selected cancer cell growth.

Indications and dosage

▶ **Testicular cancer.** *Adults:* 50 to 100 mg/m² I.V. on 5 consecutive days q 3 to 4 weeks; or 100 mg/m² on days 1, 3, and 5 q 3 to 4 weeks.
▶ **Small-cell carcinoma of lung.** *Adults:* 35 mg/m²/day I.V. for 4 days; or 50 mg/m²/day I.V. for 5 days. P.O. dosage is two times I.V. dose rounded to nearest 50 mg.

Adverse reactions

CNS: peripheral neuropathy.
CV: hypotension (from rapid infusion).
GI: *nausea, vomiting, anorexia, diarrhea,* abdominal pain, *stomatitis.*
Hematologic: *anemia, myelosuppression* (dose-limiting), LEUKOPENIA, THROMBOCYTOPENIA.
Other: reversible alopecia, *anaphylaxis* (rare), phlebitis at injection site (infrequent), rash.

Interactions

Drug-drug. *Warfarin:* may further prolong PT. Monitor patient closely.

Contraindications and precautions

• Contraindicated in patients with hypersensitivity to drug.
• Drug is not recommended for use during pregnancy unless absolutely necessary because fetal harm may occur. It also is not recommended for use in breast-feeding women.
• Use cautiously in patients who have had previous cytotoxic or radiation therapy.
• Safety of drug has not been established in children.

NURSING CONSIDERATIONS

⚖ Assessment
• Obtain history of patient's underlying condition before therapy.
• Obtain baseline blood pressure before therapy, and monitor blood pressure at 30-minute intervals during infusion.
• Monitor effectiveness by noting results of follow-up diagnostic tests and overall physical status and by regularly checking tumor size and rate of growth through appropriate studies, as ordered. Know that etoposide has produced complete remission in small-cell lung cancer and testicular cancer.
• Monitor CBC, as ordered. Observe patient for signs of bone marrow suppression.
• Monitor I.V. site for possible extravasation.
• Be alert for adverse reactions and drug interactions.
• Evaluate patient's and family's knowledge of drug therapy.

⊞ Nursing diagnoses
• Altered health maintenance related to presence of neoplastic disease
• Altered protection related to drug-induced adverse hematologic reactions
• Knowledge deficit related to drug therapy

▷ Planning and implementation
• Follow institutional policy to reduce risks. Preparation and administration of parenteral form are associated with carcinogenic, mutagenic, and teratogenic risks for personnel.
P.O. use: Store capsules in refrigerator.
I.V. use: Give drug by slow I.V. infusion (over at least 30 minutes) to prevent severe hypotension. If systolic blood pressure falls below 90 mm Hg, stop infusion and notify doctor.
– Dilute drug for infusion in either D_5W or 0.9% NaCl solution to concentration of 0.2 or 0.4 mg/ml. Higher concentrations may crystallize.

– Do not administer through membrane-type in-line filter because diluent may dissolve filter.
– Know that solutions diluted to 0.2 mg/ml are stable for 96 hours at room temperature in plastic or glass unprotected from light; solutions diluted to 0.4 mg/ml are stable for 48 hours under same conditions.
• Have diphenhydramine, hydrocortisone, epinephrine, and necessary emergency equipment available to establish airway in case of anaphylaxis.
Patient teaching
• Warn patient to watch for signs of infection and bleeding. Teach patient how to take infection-control and bleeding precautions.
• Tell patient that hair loss is possible but reversible.
• Instruct patient to report discomfort, pain, or burning at I.V. insertion site.

☑ Evaluation
• Patient exhibits positive response to therapy.
• Patient's immune function returns to normal with cessation of therapy.
• Patient and family state understanding of drug therapy.

factor IX complex
(FAK-tor nighn KOM-pleks)
Bebulin VH, Konyne 80, Profilnine Heat-Treated, Proplex T

factor IX (human)
AlphaNine SD, Mononine

Pharmacologic class: blood derivative
Therapeutic class: systemic hemostatic
Pregnancy risk category: C

How supplied

Injection: vials, with diluent. Units specified on label.

Pharmacokinetics

Absorption: not applicable.
Distribution: equilibration within extravascular space takes 4 to 6 hours.
Metabolism: cleared by plasma.
Excretion: unknown. *Half-life:* about 24 hours.

Route	Onset	Peak	Duration
I.V.	Immediate	10-30 min	Unknown

Pharmacodynamics

Chemical effect: directly replaces deficient clotting factor.
Therapeutic effect: causes clotting.

Indications and dosage

▶ **Factor IX deficiency (hemophilia B or Christmas disease), anticoagulant overdosage.** *Adults and children:* units required (0.8 to 1 times body weight in kg times percentage of desired increase of factor IX level) by slow I.V. infusion or I.V. push. Dosage depends on degree of deficiency, level of factor IX desired, patient's weight, and severity of bleeding.

Adverse reactions

CNS: headache.
CV: *thromboembolic reactions, MI, DIC, pulmonary embolism,* changes in blood pressure.
GI: nausea, vomiting.
Skin: urticaria.
Other: *transient fever, chills, flushing, tingling,* **hypersensitivity reactions** (*anaphylaxis*).

Interactions

Drug-drug. *Aminocaproic acid:* increased risk of thrombosis. Avoid concomitant use.

Contraindications and precautions

• Contraindicated in patients with hepatic disease in whom there is suspicion of in-travascular coagulation or fibrinolysis. Mononine is contraindicated in patients with hypersensitivity to murine protein.
• Use cautiously in neonates and infants and in pregnant or breast-feeding women.

NURSING CONSIDERATIONS

⬛ Assessment

• Obtain assessment of patient's coagulation studies and bleeding disorder before and after therapy.
• Be alert for adverse reactions and drug interactions.
• Monitor vital signs regularly.
• Evaluate patient's and family's knowledge of drug therapy.

⬛ Nursing diagnoses

• Altered health maintenance related to underlying disorder
• Altered protection related to drug-induced intravascular hemolysis
• Knowledge deficit related to drug therapy

⬛ Planning and implementation

• As ordered, give hepatitis B vaccine before factor IX complex.
• Avoid rapid infusion. If tingling sensation, fever, chills, or headache develops, decrease flow rate and notify doctor.
• Reconstitute with 20 ml of sterile water for injection for each vial of lyophilized drug. Keep refrigerated until ready to use; warm to room temperature before reconstituting. Use within 3 hours of reconstitution. Unstable in solution. Don't shake, refrigerate, or mix solution with other I.V. solutions. Store away from heat.
• Keep in mind that risk of hepatitis, including non-A and non-B hepatitis, must be weighed against risk of not receiving drug. Because of manufacturing process, be aware that risk of HIV transmission is extremely low.
Patient teaching
• Explain drug action to patient.
• Tell patient to report adverse reactions promptly.

☑ Evaluation
• Patient is free from bleeding.
• Patient does not experience injury.
• Patient and family state understanding of drug therapy.

famciclovir
(fam-SIGH-kloh-veer)
Famvir

Pharmacologic class: synthetic acyclic guanine derivative
Therapeutic class: antiviral
Pregnancy risk category: B

How supplied
Tablets: 125 mg, 250 mg, 500 mg

Pharmacokinetics
Absorption: absolute bioavailability is 77%.
Distribution: less than 20% is bound to plasma proteins.
Metabolism: extensively metabolized in liver to active drug, penciclovir (98.5%), and other inactive metabolites.
Excretion: primarily in urine.

Route	Onset	Peak	Duration
P.O.	Unknown	≤ 1 hr	Unknown

Pharmacodynamics
Chemical effect: converted to penciclovir, which enters viral cells and inhibits DNA polymerase and viral DNA synthesis.
Therapeutic effect: inhibits viral replication. Spectrum of activity include herpes simplex types 1 and 2 and varicella-zoster viruses.

Indications and dosage
▶ **Acute herpes zoster.** *Adults:* 500 mg P.O. q 8 hours for 7 days. *In patients with reduced renal function:* if clearance is greater than or equal to 60 ml/minute, 500 mg P.O. q 8 hours; if 40 to 59 ml/minute, 500 mg P.O. q 12 hours; if 20 to 39 ml/minute, 500 mg P.O. q 24 hours; and if below 20 ml/minute, 250 mg P.O. q 48 hours. In hemodialysis patients, 250 mg P.O. after each hemodialysis session.
▶ **Recurrent episodes of genital herpes.** *Adults:* 125 mg P.O. b.i.d. for 5 days. Therapy begins as soon as symptoms occur. *In patients with reduced renal function:* if clearance is greater than or equal to 40 ml/minute, 125 mg P.O. q 12 hours; if 20 to 39 ml/minute, 125 mg P.O. q 24 hours; if below 20 ml/minute, 125 mg P.O. q 24 hours. In hemodialysis patients, 125 mg P.O. after each hemodialysis session.

Adverse reactions
CNS: *headache,* fatigue, dizziness, paresthesia, somnolence.
EENT: pharyngitis, sinusitis.
GI: diarrhea, *nausea,* vomiting, constipation, anorexia, abdominal pain.
Musculoskeletal: back pain, arthralgia.
Skin: pruritus; zoster-related signs, symptoms, and complications.

Interactions
Drug-drug. *Probenecid:* may increase plasma concentrations of famciclovir. Monitor for increased adverse effects.

Contraindications and precautions
• Contraindicated in patients with hypersensitivity to drug.
• Breast-feeding is not recommended during drug therapy.
• Use cautiously in patients with renal or hepatic impairment. Dosage adjustment may be needed. Also use cautiously in pregnant women.
• Safety of drug has not been established in children.

NURSING CONSIDERATIONS

☑ Assessment
• Obtain assessment of patient's viral infection before therapy and reassess regularly throughout therapy.

Reactions may be *common,* uncommon, *life-threatening,* or COMMON AND LIFE-THREATENING.

• Be alert for adverse reactions and drug interactions.
• Monitor patient's hydration status if adverse GI reactions occur.
• Evaluate patient's and family's knowledge of drug therapy.

🔶 **Nursing diagnoses**
• Infection related to presence of virus susceptible to famciclovir
• Risk for fluid volume deficit related to drug's adverse GI reactions
• Knowledge deficit related to drug therapy

▶ **Planning and implementation**
• Drug may be taken without regard to meals.
Patient teaching
• Teach patient how to prevent spread of infection to others.
• Urge patient to recognize and report early symptoms of herpes infection, such as tingling, itching, or pain.

☑ **Evaluation**
• Patient is free from infection.
• Patient maintains adequate hydration.
• Patient and family state understanding of drug therapy.

---

famotidine
(fam-OH-tih-deen)
Pepcid, Pepcid AC†, Pepcidine◊

Pharmacologic class: H₂-receptor antagonist
Therapeutic class: antiulcer
Pregnancy risk category: B

How supplied

Tablets: 10 mg, 20 mg, 40 mg
Powder for oral suspension: 40 mg/5 ml after reconstitution
Injection: 10 mg/ml

Pharmacokinetics
Absorption: when given orally, about 40% to 45% is absorbed.
Distribution: distributed widely to many body tissues.
Metabolism: about 30% to 35% of dose is metabolized by liver.
Excretion: most of drug is excreted unchanged in urine. *Half-life:* 2½ to 3½ hours.

Route	Onset	Peak	Duration
P.O.	≤ 1 hr	1-3 hr	10-12 hr
I.V.	≤ 1 hr	20 min	10-12 hr

Pharmacodynamics
Chemical effect: competitively inhibits action of H₂ at receptor sites of parietal cells, decreasing gastric acid secretion.
Therapeutic effect: decreases gastric acid levels and prevents heartburn.

Indications and dosage

▶ **Duodenal ulcer (short-term treatment).** *Adults:* For acute therapy, 40 mg P.O. once daily h.s. or 20 mg P.O. b.i.d. For maintenance therapy, 20 mg P.O. once daily h.s.
▶ **Benign gastric ulcer (short-term treatment).** *Adults:* 40 mg P.O. daily h.s. for 8 weeks.
▶ **Pathologic hypersecretory conditions (such as Zollinger-Ellison syndrome).** *Adults:* 20 mg P.O. q 6 hours up to 160 mg q 6 hours.
▶ **Hospitalized patients with intractable ulcerations or hypersecretory conditions or patients who cannot take oral medication.** *Adults:* 20 mg I.V. q 12 hours.
▶ **Gastroesophageal reflux disease (GERD).** *Adults:* 20 mg P.O. b.i.d. for up to 6 weeks. For esophagitis caused by GERD, 20 to 40 mg b.i.d. for up to 12 weeks.
▶ **Prevention of heartburn.** *Adults:* 10 mg P.O. 1 hour before meals.

Adverse reactions

CNS: *headache,* dizziness, vertigo, malaise, paresthesia.
EENT: tinnitus, orbital edema.
GI: diarrhea, constipation, anorexia, taste disorder, dry mouth.
GU: increased BUN and creatinine levels.
Skin: acne, dry skin, flushing.
Other: transient irritation at I.V. site, musculoskeletal pain, palpitations, fever.

Interactions

None significant.

Contraindications and precautions

• Contraindicated in patients with hypersensitivity to drug.
• Use cautiously in pregnant or breast-feeding women.
• Safety of drug has not been established in children.

NURSING CONSIDERATIONS

Assessment
• Obtain assessment of patient's GI disorder before therapy, and reassess regularly throughout therapy.
• Be alert for adverse reactions.
• Evaluate patient's and family's knowledge of drug therapy.

Nursing diagnoses
• Impaired tissue integrity related to underlying GI disorder
• Constipation related to drug's adverse effect on GI tract
• Knowledge deficit related to drug therapy

Planning and implementation
P.O. use: Give drug at bedtime or if more than one daily dose is ordered, give last dose of day at bedtime.
• Store reconstituted oral suspension below 86° F (30° C). Discard after 30 days.
I.V. use: To prepare I.V. injection, dilute 2 ml (20 mg) drug with compatible I.V. solution to total volume of either 5 or 10 ml and inject over at least 2 minutes.

Compatible solutions include sterile water for injection, 0.9% NaCl injection, D_5W or dextrose 10% in water injection, 5% sodium bicarbonate injection, and lactated Ringer's injection.
• Alternatively, give by intermittent I.V. infusion. Dilute 20 mg (2 ml) drug in 100 ml of compatible solution and infuse over 15 to 30 minutes. Solution is stable for 48 hours at room temperature after dilution.
• Store I.V. injection in refrigerator at 36° to 46° F (2° to 8° C).
• Change I.V. site if infiltration or signs of phlebitis occur. Apply warm compresses to site.
Patient teaching
• Tell patient to take drug with snack if desired. Remind him that drug is most effective if taken at bedtime. Tell patient taking 20 mg b.i.d. to take one dose at bedtime.
• With doctor's knowledge, allow patient to take antacids concomitantly, especially at beginning of therapy when pain is severe.
• Urge patient to avoid cigarette smoking because it may increase gastric acid secretion and worsen disease.
• Advise patient not to take drug for more than 8 weeks unless specifically ordered by doctor.

Evaluation
• Patient reports decrease in or relief of GI pain with drug.
• Patient regains normal bowel pattern.
• Patient and family state understanding of drug therapy.

felodipine
(feh-LOH-dih-peen)
Agon◊, Agon SR◊, Plendil, Plendil ER◊, Renedil♦

Pharmacologic class: calcium channel blocker
Therapeutic class: antihypertensive
Pregnancy risk category: C

How supplied

Tablets: 5 mg◊
Tablets (extended-release): 2.5 mg,
5 mg, 10 mg

Pharmacokinetics

Absorption: almost completely absorbed but extensive first-pass metabolism reduces absolute bioavailability to about 20%.
Distribution: over 99% bound to plasma proteins.
Metabolism: unknown, although thought to be hepatic.
Excretion: over 70% of dose appears in urine and 10% in feces as metabolites.
Half-life: 11 to 16 hours.

Route	Onset	Peak	Duration
P.O.	2-5 hr	2.5-5 hr	24 hr

Pharmacodynamics

Chemical effect: unknown; dihydropyridine derivative that prevents entry of calcium ions into vascular smooth-muscle and cardiac cells.
Therapeutic effect: lowers blood pressure.

Indications and dosage

▶ **Hypertension.** *Adults:* initially, 5 mg P.O. daily. Dosage is adjusted based on patient response, generally at intervals not less than 2 weeks. Usual dose is 2.5 to 10 mg daily; maximum recommended dosage is 20 mg daily. *In elderly patients and patients with impaired hepatic function:* 5 mg P.O. daily; dosage is adjusted as for adults. Maximum recommended dosage is 10 mg daily.

Adverse reactions

CNS: *headache,* dizziness, paresthesia, asthenia.
CV: *peripheral edema,* chest pain, palpitations.
EENT: rhinorrhea, pharyngitis.
GI: abdominal pain, nausea, constipation, diarrhea.

Musculoskeletal: muscle cramps, back pain
Respiratory: upper respiratory infection, cough.
Skin: rash, *flushing.*
Other: gingival hyperplasia.

Interactions

Drug-drug. *Anticonvulsants:* decreased plasma concentration of felodipine. Avoid concomitant use.
Cimetidine: decreased clearance of felodipine. Use lower doses of felodipine.
Metoprolol: may alter pharmacokinetics of metoprolol. No dosage adjustment appears necessary. Monitor for adverse effects.
Theophylline: may slightly decrease theophylline levels. Monitor patient's response carefully.
Drug-food. *Grapefruit juice:* increased bioavailability and effect when taken together.

Contraindications and precautions

• Contraindicated in patients with hypersensitivity to drug.
• Breast-feeding is not recommended during drug use.
• Use cautiously in patients with heart failure, particularly those receiving beta blockers, and in patients with impaired hepatic function because clearance of drug from blood is dependent on liver. Also use cautiously in pregnant women.
• Safety of drug has not been established in children.

NURSING CONSIDERATIONS

⚕ Assessment
• Obtain assessment of patient's blood pressure before therapy, and reassess regularly thereafter.
• Be alert for adverse reactions and drug interactions.
• Evaluate patient's and family's knowledge of drug therapy.

☺ **Nursing diagnoses**
• Risk for injury related to presence of hypertension
• Fluid volume excess related to drug-induced peripheral edema
• Knowledge deficit related to drug therapy

▷ **Planning and implementation**
• Know that drug may be administered without regard to food. However, a small study reported more than twofold increase of bioavailability when drug was taken with doubly concentrated grape juice as compared with water or orange juice.
Patient teaching
• Instruct patient to swallow tablets whole and not to crush or chew them.
• Tell patient to take drug even when he feels better; to watch his diet; and to check with doctor or pharmacist before taking other medications, including OTC drugs.
• Advise patient to observe good oral hygiene and to see dentist regularly.

☑ **Evaluation**
• Patient's blood pressure is normal.
• Patient does not develop complications from peripheral edema.
• Patient and family state understanding of drug therapy.

fenofibrate
(feh-noh-FIGH-brayt)
Tricor

Pharmacologic class: fibric acid derivative
Therapeutic class: antilipemic
Pregnancy risk category: C

How supplied
Capsules (micronized): 67 mg

Pharmacokinetics
Absorption: well absorbed from GI tract.

Distribution: about 99% bound to plasma proteins.
Metabolism: rapidly hydrolyzed by esterases to active metabolite, fenofibric acid.
Excretion: approximately 60% excreted in urine mainly as metabolites and 25% in feces. *Half-life:* 20 hours.

Route	Onset	Peak	Duration
P.O.	Unknown	6-8 hr	Unknown

Pharmacodynamics
Chemical effect: exact mechanism not known. Drug is thought to inhibit triglyceride synthesis, resulting in a decrease in the quantity of very-low-density lipoproteins (VLDL) released into the circulation. Drug also may stimulate the breakdown of triglyceride-rich protein.
Therapeutic effect: decreases serum triglyceride levels.

Indications and dosage
▶ **Adjunct therapy to diet for treatment of patients with very high serum triglyceride levels (type IV and V hyperlipidemia) who are at risk of pancreatitis and who do not respond adequately to a determined dietary effort.**
Adults: initially, 67 mg P.O. daily. Increase sequentially if necessary following repeat serum triglyceride levels at 4- to 8-week intervals to maximum dose of three capsules daily (201 mg).

Adverse reactions
CNS: dizziness, miscellaneous pain, asthenia, fatigue, paresthesia, insomnia, increased appetite, headache, decreased libido.
CV: *arrhythmias.*
EENT: eye irritation, eye floaters, earache, conjunctivitis, blurred vision, rhinitis, sinusitis.
GI: dyspepsia, eructation, flatulence, nausea, vomiting, abdominal pain, constipation, diarrhea.
GU: increased BUN and creatinine levels, polyuria, vaginitis.

Reactions may be *common,* uncommon, *life-threatening,* or COMMON AND LIFE-THREATENING.

Hepatic: increased ALT, AST levels.
Musculoskeletal: arthralgia.
Respiratory: cough.
Skin: pruritus, rash.
Other: decreased hemoglobin and uric acid levels, hypersensitivity reaction, *infection,* flu syndrome.

Interactions

Drug-drug. *Bile acid sequestrants:* may bind and inhibit absorption of fenofibrate. Give drug 1 hour before or 4 to 6 hours after bile acid sequestrants.
Coumarin-type anticoagulants: potentiation of anticoagulant effect. Monitor PT and INR closely. Dosage of anticoagulant may need to be reduced.
Cyclosporine, immunosuppressants, nephrotoxic agents: induced renal dysfunction may compromise the elimination of fenofibrate. Use together cautiously.
3-Hydroxy-3-methylglutaryl coenzyme A (HMG-Co A) reductase inhibitors: no data are available on the concomitant use with fenofibrate; however, because of risk of myopathy, rhabdomyolysis, and acute renal failure reported with the combined use of HMG-Co A reductase inhibitors with gemfibrozil (another fibrate derivative), these drugs should not be given together.
Drug-food. *Any food:* absorption of fenofibrate is increased when administered with food. Give drug with meals.
Drug-lifestyle. *Alcohol use:* may elevate triglycerides. Avoid concomitant use.

Contraindications and precautions

• Contraindicated in patients with preexisting gallbladder disease, hepatic dysfunction, primary biliary cirrhosis, severe renal dysfunction, unexplained persistent liver function abnormalities, or hypersensitivity to drug.
• Use cautiously in patients with history of pancreatitis.
• Safety and efficacy in children have not been established.

NURSING CONSIDERATIONS

⚗ Assessment
• Assess baseline lipid levels and liver function tests before starting therapy and periodically thereafter as ordered.
• Be alert for adverse reactions and drug interactions.
• Evaluate patient's and family's knowledge of drug.

⊕ Nursing diagnoses
• Altered nutrition: less than body requirements related to drug-induced adverse GI reactions
• Risk for infection related to adverse drug reactions
• Knowledge deficit related to drug therapy

❯ Planning and implementation
• Be aware that patients with severe renal impairment require evaluation of renal function and triglyceride levels before dose increase.
• Give drug with meals.
• Counsel patient on importance of adhering to triglyceride-lowering diet.
Patient teaching
• Advise patient to promptly report symptoms of unexplained muscle weakness, pain, or tenderness, especially if accompanied by malaise or fever.
• Inform patient to take drug with meals to optimize drug absorption.
• Advise patient to continue weight-control measures, including diet and exercise, and to reduce alcohol intake before starting drug therapy.
• Instruct patients who are also taking bile acid resins to take fenofibrate 1 hour before or 4 to 6 hours after bile acid resin.
• Advise breast-feeding patient that a decision must be made to discontinue either breast-feeding or drug therapy.

☑ Evaluation
• Patient maintains adequate nutritional intake.

- Patient remains free from infection.
- Patient and family state understanding of drug therapy.

fenoprofen calcium
(fen-uh-PROH-fen KAL-see-um)
Nalfon, Nalfon 200

Pharmacologic class: NSAID
Therapeutic class: nonnarcotic analgesic, anti-inflammatory
Pregnancy risk category: NR

How supplied
Tablets: 600 mg
Capsules: 200 mg, 300 mg

Pharmacokinetics
Absorption: absorbed rapidly and completely from GI tract.
Distribution: 99% protein-bound.
Metabolism: metabolized in liver.
Excretion: excreted chiefly in urine with small amount excreted in feces. *Half-life:* 2½ to 3 hours.

Route	Onset	Peak	Duration
P.O.	15-30 min	About 2 hr	4-6 hr

Pharmacodynamics
Chemical effect: unknown; produces anti-inflammatory, analgesic, and antipyretic effects, possibly by inhibiting prostaglandin synthesis.
Therapeutic effect: relieves pain, fever, and inflammation.

Indications and dosage
▶ **Rheumatoid arthritis and osteoarthritis.** *Adults:* 300 to 600 mg P.O. t.i.d. or q.i.d. Maximum dosage is 3.2 g daily.
▶ **Mild to moderate pain.** *Adults:* 200 mg P.O. q 4 to 6 hours, p.r.n.

Adverse reactions
CNS: *headache,* drowsiness, fatigue, nervousness, asthenia, tremor, confusion, dizziness, *somnolence.*

CV: peripheral edema, palpitations.
EENT: tinnitus, blurred vision, decreased hearing.
GI: *epigastric distress, nausea, GI bleeding,* vomiting, occult blood loss, peptic ulceration, constipation, anorexia, *dyspepsia,* flatulence.
GU: oliguria, interstitial nephritis, proteinuria, *reversible renal failure, papillary necrosis,* cystitis, hematuria.
Hematologic: prolonged bleeding time, anemia, *aplastic anemia, agranulocytosis, thrombocytopenia, hemorrhage.*
Hepatic: elevated enzymes, *hepatitis.*
Respiratory: dyspnea, upper respiratory tract infections, nasopharyngitis.
Skin: *pruritus,* rash, urticaria, *anaphylaxis,* increased diaphoresis.
Other: *angioedema.*

Interactions
Drug-drug. *Aspirin:* decreased fenoprofen half-life; may increase GI toxicity. Avoid concomitant use.
Corticosteroids: increased risk of adverse GI reactions. Avoid concomitant use.
Diuretics: decreased diuretic effectiveness. Monitor closely.
Oral anticoagulants, sulfonylureas: fenoprofen enhances pharmacologic effects of these drugs. Use together cautiously.
Phenobarbital: enhanced metabolism of fenoprofen. Monitor for lack of fenoprofen effectiveness.
Drug-lifestyle. *Alcohol use:* increased risk of adverse GI reactions. Avoid concomitant use.

Contraindications and precautions
- Contraindicated in patients with significantly impaired kidney function, hypersensitivity to drug, or history of aspirin or NSAID-induced asthma, rhinitis, or urticaria and in pregnant women.
- Breast-feeding is not recommended during drug therapy.
- Use cautiously in elderly patients and those with history of serious GI events or peptic ulcer disease, compromised cardiac function, or hypertension.

Reactions may be *common,* uncommon, *life-threatening,* or COMMON AND LIFE-THREATENING.

• Safety of drug has not been established in children.

NURSING CONSIDERATIONS

⚗ Assessment
• Assess patient's pain or inflammation before and after administration.
• Be aware that renal, hepatic, ocular, and auditory function should be checked periodically in long-term therapy.
• Be alert for adverse reactions and drug interactions.
• Evaluate patient's and family's knowledge of drug therapy.

🔛 Nursing diagnoses
• Pain related to underlying condition
• Risk for injury related to drug-induced adverse reactions
• Knowledge deficit related to drug therapy

❱ Planning and implementation
• Administer drug on empty stomach unless adverse GI reactions occur.
• Notify doctor if abnormalities in renal, hepatic, ocular, or auditory function occur because drug will need to be discontinued.
• Drug may cause false elevations in free and total serum T_3 levels as measured by Amerlex-T assay. Fenoprofen or its metabolite may cross-react with antibody used in Amerlex-M assay. Limited data suggest that drug may alter free and total T_3 concentrations determined by Corning method.
Patient teaching
• Tell patient to take drug 30 minutes before or 2 hours after meals. If adverse GI reactions occur, drug may be taken with milk or meals.
• Tell patient that full effect for arthritis may be delayed for 2 to 4 weeks.
• Warn patient to avoid driving and other hazardous activities that require alertness until adverse CNS effects of drug are known.

• Teach patient signs and symptoms of GI bleeding, and tell him to contact doctor immediately if they occur. Serious GI toxicity, including peptic ulceration and bleeding, can occur in patients taking NSAIDs despite absence of GI symptoms.

☑ Evaluation
• Patient is free from pain.
• Patient does not experience injury from adverse reactions.
• Patient and family state understanding of drug therapy.

fentanyl citrate
(FEN-tuh-nihl SIGH-trayt)
Sublimaze

fentanyl transdermal system
Duragesic-25, Duragesic-50,
Duragesic-75, Duragesic-100

fentanyl transmucosal
Fentanyl Oralet

Pharmacologic class: opioid analgesic
Therapeutic class: analgesic, adjunct to anesthesia, anesthetic
Controlled substance schedule: II
Pregnancy risk category: C

How supplied

Injection: 50 mcg/ml
Transdermal system: patches designed to release 25, 50, 75, or 100 mcg of fentanyl per hour.
Transmucosal: 100 mcg, 200 mcg, 300 mcg, 400 mcg

Pharmacokinetics

Absorption: varies with transmucosal or transdermal use.
Distribution: distributes and accumulates to adipose tissue and skeletal muscle.
Metabolism: metabolized in liver.
Excretion: excreted in urine. *Half-life:* about 3½ hours after parenteral use, 5 to

---

15 hours after transmucosal use, 18 hours after transdermal use.

Route	Onset	Peak	Duration
I.V.	1-2 min	3-5 min	0.5-1 hr
I.M.	7-15 min	20-30 min	1-2 hr
Trans-mucosal	15 min	20-30 min	Unknown
Trans-dermal	12-24 hr	1-3 days	Varies

Pharmacodynamics

Chemical effect: unknown; binds with opioid receptors in CNS, altering both perception of and emotional response to pain.
Therapeutic effect: relieves pain.

Indications and dosage

▶ **Adjunct to general anesthetic.**
Adults: for low-dose therapy, 2 mcg/kg I.V. For moderate-dose therapy, 2 to 20 mcg/kg I.V.; then 25 to 100 mcg I.V. or I.M., p.r.n. For high-dose therapy, 20 to 50 mcg/kg I.V.; then 25 mcg to one-half initial loading dose I.V. p.r.n.
Children ages 2 to 12: 2 to 3 mcg/kg I.V. or I.M. during induction and maintenance phases of general anesthesia.
▶ **Adjunct to regional anesthesia.**
Adults: 50 to 100 mcg I.M. or slow I.V. over 1 to 2 minutes.
▶ **Postoperatively.** *Adults:* 50 to 100 mcg I.M. q 1 to 2 hours, p.r.n.
▶ **Preoperatively.** *Adults:* 50 to 100 mcg I.M. 30 to 60 minutes before surgery. Alternatively, 5 mcg/kg dispensed as oralet unit, 20 to 40 minutes before desired effects are needed. *Children age 2 or older weighing below 40 kg (44 lb) and over 15 kg (33 lb):* 5 mcg/kg as an oralet lozenge. May require a dose 10 to 15 mcg/kg transmucosally.
▶ **Management of chronic pain.** *Adults:* one transdermal system applied to upper torso on area of skin that is not irritated and has not been irradiated. Therapy initiated with 25-mcg/hour system; dosage adjusted as needed and tolerated. Each system may be worn for 72 hours.

Adverse reactions

CNS: *sedation, somnolence, clouded sensorium, euphoria,* dizziness, headache, *confusion, asthenia,* nervousness, hallucinations, anxiety, depression, *seizures* (with large doses).
CV: *hypotension,* hypertension, *arrhythmias,* chest pain, *bradycardia.*
GI: *nausea, vomiting, constipation,* ileus, abdominal pain, *dry mouth.*
GU: *urine retention.*
Respiratory: *respiratory depression,* hypoventilation, dyspnea, apnea.
Skin: reaction at application site (erythema, papules, edema), *pruritus, diaphoresis.*
Other: physical dependence.

Interactions

Drug-drug. *CNS depressants, general anesthetics, hypnotics, MAO inhibitors, other narcotic analgesics, sedatives, tricyclic antidepressant:* additive effects. Use together with extreme caution. Fentanyl dose should be reduced by one-quarter to one-third. Also give above drugs in reduced dosages.
Diazepam: CV depression when given with high doses of fentanyl. Monitor patient closely.
Droperidol: hypotension and decreased pulmonary arterial pressure. Monitor patient closely.
Drug-lifestyle. *Alcohol use:* additive effects. Avoid concomitant use.

Contraindications and precautions

• Contraindicated in patients with known intolerance of drug.
• Use with caution in elderly or debilitated patients, pregnant or breast-feeding women, and patients with head injury, increased CSF pressure, COPD, decreased respiratory reserve, potentially compromised respirations, hepatic or renal disease, or bradyarrhythmias.
• Safety of drug has not been established in children under age 2.

Reactions may be *common*, uncommon, *life-threatening*, or COMMON AND LIFE-THREATENING.

NURSING CONSIDERATIONS

✍ Assessment
• Assess patient's underlying condition before therapy.
• Evaluate degree of pain relief obtained after administration.
• Periodically monitor postoperative vital signs and bladder function. Because drug decreases both rate and depth of respirations, monitoring of arterial oxygen saturation (SaO_2) may help assess respiratory depression.
• Monitor patient who develops adverse reactions to transdermal system for at least 12 hours after removal. Serum drug levels may take as long as 17 hours to decline by 50%.
• Be alert for adverse reactions and drug interactions.
• Evaluate patient's and family's knowledge of drug therapy.

⬡ Nursing diagnoses
• Pain related to underlying condition
• Ineffective breathing pattern related to respiratory depression
• Knowledge deficit related to drug therapy

❯ Planning and implementation
• For better analgesic effect, give drug before patient has intense pain.
I.V. use: Know that only staff trained in administration of I.V. anesthetics and management of their potential adverse effects should administer I.V. fentanyl.
• Drug often used I.V. with droperidol to produce neuroleptanalgesia.
I.M. use: Follow normal protocol.
Transmucosal form: Remove foil overwrap of fentanyl oralet just prior to administration.
• Instruct patient to place fentanyl oralet in mouth and suck (not chew) it.
• Remove fentanyl oralet unit using handle after it has been consumed, patient shows adequate effect, or patient shows signs of respiratory depression. Place any remaining portion in plastic overwrap

and dispose of accordingly for Schedule II drugs.
• Because of the frequency of hypoventilation associated with high doses, transmucosal doses should not exceed 15 mcg/kg (maximum 400 mcg) in children or 5 mcg/kg (maximum 400 mcg) in adults.
Transdermal form: Transdermal fentanyl is not recommended for postoperative pain.
• Dosage equivalency charts are available to calculate fentanyl transdermal dose based on daily morphine intake—for example, for every 90 mg of oral morphine or 15 mg of I.M. morphine per 24 hours, 25 mcg/hour of transdermal fentanyl is required.
• Dosage adjustments in patient using transdermal system should be made gradually. Reaching steady-state levels of new dosage may take up to 6 days; delay dosage adjustment until after at least two applications.
• Keep naloxone and resuscitation equipment available when giving drug intravenously.
• High doses can produce muscle rigidity, which can be reversed with neuromuscular blockers; however, patient must be ventilated artificially.
• Immediately report respiratory rate below 12 breaths/minute or decreased respiratory volume or SaO_2.
• When drug is used postoperatively, encourage patient to turn, cough, and deep breathe to prevent atelectasis.
• Most patients experience good control of pain for 3 days while wearing transdermal system, but a few may need new application after 48 hours. Because serum fentanyl concentration rises for first 24 hours after application, analgesic effect cannot be evaluated for first day. Be sure patient has adequate supplemental analgesic to prevent breakthrough pain.
• When reducing opioid therapy or switching to different analgesic, know transdermal system should be withdrawn

gradually. Because fentanyl serum level drops gradually after removal, give half of equianalgesic dose of new analgesic 12 to 18 hours after removal as ordered.

Patient teaching
• Teach patient proper application of transdermal patch. Clip hair at application site, but do not use razor, which may irritate skin. Wash area with clear water if necessary, but not with soaps, oils, lotions, alcohol, or other substances that may irritate skin or prevent adhesion. Dry area completely before application.
• Tell patient to remove transdermal system from package just before applying. Hold in place for 10 to 20 seconds, and be sure edges of patch adhere to patient's skin.
• Teach patient to dispose of transdermal patch by folding so adhesive side adheres to itself and then flushing it down toilet.
• Tell patient that if another patch is needed after 72 hours, apply to new site.
• Inform patient that heat from fever or environment may increase transdermal delivery and cause toxicity requiring dosage adjustment. Instruct patient to notify doctor if fever occurs or if patient will be spending time in hot climate region.

☑ **Evaluation**
• Patient is free from pain.
• Patient maintains adequate ventilation throughout drug therapy.
• Patient and family state understanding of drug therapy.

---

ferrous fumarate
(FEH-rus FYOO-muh-rayt)
Femiron†, Feostat†, Feostat Drops†, Fumasorb†, Fumerin†, Hemocyte†, Ircon†, Neo-Fer♦, Nephro-Fer†, Novofumar♦, Palafer♦, Palafer Pediatric Drops♦, Span-FF†

ferrous gluconate
Fergon*†, Ferralet†, Fertinic♦, Novoferrogluc♦

ferrous sulfate
Apo-Ferrous Sulfate♦, Feosol*†, Fer-gen-sol, Fer-In-Sol*†, Fer-In-Sol Capsules, Fer-In-Sol Drops*†, Fer-In-Sol Syrup*†, Fer-Iron Drops†, Fero-Grad♦, Fero-Gradumet†, Ferospace†, Ferralyn Lanacaps†, Ferra-TD

ferrous sulfate, dried
Mol-Iron*†, Novoferrosulfa♦, PMS Ferrous Sulfate♦, Slow-Fe†

Pharmacologic class: oral iron supplement
Therapeutic class: hematinic
Pregnancy risk category: A

How supplied

Each 100 mg of ferrous fumarate provides 33 mg of elemental iron.
Tablets†: 60 mg, 195 mg, 200 mg, 300 mg, 324 mg, 325 mg
Tablets (chewable): 100 mg†
Capsules (extended-release): 325 mg†
Oral suspension: 100 mg/5 ml†
Drops: 45 mg/0.6 ml†
Each 100 mg of ferrous gluconate provides 11.6 mg of elemental iron.
Tablets: 300 mg†, 320 mg† (contains 37 mg Fe+), 325 mg†
Capsules: 86 mg†, 325 mg†, 435 mg†
Elixir: 300 mg/5 ml (contains 35 mg Fe+)*†
Ferrous sulfate is 20% elemental iron; dried and powdered, about 32% elemental iron.
Tablets: 195 mg†, 300 mg†, 325 mg†; 200 mg (dried)
Tablets (extended-release): 160 mg (dried)†, 525 mg
Capsules: 150 mg†, 159 mg (dried), 190 mg (dried), 250 mg†, 390 mg†
Capsules (extended-release): 159 mg (dried)†, 525 mg†
Elixir: 220 mg/5 ml*†
Syrup: 90 mg/5 ml†
Solution: 300 mg/5 ml
Drops: 125 mg/ml

Pharmacokinetics

Absorption: absorbed from entire length of GI tract but primary absorption sites are duodenum and proximal jejunum. Up to 10% of iron absorbed by healthy individuals; patients with iron-deficiency anemia may absorb up to 60%. Enteric coating and some extended-release formulas have decreased absorption because they are designed to release iron past points in GI tract of highest absorption. Food may decrease absorption by 33% to 50%.

Distribution: iron is transported through GI mucosal cells directly into blood, where it is bound immediately to carrier protein, transferrin, and transported to bone marrow for incorporation into hemoglobin. Iron is highly protein-bound.

Metabolism: iron is liberated by destruction of hemoglobin, but is conserved and reused by body.

Excretion: healthy individuals lose only small amounts of iron each day. Men and postmenopausal women lose about 1 mg/day, and premenopausal women about 1.5 mg/day. The loss usually occurs in nails, hair, feces, and urine; trace amounts are lost in bile and sweat.

Route	Onset	Peak	Duration
P.O.	≤ 4 days	7-10 days	2-4 mo

Pharmacodynamics

Chemical effect: provides elemental iron, an essential component in formation of hemoglobin.

Therapeutic effect: relieves iron deficiency.

Indications and dosage

▶ **Iron deficiency. Fumarate.** *Adults:* 50 to 100 mg elemental iron P.O. t.i.d. *Children:* 4 to 6 mg/kg P.O. daily, divided into three doses.

▶ **Iron deficiency. Gluconate.** *Adults:* 325 mg P.O. q.i.d., increased to 650 mg q.i.d. as needed and tolerated. *Children*

age 2 and older: 3 mg/kg/day P.O. in three to four divided doses.

▶ **Iron deficiency. Sulfate.** *Adults:* 300 mg P.O. b.i.d. to q.i.d. Alternatively, 1 extended-release capsule (160 to 525 mg) P.O. daily to b.i.d. *Children age 2 and older:* 3 mg/kg/day P.O. in three or four divided doses.

Adverse reactions

GI: *nausea, epigastric pain, vomiting, constipation*, diarrhea, black stools, anorexia.

Other: suspension and drops may temporarily stain teeth.

Interactions

Drug-drug. *Antacids, cholestyramine resin, fluoroquinolones, levodopa, penicillamine, tetracycline, vitamin E:* decreased iron absorption. Separate doses by 2 to 4 hours.

Chloramphenicol: delayed response to iron. Watch patient carefully.

Fluoroquinolones, penicillamine, tetracyclines: Decreased GI absorption, possibly resulting in decreased serum levels or efficacy. Separate doses by 2 to 4 hours.

L-thyroxine: decreased L-thyroxine absorption. Separate doses by at least 2 hours. Monitor thyroid function.

Levodopa, methyldopa: decreased absorption and efficacy of levodopa and methyldopa. Monitor for decreased effect of these agents.

Vitamin C: may increase iron absorption. Beneficial drug interaction.

Drug-food. *Yogurt, cheese, eggs, milk, whole-grain breads, cereals, tea, coffee:* may impair oral iron absorption. Do not administer together.

Contraindications and precautions

● Contraindicated in patients with primary hemochromatosis or hemosiderosis, hemolytic anemia unless iron deficiency anemia is also present, peptic ulcer disease, regional enteritis, or ulcerative coli-

tis, and in those receiving repeated blood transfusions.
• Use cautiously on long-term basis.

NURSING CONSIDERATIONS

⏷ Assessment
• Obtain baseline assessment of patient's iron deficiency before therapy.
• Evaluate hemoglobin and hematocrit levels and reticulocyte counts during therapy, as ordered.
• Be alert for adverse reactions and drug interactions.
• Evaluate patient's and family's knowledge of drug therapy.

⊕ Nursing diagnoses
• Fatigue related to iron deficiency
• Constipation related to adverse effect of drug therapy on GI tract
• Knowledge deficit related to drug therapy

⧁ Planning and implementation
• Give tablets with juice or water, but not with milk or antacids.
• Dilute liquid preparations in juice or water, but not in milk or antacids.
• To avoid staining teeth, give suspension or elixir with straw and place drops at back of throat.
• Do not crush or allow patient to chew extended-release forms.
• Keep in mind that GI upset may be related to dose. Between-meal dosing is preferable, but can be given with some foods, although absorption may be decreased. Enteric-coated products reduce GI upset but also reduce amount of iron absorbed.
• Be aware that oral iron may turn stools black. Although this unabsorbed iron is harmless, it could mask presence of melena.
Patient teaching
• Inform parents that as few as three or four tablets can cause serious poisoning in children.

• If patient misses dose, tell him to take it as soon as he remembers but not to double-dose.
• Advise patient to avoid certain foods that may impair oral iron absorption, including yogurt, cheese, eggs, milk, whole-grain breads and cereals, tea, and coffee.
• Teach dietary measures for preventing constipation.

☑ Evaluation
• Patient reports fatigue is no longer a problem in daily life.
• Patient states appropriate measures to prevent or relieve constipation.
• Patient and family state understanding of drug therapy.

---

fexofenadine hydrochloride
(feks-oh-FEN-uh-deen high-droh-KLOR-ighd)
Allegra, Telfast◇

Pharmacologic class: H_1-receptor antagonist
Therapeutic class: antihistamine
Pregnancy risk category: C

How supplied
Capsules: 60 mg

Pharmacokinetics
Absorption: drug is rapidly absorbed.
Distribution: plasma protein binding is 60% to 70%.
Metabolism: not reported.
Excretion: approximately 80% is recovered in feces and 11% in urine. *Half-life:* 14.4 hours.

Route	Onset	Peak	Duration
P.O.	Unknown	3 hr	14 hr

Pharmacodynamics
Chemical effect: fexofenadine's principal effects are mediated through a selective inhibition of peripheral H_1 receptors.

Therapeutic effect: relieves symptoms associated with seasonal allergies.

Indications and dosages

▶ **Seasonal allergic rhinitis.** *Adults and children age 12 and older:* 60 mg P.O. b.i.d.

Adverse reactions

CNS: fatigue, drowsiness.
GI: nausea, dyspepsia.
Other: viral infection, dysmenorrhea.

Interactions

None reported.

Contraindications and precautions

• Contraindicated in patients with hypersensitivity to drug or its components.
• Use cautiously in patients with impaired renal function.
• Safety and effectiveness in children under age 12 have not been established.
• It is not known whether drug is excreted in breast milk; caution is recommended when administering drug to breast-feeding women.

NURSING CONSIDERATIONS

🔣 **Assessment**
• Assess patient's seasonal allergy symptoms before therapy and thereafter.
• Monitor for adverse reactions.
• Evaluate patient's and family's knowledge of drug therapy.

🔣 **Nursing diagnoses**
• Risk for injury related to fatigue and drowsiness associated with drug
• Altered health maintenance related to underlying condition
• Knowledge deficit related to drug therapy

🔣 **Planning and implementation**
• Be aware that patient with impaired renal function or currently on dialysis should receive a reduced daily dosage.

Patient teaching
• Advise female patient taking drug to avoid breast-feeding.
• Caution patient not to perform hazardous activities if drowsiness occurs as a result of drug use.
• Instruct patient not to exceed prescribed dosage and to take drug only during seasonal allergy symptoms.
• Warn patient to avoid alcohol and driving or other activities that require alertness until drug's CNS effects are known.
• Tell patient that coffee or tea may reduce drowsiness. Suggest sugarless gum, sugarless sour hard candy, or ice chips to relieve dry mouth.

✅ **Evaluation**
• Patient experiences limited fatigue and drowsiness associated with drug.
• Patient responds well to the drug.
• Patient and family state understanding of drug therapy.

filgrastim (granulocyte colony-stimulating factor; G-CSF)
(fil-GRAH-stem)
Neupogen

Pharmacologic class: biologic response modifier
Therapeutic class: colony stimulating factor
Pregnancy risk category: C

How supplied

Injection: 300 mcg/ml

Pharmacokinetics

Absorption: rapid absorption after S.C. administration.
Distribution: unknown.
Metabolism: unknown.
Excretion: unknown. *Half-life:* about 3½ hours.

Route	Onset	Peak	Duration
I.V.	5-60 min	24 hr	1-7 days
S.C.	5-60 min	2-8 hr	1-7 days

Pharmacodynamics

Chemical effect: glycoprotein that stimulates proliferation and differentiation of hematopoietic cells. Drug is specific for neutrophils.
Therapeutic effect: raises WBC levels.

Indications and dosage

▶ **To decrease incidence of infection in patients with nonmyeloid malignancies receiving myelosuppressive antineoplastic agents.** *Adults and children:*
5 mcg/kg/day I.V. or S.C. as single dose. Doses may be increased in increments of 5 mcg/kg for each chemotherapy cycle, depending on duration and severity of nadir of absolute neutrophil count (ANC).
▶ **To decrease incidence of infection in patients with nonmyeloid malignancies receiving myelosuppressive antineoplastic agents followed by bone marrow transplant.** *Adults and children:*
10 mcg/kg/day I.V. or S.C. at least 24 hours after cytotoxic chemotherapy and bone marrow infusion. Subsequent dosages adjusted according to neutrophil response.
▶ **Congenital neutropenia.** *Adults:*
6 mcg/kg S.C. b.i.d. Dosage adjusted according to patient's response.
▶ **Idiopathic or cyclic neutropenia.**
Adults: 5 mcg/kg S.C. daily. Dosage adjusted based on response.

Adverse reactions

CNS: *fatigue,* headache, weakness.
CV: *MI, arrhythmias,* chest pain.
GI: *nausea, vomiting, diarrhea, mucositis,* stomatitis, constipation.
GU: hematuria, proteinuria.
Hematologic: *thrombocytopenia,* leukocytosis.
Musculoskeletal: *skeletal pain*
Respiratory: dyspnea, cough.
Skin: *alopecia,* rash, cutaneous vasculitis.
Other: *fever, hypersensitivity reactions.*

Interactions

Drug-drug. *Chemotherapeutic agents:* rapidly dividing myeloid cells are potentially sensitive to cytotoxic agents. Do not use filgrastim within 24 hours before or after a chemotherapy dose. Use with caution in patients taking lithium.

Contraindications and precautions

• Contraindicated in patients who are hypersensitive to proteins derived from *Escherichia coli* or to drug or its components.
• Use cautiously in pregnant or breast-feeding women.

NURSING CONSIDERATIONS

⚕ Assessment
• Assess patient's underlying condition before therapy.
• Obtain baseline CBC and platelet counts before therapy, as ordered.
• Evaluate CBC and platelet count during therapy, as ordered.
• Be alert for adverse reactions and drug interactions.
• Ask patient about skeletal pain.
• Evaluate patient's and family's knowledge of drug therapy.

⊞ Nursing diagnoses
• Altered protection related to underlying condition or treatment
• Pain related to drug's adverse effect on skeletal muscle
• Knowledge deficit related to drug therapy

▷ Planning and implementation
I.V. use: Dilute in 50 to 100 ml of D_5W and give by intermittent infusion over 15 to 60 minutes or continuous infusion over 24 hours. If final concentration is going to be 2 to 15 mcg/ml, add albumin at 2 mg/ml (0.2%) to minimize binding of drug to plastic containers or tubing.
S.C. use: Follow normal protocol.
• Do not give drug within 24 hours of cytotoxic chemotherapy.

Reactions may be *common,* uncommon, *life-threatening,* or COMMON AND LIFE-THREATENING.

• Once dose is withdrawn, do not reenter vial. Discard unused portion. Vials are for single-dose use and contain no preservatives.
• Give daily for up to 2 weeks or until ANC has returned to 10,000/mm³ after expected chemotherapy-induced neutrophil nadir, as ordered.
• Refrigerate drug at 36° to 46° F (2° to 8° C). Do not freeze; avoid shaking. Store at room temperature for maximum of 6 hours; discard after 6 hours.

Patient teaching
• Teach patient how to administer drug and how to dispose of used needles, syringes, drug containers, and unused medicine.
• Tell patient to report bruising or spontaneous bleeding, such as frequent nosebleeds.
• Teach patient how to manage skeletal pain.

☑ **Evaluation**
• Patient's WBC count is normal.
• Patient reports skeletal pain is bearable or relieved with analgesic administration and comfort measures.
• Patient and family state understanding of drug therapy.

---

finasteride
(fin-ES-teh-righd)
Proscar, Propecia

Pharmacologic class: steroid (synthetic 4-azasteroid) derivative
Therapeutic class: androgen synthesis inhibitor
Pregnancy risk category: X

How supplied

Tablets: 1 mg, 5 mg

Pharmacokinetics

Absorption: not clearly defined, although average bioavailability was 63% in one study.

Distribution: about 90% bound to plasma proteins; crosses blood-brain barrier.
Metabolism: extensively metabolized by liver.
Excretion: 39% of dose is excreted in urine as metabolites; 57% in feces.

Route	Onset	Peak	Duration
P.O.	Unknown	1-2 hr	About 2 wk

Pharmacodynamics

Chemical effect: competitively inhibits steroid 5-reductase, an enzyme responsible for formation of potent androgen 5-dihydrotestosterone (DHT) from testosterone. Because DHT influences development of prostate gland, decreasing levels of this hormone in adult males should relieve symptoms associated with BPH. In men with male pattern baldness, the balding scalp contains miniaturized hair follicles and increased amounts of DHT. Finasteride decreases scalp and serum DHT concentrations in these men.
Therapeutic effect: relieves symptoms of BPH and reduces hair loss and promotes hair growth.

Indications and dosage

▶ **Symptomatic BPH.** *Adults:* 5 mg P.O. daily.
▶ **Male pattern baldness (androgenetic alopecia).** *Adult men only:* 1 mg P.O. daily.

Adverse reactions

GU: impotence, decreased volume of ejaculate.
Other: decreased libido.

Interactions

Drug-drug. *Theophylline:* may increase theophylline clearance and decrease theophylline half-life. Monitor theophylline levels.

Contraindications and precautions

• Contraindicated in patients with hypersensitivity to drug.

• Drug is not indicated for use in women or children.

NURSING CONSIDERATIONS

☕ Assessment
• Before therapy, assess patient's BPH and evaluate him for conditions that might mimic BPH, including hypotonic bladder; prostate cancer, infection, or stricture; or relevant neurologic conditions. Carefully monitor patient who has large residual urine volume or severely diminished urine flow. These patients may not be candidates for finasteride therapy.
• Evaluate patient for improvement in BPH symptoms.
• Anticipate periodic digital rectal examinations.
• Be alert for adverse reactions and drug interactions.
• Carefully evaluate sustained increases in serum prostate-specific antigen levels, which could indicate noncompliance.
• Evaluate patient's and family's knowledge of drug therapy.

⊕ Nursing diagnoses
• Altered urinary elimination related to BPH
• Altered sexuality patterns related to drug-induced impotence
• Knowledge deficit related to drug therapy

⟩ Planning and implementation
• Because it's impossible to identify which patients will respond to finasteride, know that minimum of 6 months of therapy may be necessary.
Patient teaching
• Warn female patient who is or may become pregnant not to handle crushed tablets because of risk of adverse effects on male fetus.
• Caution male patient whose sexual partner is or may become pregnant to discontinue drug or take precautions to avoid exposing her to his semen.

• Reassure patient that although drug may decrease volume of ejaculate, it doesn't appear to impair normal sexual function. However, impotence and decreased libido have occurred in fewer than 4% of patients.
• Tell patient taking drug for male pattern baldness that he may not notice any results until 3 months or longer of use.

☑ Evaluation
• Patient's BPH symptoms diminish.
• Patient states appropriate ways to manage sexual dysfunction.
• Patient and family state understanding of drug therapy.

---

flavoxate hydrochloride
(flah-VOKS-ayt high-droh-KLOR-ighd)
Urispas

Pharmacologic class: flavone derivative
Therapeutic class: urinary tract spasmolytic
Pregnancy risk category: B

How supplied
Tablets: 100 mg

Pharmacokinetics
Absorption: absorbed well from GI tract.
Distribution: unknown.
Metabolism: unknown.
Excretion: excreted in urine.

Route	Onset	Peak	Duration
P.O.	Unknown	≤ 2 hr	Unknown

Pharmacodynamics
Chemical effect: produces direct spasmolytic effect on smooth muscles of urinary tract and provides some local anesthesia and analgesia.
Therapeutic effect: relieves urinary tract symptoms.

Reactions may be *common*, uncommon, *life-threatening*, or COMMON AND LIFE-THREATENING.

Indications and dosage

▶ **Symptomatic relief of dysuria, urinary frequency and urgency, nocturia, incontinence, and suprapubic pain associated with urologic disorders.** *Adults and children over age 12:* 100 to 200 mg P.O. t.i.d. or q.i.d.

Adverse reactions

CNS: *confusion* (especially in elderly patients), nervousness, dizziness, headache, drowsiness.
CV: tachycardia, palpitations.
EENT: *blurred vision,* disturbed eye accommodation, increased ocular tension.
GI: dry mouth, nausea, vomiting.
GU: dysuria.
Hematologic: eosinophilia, *leukopenia.*
Skin: urticaria, dermatoses.
Other: fever.

Interactions

Drug-lifestyle. *Exercise, hot weather:* may precipitate heat stroke. Take precautions to avoid becoming overheated.

Contraindications and precautions

• Contraindicated in patients with pyloric or duodenal obstruction, obstructive intestinal lesions or ileus, achalasia, GI hemorrhage, or obstructive uropathies of lower urinary tract.
• Use cautiously in patients suspected of having glaucoma and in pregnant or breast-feeding women.
• Safety of drug has not been established in children age 12 and younger.

NURSING CONSIDERATIONS

Assessment
• Assess patient's urinary function before therapy, and reassess regularly thereafter.
• Check history for other drug use before giving drugs with adverse anticholinergic reactions. Such reactions may be intensified by flavoxate.
• Be alert for adverse reactions.
• Evaluate patient's and family's knowledge of drug therapy.

Nursing diagnoses
• Altered urinary elimination related to underlying GU disorder
• Risk for injury related to drug-induced adverse reactions
• Knowledge deficit related to drug therapy

Planning and implementation
• Dosage may be reduced if symptoms improve.
Patient teaching
• Warn patient to avoid hazardous activities until CNS effects of drug are known.
• Tell patient to notify doctor of adverse reactions or persistent symptoms.

Evaluation
• Patient regains normal urinary elimination pattern.
• Patient does not experience injury from adverse reactions.
• Patient and family state understanding of drug therapy.

flecainide acetate
(FLEH-kay-nighd AS-ih-tayt)
Tambocor

Pharmacologic class: benzamide derivative
Therapeutic class: antiarrhythmic
Pregnancy risk category: C

How supplied

Tablets: 50 mg, 100 mg, 150 mg
Injection: 10 mg/ml ◊

Pharmacokinetics

Absorption: rapidly and almost completely absorbed from GI tract; bioavailability is 85% to 90%.
Distribution: thought to be well distributed throughout body. Only about 40% binds to plasma proteins.
Metabolism: metabolized in liver to inactive metabolites. About 30% of oral dose escapes metabolism.

Excretion: excreted in urine. *Half-life:* about 20 hours.

Route	Onset	Peak	Duration
P.O.	Unknown	2-3 hr	Unknown
I.V.	Immediate	Immediate	Unknown

Pharmacodynamics

Chemical effect: decreases excitability, conduction velocity, and automaticity as result of slowed atrial, AV node, His-Purkinje system, and intraventricular conduction and causes slight but significant prolongation of refractory periods in these tissues.
Therapeutic effect: restores normal sinus rhythm.

Indications and dosage

▶ **Paroxysmal supraventricular tachycardia, paroxysmal atrial fibrillation or flutter in patients without structural heart disease; life-threatening ventricular arrhythmias, such as sustained ventricular tachycardia.** *Adults:* for paroxysmal supraventricular tachycardia, 50 mg P.O. q 12 hours. Increased in increments of 50 mg b.i.d. q 4 days until efficacy is achieved. Maximum daily dosage is 300 mg. In patients with renal impairment (creatinine clearance 35 ml/minute), initial dosage is 100 mg once daily or 50 mg b.i.d. For life-threatening ventricular arrhythmias, 100 mg P.O. q 12 hours. Increase in increments of 50 mg b.i.d. q 4 days until efficacy is achieved. Maximum dosage is 400 mg daily for most patients. Initial dosage for patients with heart failure is 50 mg P.O. q 12 hours. Where available, flecainide may be given to adults by I.V. injection: 2 mg/kg I.V. push over not less than 10 minutes; or dilute dose and give as infusion.

Adverse reactions

CNS: *dizziness, headache,* fatigue, tremor, anxiety, insomnia, depression, malaise, paresthesia, ataxia, vertigo, *light-headedness, syncope,* asthenia.

CV: *new or worsened arrhythmias,* chest pain, *heart failure, cardiac arrest,* palpitations.
EENT: *blurred vision and other visual disturbances.*
GI: nausea, constipation, abdominal pain, dyspepsia, vomiting, diarrhea, anorexia.
Other: *dyspnea,* edema, skin rash, flushing, fever.

Interactions

Drug-drug. *Amiodarone, cimetidine:* altered pharmacokinetics. Watch for toxicity.
Cardiac glycosides: may increase plasma digoxin levels by 15% to 25%. Monitor serum digoxin levels.
Disopyramide, verapamil: negative inotropic properties may be additive with flecainide; avoid concurrent administration.
Propranolol, other beta blockers: both flecainide and propranolol plasma levels increase by 20% to 30%. Monitor for propranolol and flecainide toxicity.
Urine acidifying and alkalinizing agents: extremes of urine pH may substantially alter excretion of flecainide. Monitor for flecainide toxicity or decreased effectiveness.
Drug-lifestyle. *Smoking:* lowered flecainide serum concentrations. Monitor closely.

Contraindications and precautions

• Contraindicated in patients with cardiogenic shock or hypersensitivity to drug and in those with preexisting second- or third-degree AV block or right bundle branch block when associated with left hemiblock (in absence of artificial pacemaker).
• Breast-feeding is not recommended during drug use.
• Use cautiously in patients with preexisting heart failure, cardiomyopathy, severe renal or hepatic disease, prolonged QT interval, sick sinus syndrome, or

---

Reactions may be *common,* uncommon, *life-threatening,* or COMMON AND LIFE-THREATENING.

blood dyscrasia. Also use cautiously in pregnant women.
• Safety of drug has not been established in children.

NURSING CONSIDERATIONS

🔍 Assessment
• Obtain assessment of patient's arrhythmia before therapy.
• Monitor effectiveness by continuous ECG monitoring initially; long-term oral administration requires regular ECG readings.
• Monitor serum flecainide levels, especially in patient with renal failure or heart failure. Therapeutic levels range from 0.2 to 1 mcg/ml. Incidence of adverse effects increases when trough blood levels exceed 1 mcg/ml.
• Monitor serum potassium levels regularly.
• Be alert for adverse reactions and drug interactions.
• Evaluate patient's and family's knowledge of drug therapy.

🔷 Nursing diagnoses
• Decreased cardiac output related to underlying arrhythmia
• Altered protection related to drug-induced new arrhythmias
• Knowledge deficit related to drug therapy

▷ Planning and implementation
• When used to prevent ventricular arrhythmias, flecainide should be reserved for patient with documented life-threatening arrhythmias.
• Check that pacing threshold was determined 1 week before and after initiating therapy in patient with pacemaker because flecainide can alter endocardial pacing thresholds.
• Correct hypokalemia or hyperkalemia as ordered before giving flecainide because these electrolyte disturbances may alter effect of flecainide.
P.O. use: Follow normal protocol.

I.V. use: When administering by I.V. push, give over at least 10 minutes. For I.V. infusion, mix only with D_5W.
• Dosage adjustments should be made only once every 3 to 4 days.
• Twice-daily dosing for flecainide enhances patient compliance.
• Because of flecainide's long half-life, its full effect may take 3 to 5 days. Give concomitant I.V. lidocaine as ordered for first several days.
• Keep emergency equipment nearby.
• If ECG disturbances occur, withhold drug, obtain rhythm strip, and notify doctor immediately.
Patient teaching
• Stress importance of taking oral drug exactly as prescribed.
• Warn patient against hazardous activities that require alertness or good vision if adverse CNS or visual reactions occur.
• Tell patient to limit fluid and sodium intake to minimize heart failure or fluid retention and to weigh himself daily. Urge him to report sudden weight gain promptly.

☑ Evaluation
• Patient regains normal cardiac output with abolishment of underlying arrhythmia after drug therapy.
• Patient does not develop new arrhythmias.
• Patient and family state understanding of drug therapy.

floxuridine
(floks-YOOR-eh-deen)
FUDR

Pharmacologic class: antimetabolite (cell cycle–phase specific, S phase)
Therapeutic class: antineoplastic
Pregnancy risk category: D

How supplied
Injection: 500-mg vials (50 mg/ml in 10-ml vials or 100 mg/ml in 5-ml vials)

Pharmacokinetics

Absorption: not applicable.
Distribution: drug crosses blood-brain barrier to limited extent.
Metabolism: metabolized to fluorouracil in liver.
Excretion: about 60% excreted through lungs as carbon dioxide; small amount excreted by kidneys as unchanged drug and metabolites.

Route	Onset	Peak	Duration
Intra-arterial	Unknown	Unknown	Unknown

Pharmacodynamics

Chemical effect: inhibits DNA synthesis.
Therapeutic effect: hinders growth of GI adenocarcinoma cells that have spread to liver.

Indications and dosage

▶ **GI adenocarcinoma metastatic to liver.** *Adults:* 0.1 to 0.6 mg/kg daily by intra-arterial infusion for 14 to 21 days or until toxicity occurs; or 0.4 to 0.6 mg/kg daily into hepatic artery.

Adverse reactions

CNS: malaise, weakness, headache, lethargy, disorientation, confusion, euphoria.
CV: *myocardial ischemia,* angina.
EENT: blurred vision, nystagmus, photophobia, epistaxis.
GI: *anorexia, stomatitis, abdominal pain, nausea, vomiting, diarrhea, bleeding, enteritis,* GI ulceration, intra- and extrahepatic biliary sclerosis, acalculous cholecystitis.
Hematologic: *leukopenia, anemia, thrombocytopenia, agranulocytosis.*
Skin: *erythema,* dermatitis, pruritus, rash, *alopecia,* photosensitivity.
Other: *anaphylaxis,* thrombophlebitis, fever.

Interactions

Drug-lifestyle. *Sun exposure:* may increase skin reaction. Take precautions.

Contraindications and precautions

• Contraindicated in patients with poor nutritional state, bone marrow suppression, or serious infection.
• Drug is not recommended for use in pregnant or breast-feeding women.
• Use cautiously following high-dose pelvic radiation therapy or use of alkylating agents, and in patients with impaired hepatic or renal function.
• Safety of drug has not been established in children.

NURSING CONSIDERATIONS

⚕ Assessment
• Obtain assessment of patient's neoplastic disorder before therapy, and reassess regularly throughout therapy.
• Monitor fluid intake and output, CBC, and renal and hepatic function.
• Be alert for adverse reactions.
• Evaluate patient's and family's knowledge of drug therapy.

Nursing diagnoses
• Altered health maintenance related to drug therapy
• Altered protection related to immunosuppression
• Knowledge deficit related to drug therapy

Planning and implementation
• Follow institutional policy to reduce risks. Preparation and administration of parenteral form are associated with carcinogenic, mutagenic, and teratogenic risks for personnel.
• Reconstitute with sterile water for injection. To prepare infusion, dilute in D_5W or 0.9% NaCl solution.
• Use infusion pump with intra-arterial infusions.
• Check line for bleeding, blockage, displacement, or leakage.
• Refrigerated solution is stable for no more than 2 weeks.
• Know that use of antacid eases but won't prevent GI distress.

Reactions may be *common*, uncommon, *life-threatening*, or COMMON AND LIFE-THREATENING.

• Notify doctor immediately of severe adverse skin and GI reactions.

• Discontinue drug and notify doctor if WBC count falls below 3,500/mm³ or if platelet count falls below 100,000/mm³.

Patient teaching
• Warn patient to watch for signs of infection and bleeding. Teach infection-control and bleeding precautions.

• Advise female patient of childbearing age to avoid becoming pregnant during therapy and to consult with doctor before becoming pregnant.

• Instruct patient to notify doctor if adverse reactions occur.

🔳 **Evaluation**
• Patient exhibits positive response to drug therapy.

• Patient does not develop infection or bleeding complications.

• Patient and family state understanding of drug therapy.

fluconazole
(floo-KON-uh-zohl)
Diflucan

Pharmacologic class: bis-triazole derivative
Therapeutic class: antifungal
Pregnancy risk category: C

How supplied

Tablets: 50 mg, 100 mg, 150 mg, 200 mg
Powder for oral suspension: 10 mg/ml
Injection: 200 mg/100 ml, 400 mg/200 ml

Pharmacokinetics

Absorption: rapid and complete after P.O. administration.

Distribution: well distributed to various sites, including CNS, saliva, sputum, blister fluid, urine, normal skin, nails, and blister skin. Drug is 12% protein-bound.

Metabolism: partially metabolized.

Excretion: primarily excreted by kidneys; over 80% excreted unchanged in urine.

Route	Onset	Peak	Duration
P.O.	Unknown	1-2 hr	Unknown
I.V.	Immediate	Immediate	Unknown

Pharmacodynamics

Chemical effect: inhibits fungal cytochrome P-450, an enzyme responsible for fungal sterol synthesis, and weakens fungal cell walls.

Therapeutic effect: hinders fungal growth. Spectrum of activity includes *Cryptococcus neoformans, Candida* species (including systemic *C. albicans*), *Aspergillus flavus, Aspergillus fumigatus, Coccidioides immitis,* and *Histoplasma capsulatum.*

Indications and dosage

▶ **Oropharyngeal and esophageal candidiasis.** *Adults:* 200 mg P.O. or I.V. on first day, followed by 100 mg once daily. Higher doses (up to 400 mg daily) have been used for esophageal disease. Patients should continue drug for 2 weeks after symptoms resolve. *Children:* 6 mg/kg P.O. or I.V. on first day, followed by 3 mg/kg once daily for at least 2 weeks.

▶ **Vulvovaginal candidiasis.** *Adults:* 150 mg P.O. as a single dose.

▶ **Systemic candidiasis.** *Adults:* 400 mg P.O. or I.V. on first day, followed by 200 mg once daily. Treatment should continue for at least 4 weeks or for 2 weeks after symptoms resolve. *Children:* 6 to 12 mg/kg/day P.O. or I.V.

▶ **Cryptococcal meningitis.** *Adults:* 400 mg P.O. or I.V. on first day, followed by 200 mg once daily. Higher doses (up to 400 mg daily) may be used. Treatment should continue for 10 to 12 weeks after CSF cultures are negative. *Children:* 12 mg/kg/day P.O. or I.V. on first day, followed by 6 mg/kg/daily for 10 to 12 weeks after CSF culture becomes negative.

▶ **Prevention of candidiasis in bone marrow transplant.** *Adults:* 400 mg. P.O. or I.V. once daily. Start prophylaxis several days before anticipated granulocytopenia. Continue therapy for 7 days after neutrophil count rises above 1,000 cells/mm³.

▶ **Suppression of relapse of cryptococcal meningitis in patients with AIDS.** *Adults:* 200 mg P.O. or I.V. daily. *Children:* 3 to 6 mg/kg/day P.O. *In patients with renal failure:* if creatinine clearance is below 50 ml/minute, dosage is reduced by 50% in patients not receiving dialysis. Patients receiving hemodialysis should receive 100% of usual dose after each session.

Adverse reactions

CNS: headache.
GI: *nausea,* vomiting, abdominal pain, diarrhea.
Hepatic: *hepatotoxicity* (rare), elevated liver enzymes.
Skin: rash, *Stevens-Johnson syndrome* (rare).
Other: *anaphylaxis.*

Interactions

Drug-drug. *Cyclosporine, phenytoin:* may increase plasma concentrations of these drugs. Monitor serum cyclosporine or phenytoin levels.
Isoniazid, phenytoin, rifampin, valproic acid, oral sulfonylureas: increased risk of elevated hepatic transaminases. Monitor closely.
Oral antidiabetic agents (tolbutamide, glyburide, glipizide): may increase plasma concentrations of these drugs. Monitor for enhanced hypoglycemic effect.
Rifampin: enhanced metabolism of fluconazole. Monitor for lack of response.
Theophylline: decreased theophylline clearance. Monitor serum levels.
Warfarin: increased risk of bleeding. Monitor PT and INR.
Zidovudine: zidovudine activity may be increased. Monitor closely.
Drug-food. *Caffeine:* may increase caffeine plasma levels. Ofloxacin and lomefloxacin are alternate drugs.

Contraindications and precautions

• Contraindicated in patients with hypersensitivity to drug.
• Drug is not recommended for use in breast-feeding women.
• Although no information exists regarding cross-sensitivity, use cautiously in patients with hypersensitivity to other antifungal azole compounds. Also use cautiously in pregnant women.

NURSING CONSIDERATIONS

Assessment
• Obtain assessment of patient's fungal infection before therapy, and reassess regularly throughout therapy.
• Periodically monitor liver function during prolonged therapy, as ordered. Although adverse hepatic effects are rare, they can be serious.
• Be alert for adverse reactions and drug interactions.
• Monitor patient's hydration status if adverse GI reactions occur.
• Evaluate patient's and family's knowledge of drug therapy.

Nursing diagnoses
• Infection related to presence of susceptible fungi
• Risk for fluid volume deficit related to adverse GI reactions
• Knowledge deficit related to drug therapy

Planning and implementation
P.O. use: Follow normal protocol.
I.V. use: Do not remove protective overwrap from I.V. bags of fluconazole until just before use, to ensure product sterility. Plastic container may show some opacity from moisture absorbed during sterilization. This is normal, will not affect drug, and will diminish over time.
– Administer by continuous infusion at rate not to exceed 200 mg/hour. Use infusion pump. To prevent air embolism, do not connect in series with other infusions. Do not add any other drugs to solution.

• If patient develops mild rash, monitor closely. Discontinue drug if lesions progress, and notify doctor.
Patient teaching
• Urge patient to adhere to regimen and to return for follow-up.
• Tell patient to report adverse reactions to doctor.

☑ **Evaluation**
• Patient is free from infection.
• Patient maintains adequate hydration.
• Patient and family state understanding of drug therapy.

flucytosine (5-fluorocytosine, 5-FC)
(floo-SIGH-toh-seen)
Ancobon, Ancotil◊

Pharmacologic class: fluorinated pyrimidine
Therapeutic class: antifungal
Pregnancy risk category: C

How supplied
Capsules: 250 mg, 500 mg

Pharmacokinetics
Absorption: from 75% to 90% of dose is absorbed; food decreases absorption rate.
Distribution: distributed widely into liver, kidneys, spleen, heart, bronchial secretions, joints, peritoneal fluid, and aqueous humor. CSF levels vary from 60% to 100% of serum levels. Drug is 2% to 4% bound to plasma proteins.
Metabolism: only small amounts of drug are metabolized.
Excretion: about 75% to 95% excreted unchanged in urine; less than 10% excreted unchanged in feces. *Half-life:* 2½ to 6 hours.

Route	Onset	Peak	Duration
P.O.	Unknown	1-2 hr	Unknown

Pharmacodynamics
Chemical effect: unknown; appears to penetrate fungal cells—where it is converted to fluorouracil, a known metabolic antagonist—and cause defective protein synthesis.
Therapeutic effect: hinders fungal growth. Spectrum of activity includes some strains of *Cryptococcus* and *Candida.*

Indications and dosage
▶ **Severe fungal infections caused by susceptible strains of *Candida* (including septicemia, endocarditis, urinary tract and pulmonary infections) and *Cryptococcus* (meningitis, pulmonary infection, and possible urinary tract infections).** *Adults and children weighing over 50 kg (110 lb):* 50 to 150 mg/kg daily P.O. in divided doses given q 6 hours. *Adults and children below 50 kg:* 1.5 to 4.5 g/m²/day P.O. in four divided doses. Severe infections may require doses up to 250 mg/kg.

Adverse reactions
CNS: dizziness, confusion, headache, vertigo, sedation, fatigue, weakness, hallucinations, psychosis, ataxia, hearing loss, paresthesia, parkinsonism, peripheral neuropathy.
CV: *cardiac arrest.*
GI: nausea, vomiting, diarrhea, abdominal pain, dry mouth, duodenal ulcer, *hemorrhage,* ulcerative colitis.
GU: azotemia, elevated BUN and creatinine levels, crystalluria, *renal failure.*
Hematologic: anemia, eosinophilia, *leukopenia, bone marrow suppression, thrombocytopenia, agranulocytosis, aplastic anemia.*
Hepatic: elevated liver enzymes (ALT, AST); elevated serum alkaline phosphatase, jaundice.
Respiratory: *respiratory arrest,* chest pain, dyspnea.
Skin: occasional rash, pruritus, urticaria, photosensitivity.
Other: hypoglycemia, hypokalemia.

Interactions

Drug-drug. *Amphotericin B:* synergistic effects and possibly enhanced toxicity when used together. Monitor patient.

Contraindications and precautions

• Contraindicated in patients with hypersensitivity to drug.
• Use with extreme caution in those with impaired hepatic or renal function or bone marrow suppression.
• Use cautiously in pregnant women.

NURSING CONSIDERATIONS

▨ Assessment
• Obtain assessment of patient's fungal infection before therapy, and reassess regularly throughout therapy.
• Before therapy, obtain hematologic tests and renal and liver function studies. Ensure that susceptibility tests establishing that organism is flucytosine-sensitive are on chart.
• Monitor blood, liver, and renal function studies frequently; obtain susceptibility tests weekly, as ordered, to monitor drug resistance.
• If possible, regularly perform blood level assays of drug, as ordered, to maintain flucytosine at therapeutic level (25 to 120 mcg/ml). Higher blood levels may be toxic.
• Be alert for adverse reactions and drug interactions.
• Monitor patient's hydration status if adverse GI reactions occur.
• Evaluate patient's and family's knowledge of drug therapy.

⊞ Nursing diagnoses
• Infection related to presence of susceptible fungi
• Risk for fluid volume deficit related to adverse GI reactions
• Knowledge deficit related to drug therapy

▣ Planning and implementation
• Give capsules over 15 minutes to reduce adverse GI reactions.
Patient teaching
• Inform patient that therapeutic response may take weeks or months.
• Tell patient how to take capsules.
• Warn patient to avoid hazardous activities requiring mental alertness if adverse CNS reactions occur.

☑ Evaluation
• Patient is free from infection.
• Patient maintains adequate hydration throughout drug therapy.
• Patient and family state understanding of drug therapy.

---

fludarabine phosphate
(floo-DAR-uh-been FOS-fayt)
Fludara

Pharmacologic class: antimetabolite
Therapeutic class: antineoplastic
Pregnancy risk category: D

How supplied

Powder for injection: 50 mg

Pharmacokinetics

Absorption: not applicable.
Distribution: unknown.
Metabolism: rapidly dephosphorylated and then phosphorylated intracellularly to its active metabolite.
Excretion: 23% is excreted in urine as unchanged active metabolite. *Half-life:* about 10 hours.

Route	Onset	Peak	Duration
I.V.	7-21 hr	Unknown	Unknown

Pharmacodynamics

Chemical effect: unknown; actions may be multifaceted. After conversion to its active metabolite, fludarabine interferes with DNA synthesis by inhibiting DNA

---

polymerase alpha, ribonucleotide reductase, and DNA primase.
Therapeutic effect: kills susceptible cancer cells.

Indications and dosage

▶ **B-cell chronic lymphocytic leukemia (CLL) in patients who either have not responded or have responded inadequately to at least one standard alkylating agent regimen.** *Adults:* 25 mg/m² I.V. over 30 minutes for 5 consecutive days. Cycle repeated q 28 days.

Adverse reactions

CNS: diaphoresis, *fatigue, malaise, weakness, paresthesia,* headache, peripheral neuropathy, sleep disorder, depression, cerebellar syndrome, *CVA,* transient ischemic attack, agitation, *confusion; coma, death* (with very high doses).
CV: *edema,* angina, phlebitis, *arrhythmias, heart failure, MI,* supraventricular tachycardia, deep venous thrombosis, *aneurysm, hemorrhage.*
EENT: *visual disturbances,* hearing loss, delayed blindness (with high doses), sinusitis, pharyngitis, epistaxis.
GI: *nausea, vomiting, diarrhea,* constipation, *anorexia,* stomatitis, *GI bleeding,* esophagitis, mucositis.
GU: dysuria, *urinary infection,* urinary hesitancy, proteinuria, hematuria, *renal failure.*
Hematologic: *hemolytic anemia,* MYELOSUPPRESSION.
Hepatic: *liver failure,* cholelithiasis.
Musculoskeletal: myalgia.
Respiratory: *cough, pneumonia, dyspnea, upper respiratory infection,* allergic pneumonitis, hemoptysis, hypoxia, bronchitis.
Skin: alopecia, *rash,* pruritus, seborrhea.
Other: *fever, chills,* INFECTION, pain, tumor lysis syndrome, *anaphylaxis,* hyperglycemia, dehydration, hyperuricemia, hyperphosphatemia.

Interactions

Drug-drug. *Other myelosuppressants:* increased toxicity. Avoid concomitant use.
Pentostatin: concurrent use increases risk of pulmonary toxicity. Avoid concomitant administration.

Contraindications and precautions

• Contraindicated in patients with hypersensitivity to drug or its components.
• Use with extreme caution and only when necessary in pregnant women.
• Use cautiously in patients with renal insufficiency.
• Safety of drug has not been established in breast-feeding women and in children.

NURSING CONSIDERATIONS

⚐ Assessment
• Assess patient's underlying condition before therapy, and reassess regularly thereafter.
• Know that careful hematologic monitoring is required, especially of neutrophil and platelet counts. Bone marrow suppression can be severe.
• Be alert for adverse reactions and drug interactions.
• Evaluate patient's and family's knowledge of drug therapy.

⚐ Nursing diagnoses
• Altered health maintenance related to presence of leukemia
• Altered protection related to drug-induced immunosuppression
• Knowledge deficit related to drug therapy

⚐ Planning and implementation
• Follow institutional policy to reduce risks. Preparation and administration of parenteral form are associated with mutagenic, teratogenic, and carcinogenic risks for personnel.
• To prepare solution, add 2 ml of sterile water for injection to solid cake of drug. Dissolution should occur within 15 sec-

onds; each milliliter will contain 25 mg of drug. Dilute further in 100 or 125 ml of D$_5$W or 0.9% NaCl injection. Use within 8 hours of reconstitution.
• Optimal duration of therapy is not yet determined. Current recommendations suggest three additional cycles after achieving maximal response before discontinuing therapy.
• Store drug in refrigerator at 36° to 46° F (2° to 8° C).
Patient teaching
• Warn patient to watch for signs of infection and bleeding.
• Advise female patient of childbearing age to avoid becoming pregnant during therapy and to consult with doctor before becoming pregnant.
• Tell patient to notify doctor if adverse reactions occur.

☑ **Evaluation**
• Patient exhibits positive response to fludarabine therapy.
• Patient does not develop serious infections or bleeding complications.
• Patient and family state understanding of drug therapy.

fludrocortisone acetate
(floo-droh-KOR-tuh-sohn AS-ih-tayt)
Florinef

Pharmacologic class: mineralocorticoid, glucocorticoid
Therapeutic class: mineralocorticoid replacement therapy
Pregnancy risk category: C

How supplied
Tablets: 0.1 mg

Pharmacokinetics
Absorption: absorbed readily from GI tract.
Distribution: distributed to muscle, liver, skin, intestines, and kidneys. It is exten-sively bound to plasma proteins. Only unbound portion is active.
Metabolism: metabolized in liver to inactive metabolites.
Excretion: excreted in urine; insignificant quantities are excreted in feces.
Half-life: 18 to 36 hours.

Route	Onset	Peak	Duration
P.O.	Varies	Varies	1-2 days

Pharmacodynamics
Chemical effect: increases sodium reabsorption and potassium and hydrogen secretion at nephrons' distal convoluted tubule.
Therapeutic effect: increases sodium levels and decreases potassium and hydrogen levels.

Indications and dosage
▶ **Adrenal insufficiency (partial replacement), adrenogenital syndrome.**
Adults: 0.1 to 0.2 mg P.O. daily.

Adverse reactions
CV: *sodium and water retention,* hypertension, cardiac hypertrophy, edema, *heart failure.*
Skin: bruising, diaphoresis, urticaria, allergic rash.
Other: hypokalemia.

Interactions
Drug-drug. *Barbiturates, phenytoin, rifampin:* increased clearance of fludrocortisone acetate. Monitor for effect.
Potassium-depleting drugs (such as thiazide diuretics): enhanced potassiumwasting effects of fludrocortisone. Monitor serum potassium levels.
Drug-food. *Sodium-containing medications or foods:* may increase blood pressure. Sodium intake may need to be adjusted.

Contraindications and precautions
• Contraindicated in patients with systemic fungal infections or hypersensitivity to drug.

Reactions may be *common,* uncommon, *life-threatening,* or COMMON AND LIFE-THREATENING.

• Use cautiously in patients with hypo-thyroidism, cirrhosis, ocular herpes simplex, emotional instability and psychotic tendencies, nonspecific ulcerative colitis, diverticulitis, fresh intestinal anastomoses, active or latent peptic ulcer, renal insufficiency, hypertension, osteoporosis, and myasthenia gravis.
• Long-term use in children may delay growth and maturation.

NURSING CONSIDERATIONS

⚕ Assessment
• Assess patient's underlying condition before therapy, and reassess regularly thereafter.
• Monitor patient's blood pressure, weight, and serum electrolyte levels.
• Be alert for adverse reactions and drug interactions.
• Evaluate patient's and family's knowledge of drug therapy.

⊞ Nursing diagnoses
• Altered health maintenance related to underlying adrenal condition
• Fluid volume excess related to drug-induced adverse reactions
• Knowledge deficit related to drug therapy

▧ Planning and implementation
• Drug is used with cortisone or hydrocortisone in patients with adrenal insufficiency.
• If hypertension occurs, notify doctor, who may lower dosage by 50%.
• Be aware that potassium supplements may be needed.
Patient teaching
• Tell patient to notify doctor of worsened symptoms, such as hypotension, weakness, cramping, and palpitations.
• Warn patient that mild peripheral edema is common.

☑ Evaluation
• Patient's health is improved.

• Patient does not develop sodium and water retention.
• Patient and family state understanding of drug therapy.

---

flumazenil
(floo-MAZ-ih-nil)
Romazicon

Pharmacologic class: benzodiazepine antagonist
Therapeutic class: antidote
Pregnancy risk category: C

How supplied
Injection: 0.1 mg/ml in 5- and 10-ml multiple-dose vials

Pharmacokinetics
Absorption: not applicable.
Distribution: redistributes rapidly; 50% bound to plasma proteins.
Metabolism: metabolized by liver. Ingestion of food during I.V. infusion enhances extraction of drug from plasma, probably by increasing hepatic blood flow.
Excretion: about 90% to 95% appears in urine as metabolites; remainder excreted in feces. *Half-life:* about 54 minutes.

Route	Onset	Peak	Duration
I.V.	Unknown	Unknown	Unknown

Pharmacodynamics
Chemical effect: competitively inhibits actions of benzodiazepines on gamma-aminobutyric acid–benzodiazepine receptor complex.
Therapeutic effect: awakens patient from sedative effects of benzodiazepines.

Indications and dosage
▶ **Complete or partial reversal of sedative effects of benzodiazepines after anesthesia or short diagnostic procedures (conscious sedation).** *Adults:* initially, 0.2 mg I.V. over 15 seconds. If pa-

---

tient does not reach desired level of consciousness after 45 seconds, dose is repeated. Repeated at 1-minute intervals until cumulative dose of 1 mg has been given (initial dose plus four additional doses), if needed. Most patients respond after 0.6 to 1 mg of drug. In case of resedation, dosage may be repeated after 20 minutes; however, no more than 1 mg should be given at any one time and no more than 3 mg/hour.

▶ **Suspected benzodiazepine overdose.** *Adults:* initially, 0.2 mg I.V. over 15 seconds. If patient does not reach desired level of consciousness after 30 seconds, 0.3 mg is administered over 30 seconds. If patient still does not respond adequately, 0.5 mg is administered over 30 seconds; 0.5-mg doses are repeated as needed at 1-minute intervals until cumulative dose of 3 mg has been given. Most patients suffering from benzodiazepine overdose respond to cumulative doses between 1 and 3 mg; rarely, patients who respond partially after 3 mg may require additional doses. No more than 5 mg over 5 minutes should be given initially. Sedation that persists after this dosage is unlikely to be caused by benzodiazepines. In case of resedation, dosage may be repeated after 20 minutes; however, no more than 1 mg should be given at any one time and no more than 3 mg/hour.

Adverse reactions

CNS: *diaphoresis, dizziness, abnormal or blurred vision, headache,* **seizures,** agitation, emotional lability, tremor, insomnia.
CV: *arrhythmias,* cutaneous vasodilation, palpitations.
GI: *nausea, vomiting.*
Respiratory: dyspnea, hyperventilation.
Other: *pain at injection site.*

Interactions

Drug-drug. *Antidepressants; drugs that can cause seizures or arrhythmias:* seizures or arrhythmias can develop after effect of benzodiazepine overdose is re-

moved. Use with caution, if at all, in cases of mixed overdose.

Contraindications and precautions

• Contraindicated in patients hypersensitive to drug or benzodiazepines; in patients who show evidence of serious cyclic antidepressant overdose; and in those who received benzodiazepine to treat potentially life-threatening condition (such as status epilepticus).
• Use cautiously in patients at high risk for developing seizures; patients who recently have received multiple doses of parenteral benzodiazepine; patients displaying signs of seizure activity; patients who may be at risk for unrecognized benzodiazepine dependence, such as intensive care unit patients; patients with head injury; psychiatric or alcohol-dependent patients; and in pregnant or breast-feeding women.
• Safety of drug has not been established in children.

NURSING CONSIDERATIONS

🔖 Assessment
• Obtain assessment of patient's sedation before therapy.
• Assess patient's level of consciousness frequently.
• Be alert for adverse reactions and drug interactions.
• Monitor patient closely for resedation that may occur after reversal of benzodiazepine effects; flumazenil's duration of action is shorter than that of all benzodiazepines. Monitor closely after long-acting benzodiazepines, such as diazepam, or high doses of short-acting benzodiazepines, such as 10 mg of midazolam. In most cases, severe resedation is unlikely in patient who fails to show signs of resedation 2 hours after 1-mg dose of flumazenil.
• Monitor patient's ECG for evidence of arrhythmias.
• Evaluate patient's and family's knowledge of drug therapy.

Reactions may be *common,* uncommon, *life-threatening*, or COMMON AND LIFE-THREATENING.

Nursing diagnoses
• Altered protection related to sedated state
• Decreased cardiac output related to drug-induced seizures
• Knowledge deficit related to drug therapy

Planning and implementation
• Administer drug by direct injection or dilute with compatible solution. Discard within 24 hours unused drug that has been drawn into syringe or diluted.
• Administer drug into I.V. line in large vein with free-flowing I.V. solution to minimize pain at injection site. Compatible solutions include D_5W, lactated Ringer's injection, and 0.9% NaCl.
• Notify doctor if arrhythmias or other adverse reactions occur and be prepared to treat accordingly.
Patient teaching
• Warn patient not to perform hazardous activities, such as operating heavy equipment or driving, within 24 hours of procedure.
• Tell patient to avoid alcohol, CNS depressants, and OTC drugs for 24 hours.
• Give family members important instructions or provide patient with written instructions. Do not expect patient to recall information given in postprocedure period.

Evaluation
• Patient is awake and alert.
• Patient maintains adequate cardiac output.
• Patient and family state understanding of drug therapy.

flunisolide
(floo-NIH-soh-lighd)
AeroBid, AeroBid-M, Bronalide♦ (oral inhalant); Nasalide, Rhinalar Nasal Mist◊ (nasal inhalant)

Pharmacologic class: glucocorticoid

Therapeutic class: anti-inflammatory, antiasthmatic
Pregnancy risk category: C

How supplied
Oral inhalant: 250 mcg/metered spray (at least 100 metered inhalations/container)
Nasal inhalant: 25 mcg/metered spray, 200 doses/bottle◊
Nasal solution: 0.25 mg/ml in pump spray bottle

Pharmacokinetics
Absorption: about 50% of nasally inhaled dose is absorbed systemically. After oral inhalation, about 70% of dose is absorbed from lungs and GI tract. Only about 20% of orally inhaled dose reaches systemic circulation unmetabolized because of extensive metabolism in liver.
Distribution: unknown after intranasal use. After oral inhalation, 10% to 25% of drug is distributed to lungs; remainder is deposited in mouth and swallowed. No evidence exists of tissue storage of drug or its metabolites. When absorbed, it is 50% bound to plasma proteins.
Metabolism: drug that is swallowed undergoes rapid metabolism in liver or GI tract to variety of metabolites, one of which has glucocorticoid activity. Flunisolide and its active metabolite are eventually conjugated in liver to inactive metabolites.
Excretion: unknown for inhalation routes.

Route	Onset	Peak	Duration
Nasal or oral inhalation	1-4 wk	Unknown	Unknown

Pharmacodynamics
Chemical effect: unknown; may stabilize leukocyte lysosomal membranes.
Therapeutic effect: relieves inflammation.

---

*Liquid form contains alcohol   **May contain tartrazine   ♦Canada   ◊Australia   †OTC

Indications and dosage

Oral inhalant
▶ **Steroid-dependent asthma.** *Adults and children age 6 and over:* 2 inhalations (500 mcg) b.i.d. Maximum daily dose is 4 inhalations b.i.d.
Nasal inhalant
▶ **Symptoms of seasonal or perennial rhinitis.** *Adults:* starting dose is 2 sprays (50 mcg) in each nostril b.i.d. Total daily dosage is 200 mcg. If necessary, dosage may be increased to 2 sprays in each nostril t.i.d. Maximum total daily dosage is 8 sprays in each nostril (400 mcg daily). *Children ages 6 to 14:* starting dose is 1 spray (25 mcg) in each nostril t.i.d. or 2 sprays (50 mcg) in each nostril b.i.d. Total daily dosage is 150 to 200 mcg. Maximum total daily dosage is 4 sprays in each nostril (200 mcg daily).

Adverse reactions

CNS: headache, dizziness, irritability, nervousness.
CV: chest pain, edema, palpitations.
EENT: watery eyes, throat irritation, hoarseness, nasopharyngeal fungal infections, *sore throat, nasal congestion; mild, transient nasal burning and stinging,* nasal congestion, nasopharyngeal fungal infection, burning, stinging, dryness, sneezing, watery eyes, epistaxis (with nasal inhalant).
GI: *nausea, vomiting,* dry mouth, *unpleasant taste, upset stomach,* abdominal pain, decreased appetite, *diarrhea.*
Respiratory: *upper respiratory tract infection.*
Skin: pruritus, rash.
Other: *cold symptoms, flu,* fever.

Interactions

None significant.

Contraindications and precautions

• Contraindicated in patients with status asthmaticus, respiratory infections, or hypersensitivity to drug.

• Nasal inhalant should not be used in presence of untreated localized infection involving nasal mucosa.
• Use nasal inhalant cautiously, if at all, in patients with active or quiescent respiratory tract tubercular infections or with untreated fungal, bacterial, or systemic viral or ocular herpes simplex infections. Also use cautiously in patients who recently have had nasal septal ulcers, nasal surgery, or nasal trauma.
• Use cautiously in pregnant or breastfeeding women.
• Safety of drug has not been established in children under age 6.

NURSING CONSIDERATIONS

Assessment
• Assess patient's underlying condition before therapy, and reassess regularly thereafter.
• Be alert for adverse reactions and drug interactions.
• Evaluate patient's and family's knowledge of drug therapy.

Nursing diagnoses
• Altered health maintenance related to underlying condition
• Altered tissue integrity related to adverse EENT reactions
• Knowledge deficit related to drug therapy

Planning and implementation
Oral inhalation use: Not recommended in patients with asthma controlled by bronchodilators or other noncorticosteroids alone, or in those with nonasthmatic bronchial diseases.
– Spacer device may help to ensure proper dosage administration.
Nasal inhalation use: Flunisolide is not effective for acute exacerbations of rhinitis. Decongestants or antihistamines may be needed.
– To instill, shake container before using; have patient blow nose to clear nasal passages; have patient tilt head slightly for-

ward. Insert nozzle into nostril, pointing away from septum. Hold other nostril closed, and then have patient inspire gently and spray. Next, shake container again and repeat in other nostril. Clean nosepiece with warm water if it becomes clogged.
• Store drug between 36° and 86° F (2° and 30° C).
• Withdraw drug slowly, as ordered, in patient who has received long-term oral corticosteroid therapy.
• After withdrawal of systemic corticosteroids, patient still may need supplementation of systemic steroids if he shows signs and symptoms of adrenal insufficiency when exposed to trauma, surgery, or infections.
Patient teaching
Oral inhalant
• Warn patient that drug doesn't relieve acute asthma attacks.
• Advise patient to ensure delivery of proper dose by gently warming canister to room temperature before using. Some patients carry canister in pocket to keep it warm.
• Tell patient who also is using bronchodilator to use it several minutes before flunisolide.
• Instruct patient to allow 1 minute to elapse before repeating inhalations and to hold breath for few seconds to enhance drug action.
• Teach patient to keep inhaler clean and unobstructed. Wash with warm water and dry thoroughly after use.
• Teach patient to check mucous membranes frequently for signs of fungal infection.
• Advise patient to prevent oral fungal infections by gargling or rinsing mouth with water after each inhaler use. Caution patient not to swallow water.
Nasal inhalant
• Explain that drug's therapeutic effects, unlike those of decongestants, are not immediate. Most patients achieve benefit within a few days, but some may require 2 to 3 weeks.

• Advise patient to use drug regularly, as prescribed, because its effectiveness depends on regular use.
• Teach patient how to instill drug.
• Warn patient not to exceed recommended dosage to avoid suppression of hypothalamic-pituitary-adrenal function.
• Tell patient to stop drug and notify doctor if symptoms persist after 3 weeks.

☑ **Evaluation**
• Patient's health improves.
• Patient maintains upper airway and buccal tissue integrity.
• Patient and family state understanding of drug therapy.

fluorouracil
(5-fluorouracil, 5-FU)
(floo-roh-YOOR-uh-sil)
Adrucil, Efudex, Fluoroplex

Pharmacologic class: antimetabolite (cell cycle–phase specific, S phase)
Therapeutic class: antineoplastic
Pregnancy risk category: D

How supplied
Injection: 50 mg/ml
Cream: 1%, 5%
Topical solution: 1%, 2%, 5%

Pharmacokinetics
Absorption: unknown for topical forms.
Distribution: distributes widely into all areas of body water and tissues; crosses blood-brain barrier.
Metabolism: small amount converted in tissues to active metabolite with majority of drug degraded in liver.
Excretion: metabolites primarily excreted through lungs as carbon dioxide; small portion excreted in urine as unchanged drug.

Route	Onset	Peak	Duration
I.V., topical	Unknown	Unknown	Unknown

Pharmacodynamics

Chemical effect: inhibits DNA synthesis.
Therapeutic effect: inhibits cell growth
of selected cancers.

Indications and dosage

▶ **Colon, rectal, breast, stomach, and
pancreatic cancers.** *Adults:* 12 mg/kg
I.V. daily for 4 days; if no toxicity, give
6 mg/kg on 6th, 8th, 10th, and 12th day;
then single weekly maintenance dose of
10 to 15 mg/kg I.V. begun after toxicity
(if any) from initial course has subsided.
(Dosages recommended based on lean
body weight.) Maximum single recommended dose is 800 mg.
▶ **Palliative treatment of advanced colorectal cancer.** *Adults:* 425 mg/m² I.V.
daily for 5 consecutive days. Given with
20 mg/m² of leucovorin I.V. Repeated at
4-week intervals for two additional
courses; then repeated at intervals of 4 to
5 weeks if tolerated.
▶ **Multiple actinic (solar) keratoses;
superficial basal cell carcinoma.**
Adults: apply cream or topical solution
b.i.d.

Adverse reactions

CNS: acute cerebellar syndrome, ataxia,
confusion, disorientation, euphoria,
headache, nystagmus, *weakness, malaise.*
CV: *myocardial ischemia,* angina.
EENT: epistaxis, photophobia, lacrimation, lacrimal duct stenosis, visual
changes.
GI: *stomatitis, GI ulcer* (may precede
leukopenia), *nausea and vomiting, diarrhea, anorexia,* GI bleeding.
Hematologic: *leukopenia, thrombocytopenia, agranulocytosis,* anemia; WBC
count nadir 9 to 14 days after first dose;
platelet count nadir in 7 to 14 days.
Skin: *reversible alopecia, dermatitis,
erythema, scaling, pruritus,* contact dermatitis, nail changes, pigmented palmar
creases; erythematous, desquamative rash
of hands and feet with long-term use
("hand-foot syndrome"), photosensitivity.

Other: *pain, burning,* soreness, suppura-
tion, swelling (with topical use); *anaphylaxis,* thrombophlebitis.

Interactions

Drug-drug. *Leucovorin calcium, prior
treatment with alkylating agents:* increased toxicity of fluorouracil. Use with
extreme caution.
Drug-lifestyle. *Sun exposure:* photosensitivity reactions may occur. Take precautions.

Contraindications and precautions

• Contraindicated in patients with hypersensitivity to drug, poor nutrition, bone
marrow suppression (WBC counts of
5,000/mm³ or less or platelet counts of
100,000/mm³ or less), or potentially serious infections and in those who have had
major surgery within previous month.
• Drug is not recommended for use in
pregnant or breast-feeding women.
• Use cautiously after high-dose pelvic
radiation therapy or use of alkylating
agents or in patients with impaired hepatic or renal function or widespread neoplastic infiltration of bone marrow.
• Safety of drug has not been established
in children.

NURSING CONSIDERATIONS

🔳 **Assessment**
• Assess patient's condition before therapy, and reassess regularly thereafter.
• Monitor fluid intake and output, CBC,
platelet count, and renal and hepatic
function tests, as ordered.
• Be alert for adverse reactions and drug
interactions.
• Be aware that fluorouracil toxicity may
be delayed for 1 to 3 weeks.
• Monitor patient receiving topical form
for serious adverse reactions. Ingestion
and systemic absorption may cause
leukopenia, thrombocytopenia, stomatitis, diarrhea, or GI ulceration, bleeding,
and hemorrhage. Application to large ul-

---

cerated areas may cause systemic toxicity.
• Watch for stomatitis or diarrhea (signs of toxicity).
• Evaluate patient's and family's knowledge of drug therapy.

🔢 **Nursing diagnoses**
• Altered health maintenance related to underlying neoplastic condition
• Altered protection related to adverse hematologic reactions
• Knowledge deficit related to drug therapy

⧉ **Planning and implementation**
• Follow institutional policy to reduce risks. Preparation and administration of parenteral form are associated with carcinogenic, mutagenic, and teratogenic risks for personnel.
• Drug sometimes is ordered as 5-fluorouracil or 5-FU. The numeral 5 is part of drug name and should not be confused with dosage units.
• Give antiemetic, as ordered, before administering parenteral form of drug to reduce nausea.
I.V. use: Drug may be administered by direct injection without dilution. For I.V. infusion, drug may be diluted with D₅W, sterile water for injection, or 0.9% NaCl injection. Infuse slowly over 2 to 8 hours.
– Don't use cloudy solution. If crystals form, redissolve by warming.
– Use plastic I.V. containers for administering continuous infusions. Solution is more stable in plastic I.V. bags than in glass bottles.
Topical use: Apply with caution near eyes, nose, and mouth.
– Avoid occlusive dressings because they increase risk of inflammatory reactions in adjacent normal skin.
– Wash hands immediately after handling topical form of medication.
– Expect to use 1% topical concentration on face. Higher concentrations are used for thicker-skinned areas or resistant lesions.

– Expect to use 5% topical strength for superficial basal cell carcinoma confirmed by biopsy.
• Don't refrigerate fluorouracil.
• Use sodium hypochlorite 5% (household bleach) to inactivate drug in event of spill.
• Discontinue drug if diarrhea occurs, and notify doctor.
• Consider protective isolation if WBC count is less than 2,000/mm³.
Patient teaching
• Warn patient that alopecia may occur, but is reversible.
• Caution patient to avoid prolonged exposure to sunlight or ultraviolet light when topical form is used.
• Tell patient to use sunblock to avoid inflammatory erythematous dermatitis. Long-term use of drug is associated with erythematous, desquamative rash of hands and feet. May be treated with pyridoxine (50 to 150 mg P.O. daily) for 5 to 7 days.
• Warn patient that topically treated area may be unsightly during therapy and for several weeks after. Full healing may take 1 or 2 months.

☑ **Evaluation**
• Patient exhibits positive response to fluorouracil therapy.
• Patient does not develop serious adverse hematologic reactions.
• Patient and family state understanding of drug therapy.

fluoxetine hydrochloride
(floo-OKS-eh-teen high-droh-KLOR-ighd)
Prozac, Prozac-20 ◇

Pharmacologic class: serotonin uptake inhibitor
Therapeutic class: antidepressant
Pregnancy risk category: B

How supplied

Pulvules: 10 mg, 20 mg
Oral solution: 20 mg/5 ml

Pharmacokinetics

Absorption: well absorbed after oral administration.
Distribution: apparently highly protein-bound (about 95%).
Metabolism: metabolized primarily in liver to active metabolites.
Excretion: excreted by kidneys. *Half-life:* 2 to 3 days.

Route	Onset	Peak	Duration
P.O.	1-4 wk	6-8 hr	Unknown

Pharmacodynamics

Chemical effect: unknown; presumed to be linked to its inhibition of CNS neuronal uptake of serotonin.
Therapeutic effect: relieves depression and obsessive-compulsive behaviors.

Indications and dosage

▶ **Depression, obsessive-compulsive disorder.** *Adults:* initially, 20 mg P.O. in morning; dosage increased according to patient response. May be given b.i.d. in morning and at noon. Maximum dosage is 80 mg/day.
▶ **Treatment of binge-eating and vomiting behaviors in patients with moderate to severe bulimia nervosa.** *Adults:* 60 mg/day P.O. in the morning.

Adverse reactions

CNS: *nervousness, anxiety, insomnia, headache, drowsiness,* fatigue, tremor, dizziness, asthenia.
CV: palpitations, hot flashes.
EENT: nasal congestion, pharyngitis, cough, sinusitis.
GI: *nausea, diarrhea, dry mouth, anorexia,* dyspepsia, constipation, abdominal pain, vomiting, flatulence, increased appetite.
GU: sexual dysfunction.
Respiratory: upper respiratory infection, respiratory distress.
Skin: rash, pruritus, urticaria.
Other: flulike syndrome, muscle pain, weight loss, fever.

Interactions

Drug-drug. *Cyproheptadine:* may reverse or decrease pharmacologic effect. Monitor patient closely.
Flecainide, carbamazepine, vinblastine: increased serum levels of these drugs. Monitor serum levels and patient for adverse effects.
Insulin, oral antidiabetic agents: altered blood glucose levels and possible altered requirements for antidiabetic medication. Adjust dosage as ordered.
Lithium, tricyclic antidepressants: risk of increased adverse CNS effects. Avoid concomitant use.
Phenytoin: increased plasma phenytoin levels and risk of toxicity. Monitor serum phenytoin levels and adjust dosage as ordered.
Tryptophan: increased toxic reaction exhibited by agitation, GI distress, and restlessness. Do not use together.
Warfarin, other highly protein-bound agents: may increase plasma levels of fluoxetine or other highly protein-bound drugs. Monitor closely.
Drug-lifestyle. *Alcohol use:* increased CNS depression. Avoid concomitant use.

Contraindications and precautions

• Contraindicated in patients hypersensitive to drug and in those taking MAO inhibitors within 14 days of starting therapy.
• Drug is not recommended for use in breast-feeding women.
• Use cautiously in patients at high risk for suicide; in those with history of hepatic, renal, or CV disease, diabetes mellitus, or history of seizures; and in pregnant women.
• Safety of drug has not been established in children.

NURSING CONSIDERATIONS

▨ **Assessment**
• Obtain assessment of patient's condition before therapy, and reassess regularly throughout therapy.

Reactions may be *common*, uncommon, *life-threatening*, or COMMON AND LIFE-THREATENING.

• Be alert for adverse reactions and drug interactions.
• Evaluate patient's and family's knowledge of drug therapy.

⊞ Nursing diagnoses
• Ineffective individual coping related to patient's underlying condition
• Sleep pattern disturbance related to drug-induced insomnia
• Knowledge deficit related to drug therapy

▶ Planning and implementation
• Elderly or debilitated patients and patients with renal or hepatic dysfunction may require lower dosages or less frequent dosing.
• Administer drug in morning to prevent insomnia.
• Use antihistamines or topical corticosteroids as ordered to treat rashes or pruritus.
Patient teaching
• Tell patient to avoid taking drug in afternoon because fluoxetine commonly causes nervousness and insomnia.
• Warn patient to avoid hazardous activities that require alertness and psychomotor coordination until CNS effects of drug are known.
• Advise patient to consult doctor before taking any other prescription or OTC medications.
• Warn patient to avoid food high in tryptophan, including meats, poultry, fish, liver, kidney, eggs, nuts, peanut butter, broad beans, and wheat germ.

☑ Evaluation
• Patient behavior and communication indicate improvement of depression with drug therapy.
• Patient does not experience insomnia with drug use.
• Patient and family state understanding of drug therapy.

fluoxymesterone
(floo-oks-ee-MES-tuh-rohn)
Android-F, Halotestin**

Pharmacologic class: androgen
Therapeutic class: androgen replacement, antineoplastic
Controlled substance schedule: III
Pregnancy risk category: X

How supplied
Tablets: 2 mg, 5 mg, 10 mg

Pharmacokinetics
Drug has primarily hepatic metabolism. Other data unknown.

Route	Onset	Peak	Duration
P.O.	Unknown	Unknown	Unknown

Pharmacodynamics
Chemical effect: stimulates target tissues to develop normally in androgen-deficient men. It also exerts inhibitory, antiestrogenic effects on hormone-responsive breast tumors and metastases.
Therapeutic effect: stimulates puberty, reverses testicular deficiency, and inhibits estrogenic effects on breast tumors and metastases.

Indications and dosage
▶ **Hypogonadism from testicular deficiency.** *Adults:* 5 to 20 mg P.O. daily.
▶ **Delayed puberty.** *Adolescents:* highly individualized; duration of therapy 4 to 6 months.
▶ **Palliation of breast cancer in women.** *Adults:* 10 to 40 mg P.O. daily in divided doses. All dosages individualized and reduced to minimum when effect is noted.

Adverse reactions
CNS: headache, anxiety, depression, paresthesia, sleep apnea syndrome.
CV: edema.
GI: nausea.

GU: *hypoestrogenic effects in women (flushing; diaphoresis; vaginitis including itching, dryness, and burning; vaginal bleeding; nervousness; emotional lability; menstrual irregularities);* excessive hormonal effects in men (prepubertal—premature epiphyseal closure, *acne,* priapism, *growth of body and facial hair,* phallic enlargement; postpubertal—testicular atrophy, oligospermia, decreased ejaculate, impotence, gynecomastia, epididymitis).

Hematologic: polycythemia, elevated serum lipid levels, suppression of clotting factors.

Hepatic: reversible jaundice, peliosis hepatis, elevated liver enzyme levels, *liver cell tumors.*

Skin: hypersensitivity skin manifestations.

Other: hypercalcemia; androgenic effects in women (acne, edema, *weight gain, hirsutism,* hoarseness, clitoral enlargement, *decrease in breast size,* changes in libido, male pattern baldness, *oily skin or hair).*

Interactions

Drug-drug. *Hepatotoxic drugs:* increased risk of hepatotoxicity. Monitor closely.

Insulin, oral antidiabetic agents: altered dosage requirements. Monitor blood glucose levels in diabetic patients.

Oral anticoagulants: altered dosage requirements. Monitor PT and INR.

Contraindications and precautions

• Contraindicated in patients with hypersensitivity to drug; in males with breast cancer or prostate cancer; in those with cardiac, hepatic, or renal decompensation; and in pregnant or breast-feeding women.

• Use cautiously in prepubertal males and in patients with BPH and aspirin sensitivity.

NURSING CONSIDERATIONS

⚗ Assessment

• Assess patient's underlying condition before therapy and regularly thereafter.

• When used in breast cancer, subjective effects may not occur for about 1 month; objective effects on clinical symptoms may take 3 months.

• Semen evaluation is performed routinely every 3 to 4 months, especially in adolescent males.

• Be alert for adverse reactions and drug interactions.

• Watch for symptoms of jaundice and evaluate hepatic function.

• Monitor male patient for excessive sexual stimulation or priapism.

• Monitor patient for hypercalcemia. Symptoms may be difficult to distinguish from symptoms associated with condition being treated, unless anticipated and thought of as symptom cluster. Hypercalcemia is particularly likely to occur in patient with metastatic breast cancer and may indicate bone metastases.

• Evaluate patient's and family's knowledge of drug therapy.

⊞ Nursing diagnoses

• Sexual dysfunction related to hormonal dysfunction

• Body image disturbance related to adverse androgenic reactions

• Knowledge deficit related to drug therapy

▶ Planning and implementation

• Administer drug with food if adverse GI reactions occur.

• Dosage adjustment may reverse hepatic dysfunction. If liver function test results are abnormal, notify doctor as therapy should be stopped.

• Report signs of virilization or menstrual irregularities to doctor.

Patient teaching

• Tell patient to take drug with food or meals if GI upset occurs.

Reactions may be *common,* uncommon, *life-threatening,* or COMMON AND LIFE-THREATENING.

• Make sure patient understands importance of using effective nonhormonal contraceptive during therapy.
• Advise female patient to wash after intercourse to decrease risk of vaginitis. Instruct her to wear only cotton underwear.
• Tell female patient to report menstrual irregularities and to discontinue therapy pending etiologic determination.
• Explain to patient taking drug for palliation of breast cancer that virilization usually occurs. Give emotional support. Tell patient to report androgenic effects. Stopping drug will prevent further changes but will probably not reverse existing effects.

☑ **Evaluation**
• Patient's underlying condition exhibits improvement.
• Patient states acceptance of body image changes caused by drug.
• Patient and family state understanding of drug therapy.

fluphenazine decanoate
(floo-FEN-uh-zeen deh-kuh-NOH-ayt)
Modecate♦◇, Modecate Concentrate♦, Prolixin Decanoate

fluphenazine enanthate
Moditen Enanthate♦, Prolixin Enanthate

fluphenazine hydrochloride
Anatensol◇*, Apo-Fluphenazine♦, Moditen HCl♦, Moditen HCl-H.P.♦, Permitil* **, Permitil Concentrate, Prolixin* **, Prolixin Concentrate

Pharmacologic class: phenothiazine (piperazine derivative)
Therapeutic class: antipsychotic
Pregnancy risk category: NR

How supplied
fluphenazine decanoate
Depot injection: 25 mg/ml

fluphenazine enanthate
Depot injection: 25 mg/ml
fluphenazine hydrochloride
Tablets: 1 mg, 2.5 mg, 5 mg, 10 mg
Oral concentrate: 5 mg/ml (contains 1% alcohol)
Elixir: 2.5 mg/5 ml (with 14% alcohol)
I.M. injection: 2.5 mg/ml

Pharmacokinetics
Absorption: rate and extent of absorption vary with route of administration; oral tablet absorption is erratic and variable.
Distribution: distributed widely into body. CNS concentrations are usually higher than those in plasma. Drug is 91% to 99% protein-bound.
Metabolism: metabolized extensively by liver, but no active metabolites are formed.
Excretion: most of drug excreted in urine; some excreted in feces by way of biliary tract.

Route	Onset	Peak	Duration
P.O.	≤ 1 hr	0.5 hr	6-8 hr
I.M., S.C.	1-3 days	Unknown	1-6 wk

Pharmacodynamics
Chemical effect: unknown; may block dopamine receptors in brain.
Therapeutic effect: relieves psychotic signs and symptoms.

Indications and dosage
▶ **Psychotic disorders.** *Adults:* initially, 0.5 to 10.0 mg hydrochloride P.O. daily in divided doses q 6 to 8 hours; may increase cautiously to 20 mg. Higher doses (50 to 100 mg) have been given. Maintenance dosage is 1 to 5 mg P.O. daily. I.M. doses are one-third to one-half of oral doses. Use lower dosages for elderly patients (1.0 to 2.5 mg daily). Alternatively, 12.5 to 25 mg of long-acting esters (decanoate or enanthate) I.M. or S.C. q 1 to 6 weeks; maintenance dosage is 25 to 100 mg, p.r.n.

---

*Liquid form contains alcohol   **May contain tartrazine   ♦Canada   ◇ Australia   †OTC

Adverse reactions

CNS: *extrapyramidal reactions, tardive dyskinesia,* sedation, pseudoparkinsonism, EEG changes, drowsiness, *seizures,* dizziness.
CV: orthostatic hypotension, tachycardia, ECG changes.
EENT: ocular changes, *blurred vision,* nasal congestion.
GI: *dry mouth, constipation.*
GU: *urine retention,* dark urine, menstrual irregularities, gynecomastia, inhibited ejaculation.
Hematologic: *leukopenia, agranulocytosis, aplastic anemia,* eosinophilia, *hemolytic anemia.*
Hepatic: cholestatic jaundice, abnormal liver function test results.
Skin: *mild photosensitivity,* allergic reactions.
Other: weight gain; increased appetite; rarely, *neuroleptic malignant syndrome.*
After abrupt withdrawal of long-term therapy: gastritis, nausea, vomiting, dizziness, tremor, feeling of warmth or cold, diaphoresis, tachycardia, headache, insomnia.

Interactions

Drug-drug. *Antacids:* inhibited absorption of oral phenothiazines. Separate doses by at least 2 hours.
Anticholinergics: increased anticholinergic effects. Avoid concomitant use.
Barbiturates, lithium: may decrease phenothiazine effect. Observe patient.
Centrally acting antihypertensives: decreased antihypertensive effect. Monitor blood pressure.
CNS depressants: increased CNS depression. Avoid concomitant use.
Drug-lifestyle. *Alcohol use:* increased CNS depression. Avoid concomitant use.
Sun exposure: increased risk of photosensitivity. Avoid prolonged or unprotected exposure to sun.

Contraindications and precautions

• Contraindicated in patients with CNS depression, bone marrow suppression or other blood dyscrasia, subcortical damage, liver damage, or hypersensitivity and in those experiencing coma.
• Use cautiously in elderly or debilitated patients, pregnant or breast-feeding women, and those with pheochromocytoma, severe CV disease (may cause sudden drop in blood pressure), peptic ulcer, exposure to extreme heat or cold (including antipyretic therapy) or phosphorous insecticides, respiratory disorder, hypocalcemia, seizure disorder (may lower seizure threshold), severe reactions to insulin or electroconvulsive therapy, mitral insufficiency, glaucoma, or prostatic hyperplasia. Use parenteral form cautiously in asthmatic patients and patients allergic to sulfites.

NURSING CONSIDERATIONS

Assessment
• Assess patient's condition before therapy and regularly thereafter.
• Monitor therapy with weekly bilirubin tests during first month; periodic blood tests (CBC and liver function); and periodic renal function and ophthalmic tests (long-term use).
• Be alert for adverse reactions and drug interactions.
• Monitor patient for tardive dyskinesia, which may occur after prolonged use. It may not appear until months or years later and may disappear spontaneously or persist for life despite discontinuation of drug.
• Evaluate patient's and family's knowledge of drug therapy.

Nursing diagnoses
• Impaired thought processes related to psychosis
• Impaired physical mobility related to extrapyramidal reactions
• Knowledge deficit related to drug therapy

Reactions may be *common,* uncommon, *life-threatening,* or COMMON AND LIFE-THREATENING.

▶ Planning and implementation
P.O. use: Prolixin concentrate and Permitil concentrate are 10 times more concentrated than Prolixin elixir (5 mg/ml vs. 0.5 mg/ml). Check dosage order carefully.
– Dilute liquid concentrate with water, fruit juice, milk, or semisolid food just before administration.
I.M. and S.C. use: For long-acting forms (decanoate and enanthate), which are oil preparations, use dry needle of at least 21G. Allow 24 to 96 hours for onset of action. Note and report adverse reactions in patient taking these drug forms.
• Oral liquid and parenteral forms can cause contact dermatitis. Wear gloves when preparing solutions, and avoid contact with skin and clothing.
• Protect medication from light. Slight yellowing of injection or concentrate is common; does not affect potency. Discard markedly discolored solutions.
• Withhold dose and notify doctor if patient develops symptoms of blood dyscrasia (fever, sore throat, infection, cellulitis, weakness) or persistent extrapyramidal reactions (longer than a few hours), especially in a pregnant woman or child.
• Acute dystonic reactions may be treated with diphenhydramine.
• Do not withdraw drug abruptly unless severe adverse reactions occur.
Patient teaching
• Warn patient to avoid activities that require alertness and psychomotor coordination until CNS effects of drug are known.
• Tell patient to avoid alcohol during therapy.
• Advise patient to relieve dry mouth with sugarless gum or hard candy.
• Have patient report urine retention or constipation.
• Tell patient to use sunblock and to wear protective clothing.
• Inform patient that drug may discolor urine.
• Stress importance of not discontinuing drug suddenly.

☑ Evaluation
• Patient demonstrates decrease in psychotic behavior.
• Patient maintains pretreatment physical mobility.
• Patient and family state understanding of drug therapy.

flurazepam hydrochloride
(floo-RAH-zuh-pam high-droh-KLOR-ighd)
Apo-Flurazepam ◆, Dalmane, Novo-Flupam ◆

Pharmacologic class: benzodiazepine
Therapeutic class: sedative-hypnotic agent
Controlled substance schedule: IV
Pregnancy risk category: X

How supplied
Capsules: 15 mg, 30 mg

Pharmacokinetics
Absorption: absorbed rapidly through GI tract.
Distribution: distributed widely throughout body; about 97% bound to plasma protein.
Metabolism: metabolized in liver to active metabolite desalkylflurazepam.
Excretion: excreted in urine. *Half-life:* 50 to 100 hours.

Route	Onset	Peak	Duration
P.O.	Unknown	0.5-1 hr	Unknown

Pharmacodynamics
Chemical effect: unknown; may act on limbic system, thalamus, and hypothalamus of CNS to produce hypnotic effects.
Therapeutic effect: promotes sleep and calmness.

Indications and dosage
▶ **Insomnia.** *Adults:* 15 to 30 mg P.O. h.s. Dose repeated once, p.r.n.

Adverse reactions

CNS: *daytime sedation, dizziness, drowsiness, disturbed coordination,* lethargy, confusion, *headache,* light-headedness, nervousness, hallucinations, staggering, ataxia, disorientation, *coma.*
GI: nausea, vomiting, heartburn, diarrhea, abdominal pain.
Hepatic: elevated liver enzymes.
Other: physical or psychological dependence.

Interactions

Drug-drug. *Cimetidine:* increased sedation. Monitor carefully.
CNS depressants, including narcotic analgesics: excessive CNS depression. Use together cautiously.
Digoxin: digoxin serum levels may increase, resulting in toxicity. Monitor closely.
Disulfiram, isoniazid, oral contraceptives: decreased metabolism of benzodiazepines, leading to toxicity. Monitor closely.
Phenytoin: increased phenytoin levels. Monitor for toxicity.
Rifampin: enhanced metabolism of benzodiazepines. Monitor for decreased effectiveness.
Theophylline: antagonist with flurazepam. Monitor for decreased effectiveness.
Drug-lifestyle. *Alcohol use:* excessive CNS and respiratory depression. Use together cautiously.
Smoking: enhanced metabolism of benzodiazepines. Avoid concomitant use.

Contraindications and precautions

• Contraindicated in patients with hypersensitivity to drug and in pregnant women.
• Drug is not recommended for use in breast-feeding women.
• Use cautiously in patients with impaired hepatic or renal function, chronic pulmonary insufficiency, mental depression, suicidal tendencies, or history of drug abuse.

• Safety of drug has not been established in children under age 15.

NURSING CONSIDERATIONS

⚖ Assessment
• Assess patient's sleep patterns and CNS status before therapy.
• Evaluate patient's ability to sleep. Drug is more effective on second, third, and fourth nights of use.
• Be alert for adverse reactions and drug interactions.
• Evaluate patient's and family's knowledge of drug therapy.

⊞ Nursing diagnoses
• Sleep pattern disturbance related to underlying patient problem
• Risk for trauma related to drug-induced adverse CNS reactions
• Knowledge deficit related to drug therapy

❯ Planning and implementation
• Before leaving bedside, make sure patient has swallowed capsule.
Patient teaching
• Encourage patient to continue drug, even if it doesn't relieve insomnia on first night.
• Warn patient to avoid activities that require alertness or physical coordination. For inpatient, supervise walking and raise bed rails, particularly for elderly patient.
• Advise patient that physical and psychological dependence is possible with long-term use.

☑ Evaluation
• Patient notes drug-induced sleep.
• Patient's safety is maintained.
• Patient and family state understanding of drug therapy.

Reactions may be *common*, uncommon, *life-threatening*, or COMMON AND LIFE-THREATENING.

flurbiprofen
(flur-bih-PROH-fen)
Ansaid, Apo-Flurbiprofen♦, Froben♦,
Froben SR♦, Novo-Flurprofen♦,
Nu-Flurbiprofen♦

Pharmacologic class: NSAID, phenyl-
alkanoic acid derivative
Therapeutic class: antiarthritic
Pregnancy risk category: B

How supplied

Tablets: 50 mg, 100 mg
Capsules (extended-release)♦: 200 mg

Pharmacokinetics

Absorption: well absorbed. Administering with food alters rate, but not extent, of absorption.
Distribution: highly bound to plasma
proteins.
Metabolism: metabolized primarily in
liver.
Excretion: excreted primarily in urine.
Half-life: 6½ hours.

Route	Onset	Peak	Duration
P.O.	Unknown	About 2 hr	Unknown

Pharmacodynamics

Chemical effect: unknown; possibly inhibits prostaglandin synthesis.
Therapeutic effect: relieves pain.

Indications and dosage

▶ **Rheumatoid arthritis and osteoarthritis.** *Adults:* 200 to 300 mg P.O. daily,
divided b.i.d. to q.i.d. Where available,
patients maintained on 200 mg daily may
switch to one 200-mg extended-release
capsule P.O. daily, taken in evening after
food.

Adverse reactions

CNS: *headache,* anxiety, insomnia, increased reflexes, tremors, amnesia, asthenia, drowsiness, malaise, depression,
dizziness.

CV: *edema, heart failure,* hypertension,
vasodilation.
EENT: rhinitis, tinnitus, visual changes,
epistaxis.
GI: *dyspepsia, diarrhea, abdominal
pain, nausea,* constipation, *bleeding,* flat-
ulence, vomiting.
GU: *symptoms suggesting urinary tract
infection,* hematuria, interstitial nephritis,
renal failure.
Hematologic: *thrombocytopenia, neu-
tropenia,* anemia, *aplastic anemia.*
Hepatic: elevated liver enzymes, jaundice.
Respiratory: asthma.
Skin: rash, photosensitivity, urticaria.
Other: *angioedema,* weight changes.

Interactions

Drug-drug. *Aspirin:* decreased flurbiprofen levels. Concomitant use is not recommended.
Beta blockers: antihypertensive effect of
beta blockers may be impaired. Monitor
blood pressure.
Cyclosporine: increased risk of nephrotoxicity. Monitor patient closely.
Diuretics: possible decreased diuretic effect. Monitor patient closely.
Lithium: serum lithium levels may be increased. Monitor levels.
Methotrexate: increased risk of methotrexate toxicity. Monitor closely.
Oral anticoagulants: increased bleeding
tendency. Monitor patient.
Drug-lifestyle. *Alcohol use:* increased
risk of adverse GI reactions. Avoid concomitant use.
Sun exposure: photosensitivity reactions
may occur. Take precautions.

Contraindications and precautions

• Contraindicated in patients with hypersensitivity to drug, history of aspirin- or
NSAID-induced asthma, urticaria, or other allergic-type reactions.
• Drug is not recommended for use in
breast-feeding women or during third
trimester of pregnancy.
• Use cautiously in patients with history
of peptic ulcer disease, hepatic dysfunc-

tion, cardiac disease, or other conditions associated with fluid retention or impaired renal function. Also use cautiously in pregnant women in first and second trimesters.
• Safety of drug has not been established in children.

NURSING CONSIDERATIONS

⚕ Assessment
• Assess patient's arthritis before therapy and regularly thereafter.
• Know that patient receiving long-term therapy should have periodic liver function studies, eye examinations, and hematocrit determinations.
• Be alert for adverse reactions and drug interactions.
• Evaluate patient's and family's knowledge of drug therapy.

⊞ Nursing diagnoses
• Pain related to presence of arthritis
• Diarrhea related to drug-induced adverse effect
• Knowledge deficit related to drug therapy

▶ Planning and implementation
• Be aware that elderly or debilitated patient or patient with hepatic or renal dysfunction should be monitored closely and probably should receive lower doses.
• Give drug with food, milk, or antacid if GI upset occurs.
Patient teaching
• Tell patient to take drug with food, milk, or antacid if GI upset occurs.
• Tell patient taking extended-release capsule to swallow it whole and not to crush, chew, or break it open.
• Advise patient to avoid hazardous activities that require mental alertness until CNS effects are known.
• Serious GI toxicity, including peptic ulceration and bleeding, can occur in patients taking NSAIDs despite absence of GI symptoms. Teach signs and symptoms

of GI bleeding, and tell patient to contact doctor immediately if they occur.

☑ Evaluation
• Patient is free from pain.
• Patient regains normal bowel pattern.
• Patient and family state understanding of drug therapy.

---

flutamide
(FLOO-tuh-mighd)
Euflex♦, Eulexin

Pharmacologic class: nonsteroidal antiandrogen
Therapeutic class: antineoplastic
Pregnancy risk category: D

How supplied
Capsules: 125 mg, 250 mg♦

Pharmacokinetics
Absorption: absorbed rapidly and completely.
Distribution: studies in animals show that drug concentrates in prostate. Drug and its active metabolite are about 95% protein-bound.
Metabolism: over 97% of drug is metabolized rapidly, with at least six metabolites identified.
Excretion: over 95% excreted in urine.
Half-life: 6 hours.

Route	Onset	Peak	Duration
P.O.	Unknown	2 hr	Unknown

Pharmacodynamics
Chemical effect: inhibits androgen uptake or prevents androgen binding in cell nuclei in target tissues.
Therapeutic effect: hinders prostatic cancer cell activity.

Indications and dosage
▶ **Metastatic prostatic carcinoma (stage D₂).** *Adults:* 250 mg P.O. q 8 hours. Used with luteinizing

---

Reactions may be *common*, uncommon, *life-threatening*, or COMMON AND LIFE-THREATENING.

hormone–releasing hormone analogues such as leuprolide acetate.

Adverse reactions
CNS: drowsiness, confusion, depression, anxiety, nervousness, paresthesia.
CV: peripheral edema, hypertension.
GI: *diarrhea, nausea, vomiting,* anorexia.
GU: *impotence, loss of libido.*
Hematologic: *thrombocytopenia, leukopenia,* anemia, *hemolytic anemia.*
Hepatic: elevated liver enzyme levels, *hepatitis,* encephalopathy.
Skin: rash, photosensitivity.
Other: *hot flashes,* gynecomastia.

Interactions
Drug-drug. *Warfarin:* may increase PT. Monitor patient's PT and INR.
Drug-lifestyle. *Sun exposure:* may cause sensitivity reactions. Warn patient to take appropriate precautions.

Contraindications and precautions
• Contraindicated in patients hypersensitive to drug.
• Drug is not indicated for use in female patients.
• Safety of drug has not been established in male children.

NURSING CONSIDERATIONS

▨ Assessment
• Obtain assessment of patient's prostatic cancer before therapy.
• Monitor liver function tests periodically, as ordered.
• Be alert for adverse reactions.
• Monitor hydration status if adverse GI reactions occur.
• Evaluate patient's and family's knowledge of drug therapy.

▣ Nursing diagnoses
• Altered health maintenance related to presence of prostatic cancer
• Risk for fluid volume deficit related to adverse GI reactions

• Knowledge deficit related to drug therapy

▧ Planning and implementation
• Drug may be given without regard to meals.
• Give drug with luteinizing hormone–releasing antagonist (such as leuprolide acetate), as ordered.
Patient teaching
• Make sure patient knows that flutamide must be taken continuously with agent used for medical castration (such as leuprolide acetate) to allow full benefit of therapy. Leuprolide suppresses testosterone production while flutamide inhibits testosterone action at cellular level. Together they can impair growth of androgen-responsive tumors. Advise patient not to discontinue either drug.
• Tell patient to notify doctor if adverse reactions occur.

▨ Evaluation
• Patient responds well to drug.
• Patient maintains adequate hydration throughout drug therapy.
• Patient and family state understanding of drug therapy.

fluvastatin sodium
(floo-vuh-STAH-tin SOH-dee-um)
Lescol

Pharmacologic class: hydroxymethylglutaryl-coenzyme A (HMG-CoA)
Therapeutic class: cholesterol inhibitor
Pregnancy risk category: X

How supplied
Capsules: 20 mg, 40 mg

Pharmacokinetics
Absorption: absorbed rapidly and virtually completely (98%) after oral administration on empty stomach.
Distribution: more than 98% bound to plasma proteins.

Metabolism: completely metabolized in liver.
Excretion: about 5% excreted in urine, 90% in feces.

Route	Onset	Peak	Duration
P.O.	Unknown	Unknown	Unknown

Pharmacodynamics

Chemical effect: inhibits 3-hydroxy-3-methylglutaryl coenzyme A reductase. This enzyme is early (and rate-limiting) step in synthetic pathway of cholesterol.
Therapeutic effect: lowers blood low-density lipoprotein (LDL) and cholesterol levels.

Indications and dosage

▶ **Reduction of LDL and total cholesterol levels in patients with primary hypercholesterolemia (types IIa and IIb) or to slow progression of coronary atherosclerosis in patients with coronary artery disease.** *Adults:* initially, 20 to 40 mg P.O. h.s. Increase dosage as needed to maximum of 80 mg daily (given in divided doses).

Adverse reactions

CNS: headache, fatigue, dizziness, insomnia.
GI: dyspepsia, diarrhea, nausea, vomiting, abdominal pain, constipation, flatulence, tooth disorder.
Hematologic: *thrombocytopenia, leukopenia, hemolytic anemia.*
Hepatic: increased liver enzyme levels.
Musculoskeletal: arthropathy, muscle pain.
Respiratory: sinusitis, *upper respiratory infection*, rhinitis, cough, pharyngitis, bronchitis.
Skin: *hypersensitivity reactions* (rash, pruritus).

Interactions

Drug-drug. *Cholestyramine, colestipol:* may bind with fluvastatin in GI tract and decrease absorption. Separate administration times by at least 4 hours.

Cimetidine, omeprazole, ranitidine: decreased fluvastatin metabolism. Monitor for enhanced effects.
Cyclosporine and other immunosuppressants, erythromycin, gemfibrozil, niacin: possible increased risk of polymyositis and rhabdomyolysis. Avoid concomitant use.
Digoxin: may alter digoxin pharmacokinetics. Monitor serum digoxin levels carefully.
Rifampin: enhanced fluvastatin metabolism and decreased plasma levels. Monitor for lack of effect.
Warfarin: increased anticoagulant effect with bleeding. Monitor patient.
Drug-lifestyle. *Alcohol use:* increased risk of hepatotoxicity. Avoid concomitant use.

Contraindications and precautions

• Contraindicated in patients hypersensitive to drug, in those with active liver disease or conditions associated with unexplained persistent elevations of serum transaminase levels, in pregnant or breast-feeding women, and in women of childbearing age unless there is no risk of pregnancy.
• Use cautiously in patients with severe renal impairment with history of liver disease or heavy alcohol use.
• Safety of drug has not been established in children under age 18.

NURSING CONSIDERATIONS

☑ Assessment
• Assess patient's blood LDL and cholesterol before therapy, and evaluate regularly thereafter.
• Be aware that liver function tests should be performed periodically.
• Be alert for adverse reactions and drug interactions.
• Evaluate patient's and family's knowledge of drug therapy.

◐ Nursing diagnoses
• Risk for injury related to elevated LDL and cholesterol blood levels

Reactions may be *common*, uncommon, *life-threatening*, or COMMON AND LIFE-THREATENING.

• Diarrhea related to drug's adverse effect on GI tract
• Knowledge deficit related to drug therapy

▷ **Planning and implementation**
• Drug should be initiated only after diet and other nonpharmacologic therapies have proven ineffective.
• Give drug at bedtime to enhance effectiveness.
• Institute standard low-cholesterol diet during therapy.
Patient teaching
• Tell patient that drug may be taken without regard to meals; efficacy is enhanced if taken in evening.
• Teach patient about proper dietary management, weight control, and exercise. Explain their importance in controlling serum lipid levels.
• Warn him to restrict alcohol use.
• Tell patient to inform doctor of any adverse reactions, particularly muscle aches and pains.

☑ **Evaluation**
• Patient's blood LDL and cholesterol levels are within normal limits.
• Patient regains normal bowel pattern.
• Patient and family state understanding of drug therapy.

fluvoxamine maleate
(floo-VOKS-uh-meen MAL-ee-ayt)
Luvox

Pharmacologic class: serotonin reuptake inhibitor
Therapeutic class: antidepressant
Pregnancy risk category: C

How supplied
Tablets: 25 mg, 50 mg, 100 mg

Pharmacokinetics
Absorption: unknown.
Distribution: 77% protein-bound.

Metabolism: metabolized in liver.
Excretion: excreted in urine. *Half-life:* 16.9 hours.

Route	Onset	Peak	Duration
P.O.	Unknown	3-8 hr	Unknown

Pharmacodynamics
Chemical effect: unknown; selectively inhibits neuronal uptake of serotonin, which is thought to improve obsessive-compulsive disorders.
Therapeutic effect: relieves obsessive-compulsive behavior.

Indications and dosage
▶ **Obsessive-compulsive disorder.**
Adults: initially, 50 mg P.O. daily h.s. Increased in 50-mg increments q 4 to 7 days until maximum benefit achieved. Maximum daily dosage is 300 mg. Total daily doses of more than 100 mg should be given in two divided doses. *Children ages 8 to 17:* 25 mg P.O. daily h.s. Dose may be increased in 25-mg increments q 4 to 7 days as tolerated until maximum benefit achieved. Maximum daily dosage is 200 mg. Total daily doses exceeding 50 mg should be given in two divided doses.

Adverse reactions
CNS: *headache, asthenia, somnolence, insomnia, nervousness,* dizziness, tremor, anxiety, hypertonia, *agitation,* depression, CNS stimulation, taste perversion.
CV: palpitations, vasodilation.
EENT: amblyopia.
GI: *nausea, diarrhea, constipation, dyspepsia,* anorexia, *vomiting,* flatulence, tooth disorder, dysphagia, *dry mouth.*
GU: decreased libido, abnormal ejaculation, urinary frequency, impotence, anorgasmia, urine retention.
Respiratory: upper respiratory tract infection, dyspnea, yawning.
Skin: sweating.
Other: flulike syndrome, chills.

Interactions

Drug-drug. *Astemizole:* may cause decreased metabolism, leading to increased levels of these antihistamines and cardiotoxicity. Avoid concomitant use.
Benzodiazepines, theophylline, warfarin: reduced clearance of these drugs by fluvoxamine. Use together cautiously (except for diazepam, which should not be administered together with fluvoxamine). Dosage adjustments may be necessary.
Carbamazepine, clozapine, methadone, metopranolol, propranolol, tricyclic antidepressants: elevated serum levels of these drugs caused by fluvoxamine. Use together cautiously. Monitor patient closely for adverse reactions. Dosage adjustments may be necessary.
Diltiazem: bradycardia may occur. Monitor heart rate.
Lithium, tryptophan: may enhance effects of fluvoxamine. Use together cautiously.
MAO inhibitors: may cause severe excitation, hyperpyrexia, myoclonus, delirium, and coma. Avoid concomitant use.
Drug-lifestyle. *Smoking:* decreased effectiveness of drug. Advise patient that smoking may decrease effectiveness of drug.

Contraindications and precautions

• Contraindicated in patients with hypersensitivity to drug or other phenylpiperazine antidepressants and within 14 days of MAO inhibitor therapy.
• Drug is not recommended for use in breast-feeding women.
• Use cautiously in patients with hepatic dysfunction, concomitant conditions that may affect hemodynamic responses or metabolism, or history of mania or seizures. Also use cautiously in pregnant women.
• Safety of drug has not been established in children younger than age 8.

⚗ Assessment

• Assess patient's condition before therapy, and reassess regularly thereafter. Several weeks of therapy may be needed before positive response occurs.
• Be alert for adverse reactions and drug interactions.
• Evaluate patient's and family's knowledge of drug therapy.

⊞ Nursing diagnoses

• Ineffective individual coping related to underlying condition
• Diarrhea related to drug's adverse effect on GI tract
• Knowledge deficit related to drug therapy

❯ Planning and implementation

• At least 14 days should elapse after stopping fluvoxamine before patient is started on MAO inhibitor, and at least 14 days should elapse before patient is started on fluvoxamine after MAO inhibitor therapy has been discontinued.
• Give drug at bedtime.
Patient teaching
• Warn patient not to engage in hazardous activity until drug's CNS effects are known.
• Advise patient to avoid alcoholic beverages during drug therapy.
• Alert patient that smoking may decrease effectiveness of drug.
• Instruct female patient who becomes pregnant or intends to become pregnant to notify doctor.
• Tell patient who develops rash, hives, or related allergic reaction to notify doctor.
• Inform patient that several weeks of therapy may be required to obtain full antidepressant effect. Once improvement is seen, advise patient not to discontinue drug unless ordered.
• Advise patient to check with doctor before taking OTC medications; drug interactions can occur.

Reactions may be *common*, uncommon, *life-threatening*, or COMMON AND LIFE-THREATENING.

✓ Evaluation
- Patient's obsessive-compulsive behaviors are diminished.
- Patient regains normal bowel patterns.
- Patient and family state understanding of drug therapy.

---

folic acid (vitamin B₉)
(FOH-lek AS-id)
Apo-Folic♦, Folvite, Novo-Folacid♦

Pharmacologic class: folic acid derivative
Therapeutic class: vitamin supplement
Pregnancy risk category: NR

How supplied
Tablets: 0.4 mg, 0.8 mg, 1 mg
Injection: 10-ml vials (5 mg/ml with 1.5% benzyl alcohol or 10 mg/ml with 1.5% benzyl alcohol and 0.2% EDTA)

Pharmacokinetics
Absorption: absorbed rapidly from GI tract, mainly from proximal part of small intestine, when administered orally. Absorption unknown after S.C. or I.M. administration.
Distribution: distributed into all body tissues; liver contains about half of total body folate stores. Folate is concentrated actively in CSF.
Metabolism: metabolized in liver.
Excretion: excess folate is excreted unchanged in urine; small amounts of folic acid have been recovered in feces. About 0.05 mg/day of normal body folate stores is lost by combination of urinary and fecal excretion and oxidative cleavage of molecule.

Route	Onset	Peak	Duration
P.O., S.C., I.M.	Unknown	30-60 min	Unknown

Pharmacodynamics
Chemical effect: stimulates normal erythropoiesis and nucleoprotein synthesis.

Therapeutic effect: nutritional supplement.

Indications and dosage
▶ **RDA.** *Neonates and infants to age 6 months:* 25 mcg. *Infants ages 6 months to 1 year:* 35 mcg. *Children ages 1 to 3:* 50 mcg. *Children ages 4 to 6:* 75 mcg. *Children ages 7 to 11:* 100 mcg. *Children ages 11 to 14:* 150 mcg. *Males age 15 and over:* 200 mcg. *Females age 15 and over:* 180 mcg. *Pregnant women:* 400 mcg. *Breast-feeding women (first 6 months):* 280 mcg. *Breast-feeding women (second 6 months):* 260 mcg.
▶ **Megaloblastic or macrocytic anemia secondary to folic acid or other nutritional deficiency, hepatic disease, alcoholism, intestinal obstruction, excessive hemolysis.** *Adults and children over age 4:* 0.4 mg to 1 mg P.O., S.C., or I.M. daily. After anemia secondary to folic acid deficiency is corrected, proper diet and RDA supplements are necessary to prevent recurrence. *Children under age 4:* up to 0.3 mg P.O., S.C., or I.M. daily. *Pregnant and breast-feeding women:* 0.8 mg P.O., S.C., or I.M. daily.
▶ **Prevention of megaloblastic anemia in pregnancy and fetal damage.** *Adults:* up to 1 mg P.O., S.C., or I.M. daily throughout pregnancy.
▶ **Nutritional supplement.** *Adults:* 0.1 mg P.O., S.C., or I.M. daily. *Children:* 0.05 mg P.O. daily.
▶ **To test folic acid deficiency in patients with megaloblastic anemia without masking pernicious anemia.** *Adults and children:* 0.1 to 0.2 mg P.O. or I.M. for 10 days, with diet low in folate and vitamin B₁₂.
▶ **Tropical sprue.** *Adults:* 3 to 15 mg P.O. daily.

Adverse reactions
CNS: general malaise.
GI: anorexia, nausea, flatulence, bitter taste.
Respiratory: *bronchospasm.*

Skin: allergic reactions (rash, pruritus, erythema).

Interactions

Drug-drug. *Aminosalicylic acid, chloramphenicol, methotrexate, sulfasalazine, trimethoprim:* antagonism of folic acid. Monitor for decreased folic acid effect. Use together cautiously.
Anticonvulsants (such as phenobarbital, phenytoin): increased anticonvulsant metabolism and decreased blood levels of anticonvulsants. Monitor closely.

Contraindications and precautions

• Contraindicated in patients with B_{12} deficiency or undiagnosed anemia.

NURSING CONSIDERATIONS

⚗ Assessment
• Obtain assessment of patient's folic acid deficiency before therapy.
• Evaluate CBC and assess patient's physical status throughout therapy.
• Be alert for adverse reactions and drug interactions.
• Evaluate patient's and family's knowledge of drug therapy.

⊞ Nursing diagnoses
• Altered nutrition: less than body requirements related to presence of folic acid deficiency
• Knowledge deficit related to drug therapy

⧁ Planning and implementation
• Be aware that patient with small-bowel resection and intestinal malabsorption may require parenteral administration route.
P.O. and S.C. use: Follow normal protocol.
I.M. use: Don't mix with other medications in same syringe for I.M. injections. Follow normal protocol.
• Protect from light and heat; store at room temperature.

• Be aware that concurrent folic acid and vitamin B_{12} therapy may be used if supported by diagnosis.
• Ensure that patient is getting properly balanced diet.
Patient teaching
• Teach patient proper nutrition to prevent recurrence of anemia.
• Tell patient to report hypersensitivity reactions or breathing difficulty.

☑ Evaluation
• Patient's CBC is normal.
• Patient and family state understanding of drug therapy.

foscarnet sodium (phosphonoformic acid)
(fos-KAR-net SOH-dee-um)
Foscavir

Pharmacologic class: pyrophosphate analogue
Therapeutic class: antiviral
Pregnancy risk category: C

How supplied

Injection: 24 mg/ml in 250- and 500-ml bottles

Pharmacokinetics

Absorption: not applicable.
Distribution: unknown.
Metabolism: unknown.
Excretion: about 80% to 90% appears unchanged in urine. *Half-life:* about 3 hours.

Route	Onset	Peak	Duration
I.V.	Immediate	Immediate	Unknown

Pharmacodynamics

Chemical effect: inhibits all known herpesviruses in vitro by blocking pyrophosphate binding site on DNA polymerases and reverse transcriptases.
Therapeutic effect: inhibits herpesvirus activity.

Indications and dosage

▶ **CMV retinitis in patients with AIDS.**
Adults: initially, in patients with normal renal function, either 60 mg/kg I.V. over 1 hour q 8 hours for 2 to 3 weeks, depending on clinical response or 90 mg/kg I.V. q. 12 hours administered over 1.5 to 2 hours for 2 to 3 weeks, depending on clinical response. Follow with maintenance infusion of 90 mg/kg/day I.V. administered over 2 hours; dose may be increased as needed and tolerated to 120 mg/kg daily if disease progresses.
▶ **Mucocutaneous acyclovir-resistant HSV infections.** *Adults:* 40 mg/kg I.V. infused over minimum of 1 hour, either q 8 or q 12 hours for 2 to 3 weeks or until healed.

Adverse reactions

CNS: *headache, seizures, fatigue, malaise, asthenia, paresthesia, dizziness, hypesthesia, neuropathy,* tremor, ataxia, generalized spasms, dementia, stupor, sensory disturbances, **meningitis,** aphasia, abnormal coordination, EEG abnormalities, depression, confusion, anxiety, insomnia, somnolence, nervousness, amnesia, agitation, aggressive reaction.
CV: *hypertension, palpitations, ECG abnormalities, sinus tachycardia,* cerebrovascular disorder, *first-degree AV block, hypotension, flushing,* edema.
EENT: visual disturbances, taste perversion, eye pain, conjunctivitis, sinusitis, pharyngitis, rhinitis.
GI: *nausea, diarrhea, vomiting, abdominal pain, anorexia,* constipation, dysphagia, **rectal hemorrhage,** dry mouth, melena, flatulence, ulcerative stomatitis, **pancreatitis.**
GU: *abnormal renal function, decreased creatinine clearance and increased serum creatinine levels, albuminuria, dysuria, polyuria, urethral disorder, urine retention, urinary tract infection,* **acute renal failure,** candidiasis.
Hematologic: anemia, granulocytopenia, **leukopenia, bone marrow suppression, thrombocytopenia,** platelet abnormalities, thrombocytosis, WBC count abnormalities, lymphadenopathy.
Metabolic: hypokalemia, hypomagnesemia, hypophosphatemia or hyperphosphatemia, hypocalcemia, hyponatremia.
Musculoskeletal: leg cramps, arthralgia, myalgia.
Respiratory: *cough, dyspnea,* pneumonitis, sinusitis, pharyngitis, rhinitis, respiratory insufficiency, pulmonary infiltration, stridor, pneumothorax, **bronchospasm,** hemoptysis, flulike symptoms.
Skin: *rash, increased sweating,* pruritus, skin ulceration, erythematous rash, seborrhea, skin discoloration, facial edema.
Other: *death, fever,* pain, **sepsis,** rigors, inflammation, pain at infusion site, lymphoma-like disorder, sarcoma, back or chest pain, abnormal hepatic function, bacterial or fungal infections, abscess, increased liver enzymes.

Interactions

Drug-drug. *Nephrotoxic drugs (such as amphotericin B, aminoglycosides):* increased risk of nephrotoxicity. Avoid concomitant use.
Pentamidine: increased risk of nephrotoxicity; severe hypocalcemia has also been reported. Don't use together.
Zidovudine: possible increased incidence or severity of anemia. Monitor blood counts.

Contraindications and precautions

• Contraindicated in patients with hypersensitivity to drug.
• Use cautiously and with reduced dosage in patients with abnormal renal function as ordered because it will result in accumulation of drug and enhanced toxicity. Because foscarnet is nephrotoxic, it has potential to worsen renal impairment. Some degree of nephrotoxicity occurs in most patients treated with drug. Also use cautiously in pregnant or breastfeeding women.
• Safety of drug has not been established in children.

NURSING CONSIDERATIONS

⏣ Assessment
• Assess patient's infection before therapy and regularly thereafter.
• Obtain serum electrolyte levels and creatinine clearance before beginning therapy, as ordered.
• Monitor creatinine clearance two to three times weekly during induction and at least once every 1 to 2 weeks during maintenance.
• Because drug can adversely affect potassium, calcium, magnesium, and phosphorus, monitor levels using schedule similar to that established for creatinine clearance.
• Drug is associated with dose-related transient decrease in ionized serum calcium, which may not be reflected in laboratory values. Assess for tetany and seizures associated with abnormal electrolyte levels.
• Monitor patient's hemoglobin and hematocrit levels. Anemia is common (in up to 33% of patients treated with drug). It may be severe enough to require transfusions.
• Be alert for adverse reactions and drug interactions.
• Evaluate patient's and family's knowledge of drug therapy.

⏣ Nursing diagnoses
• Infection related to presence of herpesvirus susceptible to drug
• Sensory or perceptual (tactile) alteration related to drug's adverse effect
• Knowledge deficit related to drug therapy

⏣ Planning and implementation
• Use infusion pump to administer drug over minimum of at least 1 hour. To minimize renal toxicity, ensure adequate hydration before and during infusion.
• Do not exceed recommended dosage, infusion rate, or frequency of administration. All doses must be individualized based on patient's renal function.

• Because drug is highly toxic and toxicity is probably dose-related, keep in mind that lowest effective maintenance dose should be used.
• Dosage must be adjusted when creatinine clearance is below 1.5 ml/minute/kg. If creatinine clearance falls below 0.4 ml/minute/kg, drug should be discontinued.
Patient teaching
• Advise patient to report perioral tingling, numbness in extremities, and paresthesia.

⏣ Evaluation
• Patient is free from infection.
• Patient does not exhibit adverse neurologic reactions.
• Patient and family state understanding of drug therapy.

fosinopril sodium
(foh-SIN-oh-pril SOH-dee-um)
Monopril

Pharmacologic class: ACE inhibitor
Therapeutic class: antihypertensive
Pregnancy risk category: C (D in second and third trimesters)

How supplied
Tablets: 10 mg, 20 mg

Pharmacokinetics
Absorption: absorbed slowly through GI tract, primarily by way of proximal small intestine.
Distribution: greater than 95% protein-bound.
Metabolism: hydrolyzed primarily in liver and gut.
Excretion: 50% excreted in urine; remainder, in feces. *Half-life:* 11½ hours.

Route	Onset	Peak	Duration
P.O.	≤ 1 hr	2-6 hr	About 24 hr

Pharmacodynamics

Chemical effect: antihypertensive action not clearly defined. Inhibits ACE, preventing conversion of angiotensin I to angiotensin II, a potent vasoconstrictor. Reduced formation of angiotensin II decreases peripheral arterial resistance, thus decreasing aldosterone secretion.
Therapeutic effect: lowers blood pressure.

Indications and dosage

► **Hypertension.** *Adults:* initially, 10 mg P.O. daily. Dosage is adjusted based on blood pressure response at peak and trough levels. Usual dosage is 20 to 40 mg, up to 80 mg daily. Dosage is divided if needed.
► **Adjunctive therapy for treatment of heart failure.** *Adults:* initially, 10 mg P.O. once daily. Dosage should be increased over several weeks to maximum dosage that is tolerable but no greater than 40 mg P.O. daily.

Adverse reactions

CNS: headache, dizziness, fatigue, syncope, paresthesia, sleep disturbance, *CVA.*
CV: chest pain, angina, *MI,* rhythm disturbances, palpitations, hypotension, orthostatic hypotension.
EENT: tinnitus, sinusitis.
GI: nausea, vomiting, diarrhea, *pancreatitis,* dry mouth, abdominal distention, abdominal pain, constipation.
GU: sexual dysfunction, decreased libido, renal insufficiency.
Hepatic: *hepatitis.*
Musculoskeletal: arthralgia, musculoskeletal pain, myalgia.
Respiratory: *dry, persistent, tickling, nonproductive cough; bronchospasm.*
Skin: urticaria, rash, photosensitivity, pruritus.
Other: *angioedema,* gout, hyperkalemia.

Interactions

Drug-drug. *Antacids:* may impair absorption. Separate administration times by at least 2 hours.

Diuretics, other antihypertensives: risk of excessive hypotension. Diuretic may need to be discontinued or fosinopril dosage lowered.
Lithium: increased serum lithium levels and lithium toxicity. Avoid concomitant use.
Potassium-sparing diuretics, potassium supplements, sodium substitutes containing potassium: risk of hyperkalemia. Monitor during concomitant use.
Drug-food. *Salt substitutes containing potassium:* risk of hyperkalemia. Monitor closely during concomitant use.

Contraindications and precautions

• Contraindicated in patients with hypersensitivity to drug or other ACE inhibitors and in breast-feeding women.
• Use with extreme caution and only when necessary in pregnant women to prevent fetal harm.
• Use cautiously in patients with impaired renal or hepatic function.
• Safety of drug has not been established in children.

NURSING CONSIDERATIONS

🔢 **Assessment**
• Assess blood pressure before therapy and regularly thereafter.
• Assess renal and hepatic function before and during therapy.
• Monitor potassium intake and serum potassium level. Diabetic patients, those with impaired renal function, and those receiving drugs that can increase serum potassium may develop hyperkalemia.
• Other ACE inhibitors have been associated with agranulocytosis and neutropenia. Monitor CBC with differential counts before therapy, every 2 weeks for first 3 months of therapy, and periodically thereafter.
• Monitor patient's hydration status if adverse GI reactions occur.
• Evaluate patient's and family's knowledge of drug therapy.

⊞ Nursing diagnoses
• Risk for injury related to presence of hypertension
• Risk for fluid volume deficit related to adverse GI reactions
• Knowledge deficit related to drug therapy

▶ Planning and implementation
• Drug may be taken without regard to meals. However, taking drug with food slows absorption of drug.
Patient teaching
• Tell patient to avoid sodium substitutes; these products may contain potassium, which can cause hyperkalemia in patient taking this drug.
• Advise patient to report signs of infection (such as fever and sore throat); easy bruising or bleeding; swelling of tongue, lips, face, eyes, mucous membranes, or extremities; difficulty swallowing or breathing; and hoarseness.
• Tell patient to use caution in hot weather and during exercise. Inadequate fluid intake, vomiting, diarrhea, and excessive perspiration can lead to light-headedness and syncope.
• Tell female patient to notify doctor if pregnancy occurs. Drug will probably need to be discontinued.

✓ Evaluation
• Patient's blood pressure is normal.
• Patient maintains adequate hydration throughout drug therapy.
• Patient and family state understanding of drug therapy.

---

fosphenytoin sodium
(fahs-FEN-eh-toyn SOH-dee-um)
Cerebyx

Pharmacologic class: prodrug of phenytoin
Therapeutic class: anticonvulsant
Pregnancy risk category: D

How supplied
Injection: 2 ml (150 mg fosphenytoin sodium equivalent to 100 mg phenytoin sodium), 10 ml (750 mg fosphenytoin sodium equivalent to 500 mg phenytoin sodium)

Pharmacokinetics
Absorption: completely absorbed following I.M. and I.V. use.
Distribution: widely throughout body; 95% plasma protein–bound.
Metabolism: in liver.
Excretion: in urine.

Route	Onset	Peak	Duration
I.V.	Unknown	Immediate	Unknown
I.M.	Unknown	30 min	Unknown

Pharmacodynamics
Chemical effect: because fosphenytoin is a prodrug of phenytoin, its anticonvulsant action is the same. Phenytoin is thought to stabilize neuronal membranes and limit seizure activity.
Therapeutic effect: prevents and controls seizures.

Indications and dosage
▶ **Status epilepticus.** *Adults:* 15 to 20 mg phenytoin sodium equivalent (PE)/kg I.V. at 100 to 150 mg PE/minute as loading dose; then 4 to 6 mg PE/kg/day I.V. as maintenance dose. (Phenytoin may be used instead of fosphenytoin as maintenance, using the appropriate dose.)
▶ **Prevention and treatment of seizures during neurosurgery (nonemergent loading or maintenance dosing).** *Adults:* loading dose of 10 to 20 mg PE/kg I.M. or I.V. at infusion rate not exceeding 150 mg PE/minute. Maintenance dose is 4 to 6 mg PE/kg/day I.V. or I.M.
▶ **Short-term substitution for oral phenytoin therapy.** *Adults:* same total daily dosage equivalent as oral phenytoin sodium therapy given as a single daily dose I.M. or I.V. at infusion rate not ex-

ceeding 150 mg PE/minute. Some patients may require more frequent dosing.

Adverse reactions

CNS: increased or decreased reflexes, speech disorders, dysarthria, asthenia, *intracranial hypertension*, thinking abnormalities, nervousness, hypesthesia, extrapyramidal syndrome, brain edema, headache, *nystagmus, dizziness, somnolence, ataxia,* stupor, incoordination, paresthesia, tremor, agitation, vertigo.
CV: hypertension, vasodilation, tachycardia, hypotension.
GI: constipation, taste perversion.
Hematologic: *thrombocytopenia, leukopenia, agranulocytosis, granulocytopenia, pancytopenia.*
Musculoskeletal: back pain, myasthenia, pelvic pain.
Respiratory: pneumonia.
Skin: ecchymosis, injection site reaction and pain, rash, *pruritus.*
Other: lymphadenopathy, hypokalemia, hyperglycemia, accidental injury, infection, chills.

Interactions

Most significant drug interactions expected to occur are those that are commonly seen with phenytoin.
Drug-drug. *Amiodarone, chloramphenicol, chlordiazepoxide, cimetidine, diazepam, dicumarol, disulfiram, estrogens, ethosuximide, fluoxetine, H_2-antagonists, halothane, isoniazid, methylphenidate, phenothiazines, phenylbutazone, salicylates, succinimides, sulfonamides, tolbutamide, trazodone:* may increase plasma phenytoin levels and thus its therapeutic effects. Use together cautiously.
Carbamazepine, reserpine: may decrease plasma phenytoin levels. Monitor patient.
Coumarin, digitoxin, doxycycline, estrogens, furosemide, oral contraceptives, rifampin, quinidine, theophylline, vitamin D: efficacy may be decreased by phenytoin owing to increased hepatic metabolism. Monitor closely.

Phenobarbital, valproic acid, sodium valproate: may increase or decrease plasma phenytoin levels. Monitor patient.
Tricyclic antidepressants: may lower seizure threshold and require adjustments in phenytoin dosage. Use cautiously.
Drug-lifestyle. *Acute alcohol use:* may increase plasma phenytoin levels and thus its therapeutic effects. Use together cautiously.
Chronic alcohol use: may decrease plasma phenytoin levels. Monitor patient.

Contraindications and precautions

• Contraindicated in patients with sinus bradycardia, SA block, second- or third-degree AV block, Adams-Stokes syndrome, and hypersensitivity to drug or its components, phenytoin, or other hydantoins.

NURSING CONSIDERATIONS

🔍 Assessment
• Do not give drug I.M. for status epilepticus because therapeutic phenytoin levels may not occur as rapidly as with I.V. administration.
• Know that after drug administration, phenytoin levels should not be monitored until about 2 hours after the end of I.V. infusion or 4 hours after I.M. administration.
• Evaluate patient's and family's knowledge of drug therapy.

🔲 Nursing diagnoses
• Risk for trauma related to seizures
• Knowledge deficit related to drug therapy

▶ Planning and implementation
• Know that drug should always be prescribed and dispensed in phenytoin sodium equivalent units (PE). Do not make any adjustments in the recommended doses when substituting fosphenytoin for phenytoin, and vice versa.
I.V. use: Before I.V. infusion, dilute drug in D_5W or 0.9% NaCl for injection to a

level ranging from 1.5 to 25 mg PE/ml. Do not exceed rate of 150 mg PE/minute. – Monitor patient's ECG, blood pressure, and respiration throughout period when maximal serum phenytoin levels occur— about 10 to 20 minutes after end of fosphenytoin infusion.

I.M. use: Know that I.M. use generates systemic phenytoin levels similar to oral phenytoin sodium, allowing essentially interchangeable use when ordered.

• Know that abrupt withdrawal of drug may cause status epilepticus.

Patient teaching
• Warn patient that sensory disturbances may occur with I.V. use.
• Instruct patient to immediately report adverse reactions, especially rash.
• Warn patient not to stop drug abruptly or adjust dosage without consulting doctor.
• Inform women that breast-feeding is not recommended.

☑ **Evaluation**
• Patient is free from seizure activity.
• Patient and family state understanding of drug therapy.

---

furosemide (frusemide♦◊)
(fyoo-ROH-seh-mighd)
Apo-Furosemide♦, Furoside♦, Lasix*, Lasix Special♦, Myrosemide*, Novosemide♦, Urex◊, Urex-M◊, Uritol♦

Pharmacologic class: loop diuretic
Therapeutic class: diuretic, antihypertensive
Pregnancy risk category: C

How supplied

Tablets: 20 mg, 40 mg, 80 mg, 500 mg♦◊
Oral solution: 40 mg/5 ml, 10 mg/ml
Injection: 10 mg/ml

Pharmacokinetics

Absorption: about 60% absorbed from GI tract after oral administration; unknown after I.M. use.
Distribution: about 95% plasma protein–bound.
Metabolism: metabolized minimally by liver.
Excretion: about 50% to 80% excreted in urine. *Half-life:* about 30 minutes.

Route	Onset	Peak	Duration
P.O.	20-60 min	1-2 hr	6-8 hr
I.V.	About 5 min	≤ 30 min	2 hr
I.M.	Unknown	Unknown	Unknown

Pharmacodynamics

Chemical effect: inhibits sodium and chloride reabsorption at proximal and distal tubules and ascending loop of Henle.
Therapeutic effect: promotes water and sodium excretion.

Indications and dosage

▶ **Acute pulmonary edema.** *Adults:* 40 mg I.V. injected slowly over 1 to 2 minutes; then 80 mg I.V. in 1 to 1½ hours, if needed.
▶ **Edema.** *Adults:* 20 to 80 mg P.O. daily in a.m., second dose in 6 to 8 hours; carefully titrated up to 600 mg daily if needed. Or, 20 to 40 mg I.M. or I.V., increased by 20 mg q 2 hours until desired response is achieved. Give I.V. dose slowly over 1 to 2 minutes. *Infants and children:* 2 mg/kg P.O. daily, increased by 1 to 2 mg/kg in 6 to 8 hours if needed; carefully titrated up to 6 mg/kg daily if needed.
▶ **Hypertension.** *Adults:* 40 mg P.O. b.i.d. Dosage adjusted according to response.

Adverse reactions

CNS: vertigo, headache, dizziness, paresthesia, restlessness, weakness.
CV: volume depletion and dehydration, orthostatic hypotension.

Reactions may be *common*, uncommon, *life-threatening*, or COMMON AND LIFE-THREATENING.

EENT: transient deafness (with too-rapid I.V. injection), blurred or yellow vision.
GI: abdominal discomfort and pain, diarrhea, anorexia, nausea, vomiting, constipation, *pancreatitis.*
GU: nocturia, polyuria, frequent urination, oliguria.
Hematologic: *agranulocytosis, leukopenia, thrombocytopenia,* azotemia, anemia, *aplastic anemia.*
Hepatic: *hepatic dysfunction,* increased cholesterol levels.
Metabolic: hypokalemia, hypochloremic alkalosis, asymptomatic hyperuricemia, gout, fluid and electrolyte imbalances, including dilutional hyponatremia, hypocalcemia, hypomagnesemia, hyperglycemia, and impairment of glucose tolerance.
Musculoskeletal: muscle spasm.
Skin: dermatitis, purpura, photosensitivity.
Other: fever, transient pain (at I.M. injection site); thrombophlebitis (with I.V. use).

Interactions

Drug-drug. *Aminoglycoside antibiotics, cisplatin:* potentiated ototoxicity. Use together cautiously.
Antidiabetic agents: decreased hypoglycemic effects. Monitor blood glucose levels.
Antihypertensives: increased risk of hypotension. Use together cautiously.
Corticosteroids, corticotropin, amphotericin B, metolazone: increased risk of hypokalemia. Monitor potassium levels closely.
Cardiac glycosides, neuromuscular blocking agents: increased toxicity of these agents from furosemide-induced hypokalemia. Monitor potassium levels closely.
Ethacrynic acid: may increase risk of ototoxicity. Do not use concomitantly.
Lithium: decreased lithium excretion, resulting in lithium toxicity. Monitor lithium level.

NSAIDs: inhibited diuretic response. Use together cautiously.
Salicylates: may cause salicylate toxicity. Use together cautiously.
Sucralfate: may reduce diuretic and antihypertensive effect.
Drug-lifestyle. *Sun exposure:* photosensitivity reactions may occur. Take precautions.

Contraindications and precautions

• Contraindicated in patients with anuria or history of hypersensitivity to drug.
• Drug is not recommended for use in breast-feeding women.
• Use cautiously in patients with hepatic cirrhosis.
• Use in pregnant women only if benefits outweigh risks.

NURSING CONSIDERATIONS

Assessment
• Obtain assessment of patient's underlying condition before therapy.
• Monitor weight, peripheral edema, breath sounds, blood pressure, fluid intake and output, and serum electrolyte, blood glucose, BUN, and carbon dioxide levels.
• Monitor blood uric acid, especially in patient with history of gout.
• Be alert for adverse reactions and drug interactions.
• Evaluate patient's and family's knowledge of drug therapy.

Nursing diagnoses
• Fluid volume excess related to presence of edema
• Altered urinary elimination related to diuretic therapy
• Knowledge deficit related to drug therapy

Planning and implementation
P.O. and I.M. use: Administer P.O. and I.M. doses in morning to prevent nocturia. Give second doses in early afternoon.

I.V. use: Give drug by direct injection over 1 to 2 minutes. Alternatively, dilute with D_5W, 0.9% NaCl solution, or lactated Ringer's solution, and infuse no faster than 4 mg/minute to avoid ototoxicity. Use prepared infusion solution within 24 hours.
• Store tablets in light-resistant container to prevent discoloration. Don't use discolored (yellow) injectable preparation. Refrigerate oral furosemide solution to ensure drug stability.
• Notify doctor if oliguria or azotemia develops or increases.
Patient teaching
• Advise patient to stand slowly to prevent dizziness, and to avoid alcohol and strenuous exercise in hot weather.
• Instruct patient to report ringing in ears, severe abdominal pain, or sore throat and fever; may indicate furosemide toxicity.
• Discourage patient from storing different drugs in same container, because this increases risk of errors. The most popular strengths of furosemide and digoxin are white tablets of similar size.
• Tell patient to check with doctor before taking OTC medications.

☑ **Evaluation**
• Patient is free from edema.
• Patient demonstrates adjustment of lifestyle to deal with altered patterns of urinary elimination.
• Patient and family state understanding of drug therapy.

gabapentin
(geh-buh-PEN-tin)
Neurontin

Pharmacologic class: 1-aminomethyl cyclohexoneacetic acid

Therapeutic class: anticonvulsant
Pregnancy risk category: C

How supplied
Capsules: 100 mg, 300 mg, 400 mg

Pharmacokinetics
Absorption: drug's bioavailability is not dose proportional but averages about 60%.
Distribution: drug circulates largely unbound to plasma protein.
Metabolism: not appreciably metabolized.
Excretion: excreted by kidneys as unchanged drug. *Half-life:* 5 to 7 hours.

Route	Onset	Peak	Duration
P.O.	Unknown	Unknown	Unknown

Pharmacodynamics
Chemical effect: unknown; although structurally related to gamma-amino butyric acid (GABA), drug doesn't interact with GABA receptors and isn't converted metabolically into GABA or a GABA agonist.
Therapeutic effect: prevents and treats partial seizures.

Indications and dosage
▶ **Adjunct treatment of partial seizures with and without secondary generalization in adults with epilepsy.**
Adults: initially 300 mg P.O. h.s. on day 1; 300 mg P.O. b.i.d. on day 2; then 300 mg P.O. t.i.d. on day 3. Dosage increased as needed and tolerated to 1,800 mg daily in divided doses. Dosages up to 3,600 mg daily have been well tolerated. *In patients with renal failure:* if creatinine clearance is over 60 ml/minute, 400 mg P.O. t.i.d.; if creatinine clearance is 30 to 60 ml/minute, 300 mg P.O. b.i.d.; if creatinine clearance is 15 to 30 ml/minute, 300 mg P.O. daily; if creatinine clearance is below 15 ml/minute, 300 mg P.O. every other day. Patients on dialysis should receive loading dose of 300 to 400 mg P.O.; then 200 to 300 mg P.O. following q 4 hours of hemodialysis.

Adverse reactions

CNS: *somnolence, dizziness, ataxia, fatigue, nystagmus, tremor,* nervousness, dysarthria, amnesia, depression, abnormal thinking, twitching, abnormal coordination.
CV: peripheral edema, vasodilation.
EENT: *diplopia, rhinitis,* pharyngitis, dry throat, coughing, *amblyopia.*
GI: nausea, vomiting, dyspepsia, dry mouth, constipation.
GU: impotence.
Hematologic: *leukopenia,* decreased WBC count.
Musculoskeletal: back pain, myalgia, fractures.
Skin: pruritus, abrasion.
Other: dental abnormalities, increased appetite, weight gain.

Interactions

Drug-drug. *Antacids:* decreased absorption of gabapentin. Separate administration times by at least 2 hours.

Contraindications and precautions

• Contraindicated in patients hypersensitive to drug.
• Use cautiously in pregnant women.
• Safety of drug has not been established in breast-feeding women or in children younger than age 12.

NURSING CONSIDERATIONS

⚖ Assessment
• Assess patient's disorder before therapy and regularly thereafter.
• Routine monitoring of plasma drug levels is not necessary. Drug does not appear to alter plasma levels of other anticonvulsants.
• Be alert for adverse reactions and drug interactions.
• Evaluate patient's and family's knowledge of drug therapy.

⊞ Nursing diagnoses
• Risk for trauma related to seizures

• Risk for injury related to drug-induced adverse CNS reactions
• Knowledge deficit related to drug therapy

▶ Planning and implementation
• Give first dose at bedtime to minimize drowsiness, dizziness, fatigue, and ataxia.
• If gabapentin is discontinued or alternative drug is substituted, do so gradually over at least 1 week as ordered to minimize risk of precipitating seizures. Do not suddenly withdraw other anticonvulsants in patient starting gabapentin therapy.
• Drug may cause false-positive tests for urine protein when Ames-N-Multistix SG dipstick test is used.
• Institute seizure precautions.
Patient teaching
• Tell patient to take drug without regard to meals.
• Warn patient to avoid driving or operating heavy machinery until drug's CNS effects are known.

☑ Evaluation
• Patient is free from seizures.
• Patient does not experience injury from adverse CNS reactions.
• Patient and family state understanding of drug therapy.

ganciclovir
(jan-SIGH-kloh-veer)
Cytovene

Pharmacologic class: synthetic nucleoside
Therapeutic class: antiviral
Pregnancy risk category: C

How supplied

Capsules: 250 mg, 500 mg
Injection: 500 mg/vial

Pharmacokinetics

Absorption: poorly absorbed after oral administration. Bioavailability is about 5% under fasting conditions.

Distribution: preferentially concentrates within CMV-infected cells; only 2% to 3% protein-bound.
Metabolism: over 90% of drug is not metabolized.
Excretion: mostly excreted unchanged.
Half-life: about 3 hours.

Route	Onset	Peak	Duration
P.O.	Unknown	Unknown	Unknown
I.V.	Immediate	Immediate	Unknown

Pharmacodynamics

Chemical effect: unknown; may inhibit viral DNA synthesis of CMV.
Therapeutic effect: inhibits CMV.

Indications and dosage

▶ **Treatment of CMV retinitis in immunocompromised patients, including those with AIDS.** *Adults:* induction treatment—5 mg/kg I.V. q 12 hours for 14 to 21 days (normal renal function); maintenance treatment—5 mg/kg I.V. daily for 7 days weekly, or 6 mg/kg I.V. daily for 5 days weekly. Alternatively, following induction treatment, 1,000 mg P.O. t.i.d. with food. Dosage is adjusted for patients with impaired renal function and is based on creatinine clearance levels.
▶ **Prevention of CMV disease in transplant recipients at risk for CMV disease.** 5 mg/kg I.V. q 12 hours for 7 to 14 days, followed by 5 mg/kg once daily 7 days weekly or 6 mg/kg once daily 5 days weekly. Alternatively, 1,000 mg P.O. t.i.d. with food. Duration of treatment with I.V. ganciclovir in transplant recipients depends on duration and degree of immunosuppression.
▶ **Prevention of CMV disease in patients with advanced HIV infection at risk for development of CMV disease.** 1,000 mg P.O. t.i.d. with food.

Adverse reactions

CNS: altered dreams, confusion, ataxia, dizziness, headache, *seizures, coma,* behavioral changes.
CV: *arrhythmias,* hypotension, hypertension.
EENT: retinal detachment (in CMV retinitis patients).
GI: nausea, vomiting, diarrhea, anorexia.
GU: hematuria, increased serum creatinine levels.
Hematologic: *thrombocytopenia, agranulocytosis, leukopenia.*
Hepatic: abnormal liver function tests results.
Other: inflammation, pain, phlebitis (at injection site).

Interactions

Drug-drug. *Cytotoxic agents:* increased toxic effects, especially hematologic effects and stomatitis. Monitor closely.
Imipenem/cilastatin: heightened seizure activity with concomitant use. Monitor closely.
Immunosuppressants (such as azathioprine, corticosteroids, cyclosporine): enhanced immune and bone marrow suppression. Use together cautiously.
Probenecid: increased ganciclovir blood levels. Monitor closely.
Zidovudine: increased incidence of granulocytopenia with concurrent use. Monitor closely.

Contraindications and precautions

• Contraindicated in patients hypersensitive to drug and in those with absolute neutrophil count below 500/mm³ or platelet count below 25,000/mm³.
• Drug not recommended for use in breast-feeding women.
• Use cautiously and in reduced dosage in patients with renal dysfunction and in pregnant women.
• Safety of drug has not been established in children.

NURSING CONSIDERATIONS

Assessment
• Assess patient's condition before therapy and regularly thereafter.

• Obtain neutrophil and platelet counts every 2 days during twice-daily ganciclovir dosing and at least weekly thereafter, as ordered.
• Monitor hydration status if adverse GI reactions occur with oral drug.
• Be alert for adverse reactions and drug interactions.
• Evaluate patient's and family's knowledge of drug therapy.

🔆 Nursing diagnoses
• Infection related to CMV retinitis
• Altered protection related to adverse hematologic reactions
• Knowledge deficit related to drug therapy.

▶ Planning and implementation
P.O. use: Give drug with food.
I.V. use: Reconstitute with 10 ml sterile water for injection. Shake vial to dissolve drug. Further dilute appropriate dose in 0.9% NaCl, D₅W, Ringer's lactate or Ringer's solution (typically 100 ml) and infuse over 1 hour. Infusion concentrations greater than 10 mg/ml are not recommended.
– Administer drug over at least 1 hour. Faster infusions will result in increased toxicity. Use infusion pump. Do not administer as I.V. bolus.
– Use caution when preparing solution, which is alkaline.
• Do not administer drug S.C. or I.M.— severe tissue irritation could result.
• Encourage fluid intake; ganciclovir infusion therapy should be accompanied by adequate hydration.
• Alert doctor to signs of renal failure because the dosage will need adjustment.
Patient teaching
• Tell patient to take oral form of drug with food.
• Stress importance of drinking adequate fluid throughout therapy.
• Advise patient to alert nurse if pain or discomfort occurs at I.V. site.

• Instruct patient about infection-control and bleeding precautions.

✔ Evaluation
• Patient is free from infection.
• Patient does not experience serious adverse hematologic reactions.
• Patient and family state understanding of drug therapy.

---

gemfibrozil
(jem-FIGH-broh-zil)
Lopid

Pharmacologic class: fibric acid derivative
Therapeutic class: antilipemic
Pregnancy risk category: C

How supplied
Tablets: 600 mg
Capsules: 300 mg

Pharmacokinetics
Absorption: well absorbed from GI tract.
Distribution: 95% protein-bound.
Metabolism: metabolized by liver.
Excretion: excreted primarily in urine, with some excretion in feces. *Half-life:* about 1.25 hours. Biological half-life is considerably longer, as a result of enterohepatic circulation and reabsorption in the GI tract.

Route	Onset	Peak	Duration
P.O.	2-5 days	> 4 wk	Unknown

Pharmacodynamics
Chemical effect: inhibits peripheral lipolysis and also reduces triglyceride synthesis in liver.
Therapeutic effect: lowers serum triglyceride levels and raises high-density lipoprotein (HDL) levels.

Indications and dosage
▶ **Type IV and V hyperlipidemia unresponsive to diet and other drugs; re-**

duction of risk of coronary heart disease in patients with type IIb hyperlipidemia who cannot tolerate or who are refractory to treatment with bile acid sequestrants or niacin. *Adults:* 1,200 mg P.O. daily in two divided doses, 30 minutes before morning and evening meals. If no benefit is seen after 3 months of therapy, drug should be discontinued.

Adverse reactions

CNS: blurred vision, headache, dizziness.
GI: *abdominal and epigastric pain, diarrhea, nausea,* vomiting, flatulence.
Hematologic: *anemia, leukopenia, thrombocytopenia.*
Hepatic: bile duct obstruction, elevated liver enzymes.
Skin: rash, dermatitis, pruritus.
Other: painful extremities.

Interactions

Drug-drug. *HMG-CoA reductase inhibitors:* myopathy with rhabdomyolysis has been reported. Don't use together.
Oral anticoagulants: gemfibrozil may enhance clinical effects of oral anticoagulants. Monitor patient.

Contraindications and precautions

• Contraindicated in patients with hepatic or severe renal dysfunction (including primary biliary cirrhosis), preexisting gallbladder disease, or hypersensitivity to drug.
• Use cautiously in pregnant women.
• Safety of drug has not been established in breast-feeding women or in children.

NURSING CONSIDERATIONS

⚕ Assessment
• Assess patient's serum triglyceride and HDL levels before therapy and regularly thereafter.
• Know that periodic CBCs and liver function tests should be performed during first 12 months of therapy.
• Be alert for adverse reactions and drug interactions.

• Evaluate patient's and family's knowledge of drug therapy.

⚕ Nursing diagnoses
• High risk for injury related to elevated blood lipids and cholesterol levels
• Diarrhea related to drug's adverse effect on GI tract
• Knowledge deficit related to drug therapy

⚕ Planning and implementation
• Administer drug 30 minutes before breakfast and dinner.
• Ensure that patient is following standard low-cholesterol diet.
Patient teaching
• Instruct patient to take drug 30 minutes before breakfast and dinner.
• Teach patient dietary management of serum lipids (restricting total fat and cholesterol intake) and measures to control other cardiac disease risk factors. If appropriate, suggest weight control, exercise, and smoking cessation programs.
• Advise patient to avoid driving or other potentially hazardous activities until drug's CNS effects are known.
• Tell patient to observe bowel movements and to report signs of steatorrhea or bile duct obstruction.

⚕ Evaluation
• Patient's blood triglyceride and cholesterol levels are normal.
• Patient regains normal bowel patterns.
• Patient and family state understanding of drug therapy.

gentamicin sulfate
(jen-tuh-MIGH-sin SUL-fayt)
Cidomycin♦, Garamycin, Gentamicin Sulfate ADD-Vantage, Jenamicin

Pharmacologic class: aminoglycoside
Therapeutic class: antibiotic
Pregnancy risk category: NR

How supplied

Injection: 40 mg/ml (adult), 10 mg/ml (pediatric), 2 mg/ml (intrathecal)
I.V. infusion (premixed): 40 mg, 60 mg, 70 mg, 80 mg, 90 mg, 100 mg, available in 0.9% NaCl solution

Pharmacokinetics

Absorption: unknown after I.M. administration.
Distribution: distributed widely. CSF penetration is low even in patients with inflamed meninges. Protein-binding is minimal.
Metabolism: not metabolized.
Excretion: excreted primarily in urine; small amounts may be excreted in bile.
Half-life: 2 to 3 hours.

Route	Onset	Peak	Duration
I.V.	Immediate	30-90 min	Unknown
I.M.	Unknown	30-90 min	Unknown
Intrathecal	Unknown	Unknown	Unknown

Pharmacodynamics

Chemical effect: inhibits protein synthesis by binding to ribosomes.
Therapeutic effect: kills susceptible bacteria (many aerobic gram-negative organisms and some aerobic gram-positive organisms). Drug may act against some aminoglycoside-resistant bacteria.

Indications and dosage

▶ **Serious infections caused by sensitive strains of** *Pseudomonas aeruginosa, Escherichia coli, Proteus, Klebsiella, Serratia, Enterobacter, Citrobacter, Staphylococcus. Adults:* 3 mg/kg daily in divided doses I.M. or I.V. infusion q 8 hours (in 50 to 200 ml of 0.9% NaCl solution or D$_5$W infused over 30 minutes to 2 hours). For life-threatening infections, patient may receive up to 5 mg/kg daily in three to four divided doses. *Children:* 2 to 2.5 mg/kg q 8 hours I.M. or by I.V. infusion. *Neonates over 1 week or infants:* 7.5 mg/kg daily in divided doses q 8 hours. *Neonates under 1*

week and preterm infants: 2.5 mg/kg I.V. q 12 hours.
▶ **Meningitis.** *Adults:* systemic therapy as above; 4 to 8 mg intrathecally daily also may be used. *Children and infants over age 3 months:* systemic therapy as above; 1 to 2 mg intrathecally daily may also be used.
▶ **Endocarditis prophylaxis for GI or GU procedure or surgery.** *Adults:* 1.5 mg/kg I.M. or I.V. 30 to 60 minutes before procedure or surgery and q 8 hours after, for two doses. Given separately with aqueous penicillin or ampicillin. *Children:* 2 mg/kg I.M. or I.V. 30 to 60 minutes before procedure or surgery and q 8 hours after, for two doses. Given separately with aqueous penicillin G or ampicillin G.
▶ **Posthemodialysis to maintain therapeutic blood levels.** *Adults:* 1 to 1.7 mg/kg I.M. or by I.V. infusion after each dialysis. *Children:* 2 mg/kg I.M. or by I.V. infusion after each dialysis.

Adverse reactions

CNS: headache, lethargy, numbness, peripheral neuropathy, *seizures.*
EENT: *ototoxicity* (tinnitus, vertigo, hearing loss).
GU: *nephrotoxicity* (cells or casts in urine; oliguria; proteinuria; decreased creatinine clearance; increased BUN, nonprotein nitrogen, and serum creatinine levels).
Hematologic: *thrombocytopenia, leukopenia, agranulocytosis.*
Other: hypersensitivity reactions.

Interactions

Drug-drug. *Acyclovir, amphotericin B, cisplatin, methoxyflurane, other aminoglycosides, vancomycin:* increased ototoxicity and nephrotoxicity. Use together cautiously.
Cephalothin: increased nephrotoxicity. Use together cautiously.
Dimenhydrinate: may mask symptoms of ototoxicity. Use with caution.

General anesthetics, neuromuscular blockers: may potentiate neuromuscular blockade. Monitor closely.
Indomethacin: may increase serum peak and trough levels of gentamicin. Monitor serum gentamicin levels.
I.V. loop diuretics (such as furosemide): increased ototoxicity. Use cautiously.
Parenteral penicillins (such as ampicillin, ticarcillin): gentamicin inactivation in vitro. Don't mix together.

Contraindications and precautions

• Contraindicated in patients with hypersensitivity to drug or other aminoglycosides.
• Use cautiously in patients with impaired renal function or neuromuscular disorders and in neonates, infants, and the elderly.

NURSING CONSIDERATIONS

⚗ Assessment
• Assess patient's infection before therapy and regularly thereafter.
• Obtain specimen for culture and sensitivity tests before first dose.
• Evaluate patient's hearing before therapy and regularly thereafter.
• Weigh patient and review baseline renal function studies before therapy and then regularly during therapy.
• Obtain blood for peak drug level 1 hour after I.M. injection and 30 minutes to 1 hour after I.V. infusion; for trough levels, draw blood just before next dose. Don't collect blood in heparinized tube because heparin is incompatible with aminoglycosides.
• Be aware that peak blood levels above 12 mcg/ml and trough levels above 2 mcg/ml may be associated with higher incidence of toxicity.
• Be alert for adverse reactions and drug interactions.
• Evaluate patient's and family's knowledge of drug therapy.

✛ Nursing diagnoses
• Infection related to presence of susceptible bacteria
• Altered urinary elimination related to nephrotoxicity
• Knowledge deficit related to drug therapy

▶ Planning and implementation
I.V. use: When giving drug by intermittent I.V. infusion, dilute with 50 to 200 ml of D_5W or 0.9% NaCl injection and infuse over 30 minutes to 2 hours. After infusion, flush line with 0.9% NaCl solution or D_5W.
I.M. use: Administer drug deep into large muscle mass (gluteal or midlateral thigh); rotate injection sites. Do not inject more than 2 g of drug per site.
Intrathecal use: Use preservative-free formulations of gentamicin when using intrathecal route.
• Know that hemodialysis (8 hours) removes up to 50% of drug from blood.
• Notify doctor of signs of decreasing renal function or changes in hearing.
• Know that therapy usually continues for 7 to 10 days. If no response occurs in 3 to 5 days, therapy may be stopped and new specimens obtained for culture and sensitivity testing.
• Encourage adequate fluid intake; patient should be well hydrated while taking drug to minimize chemical irritation of renal tubules.
Patient teaching
• Instruct patient to notify doctor if adverse reactions, such as changes in hearing, occur.
• Emphasize importance of fluid intake of at least 2,000 ml/day if not contraindicated.

✔ Evaluation
• Patient is free from infection.
• Patient maintains normal renal function throughout drug therapy.
• Patient and family state understanding of drug therapy.

---

glimepiride
(gligh-MEH-peh-righd)
Amaryl

Pharmacologic class: sulfonylurea
Therapeutic class: antidiabetic
Pregnancy risk category: C

How supplied

Tablets: 1 mg, 2 mg, 4 mg

Pharmacokinetics

Absorption: completely absorbed.
Distribution: 99.5% protein-bound.
Metabolism: completely metabolized.
Excretion: in urine and feces.

Route	Onset	Peak	Duration
P.O.	Within 1 hr	2-3 hr	Unknown

Pharmacodynamics

Chemical effect: stimulates release of insulin from pancreatic beta cells; increases sensitivity of peripheral tissues to insulin.
Therapeutic effect: lowers blood glucose levels.

Indications and dosage

► **Adjunct to diet and exercise to lower blood glucose in patients with type 2 (non-insulin-dependent) diabetes mellitus whose hyperglycemia cannot be managed by diet and exercise alone.** *Adults:* initially, 1 to 2 mg P.O. once daily with first main meal of day; usual maintenance dosage is 1 to 4 mg P.O. once daily. After reaching dose of 2 mg, dosage increased in increments not exceeding 2 mg q 1 to 2 weeks, based on patient's blood glucose response. Maximum dosage is 8 mg/day.
► **Adjunct to insulin therapy in patients with type 2 (non-insulin-dependent) diabetes mellitus whose hyperglycemia cannot be managed by diet and exercise in conjunction with oral hypoglycemic agents.** *Adults:* 8 mg P.O. once daily with first main meal of day; use in combination with low-dose insulin. Adjust insulin upward weekly as needed, based on patient's blood glucose response.
Note: In patients with renal impairment: initially, 1 mg P.O. once daily with first main meal of day, followed by appropriate dose, titrated as needed.

Adverse reactions

CNS: dizziness, asthenia, headache.
EENT: changes in accommodation.
GI: nausea.
Hematologic: leukopenia, hemolytic anemia, *agranulocytosis, thrombocytopenia, aplastic anemia, pancytopenia.*
Hepatic: cholestatic jaundice, elevated transaminase levels.
Metabolic: hypoglycemia.
Skin: allergic skin reactions (pruritus, erythema, urticaria, and morbilliform or maculopapular eruptions).

Interactions

Drug-drug. *Beta blockers:* may mask symptoms of hypoglycemia. Monitor glucose levels carefully.
Drugs that produce hyperglycemia, other diuretics: may lead to loss of glucose control. Adjust dosage as ordered.
Insulin: concomitant use may increase potential for hypoglycemia.
NSAIDs, other drugs that are highly protein-bound: may potentiate hypoglycemic action of sulfonylureas like glimepiride.
Drug-lifestyle. *Alcohol use:* altered glycemic control, most commonly hypoglycemia. May cause disulfiram-like reaction. Avoid concomitant use.

Contraindications and precautions

• Contraindicated in patients with diabetic ketoacidosis or hypersensitivity to drug.
• Use cautiously in debilitated or malnourished patients and in those with adrenal, pituitary, hepatic, or renal insufficiency.

---

*Liquid form contains alcohol   **May contain tartrazine   ♦Canada   ◊Australia   †OTC

NURSING CONSIDERATIONS

⚖ Assessment
• Monitor fasting blood glucose periodically to determine therapeutic response. Also monitor glycosylated hemoglobin, usually every 3 to 6 months, to more precisely assess long-term glycemic control.
• Evaluate patient's and family's knowledge of drug therapy.

⊞ Nursing diagnoses
• Altered health maintenance related to hyperglycemia
• Risk for injury related to drug-induced hypoglycemia
• Knowledge deficit related to drug therapy

≫ Planning and implementation
• Know that oral hypoglycemic agents have been linked with an increased risk of CV mortality compared with diet alone or with diet and insulin therapy.
• Do not give drug to breast-feeding women.

Patient teaching
• Tell patient to take drug with first meal of day.
• Stress importance of adhering to diet, weight-reduction, exercise, and personal-hygiene programs. Explain to patient and family how to self-monitor blood glucose levels, and teach them signs, symptoms, and treatment of hyperglycemia and hypoglycemia.
• Advise patient to carry medical identification about his condition.
• Advise woman planning pregnancy to consult doctor before becoming pregnant.
• Instruct patient to avoid alcohol consumption while on drug therapy.

☑ Evaluation
• Patient's blood glucose level is normal.
• Patient recognizes hypoglycemia early and treats it before injury occurs.
• Patient and family state understanding of drug therapy.

glipizide
(GLIGH-peh-zighd)
Glucotrol, Glucotrol XL, Minidiab◇

Pharmacologic class: sulfonylurea
Therapeutic class: antidiabetic
Pregnancy risk category: C

How supplied
Tablets: 5 mg, 10 mg
Tablets (extended-release): 5 mg, 10 mg

Pharmacokinetics
Absorption: absorbed rapidly and completely from GI tract.
Distribution: distributed within extracellular fluid; about 92% to 99% protein-bound.
Metabolism: metabolized by liver to inactive metabolites.
Excretion: primarily in urine; small amounts in feces. *Half-life:* 2 to 4 hours.

Route	Onset	Peak	Duration
P.O.	15-30 min	1-3 hr	10-16 hr

Pharmacodynamics
Chemical effect: may stimulate insulin release from pancreas, reduce glucose output by liver, and increase peripheral sensitivity to insulin.
Therapeutic effect: lowers blood glucose levels.

Indications and dosage

▶ **Adjunct to diet to lower blood glucose level in patients with type 2 (non-insulin-dependent) diabetes mellitus.**
Adults: initially, 5 mg P.O. daily before breakfast. Elderly patients or those with liver disease may be started on 2.5 mg. Maximum once-daily dosage is 15 mg. Maximum recommended total daily dosage is 40 mg. **Extended-release tablets.** *Adults:* 5 mg P.O. daily. Titrate in 5-mg increments q 3 months depending on level of glycemic control. Maximum daily dosage for these tablets is 20 mg.

Reactions may be *common*, uncommon, *life-threatening*, or COMMON AND LIFE-THREATENING.

▶ **To replace insulin therapy.** *Adults:* if insulin dosage is more than 20 units daily, patient is started at usual dosage in addition to 50% of insulin. If insulin dosage is less than 20 units, insulin may be discontinued.

Adverse reactions

CNS: dizziness.
GI: nausea, vomiting, constipation.
Hematologic: *agranulocytosis, thrombocytopenia, aplastic anemia.*
Hepatic: cholestatic jaundice.
Metabolic: *hypoglycemia.*
Skin: rash, pruritus, facial flushing.

Interactions

Drug-drug. *Anabolic steroids, chloramphenicol, clofibrate, guanethidine, MAO inhibitors, phenylbutazone, probenecid, salicylates, sulfonamides:* increased hypoglycemic activity. Monitor blood glucose level.
Beta blockers, clonidine: prolonged hypoglycemic effect and masked symptoms of hypoglycemia. Use together cautiously.
Corticosteroids, glucagon, rifampin, thiazide diuretics: decreased hypoglycemic response. Monitor blood glucose level.
Hydantoins: increased blood levels of hydantoins. Monitor blood levels.
Oral anticoagulants: increased hypoglycemic activity or enhanced anticoagulant effect. Monitor blood glucose levels and PT and INR.
Drug-lifestyle. *Alcohol use:* altered glycemic control, most commonly hypoglycemia. May also cause disulfiram-like reaction. Avoid concomitant use.

Contraindications and precautions

• Contraindicated in patients with diabetic ketoacidosis or hypersensitivity to drug and in pregnant or breast-feeding women.
• Use cautiously in patients with renal and hepatic disease and in debilitated, malnourished, or elderly patients.
• Safety of drug has not been established in children because of the rare occurrence

of type 2 diabetes mellitus in this population.

NURSING CONSIDERATIONS

ᴴ Assessment
• Assess blood glucose level before therapy and regularly thereafter.
• Patients transferring from insulin therapy to oral antidiabetic agent require blood glucose monitoring at least three times daily before meals.
• During periods of increased stress, such as infection, fever, surgery, or trauma, patient may require insulin therapy. Monitor patient closely for hyperglycemia in these situations.
• Be alert for adverse reactions and drug interactions.
• Evaluate patient's and family's knowledge of drug therapy.

ᴴ Nursing diagnoses
• Altered health maintenance related to hyperglycemia
• Risk for injury related to drug-induced hypoglycemia
• Knowledge deficit related to drug therapy

ᴴ Planning and implementation
• Give drug about 30 minutes before meals.
• Some patients taking drug may attain effective control on once-daily regimen; others show better response with divided dosing.
• Treat hypoglycemic reaction with oral form of rapid-acting carbohydrates if patient can swallow or with glucagon or I.V. glucose if patient can't swallow or is comatose. Follow up treatment with complex carbohydrate snack when patient is awake, and determine cause of reaction.
• Be sure that adjunct therapies, such as diet and exercise, are being used appropriately.
Patient teaching
• Instruct patient about nature of disease; importance of following therapeutic regi-

men; adhering to specific diet, weight reduction, exercise, and personal hygiene programs; and avoiding infection. Explain how and when to monitor blood glucose level, and teach recognition and treatment of hypoglycemia and hyperglycemia.

• Tell patient not to change dosage without doctor's consent and to report abnormal blood or urine glucose test results.

• Advise patient not to take other medications, including OTC drugs, without first checking with doctor.

• Instruct patient to avoid alcohol consumption during drug therapy.

• Advise patient to carry medical identification at all times.

☑ **Evaluation**

• Patient's blood glucose level is normal with drug therapy.

• Patient does not experience hypoglycemia.

• Patient and family state understanding of drug therapy.

glucagon
(GLOO-kuh-gon)

Pharmacologic class: pancreatic hormone
Therapeutic class: antihypoglycemic
Pregnancy risk category: B

How supplied

Powder for injection: 1 mg (1 unit)/vial, 10 mg (10 units)/vial

Pharmacokinetics

Absorption: unknown.
Distribution: unknown.
Metabolism: drug is degraded extensively by liver, in kidneys and plasma, and at its tissue receptor sites in plasma membranes.
Excretion: excreted by kidneys. *Half-life:* 3 to 10 minutes.

Route	Onset	Peak	Duration
I.V., I.M., S.C.	Almost immediate	≤ 30 min	1-2 hr

Pharmacodynamics

Chemical effect: promotes catalytic depolymerization of hepatic glycogen to glucose.
Therapeutic effect: raises blood glucose level.

Indications and dosage

▶ **Hypoglycemia.** *Adults and children weighing over 20 kg (44 lb):* 1 mg I.V., I.M., or S.C. *Children weighing 20 kg or less:* 0.5 mg I.V., I.M., or S.C. *Note:* May repeat in 15 minutes if necessary. I.V. glucose must be given if patient fails to respond. When patient responds, supplemental carbohydrate needs to be given promptly.

▶ **Diagnostic aid for radiologic examination.** *Adults:* 0.25 to 2 mg I.V. or I.M. before initiation of radiologic procedure.

Adverse reactions

GI: nausea, vomiting.
Other: hypersensitivity reactions (*bronchospasm,* rash, dizziness, lightheadedness).

Interactions

Drug-drug. *Oral anticoagulants:* anticoagulant effect may be increased. Monitor PT and INR closely.
Phenytoin: inhibited glucagon-induced insulin release. Use cautiously.

Contraindications and precautions

• Contraindicated in patients with pheochromocytoma or hypersensitivity to drug.

• Use cautiously in patients with history of insulinoma or pheochromocytoma.

NURSING CONSIDERATIONS

☑ **Assessment**

• Assess patient's blood glucose level before therapy and after drug administration.

• Be alert for adverse reactions and drug interactions.

• Monitor patient's hydration status if vomiting occurs.

• Evaluate patient's and family's knowledge of drug therapy.

⊞ **Nursing diagnoses**
• Risk for injury related to patient's hypoglycemia
• Risk for fluid-volume deficit related to drug-induced vomiting
• Knowledge deficit related to drug therapy

▷ **Planning and implementation**
• Reconstitute 1-unit vial with 1 ml of diluent; reconstitute 10-unit vial with 10 ml of diluent. Use only diluent supplied by manufacturer when preparing doses of 2 mg or less. For larger doses, dilute with sterile water for injection.
I.V. use: For I.V. drip infusion, use dextrose solution, which is compatible with glucagon; drug forms precipitate in chloride solutions. Inject directly into vein or into I.V. tubing of free-flowing compatible solution over 2 to 5 minutes. Interrupt primary infusion during glucagon injection if using same I.V. line.
I.M. and S.C. use: Follow normal protocol.
• Arouse patient from coma as quickly as possible and give additional carbohydrates orally to prevent secondary hypoglycemic reactions.
• Notify doctor that patient's hypoglycemic episode required glucagon use. Be prepared to provide emergency intervention if patient does not respond to glucagon administration. Unstable hypoglycemic diabetic patient may not respond to glucagon; give dextrose I.V. instead as ordered.
• Notify doctor if patient cannot retain some form of sugar for 1 hour because of nausea or vomiting.
Patient teaching
• Instruct patient and family in proper drug administration.
• Teach them to recognize hypoglycemia, and tell them to notify doctor immediately in emergencies.

☑ **Evaluation**
• Patient's blood glucose level returns to normal.
• Patient remains well hydrated.
• Patient and family state understanding of drug therapy.

glyburide (glibenclamide)
(GLIGH-byoo-righd)
Albert Glyburide♦, Apo-Glyburide♦, DiaBeta**, Euglucon♦, Gen-Glybe♦, Glynase PresTab, Micronase, Novo-Glyburide♦, Nu-Glyburide♦

Pharmacologic class: sulfonylurea
Therapeutic class: antidiabetic
Pregnancy risk category: B

How supplied
Tablets: 1.25 mg, 2.5 mg, 5 mg
Tablets (micronized): 1.5 mg, 3 mg, 6 mg

Pharmacokinetics
Absorption: absorbed almost completely from GI tract.
Distribution: unknown, although it is 99% protein-bound.
Metabolism: metabolized completely by liver to inactive metabolites.
Excretion: excreted as metabolites in urine and feces in equal proportions.
Half-life: 10 hours.

Route	Onset	Peak	Duration
P.O.	1-4 hr	2-4 hr	24 hr

Pharmacodynamics
Chemical effect: unknown; may stimulate insulin release from pancreas, reduce glucose output by liver, increase peripheral sensitivity to insulin, and cause mild diuresis.
Therapeutic effect: lowers blood glucose levels.

Indications and dosage

▶ **Adjunct to diet to lower blood glucose level in patients with type 2 (non-insulin-dependent) diabetes mellitus.**
Adults: initially, 1.25 to 5 mg regular tablets P.O. once daily with breakfast; for maintenance, 1.25 to 20 mg daily as single dose or in divided doses. Or initially, 0.75 to 3 mg micronized formulation P.O. daily; for maintenance, 0.75 to 12 mg P.O. daily in single or divided doses.
▶ **To replace insulin therapy.** *Adults:* initially, if insulin dosage is more than 40 units daily, 5 mg regular tablets or 3 mg micronized formulation P.O. once daily in addition to 50% of insulin dosage. If insulin dosage is 20 to 40 units daily, 5 mg regular tablets or 3 mg micronized formulation P.O. once daily with abrupt insulin discontinuation. If insulin dosage is less than 20 units daily, 2.5 to 5 mg regular tablets or 1.5 to 3 mg micronized formulation P.O. once daily with abrupt insulin discontinuation.

Adverse reactions

GI: nausea, epigastric fullness, heartburn.
Hematologic: *agranulocytosis, thrombocytopenia, aplastic anemia.*
Hepatic: cholestatic jaundice.
Metabolic: *hypoglycemia.*
Skin: rash, pruritus, facial flushing.

Interactions

Drug-drug. *Anabolic steroids, chloramphenicol, clofibrate, guanethidine, MAO inhibitors, phenylbutazone, salicylates, sulfonamides:* increased hypoglycemic activity. Monitor blood glucose level.
Beta blockers, clonidine: prolonged hypoglycemic effect and masked symptoms of hypoglycemia. Use together cautiously.
Corticosteroids, glucagon, rifampin, thiazide diuretics: decreased hypoglycemic response. Monitor blood glucose level.
Hydantoins: increased blood levels of hydantoins. Monitor blood levels.
Oral anticoagulants: increased hypoglycemic activity or enhanced anticoagu-

lant effect. Monitor blood glucose level and PT and INR.
Drug-lifestyle. *Alcohol use:* altered glycemic control, most commonly hypoglycemia. May also cause disulfiram-like reaction. Avoid concomitant use.

Contraindications and precautions

• Contraindicated in patients with diabetic ketoacidosis or hypersensitivity to drug, in pregnant or breast-feeding women, and in children.
• Use cautiously in patients with hepatic or renal impairment, in debilitated, malnourished, or elderly patients.

NURSING CONSIDERATIONS

▨ Assessment

• Assess blood glucose level before therapy and regularly thereafter.
• Patient transferring from insulin therapy to oral antidiabetic agent requires blood glucose monitoring at least three times daily before meals.
• During periods of increased stress, such as infection, fever, surgery, or trauma, patient may require insulin therapy. Monitor patient closely for hyperglycemia in these situations.
• Be alert for adverse reactions and drug interactions.
• Evaluate patient's and family's knowledge of drug therapy.

▣ Nursing diagnoses

• Altered health maintenance related to hyperglycemia
• Risk for injury related to drug-induced hypoglycemia
• Knowledge deficit related to drug therapy

▶ Planning and implementation

• Micronized glyburide (Glynase PresTab) contains drug in smaller particle size and is not bioequivalent to regular tablets. Dose for patient who has been taking Micronase or DiaBeta needs to be retitrated.

Reactions may be *common*, uncommon, *life-threatening*, or COMMON AND LIFE-THREATENING.

• Although most patients take glyburide once daily, patient taking more than 10 mg daily may achieve better results with twice-daily dosage.
• Treat hypoglycemic reaction with oral form of rapid-acting carbohydrates if patient can swallow or with glucagon or I.V. glucose if patient can't swallow or is comatose. Follow up treatment with complex carbohydrate snack when patient is awake, and determine cause of reaction.
• Be sure that adjunct therapy, such as diet and exercise, is being used appropriately.
Patient teaching
• Instruct patient about nature of disease; importance of following therapeutic regimen; adhering to specific diet, weight reduction, exercise, and personal hygiene programs; and avoiding infection. Explain how and when to monitor blood glucose level, and teach recognition and treatment of hypoglycemia and hyperglycemia.
• Tell patient not to change dosage without doctor's consent and to report abnormal blood or urine glucose test results.
• Advise patient not to take other medications, including OTC drugs, without first checking with doctor.
• Instruct patient to avoid alcohol consumption during drug therapy.
• Advise patient to carry medical identification at all times.

☑ Evaluation
• Patient's blood glucose level is normal with drug therapy.
• Patient does not experience hypoglycemia.
• Patient and family state understanding of drug therapy.

glycerin
(GLIH-seh-rin)
Fleet Babylax†, Fleet†, Sani-Supp†

Pharmacologic class: trihydric alcohol
Therapeutic class: laxative (osmotic)
Pregnancy risk category: NR

How supplied
Enema (pediatric): 4 ml/applicator†
Suppositories: adult, children, and infant sizes†

Pharmacokinetics
Absorption: suppositories are absorbed poorly.
Distribution: distributed locally.
Metabolism: unknown.
Excretion: excreted in feces.

Route	Onset	Peak	Duration
P.R.	15-60 min	15-60 min	15-60 min

Pharmacodynamics
Chemical effect: hyperosmolar laxative that draws water from tissues into feces to stimulate evacuation.
Therapeutic effect: promotes stool evacuation.

Indications and dosage
▶ **Constipation.** *Adults and children age 6 and over:* 2 to 3 g as rectal suppository or 5 to 15 ml as enema. *Children under age 6:* 1 to 1.7 g as rectal suppository; or 2 to 5 ml as enema.

Adverse reactions
GI: *cramping pain,* rectal discomfort, hyperemia of rectal mucosa.

Interactions
None significant.

Contraindications and precautions
• Contraindicated in patients hypersensitive to drug and in those with intestinal obstruction, undiagnosed abdominal pain, vomiting or other signs of appendicitis, fecal impaction, or acute surgical abdomen.

NURSING CONSIDERATIONS

☒ Assessment
• Obtain assessment of patient's constipation before therapy.

• Monitor effectiveness by noting patient's response after drug administration.
• Be alert for adverse GI reactions.
• Evaluate patient's and family's knowledge of drug therapy.

🔲 **Nursing diagnoses**
• Constipation related to interruption of normal pattern of elimination
• Pain related to abdominal cramping
• Knowledge deficit related to drug therapy

▶ **Planning and implementation**
• Know that drug is used mainly to reestablish proper toilet habits in laxative-dependent patient.
• Be aware that drug must be retained for at least 15 minutes; usually acts within 1 hour. Entire suppository need not melt to be effective.
• Notify doctor if drug is not effective.
Patient teaching
• Warn patient that abdominal cramping may occur but will subside when bowel is emptied.

☑ **Evaluation**
• Patient reports return of normal bowel pattern of elimination.
• Patient states that abdominal cramping is transient.
• Patient and family state understanding of drug therapy.

glycopyrrolate
(gligh-koh-PEER-uh-layt)
Robinul, Robinul Forte

Pharmacologic class: anticholinergic
Therapeutic class: antimuscarinic, GI antispasmodic
Pregnancy risk category: B

How supplied
Tablets: 1 mg, 2 mg
Injection: 0.2 mg/ml

Pharmacokinetics
Absorption: poorly absorbed from GI tract after oral use. Rapidly absorbed after I.M. use. Unknown after S.C. use.
Distribution: rapidly distributed; does not cross blood-brain barrier or enter CNS.
Metabolism: unknown.
Excretion: small amounts eliminated in urine as unchanged drug and metabolites; most excreted unchanged in feces or bile.
Half-life: 1.7 hours.

Route	Onset	Peak	Duration
P.O.	Unknown	Unknown	Unknown
I.V.	Unknown	Unknown	3-7 hr
I.M.	15-30 min	30-45 min	3-7 hr
S.C.	15-30 min	Unknown	3-7 hr

Pharmacodynamics
Chemical effect: inhibits cholinergic (muscarinic) actions of acetylcholine on autonomic effectors innervated by postganglionic cholinergic nerves.
Therapeutic effect: diminishes secretions and GI motility and blocks drug-induced cholinergic effects.

Indications and dosage
▶ **Blockade of adverse cholinergic effects caused by anticholinesterase agents used to reverse neuromuscular blockade.** *Adults and children:* 0.2 mg I.V. for each 1 mg neostigmine or 5 mg of pyridostigmine. May be given I.V. without dilution or may be added to dextrose injection and given by infusion.
▶ **Preoperatively to diminish secretions and block cardiac vagal reflexes.** *Adults and children age 2 and older:* 0.0044 mg/kg of body weight I.M. 30 to 60 minutes before anesthesia. *Children under age 2:* up to 0.0088 mg/kg I.M. 30 to 60 minutes before anesthesia.
▶ **Adjunct therapy in peptic ulcerations and other GI disorders.** *Adults:* 1 to 2 mg P.O. t.i.d. or 0.1 mg I.M. t.i.d. or q.i.d. Dosage must be individualized. Maximum P.O. dosage is 8 mg/day.

Adverse reactions

CNS: disorientation, irritability, incoherence, weakness, nervousness, drowsiness, dizziness, headache, confusion or excitement (in elderly patients).
CV: palpitations, tachycardia, paradoxical bradycardia.
EENT: *dilated pupils, blurred vision,* loss of taste, photophobia, increased intraocular pressure.
GI: abdominal distention, *constipation,* difficulty swallowing, *dry mouth,* nausea, vomiting, epigastric distress.
GU: *urinary hesitancy, urine retention,* impotence.
Respiratory: *bronchial plugging.*
Skin: urticaria, decreased sweating or anhidrosis, other dermal manifestations.
Other: burning at injection site, fever, *anaphylaxis.*

Interactions

Drug-drug. *Amantadine, antihistamines, antiparkinson agents, disopyramide, glutethimide, meperidine, phenothiazines, procainamide, quinidine, tricyclic antidepressants:* additive adverse effects. Avoid concomitant use.
Antacids: decreased absorption of oral anticholinergics. Separate administration times by 2 to 3 hours.
Ketoconazole: anticholinergics may interfere with ketoconazole absorption. Avoid concomitant use.
Methotrimeprazine: anticholinergics may enhance risk of extrapyramidal reactions. Avoid concomitant use.

Contraindications and precautions

• Contraindicated in patients with glaucoma, obstructive uropathy, obstructive disease of GI tract, myasthenia gravis, paralytic ileus, intestinal atony, unstable CV status in acute hemorrhage, severe ulcerative colitis, toxic megacolon, or hypersensitivity to drug.
• Drug not recommended for use in breast-feeding women.
• Use cautiously in patients with autonomic neuropathy, hyperthyroidism, coronary artery disease, arrhythmias, heart failure, hypertension, hiatal hernia, hepatic or renal disease, or ulcerative colitis; in pregnant women; and in patients in hot or humid environments (to prevent drug-induced heatstroke).

NURSING CONSIDERATIONS

Assessment
• Assess patient's condition before therapy and regularly thereafter.
• Be alert for adverse reactions and drug interactions.
• Evaluate patient's and family's knowledge of drug therapy.

Nursing diagnoses
• Altered health maintenance related to patient's underlying condition
• Urinary retention related to drug's adverse effect on urinary system
• Knowledge deficit related to drug therapy

Planning and implementation
• Be aware that elderly patients typically receive smaller dosages.
P.O. use: Administer drug 30 minutes to 1 hour before meals.
I.V. use: Give by direct injection without dilution. Alternatively, inject into I.V. line containing free-flowing solution.
– Don't mix with I.V. solution containing sodium bicarbonate or alkaline solutions with pH above 6. Alkaline drugs, such as barbiturates (thiopental, methohexital, secobarbital, pentobarbital), chloramphenicol, dexamethasone, dimenhydrinate, diazepam, methylprednisolone, and pentazocine, are incompatible with glycopyrrolate.
I.M. and S.C. use: Follow normal protocol.
• Check all dosages carefully; slight overdose can lead to toxicity.
• Notify doctor of urine retention; be prepared to catheterize patient.

Patient teaching
● Warn patient to avoid activities that require alertness until drug's CNS effects are known.
● Advise patient to report signs of urinary hesitancy or urine retention.

☑ Evaluation
● Patient responds well to drug.
● Patient regains normal voiding pattern.
● Patient and family state understanding of drug therapy.

---

gonadorelin acetate
(goh-nah-doh-REH-lin AS-ih-tayt)
Lutrepulse

Pharmacologic class: gonadotropin-releasing hormone (GnRH)
Therapeutic class: fertility agent
Pregnancy risk category: B

How supplied
Injection: 0.8 mg/10 ml, 3.2 mg/10 ml vials; supplied as kit with I.V. supplies and ambulatory infusion pump

Pharmacokinetics
Absorption: not applicable.
Distribution: has low plasma volume of distribution and high rate of clearance from plasma.
Metabolism: rapidly metabolized.
Excretion: excreted primarily in urine.
Half-life: initial, 2 to 10 minutes; terminal, 10 to 40 minutes.

Route	Onset	Peak	Duration
I.V.	Unknown	Unknown	Unknown

Pharmacodynamics
Chemical effect: mimics action of GnRH, which results in synthesis and release of luteinizing hormone (LH) from anterior pituitary gland. LH then acts on reproductive organs to regulate hormone synthesis.
Therapeutic effect: induces ovulation.

Indications and dosage
▶ **Induction of ovulation in women with primary hypothalamic amenorrhea.** *Adults:* 5 mcg I.V. q 90 minutes for 21 days. If no response follows three treatment intervals, increase dosage as ordered.

Adverse reactions
GU: multiple pregnancy, ovarian hyperstimulation.
Skin: hematoma, local infection, inflammation, mild phlebitis.

Interactions
Drug-drug. *Ovarian-stimulating drugs:* additive effects. Avoid concomitant use.

Contraindications and precautions
● Contraindicated in patients hypersensitive to drug, in women with conditions that could be complicated by pregnancy (such as prolactinoma), in those who are anovulatory from any cause other than hypothalamic disorder, and in those with ovarian cysts.
● Safety of drug has not been established in adolescent girls.

NURSING CONSIDERATIONS

☒ Assessment
● Obtain assessment of patient's underlying condition before therapy.
● Monitor effectiveness by ensuring patient has regular pelvic examinations, midluteal phase serum progesterone determinations, and pelvic ultrasound on days 7 and 14 after establishment of baseline scan.
● Closely monitor patient response; this is critical to ensure adequate ovarian stimulation without hyperstimulation (sudden ovarian enlargement, ascites, or pleural effusion).
● Be alert for adverse reactions.
● Inspect I.V. site at each visit, noting signs of infection.
● Evaluate patient's and family's knowledge of drug therapy.

Reactions may be *common*, uncommon, *life-threatening*, or COMMON AND LIFE-THREATENING.

⊕ Nursing diagnoses
- Sexual dysfunction related to underlying condition
- Risk for infection related to prolonged need for I.V. site
- Knowledge deficit related to drug therapy

≥ Planning and implementation
- To mimic naturally occurring hormone, administer gonadorelin in pulsatile fashion with available ambulatory infusion pump. Set pulse period at 1 minute (infuse drug over 1 minute) and pulse interval at 90 minutes.
- To administer 2.5 mcg/pulse, reconstitute 0.8-mg vial with 8 ml of supplied diluent and set pump to deliver 25 microliters/pulse. To administer 5 mcg/pulse, use same dosage strength and dilution but set pump to deliver 50 microliters/pulse.
- Some patients may require higher I.V. doses. To give 10 mcg/pulse, reconstitute 3.2-mg vial with 8 ml of supplied diluent and set pump to deliver 25 microliters/pulse. To give 20 mcg/pulse, use same dosage strength and dilution but set pump to deliver 50 microliters/pulse.
- Be aware that cannula and I.V. site should be changed every 48 hours.

Patient teaching
- Inform patient that multiple pregnancy is possible (incidence is about 12%). Close monitoring of dosage, as well as ovarian ultrasonography to monitor drug response, is necessary.
- Instruct patient about proper aseptic technique and care of I.V. site. Cannula and I.V. site should be changed every 48 hours. Written instructions are available for patients.
- Teach patient to recognize and report hypersensitivity reactions (hives, wheezing, difficulty breathing); anaphylaxis has been reported with similar drugs.
- Advise patient to report signs of infection, hematoma, inflammation, or phlebitis at injection site, as well as severe abdominal pain, bloating, swelling of hands or feet, nausea, vomiting, diar-

rhea, substantial weight gain, or shortness of breath.
- Encourage patient to adhere to monitoring schedule required by therapy. Regular pelvic examinations, midluteal phase serum progesterone determinations, and multiple ovarian ultrasound scans are needed.

☑ Evaluation
- Patient ovulates during therapy.
- Patient is free from infection.
- Patient and family state understanding of drug therapy.

goserelin acetate
(GOH-seh-reh-lin AS-ih-tayt)
Zoladex, Zoladex 3-Month

Pharmacologic class: synthetic decapeptide
Therapeutic class: luteinizing hormone–releasing hormone (LHRH; GnRH) analogue
Pregnancy risk category: X

How supplied
Implants: 3.6 mg, 10.8 mg

Pharmacokinetics
Absorption: slowly absorbed from implant site.
Distribution: unknown.
Metabolism: unknown.
Excretion: route unknown. *Half-life:* about 4.2 hours.

Route	Onset	Peak	Duration
S.C.	2-4 wk	12-15 days	Throughout therapy

Pharmacodynamics
Chemical effect: LHRH analogue that acts on pituitary to decrease release of follicle-stimulating hormone and luteinizing hormone, resulting in dramatically lowered serum levels of sex hormones.

Therapeutic effect: decreases effects of sex hormones on tumor growth in prostate gland and tissue growth in uterus.

Indications and dosage

▶ **Palliative treatment of advanced carcinoma of prostate; endometriosis and advanced breast carcinoma.** *Adults:* 1 implant S.C. q 28 days into upper abdominal wall for 6 months. For endometriosis, maximum duration of therapy is 6 months.

▶ **Palliative treatment of advanced carcinoma of the prostate.** *Adult males:* 1 (10.8 mg) implant S.C. q 12 weeks into upper abdominal wall.

▶ **Endometrial thinning prior to endometrial ablation for dysfunctional uterine bleeding.** *Adults:* one or two 3.6-mg implants S.C. into upper abdominal wall. Each implant should be given 4 weeks apart.

Adverse reactions

CNS: lethargy, pain (worsened in first 30 days), dizziness, insomnia, anxiety, depression, headache, chills, emotional lability.
CV: edema, *heart failure, arrhythmias, CVA,* hypertension, *MI,* peripheral vascular disorder, chest pain.
GI: nausea, vomiting, diarrhea, constipation, ulcer.
GU: *impotence, sexual dysfunction, lower urinary tract symptoms,* renal insufficiency, urinary obstruction, urinary tract infection, amenorrhea, vaginal dryness.
Hematologic: anemia.
Respiratory: COPD, upper respiratory tract infection.
Skin: rash, diaphoresis.
Other: *hot flashes,* gout, hyperglycemia, weight increase, breast swelling and tenderness, changes in breast size, loss of bone mineral density (in women), fever.

Interactions

None reported.

Contraindications and precautions

● Contraindicated in patients with hypersensitivity to LHRH, LHRH agonist analogues, or goserelin acetate, and in pregnant or breast-feeding women. The 10.8-mg implant is contraindicated for use in women.
● Use cautiously in patients with risk factors for osteoporosis, such as family history of osteoporosis, chronic alcohol or tobacco abuse, or use of drugs that affect bone density.
● Drug should not be used in children.

NURSING CONSIDERATIONS

⚏ Assessment
● Assess patient's condition before therapy and regularly thereafter.
● Before administering to female patient, rule out pregnancy.
● When used for prostate cancer, be aware that LHRH analogues such as goserelin may initially worsen symptoms because drug initially increases testosterone serum levels. Some patients may experience increased bone pain. Rarely, disease exacerbation (spinal cord compression or ureteral obstruction) has occurred.
● Be alert for adverse reactions.
● Evaluate patient's and family's knowledge of drug therapy.

⊕ Nursing diagnoses
● Altered health maintenance related to underlying condition
● Pain related to drug's adverse effect
● Knowledge deficit related to drug therapy

❯ Planning and implementation
● Drug should be administered under supervision of doctor.
● Administer drug into upper abdominal wall using aseptic technique. After cleaning area with alcohol swab (and injecting local anesthetic), stretch patient's skin with one hand while grasping barrel of syringe with the other. Insert needle into

subcutaneous fat; then change direction of needle so that it parallels abdominal wall. Needle should then be pushed in until hub touches patient's skin; then withdrawn about 1 cm (this creates gap for drug to be injected) before depressing plunger completely.
• To avoid need for new syringe and injection site, do not aspirate after inserting needle.
• Implant comes in preloaded syringe. If package is damaged, do not use syringe. Make sure drug is visible in translucent chamber.
• After implantation, area requires bandage after needle is withdrawn.
• Be prepared to schedule patient for ultrasound to locate goserelin implants if they require removal.
• Notify doctor of adverse reactions and provide supportive care as indicated and ordered.
Patient teaching
• Advise patient to report every 28 days for new implant. A delay of a couple of days is permissible.
• Tell female patients to use nonhormonal form of contraception during treatment. Caution her about significant risks to fetus should pregnancy occur.
• Tell patient to call doctor if menstruation persists or if breakthrough bleeding occurs. Menstruation should stop during treatment.
• After therapy ends, inform patient that she may experience delayed return of menses. Persistent amenorrhea is rare.
• Warn patient that pain may occur.

☑ **Evaluation**
• Patient responds well to drug.
• Patient does not experience pain.
• Patient and family state understanding of drug therapy.

granisetron hydrochloride
(grah-NEEZ-eh-trohn high-droh-KLOR-ighd)
Kytril

Pharmacologic class: selective 5-hydroxytryptamine (5-HT3) receptor antagonist
Therapeutic class: antiemetic, antinauseant
Pregnancy risk category: B

How supplied
Tablets: 1 mg
Injection: 1 mg/ml

Pharmacokinetics
Absorption: unknown after oral administration.
Distribution: distributed freely between plasma and RBCs; plasma protein–binding about 65%.
Metabolism: metabolized by liver.
Excretion: excreted in urine and feces.

Route	Onset	Peak	Duration
P.O., I.V.	Unknown	Unknown	Unknown

Pharmacodynamics
Chemical effect: located in CNS at area postrema (chemoreceptor trigger zone) and in peripheral nervous system on nerve terminals of vagus nerve. Drug's blocking action may occur at both sites.
Therapeutic effect: prevents nausea and vomiting from chemotherapy.

Indications and dosage
▶ **Prevention of nausea and vomiting associated with emetogenic cancer chemotherapy.** *Adults and children ages 2 to 16:* 10 mcg/kg I.V. infused over 5 minutes. Begin infusion within 30 minutes before administration of chemotherapy. Alternatively, 1 mg P.O. up to 1 hour before chemotherapy. Dosage repeated 12 hours later.

Adverse reactions

CNS: *headache, asthenia,* somnolence.
CV: hypertension.
GI: diarrhea, constipation.
Hematologic: *thrombocytopenia.*
Other: taste disorder, fever.

Interactions

None significant.

Contraindications and precautions

• Contraindicated in patients hypersensitive to drug.
• Use cautiously in pregnant or breastfeeding women.

NURSING CONSIDERATIONS

⚚ Assessment
• Assess patient's chemotherapy and GI reactions before therapy.
• Monitor for nausea and vomiting.
• Be alert for adverse reactions.
• Monitor hydration status if drug is ineffective or diarrhea occurs.
• Evaluate patient's and family's knowledge of drug therapy.

⊕ Nursing diagnoses
• Risk for fluid volume deficit related to nausea and vomiting
• Pain related to drug-induced headache
• Knowledge deficit related to drug therapy

⊠ Planning and implementation
P.O. use: Administer drug 1 hour before chemotherapy; repeat in 12 hours.
I.V. use: Dilute drug with 0.9% NaCl injection or D_5W to volume of 20 to 50 ml. Infuse over 5 minutes beginning within 30 minutes before initiating chemotherapy, and only on day(s) chemotherapy is given. Diluted solutions are stable for 24 hours at room temperature.
– Do not mix with other drugs; data regarding compatibility is limited.
• Alert doctor if patient experiences nausea or vomiting.

Patient teaching
• Tell patient to notify doctor if adverse drug reactions occur.

☑ Evaluation
• Patient does not experience nausea or vomiting with chemotherapy.
• Patient's headache is relieved with mild analgesic.
• Patient and family state understanding of drug therapy.

grepafloxacin hydrochloride
(greh-peh-FLOKS-uh-sin high-droh-KLOR-ighd)
Raxar

Pharmacologic class: fluoroquinolone
Therapeutic class: antibiotic
Pregnancy risk category: C

How supplied

Tablets: 200 mg (base)

Pharmacokinetics

Absorption: rapid and extensive following oral administration. Absolute bioavailability is about 70%.
Distribution: widely distributed into extravascular spaces. Only 50% bound to plasma protein.
Metabolism: metabolized primarily by the liver.
Excretion: elimination occurs primarily by biliary excretion and hepatic metabolism. About 50% is excreted in feces and 38% in urine. *Half-life:* 16 hours.

Route	Onset	Peak	Duration
P.O.	Unknown	2-3 hr	Unknown

Pharmacodynamics

Chemical effect: exact mechanism unknown, but bactericidal effects may result from drug inhibiting bacterial DNA gyrase and preventing replication in susceptible bacteria.

Reactions may be *common*, uncommon, **life-threatening**, or COMMON AND LIFE-THREATENING.

Therapeutic effect: inhibits bacterial cell growth.

Indications and dosage

▶ **Acute bacterial exacerbations of chronic bronchitis caused by susceptible strains of** *Haemophilus influenzae,* *Streptococcus pneumoniae,* **or** *Moraxella catarrhalis.* *Adults:* 400 or 600 mg P.O. once daily for 10 days.

▶ **Community-acquired pneumonia caused by susceptible strains of** *H. influenzae, S. pneumoniae, M. catarrhalis,* **or** *Mycoplasma pneumoniae.* *Adults:* 600 mg P.O. once daily for 10 days.

▶ **Uncomplicated gonorrhea (urethral in males and endocervical and rectal in females) caused by** *Neisseria gonorrhoeae.* *Adults:* 400 mg P.O. as a single dose.

▶ **Nongonococcal urethritis and cervicitis caused by** *Chlamydia trachomatis.* *Adults:* 400 mg P.O. once daily for 7 days.

Adverse reactions

CNS: asthenia, dizziness, headache, insomnia, pain, nervousness, somnolence.
GI: abdominal pain, anorexia, constipation, *nausea,* diarrhea, dry mouth, dyspepsia, *taste perversion,* vomiting.
GU: leukorrhea, vaginitis.
Skin: pruritus, photosensitivity reactions, rash.
Other: infection.

Interactions

Drug-drug. *Antacids, metal cations, multivitamins, sucralfate:* chelates with antacids containing aluminum, magnesium, calcium, or sucralfate or multiple vitamins containing zinc to substantially interfere with absorption of grepafloxacin. Do not give these agents within 4 hours before or after grepafloxacin administration.
Antidiabetic agents: disturbances of blood glucose, including hyperglycemia and hypoglycemia, have been reported in patients given grepafloxacin concomitantly with an antidiabetic agent. Monitor serum glucose level closely.
Astemizole, cisapride, cyclosporine, midazolam, triazolam: possible interaction with grepafloxacin. Monitor patient if given concurrently.
NSAIDs: concomitant administration may increase risk of CNS stimulation and seizures. Use with caution.
Theophylline: serum theophylline concentrations increase when grepafloxacin is initiated in patients maintained on theophylline. When initiating a multiday course of grepafloxacin in patients maintained on theophylline, give half the maintenance dose of theophylline for the period of concurrent therapy. Monitor theophylline serum concentrations.
Warfarin: may enhance effects of warfarin. Monitor INR.
Drug-food. *Caffeine:* grepafloxacin interferes with metabolism of caffeine and may enhance its effects. Use together cautiously.
Dairy products: can decrease absorption of grepafloxacin. Do not give drug with dairy products.
Drug-lifestyle. *Sun exposure:* photosensitivity reactions may occur. Take precautions. Stop drug if reactions occur.

Contraindications and precautions

• Contraindicated in patients with hypersensitivity to drug or other quinolones, hepatic failure, or known QT prolongation and in those receiving concomitant therapy with medications known to produce an increase in the QT interval or torsades de pointes.
• Use cautiously in patients with known or suspected CNS disorders that predispose patient to seizures. Drug is not recommended for patients with proarrhythmic conditions.
• Safety and efficacy in children under age 18 have not been established.
• Safety in pregnant and breast-feeding patients has not been established.

NURSING CONSIDERATIONS

⚖ Assessment
• Assess patient's underlying condition before drug therapy.
• Obtain culture and sensitivity tests as ordered before starting drug therapy.
• Monitor patient for serious adverse effects. Discontinue drug and notify doctor at first sign of allergic reaction.
• Evaluate patient's and family's knowledge of drug therapy.

🔢 Nursing diagnoses
• Risk for impaired physical mobility related to drug adverse effects
• Risk for impaired skin integrity related to possible photosensitivity reactions
• Knowledge deficit related to drug therapy

▶ Planning and implementation
• Be alert for and report diarrhea, pain, inflammation, or rupture of a tendon.
• Initiate drug therapy pending results of culture and sensitivity tests.
• Test patients being treated for gonorrhea for syphilis at time of diagnosis and for 3 months after treatment, as ordered.
• Discontinue drug and notify doctor if allergic reactions or phototoxicity occurs.
Patient teaching
• Tell patient that drug may be taken with or without meals.
• Instruct patient to drink plenty of fluids.
• Inform patient that drug may increase effects of caffeine.
• Tell patient to stop drug at first sign of rash, hives, rapid heartbeat, or difficulty breathing or swallowing.
• Warn patient to avoid hazardous activities until effects of drug are known.
• Tell patient to avoid excessive sunlight or artificial ultraviolet light during drug therapy.
• Inform patient to stop drug, sit and rest, and notify doctor immediately if pain, inflammation, or rupture of tendon occurs.

☑ Evaluation
• Patient does not experience impaired physical mobility.
• Patient maintains skin integrity.
• Patient and family state understanding of drug therapy.

griseofulvin microsize
(gris-ee-oh-FUHL-vin MIGH-kroh-sighz)
Fulcin◊, Fulvicin-U/F, Grifulvin V, Grisactin, Grisovin◊, Grisovin-FP

griseofulvin ultramicrosize
Fulvicin P/G, Grisactin Ultra, Gris-PEG

Pharmacologic class: Penicillium antibiotic
Therapeutic class: antifungal
Pregnancy risk category: NR

How supplied
griseofulvin microsize
Tablets: 250 mg, 500 mg
Capsules: 125 mg, 250 mg
Oral suspension: 125 mg/5 ml
griseofulvin ultramicrosize
Tablets: 125 mg, 165 mg, 250 mg, 330 mg

Pharmacokinetics
Absorption: absorbed primarily in duodenum; varies among individuals. Ultramicrosize preparations are absorbed almost completely; microsize absorption ranges from 25% to 70% and may be increased by giving with high-fat meal.
Distribution: drug concentrates in skin, hair, nails, fat, liver, and skeletal muscle; tightly bound to new keratin.
Metabolism: metabolized in liver.
Excretion: about 50% excreted in urine, 33% in feces, less than 1% unchanged in urine; also excreted in perspiration. *Half-life:* 9 to 24 hours.

Route	Onset	Peak	Duration
P.O.	Unknown	4-8 hr	Unknown

Pharmacodynamics

Chemical effect: arrests fungal cell activity by disrupting its mitotic spindle structure.
Therapeutic effect: inhibits fungal cell growth. Spectrum of activity includes *Trichophyton, Microsporum,* and *Epidermophyton.*

Indications and dosage

▶ **Ringworm infections of skin, hair, nails (tinea corporis, tinea capitis) when caused by *Trichophyton, Microsporum,* or *Epidermophyton.*** *Adults:* 500 mg (microsize) P.O. daily in single or divided doses. Severe infections may require up to 1 g daily. Alternatively, 330 to 375 mg ultramicrosize daily in single or divided doses.
▶ **Tinea pedis and tinea unguium.** *Adults:* 0.75 to 1 g (microsize) P.O. daily. Alternatively, 660 to 750 mg ultramicrosize P.O. daily in divided doses. *Children:* 11 mg/kg/day (microsize) P.O. Alternatively, 7.3 mg/kg/day (ultramicrosize).

Adverse reactions

CNS: headache (early in treatment), transient decrease in hearing, fatigue with large doses, occasional mental confusion, impaired performance of routine activities, psychotic symptoms, dizziness, insomnia.
GI: nausea, vomiting, excessive thirst, flatulence, diarrhea, *bleeding.*
Hematologic: leukopenia, *agranulocytosis* (requires discontinuation of drug), porphyria.
Hepatic: *hepatic toxicity.*
Skin: rash, urticaria, photosensitivity, *toxic epidermal necrolysis* (rare).
Other: estrogen-like effects in children, oral thrush, hypersensitivity reactions (rash, *angioedema,* serum sickness–like reactions), lupuslike syndrome or exacerbation of existing lupus erythematosus.

Interactions

Drug-drug. *Coumarin anticoagulants:* decreased effectiveness. Monitor PT and INR when used concurrently.

Cyclosporine: cyclosporine levels may be reduced, resulting in decreased pharmacologic effects. Avoid concomitant use.
Oral contraceptives: decreased effectiveness. Suggest alternate methods of contraception.
Phenobarbital: decreased griseofulvin blood levels as a result of decreased absorption or increased metabolism. Avoid using together or administer griseofulvin t.i.d.
Drug-food. *High-fat meals:* increased absorption. Administer together.
Drug-lifestyle. *Alcohol use:* may cause tachycardia, diaphoresis, and flushing. Avoid concomitant use.

Contraindications and precautions

● Contraindicated in patients with porphyria, hepatocellular failure, or hypersensitivity to drug.
● Also contraindicated in pregnant women or women who intend to become pregnant during therapy.
● Use cautiously in penicillin-sensitive patients because griseofulvin is penicillin derivative.
● Safety of drug has not been established in breast-feeding women.

NURSING CONSIDERATIONS

⚕ Assessment
● Obtain assessment of patient's fungal infection before therapy.
● Monitor for improvement of signs and symptoms and for laboratory confirmation of complete eradication of organism.
● Assess hematologic, renal, and hepatic function periodically during prolonged therapy, as ordered.
● Be alert for adverse reactions and drug interactions.
● Evaluate patient's and family's knowledge of drug therapy.

⊞ Nursing diagnoses
● Infection related to presence of susceptible fungi

• Altered protection related to drug-induced granulocytopenia
• Knowledge deficit related to drug therapy

❯ **Planning and implementation**
• Because of potential toxicity, drug is used only when topical treatment fails to arrest mycotic disease.
• Obtain laboratory tests as ordered to confirm diagnosis of infecting organism. Continue drug until clinical and laboratory examinations confirm complete eradication.
• Because griseofulvin ultramicrosize is dispersed in polyethylene glycol, it is absorbed more rapidly and completely than microsize preparations and is effective at one-half to two-thirds the usual griseofulvin dose.
• Give after high-fat meal to enhance absorption and minimize GI distress.
• Keep in mind that effective treatment of tinea pedis may require concomitant use of topical agent.
• Notify doctor immediately of granulocytopenia, which requires discontinuation of drug.
Patient teaching
• Advise patient that prolonged treatment may be needed to control infection and prevent relapse, even if symptoms abate in first few days. Tell him to keep skin clean and dry and to maintain good hygiene.
• Instruct female patient not to become pregnant while on drug therapy.
• Caution patient to avoid intense sunlight.
• Instruct patient to avoid alcohol consumption while on drug therapy.
• Instruct patient to take drug after high-fat meal.
• Warn patient to avoid hazardous activities that require alertness if adverse CNS reactions occur.

☑ **Evaluation**
• Patient's infection is alleviated.

• Patient's CBC remains within normal limits.
• Patient and family state understanding of drug therapy.

---

guaifenesin
(glyceryl guaiacolate)
(gwah-FEH-nih-sin)
Anti-Tuss*†, Balminil Expectorant♦, Breonesin†, Gee-Gee†, GG-Cen*†, Glyate*†, Glycotuss†, Glytuss†, Guiatuss*†, Halotussin, Humibid L.A.†, Hytuss†, Hytuss-2X†, Naldecon Senior EX†, Resyl♦†, Robitussin*†, Scot-Tussin Expectorant†

Pharmacologic class: propanediol derivative
Therapeutic class: expectorant
Pregnancy risk category: C

How supplied

Tablets: 100 mg†, 200 mg†
Capsules: 200 mg†
Capsules (extended-release): 300 mg
Solution: 100 mg/ ml*†, 200 mg/5 ml*†

Pharmacokinetics

Unknown.

Route	Onset	Peak	Duration
P.O.	Unknown	Unknown	Unknown

Pharmacodynamics

Chemical effect: increases production of respiratory tract fluids to help liquefy and reduce viscosity of tenacious secretions.
Therapeutic effect: thins respiratory secretions for easier removal.

Indications and dosage

▶ **Expectorant.** *Adults and children age 12 and over:* 200 to 400 mg P.O. q 4 hours, or 600 to 1,200 mg extended-release capsules q 12 hours. Maximum dosage is 2,400 mg daily. *Children ages 2 to 6:* 50 to 100 mg P.O. q 4 hours. Maximum dosage is 600 mg daily.

Reactions may be *common*, uncommon, *life-threatening*, or COMMON AND LIFE-THREATENING.

Children ages 6 to 12: 100 to 200 mg
P.O. q 4 hours. Maximum dosage is
1,200 mg daily.

Adverse reactions

CNS: drowsiness.
GI: stomach pain, diarrhea, vomiting,
nausea (with large doses).
Skin: rash.

Interactions

Drug-drug. *Heparin:* increased risk of
bleeding. Use together cautiously.

Contraindications and precautions

• Contraindicated in patients hypersensitive to drug.
• Use cautiously in pregnant women.
• Safety of drug has not been established
in breast-feeding women.

NURSING CONSIDERATIONS

⚕ Assessment
• Assess patient's sputum production before and after drug administration.
• Be alert for adverse reactions and drug
interactions.
• Monitor patient's hydration status if adverse GI reactions occur.
• Evaluate patient's and family's knowledge of drug therapy.

⊞ Nursing diagnoses
• Ineffective airway clearance related to
underlying condition
• Risk for fluid volume deficit related to
adverse GI reactions
• Knowledge deficit related to drug
therapy

⊠ Planning and implementation
• Administer drug with glass of water.
• Know that drug may interfere with laboratory tests for 5-hydroxyindoleacetic
acid and vanillylmandelic acid.
Patient teaching
• Inform patient that persistent cough
may indicate a serious condition. Tell
him to contact doctor if cough lasts

longer than 1 week, recurs frequently, or
is associated with high fever, rash, or severe headache.
• Advise patient to take each dose with
glass of water; increasing fluid intake
may prove beneficial.
• Encourage patient to perform deep-breathing exercises.

☑ Evaluation
• Patient's lungs are clear and respiratory
secretions are normal.
• Patient maintains adequate hydration.
• Patient and family state understanding
of drug therapy.

---

guanabenz acetate
(GWAH-nuh-benz AS-ih-tayt)
Wytensin

Pharmacologic class: centrally acting
antiadrenergic
Therapeutic class: antihypertensive
Pregnancy risk category: C

How supplied

Tablets: 4 mg, 8 mg

Pharmacokinetics

Absorption: 70% to 80% absorbed from
GI tract.
Distribution: appears to be distributed
widely into body; about 90% protein-bound.
Metabolism: metabolized extensively in
liver.
Excretion: excreted primarily in urine, remainder in feces. *Half-life:* about 6 hours.

Route	Onset	Peak	Duration
P.O.	≤ 1 hr	2-5 hr	About 12 hr

Pharmacodynamics

Chemical effect: unknown; may be due
to central alpha-adrenergic stimulation,
which results in decreased sympathetic
outflow to heart, kidneys, and peripheral
vasculature.

Therapeutic effect: lowers blood pressure.

Indications and dosage

▶ **Hypertension.** *Adults:* initially, 2 to 4 mg P.O. b.i.d. Dosage increased in increments of 4 to 8 mg/day q 1 to 2 weeks. Maximum daily dosage is 32 mg b.i.d. To ensure overnight blood pressure control, give last dose h.s.

Adverse reactions

CNS: *drowsiness, sedation, dizziness,* weakness, headache, ataxia, depression.
CV: *rebound hypertension.*
GI: *dry mouth.*
GU: sexual dysfunction.

Interactions

Drug-drug. *CNS depressants:* may cause increased sedation. Use together cautiously.
MAO inhibitors, tricyclic antidepressants: may decrease antihypertensive effect. Monitor patient closely.

Contraindications and precautions

● Contraindicated in patients with hypersensitivity to drug.
● Drug not recommended for use in breast-feeding women.
● Use cautiously in patients with severe coronary insufficiency, recent MI, cerebrovascular disease, or severe hepatic or renal failure. Also use cautiously in elderly patients and pregnant women.
● Safety of drug has not been established in children.

NURSING CONSIDERATIONS

⚷ Assessment
● Assess blood pressure before therapy and regularly thereafter.
● Be alert for adverse reactions and drug interactions.
● Evaluate patient's and family's knowledge of drug therapy.

⊡ Nursing diagnoses
● Risk for injury related to presence of hypertension
● Risk for trauma related to drug-induced adverse reactions
● Knowledge deficit related to drug therapy

⧉ Planning and implementation
● Give last dose of day just before sleep to help ensure adequate blood pressure control.
● Don't discontinue drug abruptly because rebound hypertension may occur.
● Know that thiazide diuretics may be used concomitantly to treat hypertension.
Patient teaching
● Caution patient that abrupt discontinuation of drug may cause rebound hypertension.
● Advise patient to avoid hazardous tasks that require alertness until drug's CNS effects are known.
● Inform patient that orthostatic hypotension can be minimized by rising slowly and avoiding sudden position changes. Dry mouth can be relieved with chewing gum, sour hard candy, or ice chips.
● Warn patient that tolerance to alcohol or other CNS depressants may be diminished.

☑ Evaluation
● Patient's blood pressure is within normal limits.
● Patient does not experience trauma from adverse reactions.
● Patient and family state understanding of drug therapy.

guanfacine hydrochloride
(GWAHN-fuh-seen high-droh-KLOR-ighd)
Tenex

Pharmacologic class: centrally acting antiadrenergic
Therapeutic class: antihypertensive
Pregnancy risk category: B

How supplied

Tablets: 1 mg, 2 mg

Pharmacokinetics

Absorption: absorbed well and completely and is about 80% bioavailable.
Distribution: thought to be highly distributed; about 70% protein-bound.
Metabolism: metabolized in liver.
Excretion: excreted in urine. *Half-life:* about 17 hours.

Route	Onset	Peak	Duration
P.O.	Unknown	1-4 hr	24 hr

Pharmacodynamics

Chemical effect: unknown; may inhibit central vasomotor center, decreasing sympathetic outflow to heart, kidneys, and peripheral vasculature.
Therapeutic effect: lowers blood pressure.

Indications and dosage

▶ **Hypertension.** *Adults:* initially, 1 mg P.O. daily h.s. Dosage may be increased to 2 mg P.O. h.s. after 3 to 4 weeks, as needed. Dosage may be further increased to 3 mg P.O. h.s. after additional 3 to 4 weeks, as needed. Average dosage is 1 to 3 mg daily.

Adverse reactions

CNS: *drowsiness, dizziness,* fatigue, headache, insomnia.
CV: bradycardia, orthostatic hypotension, rebound hypertension.
GI: *constipation,* diarrhea, nausea, *dry mouth.*
Skin: dermatitis, pruritus.

Interactions

Drug-drug. *CNS depressants:* potential for increased sedation. Avoid concomitant use.

Contraindications and precautions

• Contraindicated in patients with hypersensitivity to drug.

• Use cautiously in patients with severe coronary insufficiency, cerebrovascular disease, recent MI, or chronic renal or hepatic insufficiency, and in pregnant women.
• Safety of drug has not been established in breast-feeding women or in children.

NURSING CONSIDERATIONS

Assessment
• Assess blood pressure before therapy and regularly thereafter.
• Be alert for adverse reactions. Incidence and severity increase with higher dosages.
• Evaluate patient's and family's knowledge of drug therapy.

Nursing diagnoses
• Risk for injury related to presence of hypertension
• Constipation related to adverse effects on GI tract
• Knowledge deficit related to drug therapy

Planning and implementation
• Give daily dosage at bedtime to minimize daytime drowsiness.
• Know that drug may be used alone or with diuretic.
Patient teaching
• Tell patient not to discontinue therapy abruptly. Rebound hypertension is less common than with similar drugs but may occur.
• Advise patient to avoid activities that require alertness until response to drug is established.
• Instruct patient to check with doctor before taking other OTC medications.

Evaluation
• Patient's blood pressure is normal.
• Patient's bowel pattern is normal.
• Patient and family state understanding of drug therapy.

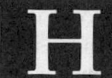

Route	Onset	Peak	Duration
P.O.	Unknown	3-6 hr	Unknown
I.M.	Unknown	10-20 min (lactate); 3-9 days (decanoate)	Unknown

haloperidol
(hal-oh-PER-uh-dol)
Apo-Haloperidol♦, Haldol**,
Novo-Peridol♦, Peridol♦,
PMS Haloperidol, Serenace◇

haloperidol decanoate
Haldol Decanoate, Haldol LA♦

haloperidol lactate
Haldol

Pharmacologic class: butyrophenone
Therapeutic class: antipsychotic
Pregnancy risk category: C

How supplied
haloperidol
Tablets: 0.5 mg, 1 mg, 2 mg, 5 mg,
10 mg, 20 mg
haloperidol decanoate
Injection: 50 mg/ml, 100 mg/ml
haloperidol lactate
Oral concentrate: 2 mg/ml
Injection: 5 mg/ml

Pharmacokinetics
Absorption: about 60% of oral dose absorbed; about 70% of I.M. dose absorbed
within 30 minutes.
Distribution: distributed widely, with
high concentrations in adipose tissue;
91% to 99% protein-bound.
Metabolism: metabolized extensively by
liver.
Excretion: about 40% excreted in urine
within 5 days; about 15% excreted in feces by way of biliary tract. *Half-life:*
P.O., 24 hours; I.M., 21 hours.

Pharmacodynamics
Chemical effect: may block postsynaptic
dopamine receptors in brain.
Therapeutic effect: decreases psychotic
behaviors.

Indications and dosage
▶ **Psychotic disorders.** *Adults and children age 12 and older:* dosage varies for
each patient. Initial range, 0.5 to 5 mg
P.O. b.i.d. or t.i.d.; or 2 to 5 mg I.M. q 4
to 8 hours although q 1 hour administration may be needed q until control is obtained. Maximum dosage is 100 mg P.O.
daily. *Children ages 3 to 12:* 0.05 to
0.15 mg/kg/day P.O. given b.i.d. or t.i.d.
Severely disturbed children may require
higher doses.
▶ **Chronic psychotic patients who require prolonged therapy.** *Adults:* 50 to
100 mg I.M. decanoate q 4 weeks.
▶ **Nonpsychotic behavior disorders.**
Children ages 3 to 12 : 0.05 to
0.075 mg/kg/day P.O. b.i.d. or t.i.d.
Maximum daily dosage is 6 mg.
▶ **Tourette syndrome.** *Adults:* 0.5 to
5 mg P.O. b.i.d., t.i.d., or p.r.n. *Children
ages 3 to 12:* 0.05 to 0.075 mg/kg/day
P.O. b.i.d. or t.i.d.

Adverse reactions
CNS: *severe extrapyramidal reactions,
tardive dyskinesia,* sedation, **seizures.**
CV: CV effects (low incidence with ther-
apeutic dosages).
EENT: *blurred vision.*
GU: urine retention, menstrual irregulari-
ties, gynecomastia.
Hematologic: transient leukopenia and
leukocytosis.
Hepatic: altered liver function tests,
jaundice.
Skin: rash.

Reactions may be *common*, uncommon, *life-threatening*, or COMMON AND LIFE-THREATENING.

Other: *neuroleptic malignant syndrome* (rare).

Interactions

Drug-drug. *Carbamazepine:* may decrease haloperidol serum concentrations. Monitor patient.
CNS depressants: increased CNS depression. Avoid concomitant use.
Fluoxetine: possibility of severe extrapyramidal reaction when administered with haloperidol. Avoid concomitant use.
Lithium: lethargy and confusion with high doses. Monitor patient.
Methyldopa: symptoms of dementia or psychosis. Monitor patient.
Phenytoin: haloperidol serum concentrations may be decreased. Monitor patient.
Drug-lifestyle. *Alcohol use:* increased CNS depression. Avoid concomitant use.

Contraindications and precautions

• Contraindicated in patients with hypersensitivity to drug or in those experiencing parkinsonism, coma, or CNS depression.
• Drug use is not recommended in breast-feeding women.
• Safety of drug has not been established in pregnant women.
• Use cautiously in elderly and debilitated patients; in patients with history of seizures or EEG abnormalities, severe CV disorders, allergies, glaucoma, or urine retention; and with anticonvulsant, anticoagulant, antiparkinsonian, or lithium medications.

NURSING CONSIDERATIONS

Assessment
• Assess patient's disorder before therapy and regularly thereafter.
• Be alert for adverse reactions and drug interactions.
• Monitor patient for tardive dyskinesia. It may occur after prolonged use. It may not appear until months or years later and may disappear spontaneously or persist for life despite discontinuation of drug.

• Evaluate patient's and family's knowledge of drug therapy.

Nursing diagnoses
• Impaired thought processes related to underlying condition
• Impaired physical mobility related to extrapyramidal effects
• Knowledge deficit related to drug therapy

Planning and implementation
P.O. use: Follow normal protocol.
I.M. use: Give drug by deep I.M. injection in gluteal region using a 21G needle. Maximum volume of injection should not exceed 3 ml.
• Know that elderly patient usually requires lower initial doses and more gradual dosage titration.
• Do not administer decanoate I.V.
• When changing from tablets to injection, patient should be given 10 to 15 times oral dose once monthly (maximum 100 mg).
• Protect drug from light. Slight yellowing of injection or concentrate is common; does not affect potency. Discard markedly discolored solutions.
• Do not stop drug abruptly unless required by severe adverse reactions.
• Acute dystonic reactions may be treated with diphenhydramine.
Patient teaching
• Warn patient to avoid activities that require alertness and psychomotor coordination until CNS effects of drug are known.
• Tell patient to avoid alcohol while taking drug.
• Tell patient to relieve dry mouth with sugarless gum or hard candy.
• Instruct patient to take drug exactly as prescribed and not to double doses to compensate for missed ones.

Evaluation
• Patient demonstrates decreased psychotic behavior.
• Patient maintains physical mobility.

• Patient and family state understanding of drug therapy.

heparin calcium
(HEH-puh-rin KAL-see-um)
Calcilean♦, Calciparine♦ ◇, Uniparin-Ca◇

heparin sodium
Hepalean♦, Heparin Leo♦, Heparin Lock Flush Solution (with Tubex), Hep-Lock, Liquaemin Sodium, Uniparin◇

Pharmacologic class: anticoagulant
Therapeutic class: anticoagulant
Pregnancy risk category: C

How supplied
Products are derived from beef lung or porcine intestinal mucosa.
heparin calcium
Ampule: 12,500 units/0.5 ml; 20,000 units/0.8 ml
Syringe: 5,000 units/0.2 ml
heparin sodium
Carpuject: 5,000 units/ml
Disposable syringes: 1,000 units/ml, 2,500 units/ml, 5,000 units/ml, 7,500 units/ml, 10,000 units/ml, 15,000 units/ml, 20,000 units/ml, 40,000 units/ml
Premixed I.V. solutions: 1,000 units in 500 ml of 0.9% NaCl solution; 2,000 units in 1,000 ml of 0.9% NaCl solution; 12,500 units in 250 ml of 0.45% NaCl solution; 25,000 units in 250 ml of 0.45% NaCl solution; 25,000 units in 500 ml of 0.45% NaCl solution; 10,000 units in 100 ml of D_5W; 12,500 units in 250 ml of D_5W; 25,000 units in 250 ml D_5W; 25,000 units in 500 ml D_5W; 20,000 units in 500 ml of D_5W
Unit-dose ampules: 1,000 units/ml, 5,000 units/ml, 10,000 units/ml
Vials: 1,000 units/ml, 2,500 units/ml, 5,000 units/ml, 7,500 units/ml, 10,000 units/ml, 15,000 units/ml, 20,000 units/ml, 40,000 units/ml

heparin sodium flush
Disposable syringes: 10 units/ml, 100 units/ml
Vials: 10 units/ml, 100 units/ml

Pharmacokinetics
Absorption: absorbed after S.C. administration.
Distribution: extensively bound to lipoprotein, globulins, and fibrinogen.
Metabolism: thought to be removed by reticuloendothelial system, with some metabolism occurring in liver.
Excretion: small amount excreted in urine as unchanged drug. *Half-life:* 1 to 2 hours. Half-life is dose-dependent and nonlinear and may be disproportionately prolonged at higher doses.

Route	Onset	Peak	Duration
I.V.	Immediate	Unknown	Unknown
S.C.	20-60 min	2-4 hr	Unknown

Pharmacodynamics
Chemical effect: accelerates formation of antithrombin III-thrombin complex and deactivates thrombin, preventing conversion of fibrinogen to fibrin.
Therapeutic effect: decreases ability of blood to clot.

Indications and dosage
Heparin dosing is highly individualized, depending upon disease state, age, and renal and hepatic status.
► **Deep vein thrombosis, pulmonary embolism.** *Adults:* initially, 10,000 units I.V. push, then adjusted according to PTT and give I.V. q 4 to 6 hours (5,000 to 10,000 units); or 5,000 units I.V. bolus, then 20,000 to 40,000 units in 24 hours by I.V. infusion pump. Hourly rate adjusted 4 to 6 hours after bolus dose according to PTT. *Children:* initially, 50 units/kg I.V. drip. Maintenance dosage is 100 units/kg I.V. drip q 4 hours. Constant infusion: 20,000 units/m² daily. Dosages adjusted according to PTT.
► **Embolism prophylaxis.** *Adults:* 5,000 units S.C. q 8 to 12 hours. In surgi-

cal patients, first dose given 2 hours before procedure; followed with 5,000 units S.C. q 8 to 12 hours for 5 to 7 days or until patient is fully ambulatory.
► **Open-heart surgery.** *Adults:* (total body perfusion) 150 to 400 units/kg continuous I.V infusion.
► **DIC.** *Adults:* 50 to 100 units/kg I.V. q 4 hours as a single injection or constant infusion. Discontinue if no improvement in 4 to 8 hours. *Children:* 25 to 50 units/kg I.V. q 4 hours, as a single injection or constant infusion. Discontinue if no improvement in 4 to 8 hours.
► **Patency maintenance of I.V. indwelling catheters.** *Adults:* 10 to 100 units I.V. flush. Use sufficient volume to fill device. Not intended for therapeutic use.

Adverse reactions

Hematologic: *hemorrhage* (with excessive dosage), *overly prolonged clotting time,* **thrombocytopenia.**
Skin: irritation, mild pain, hematoma, ulceration, cutaneous or subcutaneous necrosis.
Other: *"white clot'" syndrome; hypersensitivity reactions,* including chills, fever, pruritus, rhinitis, burning of feet, conjunctivitis, lacrimation, arthralgia, urticaria, *anaphylactoid reactions.*

Interactions

Drug-drug. *Oral anticoagulants:* increased additive anticoagulation. Monitor PT, INR, and PTT.
Salicylates, other antiplatelet agents: increased anticoagulant effect. Don't use together.
Thrombolytics: increased risk of hemorrhage. Monitor closely.

Contraindications and precautions

• Contraindicated in patients hypersensitive to drug.
• Conditionally contraindicated in patients with active bleeding; blood dyscrasia; or bleeding tendencies, such as hemophilia, thrombocytopenia, or hepatic

disease with hypoprothrombinemia; suspected intracranial hemorrhage; suppurative thrombophlebitis; inaccessible ulcerative lesions (especially of GI tract) and open ulcerative wounds; extensive denudation of skin; ascorbic acid deficiency and other conditions causing increased capillary permeability; during or after brain, eye, or spinal cord surgery; during spinal tap or spinal anesthesia; during continuous tube drainage of stomach or small intestine; in subacute bacterial endocarditis; shock; advanced renal disease; threatened abortion; severe hypertension. Although use of heparin is clearly hazardous in these conditions, its risk versus its benefits must be evaluated.
• Use cautiously during menses; in patients with mild hepatic or renal disease, alcoholism, or occupations with risk of physical injury; immediately postpartum; and in patients with history of allergies, asthma, or GI ulcerations.
• Know that when patient requires anticoagulation during pregnancy, most clinicians use heparin.

NURSING CONSIDERATIONS

Assessment
• Obtain assessment of patient's underlying condition before therapy.
• Draw blood to establish baseline coagulation parameters before therapy.
• Monitor effectiveness by measuring PTT carefully and regularly. Anticoagulation present when PTT values are 1½ to 2 times control values.
• During intermittent I.V. therapy, always draw blood 30 minutes before next dose to avoid falsely elevated PTT. Blood for PTT may be drawn 8 hours after initiation of continuous I.V. heparin therapy. Blood for PTT should never be drawn from I.V. tubing of heparin infusion or from infused vein; falsely elevated PTT will result. Always draw blood from opposite arm.
• Be alert for adverse reactions and drug interactions.

• Monitor platelet counts regularly. Thrombocytopenia caused by heparin may be associated with a type of arterial thrombosis known as "white clot" syndrome.
• Know that concentrated heparin solutions (greater than 100 units/ml) can irritate blood vessels.
• Evaluate patient's and family's knowledge of drug therapy.

❂ **Nursing diagnoses**
• Risk for injury related to potential for thrombosis or emboli development from underlying condition
• Altered protection related to increased bleeding risks
• Knowledge deficit related to drug therapy

▶ **Planning and implementation**
• Check order and vial carefully. Heparin comes in various concentrations.
I.V. use: Administer drug I.V. using infusion pump to provide maximum safety because of long-term effect and irregular absorption when given S.C. Check constant I.V. infusions regularly, even when pumps are in good working order, to prevent overdosage or underdosage.
– Do not skip dose or "catch up" with I.V. containing heparin. If I.V. is out, restart it as soon as possible and reschedule bolus dose immediately.
– Never piggyback other drugs into infusion line while heparin infusion is running. Many antibiotics and other drugs deactivate heparin. Never mix any drug with heparin in syringe when bolus therapy is used.
S.C. use: Give low-dose injections sequentially between iliac crests in lower abdomen deep into S.C. fat. Inject drug S.C. slowly into fat pad. Leave needle in place for 10 seconds after injection; then withdraw. Don't massage after S.C. injection, and watch for bleeding at injection site. Alternate sites every 12 hours— right for morning, left for evening.

• Know that drug requirements are higher in early phases of thrombogenic diseases and febrile states; lower when patient's condition stabilizes.
• Be aware that elderly patient should usually start at lower doses.
• Place notice above patient's bed to inform I.V. team or laboratory personnel to apply pressure dressings after taking blood.
• Institute bleeding precautions.
• Avoid excessive I.M. injections of other drugs to prevent or minimize hematomas. If possible, don't give I.M. injections at all.
• To treat severe heparin calcium or heparin sodium overdose, use protamine sulfate, a heparin antagonist, as ordered. Dosage is based on dose of heparin, its route of administration, and time elapsed since it was given. As a general rule, 1 to 1.5 units of protamine/100 units of heparin is given if only a few minutes have elapsed; 0.5 to 0.75 mg protamine/100 units heparin if 30 to 60 minutes have elapsed; 0.25 to 0.375 mg protamine/100 units heparin if 2 hours or more have elapsed.
• Abrupt withdrawal may cause increased coagulability, and heparin therapy is usually followed by oral anticoagulants for prophylaxis.
Patient teaching
• Instruct patient and family to watch for signs of bleeding and to notify doctor immediately if they occur.
• Tell patient to avoid OTC medications containing aspirin, other salicylates, or drugs that may interact with heparin.

☑ **Evaluation**
• Patient's PTT is reflective of goal of heparin therapy.
• Patient does not experience injury from bleeding.
• Patient and family state understanding of drug therapy.

---

hepatitis B immune globulin, human

(hep-uh-TIGH-tus bee ih-MYOON GLOH-byoo-lin, HYOO-mun)

H-BIG, HyperHep

Pharmacologic class: immune serum
Therapeutic class: hepatitis B prophylaxis
Pregnancy risk category: C

How supplied

Injection: 1-ml, 4-ml, 5-ml vials

Pharmacokinetics

Absorption: absorbed slowly after I.M. injection.
Distribution: unknown.
Metabolism: unknown.
Excretion: unknown. *Half-life:* antibodies to HBsAg, 21 days.

Route	Onset	Peak	Duration
I.M.	1-6 days	3-11 days	≥ 2 mo

Pharmacodynamics

Chemical effect: provides passive immunity to hepatitis B.
Therapeutic effect: prevents hepatitis B.

Indications and dosage

▶ **Hepatitis B exposure in high-risk patients.** *Adults and children:* 0.06 ml/kg I.M. within 7 days after exposure (preferably within first 24 hours). Dosage repeated 28 days after exposure if patient refuses hepatitis B vaccine. *Neonates born to patients who test positive for hepatitis B surface antigen (HBsAg):* 0.5 ml I.M. within 12 hours of birth.

Adverse reactions

Skin: urticaria; *pain, tenderness* (at injection site).
Other: *anaphylaxis, angioedema.*

Interactions

Drug-drug. *Live-virus vaccines:* may interfere with response to live-virus vaccines. Defer routine immunization for 3 months.

Contraindications and precautions

• Contraindicated in patients with history of anaphylactic reactions to immune serum.
• Use cautiously in pregnant women.
• Information on distribution of drug into breast milk is not available.

NURSING CONSIDERATIONS

⚕ Assessment
• Assess patient's allergies and reaction to immunizations before therapy.
• Monitor effectiveness by checking patient's antibody titers.
• Be alert for anaphylaxis.
• Evaluate patient's and family's knowledge of drug therapy.

⊞ Nursing diagnoses
• Altered protection related to lack of immunity to hepatitis B
• Knowledge deficit related to drug therapy

▷ Planning and implementation
• Inject drug into anterolateral aspect of thigh or deltoid muscle areas in older children and adults; inject into anterolateral aspect of thigh for neonates and children under age 3.
• Make sure epinephrine 1:1,000 is available in case anaphylaxis occurs.
• For postexposure prophylaxis (for example, needle stick, direct contact), know that drug is usually given with hepatitis B vaccine.
Patient teaching
• Instruct patient to report respiratory difficulty immediately.

☑ Evaluation
• Patient exhibits passive immunity to hepatitis B.
• Patient and family state understanding of drug therapy.

hetastarch
(HET-uh-starch)
Hespan

Pharmacologic class: amylopectin derivative
Therapeutic class: plasma volume expander
Pregnancy risk category: C

How supplied
Injection: 500 ml (6 g/100 ml in 0.9% NaCl solution)

Pharmacokinetics
Absorption: not applicable.
Distribution: distributed in blood plasma.
Metabolism: hetastarch molecules larger than 50,000 molecular weight are slowly enzymatically degraded to molecules that can be excreted.
Excretion: 40% of hetastarch molecules smaller than 50,000 molecular weight are excreted in urine within 24 hours. Hetastarch molecules that are not hydroxyethylated are slowly degraded to glucose.
Half-life: 17 to 48 days.

Route	Onset	Peak	Duration
I.V.	Immediate	Immediate	Unknown

Pharmacodynamics
Chemical effect: expands plasma volume.
Therapeutic effect: reverses fluid volume deficit.

Indications and dosage
▶ **Plasma expander.** *Adults:* 500 to 1,000 ml I.V., depending on amount of blood lost and resultant hemoconcentration. Total dosage usually not to exceed 1,500 ml/day. Up to 20 ml/kg hourly may be used in hemorrhagic shock.

Adverse reactions
CNS: headaches.
CV: peripheral edema of lower extremities.
EENT: periorbital edema.
GI: nausea, vomiting.
Skin: urticaria.
Other: wheezing, mild fever, *hypersensitivity reactions.*

Interactions
None significant.

Contraindications and precautions
• Contraindicated in patients with severe bleeding disorders, severe heart failure, or renal failure with oliguria and anuria.
• Women receiving hetastarch should temporarily discontinue breast-feeding.
• Use cautiously in pregnant women.
• Safety of drug has not been established in children.

NURSING CONSIDERATIONS

⚕ Assessment
• Obtain assessment of patient's underlying condition before therapy.
• Monitor for improvement in underlying condition. Assess vital signs and cardiopulmonary status.
• To avoid circulatory overload, monitor patient with impaired renal function carefully.
• Monitor CBC, total leukocyte and platelet counts, leukocyte differential count, hemoglobin, hematocrit, PT, INR, PTT, and electrolyte, BUN, and creatinine levels.
• Be alert for adverse reactions.
• Evaluate patient's and family's knowledge of drug therapy.

⊞ Nursing diagnoses
• Fluid volume deficit related to underlying condition
• Altered health maintenance related to hypersensitivity reaction
• Knowledge deficit related to drug therapy

▷ Planning and implementation
• Know that hetastarch is *not* a substitute for blood or plasma.

Reactions may be *common*, uncommon, *life-threatening*, or COMMON AND LIFE-THREATENING.

• When used in continuous-flow centrifugation, be aware that leukapheresis ratio is usually 1 part hetastarch to 8 parts venous whole blood.
• Discard partially used bottles.
• Discontinue drug if allergic or sensitivity reactions occur and notify doctor. If necessary, administer antihistamine as ordered.

Patient teaching
• Inform patient about need for drug.
• Tell patient to report difficulty breathing.

☑ **Evaluation**
• Patient regains normal fluid volume after drug therapy.
• Patient does not develop hypersensitivity reaction to drug.
• Patient and family state understanding of drug therapy.

hyaluronidase
(high-el-yoo-RON-ih-dayz)
Wydase

Pharmacologic class: protein enzyme
Therapeutic class: adjunct agent to increase absorption and dispersion of injected drugs
Pregnancy risk category: C

How supplied

Injection: 150 units/vial, 1,500 units/vial; 150 units/ml in 1-ml, 10-ml vials

Pharmacokinetics

Unknown.

Route	Onset	Peak	Duration
S.C.	Unknown	Unknown	Unknown

Pharmacodynamics

Chemical effect: hydrolyzes hyaluronic acid, promoting diffusion of fluids in tissues.

Therapeutic effect: increases fluid diffusion.

Indications and dosage

▶ **Adjunct to increase absorption and dispersion of other injected drugs.**
Adults and children: 150 units added to solution containing other medication.
▶ **Hypodermoclysis.** *Adults and children over age 3:* 150 units injected S.C. before clysis or injected into clysis tubing near needle for each 1,000 ml clysis solution.
▶ **Excretory urography when contrast medium is given S.C.** *Adults and children:* with patient in prone position, 75 units S.C. over each scapula, followed by injection of contrast medium at same sites.

Adverse reactions

Skin: rash, urticaria, irritation.

Interactions

Drug-drug. *Local anesthetics:* increased potential for toxic local reaction. Use together cautiously.

Contraindications and precautions

• Contraindicated in patients with hypersensitivity to drug.
• Use cautiously in pregnant women.
• Distribution of drug into human breast milk is not known.

NURSING CONSIDERATIONS

☙ **Assessment**
• Assess patient's condition before therapy and regularly thereafter.
• Perform skin test for sensitivity, as ordered. Avoid injecting into diseased areas (may spread infection), and observe injection site for local reactions.
• Be alert for adverse reactions and drug interactions.
• Evaluate patient's and family's knowledge of drug therapy.

⊞ Nursing diagnoses
- Altered health maintenance related to underlying condition
- Knowledge deficit related to drug therapy

▶ Planning and implementation
- Do not inject into acutely inflamed or cancerous areas.
- Be aware that drug is not recommended for I.V. use.
- For child, add 15 units to each 100 ml of solution. Drip rate of solution to which hyaluronidase was added to should not exceed 2 ml/minute.
- Don't add to solutions containing epinephrine and heparin. Hyaluronidase is incompatible with these drugs.
- In patients with hypodermoclysis, be prepared to adjust dosage, rate of injection, and type of solution based on patient response.
- Protect drug from heat. Do not use cloudy or discolored solution.
- Avoid getting solution in eyes; if this occurs, flush with water at once.

Patient teaching
- Instruct patient to report skin reactions.

☑ Evaluation
- Patient shows improved health.
- Patient and family state understanding of drug therapy.

---

hydralazine hydrochloride
(high-DRAL-uh-zeen
high-droh-KLOR-ighd)
Alphapress◇, Apresoline**,
Novo-Hylazin♦

Pharmacologic class: peripheral vasodilator
Therapeutic class: antihypertensive
Pregnancy risk category: C

How supplied

Tablets: 10 mg, 25 mg, 50 mg, 100 mg
Injection: 20 mg/ml

Pharmacokinetics
Absorption: absorbed rapidly from GI tract. Food enhances absorption. Degree of absorption is unknown after I.M. administration.
Distribution: distributed widely throughout body; about 88% to 90% protein-bound.
Metabolism: metabolized extensively in GI mucosa and liver.
Excretion: excreted primarily in urine; about 10% of oral dose is excreted in feces. *Half-life:* 3 to 7 hours.

Route	Onset	Peak	Duration
P.O.	20-30 min	1-2 hr	3-8 hr
I.V.	≤ 5 min	15-30 min	3-8 hr
I.M.	Unknown	Unknown	3-8 hr

Pharmacodynamics
Chemical effect: unknown. A direct-acting vasodilator, its predominant effect relaxes arteriolar smooth muscle.
Therapeutic effect: lowers blood pressure.

Indications and dosage

▶ **Essential hypertension (orally, alone, or in combination with other antihypertensives); severe essential hypertension (parenterally, to lower blood pressure quickly).** *Adults:* **P.O.** —initially, 10 mg P.O. q.i.d.; gradually increased to 50 mg q.i.d., as needed. Maximum recommended dosage is 200 mg daily, but some patients may require 300 to 400 mg daily. **I.V.**—10 to 20 mg given slowly and repeated as necessary. Switched to oral antihypertensives as soon as possible. **I.M.**—10 to 50 mg, repeated as necessary. Switched to oral form as soon as possible.

Adverse reactions

CNS: peripheral neuritis, *headache,* dizziness.
CV: orthostatic hypotension, tachycardia, arrhythmias, angina, palpitations, sodium retention.
GI: nausea, vomiting, diarrhea, anorexia.

Reactions may be *common,* uncommon, *life-threatening,* or COMMON AND LIFE-THREATENING.

Hematologic: neutropenia, leukopenia, *agranulocytopenia.*
Skin: rash.
Other: *lupuslike syndrome* (especially with high doses), *weight gain.*

Interactions

Drug-drug. *Diazoxide, MAO inhibitors:* may cause severe hypotension. Use together cautiously.
Indomethacin: pharmacologic effects of hydralazine may be decreased. Monitor patient.
Metoprolol, propranolol (beta blockers): serum levels of either drug may be increased. Avoid concurrent use.

Contraindications and precautions

• Contraindicated in patients with coronary artery disease, mitral valvular rheumatic heart disease, or hypersensitivity to drug.
• Use cautiously in patients with suspected cardiac disease, CVA, or severe renal impairment and in those taking other antihypertensives. Also use cautiously in pregnant women.
• Safety of drug has not been established in breast-feeding women or in children.

NURSING CONSIDERATIONS

Assessment
• Assess blood pressure before therapy and regularly thereafter.
• Monitor CBC, lupus erythematosus cell preparation, and antinuclear antibody titer determination during long-term therapy, as ordered.
• Be alert for adverse reactions and drug interactions.
• Evaluate patient's and family's knowledge of drug therapy.

Nursing diagnoses
• Risk for injury related to presence of hypertension
• Fluid volume excess related to sodium retention

• Knowledge deficit related to drug therapy

Planning and implementation
P.O. use: Give drug with meals to increase absorption.
I.V. use: Give drug slowly and repeat as necessary, generally every 4 to 6 hours.
– Know that hydralazine will undergo color changes in most infusion solutions; these color changes do not indicate loss of potency.
– Drug is compatible with 0.9% NaCl, Ringer's and lactated Ringer's solutions, and several other common I.V. solutions. Drug may undergo reaction with dextrose. Manufacturer does not recommend mixing drug in infusion solutions. Check with pharmacist for additional compatibility information.
I.M. use: Follow normal protocol.
• Some clinicians combine hydralazine therapy with diuretics and beta blockers to decrease sodium retention and tachycardia and to prevent anginal attacks.
• Compliance may be improved by giving drug twice daily. Check with doctor.
Patient teaching
• Instruct patient to take oral form with meals to increase absorption.
• Inform patient that orthostatic hypotension can be minimized by rising slowly and avoiding sudden position changes.
• Tell patient not to discontinue drug suddenly but to call doctor if unpleasant adverse reactions occur.
• Tell patient to limit sodium intake.

Evaluation
• Patient's blood pressure is normal.
• Fluid retention does not develop.
• Patient and family state understanding of drug therapy.

---

hydrochlorothiazide

(high-droh-klor-oh-THIGH-uh-zighd)
Apo-Hydro♦, Dichlotride◊, Diuchlor H♦,
Esidrix, Ezide, Hydro-chlor, Hydro-D,
HydroDIURIL, Hydro-Par, Neo-Codema♦,
Novo-Hydrazide♦, Oretic, Urozide♦

Pharmacologic class: thiazide diuretic
Therapeutic class: diuretic, anti-
hypertensive
Pregnancy risk category: D

How supplied

Tablets: 25 mg, 50 mg, 100 mg
Oral solution: 10 mg/ml, 50 mg/5 ml,
100 mg/ml

Pharmacokinetics

Absorption: absorbed from GI tract. Rate
and extent of absorption vary with differ-
ent formulations of drug.
Distribution: unknown.
Metabolism: none.
Excretion: excreted unchanged in urine.

Route	Onset	Peak	Duration
P.O.	2 hr	4-6 hr	6-12 hr

Pharmacodynamics

Chemical effect: increases sodium and
water excretion by inhibiting sodium and
chloride reabsorption in nephron's distal
segment.
Therapeutic effect: promotes sodium and
water excretion and lowers blood pressure.

Indications and dosage

▶ **Edema.** *Adults:* 25 to 100 mg P.O. daily or intermittently. *Children ages 2 to 12:*
37.5 to 100 mg P.O. daily in two divided
doses. *Children ages 6 months to 2:* 12.5
to 37.5 mg P.O. daily in two divided doses. *Infants under age 6 months:* up to
3.3 mg/kg P.O. daily in two divided doses.
▶ **Hypertension.** *Adults:* 25 to 50 mg
P.O. daily as single dose or divided b.i.d.
Daily dosage increased or decreased according to blood pressure. Dosages above
50 mg/day are not required when combined with other antihypertensives.

Adverse reactions

CV: volume depletion and dehydration,
orthostatic hypotension.
GI: anorexia, nausea, pancreatitis.
GU: nocturia, polyuria, frequent urination, *renal failure.*
Hematologic: *aplastic anemia, agranulocytosis,* leukopenia, *thrombocytopenia.*
Hepatic: hepatic encephalopathy.
Metabolic: hypokalemia; asymptomatic
hyperuricemia; hyperglycemia and impairment of glucose tolerance; fluid and
electrolyte imbalances, including dilutional hyponatremia and hypochloremia,
metabolic alkalosis, hypercalcemia; gout.
Skin: dermatitis, photosensitivity, rash.
Other: *anaphylactic reactions,* hypersensitivity reactions, such as pneumonitis
and vasculitis.

Interactions

Drug-drug. *Antidiabetic agents:* decreased effectiveness of hypoglycemic
agents; dosage adjustments may be necessary. Monitor blood glucose levels.
Antihypertensive agents: additive antihypertensive effect. Use together cautiously.
Barbiturates, opiates: increased orthostatic hypotensive effect. Monitor closely.
Cardiac glycosides: increased risk of digitalis toxicity from hydrochlorothiazide-
induced hypokalemia. Monitor potassium
and cardiac glycoside levels.
Cholestyramine, colestipol: decreased intestinal absorption of thiazides. Separate
doses.
Diazoxide: increased antihypertensive,
hyperglycemic, and hyperuricemic effects. Use together cautiously.
Lithium: decreased lithium excretion, increasing risk of lithium toxicity. Monitor
lithium level.
NSAIDs: increased risk of NSAID-
induced renal failure. Monitor closely.
Drug-lifestyle. *Alcohol use:* increased
orthostatic hypotensive effect. Avoid concomitant use.

Reactions may be *common*, uncommon, *life-threatening*, or COMMON AND LIFE-THREATENING.

Sun exposure: increased sensitivity to sun. Use appropriate precautions when exposed to sun.

Contraindications and precautions

• Contraindicated in patients with anuria or hypersensitivity to other thiazides or other sulfonamide derivatives.
• Drug is not recommended for use in pregnant women because fetal harm may occur.
• Use cautiously in patients with severe renal disease, impaired hepatic function, and progressive hepatic disease.
• Safety of drug has not been established for breast-feeding women.

NURSING CONSIDERATIONS

⚞ Assessment
• Assess patient's edema or blood pressure before starting therapy.
• Monitor effectiveness by regularly checking blood pressure, urine output, and weight. In patient with hypertension, know that therapeutic response may be delayed several days.
• Monitor serum electrolyte levels.
• Monitor serum creatinine and BUN levels regularly. Drug is not as effective if these levels are more than twice normal.
• Monitor blood uric acid levels, especially in patient with history of gout.
• Be alert for adverse reactions and drug interactions.
• Evaluate patient's and family's knowledge of drug therapy.

⚛ Nursing diagnoses
• Altered health maintenance related to presence of edema or hypertension
• Altered urinary elimination related to diuretic effect of drug
• Knowledge deficit related to drug therapy

❯ Planning and implementation
• Give drug in morning to prevent nocturia. Administer drug with food if nausea occurs.

• Drug may be used with potassium-sparing diuretic to prevent potassium loss.
Patient teaching
• Advise patient to take drug with food to minimize GI upset.
• Caution patient to avoid sudden posture changes and to rise slowly to avoid orthostatic hypotension.
• Instruct patient to avoid alcohol consumption during drug therapy.
• Advise patient to use sunblock to prevent photosensitivity reactions.
• Tell patient to check with doctor before taking OTC medications.

☑ Evaluation
• Patient's blood pressure is normal and no edema is present.
• Patient demonstrates adjustment of lifestyle to deal with altered patterns of urinary elimination.
• Patient and family state understanding of drug therapy.

hydrocortisone
(high-droh-KOR-tuh-sohn)
Cortef, Cortenema, Hydrocortone

hydrocortisone acetate
Cortifoam, Hydrocortone Acetate

hydrocortisone cypionate
Cortef

hydrocortisone sodium phosphate
Hydrocortone Phosphate

hydrocortisone sodium succinate
A-hydroCort, Solu-Cortef

Pharmacologic class: glucocorticoid, mineralocorticoid
Therapeutic class: adrenocorticoid replacement
Pregnancy risk category: NR

How supplied

hydrocortisone
Tablets: 5 mg, 10 mg, 20 mg
Enema: 100 mg/60 ml
hydrocortisone acetate
Injection: 25 mg/ml*, 50 mg/ml* suspension
Enema: 10% aerosol foam (provides 90 mg/application)
Suppositories: 25 mg
hydrocortisone cypionate
Oral suspension: 10 mg/5 ml
hydrocortisone sodium phosphate
Injection: 50 mg/ml solution
hydrocortisone sodium succinate
Injection: 100 mg/vial*, 250 mg/vial*, 500 mg/vial*, 1,000 mg/vial*

Pharmacokinetics

Absorption: absorbed rapidly after oral use. Variable absorption after I.M. or intra-articular injection. Unknown after rectal use.
Distribution: distributed to muscle, liver, skin, intestines, and kidneys. Drug is bound extensively to plasma proteins. Only unbound portion is active.
Metabolism: metabolized in liver.
Excretion: inactive metabolites and small amounts of unmetabolized drug excreted in urine; insignificant quantities excreted in feces. *Half-life:* 8 to 12 hours.

Route	Onset	Peak	Duration
All routes	Varies	Varies	Varies

Pharmacodynamics

Chemical effect: not clearly defined; decreases inflammation, mainly by stabilizing leukocyte lysosomal membranes; suppresses immune response; stimulates bone marrow; and influences nutrient metabolism.
Therapeutic effect: reduces inflammation, suppresses immune function, raises adrenocorticoid hormonal levels.

Indications and dosage

▶ **Severe inflammation, adrenal insufficiency.** *Adults:* 5 to 30 mg P.O. b.i.d.,

t.i.d., or q.i.d. (as much as 80 mg q.i.d. may be given in acute situations); or initially, 100 to 500 mg succinate I.M. or I.V., and then 50 to 100 mg I.M., as indicated; or 15 to 240 mg phosphate I.V., I.M., or S.C. q 12 hours; or 10 to 75 mg acetate into joints or soft tissue. Dosage varies with size of joint. Local anesthetics are often injected with dose.
▶ **Shock.** *Adults:* initially, 50 mg/kg succinate I.V. repeated in 4 hours. Repeat dosage q 24 hours, p.r.n. Alternatively, 0.5 to 2 g I.V. q 2 to 6 hours, p.r.n. *Children:* 0.16 to 1 mg/kg or 6 to 30 mg/m^2 phosphate I.M. or succinate I.M. or I.V. daily or b.i.d.
▶ **Adjunct for ulcerative colitis and proctitis.** *Adults:* 1 enema (100 mg) P.R. nightly for 21 days.

Adverse reactions

Most adverse reactions are dose- or duration-dependent.
CNS: *euphoria, insomnia,* psychotic behavior, pseudotumor cerebri, *seizures.*
CV: *heart failure,* hypertension, edema, *arrhythmias, thromboembolism.*
EENT: cataracts, glaucoma.
GI: *peptic ulceration,* GI irritation, increased appetite, pancreatitis.
Metabolic: possible hypokalemia, hyperglycemia, and carbohydrate intolerance.
Musculoskeletal: muscle weakness, growth suppression in children, osteoporosis.
Skin: delayed wound healing, acne, various skin eruptions, easy bruising.
Other: hirsutism, susceptibility to infections; *acute adrenal insufficiency with increased stress (infection, surgery, or trauma) or abrupt withdrawal after long-term therapy.*
After abrupt withdrawal: rebound inflammation, fatigue, weakness, arthralgia, fever, dizziness, lethargy, depression, fainting, orthostatic hypotension, dyspnea, anorexia, hypoglycemia. *After prolonged use, sudden withdrawal may be fatal.*

Reactions may be *common*, uncommon, *life-threatening*, or COMMON AND LIFE-THREATENING.

Interactions

Drug-drug. *Aspirin, indomethacin, other NSAIDs:* increased risk of GI distress and bleeding. Give together cautiously.
Barbiturates, phenytoin, rifampin: decreased corticosteroid effect. Increase corticosteroid dosage, as ordered.
Live-attenuated virus vaccines, other toxoids and vaccines: decreased antibody response and increased risk of neurologic complications. Avoid concomitant use.
Oral anticoagulants: altered dosage requirements. Monitor PT and INR closely.
Potassium-depleting drugs (such as thiazide diuretics): enhanced potassium-wasting effects of hydrocortisone. Monitor potassium levels.
Skin-test antigens: decreased response. Defer skin testing until therapy is completed.

Contraindications and precautions

• Contraindicated in patients allergic to drug or its components, in those with systemic fungal infections, and in premature infants (succinate).
• Drug use is not recommended in high doses for breast-feeding women.
• Use with extreme caution in patients with recent MI.
• Use cautiously in patients with GI ulcer, renal disease, hypertension, osteoporosis, diabetes mellitus, hypothyroidism, cirrhosis, diverticulitis, nonspecific ulcerative colitis, recent intestinal anastomoses, thromboembolic disorders, seizures, myasthenia gravis, heart failure, tuberculosis, ocular herpes simplex, emotional instability, and psychotic tendencies. Also use cautiously in pregnant women.
• Chronic use in children may delay growth and maturation.

NURSING CONSIDERATIONS

🕮 Assessment
• Assess patient's condition before therapy and regularly thereafter.

• Monitor patient's weight, blood pressure, and serum electrolyte levels.
• Monitor for stress. Fever, trauma, surgery, and emotional problems may increase adrenal insufficiency.
• Periodic measurement of growth and development may be necessary during high-dose or prolonged therapy in child.
• Be alert for adverse reactions and drug interactions.
• Evaluate patient's and family's knowledge of drug therapy.

🕮 Nursing diagnoses
• Altered health maintenance related to underlying condition
• Altered protection related to immunosuppression
• Knowledge deficit related to drug therapy

🕮 Planning and implementation
• For better results and less toxicity, give once-daily dose in morning.
P.O. use: Give oral dose with food when possible.
I.V. use: Do not use acetate or suspension form for I.V. use. When administering as direct injection, inject directly into vein or I.V. line containing free-flowing compatible solution over 30 seconds to several minutes. When administering as intermittent or continuous infusion, dilute solution according to manufacturer's instructions and give over prescribed duration. If used for continuous infusion, change solution every 24 hours.
– Hydrocortisone sodium phosphate may be added directly to D_5W or 0.9% NaCl for I.V. administration.
– Reconstitute hydrocortisone sodium succinate with bacteriostatic water or bacteriostatic NaCl solution before adding to I.V. solutions. When giving by direct I.V. injection, inject over at least 30 seconds. For infusion, dilute with D_5W, 0.9% NaCl, or dextrose 5% in 0.9% NaCl to concentration of 1 mg/ml or less.

I.M. use: Give I.M. injection deeply into gluteal muscle. Rotate injection sites to prevent muscle atrophy.

P.R. use: Enema may produce same systemic effects as other forms of hydrocortisone. If therapy must exceed 21 days, discontinue gradually by reducing administration to every other night for 2 or 3 weeks, as ordered.

• Avoid S.C. injection because atrophy and sterile abscesses may occur.

• Do not confuse Solu-Cortef with Solu-Medrol (methylprednisolone sodium succinate).

• Know that injectable forms are not used for alternate-day therapy.

• High-dose therapy is usually not continued beyond 48 hours.

• Always titrate to lowest effective dose and gradually reduce dosage after long-term therapy, as ordered.

• Administer potassium supplements, as ordered.

• Notify doctor if signs and symptoms of adrenal insufficiency appear. Dosage may need to be increased.

• Notify doctor of adverse reactions. Provide supportive care as indicated and ordered.

Patient teaching
• Teach patient signs of early adrenal insufficiency: fatigue, muscular weakness, joint pain, fever, anorexia, nausea, dyspnea, dizziness, and fainting.

• Instruct patient to carry card identifying need for supplemental systemic glucocorticoids during stress.

• Tell patient not to discontinue drug abruptly or without doctor's consent.

• Warn patient on long-term therapy about cushingoid symptoms and to report sudden weight gain or swelling to doctor. Also advise him to consider exercise or physical therapy, to ask his doctor about vitamin D or calcium supplements, and to have periodic ophthalmic examinations.

• Caution patient about easy bruising.

☑ **Evaluation**
• Patient's condition improves.
• Serious complications related to drug-induced immunosuppression do not develop.
• Patient and family state understanding of drug therapy.

hydromorphone hydrochloride (dihydromorphinone hydrochloride)

(high-droh-MOR-fohn
high-droh-KLOR-ighd)
Dilaudid, Dilaudid-HP, HydroStat

Pharmacologic class: opioid
Therapeutic class: analgesic, antitussive
Controlled substance schedule: II
Pregnancy risk category: C

How supplied

Tablets: 1 mg, 2 mg, 3 mg, 4 mg, 8 mg
Injection: 1 mg/ml, 2 mg/ml, 4 mg/ml, 10 mg/ml
Suppositories: 3 mg
Syrup: 1 mg/5 ml
Liquid: 5 mg/5 ml

Pharmacokinetics

Absorption: well absorbed after oral, rectal, or parenteral administration.
Distribution: unknown.
Metabolism: metabolized primarily in liver.
Excretion: excreted primarily in urine.
Half-life: 2.6 to 4 hours.

Route	Onset	Peak	Duration
P.O.	30 min	1.5-2 hr	4-5 hr
I.V.	10-15 min	15-30 min	2-3 hr
I.M.	15 min	30-60 min	4-5 hr
S.C.	15 min	30-90 min	4 hr
P.R.	Unknown	Unknown	4 hr

Pharmacodynamics

Chemical effect: binds with opioid receptors in CNS, altering perception of and emotional response to pain.

Suppresses cough reflex by direct action on cough center in medulla.
Therapeutic effect: relieves pain and cough.

Indications and dosage

▶ **Moderate to severe pain.** *Adults:* 2 to 4 mg P.O. q 4 to 6 hours, p.r.n.; or 1 to 2 mg I.M., S.C., or I.V. (slowly over at least 2 to 3 minutes) q 4 to 6 hours p.r.n.; or 3 mg rectal suppository q 6 to 8 hours p.r.n.
▶ **Cough.** *Adults:* 1 teaspoon (5 ml = 1 mg) P.O. q 3 to 4 hours p.r.n.

Adverse reactions

CNS: *sedation, somnolence, clouded sensorium,* dizziness, *euphoria, **seizures*** (with large doses).
CV: hypotension, bradycardia.
EENT: blurred vision, diplopia, nystagmus.
GI: nausea, vomiting, constipation, ileus.
GU: urine retention.
Respiratory: ***respiratory depression, bronchospasm.***
Other: induration (with repeated S.C. injections), physical dependence.

Interactions

Drug-drug. *CNS depressants, general anesthetics, hypnotics, MAO inhibitors, other narcotic analgesics, sedatives, tranquilizers, tricyclic antidepressants:* additive effects. Use together with extreme caution. Reduce hydromorphone dose and monitor patient response.
Drug-lifestyle. *Alcohol use:* additive effects. Avoid concomitant use.

Contraindications and precautions

- Contraindicated in patients with intracranial lesions associated with increased intracranial pressure, hypersensitivity to drug, and whenever ventilator function is depressed, such as in status asthmaticus, COPD, cor pulmonale, emphysema, and kyphoscoliosis.
- Use with extreme caution in patients with hepatic or renal disease, hypothyroidism, Addison's disease, prostatic hypertrophy, or urethral stricture.
- Use with caution in elderly or debilitated patients and in pregnant or breast-feeding women.

NURSING CONSIDERATIONS

Assessment
- Assess patient's pain or cough before and after drug administration.
- Respiratory depression and hypotension can occur with I.V. administration. Monitor respiratory and circulatory status constantly.
- Be aware that drug may worsen or mask gallbladder pain.
- Be aware that drug is a commonly abused narcotic.
- Be alert for adverse reactions and drug interactions.
- Evaluate patient's and family's knowledge of drug therapy.

Nursing diagnoses
- Pain related to underlying condition
- Ineffective breathing pattern related to respiratory depression
- Knowledge deficit related to drug therapy

Planning and implementation
- For better analgesic effect, give drug before patient has intense pain.
- Dilaudid-HP, a highly concentrated form (10 mg/ml), may be administered in smaller volumes to prevent discomfort associated with large-volume I.M. or S.C. injections. Check dosage carefully.

P.O., I.M., and P.R. use: Follow normal protocol.
I.V. use: Give drug by direct injection over no less than 2 minutes. For infusion, drug may be mixed in D_5W, 0.9% NaCl, dextrose 5% in 0.9% NaCl, dextrose 5% in 0.45% NaCl, or Ringer's or lactated Ringer's solutions.
S.C. use: Rotate injection sites to avoid induration with S.C. injection.

• Keep resuscitation equipment and narcotic antagonist (naloxone) available.
• Postoperatively, encourage patient turning, coughing, and deep breathing to avoid atelectasis.
Patient teaching
• Caution ambulatory patient about getting out of bed or walking. Warn outpatient to avoid activities that require mental alertness until drug's CNS effects are known.
• Suggest measures to prevent constipation during maintenance therapy.
• Encourage patient to ask for drug before pain becomes severe.
• Tell patient or family caregiver to notify health care professional if patient's respiratory rate decreases.
• Instruct patient to avoid alcohol consumption during drug therapy.

☑ **Evaluation**
• Patient is free from pain.
• Patient maintains adequate breathing patterns.
• Patient and family state understanding of drug therapy.

---

hydroxychloroquine sulfate
(high-droks-ee-KLOR-oh-kwin SUL-fayt)
Plaquenil

Pharmacologic class: 4-aminoquinoline
Therapeutic class: antimalarial, antiinflammatory
Pregnancy risk category: NR

How supplied

Tablets: 200 mg (155-mg base)

Pharmacokinetics

Absorption: absorbed readily and almost completely.
Distribution: concentrates in liver, spleen, kidneys, heart, and brain and is strongly bound in melanin-containing cells. Drug is bound to plasma proteins.
Metabolism: metabolized by liver.

Excretion: most excreted unchanged in urine. *Half-life:* 32 to 50 days.

Route	Onset	Peak	Duration
P.O.	Unknown	2-4.5 hr	Unknown

Pharmacodynamics

Chemical effect: unknown; may bind to and alter properties of DNA in susceptible organisms.
Therapeutic effect: prevents or hinders growth of *Plasmodium malariae, P. ovale, P. vivax,* and *P. falciparum.* Also relieves inflammation.

Indications and dosage

▶ **Suppressive prophylaxis of malaria attacks caused by *P. vivax, P. malariae, P. ovale,* and susceptible strains of *P. falciparum.*** *Adults and children:* for suppression—5 mg (base)/kg P.O. (not to exceed 310 mg) weekly on same day of week (begin 2 weeks before entering and continue for 8 weeks after leaving endemic area). If not started before exposure, initial dose is doubled (620 mg for adults, 10 mg/kg for children) in two divided doses P.O. 6 hours apart.
▶ **Acute malarial attacks.** *Adults:* initially, 800 mg (sulfate) P.O., then 400 mg (sulfate) after 6 to 8 hours, then 400 mg (sulfate) daily for 2 days (total 2 g sulfate salt). *Children:* initial dose, 10 mg base/kg (up to 620 mg base); second dose, 5 mg base/kg (up to 310 mg base) 6 hours after first dose; third dose, 5 mg base/kg 18 hours after second dose; fourth dose, 5 mg base/kg 24 hours after third dose.
▶ **Lupus erythematosus (chronic discoid and systemic).** *Adults:* 400 mg (sulfate) P.O. daily or b.i.d., continued for several weeks or months, depending on response. Prolonged maintenance dosage—200 to 400 mg (sulfate) daily.
▶ **Rheumatoid arthritis.** *Adults:* initially, 400 to 600 mg (sulfate) P.O. daily. When response occurs (usually in 4 to 12 weeks), dosage is cut in half.

Reactions may be *common,* uncommon, *life-threatening,* or COMMON AND LIFE-THREATENING.

Adverse reactions

CNS: irritability, nightmares, ataxia, *seizures,* psychic stimulation, toxic psychosis, vertigo, nystagmus, lassitude, fatigue, dizziness, hypoactive deep tendon reflexes, skeletal muscle weakness.
EENT: visual disturbances (blurred vision; difficulty in focusing; reversible corneal changes; typically irreversible, sometimes progressive or delayed retinal changes, such as narrowing of arterioles; macular lesions; pallor of optic disk; optic atrophy; visual field defects; patchy retinal pigmentation, commonly leading to blindness), ototoxicity (irreversible nerve deafness, tinnitus, labyrinthitis).
GI: anorexia, abdominal cramps, diarrhea, nausea, vomiting.
Hematologic: *agranulocytosis, leukopenia, thrombocytopenia, aplastic anemia; hemolysis* (in patients with G6PD deficiency).
Skin: pruritus, lichen planus eruptions, skin and mucosal pigmentary changes, pleomorphic skin eruptions.
Other: weight loss, alopecia, bleaching of hair.

Interactions

Drug-drug. *Aluminum and magnesium salts, kaolin:* decreased GI absorption. Separate administration times.
Cimetidine: decreased hepatic metabolism of hydroxychloroquine. Monitor for toxicity.

Contraindications and precautions

• Contraindicated in patients with retinal or visual field changes, porphyria, or hypersensitivity to drug, and in long-term therapy for children.
• Use with extreme caution in patients with severe GI, neurologic, or blood disorders.
• Use cautiously in patients with hepatic disease or alcoholism because drug concentrates in liver, and in those with G6PD deficiency or psoriasis because drug may exacerbate these conditions. Also use cautiously in pregnant women.

• Safety of drug has not been established in breast-feeding women.

NURSING CONSIDERATIONS

☢ Assessment
• Assess patient's condition before therapy and regularly thereafter.
• Ensure baseline and periodic ophthalmic examinations are performed. Check periodically for ocular muscle weakness after long-term use.
• Obtain audiometric examinations before, during, and after therapy, especially if long-term.
• Monitor CBCs and liver function studies periodically during long-term therapy, as ordered.
• Assess patient for overdose, which can quickly lead to toxic symptoms: headache, drowsiness, visual disturbances, CV collapse, and seizures, followed by cardiopulmonary arrest. Children are extremely susceptible to toxicity; long-term treatment should be avoided.
• Be alert for adverse reactions and drug interactions.
• Evaluate patient's and family's knowledge of drug therapy.

✛ Nursing diagnoses
• Infection related to susceptible organisms
• Sensory or perceptual alterations (visual and auditory) related to drug's adverse reactions
• Knowledge deficit related to drug therapy

▶ Planning and implementation
• Give drug right before or after meals on same day of each week.
• Notify doctor immediately of severe blood disorder not attributable to disease under treatment. Blood reaction may require discontinuation.
Patient teaching
• Advise patient to take drug immediately before or after meals on same day each

week to enhance compliance for prophylaxis.
• Warn patient to avoid hazardous activities if adverse CNS or visual disturbances occur.
• Tell patient to promptly report visual or auditory changes.

☑ **Evaluation**
• Patient is free from infection.
• Patient maintains normal visual and auditory function.
• Patient and family state understanding of drug therapy.

hydroxyprogesterone caproate
(high-droks-ee-proh-JES-ter-ohn KAP-roh-ayt)
Hylutin

Pharmacologic class: progestin
Therapeutic class: progestin, antineoplastic
Pregnancy risk category: X

How supplied

Injection: 125 mg/ml, 250 mg/ml

Pharmacokinetics

Absorption: absorbed slowly after I.M. administration.
Distribution: unknown.
Metabolism: primarily hepatic.
Excretion: primarily renal.

Route	Onset	Peak	Duration
I.M.	Unknown	Unknown	Unknown

Pharmacodynamics

Chemical effect: suppresses ovulation, possibly by inhibiting pituitary gonadotropin secretion, and forms thick cervical mucus.
Therapeutic effect: inhibits growth of progestin-sensitive uterine cancer tissue and suppresses ovulation.

Indications and dosage

► **Amenorrhea, uterine bleeding.**
Adults: 375 mg I.M. q 4 weeks. Stop after four cycles.
► **Palliative treatment of advanced inoperable endometrial cancer.** *Adults:* 1 g I.M. up to seven times weekly.

Adverse reactions

CNS: dizziness, migraine, lethargy, depression.
CV: hypertension, thrombophlebitis, *thromboembolism, CVA, pulmonary embolism,* edema.
GI: nausea, vomiting, abdominal cramps.
GU: breakthrough bleeding, dysmenorrhea, amenorrhea, cervical erosion, abnormal secretions, uterine fibromas, vaginal candidiasis.
Hepatic: cholestatic jaundice.
Skin: melasma, rash; local irritation and pain at injection site.
Other: breast tenderness, enlargement, or secretion; decreased libido; hyperglycemia.

Interactions

Drug-drug. *Barbiturates, carbamazepine, rifampin:* decreased progestin effects. Monitor for diminished therapeutic response.
Bromocriptine: may cause amenorrhea, interfering with bromocriptine's effects. Avoid concomitant use.
Corticosteroids: possible enhanced effects. Monitor closely.
Dantrolene, other hepatotoxic drugs: increased risk of hepatotoxicity. Monitor closely.
Oral anticoagulants: dosage adjustments may be necessary. Monitor PT and INR.

Contraindications and precautions

• Contraindicated in patients with thromboembolic disorders, cerebral apoplexy, breast or genital organ cancer, undiagnosed abnormal vaginal bleeding, severe hepatic disease, missed abortion, or hypersensitivity to drug and in pregnant women.

Reactions may be *common*, uncommon, *life-threatening*, or COMMON AND LIFE-THREATENING.

- Drug is not recommended for use in breast-feeding women.
- Use cautiously in patients with diabetes mellitus, seizure disorder, migraine, cardiac or renal disease, asthma, mental depression, or impaired liver function.
- Safety of drug has not been established in children.

NURSING CONSIDERATIONS

Assessment
- Assess patient's condition before therapy and regularly thereafter.
- Be alert for adverse reactions and drug interactions.
- Evaluate patient's and family's knowledge of drug therapy.

Nursing diagnoses
- Sexual dysfunction related to underlying condition
- Fluid volume excess related to drug-induced edema
- Knowledge deficit related to drug therapy

Planning and implementation
- Drug should not be used to induce withdrawal bleeding or as pregnancy test; drug may cause birth defects and masculinization of female fetus.
- Give oil solutions (sesame oil and castor oil) via deep I.M. injection in gluteal muscle. Rotate injection sites to prevent muscle atrophy.
- Withhold drug and notify doctor if pulmonary embolism is suspected; provide supportive care as indicated.

Patient teaching
- Instruct patient to read package insert explaining possible adverse effects of progestin before receiving first dose. Also, provide verbal explanation.
- Tell patient to report unusual symptoms immediately and to stop drug and call doctor if visual disturbances or migraine occurs.
- Warn patient that edema and weight gain are likely. Tell her to monitor weight routinely. Recommend sodium-restricted diet, as needed.
- Instruct patient to report breast pain or tenderness, vaginal discharge or bleeding, and swelling of hands or feet.
- Teach her how to perform routine breast self-examination.
- Inform her that normal menstrual cycle may not resume for 2 to 3 months after drug is stopped.

Evaluation
- Patient's sexual dysfunction is resolved.
- Patient does not exhibit serious fluid excess.
- Patient and family state understanding of drug therapy.

hydroxyurea
(high-droks-ee-yoo-REE-uh)
Hydrea**

Pharmacologic class: antimetabolite (cell cycle–phase specific, S phase)
Therapeutic class: antineoplastic
Pregnancy risk category: NR

How supplied
Capsules: 500 mg

Pharmacokinetics
Absorption: well absorbed. Serum levels are higher with a large, single dose than with divided doses.
Distribution: crosses blood-brain barrier.
Metabolism: about 50% of dose is degraded in liver.
Excretion: 50% of drug excreted in urine as unchanged drug; metabolites excreted through lungs as carbon dioxide and in urine as urea. *Half-life:* 3 to 4 hours.

Route	Onset	Peak	Duration
P.O.	Unknown	2 hr	Unknown

Pharmacodynamics
Chemical effect: unknown; thought to inhibit DNA synthesis.

Therapeutic effect: hinders selected cancer cell growth.

Indications and dosage

▶ **Melanoma; resistant chronic myelocytic leukemia; recurrent, metastatic, or inoperable ovarian cancer; head and neck cancers.** *Adults:* 80 mg/kg P.O. as single dose q 3 days; or 20 to 30 mg/kg P.O. as single daily dose.

Adverse reactions

CNS: drowsiness, hallucinations, *seizures.*
GI: anorexia, nausea, vomiting, diarrhea, stomatitis.
GU: increased BUN and serum creatinine levels.
Hematologic: *leukopenia, thrombocytopenia,* anemia, *megaloblastosis; bone marrow suppression* (dose-limiting and dose-related; with rapid recovery).
Metabolic: hyperuricemia.
Skin: rash, pruritus.

Interactions

Drug-drug. *Cytotoxic drugs, radiation therapy:* enhanced toxicity of hydroxyurea. Use together cautiously.

Contraindications and precautions

• Contraindicated in patients with marked bone marrow depression or hypersensitivity to drug.
• Drug use is not recommended in pregnant or breast-feeding women.
• Use cautiously in patients with renal dysfunction.
• Safety of drug has not been established in children.

NURSING CONSIDERATIONS

⚕ Assessment
• Assess patient's condition before therapy and regularly thereafter.
• Measure CBC, BUN, uric acid, and serum creatinine levels, as ordered.

• Auditory and visual hallucinations and hematologic toxicity increase with decreased renal function.
• Concomitant radiation therapy may increase incidence or severity of GI distress or stomatitis.
• Be alert for adverse reactions and drug interactions.
• Evaluate patient's and family's knowledge of drug therapy.

⊕ Nursing diagnoses
• Altered health maintenance related to presence of neoplastic disease
• Altered protection related to adverse hematologic reactions
• Knowledge deficit related to drug therapy

⟫ Planning and implementation
• Keep patient hydrated.
• Be aware that dosage modification may be required after chemotherapy or radiation therapy.
Patient teaching
• Tell patient who can't swallow capsules to empty contents into water and take immediately.
• Warn patient to watch for signs of infection (fever, sore throat, fatigue) and bleeding (easy bruising, nosebleeds, bleeding gums, melena). Instruct patient to take infection-control and bleeding precautions. Tell patient to take temperature daily.
• Advise female patient of childbearing age to avoid becoming pregnant during therapy and to consult with doctor before becoming pregnant.

☑ Evaluation
• Patient responds well to drug therapy.
• Serious infections or bleeding complications do not develop.
• Patient and family state understanding of drug therapy.

Reactions may be *common*, uncommon, *life-threatening*, or COMMON AND LIFE-THREATENING.

hydroxyzine embonate◇
(high-DROKS-ih-zeen EM-boh-nayt)
Atarax

hydroxyzine hydrochloride
Apo-Hydroxyzine♦, Atarax*, Evista,
Hydroxacen, Hyzine-50, Multipax♦,
Novo-Hydroxyzin♦, Quiess, Vistacon-50,
Vistaject-25, Vistaject-50, Vistaril,
Vistazine 50

hydroxyzine pamoate
Hy-Pam, Vamate, Vistaril

Pharmacologic class: antihistamine
(piperazine derivative)
Therapeutic class: antianxiety, sedative,
antipruritic, antiemetic, antispasmodic
Pregnancy risk category: NR

How supplied
hydroxyzine embonate◇
Capsules: 25 mg, 50 mg
hydroxyzine hydrochloride
Tablets: 10 mg, 25 mg, 50 mg, 100 mg
Capsules: 10 mg♦◇, 25 mg♦◇,
50 mg♦◇
Syrup: 10 mg/5 ml
Injection: 25 mg/ml, 50 mg/ml
hydroxyzine pamoate
Capsules: 25 mg, 50 mg, 100 mg
Oral suspension: 25 mg/5 ml

Pharmacokinetics
Absorption: absorbed rapidly and completely after oral administration. Unknown for I.M. administration.
Distribution: unknown.
Metabolism: metabolized almost completely in liver.
Excretion: metabolites excreted primarily in urine; small amounts of drug and
metabolites excreted in feces. *Half-life:* 3
hours.

Route	Onset	Peak	Duration
P.O.	15-30 min	About 2 hr	4-6 hr
I.M.	Unknown	Unknown	4-6 hr

Pharmacodynamics
Chemical effect: unknown; may suppress
activity in key regions of subcortical area
of CNS.
Therapeutic effect: relieves anxiety and
itching, promotes calmness, and alleviates nausea and vomiting.

Indications and dosage
▶ **Anxiety.** *Adults:* 50 to 100 mg P.O.
q.i.d. *Children under age 6:* 50 mg P.O.
daily in divided doses. *Children age 6
and over:* 50 to 100 mg P.O. daily in divided doses.
▶ **Preoperative and postoperative adjunct therapy.** *Adults:* 25 to 100 mg I.M.
q 4 to 6 hours. *Children:* 1.1 mg/kg I.M.
q 4 to 6 hours.
▶ **Pruritus due to allergies.** *Adults:*
25 mg P.O. t.i.d. or q.i.d. *Children under
age 6:* 50 mg P.O. daily in divided doses.
Children age 6 and over: 50 to 100 mg
P.O. daily in divided doses.
▶ **Psychiatric and emotional emergencies, including acute alcoholism.** *Adults:*
50 to 100 mg I.M. q 4 to 6 hours, p.r.n.
▶ **Nausea and vomiting (excluding
nausea and vomiting of pregnancy).**
Adults: 25 to 100 mg I.M. *Children:*
1.1 mg/kg I.M.
▶ **Prepartum and postpartum adjunct
therapy.** *Adults:* 25 to 100 mg I.M.

Adverse reactions
CNS: *drowsiness,* involuntary motor activity.
GI: *dry mouth.*
Other: marked discomfort (at I.M. injection site), *hypersensitivity reactions*
(wheezing, dyspnea, chest tightness).

Interactions
Drug-drug. *CNS depressants:* increased
CNS depression. Avoid concomitant use.
Drug-lifestyle. *Alcohol use:* increased
CNS depression. Avoid concomitant use.

Contraindications and precautions
● Contraindicated in patients hypersensitive to drug and during early pregnancy.

---

*Liquid form contains alcohol   **May contain tartrazine   ♦Canada   ◇Australia   †OTC

• Safety of drug has not been established in breast-feeding women.

NURSING CONSIDERATIONS

⚖ Assessment
• Assess patient's condition before therapy and regularly thereafter.
• Be alert for adverse reactions and drug interactions.
• Evaluate patient's and family's knowledge of drug therapy.

✛ Nursing diagnoses
• Altered health maintenance related to underlying condition
• Risk for injury related to adverse CNS reactions
• Knowledge deficit related to drug therapy

▷ Planning and implementation
• Dosage should be reduced in elderly or debilitated patients.
P.O. use: Follow normal protocol.
I.M. use: Parenteral form (hydroxyzine hydrochloride) for I.M. use only; never administer drug I.V. Z-track injection method is preferred.
– Aspirate I.M. injection carefully to prevent inadvertent intravascular injection. Inject deeply into large muscle mass.
• Drug may cause false elevations of urine 17-hydroxycorticosteroids, depending on test method used.
Patient teaching
• Warn patient to avoid hazardous activities until CNS effects of drug are known.
• Tell patient to avoid alcohol during drug therapy.
• Suggest sugarless hard candy or gum to relieve dry mouth.

✓ Evaluation
• Patient exhibits improved health.
• Patient does not experience injury.
• Patient and family state understanding of drug therapy.

ibuprofen
(igh-byoo-PROH-fen)
Aches-N-Pain†, ACT-3◊, Advil†, Apo-Ibuprofen♦, Brufen◊, Children's Advil, Excedrin IB Caplets†, Excedrin-IB Tablets†, Genpril Caplets†, Genpril Tablets†, Haltran†, Ibuprin†, Ibuprohm Caplets†, Ibuprohm Tablets†, Ibu-Tab†, Inflam◊, Medipren Caplets†, Medipren Tablets†, Midol IB, Motrin, Motrin IB Caplets†, Motrin IB Tablets†, Novo-Profen♦, Nuprin Caplets†, Nuprin Tablets†, Nurofen◊, Pamprin-IB, Pedia Profen, Rafen◊, Rufen, Saleto-200, Saleto-400, Saleto-600, Saleto-800, Trendar†

Pharmacologic class: NSAID
Therapeutic class: nonnarcotic analgesic, antipyretic, anti-inflammatory
Pregnancy risk category: NR

How supplied
Tablets: 200 mg†, 300 mg, 400 mg, 600 mg, 800 mg
Tablets (chewable): 50 mg, 100 mg
Caplets: 100 mg, 200 mg†
Oral suspension: 100 mg/5 ml
Oral drops: 40 mg/ml

Pharmacokinetics
Absorption: absorbed rapidly and completely from GI tract when administered orally.
Distribution: highly protein-bound.
Metabolism: undergoes biotransformation in liver.
Excretion: excreted mainly in urine, with some biliary excretion. *Half-life:* 2 to 4 hours.

Route	Onset	Peak	Duration
P.O.	≤ 30 min	2-4 hr	≥ 4 hr

Pharmacodynamics

Chemical effect: unknown; produces anti-inflammatory, analgesic, and antipyretic effects, possibly by inhibiting prostaglandin synthesis.
Therapeutic effect: relieves pain, fever, and inflammation.

Indications and dosage

▶ **Rheumatoid or osteoarthritis, arthritis.** *Adults:* 300 to 800 mg P.O. t.i.d. or q.i.d. not to exceed 3.2 g/day.
▶ **Mild to moderate pain, dysmenorrhea.** *Adults:* 400 mg P.O. q 4 to 6 hours, p.r.n.
▶ **Fever.** *Adults:* 200 to 400 mg P.O. q 4 to 6 hours, p.r.n. Do not exceed 1.2 g daily or give longer than 3 days. *Children ages 6 months to 12 years:* if fever is below 102.5°F (39.2°C), recommended dose is 5 mg/kg P.O. q 6 to 8 hours p.r.n. Treat higher fevers with 10 mg/kg P.O. q 6 to 8 hours p.r.n. Do not exceed 40 mg/kg daily.

Adverse reactions

CNS: *headache, drowsiness, dizziness,* cognitive dysfunction, aseptic meningitis.
CV: *peripheral edema,* hypertension, *heart failure.*
EENT: visual disturbances, *tinnitus.*
GI: *epigastric distress, nausea, occult blood loss, peptic ulceration.*
GU: reversible renal failure.
Hematologic: prolonged bleeding time, anemia, *neutropenia, pancytopenia, thrombocytopenia, aplastic anemia,* leukopenia, *agranulocytosis.*
Hepatic: elevated enzymes.
Respiratory: *bronchospasm.*
Skin: pruritus, rash, urticaria, photosensitivity, *Stevens-Johnson syndrome.*
Other: edema.

Interactions

Drug-drug. *Antihypertensives, furosemide, thiazide diuretics:* ibuprofen may decrease effectiveness of diuretics or antihypertensives. Monitor patient.
Aspirin: may decrease serum levels of ibuprofen. Avoid concomitant use.

Aspirin, corticosteroids: increased risk of adverse GI reactions. Avoid concomitant use.
Cyclosporine: nephrotoxicity of both agents may be increased. Avoid concomitant use.
Digoxin, hydantoins: may increase serum levels of these drugs. Monitor closely.
Lithium, oral anticoagulants: may increase plasma levels or effects of these drugs. Monitor for toxicity.
Methotrexate: risk of methotrexate toxicity may be increased. Monitor closely.
Probenecid: probenecid may increase concentration and possibly toxicity of NSAIDs. Monitor closely.
Drug-lifestyle. *Alcohol use:* increased risk of adverse GI reactions. Avoid concomitant use.
Sun exposure: may cause photosensitivity reactions. Take appropriate precautions.

Contraindications and precautions

• Contraindicated in patients with hypersensitivity to drug, syndrome of nasal polyps, angioedema, and bronchospastic reactivity to aspirin or other NSAIDs.
• Drug use is not recommended in pregnant or breast-feeding women.
• Use cautiously in patients with GI disorders, history of peptic ulcer disease, hepatic or renal disease, cardiac decompensation, hypertension, or known intrinsic coagulation defects.

NURSING CONSIDERATIONS

⚗ Assessment
• Obtain assessment of patient's underlying condition before drug therapy.
• Monitor for relief from pain, fever, or inflammation. Full effects in arthritis may take 2 to 4 weeks.
• Check renal and hepatic function periodically in long-term therapy.
• Be alert for adverse reactions and drug interactions.
• Evaluate patient's and family's knowledge of drug therapy.

⊕ Nursing diagnoses
• Pain related to underlying condition
• Risk for injury related to drug-induced adverse reactions
• Knowledge deficit related to drug therapy

▶ Planning and implementation
• Give with meals or milk to reduce adverse GI reactions.
• Notify doctor if drug is ineffective.
• Stop drug if renal or hepatic abnormalities occur, and notify doctor.
Patient teaching
• Tell patient to take drug with meals or milk to reduce adverse GI reactions.
• Instruct patient not to exceed 1.2 g daily, give to children under age 12, or self-medicate for extended periods without consulting doctor.
• Caution patient that concomitant use with aspirin, alcohol, or corticosteroids may increase risk of adverse GI reactions.
• Serious GI toxicity, including peptic ulceration and bleeding, can occur in patients taking NSAIDs despite absence of GI symptoms. Teach patient to recognize and report signs and symptoms of GI bleeding.
• Instruct patient to avoid alcohol consumption during drug therapy.
• Instruct patient to use sunblock, wear protective clothing, and avoid prolonged exposure to the sun.

☑ Evaluation
• Patient is free from pain.
• Patient does not experience injury from adverse reactions.
• Patient and family state understanding of drug therapy.

---

ibutilide fumarate
(igh-BYOO-tih-lighd FYOO-muh-rayt)
Corvert

Pharmacologic class: ibutilide derivative

Therapeutic class: supraventricular anti-arrhythmic
Pregnancy risk category: C

How supplied
Injection: 0.1 mg/ml

Pharmacokinetics
Absorption: not applicable.
Distribution: highly distributed; about 40% protein-bound.
Metabolism: not clearly defined.
Excretion: excreted in urine and feces.
Half-life: averages about 6 hours.

Route	Onset	Peak	Duration
I.V.	Unknown	Unknown	Unknown

Pharmacodynamics
Chemical effect: prolongs action potential in isolated cardiac myocyte and increases atrial and ventricular refractoriness; has predominantly class III properties.
Therapeutic effect: restores normal sinus rhythm.

Indications and dosage
▶ **Rapid conversion of recent atrial fibrillation or atrial flutter to sinus rhythm.** *Adults weighing 60 kg (132 lb) or more:* 1 mg I.V. infused over 10 minutes. *Adults weighing under 60 kg:* 0.01 mg/kg I.V. infused over 10 minutes. *Note:* Infusion should be stopped if arrhythmia is terminated or if sustained or nonsustained ventricular tachycardia or marked prolongation of QT or QTc develops. If arrhythmia does not terminate within 10 minutes after infusion ends, a second 10-minute infusion of equal strength may be administered.

Adverse reactions
CNS: headache.
CV: ventricular extrasystoles, nonsustained ventricular tachycardia, hypotension, bundle branch block, *sustained ventricular tachycardia,* AV block, hyperten-

---

sion, QT segment prolongation, bradycardia, palpitation, tachycardia.
GI: nausea.

Interactions

Drug-drug. *Class Ia antiarrhythmics
(such as disopyramide, procainamide,
quinidine), other class III drugs (such as
amiodarone, sotalol):* increased potential
for prolonged refractoriness. Avoid concomitant administration; wait at least 5
half-lives before and 4 hours after giving
ibutilide.
Digoxin: supraventricular arrhythmias
may mask cardiotoxicity associated with
excessive digoxin levels. Use cautiously.
*H_1-receptor antagonist antihistamines,
phenothiazines, tetracyclic antidepressants, tricyclic antidepressants, other
drugs that prolong QT interval:* increased
risk for proarrhythmia. Monitor patient
closely.

Contraindications and precautions

• Contraindicated in patients with hypersensitivity to drug or its components.
• Drug is not recommended for use in patients with history of polymorphic ventricular tachycardia, such as torsades de
pointes, and in breast-feeding women.
• Use cautiously in patients with hepatic
or renal dysfunction (usually, no dosage
adjustments are necessary) and in pregnant women.
• Safety of drug has not been established
in breast-feeding women and in children.

NURSING CONSIDERATIONS

🔟 Assessment
• Assess patient's arrhythmia before therapy.
• Monitor ECG continuously during therapy and for at least 4 hours afterward (or
until QTc returns to baseline) because
drug can induce or worsen ventricular arrhythmias. Longer monitoring is required
if ECG shows arrhythmic activity.
• Be alert for adverse reactions and drug
interactions.

• Evaluate patient's and family's knowledge of drug therapy.

🔳 Nursing diagnoses
• Decreased cardiac output related to arrhythmia
• Risk for injury related to life-threatening arrhythmia
• Knowledge deficit related to drug
therapy

▶ Planning and implementation
• Know that drug should be administered
only by skilled personnel, with proper
equipment and facilities (cardiac monitoring, intracardiac pacing, cardioverter/
defibrillator, and medication for treatment
of sustained ventricular tachycardia)
available during and after administration.
• Be aware that hypokalemia and hypomagnesemia should be corrected before
therapy to reduce potential for proarrhythmia.
• Drug may be administered undiluted or
diluted in 50 ml of diluent. It may be
added to 0.9% NaCl for injection or 5%
dextrose injection before infusion.
Contents of one 10-ml vial (0.1 mg/ml)
may be added to a 50-ml infusion bag to
form admixture of about 0.017 mg/ml
ibutilide fumarate. Strict adherence to
aseptic technique must be used. Drug is
compatible with polyvinyl chloride plastic bags or polyolefin bags.
• Admixtures with approved diluents are
chemically and physically stable for 24
hours at room temperature or 48 hours if
refrigerated.
• Inspect parenteral drugs for particles
and discoloration before administration.
Patient teaching
• Tell patient to report adverse reactions
promptly.
• Instruct him to alert nurse if he feels
discomfort at injection site.

☑ Evaluation
• Patient regains normal sinus rhythm.
• Life-threatening arrhythmia does not
develop.

• Patient and family state understanding of drug therapy.

idarubicin hydrochloride
(igh-duh-ROO-bih-sin high-droh-KLOR-ighd)
Idamycin, Idamycin PFS

Pharmacologic class: antibiotic antineoplastic
Therapeutic class: antineoplastic
Pregnancy risk category: D

How supplied

Powder for injection: 1 mg/ml available in 5-, 10-, or 20-mg vials

Pharmacokinetics

Absorption: not applicable.
Distribution: drug is highly lipophilic and tissue-bound (97%), with highest concentrations in nucleated blood and bone marrow cells.
Metabolism: extensive extrahepatic metabolism is indicated. Metabolite has cytotoxic activity.
Excretion: primarily biliary excretion, minimally by kidneys. *Half-life:* 20 to 22 hours.

Route	Onset	Peak	Duration
I.V.	Unknown	≤ 3 min	Unknown

Pharmacodynamics

Chemical effect: may inhibit nucleic acid synthesis by intercalation and interacts with enzyme topoisomerase II.
Therapeutic effect: hinders growth of susceptible cancer cells.

Indications and dosage

Dosage and indications may vary. Check current literature for recommended protocol.
▶ **Acute myeloid leukemia, including FAB (French-American-British) classifications M1 through M7, in combination with other approved antileukemic agents.** *Adults:* 12 mg/m²/day for 3 days by slow I.V. injection (over 10 to 15 minutes) in combination with 100 mg/m²/day of cytarabine for 7 days by continuous I.V. infusion or cytarabine as 25 mg/m² bolus followed by 200 mg/m²/day for 5 days by continuous infusion. A second course may be administered if needed. If patients experience severe mucositis, administration is delayed until recovery is complete. Dosage reduced by 25%. Dosage should also be reduced in patients with hepatic or renal impairment. Idarubicin should not be given if bilirubin level is above 5 mg/dl.

Adverse reactions

CNS: headache, changed mental status, peripheral neuropathy, *seizures.*
CV: *heart failure,* atrial fibrillation, chest pain, *MI,* asymptomatic decline in left ventricular ejection fraction, *myocardial insufficiency, arrhythmias,* HEMORRHAGE, *myocardial toxicity.*
GI: *nausea, vomiting,* cramps, diarrhea, *mucositis, severe enterocolitis with perforation (rare).*
GU: decreased renal function.
Hematologic: *myelosuppression.*
Hepatic: changes in hepatic function.
Skin: rash, urticaria, bullous erythrodermatous rash on palms and soles, hives at injection site; erythema (at previously irradiated sites); tissue necrosis (at injection site if extravasation occurs).
Other: INFECTION, alopecia, fever, hyperuricemia, *hypersensitivity reactions.*

Interactions

Drug-drug. *Alkaline solutions, heparin:* incompatible. Idarubicin should not be mixed with other drugs unless specific compatibility data are available.

Contraindications and precautions

• No known contraindications. Drug is not recommended for use in pregnant or breast-feeding women.
• Use with extreme caution in patients with bone marrow suppression induced

---

Reactions may be *common,* uncommon, *life-threatening,* or COMMON AND LIFE-THREATENING.

by previous drug therapy or radiotherapy, or in patients with hepatic or renal function impairment.
• Safety of drug has not been established in children.

NURSING CONSIDERATIONS

🔲 Assessment
• Assess patient's condition before therapy and regularly thereafter.
• Assess patient for systemic infection, which should be controlled before therapy begins.
• Monitor hepatic and renal function tests and CBC frequently, as ordered.
• Be alert for adverse reactions and drug interactions.
• Evaluate patient's and family's knowledge of drug therapy.

🔲 Nursing diagnoses
• Altered health maintenance related to presence of underlying condition
• Altered protection related to adverse hematologic reactions
• Knowledge deficit related to drug therapy

🔲 Planning and implementation
• Follow institutional policy to reduce risks. Preparation and administration of parenteral form are associated with carcinogenic, mutagenic, and teratogenic risks for personnel.
• Take appropriate preventive measures (including adequate hydration) before starting treatment.
• Reconstitute to final concentration of 1 mg/ml using 0.9% NaCl injection without preservatives. Add 5 ml to 5-mg vial or 10 ml to 10-ml vial. *Do not use bacteriostatic NaCl.* Vial is under negative pressure.
• Administer over 10 to 15 minutes into free-flowing I.V. infusion of 0.9% NaCl or 5% dextrose solution that is running into large vein.
• Know that reconstituted solutions are stable for 3 days (72 hours) at room temperature (59°to 86°F [15°to 30°C]); 7 days if refrigerated. Label unused solutions with "CHEMOTHERAPY HAZARD" label.
• Hyperuricemia may result from rapid lysis of leukemic cells. Allopurinol may be ordered.
• If extravasation occurs, discontinue infusion immediately and notify doctor. Treat with intermittent ice packs—30 minutes immediately, and then 30 minutes four times daily for 4 days.
Patient teaching
• Teach patient to recognize and report signs of extravasation, infection, and bleeding.
• Advise patient that red urine for several days is normal and does not indicate blood in urine.
• Advise female patient of childbearing age to use a reliable contraceptive during therapy and to consult with doctor before becoming pregnant.

🔲 Evaluation
• Patient responds well to drug.
• Serious adverse hematologic reactions do not develop.
• Patient and family state understanding of drug therapy.

Ifosfamide
(igh-FOHS-fuh-mighd)
IFEX

Pharmacologic class: alkylating agent (cell cycle–phase nonspecific)
Therapeutic class: antineoplastic
Pregnancy risk category: D

How supplied

Injection: 1 g (supplied with 200-mg ampule of mesna), 2 g♦, 3 g (supplied with 400-mg ampule of mesna)

Pharmacokinetics

Exhibits dose-dependent pharmacokinetics.
Absorption: not applicable.

Distribution: drug crosses blood-brain barrier but its metabolites do not; therefore alkylating activity does not occur in CSF.
Metabolism: about 50% of dose is metabolized in liver.
Excretion: excreted primarily in urine.
Half-life: about 14 hours.

Route	Onset	Peak	Duration
I.V.	Unknown	Unknown	Unknown

Pharmacodynamics

Chemical effect: cross-links strands of cellular DNA and interferes with RNA transcription, causing growth imbalance that leads to cell death.
Therapeutic effect: causes death of testicular cancer cells.

Indications and dosage

▶ **Testicular cancer.** *Adults:* 1.2 g/m²/day I.V. for 5 consecutive days. Repeated q 3 weeks or after patient recovers from hematologic toxicity.

Adverse reactions

CNS: *lethargy, somnolence, confusion, depressive psychosis,* **coma, seizures,** *ataxia.*
GI: *nausea, vomiting.*
GU: *hemorrhagic cystitis* (dose-limiting, occurring in up to 50% of patients), *hematuria,* **nephrotoxicity.**
Hematologic: *leukopenia, thrombocytopenia, myelosuppression.*
Hepatic: elevated liver enzyme levels.
Other: *alopecia.*

Interactions

Drug-drug. *Allopurinol:* may produce excessive ifosfamide effect by prolonging half-life. Monitor for enhanced toxicity.
Anticoagulants, aspirin: increased risk of bleeding. Avoid concomitant use.
Barbiturates, chloral hydrate, phenytoin: may increase ifosfamide toxicity by inducing hepatic enzymes that hasten formation of toxic metabolites. Monitor closely.
Corticosteroids: may inhibit hepatic enzymes, reducing ifosfamide's effect.

Monitor for enhanced ifosfamide toxicity if concurrent steroid dosage is suddenly reduced or discontinued.
Myelosuppressants: enhanced hematologic toxicity. Dosage adjustment may be necessary.

Contraindications and precautions

• Contraindicated in patients with severely depressed bone marrow function or hypersensitivity to drug.
• Use of drug in unlabeled conditions is not recommended in pregnant or breast-feeding women.
• Use cautiously in patients with renal impairment or compromised bone marrow reserve as indicated by leukopenia, granulocytopenia, extensive bone marrow metastases, prior radiation therapy, or prior therapy with cytotoxic agents.
• Safety of drug has not been established in children.

NURSING CONSIDERATIONS

☞ Assessment
• Assess patient's condition before therapy and regularly thereafter.
• Obtain urinalysis before each dose. If microscopic hematuria is present, patient should be evaluated for hemorrhagic cystitis. Dosage adjustments of mesna may be necessary.
• Monitor CBC and renal and liver function tests, as ordered.
• Be alert for adverse reactions and drug interactions.
• Assess patient for mental status changes; dosage may have to be decreased.
• Evaluate patient's and family's knowledge of drug therapy.

☷ Nursing diagnoses
• Altered health maintenance related to presence of cancer
• Altered protection related to adverse hematologic reactions
• Knowledge deficit related to drug therapy

Reactions may be *common,* uncommon, *life-threatening,* or COMMON AND LIFE-THREATENING.

▶ Planning and implementation

• Administer antiemetics, as ordered, before giving ifosfamide to help decrease nausea.

• Follow institutional policy to reduce risks. Preparation and administration of parenteral form are associated with carcinogenic, mutagenic, and teratogenic risks for personnel.

• Reconstitute each gram of drug with 20 ml of diluent to yield solution of 50 mg/ml. Use sterile water for injection or bacteriostatic water for injection. Solutions may then be further diluted with sterile water, dextrose 2.5% or 5% in water, 0.45% or 0.9% NaCl injection, 5% dextrose and 0.9% NaCl injection, or lactated Ringer's injection.

• Infuse each dose over at least 30 minutes.

• As ordered, administer ifosfamide with protecting agent (mesna) to prevent hemorrhagic cystitis. Mesna must be given concomitantly with or before ifosfamide to prevent cystitis. Adequate fluid intake (2 L/day, either P.O. or I.V.) is essential.

• Know that ifosfamide and mesna are physically compatible and may be mixed in same I.V. solution.

• Keep in mind that reconstituted solution is stable for 1 week at room temperature or 6 weeks refrigerated. However, use solution within 6 hours if drug was reconstituted with sterile water without preservative (such as benzyl alcohol or parabens).

• Don't give drug at bedtime; infrequent voiding during night may increase possibility of cystitis. If cystitis develops, discontinue drug and notify doctor.

• Be aware that bladder irrigation with 0.9% NaCl solution may decrease possibility of cystitis.

• Institute infection-control and bleeding precautions.

Patient teaching

• Tell patient to void frequently to minimize contact of drug and its metabolites with bladder mucosa.

• Warn patient to watch for signs of infection (fever, sore throat, fatigue) and bleeding (easy bruising, nosebleeds, bleeding gums, melena). Teach patient about infection-control and bleeding precautions. Tell him to take temperature daily.

• Instruct patient to avoid OTC medications containing aspirin.

• Stress importance of adequate fluid intake when drug is administered. Explain that it may help prevent hemorrhagic cystitis.

• Warn patient that hyperpigmentation may occur.

☑ Evaluation

• Patient responds well to drug.

• Serious infections or bleeding complications do not develop.

• Patient and family state understanding of drug therapy.

imipenem/cilastatin
(im-ih-PEN-em/sigh-luh-STAT-in)
Primaxin IM, Primaxin IV

Pharmacologic class: carbapenem (thienamycin class); beta-lactam antibiotic
Therapeutic class: antibiotic
Pregnancy risk category: C

How supplied

Injection: 250-mg, 500-mg, 750-mg vials
Powder for injection: 500 mg

Pharmacokinetics

Absorption: imipenem is about 75% bioavailable and cilastatin is about 95% bioavailable after I.M. use.
Distribution: distributed rapidly and widely. About 20% of imipenem is protein-bound; 40% of cilastatin is protein-bound.
Metabolism: imipenem is metabolized by kidney dehydropeptidase I, resulting in low urine concentrations. Cilastatin inhibits this enzyme, thereby reducing imipenem's metabolism.

Excretion: about 70% excreted unchanged by kidneys. *Half-life:* 1 hour after I.V. dose; 2 to 3 hours after I.M. dose.

Route	Onset	Peak	Duration
I.V.	Unknown	Immediate	Unknown
I.M.	Unknown	Unknown	Unknown

Pharmacodynamics

Chemical effect: imipenem is bactericidal and inhibits bacterial cell-wall synthesis. Cilastatin inhibits enzymatic breakdown of imipenem in kidneys, making it effective in urinary tract. *Therapeutic effect:* kills susceptible organisms. Spectrum of activity includes many gram-positive, gram-negative, and anaerobic bacteria, including *Staphylococcus* and *Streptococcus* species, *Escherichia coli, Klebsiella, Proteus, Enterobacter* species, *Pseudomonas aeruginosa,* and *Bacteroides* species, including *B. fragilis.*

Indications and dosage

▶ **Mild to moderate lower respiratory tract, skin to skin structure, and gynecologic infections.** *Adults weighing at least 70 kg (154 lb):* 500 to 750 mg I.M. q 12 hours. Alternatively, 250 to 500 mg I.V. q 6 hours. Maximum daily I.V. dosage is 50 mg/kg/day or 4 g/day, whichever is less. *Children age 3 months and older:* 15 to 25 mg/kg I.V. q 6 hours. Maximum daily dose for fully susceptible organisms is 2 g/day, and for infection with moderately susceptible organisms is 4 g/day (based on adult studies). *Infants ages 4 weeks to 3 months and weighing at least 1.5 kg (3.3 lb):* 25 mg/kg I.V. q 6 hours. *Neonates ages 1 to 4 weeks and weighing at least 1.5 kg:* 25 mg/kg I.V. q 8 hours. *Neonates age less than 1 week and weighing at least 1.5 kg:* 25 mg/kg I.V. q 12 hours.

▶ **Mild to moderate intra-abdominal infections.** *Adults:* 750 mg I.M. q 12 hours. *Children ages 3 months and older:* 15 to 25 mg/kg I.V. q 6 hours. Maximum daily dosage for fully susceptible organisms is 2 g/day, and for infection with moderately susceptible organisms is 4 g/day (based on adult studies). *Infants ages 4 weeks to 3 months and weighing at least 1.5 kg (3.3 lb):* 25 mg/kg I.V. q 6 hours. *Neonates ages 1 to 4 weeks and weighing at least 1.5 kg:* 25 mg/kg I.V. q 8 hours. *Neonates age less than 1 week and weighing at least 1.5 kg:* 25 mg/kg I.V. q 12 hours.

▶ **Serious infections of lower respiratory and urinary tracts, intra-abdominal and gynecologic infections, bacterial septicemia, bone and joint infections, skin and soft-tissue infections, and endocarditis.** *Adults weighing at least 70 kg (154 lb):* 500 mg I.V. q 6 hours or 1 g q 6 to 8 hours by I.V. infusion. Maximum daily dosage is 50 mg/kg/day or 4 g/day, whichever is less. For the treatment of infections (other than CNS infections) in children: *Children age 3 months and older:* 15 to 25 mg/kg I.V. q 6 hours. Maximum daily dosage for fully susceptible organisms is 2 g/day, and for infection with moderately susceptible organisms is 4 g/day (based on adult studies). *Infants ages 4 weeks to 3 months and weighing at least 1.5 kg (3.3 lb):* 25 mg/kg I.V. q 6 hours. *Neonates ages 1 to 4 weeks and weighing at least 1.5 kg:* 25 mg/kg I.V. q 8 hours. *Neonates age less than 1 week and weighing at least 1.5 kg:* 25 mg/kg I.V. q 12 hours.

Adverse reactions

CNS: *seizures,* dizziness, somnolence.
CV: hypotension.
GI: nausea, vomiting, diarrhea, *pseudomembranous colitis.*
Skin: rash, urticaria, pruritus.
Other: *hypersensitivity reactions (anaphylaxis);* thrombophlebitis, pain at injection site, fever, transient increases in liver enzymes.

Interactions

Drug-drug. *Beta-lactam antibiotics:* possible in vitro antagonism. Avoid concomitant use.

Reactions may be *common*, uncommon, *life-threatening*, or COMMON AND LIFE-THREATENING.

Cyclosporine: CNS adverse effects of both agents may be increased possibly because of additive or synergistic toxicity. Avoid concomitant use.
Ganciclovir: may cause seizures. Avoid concomitant use.
Probenecid: increased serum concentrations of cilastatin. Avoid concomitant use.

Contraindications and precautions

• Contraindicated in patients with hypersensitivity to drug.
• Use cautiously in pregnant or breastfeeding women, in patients allergic to penicillins or cephalosporins, and in those with history of seizure disorders, especially if they also have compromised renal function.
• I.M. safety and efficacy in children under age 12 have not been established.
• I.V. use is not recommended in children with CNS infections because of risk of seizures; also not recommended in children weighing under 30 kg (66 lb) with impaired renal function because no data are available.

NURSING CONSIDERATIONS

▩ Assessment

• Assess patient's infection before therapy and regularly thereafter.
• Obtain urine specimen for culture and sensitivity tests before first dose. Therapy may begin pending results.
• Be alert for adverse reactions and drug interactions.
• Monitor patient's hydration status if adverse GI reactions occur.
• Evaluate patient's and family's knowledge of drug therapy.

▩ Nursing diagnoses

• Infection related to presence of susceptible organisms
• Risk for fluid volume deficit related to adverse GI reactions
• Knowledge deficit related to drug therapy

▧ Planning and implementation

I.V. use: Don't administer drug by direct I.V. bolus injection. Each 250- or 500-mg dose should be given by I.V. infusion over 20 to 30 minutes. Each 1-g dose should be infused over 40 to 60 minutes. If nausea occurs, infusion may be slowed.
– When reconstituting powder, shake until solution is clear. Solutions may range from colorless to yellow, and variations of color within this range do not affect drug's potency. After reconstitution, solution is stable for 10 hours at room temperature and for 48 hours when refrigerated.
I.M. use: Follow normal protocol.
• Patients who have impaired renal function or who weigh under 70 kg (154 lb) may need lower dose or longer intervals between doses.
• If seizures develop and persist, despite anticonvulsants, notify doctor who may discontinue drug.
Patient teaching
• Instruct patient to report adverse reactions because supportive therapy may be needed.
• Warn patient about pain at injection site.

▨ Evaluation

• Patient is free from infection.
• Patient maintains adequate hydration throughout therapy.
• Patient and family state understanding of drug therapy.

imipramine hydrochloride

(ih-MIP-ruh-meen high-droh-KLOR-ighd)
Apo-Imipramine♦, Impril♦, Janimine**, Melipramine◊, Norfranil, Novopramine♦, Tipramine, Tofranil**

imipramine pamoate

Tofranil-PM**

Pharmacologic class: dibenzazepine tricyclic antidepressant
Therapeutic class: antidepressant

Pregnancy risk category: NR

How supplied

imipramine hydrochloride
Tablets: 10 mg, 25 mg, 50 mg
Injection: 12.5 mg/ml
imipramine pamoate
Capsules: 75 mg, 100 mg, 125 mg,
150 mg

Pharmacokinetics

Absorption: absorbed rapidly from GI
tract after oral use and rapidly from muscle tissue after I.M. use.
Distribution: distributed widely into
body, including CNS. Drug is 90% protein-bound.
Metabolism: metabolized by liver. A significant first-pass effect may explain variability of serum concentrations in different patients taking same dose.
Excretion: most of drug is excreted in
urine.

Route	Onset	Peak	Duration
P.O.	Unknown	1-2 hr	Unknown
I.M.	Unknown	30 min	Unknown

Pharmacodynamics

Chemical effect: increases amount of
norepinephrine, serotonin, or both in
CNS by blocking their reuptake by presynaptic neurons.
Therapeutic effect: relieves depression
and childhood enuresis (hydrochloride
formulation only).

Indications and dosage

▶ **Depression.** *Adults:* 75 to 100 mg P.O.
or I.M. daily in divided doses, increased
in 25- to 50-mg increments to maximum
dosage; or 25 mg P.O. daily, increased in
25-mg increments every other day. Alternatively, entire dosage may be given h.s.
(I.M. route rarely used.) Maximum dosage: 200 mg/day for outpatients, 300 mg/
day for inpatients, 100 mg/day for elderly
patients.
▶ **Childhood enuresis.** *Children age 6
and older:* 25 mg P.O. 1 hour before bed-

time. If no response within 1 week,
dosage may be increased to 50 mg nightly for children under age 12 or 75 mg
nightly for children age 12 and older.
Maximum dosage should not exceed
2.5 mg/kg/day.

Adverse reactions

CNS: *drowsiness, dizziness,* excitation,
tremors, weakness, confusion, headache,
nervousness, EEG changes, *seizures,* extrapyramidal reactions.
CV: *orthostatic hypotension, tachycardia, ECG changes,* hypertension, *MI,
stroke, arrhythmias, heart block.*
EENT: *blurred vision, tinnitus, mydriasis.*
GI: *dry mouth, constipation,* nausea,
vomiting, anorexia, paralytic ileus.
GU: *urine retention,* impotence, testicular swelling.
Metabolic: hypoglycemia, hyperglycemia.
Skin: rash, urticaria, photosensitivity.
Other: *diaphoresis,* SIADH, *hypersensitivity,* gynecomastia (in men), galactorrhea and breast enlargement (in women),
altered libido.
**After abrupt withdrawal of long-term
therapy:** nausea, headache, malaise
(does not indicate addiction).

Interactions

Drug-drug. *Barbiturates, CNS depressants:* enhanced CNS depression. Avoid
concomitant use.
Cimetidine, methylphenidate: may increase imipramine serum levels. Monitor
for adverse reactions.
Clonidine, epinephrine, norepinephrine:
increased hypertensive effect. Use with
caution.
Fluoxetine: may increase the pharmacologic and toxic effects of tricyclic antidepressants; symptoms may persist several
weeks after the discontinuation of fluoxetine. Monitor closely.
MAO inhibitors: may cause hyperpyretic
crisis, severe seizures, and fatalities.
Avoid concomitant use.
Drug-lifestyle. *Alcohol use:* enhanced
CNS depression. Avoid concomitant use.

Smoking: may lower plasma concentrations of imipramine. Monitor for lack of effect.
Sun exposure: increased risk of photosensitivity. Take appropriate precautions.

Contraindications and precautions

• Contraindicated during acute recovery phase of MI, in patients with hypersensitivity to drug, and in those receiving MAO inhibitors.
• Drug use is not recommended in pregnant or breast-feeding women.
• Use with extreme caution in patients at risk for suicide; in patients with history of urine retention or angle-closure glaucoma, increased intraocular pressure, CV disease, impaired hepatic function, hyperthyroidism, history of seizure disorder, or impaired renal function; and in patients receiving thyroid medications. Injectable form contains sulfites, which may cause allergic reactions in hypersensitive patients.
• Safety of drug has not been established for treating depression in children.

NURSING CONSIDERATIONS

Assessment
• Assess patient's condition before therapy and regularly thereafter.
• Be alert for adverse reactions and drug interactions.
• Evaluate patient's and family's knowledge of drug therapy.

Nursing diagnoses
• Ineffective individual coping related to depression
• Knowledge deficit related to drug therapy

Planning and implementation
• Be aware that reduced dosage in elderly or debilitated patients, adolescents, and patients with aggravated psychotic symptoms is necessary.
P.O. use: Although doses have been administered up to four times daily, patients may receive entire daily dosage at one time because of drug's long action.
I.M. use: Follow normal protocol.
• Do not withdraw drug abruptly.
• Be aware that drug is associated with high incidence of orthostatic hypotension. Check sitting and standing blood pressures after initial dose.
• Because of hypertensive episodes during surgery in patients receiving tricyclic antidepressants, be aware that drug should be gradually discontinued several days before surgery.
• If signs of psychosis occur or increase, notify doctor and expect doctor to reduce dosage.

Patient teaching
• Advise patient to take full dose at bedtime but warn about possible morning orthostatic hypotension.
• Suggest taking drug with food or milk if it causes stomach upset.
• Suggest relieving dry mouth with sugarless chewing gum or hard candy. Encourage good dental prophylaxis because persistent dry mouth may lead to increased incidence of dental caries.
• Tell patient to avoid alcohol and smoking during drug therapy.
• Warn patient to avoid hazardous activities until CNS effects of drug are known.
• Warn patient not to stop taking drug suddenly.
• Advise patient to consult doctor before taking other prescription or OTC medications.
• Advise patient to use sunblock, wear protective clothing, and avoid prolonged exposure to sunlight to prevent photosensitivity reactions.

Evaluation
• Patient behavior and communication show diminished depression.
• Patient and family state understanding of drug therapy.

---

*Liquid form contains alcohol   **May contain tartrazine   ◆Canada   ◇Australia   †OTC

immune globulin intramuscular (gamma globulin, IG, IGIM)
(ih-MYOON GLOH-byoo-lin
in-truh-MUS-kyoo-ler)
Gamastan, Gammar

immune globulin intravenous (IGIV)
Gamimune N, Gammagard S/D,
Gammar-IV, Iveegam, Polygam,
Sandoglobulin, Venoglobulin-I

Pharmacologic class: immune serum
Therapeutic class: immune serum
Pregnancy risk category: C

How supplied
immune globulin intramuscular
Injection: 2-ml, 10-ml vials
immune globulin intravenous
Injection: 5% in 10-ml, 50-ml, 100-ml,
250-ml vials (Gamimune N); 10% in
10-ml, 50-ml, 100-ml, 200-ml (Gam-
mimune N) vials
Powder for injection: 50 mg protein/ml
in 0.5-g, 2.5-g, 5-g, 10-g vials
(Gammagard); 2.5-g vials (Gammar-IV);
500-mg and 1-g vials (Iveegam); 1-g,
3-g, 6-g vials (Sandoglobulin); 2.5-g, 5-g
vials (Venoglobulin-I)

Pharmacokinetics
Absorption: absorbed slowly after I.M.
administration.
Distribution: distributes evenly between
intravascular and extravascular spaces.
Metabolism: unknown.
Excretion: unknown. *Half-life:* 21 to 24
days in immunocompetent patients.

Route	Onset	Peak	Duration
I.V.	Immediate	Immediate	Unknown
I.M.	Unknown	2-5 days	Unknown

Pharmacodynamics
Chemical effect: provides passive immunity by increasing antibody titer. The primary component is IgG.

Therapeutic effect: helps prevent infections.

Indications and dosage
▶ **Agammaglobulinemia or hypogam-
maglobulinemia.** *Adults:* 30 to 50 ml I.M.
monthly. Alternatively, 100 to 200 mg/kg
I.V. (Gamimune N) monthly. Infused at
0.01 to 0.02 ml/kg/minute for 30 minutes.
If no discomfort, rate increased to maximum of 0.08 ml/kg/minute. For Sandoglobulin, 200 mg/kg I.V. monthly. Infused
at 0.5 to 1 ml/minute. After 15 to 30 minutes, infusion rate increased to 1.5 to
2.5 ml/minute. *Children:* 20 to 40 ml I.M.
monthly.
▶ **Hepatitis A exposure.** *Adults and
children:* 0.02 ml/kg I.M. as soon as possible after exposure. Up to 0.06 ml/kg
may be given q 4 to 6 months if exposure
will be 3 months or longer.
▶ **Measles exposure.** *Adults and children:* 0.25 ml/kg I.M. within 6 days after
exposure.
▶ **Modification of measles.** *Adults and
children:* 0.5 ml/kg I.M. within 6 days after exposure.
▶ **Prophylaxis in primary immunodefi-
ciencies.** *Adults and children:* 100 to
200 mg/kg by I.V. infusion monthly
(Gamimune N only). Infusion rate is 0.01
to 0.02 ml/kg/minute for 30 minutes. If
no discomfort, rate increased to maximum of 0.08 ml/kg/minute.
▶ **Idiopathic thrombocytopenic purpura.** *Adults:* 0.4 g/kg Gamimune N or
Sandoglobulin I.V. for 5 consecutive days
or 1,000 mg/kg Gammagard. Additional
doses may be given based on response.
Up to three doses given (every other day)
if necessary. Or, Venoglobulin-I up to
2,000 mg/kg daily for 2 to 7 days.

Adverse reactions
CNS: headache, malaise.
GI: nausea, vomiting.
GU: nephrotic syndrome.
Skin: urticaria.
Other: pain, erythema, muscle stiffness
at injection site, *anaphylaxis,* fever.

Reactions may be *common,* uncommon, *life-threatening,* or COMMON AND LIFE-THREATENING.

Interactions

Drug-drug. *Live-virus vaccines:* antibodies within the vaccine may interfere with drug therapy. Don't give within 3 months after administration of immune globulin.

Contraindications and precautions

• Contraindicated in patients hypersensitive to drug.
• Use with caution in pregnant or breastfeeding women.
• I.M. administration contraindicated in patients with severe thrombocytopenia or other coagulation disorders that contraindicate I.M. administration.

NURSING CONSIDERATIONS

Assessment
• Obtain history of allergies and reaction to immunizations.
• Observe patient for signs of anaphylaxis immediately after injection.
• Inspect injection site for local reactions.
• Monitor effectiveness by checking antibody titers after immunization.
• Be alert for adverse reactions and drug interactions.
• Evaluate patient's and family's knowledge of drug therapy.

Nursing diagnoses
• Altered protection related to lack of or decreased immunity
• Ineffective breathing pattern related to anaphylaxis
• Knowledge deficit related to drug therapy

Planning and implementation
I.V. use: I.V. products are not interchangeable. Gammagard requires filter, which is supplied by manufacturer.
– Most adverse effects are related to rapid infusion rate. Infuse slowly.
I.M. use: When giving I.M., use gluteal region. Doses over 10 ml should be divided and injected into several muscle sites to reduce local pain and discomfort.

• Know that immune globulin should not be given for prophylaxis against hepatitis A if 6 weeks or more have elapsed since exposure or after onset of clinical illness.
• Make sure epinephrine 1:1,000 is available in case of anaphylaxis.
Patient teaching
• Instruct patient to report respiratory difficulty immediately.

Evaluation
• Patient exhibits increased passive immunity.
• Patient demonstrates no signs of anaphylaxis.
• Patient and family state understanding of drug therapy.

indapamide
(in-DAP-uh-mighd)
Lozide♦, Lozol, Natrilix◊

Pharmacologic class: thiazide-like diuretic
Therapeutic class: diuretic, antihypertensive
Pregnancy risk category: B

How supplied
Tablets: 1.25 mg, 2.5 mg

Pharmacokinetics
Absorption: absorbed completely from GI tract.
Distribution: distributes widely into body tissues as result of its lipophilicity; 71% to 79% plasma protein-bound.
Metabolism: undergoes significant hepatic metabolism.
Excretion: primarily excreted in urine; smaller amounts excreted in feces. *Half-life:* about 14 hours.

Route	Onset	Peak	Duration
P.O.	1-2 hr	≤ 2 hr	≤ 36 hr

Pharmacodynamics

Chemical effect: unknown; probably inhibits sodium reabsorption in nephron's distal segment. Also has direct vasodilating effect that may be result of calcium channel-blocking action.
Therapeutic effect: promotes water and sodium excretion and lowers blood pressure. •

Indications and dosage

Edema. *Adults:* initially, 2.5 mg P.O. daily in morning. Increased to 5 mg daily after 1 week, if needed.
Hypertension. *Adults:* initially, 1.25 mg P.O. daily in morning. Increased to 2.5 mg daily after 4 weeks, if needed. Increased to 5 mg daily after 4 more weeks, if needed.

Adverse reactions

CNS: headache, irritability, nervousness, dizziness, light-headedness, weakness.
CV: volume depletion and dehydration, orthostatic hypotension.
GI: anorexia, nausea, pancreatitis.
GU: nocturia, polyuria, frequent urination.
Metabolic: hypokalemia; asymptomatic hyperuricemia; fluid and electrolyte imbalances, including dilutional hyponatremia and hypochloremia, metabolic alkalosis; gout.
Musculoskeletal: muscle cramps and spasms.
Skin: dermatitis, photosensitivity, rash.

Interactions

Drug-drug. *Cardiac glycosides:* increased risk of digoxin toxicity from indapamide-induced hypokalemia. Monitor potassium and digoxin levels.
Diazoxide: increased antihypertensive, hyperglycemic, and hyperuricemic effects. Use together cautiously.
NSAIDs: increased risk of NSAID-induced renal failure. Monitor patient for signs of renal failure.

Contraindications and precautions

• Contraindicated in patients with anuria or hypersensitivity to other sulfonamide-derived drugs.
• Use cautiously in patients with severe renal disease, impaired hepatic function, and progressive hepatic disease.
• Use cautiously in pregnant women.
• Safety of drug has not been established in breast-feeding women or in children.

NURSING CONSIDERATIONS

⚕ Assessment
• Obtain assessment of patient's underlying condition before therapy.
• Monitor effectiveness by assessing fluid intake and output, weight, and blood pressure. In patient with hypertension, be aware that therapeutic response may be delayed several days.
• Monitor serum electrolytes and blood glucose.
• Monitor serum creatinine and BUN levels regularly. Drug is not as effective if these levels are more than twice normal.
• Monitor blood uric acid levels, especially in patient with history of gout.
• Be alert for adverse reactions and drug interactions.
• Evaluate patient's and family's knowledge of drug therapy.

⚕ Nursing diagnoses
• Risk for injury related to presence of hypertension
• Fluid volume excess related to presence of edema
• Knowledge deficit related to drug therapy

⚕ Planning and implementation
• To prevent nocturia, give drug in morning.
• Know that drug may be used with potassium-sparing diuretic to prevent potassium loss.

Reactions may be *common*, uncommon, *life-threatening*, or COMMON AND LIFE-THREATENING.

Patient teaching
• Advise patient to avoid sudden postural changes and to rise slowly to avoid orthostatic hypotension.
• Advise patient to use sunblock to prevent photosensitivity reactions.
• Teach patient to monitor fluid volume by recording daily weight and intake and output.
• Tell patient to avoid high-sodium foods and to choose high-potassium foods.
• Advise patient to take drug early in day to avoid nocturia.

☑ **Evaluation**
• Patient's blood pressure is normal.
• Patient is free from edema.
• Patient and family state understanding of drug therapy.

indinavir sulfate
(in-DIH-nuh-veer SUL-fayt)
Crixivan

Pharmacologic class: protease inhibitor
Therapeutic class: antiviral
Pregnancy risk category: C

How supplied
Capsules: 200 mg, 400 mg

Pharmacokinetics
Absorption: rapidly absorbed.
Distribution: 60% bound to plasma proteins.
Metabolism: by liver and kidneys.
Excretion: excreted in urine.

Route	Onset	Peak	Duration
P.O.	Unknown	< 1 hr	1-8 hr

Pharmacodynamics
Chemical effect: binds to protease active sites and inhibits its activity.
Therapeutic effect: prevents cleavage of the viral polyproteins, resulting in the formation of immature noninfectious viral particles.

Indications and dosage
▶ **Treatment of patients with HIV infection when antiretroviral therapy is warranted.** *Adults:* 800 mg P.O. q 8 hours. Dosage reduced to 600 mg P.O. q 8 hours in mild to moderate hepatic insufficiency resulting from cirrhosis.

Adverse reactions
CNS: headache, insomnia, dizziness, malaise, somnolence, asthenia, fatigue.
EENT: taste perversion.
GI: abdominal pain, *nausea,* diarrhea, vomiting, acid regurgitation, anorexia, dry mouth.
GU: nephrolithiasis.
Hematologic: decreased hemoglobin or neutrophil count.
Hepatic: *hyperbilirubinemia;* elevation in ALT, AST, and serum amylase levels.
Musculoskeletal: flank pain, back pain.

Interactions
Drug-drug. *Astemizole, cisapride, midazolam, triazolam:* possibly inhibits metabolism of these drugs. Do not administer concurrently.
Didanosine: possible degradation of didanosine. If given concomitantly with indinavir, administer at least 1 hour apart on an empty stomach.
Ketoconazole: increases plasma concentration of indinavir.
Rifabutin: increases plasma concentrations. Reduce dosage of rifabutin by 50% if administered concomitantly with indinavir.
Rifampin: markedly diminishes plasma concentrations of indinavir. Avoid concomitant use.
Drug-food. *Any food:* substantially decreases absorption of oral indinavir. Take drug on an empty stomach.

Contraindications and precautions
• Contraindicated in patients with hypersensitivity to drug.
• Use cautiously in patients with hepatic insufficiency resulting from cirrhosis.

NURSING CONSIDERATIONS

⚕ Assessment
• Monitor for adverse reactions and drug interactions.
• Evaluate patient's and family's knowledge of drug therapy.

⊞ Nursing diagnoses
• Infection related to presence of virus
• Risk for fluid volume deficit related to effect on kidneys
• Knowledge deficit related to drug therapy

⊠ Planning and implementation
• Be aware that patient should maintain adequate hydration (at least 48 oz or 1.5 L of fluids q 24 hours while on indinavir).
Patient teaching
• Instruct patient to use barrier protection during sexual intercourse.
• Advise patient that if a dose is missed, he should take the next dose at regular, scheduled time and not double the dose.
• Instruct patient to take drug on an empty stomach with water 1 hour before or 2 hours after a meal.
• Instruct patient to store capsules in the original container and to keep desiccant in the bottle.
• Instruct patient to drink at least 48 oz of fluid daily.
• Advise HIV-positive woman to avoid breast-feeding to prevent transmitting virus to infant.

⚕ Evaluation
• Patient's health improves because of diminished signs and symptoms of underlying condition with use of drug.
• Patient maintains adequate hydration.
• Patient and family state understanding of drug therapy.

indomethacin
(in-doh-METH-uh-sin)
Apo-Indomethacin♦, Arthrexin◇, Indameth, Indochron E-R, Indocid♦◇, Indocid SR♦, Indocin, Indocin SR, Novo-Methacin♦

indomethacin sodium trihydrate
Indameth, Indocid P.D.A.♦, Indocin I.V.

Pharmacologic class: NSAID
Therapeutic class: nonnarcotic analgesic, antipyretic, anti-inflammatory
Pregnancy risk category: NR

How supplied

indomethacin
Capsules: 25 mg, 50 mg
Capsules (sustained-release): 75 mg
Oral suspension: 25 mg/5 ml
Suppositories: 50 mg
indomethacin sodium trihydrate
Injection: 1-mg vials

Pharmacokinetics

Absorption: absorbed rapidly and completely from GI tract after oral and rectal administration.
Distribution: highly protein-bound.
Metabolism: metabolized in liver.
Excretion: excreted mainly in urine, with some biliary excretion.

Route	Onset	Peak	Duration
P.O.	2-3 hr	1-4 hr	4-6 hr
I.V.	Immediate	Immediate	Unknown
P.R.	2-4 hr	Unknown	4-6 hr

Pharmacodynamics

Chemical effect: unknown; produces anti-inflammatory, analgesic, and antipyretic effects, possibly by inhibiting prostaglandin synthesis.
Therapeutic effect: relieves pain, fever, and inflammation.

Indications and dosage

▶ **Moderate to severe rheumatoid or osteoarthritis, ankylosing spondylitis.**

Adults: 25 mg P.O. b.i.d. or t.i.d. with food or antacids, increased by 25 mg or 50 mg daily q 7 days up to 200 mg daily; or 50 mg P.R. q.i.d. Alternatively, 75 mg sustained-release capsules P.O. to start, in morning or h.s., followed, if necessary, by another 75 mg b.i.d.

▶ **Acute gouty arthritis.** *Adults:* 50 mg P.O. t.i.d. Dose reduced as soon as possible; then discontinued. Don't use sustained-release capsules for this condition.

▶ **Acute painful shoulders (bursitis or tendinitis).** *Adults:* 75 to 150 mg P.O. daily b.i.d. or t.i.d. with food or antacids for 7 to 14 days.

▶ **To close hemodynamically significant patent ductus arteriosus in premature infants (I.V. form only).** *Neonates under 48 hours:* 0.2 mg/kg I.V. followed by two doses of 0.1 mg/kg at 12- to 24-hour intervals. *Neonates ages 2 to 7 days:* 0.2 mg/kg I.V. followed by two doses of 0.2 mg/kg at 12- to 24-hour intervals. *Neonates over age 7 days:* 0.2 mg/ kg I.V. followed by two doses of 0.25 mg/ kg at 12- to 24-hour intervals.

Adverse reactions

P.O. and P.R. form:
CNS: *headache, dizziness,* depression, drowsiness, confusion, peripheral neuropathy, *seizures,* psychic disturbances, syncope, *vertigo.*
CV: hypertension, *edema,* **heart failure.**
EENT: blurred vision, corneal and retinal damage, hearing loss, tinnitus.
GI: *nausea, vomiting,* anorexia, *diarrhea, peptic ulceration,* **GI bleeding,** pancreatitis.
GU: hematuria, *acute renal failure.*
Hematologic: *hemolytic anemia, aplastic anemia, agranulocytosis,* leukopenia, *thrombocytopenic purpura,* iron-deficiency anemia.
Hepatic: elevated enzymes.
Skin: pruritus, urticaria, *Stevens-Johnson syndrome.*
Other: hypersensitivity (rash, respiratory distress, *anaphylaxis, angioedema*), hyperkalemia.

I.V. form:
GI: *bleeding,* vomiting.
GU: *renal dysfunction, azotemia.*
Hematologic: decreased platelet aggregation.
Other: *hyponatremia, hyperkalemia, hypoglycemia,* hypersensitivity (rash, respiratory distress, *anaphylaxis, angioedema*).

Interactions

Drug-drug. *Aminoglycosides, cyclosporine, methotrexate:* indomethacin may enhance toxicity of these agents. Avoid concomitant use.
Antihypertensive agents: reduced antihypertensive effect. Monitor closely.
Aspirin: decreased blood levels of indomethacin. Avoid concomitant use.
Corticosteroids: increased risk of GI toxicity. Don't use together.
Diflunisal, probenecid: decreased indomethacin excretion; watch for increased incidence of indomethacin adverse reactions.
Digoxin: indomethacin may prolong half-life of digoxin. Use together cautiously.
Dipyridamole: enhanced fluid retention. Avoid concomitant use.
Furosemide, thiazide diuretics: impaired response to both drugs. Avoid using together if possible.
Lithium: increased plasma lithium levels. Monitor for toxicity.
Triamterene: possible nephrotoxicity. Monitor closely.
Drug-lifestyle. *Alcohol use:* increased risk of GI toxicity. Avoid concomitant use.

Contraindications and precautions

● Contraindicated in patients hypersensitive to drug; in those with history of aspirin- or NSAID-induced asthma, rhinitis, or urticaria; and in pregnant, or breast-feeding patients. Also contraindicated in infants with untreated infection, active bleeding, coagulation defects or thrombocytopenia, congenital heart disease in whom patency of ductus arteriosus is nec-

essary for satisfactory pulmonary or systemic blood flow, necrotizing enterocolitis, or impaired renal function. Suppositories contraindicated in patients with history of proctitis or recent rectal bleeding.
• Because of its high incidence of adverse effects during chronic use, indomethacin should not be used routinely as analgesic or antipyretic.
• Drug use is not recommended in pregnant or breast-feeding women.
• Use cautiously in elderly patients and in those with epilepsy, parkinsonism, hepatic or renal disease, CV disease, infection, mental illness or depression, or history of GI disease.

NURSING CONSIDERATIONS

Assessment
• Assess patient's condition before therapy and regularly thereafter.
• Monitor carefully for bleeding and for reduced urine output with I.V. administration.
• Be alert for adverse reactions and drug interactions.
• Evaluate patient's and family's knowledge of drug therapy.

Nursing diagnoses
• Pain related to underlying condition
• Risk for injury related to adverse reactions
• Knowledge deficit related to drug therapy

Planning and implementation
P.O. use: Administer drug with food, milk, or antacid if GI upset occurs.
I.V. use: Reconstitute powder for injection with sterile water for injection or 0.9% NaCl. For each 1-mg vial, add 1 ml of diluent for solution containing 1 mg/ml; add 2 ml of diluent to yield solution containing 0.5 mg/ml. Give by direct injection over 5 to 10 seconds.
– Use only preservative-free diluents to prepare I.V. injection. Never use diluents containing benzyl alcohol because this

has been associated with fatal gasping syndrome in neonates. Because injection contains no preservatives, reconstitute immediately before administration, and discard unused solution.
– Don't administer second or third scheduled I.V. dose if anuria or marked oliguria is evident; instead, notify doctor.
P.R. use: Follow normal protocol.
• Be aware that if ductus arteriosus reopens, second course of one to three doses may be given. If ineffective, surgery may be necessary.
• Discontinue drug if bleeding or reduced urine output occurs and notify doctor.
• Drug may enhance hypothalamic-pituitary-adrenal axis response to dexamethasone suppression test. Inform laboratory personnel that patient is taking indomethacin.
• Notify doctor if drug is ineffective.
Patient teaching
• Tell patient to take oral form of drug with food, milk, or antacid if GI upset occurs.
• Alert patient that concomitant use of oral form with aspirin, alcohol, or corticosteroids may increase risk of adverse GI reactions.
• Teach patient to recognize and report signs and symptoms of GI bleeding. Serious GI toxicity, including peptic ulceration and bleeding, can occur in patients taking oral NSAIDs despite absence of GI symptoms.
• Instruct patient to avoid alcohol consumption during drug therapy.
• Tell patient to notify doctor immediately of visual or hearing changes. Patient on long-term oral therapy should have regular eye examinations, hearing tests, CBC, and renal function tests to monitor for toxicity.
• Advise patient to avoid hazardous activities if adverse CNS reactions occur.

Evaluation
• Patient is free from pain.

• Patient does not experience injury from adverse reactions.
• Patient and family state understanding of drug therapy.

---

insulins

(IN-suh-linz)

insulin analog injection

Humalog

insulin injection (regular insulin, crystalline zinc insulin)

Actrapid HM◇, Actrapid HM Penfill◇, Actrapid MC◇, Actrapid MC Penfill◇, Humulin R†, Hypurin Neutral◇, Insulin 2 Neutral◇, Novolin R†, Novolin R PenFill†, Pork Regular Iletin II†, Regular (Concentrated) Iletin II, Regular Iletin I†, Regular Purified Pork Insulin†, Velosulin Human◇, Velosulin Insuject◇

insulin zinc suspension (lente)

Humulin L†, Lente Iletin II†, Lente Insulin†, Lente MC◇, Lente Purified Pork Insulin†, Monotard HM◇, Monotard MC◇, Novolin L†

insulin zinc suspension, extended (ultralente)

Humulin U†, Insulin Analog Injection Humalog, Ultralente Insulin†, Ultratard HM◇, Ultratard MC◇

insulin zinc suspension, prompt (semilente)

Semilente MC◇

isophane insulin suspension (neutral protamine Hagedorn insulin, NPH)

Humulin N†, Humulin NPH◇, Hypurin Isophane◇, Insulatard◇, Insulatard Human♦, Isotard MC◇, Novolin N†, Novolin N PenFill†, NPH Insulin†, NPH Purified Pork†, Pork NPH Iletin II†, Protaphane HM◇, Protaphane HM Penfill◇, Protaphane MC◇

isophane insulin suspension with insulin injection

Actraphane HM◇, Actraphane HM Penfill◇, Actraphane MC◇, Humulin 50/50†, Humulin 70/30†, Novolin 70/30, Novolin 70/30 PenFill†

protamine zinc suspension (PZI)

Protamine Zinc Insulin MC◇

Pharmacologic class: pancreatic hormone
Therapeutic class: antidiabetic
Pregnancy risk category: NR

How supplied

insulin injection
Injection (human): 100 units/ml (Actrapid HM◇, Humulin R†, Novolin R†, Humalog (lispro), Velosulin Human◇); 100 units/ml in 1.5-ml cartridge system† (Actrapid HM Penfill◇, Novolin R PenFill†)
Injection (from pork): 100 units/ml†
Injection (purified beef): 100 units/ml (Hypurin Neutral◇, Insulin 2◇)
Injection (purified pork): 100 units/ml (Actrapid MC◇, Pork Regular Iletin II†, Regular Purified Pork Insulin†); 100 units/ml in 1.5-ml cartridge system◇ (Actrapid MC Penfill◇); 100 units/ml in 2-ml cartridge system◇; 500 units/ml (Regular [Concentrated] Iletin II)
insulin zinc suspension, prompt
Injection (purified pork): 100 units/ml† (Semilente MC◇)
isophane insulin suspension
Injection (from beef): 100 units/ml† (NPH Insulin†)
Injection (human, recombinant): 100 units/ml (Humulin N†, Humulin NPH◇, Insulatard Human♦, Novolin N†, Protaphane HM◇); 100 units/ml in 1.5-ml cartridge system (Protaphane HM PenFill◇, Novolin N PenFill†)
Injection (purified beef): 100 units/ml (Hypurin Isophane◇, Isotard MC◇)
Injection (purified pork): 100 units/ml (Insulatard◇, NPH Purified Pork†, Pork NPH Iletin II, Protaphane MC◇)

**isophane insulin suspension 50%
with insulin injection 50%**
Injection (human): 100 units/ml
(Humulin 50/50†)
**isophane insulin suspension 70%
with insulin injection 30%**
Injection (human): 100 units/ml
(Actraphane HM◊, Humulin 70/30†,
Novolin 70/30†); 100 units/ml in 1.5-ml
cartridge system (Actraphane HM
Penfill◊, Novolin 70/30 PenFill†)
Injection (purified pork): 100 units/ml
(Actraphane MC◊)
insulin zinc suspension
Injection (from beef): 100 units/ml
(Lente Insulin†, Lente MC◊)
Injection (purified beef): 100 units/ml
(Lente MC◊)
Injection (purified pork): 100 units/ml
(Lente Iletin II†, Monotard MC◊, Lente
Purified Pork Insulin†)
Injection (human): 100 units/ml†
(Humulin L†, Monotard HM◊,
Novolin L†)
protamine zinc suspension
Injection (purified pork): Protamine
Zinc Insulin MC◊
insulin zinc suspension, extended
Injection (from beef): 100 units/ml†
(Ultralente Insulin†)
Injection (human): 100 units/ml
(Ultratard HM◊, Humulin U†)
Injection (purified pork): 100 units/ml◊
(Ultratard MC◊)

Pharmacokinetics

Absorption: highly variable after S.C. administration depending on insulin type and injection site.
Distribution: distributed widely throughout body.
Metabolism: some is bound and inactivated by peripheral tissues, but most appears to be degraded in liver and kidneys.
Excretion: filtered by renal glomeruli; undergoes some tubular reabsorption.
Half-life: about 9 minutes after I.V. administration.

Route	Onset	Peak	Duration
I.V.	≤ 0.5 hr	0.25-0.5 hr	0.5-1 hr
S.C.	0.25-8 hr	2-30 hr	5-36 hr

Pharmacodynamics

Chemical effect: increases glucose transport across muscle and fat cell membranes to reduce blood glucose level. Promotes conversion of glucose to its storage form, glycogen; triggers amino acid uptake and conversion to protein in muscle cells and inhibits protein degradation; stimulates triglyceride formation and inhibits release of free fatty acids from adipose tissue; and stimulates lipoprotein lipase activity, which converts circulating lipoproteins to fatty acids.
Therapeutic effect: lowers blood glucose levels.

Indications and dosage

▶ **Diabetic ketoacidosis (use regular insulin only).** *Adults:* 0.15 units/kg as I.V. bolus, followed by 0.1 units/kg/hour by continuous infusion. Continue infusion until blood glucose level drops to 250 mg/dl; then S.C. insulin started with dosage and dosage interval adjusted according to patient's blood glucose concentrations. Alternatively, 50 to 100 units I.V. and 50 to 100 units S.C. immediately; then additional doses q 1 to 2 hours based on blood glucose levels. *Children:* 0.1 unit/kg as I.V. bolus, then 0.1 unit/kg hourly by continuous infusion until blood glucose level drops to 250 mg/dl; then S.C. insulin started. Alternatively, 0.5 to 1 unit/kg in two divided doses, one I.V. and the other S.C., followed by 0.5 to 1 unit/kg I.V. q 1 to 2 hours based on blood glucose levels.
▶ **Type 1 diabetes mellitus (insulin-dependent), adjunct to type 2 diabetes mellitus (non-insulin-dependent) inadequately controlled by diet and oral antidiabetic agents.** *Adults and children:* therapeutic regimen is prescribed by doctor and adjusted based on patient's blood glucose levels.

Adverse reactions

Skin: urticaria, itching, swelling, redness, stinging, warmth (at injection site). **Other:** *lipoatrophy, lipohypertrophy,* hypersensitivity reactions, **anaphylaxis,** rash), **hypoglycemia,** hyperglycemia (rebound, or Somogyi, effect).

Interactions

Drug-drug. *AIDS antivirals, corticosteroids, dextrothyroxine, epinephrine, thiazide diuretics:* diminished insulin response. Monitor for hyperglycemia.
Anabolic steroids, beta blockers, clofibrate, fenfluramine, guanethidine, MAO inhibitors, salicylates, tetracycline: prolonged hypoglycemic effect. Monitor blood glucose level carefully.
Diazoxide, phenytoin (high doses): may inhibit endogenous insulin secretion and may cause hypoglycemia in diabetic patients. Carefully adjust insulin dosage.
Oral contraceptives: may decrease glucose tolerance in diabetic patients. Monitor blood glucose levels and adjust insulin dosage carefully.
Drug-lifestyle. *Alcohol use:* hypoglycemic effect. Avoid concomitant use.
Marijuana use: may increase serum glucose concentrations.
Smoking: may increase glucose concentrations and decrease response to insulin administration.

Contraindications and precautions

● No known contraindications.
● Know that insulin is drug of choice to treat diabetes in pregnant and breastfeeding women.

NURSING CONSIDERATIONS

⚡ Assessment
● Assess patient's blood glucose level before therapy and regularly thereafter. Monitor levels more frequently if patient is under stress, unstable, pregnant, or recently diagnosed.
● Monitor patient's hemoglobin A_{1c} regularly, as ordered.

● Monitor urine ketone levels when blood glucose levels are elevated.
● Be alert for adverse reactions and drug interactions.
● Monitor injection sites for local reactions.
● Evaluate patient's and family's knowledge of drug therapy.

⊕ Nursing diagnoses
● Altered health maintenance related to hyperglycemia
● Risk for injury related to drug-induced hypoglycemia
● Knowledge deficit related to drug therapy

❯ Planning and implementation
● Know that regular insulin is used in patients with circulatory collapse, diabetic ketoacidosis, or hyperkalemia. Do not use regular insulin concentrated (500 units/ml) I.V. Do not use intermediate- or long-acting insulins for coma or other emergency requiring rapid drug action.
● Dosage is always expressed in USP units. Use only syringes calibrated for particular concentration of insulin administered. U-500 insulin must be administered with U-100 syringe because no syringes are made for this strength.
● Be aware that insulin resistance may develop and large insulin doses are needed to control symptoms of diabetes in these patients. U-500 insulin is available as Regular (Concentrated) Iletin II for such patients. Although every pharmacy may not normally stock it, it is readily available. Nurses should give hospital pharmacy sufficient notice before needing to refill in-house prescription. Never store U-500 insulin in same area with other insulin preparations because of danger of severe overdose if given accidentally to other patients.
● To mix insulin suspension, swirl vial gently or rotate between palms or between palm and thigh. Don't shake vigorously: this causes bubbling and air in syringe.

• Know that Humalog insulin has a rapid onset of action and should be given 15 minutes before meals.

• Know lente, semilente, and ultralente insulins may be mixed in any proportion.

• Know that regular insulin may be mixed with NPH or lente insulins in any proportion.

• Note that switching from separate injections to prepared mixture may alter patient response. Whenever NPH or lente is mixed with regular insulin in same syringe, give immediately to avoid loss of potency.

• Don't use insulin that changes color or becomes clumped or granular.

• Check expiration date on vial before using contents.

I.V. use: Only administer regular insulin I.V. Inject directly at ordered rate into vein, through intermittent infusion device, or into port close to I.V. access site. Intermittent infusion is not recommended. If given by continuous infusion, infuse drug diluted in 0.9% NaCl at prescribed rate.

S.C. use: Know that usual administration route is S.C. Pinch fold of skin with fingers at least 3″ apart and insert needle at 45- to 90-degree angle.

– Press but do not rub site after injection. Rotate injection sites and chart to avoid overuse of one area. Know that diabetic patients may achieve better control if injection site is rotated within same anatomic region.

– Know that ketosis-prone type I, severely ill, and newly diagnosed diabetic patients with very high blood glucose levels may require hospitalization and I.V. treatment with regular fast-acting insulin.

• Store drug in cool area. Refrigeration is desirable but not essential, except with regular insulin (concentrated).

• Notify doctor of sudden changes in blood glucose levels, dangerously high or low levels, or ketosis.

• Be prepared to provide supportive measures if diabetic ketoacidosis or hyper-glycemic hyperosmolar nonketotic coma occurs.

• Treat hypoglycemic reaction with oral form of rapid-acting glucose if patient can swallow or with glucagon or I.V. glucose if patient cannot be roused. Follow with complex carbohydrate snack when patient is awake, and determine cause of reaction.

• Be sure that other treatments, such as diet and exercise programs, are being used appropriately. Expect to adjust insulin dosage when other aspects of regimen are altered.

• Discuss how to deal with issues of noncompliance with doctor.

• Treat lipoatrophy or lipohypertrophy according to prescribed protocol.

Patient teaching

• Tell patient that therapy relieves symptoms but doesn't cure disease.

• Instruct patient about nature of disease; importance of following therapeutic regimen; adhering to specific diet, weight reduction, exercise, and personal hygiene program; and avoiding infection. Review timing of injections and eating, and explain that meals must not be omitted.

• Stress that accuracy of measurement is very important, especially with regular insulin concentrated. Aids, such as magnifying sleeve or dose magnifier, may improve accuracy. Instruct patient and family how to measure and administer insulin.

• Advise patient not to alter order of mixing insulins or change model or brand of syringe or needle.

• Teach that self-monitoring of blood glucose levels and urine ketone tests are essential guides to dosage and success of therapy. It's important to recognize hypoglycemic symptoms because insulin-induced hypoglycemia is hazardous and may cause brain damage if prolonged; most adverse effects are self-limiting and temporary.

• Teach patient about proper use of equipment for self-monitoring of blood glucose levels.

• Instruct patient to avoid alcohol consumption during drug therapy.
• Advise patient not to smoke within 30 minutes after insulin injection. Smoking decreases absorption.
• Tell patient that marijuana use may increase insulin requirements.
• Advise patient to carry medical identification at all times, to carry ample insulin supply and syringes on trips, to have carbohydrates (lump of sugar or candy) on hand for emergencies, and to note time zone changes for dose schedule when traveling.

☑ **Evaluation**
• Patient's blood glucose level is normal.
• Patient does not experience injury from drug-induced hypoglycemia.
• Patient and family state understanding of drug therapy.

interferon alfa-2a, recombinant (rIFN-A)
(in-ter-FEER-on AL-fuh too-ay ree-COM-bih-nent)
Roferon-A

interferon alfa-2b, recombinant (IFN-alpha 2)
Intron-A

Pharmacologic class: biological response modifier
Therapeutic class: antineoplastic
Pregnancy risk category: C

How supplied

alfa-2a
Injection: 3 million IU/vial; 6 million IU/ml; 9 million IU/ml; 18 and 36 million IU/multiple-dose vial
Sterile powder for injection: 18 million IU/vial
alfa-2b
Injection: 3 million IU/vial with diluent, 5 million IU/vial with diluent, 10 mil-

lion IU/vial with diluent, 18 million IU/vial with diluent, 25 million IU/vial with diluent, 50 million IU/vial with diluent

Pharmacokinetics
Absorption: more than 80% absorbed after I.M. or S.C. injection.
Distribution: not applicable.
Metabolism: drug appears to be metabolized in liver and kidney.
Excretion: reabsorbed from glomerular filtrate with minor biliary elimination.

Route	Onset	Peak	Duration
I.M.	Unknown	3.8 hr	Unknown
S.C.	Unknown	7.3 hr	Unknown
Intralesional	Unknown	Unknown	Unknown

Pharmacodynamics
Chemical effect: unknown; appears to involve direct antiproliferative action against tumor cells or viral cells to inhibit replication and modulation of host immune response by enhancing phagocytic activity of macrophages and by augmenting specific cytotoxicity of lymphocytes for target cells.
Therapeutic effect: inhibits growth of selected tumor cells and viral cells.

Indications and dosage
▶ **Hairy-cell leukemia. alfa-2a.** *Adults:* for induction, 3 million units S.C. or I.M. daily for 16 to 24 weeks. For maintenance, 3 million units S.C. or I.M. three times weekly. **alfa-2b.** *Adults:* 2 million units/m² I.M. or S.C., three times weekly for up to 6 months.
▶ **AIDS-related Kaposi's sarcoma. alfa-2a.** *Adults:* for induction, 36 million units S.C. or I.M. daily for 10 to 12 weeks. For maintenance, 36 million units S.C. or I.M. three times weekly. **alfa-2b.** *Adults:* 30 million units/m² S.C. or I.M. three times weekly.
▶ **Condylomata acuminata (genital or venereal warts). alfa-2b.** *Adults:* 1 mil-

lion units/lesion intralesionally three times weekly for 3 weeks.

▶ **Chronic hepatitis B. alfa-2b.** *Adults:* 30 to 35 million units weekly I.M. or S.C., administered either as 5 million units daily or 10 million units three times weekly, for 16 weeks.

▶ **Chronic hepatitis C. alfa-2a and alfa-2b.** *Adults:* 3 million units I.M. or S.C. three times weekly.

▶ **Chronic myelogenous leukemia (CML, chronic phase Ph positive). alfa-2a.** *Adults:* initial dose of 9 million units daily administered S.C. or I.M. Optimal maintenance dosage and duration of therapy have not been determined. See package insert for specific recommendations.

▶ **Malignant melanoma. alfa-2b.** *Adults:* initial dose of 20 million IU/ m² I.V. on 5 consecutive days weekly for 4 weeks. Maintenance dosage is 10 million IU/m² S.C. three times weekly for 48 weeks.

Adverse reactions

CNS: *dizziness,* confusion, paresthesia, numbness, lethargy, depression, nervousness, difficulty in thinking or concentrating, insomnia, sedation, apathy, anxiety, irritability, fatigue, vertigo, gait disturbances, poor coordination.
CV: hypotension, chest pain, *arrhythmias,* palpitations, syncope, *heart failure,* hypertension, edema, *MI.*
EENT: visual disturbances, dryness or inflammation of oropharynx, rhinorrhea, sinusitis, conjunctivitis, earache, eye irritation, rhinitis.
GI: *anorexia, nausea, diarrhea,* vomiting, abdominal fullness, abdominal pain, flatulence, constipation, hypermotility, gastric distress, dysgeusia.
GU: transient impotence.
Hematologic: *leukopenia, mild thrombocytopenia.*
Hepatic: *hepatitis.*
Respiratory: coughing, dyspnea, tachypnea.

Skin: *rash,* dryness, *pruritus,* partial alopecia, urticaria, flushing.
Other: inflammation (at injection site; rare), flulike syndrome (fever, fatigue, myalgia, headache, chills, arthralgia), diaphoresis, hot flashes, excessive salivation, cyanosis.

Interactions

Drug-drug. *Aminophylline, theophylline:* may reduce theophylline clearance. Monitor serum levels.
Cardiotoxic, hematotoxic, or neurotoxic drugs: effects of previously or concurrently administered drugs may be increased by interferons. Monitor closely.
CNS depressants: enhanced CNS effects. Avoid concomitant use.
Interleukin-2: increased potential risk of renal failure from interleukin-2. Monitor closely.
Live-virus vaccine: increased risk of adverse reactions and decreased antibody response. Don't use together.
Zidovudine: may be synergistic adverse effects between alfa-2b and zidovudine. Carefully monitor WBC count.
Drug-lifestyle. *Alcohol use:* increased risk of GI bleeding. Avoid concomitant use.

Contraindications and precautions

• Contraindicated in patients hypersensitive to drug or to mouse immunoglobulin.
• Drug is not recommended for use in breast-feeding women.
• Use cautiously in patients with severe hepatic or renal function impairment, seizure disorders, compromised CNS function, cardiac disease, or myelosuppression. Also use cautiously in pregnant women.
• Safety of drug has not been established in children.

NURSING CONSIDERATIONS

🔧 **Assessment**
• Assess patient's condition before therapy and regularly thereafter.

• Obtain allergy history. Drug contains phenol as preservative and serum albumin as stabilizer.
• At beginning of therapy, assess for flulike symptoms, which tend to diminish with continued therapy.
• Monitor blood studies, as ordered. Interferons may decrease hemoglobin, hematocrit, WBC count, platelet count, and neutrophil count; increase PT and PTT; and increase serum levels of AST, ALT, lactate dehydrogenase, alkaline phosphatase, calcium, phosphorus, and fasting glucose, which are dose-related and reversible. Recovery occurs within several days or weeks after withdrawal.
• Be alert for adverse reactions and drug interactions.
• Evaluate patient's and family's knowledge of drug therapy.

Nursing diagnoses
• Altered health maintenance related to underlying condition
• Risk for injury related to drug-induced adverse CNS reactions
• Knowledge deficit related to drug therapy

Planning and implementation
• Premedicate patient with acetaminophen to minimize flulike symptoms.
• Administer drug at bedtime to minimize daytime drowsiness.
• Make sure patient is well hydrated, especially during initial stages of treatment.
• Know that different brands of interferon may not be equivalent and may require different dosage.
I.M. use: Follow normal protocol.
S.C. use: Use S.C. administration route in patients whose platelet count is below 50,000/mm³.

Intralesional use: When administering interferon alfa-2b for condylomata acuminata, use only 10-million-IU vial because dilution of other strengths required for intralesional use results in hypertonic solution. Do not reconstitute 10-million-IU vial with more than 1 ml of diluent. Use tuberculin or similar syringe and 25G to 30G needle. Don't inject too deeply beneath lesion or too superficially. As many as five lesions can be treated at one time. To ease discomfort, administer drug in evening with acetaminophen.
• Refrigerate drug.
• Notify doctor of severe adverse reactions, which may require dosage reduction or discontinuation.
• Use with blood dyscrasia-causing medications, bone marrow suppressant, or radiation therapy may increase bone marrow suppressant effects. Dosage reduction may be required.

Patient teaching
• Advise patient that laboratory tests will be performed before and periodically during therapy. Tests include CBC with differential, platelet count, blood chemistry and electrolyte studies, liver function tests, and, if patient has preexisting cardiac disorder or advanced stages of cancer, ECGs.
• Instruct patient in proper oral hygiene during treatment because bone marrow suppressant effects of interferon may lead to microbial infection, delayed healing, and gingival bleeding. This drug may also decrease salivary flow.
• Emphasize need to follow doctor's instructions about taking and recording temperature, and how and when to take acetaminophen.
• Advise patient to check with doctor for instructions after missing dose.
• Tell patient that drug may cause temporary loss of some hair, which should return when therapy ends.
• Teach patient how to prepare and administer drug and how to dispose of used needles, syringes, containers, and unused medication. Give him a copy of information for patients included with product and ensure that he understands it. Also provide information on drug stability.
• Warn patient not to receive any immunization without doctor's approval and to avoid contact with people who have taken oral polio vaccine. Concurrent use

with live-virus vaccine may potentiate replication of vaccine virus, increase adverse reactions, and decrease patient's antibody response. Patients are at increased risk for infection during therapy.
• Instruct patient to avoid alcohol consumption during drug therapy.

☑ Evaluation
• Patient shows improved health.
• Patient does not experience injury from adverse CNS reactions.
• Patient and family state understanding of drug therapy.

---

interferon alfa-n3
(in-ter-FEER-on AL-fuh en-three)
Alferon N

Pharmacologic class: biological response modifier
Therapeutic class: antiviral
Pregnancy risk category: C

How supplied

Injection: 5 million units/ml in 1-ml vials

Pharmacokinetics

Unknown.

Route	Onset	Peak	Duration
Intra-lesional	Unknown	Unknown	Unknown

Pharmacodynamics

Chemical effect: attaches to membrane receptors and causes cellular changes, including increased protein synthesis.
Therapeutic effect: inhibits growth of selected viral cells.

Indications and dosage

▶ **Condylomata acuminata (genital or venereal warts).** *Adults:* 0.05 ml/wart by intralesional injection. Treatment usually continues twice weekly for up to 8

weeks. Dosage should not exceed 0.5 ml (2.5 million units) per session.

Adverse reactions

CNS: dizziness, light-headedness.
GI: dyspepsia, heartburn, vomiting, nausea.
Other: *acute hypersensitivity reactions with mild to moderate flulike syndrome (myalgia, fever, headache), arthralgia, back pain, malaise.*

Interactions

None reported.

Contraindications and precautions

• Contraindicated in patients hypersensitive to interferon-alfa and in those with history of anaphylactic reactions to murine immunoglobulin, egg protein, or neomycin.
• Use of drug is not recommended in breast-feeding women.
• Use cautiously in pregnant women and in patients with debilitating illnesses (uncontrolled heart failure, unstable angina, severe pulmonary disease, coagulation disorders, seizure disorders, severe myelosuppression, or diabetes mellitus with ketoacidosis) because of association of interferon with flulike syndrome.
• Safety of drug has not been established in children.

NURSING CONSIDERATIONS

☒ Assessment
• Assess patient's condition before therapy and regularly thereafter.
• Be alert for adverse reactions.
• Evaluate patient's and family's knowledge of drug therapy.

⊕ Nursing diagnoses
• Impaired skin integrity related to lesions induced by condylomata acuminata
• Pain related to interferon-induced headache, backache, and arthralgia
• Knowledge deficit related to drug therapy

Reactions may be *common*, uncommon, *life-threatening*, or COMMON AND LIFE-THREATENING.

▷ Planning and implementation

• Inject each lesion at base of wart, using 30G needle.
• Although anaphylaxis hasn't been reported, be prepared to treat acute hypersensitivity reactions.
• Administer acetaminophen for flulike symptoms and pain.

Patient teaching
• Teach patient to recognize and report symptoms of hypersensitivity: urticaria, tightness of chest, wheezing, shortness of breath.
• Explain that warts will continue to disappear after completion of 8 weeks of therapy and discontinuation of drug.
• Teach patient good hand-washing technique. Caution him to avoid scratching, rubbing, or picking lesions or warts.

☑ Evaluation

• Patient shows reduction in or elimination of lesions or warts.
• Patient is free from pain.
• Patient and family state understanding of drug therapy.

interferon beta-1b, recombinant
(in-ter-FEER-on BAY-tuh wun bee ree-COM-bih-nent)
Betaseron

Pharmacologic class: biological response modifier
Therapeutic class: antiviral/immunoregulator
Pregnancy risk category: C

How supplied

Powder for injection: 9.6 million IU (0.3 mg)-beta 1b

Pharmacokinetics

Unknown.

Route	Onset	Peak	Duration
S.C.	Unknown	Unknown	Unknown

Pharmacodynamics

Chemical effect: attaches to membrane receptors and causes cellular changes, including increased protein synthesis.
Therapeutic effect: decreases exacerbations in multiple sclerosis.

Indications and dosage

▶ **To reduce frequency of exacerbations in patients with relapsing-remitting multiple sclerosis.** *Adults:* 8 million IU (0.25 mg) S.C. every other day.

Adverse reactions

CNS: depression, anxiety, emotional lability, depersonalization, *malaise, suicidal tendencies,* confusion, somnolence, *seizures,* headache, dizziness.
CV: *hemorrhage.*
EENT: laryngitis.
GI: *nausea, diarrhea, constipation.*
GU: *menstrual disorders (bleeding or spotting, early or delayed menses, decreased days of menstrual flow, menorrhagia).*
Hematologic: *decreased WBC and absolute neutrophil counts.*
Hepatic: elevated ALT levels, elevated bilirubin levels.
Respiratory: dyspnea.
Other: *flulike symptoms (fever, chills, myalgia, diaphoresis),* breast pain, *pelvic pain; lymphadenopathy, hypersensitivity reaction; inflammation, pain, necrosis* (at injection site).

Interactions

None significant.

Contraindications and precautions

• Contraindicated in patients hypersensitive to interferon beta or human albumin.
• Drug is not recommended in pregnant or breast-feeding women. It is not known if drug is excreted in breast milk.
• Use cautiously in women of childbearing age.
• Safety of drug has not been established in children.

*Liquid form contains alcohol   **May contain tartrazine   ♦Canada   ◇Australia   †OTC

NURSING CONSIDERATIONS

⚕ Assessment
• Obtain assessment of patient's underlying condition before therapy.
• Monitor frequency of exacerbations after drug therapy begins.
• Monitor WBC counts, platelet counts and blood chemistries, including liver function tests.
• Be alert for adverse reactions.
• Monitor for depression and suicidal ideation.
• Evaluate patient's and family's knowledge of drug therapy.

⚙ Nursing diagnoses
• Altered health maintenance related to exacerbations of multiple sclerosis
• Risk for injury related to drug-induced adverse CNS reactions
• Knowledge deficit related to drug therapy

▶ Planning and implementation
• Premedicate patient with acetaminophen, as ordered, to minimize flulike symptoms.
• To reconstitute, inject 1.2 ml of supplied diluent (0.54% NaCl injection) into vial and gently swirl to dissolve drug. Do not shake. Reconstituted solution will contain 8 million IU (0.25 mg)/ml. Discard vials that contain particles or discolored solution.
• Inject immediately after preparation.
• Rotate injection sites to minimize local reactions.
Patient teaching
• Warn female patient of childbearing age about dangers to fetus. If patient becomes pregnant during therapy, tell her to notify doctor promptly.
• Teach patient how to self-administer S.C. injections, including solution preparation, use of aseptic technique, rotation of injection sites, and equipment disposal. Periodically reevaluate patient's technique.

• Advise patient to take drug at bedtime to minimize mild flulike symptoms.
• Advise patient to report thoughts of depression or suicidal ideation.

⚕ Evaluation
• Patient exhibits decreased frequency of exacerbations.
• Patient does not experience injury from adverse CNS reactions.
• Patient and family state understanding of drug therapy.

interferon gamma-1b
(in-ter-FEER-on GAH-muh wun bee)
Actimmune

Pharmacologic class: biological response modifier
Therapeutic class: antineoplastic
Pregnancy risk category: C

How supplied

Injection: 100 mcg (3 million units)/vial

Pharmacokinetics

Absorption: about 90% is absorbed after S.C. administration.
Distribution: unknown.
Metabolism: unknown.
Excretion: unknown. *Half-life:* 5.9 hours.

Route	Onset	Peak	Duration
S.C.	Unknown	≤ 7 hr	Unknown

Pharmacodynamics

Chemical effect: acts as interleukin-type lymphokine. It has potent phagocyte-activating properties and enhances oxidative metabolism of tissue macrophages.
Therapeutic effect: promotes phagocyte activity.

Indications and dosage

▶ **Chronic granulomatous disease.**
Adults with body surface area over 0.5 m²: 50 mcg/m² (1.5 million units/m²) S.C. three times weekly, preferably h.s.

Preferred injection site is the deltoid or anterior thigh. *Adults with body surface area of 0.5 m² or less:* 1.5 mcg/kg/dose S.C. three times weekly.

Adverse reactions

CNS: *fatigue, decreased mental status, gait disturbance.*
GI: *nausea, vomiting, diarrhea.*
Hematologic: *neutropenia, thrombocytopenia.*
Hepatic: elevated liver enzyme levels (at high doses).
Skin: rash.
Other: erythema, tenderness (at injection site); flulike syndrome (headache, fever, chills, myalgia, arthralgia).

Interactions

Drug-drug. *Myelosuppressive agents:* possible additive myelosuppression. Monitor closely.
Zidovudine: increased plasma levels of zidovudine. Dosage adjustments are necessary when used at same time.

Contraindications and precautions

• Contraindicated in patients hypersensitive to drug or to genetically engineered products derived from *Escherichia coli.*
• Drug is not recommended for use in breast-feeding women.
• Use cautiously in pregnant women and in patients with cardiac disease, compromised CNS function, or seizure disorders.
• Safety of drug has not been established in children under age 18.

NURSING CONSIDERATIONS

ᴁ Assessment
• Assess patient's condition before therapy and regularly thereafter.
• Be alert for adverse reactions and drug interactions.
• Monitor patient's hydration status if adverse GI reactions occur.
• Evaluate patient's and family's knowledge of drug therapy.

⊞ Nursing diagnoses
• Altered health maintenance related to underlying condition
• Risk for fluid volume deficit related to adverse GI reactions
• Knowledge deficit related to drug therapy

⊠ Planning and implementation
• Premedicate with acetaminophen to minimize symptoms at beginning of therapy. Flulike symptoms tend to diminish with continued therapy.
• Discard unused portion. Each vial is for single-dose use only and does not contain preservative.
• Give drug at bedtime to reduce discomfort from flulike symptoms.
• Refrigerate drug immediately. Vials must be stored at 36°to 46°F (2°to 8°C); do not freeze. Do not shake vial; avoid excessive agitation. Discard vials that have been left at room temperature for more than 12 hours.
Patient teaching
• Teach patient how to administer drug and how to dispose of used needles, syringes, containers, and unused medication. Give him a copy of information for patients included with product and ensure that he understands it.
• Instruct patient to notify doctor if adverse reactions occur.

⊠ Evaluation
• Patient responds well to drug.
• Patient maintains adequate hydration.
• Patient and family state understanding of drug therapy.

iodoquinol
(igh-oh-doh-KWIN-ohl)
Diodoquin♦, Diquinol, Yodoxin

Pharmacologic class: iodine derivative
Therapeutic class: antiprotozoal
Pregnancy risk category: C

How supplied

Tablets: 210 mg, 650 mg
Powder: 25 g

Pharmacokinetics

Absorption: poorly absorbed; exerts effects locally in lower GI tract.
Distribution: unknown.
Metabolism: unknown.
Excretion: excreted primarily in feces; less than 10% in urine.

Route	Onset	Peak	Duration
P.O.	Unknown	Unknown	Unknown

Pharmacodynamics

Chemical effect: unknown; has amebicidal activity in intestinal lumen.
Therapeutic effect: hinders amebiasis activity. Spectrum of activity includes trophozoites of *Entamoeba histolytica.*

Indications and dosage

▶ **Intestinal amebiasis.** *Adults:* 630 to 650 mg P.O. t.i.d. after meals for 20 days. Total daily dosage should not exceed 2 g. *Children:* usual dosage is 30 to 40 mg/kg of body weight daily in two to three divided doses for 20 days. Additional doses should not be repeated for 2 to 3 weeks.

Adverse reactions

CNS: neurotoxicity (dose-related), dysesthesia, weakness, vertigo, malaise, headache, agitation, retrograde amnesia, ataxia, *peripheral neuropathy.*
EENT: *optic neuritis,* optic atrophy, loss of vision.
GI: anorexia, nausea, vomiting, abdominal cramps, diarrhea, increased motility, constipation, epigastric burning and pain, gastritis, anal irritation and itching.
Hematologic: *agranulocytosis.*
Skin: pruritus, hives, papular and pustular eruptions, urticaria, discoloration of hair and nails.
Other: thyroid enlargement, fever, chills, generalized furunculosis, alopecia.

Interactions

None significant.

Contraindications and precautions

• Contraindicated in patients with hypersensitivity to 8-hydroxyquinoline derivatives or iodine-containing preparations. Iodoquinol causes liver damage in such patients. Also contraindicated in patients with hepatic or renal disease or preexisting optic neuropathy.
• Use cautiously in patients with thyroid diseases and in pregnant or breast-feeding women.

NURSING CONSIDERATIONS

▨ Assessment

• Obtain assessment of patient's infection before therapy.
• Monitor effectiveness by checking stools for organism. Send warm specimens to laboratory for analysis.
• Be alert for adverse reactions.
• Watch for diarrhea during first 2 or 3 days.
• Evaluate patient's and family's knowledge of drug therapy.

▣ Nursing diagnoses

• Infection related to presence of susceptible organisms
• Sensory or perceptual (visual) alterations related to drug's adverse effect on eye structure
• Knowledge deficit related to drug therapy

▶ Planning and implementation

• If patient has difficulty swallowing, crush tablets and mix with applesauce or chocolate syrup.
• Notify doctor if diarrhea continues beyond 3 days.
• Be aware that iodoquinol may interfere with thyroid function tests for up to 6 months after discontinuation.

Reactions may be *common*, uncommon, *life-threatening*, or COMMON AND LIFE-THREATENING.

Photoguide to tablets and capsules

This photoguide provides full-color photographs of some of the most commonly prescribed tablets and capsules in the United States. Shown in actual size, the drugs are organized alphabetically by trade or generic name for quick reference.

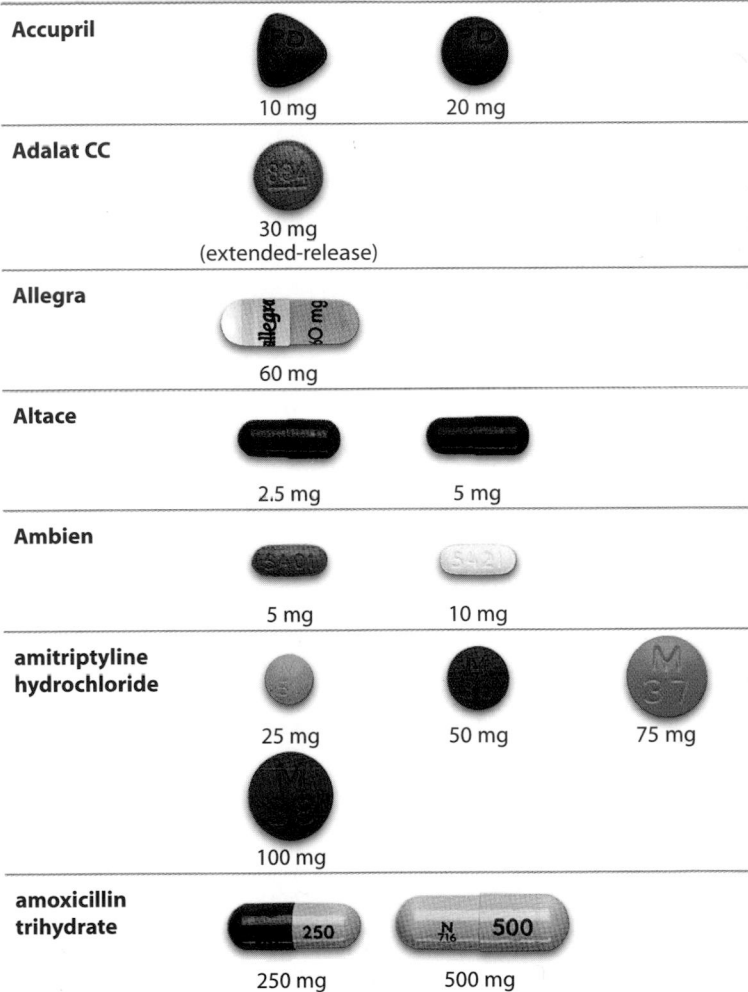

Accupril	10 mg	20 mg	
Adalat CC	30 mg (extended-release)		
Allegra	60 mg		
Altace	2.5 mg	5 mg	
Ambien	5 mg	10 mg	
amitriptyline hydrochloride	25 mg	50 mg	75 mg
	100 mg		
amoxicillin trihydrate	250 mg	500 mg	

Springhouse Nurse's Drug Guide, Third Edition, Springhouse Corporation, Springhouse, Pa.

Amoxil

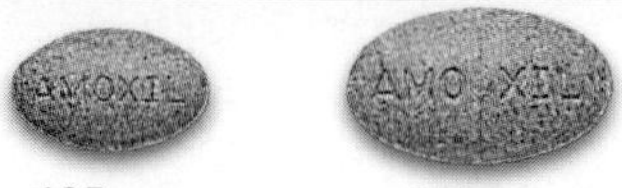

125 mg
(chewable)

250 mg
(chewable)

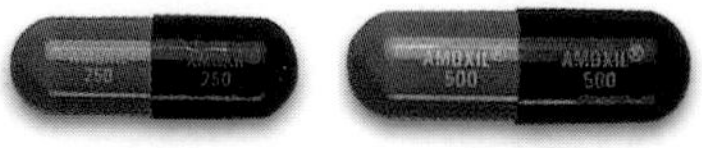

250 mg

500 mg

atenolol

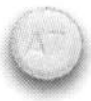

25 mg

Ativan

0.5 mg

1 mg

Augmentin

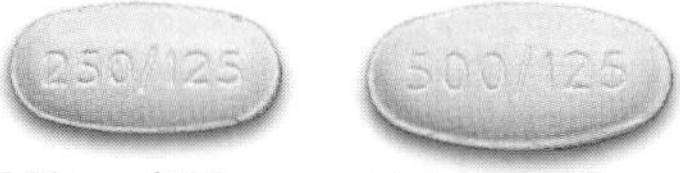

250 mg/125 mg

500 mg/125 mg

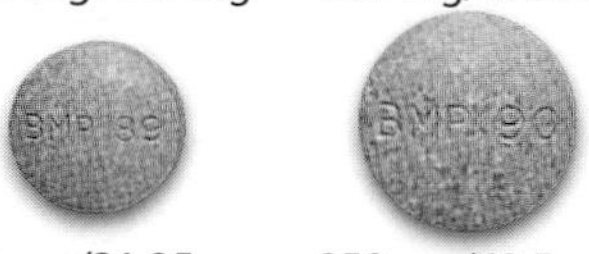

125 mg/31.25 mg
(chewable)

250 mg/62.5 mg
(chewable)

Axid

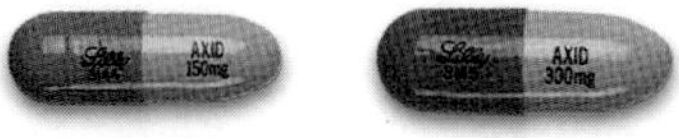

150 mg

300 mg

Biaxin

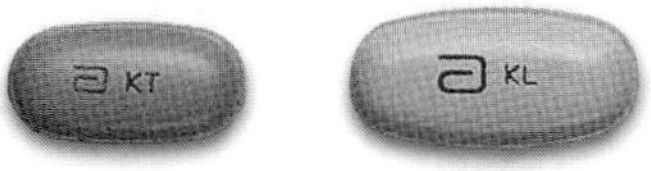

250 mg

500 mg

Bumex

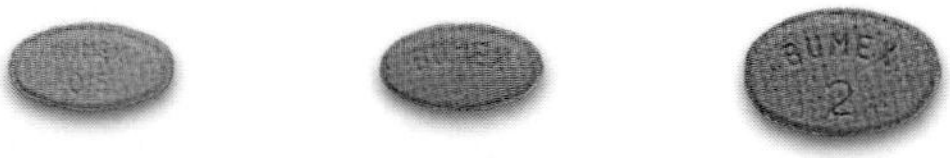

0.5 mg

1 mg

2 mg

BuSpar

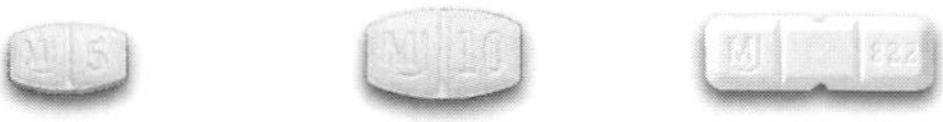

5 mg

10 mg

15 mg

Calan

40 mg   80 mg   120 mg

Capoten

12.5 mg   25 mg

Carafate

1 g

Cardizem

30 mg   60 mg   90 mg

Cardizem CD
(extended-release)

120 mg   180 mg   240 mg

Cardura

1 mg   2 mg   4 mg

Ceclor

250 mg   500 mg

Ceftin

250 mg   500 mg

Cefzil

250 mg

cephalexin

250 mg   500 mg

cimetidine

300 mg   400 mg

Cipro

250 mg   500 mg   750 mg

Claritin

10 mg

Compazine

5 mg   10 mg

Cordarone

200 mg

Coreg

3.125 mg   6.25 mg   12.5 mg

25 mg

Coumadin

1 mg   2 mg   2.5 mg

5 mg   7.5 mg   10 mg

Cozaar

25 mg   50 mg

**cyclobenzaprine
hydrochloride**

10 mg

Darvocet-N 100

100 mg/650 mg

Daypro

600 mg

Deltasone

2.5 mg   5 mg   10 mg

20 mg

Depakote
(delayed-release)

125 mg   250 mg   500 mg

Depakote Sprinkle

125 mg

DiaBeta

1.25 mg   2.5 mg   5 mg

Diflucan

100 mg   150 mg   200 mg

Dilacor XR

180 mg   240 mg

Dilantin Infatabs

50 mg

Dilantin Kapseals

30 mg   100 mg

doxepin hydrochloride

75 mg

Duricef

500 mg

Dyazide

25 mg/37.5 mg

E.E.S.

400 mg

Effexor

25 mg	37.5 mg	50 mg
75 mg	100 mg	

E-Mycin
(delayed-release)

250 mg	333 mg

Ery-Tab
(delayed-release)

250 mg	333 mg

Erythrocin Stearate Filmtab

250 mg

Erythromycin Base Filmtab

250 mg	500 mg

Estrace

1 mg	2 mg

Fiorinal with Codeine

325 mg aspirin, 50 mg butalbital, 40 mg caffeine, 30 mg codeine phosphate

Floxin

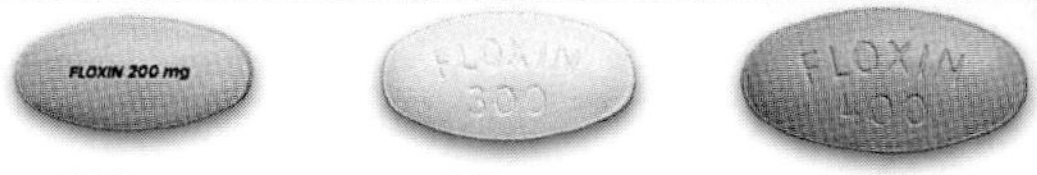

| 200 mg | 300 mg | 400 mg |

Fosamax

| 10 mg | 40 mg |

furosemide

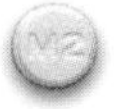

20 mg

glipizide

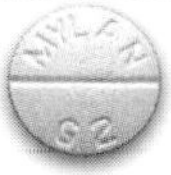

10 mg

Glucophage

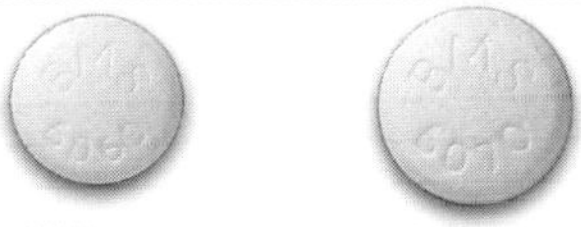

| 500 mg | 850 mg |

Glucotrol

| 5 mg | 10 mg |

Glucotrol XL

| 5 mg | 10 mg |

Glynase

| 3 mg | 6 mg |

hydrocodone bitartrate and acetaminophen

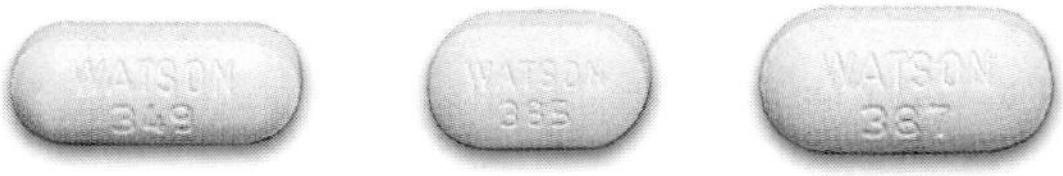

| 5 mg/500 mg | 7.5 mg/500 mg | 7.5 mg/750 mg |

Hytrin

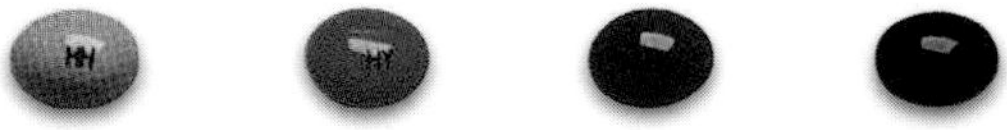

| 1 mg | 2 mg | 5 mg | 10 mg |

ibuprofen

IBU 400	IBU 600	IBU 800
400 mg	600 mg	800 mg

Inderal

10 mg	20 mg	40 mg

60 mg

K-Dur

10 mEq	20 mEq

Klonopin

0.5 mg	1 mg	2 mg

Lanoxin

0.125 mg	0.25 mg

Lasix

20 mg	40 mg

Levoxyl

0.025 mg	0.05 mg	0.075 mg
0.088 mg	0.1 mg	0.112 mg
0.125 mg	0.137 mg	0.15 mg
0.175 mg	0.2 mg	0.3 mg

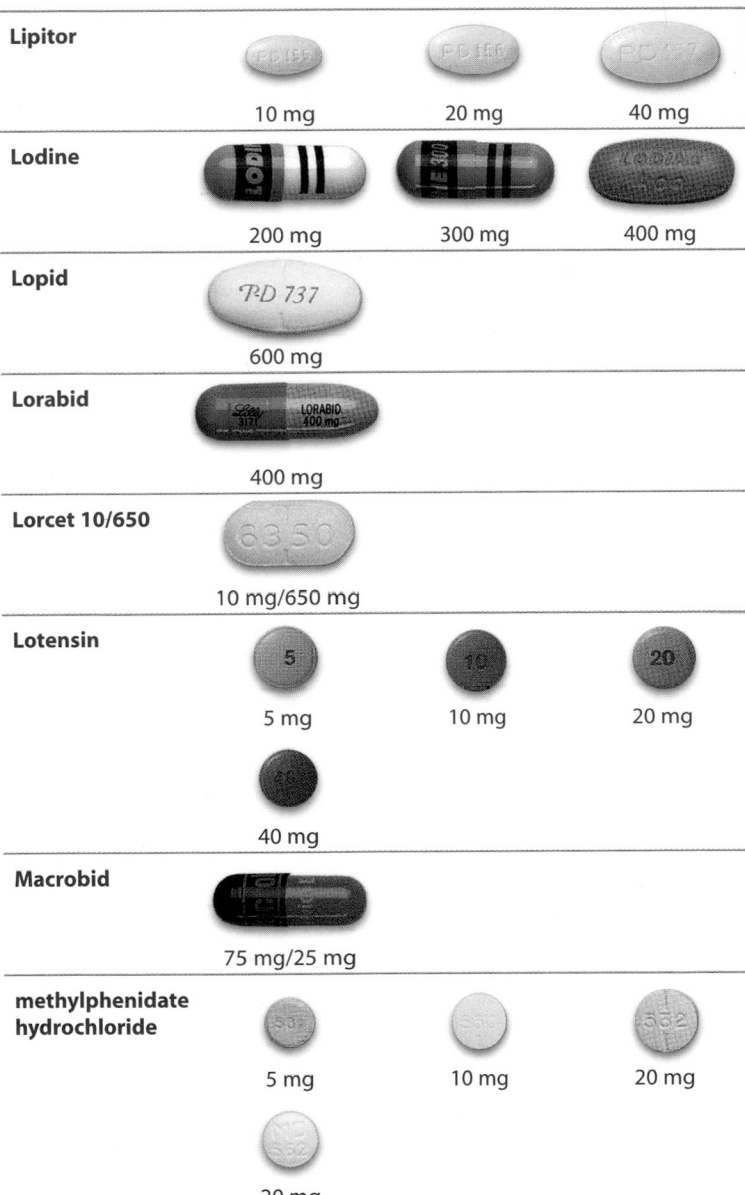

Lipitor

10 mg   20 mg   40 mg

Lodine

200 mg   300 mg   400 mg

Lopid

600 mg

Lorabid

400 mg

Lorcet 10/650

10 mg/650 mg

Lotensin

5 mg   10 mg   20 mg

40 mg

Macrobid

75 mg/25 mg

methylphenidate hydrochloride

5 mg   10 mg   20 mg

20 mg
(extended-release)

Mevacor

| 10 mg | 20 mg | 40 mg |

Micronase

| 2.5 mg | 5 mg |

Motrin

| 400 mg | 600 mg | 800 mg |

Naprosyn

| 250 mg | 375 mg | 500 mg |

naproxen

| 375 mg | 500 mg |

Nitrostat

| 0.3 mg | 0.4 mg | 0.6 mg |

Nolvadex

| 10 mg |

nortriptyline hydrochloride

| 10 mg | 25 mg | 50 mg |

Norvasc

| 5 mg | 10 mg |

Oruvail

| 100 mg | 150 mg | 200 mg |

Pamelor

10 mg   25 mg   50 mg

75 mg

Paxil

20 mg   30 mg

PCE

333 mg   500 mg

Pepcid

20 mg   40 mg

Percocet

5 mg/325 mg

potassium chloride

10 mEq
(extended-release)

Pravachol

10 mg   20 mg   40 mg

Premarin

0.3 mg   0.625 mg   0.9 mg

1.25 mg   2.5 mg

Prevacid

15 mg | 30 mg

Prilosec

10 mg | 20 mg

Prinivil

5 mg | 10 mg | 20 mg

Procardia XL
(extended-release)

30 mg | 60 mg | 90 mg

propoxyphene napsylate with acetaminophen

100 mg/650 mg

Propulsid

10 mg

Provera

2.5 mg | 5 mg | 10 mg

Prozac

10 mg | 20 mg

Relafen

500 mg | 750 mg

Risperdal

1 mg | 2 mg | 3 mg

4 mg

Roxicet

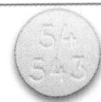

5 mg/325 mg

Sinemet

 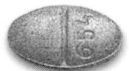

10 mg/100 mg   25 mg/250 mg

Sinemet CR

25 mg/100 mg
(extended-release)

Slo-bid Gyrocaps
(extended-release)

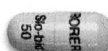   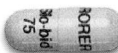   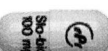

50 mg   75 mg   100 mg

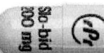   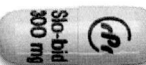

200 mg   300 mg

Sumycin

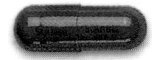

250 mg

Synthroid

25 mcg   50 mcg   75 mcg

88 mcg   100 mcg   112 mcg

125 mcg   150 mcg   175 mcg

200 mcg   300 mcg

Tagamet

        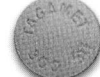

200 mg   300 mg

Tenormin

| 25 mg | 50 mg | 100 mg |

Theo-Dur
(extended-release)

| 100 mg | 200 mg | 300 mg |

450 mg

Ticlid

250 mg

Toprol XL

| 50 mg | 100 mg | 200 mg |

Toradol

10 mg

Trental

400 mg

Trimox

| 250 mg | 500 mg |

Tylenol with Codeine No. 3

300 mg/30 mg

Ultram

50 mg

Valium

| 2 mg | 5 mg | 10 mg |

Vasotec

2.5 mg   5 mg   10 mg

20 mg

Veetids

250 mg   500 mg

**verapamil
hydrochloride**

180 mg
(sustained-release)

Verelan
(sustained-release)

120 mg   240 mg

Vicodin

5 mg/500 mg

Vicodin ES

7.5 mg/750 mg

Xanax

0.25 mg   0.5 mg   1 mg

Zantac

150 mg   300 mg

Zantac EFFERdose

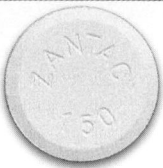

150 mg

Zestril

5 mg

10 mg

20 mg

40 mg

Zithromax

250 mg

Zocor

5 mg

10 mg

20 mg

Zoloft

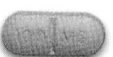

50 mg

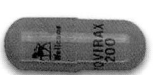

100 mg

Zovirax

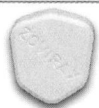

200 mg

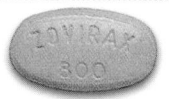

400 mg

800 mg

Zyrtec

5 mg

10 mg

Patient teaching
• Recommend that patient have periodic ophthalmic examinations during treatment.
• Advise patient not to discontinue drug prematurely. Tell him to notify doctor if rash occurs.
• To help prevent reinfestation, emphasize personal hygiene, especially good hand-washing technique. Encourage patient not to prepare food for others until stools are negative.

☑ **Evaluation**
• Patient is free from infection.
• Visual complications do not develop.
• Patient and family state understanding of drug therapy.

ipecac syrup
(IH-pee-kak SIH-rup)
Pharmacologic class: alkaloid emetic
Therapeutic class: emetic
Pregnancy risk category: C

How supplied

*Syrup:** 70 mg powdered ipecac/ml (contains glycerin 10% and alcohol 1% to 2.5%)†

Pharmacokinetics

Absorption: absorbed in significant amounts mainly when it does not produce emesis.
Distribution: unknown.
Metabolism: unknown.
Excretion: slowly excreted in urine.

Route	Onset	Peak	Duration
P.O.	20-30 min	Unknown	20-25 min

Pharmacodynamics

Chemical effect: induces vomiting by acting locally on gastric mucosa and centrally on the chemoreceptor trigger zone.
Therapeutic effect: induces vomiting.

Indications and dosage

▶ **To induce vomiting in poisoning.**
Adults and children age 12 and older: 30 ml P.O., followed by 200 to 300 ml of water. *Children ages 6 months to 1 year:* 5 ml P.O., followed by 100 to 200 ml of water or milk. If necessary, repeat dose once after 20 minutes. *Children ages 1 to 12:* 15 ml P.O., followed by about 200 ml of water or milk.

Adverse reactions

CNS: depression.
CV: *arrhythmias,* bradycardia, hypotension, atrial fibrillation, *fatal myocarditis* (after excessive dose).
GI: diarrhea.

Interactions

Drug-drug. *Activated charcoal:* neutralized emetic effect. Don't give together; may give activated charcoal after vomiting.

Contraindications and precautions

• Contraindicated in semicomatose or unconscious patients, or in those with severe inebriation, seizures, shock, or loss of gag reflex. Do not use if strychnine corrosives such as alkalies and strong acids, or petroleum distillates have been ingested.

NURSING CONSIDERATIONS

⚎ **Assessment**
• Obtain assessment of patient's substance ingestion before therapy.
• Monitor effectiveness by observing patient for vomiting. Know that ipecac syrup usually induces vomiting within 20 to 30 minutes. In antiemetic toxicity, ipecac syrup is usually effective if less than 1 hour has passed since ingestion of antiemetic.
• Be aware that no systemic toxicity occurs with doses of 30 ml or less.
• Monitor blood pressure, ECG, and fluid and electrolyte balance.

• Be alert for adverse reactions and drug interactions.
• Evaluate patient's and family's knowledge of drug therapy.

✣ Nursing diagnoses
• Altered health maintenance related to ingestion of poisonous substance
• Decreased cardiac output related to adverse cardiac reactions
• Knowledge deficit related to drug therapy

⊠ Planning and implementation
• Unless advised otherwise by poison control center, don't give after ingestion of petroleum distillates (for example, kerosene, gasoline) or volatile oils; retching and vomiting may cause aspiration and lead to bronchospasm, pulmonary edema, or aspiration pneumonitis. Vegetable oil will delay absorption of these substances. Don't give after ingestion of caustic substances, such as lye; additional injury to esophagus and mediastinum can occur.
• Clearly indicate ipecac *syrup,* not single word "ipecac," to avoid confusion with fluid extract, which is 14 times more concentrated and, if inadvertently used instead of syrup, may cause death. Fluid extract is no longer commercially available in United States.
• Follow dose with 200 to 300 ml of water.
• If two doses do not induce vomiting, be prepared for gastric lavage.
• Position patient on side to prevent aspiration of vomitus. Have airway and suction equipment nearby.
Patient teaching
• Recommend that parents keep 1 oz (30 ml) of syrup available in home for use in emergency when child reaches age 1.

✓ Evaluation
• Patient regains health after elimination of poisonous substance.
• Patient's cardiac output remains adequate.

• Patient and family state understanding of drug therapy.

---

ipratropium bromide
(ip-ruh-TROH-pee-um BROH-mighd)
Atrovent

Pharmacologic class: anticholinergic
Therapeutic class: bronchodilator
Pregnancy risk category: B

How supplied
Inhaler: each metered dose supplies 18 mcg
Solution (for nebulizer): 0.025% (250 mcg/ml)◊, 0.02% (200 mcg/ml)
Nasal spray: 0.03% (21 mcg), 0.06% (42 mcg)

Pharmacokinetics
Absorption: drug is not readily absorbed into systemic circulation.
Distribution: not applicable.
Metabolism: small amount that is absorbed is metabolized in liver.
Excretion: absorbed drug excreted in urine and bile; remainder excreted unchanged in feces. *Half-life:* about 2 hours.

Route	Onset	Peak	Duration
Inhalation	5-15 min	1-2 hr	3-6 hr

Pharmacodynamics
Chemical effect: inhibits vagally mediated reflexes by antagonizing acetylcholine.
Therapeutic effect: relieves bronchospasms and symptoms of seasonal allergic rhinitis.

Indications and dosage
▶ **Bronchospasm associated with COPD.** *Adults:* 1 to 2 inhalations q.i.d. Additional inhalations may be needed. However, total inhalations should not exceed 12 in 24 hours. Alternatively, use inhalation solution, where available, giving

---

Reactions may be *common,* uncommon, *life-threatening,* or COMMON AND LIFE-THREATENING.

up to 500 mcg every 6 to 8 hours via oral nebulizer.
▶ **Rhinorrhea associated with allergic and nonallergic perennial rhinitis (0.03% nasal spray).** *Adults and children age 6 and older:* 2 sprays in each nostril b.i.d. or t.i.d (total dosage 168 to 252 mcg/day).
▶ **Rhinorrhea associated with the common cold (0.06% nasal spray).** *Adults and children age 12 and over:* 2 sprays per nostril t.i.d. or q.i.d. (total dosage 504 to 672 mcg/day). *Children ages 5 to 11:* 2 sprays (84 mcg) per nostril t.i.d. (total dosage 504 mcg/day).

Adverse reactions

CNS: nervousness, dizziness, headache.
CV: palpitations.
EENT: cough, blurred vision, epistaxis.
GI: nausea, GI distress, dry mouth.
Respiratory: *upper respiratory tract infection, bronchitis, bronchospasm.*
Skin: rash.

Interactions

Drug-drug. *Anticholinergics:* increased anticholinergic effects. Avoid concomitant use.
Cromolyn sodium: will form precipitate if mixed in same nebulizer. Don't use together.

Contraindications and precautions

• Contraindicated in patients with hypersensitivity to drug or to atropine or its derivatives and in those with history of hypersensitivity to soyalecithin or related food products such as soybeans and peanuts.
• Use cautiously in patients with angle-closure glaucoma, prostatic hyperplasia, or bladder-neck obstruction and in pregnant or breast-feeding women.
• Safety of drug has not been established in children under age 6 for rhinorrhea associated with allergic and non-allergic perennial rhinitis.

• The safety and efficacy of use beyond 4 days in patients treated for rhinorrhea associated with the common cold has not been established.

NURSING CONSIDERATIONS

☙ Assessment
• Assess patient's condition before and after drug administration.
• Be alert for adverse reactions and drug interactions.
• Evaluate patient's and family's knowledge of drug therapy.

⊕ Nursing diagnoses
• Ineffective breathing pattern related to patient's underlying condition
• Pain related to drug-induced headache
• Knowledge deficit related to drug therapy

⧐ Planning and implementation
• Drug is not effective for treatment of acute episodes of bronchospasm when rapid response is required.
• Know that total inhalations should not exceed 12 in 24 hours and total nasal sprays should not exceed 8 in each nostril in 24 hours.
• If more than one inhalation is ordered, 2 minutes should elapse between inhalations. If more than one type of inhalant is ordered, always give bronchodilator first and wait 5 minutes before giving the other.
• Be sure to give medication on time to ensure maximal effect.
• Notify doctor if bronchospasms are not relieved with drug.
Patient teaching
• Warn patient that drug is not effective for treating acute episodes of bronchospasm where rapid response is required.
• Give patient these instructions for using metered-dose inhaler: Clear nasal passages and throat. Breathe out, expelling as much air from lungs as possible. Place mouthpiece well into mouth as dose from inhaler is released, and inhale deeply.

---

*Liquid form contains alcohol   **May contain tartrazine   ♦Canada   ◊ Australia   †OTC

Hold breath for several seconds, remove mouthpiece, and exhale slowly.
• Tell patient to avoid accidentally spraying into eyes. Temporary blurring of vision may result.
• If more than one inhalation is ordered, tell patient to wait at least 2 minutes before repeating procedure.
• Tell patient also using steroid inhaler to use ipratropium first, then wait about 5 minutes before using steroid. This allows bronchodilator to open air passages for maximum effectiveness.
• Tell patient to take missed dose as soon as remembered, unless it's almost time for next dose. In that case, skip missed dose. Do not double-dose.
• Advise patient to use sugarless hard candy or gum or saliva substitute to relieve dry mouth.

☑ **Evaluation**
• Patient's bronchospasms are relieved.
• Patient's drug-induced headache is relieved with mild analgesic.
• Patient and family state understanding of drug therapy.

---

irbesartan
(ir-buh-SAR-tun)
Avapro

Pharmacologic class: angiotensin II receptor antagonist
Therapeutic class: antihypertensive
Pregnancy risk category: C (D in second and third trimesters)

How supplied

Tablets: 75 mg, 150 mg, 300 mg

Pharmacokinetics

Absorption: rapid and complete with an average absolute bioavailability of 60% to 80%.
Distribution: widely distributed into body tissues; 90% bound to plasma proteins.

Metabolism: metabolized primarily by conjugation and oxidation.
Excretion: excreted by biliary and renal routes. Approximately 20% is recovered in urine and rest is recovered in feces.
Half-life: 11 to 15 hours.

Route	Onset	Peak	Duration
P.O.	Unknown	1.5-2 hr	24 hr

Pharmacodynamics

Chemical effect: inhibits the vasoconstricting and aldosterone-secreting effects of angiotensin II by selectively blocking binding of angiotension II to its receptor sites that are found in many tissues.
Therapeutic effect: lowers blood pressure.

Indications and dosages

▶ **Hypertension.** *Adults:* initially 150 mg P.O. daily, increased to a maximum of 300 mg daily if necessary.

Adverse reactions

CNS: fatigue, anxiety, dizziness, headache.
CV: chest pain, edema, tachycardia.
EENT: pharyngitis, rhinitis, sinus abnormality.
GI: diarrhea, dyspepsia, abdominal pain, nausea, vomiting.
GU: urinary tract infection.
Musculoskeletal: musculoskeletal trauma or pain.
Respiratory: upper respiratory infection.
Skin: rash.

Interactions

None reported.

Contraindications and precautions

• Contraindicated in patients hypersensitive to drug or its components.
• Use in pregnancy can cause injury and death to the developing fetus. When pregnancy is detected, drug should be discontinued as soon as possible.

Reactions may be *common*, uncommon, *life-threatening*, or COMMON AND LIFE-THREATENING.

• Use cautiously in volume- or salt-depleted patients, in patients with impaired renal function, or renal artery stenosis.

NURSING CONSIDERATIONS

Assessment
• Monitor patient's blood pressure regularly.
• Monitor patient's electrolytes and assess patient for volume or salt depletion prior to initiation of drug therapy.
• Assess whether female patients of childbearing age are using effective birth control methods prior to taking this medication because of the potential danger of the drug to the fetus.
• Evaluate patient's and family's knowledge of drug therapy.

Nursing diagnoses
• Risk for hypotension in volume- or salt-depleted patients
• Risk of injury related to the presence of hypertension
• Knowledge deficit related to drug therapy

Planning and implementation
• Know that drug may be administered with a diuretic or other antihypertensive if necessary for control of blood pressure.
• If patient becomes hypotensive, place in a supine position and give an I.V. infusion of 0.9% NaCl solution, as ordered.
Patient teaching
• Warn female patient of childbearing age about consequences of exposure of the fetus to drug. Tell her to call doctor immediately if pregnancy is suspected.
• Tell patient that drug may be taken once daily with or without food.
• Instruct patient to avoid driving and hazardous activities until CNS effects are known.

Evaluation
• Patient does not experience hypotension as a result of volume- or salt-depletion.

• Patient's blood pressure remains within normal limits and no injury is suffered as a result of drug therapy.
• Patient and family state understanding of drug therapy.

iron dextran
(IGH-ern DEKS-tran)
DexFerrum, Dexiron♦, InFeD

Pharmacologic class: parenteral iron supplement
Therapeutic class: hematinic
Pregnancy risk category: NR

How supplied
1 ml iron dextran provides 50 mg elemental iron.
Injection: 50 mg elemental iron/ml

Pharmacokinetics
Absorption: I.M. doses are absorbed in two stages: 60% after 3 days and up to 90% by 3 weeks. Remainder is absorbed over several months or longer.
Distribution: during first 3 days, local inflammation facilitates passage of drug into lymphatic system; drug is then ingested by macrophages, which enter lymph and blood.
Metabolism: drug is cleared from plasma by reticuloendothelial cells of liver, spleen, and bone marrow.
Excretion: trace amounts excreted in urine, bile, and feces. *Half-life:* 6 hours.

Route	Onset	Peak	Duration
I.V., I.M.	Unknown	Unknown	Unknown

Pharmacodynamics
Chemical effect: provides elemental iron, a component of hemoglobin.
Therapeutic effect: increases plasma iron concentration, an essential component of hemoglobin.

Indications and dosage

▶ **Iron-deficiency anemia.** *Adults and children:* dosage is individualized and based on patient's weight and hemoglobin level. I.M. or I.V. test dose required before administration. **I.M. (by Z-track method):** 0.5 ml test dose injected. If no reactions occur, daily dosage should ordinarily not exceed 0.5 ml (25 mg) for infants weighing under 5 kg (11 lb); 1 ml (50 mg) for children weighing under 10 kg (22 lb); 2 ml (100 mg) for heavier children and adults. **I.V.:** 0.5 ml test dose injected over 30 seconds. If no reactions occur in 1 hour, remainder of therapeutic dose I.V. is given. Therapeutic dose repeated I.V. daily. Single dose should not exceed 100 mg. Give slowly (1 ml/minute).

Adverse reactions

CNS: headache, transitory paresthesia, arthralgia, myalgia, dizziness, malaise, syncope.
CV: chest pain, chest tightness, shock, hypertension, arrhythmias, *hypotensive reaction, peripheral vascular flushing with overly rapid I.V. administration, tachycardia.*
GI: nausea, vomiting, metallic taste, transient loss of taste, abdominal pain, diarrhea.
Respiratory: *bronchospasm.*
Skin: rash, urticaria.
Other: *soreness, inflammation, brown skin discoloration* (at I.M. injection site); *local phlebitis* (at I.V. injection site); sterile abscess, necrosis, atrophy, fibrosis, *anaphylaxis,* delayed sensitivity reactions.

Interactions

None significant.

Contraindications and precautions

• Contraindicated in patients with acute infectious renal disease, anemia disorders except iron-deficiency anemia, or hypersensitivity to drug.

• Use with extreme caution in patients with serious hepatic impairment, rheumatoid arthritis, and other inflammatory diseases because these patients may be at higher risk for certain delays and reactions.
• Use cautiously in patients with history of significant allergies or asthma.

NURSING CONSIDERATIONS

⚕ Assessment
• Obtain assessment of patient's iron deficiency before therapy.
• Monitor effectiveness by evaluating hemoglobin concentration, hematocrit, and reticulocyte count, and monitor patient's health status.
• Be alert for adverse reactions and drug interactions.
• Observe patient for delayed reactions (1 to 2 days), which may include arthralgia, backache, chills, dizziness, headache, malaise, fever, myalgia, nausea, and vomiting.
• Evaluate patient's and family's knowledge of drug therapy.

⚑ Nursing diagnoses
• Altered health maintenance related to iron deficiency
• Risk for injury related to potential drug-induced anaphylaxis
• Knowledge deficit related to drug therapy

❯ Planning and implementation
• Do not administer iron dextran concomitantly with oral iron preparations.
• Keep in mind that I.M. or I.V. injections of iron are recommended only for patients for whom oral administration is impossible or ineffective.
I.V. use: Check institutional policy before administering I.V.
– Use I.V. in these situations: Insufficient muscle mass for deep I.M. injection; impaired absorption from muscle as a result of stasis or edema; possibility of uncon-

---

trolled I.M. bleeding from trauma (as may occur in hemophilia); and with massive and prolonged parenteral therapy (as may be necessary in chronic substantial blood loss).
– Upon completion of I.V. dose, flush vein with 10 ml of 0.9% NaCl solution. The patient should rest 15 to 30 minutes after I.V. administration.
I.M. use: Inject deeply into upper outer quadrant of buttock—never into arm or other exposed area—with 2″ to 3″, 19G or 20G needle. Use Z-track method to avoid leakage into S.C. tissue and staining of skin.
• Minimize skin staining by using separate needle to withdraw drug from its container.
• Keep epinephrine and resuscitation equipment readily available to treat anaphylaxis.
Patient teaching
• Warn patient to avoid OTC vitamins that include iron.
• Teach patient to recognize and report symptoms of reaction or toxicity.

☑ Evaluation
• Patient's hemoglobin, hematocrit, and reticulocyte counts are normal.
• Patient does not experience anaphylaxis.
• Patient and family state understanding of drug therapy.

isoetharine hydrochloride
**(igh-soh-ETH-ah-reen
high-droh-KLOR-ighd)**
Arm-a-Med Isoetharine, Bronkosol

isoetharine mesylate
Bronkometer

Pharmacologic class: adrenergic
Therapeutic class: bronchodilator
Pregnancy risk category: NR

How supplied
Aerosol inhaler: 340 mcg/metered spray
Nebulizer inhaler: 0.062%, 0.08%, 0.1%, 0.125%, 0.167%, 0.17%, 0.2%, 0.25%, 0.5%, 1% solution

Pharmacokinetics
Absorption: absorbed rapidly from respiratory tract.
Distribution: distributed widely throughout body.
Metabolism: metabolized in lungs, liver, GI tract, and other tissues.
Excretion: excreted in urine.

Route	Onset	Peak	Duration
Inhalation	1-6 min	15-60 min	1-4 hr

Pharmacodynamics
Chemical effect: relaxes bronchial smooth muscle by acting on beta$_2$-adrenergic receptors.
Therapeutic effect: relieves bronchospasms.

Indications and dosage
▶ **Bronchial asthma and reversible bronchospasm that may occur with bronchitis and emphysema.** *Adults:* hydrochloride form—administered by hand nebulizer, oxygen aerosolization, or IPPB; use chart below.

Method	Dose	Dilutions
Hand nebulizer	3 to 7 inhalations	Undiluted
Oxygen aerosolization	0.5 ml	1:3 with saline
IPPB	0.5 ml	1:3 with saline

mesylate form—1 to 2 inhalations. Occasionally, more may be required.

Adverse reactions
CNS: *tremor, headache,* dizziness, excitement.
CV: *palpitations,* increased heart rate, alterations in blood pressure.
GI: nausea, vomiting.

Interactions

Drug-drug. *Cardiac glycosides, cyclopropane, halogenated inhalation anesthetics, levodopa:* increased risk of arrhythmias. Monitor closely.
Epinephrine, other sympathomimetic agents: may cause excessive tachycardia. Should not be used together with isoetharine.
Propranolol, other beta blockers: blocked bronchodilating effect of isoetharine. Monitor patient carefully.

Contraindications and precautions

• Contraindicated in patients with hypersensitivity to drug.
• Use cautiously in pregnant or breast-feeding women and in those with hyperthyroidism, hypertension, coronary disease, or hypersensitivity to sympathomimetics.
• Although isoetharine has minimal effects on heart, it should be used cautiously in patients receiving general anesthetics that sensitize myocardium to sympathomimetic drugs.
• Safety of drug has not been established in children.

NURSING CONSIDERATIONS

⚕ Assessment

• Assess patient's respiratory condition before therapy.
• Monitor effectiveness by auscultating lungs, noting respiratory rate and results of laboratory studies, such as arterial blood gases.
• Be alert for adverse reactions and drug interactions.
• Monitor for severe paradoxical bronchoconstriction after excessive use.
• Monitor patient's hydration status if adverse GI reactions occur.
• Evaluate patient's and family's knowledge of drug therapy.

⊞ Nursing diagnoses

• Ineffective breathing pattern related to respiratory condition

• Risk for fluid volume deficit related to adverse GI reactions
• Knowledge deficit related to drug therapy

⊠ Planning and implementation

• If bronchodilator is administered by inhalant and more than one inhalation is ordered, 2 minutes should elapse between inhalations. If more than one type of inhalant is ordered, always administer bronchodilator first and wait 5 minutes before administering the other.
• If bronchoconstriction occurs, discontinue immediately and notify doctor.
Patient teaching
• Give patient the following instructions for using metered-dose inhaler:
– Clear nasal passages and throat.
– Breathe out, expelling as much air from lungs as possible.
– Place mouthpiece well into mouth as dose from inhaler is released, and inhale deeply.
– Hold breath for several seconds, remove mouthpiece, and exhale slowly.
• If more than one inhalation is ordered, tell patient to wait at least 2 minutes before repeating procedure.
• Tell patient also using steroid inhaler to use bronchodilator first, then wait about 5 minutes before using steroid. This allows bronchodilator to open air passages for maximum effectiveness.
• Because of oxidation of drug when diluted with water, pink sputum mimicking hemoptysis may occur after inhaling isoetharine solution. Tell patient not to be concerned.
• Warn patient that excessive use can lead to decreased effectiveness.

☑ Evaluation

• Patient reports relief from respiratory symptoms.
• Patient maintains adequate hydration.
• Patient and family state understanding of drug therapy.

isoniazid (isonicotinic acid hydride INH)
(igh-soh-NIGH-uh-sid)
Isotamine♦, Laniazid, Nydrazid**,
PMS Isoniazid♦

Pharmacologic class: isonicotinic acid hydrazine
Therapeutic class: antitubercular
Pregnancy risk category: C

How supplied

Tablets: 50 mg, 100 mg, 300 mg
Oral solution: 50 mg/5 ml
Injection: 100 mg/ml

Pharmacokinetics

Absorption: absorbed completely and rapidly from GI tract after oral administration. Also absorbed readily after I.M. injection.
Distribution: distributed widely into body tissues and fluids.
Metabolism: drug is inactivated primarily in liver. Rate of metabolism varies individually; fast acetylators metabolize drug five times as rapidly as others. About 50% of blacks and whites are slow acetylators of drug, whereas over 80% of Chinese, Japanese, and Eskimos are fast acetylators.
Excretion: excreted primarily in urine; some drug excreted in saliva, sputum, feces, and breast milk. *Half-life:* 1 to 4 hours.

Route	Onset	Peak	Duration
P.O., I.M.	Unknown	1-2 hr	Unknown

Pharmacodynamics

Chemical effect: appears to inhibit cell-wall biosynthesis by interfering with lipid and DNA synthesis.
Therapeutic effect: kills susceptible bacteria: *Mycobacterium tuberculosis, Mycobacterium bovis,* and some strains of *Mycobacterium kansasii.*

Indications and dosage

▶ **Actively growing tubercle bacilli.**
Adults: 5 mg/kg P.O. or I.M. daily in single dose, up to 300 mg/day, continued for 6 months to 2 years. *Infants and children:* 10 mg/kg P.O. or I.M. daily in single dose, up to 300 mg/day, continued for 18 months to 2 years. Concomitant administration of at least one other antitubercular drug is recommended.
▶ **Prevention of tubercle bacilli in those closely exposed to tuberculosis or those with positive skin test whose chest X-rays and bacteriologic studies are consistent with nonprogressive tuberculosis.** *Adults:* 300 mg P.O. daily in single dose, for 6 months to 1 year. *Infants and children:* 10 mg/kg P.O. daily in single dose, up to 300 mg/day, for 1 year.

Adverse reactions

CNS: *peripheral neuropathy* (especially in patients who are malnourished, alcoholic, diabetic, or slow acetylators), usually preceded by paresthesia of hands and feet; psychosis, *seizures.*
GI: nausea, vomiting, epigastric distress, constipation, mouth dryness.
Hematologic: *agranulocytosis,* hemolytic anemia, *aplastic anemia,* eosinophilia, leukopenia, neutropenia, *thrombocytopenia,* methemoglobinemia, pyridoxine-responsive hypochromic anemia.
Hepatic: *hepatitis* (occasionally severe and sometimes fatal, especially in elderly patients).
Metabolic: hyperglycemia, metabolic acidosis.
Other: rheumatic syndrome and lupus-like syndrome, *hypersensitivity reactions* (fever, rash, lymphadenopathy, vasculitis); irritation (at I.M. injection site).

Interactions

Drug-drug. *Acetaminophen:* increased hepatotoxic effects of acetaminophen. Do not administer together.
Aluminum-containing antacids and laxatives: may decrease rate and amount of

isoniazid absorbed. Give isoniazid at least 1 hour before antacid or laxative.
Carbamazepine: increased risk of isoniazid hepatotoxicity. Use together cautiously.
Carbamazepine, phenytoin: increased plasma levels of these anticonvulsants. Monitor closely.
Corticosteroids: may decrease therapeutic effect of isoniazid. Monitor need for larger isoniazid dose.
Cyclosporine: in combination with isoniazid may result in increased cyclosporine CNS side effects. Monitor closely.
Disulfiram: may cause neurologic symptoms, including changes in behavior and coordination. Avoid concomitant use.
Ketoconazole: decreased concentrations of ketoconazole. Monitor closely.
Oral anticoagulants: anticoagulant activity may be enhanced by concurrent isoniazid.
Rifampin: isoniazid combination may result in a higher ratio of hepatotoxicity than with either agent alone.
Theophylline: increased serum levels of theophylline. Monitor serum levels closely. Dosage adjustment of theophylline may be needed.
Drug-food. *Any food:* significantly decreased absorption. Take drug on an empty stomach.
Drug-lifestyle. *Alcohol use:* may be associated with increased incidence of isoniazid-related hepatitis. Avoid concomitant use.

Contraindications and precautions

• Contraindicated in patients with acute hepatic disease or isoniazid-associated liver damage.
• Use cautiously in patients with chronic non-isoniazid-associated liver disease, seizure disorders (especially in those taking phenytoin), severe renal impairment, or chronic alcoholism; in elderly patients; and in pregnant or breast-feeding women.

NURSING CONSIDERATIONS

✒ Assessment
• Obtain assessment of patient's infection before therapy.
• Monitor for improvement, and evaluate culture and sensitivity tests.
• Be alert for adverse reactions and drug interactions.
• Monitor hepatic function closely for changes.
• Monitor patient for paresthesia of hands and feet, which usually precede peripheral neuropathy, especially in patients who are malnourished, alcoholic, or diabetic, or who are slow acetylators.
• Evaluate patient's and family's knowledge of drug therapy.

⊞ Nursing diagnoses
• Infection related to presence of susceptible bacteria
• Sensory or perceptual alterations (tactile) related to drug-induced peripheral neuropathy
• Knowledge deficit related to drug therapy

▶ Planning and implementation
P.O. use: Give drug 1 hour before or 2 hours after meals to avoid decreased absorption of drug.
I.M. use: Follow normal protocol. Switch from P.O. form as soon as possible.
• Be aware that isoniazid should always be administered with other antitubercular agents to prevent development of resistant organisms.
• Administer pyridoxine, as ordered, to prevent peripheral neuropathy, especially in malnourished patients.
Patient teaching
• Tell patient to take drug as prescribed; warn against discontinuing drug without doctor's consent.
• Advise patient to take with food if GI irritation occurs.
• Instruct patient to avoid alcohol consumption during drug therapy.

Reactions may be *common*, uncommon, *life-threatening*, or COMMON AND LIFE-THREATENING.

• Tell patient to notify doctor immediately if symptoms of liver impairment occur (loss of appetite, fatigue, malaise, jaundice, dark urine).
• Urge patient to comply with treatment, which may take months or years.

☑ **Evaluation**
• Patient is free from infection.
• Patient maintains normal peripheral nervous system function.
• Patient and family state understanding of drug therapy.

isoproterenol (isoprenaline)
(igh-soh-proh-TEER-uh-nol)
Dispos-a-Med Isoproterenol, Isuprel

isoproterenol hydrochloride
Isuprel, Isuprel Glossets, Isuprel Mistometer, Norisodrine

isoproterenol sulfate
Medihaler-Iso

Pharmacologic class: adrenergic
Therapeutic class: bronchodilator, cardiac stimulant
Pregnancy risk category: C

How supplied

isoproterenol
Nebulizer inhaler: 0.25%, 0.5%, 1%
isoproterenol hydrochloride
Tablets (S.L.): 10 mg, 15 mg
Aerosol inhaler: 131 mcg/metered spray
Injection: 20 mcg/ml, 200 mcg/ml
isoproterenol sulfate
Aerosol inhaler: 80 mcg/metered spray

Pharmacokinetics

Absorption: variable and often unreliable after S.L. administration. Rapid after oral inhalation.
Distribution: distributed widely throughout body.

Metabolism: by conjugation in GI tract and by enzymatic reduction in liver, lungs, and other tissues.
Excretion: primarily in urine.

Route	Onset	Peak	Duration
P.O., inhalation	2-5 min	Unknown	0.5-2 hr
I.V.	Immediate	Unknown	< 1 hr
S.L.	15-30 min	Unknown	1-2 hr

Pharmacodynamics

Chemical effect: relaxes bronchial smooth muscle by acting on beta$_2$-adrenergic receptors. As cardiac stimulant, acts on beta$_1$-adrenergic receptors in heart.
Therapeutic effect: relieves bronchospasms and heart block and restores normal sinus rhythm after ventricular arrhythmia is present.

Indications and dosage

▶ **Bronchial asthma and reversible bronchospasm.** *Adults:* 10 to 15 mg hydrochloride S.L. q 6 to 8 hours. Daily S.L. dosage should not exceed 60 mg. *Children:* 5 to 10 mg hydrochloride S.L. q 8 hours. Daily S.L. dosage should not exceed 30 mg.
▶ **Bronchospasm.** *Adults and children:* acute dyspneic episodes: 1 inhalation of sulfate form initially. Repeated if needed after 2 to 5 minutes. Maintenance dosage is 1 to 2 inhalations q.i.d. to six times daily. Repeated once more 10 minutes after second dose. No more than three doses should be given for each attack.
▶ **Bronchospasm in COPD.** Administered by IPPB or for nebulization by compressed air or oxygen. *Adults:* 2 ml of 0.125% or 2.5 ml of 0.1% solution (prepared by diluting 0.5 ml of 0.5% solution to 2 or 2.5 ml or by diluting 0.25 ml of 1% solution to 2 or 2.5 ml with water or 0.45% or 0.9% NaCl solution) up to five times daily. *Children:* 2 ml of 0.125% solution or 2.5 ml of 0.1% solution up to five times daily.
▶ **Heart block and ventricular arrhythmias.** *Adults:* (hydrochloride) initially,

0.02 to 0.06 mg I.V. Subsequent doses 0.01 to 0.2 mg I.V. or 5 mcg/minute I.V.; or 0.2 mg I.M. initially, then 0.02 to 1 mg, p.r.n. *Children:* (hydrochloride) half of initial adult dose may be given.

▶ **Shock.** *Adults and children:* (hydrochloride) 0.5 to 5 mcg/minute by continuous I.V. infusion. Usual concentration is 1 mg (5 ml) in 500 ml D_5W. Rate adjusted according to heart rate, CVP, blood pressure, and urine flow.

Adverse reactions

CNS: *headache,* mild tremor, weakness, dizziness, nervousness, insomnia, *Stokes-Adams seizures.*
CV: *palpitations, tachycardia, anginal pain,* **cardiac arrest,** *blood pressure may rise and then fall,* **arrhythmias.**
GI: nausea, vomiting.
Metabolic: hyperglycemia.
Respiratory: *bronchospasm.*
Other: diaphoresis, flushing of face.

Interactions

Drug-drug. *Epinephrine, other sympathomimetics:* increased risk of arrhythmias. Avoid concomitant use.
Propranolol, other beta blockers: blocked bronchodilating effect of isoproterenol. Monitor patient carefully if used together.

Contraindications and precautions

• Contraindicated in patients with tachycardia caused by digitalis intoxication; preexisting arrhythmias (other than those that may respond to treatment with isoproterenol); or angina pectoris.
• Use cautiously in elderly patients; in patients with renal or CV disease, coronary insufficiency, diabetes, hyperthyroidism, or history of sensitivity to sympathomimetic amines; in pregnant or breast-feeding women; and in children.

NURSING CONSIDERATIONS

⚕ **Assessment**
• Obtain assessment of patient's underlying condition before therapy.

• Monitor cardiopulmonary status frequently.
• Be alert for adverse reactions and drug interactions.
• Keep in mind that this drug may aggravate ventilation and perfusion abnormalities; even while ease of breathing is improved, arterial oxygen tension may fall paradoxically.
• Evaluate patient's and family's knowledge of drug therapy.

⊕ **Nursing diagnoses**
• Altered health maintenance related to underlying condition
• Risk for injury related to drug-induced adverse reactions
• Knowledge deficit related to drug therapy

▷ **Planning and implementation**
• Know that drug is not substitute for blood or fluid volume deficit. Volume deficit should be corrected before administering vasopressors.
• Do not use injection or inhalation solution if it is discolored or contains precipitate.
P.O. and S.L. use: Follow normal protocol.
I.V. use: Give drug by direct injection or I.V. infusion. For infusion, drug may be diluted with most common I.V. solutions. However, do not use with sodium bicarbonate injection; drug decomposes rapidly in alkaline solutions.
– If heart rate exceeds 110 beats/minute with I.V. infusion, notify doctor. Doses sufficient to increase heart rate to more than 130 beats/minute may induce ventricular arrhythmias.
– When administering I.V. isoproterenol to treat shock, closely monitor blood pressure, CVP, ECG, arterial blood gas measurements, and urine output. Carefully adjust infusion rate according to these measurements, as ordered. Use continuous infusion pump to regulate flow rate.

Inhalation use: If drug is administered by inhalation with oxygen, be sure oxygen concentration will not suppress respiratory drive.
– Follow same instructions for metered powder nebulizer, although deep inhalation is not necessary.
• Notify doctor if adverse reactions occur. Dosage adjustment or discontinuation of drug may be required.
• Stop drug immediately if precordial distress or anginal pain occurs.
Patient teaching
• Teach patient how to take S.L. form of drug: Tell him to hold tablet under tongue until it dissolves and is absorbed and not to swallow saliva until that time.
• Give patient the following instructions for using metered-dose inhaler:
– Clear nasal passages and throat.
– Breathe out, expelling as much air from lungs as possible.
– Place mouthpiece well into mouth as dose from inhaler is released, and inhale deeply.
– Hold breath for several seconds, remove mouthpiece, and exhale slowly.
• If more than one inhalation is ordered, tell patient to wait at least 2 minutes before repeating procedure.
• Tell patient also using steroid inhaler to use bronchodilator first, then wait about 5 minutes before using steroid. This allows bronchodilator to open air passages for maximum effectiveness.
• Warn patient using oral inhalant that this drug may turn sputum and saliva pink.
• Instruct patient taking drug S.L. to rinse mouth with water between doses. This will also help prevent dryness of oropharynx.
• Tell patient to stop drug and notify doctor if chest tightness or dyspnea occurs.
• Warn patient against overuse of drug. Tell him that tolerance can develop.
• Tell patient to reduce caffeine intake during drug therapy.

☑ Evaluation
• Patient exhibits improved health.
• Patient does not experience injury from adverse reactions.
• Patient and family state understanding of drug therapy.

isosorbide dinitrate
(igh-soh-SOR-bighd digh-NIGH-trayt)
Apo-ISDN♦, Cedocard SR♦, Coronex♦, Dilatrate-SR, Iso-Bid, Isonate, Isorbid, Isordil, Isotrate, Novosorbide♦, Sorbitrate, Sorbitrate SA

isosorbide mononitrate
IMDUR, ISMO, Monoket

Pharmacologic class: nitrate
Therapeutic class: antianginal, vasodilator
Pregnancy risk category: C

How supplied

isosorbide dinitrate
Tablets: 5 mg, 10 mg, 20 mg, 30 mg, 40 mg
Tablets (chewable): 5 mg, 10 mg
Tablets (S.L.): 2.5 mg, 5 mg, 10 mg
Tablets (sustained-release): 40 mg
Capsules: 40 mg
Capsules (sustained-release): 40 mg
isosorbide mononitrate
Tablets: 10 mg, 20 mg
Tablets (extended-release): 60 mg

Pharmacokinetics

Absorption: dinitrate is well absorbed from GI tract but undergoes first-pass metabolism, resulting in bioavailability of about 50% (depending on dosage form used). Mononitrate is also absorbed well, with almost 100% bioavailability.
Distribution: distributed widely throughout body.
Metabolism: metabolized in liver to active metabolites.

Excretion: excreted in urine. *Half-life:* dinitrate oral, 5 to 6 hours; sublingual, 2 hours; mononitrate, about 5 hours.

Route	Onset	Peak	Duration
P.O.	2-60 min	2-60 min	1-12 hr
S.L.	2-5 min	2-5 min	1-2 hr

Pharmacodynamics

Chemical effect: may reduce cardiac oxygen demand by decreasing left ventricular end-diastolic pressure (preload) and, to lesser extent, systemic vascular resistance (afterload). Drug also may increase blood flow through collateral coronary vessels. Most of isosorbide dinitrate's activity is attributed to its active metabolite, isosorbide mononitrate. *Therapeutic effect:* relieves anginal pain.

Indications and dosage

► **Acute anginal attacks (S.L. and chewable tablets of isosorbide dinitrate only), prophylaxis in situations likely to cause anginal attacks.** *Adults:* S.L. form—2.5 to 5 mg under tongue for prompt relief of anginal pain, repeated q 5 to 10 minutes (maximum of three doses for each 30-minute period). For prophylaxis, 2.5 to 10 mg q 2 to 3 hours. **Chewable form**—5 to 10 mg p.r.n. for acute attack or q 2 to 3 hours for prophylaxis, but only after initial test dose of 5 mg to determine risk of severe hypotension. **P.O. form (isosorbide dinitrate)**— 30 mg P.O. t.i.d. or q.i.d. for prophylaxis only (use smallest effective dose); 40 mg P.O. (sustained-release form) q 6 to 12 hours. **P.O. form (isosorbide mononitrate)**—for prophylaxis only, 20 mg P.O. b.i.d. with doses 7 hours apart and first dose upon awakening. For sustained-release form, 30 to 60 mg P.O. once daily on arising; after several days, dosage may be increased to 120 mg once daily; rarely, 240 mg may be required.

Adverse reactions

CNS: *headache, sometimes with throbbing; dizziness;* weakness.

CV: orthostatic hypotension, tachycardia, palpitations, ankle edema, fainting.
GI: nausea, vomiting.
Skin: cutaneous vasodilation, *flushing.*
Other: hypersensitivity reactions, sublingual burning.

Interactions

Drug-drug. *Antihypertensives:* possibly increased hypotensive effects. Monitor closely during initial therapy.
Drug-lifestyle. *Alcohol use:* may increase hypotension. Avoid concomitant use.

Contraindications and precautions

• Contraindicated in patients with hypersensitivity or idiosyncrasy to nitrates; severe hypotension; shock; or acute MI with low left ventricular filling pressure.
• Use cautiously in patients with blood volume depletion (such as that resulting from diuretic therapy) or mild hypotension and in pregnant or breast-feeding women.
• Safety of drug has not been established in children.

NURSING CONSIDERATIONS

Assessment
• Assess patient's angina before therapy and regularly thereafter.
• Monitor blood pressure, heart rate and rhythm, and intensity and duration of drug response.
• Be alert for adverse reactions and drug interactions.
• Evaluate patient's and family's knowledge of drug therapy.

Nursing diagnoses
• Pain related to angina
• Risk for injury related to drug-induced adverse reactions
• Knowledge deficit related to drug therapy

Reactions may be *common*, uncommon, *life-threatening*, or COMMON AND LIFE-THREATENING.

▷ Planning and implementation
• Know that to prevent development of tolerance, nitrate-free interval of 8 to 12 hours per day has been recommended. The dosage regimen for isosorbide mononitrate (one tablet upon awakening with second dose in 7 hours, or one extended-release tablet daily) is intended to minimize nitrate tolerance by providing substantial nitrate-free interval.

P.O. use: Administer drug on empty stomach, either 30 minutes before or 1 to 2 hours after meals, and have patient swallow oral tablets whole. Have patient chew chewable tablets thoroughly before swallowing.

S.L. use: Administer drug at first sign of anginal attack. Have patient wet tablet with saliva, place it under his tongue until completely absorbed, and sit down and rest. Dose may be repeated every 10 to 15 minutes for maximum of three doses.
• Do not discontinue drug abruptly as coronary vasospasm may occur.
• Store drug in cool place, in tightly closed container, away from light.
• Notify doctor immediately if patient does not experience pain relief.

Patient teaching
• Caution patient to take drug regularly, as prescribed, and to keep it accessible at all times.
• Advise patient that abrupt discontinuation causes coronary vasospasm.
• Tell patient to take S.L. tablet at first sign of attack. Tablet should be wet with saliva and placed under tongue until completely absorbed, and patient should sit down and rest until pain subsides. Dose may be repeated every 10 to 15 minutes for maximum of three doses. If drug doesn't provide relief, medical help should be obtained promptly.
• Tell patient who complains of tingling sensation with drug placed S.L. to try holding tablet in buccal pouch.
• Warn patient not to confuse S.L. with oral form.
• Teach patient taking oral form to take tablet on empty stomach, either 30 min-

utes before or 1 to 2 hours after meals and to swallow tablet whole or chew chewable tablet thoroughly before swallowing
• Tell patient to minimize orthostatic hypotension by changing to upright position slowly. Tell him to go up and down stairs carefully and to lie down at first sign of dizziness.
• Instruct patient to avoid alcohol consumption during drug therapy.
• Tell patient to store drug in cool place, in tightly closed container, away from light.

☑ Evaluation
• Patient is free from pain.
• Patient does not experience injury from adverse reactions.
• Patient and family state understanding of drug therapy.

---

isotretinoin
(igh-soh-TREH-tih-noyn)
Accutane, Accutane Roche♦,
Roaccutane◇

Pharmacologic class: retinoic acid derivative
Therapeutic class: antiacne
Pregnancy risk category: X

How supplied
Capsules: 10 mg, 20 mg, 40 mg

Pharmacokinetics
Absorption: absorbed rapidly from GI tract.
Distribution: distributed widely in body; 99.9% protein-bound, primarily to albumin.
Metabolism: metabolized in liver and possibly in gut wall.
Excretion: unknown.

Route	Onset	Peak	Duration
P.O.	Unknown	About 3 hr	Unknown

Pharmacodynamics

Chemical effect: unknown; thought to normalize keratinization, reversibly decrease size of sebaceous glands, and alter composition of sebum to less viscous form that is less likely to cause follicular plugging.
Therapeutic effect: improves skin integrity.

Indications and dosage

▶ **Severe recalcitrant nodular acne unresponsive to conventional therapy.**
Adults and adolescents: 0.5 to 2 mg/kg P.O. daily in two divided doses for 15 to 20 weeks.

Adverse reactions

CNS: headache, fatigue, *pseudotumor cerebri* (benign intracranial hypertension).
EENT: *conjunctivitis,* corneal deposits, dry eyes, visual disturbances.
GI: nonspecific GI symptoms, gum bleeding and inflammation, nausea, vomiting.
Hematologic: anemia, elevated platelet count.
Hepatic: elevated AST, ALT, and alkaline phosphatase levels.
Metabolic: *hypertriglyceridemia,* hyperglycemia.
Musculoskeletal: *musculoskeletal pain (skeletal hyperostosis).*
Skin: *cheilosis, rash, dry skin,* peeling of palms and toes, skin infection, photosensitivity.
Other: thinning of hair.

Interactions

Drug-drug. *Carbamazepine:* coadministration has resulted in reduced carbamazepine plasma levels. Monitor patient for loss of therapeutic effects.
Tetracyclines: increased risk of pseudotumor cerebri. Avoid concomitant use.
Vitamin A, products containing vitamin A: increased toxic effects of isotretinoin. Don't use together without doctor's permission.

Drug-food. *Any food:* enhanced absorption of drug.
Drug-lifestyle. *Alcohol use:* increased risk of hypertriglyceridemia.
Sun exposure: increased photosensitivity reactions.

Contraindications and precautions

• Contraindicated in women of childbearing age unless patient has had negative serum pregnancy test within 2 weeks before beginning therapy; will begin drug therapy on second or third day of next menstrual period; and will comply with stringent contraceptive measures for 1 month before therapy, during therapy, and for at least 1 month after therapy. *Severe fetal abnormalities may occur if used during pregnancy.*
• Also contraindicated in patients hypersensitive to parabens, which are used as preservatives.
• Drug is not recommended for use in breast-feeding women.
• Safety of drug has not been established in children under age 12.

NURSING CONSIDERATIONS

Assessment
• Assess patient's skin before therapy and regularly thereafter.
• Obtain baseline serum lipid studies and liver function tests before therapy, as ordered. Monitor at regular intervals until response to drug is established (usually about 4 weeks).
• Monitor CK levels in patients who engage in vigorous physical activity.
• Be alert for adverse reactions and drug interactions.
• Most adverse reactions appear to be dose-related, occurring at dosages greater than 1 mg/kg daily. They are generally reversible when therapy is discontinued or dosage is reduced.
• Evaluate patient's and family's knowledge of drug therapy.

⊕ **Nursing diagnoses**
● Altered skin integrity related to underlying skin condition
● Impaired tissue integrity related to adverse reactions
● Knowledge deficit related to drug therapy

≫ **Planning and implementation**
● Anticipate second course of therapy, if needed, not to start for at least 8 weeks after completion of first course because improvement may continue after withdrawal of drug.
● Give drug with meals or shortly thereafter to enhance absorption.
● Patient who experiences headache, nausea and vomiting, or visual disturbances should be screened for papilledema. Signs and symptoms of pseudotumor cerebri require immediate discontinuation of therapy and prompt neurologic intervention.
Patient teaching
● Advise patient to take drug with milk, a meal, or shortly after meals to ensure adequate absorption.
● Tell patient to report immediately visual disturbances and bone, muscle, or joint pain.
● Warn patient that contact lenses may feel uncomfortable during drug therapy.
● Warn patient against using abrasives, medicated soaps and cleansers, acne preparations containing peeling agents, and topical alcohol preparations (including cosmetics, after-shave, cologne) because these agents cause cumulative irritation or excessive drying of skin.
● Instruct patient to avoid alcohol consumption during drug therapy.
● Tell patient to avoid prolonged exposure to sun, to use sunblock, and to wear protective clothing.

☑ **Evaluation**
● Patient exhibits improved skin condition.
● Patient is free from conjunctivitis, corneal deposits, and dry eyes.

● Patient and family state understanding of drug therapy.

---

isradipine
(is-RAH-deh-peen)
DynaCirc

Pharmacologic class: calcium channel blocker
Therapeutic class: antihypertensive
Pregnancy risk category: C

How supplied
Capsules: 2.5 mg, 5 mg

Pharmacokinetics
Absorption: 90% to 95% absorbed after oral administration.
Distribution: 95% is bound to plasma protein.
Metabolism: completely metabolized before elimination with extensive first-pass metabolism.
Excretion: 60% to 65% of drug excreted in urine; 25% to 30% in feces. *Half-life:* about 8 hours.

Route	Onset	Peak	Duration
P.O.	≤ 20 min	≤ 1.5 hr	12 hr

Pharmacodynamics
Chemical effect: inhibits calcium ion influx across cardiac and smooth-muscle cells and may decrease arteriolar resistance and blood pressure.
Therapeutic effect: lowers blood pressure.

Indications and dosage
▶ **Essential hypertension.** *Adults:* initially, 2.5 mg P.O. b.i.d., alone or with thiazide diuretic. Dosage increased by gradual titration. If response is inadequate after first 2 to 4 weeks, dosage increased by 5 mg daily at 2- to 4-week intervals to maximum of 20 mg daily.

Adverse reactions

CNS: dizziness.
CV: edema, flushing, palpitations, tachycardia, orthostatic hypotension.
GI: nausea, diarrhea.
GU: frequent urination.
Respiratory: dyspnea.
Skin: rash.

Interactions

Drug-drug. *Cimetidine:* increases levels of isradipine. Monitor for increased effects.
Fentanyl anesthesia: severe hypotension has been reported with concomitant use of beta blocker and calcium channel blocker. Avoid concomitant use.
Rifampin: reduced isradipine effects. Monitor closely.

Contraindications and precautions

• Contraindicated in patients with hypersensitivity to drug.
• Use cautiously in patients with heart failure, especially if combined with beta blocker, and in pregnant or breast-feeding women.
• Safety of drug has not been established in children.

NURSING CONSIDERATIONS

⚕ Assessment
• Assess blood pressure before therapy and regularly thereafter.
• Be alert for adverse reactions and drug interactions.
• Monitor patient's hydration status if adverse GI reactions occur.
• Evaluate patient's and family's knowledge of drug therapy.

⚙ Nursing diagnoses
• Risk for injury related to presence of hypertension
• Risk for fluid volume deficit related to adverse GI reactions
• Knowledge deficit related to drug therapy

⊠ Planning and implementation
• Drug may be given without regard to meals. However, giving drug with food slows absorption of drug.
• Before surgery, inform anesthesiologist that patient is taking calcium channel blocker.
Patient teaching
• Explain that patient may note increased need to void because drug has some diuretic activity.
• Instruct patient to notify doctor of adverse reactions or significant changes in blood pressure.

☑ Evaluation
• Patient's blood pressure is normal.
• Patient maintains normal hydration.
• Patient and family state understanding of drug therapy.

itraconazole
(ih-truh-KAHN-uh-zohl)
Sporanox

Pharmacologic class: synthetic triazole
Therapeutic class: antifungal
Pregnancy risk category: C

How supplied

Capsules: 100 mg

Pharmacokinetics

Absorption: oral bioavailability is maximal when taken with food. Absolute oral bioavailability is 55%.
Distribution: plasma protein binding of itraconazole is 99.8%; that of its metabolite, hydroxyitraconazole, 99.5%.
Metabolism: extensively metabolized by liver into large number of metabolites, including hydroxyitraconazole, the major metabolite.
Excretion: excreted in feces and urine.

Route	Onset	Peak	Duration
P.O.	Unknown	Unknown	Unknown

Reactions may be *common*, uncommon, *life-threatening*, or COMMON AND LIFE-THREATENING.

Pharmacodynamics

Chemical effect: interferes with fungal cell-wall synthesis by inhibiting formation of ergosterol and increasing cell-wall permeability.
Therapeutic effect: hinders fungal activity. Spectrum of activity includes *Aspergillus* species and *Blastomyces dermatitidis.*

Indications and dosage

▶ **Pulmonary and extrapulmonary blastomycosis; histoplasmosis.** *Adults:* 200 mg P.O. daily. Dosage increased as needed and tolerated in 100-mg increments to maximum of 400 mg daily. Dosages that exceed 200 mg daily should be given in two divided doses. Treatment should continue for minimum of 3 months. In life-threatening illness, loading dose of 200 mg t.i.d. is administered for 3 days.
▶ **Aspergillosis.** *Adults:* 200 to 400 mg P.O. daily.
▶ **Onychomycosis for toenails with or without fingernail involvement.** *Adults:* 200 mg once daily for 12 weeks.
▶ **Onychomycosis for fingernails only.** *Adults:* 2 treatment phases each consisting of 200 mg P.O. b.i.d. for 1 week. Phases are separated by a 3-week period without drug.

Adverse reactions

GI: nausea, vomiting, diarrhea, abdominal pain, anorexia.
Skin: rash, pruritus.
Other: edema, fatigue, fever, malaise.

Interactions

Drug-drug. *Antacids, H₂-receptor antagonists, phenytoin, rifampin:* possible lowered itraconazole plasma levels. Avoid concomitant use.
Astemizole: inhibited metabolism of these antihistamines, resulting in elevated blood levels and risk of serious cardiac toxicity. Never administer together.

Cyclosporine, digoxin: possible increased plasma levels of these drugs. Monitor plasma levels closely.
Isoniazid: may decrease plasma levels of itraconazole. Monitor closely.
Oral anticoagulants: possible enhanced anticoagulant effects. Monitor PT and INR closely.
Oral antidiabetic agents: similar antifungals have caused hypoglycemia. Monitor blood glucose levels.

Contraindications and precautions

• Contraindicated in patients with hypersensitivity to drug; in those receiving astemizole, cisapride, oral triazolam, or oral midazolam; and in breast-feeding women (drug is excreted in breast milk).
• Use cautiously in patients with hypochlorhydria (they may not absorb drug as readily as patients with normal gastric acidity), in HIV-infected patients (hypochlorhydria can accompany HIV infection), and in pregnant women.
• Safety of drug has not been established in children.

NURSING CONSIDERATIONS

⬛ Assessment
• Assess patient's infection before therapy and regularly thereafter.
• Monitor liver function tests.
• Be alert for adverse reactions and drug interactions.
• Evaluate patient's and family's knowledge of drug therapy.

⬛ Nursing diagnoses
• Infection related to presence of susceptible fungi
• Risk for fluid volume deficit related to adverse reactions
• Knowledge deficit related to drug therapy

⬛ Planning and implementation
• Administer drug with food.
• Report signs and symptoms of liver disease and abnormal liver tests.

Patient teaching
• Teach patient to recognize and report signs and symptoms of liver disease (anorexia, dark urine, pale stools, unusual fatigue, or jaundice).
• Tell patient to take drug with food to ensure maximal absorption.

☑ **Evaluation**
• Patient is free from infection.
• Patient maintains adequate fluid balance.
• Patient and family state understanding of drug therapy.

kanamycin sulfate
(kan-uh-MIGH-sin SUL-fayt)
Kantrex

Pharmacologic class: aminoglycoside
Therapeutic class: antibiotic
Pregnancy risk category: D

How supplied

Capsules: 500 mg
Injection: 37.5 mg/ml (pediatric), 250 mg/ml, 333 mg/ml

Pharmacokinetics

Absorption: absorbed poorly after oral administration (absorption enhanced in patients with impaired GI motility or mucosal ulcerations); unknown after I.M. administration.
Distribution: distributed widely in body. CSF penetration is low, even in patients with inflamed meninges. Protein binding is minimal.
Metabolism: none.
Excretion: excreted primarily in urine; small amounts may be excreted in bile.
Half-life: 2 to 4 hours.

Route	Onset	Peak	Duration
P.O.	Unknown	Unknown	8-12 hr
I.V.	Immediate	Immediate	8-12 hr
I.M.	Unknown	1 hr	8-12 hr

Pharmacodynamics

Chemical effect: inhibits protein synthesis by binding directly to 30S ribosomal subunit.
Therapeutic effect: kills susceptible bacteria: many aerobic gram-negative organisms and some aerobic gram-positive organisms.

Indications and dosage

▶ **Serious infections caused by sensitive strains of** *Escherichia coli, Proteus, Enterobacter aerogenes, Klebsiella pneumoniae, Serratia marcescens, Mycobacterium, Acinetobacter. Adults and children with normal renal function:* 15 mg/kg/day divided q 8 to 12 hours I.M. or I.V. Maximum daily dosage is 1.5 g. *Neonates:* 15 mg/kg/day divided q 12 hours I.M. or I.V.
▶ **Adjunct treatment in hepatic coma.** *Adults:* 8 to 12 g P.O. daily in divided doses.
▶ **Preoperative bowel sterilization.** *Adults:* 1 g P.O. q hour for four doses, then q 4 hours for four doses; or 1 g P.O. q hour for four doses, then q 6 hours for 36 to 72 hours.
▶ **Intraperitoneal irrigation.** 500 mg in 20 ml sterile distilled water instilled via catheter into wound after patient has recovered from anesthesia and neuromuscular blocker effects.
▶ **Wound irrigation.** 0.25% solution.

Adverse reactions

CNS: headache, lethargy, *neuromuscular blockade.*
EENT: ototoxicity (tinnitus, vertigo, hearing loss).
GU: nephrotoxicity (cells or casts in urine, oliguria, proteinuria, decreased creatinine clearance, increased BUN and serum creatinine levels).

Reactions may be *common*, uncommon, *life-threatening*, or COMMON AND LIFE-THREATENING.

Other: hypersensitivity reactions *(anaphylaxis).*

Interactions

Drug-drug. *Acyclovir, amphotericin B, cisplatin, methoxyflurane, other aminoglycosides, vancomycin:* increased nephrotoxicity. Don't use together.
Cephalothin: increased nephrotoxicity. Use together cautiously.
Dimenhydrinate: may mask symptoms of ototoxicity. Use with caution.
General anesthetics, neuromuscular blocking agents: may potentiate neuromuscular blockade. Monitor closely.
I.V. loop diuretics (such as furosemide): increased ototoxicity. Use cautiously.
Parenteral penicillins (such as ticarcillin): kanamycin inactivation in vitro. Don't mix together.

Contraindications and precautions

• Contraindicated for oral use in patients with intestinal obstruction, systemic infection, or hypersensitivity to drug or other aminoglycosides.
• Drug is not recommended for use in pregnant women.
• Use cautiously in patients with impaired renal function or neuromuscular disorders; in elderly patients; and in breast-feeding women.

NURSING CONSIDERATIONS

🗓 Assessment
• Assess patient's infection before therapy and regularly thereafter.
• Obtain specimen for culture and sensitivity tests before giving first dose. Therapy may begin pending results.
• Evaluate patient's hearing before and during therapy.
• Weigh patient and review baseline renal function studies before therapy and regularly during therapy.
• Be alert for adverse reactions and drug interactions.
• Obtain peak and trough levels as ordered. Be aware that peak blood levels

over 30 mcg/ml and trough levels over 10 mcg/ml may be associated with increased incidence of toxicity.
• Evaluate patient's and family's knowledge of drug therapy.

🗓 Nursing diagnoses
• Infection related to presence of susceptible bacteria
• Altered urinary elimination related to drug-induced nephrotoxicity
• Knowledge deficit related to drug therapy

❯ Planning and implementation
P.O. use: Follow normal protocol.
I.V. use: Dilute 500 mg of drug per 200 ml of 0.9% NaCl solution or D_5W; infuse over 30 to 60 minutes.
I.M. use: Inject deeply into upper outer quadrant of buttocks. Rotate injection sites.
Local use: Follow doctor's instructions when using as irrigation.
• Know that if no response occurs in 3 to 5 days, therapy may be stopped and new specimens obtained for culture and sensitivity testing.
• Encourage adequate fluid intake; patient should be well hydrated while taking drug to minimize chemical irritation of renal tubules.
Patient teaching
• Instruct patient to drink 2,000 ml of fluid daily if not contraindicated.
• Tell patient to report change in hearing or urinary elimination pattern immediately.
• Tell patient to call doctor if infection worsens or does not improve.

🗹 Evaluation
• Patient is free from infection.
• Patient maintains normal urinary elimination pattern.
• Patient and family state understanding of drug therapy.

---

kaolin and pectin mixtures
(KAY-oh-lin and PEK-tin MIX-tyers)
Donnagel-MB* ♦, Kaolin w/Pectin†,
Kao-Spen, Kapectolin†, K-C†, K-P†

Pharmacologic class: absorbent
Therapeutic class: antidiarrheal
Pregnancy risk category: NR

How supplied

Oral suspension: 5.2 g kaolin and
260 mg pectin per 30 ml† (Kao-Spen, K-
C†, K-P†); 90 g kaolin and 2 g pectin per
30 ml† (Kapectolin†, Kaolin w/pectin†);
6 g kaolin and 143 mg pectin per 30 ml†,
with 3.8% ethanol (Donnagel-MB* ♦)

Pharmacokinetics

Absorption: none.
Distribution: none.
Metabolism: none.
Excretion: excreted in feces.

Route	Onset	Peak	Duration
P.O.	Unknown	Unknown	Unknown

Pharmacodynamics

Chemical effect: decreases stool's fluid
content, although *total* water loss seems
to remain same.
Therapeutic effect: alleviates diarrhea.

Indications and dosage

▶ **Mild, nonspecific diarrhea.** *Adults:*
60 to 120 ml regular-strength suspension
P.O. after each bowel movement. *Children ages 3 to 6:* 15 to 30 ml regular-
strength P.O. after each bowel movement.
Children ages 6 to 12: 30 to 60 ml regular-strength P.O. after each bowel movement. *Children over age 12:* 60 ml regular-strength P.O. after each bowel movement.

Adverse reactions

GI: constipation, drug absorption of nutrients, other drugs, and enzymes; fecal
impaction or ulceration (in infants and elderly or debilitated patients after chronic
use).

Interactions

Drug-drug. *Orally administered drugs:*
absorption may occur. Separate administration times by at least 2 to 3 hours.

Contraindications and precautions

• No known contraindications.
• Use cautiously in pregnant women.

NURSING CONSIDERATIONS

⚿ Assessment
• Obtain assessment of patient's bowel
patterns before and after therapy.
• Be alert for adverse GI reactions and
drug interactions.
• Evaluate patient's and family's knowledge of drug therapy.

⊕ Nursing diagnoses
• Diarrhea related to underlying condition
• Constipation related to chronic use of
drug
• Knowledge deficit related to drug
therapy

▷ Planning and implementation
• Read label carefully. Check dosage and
strength.
• Administer dose after each loose bowel
movement.
• Do not use in place of specific therapy
for underlying cause of diarrhea.
Patient teaching
• Warn patient not to use drug to replace
therapy for underlying cause.
• Advise patient not to use drug for more
than 2 days.

☑ Evaluation
• Patient reports decrease in or absence
of loose stools.
• Patient does not have constipation.
• Patient and family state understanding
of drug therapy.

Reactions may be *common*, uncommon, **life-threatening**, or COMMON AND LIFE-THREATENING.

ketoconazole
(kee-toh-KAHN-uh-zohl)
Nizoral

Pharmacologic class: imidazole
derivative
Therapeutic class: antifungal
Pregnancy risk category: C

How supplied
Tablets: 200 mg

Pharmacokinetics
Absorption: decreased by raised gastric
pH and may be increased in extent and
consistency by food.
Distribution: distributed into bile, saliva,
cerumen, synovial fluid, and sebum. CSF
penetration is erratic and considered minimal. Drug is 84% to 99% bound to plasma proteins.
Metabolism: metabolized in liver.
Excretion: excreted primarily in feces,
with smaller amount excreted in urine.
Half-life: 8 hours.

Route	Onset	Peak	Duration
P.O.	Unknown	1-2 hr	Unknown

Pharmacodynamics
Chemical effect: inhibits purine transport
and DNA, RNA, and protein synthesis;
increases cell wall permeability, making
fungus more susceptible to osmotic pressure.
Therapeutic effect: kills susceptible fungi or hinders growth. Spectrum of activity includes most pathogenic fungi.

Indications and dosage
► **Systemic candidiasis, chronic muco-
candidiasis, oral thrush, candiduria,
coccidioidomycosis, histoplasmosis,
chromomycosis, and paracoccidioidomycosis; severe cutaneous dermatophyte infections resistant to therapy
with topical or oral griseofulvin.** *Adults
and children weighing over 40 kg (88 lb):*
initially, 200 mg P.O. daily in single
dose. Dosage may be increased to
400 mg once daily in patients who don't
respond to lower dosage. *Children age 2
and older:* 3.3 to 6.6 mg/kg P.O. daily as
single dose.

Adverse reactions
CNS: headache, nervousness, dizziness,
suicidal tendencies.
GI: *nausea, vomiting,* abdominal pain,
diarrhea, constipation.
Hematologic: *thrombocytopenia.*
Hepatic: elevated liver enzymes, *fatal
hepatotoxicity.*
Skin: itching.
Other: gynecomastia with tenderness.

Interactions
Drug-drug. *Antacids, anticholinergics,
H₂ blockers:* decreased absorption of ketoconazole. Wait at least 2 hours after ketoconazole dose before administering
these drugs.
Astemizole, cisapride: may increase plasma levels of these drugs, precipitating
CV events. Monitor closely.
Corticosteroids: corticosteroid bioavailability may be increased and clearance
may be decreased, possibly resulting in
toxicity. Monitor closely.
*Cyclosporine, methylprednisolone, tacro-
limus:* increased serum concentrations
may occur. Dosage adjustment of these
drugs may be required. Monitor closely.
Isoniazid, rifampin: increased ketoconazole metabolism. Monitor for decreased
antifungal effect.
Oral anticoagulants: anticoagulant response may be enhanced. Monitor PT
and INR.
Oral midazolam, triazolam: elevated plasma concentrations of these drugs, which
may potentiate or prolong the sedative or
hypnotic effects. Avoid concomitant use.

Contraindications and precautions
• Contraindicated in patients with hypersensitivity to drug and in those taking
astemizole, cisapride, oral midazolam or
oral triazolam.

• Breast-feeding women should seek alternative feeding methods during drug therapy.
• Use cautiously in patients with hepatic disease, in those taking other hepatotoxic drugs, and in pregnant women.

NURSING CONSIDERATIONS

🔢 Assessment
• Assess patient's infection before therapy and regularly thereafter.
• Evaluate laboratory studies for eradication of fungi.
• Be alert for adverse reactions and drug interactions.
• Monitor patient's hydration status if adverse GI reactions occur.
• Evaluate patient's and family's knowledge of drug therapy.

🔢 Nursing diagnoses
• Infection related to presence of susceptible fungi
• Risk for fluid volume deficit related to adverse GI reactions
• Knowledge deficit related to drug therapy

🔢 Planning and implementation
• Because of potential for serious hepatotoxicity, be aware that drug should not be used for less serious conditions, such as fungus infections of skin or nails.
• To minimize nausea, divide daily dosage into two doses. Taking with meals also helps to decrease nausea.
• Have patient dissolve each tablet in 4 ml aqueous solution of 0.2 N hydrochloric acid and have patient sip mixture through straw to avoid contact with teeth. Have patient drink full glass (8 oz) of water afterward.
Patient teaching
• Instruct patient to dissolve each tablet in 4 ml aqueous solution of 0.2 N hydrochloric acid, sip mixture through a glass or plastic straw (to avoid contact with teeth), and drink a glass of water because

ketoconazole requires gastric acidity for dissolution and absorption.
• Make sure patient understands that treatment should be continued until all clinical and laboratory tests indicate that active fungal infection has subsided. If drug is discontinued too soon, infection will recur. Minimum treatment for candidiasis is 7 to 14 days; for other systemic fungal infections, 6 months; for resistant dermatophyte infections, at least 4 weeks.
• Reassure patient that nausea will subside.

🔢 Evaluation
• Patient is free from infection.
• Patient maintains adequate hydration.
• Patient and family state understanding of drug therapy.

ketoprofen
(kee-toh-PROH-fen)
Actron caplets†, Apo-Keto♦,
Apo-Keto-E♦, Novo-Keto-EC♦, Orudis,
Orudis E♦, Orudis KT†, Orudis SR♦◊,
Oruvail, Rhodis♦, Rhodis-EC♦

Pharmacologic class: NSAID
Therapeutic class: nonnarcotic analgesic, antipyretic, anti-inflammatory
Pregnancy risk category: B

How supplied

Tablets: 12.5 mg†
Tablets (sustained-release): 200 mg♦
Tablets (enteric-coated): 50 mg♦,
100 mg♦
Capsules (extended-release): 100 mg,
150 mg, 200 mg
Capsules: 25 mg, 50 mg, 75 mg
Suppositories: 100 mg♦

Pharmacokinetics

Absorption: absorbed rapidly and completely from GI tract.
Distribution: highly protein-bound.
Metabolism: metabolized extensively in liver.

Reactions may be *common*, uncommon, *life-threatening*, or COMMON AND LIFE-THREATENING.

Excretion: excreted in urine.

Route	Onset	Peak	Duration
P.O., P.R.	1-2 hr	0.5-2 hr	3-4 hr

Pharmacodynamics

Chemical effect: may inhibit prostaglandin synthesis.
Therapeutic effect: relieves pain, fever, and inflammation.

Indications and dosage

▶ **Rheumatoid arthritis and osteoarthritis.** *Adults:* 75 mg t.i.d. or 50 mg q.i.d. or 200 mg as sustained-release tablet once daily. Maximum dosage is 300 mg/day. Alternatively, where suppository is available, 100 mg P.R. b.i.d.; or 1 suppository h.s. (with oral ketoprofen during day).
▶ **Mild to moderate pain; dysmenorrhea.** *Adults:* 25 to 50 mg P.O. q 6 to 8 hours p.r.n.
▶ **Minor aches and pain or fever.** *Adults:* 12.5 mg with full glass of water q 4 to 6 hours. Do not exceed 25 mg in 4 hours or 75 mg in a 24-hour period. Do not give to children under age 16 unless directed by doctor.

Adverse reactions

CNS: *headache,* dizziness, *CNS excitation* or depression.
EENT: tinnitus, visual disturbances.
GI: *nausea, abdominal pain, diarrhea, constipation, flatulence,* **peptic ulceration,** anorexia, vomiting, stomatitis.
GU: *nephrotoxicity, elevated BUN.*
Hematologic: prolonged bleeding time, *thrombocytopenia, agranulocytosis.*
Hepatic: elevated liver enzymes.
Respiratory: dyspnea, *bronchospasm, laryngeal edema.*
Skin: rash, photosensitivity, *exfoliative dermatitis.*

Interactions

Drug-drug. *Anticoagulants:* may increase anticoagulant effect. Monitor PT and INR.

Aspirin, corticosteroids: increased risk of adverse GI reactions. Avoid concomitant use.
Aspirin, probenecid: increased plasma levels of ketoprofen. Avoid concomitant use.
Hydrochlorothiazide, other diuretics: decreased diuretic effectiveness. Monitor for lack of effect.
Lithium, methotrexate: increased levels of these drugs, leading to toxicity. Monitor closely.
Oral anticoagulants: increased risk of bleeding. Monitor closely.
Drug-lifestyle. *Alcohol use:* increased risk of GI toxicity. Avoid concomitant use.
Sun exposure: may cause photosensitivity reactions. Take appropriate precautions.

Contraindications and precautions

• Contraindicated in patients with hypersensitivity to drug or history of aspirin- or NSAID-induced asthma, urticaria, or other allergic-type reactions.
• Avoid use of drug during third trimester of pregnancy. Drug is not recommended for use in breast-feeding women.
• Use cautiously in patients with history of peptic ulcer disease, renal dysfunction, hypertension, heart failure, or fluid retention.
• Safety of drug has not been established in children.
• Do not give to children under age 16 unless directed by doctor.

NURSING CONSIDERATIONS

⚏ Assessment
• Assess patient's pain before and after drug administration. Full effect may not occur for 2 to 4 weeks.
• Check renal and hepatic function every 6 months or as indicated and ordered during long-term therapy.
• Be alert for adverse reactions and drug interactions.
• Monitor patient's hydration status if adverse GI reactions occur.
• Evaluate patient's and family's knowledge of drug therapy.

---

*Liquid form contains alcohol   **May contain tartrazine   ♦Canada   ◇ Australia   †OTC

✥ Nursing diagnoses
• Pain related to underlying condition
• Risk for fluid volume deficit related to adverse GI reactions
• Knowledge deficit related to drug therapy

▷ Planning and implementation
P.O. use: Know that sustained-release dosage form is not recommended for patients in acute pain.
– Administer drug on empty stomach unless GI upset occurs.
P.R. use: Follow normal protocol.
• Inform laboratory personnel that patient is taking ketoprofen. Drug may interfere with some laboratory determinations of blood glucose and serum iron levels, depending on testing method used.
Patient teaching
• Inform patient to take drug 30 minutes before or 2 hours after meals. If adverse GI reactions occur, patient may take drug with milk or meals.
• Tell patient that full therapeutic effect may be delayed for 2 to 4 weeks.
• Instruct patient to report visual or auditory adverse reactions immediately.
• Teach patient to recognize and immediately report signs and symptoms of GI bleeding. Also explain that serious GI toxicity, including peptic ulceration and bleeding, can occur in patients taking NSAIDs despite absence of GI symptoms.
• Alert patient that concomitant use with aspirin, alcohol, or corticosteroids may increase risk of adverse GI reactions.
• Advise patient to use sunblock, wear protective clothing, and avoid prolonged exposure to sunlight. This drug has been associated with photosensitivity reactions.

✓ Evaluation
• Patient is free from pain.
• Patient maintains normal hydration status.
• Patient and family state understanding of drug therapy.

ketorolac tromethamine
(KEE-toh-roh-lak troh-METH-uh-meen)
Toradol

Pharmacologic class: NSAID
Therapeutic class: analgesic
Pregnancy risk category: C

How supplied

Tablets: 10 mg
Injection: 15 mg/ml, 30 mg/ml

Pharmacokinetics

Absorption: completely absorbed after I.M. use. After oral use, food delays absorption but does not decrease total amount absorbed.
Distribution: over than 99.9% protein-bound.
Metabolism: metabolized primarily in liver.
Excretion: more than 90% excreted in urine; remainder, in feces. *Half-life:* 3.8 to 6.3 hours.

Route	Onset	Peak	Duration
P.O.	30-60 min	30-60 min	6-8 hr
I.V.	Immediate	Immediate	8 hr
I.M.	≤ 10 min	30-60 min	6-8 hr

Pharmacodynamics

Chemical effect: unknown; may inhibit prostaglandin synthesis.
Therapeutic effect: relieves pain.

Indications and dosage

▶ **Short-term management of pain.**
Adults under age 65: dosage based on patient response. Initially, 60 mg I.M. or 30 mg I.V. as single dose, or multiple doses of 30 mg I.M. or I.V. q 6 hours. Maximum daily dosage is 120 mg. To switch to oral dosing, initially 20 mg P.O., then 10 mg P.O. q 4 to 6 hours, p.r.n., up to 40 mg/day. *Adults age 65 or older, renally impaired patients, and those weighing under 50 kg (110 lb):* initially, 30 mg I.M. or 15 mg I.V. as single dose, or multiple doses of 15 mg I.M. or I.V. q 6 hours.

Maximum daily dosage is 60 mg. To switch to oral dosing, 10 mg P.O. q 4 to 6 hours, p.r.n., up to 40 mg/day.
Note: Combined use of drug not to exceed 5 days.

Adverse reactions

CNS: drowsiness, sedation, dizziness, headache, sweating.
CV: edema, hypertension, palpitations, arrhythmias.
GI: *nausea, dyspepsia, GI pain,* diarrhea, *peptic ulceration.*
GU: *acute renal failure.*
Hematologic: decreased platelet adhesion, purpura, *thrombocytopenia.*
Metabolic: hyperkalemia.
Respiratory: *bronchospasm.*
Other: pain (at injection site).

Interactions

Drug-drug. *Antihypertensives, diuretics:* decreased effectiveness. Monitor closely.
Lithium: increased lithium levels. Monitor closely.
Methotrexate: decreased methotrexate clearance and increased toxicity. Don't use together.
Salicylates, warfarin: ketorolac may increase levels of free (unbound) salicylates or warfarin in blood. Clinical significance is unknown.

Contraindications and precautions

• Contraindicated in patients with hypersensitivity to drug or history of syndrome of nasal polyps, angioedema, bronchospastic reactivity, or allergic reactions to aspirin or other NSAIDs.
• Also contraindicated in patients currently receiving aspirin or other NSAIDs; in those with advanced renal impairment; and in those at risk for renal failure as a result of volume depletion.
• Contraindicated in patients with suspected or confirmed cerebrovascular bleeding, hemorrhage diathesis, and incomplete hemostasis, and in those at high risk of bleeding.

• Contraindicated for intrathecal or epidural administration because of its alcohol content.
• Use cautiously in patients with hepatic or renal impairment, history of serious GI events or peptic ulcer disease, or cardiac decompensation, hypertension, or coagulation disorders; during perioperative period, in pregnancy, and during labor and delivery.
• Use with caution in breast-feeding patients. Trace amounts of drug have been detected in breast milk.
• Safety of drug has not been established in children.

NURSING CONSIDERATIONS

Assessment
• Obtain assessment of patient's pain before and after drug administration.
• Be alert for adverse reactions and drug interactions.
• Evaluate patient's and family's knowledge of drug therapy.

Nursing diagnoses
• Pain related to underlying condition
• Risk for injury related to drug-induced adverse CNS reactions
• Knowledge deficit related to drug therapy

Planning and implementation
P.O. use: When switching from injectable to oral form, know that total dosage of 120 mg of drug on day of transition should not be exceeded, including maximum of 40 mg P.O.
I.V. use: I.V. bolus must be given over at least 15 seconds.
I.M. use: I.M. administration may cause pain at injection site. Holding pressure over site for 15 to 30 seconds after injection may minimize local effects.
• Notify doctor if pain persists or worsens.
Patient teaching
• Teach patient to recognize and immediately report signs and symptoms of GI bleeding. Also explain that serious GI tox-

icity, including peptic ulceration and bleeding, can occur in patient taking oral NSAIDs despite absence of GI symptoms.
• Advise patient to report persistent or worsening pain.
• Explain that drug is intended for short-term use only.

☑ **Evaluation**
• Patient is free from pain.
• Patient does not experience injury from adverse reactions.
• Patient and family state understanding of drug therapy.

labetalol hydrochloride
(lah-BAY-tuh-lol high-droh-KLOR-ighd)
Normodyne, Presolol◇, Trandate

Pharmacologic class: alpha-adrenergic and beta blocker
Therapeutic class: antihypertensive
Pregnancy risk category: C

How supplied

Tablets: 100 mg, 200 mg, 300 mg
Injection: 5 mg/ml

Pharmacokinetics

Absorption: 90% to 100% absorbed with P.O. administration; however, drug undergoes extensive first-pass metabolism in liver and only about 25% of P.O. dose reaches systemic circulation unchanged.
Distribution: distributed widely throughout body; about 50% protein-bound.
Metabolism: drug administered P.O. metabolized extensively in liver and, possibly, GI mucosa.
Excretion: about 5% excreted unchanged in urine; remainder excreted as metabolites in urine and feces. *Half-life:* about

5½ hours after I.V. dose; 6 to 8 hours after P.O. dose.

Route	Onset	Peak	Duration
P.O.	≤ 20 min	2-4 hr	12-24 hr
I.V.	≤ 2-5 min	5 min	2-4 hr

Pharmacodynamics

Chemical effect: unknown; may be related to reduced peripheral vascular resistance as result of alpha-adrenergic blockade.
Therapeutic effect: lowers blood pressure.

Indications and dosage

▶ **Hypertension.** *Adults:* 100 mg P.O. b.i.d. with or without diuretic. If needed, dosage is increased to 200 mg b.i.d. after 2 days. Further increases may be made q 2 to 3 days until optimum response is reached. Usual maintenance dosage is 200 to 400 mg b.i.d.
▶ **Severe hypertension, hypertensive emergencies.** *Adults:* 200 mg diluted in 160 ml of D₅W, infused at 2 mg/minute until satisfactory response is obtained, then infusion stopped. Dose may be repeated q 6 to 12 hours. Alternatively, administered by repeated I.V. injection: initially, 20 mg I.V. slowly over 2 minutes. Then repeat injections of 40 to 80 mg q 10 minutes until maximum dosage of 300 mg is reached, p.r.n.

Adverse reactions

CNS: vivid dreams, fatigue, headache, transient scalp tingling.
CV: *orthostatic hypotension and dizziness,* peripheral vascular disease, bradycardia, **ventricular arrhythmias.**
EENT: nasal stuffiness.
GI: nausea, vomiting, diarrhea.
GU: sexual dysfunction, urine retention.
Respiratory: increased airway resistance.
Skin: rash.

Reactions may be *common,* uncommon, *life-threatening,* or COMMON AND LIFE-THREATENING.

Interactions

Drug-drug. *Cimetidine:* may enhance labetalol's effect. Give together cautiously.
Halothane: additive hypotensive effect. Monitor blood pressure.
Insulin, oral antidiabetic agents: can alter dosage requirements in previously stabilized diabetic patients. Observe patient carefully.

Contraindications and precautions

• Contraindicated in patients with bronchial asthma, overt cardiac failure, greater than first-degree heart block, cardiogenic shock, severe bradycardia, other conditions associated with severe and prolonged hypotension, or hypersensitivity to drug.
• Use cautiously in pregnant or breastfeeding women and in patients with heart failure, hepatic failure, chronic bronchitis, emphysema, preexisting peripheral vascular disease, or pheochromocytoma.
• Safety of drug has not been established in children.

NURSING CONSIDERATIONS

Assessment
• Obtain history of patient's hypertension before therapy.
• Monitor blood pressure frequently. Drug masks common signs of shock.
• When administered I.V. for hypertensive emergencies, labetalol produces rapid, predictable fall in blood pressure within 5 to 10 minutes.
• Be alert for adverse reactions and drug interactions.
• Evaluate patient's and family's knowledge of drug therapy.

Nursing diagnoses
• Altered health maintenance related to presence of hypertension
• Risk for trauma related to drug-induced hypotension
• Knowledge deficit related to drug therapy

Planning and implementation
P.O. use: If dizziness occurs, ask doctor if patient may take dose at bedtime or take smaller doses t.i.d. to help minimize this reaction.
I.V. use: Administer injection with infusion-control device. Monitor blood pressure q 5 minutes for 30 minutes, then q 30 minutes for 2 hours, then hourly for 6 hours. Patient should remain in supine position for 3 hours after infusion.
– Sodium bicarbonate injection is incompatible with I.V. labetalol.
Patient teaching
• Tell patient that abrupt discontinuation of therapy can exacerbate angina and precipitate MI.
• Inform patient that dizziness can be minimized by rising slowly and avoiding sudden position changes.

Evaluation
• Patient's blood pressure is normal.
• Patient does not experience trauma caused by drug-induced hypotension.
• Patient and family state understanding of drug therapy.

lactulose
(LAK-tyoo-lohs)
Cephulac, Cholac, Chronulac, Constilac, Duphalac, Enulose, Lac-Dol◊, Portalac

Pharmacologic class: disaccharide
Therapeutic class: laxative
Pregnancy risk category: B

How supplied
Syrup: 10 g/15 ml

Pharmacokinetics
Absorption: absorbed minimally.
Distribution: distributed locally, primarily in colon.
Metabolism: metabolized by colonic bacteria (absorbed portion is not metabolized).
Excretion: most excreted in feces; absorbed portion excreted in urine.

Route	Onset	Peak	Duration
P.O.	24-48 hr	Varies	Varies

Pharmacodynamics

Chemical effect: produces osmotic effect in colon. Resulting distention promotes peristalsis. Lactulose also decreases blood ammonia, probably as result of bacterial degradation, which lowers pH of colon contents.
Therapeutic effect: relieves constipation.

Indications and dosage

▶ **Constipation.** *Adults:* 10 to 20 g (15 to 30 ml) P.O. daily.
▶ **Prevention and treatment of hepatic encephalopathy, including hepatic pre-coma and coma in patients with severe hepatic disease.** *Adults:* initially, 20 to 30 g (30 to 45 ml) P.O. t.i.d. or q.i.d. until two or three soft stools are produced daily. Usual dosage is 60 to 100 g daily in divided doses. Alternatively, 200 g (300 ml) diluted with 700 ml of water or saline solution and administered as retention enema q 4 to 6 hours, p.r.n.

Adverse reactions

GI: *abdominal cramps, belching, diarrhea, gaseous distention, flatulence.*
Other: hypernatremia.

Interactions

Drug-drug. *Antacids, antibiotics, orally administered neomycin:* decreased effectiveness of lactulose. Avoid concomitant use.

Contraindications and precautions

• Contraindicated in patients on low-galactose diet.
• Use cautiously in patients with diabetes mellitus.

NURSING CONSIDERATIONS

🏵 Assessment

• Assess patient's condition before therapy and regularly thereafter.
• Monitor serum sodium levels.

• Be alert for adverse reactions and drug interactions.
• Evaluate patient's and family's knowledge of drug therapy.

🏵 Nursing diagnoses

• Constipation related to underlying condition
• Knowledge deficit related to drug therapy

▷ Planning and implementation

• Be prepared to replace fluid loss.
• Store drug at room temperature, preferably below 86° F (30° C). Don't freeze.
Patient teaching
• Advise patient to dilute drug with juice or water or to take it with food to improve taste.

🏵 Evaluation

• Patient's constipation is relieved.
• Patient and family state understanding of drug therapy.

---

lamotrigine
(lah-MOH-trigh-jeen)
Lamictal

Pharmacologic class: phenytriazine
Therapeutic class: anticonvulsant
Pregnancy risk category: C

How supplied

Tablets: 25 mg, 100 mg, 150 mg, 200 mg

Pharmacokinetics

Absorption: rapidly and completely absorbed after P.O. administration with negligible first-pass metabolism.
Distribution: 55% protein-bound.
Metabolism: predominantly by glucuronic acid conjugation.
Excretion: excreted primarily in urine.
Half-life: 14.4 to 70.3 hours, depending on dosage schedule and use of other anticonvulsants.

Reactions may be *common,* uncommon, *life-threatening*, or COMMON AND LIFE-THREATENING.

Route	Onset	Peak	Duration
P.O.	Unknown	1.4-4.8 hr	Unknown

Pharmacodynamics

Chemical effect: unknown; may inhibit release of glutamate and aspartate, excitatory neurotransmitters in brain, through action at sodium channels.
Therapeutic effect: prevents partial seizure activity.

Indications and dosage

▶ **Adjunct therapy in treatment of partial seizures caused by epilepsy.**
Adults: 50 mg P.O. daily for 2 weeks, followed by 100 mg daily in two divided doses for 2 weeks. Usual maintenance dosage is 300 to 500 mg P.O. daily in two divided doses. For patients also taking valproic acid, 25 mg P.O. every other day for 2 weeks, followed by 25 mg P.O. daily for 2 weeks. Thereafter, no more than 150 mg P.O. daily in two divided doses.

Adverse reactions

CNS: *dizziness, headache, ataxia, somnolence,* incoordination, insomnia, tremors, depression, anxiety, *seizures,* irritability, speech disorder, decreased memory, aggravated reaction, concentration disturbance, sleep disorder, emotional lability, vertigo, malaise, mind racing, *suicide attempts.*
CV: palpitations.
EENT: *diplopia, blurred vision,* vision abnormality, nystagmus, rhinitis, pharyngitis.
GI: *nausea, vomiting,* diarrhea, dyspepsia, abdominal pain, constipation, tooth disorder, anorexia, dry mouth.
GU: dysmenorrhea, vaginitis, amenorrhea.
Musculoskeletal: dysarthria, muscle spasm, neck pain.
Respiratory: cough, dyspnea.
Skin: *Stevens-Johnson syndrome, toxic epidermal necrolysis, rash,* pruritus, hot flashes, alopecia, acne.
Other: flulike syndrome, fever, infection, chills.

Interactions

Drug-drug. *Acetaminophen:* serum lamotrigine concentrations may be reduced decreasing therapeutic effects. Monitor patient.
Carbamazepine, phenobarbital, phenytoin, primidone: decrease lamotrigine's steady-state concentrations. Monitor patient closely.
Folate inhibitors (such as co-trimoxazole, methotrexate): lamotrigine inhibits dihydrofolate reductase, an enzyme involved in folic acid synthesis; may have additive effect. Monitor patient closely.
Valproic acid: decreases lamotrigine's clearance, which increases drug's steady-state concentrations. Monitor patient closely for toxicity.
Drug-lifestyle. *Sun exposure:* photosensitivity reactions may occur. Take precautions.

Contraindications and precautions

• Contraindicated in patients with hypersensitivity to drug and in children under age 16.
• Use of drug in breast-feeding women is not recommended.
• Use cautiously in patients with renal, hepatic, or cardiac impairment and in pregnant women.

NURSING CONSIDERATIONS

Assessment
• Obtain history of patient's seizure disorder before therapy.
• Evaluate patient for reduction in frequency and duration of seizures after therapy begins. Check adjunct anticonvulsant's serum levels periodically, as ordered.
• Evaluate patient's and family's knowledge of drug therapy.

Nursing diagnoses
• Risk for trauma related to seizures
• Risk for impaired skin integrity related to dermatologic reactions
• Knowledge deficit related to drug therapy

⟩⟩ Planning and implementation
• Drug dose should be lowered if it is added to multidrug regimen that includes valproic acid.
• Know that lowered maintenance dosage should be used in patients with severe renal impairment.
• Drug should not be discontinued abruptly to prevent increased seizure frequency. Instead, drug should be tapered over at least 2 weeks.
• Know that rash may be life-threatening. Stop drug and notify doctor at first sign of rash, unless it is not drug-related.
Patient teaching
• Inform patient that lamotrigine may cause rash. Combination therapy of valproic acid and lamotrigine appears to be more likely to precipitate serious rash. Tell patient to report rash or signs or symptoms of hypersensitivity promptly because they could be serious enough to warrant discontinuation of drug.
• Instruct patient to avoid prolonged exposure to the sun, and to use sunblock and wear protective clothing.
• Warn patient not to engage in hazardous activity until drug's CNS effects are known.

☑ Evaluation
• Patient is seizure-free.
• Drug-induced skin impairment does not develop.
• Patient and family state understanding of drug therapy.

---

lansoprazole
(lan-soh-PRAY-zohl)
Prevacid

Pharmacologic class: substituted benzimidazole
Therapeutic class: antiulcer agent
Pregnancy risk category: B

How supplied
Capsules (delayed-release): 15 mg, 30 mg

Pharmacokinetics
Absorption: absorbed rapidly.
Distribution: 97% bound to plasma proteins.
Metabolism: metabolized extensively in liver.
Excretion: excreted primarily in feces, minimally in urine. *Half-life:* less than 2 hours.

Route	Onset	Peak	Duration
P.O.	Unknown	1.7 hr	> 24 hr

Pharmacodynamics
Chemical effect: inhibits activity of proton pump and binds to hydrogen or potassium adenosine triphosphatase, located at secretory surface of gastric parietal cells.
Therapeutic effect: decreases gastric acid formation.

Indications and dosage
▶ **Short-term treatment of active duodenal ulcer.** *Adults:* 15 mg P.O. daily before meals for 4 weeks.
▶ **Maintenance of healed duodenal ulcers.** *Adults:* 15 mg P.O. once daily.
▶ **Short-term treatment of erosive esophagitis.** *Adults:* 30 mg P.O. daily before meals for up to 8 weeks. If healing does not occur, additional 8 weeks of therapy may be given. Maintenance dosage for healing is 15 mg P.O. daily.
▶ **Short-term treatment of active benign gastric ulcer.** *Adults:* 30 mg P.O. once daily for up to 8 weeks.
▶ *Helicobacter pylori* **eradication to reduce risk of duodenal ulcer recurrence. Triple therapy.** *Adults:* 30 mg P.O. lansoprazole with 500 mg P.O. clarithromycin and 1 g P.O. amoxicillin, each given q 12 hours for 14 days.
▶ **Dual therapy:** *Adults:* 30 mg P.O. lansoprazole with 1 g P.O. amoxicillin each given q 8 hours for 14 days.

▶ **Long-term treatment of pathological hypersecretory conditions, including Zollinger-Ellison syndrome.** *Adults:* initially, 60 mg P.O. once daily. Dosage increased as needed. Daily dosages of more than 120 mg should be given in divided doses.

▶ **Short-term treatment of symptomatic gastroesophageal reflux disease (GERD).** *Adults:* 15 mg P.O. daily for up to 8 weeks.

Adverse reactions

GI: diarrhea, nausea, abdominal pain.

Interactions

Drug-drug. *Ampicillin esters, digoxin, iron salts, ketoconazole:* lansoprazole may interfere with absorption. Monitor patient closely.
Sucralfate: delays lansoprazole absorption. Give lansoprazole at least 30 minutes before sucralfate.
Theophylline: may cause mild increase in theophylline clearance. Use together cautiously. Dosage adjustment of theophylline may be necessary when lansoprazole is started or stopped.

Contraindications and precautions

• Contraindicated in patients hypersensitive to drug.
• Drug is not recommended for use in breast-feeding women.
• Use cautiously in pregnant women.
• Safety of drug has not been established in children.

NURSING CONSIDERATIONS

☡ Assessment
• Assess patient's condition before therapy and regularly thereafter.
• Be alert for adverse reactions and drug interactions.
• Evaluate patient's and family's knowledge of drug therapy.

✥ Nursing diagnoses
• Impaired tissue integrity related to underlying condition
• Altered health maintenance related to drug-induced adverse reactions
• Knowledge deficit related to drug therapy

❯ Planning and implementation
• Give drug on empty stomach.
• Dosage adjustment may be necessary for patients with severe liver disease.
• Drug should not be used as maintenance therapy for patient with duodenal ulcer or erosive esophagitis.
• Notify doctor if adverse reactions occur, and be prepared to provide supportive care.
Patient teaching
• Instruct patient to take drug before eating. Caution him not to open, chew, or crush capsules. The capsules should be swallowed whole.
• Instruct patient to notify doctor if adverse reactions occur.

☑ Evaluation
• Patient regains normal GI tissue integrity.
• Patient does not experience serious adverse reactions.
• Patient and family state understanding of drug therapy.

leflunomide
(leh-FLOO-noh-mighd)
Arava

Pharmacologic class: pyrimidine synthesis inhibitor
Therapeutic class: immunomodulatory agent
Pregnancy risk category: X

How supplied

Tablets: 10 mg, 20 mg, 100 mg

Pharmacokinetics

Absorption: 80% of dose is absorbed following oral administration.
Distribution: extensively bound to albumin; has low volume of distribution.
Metabolism: primary route of metabolism has not been identified.
Excretion: excreted renally as well as by direct biliary elimination; 43% excreted in urine, 48% eliminated in feces.

Route	Onset	Peak	Duration
P.O.	Unknown	6-12 hr	Unknown

Pharmacodynamics

Chemical effect: inhibits dihydroorotate dehydrogenase, an enzyme involved in pyrimidine synthesis, and has antiproliferative activity and anti-inflammatory effects.
Therapeutic effect: reduces pain and inflammation related to rheumatoid arthritis.

Indications and dosage

▶ **Treatment of active rheumatoid arthritis to reduce signs and symptoms and to retard structural damage as evidenced by X-ray erosions and joint space narrowing.** *Adults:* 100 mg P.O. q 24 hours for 3 days followed by 20 mg (maximum daily dosage) P.O. q 24 hours. Dosage may be decreased to 10 mg daily if higher dosage is not well-tolerated.

Adverse reactions

CNS: asthenia, dizziness, headache, paresthesia, malaise, migraine, sleep disorder, vertigo, neuritis, anxiety, depression, insomnia, neuralgia.
CV: angina pectoris, *hypertension,* chest pain, palpitation, tachycardia, vasculitis, vasodilation, varicose veins.
EENT: pharyngitis, rhinitis, sinusitis, epistaxis, mouth ulcer, oral candidiasis, enlarged salivary gland, stomatitis, tooth disorder, dry mouth, blurred vision, cataract, conjunctivitis, eye disorder, gingivitis, taste perversion.

GI: anorexia, *diarrhea,* dyspepsia, gastroenteritis, nausea, abdominal pain, vomiting, cholelithiasis, colitis, constipation, esophagitis, flatulence, gastritis, melena.
GU: urinary tract infection, albuminuria, cystitis, dysuria, hematuria, menstrual disorder, pelvic pain, vaginal candidiasis, prostate disorder, urinary frequency.
Hematologic: anemia, ecchymosis, hyperlipidemia.
Hepatic: elevated liver enzymes.
Metabolic: diabetes mellitus, fever, hyperglycemia, hyperthyroidism, hypokalemia.
Musculoskeletal: arthrosis, back pain, bursitis, muscle cramps, myalgia, bone necrosis, bone pain, arthralgia, leg cramps, joint disorder, neck pain, synovitis, tendon rupture, tenosynovitis.
Respiratory: bronchitis, increased cough, pneumonia, *respiratory infection,* asthma, dyspnea, lung disorder.
Skin: *alopecia,* eczema, pruritus, *rash,* dry skin, acne, contact dermatitis, fungal dermatitis, hair discoloration, hematoma, herpes simplex, herpes zoster, nail disorder, skin nodule, subcutaneous nodule, maculopapular rash, skin disorder, skin discoloration, skin ulcer.
Other: allergic reaction, flulike syndrome, injury or accident, pain, weight loss, abscess, cyst, hernia, peripheral edema, increased sweating, increased creatine phosphokinase.

Interactions

Drug-drug. *Cholestyramine, charcoal:* decreased plasma concentrations of leflunomide. Sometimes used for this effect in overdose.
Methotrexate, other hepatotoxic drugs: increased risk of hepatotoxicity. Monitor liver enzymes, as ordered.
NSAIDs (diclofenac, ibuprofen): increased levels of NSAIDs. Clinical significance unknown.
Rifampin: increased active leflunomide metabolite level. Use caution with concomitant administration.

Reactions may be *common,* uncommon, *life-threatening,* or COMMON AND LIFE-THREATENING.

Tolbutamide: increased levels of tolbutamide. Clinical significance unknown.

Contraindications and precautions

• Contraindicated in patients with known hypersensitivity to drug or its components and in women who are or may become pregnant or who are breast-feeding.
• Drug is not recommended in patients with hepatic insufficiency, hepatitis B or C, severe immunodeficiency, bone marrow dysplasia, or severe uncontrolled infections.
• Vaccination with live vaccines is not recommended. Long half-life of drug should be considered when contemplating administration of a live vaccine after stopping drug treatment.
• Drug is not recommended for use in children under age 18 and in men attempting to father a child.
• Use cautiously in patients with renal insufficiency.
• Know that there is an increased risk of malignancy, particularly lymphoproliferative disorders, with use of some immunosuppression drugs, including leflunomide.

NURSING CONSIDERATIONS

Assessment
• Assess patient's condition before therapy and regularly thereafter.
• Be alert for adverse reactions and drug interactions.
• Monitor liver enzymes (ALT and AST) before starting therapy and monthly thereafter until stable. Frequency can then be decreased based on clinical situation.
• Evaluate patient's and family's knowledge of drug therapy.

Nursing diagnoses
• Altered health maintenance related to underlying disease.
• Knowledge deficit related to drug therapy.

Planning and implementation
• Drug can cause fetal harm when given to pregnant women. Discontinue drug in women planning to become pregnant and notify doctor.
• Know that drug should be discontinued in men planning to father a child. Tell patient to follow recommended leflunomide removal protocol (cholestyramine 8 g, P.O. t.i.d. for 11 days).
Patient teaching
• Explain need and frequency of required blood test monitoring.
• Instruct patient to use contraceptive measures during drug therapy and until it has been determined that drug is no longer active.
• Advise patient to notify doctor immediately if pregnancy is suspected.
• Advise breast-feeding patient to discontinue breast-feeding during drug therapy.
• Inform patient that aspirin, other NSAIDs, and low-dose corticosteroids may be continued during treatment; however, combined use of drug with antimalarials, I.M. or oral gold, penicillamine, azathioprine, or methotrexate has not been adequately studied.

Evaluation
• Patient has improvement in symptoms of rheumatoid arthritis.
• Patient and family state understanding of drug therapy.

leucovorin calcium (citrovorum factor, folinic acid)
(loo-koh-VOR-in KAL-see-um)
Wellcovorin

Pharmacologic class: formyl derivative (active reduced form of folic acid)
Therapeutic class: vitamin; antidote
Pregnancy risk category: C

How supplied

Tablets: 5 mg, 10 mg, 15 mg, 25 mg

Injection: 1-ml ampule (3 mg/ml with 0.9% benzyl alcohol)
Powder for injection: 50 mg/vial, 100 mg/vial, 350 mg/vial

Pharmacokinetics

Absorption: absorbed rapidly after P.O. administration.
Distribution: distributed throughout body; liver contains about one-half of total body folate stores.
Metabolism: metabolized in liver.
Excretion: excreted by kidneys. *Half-life:* 6.2 hours.

Route	Onset	Peak	Duration
P.O.	20-30 min	2-3 hr	3-6 hr
I.V.	5 min	< 1 hr	3-6 hr
I.M.	10-20 min	≤ 10 min	3-6 hr

Pharmacodynamics

Chemical effect: readily converts to other folic acid derivatives.
Therapeutic effect: raises folic acid level in body.

Indications and dosage

▶ **Overdose of folic acid antagonist.** *Adults and children:* P.O., I.M., or I.V. dose equivalent to weight of antagonist given.
▶ **Rescue after high methotrexate dose in treatment of cancer.** *Adults and children:* 10 mg/m^2 P.O., I.M., or I.V. q 6 hours until methotrexate level falls below 5 × 10^{-8} M.
▶ **Megaloblastic anemia caused by congenital enzyme deficiency.** *Adults and children:* 3 to 6 mg I.M. daily, then 1 mg P.O. or I.M. daily for life.
▶ **Folate-deficient megaloblastic anemia.** *Adults and children:* up to 1 mg P.O. or I.M daily. Duration of treatment depends on hematologic response.
▶ **Treatment of hematologic toxicity caused by pyrimethamine or trimethoprim therapy.** *Adults and children:* 5 to 15 mg P.O. or I.M. daily.
▶ **Palliative treatment of advanced colorectal carcinoma.** *Adults:* 20 mg/m^2 I.V., followed by fluorouracil, for 5 consecutive days. Repeated q 4 weeks for two additional courses, then q 4 to 5 weeks, if tolerated.

Adverse reactions

Respiratory: *bronchospasm.*
Skin: *hypersensitivity reactions* (rash, pruritus, erythema).

Interactions

Drug-drug. *Anticonvulsants:* may decrease effectiveness of these agents. Monitor closely.
Fluorouracil: may enhance fluorouracil toxicity. Avoid concomitant use.
Methotrexate: may decrease efficacy of intrathecal methotrexate. Avoid concomitant use.

Contraindications and precautions

• Contraindicated in patients with pernicious anemia and other megaloblastic anemias secondary to lack of vitamin B$_{12}$.

NURSING CONSIDERATIONS

▨ Assessment
• Assess patient's condition before therapy and regularly thereafter.
• Monitor serum creatinine level daily to detect renal dysfunction.
• Be alert for adverse reactions and drug interactions.
• Monitor patient for rash, wheezing, pruritus, and urticaria, which can be signs of drug allergy.
• Evaluate patient's and family's knowledge of drug therapy.

⊕ Nursing diagnoses
• Altered health maintenance related to underlying conditions
• Knowledge deficit related to drug therapy

▧ Planning and implementation
P.O. and I.M. use: Follow normal protocol.

Reactions may be *common,* uncommon, *life-threatening,* or COMMON AND LIFE-THREATENING.

I.V. use: When using powder for injection, reconstitute 50-mg vial with 5 ml, 100-mg vial with 10 ml, or 350-mg vial with 17 ml of sterile water or bacteriostatic water for injection. When doses are greater than 10 mg/m^2, don't use diluents containing benzyl alcohol.
– Don't exceed 160 mg/minute when giving by direct injection.
• Do not confuse leucovorin (folinic acid) with folic acid.
• Follow leucovorin rescue schedule and protocol closely to maximize therapeutic response.
• Do not give simultaneously with systemic methotrexate.
• Protect drug from light and heat, especially reconstituted parenteral forms.
Patient teaching
• Tell patient reason for drug use.

☑ Evaluation
• Patient's condition improves.
• Patient and family state understanding of drug therapy.

leuprolide acetate
(loo-PROH-lighd AS-ih-tayt)
Leupron for Pediatric use, Lucrin◇, Lupron, Lupron Depot, Lupron Depot-Ped, Lupron Depot-3 Month, Lupron Depot-4 Month

Pharmacologic class: gonadotropin-releasing hormone
Therapeutic class: antineoplastic, luteinizing hormone-releasing hormone analogue
Pregnancy risk category: X

How supplied

Injection: 5 mg/ml in 2.8-ml multiple-dose vial
Depot injection:
Lupron Depot. 3.75 mg, 7.5 mg
Lupron Depot-Ped. 7.5 mg, 11.25 mg, 15 mg

Lupron Depot-3 month. 11.25 mg, 22.5 mg
Lupron Depot-4 month. 30 mg

Pharmacokinetics

Absorption: after S.C. administration, drug is rapidly and completely absorbed; unknown for I.M. use.
Distribution: unknown; about 7% to 15% bound to plasma proteins.
Metabolism: unknown.
Excretion: unknown. *Half-life:* 3 hours.

Route	Onset	Peak	Duration
I.M., S.C.	Unknown	1-2 mo	4-12 wk

Pharmacodynamics

Chemical effect: initially stimulates but then inhibits release of follicle-stimulating hormone and luteinizing hormone, resulting in testosterone suppression.
Therapeutic effect: hinders prostatic cancer cell growth and eases signs and symptoms of endometriosis.

Indications and dosage

▶ **Advanced prostate cancer.** *Adults:* 1 mg S.C. daily. Alternatively, 7.5 mg I.M. (depot injection) monthly; or 22.5 mg I.M. q 3 months (84 days); or 30 mg I.M. q 4 months (4 weeks, depot).
▶ **Endometriosis.** *Adults:* 3.75 mg I.M. (depot injection only) as single injection once monthly for up to 6 months.
▶ **Central precocious puberty.**
Children: initially, 0.3 mg/kg (minimum 7.5 mg) I.M. (depot injection only) as single injection q 4 weeks. Dosage may be increased in increments of 3.75 mg q 4 weeks, if needed. Alternatively, (injection form) 50 mcg/kg/day S.C. If total downregulation is not achieved, titrate dosage upward by 10 mcg/kg/day. This becomes the maintenance dosage. Therapy should be discontinued before female child reaches age 11 and before male child reaches age 12.

Adverse reactions

CNS: dizziness, depression, headache.

CV: *arrhythmias,* angina, *MI,* peripheral edema.
GI: nausea, vomiting.
Hepatic: elevated liver enzyme levels.
Respiratory: pulmonary embolism.
Other: transient bone pain (during first week of treatment), *hot flashes,* decreased libido, skin reactions (at injection site), gynecomastia, impotence.

Interactions
None significant.

Contraindications and precautions
• Contraindicated in patients hypersensitive to drug or other gonadotropin-releasing hormone analogues, in pregnant or breast-feeding women, and in women with undiagnosed vaginal bleeding.
• Use cautiously in patients hypersensitive to benzyl alcohol.
• Know that 30-mg depot formulation is contraindicated in women.

NURSING CONSIDERATIONS

Assessment
• Assess patient's condition before therapy and regularly thereafter.
• Be alert for adverse reactions.
• Evaluate patient's and family's knowledge of drug therapy.

Nursing diagnoses
• Altered health maintenance related to underlying condition
• Altered thought processes related to drug-induced depression
• Knowledge deficit related to drug therapy

Planning and implementation
• Never administer drug by I.V. injection.
I.M. use: Know that once-monthly depot injection should be administered under medical supervision. Use supplied diluent to reconstitute drug (extra diluent is provided and should be discarded). Draw 1 ml into syringe with 22G needle. (When preparing Lupron Depot-3 Month

22.5 mg, use a 23G or larger needle.) Withdraw 1.5 ml from ampule for the 3-month formulation. Inject into vial; then shake well. Suspension will appear milky. Although suspension is stable for 24 hours after reconstitution, it contains no bacteriostatic agent. Use immediately.
– When using prefilled dual-chamber syringes: Prepare for injection by screwing white plunger into end stopper until stopper begins to turn. Remove and discard tab around base of needle. Hold syringe upright and release diluent by slowly pushing plunger until first stopper is at blue line in middle of barrel. Gently shake syringe to form a uniform milky suspension. If particles adhere to stopper, tap syringe against finger. Remove needle guard and advance plunger to expel air from syringe. Inject entire contents I.M. as for a normal injection.
S.C. use: Follow normal protocol.
• Know that leuprolide is nonsurgical alternative to orchiectomy for prostate cancer.
• Know that a fractional dose of drug formulated to give q 3 months is not equivalent to same dose of once-monthly formulation.
Patient teaching
• Before starting therapy in child for central precocious puberty, ensure that parents understand importance of continuous therapy.
• Carefully instruct patient who will self-administer S.C. injection about proper administration techniques, and advise him to use only syringes provided by manufacturer.
• Advise patient that if another syringe must be substituted, a low-dose insulin syringe (U-100, 0.5 ml) may be an appropriate choice.
• Advise patient to store drug at room temperature, protected from light and sources of heat.
• Reassure patient with history of undesirable effects from other endocrine ther-

---

Reactions may be *common,* uncommon, *life-threatening,* or COMMON AND LIFE-THREATENING.

apies that leuprolide is much easier to tolerate.
• Reassure patient that these effects are transient and will disappear after about 1 week. Worsening of prostate cancer symptoms may occur when therapy is initiated.

☑ Evaluation
• Patient exhibits improvement in underlying condition.
• Patient demonstrates pretreatment thought processes.
• Patient and family state understanding of drug therapy.

levamisole hydrochloride
(lee-VUH-mee-sohl high-droh-KLOR-ighd)
Ergamisol

Pharmacologic class: immunomodulator
Therapeutic class: antineoplastic
Pregnancy risk category: C

How supplied
Tablets: 50 mg (base)

Pharmacokinetics
Absorption: rapidly absorbed from GI tract.
Distribution: unknown.
Metabolism: extensively metabolized by liver.
Excretion: excreted primarily in urine, with some excretion in feces. *Half-life:* 3 to 4 hours.

Route	Onset	Peak	Duration
P.O.	Unknown	1.5-2 hr	Unknown

Pharmacodynamics
Chemical effect: unknown; appears to restore depressed immune function and may potentiate actions of monocytes and macrophages and enhance T-cell responses.

Therapeutic effect: increases immune response.

Indications and dosage
▶ **Adjuvant treatment of Dukes' stage C colon cancer (with fluorouracil) after surgical resection.** *Adults:* 50 mg P.O. q 8 hours for 3 days. Therapy begun no sooner than 7 days and no later than 30 days after surgery, provided that patient is out of hospital, ambulating, and maintaining normal oral nutrition; has well-healed wounds; and has recovered from any postoperative complications. Fluorouracil (450 mg/m^2/day I.V.) is given for 5 days concomitant with 3-day course of levamisole starting 21 to 34 days after surgery. Maintenance dosage is 50 mg P.O. q 8 hours for 3 days q 2 weeks for 1 year. Given in conjunction with fluorouracil maintenance therapy (450 mg/m^2/day by rapid I.V. push, once a week beginning 28 days after initial 5-day course) for 1 year.

Adverse reactions
CNS: *dizziness, headache, paresthesias, somnolence, depression, nervousness, insomnia, anxiety, fatigue.*
CV: chest pain, edema.
EENT: blurred vision, conjunctivitis, *stomatitis, altered sense of taste and smell.*
GI: *nausea, diarrhea, vomiting, anorexia, abdominal pain, constipation, flatulence, dyspepsia.*
Hematologic: agranulocytosis, *leukopenia, thrombocytopenia.*
Skin: *dermatitis, exfoliative dermatitis,* pruritus, urticaria.
Other: hyperbilirubinemia, rigors, *alopecia, infection, fever, arthralgia, myalgia.*

Interactions
Drug-drug. *Phenytoin:* plasma levels may be elevated when administered with levamisole and fluorouracil. Monitor phenytoin plasma levels.

---

*Liquid form contains alcohol   **May contain tartrazine   ◆Canada   ◇ Australia   †OTC

Drug-lifestyle. *Alcohol use:* may precipitate disulfiram-like reaction. Avoid concomitant use.

Contraindications and precautions

• Contraindicated in patients hypersensitive to drug.
• Use cautiously in pregnant women.
• Safety of drug in breast-feeding women and in children has not been established.

NURSING CONSIDERATIONS

☰ Assessment
• Assess patient's condition before therapy and regularly thereafter.
• Obtain baseline CBC with differential, platelet count, electrolyte levels, and liver function studies, as ordered, immediately before starting therapy.
• Obtain CBC with differential and platelet count at weekly intervals, as ordered, before treatment with fluorouracil. Obtain electrolyte levels and liver function studies every 3 months for 1 year, as ordered.
• Be alert for adverse reactions and drug interactions.
• Evaluate patient's and family's knowledge of drug therapy.

⊞ Nursing diagnoses
• Altered health maintenance related to underlying condition
• Altered protection related to adverse hematologic reactions
• Knowledge deficit related to drug therapy

⊠ Planning and implementation
• Be aware that if levamisole therapy begins 7 to 20 days after surgery, fluorouracil should be started with second course of levamisole therapy. It should begin no sooner than 21 days and no later than 35 days after surgery. If levamisole is deferred until 21 to 30 days after surgery, fluorouracil therapy should begin with first course of levamisole.

• Know that dosage modifications are based on hematologic parameters. If WBC count is between $2,500/mm^3$ and $3,500/mm^3$, don't administer fluorouracil, as ordered, until WBC count is above $3,500/mm^3$. When fluorouracil is restarted, reduce dosage by 20%, as ordered. If WBC count stays below $2,500/mm^3$ for more than 10 days after fluorouracil is withdrawn, discontinue levamisole, as ordered. If platelet count is below $100,000/mm^3$, know that therapy with both fluorouracil and levamisole should be discontinued and the doctor notified.
• Don't exceed recommended doses. Higher doses are associated with greater incidence of agranulocytosis.
• Promptly report development of stomatitis or diarrhea. If either occurs during initial course of fluorouracil therapy, drug is discontinued and then weekly fluorouracil therapy is begun 28 days after start of initial course. If stomatitis or diarrhea develops during weekly doses of fluorouracil, fluorouracil therapy is deferred until these symptoms subside. Then fluorouracil therapy is started at reduced dosages (decreased by 20%).
Patient teaching
• Instruct patient to report stomatitis, diarrhea, or flulike symptoms, such as fever and chills.
• Advise patient to use soft toothbrush and electric razor to avoid trauma and excessive bleeding.
• Instruct patient to avoid alcohol consumption during drug therapy.
• Tell patient to avoid exposure to people with infection.

☑ Evaluation
• Patient responds well to therapy.
• Patient regains normal hematologic parameters.
• Patient and family state understanding of drug therapy.

Reactions may be *common,* uncommon, *life-threatening*, or COMMON AND LIFE-THREATENING.

levocarnitine (L-carnitine)
(lee-voh-KAR-nuh-teen)
Carnitor, L-Carnitine

Pharmacologic class: amino acid derivative
Therapeutic class: nutritional supplement
Pregnancy risk category: B

How supplied
Tablets: 330 mg
Capsules: 250mg
Oral liquid: 100 mg/ml
Injection: 1 g/5 ml

Pharmacokinetics
Absorption: unknown after P.O. administration.
Distribution: not bound to plasma proteins or albumin.
Metabolism: metabolized to major metabolites, trimethylamine *N*-oxide and gamma butyrobetaine.
Excretion: excreted primarily in urine; small amount excreted in feces.

Route	Onset	Peak	Duration
P.O., I.V.	Unknown	Unknown	Unknown

Pharmacodynamics
Chemical effect: facilitates transport of fatty acids (used to produce energy) into cellular mitochondria.
Therapeutic effect: relieves signs and symptoms of carnitine deficiency.

Indications and dosage
▶ **Primary and secondary systemic carnitine deficiency.** *Adults:* 990 mg P.O. b.i.d. or t.i.d. Alternatively, 10 to 30 ml (1 to 3 g) of oral liquid daily. *Children:* 50 to 100 mg/kg/day P.O. in divided doses. All dosages depend on clinical response. Higher dosages may be given. For children, maximum dosage is 3 g/day.
▶ **Acute and chronic treatment of secondary carnitine deficiency.** *Adults:* 50 mg/kg/day, divided and given I.V. slowly over 2 to 3 minutes q 3 to 4 hours.

Adverse reactions
GI: *nausea, vomiting, cramps, diarrhea.*
Other: body odor.

Interactions
Drug-drug. *L-carnitine (sold as vitamin B_T):* inhibition of levocarnitine and possible deficiency. Avoid concomitant use.
Valproic acid: increases requirement for carnitine. Adjust dosage as ordered.
Drug-lifestyle. *Any food:* decreased GI upset. Give with food.

Contraindications and precautions
• No known contraindications.
• Drug is not recommended for use in breast-feeding women.
• Use cautiously in pregnant women.

NURSING CONSIDERATIONS

⚕ Assessment
• Obtain history of patient's underlying condition before therapy.
• Monitor blood chemistry and plasma drug levels periodically, as ordered, as well as vital signs and patient's overall condition.
• Monitor patient's tolerance during first week of therapy and after increasing dosage, as ordered.
• Be alert for adverse reactions and drug interactions.
• Monitor patient's hydration status if adverse GI reactions occur.
• Evaluate patient's and family's knowledge of drug therapy.

▣ Nursing diagnoses
• Fatigue related to carnitine deficiency
• Risk for fluid volume deficit related to drug-induced adverse GI reactions
• Knowledge deficit related to drug therapy

▷ Planning and implementation
P.O. use: Give enteral liquid alone or dissolve in drinks or liquid food.

---

*Liquid form contains alcohol   **May contain tartrazine   ♦Canada   ◊Australia   †OTC

– Space doses evenly every 3 to 4 hours, and give drug with or after meals, if possible.

– Use contents of containers of liquid immediately after opening; discard unused contents.

– Do not refrigerate solution.

I.V. use: Administer drug slowly over 2 to 3 minutes.

Patient teaching
• Tell patient to consume oral liquid slowly to minimize GI distress. If GI intolerance persists, dosage may have to be reduced.
• Instruct patient to dissolve drug in drink or liquid food or take with meals to reduce GI upset.
• Warn patient to avoid "vitamin B$_T$" in health food stores because it interacts with drug and renders it ineffective.
• Caution patient not to share drug with others. Some people have used it to improve athletic performance.

☑ Evaluation
• Patient's energy level is increased.
• Patient maintains adequate hydration throughout therapy.
• Patient and family state understanding of drug therapy.

levodopa
(lee-voh-DOH-puh)
Dopar, Larodopa

Pharmacologic class: precursor of dopamine
Therapeutic class: antiparkinsonian agent
Pregnancy risk category: C

How supplied

Tablets: 100 mg, 250 mg, 500 mg
Capsules: 100 mg, 250 mg, 500 mg

Pharmacokinetics

Absorption: absorbed rapidly from small intestine by active amino acid transport system, with 30% to 50% reaching general circulation.

Distribution: distributed widely to most body tissues but not to CNS, which receives less than 1% of dose because of extensive metabolism in periphery.

Metabolism: 95% of levodopa is converted to dopamine in lumen of stomach and intestines and on first pass through liver.

Excretion: excreted primarily in urine.

Half-life: 1 to 3 hours.

Route	Onset	Peak	Duration
P.O.	3 wk-6 mo	1-3 hr	About 5 hr (but varies greatly)

Pharmacodynamics

Chemical effect: unknown; may be decarboxylated to dopamine, countering dopamine depletion in extrapyramidal centers.

Therapeutic effect: relieves signs and symptoms of parkinsonism.

Indications and dosage

▶ **Idiopathic parkinsonism, postencephalitic parkinsonism, and symptomatic parkinsonism after carbon monoxide or manganese intoxication or in association with cerebral arteriosclerosis.** *Adults and children over age 12:* initially, 0.5 to 1.0 g P.O. daily divided in two or more doses with food; increased by no more than 0.75 g daily q 3 to 7 days until usual optimal daily dosage of 3 to 6 g is reached. Dosage must not exceed 8 g daily. Dosage carefully adjusted to patient requirements, tolerance, and response. Higher dosage requires close supervision.

Adverse reactions

CNS: *aggressive behavior; choreiform, dystonic, and dyskinetic movements; involuntary grimacing, head movements, myoclonic body jerks,* **seizures,** *ataxia, tremors, muscle twitching; bradykinetic episodes; psychiatric disturbances; memory loss, mood changes, nervousness,*

*anxiety, disturbing dreams, euphoria, malaise, fatigue; severe depression, **suicidal tendencies,** dementia, delirium, hallucinations* (may necessitate reduction or withdrawal of drug).
CV: *orthostatic hypotension,* cardiac irregularities, flushing, hypertension, phlebitis.
EENT: blepharospasm, blurred vision, diplopia, mydriasis or miosis, widening of palpebral fissures, activation of latent Horner's syndrome, oculogyric crises, nasal discharge.
GI: dry mouth, excessive salivation, bitter taste, *nausea, vomiting, anorexia,* weight loss, constipation, flatulence, diarrhea, epigastric pain.
GU: urinary frequency, urine retention, incontinence, darkened urine, excessive and inappropriate sexual behavior, priapism.
Hematologic: *hemolytic anemia, leukopenia, agranulocytosis.*
Hepatic: hepatotoxicity.
Other: dark perspiration, hyperventilation, hiccups.

Interactions

Drug-drug. *Antacids:* increased absorption of levodopa. Administer antacids 1 hour after levodopa.
Anticholinergics: increased gastric deactivation and decreased intestinal absorption of levodopa may occur. Avoid concomitant use.
Benzodiazepine: levodopa's therapeutic value may be attenuated. Monitor closely.
Furazolidone, MAO inhibitors, procarbazine: risk of severe hypertension. Avoid concomitant use.
Inhalational halogen anesthetics, sympathomimetic agents: increased risk of arrhythmias. Monitor patient closely.
Metoclopramide: accelerated gastric emptying of levodopa. Give metoclopramide 1 hour after levodopa.
Papaverine, phenothiazines and other antipsychotics, phenytoin, rauwolfia alkaloids: decreased levodopa effect. Use together cautiously.

Pyridoxine: reversal of antiparkinsonian effects. Check vitamin preparations and nutritional supplements for pyridoxine (vitamin B_6) content. Don't give together.
Tricyclic antidepressants: delayed absorption and decreased bioavailability of levodopa may occur. Hypertensive episodes have occurred. Monitor closely.
Drug-food. *Foods high in protein:* decreased absorption of levodopa. Don't give with foods high in protein.
Drug-lifestyle. *Cocaine use:* increased risk of arrhythmias. Don't use together.

Contraindications and precautions

• Contraindicated in concurrent therapy with MAO inhibitors within 14 days and in patients with hypersensitivity to drug, acute angle-closure glaucoma, melanoma, or undiagnosed skin lesions.
• Drug should not be used in breast-feeding women.
• Use cautiously in patients with severe CV, renal, hepatic, or pulmonary disorder; peptic ulcer; psychiatric illness; MI with residual arrhythmias; bronchial asthma; emphysema; or endocrine disease and in pregnant women.
• Safety of drug has not been established in children age 12 and younger.

NURSING CONSIDERATIONS

▨ Assessment

• Assess patient's condition before therapy and regularly thereafter.
• Observe and monitor vital signs, especially while adjusting dosage.
• Know that patient receiving long-term therapy should be tested regularly for diabetes and acromegaly; periodically monitor kidney, liver, and hematopoietic function, as ordered.
• Be alert for adverse reactions and drug interactions.
• Evaluate patient's and family's knowledge of drug therapy.

---

*Liquid form contains alcohol   **May contain tartrazine   ◆Canada   ◇Australia   †OTC

⊕ Nursing diagnoses
• Impaired physical mobility related to presence of parkinsonism
• Altered thought processes related to drug-induced adverse reactions
• Knowledge deficit related to drug therapy

⊳ Planning and implementation
• To minimize GI upset, give drug with food. However, be aware that high-protein meals can impair absorption and reduce effectiveness.
• Know that patient who must undergo surgery should continue levodopa as long as oral intake is permitted, usually 6 to 24 hours before surgery. Drug should be resumed as soon as patient is able to take oral medication.
• Protect drug from heat, light, and moisture. If preparation darkens, it has lost potency and should be discarded.
• Report significant changes in vital signs.
• Be aware that muscle twitching and blepharospasm (twitching of eyelids) may be early signs of drug overdose; report immediately.
• Know that doctor-supervised period of drug discontinuance (called a drug holiday) may reestablish effectiveness of lower dosage regimen.
• Be aware that Coombs' test occasionally becomes positive during extended use. Expect elevated uric acid levels with colorimetric method but not with urate oxidase.
• Know that alkaline phosphatase, AST, ALT, LD, bilirubin, BUN, and protein-bound iodine levels show transient elevations in patient receiving levodopa; WBC count, hemoglobin, and hematocrit show occasional reductions.
• Depending on reagent and test method used, expect possible false-positive increases in uric acid, urine ketone, urine catecholamine, and urine vanillylmandelic acid levels.
• False-positive tests for urine glucose can occur if reagents using copper sulfate are used; false-negative results can occur with tests that use glucose enzymatic methods. An accurate measure can be obtained if paper strip is only partially immersed in urine sample. Urine migrates up strip, as with ascending chromatographic system. Read only top of strip.

Patient teaching
• Advise patient to take drug with food but to avoid taking it with high-protein meals. If patient has difficulty swallowing pills, tell him or family to crush tablets and mix with applesauce or baby food.
• Warn patient and family not to increase dosage without doctor's orders.
• Warn patient of possible dizziness and orthostatic hypotension, especially at start of therapy. Tell patient to change position slowly and dangle legs before getting out of bed. Elastic stockings may control this reaction.
• Advise patient and family that multivitamin preparations, fortified cereals, and certain OTC medications may contain pyridoxine (vitamin B_6), which can block effects of levodopa.
• Advise patient of potential for arrhythmias if using cocaine in conjunction with drug.

☑ Evaluation
• Patient exhibits improved physical mobility.
• Patient maintains normal thought process.
• Patient and family state understanding of drug therapy.

---

levonorgestrel
(lee-voh-nor-JES-trel)
Norplant System

Pharmacologic class: progestin
Therapeutic class: contraceptive
Pregnancy risk category: X

How supplied

Implants: 36 mg/capsule; each kit contains six capsules

Pharmacokinetics

Absorption: 100% bioavailable.
Distribution: bound by circulating protein sex hormone-binding globulin (SHBG).
Metabolism: metabolized by liver.
Excretion: metabolites excreted in urine.

Route	Onset	Peak	Duration
Subdermal	≤ 24 hr	≤ 24 hr	About 5 yr

Pharmacodynamics

Chemical effect: slowly releases synthetic progestin levonorgestrel into bloodstream. How progestins provide contraception is not understood, but they alter mucus covering cervix, prevent implantation of egg and, in some patients, prevent ovulation.
Therapeutic effect: prevents pregnancy.

Indications and dosage

▶ **Prevention of pregnancy.** *Women:* six capsules implanted subdermally in midportion of upper arm, about 8 cm above elbow crease, during first 7 days of onset of menses. Capsules are placed fanlike, 15 degrees apart (total of 75 degrees). Contraceptive efficacy lasts for 5 years.

Adverse reactions

CNS: headache, nervousness, dizziness.
GI: nausea, *abdominal discomfort*, appetite change.
GU: *amenorrhea, many days of bleeding or prolonged bleeding, spotting, irregular onset of bleeding, frequent onset of bleeding, scanty bleeding, cervicitis, vaginitis, leukorrhea.*
Skin: dermatitis, acne, hirsutism, hypertrichosis, scalp hair loss; infection, transient pain or itching (at implant site).
Other: adnexal enlargement, mastalgia, weight gain, *musculoskeletal pain, removal difficulty, breast discharge.*

Interactions

Drug-drug. *Carbamazepine, phenytoin, rifampin:* may reduce contraceptive efficacy of levonorgestrel implants. Avoid concomitant use.

Drug-food. *Caffeine:* may increase serum caffeine concentrations. Monitor effects.
Drug-lifestyle. *Smoking:* increased risk of adverse CV effects. Advise patient to stop smoking.

Contraindications and precautions

• Contraindicated in patients with active thrombophlebitis or thromboembolic disorders, undiagnosed abnormal genital bleeding, acute liver disease, malignant or benign liver tumors, known or suspected breast cancer, or known or suspected pregnancy.
• Use cautiously in patients with hyperlipidemia or history of depression and in diabetic or prediabetic patients.
• Little is known about effects of drug in breast-feeding women.

NURSING CONSIDERATIONS

Assessment

• Obtain pregnancy test before therapy and retest if pregnancy is suspected.
• Closely monitor patient with condition that may be aggravated by fluid retention because steroid hormones may cause fluid retention.
• Be alert for adverse reactions and drug interactions.
• Evaluate patient's and family's knowledge of drug therapy.

Nursing diagnoses

• Health-seeking behavior related to desire to prevent pregnancy
• Pain related to drug-induced adverse reactions
• Knowledge deficit related to drug therapy

Planning and implementation

• During insertion, pay special attention to asepsis and correct placement of capsules; use careful technique to minimize tissue trauma.
• Be aware that laboratory tests for SHBG and T_4 concentrations may show

decreased values; for T_3 uptake, increased values.

• Expect implants to be removed if active thrombophlebitis or thromboembolic disease develops or if the patient will be immobilized for a long time.

• If jaundice develops, expect implants to be removed because steroid hormone metabolism is impaired in patients with liver failure.

• Although retinal thrombosis after use of oral contraceptives has been reported, no similar incidents have been documented after use of implant system. However, patients with sudden, unexplained vision problems, including users of contact lenses in whom vision changes or changes in lens tolerance develop, should be immediately evaluated by an ophthalmologist.

Patient teaching

• Tell patient to report to doctor immediately if implant capsule falls out (before skin heals over implant). Efficacy may be impaired.

• Warn patient that missed menstrual periods are not accurate indicators of early pregnancy because drug may induce amenorrhea. Advise patient that 6 weeks or more of amenorrhea (after pattern of regular menstrual periods) could indicate pregnancy. If pregnancy is confirmed, implants must be removed.

• Encourage regular (at least annual) physical examinations.

• Inform patient that most patients develop variations in menstrual bleeding patterns, including irregular bleeding, prolonged bleeding, spotting, and amenorrhea. These irregularities usually diminish over time.

• Instruct patient to avoid caffeine consumption and smoking while on drug therapy.

☑ **Evaluation**

• Patient does not become pregnant.

• Patient is free from pain.

• Patient and family state understanding of drug therapy.

levothyroxine sodium (T_4-thyroxine sodium)
(lee-voh-thigh-ROKS-een SOH-dee-um)
Levo-T, Levothroid, Levoxyl, Oroxine◇, Synthroid**

Pharmacologic class: thyroid hormone
Therapeutic class: thyroid hormone replacement agent
Pregnancy risk category: A

How supplied

Tablets: 0.025 mg, 0.05 mg, 0.075 mg, 0.088 mg, 0.1 mg, 0.112 mg, 0.125 mg, 0.137 mg, 0.15 mg, 0.175 mg, 0.2 mg, 0.3 mg
Injection: 200 mcg/vial, 500 mcg/vial

Pharmacokinetics

Absorption: well absorbed from GI tract after P.O. administration.
Distribution: distributed widely; 99% protein-bound.
Metabolism: metabolized in peripheral tissues, primarily in liver, kidneys, and intestines.
Excretion: 20% to 40% excreted in feces. *Half-life:* 6 to 7 days.

Route	Onset	Peak	Duration
P.O., I.V., I.M.	24 hr	3-4 wk	1-3 wk

Pharmacodynamics

Chemical effect: not fully defined; stimulates metabolism by accelerating rate of cellular oxidation.
Therapeutic effect: raises thyroid hormone levels in body.

Indications and dosage

▶ **Cretinism.** *Children under age 1:* initially, 0.025 to 0.05 mg P.O. daily, increased to 0.05 mg P.O. in 4 to 6 weeks, as needed.

▶ **Myxedema coma.** *Adults:* 300 to 500 mcg I.V.; if no response in 24 hours, give an additional 100 to 300 mcg I.V. in 48 hours, followed by parenteral mainte-

nance dosage of 50 to 200 mcg I.V. daily. Patient should be switched to oral maintenance as soon as possible.
▶ **Thyroid hormone replacement.**
Adults: initially, 0.025 to 0.05 mg P.O. daily, increased by 0.025 mg P.O. q 2 to 4 weeks until desired response occurs. Maintenance dosage is 0.1 to 0.2 mg P.O. daily. May administer I.V. or I.M. when P.O. ingestion is precluded for long periods. Dosage adjustment may be necessary. *Adults over age 65:* 0.0125 to 0.025 mg P.O. daily. Increased by 0.0125 to 0.025 mg at 3- to 8-week intervals, depending on response. *Children:* initially, 0.025 to 0.075 mg in children younger than age 1 or 3 to 5 mcg/kg in children age 1 and older P.O. daily, gradually increased by 0.025 to 0.05 mg q 2 to 4 weeks until desired response occurs.

Adverse reactions

Adverse reactions to thyroid hormones are extensions of their pharmacologic properties and reflect patient sensitivity to them.
CNS: headache, *nervousness, insomnia, tremors.*
CV: *tachycardia, palpitations, arrhythmias,* angina pectoris, hypertension, *cardiac arrest.*
GI: appetite change, nausea, diarrhea.
GU: menstrual irregularities.
Other: leg cramps, weight loss, diaphoresis, heat intolerance, fever.

Interactions

Drug-drug. *Cholestyramine, colestipol:* impaired levothyroxine absorption. Separate doses by 4 to 5 hours.
Insulin, oral antidiabetic agents: altered serum glucose levels. Monitor blood glucose levels. Dosage adjustments may be necessary.
I.V. phenytoin: free thyroid released. Monitor for tachycardia.
Oral anticoagulants: altered PT. Monitor PT and INR. Dosage adjustments may be necessary.

Sympathomimetics (such as epinephrine): increased risk of coronary insufficiency. Monitor patient closely.

Contraindications and precautions

• Contraindicated in patients with acute MI uncomplicated by hypothyroidism, untreated thyrotoxicosis, uncorrected adrenal insufficiency, or hypersensitivity to drug.
• Use with extreme caution in patients with angina pectoris, hypertension, other CV disorders, renal insufficiency, or ischemia and in the elderly.
• Rapid replacement in patients with arteriosclerosis may precipitate angina, coronary occlusion, or CVA. Use cautiously in these patients.
• Use cautiously in patients with diabetes mellitus, diabetes insipidus, or myxedema and in breast-feeding women.

NURSING CONSIDERATIONS

⚏ Assessment
• Assess patient's condition before therapy and regularly thereafter. Normal serum levels of T_4 should occur within 24 hours, followed by threefold increase in serum T_3 in 3 days.
• Be alert for adverse reactions and drug interactions.
• In patients with coronary artery disease who must receive thyroid hormone, observe carefully for possible coronary insufficiency.
• Evaluate patient's and family's knowledge of drug therapy.

⚏ Nursing diagnoses
• Altered health maintenance related to presence of hypothyroidism
• Risk for injury related to drug-induced adverse reactions
• Knowledge deficit related to drug therapy

⚏ Planning and implementation
• Know that thyroid hormone replacement requirements are about 25% lower in patients over age 60 than in young adults.

• Be aware that patients with adult hypothyroidism are unusually sensitive to thyroid hormone. Patient should be started at lowest dosage and titrated to higher dosages based on symptoms and laboratory data until euthyroid state is reached. **P.O. use:** When changing from levothyroxine to liothyronine, levothyroxine should be stopped and liothyronine begun. Dosage increased in small increments after residual effects of levothyroxine disappear. When changing from liothyronine to levothyroxine, levothyroxine is started several days before withdrawing liothyronine to avoid relapse. **I.V. use:** Prepare I.V. dose immediately before injection. Do not mix with other solutions. Inject into vein over 1 to 2 minutes. **I.M. use:** Follow normal protocol. • Thyroid hormones alter thyroid function test results. Patients taking these hormones usually require decreased anticoagulant dosage. • Patients taking levothyroxine who need to have radioactive iodine uptake studies performed must discontinue drug 4 weeks before test. *Patient teaching* • Stress importance of compliance. Tell patient to take thyroid hormones at same time each day, preferably before breakfast, to maintain constant hormone levels. Suggest morning dosage to prevent insomnia. • Warn patient (especially elderly patient) to notify doctor at once of chest pain, palpitations, sweating, nervousness, shortness of breath, or other signs of overdose or aggravated CV disease. • Advise patient who has achieved stable response not to change brands. • Tell patient to report unusual bleeding and bruising.

☑ **Evaluation** • Patient's thyroid hormone levels are normal. • Patient does not experience injury.

• Patient and family state understanding of drug therapy.

lidocaine hydrochloride (lignocaine hydrochloride)
(LIGH-doh-kayn high-droh-KLOR-ighd)
LidoPen Auto-Injector, Xylocaine, Xylocard♦ ◊

Pharmacologic class: amide derivative
Therapeutic class: ventricular antiarrhythmic
Pregnancy risk category: B

How supplied

Injection (for I.M. use): 300 mg/3 ml automatic injection device
Injection (for direct I.V. use): 1% (10 mg/ml), 2% (20 mg/ml)
Injection (for I.V. admixtures): 4% (40 mg/ml), 10% (100 mg/ml), 20% (200 mg/ml)
Infusion (premixed): 0.2% (2 mg/ml), 0.4% (4 mg/ml), 0.8% (8 mg/ml)

Pharmacokinetics

Absorption: nearly complete after I.M. administration.
Distribution: distributed widely, especially to adipose tissue.
Metabolism: most of drug metabolized in liver to two active metabolites.
Excretion: less than 10% excreted in urine unchanged. *Half-life:* ½ to 2 hours (may be prolonged in patients with heart failure or hepatic disease).

Route	Onset	Peak	Duration
I.V.	Immediate	30-60 min (no bolus)	10-20 min
I.M.	5-15 min	10 min	60 min

Pharmacodynamics

Chemical effect: decreases depolarization, automaticity, and excitability in ventricles during diastolic phase by direct action on tissues.

Therapeutic effect: abolishes ventricular arrhythmias.

Indications and dosage

▶ **Ventricular arrhythmias resulting from MI, cardiac manipulation, or cardiac glycosides.** *Adults:* 50 to 100 mg (1.0 to 1.5 mg/kg) by I.V. bolus at 25 to 50 mg/minute. Half this amount is given to elderly patients or patients under 50 kg (110 lb) and to those with heart failure or hepatic disease. Bolus dose is repeated q 3 to 5 minutes until arrhythmias subside or adverse reactions develop. Don't exceed 300-mg total bolus during 1-hour period. Simultaneously, constant infusion of 20 to 50 mcg/kg/minute (1 to 4 mg/minute) is begun. If single bolus has been given, smaller bolus dose may be repeated 5 to 10 minutes after start of infusion to maintain therapeutic serum level. After 24 hours of continuous infusion, rate is decreased by one-half. Alternatively, 200 to 300 mg I.M., followed by second I.M. dose 60 to 90 minutes later, if needed. *Children:* 1 mg/kg by I.V. bolus, followed by infusion of 20 to 50 mcg/kg/minute.

Adverse reactions

CNS: *confusion, tremors,* lethargy, somnolence, *stupor, restlessness,* slurred speech, euphoria, depression, *light-headedness,* paresthesia, muscle twitching, *seizures, respiratory arrest.*
CV: *hypotension,* bradycardia, *new or worsened arrhythmias, cardiac arrest.*
EENT: *tinnitus, blurred or double vision.*
Other: *anaphylaxis,* soreness at injection site, cold sensation, *status asthmaticus,* diaphoresis.

Interactions

Drug-drug. *Beta blockers, cimetidine:* decreased metabolism of lidocaine. Monitor for toxicity.
Phenytoin, procainamide, propranolol, quinidine: additive cardiac depressant effects. Monitor patient.

Succinylcholine: prolongation of neuromuscular blockage may occur. Monitor for increased effects.
Tocainide: concomitant use may cause an increased incidence of adverse reactions. Avoid concomitant use.
Drug-lifestyle. *Smoking:* may increase metabolism of lidocaine. Monitor closely.

Contraindications and precautions

• Contraindicated in patients with hypersensitivity to amide-type local anesthetics, Adams-Stokes syndrome, Wolff-Parkinson-White syndrome, or severe degrees of SA, AV, or intraventricular block in absence of artificial pacemaker.
• Use cautiously in patients with complete or second-degree heart block or sinus bradycardia, in elderly patients, in those with heart failure or renal or hepatic disease, and in those weighing below 50 kg. Reduced dosage in these patients is required.
• Safety of drug has not been established in children and in breast-feeding women.

NURSING CONSIDERATIONS

🔆 **Assessment**
• Assess patient's condition before therapy and regularly thereafter.
• Know that patient receiving infusion must be on cardiac monitor and be attended *at all times.*
• Monitor patient's response, especially ECG, blood pressure, and serum electrolyte, BUN, and creatinine levels, as ordered.
• Monitor therapeutic serum levels, as ordered. Therapeutic serum levels are 2 to 5 mcg/ml.
• Be alert for adverse reactions and drug interactions.
• Monitor patient for toxicity. Seizures may be first clinical sign. Severe reactions usually are preceded by somnolence, confusion, and paresthesias.
• Evaluate patient's and family's knowledge of drug therapy.

🕮 Nursing diagnoses

• Decreased cardiac output related to presence of ventricular arrhythmia
• Altered thought processes related to adverse CNS reactions
• Knowledge deficit related to drug therapy

▷ Planning and implementation

I.V. use: Use infusion-control device for administering infusion precisely. Do not exceed infusion rate of 4 mg/minute; faster rate greatly increases risk of toxicity.

I.M. use: Give I.M. injections in deltoid muscle only.

– Remind doctor to test isoenzymes if I.M. route is prescribed in patients with suspected MI. This is necessary because patients who received I.M. lidocaine show sevenfold increase in serum CK level. Such an increase originates in skeletal muscle, not cardiac muscle.

• If signs of toxicity (such as dizziness) occur, stop drug at once and notify doctor. Continued infusion could lead to seizures and coma. Give oxygen by way of nasal cannula, if not contraindicated. Keep oxygen and cardiopulmonary resuscitation equipment available.

• Discontinue drug and notify doctor if arrhythmias worsen or if ECG changes, such as widening QRS complex or substantially prolonged PR interval, are evident.

Patient teaching

• Explain drug's purpose.
• Tell patient or caregiver to alert nurse of adverse reactions.
• Instruct patient to avoid smoking during drug therapy.

☑ Evaluation

• Patient's cardiac output returns to normal with abolishment of ventricular arrhythmia.
• Patient maintains normal thought processes throughout therapy.
• Patient and family state understanding of drug therapy.

lincomycin hydrochloride
(lin-koh-MIGH-sin high-droh-KLOR-ighd)
Lincocin

Pharmacologic class: lincosamide
Therapeutic class: antibiotic
Pregnancy risk category: NR

How supplied

Capsules: 500 mg
Pediatric capsules: 250 mg
Injection: 300 mg/ml in 2-ml and 10-ml vials and 2-ml U-Ject

Pharmacokinetics

Absorption: with P.O. administration, only about 20% to 30% of dose is absorbed. With I.M. administration, drug is absorbed rapidly.
Distribution: well distributed in pleural, synovial, and peritoneal fluids; bone; bile; and aqueous humor. It penetrates CSF poorly. Plasma protein binding depends on concentration and ranges from about 57% to 72%.
Metabolism: metabolized partially in liver.
Excretion: excreted by renal and biliary pathways. *Half-life:* 4 to 6 hours.

Route	Onset	Peak	Duration
P.O.	Unknown	2-4 hr	Unknown
I.V.	Immediate	Immediate	Unknown
I.M.	Unknown	30 min	Unknown

Pharmacodynamics

Chemical effect: unknown; may inhibit bacterial protein synthesis by binding to 50S subunit of ribosome.
Therapeutic effect: inhibits growth of susceptible bacteria. Spectrum of activity includes *Streptococcus pneumoniae* and most staphylococci and several anaerobic gram-negative and gram-positive organisms.

Indications and dosage

▶ **Respiratory tract, skin and soft-tissue, and urinary tract infections; osteomyelitis, septicemia caused by sensitive group A beta-hemolytic streptococci, pneumococci, and staphylococci.**
Adults: 500 mg P.O. q 6 to 8 hours (not to exceed 8 g daily); or 600 mg I.M. daily or q 12 hours; or 600 mg to 1 g I.V. q 8 to 12 hours (not to exceed 8 g daily).
Children over age 1 month: 30 to 60 mg/kg P.O. daily in divided doses q 6 to 8 hours; or 10 mg/kg I.M. daily or in divided doses q 12 hours; or 10 to 20 mg/kg I.V. daily in divided doses q 6 to 8 hours.

Adverse reactions

CNS: dizziness, headache.
CV: hypotension, *cardiopulmonary arrest* (with rapid I.V. infusion).
EENT: tinnitus.
GI: nausea, vomiting, glossitis, *pseudomembranous colitis, persistent diarrhea,* abdominal cramps, stomatitis, pruritus ani.
GU: vaginitis.
Hematologic: *neutropenia, leukopenia, thrombocytopenia,* purpura, *agranulocytosis.*
Skin: rash, urticaria.
Other: hypersensitivity reactions *(anaphylaxis),* angioedema, cholestatic jaundice, pain (at injection site).

Interactions

Drug-drug. *Antidiarrheals (such as attapulgite, kaolin, pectin):* reduced oral absorption of lincomycin by as much as 90%. Avoid antidiarrheals or give at least 2 hours before lincomycin.
Neuromuscular blockers: may potentiate neuromuscular blockade. Monitor for prolonged weakness.

Contraindications and precautions

• Contraindicated in patients with hypersensitivity to lincomycin or clindamycin.
• Drug is not recommended for use in breast-feeding women.

• Use cautiously in patients with GI disorders (especially colitis), asthma or significant allergies, hepatic or renal disease, or endocrine or metabolic disorders. Also use cautiously in pregnant women.

NURSING CONSIDERATIONS

☍ Assessment
• Assess patient's infection before therapy and regularly thereafter.
• Obtain specimen for culture and sensitivity tests before first dose. Therapy may begin pending results.
• Monitor CBC and platelets.
• Monitor liver function (increased levels of alkaline phosphatase, ALT, AST, or bilirubin may occur).
• Monitor blood pressure in patient receiving drug parenterally.
• Be alert for adverse reactions and drug interactions.
• When giving I.V., check site daily for phlebitis and irritation and rotate infusion sites regularly.
• Monitor patient's hydration status if adverse GI reactions occur.
• Monitor for signs of bacterial and fungal superinfection, especially when therapy exceeds 10 days.
• Evaluate patient's and family's knowledge of drug therapy.

☍ Nursing diagnoses
• Infection related to presence of susceptible bacteria
• Risk for fluid volume deficit related to drug-induced adverse GI reactions
• Knowledge deficit related to drug therapy

▶ Planning and implementation
P.O. use: Give drug on empty stomach with full glass of water.
I.V. use: Dilute drug to 100 ml, and infuse over 1 hour. Rapid I.V. infusion may cause hypotension and syncope.
I.M. use: Inject drug deeply, and rotate injection sites. Warn patient that I.M. injection may be painful.

• Stop drug immediately if neutropenia, leukopenia, or other blood disorders develop, and notify doctor.
Patient teaching
• For best absorption, tell patient to take drug with full glass of water 1 hour before or 2 hours after meals.
• Advise patient to take drug exactly as directed, even after he feels better, and to take entire amount prescribed.
• Tell patient to report adverse reactions to doctor, especially diarrhea. Warn him not to treat diarrhea himself because it may reflect onset of antibiotic-associated pseudomembranous colitis.

☑ **Evaluation**
• Patient is free from infection.
• Patient maintains adequate hydration throughout therapy.
• Patient and family state understanding of drug therapy.

liothyronine sodium (T_3)
(lee-oh-THIGH-roh-neen SOH-dee-um)
Cytomel, Tertroxin◇, Triostat

Pharmacologic class: thyroid hormone
Therapeutic class: thyroid hormone replacement agent
Pregnancy risk category: A

How supplied

Tablets: 5 mcg, 25 mcg, 50 mcg
Injection: 10 mcg/ml

Pharmacokinetics

Absorption: 95% absorbed from GI tract.
Distribution: highly protein-bound.
Metabolism: unknown.
Excretion: unknown. *Half-life:* 1 to 2 days.

Route	Onset	Peak	Duration
P.O.	Unknown	2-3 days	About 3 days
I.V.	Unknown	Unknown	Unknown

Pharmacodynamics

Chemical effect: not clearly defined; enhances oxygen consumption by most tissues of body and increases basal metabolic rate and metabolism of carbohydrates, lipids, and proteins.
Therapeutic effect: raises thyroid hormone levels in body.

Indications and dosage

▶ **Congenital hypothyroidism.**
Children: 5 mcg P.O. daily with a 5-mcg increase q 3 to 4 days until desired response achieved.
▶ **Myxedema.** *Adults:* initially, 5 mcg P.O. daily, increased by 5 to 10 mcg q 1 to 2 weeks until daily dosage reaches 25 mcg. Then, increased by 12.5 to 25.0 mcg daily q 1 to 2 weeks. Maintenance dosage is 50 to 100 mcg daily.
▶ **Myxedema coma, precoma.** *Adults:* initially 10 to 20 mcg I.V. for patients with known or suspected CV disease; 25 to 50 mcg I.V. for those not known to have CV disease. Subsequent dosages based on patient's condition and response.
▶ **Nontoxic goiter.** *Adults:* initially, 5 mcg P.O. daily; may increase by 5 to 10 mcg daily q 1 to 2 weeks until daily dosage reaches 25 mcg. Then, increase by 12.5 to 25.0 mcg daily q 1 to 2 weeks. Usual maintenance dosage is 75 mcg daily.
▶ **Thyroid hormone replacement.** *Adults:* initially, 25 mcg P.O. daily, increased by 12.5 to 25.0 mcg q 1 to 2 weeks until satisfactory response. Usual maintenance dosage is 25 to 75 mcg daily.
▶ **T_3 suppression test to differentiate hyperthyroidism from euthyroidism.** *Adults:* 75 to 100 mcg P.O. daily for 7 days.

Adverse reactions

Adverse reactions to thyroid hormones are extensions of their pharmacologic properties and reflect patient sensitivity to them.
CNS: hyperirritability, *nervousness, insomnia, tremors,* headache.

Reactions may be *common*, uncommon, **life-threatening**, or COMMON AND LIFE-THREATENING.

CV: *tachycardia,* ***arrhythmias,*** angina pectoris, increased blood pressure, ***cardiac arrest.***
GI: diarrhea, abdominal cramps, vomiting.
Other: weight loss, heat intolerance, diaphoresis, accelerated rate of bone maturation in infants and children, menstrual irregularities.

Interactions

Drug-drug. *Cholestyramine, colestipol:* impaired liothyronine absorption. Separate doses by 4 to 5 hours.
Insulin, oral antidiabetic agents: initial thyroid replacement therapy may cause increases in insulin or oral hypoglycemic requirements. Monitor blood glucose levels. Dosage adjustments may be necessary.
I.V. phenytoin: free thyroid released. Monitor for tachycardia.
Oral anticoagulants: altered PT. Monitor PT and INR. Dosage adjustments may be necessary.
Sympathomimetics (such as epinephrine): increased risk of coronary insufficiency. Monitor patient closely.

Contraindications and precautions

• Contraindicated in patients with acute MI uncomplicated by hypothyroidism, untreated thyrotoxicosis, uncorrected adrenal insufficiency, hypersensitivity to drug.
• Use with extreme caution in elderly patients and those with angina pectoris, hypertension, other CV disorders, renal insufficiency, or ischemia.
• Rapid replacement in patients with arteriosclerosis may precipitate angina, coronary occlusion, or CVA. Use cautiously in these patients.
• Use cautiously in patients with diabetes mellitus, diabetes insipidus, or myxedema and in breast-feeding women.

NURSING CONSIDERATIONS

☑ Assessment
• Assess patient's condition before therapy and regularly thereafter.

• Monitor pulse rate and blood pressure.
• Observe patient with coronary artery disease for coronary insufficiency.
• Be alert for adverse reactions and drug interactions.
• Evaluate patient's and family's knowledge of drug therapy.

⊞ Nursing diagnoses
• Altered health maintenance related to underlying thyroid condition
• Sleep pattern disturbance related to drug-induced insomnia
• Knowledge deficit related to drug therapy

⊠ Planning and implementation
• Levothyroxine is usually preferred for thyroid hormone replacement therapy. Liothyronine may be used when rapid onset or rapidly reversible agent is desirable or in patients with impaired peripheral conversion of levothyroxine to liothyronine.
• In most patients, regulation of liothyronine dosage is difficult.
P.O. use: Give drug at same time every day, preferably in the morning to prevent insomnia.
I.V. use: Repeat dosages should be given longer than 4 hours but less than 12 hours apart. Do not give I.M. or S.C.
• Know that thyroid hormone replacement requirements are about 25% lower in patients over age 60 than in young adults.
• When changing from levothyroxine to liothyronine, levothyroxine should be stopped and liothyronine begun at low dosage and increased in small increments after residual effects of levothyroxine have disappeared. When changing from liothyronine to levothyroxine, levothyroxine is started several days before withdrawing liothyronine to avoid relapse.
• Know that thyroid hormones alter thyroid function tests. Patient taking these hormones usually requires decreased anticoagulant dosage.

• Be aware that patient taking liothyronine who needs to have radioactive iodine uptake studies performed must discontinue drug 7 to 10 days before test.

Patient teaching

• Stress importance of compliance. Tell patient to take thyroid hormones at same time each day, preferably before breakfast, to maintain constant hormone levels. Suggest morning dosage to prevent insomnia.

• Advise patient who has achieved stable response not to change brands to avoid problems with bioequivalence.

• Warn patient (especially elderly patient) to notify doctor at once if chest pain, palpitations, sweating, nervousness, or other signs of overdose occur or if signs of aggravated CV disease (chest pain, dyspnea, and tachycardia) develop.

• Tell patient to report unusual bleeding and bruising.

☑ Evaluation

• Patient's thyroid hormone levels are normal.

• Patient does not have insomnia.

• Patient and family state understanding of drug therapy.

lisinopril
(ligh-SIN-uh-pril)
Prinivil, Zestril

Pharmacologic class: ACE inhibitor
Therapeutic class: antihypertensive
Pregnancy risk category: C (D in second and third trimesters)

How supplied

Tablets: 2.5 mg, 5 mg, 10 mg, 20 mg, 40 mg

Pharmacokinetics

Absorption: variable.
Distribution: distributed widely in tissues, although only minimal amount enters brain. Plasma protein binding appears insignificant.
Metabolism: not metabolized.
Excretion: excreted unchanged in urine.
Half-life: 12 hours.

Route	Onset	Peak	Duration
P.O.	1 hr	7 hr	24 hr

Pharmacodynamics

Chemical effect: unknown; may result primarily from suppression of renin-angiotensin-aldosterone system.
Therapeutic effect: lowers blood pressure.

Indications and dosage

▶ **Hypertension.** Adults: initially, 10 mg P.O. daily. If patient is also receiving diuretic therapy, reduce initial dosage to 5 mg P.O. daily. Most patients are well controlled on 20 to 40 mg daily as single dose.

▶ **Treatment adjunct in heart failure (with diuretics and cardiac glycosides).** Adults: initially, 5 mg P.O. daily. Usual effective dosage range is 5 to 20 mg daily as single dose. In patients with hyponatremia (serum sodium below 130 mEq/L) or serum creatinine above 3 mg/dl, initiate dose at 2.5 mg P.O. once daily.

▶ **Treatment of hemodynamically stable patients within 24 hours of acute MI to improve survival.** Adults: initially, 5 mg P.O., followed by 5 mg P.O. after 24 hours, 10 mg P.O. after 48 hours, then 10 mg P.O. once daily for 6 weeks. Patients with systolic blood pressure of 120 mm Hg or less at initiation of therapy or during first 3 days after an infarct should receive reduced dosage of 2.5 mg P.O.

Adverse reactions

CNS: *dizziness, headache, fatigue,* depression, somnolence, paresthesia.
CV: hypotension, *orthostatic hypotension,* chest pain.
EENT: *nasal congestion.*

GI: *diarrhea,* nausea, dyspepsia, dysgeusia.
GU: impotence.
Hematologic: neutropenia, *agranulocytopenia.*
Respiratory: *dry, persistent, tickling, nonproductive cough.*
Skin: rash.
Other: *muscle cramps, angioedema, anaphylaxis,* decreased libido, hyperkalemia.

Interactions

Drug-drug. *Capsaicin:* may cause or exacerbate coughing associated with ACE inhibitors treatment. Monitor closely.
Diuretics: excessive hypotension. Monitor blood pressure.
Indomethacin: attenuated hypotensive effect. Monitor blood pressure.
Insulin, oral antidiabetic agents: risk of hypoglycemia, especially when lisinopril starts. Monitor closely.
Lithium: increased serum lithium levels. Monitor for toxicity.
Potassium-sparing diuretics, potassium supplements: hyperkalemia. Monitor potassium level.
Thiazide diuretics: attenuation of potassium loss caused by thiazide diuretics. Discontinue diuretics 2 to 3 days before lisinopril therapy or reduce lisinopril dosage to 5 mg P.O. once daily, as ordered.
Drug-food. *Potassium-containing salt substitutes*: possible hyperkalemia. Monitor closely.

Contraindications and precautions

• Contraindicated in patients with hypersensitivity to ACE inhibitors or history of angioedema related to previous treatment with ACE inhibitor and in pregnant women.
• Use cautiously in patients with impaired kidney function; dosage adjustment is required. Also use cautiously in patients at risk for hyperkalemia (presence of renal insufficiency or diabetes or use of drugs that raise potassium level) and in breast-feeding women.
• Safety of drug has not been established in children.

NURSING CONSIDERATIONS

✎ Assessment
• Assess patient's condition before therapy and regularly thereafter. Beneficial effects of drug may require several weeks of therapy.
• Monitor WBC with differential counts before therapy, every 2 weeks for first 3 months of therapy, and periodically thereafter.
• Be alert for adverse reactions and drug interactions.
• Evaluate patient's and family's knowledge of drug therapy.

⊕ Nursing diagnoses
• Risk for injury related to presence of hypertension
• Decreased cardiac output related to drug-induced hypotension
• Knowledge deficit related to drug therapy

❯ Planning and implementation
• If drug does not control blood pressure, diuretics may be added.
Patient teaching
• Advise patient to report signs or symptoms of angioedema (including laryngeal edema), such as swelling of face, eyes, lips, or tongue, or breathing difficulty.
• Tell patient that light-headedness may occur, especially during first few days of therapy. Tell him to rise slowly to minimize this effect and to report symptoms to doctor. If syncope occurs, tell patient to stop taking drug and call doctor immediately.
• Tell patient not to discontinue drug suddenly but to call doctor if adverse reactions occur.
• Advise patient to report signs of infection, such as fever and sore throat.

• Tell female patient to notify doctor if pregnancy occurs. Drug will need to be discontinued.

☑ **Evaluation**
• Patient's blood pressure is within normal limits.
• Patient maintains adequate cardiac output throughout therapy.
• Patient and family state understanding of drug therapy.

lithium carbonate
(LITH-ee-um KAR-buh-nayt)
Carbolith♦, Duralith♦, Eskalith, Eskalith CR, Lithane**, Lithicarb◇, Lithizine♦, Lithobid, Lithonate, Lithotabs

lithium citrate
Cibalith-S*

Pharmacologic class: alkali metal
Therapeutic class: antimanic agent
Pregnancy risk category: D

How supplied

lithium carbonate
Tablets: 300 mg (300 mg = 8.12 mEq lithium)
Tablets (controlled-release): 300 mg, 450 mg
Capsules: 150 mg, 300 mg, 600 mg
lithium citrate
Syrup (sugarless): 8 mEq (of lithium) per 5 ml
Note: 5 ml of lithium citrate (liquid) contains 8 mEq lithium, equal to 300 mg of lithium carbonate.

Pharmacokinetics

Absorption: rate and extent vary with dosage form; absorption is complete within 8 hours of P.O. use.
Distribution: distributed widely in body; concentrations in thyroid gland, bone, and brain tissue exceed serum levels.
Metabolism: not metabolized.

Excretion: 95% excreted unchanged in urine. *Half-life:* 18 hours (adolescents) to 36 hours (elderly).

Route	Onset	Peak	Duration
P.O.	1-3 wk	0.5-3 hr	Unknown

Pharmacodynamics

Chemical effect: unknown; probably alters chemical transmitters in CNS, possibly by interfering with ionic pump mechanisms in brain cells, and may compete with sodium ions.
Therapeutic effect: prevents or controls mania.

Indications and dosage

▶ **Prevention or control of mania.**
Adults: 300 to 600 mg P.O. up to q.i.d., increasing on basis of blood levels to achieve optimal dosage, usually 1,800 mg/day. Recommended therapeutic lithium blood levels: 1 to 1.5 mEq/L for acute mania; 0.6 to 1.2 mEq/L for maintenance therapy; and 2 mEq/L as maximum dosage.

Adverse reactions

CNS: tremors, drowsiness, headache, confusion, restlessness, dizziness, psychomotor retardation, stupor, lethargy, *coma,* blackouts, *epileptiform seizures,* EEG changes, worsened organic mental syndrome, impaired speech, ataxia, muscle weakness, incoordination.
CV: *reversible ECG changes, arrhythmias,* hypotension, *peripheral vascular collapse* (rare).
EENT: tinnitus, blurred vision.
GI: dry mouth, metallic taste, nausea, vomiting, anorexia, diarrhea, thirst, abdominal pain, flatulence, indigestion.
GU: polyuria, glycosuria, *renal toxicity* with long-term use, decreased creatinine clearance, albuminuria.
Hematologic: *leukocytosis with leukocyte count of 14,000 to 18,000/mm³* (reversible).
Metabolic: transient hyperglycemia, goiter, hypothyroidism (lowered T_3, T_4, and

---

Reactions may be *common,* uncommon, *life-threatening*, or COMMON AND LIFE-THREATENING.

protein-bound iodine but elevated ^{131}I [radioactive iodine] uptake), hyponatremia.
Skin: pruritus, rash, diminished or absent sensation, drying and thinning of hair, psoriasis, acne, alopecia.
Other: ankle and wrist edema.

Interactions

Drug-drug. *Aminophylline, sodium bicarbonate, urine alkalinizers:* increased lithium excretion. Avoid salt loads and monitor lithium levels.
Carbamazepine, indomethacin, methyldopa, piroxicam, probenecid: increased effect of lithium. Monitor for lithium toxicity.
Diuretics: increased reabsorption of lithium by kidneys with possible toxic effect. Use with extreme caution, and monitor lithium and electrolyte levels (especially sodium).
Fluoxetine: increased lithium serum levels.
Neuroleptics: may cause encephalopathy. Watch for signs and symptoms (lethargy, tremors, extrapyramidal symptoms), and stop drug if they occur.
Neuromuscular blockers: may cause prolonged paralysis or weakness. Monitor patient closely.
Thyroid hormones: may induce hypothyroidism. Monitor thyroid function.

Contraindications and precautions

• Contraindicated if therapy cannot be closely monitored.
• Drug should not be used in pregnant or breast-feeding women.
• Drug is not recommended for use in children under age 12.
• Use with extreme caution in patients receiving neuroleptics, neuromuscular blockers, or diuretics; in elderly or debilitated patients; and in patients with thyroid disease, seizure disorder, renal or CV disease, severe debilitation or dehydration, or sodium depletion.

NURSING CONSIDERATIONS

▨ Assessment
• Assess patient's condition before therapy and regularly thereafter. Expect delay of 1 to 3 weeks before drug's beneficial effects are noticed.
• Monitor baseline ECG, thyroid and kidney studies, and electrolyte levels, as ordered. Monitor lithium blood levels 8 to 12 hours after first dose, usually before morning dose, two or three times weekly in first month, then weekly to monthly during maintenance therapy.
• Know that with blood levels of lithium below 1.5 mEq/L, adverse reactions usually remain mild.
• Check urine-specific gravity and report level below 1.005, which may indicate diabetes insipidus.
• Be aware that lithium may alter glucose tolerance in diabetic patient. Monitor blood glucose level closely.
• Perform outpatient follow-up of thyroid and kidney function every 6 to 12 months. Palpate thyroid to check for enlargement.
• Be alert for adverse reactions and drug interactions.
• Evaluate patient's and family's knowledge of drug therapy.

⊞ Nursing diagnoses
• Altered thought processes related to presence of manic disorder
• Altered health maintenance related to drug-induced endocrine dysfunction
• Knowledge deficit related to drug therapy

▷ Planning and implementation
• Be aware that determination of lithium blood concentration is crucial to safe use of drug. Drug should not be used in patients who can't have regular lithium blood level checks.
• Give with plenty of water and after meals to minimize GI reactions.
• Before leaving bedside, make sure patient has swallowed medication.

• Notify doctor if patient's behavior has not improved in 3 weeks or if it worsens.
Patient teaching
• Tell patient to take drug with plenty of water and after meals to minimize GI upset.
• Explain that lithium has narrow therapeutic margin of safety. A blood level that is even slightly high can be dangerous.
• Warn patient and family to watch for signs of toxicity (diarrhea, vomiting, tremors, drowsiness, muscle weakness, ataxia) and to expect transient nausea, polyuria, thirst, and discomfort during first few days. Tell patient to withhold one dose and call doctor if toxic symptoms appear but not to stop drug abruptly.
• Warn ambulatory patient to avoid activities that require alertness and good psychomotor coordination until CNS effects of drug are known.
• Tell patient not to switch brands or take other prescription or OTC drugs without doctor's approval.
• Inform patient that he should carry a medical identification card.

☑ **Evaluation**
• Patient exhibits improved behavior and thought processes.
• Patient maintains normal endocrine function throughout therapy.
• Patient and family state understanding of drug therapy.

lomefloxacin hydrochloride
(loh-muh-FLOKS-uh-sin high-droh-KLOR-ighd)
Maxaquin

Pharmacologic class: fluoroquinolone
Therapeutic class: broad-spectrum antibiotic
Pregnancy risk category: C

How supplied
Tablets (film-coated): 400 mg

Pharmacokinetics
Absorption: absorbed rapidly from GI tract; absolute bioavailability is 95% to 98%. Food impairs absorption by reducing total amount absorbed and slowing absorption rate.
Distribution: 10% bound to plasma proteins.
Metabolism: metabolized in liver.
Excretion: most of drug excreted in urine; about 10% excreted in feces. *Half-life:* 8 hours.

Route	Onset	Peak	Duration
P.O.	Unknown	1.5 hr	Unknown

Pharmacodynamics
Chemical effect: inhibits bacterial DNA gyrase, an enzyme necessary for bacterial replication (bactericidal).
Therapeutic effect: inhibits bacterial growth. Spectrum of activity includes *Escherichia coli, Haemophilus influenzae, Klebsiella pneumoniae, Moraxella (Branhamella) catarrhalis, Proteus mirabilis, Pseudomonas aeruginosa, Staphylococcus saprophyticus* and, possibly, *Citrobacter diversus* or *Enterobacter cloacae.*

Indications and dosage
▶ **Acute bacterial exacerbations of chronic bronchitis caused by *H. influenzae* or *M. catarrhalis.** Adults:*
400 mg P.O. daily for 10 days.
▶ **Uncomplicated urinary tract infections (cystitis) caused by *E. coli, K. pneumoniae, P. mirabilis,* or *S. saprophyticus.** Adults:* 400 mg P.O. daily for 10 days.
▶ **Complicated urinary tract infections caused by *E. coli, K. pneumoniae, P. mirabilis,* or *P. aeruginosa*; possibly effective against infections caused by *C. diversus* or *E. cloacae.** Adults:* 400 mg P.O. daily for 14 days.
▶ **Prophylaxis of infections after transurethral surgical procedures.** *Adults:* 400 mg P.O. as single dose 2 to 6 hours before surgery. Patients with creati-

nine clearance of 10 to 40 ml/minute should receive loading dose of 400 mg P.O. on first day, followed by 200 mg daily for duration of therapy. Hemodialysis removes negligible amounts of drug.

Adverse reactions

CNS: *dizziness, headache,* abnormal dreams, fatigue, malaise, asthenia, agitation, anxiety, confusion, depersonalization, depression, insomnia, nervousness, somnolence, *seizures, coma,* hyperkinesia, tremors, vertigo, paresthesias.
CV: flushing, hypotension, hypertension, edema, syncope, arrhythmia, tachycardia, bradycardia, extrasystoles, cyanosis, angina pectoris, *MI, cardiac failure, pulmonary embolisms,* cerebrovascular disorder, cardiomyopathy, phlebitis.
EENT: epistaxis, abnormal vision, conjunctivitis, eye pain, earache, tinnitus.
GI: *diarrhea, nausea,* anorexia, increased appetite, tongue discoloration, dry mouth, abdominal pain, dyspepsia, vomiting, flatulence, constipation, inflammation, dysphagia, bleeding.
GU: dysuria, hematuria, anuria, epididymitis, orchitis, vaginal moniliasis, perineal pain, intermenstrual bleeding, leukorrhea, vaginitis.
Hematologic: thrombocythemia, *thrombocytopenia,* lymphadenopathy, increased fibrinolysis.
Respiratory: cough, dyspnea, chest pain, *bronchospasm,* respiratory disorder, respiratory infection, increased sputum, stridor.
Skin: pruritus, skin disorder, skin exfoliation, eczema, rash, urticaria, *photosensitivity.*
Other: *anaphylaxis,* arthralgia, myalgia, increased diaphoresis, taste perversion, leg cramps, thirst, back pain, chills, allergic reaction, facial edema, influenza-like symptoms, decreased heat tolerance, hypoglycemia, elevated liver enzyme levels, gout.

Interactions

Drug-drug. *Antacids, sucralfate:* impaired absorption after binding with lomefloxacin in GI tract. Give no less than 4 hours before or 2 hours after dose. *Antineoplastic agents:* fluoroquinolone serum levels may be decreased. Monitor patient.
Cimetidine: increased half-life of other fluoroquinolones when administered to patient taking cimetidine; lomefloxacin has not been tested. Monitor for toxicity.
Cyclosporine, warfarin: increased effects on serum levels when combined with other fluoroquinolones; lomefloxacin has not been tested. Monitor for toxicity.
Probenecid: decreased excretion of lomefloxacin. Monitor for toxicity.
Drug-lifestyle. *Sun exposure:* photosensitivity reactions may occur.

Contraindications and precautions

● Contraindicated in patients with hypersensitivity to drug or other fluoroquinolones.
● Drug is not recommended for use in breast-feeding women.
● Use cautiously in patients with known or suspected CNS disorders, such as seizure disorder or cerebral arteriosclerosis, that may predispose patient to seizures.
● Safety of drug has not been established in children.

NURSING CONSIDERATIONS

Assessment
● Assess patient's infection before therapy and regularly thereafter.
● Obtain culture and sensitivity tests before first dose. Therapy may begin pending test results.
● Be alert for adverse reactions and drug interactions.
● Monitor patient's hydration status if adverse GI reactions occur.
● Evaluate patient's and family's knowledge of drug therapy.

⬚ Nursing diagnoses
• Infection related to presence of susceptible bacteria
• Risk for fluid volume deficit related to drug-induced adverse GI reactions
• Knowledge deficit related to drug therapy

⬚ Planning and implementation
• Administer drug on empty stomach.
• Keep in mind that prolonged use may result in overgrowth of organisms resistant to lomefloxacin.
Patient teaching
• Advise patient that hypersensitivity reactions may occur even after first dose. If rash or other allergic reaction occurs, tell patient to stop taking drug and notify doctor.
• Warn patient to refrain from driving and performing other hazardous tasks until CNS effects of drug are known. Drug may cause dizziness or light-headedness.
• Advise patient to wear protective clothing, use sunblock, and avoid prolonged exposure to sunlight during treatment and for a few days after therapy ends. If sunburn occurs, tell him to call doctor promptly.

⬚ Evaluation
• Patient is free from infection.
• Patient maintains adequate hydration throughout therapy.
• Patient and family state understanding of drug therapy.

---

lomustine (CCNU)
(loh-MUH-steen)
CeeNU

Pharmacologic class: alkylating agent, nitrosourea (cell cycle-phase nonspecific)
Therapeutic class: antineoplastic
Pregnancy risk category: D

How supplied
Capsules: 10 mg, 40 mg, 100 mg, dose pack (two 10-mg, two 40-mg, two 100-mg capsules)

Pharmacokinetics
Absorption: absorbed rapidly and well across GI tract after P.O. use.
Distribution: distributed widely in body tissues and crosses blood-brain barrier to significant extent.
Metabolism: metabolized rapidly and extensively in liver.
Excretion: metabolites excreted primarily in urine with smaller amounts excreted in feces and through lungs. *Half-life:* 1 to 2 days.

Route	Onset	Peak	Duration
P.O.	Unknown	Unknown	Unknown

Pharmacodynamics
Chemical effect: cross-links strands of cellular DNA and interferes with RNA transcription.
Therapeutic effect: kills selected cancer cells.

Indications and dosage
▶ **Brain tumor, Hodgkin's disease.**
Adults and children: 100 to 130 mg/m^2 P.O. as single dose q 6 weeks. Dosage reduced according to degree of bone marrow suppression. Repeat doses should not be given until WBC count is more than 4,000/mm^3 and platelet count is more than 100,000/mm^3.

Adverse reactions
GI: *nausea, vomiting* (beginning within 4 to 5 hours); stomatitis.
GU: *nephrotoxicity,* progressive azotemia, *renal failure.*
Hematologic: anemia; leukopenia (delayed up to 6 weeks, lasting 1 to 2 weeks); *thrombocytopenia* (delayed up to 4 weeks, lasting 1 to 2 weeks); *bone marrow suppression* (delayed up to 6 weeks).
Hepatic: *hepatotoxicity.*

Reactions may be *common*, uncommon, *life-threatening*, or COMMON AND LIFE-THREATENING.

Respiratory: *pulmonary fibrosis*.
Other: *secondary malignant disease*.

Interactions

Drug-drug. *Anticoagulants, aspirin:* increased bleeding risk. Avoid concomitant use.

Contraindications and precautions

• Contraindicated in patients with hypersensitivity to drug.
• Drug is not recommended for use in pregnant or breast-feeding women.
• Use cautiously in patients with decreased platelet, WBC, or RBC count and in those receiving other myelosuppressant drugs.

NURSING CONSIDERATIONS

Assessment
• Assess patient's condition before therapy and regularly thereafter.
• Monitor CBC weekly, as ordered; bone marrow toxicity is delayed.
• Periodically monitor liver function tests, as ordered.
• Be alert for adverse reactions and drug interactions.
• Evaluate patient's and family's knowledge of drug therapy.

Nursing diagnoses
• Altered health maintenance related to presence of neoplastic disease
• Altered protection related to adverse hematologic reactions
• Knowledge deficit related to drug therapy

Planning and implementation
• Give antiemetic before administering drug to avoid nausea, as ordered.
• Give 2 to 4 hours after meals; drug is more completely absorbed if taken when stomach is empty.
• Know that drug administration is repeated only when CBC results reveal safe hematologic parameters.

• Institute infection-control and bleeding precautions.
Patient teaching
• Warn patient to watch for signs of infection (fever, sore throat, fatigue) and bleeding (easy bruising, nosebleeds, bleeding gums, melena) and to take temperature daily.
• Instruct patient to avoid OTC products containing aspirin.
• Advise female patient of childbearing age to avoid becoming pregnant during therapy and to consult with doctor before becoming pregnant.

Evaluation
• Patient responds well to therapy.
• Patient regains normal hematologic function.
• Patient and family state understanding of drug therapy.

loperamide
(loh-PEH-ruh-mighd)
Imodium, Imodium A-D†

Pharmacologic class: piperidine derivative
Therapeutic class: antidiarrheal
Pregnancy risk category: B

How supplied

Tablets: 2 mg
Capsules: 2 mg
Oral liquid: 1 mg/5 ml†

Pharmacokinetics

Absorption: absorbed poorly from GI tract.
Distribution: unknown.
Metabolism: metabolized in liver.
Excretion: excreted primarily in feces; less than 2% excreted in urine. *Half-life:* 9.1 to 14.4 hours.

Route	Onset	Peak	Duration
P.O.	Unknown	2.5-5 hr	24 hr

Pharmacodynamics

Chemical effect: inhibits peristaltic activity, prolonging transit of intestinal contents.
Therapeutic effect: relieves diarrhea.

Indications and dosage

▶ **Acute, nonspecific diarrhea.** *Adults and children over age 12:* initially, 4 mg P.O., then 2 mg after each unformed stool. Maximum dosage is 16 mg daily. *Children ages 8 to 12:* 10 ml (2 mg) t.i.d. P.O. on first day. (Subsequent doses of 5 ml (1 mg)/10 kg (22 lb) of body weight may be given after each unformed stool.) Maximum dosage is 6 mg daily. *Children ages 6 to 8:* 10 ml (2 mg) P.O. b.i.d. on first day. Report persistent diarrhea. *Children ages 2 to 6:* 5 ml (1 mg) P.O. t.i.d. on first day. Report persistent diarrhea.
▶ **Chronic diarrhea.** *Adults:* initially, 4 mg P.O., then 2 mg after each unformed stool until diarrhea subsides. Dosage adjusted to individual response.
▶ **Acute diarrhea including traveler's diarrhea (OTC).** *Adults:* 4 mg after first loose bowel movement followed by 2 mg after each subsequent loose bowel movement but no more than 8 mg/day for no more than 2 days.

Adverse reactions

CNS: drowsiness, fatigue, dizziness.
GI: dry mouth; abdominal pain, distention, or discomfort; *constipation;* nausea; vomiting.
Skin: rash, *hypersensitivity reactions.*

Interactions

None significant.

Contraindications and precautions

• Contraindicated in patients with hypersensitivity and when constipation must be avoided. Also contraindicated in children younger than age 2.
• Use cautiously in patients with hepatic disease and in pregnant or breast-feeding women.

• Over the counter use: bloody diarrhea; body temperature over 101°F (38°C).

NURSING CONSIDERATIONS

📧 Assessment

• Assess patient's diarrhea before therapy and regularly thereafter.
• Be alert for adverse reactions.
• Monitor children closely for CNS effects because they may be more sensitive than adults to such effects.
• Monitor patient's hydration status if adverse GI reactions occur.
• Evaluate patient's and family's knowledge of drug therapy.

🔹 Nursing diagnoses

• Diarrhea related to underlying condition
• Risk for fluid volume deficit related to drug-induced adverse GI reactions
• Knowledge deficit related to drug therapy

▶ Planning and implementation

• Notify doctor if acute abdominal signs occur or drug is ineffective.
• If drug is given by nasogastric tube, flush tube to clear it and ensure drug's passage to stomach.
Patient teaching
• Advise patient not to exceed recommended dosage.
• Tell patient with acute diarrhea to discontinue drug and seek medical attention if no improvement occurs within 48 hours; for chronic diarrhea, tell him to notify doctor and discontinue drug if no improvement occurs after giving 16 mg daily for at least 10 days.
• Advise patient to stop taking drug immediately if abdominal distention or other symptoms develop in acute colitis, and to notify doctor.

📋 Evaluation

• Patient's diarrhea is relieved.
• Patient maintains adequate hydration throughout therapy.

Reactions may be *common,* uncommon, *life-threatening*, or COMMON AND LIFE-THREATENING.

• Patient and family state understanding of drug therapy.

loracarbef
(loh-ruh-KAR-bef)
Lorabid

Pharmacologic class: synthetic beta-lactam antibiotic of carbacephem class
Therapeutic class: antibiotic
Pregnancy risk category: B

How supplied

Pulvules: 200 mg, 400 mg
Powder for oral suspension: 100 mg/5 ml, 200 mg/5 ml in 50-ml, 75-ml and 100-ml bottles

Pharmacokinetics

Absorption: about 90% absorbed from GI tract. Absorption of suspension is greater than that of capsule.
Distribution: about 25% of circulating drug is bound to plasma proteins.
Metabolism: does not appear to be metabolized.
Excretion: excreted primarily in urine.
Half-life: about 1 hour.

Route	Onset	Peak	Duration
P.O.	Unknown	0.5-1 hr	Unknown

Pharmacodynamics

Chemical effect: inhibits cell-wall synthesis, promoting osmotic instability; usually bactericidal.
Therapeutic effect: kills susceptible bacteria. Spectrum of activity includes gram-positive aerobes, such as *Staphylococcus aureus, Staphylococcus saprophyticus, Streptococcus pneumoniae,* and *Streptococcus pyogenes,* and gram-negative aerobes, such as *Escherichia coli, Haemophilus influenzae,* and *Moraxella (Branhamella) catarrhalis.*

Indications and dosage

▶ **Secondary bacterial infections of acute bronchitis.** *Adults:* 200 to 400 g P.O. q 12 hours for 7 days.
▶ **Acute bacterial exacerbations of chronic bronchitis.** *Adults:* 400 mg P.O. q 12 hours for 7 days.
▶ **Pneumonia.** *Adults:* 400 mg P.O. q 12 hours for 14 days.
▶ **Pharyngitis, sinusitis, tonsillitis.** *Adults:* 200 to 400 mg P.O. q 12 hours for 10 days. *Children:* 15 mg/kg P.O. daily in divided doses q 12 hours for 10 days.
▶ **Acute otitis media.** *Children:* 30 mg/kg (oral suspension) P.O. daily in divided doses q 12 hours for 10 days.
▶ **Uncomplicated skin and skin-structure infections.** *Adults:* 200 mg P.O. q 12 hours for 7 days.
▶ **Impetigo.** *Children:* 15 mg/kg P.O. daily in divided doses q 12 hours for 7 days.
▶ **Uncomplicated cystitis.** *Adults:* 200 mg P.O. daily for 7 days.
▶ **Uncomplicated pyelonephritis.** *Adults:* 400 mg P.O. q 12 hours for 14 days. Patients with creatinine clearance 50 ml/minute/1.73 m^2 or more don't require dose and interval changes. Patients with creatinine clearance of 10 to 49 ml/minute/1.73 m^2 should receive half of usual dose at same interval; with creatinine clearance below 10 ml/minute/1.73 m^2, usual dose q 3 to 5 days. Hemodialysis patients require another dose after dialysis.

Adverse reactions

CNS: headache, somnolence, nervousness, insomnia, dizziness.
CV: vasodilation.
GI: diarrhea, nausea, vomiting, abdominal pain, anorexia, *pseudomembranous colitis.*
GU: vaginal candidiasis.
Hematologic: *transient thrombocytopenia, leukopenia,* eosinophilia.
Skin: rash, urticaria, pruritus, *erythema multiforme.*

Other: hypersensitivity reactions, including *anaphylaxis;* transient elevations in AST, ALT, alkaline phosphatase, BUN, and creatinine levels.

Interactions

Drug-drug. *Probenecid:* decreased excretion of loracarbef, causing increased plasma levels. Monitor for toxicity.
Drug-food. *Any food:* decreased absorption. Give drug 1 hour before or 2 hours after meals.

Contraindications and precautions

• Contraindicated in patients with diarrhea caused by pseudomembranous colitis or hypersensitivity to drug or other cephalosporins.
• Use cautiously in pregnant or breast-feeding women.
• Safety and efficacy have not been established in infants under age 6 months.

NURSING CONSIDERATIONS

Assessment
• Assess patient's infection before therapy and regularly thereafter.
• Obtain specimen for culture and sensitivity tests before giving first dose. Therapy may begin pending test results.
• Be alert for adverse reactions and drug interactions.
• Watch for seizures. Beta-lactam antibiotics may trigger seizures in susceptible patients, especially when given without dosage modification to those with renal impairment.
• Monitor patient's hydration status if adverse GI reactions occur.
• Evaluate patient's and family's knowledge of drug therapy.

Nursing diagnoses
• Infection related to presence of susceptible bacteria
• Risk for fluid volume deficit related to drug-induced adverse GI reactions
• Knowledge deficit related to drug therapy

Planning and implementation
• To reconstitute powder for oral suspension, add 30 ml of water in two portions to 50-ml bottle or 60 ml of water in two portions to 100-ml bottle. Shake after each addition.
• After reconstitution, store oral suspension for 14 days at room temperature (59° to 86° F [15° to 30° C]).
• If seizures occur, stop drug and tell doctor. Give anticonvulsants, as ordered.
• Know that 40% to 75% of patients receiving cephalosporins show false-positive direct Coombs' test; only some indicate hemolytic anemia.
Patient teaching
• Tell patient to take drug on an empty stomach, at least 1 hour before or 2 hours after meals.
• Tell patient to shake container of suspension well before measuring dosage.
• Tell patient to take drug exactly as prescribed.
• Instruct patient to discard unused portion after 14 days.

Evaluation
• Patient is free from infection.
• Patient maintains adequate hydration throughout therapy.
• Patient and family state understanding of drug therapy.

loratadine
(loo-RAH-tuh-deen)
Claratyne◇, Claritin

Pharmacologic class: tricyclic antihistamine
Therapeutic class: antihistamine
Pregnancy risk category: B

How supplied

Tablets: 10 mg
Tablets (rapidly disintegrating): 10 mg
Syrup: 1 mg/ml

Pharmacokinetics

Absorption: readily absorbed. Food may delay peak plasma concentration by 1 hour.
Distribution: does not readily cross blood-brain barrier; about 97% bound to plasma protein.
Metabolism: extensively metabolized, although specific enzyme systems responsible for metabolism have not been identified.
Excretion: about 80% distributed equally between urine and feces. *Half-life:* 8.4 hours.

Route	Onset	Peak	Duration
P.O.	1 hr	4-6 hr	24 hr

Pharmacodynamics

Chemical effect: blocks effects of histamine at H_1-receptor sites. Loratadine is a nonsedating antihistamine; its chemical structure prevents entry into CNS.
Therapeutic effect: relieves allergy symptoms.

Indications and dosage

▶ **Symptomatic treatment of seasonal allergic rhinitis.** *Adults and children age 12 and over:* 10 mg P.O. daily. *Children ages 6 to 11:* 10 mg (10 ml) once daily. Dosage for patients with hepatic failure or renal insufficiency is 10 mg P.O. every other day.

Adverse reactions

CNS: headache, somnolence, fatigue.
GI: dry mouth.

Interactions

Drug-drug. *Erythromycin:* increased loratadine plasma concentrations. Monitor patient closely.
Drug-lifestyle. *Sun exposure:* photosensitivity reactions may occur. Take precautions.

Contraindications and precautions

• Contraindicated in patients with hypersensitivity to drug.

• Drug is not recommended for use in breast-feeding women.
• Use in pregnant women only when absolutely necessary.
• Use cautiously in patients with hepatic impairment.
• Safety of drug has not been established in children younger than age 6.

NURSING CONSIDERATIONS

⬛ Assessment
• Assess patient's condition before therapy and regularly thereafter.
• Be alert for adverse reactions and drug interactions.
• Evaluate patient's and family's knowledge of drug therapy.

⬛ Nursing diagnoses
• Altered health maintenance related to underlying allergy condition
• Fatigue related to drug's adverse effect on body
• Knowledge deficit related to drug therapy

⬛ Planning and implementation
• Give drug on empty stomach.
• Notify doctor if drug is ineffective.
Patient teaching
• Tell patient to take drug at least 2 hours after meal, to avoid eating for at least 1 hour after taking drug, and to take it only once daily.
• Tell patient to contact doctor if symptoms persist or worsen.
• Advise patient to stop taking drug 4 days before allergy skin tests to preserve accuracy of tests.
• Instruct patient to avoid prolonged exposure to the sun, to wear sunblock and protective clothing while on drug therapy.
• Review coping strategies for handling fatigue.

⬛ Evaluation
• Patient states that allergy symptoms are relieved.

• Patient describes coping strategies for handling fatigue.
• Patient and family state understanding of drug therapy.

lorazepam
(loo-RAZ-eh-pam)
Apo-Lorazepam♦, Ativan, Lorazepam Intensol, Novo-Lorazem♦, Nu-Loraz♦

Pharmacologic class: benzodiazepine
Therapeutic class: antianxiety agent, sedative-hypnotic
Controlled substance schedule: IV
Pregnancy risk category: NR

How supplied

Tablets: 0.5 mg, 1 mg, 2 mg
Tablets (S.L.): 0.5 mg♦, 1 mg♦, 2 mg♦
Oral solution (concentrated): 2 mg/ml
Injection: 2 mg/ml, 4 mg/ml

Pharmacokinetics

Absorption: well absorbed through GI tract after P.O. administration; unknown after I.M. administration.
Distribution: distributed widely throughout body; about 85% protein-bound.
Metabolism: metabolized in liver.
Excretion: excreted in urine. *Half-life:* 10 to 20 hours.

Route	Onset	Peak	Duration
P.O.	1 hr	2 hr	12-24 hr
I.V.	1-5 min	1-1.5 hr	6-8 hr
I.M.	15-30 min	1-1.5 hr	6-8 hr

Pharmacodynamics

Chemical effect: unknown; probably stimulates gamma-aminobutyric receptors in ascending reticular activating system.
Therapeutic effect: relieves anxiety and promotes calmness and sleep.

Indications and dosage

▶ **Anxiety.** *Adults:* 2 to 6 mg P.O. daily in divided doses. Maximum dosage is 10 mg daily.

▶ **Insomnia due to anxiety.** *Adults:* 2 to 4 mg P.O. h.s.
▶ **Premedication before operative procedure.** *Adults:* 0.05 mg/kg I.M. 2 hours before procedure. Total dosage should not exceed 4 mg. Alternatively, 2 mg total or 0.044 mg/kg I.V., whichever is smaller. Larger doses up to 0.05 mg/kg I.V. up to total of 4 mg may be required.

Adverse reactions

CNS: *drowsiness, lethargy, hangover,* fainting, anterograde amnesia, restlessness, psychosis.
CV: transient hypotension.
EENT: visual disturbances.
GI: dry mouth, abdominal discomfort.
GU: incontinence, urine retention.
Other: *acute withdrawal syndrome* (after sudden discontinuation in physically dependent people).

Interactions

Drug-drug. *CNS depressants:* increased CNS depression. Avoid concomitant use.
Digoxin: may increase serum levels of digoxin, increasing toxicity. Monitor patient closely.
Drug-lifestyle. *Alcohol use:* increased CNS depression. Monitor patient.
Smoking: decreased effectiveness of benzodiazepines. Monitor closely.

Contraindications and precautions

• Contraindicated in patients with acute angle-closure glaucoma or hypersensitivity to drug, other benzodiazepines, or its vehicle (used in parenteral dosage form).
• Avoid using in pregnant women, especially during first trimester, and in breast-feeding women.
• Use cautiously in patients with pulmonary, renal, or hepatic impairment. Also use cautiously in elderly, acutely ill, or debilitated patients.
• Safety of drug has not been established in children.

Reactions may be *common*, uncommon, *life-threatening*, or COMMON AND LIFE-THREATENING.

NURSING CONSIDERATIONS

⚘ Assessment
• Assess patient's condition before therapy and regularly thereafter.
• Check respirations every 5 to 15 minutes and before each repeated I.V. dose.
• Monitor liver, kidney, and hematopoietic function studies periodically in patient receiving repeated or prolonged therapy, as ordered.
• Be alert for adverse reactions and drug interactions.
• Evaluate patient's and family's knowledge of drug therapy.

⊞ Nursing diagnoses
• Anxiety related to underlying condition
• Risk for injury related to drug-induced adverse CNS effects
• Knowledge deficit related to drug therapy

▶ Planning and implementation
• Know that dosage should be reduced in elderly or debilitated patients. Preoperative I.V. dose not to exceed 2 mg in patients older than age 50.
P.O. use: Follow normal protocol.
I.V. use: Give drug slowly, at rate not exceeding 2 mg/minute. Dilute with equal volume of sterile water for injection, 0.9% NaCl injection, or dextrose 5% injection.
I.M. use: Inject drug deeply into muscle mass. Don't dilute.
• Have emergency resuscitation equipment and oxygen available.
• Refrigerate parenteral form to prolong shelf life.
• Know that possibility of abuse and addiction exists. Do not withdraw drug abruptly after long-term use; withdrawal symptoms may occur.
Patient teaching
• Warn patient to avoid hazardous activities until CNS effects of drug are known.
• Tell patient to avoid alcohol consumption and smoking during drug therapy.
• As premedication before surgery, lorazepam provides substantial preoperative amnesia. Patient teaching requires extra care to ensure adequate recall. Provide written materials or inform family member, if possible.

☑ Evaluation
• Patient is less anxious.
• Patient does not experience injury as result of adverse CNS reactions.
• Patient and family state understanding of drug therapy.

losartan potassium
(loh-SAR-tan poh-TAH-see-um)
Cozaar

Pharmacologic class: angiotensin II receptor antagonist
Therapeutic class: antihypertensive
Pregnancy risk category: C (D in second and third trimesters)

How supplied
Tablets: 25 mg, 50 mg

Pharmacokinetics
Absorption: absorbed well and undergoes extensive first-pass metabolism; systemic bioavailability of drug is about 33%.
Distribution: highly bound to plasma proteins.
Metabolism: cytochrome P-450 2C9 and 3A4 are involved in biotransformation of losartan to its metabolites.
Excretion: excreted primarily in feces with smaller amount excreted in urine.
Half-life: about 2 hours.

Route	Onset	Peak	Duration
P.O.	Unknown	1-4 hr	Unknown

Pharmacodynamics
Chemical effect: inhibits vasoconstricting and aldosterone-secreting effects of angiotensin II by selectively blocking binding of angiotensin II to its receptor sites that are found in many tissues, in-

cluding vascular smooth muscle and adrenal glands.
Therapeutic effect: lowers blood pressure.

Indications and dosage

▶ **Hypertension.** *Adults:* initially, 25 to 50 mg P.O. daily. Maximum daily dosage is 100 mg in one or two divided doses.

Adverse reactions

CNS: dizziness, insomnia.
GI: diarrhea, dyspepsia.
Musculoskeletal: muscle cramps, myalgia, back or leg pain.
Respiratory: nasal congestion, cough, upper respiratory tract infection, sinus disorder, sinusitis.

Interactions

None significant.

Contraindications and precautions

• Contraindicated in patients with hypersensitivity to drug.
• Breast-feeding is not recommended during drug therapy.
• Drug should be used in pregnant women only when absolutely necessary. Drug acts directly on renin-angiotensin system and can cause fetal and neonatal morbidity and death. These problems have not been detected when exposure has been limited to first trimester.
• Use cautiously in patients with impaired kidney or liver function.
• Safety of drug has not been established in children.

NURSING CONSIDERATIONS

🔬 Assessment

• Assess patient's blood pressure before therapy and regularly thereafter. Know that when drug is used alone, effect on blood pressure is notably less in black patients than those of other races.
• Regularly assess patient's kidney function (by way of serum creatinine and BUN levels), as ordered. Be aware that

patients with severe heart failure whose kidney function depends on angiotensin-aldosterone system have experienced acute renal failure during ACE inhibitor therapy. Manufacturer of losartan states that drug would be expected to do same. Closely monitor patient, especially during first few weeks of therapy.
• Be alert for adverse reactions.
• Monitor for symptomatic hypotension in patient taking a diuretic.
• Evaluate patient's and family's knowledge of drug therapy.

🔷 Nursing diagnoses

• Risk for injury related to presence of hypertension
• Sleep pattern disturbance related to drug-induced insomnia
• Knowledge deficit related to drug therapy

▶ Planning and implementation

• Know that lowest dosage (25 mg) should be used initially in patients with impaired liver function and in those with volume depletion (such as those receiving diuretics).
• Drug can be used alone or with other antihypertensives.
• If antihypertensive effect measured by serum trough level of drug, using once-daily dosing, is inadequate, twice-daily regimen using same total daily dosage or increase in dosage may give better response.
• Administer once-daily dosing in morning to prevent insomnia.
• If pregnancy is suspected, notify doctor because drug should probably be discontinued.

Patient teaching

• Tell patient to avoid sodium substitutes; these products may contain potassium, which can cause hyperkalemia in patients taking losartan.
• Inform female patient of childbearing age about consequences of second- and third-trimester exposure to losartan, and

---

instruct her to notify doctor immediately if pregnancy occurs or is suspected.

☑ Evaluation
• Patient's blood pressure is normal.
• Patient states that insomnia has not occurred.
• Patient and family state understanding of drug therapy.

lovastatin (mevinolin)
(loh-vuh-STAH-tin)
Mevacor

Pharmacologic class: lactone
Therapeutic class: cholesterol-lowering agent
Pregnancy risk category: X

How supplied
Tablets: 10 mg, 20 mg, 40 mg

Pharmacokinetics
Absorption: about 30% absorbed. Administration with food improves plasma concentrations of total inhibitors by about 30%.
Distribution: less than 5% of dose reaches systemic circulation because of extensive first-pass hepatic extraction; liver is drug's principal site of action. Drug and its principal metabolite are more than 95% bound to plasma proteins.
Metabolism: metabolized in liver.
Excretion: about 80% excreted in feces, about 10% in urine. *Half-life:* 3 hours.

Route	Onset	Peak	Duration
P.O.	Unknown	2-6 hr	4-6 wk

Pharmacodynamics
Chemical effect: inhibits 3-hydroxy-3-methylglutaryl coenzyme A reductase. This enzyme is early (and rate-limiting) step in synthetic pathway of cholesterol.
Therapeutic effect: lowers low-density lipoprotein (LDL) and total cholesterol levels.

Indications and dosage
▶ **Reduction of LDL and total cholesterol levels in patients with primary hypercholesterolemia (types IIa and IIb).** *Adults:* initially, 20 mg P.O. once daily with evening meal. For patients with severely elevated cholesterol levels (for example, over 300 mg/dl), initial dose is 40 mg. Recommended daily dosage range is 20 to 80 mg in single or divided doses.

Adverse reactions
CNS: headache, dizziness, peripheral neuropathy.
EENT: blurred vision.
GI: constipation, diarrhea, dyspepsia, flatulence, abdominal pain or cramps, heartburn, dysgeusia, nausea.
Skin: rash, pruritus.
Other: muscle cramps, myalgia, myositis, *rhabdomyolysis,* elevated serum transaminase levels, abnormal liver function test results.

Interactions
Drug-drug. *Bile acid sequestrants*: a decrease in lovastatin bioavailability may occur. Administer separately.
Cyclosporine or other immunosuppressants, erythromycin, gemfibrozil, niacin: possible increased risk of polymyositis and rhabdomyolysis. Maximum recommended lovastatin dosage is 20 mg daily. Monitor patient closely.
Digoxin: slight elevation in digoxin levels is possible. Monitor patient.
Isradipine: isradipine may increase clearance of lovastatin and its metabolites by increasing hepatic blood flow. Monitor for loss of therapeutic effect.
Itraconazole: coadministration increased HMG-COA reductase inhibitor levels about 20 fold in normal volunteers; probably because of enzyme inhibition of competition. Temporarily interrupt HMG-COA reductase inhibitors if systemic azole antifungals are needed.
Oral anticoagulants: lovastatin may enhance clinical effects of oral anticoagulants. Monitor patient closely.

Drug-lifestyle. *Alcohol use:* increased risk of hepatotoxicity. Avoid concomitant use.

Contraindications and precautions

• Contraindicated in patients with hypersensitivity to drug, in those with active liver disease or conditions associated with unexplained persistent elevations of serum transaminase levels, in pregnant or breast-feeding women, and in women of childbearing age unless there is no risk of pregnancy.
• Use cautiously in patients who consume substantial quantities of alcohol or have history of liver disease.
• Safety of drug has not been established in children.

NURSING CONSIDERATIONS

Assessment
• Obtain history of patient's lipoprotein and cholesterol levels before therapy and reassess regularly thereafter.
• Be aware that liver function tests should be performed at start of therapy and periodically thereafter.
• Be alert for adverse reactions and drug interactions.
• Evaluate patient's and family's knowledge of drug therapy.

Nursing diagnoses
• Risk for injury related to underlying condition
• Pain related to drug-induced adverse musculoskeletal reactions
• Knowledge deficit related to drug therapy

Planning and implementation
• Know that drug therapy should be initiated only after diet and other nonpharmacologic therapies have proved ineffective. Patient should be on standard low-cholesterol diet during therapy.
• Administer drug with evening meal; absorption is enhanced and cholesterol biosynthesis is greater in evening.

Patient teaching
• Instruct patient to take drug with evening meal.
• Teach patient dietary management of serum lipids (restricting total fat and cholesterol intake) and measures to control other cardiac disease risk factors. If appropriate, recommend weight control, exercise, and smoking cessation programs.
• Advise patient to have periodic eye examinations.
• Tell patient to store drug at room temperature in light-resistant container.
• Instruct patient to avoid alcohol consumption during drug therapy.
• Inform female patient that drug is contraindicated during pregnancy. Advise her to notify doctor immediately if pregnancy occurs.

Evaluation
• Patient's LDLs and cholesterol are within normal limits.
• Patient states that musculoskeletal pain does not occur.
• Patient and family state understanding of drug therapy.

loxapine hydrochloride
(LOKS-uh-peen high-droh-KLOR-ighd)
Loxapac♦, Loxitane C, Loxitane IM

loxapine succinate
Loxapac♦, Loxitane

Pharmacologic class: dibenzoxazepine
Therapeutic class: antipsychotic
Pregnancy risk category: NR

How supplied

loxapine hydrochloride
Oral concentrate: 25 mg/ml
Injection: 50 mg/ml
loxapine succinate
Capsules: 5 mg, 10 mg, 25 mg, 50 mg
Tablets: 5 mg♦, 10 mg♦, 25 mg♦, 50 mg♦

Reactions may be *common*, uncommon, *life-threatening*, or COMMON AND LIFE-THREATENING.

Pharmacokinetics

Absorption: absorbed rapidly and completely from GI tract.
Distribution: distributed widely in body; 91% to 99% protein-bound.
Metabolism: metabolized extensively by liver.
Excretion: most of drug excreted as metabolites in urine; some excreted in feces. **Half-life:** P.O. form, 3 to 4 hours; I.M. form, 12 hours.

Route	Onset	Peak	Duration
P.O.	30 min	1.5-3 hr	≤ 2 hr
I.M.	30 min	1.5-3 hr	≤ 12 hr

Pharmacodynamics

Chemical effect: unknown; probably blocks postsynaptic dopamine receptors in brain.
Therapeutic effect: relieves psychotic symptoms.

Indications and dosage

▶ **Psychotic disorders.** *Adults:* 10 mg P.O. b.i.d. to q.i.d., rapidly increasing to 60 to 100 mg P.O. daily for most patients (dosage varies from patient to patient); or 12.5 to 50 mg I.M. q 4 to 6 hours or longer, both dose and interval depending on patient response. Maximum dosage is 250 mg daily.

Adverse reactions

CNS: *extrapyramidal reactions* (moderate incidence), *sedation* (moderate incidence), *tardive dyskinesia,* **seizures,** pseudoparkinsonism, EEG changes, dizziness.
CV: *orthostatic hypotension,* tachycardia, ECG changes.
EENT: *blurred vision.*
GI: *dry mouth, constipation.*
GU: *urine retention,* dark urine, menstrual irregularities, gynecomastia.
Hematologic: *leukopenia, agranulocytosis, thrombocytopenia.*
Skin: *mild photosensitivity,* allergic reactions.
Other: weight gain, increased appetite, **neuroleptic malignant syndrome.**

Interactions

Drug-drug. *CNS depressants:* increased CNS depression. Avoid concomitant use.
Drug-lifestyle. *Alcohol use:* increased CNS depression. Avoid concomitant use.

Contraindications and precautions

• Contraindicated in patients with hypersensitivity to dibenzoxazepines and in patients experiencing coma, severe CNS depression, or drug-induced depressed states.
• Drug is not recommended for use in breast-feeding women.
• Use with extreme caution in those with seizure disorder, CV disorder, glaucoma, or history of urine retention.
• Safety of drug has not been established in children and in pregnant women.

NURSING CONSIDERATIONS

Assessment
• Assess patient's condition before therapy and regularly thereafter.
• Assess blood pressure before therapy and monitor regularly.
• Be alert for adverse reactions and drug interactions.
• Monitor patient for tardive dyskinesia. It may occur after prolonged use. It may not appear until months or years later and may disappear spontaneously or persist for life despite discontinuation of drug.
• Evaluate patient's and family's knowledge of drug therapy.

Nursing diagnoses
• Altered thought processes related to underlying psychotic condition
• Impaired physical mobility related to drug-induced extrapyramidal symptoms
• Knowledge deficit related to drug therapy

Planning and implementation
P.O. use: Dilute liquid concentrate with orange or grapefruit juice just before giving.
I.M. use: Follow normal protocol.

---

*Liquid form contains alcohol   **May contain tartrazine   ◆Canada   ◇Australia   †OTC

• Acute dystonic reactions may be treated with diphenhydramine.

Patient teaching

• Warn patient to avoid activities that require alertness and good psychomotor coordination until CNS effects of drug are known.

• Tell patient to avoid alcohol consumption.

• Advise patient to get up slowly to avoid orthostatic hypotension.

• Tell patient to relieve dry mouth with sugarless gum or hard candy.

• Tell patient that periodic eye examinations are recommended.

☑ Evaluation

• Patient demonstrates decrease in psychotic behavior.

• Patient maintains physical mobility throughout therapy.

• Patient and family state understanding of drug therapy.

---

lymphocyte immune globulin (antithymocyte globulin [equine], ATG)

(LIM-foh-sight ih-MYOON GLOH-byoo-lin)
Atgam

Pharmacologic class: immunoglobulin
Therapeutic class: immunosuppressant
Pregnancy risk category: C

How supplied

Injection: 50 mg of equine IgG/ml in 5-ml ampules

Pharmacokinetics

Absorption: not applicable.
Distribution: unknown.
Metabolism: unknown.
Excretion: about 1% excreted in urine, principally as unchanged drug. *Half-life:* about 6 days.

Route	Onset	Peak	Duration
I.V.	Unknown	5 days	Unknown

Pharmacodynamics

Chemical effect: unknown; inhibits cell-mediated immune responses by either altering T-cell function or eliminating antigen-reactive T cells.
Therapeutic effect: prevents or relieves signs and symptoms of renal allograft rejection; also relieves signs and symptoms of aplastic anemia.

Indications and dosage

► **Prevention of acute renal allograft rejection.** *Adults and children:* 15 mg/kg I.V. daily for 14 days, followed by alternate-day dosing for 14 days. First dose should be given within 24 hours of transplantation.

► **Treatment of acute renal allograft rejection.** *Adults and children:* 10 to 15 mg/kg I.V. daily for 14 days, followed by alternate-day dosing for 14 days. Therapy should be initiated when rejection is diagnosed.

► **Aplastic anemia.** *Adults:* 10 to 20 mg/kg I.V. daily for 8 to 14 days. Additional alternate-day therapy up to total of 21 doses can be administered.

Adverse reactions

CNS: malaise, *seizures,* headache.
CV: *hypotension, chest pain,* thrombophlebitis, tachycardia, edema, iliac vein obstruction, renal artery stenosis.
EENT: *laryngospasm.*
GI: *nausea, vomiting,* diarrhea, hiccups, epigastric pain, abdominal distention, stomatitis.
Hematologic: *leukopenia, thrombocytopenia,* hemolysis, *aplastic anemia.*
Hepatic: elevated liver enzyme levels.
Respiratory: *dyspnea, pulmonary edema.*
Other: febrile reactions, serum sickness, *anaphylaxis,* rash, infection, arthralgia, night sweats, lymphadenopathy, hyperglycemia.

Interactions

Drug-drug. *Muromonab-CD3:* increased risk of infection. Monitor patient closely.

Reactions may be *common,* uncommon, *life-threatening*, or COMMON AND LIFE-THREATENING.

Contraindications and precautions

• Contraindicated in patients hypersensitive to drug. An intradermal skin test is recommended at least 1 hour before first dose. Marked local swelling or erythema larger than 10 mm indicates increased potential for severe systemic reaction, such as anaphylaxis. Severe reactions to skin test, such as hypotension, tachycardia, dyspnea, generalized rash, or anaphylaxis, usually preclude further administration.

• Drug is not recommended for use in breast-feeding women.

• Use cautiously in pregnant women. Also use cautiously in patients receiving additional immunosuppressive therapy (such as corticosteroids and azathioprine) because of increased potential for infection.

NURSING CONSIDERATIONS

Assessment

• Assess patient's condition before therapy and regularly thereafter.

• Be alert for adverse reactions and drug interactions.

• Evaluate patient's and family's knowledge of drug therapy.

Nursing diagnoses

• Altered health maintenance related to underlying condition

• Altered protection related to adverse hematologic reactions

• Knowledge deficit related to drug therapy

Planning and implementation

• Do not dilute ATG concentrate with dextrose solutions or solutions with low salt concentration because precipitate may form. The proteins in ATG can be denatured by air. ATG is unstable in acidic solutions.

• Know that ATG solutions must be filtered during administration; filters with pore sizes of 0.2 to 5.0 microns have been used.

• Dilute concentrated drug for injection before administration. Dilute required dose in 250 to 1,000 ml of 0.45% or 0.9% NaCl injection. Final concentration of drug should not exceed 1 mg/ml. When adding ATG to infusion solution, make sure container is inverted so that drug does not contact air inside container. Gently rotate or swirl container to mix contents; do not shake because this may cause excessive foaming or denature drug protein. Infuse with in-line filter with pore size of 0.2 to 1.0 micron over no less than 4 hours (most institutions infuse over 4 to 8 hours).

• Do not use solutions that are more than 12 hours old, including actual infusion time.

• Refrigerate drug at 35° to 47° F (2° to 8° C). Do not freeze. ATG concentrate is heat-sensitive.

Patient teaching

• Warn patient that febrile reaction is likely. Instruct him to report adverse drug effects.

• Instruct patient to take infection-control and bleeding precautions.

Evaluation

• Patient responds well to therapy.

• Patient does not experience serious adverse hematologic reactions.

• Patient and family state understanding of drug therapy.

lypressin
(ligh-PREH-sin)
Diapid

Pharmacologic class: posterior pituitary hormone
Therapeutic class: antidiuretic hormone
Pregnancy risk category: B

How supplied

Nasal spray: 0.185 mg/ml

Pharmacokinetics

Absorption: rapid from nasal mucosa.

Distribution: distributed in extracellular fluid.
Metabolism: metabolized by kidneys.
Excretion: small amount excreted in urine. *Half-life:* about 15 minutes.

Route	Onset	Peak	Duration
Intranasal	≤ 1 hr	0.5-2 hr	3-4 hr

Pharmacodynamics

Chemical effect: increases permeability of renal tubular epithelium to adenosine monophosphate and water; epithelium promotes reabsorption of water and produces concentrated urine (ADH effect).
Therapeutic effect: promotes water retention.

Indications and dosage

▶ **Nonnephrogenic diabetes insipidus.**
Adults and children: 1 or 2 sprays (about 2 USP posterior pituitary pressor units/spray) in either or both nostrils q.i.d. and additional dose h.s., if needed, to prevent nocturia. If usual dosage is inadequate, frequency is increased rather than number of sprays.

Adverse reactions

CNS: headache, dizziness.
EENT: nasal congestion or ulceration, irritation or pruritus of nasal passages, rhinorrhea, conjunctivitis.
GI: heartburn because of drip of excess spray into pharynx, abdominal cramps, frequent bowel movements.
GU: possible transient fluid retention (with overdose).
Skin: hypersensitivity reaction.

Interactions

Drug-drug. *Carbamazepine, chlorpropamide:* potentiates ADH and may potentiate effects of lypressin. Use together with caution.

Contraindications and precautions

• Contraindicated in patients hypersensitive to drug.

• Use cautiously in patients with coronary artery disease, hypertension, allergic rhinitis, or upper airway infection and in pregnant or breast-feeding women.

NURSING CONSIDERATIONS

Assessment
• Assess patient's condition before therapy and regularly thereafter.
• Test patients sensitive to ADH for sensitivity to lypressin, as ordered, before therapy.
• Be alert for adverse reactions.
• Evaluate patient's and family's knowledge of drug therapy.

Nursing diagnoses
• Fluid volume deficit related to underlying condition
• Impaired tissue integrity related to drug-induced nasal irritation
• Knowledge deficit related to drug therapy

Planning and implementation
• Know that drug is particularly useful if diabetes insipidus is unresponsive to other therapy or if ADH of animal origin causes adverse reactions.
• To administer uniform, well-diffused spray, hold bottle upright with patient in vertical position holding head upright.
• Nasal congestion, allergic rhinitis, or upper respiratory tract infection may diminish absorption and require larger dose or adjunct therapy.
Patient teaching
• Warn patient that drug is for topical application to nasal mucosa and should not be inhaled. Inhalation may cause tightness in chest, coughing, and transient dyspnea.
• Instruct patient to clear nasal passage before administering drug. Teach him how to administer it.
• Advise patient to carry a medical identification card at all times.

Reactions may be *common,* uncommon, ***life-threatening,*** or COMMON AND LIFE-THREATENING.

☑ **Evaluation**
• Patient has normal fluid status.
• Patient does not develop serious nasal irritation.
• Patient and family state understanding of drug therapy.

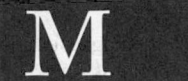

magaldrate
(aluminum-magnesium complex)
(muh-GAL-drayt)
Isopan, Lowsium†, Riopan†

Pharmacologic class: aluminum-magnesium salt
Therapeutic class: antacid
Pregnancy risk category: NR

How supplied

Tablets: 480 mg†
Tablets (chewable): 480 mg†
Oral suspension: 540 mg/5 ml†,
1,080 mg/5 ml†

Pharmacokinetics

Absorption: may be absorbed systemically, posing risk to patient with renal failure. Absorption is unrelated to mechanism of action.
Distribution: primarily local.
Metabolism: none.
Excretion: excreted in feces.

Route	Onset	Peak	Duration
P.O.	≤ 20 min	Unknown	20-60 min (fasting); 3 hr (non-fasting)

Pharmacodynamics

Chemical effect: reduces total acid load in GI tract, elevates gastric pH to reduce pepsin activity, strengthens gastric mu-

cosal barrier, and increases esophageal sphincter tone.
Therapeutic effect: soothes stomach upset.

Indications and dosage

▶ **Antacid.** *Adults:* 540 to 1,080 mg (5 to 10 ml) of suspension P.O. with water between meals and h.s.; or 480- to 960-mg tablets (1 or 2 tablets) P.O. with water between meals and h.s.; or 480- to 960-mg chewable tablets (1 or 2 tablets) P.O., chewed before swallowing, between meals and h.s.

Adverse reactions

GI: mild constipation or diarrhea.

Interactions

Drug-drug. *Allopurinol, antibiotics (including fluoroquinolones and tetracyclines), diflunisal, digoxin, iron, isoniazid, penicillamine, phenothiazines, quinidine:* decreased pharmacologic effect possible because of impaired absorption. Separate administration times.
Enteric-coated drugs: may release prematurely in stomach. Separate doses by at least 1 hour.

Contraindications and precautions

• Contraindicated in patients with severe renal disease.
• Use cautiously in patients with mild renal impairment and in pregnant or breastfeeding women.

NURSING CONSIDERATIONS

☑ **Assessment**
• Assess patient's condition before therapy and regularly thereafter.
• Record amount and consistency of stools.
• Monitor serum magnesium level in patient with mild renal impairment. Symptomatic hypermagnesemia usually occurs only in severe renal failure.
• Be alert for adverse reactions and drug interactions.

- Evaluate patient's and family's knowledge of drug therapy.

⊞ **Nursing diagnoses**
- Pain related to gastric hyperacidity
- Diarrhea related to drug-induced adverse GI reactions
- Knowledge deficit related to drug therapy

❯ **Planning and implementation**
- Shake suspension well. Give with water to facilitate passage.
- When giving through nasogastric tube, make sure tube is placed properly and is patent. After instilling drug, flush tube with water to ensure passage to stomach and to clear tube.
- Be aware that drug has very low sodium content and is acceptable for patient on restricted sodium intake.
Patient teaching
- Advise patient not to take drug indiscriminately or to switch antacids without doctor's advice.

✓ **Evaluation**
- Patient states that pain is relieved.
- Patient maintains normal bowel patterns throughout therapy.
- Patient and family state understanding of drug therapy.

---

magnesium chloride
(mag-NEE-see-um KLOR-ighd)
Slow-Mag†

magnesium sulfate

Pharmacologic class: magnesium salt
Therapeutic class: anticonvulsant, electrolyte supplement, antiarrhythmic
Pregnancy risk category: NR

How supplied

magnesium chloride
Tablets (delayed-release): 64 mg

magnesium sulfate
Injectable solutions: 10%, 12.5%, 25%, 50% in 2-ml, 5-ml, 10-ml, 20-ml, and 30-ml ampules, vials, and prefilled syringes

Pharmacokinetics

Absorption: 35% to 40% of P.O. dose is absorbed through GI tract. High-fat diets may interfere with absorption.
Distribution: about 30% of magnesium is bound intracellularly to proteins and energy-rich phosphates.
Metabolism: unknown.
Excretion: parenteral dose excreted primarily in urine; P.O. dose excreted in urine and feces.

Route	Onset	Peak	Duration
P.O.	Unknown	4 hr	4-6 hr
I.V., I.M.	Unknown	Unknown	4-6 hr

Pharmacodynamics

Chemical effect: replaces and maintains magnesium levels; as anticonvulsant, reduces muscle contractions by interfering with release of acetylcholine at myoneural junction.
Therapeutic effect: raises magnesium levels, alleviates seizure activity, and restores normal sinus rhythm.

Indications and dosage

▶ **Mild hypomagnesemia.** *Adults:* 1 g I.M. q 6 hours for four doses, depending on serum magnesium level.
▶ **Severe hypomagnesemia (serum magnesium level 0.8 mEq/L or less with symptoms).** *Adults:* 5 g I.V. in 1 L of solution over 3 hours. Subsequent doses depend on serum magnesium level.
▶ **Magnesium supplementation.** *Adults:* 2 tablets magnesium chloride P.O. daily.
▶ **Magnesium supplementation in total parenteral nutrition (TPN).** *Adults:* 4 to 24 mEq I.V. daily added to TPN solution. *Infants:* 2 to 10 mEq I.V. daily added to TPN solution. Each 2 ml of 50% solution contains 1 g, or 8.12 mEq, magnesium sulfate.

Reactions may be *common*, uncommon, *life-threatening*, or COMMON AND LIFE-THREATENING.

▶ **Hypomagnesemic seizures.** *Adults:* 1 to 2 g of 10% solution I.V. over 15 minutes, then 1 g I.M. q 4 to 6 hours, based on patient's response and serum magnesium level.

▶ **Seizures secondary to hypomagnesemia in acute nephritis.** *Children:* 0.2 ml/kg of 50% solution I.M. q 4 to 6 hours, p.r.n., or 100 mg/kg of 10% solution I.V. very slowly. Titrate dosage according to serum magnesium level and seizure response.

▶ **Paroxysmal atrial tachycardia unresponsive to other treatments.** *Adults:* 3 to 4 g I.V. of 10% solution over 30 seconds with close monitoring of ECG.

Adverse reactions

CNS: *weak or absent deep tendon reflexes* (with toxicity), flaccid paralysis, hypothermia, drowsiness, hypocalcemia (perioral paresthesia, twitching carpopedal spasm, tetany, and seizures).
CV: slow, weak pulse; *arrhythmias* (caused by hypocalcemia); *hypotension, circulatory collapse.*
Respiratory: *respiratory paralysis.*
Skin: diaphoresis, flushing.
Other: hypocalcemia.

Interactions

Drug-drug. *Cardiac glycosides:* possible serious cardiac conduction changes. Administer with extreme caution.
Neuromuscular blockers: possible increased neuromuscular blockage. Use cautiously.
Nitrofurantoin, penicillamine, tetracyclines: decreased bioavailability with oral magnesium supplements. Separate administration times by 2 to 3 hours.

Contraindications and precautions

● Contraindicated in patients with myocardial damage or heart block and in women who are in actively progressing labor.
● Use parenteral magnesium with extreme caution in patients with impaired kidney function.

NURSING CONSIDERATIONS

Assessment
● Assess patient's condition before therapy and regularly thereafter.
● When administering I.V. for severe hypomagnesemia, watch for respiratory depression and signs of heart block. Respirations should be more than 16 breaths/minute before dose is given.
● Check serum magnesium level after repeated doses.
● Monitor patient's fluid intake and output. Output should be 100 ml or more during 4-hour period before dose.
● Be alert for adverse reactions and drug interactions.
● Evaluate patient's and family's knowledge of drug therapy.

Nursing diagnoses
● Altered health maintenance related to underlying condition
● Risk for injury related to drug-induced adverse reactions
● Knowledge deficit related to drug therapy

Planning and implementation
P.O. use: Follow normal protocol.
I.V. use: Inject I.V. bolus dose slowly, using infusion pump for continuous infusion if available, to avoid respiratory or cardiac arrest. Maximum infusion rate should not exceed 150 mg/minute. Rapid drip causes feeling of heat.
– Magnesium sulfate may form precipitate when mixed with solutions containing arsenates, barium, calcium, clindamycin, ethanol, heavy metals, hydrocortisone sodium succinate, phosphates, polymyxin B sulfate, procaine, salicylates, or tartrates. Drug is also incompatible with alkalis, including carbonates and bicarbonates.
I.M. use: Undiluted 50% solutions may be administered by deep I.M. injection to adults. When administering to children, dilute solutions to 20% or less.

- Keep I.V. calcium available to reverse magnesium intoxication.
- Test knee-jerk and patellar reflexes before each additional dose. If absent, notify doctor and give no more magnesium until reflexes return; otherwise, patient may develop temporary respiratory failure and need cardiopulmonary resuscitation or I.V. administration of calcium.

Patient teaching
- Instruct patient receiving parenteral drug to report adverse reactions immediately.
- Review oral administration schedule with patient. Tell him not to take more than prescribed.

✔ **Evaluation**
- Patient exhibits positive response to drug administration.
- Patient does not experience injury from adverse reactions.
- Patient and family state understanding of drug therapy.

---

magnesium citrate (citrate of magnesia)
(mag-NEE-see-um SIH-trayt)
Citroma†, Citro-Mag♦

magnesium hydroxide (milk of magnesia)
Milk of Magnesia†, Phillips' Milk of Magnesia†

magnesium sulfate (epsom salts)

Pharmacologic class: magnesium salt
Therapeutic class: saline laxative
Pregnancy risk category: NR

How supplied

magnesium citrate
Oral solution: about 168 mEq magnesium/240 ml†
magnesium hydroxide
Oral suspension: 7% to 8.5% (about 80 mEq magnesium/30 ml)†

magnesium sulfate
Granules: about 40 mEq magnesium/5 g†

Pharmacokinetics
Absorption: about 15% to 30% may be absorbed systemically (posing risk to patients with renal failure).
Distribution: unknown.
Metabolism: unknown.
Excretion: unabsorbed drug excreted in feces; absorbed drug excreted rapidly in urine.

Route	Onset	Peak	Duration
P.O.	0.5-3 hr	Varies	Varies

Pharmacodynamics
Chemical effect: produces osmotic effect in small intestine by drawing water into intestinal lumen.
Therapeutic effect: relieves constipation.

Indications and dosage
▶ **Constipation; to evacuate bowel before surgery. Magnesium citrate.** *Adults and children age 12 and older:* 11 to 25 g P.O. daily as single dose or divided. *Children ages 6 to 11:* 5.5 to 12.5 g P.O. daily as single dose or divided. *Children ages 2 to 5:* 2.7 to 6.25 g P.O. daily as single dose or divided. **Magnesium hydroxide.** *Adults and children age 12 and older:* 2.4 to 4.8 g (30 to 60 ml) P.O. daily as single dose or divided. *Children ages 6 to 11:* 1.2 to 2.4 g (15 to 30 ml) P.O. daily as single dose or divided. *Children ages 2 to 5:* 0.4 to 1.2 g (5 to 15 ml) P.O. daily as single dose or divided. **Magnesium sulfate.** *Adults and children age 12 and older:* 10 to 30 g P.O. daily as single dose or divided. *Children ages 6 to 11:* 5 to 10 g P.O. daily as single dose or divided. *Children ages 2 to 5:* 2.5 to 5.0 g P.O. daily as single dose or divided.
▶ **Antacid. Magnesium hydroxide.** *Adults:* 5 to 15 ml P.O. t.i.d. or q.i.d.

Reactions may be *common*, uncommon, *life-threatening*, or COMMON AND LIFE-THREATENING.

Adverse reactions

GI: *abdominal cramping, nausea, diarrhea;* laxative dependence (with long-term or excessive use).
Other: fluid and electrolyte disturbances (with daily use).

Interactions

Drug-drug. *Orally administered drugs:* impaired absorption. Separate administration times.

Contraindications and precautions

• Contraindicated in patients with abdominal pain, nausea, vomiting, other symptoms of appendicitis or acute surgical abdomen, myocardial damage, heart block, imminent delivery, fecal impaction, rectal fissures, intestinal obstruction or perforation, or renal disease.
• Use cautiously in patients with rectal bleeding and in pregnant or breast-feeding women.

NURSING CONSIDERATIONS

⚙ Assessment
• Assess patient's condition before therapy and regularly thereafter.
• Before giving for constipation, determine if patient has adequate fluid intake, exercise, and diet.
• Monitor serum electrolyte levels, as ordered, during prolonged use. Magnesium may accumulate in patient with renal insufficiency.
• Be alert for adverse reactions and drug interactions.
• Evaluate patient's and family's knowledge of drug therapy.

⚙ Nursing diagnoses
• Constipation related to underlying condition
• Diarrhea related to therapy
• Knowledge deficit related to drug therapy

⟩ Planning and implementation
• Time drug administration so that it doesn't interfere with scheduled activities or sleep.
• Chill magnesium citrate before use to make it more palatable.
• Shake suspension well. Give with large amount of water when used as laxative. When administering through nasogastric tube, make sure tube is placed properly and is patent. After instilling drug, flush tube with water to ensure passage to stomach and maintain tube patency.
• Drug is for short-term therapy.
• Magnesium sulfate is more potent than other saline laxatives.
Patient teaching
• Teach patient about dietary sources of bulk, which include bran and other cereals, fresh fruit, and vegetables.
• Warn patient that frequent or prolonged use may cause dependence.

☑ Evaluation
• Patient's constipation is relieved.
• Diarrhea does not develop.
• Patient and family state understanding of drug therapy.

magnesium oxide
(mag-NEE-see-um OKS-ighd)
Mag-Ox 400†, Maox†, Uro-Mag†

Pharmacologic class: magnesium salt
Therapeutic class: antacid, laxative
Pregnancy risk category: NR

How supplied

Tablets: 400 mg†, 420 mg†
Capsules: 140 mg†
Oral suspension: 7.75%†

Pharmacokinetics

Absorption: small amount absorbed from GI tract.
Distribution: unknown.
Metabolism: none.

Excretion: unabsorbed drug excreted in feces; absorbed drug excreted in urine.

Route	Onset	Peak	Duration
P.O.	20 min	Unknown	20-60 min (fasting); 3 hr (non-fasting)

Pharmacodynamics

Chemical effect: reduces total acid load in GI tract, elevates gastric pH to reduce pepsin activity, strengthens gastric mucosal barrier, and increases esophageal sphincter tone.
Therapeutic effect: soothes stomach upset, relieves constipation, and raises serum magnesium level.

Indications and dosage

▶ **Antacid.** *Adults:* 140 mg P.O. with water or milk after meals and h.s.
▶ **Laxative.** *Adults:* 4 g P.O. with water or milk, usually h.s.
▶ **Oral replacement therapy in mild hypomagnesemia.** *Adults:* 400 to 840 mg P.O. daily. Monitor serum magnesium response.

Adverse reactions

GI: *diarrhea,* nausea, abdominal pain.
Metabolic: hypermagnesemia.

Interactions

Drug-drug. *Allopurinol, antibiotics (including fluoroquinolones and tetracyclines), diflunisal, digoxin, iron, isoniazid, penicillamine, phenothiazines, quinidine:* decreased pharmacologic effect possibly because of impaired absorption. Separate administration times.
Enteric-coated drugs: may release prematurely in stomach. Separate doses by at least 1 hour.

Contraindications and precautions

• Contraindicated in patients with severe renal disease.

• Use cautiously in patients with mild renal impairment and in pregnant or breast-feeding women.

NURSING CONSIDERATIONS

⚏ Assessment
• Assess patient's condition before therapy and regularly thereafter.
• Monitor serum magnesium level. With prolonged use and some renal impairment, watch for symptoms of hypermagnesemia (hypotension, nausea, vomiting, depressed reflexes, respiratory depression, and coma).
• Be alert for adverse reactions and drug interactions.
• Evaluate patient's and family's knowledge of drug therapy.

⚏ Nursing diagnoses
• Altered health maintenance related to underlying condition
• Risk for injury related to potential for hypermagnesemia
• Knowledge deficit related to drug therapy

⚏ Planning and implementation
• When using as laxative, do not give other oral drugs 1 to 2 hours before or after treatment.
• If diarrhea occurs, be prepared to suggest alternative preparation.
Patient teaching
• Advise patient not to take drug indiscriminately or to switch antacids without doctor's advice.

⚏ Evaluation
• Patient responds well to therapy.
• Patient maintains normal serum magnesium level throughout therapy.
• Patient and family state understanding of drug therapy.

Reactions may be *common*, uncommon, *life-threatening*, or COMMON AND LIFE-THREATENING.

magnesium sulfate
(mag-NEE-see-um SUL-fayt)

Pharmacologic class: mineral/electrolyte
Therapeutic class: anticonvulsant
Pregnancy risk category: A

How supplied

Injection: 4%, 8%, 10%, 12.5%, 25%, 50%
Injection solution: 1% in 5% dextrose, 2% in 5% dextrose

Pharmacokinetics

Absorption: unknown after I.M. administration.
Distribution: distributed widely throughout body.
Metabolism: none.
Excretion: excreted unchanged in urine.

Route	Onset	Peak	Duration
I.V.	1-2 min	Almost immediate	About 30 min
I.M.	1 hr	Unknown	3-4 hr

Pharmacodynamics

Chemical effect: unknown; may decrease acetylcholine released by nerve impulses, but its anticonvulsant mechanism is unknown.
Therapeutic effect: prevents or controls seizures, raises serum magnesium levels, stops paroxysmal atrial tachycardia, and alleviates selected symptoms of acute nephritis in children.

Indications and dosage

▶ **Prevention or control of seizures in preeclampsia or eclampsia.** *Women:* initially, 4 g I.V. in 250 ml of D₅W and 4 to 5 g deep I.M. each buttock; then 4 g deep I.M. into alternate buttock q 4 hours, p.r.n. Alternatively, 4 g I.V. loading dose, followed by 1 to 2 g hourly as I.V. infusion.
▶ **Hypomagnesemia.** *Adults:* 1 g I.M. q 6 hours for four doses for mild deficien-

cy; up to 250 mg/kg I.M. over 4-hour period for severe deficiency.
▶ **Seizures, hypertension, and encephalopathy associated with acute nephritis in children.** *Children:* 0.2 ml/kg of 50% solution I.M. q 4 to 6 hours, p.r.n. For severe symptoms, 100 to 200 mg/kg I.V. very slowly over 1 hour with one-half of dose administered in first 15 to 20 minutes. Dosage titrated according to serum magnesium level and seizure response.
▶ **Management of paroxysmal atrial tachycardia.** *Adults:* 3 to 4 g I.V. over 30 seconds.
▶ **Management of life-threatening ventricular arrhythmias, such as sustained ventricular tachycardia or torsades de pointes.** *Adults:* 2 to 6 g I.V. over several minutes, followed by continuous infusion of 3 to 20 mg/minute for 5 to 48 hours. Dosage and duration of therapy based on patient response and serum magnesium level.

Adverse reactions

CNS: drowsiness, *depressed reflexes,* flaccid paralysis, hypothermia.
CV: *hypotension, flushing,* **circulatory collapse,** depressed cardiac function, **heart block.**
Other: diaphoresis, *respiratory paralysis,* hypocalcemia.

Interactions

Drug-drug. *Anesthetics, CNS depressants:* may cause additive CNS depression. Use cautiously.
Cardiac glycosides: concomitant use may exacerbate arrhythmias. Use together cautiously.
Neuromuscular blockers: may increase neuromuscular blockade. Use cautiously.

Contraindications and precautions

• Parenteral administration contraindicated in patients with heart block or myocardial damage.
• Drug is not recommended for use in breast-feeding women.

• Use cautiously in patients with impaired kidney function and in women who are in labor.

NURSING CONSIDERATIONS

⚕ Assessment
• Assess patient's condition before therapy and regularly thereafter.
• Monitor vital signs every 15 minutes when giving drug I.V.
• Watch for respiratory depression and signs of heart block. Respirations should be about 16 breaths/minute before each dose.
• Monitor fluid intake and output. Output should be 100 ml or more in 4-hour period before each dose.
• Be alert for adverse reactions and drug interactions.
• Check serum magnesium level after repeated doses. Disappearance of knee-jerk and patellar reflexes is sign of pending magnesium toxicity. Signs of hypermagnesemia begin to appear at serum levels of 4 mEq/L.
• Observe neonate for signs of magnesium toxicity, including neuromuscular or respiratory depression, when giving I.V. form to toxemic mother within 24 hours before delivery.
• Evaluate patient's and family's knowledge of drug therapy.

⚎ Nursing diagnoses
• Altered health maintenance related to underlying condition
• Risk for injury related to drug-induced adverse reactions
• Knowledge deficit related to drug therapy

▷ Planning and implementation
I.V. use: If necessary, dilute to maximum concentration of 20%. Infuse no faster than 150 mg/minute (1.5 ml/minute of 10% solution or 0.75 ml/minute of 20% solution). Drug is compatible with D₅W.

– Maximum infusion rate is 150 mg/minute. Rapid drip induces uncomfortable feeling of heat.
I.M. use: Follow normal protocol.
• Keep I.V. calcium gluconate available to reverse magnesium intoxication; use cautiously in patients undergoing digitalization because of danger of arrhythmias.
• If used to treat seizures, institute appropriate seizure precautions.
Patient teaching
• Stress importance of reporting adverse reactions immediately.

☑ Evaluation
• Patient responds well to therapy.
• Patient does not experience injury.
• Patient and family state understanding of drug therapy.

mannitol
(MAN-ih-tol)
Osmitrol

Pharmacologic class: osmotic diuretic
Therapeutic class: diuretic, diagnostic and treatment nephrotic agent, treatment of drug intoxication, reduction of intracranial or intraocular pressure
Pregnancy risk category: C

How supplied
Injection: 5%, 10%, 15%, 20%, 25%

Pharmacokinetics
Absorption: not applicable.
Distribution: remains in extracellular compartment; does not cross blood-brain barrier.
Metabolism: metabolized minimally to glycogen in liver.
Excretion: excreted in urine. *Half-life:* about 100 minutes.

Route	Onset	Peak	Duration
I.V.	30-60 min	≤ 1 hr	6-8 hr

Reactions may be *common*, uncommon, *life-threatening*, or COMMON AND LIFE-THREATENING.

Pharmacodynamics

Chemical effect: increases osmotic pressure of glomerular filtrate, inhibiting tubular reabsorption of water and electrolytes. This elevates blood plasma osmolality, enhancing water flow into extracellular fluid.

Therapeutic effect: increases water excretion, decreases intracranial or intraocular pressure, prevents or treats kidney dysfunction, and alleviates drug intoxication.

Indications and dosage

▶ **Test dose for marked oliguria or suspected inadequate kidney function.**
Adults and children over age 12:
200 mg/kg or 12.5 g as 15% or 20% I.V. solution over 3 to 5 minutes. Response is adequate if 30 to 50 ml urine/hour is excreted over 2 to 3 hours; if response is inadequate, second test dose is given. If still no response after second dose, drug should not be continued.

▶ **Oliguria.** *Adults and children over age 12:* 100 g I.V. as 15% to 20% solution over 90 minutes to several hours.

▶ **Prevention of oliguria or acute renal failure.** *Adults and children over age 12:* 50 to 100 g I.V. of concentrated solution, followed by 5% to 10% solution. Exact concentration determined by fluid requirements.

▶ **Edema; ascites caused by renal, hepatic, or cardiac failure.** *Adults and children over age 12:* 100 g I.V. as 10% to 20% solution over 2 to 6 hours.

▶ **Reduction of intraocular or intracranial pressure.** *Adults and children over age 12:* 1.5 to 2.0 g/kg as 15% to 25% I.V. solution over 30 to 60 minutes.

▶ **Diuresis in drug intoxication.** *Adults and children over age 12:* 25-g loading dose followed by an infusion maintaining 100- to 500-ml urine output/hour and positive fluid balance.

▶ **Irrigating solution during transurethral resection of prostate.**
Adults: 2.5% solution, p.r.n.

Adverse reactions

CNS: headache, confusion, *seizures.*
CV: transient expansion of plasma volume during infusion, causing circulatory overload and *heart failure;* tachycardia; angina-like chest pain.
EENT: blurred vision, rhinitis.
GI: thirst, nausea, vomiting, *diarrhea.*
GU: urine retention.
Metabolic: fluid and electrolyte imbalance, water intoxication, cellular dehydration.

Interactions

Drug-drug. *Lithium:* increased urinary excretion of lithium. Monitor patient closely.

Contraindications and precautions

• Contraindicated in patients with hypersensitivity to drug and in those with anuria, severe pulmonary congestion, frank pulmonary edema, severe heart failure, severe dehydration, metabolic edema, progressive renal disease or dysfunction, or active intracranial bleeding except during craniotomy.
• Use of drug not recommended in breast-feeding women.
• Use cautiously in pregnant women.

NURSING CONSIDERATIONS

☑ Assessment

• Assess patient's condition before therapy and regularly thereafter.
• Monitor vital signs, including central venous pressure, and fluid intake and output hourly. Insert urethral catheter in comatose or incontinent patient because therapy is based on strict evaluation of fluid intake and output. In patient with urethral catheter, use hourly urometer collection bag to facilitate accurate evaluation.
• Monitor weight, kidney function, and serum and urine sodium and potassium levels daily.
• Be alert for adverse reactions and drug interactions.

• Evaluate patient's and family's knowledge of drug therapy.

⊞ Nursing diagnoses
• Altered health maintenance related to underlying condition
• Risk for fluid volume deficit related to drug-induced adverse GI reactions
• Knowledge deficit related to drug therapy

⊵ Planning and implementation
• To redissolve crystallized solution (occurs at low temperatures or in concentrations greater than 15%), warm bottle in hot water bath and shake vigorously. Cool to body temperature before giving. Do not use solution with undissolved crystals.
• Give as intermittent or continuous infusion at prescribed rate, using in-line filter and infusion pump. Direct injection is not recommended. Check I.V. line patency at infusion site before and during administration.
• Avoid infiltration; if it occurs, observe for inflammation, edema, and necrosis.
• For maximum intraocular pressure reduction before surgery, give 1 to 1½ hours preoperatively, as ordered.
• When used as irrigating solution for prostate surgery, keep in mind that concentrations of 3.5% or greater are needed to avoid hemolysis.
• Notify doctor immediately if increasing oliguria or adverse reactions occur.
Patient teaching
• Tell patient he may feel thirsty or experience mouth dryness, and emphasize importance of drinking only amount of fluid provided.
• Instruct patient to immediately report pain in chest, back, or legs or shortness of breath.

☑ Evaluation
• Patient responds well to mannitol.
• Patient maintains adequate hydration throughout therapy.
• Patient and family state understanding of drug therapy.

maprotiline hydrochloride
(ma-PROH-tih-leen high-droh-KLOR-ighd)
Ludiomil

Pharmacologic class: tricyclic antidepressant
Therapeutic class: antidepressant
Pregnancy risk category: B

How supplied
Tablets: 25 mg, 50 mg, 75 mg

Pharmacokinetics
Absorption: absorbed slowly but completely from GI tract.
Distribution: distributed widely in body, including CNS; 88% protein-bound.
Metabolism: metabolized slowly by liver; significant first-pass effect may account for variability of serum concentrations in different patients taking same dosage.
Excretion: most of drug excreted in urine; 30% excreted in feces. *Half-life:* averages 61 hours.

Route	Onset	Peak	Duration
P.O.	1-3 wk	12 hr	Unknown

Pharmacodynamics
Chemical effect: unknown; probably increases amount of norepinephrine, serotonin, or both in CNS by blocking their reuptake by presynaptic neurons.
Therapeutic effect: relieves depression.

Indications and dosage
▶ **Depression.** *Adults:* initially, 75 mg P.O. daily for patients with mild to moderate depression, increased to 150 mg daily, if needed. Maximum dosage is 225 mg daily.

Adverse reactions
CNS: *drowsiness, dizziness,* excitation, *seizures,* tremors, weakness, confusion, headache, nervousness, extrapyramidal reactions.

Reactions may be *common,* uncommon, *life-threatening*, or COMMON AND LIFE-THREATENING.

CV: *orthostatic hypotension, tachycardia, ECG changes.*
EENT: *blurred vision,* tinnitus, mydriasis.
GI: dry mouth, *constipation,* nausea, vomiting, anorexia, paralytic ileus.
GU: *urine retention.*
Skin: rash, urticaria, photosensitivity.
Other: *diaphoresis,* hypersensitivity reaction.
After abrupt withdrawal of long-term therapy: nausea, headache, malaise (does not indicate addiction).

Interactions

Drug-drug. *Anticholinergics:* additive atropine-like effects may occur. Monitor patient.
Barbiturates: decreased maprotiline serum levels. Monitor for decreased antidepressant effect.
Cimetidine, methylphenidate: may increase maprotiline serum levels. Monitor for adverse reactions.
Clonidine, epinephrine, norepinephrine: increased hypertensive effect. Use with caution.
CNS depressants: enhanced CNS depression. Avoid concomitant use.
Guanethidine: maprotiline may block the pharmacologic effects of guanethidine. Monitor closely.
MAO inhibitors: may cause severe excitation, hyperpyrexia, or seizures, usually with high dosage. Use with caution.
Phenothiazines: risk of seizures may be increased with concomitant use. Monitor closely.
Thyroid hormones: possible enhanced potential for CV toxicity of maprotiline. Use cautiously together.
Drug-lifestyle. *Alcohol use:* enhanced CNS depression. Avoid concomitant use.

Contraindications and precautions

• Contraindicated during acute recovery phase of MI, in patients with seizure disorders or hypersensitivity to drug, or within 14 days of MAO inhibitor therapy.

• Use with extreme caution in patients with history of MI or CV disease.
• Use cautiously in patients with suicidal tendency, increased intraocular pressure, or history of urine retention or angle-closure glaucoma and in pregnant or breast-feeding women.
• Safety of drug has not been established in children.

NURSING CONSIDERATIONS

Assessment
• Assess patient's depression before therapy and regularly thereafter.
• Be alert for adverse reactions and drug interactions.
• Evaluate patient's and family's knowledge of drug therapy.

Nursing diagnoses
• Altered thought processes related to presence of depression
• Constipation related to drug-induced adverse GI reactions
• Knowledge deficit related to drug therapy

Planning and implementation
• Know that dosage needs to be reduced in elderly or debilitated patients and in adolescents.
• Because maprotiline shares toxic potentials with tricyclic antidepressants and may cause hypertensive episodes during surgery, know that dosage should be gradually discontinued several days before surgery.
• If signs of depression are not improved or increase, notify doctor.
Patient teaching
• Warn patient to avoid activities that require alertness and good psychomotor coordination until CNS effects of drug are known.
• Advise patient to take full dose at bedtime, but warn him of possible morning orthostatic hypotension.
• Tell patient to avoid alcohol consumption during drug therapy.

- Warn patient not to withdraw drug suddenly.
- Advise patient to consult the doctor before taking other drugs.
- Advise patient to use sunblock, wear protective clothing, and avoid prolonged exposure to sunlight.
- Advise patient about measures to prevent constipation.

☑ **Evaluation**
- Patient behavior and communication indicate diminished depression.
- Patient maintains normal bowel patterns throughout therapy.
- Patient and family state understanding of drug therapy.

mebendazole
(meh-BEN-duh-zohl)
Vermox

Pharmacologic class: benzimidazole
Therapeutic class: anthelmintic
Pregnancy risk category: C

How supplied

Tablets (chewable): 100 mg
Oral suspension: 100 mg/5 ml ◊

Pharmacokinetics

Absorption: about 5% to 10% of dose is absorbed; varies widely among patients.
Distribution: highly bound to plasma proteins.
Metabolism: metabolized to inactive metabolites.
Excretion: mostly excreted in feces; 2% to 10% excreted in urine. *Half-life:* 3 to 9 hours.

Route	Onset	Peak	Duration
P.O.	Unknown	2-5 hr	Varies

Pharmacodynamics

Chemical effect: selectively and irreversibly inhibits uptake of glucose and other nutrients in susceptible helminths.

Therapeutic effect: kills helminth infestation.

Indications and dosage

▶ **Pinworm.** *Adults and children over age 2:* 100 mg P.O. as single dose. If infection persists 3 weeks later, treatment is repeated.
▶ **Roundworm, whipworm, hookworm.** *Adults and children over age 2:* 100 mg P.O. b.i.d. for 3 days. If infection persists 3 weeks later, treatment is repeated.

Adverse reactions

GI: transient abdominal pain, diarrhea (in massive infection).

Interactions

Drug-drug. *Carbamazepine, hydantoins:* may reduce plasma levels of concomitant mebendazole, possibly decreasing its therapeutic effect. Monitor patient.
Cimetidine: increased plasma concentrations of mebendazole. Monitor patient closely.

Contraindications and precautions

- Contraindicated in patients with hypersensitivity to drug.
- Use cautiously in pregnant women.
- Safety of drug has not been established in breast-feeding women.

NURSING CONSIDERATIONS

☑ **Assessment**
- Assess patient's condition before therapy and regularly thereafter.
- Be alert for adverse reactions and drug interactions.
- Evaluate patient's and family's knowledge of drug therapy.

☑ **Nursing diagnoses**
- Infection related to presence of helminths
- Diarrhea related to drug-induced adverse GI reactions
- Knowledge deficit related to drug therapy

Reactions may be *common*, uncommon, **life-threatening**, or COMMON AND LIFE-THREATENING.

> **Planning and implementation**
- Know that tablets may be chewed, swallowed whole, or crushed and mixed with food.
- Administer drug to all family members, as prescribed, to decrease risk of spreading infection.
- Know that no dietary restrictions, laxatives, or enemas are necessary.

Patient teaching
- Teach patient about personal hygiene, especially good hand-washing technique. To avoid reinfection, teach patient to wash perianal area daily, to change undergarments and bedclothes daily, and to wash hands and clean fingernails before meals and after bowel movements.
- Advise patient to refrain from preparing food for others.

☑ **Evaluation**
- Patient is free from infestation.
- Patient's bowel pattern returns to normal after therapy is stopped.
- Patient and family state understanding of drug therapy.

---

mechlorethamine hydrochloride (nitrogen mustard)
(meh-klor-ETH-uh-meen high-droh-KLOR-ighd)
Mustargen

Pharmacologic class: alkylating agent (cell cycle–phase nonspecific)
Therapeutic class: antineoplastic
Pregnancy risk category: D

How supplied
Injection: 10-mg vials

Pharmacokinetics
Absorption: after intracavitary administration, drug is absorbed incompletely, probably from deactivation by body fluids in cavity.

Distribution: does not cross blood-brain barrier.
Metabolism: converted rapidly to its active form, which reacts quickly with various cellular components before being deactivated.
Excretion: metabolites excreted in urine.

Route	Onset	Peak	Duration
I.V., intra-cavitary	Sec-min	Unknown	Unknown

Pharmacodynamics
Chemical effect: cross-links strands of cellular DNA and interferes with RNA transcription, causing imbalance of growth that leads to cell death.
Therapeutic effect: kills selected cancer cells.

Indications and dosage
▶ **Polycythemia vera, chronic lymphocytic leukemia, chronic myelocytic leukemia, malignant effusions (pericardial, peritoneal, pleural), mycosis fungoides, Hodgkin's disease, lymphosarcoma, bronchogenic cancer.**
Adults: 0.4 mg/kg or 10 mg/m^2 I.V. as single dose or in divided doses of 0.1 to 0.2 mg/kg/day on 2 to 4 successive days q 3 to 6 weeks. Given through running I.V. infusion. Subsequent courses given when patient has recovered hematologically from previous course (usually 3 to 6 weeks).
▶ **Malignant effusions.** *Adults:* 0.2 to 0.4 mg/kg intracavitarily.

Adverse reactions
CNS: headache, weakness, drowsiness, vertigo.
EENT: tinnitus, *metallic taste* (immediately after dose), deafness (with high doses).
GI: *nausea, vomiting, anorexia* (beginning within minutes, lasting 8 to 24 hours).
Hematologic: *thrombocytopenia, agranulocytosis,* lymphocytopenia, nadir of myelosuppression occurring by days 4 to

10 and lasting 10 to 21 days; mild anemia begins in 2 to 3 weeks.

Skin: rash, sloughing, severe irritation (if drug extravasates or touches skin).

Other: *alopecia,* precipitation of herpes zoster, *anaphylaxis, secondary malignant disease,* hyperuricemia, *thrombophlebitis.*

Interactions

Drug-drug. *Anticoagulants, aspirin:* increased risk of bleeding. Avoid concomitant use.

Contraindications and precautions

• Contraindicated in patients with known infectious diseases or hypersensitivity to drug.
• Drug is not recommended for use in pregnant or breast-feeding women.
• Use cautiously in patients with severe anemia or depressed neutrophil or platelet count and in those who have recently undergone radiation therapy or chemotherapy.
• Safety of drug has not been established in children.

NURSING CONSIDERATIONS

Assessment
• Assess patient's condition before therapy and regularly thereafter.
• Monitor CBC and platelet counts regularly, as ordered.
• Monitor serum uric acid level, as ordered.
• Be alert for adverse reactions and drug interactions.
• Be aware that neurotoxicity increases with dose and patient age.
• Evaluate patient's and family's knowledge of drug therapy.

Nursing diagnoses
• Altered health maintenance related to presence of neoplastic disease
• Altered protection related to adverse hematologic reactions

• Knowledge deficit related to drug therapy

Planning and implementation
• Follow institutional policy to reduce risks. Preparation and administration of parenteral form are associated with carcinogenic, mutagenic, and teratogenic risks for personnel.

I.V. use: Reconstitute drug using 10 ml of sterile water for injection or 0.9% NaCl injection. Resulting solution contains 1 mg/ml of mechlorethamine. Give by direct injection into vein or into I.V. line containing free-flowing solution.
– Make sure I.V. solution doesn't infiltrate. Mechlorethamine is potent vesicant. If drug extravasates, apply cold compresses and infiltrate area with isotonic sodium thiosulfate, as ordered.

Intracavitary use: When given intracavitarily for sclerosing effect, dilute using up to 100 ml of 0.9% NaCl injection. Turn patient from side to side every 15 minutes to 1 hour to distribute drug.
• Prepare immediately before infusion. Solution is very unstable. Use within 15 minutes, and discard unused solution.
• Do not use solutions that are discolored or contain particulate matter. Do not use vials that appear to contain droplets of water.
• Dispose of equipment used in drug preparation and administration properly and according to institutional policy. Neutralize unused solution with equal volume of 5% sodium bicarbonate and 5% sodium thiosulfate.
• To prevent hyperuricemia with resulting uric acid nephropathy, know that drug may be used with adequate hydration.

Patient teaching
• Warn patient to watch for signs of infection (fever, sore throat, fatigue) and bleeding (easy bruising, nosebleeds, bleeding gums, melena). Have patient take temperature daily.
• Instruct patient to avoid OTC products containing aspirin.

Reactions may be *common*, uncommon, *life-threatening*, or COMMON AND LIFE-THREATENING.

• Advise female patient of childbearing age to avoid becoming pregnant during therapy and to consult with doctor before becoming pregnant.

☑ **Evaluation**
• Patient responds positively to drug.
• Patient regains normal hematologic parameters.
• Patient and family state understanding of drug therapy.

meclizine hydrochloride (meclozine hydrochloride)
(MEK-lih-zeen high-droh-KLOR-ighd)
Ancolan◇, Antivert, Antivert/25†, Antivert/50, Bonamine♦, Bonine†, Dizmiss†, D-Vert 15, D-Vert 30, Meni-D, Ru-Vert M

Pharmacologic class: piperazine-derivative antihistamine
Therapeutic class: antiemetic, antivertigo agent
Pregnancy risk category: B

How supplied
Tablets: 12.5 mg, 25 mg†, 50 mg
Tablets (chewable): 25 mg†
Capsules: 15 mg, 25 mg, 30 mg

Pharmacokinetics
Absorption: unknown.
Distribution: well distributed throughout body.
Metabolism: unknown, although thought to metabolize in liver.
Excretion: excreted unchanged in feces; metabolites found in urine. *Half-life:* about 6 hours.

Route	Onset	Peak	Duration
P.O.	About 1 hr	Unknown	8-24 hr

Pharmacodynamics
Chemical effect: unknown; may affect neural pathways originating in labyrinth to inhibit nausea and vomiting.

Therapeutic effect: relieves vertigo and nausea.

Indications and dosage
▶ **Vertigo.** *Adults:* 25 to 100 mg P.O. daily in divided doses. Dosage varies with patient response.
▶ **Motion sickness.** *Adults:* 25 to 50 mg P.O. 1 hour before travel, repeated daily for duration of journey.

Adverse reactions
CNS: *drowsiness,* fatigue.
EENT: blurred vision.
GI: dry mouth.

Interactions
Drug-drug. *CNS depressants:* increased drowsiness. Use together cautiously.

Contraindications and precautions
• Contraindicated in patients hypersensitive to drug.
• Use cautiously in patients with asthma, glaucoma, or prostatic hyperplasia and in breast-feeding women.
• Safety of drug has not been established in children and in pregnant women.

NURSING CONSIDERATIONS

☞ **Assessment**
• Assess patient's condition before therapy and regularly thereafter.
• Be alert for adverse reactions and drug interactions.
• Evaluate patient's and family's knowledge of drug therapy.

⊞ **Nursing diagnoses**
• Risk for injury related to vertigo
• Risk for fluid volume deficit related to motion sickness
• Knowledge deficit related to drug therapy

▶ **Planning and implementation**
• Know that tablets may be placed in mouth and allowed to dissolve without

water, or they may be chewed or swallowed whole.

• If used to prevent motion sickness, know that drug should be administered 1 hour before travel.

• Do not discontinue abruptly after long-term therapy because paradoxical reactions or sudden reversal of improved state may occur.

Patient teaching

• Advise patient to refrain from driving and performing other hazardous activities that require alertness until CNS effects of drug are known.

• Teach patient how to take drug.

• Stress importance of not stopping drug abruptly if used long term.

☑ **Evaluation**

• Patient states that vertigo is relieved.

• Patient states that motion sickness does not occur.

• Patient and family state understanding of drug therapy.

meclofenamate sodium

(mek-loh-fen-AM-ayt SOH-dee-um)
Meclomen

Pharmacologic class: NSAID
Therapeutic class: nonnarcotic analgesic, antipyretic, anti-inflammatory
Pregnancy risk category: NR

How supplied

Capsules: 50 mg, 100 mg

Pharmacokinetics

Absorption: absorbed rapidly and completely from GI tract.
Distribution: highly bound to plasma proteins.
Metabolism: metabolized in liver.
Excretion: excreted primarily in urine with some biliary excretion. *Half-life:* about 3 hours.

Route	Onset	Peak	Duration
P.O.	30 min (analgesic) 3 days (antirheumatic)	0.5-1 hr	Unknown

Pharmacodynamics

Chemical effect: unknown; produces anti-inflammatory, analgesic, and antipyretic effects, possibly by inhibiting prostaglandin synthesis.
Therapeutic effect: relieves pain, fever, and inflammation.

Indications and dosage

▶ **Rheumatoid arthritis, osteoarthritis.** *Adults:* 200 to 400 mg/day P.O. in three or four equally divided doses.
▶ **Mild to moderate pain.** *Adults:* 50 to 100 mg P.O. q 4 to 6 hours. Maximum dosage is 400 mg/day.
▶ **Dysmenorrhea, menorrhagia.** *Adults:* 100 mg P.O. t.i.d.

Adverse reactions

CNS: fatigue, malaise, insomnia, *dizziness,* nervousness, *headache.*
CV: edema.
EENT: blurred vision, eye irritation.
GI: *abdominal pain, flatulence, **peptic ulceration,*** nausea, vomiting, diarrhea, **hemorrhage.**
GU: dysuria, hematuria, nephrotoxicity, *renal failure.*
Hematologic: leukopenia, *thrombocytopenia, agranulocytosis, aplastic anemia.*
Hepatic: *hepatotoxicity.*
Skin: rash, urticaria.

Interactions

Drug-drug. *Antihypertensives, diuretics:* decreased effectiveness. Monitor patient closely.
Aspirin: decreased plasma levels of meclofenamate. Monitor for decreased effect.
Corticosteroids, other NSAIDs: increased risk of adverse GI reactions. Avoid concomitant use.

Reactions may be *common,* uncommon, *life-threatening,* or COMMON AND LIFE-THREATENING.

Oral anticoagulants: enhanced anticoagulant effect. Monitor for toxicity.
Drug-lifestyle. *Alcohol use:* increased risk of adverse GI reactions.

Contraindications and precautions

• Contraindicated in patients with hypersensitivity to drug or history of aspirin- or NSAID-induced bronchospasm, urticaria, or rhinitis.
• Use cautiously in patients with hepatic, renal, or CV disease; blood dyscrasia; or history of peptic ulcer disease and in elderly patients, who are more prone to adverse reactions.
• Drug is not recommended for use in pregnant women, especially during first and third trimesters, and in breast-feeding women.
• Safety of drug has not been established in children under age 14.

NURSING CONSIDERATIONS

Assessment
• Assess patient's condition before therapy and regularly thereafter.
• Be aware that CBC and kidney and liver function should be assessed every 6 months or as indicated in patient receiving long-term therapy.
• Be alert for adverse reactions and drug interactions.
• Evaluate patient's and family's knowledge of drug therapy.

Nursing diagnoses
• Pain related to underlying condition
• Altered tissue integrity related to drug's adverse effect on GI mucosa
• Knowledge deficit related to drug therapy

Planning and implementation
• Administer drug with food.
• Know that false-positive reactions for urine bilirubin using diazo tablet test have been reported.

• Notify doctor if serious adverse GI reactions occur or laboratory test results are abnormal.
Patient teaching
• Tell patient to take drug with food to minimize adverse GI reactions.
• Tell patient to stop taking drug and contact doctor immediately if rash, visual disturbances, or diarrhea develops.
• Caution patient that concomitant use with other NSAIDs, alcohol, or corticosteroids may increase risk of adverse GI reactions.
• Advise patient to refrain from driving or performing other hazardous activities that require mental alertness until CNS effects are known.
• Teach patient signs and symptoms of GI bleeding, and tell him to contact doctor immediately if they occur.

Evaluation
• Patient states that pain is relieved.
• Patient does not experience GI bleeding.
• Patient and family state understanding of drug therapy.

medroxyprogesterone acetate
(med-roks-ee-proh-JES-ter-ohn AS-ih-tayt)
Amen, Curretab, Cycrin, Depo-Provera, Provera

Pharmacologic class: progestin
Therapeutic class: progestin antineoplastic
Pregnancy risk category: X

How supplied

Tablets: 2.5 mg, 5 mg, 10 mg
Injection (suspension): 100 mg/ml, 150 mg/ml, 400 mg/ml

Pharmacokinetics

Absorption: slow after I.M. use; unknown for P.O. use.
Distribution: unknown.

Metabolism: primarily in liver; not well characterized.
Excretion: primarily in urine; not well characterized.

Route	Onset	Peak	Duration
P.O., I.M.	Unknown	Unknown	Unknown

Pharmacodynamics

Chemical effect: suppresses ovulation, possibly by inhibiting pituitary gonadotropin secretion, and forms thick cervical mucus.
Therapeutic effect: stops abnormal uterine bleeding, reverses secondary amenorrhea, prevents pregnancy, and hinders cancer cell growth.

Indications and dosage

▶ **Abnormal uterine bleeding caused by hormonal imbalance.** *Adults:* 5 to 10 mg P.O. daily for 5 to 10 days beginning on day 16 of menstrual cycle. If patient also has received estrogen, 10 mg P.O. daily for 10 days beginning on day 16 of cycle.
▶ **Secondary amenorrhea.** *Adults:* 5 to 10 mg P.O. daily for 5 to 10 days.
▶ **Endometrial or renal carcinoma.** *Adults:* 400 to 1,000 mg I.M. weekly.
▶ **Contraception in women.** *Adults:* 150 mg I.M. once q 3 months.

Adverse reactions

CNS: dizziness, migraine, lethargy, depression.
CV: hypertension, thrombophlebitis, *pulmonary embolism,* edema, *thromboembolism, CVA.*
GI: nausea, vomiting, abdominal cramps.
GU: breakthrough bleeding, dysmenorrhea, amenorrhea, cervical erosion, abnormal secretions, uterine fibromas, vaginal candidiasis.
Hepatic: cholestatic jaundice.
Skin: melasma, rash, pain, induration, sterile abscesses.
Other: hyperglycemia; breast tenderness, enlargement, or secretion; decreased libido.

Interactions

Drug-drug. *Aminoglutethimide, rifampin:* decreased progestin effects. Monitor for diminished therapeutic response. Tell patient to use nonhormonal contraceptive during therapy with these drugs.
Bromocriptine: may cause amenorrhea, interfering with bromocriptine's effects. Avoid concomitant use.
Drug-food. *Caffeine:* may increase serum caffeine concentrations. Monitor for effect.
Drug-lifestyle. *Smoking:* increased risk of adverse CV effects. If smoking continues, may need alternative therapy.

Contraindications and precautions

• Contraindicated in patients with hypersensitivity to drug, active thromboembolic disorders, history of thromboembolic disorders or cerebrovascular disease or apoplexy, breast cancer, undiagnosed abnormal vaginal bleeding, missed abortion, or hepatic dysfunction and in pregnant women. Tablets are also contraindicated in patients with liver dysfunction or known or suspected cancer of genital organs.
• Drug is not recommended for use in breast-feeding women.
• Use cautiously in patients with diabetes mellitus, seizure disorder, migraine, cardiac or renal disease, asthma, or depression.

NURSING CONSIDERATIONS

Assessment
• Assess patient's condition before therapy and regularly thereafter.
• Be alert for adverse reactions and drug interactions.
• Monitor injection sites for evidence of sterile abscess.
• Evaluate patient's and family's knowledge of drug therapy.

Nursing diagnoses
• Altered health maintenance related to underlying condition

Reactions may be *common,* uncommon, *life-threatening,* or COMMON AND LIFE-THREATENING.

• Fluid volume excess related to drug-induced edema
• Knowledge deficit related to drug therapy

⚡ Planning and implementation
P.O. use: Follow normal protocol.
I.M. use: Rotate injection sites to prevent muscle atrophy.
Patient teaching
• Have patient read package insert explaining possible adverse effects of progestins before administering first dose; then provide verbal explanation.
• Instruct patient to avoid caffeine products and smoking during drug therapy.
• Tell patient to report unusual symptoms immediately, and to stop drug and notify doctor if visual disturbances or migraine occurs.
• Teach female patient how to perform routine monthly breast self-examination.
• Warn patient that I.M. injection may be painful.

⚡ Evaluation
• Patient responds well to drug therapy.
• Patient does not develop fluid excess throughout drug therapy.
• Patient and family state understanding of drug therapy.

---

mefenamic acid
(mef-eh-NAM-ik AS-ihd)
Mefic◊, Ponstan♦, Ponstel

Pharmacologic class: NSAID
Therapeutic class: nonnarcotic analgesic, antipyretic, anti-inflammatory
Pregnancy risk category: C

How supplied
Capsules: 250 mg

Pharmacokinetics
Absorption: absorbed rapidly and completely from GI tract.
Distribution: highly protein-bound.

Metabolism: metabolized in liver.
Excretion: excreted mainly in urine with some biliary excretion. *Half-life:* about 2 to 4 hours.

Route	Onset	Peak	Duration
P.O.	Unknown	2-4 hr	Unknown

Pharmacodynamics
Chemical effect: unknown; produces anti-inflammatory, analgesic, and antipyretic effects, possibly by inhibiting prostaglandin synthesis.
Therapeutic effect: relieves pain, fever, and inflammation.

Indications and dosage

▶ **Mild to moderate pain, dysmenorrhea.** *Adults and children over age 14:* 500 mg P.O.; then 250 mg q 6 hours, p.r.n. Maximum therapy 1 week.

Adverse reactions
CNS: drowsiness, dizziness, nervousness, headache.
CV: edema.
EENT: blurred vision, eye irritation.
GI: nausea, vomiting, *diarrhea, peptic ulceration, pancreatitis, hemorrhage.*
GU: dysuria, hematuria, nephrotoxicity, *renal failure.*
Hematologic: leukopenia, *thrombocytopenia, agranulocytosis, aplastic anemia, hemolytic anemia.*
Hepatic: *hepatotoxicity.*
Skin: rash, urticaria.

Interactions
Drug-drug. *Antihypertensives, diuretics:* decreased effect. Monitor patient.
Aspirin, corticosteroids: increased risk of adverse GI reactions. Avoid concomitant use.
Oral anticoagulants, sulfonylureas, other drugs that are highly protein-bound: increased risk of toxicity. Monitor patient closely.
Drug-lifestyle: *Alcohol use:* increased risk of adverse GI reactions. Avoid concomitant use.

Contraindications and precautions

● Contraindicated in patients with hypersensitivity to drug; history of aspirin- or NSAID-induced bronchospasm, allergic rhinitis, or urticaria; GI ulceration or inflammation; or renal disease.

● Use cautiously in patients with hepatic or CV disease or history of peptic ulcer disease.

● Drug is not recommended for use during third trimester or in breast-feeding women.

● Safety of drug has not been established in children under age 14.

NURSING CONSIDERATIONS

⚚ Assessment

● Assess patient's condition before therapy and regularly thereafter.

● Be aware that severe hemolytic anemia may occur with prolonged use. Monitor CBC every 4 to 6 months, as ordered or as indicated.

● Be alert for adverse reactions and drug interactions.

● Evaluate patient's and family's knowledge of drug therapy.

⊕ Nursing diagnoses

● Pain related to underlying condition

● Impaired tissue integrity related to drug's adverse effect on GI mucosa

● Knowledge deficit related to drug therapy

▶ Planning and implementation

● Drug should not be administered for more than 1 week at a time because of increased risk of toxicity.

● Administer drug with food.

● Note that false-positive reactions for urine bilirubin using diazo tablet test have been reported.

Patient teaching

● Tell patient to take drug with food to minimize adverse GI reactions.

● Warn patient against performing hazardous activities that require alertness until CNS effects are known.

● Tell patient to stop drug and contact doctor immediately if rash, visual disturbances, or diarrhea develops.

● Caution patient that concomitant use with aspirin, alcohol, or corticosteroids may increase risk of adverse GI reactions.

● Teach patient to recognize and immediately report signs and symptoms of GI bleeding. Also explain that serious GI toxicity, including peptic ulceration and bleeding, can occur in patients taking NSAIDs, despite absence of GI symptoms.

☑ Evaluation

● Patient states that pain is relieved.

● Patient does not experience GI bleeding.

● Patient and family state understanding of drug therapy.

mefloquine hydrochloride
(MEF-loh-kwin high-droh-KLOR-ighd)
Lariam, Mephaquin

Pharmacologic class: quinine derivative
Therapeutic class: antimalarial
Pregnancy risk category: C

How supplied

Tablets: 250 mg

Pharmacokinetics

Absorption: well absorbed.
Distribution: concentrates in RBCs; about 98% protein-bound.
Metabolism: metabolized by liver.
Excretion: excreted primarily by liver; small amounts found in urine. *Half-life:* about 21 days.

Route	Onset	Peak	Duration
P.O.	Unknown	7-24 hr	Unknown

Pharmacodynamics

Chemical effect: unknown; may be related to its ability to form complexes with hemin.
Therapeutic effect: kills malaria-causing organisms. Spectrum of activity includes

all human types of malaria, including chloroquine-resistant malaria and strains of *Plasmodium falciparum* and *Plasmodium vivax.*

Indications and dosage

► **Acute malaria infections caused by mefloquine-sensitive strains of *P. falciparum* and *P. vivax.** Adults:* 1,250 mg P.O. as single dose. Patients with *P. vivax* infections should receive primaquine or other 8-aminoquinolones to avoid relapse after treatment of initial infection.
► **Malaria prophylaxis.** *Adults:* 250 mg P.O. once weekly. Prophylaxis should be initiated 1 week before entering endemic area and continued for 4 weeks after return. To avoid development of malaria after return from an endemic area, continue prophylaxis for 4 additional weeks.

Adverse reactions

CNS: dizziness, fatigue, syncope, headache, transient emotional disturbances (rare), *seizures.*
CV: extrasystoles.
EENT: tinnitus.
GI: loss of appetite, vomiting, *nausea, loose stools,* diarrhea, GI discomfort.
Skin: rash.
Other: fever, chills.

Interactions

Drug-drug. *Beta blockers, quinidine, quinine:* ECG abnormalities and cardiac arrest may occur. Avoid concomitant use.
Chloroquine, quinine: increased risk of seizures. Monitor patient.
Halofantrine: risk of potential fatal prolongation of QTC interval. Don't use together.
Valproic acid: decreased valproic acid blood levels and loss of seizure control at start of mefloquine therapy. Check anticonvulsant blood levels.

Contraindications and precautions

• Contraindicated in patients with hypersensitivity to mefloquine or related compounds.

• Use cautiously in patients with cardiac disease or seizure disorders and in pregnant or breast-feeding women.
• Safety of drug has not been established in children.

NURSING CONSIDERATIONS

✍ Assessment
• Assess patient's condition before therapy and regularly thereafter.
• Monitor liver function tests periodically, as ordered.
• Be alert for adverse reactions and drug interactions.
• Monitor patient's hydration status if adverse GI reactions occur.
• Evaluate patient's and family's knowledge of drug therapy.

⊞ Nursing diagnoses
• Infection related to presence of malaria organisms
• Risk of fluid volume deficit related to drug-induced adverse reactions
• Knowledge deficit related to drug therapy

⊠ Planning and implementation
• Because health risks from concomitant administration of quinine and mefloquine are great, be aware that drug therapy should not begin sooner than 12 hours after last dose of quinine or quinidine.
• Keep in mind that patients with infections caused by *P. vivax* are at high risk for relapse because drug does not eliminate hepatic phase (exoerythrocytic parasites). Follow-up therapy with primaquine is advisable.
• Give drug with food and full glass of water to minimize adverse GI reactions.
Patient teaching
• Advise patient to take drug on same day of week when using it for prophylaxis.
• Advise patient to use caution when performing hazardous activities that require alertness and coordination because dizziness, disturbed sense of balance, and neuropsychiatric reactions may occur.

• Instruct patient taking mefloquine prophylaxis to discontinue drug if he notices signs or symptoms of impending toxicity, such as unexplained anxiety, depression, confusion, or restlessness, and to notify doctor.
• Recommend to patient undergoing long-term therapy that he have periodic ophthalmologic examinations.

☑ **Evaluation**
• Patient is free from infection.
• Patient maintains adequate hydration throughout therapy.
• Patient and family state understanding of drug therapy.

megestrol acetate
(meh-JES-trol AS-ih-tayt)
Megace, Megostat ◇

Pharmacologic class: progestin
Therapeutic class: antineoplastic
Pregnancy risk category: D

How supplied

Tablets: 20 mg, 40 mg
Oral suspension: 40 mg/ml

Pharmacokinetics

Absorption: well absorbed across GI tract.
Distribution: appears to be stored in fatty tissue; highly bound to plasma proteins.
Metabolism: completely metabolized in liver.
Excretion: excreted in urine.

Route	Onset	Peak	Duration
P.O.	Unknown	Unknown	Unknown

Pharmacodynamics

Chemical effect: changes tumor's hormonal environment and alters neoplastic process. Mechanism of appetite stimulation is unknown.
Therapeutic effect: hinders cancer cell growth and increases appetite.

Indications and dosage

▶ **Breast cancer.** *Adults:* 40 mg P.O. q.i.d.
▶ **Endometrial cancer.** *Adults:* 40 to 320 mg P.O. daily in divided doses.
▶ **Treatment of anorexia, cachexia, or unexplained significant weight loss in patients with AIDS.** *Adults:* 800 mg P.O. (oral suspension) daily in divided doses; 100 to 400 mg for AIDS-related cachexia.

Adverse reactions

CV: hypertension, thrombophlebitis, *heart failure.*
GI: nausea, vomiting.
GU: breakthrough menstrual bleeding.
Respiratory: *pulmonary embolism.*
Other: weight gain, increased appetite, carpal tunnel syndrome, alopecia, hirsutism, breast tenderness.

Interactions

None significant.

Contraindications and precautions

• Contraindicated in patients hypersensitive to drug and in pregnant women.
• Use of drug is not recommended in breast-feeding women.
• Use cautiously in patients with history of thrombophlebitis.
• Safety of drug has not been established in children.

NURSING CONSIDERATIONS

☜ **Assessment**
• Assess patient's condition before therapy and regularly thereafter.
• Be alert for adverse reactions.
• Monitor patient's hydration status if adverse GI reactions occur.
• Evaluate patient's and family's knowledge of drug therapy.

❸ **Nursing diagnoses**
• Altered health maintenance related to underlying condition
• Risk for fluid volume deficit related to drug-induced adverse GI reactions

• Knowledge deficit related to drug therapy

▶ Planning and implementation
• Be aware that 2 months is adequate trial when treating cancer.
Patient teaching
• Inform patient that therapeutic response isn't immediate.
• Advise breast-feeding woman to discontinue breast-feeding during therapy because of possible infant toxicity.

▣ Evaluation
• Patient responds well to therapy.
• Patient maintains adequate hydration throughout therapy.
• Patient and family state understanding of drug therapy.

---

melphalan
(L-phenylalanine mustard)
(MEL-feh-len)
Alkeran

Pharmacologic class: alkylating agent (cell cycle-phase nonspecific)
Therapeutic class: antineoplastic
Pregnancy risk category: D

How supplied

Tablets (scored): 2 mg
Injection: 50 mg

Pharmacokinetics

Absorption: incomplete and variable from GI tract.
Distribution: distributed rapidly and widely in total body water; initially 50% to 60% bound to plasma proteins and increases to 80% to 90% over time.
Metabolism: extensively deactivated by hydrolysis.
Excretion: excreted primarily in urine.
Half-life: 2 hours.

Route	Onset	Peak	Duration
P.O., I.V.	Unknown	Unknown	Unknown

Pharmacodynamics

Chemical effect: cross-links strands of cellular DNA and interferes with RNA transcription.
Therapeutic effect: kills selected cancer cells.

Indications and dosage

▶ Multiple myeloma. *Adults:* 6 mg P.O. daily for 2 to 3 weeks; then drug stopped for up to 4 weeks or until WBC and platelet counts begin to rise again; maintenance dosage of 2 mg daily then given. *Alternative therapy:* 0.15 mg/kg P.O. daily for 7 days at 2- to 6-week intervals; or 0.25 mg/kg P.O. daily for 4 days, repeated q 4 to 6 weeks.
   Alternatively, administered I.V. to patients who can't tolerate oral therapy: 16 mg/m² given by infusion over 15 to 20 minutes q 2 week for four doses. After patient has recovered from toxicity, drug given q 4 weeks.
▶ Nonresectable advanced ovarian cancer. *Adults:* 0.2 mg/kg P.O. daily for 5 days. Repeated q 4 to 6 weeks, depending on bone marrow recovery.

Adverse reactions

Hematologic: *thrombocytopenia, leukopenia, bone marrow suppression.*
Respiratory: *pneumonitis, pulmonary fibrosis.*
Skin: dermatitis, pruritus, rash.
Other: *anaphylaxis, hypersensitivity, hepatotoxicity,* alopecia.

Interactions

Drug-drug. Anticoagulants, aspirin: increased risk of bleeding. Avoid concomitant use.
Antigout agents: decreased effectiveness. Dosage adjustments may be necessary.
Bone marrow suppressants: additive toxicity. Monitor patient closely.
Carmustine: carmustine lung toxicity threshold may be reduced. Monitor closely.
Cisplatin: cisplatin may affect melphalan kinetics by inducing renal dysfunction

---

and subsequently altering melphalan clearance. Monitor patient closely. *Cyclosporine:* an increase in the toxicity of cyclosporine, particularly nephrotoxicity, has been observed following coadministration. Use cautiously together. *Interferon alpha:* serum melphalan concentrations may be decreased. Monitor closely. *Nalidixic acid:* incidence of severe hemorrhagic necrotic enterocolitis may increase in pediatric patients. Monitor patient closely. *Vaccines:* decreased effectiveness of killed-virus vaccines and increased risk of toxicity from live-virus vaccines. Postpone routine immunization for at least 3 months after last dose of melphalan. **Drug-food.** *Any food:* decreased oral drug absorption. Separate administration times.

Contraindications and precautions

• Contraindicated in patients with hypersensitivity to drug and in those whose disease is known to be resistant to drug. Patients who are hypersensitive to chlorambucil may have cross-sensitivity to melphalan.
• Drug is not recommended for use in pregnant or breast-feeding women.
• Drug is not recommended for use in patients with severe leukopenia, thrombocytopenia, or anemia or chronic lymphocytic leukemia.
• Safety of drug has not been established in children.

NURSING CONSIDERATIONS

Assessment
• Assess patient's condition before therapy and regularly thereafter.
• Monitor serum uric acid level and CBC, as ordered.
• Be alert for adverse reactions and drug interactions.
• Evaluate patient's and family's knowledge of drug therapy.

Nursing diagnoses
• Altered health maintenance related to presence of neoplastic disease
• Altered protection related to adverse hematologic reactions
• Knowledge deficit related to drug therapy

Planning and implementation
• Follow institutional policy to reduce risks. Preparation and administration of parenteral form are associated with carcinogenic, mutagenic, and teratogenic risks for personnel.
• Dosage may need to be reduced in patient with renal impairment.
• Melphalan is drug of choice in combination with prednisone in patients with multiple myeloma.
P.O. use: Give drug on empty stomach.
I.V. use: Because drug isn't stable in solution, reconstitute immediately before administering. Reconstitute drug with 10 ml of sterile diluent supplied by manufacturer. Shake vigorously until clear solution is obtained. Resultant solution contains 5 mg of melphalan per milliliter. Immediately dilute required dose in 0.9% NaCl injection. Final concentration shouldn't exceed 0.45 mg/ml. Give I.V. infusion over 15 to 20 minutes.
– Promptly dilute and administer; reconstituted product begins to degrade within 30 minutes. After final dilution, nearly 1% of drug degrades every 10 minutes. Don't refrigerate reconstituted product because precipitate will form.
Patient teaching
• Tell patient to take oral drug on empty stomach.
• Warn patient to watch for signs of infection (fever, sore throat, fatigue) and bleeding (easy bruising, nosebleeds, bleeding gums, melena). Have patient take temperature daily.
• Instruct patient to avoid OTC products containing aspirin.
• Advise female patient of childbearing age to avoid becoming pregnant during

---

Reactions may be *common*, uncommon, *life-threatening*, or COMMON AND LIFE-THREATENING.

therapy and to consult with doctor before becoming pregnant.

☑ **Evaluation**
• Patient responds well to therapy.
• Patient regains normal hematologic function when therapy is completed.
• Patient and family state understanding of drug therapy.

menotropins
(meh-noh-TROH-pins)
Humegon, Pergonal

Pharmacologic class: gonadotropin
Therapeutic class: ovulation stimulant, spermatogenesis stimulant
Pregnancy risk category: X

How supplied

Injection: 75 international units (IU) of luteinizing hormone (LH) and 75 units of follicle-stimulating hormone (FSH) activity/ampule; 150 units of LH and 150 units of FSH activity/ampule

Pharmacokinetics

Absorption: unknown.
Distribution: unknown.
Metabolism: unknown.
Excretion: excreted in urine.

Route	Onset	Peak	Duration
I.M.	9-12 days	Unknown	Unknown

Pharmacodynamics

Chemical effect: when administered to women who have not had primary ovarian failure, mimics FSH in inducing follicular growth and LH in aiding follicular maturation.
Therapeutic effect: stimulates ovulation and fertility.

Indications and dosage

▶ **Anovulation.** *Women:* 75 units each of FSH and LH I.M. daily for 7 to 12 days, followed by 5,000 to 10,000 units of hu-

man chorionic gonadotropin (HCG) I.M. 1 day after last dose of menotropins. Repeated for one to three menstrual cycles until ovulation occurs.
▶ **Infertility with ovulation.** *Women:* 75 units each of FSH and LH I.M. daily for 7 to 12 days, followed by 5,000 to 10,000 units of HCG I.M. 1 day after last dose of menotropins. Repeated for two menstrual cycles and then increased to 150 units each of FSH and LH daily for 7 to 12 days, followed by 5,000 to 10,000 units of HCG I.M. 1 day after last dose of menotropins. Repeated for two menstrual cycles.
▶ **Infertility in men.** *Men:* Prior treatment with HCG of 5,000 units three times a week for 4 to 6 months; then 75 units each of FSH and LH I.M. three times weekly (given with 2,000 units of HCG twice weekly) for at least 4 months. If spermatogenesis does not increase, dosage increased to 150 units each of FSH and LH three times weekly (dosage of HCG remains unchanged).

Adverse reactions

CV: *CVA,* tachycardia.
GI: nausea, vomiting, diarrhea.
GU: *ovarian enlargement with pain and abdominal distention,* multiple births, ovarian hyperstimulation syndrome (sudden ovarian enlargement, ascites, or pleural effusion).
Hematologic: hemoconcentration with fluid loss into abdomen.
Respiratory: *atelectasis, acute respiratory distress syndrome, pulmonary embolism, pulmonary infarction, arterial occlusion.*
Other: fever, *gynecomastia, hypersensitivity, anaphylactic reactions.*

Interactions

None significant.

Contraindications and precautions

• Contraindicated in patients hypersensitive to drug; in women with primary ovarian failure, uncontrolled thyroid or

adrenal dysfunction, pituitary tumor, abnormal uterine bleeding, uterine fibromas, or ovarian cysts or enlargement; in pregnant women; and in men with normal pituitary function, primary testicular failure, or infertility disorders other than hypogonadotropic hypogonadism.
• Drug should not be used in breastfeeding women or children.

NURSING CONSIDERATIONS

🔧 Assessment
• Assess patient's condition before therapy and regularly thereafter.
• Be alert for adverse reactions.
• Evaluate patient's and family's knowledge of drug therapy.

🔲 Nursing diagnoses
• Sexual dysfunction related to underlying disorder
• Risk for fluid volume deficit related to drug-induced adverse reactions
• Knowledge deficit related to drug therapy

🔳 Planning and implementation
• Monitor patient closely to ensure adequate ovarian stimulation.
• Reconstitute with 1 to 2 ml of sterile 0.9% NaCl. Use immediately.
• Rotate injection sites.
Patient teaching
• Discuss risk of multiple births.
• In infertility, encourage daily intercourse from day before HCG is given until ovulation occurs.
• Tell patient that pregnancy usually occurs 4 to 6 weeks after therapy.
• Instruct patient to report immediately severe abdominal pain, bloating, swelling of hands or feet, nausea, vomiting, diarrhea, substantial weight gain, or shortness of breath.

🔲 Evaluation
• Patient or female partner becomes pregnant.

• Patient maintains adequate hydration throughout therapy.
• Patient and family state understanding of drug therapy.

---

meperidine hydrochloride (pethidine hydrochloride)
(meh-PER-uh-deen high-droh-KLOR-ighd)
Demerol

Pharmacologic class: opioid
Therapeutic class: analgesic, adjunct to anesthesia
Controlled substance schedule: II
Pregnancy risk category: NR

How supplied

Tablets: 50 mg, 100 mg
Syrup: 50 mg/ml
Injection: 10 mg/ml, 25 mg/ml, 50 mg/ml, 75 mg/ml, 100 mg/ml

Pharmacokinetics

Absorption: unknown.
Distribution: distributed widely throughout body.
Metabolism: metabolized primarily by hydrolysis in liver.
Excretion: excreted primarily in urine. Excretion enhanced by acidifying urine.
Half-life: 2.4 to 4 hours.

Route	Onset	Peak	Duration
P.O.	About 15 min	60-90 min	2-4 hr
I.V.	About 1 min	5-7 min	2-4 hr
I.M., S.C.	10-15 min	30-50 min	2-4 hr

Pharmacodynamics

Chemical effect: binds with opioid receptors in CNS, altering both perception of and emotional response to pain through unknown mechanism.
Therapeutic effect: relieves pain.

Reactions may be *common*, uncommon, *life-threatening*, or COMMON AND LIFE-THREATENING.

Indications and dosage

▶ **Moderate to severe pain.** *Adults:* 50 to 150 mg P.O., I.M., or S.C. q 3 to 4 hours, p.r.n.; or 15 to 35 mg/hour by continuous I.V. infusion. *Children:* 1.1 to 1.76 mg/kg P.O., I.M., or S.C. q 3 to 4 hours. Maximum dosage is 100 mg q 4 hours, p.r.n.
▶ **Preoperatively.** *Adults:* 50 to 100 mg I.M., I.V., or S.C. 30 to 90 minutes before surgery. *Children:* 1 to 2.2 mg/kg I.M., I.V., or S.C. up to adult dose 30 to 90 minutes before surgery.
▶ **Adjunct to anesthesia.** *Adults:* Repeated slow I.V. injections of fractional doses (i.e., 10 mg/ml); alternatively, continuous I.V. infusion of more dilute solution (1 mg/ml) titrated to needs of patient.
▶ **Obstetric analgesia.** *Adults:* 50 to 100 mg I.M. or S.C. when pain becomes regular, repeated at 1- to 3-hour intervals.

Adverse reactions

CNS: *sedation, somnolence, clouded sensorium, euphoria,* paradoxical excitement, tremors, dizziness, *seizures* (with large doses).
CV: *hypotension,* bradycardia, tachycardia, *cardiac arrest, shock.*
GI: *nausea, vomiting, constipation,* ileus.
GU: *urine retention.*
Respiratory: *respiratory depression,* respiratory arrest.
Skin: pain (at injection site), local tissue irritation and induration (after S.C. injection); phlebitis (after I.V. use).
Other: physical dependence, muscle twitching.

Interactions

Drug-drug. *CNS depressants, general anesthetics, hypnotics, other narcotic analgesics, phenothiazines, sedatives, tricyclic antidepressants:* possible respiratory depression, hypotension, profound sedation, or coma. Use together with extreme caution. Reduce meperidine dosage.
MAO inhibitors: increased CNS excitation or depression that can be severe or fatal. Don't use together.

Phenytoin: decreased serum levels of meperidine. Monitor for decreased analgesia.
Drug-lifestyle. *Alcohol use:* additive effects. Use together cautiously.

Contraindications and precautions

• Contraindicated in patients with hypersensitivity to drug and in those who have received MAO inhibitors within past 14 days.
• Use with extreme caution in patients with increased intracranial pressure, head injury, asthma, or other respiratory conditions, supraventricular tachycardias, seizures, acute abdominal conditions, hepatic or renal disease, hypothyroidism, Addison's disease, urethral stricture, or prostatic hyperplasia and in elderly or debilitated patients.
• Use with caution in pregnant or breast-feeding women.

NURSING CONSIDERATIONS

▨ **Assessment**
• Assess patient's pain before therapy and regularly thereafter.
• Be alert for adverse reactions and drug interactions.
• Meperidine and its active metabolite normeperidine accumulate in body. Monitor for increased toxic effect, especially in patient with impaired kidney function.
• Monitor respirations of neonate exposed to drug during labor.
• Monitor for withdrawal symptoms if drug is discontinued abruptly after long-term use.
• Evaluate patient's and family's knowledge of drug therapy.

▨ **Nursing diagnoses**
• Pain related to underlying condition
• Risk for injury related to drug-induced adverse reactions
• Knowledge deficit related to drug therapy

≥ Planning and implementation

• Know that drug may be used in some patients who are allergic to morphine.

• Because meperidine toxicity often appears after several days of treatment, it is not recommended for treatment of chronic pain.

P.O. use: Be aware that P.O. dose is less than half as effective as parenteral dose. Give I.M., if possible. When changing from parenteral to P.O. route, know that dosage should be increased.

– Know that syrup has local anesthetic effect. Give with full glass of water.

I.V. use: Give slowly by direct I.V. injection or slow continuous I.V. infusion. Drug is compatible with most I.V. solutions, including D₅W, 0.9% NaCl, and Ringer's or lactated Ringer's solutions.

– Drug is incompatible when mixed in same container as aminophylline, barbiturates, heparin, morphine sulfate, phenytoin, sodium bicarbonate, or sulfonamides.

I.M. use: Follow normal protocol.

S.C. use: S.C. injection is not recommended because it is painful.

• Have resuscitation equipment and naloxone available.

• Don't give if respirations are below 12 breaths/minute, if respiratory rate or depth is decreased, or if change in pupils is noted.

Patient teaching

• Warn outpatient to avoid hazardous activities until drug's CNS effects are known.

• Instruct patient to avoid alcohol consumption during drug therapy.

• Teach patient to manage adverse reactions, such as constipation.

• Tell family members to withhold drug and notify doctor if patient's respiratory rate decreases.

☑ Evaluation

• Patient is free from pain.

• Patient does not experience injury.

• Patient and family state understanding of drug therapy.

mephenytoin
(me-FEN-uh-toyn)
Mesantoin

Pharmacologic class: hydantoin derivative
Therapeutic class: anticonvulsant
Pregnancy risk category: C

How supplied

Tablets: 100 mg

Pharmacokinetics

Absorption: absorbed from GI tract.
Distribution: distributed widely throughout body.
Metabolism: metabolized in liver.
Excretion: excreted in urine. *Half-life:* about 7 hours.

Route	Onset	Peak	Duration
P.O.	Unknown	0.75-4 hr	Unknown

Pharmacodynamics

Chemical effect: unknown; probably stabilizes neuronal membranes and limits seizure activity by either increasing efflux or decreasing influx of sodium ions across cell membranes in motor cortex.
Therapeutic effect: prevents seizure activity.

Indications and dosage

▶ **Tonic-clonic, simple partial, and complex partial seizures in patients refractory to less toxic anticonvulsants.** *Adults:* 50 to 100 mg P.O. daily. Increased by 50 to 100 mg at weekly intervals. Maintenance dosage is 200 to 800 mg daily in three equally divided doses. *Children:* initially, 50 to 100 mg P.O. daily. Increased by 50 to 100 mg at weekly intervals. Maintenance dosage is 100 to 400 mg or 100 to 450 mg/m² daily in three divided doses.

Adverse reactions

CNS: ataxia, *drowsiness,* fatigue, irritability, choreiform movements, depression, tremors, sleeplessness, dizziness (usually transient).

Reactions may be *common,* uncommon, *life-threatening,* or COMMON AND LIFE-THREATENING.

EENT: conjunctivitis, diplopia, nystagmus, gingival hyperplasia (with prolonged use).
GI: nausea, vomiting (with prolonged use).
Hematologic: *leukopenia, neutropenia, agranulocytosis, thrombocytopenia, pancytopenia,* eosinophilia.
Skin: *rash, exfoliative dermatitis,* hypertrichosis, photosensitivity, *Stevens-Johnson syndrome, fatal dermatitides.*
Other: edema, dysarthria, lymphadenopathy, polyarthropathy, *pulmonary fibrosis.*

Interactions

Drug-drug. *Antihistamines, chloramphenicol, cimetidine, diazepam, disulfiram, isoniazid, phenylbutazone, salicylates, sulfamethizole, valproate:* increased mephenytoin activity and toxicity. Monitor patient closely.
Diazoxide, folic acid: decreased mephenytoin activity. Monitor patient closely.
Drug-lifestyle. *Alcohol use:* decreased mephenytoin activity. Avoid concomitant use.

Contraindications and precautions

• Contraindicated in patients with hydantoin hypersensitivity.
• Use cautiously in patients receiving other hydantoin derivatives and in pregnant women.
• Safe use in breast-feeding women has not been established.

NURSING CONSIDERATIONS

⚖ Assessment
• Assess patient's condition before therapy and regularly thereafter.
• Monitor serum levels. Therapeutic serum level of mephenytoin and its active metabolite is 25 to 40 mcg/ml.
• Monitor liver function studies with long-term use. Check CBC and platelet count before therapy and periodically thereafter, as ordered.

• Be alert for adverse reactions and drug interactions.
• Evaluate patient's and family's knowledge of drug therapy.

⊞ Nursing diagnoses
• Risk for injury related to underlying seizure condition
• Fluid volume excess related to drug-induced edema
• Knowledge deficit related to drug therapy

▷ Planning and implementation
• Alert doctor if neutrophil count falls to less than 1,600/mm³.
• Know that potentially life-threatening blood dyscrasias limit drug's usefulness.
• Never withdraw drug suddenly because seizures may worsen. Call doctor if adverse reactions develop.
Patient teaching
• Tell patient to notify doctor of fever, sore throat, bleeding, or rash.
• Advise patient to avoid hazardous activities until drug's CNS effects are known.
• Caution patient that heavy alcohol use may diminish drug's benefits.
• Advise patient to use sunblock, wear protective clothing, and avoid prolonged exposure to sunlight.
• Warn patient and parents, if appropriate, not to stop drug abruptly.

☑ Evaluation
• Patient is free from seizure activity.
• Patient does not experience edema.
• Patient and family state understanding of drug therapy.

mephobarbital
(mef-oh-BAR-bih-tahl)
Mebaral

Pharmacologic class: barbiturate
Therapeutic class: anticonvulsant, nonspecific CNS depressant
Controlled substance schedule: IV

Pregnancy risk category: D

How supplied

Tablets: 32 mg, 50 mg, 100 mg

Pharmacokinetics

Absorption: about 50% absorbed from GI tract.
Distribution: distributed widely throughout body.
Metabolism: metabolized by liver.
Excretion: excreted primarily in urine.

Route	Onset	Peak	Duration
P.O.	≥1 hr	Unknown	10-12 hr

Pharmacodynamics

Chemical effect: unknown; probably depresses monosynaptic and polysynaptic transmission in CNS and increases threshold for seizure activity in motor cortex. Some activity comes from phenobarbital, an active metabolite.
Therapeutic effect: prevents seizures and promotes calmness.

Indications and dosage

▶ **Generalized tonic-clonic or absence seizures.** *Adults:* 400 to 600 mg P.O. once daily or in divided doses. Children age 5 and over: 32 to 64 mg P.O. t.i.d. or q.i.d. *Children under age 5:* 16 to 32 mg P.O. t.i.d. or q.i.d.
▶ **Relief from anxiety, tension, apprehension.** *Adults:* 32 to 100 mg P.O. t.i.d. or q.i.d. *Children:* 16 to 32 mg P.O. t.i.d. or q.i.d.

Adverse reactions

CNS: *dizziness,* headache, *hangover,* confusion, paradoxical excitation, exacerbation of existing pain, drowsiness.
CV: hypotension, bradycardia.
GI: nausea, vomiting, epigastric pain.
Hematologic: megaloblastic anemia, ***agranulocytosis, thrombocytopenia,*** enhanced porphyria.
Respiratory: ***respiratory depression.***
Skin: urticaria, morbilliform rash, blisters, purpura, ***erythema multiforme.***

Other: allergic reactions (facial edema).

Interactions

Drug-drug. *Chloramphenicol, MAO inhibitors, valproic acid:* potentiated barbiturate effect. Monitor for increased CNS and respiratory depression.
CNS depressants, including narcotic analgesics: excessive CNS depression. Use cautiously.
Corticosteroids, digitoxin, doxycycline, estrogens and oral contraceptives, oral anticoagulants, tricyclic antidepressants: mephobarbital may enhance metabolism of these drugs. Monitor for decreased effect.
Griseofulvin: decreased absorption of griseofulvin. Monitor for decreased effectiveness of griseofulvin.
Rifampin: may decrease barbiturate levels. Monitor for decreased effect.
Drug-lifestyle. *Alcohol use:* excessive CNS depression. Use cautiously.

Contraindications and precautions

• Contraindicated in patients with porphyria or barbiturate hypersensitivity.
• Use of drug is not recommended in pregnant or breast-feeding women.
• Use cautiously in patients with acute or chronic pain; depression; suicidal tendencies; history of drug abuse; hepatic, renal, cardiac, or respiratory function impairment; myasthenia gravis; or myxedema and in elderly or debilitated patients.

NURSING CONSIDERATIONS

⚕ Assessment

• Assess patient's condition before therapy and regularly thereafter.
• Monitor phenobarbital serum levels. Therapeutic levels range from 15 to 40 mcg/ml.
• Periodically monitor CBC and BUN and creatinine levels.
• Be alert for adverse reactions and drug interactions.
• Monitor patient's hydration status if adverse GI reactions occur.

Reactions may be *common,* uncommon, *life-threatening,* or COMMON AND LIFE-THREATENING.

• Evaluate patient's and family's knowledge of drug therapy.

🔛 **Nursing diagnoses**
• Risk for injury related to underlying seizure disorder
• Risk for fluid volume deficit related to drug-induced adverse GI reactions
• Knowledge deficit related to drug therapy

▶ **Planning and implementation**
• Know that dosage should be reduced in elderly or debilitated patients because they may be more sensitive to barbiturates. Dosage also should be reduced for patients with impaired kidney or liver function.
• Never withdraw drug suddenly. Seizures may worsen. Call doctor at once if adverse reactions develop.
• Know that patient with nighttime seizures may need to take total or largest dose at night.
Patient teaching
• Instruct patient to avoid hazardous activities until drug's CNS effects are known.
• Advise adult patient with nighttime seizures to take total or largest dose at night after checking with doctor.
• Instruct patient to avoid alcohol consumption during drug therapy.
• Warn patient and parents, if appropriate, not to stop drug abruptly.
• Instruct patient to store drug in light-resistant container.
• Inform patient who uses oral contraceptives that she should consider alternate birth control methods because drug may enhance contraceptive hormone metabolism and decrease its effectiveness.
• Tell patient that drug suppresses REM sleep. When drug is discontinued, patient may experience increased dreaming.

☑ **Evaluation**
• Patient is free from seizure activity.
• Patient maintains adequate hydration throughout therapy.

• Patient and family state understanding of drug therapy.

meprobamate
(meh-PROH-bah-mayt)
Apo-Meprobamate♦, Equanil**,
Meprospan 200, Meprospan 400,
'Miltown'-200, 'Miltown'-400, '
Miltown'-600, Probate, Trancot

Pharmacologic class: carbamate
Therapeutic class: antianxiety agent
Controlled substance schedule: IV
Pregnancy risk category: NR

How supplied
Tablets: 200 mg, 400 mg, 600 mg
Capsules (sustained-release): 200 mg, 400 mg

Pharmacokinetics
Absorption: well absorbed from GI tract.
Distribution: distributed throughout body; 20% protein-bound.
Metabolism: metabolized rapidly in liver.
Excretion: excreted in urine. *Half-life:* about 10 hours.

Route	Onset	Peak	Duration
P.O.	Unknown	Unknown	Unknown

Pharmacodynamics
Chemical effect: unknown; appears to act at multiple sites in CNS.
Therapeutic effect: relieves anxiety.

Indications and dosage
▶ **Anxiety.** *Adults:* 1.2 to 1.6 g P.O. daily in three or four equally divided doses. Maximum dosage is 2.4 g daily. Alternatively, 400 to 800 mg sustained-release capsule P.O. b.i.d. *Children ages 6 to 12:* 100 to 200 mg P.O. b.i.d. or t.i.d. Or, 200 mg sustained-release capsule P.O. b.i.d. Drug is not recommended for children younger than age 6.

Adverse reactions

CNS: *drowsiness,* ataxia, dizziness, slurred speech, headache, vertigo, *seizures.*
CV: palpitation, tachycardia, hypotension*, arrhythmias.*
GI: anorexia, nausea, vomiting, diarrhea, stomatitis.
Hematologic: *aplastic anemia, thrombocytopenia, leukopenia, agranulocytosis.*
Skin: pruritus, urticaria, erythematous maculopapular rash, *hypersensitivity reactions.*
After abrupt withdrawal of long-term therapy: severe generalized tonic-clonic seizures.

Interactions

Drug-drug. *CNS depressants:* increased CNS depression. Avoid concomitant use.
Drug-lifestyle. *Alcohol use:* increased CNS depression. Avoid concomitant use.

Contraindications and precautions

• Contraindicated in patients with porphyria or hypersensitive to drug or related compounds (such as carisoprodol, mebutamate, tybamate, and carbromal).
• Use of drug should be avoided in pregnant women, especially during first trimester, and in breast-feeding women.
• Use cautiously in patients with impaired liver or kidney function, seizure disorders, or suicidal tendencies.

NURSING CONSIDERATIONS

⚎ Assessment
• Assess patient's anxiety before therapy and regularly thereafter.
• Periodically monitor CBC and kidney and liver function tests in patient receiving high doses, as ordered.
• Be alert for adverse reactions and drug interactions.
• Evaluate patient's and family's knowledge of drug therapy.

⊞ Nursing diagnoses
• Anxiety related to underlying condition

• Risk for injury related to drug-induced adverse CNS reactions
• Knowledge deficit related to drug therapy

⊇ Planning and implementation
• Be aware that dosage should be reduced in elderly or debilitated patient.
• Give drug with meals to reduce GI distress.
• Be aware that possibility of abuse and addiction exists with long-term use. Withdraw drug gradually over 2 weeks to avoid withdrawal symptoms.
• Know that drug may interfere with certain laboratory tests for urinary 17-ketogenic steroids and 17-hydroxycorticosteroids.
Patient teaching
• Tell patient to take drug with food.
• Warn patient to avoid hazardous activities until CNS effects of drug are known.
• Tell patient to avoid alcohol.
• Tell patient to report signs of hematologic toxicity: bruising or bleeding, fever, or sore throat.

☑ Evaluation
• Patient states that he is less anxious.
• Patient does not experience injury from adverse CNS reactions.
• Patient and family state understanding of drug therapy.

mercaptopurine
(6-mercaptopurine, 6-MP)
(mer-cap-toh-PYOO-reen)
Purinethol

Pharmacologic class: antimetabolite (cell cycle–phase specific, S phase)
Therapeutic class: antineoplastic
Pregnancy risk category: D

How supplied

Tablets (scored): 50 mg

Pharmacokinetics

Absorption: incomplete and variable; about 50% of dose is absorbed.
Distribution: distributed widely in total body water.
Metabolism: extensively metabolized in liver.
Excretion: excreted in urine.

Route	Onset	Peak	Duration
P.O.	Unknown	Unknown	Unknown

Pharmacodynamics

Chemical effect: inhibits RNA and DNA synthesis.
Therapeutic effect: inhibits selected cancer cell growth.

Indications and dosage

Dosage and indications may vary. Check current literature for recommended protocols.
▶ **Acute lymphoblastic leukemia (in children), acute myeloblastic leukemia, chronic myelocytic leukemia.** *Adults:* 2.5 mg/kg P.O. daily as single dose, up to 5 mg/kg/day. Maintenance dosage is 1.5 to 2.5 mg/kg/day. *Children age 5 and over:* 2.5 mg/kg P.O. daily. Maintenance dosage is 1.5 to 2.5 mg/kg/day.

Adverse reactions

GI: *nausea, vomiting, anorexia,* painful oral ulcers.
Hematologic: *leukopenia, thrombocytopenia,* anemia (may persist several days after drug is stopped).
Hepatic: biliary stasis, *jaundice, hepatotoxicity.*
Skin: rash, hyperpigmentation.
Other: hyperuricemia.

Interactions

Drug-drug. *Allopurinol:* slowed inactivation of mercaptopurine. Decrease mercaptopurine to one-fourth or one-third normal dose.
Hepatotoxic drugs: may enhance hepatotoxicity of mercaptopurine. Monitor patient closely.

Nondepolarizing neuromuscular blockers: antagonized muscle relaxant effect. Notify anesthesiologist that patient is receiving drug.
Warfarin: antagonized anticoagulant effect. Monitor PT and INR.

Contraindications and precautions

● Contraindicated in patients whose disease has resisted drug.
● Drug is not recommended for use in pregnant or breast-feeding women.

NURSING CONSIDERATIONS

☢ Assessment
● Assess patient's condition before therapy and regularly thereafter.
● Monitor blood count and serum transaminase, alkaline phosphatase, and bilirubin levels weekly during induction and monthly during maintenance, as ordered.
● Observe for signs of bleeding and infection.
● Monitor fluid intake and output and serum uric acid levels, as ordered.
● Be alert for adverse reactions and drug interactions. Adverse GI reactions are less common in children.
● Evaluate patient's and family's knowledge of drug therapy.

⊞ Nursing diagnoses
● Altered health maintenance related to presence of leukemia
● Altered protection related to drug-induced adverse hematologic reactions
● Knowledge deficit related to drug therapy

▷ Planning and implementation
● Dosage modifications may be required after chemotherapy or radiation therapy and in patient with depressed neutrophil or platelet count or impaired liver or kidney function.
● Sometimes drug is ordered as 6-mercaptopurine or 6-MP. The numeral 6

---

is part of drug name and does not signify number of dosage units.
• Regimen must continue despite nausea and vomiting. Notify doctor if adverse GI reactions occur, and obtain order for antiemetic.
• Encourage adequate fluid intake (3 L daily).
• If allopurinol is ordered, use cautiously.
• Discontinue drug if hepatic tenderness occurs and notify doctor.
Patient teaching
• Tell patient to notify doctor if vomiting occurs shortly after taking dose because antiemetic will be needed so drug therapy can continue.
• Warn patient to watch for signs of infection (fever, sore throat, fatigue) and bleeding (easy bruising, nosebleeds, bleeding gums, melena). Have patient take his temperature daily.
• Advise female patient of childbearing age to avoid becoming pregnant during therapy and to consult with doctor before becoming pregnant.

☑ **Evaluation**
• Patient responds well to therapy.
• Patient does not develop serious ill effects when hematologic studies are abnormal.
• Patient and family state understanding of drug therapy.

meropenem
(mer-oh-PEN-em)
Merrem I.V.

Pharmacologic class: synthetic broad-spectrum carbapenem antibiotic
Therapeutic class: antibiotic
Pregnancy risk category: B

How supplied

Powder for injection: 500 mg/15 ml, 500 mg/20 ml, 500 mg/100 ml, 1 g/15 ml, 1 g/30 ml, 1 g/100 ml

Pharmacokinetics
Absorption: penetrates into most body fluids and tissues including CSF.
Distribution: plasma protein binding is 2%.
Metabolism: within kidneys.
Excretion: excreted in urine.

Route	Onset	Peak	Duration
I.V.	Unknown	Within 1 hr	Unknown

Pharmacodynamics
Chemical effect: readily penetrates the cell wall of most gram-positive and gram-negative bacteria to reach penicillin binding protein targets.
Therapeutic effect: bactericidal activity results from inhibition of cell-wall synthesis.

Indications and dosage
▶ **Complicated appendicitis and peritonitis caused by viridans group streptococci,** *Escherichia coli, Klebsiella pneumoniae, Pseudomonas aeruginosa, Bacteroides fragilis, Bacteroides thetaiotaomicron,* **and** *Peptostreptococcus* **species; bacterial meningitis (children only) caused by** *Streptococcus pneumoniae, Haemophilus influenzae,* **and** *Neisseria meningitidis. Adults:* 1 g I.V. q 8 hours over 15 to 30 minutes as I.V. infusion or over about 3 to 5 minutes as I.V. bolus injection (5 to 20 ml). *Children age 3 months and older:* 20 mg/kg (intra-abdominal infection) or 40 mg/kg (bacterial meningitis) q 8 hours over 15 to 30 minutes as I.V. infusion or over about 3 to 5 minutes as I.V. bolus injection (5 to 20 ml). Maximum dosage is 2 g I.V. q 8 hours. *Children weighing over 50 kg (110 lb):* 1 g I.V. q 8 hours for intra-abdominal infections and 2 g I.V. q 8 hours for meningitis.
Note: Dosages need to be adjusted for patients with renal insufficiency or renal failure or with creatinine clearance below 51 ml/minute.

Adverse reactions
CNS: *seizures,* headache.

GI: diarrhea, nausea, vomiting, constipation, oral moniliasis, glossitis.
GU: increased creatinine or BUN levels, presence of RBCs in urine.
Hematologic: increased or decreased platelet count, increased eosinophil count, prolonged or shortened PT or PTT, positive direct or indirect Coombs' test, decreased hemoglobin or hematocrit, decreased WBC count.
Hepatic: increased levels of ALT, AST, alkaline phosphatase, LD, and bilirubin.
Respiratory: *apnea.*
Skin: rash, pruritus.
Other: *hypersensitivity reaction, anaphylaxis;* inflammation, phlebitis, thrombophlebitis (at injection site).

Interactions

Drug-drug. *Probenecid:* inhibited renal excretion of meropenem. Concomitant administration of probenecid with meropenem is not recommended.

Contraindications and precautions

• Contraindicated in patients with hypersensitivity to drug or its components or other drugs in same class and in those who have shown anaphylactic reactions to beta-lactams.

NURSING CONSIDERATIONS

Assessment
• Obtain specimen for culture and sensitivity test before giving first dose.
• Before therapy is initiated, determine whether previous hypersensitivity reactions to penicillins, cephalosporins, or other beta-lactams or to other allergens have occurred.
• Monitor patient for signs and symptoms of superinfection.
• Periodically assess organ system functions, as ordered, during prolonged therapy.

Nursing diagnoses
• Infection related to bacteria

• Risk for fluid volume deficit related to effect on kidneys
• Knowledge deficit related to drug therapy

Planning and implementation
• For I.V. bolus administration, add 10 ml of sterile water for injection to 500 mg/20-ml vial or 20 ml to 1 g/30-ml vial.
• For I.V. infusion, reconstitute infusion vials (500 mg/100 ml and 1 g/100 ml) with compatible infusion fluid. Or, reconstitute an injection vial, add resulting solution to an I.V. container, and further dilute with appropriate infusion fluid.
• Follow manufacturer's guidelines closely when using ADD-Vantage vials.
Patient teaching
• Advise breast-feeding patient of risk of drug transmission to infant.
• Instruct patient to report adverse reactions.

Evaluation
• Patient is free from infection.
• Patient maintains adequate hydration.
• Patient and family state understanding of drug therapy.

mesalamine
(mez-AL-uh-meen)
Asacol, Pentasa, Rowasa

Pharmacologic class: salicylate
Therapeutic class: anti-inflammatory
Pregnancy risk category: B

How supplied

Tablets (delayed-release): 400 mg
Capsules (controlled-release): 250 mg
Rectal suspension: 4 g/60 ml
Suppositories: 500 mg

Pharmacokinetics

Absorption: poorly absorbed with P.R. administration; P.O. tablets and capsules

are made to have delayed absorption from GI tract.
Distribution: not clearly defined.
Metabolism: undergoes acetylation, but whether this takes place at colonic or systemic sites is unknown.
Excretion: oral form primarily excreted in urine; most of rectal form excreted in feces. *Half-life:* mesalamine, 30 minutes to 1½ hours; acetylated metabolite, about 5 to 10 hours.

Route	Onset	Peak	Duration
P.O., P.R.	Unknown	3-6 hr	Unknown

Pharmacodynamics

Chemical effect: unknown; probably acts topically by inhibiting prostaglandin production in colon.
Therapeutic effect: relieves inflammation in lower GI tract.

Indications and dosage

▶ **Active mild to moderate distal ulcerative colitis, proctitis, proctosigmoiditis.** *Adults:* 800 mg P.O. (tablets) t.i.d. for total dose of 2.4 g/day for 6 weeks; 1 g P.O. (capsules) q.i.d. for total dose of 4 g up to 8 weeks; 500 mg P.R. (suppository) b.i.d. retained for 1 to 3 hours or longer, or 4 g as retention enema once daily (preferably h.s.) retained overnight (for about 8 hours). Usual course of therapy for P.R. form is 3 to 6 weeks.

Adverse reactions

CNS: headache, dizziness, fatigue, malaise.
GI: abdominal pain, cramps, discomfort, flatulence, diarrhea, rectal pain, bloating, nausea, *pancolitis.*
Skin: pruritus, rash, urticaria, hair loss.
Other: wheezing, *anaphylaxis* (rare), fever.

Interactions

None significant.

Contraindications and precautions

• Contraindicated in patients hypersensitive to drug, its components, or salicylates.
• Drug is not recommended for use in breast-feeding women.
• Use cautiously in patients with renal impairment. Nephrotoxic potential from absorbed mesalamine exists. Also use cautiously in pregnant women.

NURSING CONSIDERATIONS

☒ Assessment
• Assess patient's condition before therapy and regularly thereafter.
• Monitor periodic kidney function studies in patient on long-term therapy, as ordered.
• Because it contains potassium metabisulfite, drug may cause hypersensitivity reactions in patient sensitive to sulfites.
• Be alert for adverse reactions.
• Evaluate patient's and family's knowledge of drug therapy.

🔁 Nursing diagnoses
• Altered tissue integrity related to underlying condition
• Pain related to drug-induced adverse GI reactions
• Knowledge deficit related to drug therapy

▷ Planning and implementation
P.O. use: Have patient swallow tablets and capsules whole and not crush or chew them.
P.R. use: For maximum effectiveness, have patient retain suppository as long as possible (1 to 3 hours). When giving suspension, shake bottle before application.
Patient teaching
• Teach patient how to take oral form or administer rectal form, and instruct him to carefully follow instructions supplied with medication.
• Instruct patient to discontinue drug if he experiences fever or rash. Patient intoler-

---

ant of sulfasalazine may also be hypersensitive to mesalamine.

☑ Evaluation
• Patient reports relief from GI symptoms.
• Patient states that no new pain is experienced during therapy.
• Patient and family state understanding of drug therapy.

mesna
(MEZ-nah)
MESNEX

Pharmacologic class: thiol derivative
Therapeutic class: uroprotectant
Pregnancy risk category: B

How supplied
Injection: 100 mg/ml

Pharmacokinetics
Absorption: not applicable.
Distribution: remains in vascular compartment; doesn't distribute through tissues.
Metabolism: rapidly metabolized to mesna disulfide, its only metabolite.
Excretion: excreted in urine. *Half-life:* mesna, 0.36 hour; mesna disulfide, 1.17 hours.

Route	Onset	Peak	Duration
I.V.	Unknown	Unknown	Unknown

Pharmacodynamics
Chemical effect: prevents ifosfamide-induced hemorrhagic cystitis by reacting with urotoxic ifosfamide metabolites.
Therapeutic effect: prevents ifosfamide from adversely affecting bladder tissue.

Indications and dosage
▶ **Prophylaxis of hemorrhagic cystitis in patients receiving ifosfamide.** *Adults:* dosage varies with amount of ifosfamide administered. Usual dosage is 240 mg/m^2

as I.V. bolus with administration of ifosfamide. Dosage repeated at 4 hours and 8 hours after administration of ifosfamide.

Adverse reactions
GI: soft stools, nausea, vomiting, diarrhea, dysgeusia.
Note: Because mesna is used concomitantly with ifosfamide and other chemotherapeutic agents, it is difficult to determine adverse reactions attributable solely to mesna.

Interactions
None significant.

Contraindications and precautions
• Contraindicated in patients hypersensitive to mesna or thiol-containing compounds.
• Use cautiously in pregnant women.
• Safety of drug has not been established in children and in breast-feeding women.

NURSING CONSIDERATIONS

☷ Assessment
• Assess patient's condition before therapy and regularly thereafter.
• Up to 6% of patients may not respond to drug's protective effects.
• Monitor urine samples daily in patient receiving mesna for hematuria.
• Be alert for adverse reactions.
• Monitor patient's hydration status if adverse GI reactions occur.
• Evaluate patient's and family's knowledge of drug therapy.

⊞ Nursing diagnoses
• Risk for fluid volume deficit related to drug-induced adverse GI reactions
• Knowledge deficit related to drug therapy

⟩ Planning and implementation
• Prepare I.V. solution by diluting commercially available ampules with D$_5$W solution, dextrose 5% and 0.9% NaCl injection, 0.9% NaCl injection, or lactated

Ringer's solution to obtain final solution of 20 mg of mesna per milliliter.
• Do not mix mesna I.V. with cisplatin because they are incompatible.
• Refrigerate diluted solutions after preparation and use within 6 hours. Diluted solutions are stable for 24 hours at room temperature. After opening ampule, discard any unused drug because it decomposes quickly into inactive compound.
• Know that mesna is not effective in preventing hematuria from other causes (such as thrombocytopenia).
• Although formulated to prevent hemorrhagic cystitis from ifosfamide, drug will not protect against other toxicities associated with ifosfamide.
• Know that mesna may interfere with diagnostic tests for urine ketones.
Patient teaching
• Instruct patient to report hematuria immediately and to notify doctor of adverse GI reactions.

✓ Evaluation
• Patient maintains adequate hydration throughout therapy.
• Patient and family state understanding of drug therapy.

---

mesoridazine besylate
(mes-oh-RID-eh-zeen BES-eh-layt)
Serentil* **, Serentil Concentrate

Pharmacologic class: phenothiazine (piperidine derivative)
Therapeutic class: antipsychotic
Pregnancy risk category: NR

How supplied

Tablets: 10 mg, 25 mg, 50 mg, 100 mg
Oral concentrate: 25 mg/ml (0.6% alcohol)
Injection: 25 mg/ml

Pharmacokinetics

Absorption: erratic and variable with P.O. use; unknown with I.M. use.

Distribution: distributed widely in body; 91% to 99% protein-bound.
Metabolism: metabolized extensively by liver.
Excretion: excreted primarily in urine with some excretion in feces by way of biliary tract.

Route	Onset	Peak	Duration
P.O., I.M.	Up to several wk	Unknown	Unknown

Pharmacodynamics

Chemical effect: unknown. A piperidine phenothiazine and major sulfoxide metabolite of thioridazine, mesoridazine may block postsynaptic dopamine receptors in brain.
Therapeutic effect: relieves psychotic and alcoholic signs and symptoms.

Indications and dosage

▶ **Alcoholism.** *Adults and children over age 12:* 25 mg P.O. b.i.d. up to maximum of 200 mg daily.
▶ **Behavioral problems associated with chronic organic mental syndrome.** *Adults and children over age 12:* 25 mg P.O. t.i.d. up to maximum of 300 mg daily.
▶ **Psychoneurotic manifestations (anxiety).** *Adults and children over age 12:* 10 mg P.O. t.i.d. up to maximum of 150 mg daily.
▶ **Schizophrenia.** *Adults and children over age 12:* initially, 50 mg P.O. t.i.d. up to 400 mg/day; or 25 mg I.M. repeated in 30 to 60 minutes, p.r.n., up to 200 mg daily.

Adverse reactions

CNS: extrapyramidal reactions (low incidence), *tardive dyskinesia, sedation* (high incidence), EEG changes, dizziness.
CV: *orthostatic hypotension,* tachycardia, ECG changes.
EENT: *ocular changes, blurred vision,* retinitis pigmentosa.
GI: *dry mouth, constipation.*

Reactions may be common, uncommon, *life-threatening*, or COMMON AND LIFE-THREATENING.

GU: *urine retention,* dark urine, menstrual irregularities, gynecomastia, inhibited ejaculation.
Hematologic: *leukopenia, agranulocytosis,* hyperprolactinemia, *aplastic anemia, thrombocytopenia.*
Hepatic: cholestatic jaundice, abnormal liver function test results.
Skin: *mild photosensitivity,* allergic reactions, pain at I.M. injection site, sterile abscess.
Other: weight gain; increased appetite; rarely, *neuroleptic malignant syndrome.*
After abrupt withdrawal of long-term therapy: gastritis, nausea, vomiting, dizziness, tremors, feeling of warmth or cold, diaphoresis, tachycardia, headache, insomnia.

Interactions

Drug-drug. *Antacids:* inhibited absorption of oral phenothiazines. Separate doses by at least 2 hours.
Anticholinergics: may increase anticholinergic effects. Use together cautiously.
Barbiturates: may decrease phenothiazine effect. Observe patient.
CNS depressants: increased CNS depression. Use together cautiously.
Lithium, phenothiazine: coadministration may induce disorientation, unconsciousness and extrapyramidal symptoms. Use with caution.
Metrizamide: increased risk of seizures. Monitor closely.
Drug-lifestyle. *Alcohol use:* increased CNS depression. Avoid concomitant use.
Sun exposure: increased photosensitivity reactions. Take precautions.

Contraindications and precautions

• Contraindicated in patients with hypersensitivity to drug and in those experiencing severe CNS depression or comatose states.
• Drug is not recommended for use in breast-feeding women.
• Use cautiously in pregnant women.

• Safety of drug has not been established in children younger than age 12.

NURSING CONSIDERATIONS

⚕ Assessment
• Assess patient's condition before therapy and regularly thereafter.
• Obtain baseline measures of blood pressure before starting therapy and monitor regularly. Watch for orthostatic hypotension, especially with parenteral administration.
• Monitor therapy with weekly bilirubin tests during first month, periodic blood tests (CBC and liver function), and ophthalmologic tests (long-term use), as ordered.
• Be alert for adverse reactions and drug interactions.
• Monitor patient for tardive dyskinesia. It may occur after prolonged use. It may not appear until months or years later and may disappear spontaneously or persist for life, despite discontinuation of drug.
• Evaluate patient's and family's knowledge of drug therapy.

⊞ Nursing diagnoses
• Altered thought processes related to underlying condition
• Constipation related to drug-induced adverse GI reactions
• Knowledge deficit related to drug therapy

▷ Planning and implementation
P.O. use: Oral therapy should replace parenteral therapy as soon as possible. When oral concentrate solution is used, dilute dose with water, orange juice, or grape juice just before administration.
• Oral liquid and parenteral forms may cause contact dermatitis. Wear gloves when preparing solutions, and avoid contact with skin and clothing.
I.M. use: Administer drug deeply I.M. only in upper outer quadrant of buttocks. Massage slowly afterward to prevent sterile abscess. Injection may sting.

• Protect drug from light. Slight yellowing of injection or concentrate is common; this does not affect potency. Discard markedly discolored solutions.
• Withhold dose and notify doctor if jaundice, symptoms of blood dyscrasia (fever, sore throat, infection, cellulitis, weakness), or persistent extrapyramidal reactions (longer than a few hours) develop, especially in pregnant woman or in child.
• Acute dystonic reactions may be treated with diphenhydramine.
• Do not discontinue use of drug abruptly unless severe adverse reactions occur.

Patient teaching
• Warn patient to avoid activities that require alertness and psychomotor coordination until CNS effects of drug are known.
• Advise patient to change position slowly.
• Tell patient to avoid alcohol during drug therapy.
• Have patient report urine retention or constipation.
• Tell patient that drug may discolor urine.
• Advise patient to relieve dry mouth with sugarless gum or hard candy.
• Tell patient to avoid prolonged exposure to the sun, use sunblock, and wear protective clothing to avoid photosensitivity reactions.

☑ **Evaluation**
• Patient exhibits improved behavior.
• Patient maintains normal bowel pattern.
• Patient and family state understanding of drug therapy.

---

metaproterenol sulfate
(met-uh-proh-TER-eh-nul SUL-fayt)
Alupent, Arm-a-Med Metaproterenol, Dey-Lute Metaproterenol, Metaprel

---

Pharmacologic class: adrenergic
Therapeutic class: bronchodilator
Pregnancy risk category: C

How supplied
Tablets: 10 mg, 20 mg
Syrup: 10 mg/5 ml
Aerosol inhaler: 0.65 mg/metered spray
Nebulizer inhaler: 0.4%, 0.6%, 5% solution

Pharmacokinetics
Absorption: well absorbed.
Distribution: widely distributed.
Metabolism: extensively metabolized on first pass through liver.
Excretion: excreted in urine.

Route	Onset	Peak	Duration
P.O.	1 min	≤ 1 hr	1-4 hr
Inhalation	15 min	≤ 1 hr	2-6 hr
Nebulization	5-30 min	≤ 1 hr	2-6 hr

Pharmacodynamics
Chemical effect: relaxes bronchial smooth muscle by acting on $beta_2$-adrenergic receptors.
Therapeutic effect: improves breathing ability.

Indications and dosage
▶ **Acute episodes of bronchial asthma.**
Adults and children: 2 to 3 inhalations. Do not repeat inhalations more often than q 3 to 4 hours. Do not exceed 12 inhalations daily.
▶ **Bronchial asthma and reversible bronchospasm.** *Adults:* 20 mg P.O. q 6 to 8 hours. *Children over age 9 or weighing over 27 kg (60 lb):* 20 mg P.O. q 6 to 8 hours. *Children ages 6 to 9 or weighing below 27 kg:* 10 mg P.O. q 6 to 8 hours.
  Alternatively, by way of IPPB or nebulizer. *Adults and children age 12 and older:* by IPPB, 0.2 to 0.3 ml of 5% solution diluted in approximately 2.5 ml of 0.9% NaCl or 2.5 ml of commercially available 0.4% or 0.6% solution q 4 hours, p.r.n.; by hand-bulb nebulizer, 10 inhalations of an undiluted 5% solution. *Children ages 6 to 12:* 0.1 to 0.2 ml of 5% solution diluted in 0.9% NaCl to final volume of 3 ml q 4 hours, p.r.n.

Adverse reactions

CNS: nervousness, weakness, drowsiness, tremors.
CV: tachycardia, hypertension, palpitations; *cardiac arrest* (with excessive use).
GI: vomiting, nausea, bad taste in mouth.
Respiratory: paradoxical bronchiolar constriction (with excessive use).

Interactions

Drug-drug. *Levodopa:* risk of arrhythmias. Avoid concomitant use.
Propranolol, other beta blockers: blocked bronchodilating effect of metaproterenol. Monitor patient.

Contraindications and precautions

• Contraindicated in patients with hypersensitivity to drug or its ingredients, in use during anesthesia with cyclopropane or halogenated hydrocarbon general anesthetics, and in those with tachycardia and arrhythmias associated with tachycardia, peripheral or mesenteric vascular thrombosis, or profound hypoxia or hypercapnia.
• Use cautiously in patients with hypertension, hyperthyroidism, heart disease, diabetes, or cirrhosis; in those who are receiving cardiac glycosides; and in pregnant or breast-feeding women.

NURSING CONSIDERATIONS

Assessment
• Assess patient's condition before therapy and regularly thereafter.
• Be alert for adverse reactions and drug interactions.
• Monitor patient's hydration status if adverse GI reactions occur.
• Evaluate patient's and family's knowledge of drug therapy.

Nursing diagnoses
• Impaired gas exchange related to underlying respiratory condition
• Risk for fluid volume deficit related to drug-induced adverse GI reactions

• Knowledge deficit related to drug therapy

Planning and implementation
• Patient may use tablets and aerosol concomitantly. Monitor for toxicity.
P.O. and oral inhalation use: Follow normal protocol.
Aerosol nebulization use: Solution can be given by IPPB with drug diluted in 0.9% NaCl solution or by hand-bulb nebulizer at full strength.
Patient teaching
• Give patient the following instructions for using metered-dose inhaler:
– Clear nasal passages and throat.
– Breathe out, expelling as much air from lungs as possible.
– Place mouthpiece well into mouth as dose from inhaler is released, and inhale deeply.
– Hold breath for several seconds, remove mouthpiece, and exhale slowly. Allow 2 minutes between inhalations.
• Instruct patient to store drug in light-resistant container.
• Advise patient that metaproterenol inhalations should precede steroid inhalations (when prescribed) by 10 to 15 minutes to maximize therapy.
• Tell patient using steroid inhaler to use bronchodilator first, then wait 5 minutes before using steroid. This allows bronchodilator to open air passages for maximum effectiveness.
• If more than one inhalation of metaproterenol is ordered, tell patient to wait at least 2 minutes before repeating procedure.
• Warn patient to discontinue immediately and notify doctor if paradoxical bronchospasm occurs.
• Warn patient to notify doctor if no response is derived from dosage or to request dosage adjustments.

Evaluation
• Patient's status improves.
• Patient maintains adequate hydration.

• Patient and family state understanding of drug therapy.

---

metformin hydrochloride
(met-FOR-min high-droh-KLOR-ighd)
Glucophage

Pharmacologic class: biguanide
Therapeutic class: antidiabetic agent
Pregnancy risk category: B

How supplied
Tablets: 500 mg, 850 mg

Pharmacokinetics
Absorption: absorbed from GI tract, with food decreasing extent of absorption as well as slightly delaying rate of absorption.
Distribution: only negligibly bound to plasma proteins in contrast to sulfonylureas, which are more than 90% protein-bound.
Metabolism: not metabolized.
Excretion: excreted unchanged in urine.
Half-life: about 6.2 hours.

Route	Onset	Peak	Duration
P.O.	Unknown	Unknown	Unknown

Pharmacodynamics
Chemical effect: decreases hepatic glucose production and intestinal absorption of glucose and improves insulin sensitivity (increases peripheral glucose uptake and utilization).
Therapeutic effect: lowers blood glucose levels.

Indications and dosage
▶ **Adjunct to diet to lower blood glucose level in patients with type 2 (non-insulin-dependent) diabetes mellitus.**
Adults: initially, 500 mg P.O. b.i.d. with morning and evening meals, or 850 mg P.O. once daily with morning meal. When 500-mg dose form is used, dosage increased 500 mg weekly to maximum of 2,500 mg P.O. daily, as necessary. When 850-mg dose form is used, dosage increased 850 mg every other week to maximum of 2,550 mg P.O. daily, as necessary.

Adverse reactions
GI: diarrhea, nausea, vomiting, abdominal bloating, flatulence, anorexia.
Hematologic: megaloblastic anemia.
Skin: rash, dermatitis.
Other: *lactic acidosis,* unpleasant or metallic taste.

Interactions
Drug-drug. *Calcium channel blockers, corticosteroids, estrogens, isoniazid, nicotinic acid, oral contraceptives, phenothiazines, phenytoin, sympathomimetics, thiazide and other diuretics, thyroid agents:* may produce hyperglycemia. Monitor patient's glycemic control. Metformin dosage may need to be increased.
Cationic drugs (such as amiloride, cimetidine, digoxin, morphine, procainamide, quinidine, quinine, ranitidine, triamterene, trimethoprim, vancomycin): have potential to compete for common renal tubular transport systems, which may increase metformin plasma levels. Monitor patient's blood glucose level.
Iodinated contrast material: parenteral contrast studies with iodinated materials have been associated with lactic acidosis leading to acute renal failure. Withhold metformin for at least 48 hours prior to study, as ordered, and reinstitute after renal function has been reevaluated.
Nifedipine: increased metformin levels. Monitor patient. Metformin dosage may need to be decreased.
Drug-lifestyle. *Alcohol use:* potentiated drug's effects. Avoid concomitant use.

Contraindications and precautions
• Contraindicated in patients with renal disease, metabolic acidosis, or hypersensitivity to drug. Drug should be temporarily withheld in patients undergoing radio-

---

logic studies involving parenteral administration of iodinated contrast materials; use of such products may result in acute renal dysfunction. Drug should also be stopped if patient enters hypoxic state. Metformin should be avoided in patients with hepatic disease.

• Use of drug is not recommended in breast-feeding women.

• Use caution when giving drug to elderly, debilitated, or malnourished patients and those with adrenal or pituitary insufficiency because of increased risk of hypoglycemia.

• Safety has not been established in pregnant women and in children.

NURSING CONSIDERATIONS

🔎 Assessment

• Assess patient's blood glucose level before therapy and regularly thereafter.

• Before therapy is begun, patient's kidney function should be assessed and then reassessed at least annually. If renal impairment is detected, expect doctor to switch to different antidiabetic agent.

• Monitor patient's hematologic status for megaloblastic anemia. Patients with inadequate vitamin B_{12} or calcium intake or absorption seem predisposed to developing subnormal vitamin B_{12} levels when taking metformin. They should have serum vitamin B_{12} level determinations every 2 to 3 years.

• Be alert for adverse reactions and drug interactions.

• Monitor patient closely during times of increased stress, such as infection, fever, surgery, or trauma; insulin therapy may be required.

• Incidence of metformin-induced lactic acidosis is very low. Reported cases have occurred primarily in diabetic patients with significant renal insufficiency; with multiple, concomitant medical or surgical problems; and with multiple, concomitant drug regimens. The risk of lactic acidosis increases with the degree of renal impairment and patient's age.

• Evaluate patient's and family's knowledge of drug therapy.

🔲 Nursing diagnoses

• Altered health maintenance related to presence of hyperglycemia

• Risk for fluid volume deficit related to drug-induced adverse GI reactions

• Knowledge deficit related to drug therapy

⟩ Planning and implementation

• Know that when transferring patient from standard oral antidiabetic drugs (except chlorpropamide) to metformin, no transition period usually is necessary. When switching patient from chlorpropamide to metformin, care should be exercised during first 2 weeks of metformin therapy because prolonged retention of chlorpropamide increases risk of hypoglycemia during this time.

• Notify doctor if blood glucose level becomes elevated despite therapy.

• If patient has not responded to 4 weeks of therapy using maximum dosage, doctor may add oral sulfonylurea while continuing metformin at maximum dosage. If patient still does not respond after several months of concomitant therapy at maximum dosages, doctor may stop both agents and start insulin therapy.

• Discontinue drug immediately and notify doctor if patient develops conditions associated with hypoxemia or dehydration because of risk of lactic acidosis.

• Metformin therapy may be temporarily suspended for surgical procedure (except minor procedures not associated with restricted intake of food and fluids) and not restarted until patient's oral intake has resumed and kidney function is normal.

Patient teaching

• Tell patient to take once-daily dose with breakfast and twice-daily dose with breakfast and dinner.

• Instruct patient to stop drug and tell doctor of unexplained hyperventilation, myalgia, malaise, unusual somnolence,

---

*Liquid form contains alcohol   **May contain tartrazine   ◆Canada   ◇ Australia   †OTC

or other symptoms of early lactic acidosis.
- Warn patient to control alcohol consumption while taking drug.
- Teach patient about diabetes and the importance of following therapeutic regimen; adhering to diet, weight reduction, exercise, and hygiene programs; and avoiding infection. Explain how and when to self-monitor blood glucose level and how to differentiate between hypoglycemia and hyperglycemia.
- Tell patient not to change drug dosage without doctor's consent. Encourage patient to report abnormal blood test results.
- Advise patient not to take other medication, including OTC drugs, without checking with doctor.
- Instruct patient to carry a medical identification card.

☑ **Evaluation**
- Patient's blood glucose level is normal.
- Patient maintains adequate hydration throughout therapy.
- Patient and family state understanding of drug therapy.

---

methadone hydrochloride
(METH-eh-dohn high-droh-KLOR-ighd)
Dolophine, Methadose, Physeptone◇

Pharmacologic class: opioid
Therapeutic class: analgesic, narcotic detoxification adjunct
Controlled substance schedule: II
Pregnancy risk category: NR

How supplied

Tablets: 5 mg, 10 mg
Dispersible tablets (for methadone maintenance therapy): 40 mg
Oral solution: 5 mg/5 ml, 10 mg/5 ml, 10 mg/ml (concentrate)
Injection: 10 mg/ml

Pharmacokinetics

Absorption: well absorbed from GI tract; unknown for I.M. route.
Distribution: highly bound to tissue protein.
Metabolism: metabolized primarily in liver.
Excretion: excreted primarily in urine; metabolites excreted in feces. *Half-life:* 15 to 25 hours.

Route	Onset	Peak	Duration
P.O.	30-60 min	1.5-2 hr	4-6 hr
I.M.	10-20 min	1-2 hr	4-5 hr
S.C.	Unknown	Unknown	Unknown

Pharmacodynamics

Chemical effect: binds with opioid receptors at many sites in CNS, altering both perception of and emotional response to pain through unknown mechanism.
Therapeutic effect: relieves pain and symptoms of opioid withdrawal.

Indications and dosage

▶ **Severe pain.** *Adults:* 2.5 to 10 mg P.O., I.M., or S.C. q 3 to 4 hours, p.r.n.
▶ **Narcotic withdrawal syndrome.**
Adults: 15 to 20 mg P.O. daily (highly individualized). Maintenance dosage is 20 to 120 mg P.O. daily. Dosage adjusted as needed. Daily dosages greater than 120 mg require special state and federal approval.

Adverse reactions

CNS: *sedation, somnolence, clouded sensorium, euphoria,* dizziness, chorea, *seizures* (with large doses).
CV: *hypotension,* bradycardia, **shock, cardiac arrest.**
EENT: visual disturbances.
GI: *nausea, vomiting, constipation,* ileus.
GU: *urine retention,* decreased libido.
Respiratory: *respiratory depression, respiratory arrest.*
Skin: pain (at injection site), tissue irritation, induration (after S.C. injection), diaphoresis.
Other: physical dependence.

Reactions may be *common*, uncommon, *life-threatening*, or COMMON AND LIFE-THREATENING.

Interactions
Drug-drug. *Ammonium chloride and other urine acidifiers, phenytoin:* may reduce methadone effect. Monitor for decreased pain control.
CNS depressants, general anesthetics, hypnotics, MAO inhibitors, sedatives, tranquilizers, tricyclic antidepressants: possible respiratory depression, hypotension, profound sedation, or coma. Use together cautiously. Monitor patient.
Rifampin: withdrawal symptoms; reduced blood levels of methadone. Use together cautiously.
Drug-lifestyle. *Alcohol use:* additive effects. Use together cautiously.

Contraindications and precautions
• Contraindicated in patients with hypersensitivity to drug.
• Use with extreme caution in patients with acute abdominal conditions, severe hepatic or renal impairment, hypothyroidism, Addison's disease, prostatic hyperplasia, urethral stricture, head injury, increased intracranial pressure, or asthma or other respiratory conditions.
• Use with caution in elderly or debilitated patients and in pregnant or breast-feeding women.
• Safety of drug has not been established in children.

NURSING CONSIDERATIONS

⚖ Assessment
• Assess patient's pain or opioid dependence before and during therapy.
• Monitor patient closely because drug has cumulative effect; marked sedation can occur after repeated doses.
• Be alert for adverse reactions and drug interactions.
• Evaluate patient's and family's knowledge of drug therapy.

Nursing diagnoses
• Pain related to underlying condition
• Ineffective individual coping related to opioid dependence

• Knowledge deficit related to drug therapy

➤ Planning and implementation
P.O. use: Oral liquid form is legally required in maintenance programs. Dissolve tablets in 120 ml of orange juice or powdered citrus drink.
I.M. and S.C. use: Be aware that for parenteral use, I.M. injection is preferred. Rotate injection sites.
• Know that P.O. dose is one-half as potent as injected dose.
• Around-the-clock regimen is needed to manage severe, chronic pain.
• Know that patient treated for narcotic withdrawal syndrome usually needs further analgesic if pain control is needed.
• When used as adjunct in treating narcotic addiction, withdrawal usually is delayed and mild.
Patient teaching
• Caution ambulatory patient about getting out of bed or walking. Warn outpatient to avoid hazardous activities until drug's CNS effects are known.
• Instruct patient to avoid alcohol consumption during drug therapy.

☑ Evaluation
• Patient is free from pain.
• Patient does not exhibit opioid withdrawal symptoms.
• Patient and family state understanding of drug therapy.

methamphetamine hydrochloride
(meth-am-FET-uh-meen high-droh-KLOR-ighd)
Desoxyn, Desoxyn Gradumets

Pharmacologic class: amphetamine
Therapeutic class: CNS stimulant, short-term adjunct anorexigenic, sympathomimetic amine
Controlled substance schedule: II
Pregnancy risk category: C

How supplied

Tablets: 5 mg, 10 mg
Tablets (extended release): 5 mg, 10 mg, 15 mg**

Pharmacokinetics

Absorption: rapidly absorbed from GI tract.
Distribution: widely distributed.
Metabolism: metabolized in liver to at least seven metabolites.
Excretion: excreted in urine. *Half-life:* 4 to 5 hours.

Route	Onset	Peak	Duration
P.O.	Unknown	Unknown	≤ 24 hr

Pharmacodynamics

Chemical effect: unknown; probably promotes nerve impulse transmission by releasing stored norepinephrine from nerve terminals in brain. Main sites of activity appear to be cerebral cortex and reticular activating system. In hyperkinetic children, drug has paradoxical calming effect.
Therapeutic effect: promotes calmness in children with attention deficit disorder and causes weight loss.

Indications and dosage

▶ **Attention deficit disorder with hyperactivity.** *Children age 6 and older:* initially, 5 mg P.O. once daily or b.i.d., with 5-mg increments weekly, p.r.n. Usual effective dosage is 20 to 25 mg daily.
▶ **Short-term adjunct in exogenous obesity.** *Adults:* 2.5 to 5 mg P.O. b.i.d. to t.i.d. 30 minutes before meals; or 10- or 15-mg long-acting tablet daily before breakfast.

Adverse reactions

CNS: *nervousness, insomnia,* irritability, *talkativeness,* dizziness, headache, hyperexcitability, tremors.
CV: hypertension, hypotension, *tachycardia, palpitations,* **arrhythmias.**
EENT: blurred vision, mydriasis.

GI: dry mouth, metallic taste, nausea, vomiting, abdominal cramps, diarrhea, constipation, anorexia.
GU: impotence.
Skin: urticaria.
Other: altered libido.

Interactions

Drug-drug. *Acetazolamide, antacids, sodium bicarbonate:* increased renal reabsorption. Monitor for enhanced effects.
Ammonium chloride, ascorbic acid: decreased serum levels and increased renal excretion of methamphetamine. Monitor for decreased methamphetamine effects.
Guanethidine: amphetamines may decrease the antihypertensive effectiveness of guanethidine.
Haloperidol, phenothiazines, tricyclic antidepressants: increased CNS effects. Avoid concomitant use.
Insulin, oral antidiabetic agents: may decrease antidiabetic agent requirements. Monitor blood glucose levels.
MAO inhibitors: severe hypertension; possible hypertensive crisis. Don't use together or within 14 days after MAO inhibitor has been stopped.
Drug-food. *Caffeine-containing beverages:* may increase amphetamine and related amine effects. Avoid concomitant use.

Contraindications and precautions

• Contraindicated in patients with moderate to severe hypertension, hyperthyroidism, symptomatic CV disease, advanced arteriosclerosis, glaucoma, hypersensitivity or idiosyncrasy to sympathomimetic amines, or history of drug abuse; within 14 days of MAO inhibitor therapy; and in agitated patients.
• Drug not indicated for use in pregnant women.
• Use cautiously in patients who are elderly, debilitated, asthenic, or psychopathic or who have history of suicidal or homicidal tendencies.

Reactions may be *common,* uncommon, **life-threatening,** or COMMON AND LIFE-THREATENING.

• Safety of drug has not been established in breast-feeding women.

NURSING CONSIDERATIONS

⚕ Assessment
• Assess patient's condition before therapy and regularly thereafter.
• Be alert for adverse reactions and drug interactions.
• Evaluate patient's and family's knowledge of drug therapy.

⊞ Nursing diagnoses
• Altered health maintenance related to underlying condition
• Sleep pattern disturbance related to drug-induced insomnia
• Knowledge deficit related to drug therapy

⊠ Planning and implementation
• Drug is not the first-line treatment for obesity. Use as anorexigenic agent is prohibited in some states.
• When used for obesity, be sure patient is on weight-reduction program.
• If tolerance to anorexigenic effect develops, notify doctor because drug will need to be discontinued.
Patient teaching
• Warn patient of high potential for abuse. Advise him that drug should not be used to prevent fatigue.
• Tell patient not to crush long-acting tablets.
• Advise patient to take last dose of drug at least 6 hours before bedtime.
• Warn patient to avoid activities that require alertness or good coordination until CNS effects are known.
• Tell patient to avoid caffeine products during drug therapy.
• Instruct patient to report signs of excessive stimulation.

☑ Evaluation
• Patient exhibits positive response to methamphetamine therapy.

• Patient states that insomnia does not occur.
• Patient and family state understanding of drug therapy.

methenamine hippurate
(meth-EN-ah-meen HIP-yoo-rayt)
Hiprex**, Hip-Rex♦, Urex

methenamine mandelate
Mandelamine

Pharmacologic class: formaldehyde prodrug
Therapeutic class: urinary tract antiinfective
Pregnancy risk category: C

How supplied
methenamine hippurate
Tablets: 1 g
methenamine mandelate
Tablets: 500 mg, 1 g
Tablets (enteric-coated): 500 mg, 1 g
Tablets (film-coated): 500 mg, 1 g
Suspension: 500 mg/15 ml

Pharmacokinetics
Absorption: drug and its acid salts are readily absorbed.
Distribution: crosses placenta and enters breast milk.
Metabolism: about 10% to 25% metabolized in liver.
Excretion: most of drug excreted in urine. *Half-life:* 3 to 6 hours.

Route	Onset	Peak	Duration
P.O.	Unknown	≤1 hr	Unknown

Pharmacodynamics
Chemical effect: hydrolyzed to ammonia and to formaldehyde, causing antibacterial action against gram-positive and gram-negative organisms. Mandelic and hippuric acids, with which methenamines are combined, are also antibacterial by unknown mechanisms.

Therapeutic effect: interferes with bacterial growth of selected organisms. Spectrum of activity includes gram-positive and gram-negative organisms found in urinary tract.

Indications and dosage

▶ **Long-term prophylaxis or suppression of chronic urinary tract infections. Methenamine hippurate.** *Adults and children over age 12:* 1 g P.O. q 12 hours. *Children ages 6 to 12:* 500 mg to 1 g P.O. q 12 hours.
▶ **Urinary tract infections, infected residual urine in patients with neurogenic bladder. Methenamine mandelate.** *Adults:* 1 g P.O. q.i.d. after meals and h.s. *Children ages 6 to 12:* 500 mg P.O. q.i.d. after meals and h.s. *Children under age 6:* 18.4 mg/kg P.O. q.i.d.

Adverse reactions

GI: nausea, vomiting, diarrhea, abdominal cramps, anorexia.
GU: urinary tract irritation, dysuria, frequency, albuminuria, hematuria (with high doses).
Skin: rash.
Other: elevated liver enzyme levels.

Interactions

Drug-drug. *Acetazolamide:* antagonized methenamine effect. Use together cautiously.
Sulfamethizole, sulfonamides: forms insoluble precipitate in acid urine. Do not administer together.
Urine alkalinizing agents: inhibited methenamine action. Don't use together.

Contraindications and precautions

• Contraindicated in patients with renal insufficiency, severe hepatic disease, or severe dehydration.
• Use cautiously in elderly or debilitated patients because aspiration could cause lipid pneumonia. Also use cautiously in pregnant or breast-feeding women.

NURSING CONSIDERATIONS

⚖ Assessment

• Assess patient's urinary tract infection before therapy and regularly thereafter.
• Obtain clean-catch urine specimen for culture and sensitivity tests before therapy, and repeat as needed. Therapy may begin pending test results.
• Monitor liver function studies periodically during long-term therapy.
• Be alert for adverse reactions and drug interactions.
• Evaluate patient's and family's knowledge of drug therapy.

🔛 Nursing diagnoses

• Infection related to presence of susceptible bacteria
• Risk for fluid volume deficit related to drug-induced adverse reactions
• Knowledge deficit related to drug therapy

▷ Planning and implementation

• Maintain adequate fluid intake. Intake should be at least 1,500 ml daily.
• Maintain urine pH at 5.5 or below. Use Nitrazine paper to check pH. Large doses of ascorbic acid (12 g/day) may be needed to acidify urine.
• *Proteus* and *Pseudomonas* tend to raise urine pH; urine acidifiers are usually needed during treatment.
• Withhold dose and notify doctor if rash occurs.
• Drug interferes with fluorometric procedures for determining urine catecholamine and vanillylmandelic acid levels, causing high results.
Patient teaching
• Tell patient to take drug after meals.
• Instruct patient to limit intake of alkaline foods, such as vegetables, milk, and peanuts. Cranberry, plum, or prune juice or ascorbic acid may be used to acidify urine.
• Warn patient not to take antacids (Alka-Seltzer, sodium bicarbonate).

Reactions may be *common,* uncommon, *life-threatening,* or COMMON AND LIFE-THREATENING.

✓ Evaluation
• Patient is free from infection.
• Patient maintains adequate hydration throughout therapy.
• Patient and family state understanding of drug therapy.

---

methimazole
(meth-IH-muh-zohl)
Tapazole

Pharmacologic class: thyroid hormone antagonist
Therapeutic class: antihyperthyroid agent
Pregnancy risk category: D

How supplied
Tablets: 5 mg, 10 mg

Pharmacokinetics
Absorption: absorbed rapidly from GI tract.
Distribution: concentrates in thyroid and is not protein-bound.
Metabolism: undergoes hepatic metabolism.
Excretion: excreted primarily in urine.
Half-life: 5 to 13 hours.

Route	Onset	Peak	Duration
P.O.	≤ 5 days	0.5-1 hr	Unknown

Pharmacodynamics
Chemical effect: inhibits oxidation of iodine in thyroid gland, blocking iodine's ability to combine with tyrosine to form T_4. May also prevent coupling of monoiodotyrosine and diiodotyrosine to form T_4 and T_3.
Therapeutic effect: reduces thyroid hormone level.

Indications and dosage
▶ **Hyperthyroidism.** *Adults:* if mild, 15 mg P.O. daily; if moderately severe, 30 to 40 mg daily; if severe, 60 mg daily. Daily dose divided into three doses at 8-hour intervals. Maintenance dosage is 5 to 15 mg daily. *Children:* 0.4 mg/kg P.O. daily in divided doses q 8 hours. Maintenance dosage is 0.2 mg/kg daily in divided doses q 8 hours.

Adverse reactions
CNS: headache, drowsiness, vertigo.
EENT: loss of taste.
GI: diarrhea, nausea, vomiting (may be dose-related); salivary gland enlargement.
Hematologic: *agranulocytosis,* leukopenia, *thrombocytopenia* (appear to be dose-related); *aplastic anemia.*
Hepatic: jaundice; hepatic dysfunction (anorexia, pruritus, right upper quadrant pain, yellow skin or sclera).
Musculoskeletal: arthralgia, myalgia.
Skin: rash, urticaria, discoloration.
Other: drug-induced fever, lymphadenopathy; hypothyroidism (depression; cold intolerance; hard, nonpitting edema).

Interactions
Drug-drug. *Anticoagulants:* enhance effects due to anti-vitamin K activity attributed to drug. Monitor PT and INR as indicated.

Contraindications and precautions
• Contraindicated in patients with hypersensitivity to drug.
• Drug is not recommended for use in breast-feeding women.
• Use with extreme caution in pregnant women.

NURSING CONSIDERATIONS

✎ Assessment
• Assess patient's thyroid condition before therapy and regularly thereafter.
• Monitor thyroid function studies.
• Monitor CBC and liver function periodically, as ordered.
• Dosages higher than 30 mg/day increase risk of agranulocytosis.
• Be alert for adverse reactions.

---

*Liquid form contains alcohol   **May contain tartrazine   ◆Canada   ◇Australia   †OTC

• Evaluate patient's and family's knowledge of drug therapy.

⊞ **Nursing diagnoses**
• Altered health maintenance related to presence of hyperthyroidism
• Altered protection related to drug-induced adverse hematologic reactions
• Knowledge deficit related to drug therapy

▶ **Planning and implementation**
• Pregnant women may need less drug as pregnancy progresses. Thyroid may be added. Drug may be stopped during last weeks of pregnancy.
• Notify doctor if signs and symptoms of hypothyroidism occur because dosage may need to be adjusted.
• Stop drug and notify doctor if severe rash occurs or cervical lymph nodes become enlarged.
Patient teaching
• Tell patient to take drug with meals.
• Warn patient to immediately report fever, sore throat, or mouth sores (signs of agranulocytosis); skin eruptions (sign of hypersensitivity); and anorexia, pruritus, right upper quadrant pain, and yellow skin or sclera (signs of hepatic dysfunction).
• Tell patient to ask doctor about using iodized salt and eating shellfish.
• Warn patient against taking OTC cough medications; many contain iodine.
• Instruct patient to store drug in light-resistant container.

☑ **Evaluation**
• Patient demonstrates normal thyroid hormone level.
• Patient maintains normal hematologic parameters throughout therapy.
• Patient and family state understanding of drug therapy.

methocarbamol
(meth-oh-KAR-buh-mol)
Robaxin, Roboxin-750

Pharmacologic class: carbamate derivative of guaifenesin
Therapeutic class: skeletal muscle relaxant
Pregnancy risk category: NR

How supplied
Tablets: 500 mg, 750 mg
Injection: 100 mg/ml

Pharmacokinetics
Absorption: rapidly and completely absorbed from GI tract after P.O. administration; unknown after I.M. administration.
Distribution: widely distributed throughout body.
Metabolism: extensively metabolized in liver.
Excretion: excreted primarily in urine.
Half-life: 0.9 to 2.2 hours.

Route	Onset	Peak	Duration
P.O.	≤ 0.5 hr	≤ 2 hr	Unknown
I.V.	Immediate	Immediate	Unknown
I.M.	Unknown	Unknown	Unknown

Pharmacodynamics
Chemical effect: unknown; probably modifies central perception of pain without modifying pain reflexes.
Therapeutic effect: relieves skeletal muscle pain.

Indications and dosage
▶ **As adjunct in acute, painful musculoskeletal conditions.** *Adults:* 1.5 g P.O. q.i.d. for 2 to 3 days, then 1 g P.O. q.i.d., or not more than 500 mg (5 ml) I.M. into each gluteal region. Repeated q 8 hours, p.r.n. Or 1 to 3 g daily (10 to 30 ml) I.V. directly into vein at 3 ml/minute, or 10 ml may be added to no more than 250 ml of D_5W or 0.9% NaCl solution.

Maximum dosage is 3 g daily I.M. or I.V. for 3 consecutive days.
▶ **Supportive therapy in tetanus management.** *Adults:* 1 to 2 g by direct I.V. or 1 to 3 g as infusion q 6 hours. *Children:* 15 mg/kg I.V. q 6 hours.

Adverse reactions

CNS: drowsiness, dizziness, light-headedness, headache, syncope, mild muscle incoordination (with I.M. or I.V. use), *seizures* (with I.V. use).
CV: hypotension, bradycardia (with I.M. or I.V. use), thrombophlebitis.
GI: nausea, anorexia, GI upset, metallic taste.
GU: hematuria (with I.V. use), discoloration of urine.
Hematologic: hemolysis, decreased hemoglobin level (with I.V. use).
Skin: urticaria, pruritus, rash.
Other: extravasation (with I.V. use), fever, flushing, *anaphylactic reactions* (with I.M. or I.V. use).

Interactions

Drug-drug. *CNS depressants:* increased CNS depression. Avoid concomitant use.
Drug-lifestyle. *Alcohol use:* increased CNS depression. Avoid concomitant use.

Contraindications and precautions

• Contraindicated in patients with impaired kidney function, seizure disorder (injectable form), or hypersensitivity to drug.
• Use of drug in breast-feeding women is not recommended.
• Use cautiously in pregnant women.

NURSING CONSIDERATIONS

Assessment
• Assess patient's condition before therapy and regularly thereafter.
• Watch for orthostatic hypotension, especially with parenteral route.
• Monitor CBC periodically during prolonged therapy.

• Be alert for adverse reactions and drug interactions.
• Monitor patient's hydration status if adverse GI reactions occur.
• Evaluate patient's and family's knowledge of drug therapy.

Nursing diagnoses
• Pain related to underlying musculoskeletal condition
• Risk for fluid volume deficit related to drug-induced adverse GI reactions
• Knowledge deficit related to drug therapy

Planning and implementation
P.O. use: Give tablets with meals or milk.
– Prepare liquid by crushing tablets into water or NaCl solution. Give through nasogastric tube.
I.V. use: Dilute 10 ml of drug in not more than 250 ml of D_5W or 0.9% NaCl injection. Infuse slowly; maximum rate is 300 mg (3 ml)/minute.
– Drug irritates veins; may cause phlebitis and fainting and aggravate seizures if injected rapidly. Keep patient supine during infusion and for 15 minutes afterward. Drug is an irritant; avoid extravasation.
I.M. use: Give drug I.M. deeply into upper outer quadrant of buttocks, with maximum of 5 ml in each buttock.
• Do not give drug S.C.
• In tetanus, methocarbamol is used with tetanus antitoxin, penicillin, tracheotomy, and aggressive supportive care. Long course of I.V. methocarbamol therapy is required.
• Have epinephrine, antihistamines, and corticosteroids available.
• Drug may interfere with urine tests to determine 5-hydroxyindoleacetic acid and vanillylmandelic acid levels.
Patient teaching
• Advise patient to get up slowly after parenteral administration.

• Tell patient that urine may turn green, black, or brown.
• Advise patient to follow doctor's orders regarding physical activity.
• Warn patient to avoid activities that require alertness until drug's CNS effects are known.
• Tell patient not to combine drug with alcohol or other CNS depressants. Instruct patient to avoid alcohol consumption during drug therapy.

☑ **Evaluation**
• Patient is free from pain.
• Patient maintains adequate hydration throughout therapy.
• Patient and family state understanding of drug therapy.

---

methotrexate
(meth-oh-TREKS-ayt)
Rheumatrex

methotrexate sodium
Folex PFS, Mexate-AQ

Pharmacologic class: antimetabolite (cell cycle–phase specific, S phase)
Therapeutic class: antineoplastic
Pregnancy risk category: X

How supplied

Tablets (scored): 2.5 mg
Injection: 20-mg, 25-mg, 50-mg, 100-mg, 250-mg, 1g vials, lyophilized powder, preservative-free; 25-mg/ml vials, preservative-free solution; 2.5-mg/ml, 25-mg/ml vials, lyophilized powder, preserved

Pharmacokinetics

Absorption: P.O. absorption appears to be dose-related; lower doses are almost completely absorbed, whereas absorption of larger doses is incomplete and variable. I.M. doses are absorbed completely.
Distribution: distributed widely throughout body with highest concentrations found in kidneys, gallbladder, spleen, liver, and skin; about 50% bound to plasma protein.
Metabolism: metabolized only slightly in liver.
Excretion: excreted primarily in urine. *Half-life:* 4 hours. *Terminal half-life:* about 3 to 10 hours for patients receiving low-dose antineoplastic therapy (below 30 mg/m²). For patients on high doses, the terminal half-life is 8 to 15 hours.

Route	Onset	Peak	Duration
P.O.	Unknown	1-2 hr	Unknown
I.V., intrathecal	Unknown	Immediate	Unknown
I.M.	Unknown	0.5-1 hr	Unknown

Pharmacodynamics

Chemical effect: prevents reduction of folic acid to tetrahydrofolate by binding to dihydrofolate reductase.
Therapeutic effect: kills selected cancer cells and reduces inflammation.

Indications and dosage

▶ **Trophoblastic tumors (choriocarcinoma, hydatidiform mole).** *Adults:* 15 to 30 mg P.O. or I.M. daily for 5 days. Repeated after 1 or more weeks, based on response or toxicity.
▶ **Acute lymphoblastic and lymphatic leukemia.** *Adults and children:* 3.3 mg/m²/day P.O. or I.M. for 4 to 6 weeks or until remission occurs; then 20 to 30 mg/m² P.O. or I.M. twice weekly.
▶ **Meningeal leukemia.** *Adults and children:* 12mg/m² intrathecally or an empirical dose of 15 mg q 2 to 5 days and repeat until cell count of CSF returns to normal, then give one additional dose.
▶ **Burkitt's lymphoma (stage I or stage II).** *Adults:* 10 to 25 mg P.O. daily for 4 to 8 days with 1-week rest intervals.
▶ **Lymphosarcoma (stage III).** *Adults:* 0.625 to 2.5 mg/kg daily P.O., I.M., or I.V.
▶ **Osteosarcoma.** *Adults:* initially, 12 g/m² I.V. as 4-hour infusion. Subsequent doses 12 to 15 g/m² I.V. as 4-

---

Reactions may be *common*, uncommon, *life-threatening*, or COMMON AND LIFE-THREATENING.

hour infusion given weeks 4, 5, 6, 7, 11, 12, 15, 16, 29, 30, 44, and 45 after surgery. Given with leucovorin, 15 mg P.O. q 6 hours for 10 doses after start of methotrexate infusion.
► **Mycosis fungoides.** *Adults:* 2.5 to 10.0 mg P.O. daily, or 50 mg I.M. weekly, or 25 mg I.M. twice weekly.
► **Psoriasis.** *Adults:* 10 to 25 mg P.O., I.M., or I.V. as single weekly dose.
► **Rheumatoid arthritis.** *Adults:* initially, 7.5 mg P.O. weekly, either in single dose or divided as 2.5 mg P.O. q 12 hours for three doses once a week. Dosage may be gradually increased to maximum of 20 mg weekly.

Adverse reactions

CNS: *arachnoiditis* (within hours of intrathecal use); subacute neurotoxicity (may begin few weeks later); demyelination, *leukoencephalopathy.*
EENT: pharyngitis.
GI: *stomatitis, diarrhea,* enteritis, *intestinal perforation, nausea, vomiting.*
GU: nephropathy, *tubular necrosis, renal failure.*
Hematologic: WBC and platelet count nadirs occurring on day 7; *anemia, leukopenia, thrombocytopenia* (all dose-related).
Hepatic: *acute toxicity* (elevated transaminase level), *chronic toxicity* (cirrhosis, *hepatic fibrosis*).
Respiratory: *pulmonary fibrosis, pulmonary interstitial infiltrates,* pneumonitis.
Skin: *urticaria,* pruritus, hyperpigmentation; exposure to sun may aggravate psoriatic lesions, rash, photosensitivity.
Other: alopecia, osteoporosis (in children with long-term use), hyperuricemia, *sudden death.*

Interactions

Drug-drug. *Digoxin:* may decrease serum digoxin levels. Monitor patient closely.
Folic acid derivatives: antagonized methotrexate effect. Monitor patient.

NSAIDs, phenylbutazone, probenecid, salicylates, sulfonamides: increased methotrexate toxicity. Don't use together.
Phenytoin: may decrease serum phenytoin levels. Monitor patient.
Procarbazine: may increase hepatotoxicity of methotrexate. Monitor closely.
Vaccines: immunizations may be ineffective; risk of disseminated infection with live-virus vaccines. Consult with doctor about safe time to administer vaccine.
Drug-lifestyle. *Alcohol use:* may increase hepatotoxicity. Avoid concomitant use.
Sun exposure: photosensitivity reactions may occur. Take precautions.

Contraindications and precautions

• Contraindicated in patients hypersensitive to drug; in pregnant or breast-feeding women; and in those with psoriasis or rheumatoid arthritis who also have alcoholism, alcoholic liver, chronic liver disease, immunodeficiency syndromes, or preexisting blood dyscrasias.
• Use cautiously and at modified dosage in patients with impaired liver or kidney function, bone marrow suppression, aplasia, leukopenia, thrombocytopenia, or anemia. Also use cautiously in patients with infection, peptic ulceration, or ulcerative colitis and in very young, elderly, or debilitated patients.

NURSING CONSIDERATIONS

Assessment
• Assess patient's condition before therapy and regularly thereafter.
• Perform baseline pulmonary function tests and repeat periodically.
• Monitor fluid intake and output daily.
• Monitor serum uric acid level.
• Watch for increases in AST, ALT, and alkaline phosphatase levels—signs of hepatic dysfunction.
• Monitor CBC regularly, as ordered.
• Be alert for adverse reactions and drug interactions.

• Evaluate patient's and family's knowledge of drug therapy.

🔃 **Nursing diagnoses**
• Altered health maintenance related to underlying condition
• Altered protection related to drug-induced adverse hematologic reactions
• Knowledge deficit related to drug therapy

▶ **Planning and implementation**
• Follow institutional policy to reduce risks. Preparation and administration of parenteral form are associated with carcinogenic, mutagenic, and teratogenic risks.
P.O. and I.M. use: Follow normal protocol.
I.V. use: Give undiluted by direct injection. Or, dilute with up to 25 ml of 0.9% NaCl injection (for Folex) or 2 to 10 ml of sterile water for injection, 0.9% NaCl injection, or bacteriostatic water for injection containing parabens or benzyl alcohol (for Mexate).
Intrathecal use: Use only 20-, 50-, or 100-mg vials of powder with no preservatives. Reconstitute immediately before using with preservative-free 0.9% NaCl injection. Dilute to maximum concentration of 1 mg/ml. Use only new vials of drug and diluent.
– Reconstitute solutions without preservatives immediately before use, and discard unused drug.
• CSF volume is dependent on age, not body surface area (BSA). Using BSA for dosing when treating meningeal leukemia has resulted in low CSF methotrexate level in children and high level and neurotoxicity in adults. Alternatively, a dosing regimen that is based on age may be used. Elderly patients may require a reduced dosage because CSF volume and turnover may decrease with age.
• Have patient consume fluid intake of 2 to 3 L daily.
• Alkalinize urine, as ordered, by giving sodium bicarbonate tablets to prevent

precipitation of drug, especially with high doses. Maintain urine pH at more than 6.5. Reduce dosage, as ordered, if BUN level reaches 20 to 30 mg/dl or creatinine level reaches 1.2 to 2 mg/dl. Report BUN level over 30 mg/dl or creatinine level over 2 mg/dl, and stop use of drug.
• Rash, redness, or ulcerations in mouth or adverse pulmonary reactions may signal serious complications. Therapy may be discontinued if ulcerative stomatitis or other severe adverse GI reaction occurs or if pulmonary toxicity is detected.
• Leucovorin rescue necessary with high-dose (greater than 100 mg) protocols. Don't confuse with folic acid. This technique works against systemic toxicity but doesn't interfere with tumor cells' absorption of methotrexate.
Patient teaching
• Teach and encourage diligent mouth care to reduce risk of superinfection in mouth.
• Warn patient to avoid prolonged exposure to the sun, wear protective clothing and use highly protective sunblock.
• Tell patient to continue leucovorin rescue despite severe nausea and vomiting and to tell doctor. Parenteral leucovorin therapy may be needed.
• Warn patient to avoid conception during and immediately after therapy because of possible abortion or congenital anomalies.
• Instruct patient to avoid alcohol consumption during drug therapy.

☑ **Evaluation**
• Patient exhibits positive response to drug therapy.
• Patient does not experience serious complications when hematologic parameters are depressed during therapy.
• Patient and family state understanding of drug therapy.

Reactions may be *common*, uncommon, *life-threatening*, or COMMON AND LIFE-THREATENING.

methsuximide (mesuximide)
(meth-SUKS-ih-mighd)
Celontin

Pharmacologic class: succinimide derivative
Therapeutic class: anticonvulsant
Pregnancy risk category: NR

How supplied

Capsules: 150 mg, 300 mg

Pharmacokinetics

Absorption: absorbed from GI tract.
Distribution: widely distributed.
Metabolism: metabolized in liver.
Excretion: excreted in urine. *Half-life:* 2.6 to 4 hours.

Route	Onset	Peak	Duration
P.O.	Unknown	1-4 hr	Unknown

Pharmacodynamics

Chemical effect: unknown; may increase seizure threshold. Methsuximide reduces paroxysmal spike-and-wave pattern of absence seizures by depressing neurotransmission in motor cortex.
Therapeutic effect: prevents seizures.

Indications and dosage

▶ **Refractory absence seizures.** *Adults and children:* initially, 300 mg P.O. daily. Increased by 300 mg daily at weekly intervals, as indicated. Maximum daily dosage is 1.2 g in divided doses.

Adverse reactions

CNS: *drowsiness, ataxia, dizziness,* irritability, nervousness, headache, insomnia, confusion, depression, aggressiveness.
EENT: blurred vision, photophobia, periorbital edema.
GI: *nausea, vomiting, anorexia,* diarrhea, weight loss, abdominal or epigastric pain.
Hematologic: eosinophilia, *aplastic anemia, leukopenia,* monocytosis, *fatal blood dyscrasias, pancytopenia.*

Skin: urticaria, pruritic and erythematous rashes.

Interactions

Drug-drug. *Valproic acid:* both increases and decreases in succinimide levels have occurred. Monitor patient.

Contraindications and precautions

• Contraindicated in patients with hypersensitivity to succinimide derivatives.
• Drug is not recommended for use in breast-feeding women.
• Use with extreme caution in those with hepatic or renal dysfunction.
• Use cautiously in pregnant women.

NURSING CONSIDERATIONS

Assessment
• Assess patient's seizure disorder before therapy and regularly thereafter.
• Check CBC, urinalysis, and liver function tests periodically, as ordered.
• Monitor methsuximide level. Therapeutic serum level is 10 to 40 mcg/ml.
• Be alert for adverse reactions.
• Monitor patient's hydration status if adverse GI reactions occur.
• Evaluate patient's and family's knowledge of drug therapy.

Nursing diagnoses
• Risk for injury related to seizure activity
• Risk for fluid volume deficit related to drug-induced adverse reactions
• Knowledge deficit related to drug therapy

Planning and implementation
• Never change or withdraw drug suddenly. Abrupt withdrawal may precipitate absence seizures. Report adverse reactions promptly.
Patient teaching
• Warn patient to avoid activities that require alertness until drug's CNS effects are known.

• Tell patient to call doctor promptly if lupus-like syndrome develops.
• Warn patient and parents, if appropriate, not to stop drug abruptly.
• Caution patient that this drug may color urine pink or brown.

☑ Evaluation
• Patient is free from seizure activity.
• Patient maintains adequate hydration throughout therapy.
• Patient and family state understanding of drug therapy.

methylcellulose
(meth-il-SEL-yoo-lohs)
Citrucel†, Cologel†

Pharmacologic class: adsorbent
Therapeutic class: bulk-forming laxative
Pregnancy risk category: NR

How supplied
Powder: 2 g/heaping tablespoon†
Tablets: 500 mg†

Pharmacokinetics
Absorption: not absorbed.
Distribution: distributed locally, in intestine.
Metabolism: none.
Excretion: excreted in feces.

Route	Onset	Peak	Duration
P.O.	12-24 hr	≤ 3 days	Varies

Pharmacodynamics
Chemical effect: absorbs water and expands to increase bulk and moisture content of stool, which encourages peristalsis and bowel movement.
Therapeutic effect: relieves constipation.

Indications and dosage
▶ **Chronic constipation.** *Adults:* 1 to 3 heaping tablespoons in 8 oz (240 ml) cold water daily to t.i.d. Usual dosage up to 6 g daily (3 tablespoons). *Children*

ages 6 to 12: 1 to 1½ level tablespoons in 4 oz (120 ml) cold water daily to t.i.d. Usual dosage up to 3 g daily (1½ tablespoons).

Adverse reactions
GI: *nausea,* vomiting, diarrhea (with excessive use); esophageal, gastric, small intestinal, or colonic strictures (when drug is chewed or taken in dry form); *abdominal cramps* (especially in severe constipation); laxative dependence (with long-term or excessive use).

Interactions
None significant.

Contraindications and precautions
• Contraindicated in patients with abdominal pain, nausea, vomiting, or other symptoms of appendicitis or acute surgical abdomen and in those with intestinal obstruction or ulceration, disabling adhesions, or difficulty swallowing.
• Use cautiously in pregnant or breast-feeding women.

NURSING CONSIDERATIONS

☞ Assessment
• Assess patient's constipation before therapy and regularly thereafter.
• Before giving for constipation, determine whether patient has adequate fluid intake, exercise, and diet.
• Be alert for adverse reactions.
• Monitor patient's hydration status if adverse GI reactions occur.
• Evaluate patient's and family's knowledge of drug therapy.

☷ Nursing diagnoses
• Constipation related to underlying condition
• Risk for fluid volume deficit related to drug-induced adverse GI reactions
• Knowledge deficit related to drug therapy

⊠ Planning and implementation
• Be aware that drug is especially useful in debilitated patients and in those with postpartum constipation, irritable bowel syndrome, diverticulitis, or colostomies. Drug is also used to treat laxative abuse and to empty colon before barium enema.
Patient teaching
• Tell patient to take drug with at least 8 oz of pleasant-tasting liquid.
• Teach patient about dietary sources of bulk, which include bran and other cereals, fresh fruit, and vegetables.

☑ Evaluation
• Patient's constipation is relieved.
• Patient maintains adequate hydration throughout therapy.
• Patient and family state understanding of drug therapy.

methyldopa
(meth-il-DOH-puh)
Aldomet, Aldomet M◇, Apo-Methyldopa♦, Dopamet♦, Hydopa◇, Novo-Medopa♦, Nu-Medopa♦

methyldopate hydrochloride
Aldomet, Aldomet Ester Injection◇

Pharmacologic class: centrally acting antiadrenergic agent
Therapeutic class: antihypertensive
Pregnancy risk category: B (oral), C (IV)

How supplied
methyldopa
Tablets: 125 mg, 250 mg, 500 mg
Oral suspension: 250 mg/5 ml
methyldopate hydrochloride
Injection: 250 mg/5 ml

Pharmacokinetics
Absorption: absorbed partially from GI tract after P.O. administration.
Distribution: distributed throughout body; bound weakly to plasma proteins.

Metabolism: metabolized extensively in liver and intestinal cells.
Excretion: absorbed drug excreted in urine; unabsorbed drug excreted in feces.
Half-life: about 2 hours.

Route	Onset	Peak	Duration
P.O.	Unknown	4-6 hr	12-48 hr
I.V.	Unknown	4-6 hr	10-16 hr

Pharmacodynamics
Chemical effect: unknown; thought to involve inhibition of central vasomotor centers, thereby decreasing sympathetic outflow to heart, kidneys, and peripheral vasculature.
Therapeutic effect: lowers blood pressure.

Indications and dosage
▶ **Hypertension, hypertensive crisis.** *Adults:* **P.O.**—initially, 250 mg P.O. b.i.d. to t.i.d. in first 48 hours. Then increased as needed q 2 days. Entire daily dosage may be given in evening or h.s. Adjust dosages, as needed, if other antihypertensives are added to or deleted from therapy. Maintenance dosage is 500 mg to 2 g daily in two to four divided doses. Maximum recommended daily dosage is 3 g. **I.V.**—250 to 500 mg q 6 hours, diluted in D_5W and given over 30 to 60 minutes. Maximum dosage is 1 g q 6 hours. Switch to oral antihypertensives as soon as possible. *Children:* initially, 10 mg/kg P.O. daily in two to four divided doses; or 20 to 40 mg/kg I.V. daily in four divided doses. Increase dosage at least every 2 days until desired response occurs. Maximum daily dosage is 65 mg/kg, 2 g/m², or 3 g, whichever is least.

Adverse reactions
CNS: *sedation,* headache, asthenia, weakness, dizziness, *decreased mental acuity,* involuntary choreoathetoid movements, psychic disturbances, depression, nightmares.

CV: bradycardia, *orthostatic hypotension,* aggravated angina, *myocarditis, edema.*
EENT: *nasal congestion.*
GI: nausea, vomiting, diarrhea, pancreatitis, *dry mouth.*
Hematologic: *hemolytic anemia,* reversible agranulocytosis, *thrombocytopenia.*
Hepatic: *hepatic necrosis.*
Other: gynecomastia, galactorrhea, rash, *drug-induced fever,* impotence, *weight gain.*

Interactions

Drug-drug. *Amphetamines, norepinephrine, phenothiazines, tricyclic antidepressants:* possible hypertensive effects. Monitor patient carefully.
Barbiturates: the action of methyldopa may be reduced. Monitor patient.
Levodopa: additive hypotensive effects may increase adverse CNS reactions. Monitor patient closely.
Lithium: may increase lithium levels. Monitor for increased lithium levels.

Contraindications and precautions

• Contraindicated in patients with active hepatic disease (such as acute hepatitis), active cirrhosis, or hypersensitivity to drug. Also contraindicated if previous methyldopa therapy has been associated with liver disorders.
• Use cautiously in patients with history of impaired liver function and in breast-feeding women.

NURSING CONSIDERATIONS

☒ Assessment
• Assess patient's blood pressure before therapy and regularly thereafter.
• Monitor CBC with differential counts before therapy, every 2 weeks for first 3 months of therapy, and periodically thereafter.
• Monitor patient's Coombs' test results. In patient who has received this drug for

several months, positive reaction to direct Coombs' test indicates hemolytic anemia.
• Be alert for adverse reactions and drug interactions.
• Evaluate patient's and family's knowledge of drug therapy.

⊞ Nursing diagnoses
• Altered health maintenance related to presence of hypertension
• Risk for injury related to drug-induced adverse CNS reactions
• Knowledge deficit related to drug therapy

⊠ Planning and implementation
P.O. use: Follow normal protocol.
I.V. use: Report involuntary choreoathetoid movements; drug may be stopped.
• After dialysis, notify doctor if hypertension occurs; patient may need extra dose of methyldopa.
• Patient who needs blood transfusions should have direct and indirect Coombs' tests to prevent crossmatching problems.
Patient teaching
• Advise patient to report signs of infection, such as fever and sore throat.
• Tell patient to report adverse reactions but not to stop taking drug.
• Tell patient to check his weight daily and to report weight gain over 2.27 kg (5 lb). Diuretics can relieve sodium and water retention.
• Warn patient that drug may impair mental alertness, particularly at start of therapy. Once-daily dosage at bedtime minimizes daytime drowsiness.
• Tell patient to rise slowly and avoid sudden position changes.
• Tell patient that dry mouth can be relieved with ice chips or sugarless gum or sour hard candy.
• Advise patient that urine may turn dark in bleached toilet bowls.

☑ Evaluation
• Patient's blood pressure is normal.

Reactions may be *common,* uncommon, *life-threatening,* or COMMON AND LIFE-THREATENING.

• Patient does not experience injury as result of drug-induced adverse CNS reactions.
• Patient and family state understanding of drug therapy.

---

methylergonovine maleate
(meth-il-er-goh-NOH-veen MAL-ee-ayt)
Methergine

Pharmacologic class: ergot alkaloid
Therapeutic class: oxytocic
Pregnancy risk category: C

How supplied

Tablets: 0.2 mg
Injection: 0.2 mg/ml

Pharmacokinetics

Absorption: absorption is rapid, with 60% of P.O. dose appearing in blood; unknown after I.M. administration.
Distribution: rapidly distributed in tissues.
Metabolism: extensive first-pass metabolism precedes hepatic metabolism.
Excretion: excreted primarily in feces with small amount in urine.

Route	Onset	Peak	Duration
P.O.	5-10 min	30 min	≥ 3 hr
I.V.	Immediate	Unknown	45 min
I.M.	2-5 min	Unknown	≥ 3 hr

Pharmacodynamics

Chemical effect: increases motor activity of uterus by direct stimulation.
Therapeutic effect: prevents or stops postpartum hemorrhage.

Indications and dosage

▶ **Prevention and treatment of postpartum hemorrhage caused by uterine atony or subinvolution.** *Adults:* 0.2 mg I.M. q 2 to 4 hours; for excessive uterine bleeding or other emergencies, 0.2 mg I.V. over 1 minute while blood pressure and uterine contractions are monitored.

After initial I.M. or I.V. dose, 0.2 to 0.4 mg P.O. q 6 to 12 hours for 2 to 7 days. Dosage is decreased if severe cramping occurs.

Adverse reactions

CNS: dizziness, headache, *seizures; CVA* (with I.V. use).
CV: hypertension, transient chest pain, palpitations, peripheral vasoconstriction, gangrene, thrombophlebitis.
EENT: tinnitus.
GI: *nausea, vomiting.*
Respiratory: dyspnea.
Other: diaphoresis, hypersensitivity reactions, *uterine tetany.*

Interactions

Drug-drug. *Dopamine, I.V. oxytocin, regional anesthetics, vasoconstrictors:* excessive vasoconstriction. Use together cautiously.

Contraindications and precautions

• Contraindicated in patients with hypertension, toxemia, or sensitivity to ergot preparations and in pregnant women.
• Drug is not recommended for use in breast-feeding women.
• Use cautiously in patients with sepsis, obliterative vascular disease, or hepatic or renal disease and during last stage of labor.
• Drug is not indicated for use in children.

NURSING CONSIDERATIONS

⚕ Assessment
• Assess patient's condition before therapy and regularly thereafter.
• Monitor blood pressure, pulse rate, and uterine response; report sudden change in vital signs, frequent periods of uterine relaxation, and character and amount of vaginal bleeding.
• Monitor contractions, which may continue 3 hours or more after P.O. or I.M. administration.

- Be alert for adverse reactions and drug interactions.
- Monitor patient's hydration status if adverse GI reactions occur.
- Evaluate patient's and family's knowledge of drug therapy.

⊞ Nursing diagnoses
- Decreased cardiac output related to postpartum hemorrhage
- Risk for fluid volume deficit related to drug therapy
- Knowledge deficit related to drug therapy

⧈ Planning and implementation
P.O. and I.M. use: Follow normal protocol.
I.V. use: Drug should not be routinely given I.V. because of risk of severe hypertension and CVA. If it must be given I.V., give slowly over 1 minute with careful blood pressure monitoring. I.V. dose may be diluted to 5 ml with 0.9% NaCl solution.
- Store in tightly closed, light-resistant container. Discard if discolored.
- Store I.V. solutions below 46.4° F (8° C). Daily stock may be kept at room temperature for 60 to 90 days.
Patient teaching
- Advise patient to report adverse reactions promptly.

☑ Evaluation
- Patient's bleeding is stopped.
- Patient maintains adequate hydration throughout therapy.
- Patient and family state understanding of drug therapy.

---

methylphenidate hydrochloride
**(meth-il-FEN-ih-dayt
high-droh-KLOR-ighd)**
Ritalin, Ritalin-SR

Pharmacologic class: piperidine CNS stimulant

Therapeutic class: CNS stimulant (analeptic)
Controlled substance schedule: II
Pregnancy risk category: NR

How supplied
Tablets: 5 mg, 10 mg, 20 mg
Tablets (sustained-release): 20 mg

Pharmacokinetics
Absorption: absorbed rapidly and completely.
Distribution: unknown.
Metabolism: metabolized by liver.
Excretion: excreted in urine.

Route	Onset	Peak	Duration
P.O.	Unknown	2-5 hr	Unknown

Pharmacodynamics
Chemical effect: unknown; probably promotes nerve impulse transmission by releasing stored norepinephrine from nerve terminals in brain. Main site of activity appears to be cerebral cortex and reticular activating system. In hyperkinetic children, drug has paradoxical calming effect.
Therapeutic effect: promotes calmness and prevents sleep.

Indications and dosage
▶ **Attention deficit disorder with hyperactivity (ADDH).** *Children age 6 and older:* initial dose, 5 to 10 mg P.O. daily before breakfast and lunch with 5- to 10-mg increments weekly, as needed, up to 60 mg daily.
▶ **Narcolepsy.** *Adults:* 10 mg P.O. b.i.d. or t.i.d. 30 to 45 minutes before meals. Dosage varies with patient needs, but averages 40 to 60 mg/day.

Adverse reactions
CNS: *nervousness, insomnia,* Tourette syndrome, dizziness, headache, akathisia, dyskinesia, *seizures.*
CV: *palpitations,* angina, *tachycardia,* changes in blood pressure and pulse rate.
EENT: dry throat.

Reactions may be *common,* uncommon, *life-threatening,* or COMMON AND LIFE-THREATENING.

GI: nausea, abdominal pain, anorexia, weight loss.
Hematologic: *thrombocytopenia,* thrombocytopenic purpura, *leukopenia.*
Musculoskeletal: delayed growth.
Skin: rash, urticaria, *exfoliative dermatitis, erythema multiforme.*

Interactions

Drug-drug. *Centrally acting antihypertensives:* decreased antihypertensive effect. Monitor blood pressure.
MAO inhibitors: severe hypertension; possible hypertensive crisis. Don't use together or within 14 days after MAO inhibitor has been stopped.
Tricyclic antidepressants: increased plasma levels of these drugs. Avoid concomitant use.
Drug-food. *Caffeine:* may increase amphetamine and related amine effects. Avoid concomitant use

Contraindications and precautions

• Contraindicated in patients with glaucoma, motor tics, family history or diagnosis of Tourette syndrome, hypersensitivity to drug, or history of marked anxiety, tension, or agitation.
• Use cautiously in patients with hypertension, history of drug abuse, seizures, or EEG abnormalities and in pregnant or breast-feeding women.
• Drug is not recommended for use in children younger than age 6.

NURSING CONSIDERATIONS

⚏ Assessment
• Assess patient's condition before therapy and regularly thereafter.
• Know that drug may precipitate Tourette syndrome in children. Monitor especially at start of therapy.
• Observe for signs of excessive stimulation. Monitor blood pressure.
• Monitor results of periodic CBC, differential, and platelet counts with long-term use.

• Monitor height and weight in child on prolonged therapy. Drug may delay growth spurt, but child will attain normal height when drug is stopped.
• Monitor patient for tolerance or psychological dependence.
• Be alert for adverse reactions and drug interactions.
• Evaluate patient's and family's knowledge of drug therapy.

⊞ Nursing diagnoses
• Altered health maintenance related to underlying condition
• Sleep pattern disturbance related to drug-induced insomnia
• Knowledge deficit related to drug therapy

❱ Planning and implementation
• Drug of choice for ADDH. It is usually discontinued after puberty.
• Know that drug should not be used to prevent fatigue.
• Give at least 6 hours before bedtime to prevent insomnia. Give after meals to reduce appetite suppression.
• Ritalin SR tablets have a duration of about 8 hours and may be used in place of regular tablets when the 8-hour dosage of the SR tablets corresponds to the titrated dosage of the regular tablets.
Patient teaching
• Tell patient to swallow Ritalin SR tablets whole. Do not chew or crush them.
• Caution patient to avoid activities that require alertness until CNS effects of drug are known.
• Tell patient to avoid caffeine.
• Advise patient with seizure disorder to notify doctor if seizure occurs.
• Inform patient that he will need more rest as drug effects wear off.

☑ Evaluation
• Patient exhibits positive response to drug therapy.
• Patient does not experience insomnia during therapy.

• Patient and family state understanding of drug therapy.

methylprednisolone
(meth-il-pred-NIS-uh-lohn)
Medrol**, Meprolone

methylprednisolone acetate
depMedalone 40, depMedalone 80, Depoject-40, Depoject-80, Depo-Medrol, Depopred-40, Depopred-80, Depo-Predate 40, Depo-Predate 80, Duralone-40, Duralone-80, Medralone-40, Medralone-80

methylprednisolone sodium succinate
A-methaPred, Solu-Medrol

Pharmacologic class: glucocorticoid
Therapeutic class: anti-inflammatory, immunosuppressant
Pregnancy risk category: NR

How supplied
methylprednisolone
Tablets: 2 mg, 4 mg, 8 mg, 16 mg, 24 mg, 32 mg
methylprednisolone acetate
Injection (suspension): 20 mg/ml, 40 mg/ml, 80 mg/ml
methylprednisolone sodium succinate
Injection: 40 mg/vial, 125 mg/vial, 500 mg/vial, 1,000 mg/vial, 2,000 mg/vial

Pharmacokinetics
Absorption: absorbed readily after P.O. administration; unknown after I.M. administration.
Distribution: distributed rapidly to muscle, liver, skin, intestines, and kidneys.
Metabolism: metabolized in liver.
Excretion: excreted primarily in urine; insignificant amount excreted in feces.
Half-life: 18 to 36 hours.

Route	Onset	Peak	Duration
P.O.	Rapid	1-2 hr	30-36 hr
I.V.	Immediate	Immediate	Unknown
I.M.	6-48 hr	4-8 days	1-4 wk

Pharmacodynamics
Chemical effect: not clear; decreases inflammation, mainly by stabilizing leukocyte lysosomal membranes. Drug also suppresses immune response, stimulates bone marrow, and influences protein, fat, and carbohydrate metabolism.
Therapeutic effect: relieves inflammation and suppresses immune system function.

Indications and dosage
▶ **Severe inflammation or immunosuppression. Methylprednisolone.** *Adults:* 2 to 60 mg P.O. daily in four divided doses. **Methylprednisolone acetate.** *Adults:* 10 to 80 mg I.M. daily, or 4 to 80 mg into joint or soft tissue, p.r.n.
Methylprednisolone succinate. *Adults:* 10 to 250 mg I.M. or I.V. q 4 hours.
Children: 0.03 to 0.2 mg/kg or 1 to 6.25 mg/m² I.M. or I.V. daily in divided doses.
▶ **Shock. Methylprednisolone succinate.** *Adults:* 100 to 250 mg I.V. at 2- to 6-hour intervals; or 30 mg/kg I.V. initially, repeated q 4 to 6 hours, p.r.n. Continue therapy for 2 to 3 days or until patient is stable.

Adverse reactions
Most adverse reactions are dose- or duration-dependent.
CNS: *euphoria, insomnia,* psychotic behavior, pseudotumor cerebri.
CV: *heart failure,* hypertension, edema, *thromboembolism, fatal arrest or circulatory collapse* (after rapid administration of large I.V. doses).
EENT: cataracts, glaucoma.
GI: *peptic ulceration,* GI irritation, increased appetite, pancreatitis.
Metabolic: hypokalemia, hyperglycemia, and carbohydrate intolerance.

Reactions may be *common,* uncommon, *life-threatening*, or COMMON AND LIFE-THREATENING.

Musculoskeletal: muscle weakness, osteoporosis, growth suppression in children.
Skin: hirsutism, delayed wound healing, acne, various skin eruptions.
Other: susceptibility to infections; *acute adrenal insufficiency may occur with increased stress (infection, surgery, or trauma) or abrupt withdrawal after long-term therapy.*
After abrupt withdrawal: rebound inflammation, fatigue, weakness, arthralgia, fever, dizziness, lethargy, depression, fainting, orthostatic hypotension, dyspnea, anorexia, hypoglycemia. *After prolonged use, sudden withdrawal may be fatal.*

Interactions

Drug-drug. *Aspirin, indomethacin, other NSAIDs:* increased risk of GI distress and bleeding. Give together cautiously.
Barbiturates, phenytoin, rifampin: decreased corticosteroid effect. Increase corticosteroid dosage, as ordered.
Oral anticoagulants: altered dosage requirements. Monitor PT closely.
Potassium-depleting drugs (such as thiazide diuretics): enhanced potassium-wasting effects of methylprednisolone. Monitor serum potassium level.
Skin-test antigens: decreased response. Defer skin testing until therapy is completed.
Toxoids, vaccines: decreased antibody response and increased risk of neurologic complications. Avoid concomitant use.

Contraindications and precautions

● Contraindicated in patients allergic to drug or its components, in those with systemic fungal infections, and in premature infants (acetate and succinate).
● Use cautiously in patients with GI ulceration or renal disease, hypertension, osteoporosis, diabetes mellitus, hypothyroidism, cirrhosis, diverticulitis, nonspecific ulcerative colitis, recent intestinal anastomoses, thromboembolic disorders,

seizures, myasthenia gravis, heart failure, tuberculosis, ocular herpes simplex, emotional instability, or psychotic tendencies and in pregnant women.
● Use of drug is not recommended in breast-feeding women.

NURSING CONSIDERATIONS

☲ Assessment
● Assess patient's condition before therapy and regularly thereafter.
● Watch for enhanced response in patient with hypothyroidism or cirrhosis.
● Monitor patient's weight, blood pressure, serum electrolyte levels, and sleep patterns. Euphoria may initially interfere with sleep, but patient generally adjusts to drug after 1 to 3 weeks.
● Be alert for adverse reactions and drug interactions.
● Evaluate patient's and family's knowledge of drug therapy.

⊞ Nursing diagnoses
● Altered health maintenance related to underlying condition
● Risk for injury related to drug-induced adverse reactions
● Knowledge deficit related to drug therapy

⧁ Planning and implementation
● Know that drug may be used for alternate-day therapy.
● For better results and less risk of toxicity, give once-daily dose in morning.
P.O. use: Give P.O. dose with food when possible. Critically ill patients may require concomitant antacid or H_2-receptor antagonist therapy.
I.V. use: Give only methylprednisolone sodium succinate; never give acetate form I.V. Reconstitute according to manufacturer's directions using supplied diluent or bacteriostatic water for injection with benzyl alcohol.
– For direct injection, inject diluted drug into vein or I.V. line containing free-flowing compatible solution over at least

---

*Liquid form contains alcohol   **May contain tartrazine   ◆Canada   ◇Australia   †OTC

1 minute. For treatment of shock, give massive doses over at least 10 minutes to prevent arrhythmias and circulatory collapse. When giving as intermittent or continuous infusion, dilute solution according to manufacturer's instructions and give over prescribed duration. If used for continuous infusion, change solution every 24 hours.
– Compatible solutions include D₅W, 0.9% NaCl, and dextrose 5% in 0.9% NaCl.

I.M. use: Give I.M. injection deeply into gluteal muscle.
– Dermal atrophy may occur with large doses of acetate salt. Use multiple small injections rather than single large dose and rotate injection sites.
• Avoid S.C. injection because atrophy and sterile abscesses may occur.
• Do not confuse Solu-Medrol with Solu-Cortef (hydrocortisone sodium succinate).
• Know that manufacturers of Solu-Medrol state that drug should not be given intrathecally because severe adverse reactions have been reported.
• Don't use acetate salt when immediate onset of action is needed.
• Discard reconstituted solutions after 48 hours.
• Always titrate to lowest effective dose, as ordered.
• Administer potassium supplements, as needed.
• Gradually reduce drug dosage after long-term therapy, as ordered.

Patient teaching
• Tell patient not to discontinue drug abruptly or without doctor's consent.
• Teach patient signs of early adrenal insufficiency: fatigue, muscle weakness, joint pain, fever, anorexia, nausea, dyspnea, dizziness, and fainting.
• Instruct patient to carry a medical identification card.
• Warn patient on long-term therapy about cushingoid symptoms, and tell him to report sudden weight gain or swelling. Suggest exercise or physical therapy and

advise asking doctor about vitamin D or calcium supplements.

✓ Evaluation
• Patient exhibits positive response to drug therapy.
• Patient does not experience injury from adverse reactions.
• Patient and family state understanding of drug therapy.

---

metoclopramide hydrochloride
(met-oh-KLOH-preh-mighd high-droh-KLOR-ighd)
Apo-Metoclop♦, Clopra, Maxeran♦, Maxolon, Octamide, Octamide PFS, Pramin◊, Reclomide, Reglan

Pharmacologic class: para-aminobenzoic acid derivative
Therapeutic class: antiemetic, GI stimulant
Pregnancy risk category: B

How supplied
Tablets: 5 mg, 10 mg
Syrup: 5 mg/5 ml
Injection: 5 mg/ml

Pharmacokinetics
Absorption: after P.O. dose, absorbed rapidly and completely from GI tract; after I.M. dose, about 74% to 96% bioavailable.
Distribution: distributed to most body tissues and fluids, including brain.
Metabolism: not metabolized extensively; small amount metabolized in liver.
Excretion: excreted in urine and feces.
Half-life: 4 to 6 hours.

Route	Onset	Peak	Duration
P.O.	30-60 min	1-2 hr	1-2 hr
I.V.	1-3 min	Unknown	1-2 hr
I.M.	10-15 min	Unknown	1-2 hr

Pharmacodynamics
Chemical effect: stimulates motility of upper GI tract by increasing lower

esophageal sphincter tone and blocks dopamine receptors at chemoreceptor trigger zone.
Therapeutic effect: prevents or minimizes nausea and vomiting from chemotherapy or surgery. Also reduces gag reflex in small-bowel intubation and radiologic examinations, improves gastric emptying when diabetic gastroparesis is present, and reduces gastric reflux.

Indications and dosage

► **Prevention or reduction of nausea and vomiting induced by cisplatin and other chemotherapeutic agents.** *Adults:* 1 to 2 mg/kg I.V. 30 minutes before chemotherapy, then repeated q 2 hours for two doses, then q 3 hours for three doses.
► **Prevention or reduction of postoperative nausea and vomiting.** *Adults:* 10 to 20 mg I.M. near end of surgical procedure, repeated q 4 to 6 hours, p.r.n.
► **To facilitate small-bowel intubation and aid in radiologic examinations.** *Adults and children over age 14:* 10 mg (2 ml) I.V. as single dose over 1 to 2 minutes. *Children ages 6 to 14:* 2.5 to 5.0 mg I.V. (0.5 to 1.0 ml). *Children under age 6:* 0.1 mg/kg I.V.
► **Delayed gastric emptying secondary to diabetic gastroparesis.** *Adults:* 10 mg P.O. for mild symptoms; slow I.V. for severe symptoms 30 minutes before meals and h.s. for 2 to 8 weeks, depending on response.
► **Gastroesophageal reflux disease.** *Adults:* 10 to 15 mg P.O. q.i.d., p.r.n., 30 minutes before meals and h.s.

Adverse reactions

CNS: *restlessness, anxiety, drowsiness,* fatigue, *lassitude,* insomnia, *suicide ideation, seizures,* headache, dizziness, extrapyramidal symptoms, tardive dyskinesia, dystonic reactions, sedation.
CV: transient hypertension.
GI: nausea, bowel disturbances.
Hematologic: *agranulocytosis, neutropenia.*

Skin: rash.
Other: fever, prolactin secretion, loss of libido.

Interactions

Drug-drug. *Anticholinergics, opioid analgesics:* antagonize GI motility effects of metoclopramide. Use together cautiously.
Butyrophenones, phenothiazines: increased risk of extrapyramidal effects. Monitor patient closely.
CNS depressants: additive CNS depression. Avoid concomitant use.
Drug-lifestyle. *Alcohol use:* additive CNS depression. Avoid concomitant use

Contraindications and precautions

• Contraindicated in patients in whom stimulation of GI motility might be dangerous (such as those with hemorrhage) and in those with pheochromocytoma, seizure disorder, or hypersensitivity to drug.
• Use cautiously in patients with history of depression, Parkinson's disease, or hypertension and in pregnant or breastfeeding women.
• Safety and effectiveness have not been established for therapy that lasts over 12 weeks.

NURSING CONSIDERATIONS

⬛ Assessment
• Assess patient's condition before therapy and regularly thereafter.
• Monitor blood pressure frequently in patient receiving I.V. form of drug.
• Be alert for adverse reactions and drug interactions.
• Evaluate patient's and family's knowledge of drug therapy.

⬛ Nursing diagnoses
• Risk for fluid volume deficit related to nausea and vomiting
• Risk for injury related to drug-induced adverse CNS reactions

• Knowledge deficit related to drug therapy

⧉ Planning and implementation
P.O. use: Follow normal protocol. Dilute oral concentrate just before administration in water, juice, or carbonated beverage. Semisolid food such as applesauce ans pudding also may be used.
I.V. use: Give lower doses (10 mg or less) by direct injection over 1 to 2 minutes. Dilute doses larger than 10 mg in 50 ml of compatible diluent and infuse over at least 15 minutes. Protection from light is unnecessary if infusion mixture is given within 24 hours.
– Know that drug is compatible with D_5W, 0.9% NaCl injection, and dextrose 5% in 0.45% NaCl.
• Diphenhydramine 25 mg I.V. counteracts extrapyramidal effects associated with high drug doses.
I.M. use: Commercially available preparation may be used for I.M. injection without further dilution.
Patient teaching
• Instruct patient to avoid alcohol consumption during drug therapy.
• Advise patient to avoid activities requiring alertness for 2 hours after taking each dose.

☑ Evaluation
• Patient responds positively to drug and does not develop fluid volume deficit.
• Patient does not experience injury from adverse reactions.
• Patient and family state understanding of drug therapy.

---

metolazone
(meh-TOH-luh-zohn)
Mykrox, Zaroxolyn**

Pharmacologic class: quinazoline derivative (thiazide-like) diuretic

Therapeutic class: diuretic, antihypertensive
Pregnancy risk category: B

How supplied
Tablets (extended): 2.5 mg, 5 mg, 10 mg
Tablets (prompt): 0.5 mg

Pharmacokinetics
Absorption: about 65% absorbed in healthy subjects; in cardiac patients, absorption falls to 40%. Rate and extent vary among preparations.
Distribution: 50% to 70% erythrocyte-bound; 33% protein-bound.
Metabolism: insignificant.
Excretion: 70% to 95% excreted unchanged in urine. *Half-life:* about 14 hours.

Route	Onset	Peak	Duration
P.O.	1 hr	2-8 hr	12-24 hr

Pharmacodynamics
Chemical effect: increases sodium and water excretion by inhibiting sodium reabsorption in cortical diluting site of ascending loop of Henle.
Therapeutic effect: promotes water and sodium elimination and lowers blood pressure.

Indications and dosage
▶ **Edema in heart failure or renal disease.** *Adults:* 5 to 20 mg (extended) P.O. daily.
▶ **Hypertension.** *Adults:* 2.5 to 5.0 mg (extended) P.O. daily. Maintenance dosage determined by patient's blood pressure. Alternatively, 0.5 mg (prompt) P.O. once daily in morning, increased to 1 mg P.O. daily, p.r.n. If response is inadequate, another antihypertensive agent is added.

Adverse reactions
CNS: dizziness, headache, fatigue.
CV: volume depletion and dehydration, orthostatic hypotension.
GI: anorexia, nausea, pancreatitis.

Reactions may be *common*, uncommon, *life-threatening*, or COMMON AND LIFE-THREATENING.

GU: nocturia, polyuria, frequent urination.
Hematologic: *aplastic anemia, agranulocytosis, leukopenia, thrombocytopenia.*
Hepatic: hepatic encephalopathy.
Skin: dermatitis, photosensitivity, rash.
Other: a symptomatic hyperuricemia; hyperglycemia and glucose tolerance impairment; fluid and electrolyte imbalances, including hypokalemia, dilutional hyponatremia and hypochloremia, metabolic alkalosis, hypercalcemia; gout; muscle cramps, swelling; hypersensitivity reactions (such as pneumonitis, vasculitis).

Interactions
Drug-drug. *Barbiturates, opioids:* increased orthostatic hypotensive effect. Monitor patient closely.
Cardiac glycosides: increased risk of digitalis toxicity from metolazone-induced hypokalemia. Monitor potassium and digitalis levels.
Cholestyramine, colestipol: decreased intestinal absorption of thiazides. Separate doses.
Diazoxide: increased antihypertensive, hyperglycemic, and hyperuricemic effects. Use together cautiously.
Lithium: decreased lithium clearance, increasing risk of lithium toxicity. Monitor lithium level.
NSAIDs: increased risk of NSAID-induced renal failure. Monitor patient for signs of renal failure.
Drug-lifestyle. *Alcohol use:* increased orthostatic hypotensive effect. Take appropriate precautions.
Sun exposure: photosensitivity reactions may occur. Take appropriate precautions.

Contraindications and precautions
• Contraindicated in patients with anuria, hepatic coma or precoma, or hypersensitivity to thiazides or other sulfonamide-derived drugs.
• Use of drug is not recommended in pregnant women.

• Use cautiously in patients with impaired kidney or liver function.
• Safety of drug has not been established in breast-feeding women and in children.

NURSING CONSIDERATIONS

⚕ Assessment
• Assess patient's condition before therapy and regularly thereafter. In hypertensive patients, therapeutic response may be delayed several days.
• Unlike thiazide diuretics, drug is effective in patient with decreased kidney function.
• Monitor fluid intake and output, weight, blood pressure, and serum electrolyte levels.
• Monitor blood uric acid levels, especially in patient with history of gout.
• Be alert for adverse reactions and drug interactions.
• Evaluate patient's and family's knowledge of drug therapy.

⊞ Nursing diagnoses
• Fluid volume excess related to presence of edema
• Risk for injury related to presence of hypertension
• Knowledge deficit related to drug therapy

▶ Planning and implementation
• Give drug in morning to prevent nocturia.
• Mykrox (prompt) tablets are more rapidly and completely absorbed than other brands mimicking oral solution. Do not interchange Mykrox with Zaroxolyn (extended) tablets.
• Know that drug may be used with potassium-sparing diuretic to prevent potassium loss.
• Be aware that drug is used as adjunct in furosemide-resistant edema.
Patient teaching
• Advise patient to avoid sudden posture changes and to rise slowly to avoid orthostatic hypotension.

---

*Liquid form contains alcohol   **May contain tartrazine   ◆Canada   ◇Australia   †OTC

- Advise patient to wear protective clothing, avoid prolonged exposure to sun and to use sunblock to prevent photosensitivity reactions.
- Instruct patient to avoid alcohol consumption during drug therapy.

☑ Evaluation
- Patient does not have edema.
- Patient's blood pressure is normal.
- Patient and family state understanding of drug therapy.

metoprolol succinate
(meh-TOH-pruh-lol SUHK-seh-nayt)
Toprol-XL

metoprolol tartrate
(meh-TOH-pruh-lol TAR-trayt)
Apo-Metoprolol♦, Apo-Metoprolol (Type L)♦, Betaloc♦◇, Betaloc Durules♦, Lopresor♦, Lopresor SR♦, Lopresor, Minax◇, Novo-Metoprol♦, Nu-Metop♦

Pharmacologic class: beta blocker
Therapeutic class: antihypertensive, adjunct treatment of acute MI
Pregnancy risk category: C

How supplied

metoprolol succinate
Tablets (extended-release): 50 mg, 100 mg, 200 mg
metoprolol tartrate
Tablets: 50 mg, 100 mg
Tablets (extended-release): 100 mg♦, 200 mg♦
Injection: 1 mg/ml in 5-ml ampules

Pharmacokinetics

Absorption: absorbed rapidly and almost completely from GI tract with oral administration; food enhances absorption.
Distribution: distributed widely throughout body; about 12% bound.
Metabolism: metabolized in liver.
Excretion: about 95% excreted in urine.
Half-life: 3 to 7 hours.

Route	Onset	Peak	Duration
P.O.	≤ 15 min	1-12 hr	6-24 hr
I.V.	≤ 5 min	20 min	5-8 hr

Pharmacodynamics

Chemical effect: unknown for antihypertensive action. Drug decreases myocardial contractility, heart rate, and cardiac output; lowers blood pressure; and reduces myocardial oxygen consumption. It also depresses renin secretion.
Therapeutic effect: reduces blood pressure and anginal pain and helps to prevent myocardial tissue damage.

Indications and dosage

▶ **Hypertension. Metoprolol succinate.** *Adults:* initially, 100 to 150 mg (extended-release tablets) P.O. once daily. Dosage is adjusted as needed and tolerated at intervals of not less than 1 week to maximum of 400 mg daily. **Metoprolol tartrate.** *Adults:* 100 mg P.O. daily in single or divided doses; usual maintenance dosage is 100 to 450 mg daily.

▶ **Early intervention in acute MI. Metoprolol tartrate.** *Adults:* three 5-mg I.V. boluses q 2 minutes. Then, beginning 15 minutes after last dose, 25 to 50 mg P.O. q 6 hours for 48 hours. Maintenance dosage is 100 mg P.O. b.i.d. for 3 months to 3 years.

▶ **Angina pectoris. Metoprolol succinate.** *Adults:* initially, 100 mg (extended-release tablets) P.O. daily as single dose. Dosage increased at weekly intervals until adequate response or pronounced decrease in heart rate is seen. Daily dosage beyond 400 mg has not been studied. **Metoprolol tartrate.** *Adults:* 100 mg P.O. in two divided doses. Dosage increased at weekly intervals until adequate response or pronounced decrease in heart rate is seen. Maintenance dosage is 100 to 400 mg/day.

Adverse reactions

CNS: fatigue, lethargy, dizziness.

Reactions may be *common*, uncommon, *life-threatening*, or COMMON AND LIFE-THREATENING.

CV: *bradycardia, hypotension, heart failure, AV block,* peripheral vascular disease.
GI: nausea, vomiting, diarrhea.
Respiratory: dyspnea, *bronchospasm.*
Skin: rash.
Other: fever, arthralgia.

Interactions

Drug-drug. *Barbiturates, rifampin:* increased metabolism of metoprolol. Monitor for decreased effect.
Cardiac glycosides, diltiazem, verapamil: excessive bradycardia and increased depressant effect on myocardium. Use together cautiously.
Chlorpromazine, cimetidine, verapamil: decreased hepatic clearance. Monitor for greater beta-blocking effect.
Hydralazine: serum levels and, hence, pharmacologic effects of beta blockers and hydralazine may be enhanced. Monitor patient closely.
Indomethacin: decreased antihypertensive effect. Monitor blood pressure and adjust dosage.
Insulin, oral antidiabetic agents: can alter dosage requirements in previously stabilized diabetic patients. Observe patient carefully.
MAO inhibitors: bradycardia may develop during concurrent use. Monitor ECG and patient closely.
Drug-food. *Any food:* may increase absorption. Give together.

Contraindications and precautions

• Contraindicated in patients with hypersensitivity to drug or other beta blockers and in those with sinus bradycardia, heart block greater than first-degree, cardiogenic shock, or overt cardiac failure when used to treat hypertension or angina. When used to treat MI, drug is also contraindicated in patients with heart rate below 45 beats/minute, second- or third-degree heart block, PR interval of 0.24 second or more with first-degree heart block, systolic blood pressure under 100 mm Hg, or moderate to severe cardiac failure.
• Drug is not recommended for use in breast-feeding women.
• Use cautiously in patients with heart failure, diabetes, or respiratory or hepatic disease and in pregnant women.
• Safety of drug has not been established in children.

NURSING CONSIDERATIONS

⚖ Assessment
• Assess patient's condition before therapy and regularly thereafter.
• Monitor blood pressure frequently. Drug masks common signs of shock.
• Be alert for adverse reactions and drug interactions.
• Evaluate patient's and family's knowledge of drug therapy.

⊕ Nursing diagnoses
• Altered health maintenance related to underlying disorder
• Risk for injury related to drug-induced adverse CNS reactions
• Knowledge deficit related to drug therapy

❯ Planning and implementation
• Always check patient's apical pulse rate before giving drug. If it's slower than 60 beats/minute, withhold drug and call doctor immediately.
P.O. use: Give drug with meals because food may increase absorption.
I.V. use: Give drug undiluted by direct injection. Although mixing with other drugs should be avoided, studies have shown that metoprolol is compatible when mixed with meperidine hydrochloride or morphine sulfate or when administered with alteplase infusions at Y-site connection.
• Store drug at room temperature and protect from light. Discard solution if discolored or contains particles.

Patient teaching

• Tell patient that abrupt discontinuation of therapy can exacerbate angina and precipitate MI. Withdraw drug gradually over 1 to 2 weeks.

• Instruct patient to take oral form of drug with meals to enhance absorption.

• Advise patient to report adverse reactions to doctor.

• Warn patient to avoid performing hazardous activities until CNS effects of drug are known.

☑ **Evaluation**

• Patient responds well to therapy.

• Patient does not experience injury from adverse CNS reactions.

• Patient and family state understanding of drug therapy.

---

metronidazole

(met-roh-NIGH-duh-zohl)
Apo-Metronidazole♦, Flagyl, Metric 21, Metrogyl◇, Metrozine◇, Novo-Nidazol♦, Protostat, Trikacide♦

metronidazole hydrochloride

Flagyl I.V. RTU, Metro I.V., Novo-Nidazol♦

Pharmacologic class: nitroimidazole
Therapeutic class: antibacterial, antiprotozoal, amebicide
Pregnancy risk category: B

How supplied

Capsules: 375 mg
Tablets: 200 mg◇, 250 mg, 400 mg◇, 500 mg
Oral suspension (benzoyl metronidazole): 200 mg/5 ml◇
Injection: 500 mg/100 ml
Powder for injection: 500-mg single-dose vials

Pharmacokinetics

Absorption: about 80% of P.O. dose absorbed; food delays peak concentrations to about 2 hours.

Distribution: distributed in most body tissues and fluids; less than 20% bound to plasma proteins.
Metabolism: metabolized to active metabolite and to other metabolites.
Excretion: excreted primarily in urine; 6% to 15% in feces. *Half-life:* 6 to 8 hours (may be longer in patients with impaired liver function).

Route	Onset	Peak	Duration
P.O.	Unknown	1-2 hr	Unknown
I.V.	Immediate	Immediate	Unknown

Pharmacodynamics

Chemical effect: direct-acting trichomonacide and amebicide that works at both intestinal and extraintestinal sites.
Therapeutic effect: hinders growth of selected organisms. Spectrum of activity includes most anaerobic bacteria and protozoa, including *Bacteroides fragilis, Bacteroides melaninogenicus, Balantidium coli, Clostridium, Entamoeba histolytica, Fusobacterium, Giardia lamblia, Peptococcus, Peptostreptococcus, Trichomonas vaginalis,* and *Veillonella.*

Indications and dosage

▶ **Amebic hepatic abscess.** *Adults:* 500 to 750 mg P.O. t.i.d. for 5 to 10 days. *Children:* 35 to 50 mg/kg daily (in three doses) for 10 days.

▶ **Intestinal amebiasis.** *Adults:* 750 mg P.O. t.i.d. for 5 to 10 days. *Children:* 35 to 50 mg/kg daily (in three doses) for 10 days. Therapy followed with oral iodoquinol.

▶ **Trichomoniasis.** *Adults:* 375 mg P.O. b.i.d. for 7 days or 2 g P.O. in single dose (may give 2-g dose in two 1-g doses on same day); 4 to 6 weeks should elapse between courses of therapy. *Children:* 5 mg/kg dose P.O. t.i.d. for 7 days.

▶ **Refractory trichomoniasis.** *Adults:* 500 mg P.O. b.i.d. for 10 days.

▶ **Bacterial infections caused by anaerobic microorganisms.** *Adults:* loading dose is 15 mg/kg I.V. infused over 1 hour

---

(about 1 g for 70-kg [154-lb] adult). Maintenance dosage is 7.5 mg/kg I.V. or P.O. q 6 hours (about 500 mg for 70-kg adult). First maintenance dose should be given 6 hours after loading dose. Maximum dosage not to exceed 4 g daily.
▶ **Prevention of postoperative infection in contaminated or potentially contaminated colorectal surgery.** *Adults:* 15 mg/kg I.V. infused over 30 to 60 minutes and completed about 1 hour before surgery. Then, 7.5 mg/kg I.V. infused over 30 to 60 minutes at 6 and 12 hours after initial dose.

Adverse reactions

CNS: vertigo, headache, ataxia, incoordination, confusion, irritability, depression, restlessness, weakness, fatigue, drowsiness, insomnia, sensory neuropathy, paresthesias of extremities, psychic stimulation, *seizures,* neuropathy.
CV: ECG change (flattened T wave), edema (with I.V. RTU preparation).
GI: abdominal cramping, stomatitis, *nausea, vomiting, anorexia,* diarrhea, constipation, proctitis, dry mouth, metallic taste.
GU: darkened urine, polyuria, dysuria, pyuria, incontinence, cystitis, decreased libido, gynecomastia, dyspareunia, dryness of vagina and vulva, sense of pelvic pressure.
Hematologic: transient leukopenia, *neutropenia.*
Skin: pruritus, flushing, rash.
Other: overgrowth of nonsusceptible organisms, especially *Candida* (glossitis, furry tongue), fever; thrombophlebitis (after I.V. infusion).

Interactions

Drug-drug. *Cimetidine:* increased risk of metronidazole toxicity because of inhibited hepatic metabolism. Monitor patient.
Disulfiram: acute psychoses and confusional states. Don't use together.
Lithium: increased lithium levels, possibly resulting in toxicity. Monitor serum lithium levels closely.

Oral anticoagulants: increased anticoagulant effects. Monitor patient.
Phenobarbital, phenytoin: decreased metronidazole effectiveness because of increased hepatic clearance. Monitor patient closely.
Drug-lifestyle. *Alcohol use:* disulfiram-like reaction (nausea, vomiting, headache, cramps, flushing). Don't use together.

Contraindications and precautions

• Contraindicated in patients with hypersensitivity to drug or other nitroimidazole derivatives.
• Drug is not recommended for use in breast-feeding women.
• Use cautiously with known hepatotoxic drugs and in patients with history of blood dyscrasia or CNS disorder, retinal or visual field changes, hepatic disease, or alcoholism.

NURSING CONSIDERATIONS

▣ Assessment

• Assess patient's infection before therapy and regularly thereafter.
• Observe carefully for edema, especially in patients also receiving corticosteroids, because Flagyl I.V. RTU may cause sodium retention.
• Record number and character of stools when used in amebiasis.
• Be alert for adverse reactions and drug interactions.
• Evaluate patient's and family's understanding of drug therapy.

▣ Nursing diagnoses

• Infection related to presence of susceptible organisms
• Risk for fluid volume deficit related to drug-induced adverse GI reactions
• Knowledge deficit related to drug therapy

▶ Planning and implementation

• Be aware that metronidazole should be used only after *T. vaginalis* has been confirmed by wet smear or culture or *E. histolytica* has been identified.

Asymptomatic sexual partners of patients being treated for *T. vaginalis* infection should be treated simultaneously to avoid reinfection.

• If indicated during pregnancy for trichomoniasis, be aware that 7-day regimen is preferred over 2-g single-dose regimen.

P.O. use: Give drug with meals to minimize GI distress.

I.V. use: No preparation is necessary for RTU (ready to use). To prepare lyophilized vials of metronidazole, add 4.4 ml of sterile water for injection, bacteriostatic water for injection, sterile 0.9% NaCl injection, or bacteriostatic 0.9% NaCl injection. Reconstituted drug contains 100 mg/ml. Add contents of vial to 100 ml of D_5W, lactated Ringer's injection, or 0.9% NaCl for final concentration of 5 mg/ml. Resulting highly acidic solution must be neutralized before administering. Carefully add 5 mEq of sodium bicarbonate for each 500 mg of metronidazole. Carbon dioxide will form and may need to be vented.

– Infuse drug over at least 1 hour. Don't give I.V. push.

– Don't refrigerate neutralized diluted solution. Precipitation may occur. If Flagyl I.V. RTU is refrigerated, crystals may form. These will disappear after solution is gently warmed to room temperature.

Patient teaching

• Tell patient to avoid alcohol or alcohol-containing medications during therapy and for at least 48 hours after therapy is completed.

• Tell patient that metallic taste and dark or red-brown urine may occur.

• Instruct patient to take oral form with meals to minimize reactions.

• Instruct patient in proper hygiene.

☑ Evaluation

• Patient is free from infection.

• Patient maintains adequate hydration throughout therapy.

• Patient and family state understanding of drug therapy.

mexiletine hydrochloride
(MEKS-il-eh-teen high-droh-KLOR-ighd)
Mexitil

Pharmacologic class: lidocaine analogue, sodium channel antagonist
Therapeutic class: ventricular antiarrhythmic
Pregnancy risk category: C

How supplied

Capsules: 50 mg◊, 100 mg♦, 150 mg, 200 mg, 250 mg
Injection: 250 mg/10 ml◊

Pharmacokinetics

Absorption: about 90% absorbed from GI tract after oral use.
Distribution: distributed widely throughout body. Distribution volume declines in patients with liver disease, resulting in toxic serum drug levels with usual doses. About 50% to 60% of circulating drug is bound to plasma proteins.
Metabolism: most of drug metabolized in liver.
Excretion: excreted in urine. *Half-life:* 10 to 12 hours.

Route	Onset	Peak	Duration
P.O.	0.5-2 hr	2-3 hr	Unknown
I.V.	Immediate	Immediate	Unknown

Pharmacodynamics

Chemical effect: class Ib antiarrhythmic that blocks fast sodium channel in cardiac tissues, especially Purkinje network, without involvement of autonomic nervous system. Drug reduces rate of rise and amplitude of action potential and decreases automaticity in Purkinje fibers. It also shortens action potential and, to a

lesser extent, decreases effective refractory period in Purkinje fibers.
Therapeutic effect: abolishes ventricular arrhythmias.

Indications and dosage

▶ **Refractory life-threatening ventricular arrhythmias, including ventricular tachycardia and PVCs.** *Adults:* 200 to 400 mg P.O., followed by 200 mg q 8 hours. Dose increased q 2 to 3 days to 400 mg q 8 hours if satisfactory control is not obtained. Patients who respond well to every-12-hour schedule may be given up to 450 mg q 12 hours. Maximum daily dosage should not exceed 1,200 mg.
Where available, mexiletine may be given I.V. ◊ *Adults:* loading dose is 100 to 250 mg I.V. at rate of 25 mg/minute. Then prepare infusion solution of 250 mg of mexiletine in 500 ml of D$_5$W, and administer first 120 ml (60 mg) over 1 hour. If clinical response is inadequate, give another bolus of 200 mg over 10 to 20 minutes. Maintenance dosage is 0.5 mg/ minute (1 ml/minute of prepared solution).

Adverse reactions

CNS: *tremors, dizziness,* blurred vision, ataxia, diplopia, confusion, nystagmus, nervousness, headache.
CV: hypotension, bradycardia, widened QRS complex, *new or worsened arrhythmias,* palpitations, chest pain.
GI: nausea, vomiting.
Skin: rash.

Interactions

Drug-drug. *Antacids, atropine, narcotics:* slowed mexiletine absorption. Monitor patient.
Cimetidine: increased or decreased mexiletine blood levels. Monitor patient carefully.
Methylxanthines (such as caffeine, theophylline): reduced clearance of methylxanthines, possibly resulting in toxicity. Monitor patient.

Metoclopramide: mexiletine absorption may be accelerated. Monitor for toxicity.
Phenobarbital, phenytoin, rifampin, urine acidifiers: decreased mexiletine blood levels. Monitor patient.
Urine alkalinizers: increased mexiletine blood levels. Monitor patient.

Contraindications and precautions

• Contraindicated in patients with cardiogenic shock or preexisting second- or third-degree AV block in absence of artificial pacemaker.
• Drug is not recommended for use in breast-feeding women.
• Use cautiously in patients with preexisting first-degree heart block, ventricular pacemaker, preexisting sinus node dysfunction, intraventricular conduction disturbances, hypotension, severe heart failure, or seizure disorder and in pregnant women.
• Safety of drug has not been established in children.

NURSING CONSIDERATIONS

Assessment
• Assess patient's condition until arrhythmia is abolished.
• Monitor drug levels, as ordered. Therapeutic levels range from 0.75 to 2.0 mcg/ml.
• Be alert for adverse reactions and drug interactions.
• Monitor for toxicity. An early sign is tremors, usually fine tremor of hands. This progresses to dizziness and later to ataxia and nystagmus as drug's blood level increases. Question patient about these symptoms.
• Monitor patient's hydration status if adverse GI reactions occur.
• Evaluate patient's and family's knowledge of drug therapy.

Nursing diagnoses
• Decreased cardiac output related to presence of ventricular arrhythmia

---

• Risk for fluid volume deficit related to drug-induced adverse GI reactions
• Knowledge deficit related to drug therapy

⧉ Planning and implementation
• When changing from lidocaine to mexiletine, stop lidocaine infusion when first mexiletine dose is given. Keep infusion line open, however, until arrhythmia is controlled.
P.O. use: Give oral dose with meals or antacids to lessen GI distress.
I.V. use: Mexiletine injection is compatible with 0.9% NaCl, D_5W, 5% sodium bicarbonate, 1/6 M sodium lactate, and 10% fructose (levulose).
• If patient appears to be good candidate for every-12-hour therapy, notify doctor. Twice-daily dosage enhances compliance.
• Notify doctor of significant change in blood pressure and heart rate and rhythm.
Patient teaching
• Instruct patient taking oral form of drug to take it with food.
• Instruct patient to report adverse reactions.

☑ Evaluation
• Patient regains normal cardiac output.
• Patient maintains adequate hydration throughout therapy.
• Patient and family state understanding of drug therapy.

---

mezlocillin sodium
(mez-loh-SIL-in SOH-dee-um)
Mezlin

Pharmacologic class: extended-spectrum penicillin, acyclaminopenicillin
Therapeutic class: antibiotic
Pregnancy risk category: B

How supplied
Injection: 1 g, 2 g, 3 g, 4 g

Pharmacokinetics
Absorption: unknown after I.M. use.
Distribution: distributed widely; 16% to 42% protein-bound.
Metabolism: metabolized partially.
Excretion: excreted primarily in urine; up to 30% of dose excreted in bile. *Half-life:* 45 to 90 minutes.

Route	Onset	Peak	Duration
I.V.	Immediate	Immediate	Unknown
I.M.	Unknown	45-90 min	Unknown

Pharmacodynamics
Chemical effect: inhibits cell-wall synthesis during microorganism multiplication; bacteria resist mezlocillin by producing penicillinases—enzymes that hydrolyze mezlocillin.
Therapeutic effect: kills susceptible bacteria. Spectrum of activity includes many gram-negative bacilli, many gram-positive and gram-negative aerobic cocci, and some gram-positive bacilli.

Indications and dosage
▶ **Systemic infections caused by susceptible strains of gram-positive and especially gram-negative organisms (including *Proteus* and *Pseudomonas aeruginosa*).** *Adults:* 200 to 300 mg/kg daily I.V. or I.M. in four to six divided doses. Usual dose is 3 g q 4 hours or 4 g q 6 hours. For serious infections, up to 24 g daily may be given. *Children between ages 1 month and 12 years:* 50 mg/kg q 4 hours I.V. or I.M. Neonates weighing 2,000 g (4.4 lb) or less and age 1 week or less: 75 mg/kg I.V. q 12 hours (150 mg/kg/day). Neonates weighing 2,000 g or less and older than age 1 week: 75 mg/kg I.V. q 8 hours (225 mg/kg/day). Neonates weighing over 2,000 g and age 1 week or less: 75 mg/kg I.V. q 12 hours (150 mg/kg/day). Neonates weighing over 2,000 g and older than age 1 week: 75 mg/kg I.V. q 6 hours (300 mg/kg/day).*

Adverse reactions

CNS: neuromuscular irritability, *seizures*.
GI: nausea, diarrhea.
Hematologic: *bleeding* (with high doses), *neutropenia, thrombocytopenia,* eosinophilia, *leukopenia, hemolytic anemia*.
Skin: rash, pruritus.
Other: hypersensitivity reactions (*anaphylaxis,* edema, fever, chills, urticaria), overgrowth of nonsusceptible organisms, *hypokalemia,* pain at injection site, vein irritation, phlebitis.

Interactions

Drug-drug. *Aminoglycoside antibiotics (such as gentamicin, tobramycin):* chemically incompatible. Don't mix together in I.V. solution. Give 1 hour apart, especially in patients with renal insufficiency.
Anticoagulants: large IV doses of penicillins can increase bleeding risk of anticoagulants by prolonging bleeding time. Monitor patient.
Probenecid: increased blood levels of mezlocillin. Probenecid may be used for this purpose.
Vecuronium: may prolong neuromuscular blockage of vecuronium. Use with caution.

Contraindications and precautions

• Contraindicated in patients with hypersensitivity to drug or other penicillins.
• Use cautiously in patients with other drug allergies, especially to cephalosporins (possible cross-sensitivity), and in those with bleeding tendencies, uremia, or hypokalemia. Also use cautiously in pregnant women.
• Safety of drug has not been established in breast-feeding women.

NURSING CONSIDERATIONS

✓ Assessment

• Assess patient's infection before therapy and regularly thereafter.

• Before giving, ask patient about any allergic reactions to penicillin. A negative history of penicillin allergy is no guarantee against future reaction.
• Obtain specimen for culture and sensitivity tests before giving first dose. Therapy may begin pending results.
• Check CBC and platelet counts frequently, as ordered. Drug may cause thrombocytopenia.
• Monitor serum potassium level.
• Be alert for adverse reactions and drug interactions.
• Monitor patient's hydration status if adverse GI reactions occur.
• Evaluate patient's and family's knowledge of drug therapy.

Nursing diagnoses

• Infection related to presence of susceptible bacteria
• Risk of fluid volume deficit related to drug-induced adverse GI reactions
• Knowledge deficit related to drug therapy

Planning and implementation

I.V. use: Reconstitute vial with at least 10 ml/g of drug using sterile water for injection, D₅W, or 0.9% NaCl injection. Solutions with concentration not exceeding 10% may be given by direct injection over 3 to 5 minutes. Alternatively, dilute in 50 to 100 ml of I.V. solution and give by intermittent infusion over 30 minutes.
– Give I.V. intermittently to prevent vein irritation. Change site every 48 hours.
I.M. use: Don't give more than 2 g per injection. Inject deeply and slowly (12 to 15 seconds) into body of large muscle.
• Give drug at least 1 hour before bacteriostatic antibiotics.
• Institute seizure precautions. Patient with high serum drug levels may have seizures.
• Know that dosage should be altered in patients with impaired kidney function.

• Be aware that drug is almost always used with another antibiotic, such as gentamicin.

• Drug may interfere with positive direct antiglobulin (Coombs') test results and with certain tests for serum and urine proteins; tests that use bromphenol blue (Albustix, Albutest) are not affected.

Patient teaching

• Advise patient to promptly report adverse reactions.

☑ **Evaluation**

• Patient is free from infection.

• Patient maintains adequate hydration throughout therapy.

• Patient and family state understanding of drug therapy.

miconazole
(migh-KON-uh-zohl)
Monistat I.V.

Pharmacologic class: imidazole derivative
Therapeutic class: antifungal
Pregnancy risk category: C

How supplied

Injection: 10 mg/ml

Pharmacokinetics

Absorption: not applicable.
Distribution: penetrates inflamed joints, vitreous humor, and peritoneal cavity; more than 90% protein bound.
Metabolism: metabolized in liver.
Excretion: excreted in feces and urine.
Half-life: about 24 hours.

Route	Onset	Peak	Duration
I.V.	Immediate	Immediate	Unknown
Intrathecal	Unknown	Unknown	Unknown

Pharmacodynamics

Chemical effect: inhibits purine transport and DNA, RNA, and protein synthesis; increases cell-wall permeability, making fungus more susceptible to osmotic pressure.

Therapeutic effect: kills susceptible organisms. Spectrum of activity includes *Aspergillus flavus, Candida albicans, Candida parapsilosis, Candida tropicalis, Coccidioides immitis, Cryptococcus neoformans, Curvularia, Histoplasma capsulatum, Microsporum canis, Paracoccidioides brasiliensis, Pseudallescheria boydii, Sporothrix schenckii,* dermatophytes, and some gram-positive bacteria.

Indications and dosage

▶ **Systemic fungal infections (coccidioidomycosis, candidiasis, cryptococcosis, paracoccidioidomycosis), chronic mucocutaneous candidiasis.** *Adults:* 200 to 3,600 mg/day I.V. Dosages may vary with diagnosis and infective agent. Daily dosage may be divided over three infusions, 200 to 1,200 mg per infusion. Dilute in at least 200 ml of 0.9% NaCl. Repeated courses may be needed because of relapse or reinfection. *Children age 1 and over:* 20 to 40 mg/kg/day I.V. Do not exceed 15 mg/kg per infusion.

▶ **Fungal meningitis.** *Adults:* 20 mg intrathecally q 1 to 2 days if S.C. ventricular reservoir is used, or q 3 to 7 days if not used, as adjunct to I.V. administration.

Adverse reactions

CNS: dizziness, drowsiness.
GI: *nausea, vomiting,* diarrhea.
Hematologic: transient decreases in hematocrit, *thrombocytopenia.*
Skin: *pruritic rash.*
Other: *anaphylactoid reactions,* fever, chills, transient decrease in serum sodium level, phlebitis at injection site.

Interactions

Drug-drug. *Oral anticoagulants:* enhanced anticoagulant effect. Monitor patient.

Reactions may be *common,* uncommon, *life-threatening,* or COMMON AND LIFE-THREATENING.

Contraindications and precautions

• Contraindicated in patients with hypersensitivity to drug.
• Use cautiously in pregnant women.
• Safety of drug has not been established in breast-feeding women.

NURSING CONSIDERATIONS

⚖ **Assessment**
• Assess patient's infection before therapy and regularly thereafter.
• Monitor levels of hemoglobin, hematocrit, electrolytes, and lipids regularly. Transient elevations in serum levels of cholesterol and triglycerides may be caused by castor oil vehicle.
• Be alert for adverse reactions and drug interactions.
• Monitor patient's hydration status if adverse GI reactions occur.
• Evaluate patient's and family's knowledge of drug therapy.

⊕ **Nursing diagnoses**
• Infection related to presence of susceptible organisms
• Risk for fluid volume deficit related to drug-induced adverse GI reactions
• Knowledge deficit related to drug therapy

❯ **Planning and implementation**
• Because drug is dissolved in vehicle containing polyoxyl 35 castor oil, a substance known to cause anaphylactoid reactions, give first dose under continuous medical supervision with emergency resuscitative equipment immediately available. Subsequent doses may be administered on outpatient basis in select patients.
• Don't administer drug with meals to lessen adverse GI reactions.
• Know that premedication with antiemetic may lessen nausea and vomiting.
I.V. use: Be aware that I.V. miconazole has been replaced largely by newer drugs that are better tolerated.

– Dilute infusion with at least 200 ml of 0.9% NaCl solution and infuse over 30 to 60 minutes.
– Rapid I.V. injection of undiluted drug may produce arrhythmias.
Intrathecal use: Administer drug undiluted using S.C. intrathecal (Ommaya) reservoir. Alternatively, be aware that drug may be given by lumbar or cisternal puncture.
• In patients with fungal meningitis or urinary bladder infections, assist with supplemental intrathecal administration and bladder irrigation, respectively.
Patient teaching
• Inform patient that pruritic rash may persist for weeks after drug is discontinued. Pruritus may be controlled with diphenhydramine.
• Inform patient that therapeutic response may take weeks or months.

☑ **Evaluation**
• Patient is free from infection.
• Patient maintains adequate hydration throughout therapy.
• Patient and family state understanding of drug therapy.

midazolam hydrochloride
(MID-ayz-oh-lam high-droh-KLOR-ighd)
Hypnovel◇, Versed

Pharmacologic class: benzodiazepine
Therapeutic class: preoperative sedative, agent for conscious sedation, adjunct for induction of general anesthesia
Controlled substance schedule: IV
Pregnancy risk category: D

How supplied

Injection: 1 mg/ml, 5 mg/ml

Pharmacokinetics

Absorption: absorption after I.M. use appears to be 80% to 100%.
Distribution: drug has large volume of distribution; about 97% protein-bound.

Metabolism: metabolized in liver.
Excretion: excreted in urine. *Half-life:* 2
to 6 hours.

Route	Onset	Peak	Duration
I.V.	1.5-5 min	Rapid	2-6 hr
I.M.	≤ 15 min	15-60 min	2-6 hr

Pharmacodynamics

Chemical effect: unknown; thought to
depress CNS at limbic and subcortical
levels of brain by potentiating effects of
gamma-aminobutyric acid.
Therapeutic effect: promotes calmness
and sleep.

Indications and dosage

Know that dosage should be adjusted for
older or debilitated patients.
► **Preoperative sedation (to induce
sleepiness or drowsiness and relieve
apprehension).** *Adults under age 60:*
0.07 mg to 0.08 mg/kg I.M. about 1 hour
before surgery.
► **Conscious sedation before short diagnostic or endoscopic procedures.**
Adults under age 60: initially, small dose
not to exceed 2.5 mg I.V. administered
slowly; repeated in 2 minutes if needed in
small increments of initial dose over at
least 2 minutes to achieve desired effect.
Total dosage of up to 5 mg may be used.
Elderly: 1.5 mg or less I.M. over at least
2 minutes. If additional titration is needed, give at rate not exceeding 1 mg over 2
minutes. Total dosages exceeding 3.5 mg
are not usually necessary.
► **Induction of general anesthesia.**
Adults under age 55: 0.3 to 0.35 mg/kg
I.V. over 20 to 30 seconds if patient has
not received preanesthesia medication, or
0.15 to 0.35 mg/kg I.V. over 20 to 30 seconds if patient has received preanesthesia
medication. Additional increments of
25% of initial dose may be needed to
complete induction.

Adverse reactions

CNS: headache, oversedation, involuntary movements, combativeness, amnesia.

CV: variations in blood pressure *(hy-
potension)* and pulse rate, **cardiac arrest.**
GI: *nausea,* vomiting, *hiccups.*
Respiratory: *decreased respiratory rate,*
APNEA.
Skin: pain, tenderness (at injection site).

Interactions

Drug-drug. *CNS depressants:* may increase risk of apnea. Avoid concomitant
use.
Indinavir, ritonavir: possible prolonged
or severe sedation and respiratory depression. Monitor patient closely.
Oral contraceptives: may prolong benzodiazepine half-life. Monitor closely.
Verapamil: effects of benzodiazepine
may be increased. Monitor closely.
Drug-lifestyle. *Alcohol use:* may increase
risk of apnea. Avoid concomitant use.

Contraindications and precautions

• Contraindicated in patients with acute
angle-closure glaucoma, shock, coma,
acute alcohol intoxication, or hypersensitivity to drug.
• Drug is not recommended for use in
pregnant women.
• Use cautiously in patients with uncompensated acute illness, in elderly or debilitated patients, and in breast-feeding
women.

NURSING CONSIDERATIONS

Assessment
• Assess patient's condition before therapy and regularly thereafter.
• Monitor blood pressure, heart rate and
rhythm, respirations, airway integrity,
and arterial oxygen saturation during procedure, especially in patients premedicat-
ed with narcotics.
• Be alert for adverse reactions and drug
interactions.
• Evaluate patient's and family's knowledge of drug therapy.

Nursing diagnoses
• Anxiety related to surgery

Reactions may be *common,* uncommon, *life-threatening*, or COMMON AND LIFE-THREATENING.

• Ineffective breathing pattern related to drug's effect on respiratory system
• Knowledge deficit related to drug therapy

▶ **Planning and implementation**
• Before administering, have oxygen and resuscitation equipment available in case of severe respiratory depression. Excessive dosage or rapid infusion has been associated with respiratory arrest, particularly in elderly or debilitated patients.
• Know that midazolam may be mixed in same syringe with morphine sulfate, meperidine, atropine sulfate, or scopolamine.
I.V. use: Administer drug slowly over at least 2 minutes, and wait at least 2 minutes when titrating doses to effect.
– Take care to avoid extravasation.
I.M. use: Administer drug deeply into large muscle mass.
Patient teaching
• Drug's beneficial amnestic effect diminishes patient's recall of perioperative events. This effect requires extra caution when teaching patients. Written information, family member instruction, and follow-up contact may be required to ensure that patient has adequate information.
• Instruct patient to avoid alcohol consumption during drug therapy.

☑ **Evaluation**
• Patient exhibits calmness.
• Patient maintains adequate breathing pattern throughout therapy.
• Patient and family state understanding of drug therapy.

---

milrinone lactate
(MIL-rih-nohn LAK-tayt)
Primacor

Pharmacologic class: bipyridine phosphodiesterase inhibitor
Therapeutic class: inotropic vasodilator
Pregnancy risk category: C

How supplied
Injection: 1 mg/ml
Premixed injection: 200 mcg/ml in 100 ml 5% dextrose injection; 200 mcg/ml in 200 ml 5% dextrose injection.

Pharmacokinetics
Absorption: not applicable.
Distribution: about 70% bound to human plasma protein.
Metabolism: about 12% metabolized to glucuronide metabolite.
Excretion: about 83% excreted unchanged in urine. *Half-life:* 2.3 to 2.7 hours.

Route	Onset	Peak	Duration
I.V.	5-15 min	1-2 hr	3-6 hr

Pharmacodynamics
Chemical effect: produces inotropic action by increasing cellular levels of cAMP; produces vasodilation by relaxing vascular smooth muscle.
Therapeutic effect: relieves acute signs and symptoms of heart failure.

Indications and dosage
▶ **Short-term treatment of heart failure.** *Adults:* loading dose is 50 mcg/kg I.V., given slowly over 10 minutes, followed by continuous I.V. infusion of 0.375 to 0.75 mcg/kg/minute. Adjust infusion dose based on clinical and hemodynamic responses, as ordered. *In patients with renal failure:* clearance is 50 ml/minute or less, dosage is titrated to maximum clinical effect and not to exceed 1.13 mg/kg/day.

Adverse reactions
CNS: headache.
CV: VENTRICULAR ARRHYTHMIAS, *ventricular ectopic activity,* nonsustained ventricular tachycardia, *sustained ventricular tachycardia, ventricular fibrillation.*

Interactions
None reported.

Contraindications and precautions

• Contraindicated in patients with hypersensitivity to drug.

• Drug is not recommended for use in patients with severe aortic or pulmonic valvular disease in place of surgical correction of obstruction or during acute phase of MI.

• Use cautiously in patients with atrial flutter or fibrillation because drug slightly shortens AV node conduction time and may increase ventricular response rate. Also use cautiously in pregnant or breast-feeding women.

• Safety of drug has not been established in children.

NURSING CONSIDERATIONS

⚖ Assessment

• Assess patient's heart failure before therapy and regularly thereafter.

• Monitor fluid and electrolyte status, blood pressure, heart rate, and kidney function during therapy.

• Monitor patient's ECG continuously during therapy.

• Be alert for adverse reactions.

• Evaluate patient's and family's knowledge of drug therapy.

Nursing diagnoses

• Impaired gas exchange related to presence of heart failure

• Decreased cardiac output related to drug-induced cardiac arrhythmias

• Knowledge deficit related to drug therapy

Planning and implementation

• Be aware that milrinone is typically given with digoxin and diuretics.

• Be aware that inotropic agents may aggravate outflow tract obstruction in hypertrophic subaortic stenosis.

• Prepare I.V. infusion solution using 0.45% or 0.9% NaCl or D₅W. Prepare 100-mcg/ml solution by adding 180 ml of diluent per 20-mg (20-ml) vial, 150-mcg/ml solution by adding 113 ml of diluent per 20-mg (20-ml) vial, and 200-mcg/ml solution by adding 80 ml of diluent per 20-mg (20-ml) vial.

• Improvement of cardiac output may result in enhanced urine output. Expect dosage reduction in diuretic therapy as heart failure improves. Potassium loss may predispose patient to digitalis toxicity.

• Know that excessive decrease in blood pressure requires discontinuation or slower rate of infusion.

Patient teaching

• Tell patient to report headache; mild analgesic can be given for relief.

✔ Evaluation

• Patient exhibits adequate gas exchange as heart failure is resolved.

• Drug-induced arrhythmias do not develop during therapy.

• Patient and family state understanding of drug therapy.

mineral oil (liquid petrolatum)
(MIN-er-ul OYL)
Agoral Plain†, Fleet Enema Mineral Oil†, Kondremul†, Kondremul Plain†, Lansoyl♦, Liqui-Doss†, Milkinol†, Neo-Cultol†, Petrogalar Plain†, Zymenol†

Pharmacologic class: lubricant oil
Therapeutic class: laxative
Pregnancy risk category: C

How supplied

Emulsion: 50%†
Oral liquid: in pints, quarts, gallons†
Enema: 120 ml†, 133 ml†

Pharmacokinetics

Absorption: absorbed minimally except for emulsified drug form, which has significant absorption.
Distribution: distributed locally, primarily in colon.
Metabolism: none.
Excretion: excreted in feces.

Route	Onset	Peak	Duration
P.O., P.R.	6-8 hr	Varies	Varies

Pharmacodynamics

Chemical effect: increases water retention in stool by creating barrier between colon wall and feces that prevents colonic reabsorption of fecal water.
Therapeutic effect: relieves constipation.

Indications and dosage

▶ **Constipation, preparation for bowel studies or surgery.** *Adults and children age 12 and older:* 5 to 45 ml P.O. h.s.; or 120 ml P.R. (as enema). *Children ages 6 to 12:* 5 to 15 ml P.O. h.s.; or 30 to 60 ml P.R. (as enema). *Children ages 2 to 6:* 30 to 60 ml P.R. (as enema).

Adverse reactions

GI: *nausea,* vomiting, decreased absorption of nutrients and fat-soluble vitamins, anal pruritus, diarrhea (with excessive use), *abdominal cramps* (especially in severe constipation), slowed healing (after hemorrhoidectomy).
Respiratory: *lipid pneumonia.*
Other: laxative dependence (with long-term or excessive use).

Interactions

Drug-drug. *Docusate salts:* may increase mineral oil absorption and cause lipid pneumonia. Separate administration times.
Fat-soluble vitamins (A, D, E, and K): possible decreased absorption after prolonged administration. Monitor for deficiencies.

Contraindications and precautions

• Contraindicated in patients with abdominal pain, nausea, vomiting, or other symptoms of appendicitis or acute surgical abdomen and in those with fecal impaction or intestinal obstruction or perforation.
• Use cautiously in young children; in pregnant or breast-feeding women; in elderly or debilitated patients because of

susceptibility to lipid pneumonia through aspiration, absorption, and transport from intestinal mucosa; and in patients with rectal bleeding.

NURSING CONSIDERATIONS

⚗ Assessment
• Assess patient's condition before therapy and regularly thereafter.
• Before giving for constipation, determine if patient has adequate fluid intake, exercise, and diet.
• Be alert for adverse reactions and drug interactions.
• Evaluate patient's and family's knowledge of drug therapy.

⊞ Nursing diagnoses
• Constipation related to underlying condition
• Risk for fluid volume deficit related to drug-induced adverse GI reactions
• Knowledge deficit related to drug therapy

▷ Planning and implementation
P.O. use: Give drug on empty stomach.
– Give drug with fruit juice or carbonated drink to disguise taste.
P.R. use: Follow normal protocol.
Patient teaching
• Advise patient to take drug only at bedtime and not to take for more than 1 week.
• Warn patient of possible rectal leakage from excessive dosages.
• Teach patient about dietary sources of bulk, which include bran and other cereals, fresh fruit, and vegetables.

☑ Evaluation
• Patient regains normal bowel pattern.
• Patient maintains adequate hydration throughout therapy.
• Patient and family state understanding of drug therapy.

---

minocycline hydrochloride
(migh-noh-SIGH-kleen high-droh-KLOR-ighd)
Dynacin, Minocin*, Minomycin◊, Minomycin IV◊

Pharmacologic class: tetracycline
Therapeutic class: antibiotic
Pregnancy risk category: D

How supplied

Tablets (film-coated): 50 mg, 100 mg
Capsules: 50 mg, 100 mg
Oral suspension: 50 mg/5 ml
Injection: 100 mg

Pharmacokinetics

Absorption: 90% to 100% absorbed after oral administration.
Distribution: distributed widely in body tissues and fluids, including synovial, pleural, prostatic, and seminal fluids; bronchial secretions; saliva; and aqueous humor. CSF penetration is poor. Drug is 70% to 80% protein-bound.
Metabolism: metabolized partially.
Excretion: excreted primarily unchanged in liver. *Half-life:* 11 to 26 hours.

Route	Onset	Peak	Duration
P.O.	Unknown	1-4 hr	Unknown
I.V.	Immediate	Immediate	Unknown

Pharmacodynamics

Chemical effect: unknown; may exert bacteriostatic effect by binding to ribosomal subunit of microorganisms, inhibiting protein synthesis.
Therapeutic effect: hinders bacterial cell growth. Spectrum of activity includes many gram-negative and gram-positive organisms, *Chlamydia, Mycoplasma, Rickettsia,* and spirochetes.

Indications and dosage

▶ **Infections caused by sensitive gram-negative and gram-positive organisms, trachoma, amebiasis.** *Adults:* 200 mg I.V.; then 100 mg I.V. q 12 hours. Not to exceed 400 mg/day. Or 200 mg P.O. initially; then 100 mg P.O. q 12 hours. Some clinicians use 100 or 200 mg P.O. initially, followed by 50 mg q.i.d. *Children over age 8:* initially, 4 mg/kg P.O. or I.V., followed by 2 mg/kg P.O. q 12 hours. Given I.V. in 500- to 1,000-ml solution without calcium over 6 hours.
▶ **Gonorrhea in patients sensitive to penicillin.** *Adults:* initially, 200 mg P.O.; then 100 mg q 12 hours for at least 4 days.
▶ **Syphilis in patients sensitive to penicillin.** *Adults:* initially, 200 mg P.O.; then 100 mg q 12 hours for 10 to 15 days.
▶ **Meningococcal carrier state.** *Adults:* 100 mg P.O. q 12 hours for 5 days.
▶ **Uncomplicated urethral, endocervical, or rectal infection caused by *Chlamydia trachomatis* or *Ureaplasma urealyticum*.** Adults: 100 mg P.O. b.i.d. for at least 7 days.
▶ **Uncomplicated gonococcal urethritis in men.** *Adults:* 100 mg P.O. b.i.d. for 5 days.

Adverse reactions

CNS: *light-headedness, dizziness from vestibular toxicity;* **intracranial hypertension (pseudotumor cerebri).**
CV: pericarditis, *thrombophlebitis.*
EENT: dysphagia, glossitis.
GI: *anorexia,* epigastric distress, oral candidiasis, *nausea,* vomiting, *diarrhea,* enterocolitis, inflammatory lesions in anogenital region.
GU: increased BUN level.
Hematologic: *neutropenia,* eosinophilia, *thrombocytopenia.*
Hepatic: elevated liver enzyme levels.
Musculoskeletal: permanent discoloration of teeth, enamel defects, and bone growth retardation if used in children under age 8; superinfection.
Skin: *maculopapular and erythematous rashes, photosensitivity, increased pigmentation, urticaria.*
Other: hypersensitivity reactions (**ana-phylaxis**).

Reactions may be *common*, uncommon, *life-threatening*, or COMMON AND LIFE-THREATENING.

Interactions

Drug-drug. *Antacids (including sodium bicarbonate) and laxatives containing aluminum, magnesium, or calcium; antidiarrheals:* decreased antibiotic absorption. Give antibiotic 1 hour before or 2 hours after any of above.
Ferrous sulfate, other iron products, zinc: decreased antibiotic absorption. Give drug 3 hours after or 2 hours before iron administration.
Methoxyflurane: may cause nephrotoxicity with tetracyclines. Monitor patient carefully.
Oral anticoagulants: increased anticoagulant effect. Monitor PT and INR and adjust dosage, as ordered.
Oral contraceptives: decreased contraceptive effectiveness and increased risk of breakthrough bleeding. Use nonhormonal form of birth control.
Penicillins: may interfere with bactericidal action of penicillins. Avoid using together.
Drug-lifestyle. *Sun exposure:* photosensitivity reactions may occur. Take precautions.

Contraindications and precautions

• Contraindicated in patients with hypersensitivity to drug or other tetracyclines.
• Drug is not recommended for use in breast-feeding women.
• Use cautiously in patients with impaired kidney or liver function. Use of this drug during last half of pregnancy and in children under age 8 may cause permanent discoloration of teeth, enamel defects, and bone growth retardation.

NURSING CONSIDERATIONS

☞ Assessment
• Assess patient's infection before therapy and regularly thereafter.
• Obtain specimen for culture and sensitivity tests before giving first dose. Therapy may begin pending results.
• Be alert for adverse reactions and drug interactions.

• Monitor patient's hydration status if adverse GI reactions occur.
• Evaluate patient's and family's knowledge of drug therapy.

⊞ Nursing diagnoses
• Infection related to presence of susceptible bacteria
• Risk for fluid volume deficit related to drug-induced adverse reactions
• Knowledge deficit related to drug therapy

⊠ Planning and implementation
• Check expiration date. Outdated or deteriorated tetracyclines have been associated with reversible nephrotoxicity (Fanconi's syndrome).
• Don't expose these drugs to light or heat. Keep cap tightly closed.
P.O. use: Follow normal protocol.
I.V. use: Reconstitute 100 mg of powder with 5 ml of sterile water for injection, with further dilution of 500 to 1,000 ml for I.V. infusion. Solution is stable for 24 hours at room temperature.
– Thrombophlebitis may develop with I.V. administration of drug. Avoid extravasation. Switch to oral therapy as soon as possible.
• Drug may cause tooth discoloration in young adults. Inform doctor if brown pigmentation occurs.
• Parenteral form may cause false-positive reading of copper sulfate tests (Clinitest). All forms may cause false-negative reading of glucose enzymatic tests (Diastix).
Patient teaching
• Inform patient that drug may be taken with food, and instruct him to take drug exactly as prescribed.
• Instruct patient to take oral form of drug with full glass of water, and to avoid taking it within 1 hour of bedtime to avoid esophagitis.
• Warn patient to avoid hazardous tasks until adverse CNS effects of drug are known.

• Warn patient to avoid direct sunlight and ultraviolet light, to use a sunblock, and wear protective clothing.

☑ **Evaluation**
• Patient is free from infection.
• Patient maintains adequate hydration throughout therapy.
• Patient and family state understanding of drug therapy.

minoxidil
(migh-NOKS-uh-dil)
Loniten

Pharmacologic class: peripheral vasodilator
Therapeutic class: antihypertensive
Pregnancy risk category: C

How supplied
Tablets: 2.5 mg, 10 mg, 25 mg◇

Pharmacokinetics
Absorption: absorbed rapidly from GI tract.
Distribution: distributed widely in body tissues; not bound to plasma proteins.
Metabolism: about 90% metabolized.
Excretion: excreted primarily in urine.
Half-life: 4.2 hours.

Route	Onset	Peak	Duration
P.O.	About 30 min	≤ 1 hr	2-5 days

Pharmacodynamics
Chemical effect: unknown; produces direct arteriolar vasodilation.
Therapeutic effect: lowers blood pressure.

Indications and dosage
▶ **Severe hypertension.** *Adults:* initially, 5 mg P.O. as single dose. Effective dosage range is usually 10 to 40 mg daily. Maximum dosage is 100 mg daily. *Children under age 12:* 0.2 mg/kg P.O. (max-

imum 5 mg) as single daily dose. Effective dosage range usually is 0.25 to 1.0 mg/kg daily. Maximum dosage is 50 mg.

Adverse reactions
CV: *edema, tachycardia, pericardial effusion and tamponade,* **heart failure,** ECG changes.
Skin: rash, **Stevens-Johnson syndrome.**
Other: *hypertrichosis* (elongation, thickening, and enhanced pigmentation of fine body hair), breast tenderness, weight gain.

Interactions
Drug-drug. *Guanethidine:* severe orthostatic hypotension. Advise patient to stand up slowly.

Contraindications and precautions
• Contraindicated in patients with pheochromocytoma or hypersensitivity to drug.
• Drug is not recommended for use in breast-feeding women.
• Use cautiously in patients with impaired kidney function and after acute MI. Also use cautiously in pregnant women.

NURSING CONSIDERATIONS

☑ **Assessment**
• Obtain history of patient's blood pressure and pulse rate before therapy and reassess regularly thereafter.
• Be alert for adverse reactions and drug interactions.
• Monitor fluid intake and output and check for weight gain and edema.
• Evaluate patient's and family's knowledge of drug therapy.

☑ **Nursing diagnoses**
• Risk for injury related to presence of hypertension
• Fluid volume excess related to drug-induced edema
• Knowledge deficit related to drug therapy

Reactions may be *common,* uncommon, *life-threatening*, or COMMON AND LIFE-THREATENING.

☒ Planning and implementation
• Drug is removed by hemodialysis. Administer dose after dialysis.
• Know that drug usually is prescribed with beta blocker to control tachycardia and diuretic to counteract fluid retention.
• Notify doctor if blood pressure becomes significantly altered or pulse rate rises more than 20 beats/minute from baseline.

Patient teaching
• Make sure patient reads package insert that describes drug's adverse reactions. Provide verbal explanation.
• Teach patient how to take his own pulse and to report increases over 20 beats/minute to doctor.
• Tell patient not to suddenly stop taking drug but to call doctor if unpleasant adverse effects occur.
• Tell patient to weigh himself at least weekly and to report weight gain over 2.27 kg (5 lb).
• Inform patient that excessive hair growth commonly occurs within 3 to 6 weeks of beginning treatment. Unwanted hair can be removed by depilatory cream or by shaving. Assure patient that extra hair will disappear within 1 to 6 months of stopping minoxidil. Advise him not to discontinue drug without doctor's approval.

☑ Evaluation
• Patient's blood pressure is normal.
• Patient exhibits no evidence of edema throughout therapy.
• Patient and family state understanding of drug therapy.

mirtazapine
(mir-TAH-zuh-peen)
Remeron

Pharmacologic class: piperazinoazepine group of compounds
Therapeutic class: antidepressant
Pregnancy risk category: C

How supplied
Tablets: 15 mg, 30 mg

Pharmacokinetics
Absorption: rapidly absorbed.
Distribution: 85% bound by plasma proteins.
Metabolism: extensively in liver.
Excretion: mainly in urine; some in feces. *Mean elimination half-life:* about 20 to 40 hours.

Route	Onset	Peak	Duration
P.O.	Unknown	Within 2 hr	Unknown

Pharmacodynamics
Chemical effect: enhances central noradrenergic and serotonergic activity; potent antagonist of histamine receptors.
Therapeutic effect: relieves depression.

Indications and dosage
▶ **Depression.** Adults: initially, 15 mg P.O. h.s. Maintenance dosage is 15 to 45 mg daily. Adjust dosage at intervals of at least 1 to 2 weeks.

Adverse reactions
CNS: somnolence, dizziness, asthenia, abnormal dreams, abnormal thinking, tremors, confusion.
GI: nausea, increased appetite, dry mouth, constipation.
GU: urinary frequency.
Hematologic: *agranulocytosis* (rare).
Musculoskeletal: back pain, myalgia.
Respiratory: dyspnea.
Other: weight gain, flulike syndrome, edema, peripheral edema.

Interactions
Drug-drug. *Diazepam, other CNS depressants:* possible additive CNS effects. Avoid concomitant use.
MAO inhibitor: potentially serious, sometimes fatal reactions. Do not use drug with MAO inhibitor or within 14 days of initiating or stopping therapy with MAO inhibitor.

Drug-lifestyle. *Alcohol use:* possible additive CNS effects. Avoid concomitant use.

Contraindications and precautions

• Contraindicated in patients with hypersensitivity to drug.
• Use cautiously in patients with CV or cerebrovascular disease, seizure disorders, suicidal ideations, impaired hepatic or renal function, or history of mania or hypomania.
• Coadministration with MAO inhibitors is contraindicated.

NURSING CONSIDERATIONS

⚕ Assessment
• Stop drug and monitor patient closely if he develops a sore throat, fever, stomatitis, or other signs of infection together with a low WBC count.
• Evaluate patient's and family's knowledge of drug therapy.

⊕ Nursing diagnoses
• Altered thought processes related to adverse effects
• Risk for injury related to sedation and orthostatic hypotension
• Knowledge deficit related to drug therapy

▶ Planning and implementation
• Use cautiously when administering drug to breast-feeding women.
Patient teaching
• Warn patient to avoid hazardous activities if somnolence occurs.
• Tell patient to report signs and symptoms of infection or flulike symptoms.
• Advise patient to avoid alcohol or other CNS depressants.
• Stress importance of compliance with therapy.
• Instruct patient not to take other drugs without doctor's approval.
• Tell female patient to notify doctor of suspected pregnancy or if she is breast-feeding.

☑ Evaluation
• Patient regains normal thought processes.
• Patient does not experience injury from adverse reactions.
• Patient and family state understanding of drug therapy.

---

misoprostol
(mee-SOH-pruh-stol)
Cytotec

Pharmacologic class: prostaglandin E_1 analogue
Therapeutic class: gastric mucosal protectant
Pregnancy risk category: X

How supplied

Tablets: 100 mcg, 200 mcg

Pharmacokinetics

Absorption: absorbed rapidly from GI tract.
Distribution: highly bound to plasma proteins.
Metabolism: rapidly de-esterified to misoprostol acid, the biologically active metabolite.
Excretion: about 15% excreted in feces; balance excreted in urine. *Half-life:* 20 to 40 minutes.

Route	Onset	Peak	Duration
P.O.	30 min	10-15 min	About 3 hr

Pharmacodynamics

Chemical effect: replaces gastric prostaglandins depleted by NSAID therapy. Misoprostol also decreases basal and stimulated gastric acid secretion and may increase gastric mucus and bicarbonate production.
Therapeutic effect: protects gastric mucosa from ulcerating.

Reactions may be *common*, uncommon, *life-threatening*, or COMMON AND LIFE-THREATENING.

Indications and dosage

▶ **Prevention of NSAID-induced gastric ulcer in elderly or debilitated patients at high risk for complications from gastric ulcer and in patients with history of NSAID-induced ulcer.**
Adults: 200 mcg P.O. q.i.d. with food. If dosage isn't tolerated, decreased to 100 mcg P.O. q.i.d.

Adverse reactions

CNS: headache.
GI: *diarrhea, abdominal pain,* nausea, flatulence, dyspepsia, vomiting, constipation.
GU: hypermenorrhea, dysmenorrhea, spotting, cramps, menstrual disorders.

Interactions

Drug-drug. *Antacids:* reduced plasma levels when administered concomitantly. Not considered significant.

Contraindications and precautions

• Contraindicated in pregnant or breast-feeding women and in patients with history of allergy to prostaglandins.

NURSING CONSIDERATIONS

Assessment
• Obtain history of patient's GI condition before therapy.
• In female patient of childbearing age, ensure that negative pregnancy test is obtained within 2 weeks before therapy begins.
• Be alert for adverse reactions and drug interactions.
• Evaluate patient's and family's knowledge of drug therapy.

Nursing diagnoses
• Risk for injury related to potential for gastric ulceration
• Pain related to headache
• Knowledge deficit related to drug therapy

Planning and implementation
• Drug should not be routinely administered to women of childbearing age unless they are at high risk for development of ulcers or complications from NSAID-induced ulcers.
• Take special precautions to prevent use of drug during pregnancy. Make sure patient is fully aware of dangers of misoprostol to fetus and that she receives both verbal and written warnings regarding these dangers. Also ensure that patient can comply with effective contraceptive means.
Patient teaching
• Instruct patient not to share drug. Remind her that drug may cause miscarriage, often with potentially life-threatening bleeding.
• Advise her not to begin therapy until second or third day of next normal menstrual period.

Evaluation
• Patient remains free from signs and symptoms of gastric ulceration.
• Patient states that drug-induced headache does not occur.
• Patient and family state understanding of drug therapy.

mitomycin (mitomycin-C)
(might-oh-MIGH-sin)
Mutamycin

Pharmacologic class: antineoplastic antibiotic (cell cycle–phase nonspecific)
Therapeutic class: antineoplastic
Pregnancy risk category: NR

How supplied
Injection: 5-mg, 20-mg, 40-mg vials

Pharmacokinetics
Absorption: not applicable with I.V. administration.

Distribution: distributed widely in body tissues; does not cross blood-brain barrier.

Metabolism: metabolized by hepatic microsomal enzymes and deactivated in kidneys, spleen, brain, and heart.

Excretion: excreted primarily in urine; small portion excreted in bile and feces.

Half-life: about 50 minutes.

Route	Onset	Peak	Duration
I.V.	Unknown	Unknown	Unknown

Pharmacodynamics

Chemical effect: acts like alkylating agent, cross-linking strands of DNA. This causes imbalance of cell growth, leading to cell death.

Therapeutic effect: kills selected cancer cells.

Indications and dosage

Dosage and indications may vary. Check protocol with doctor.

▶ **Pancreatic and stomach cancers.** *Adults:* 20 mg/m² I.V. as single dose. Cycle repeated after 6 to 8 weeks, with dosage adjusted if needed based on nadir WBC and platelet counts.

Adverse reactions

GI: *nausea, vomiting,* anorexia, stomatitis.

Hematologic: THROMBOCYTOPENIA, LEUKOPENIA (may be delayed up to 8 weeks and be cumulative with successive doses), *microangiopathic hemolytic anemia.*

Respiratory: *interstitial pneumonitis.*

Other: desquamation, induration, pruritus, *pain at injection site; septicemia,* cellulitis, ulceration, sloughing (with extravasation); *reversible alopecia;* purple coloration of nail beds.

Interactions

Drug-drug. *Vinca alkaloids:* may cause acute respiratory distress. Avoid concomitant use.

Contraindications and precautions

• Contraindicated in patients hypersensitive to drug and in those with thrombocytopenia, coagulation disorder, or increase in bleeding tendency due to other causes.

• Drug is not recommended for use in pregnant or breast-feeding women.

• Safety of drug has not been established in children.

NURSING CONSIDERATIONS

☤ Assessment

• Assess patient's condition before therapy and regularly thereafter.

• Obtain CBC and blood studies, as ordered.

• Monitor kidney function tests, as ordered.

• Be alert for adverse reactions and drug interactions.

• Evaluate patient's and family's knowledge of drug therapy.

⊕ Nursing diagnoses

• Altered health maintenance related to presence of neoplastic disease

• Altered protection related to adverse hematologic reactions

• Knowledge deficit related to drug therapy

▷ Planning and implementation

• Follow institutional policy to reduce risks. Preparation and administration of parenteral form are associated with mutagenic, teratogenic, and carcinogenic risks to personnel.

• Using sterile water for injection, reconstitute 5-mg vials with 10 ml, 20-mg vials with 40 ml, and 40-mg vials with 80 ml.

• For infusion, dilute with 0.9% NaCl injection, D₅W, or sodium lactate for injection. After dilution, drug is stable for 3 hours in D₅W, 12 hours in 0.9% NaCl injection, and 24 hours in sodium lactate for injection at room temperature.

• Avoid extravasation. Stop infusion immediately if extravasation occurs because

---

Reactions may be *common,* uncommon, *life-threatening,* or COMMON AND LIFE-THREATENING.

of potential for severe ulceration and necrosis, and notify doctor.
• Never administer drug I.M. or S.C.
Patient teaching
• Instruct patient to watch for signs of infection and bleeding and to take temperature daily.
• Warn patient that alopecia may occur but assure him that it's reversible.
• Tell patient to report adverse reactions to doctor promptly.

☑ **Evaluation**
• Patient responds well to therapy.
• Patient does not develop serious complications.
• Patient and family state understanding of drug therapy.

mitotane
(MIGH-toh-tayn)
Lysodren

Pharmacologic class: chlorophenothane (DDT) analogue
Therapeutic class: antineoplastic
Pregnancy risk category: C

How supplied
Tablets (scored): 500 mg

Pharmacokinetics
Absorption: 35% to 40% absorbed across GI tract.
Distribution: widely distributed in body tissue; fatty tissue is primary storage site. Slow release of drug from fatty tissue into plasma occurs after drug is discontinued.
Metabolism: metabolized in liver and other tissue.
Excretion: excreted in urine and bile.
Half-life: 18 to 159 days.

Route	Onset	Peak	Duration
P.O.	2-3 days (steroid); ≤ 6 mo (tumor)	3-5 hr	Unknown

Pharmacodynamics
Chemical effect: unknown; thought to selectively destroy adrenocortical tissue and hinder extra-adrenal metabolism of cortisol.
Therapeutic effect: hinders adrenocortical cancer cell growth.

Indications and dosage
▶ **Inoperable adrenocortical cancer.**
Adults: initially, 2 to 6 g P.O. daily in divided doses t.i.d. or q.i.d.; increased to 9 to 10 g P.O. daily in divided doses t.i.d. or q.i.d. Dosage is adjusted until maximum tolerated dosage is achieved (varies from 2 to 19 g/day but is usually 8 to 10 g/day).

Adverse reactions
CNS: *depression, somnolence, lethargy, vertigo;* brain damage and dysfunction in long-term, high-dose therapy.
CV: hypertension.
EENT: visual disturbances.
GI: *severe nausea, vomiting,* diarrhea, anorexia.
GU: hemorrhagic cystitis.
Skin: dermatitis, maculopapular rash.
Other: hypouricemia, increased serum cholesterol level, adrenal insufficiency.

Interactions
Drug-drug. *Corticosteroids:* corticosteroid metabolism may be altered; higher doses of corticosteroids may be required. *Warfarin:* increased metabolism, which may require higher warfarin doses. Monitor PT and INR closely.

Contraindications and precautions
• Contraindicated in patients hypersensitive to drug and in those who are in shock or who have suffered trauma.
• Drug is not recommended for use in breast-feeding women.
• Use cautiously in patients with hepatic disease and in pregnant women.
• Safety of drug has not been established in children.

NURSING CONSIDERATIONS

⚗ Assessment

• Obtain history of patient's adrenocortical cancer before therapy.
• Monitor effectiveness according to reduction in pain, weakness, and anorexia.
• Assess and record behavioral and neurologic signs daily throughout therapy. Prolonged therapy has been associated with significant neurologic impairment.
• Be alert for adverse reactions.
• Monitor patient's hydration status if adverse GI reactions occur.
• Evaluate patient's and family's knowledge of drug therapy.

⚕ Nursing diagnoses

• Altered health maintenance related to presence of neoplastic disease
• Risk for fluid volume deficit related to drug-induced adverse GI reactions
• Knowledge deficit related to drug therapy

▶ Planning and implementation

• Give antiemetic before mitotane, as ordered.
• Be prepared to reduce dosage if adverse GI or skin reactions are severe.
• Use of corticosteroids may avoid acute adrenocorticoid insufficiency and is usually required. Glucocorticoid dosage should be increased in periods of stress, such as infection or trauma, as ordered.
• Know that drug distributes mostly to body fat. Obese patients may need higher dosage and have longer-lasting adverse reactions.
• Keep in mind that adequate therapeutic trial is at least 3 months, but treatment can continue if clinical benefits are observed.
• Monitor PT and INR on patient receiving mitotane and warfarin concurrently.
Patient teaching
• Warn ambulatory patient to avoid activities that require alertness and good motor coordination until CNS effects of drug are known.

• Tell patient to report adverse reactions promptly.
• For patient also receiving warfarin, instruct him to watch for and report signs of bleeding.

☑ Evaluation

• Patient responds well to therapy.
• Patient maintains adequate hydration throughout therapy.
• Patient and family state understanding of drug therapy.

mitoxantrone hydrochloride
(migh-toh-ZAN-trohn high-droh-KLOR-ighd)
Novantrone

Pharmacologic class: antibiotic antineoplastic
Therapeutic class: antineoplastic
Pregnancy risk category: D

How supplied

Injection: 2 mg/ml in 10-ml, 12.5-ml, 15-ml vials

Pharmacokinetics

Absorption: not applicable.
Distribution: 78% plasma protein-bound.
Metabolism: metabolized by liver.
Excretion: excreted by way of renal and hepatobiliary systems. *Half-life:* 5.8 days.

Route	Onset	Peak	Duration
I.V.	Unknown	Unknown	Unknown

Pharmacodynamics

Chemical effect: not fully understood; probably cell cycle-nonspecific. Drug reacts with DNA, producing cytotoxic effect.
Therapeutic effect: hinders susceptible cancer cell growth.

Reactions may be *common*, uncommon, *life-threatening*, or COMMON AND LIFE-THREATENING.

Indications and dosage

▶ **Combination initial therapy for acute nonlymphocytic leukemia.**
Adults: induction begins with 12 mg/m² I.V. daily on days 1 through 3, in combination with 100 mg/m² daily of cytarabine on days 1 through 7. A second induction may be given if response is not adequate. Maintenance therapy: 12 mg/m² on days 1 and 2, in combination with cytarabine on days 1 through 5.

Adverse reactions

CNS: *seizures,* headache.
CV: *heart failure, arrhythmias,* tachycardia.
EENT: conjunctivitis.
GI: *bleeding, abdominal pain, diarrhea, nausea, mucositis, vomiting, stomatitis.*
GU: uric acid nephropathy, *renal failure.*
Hematologic: *myelosuppression.*
Hepatic: jaundice.
Respiratory: dyspnea, cough.
Skin: petechiae, ecchymoses.
Other: alopecia, hyperuricemia.

Interactions

None significant.

Contraindications and precautions

• Contraindicated in patients hypersensitive to drug.
• Drug is not recommended for use in pregnant or breast-feeding women.
• Use cautiously in patients with prior exposure to anthracyclines or other cardiotoxic drugs.
• Safety of drug has not been established in children.

NURSING CONSIDERATIONS

Assessment
• Assess patient's condition before therapy and regularly thereafter.
• Monitor hematologic and laboratory chemistry parameters, as ordered.
• Be aware that left ventricular ejection fraction should be monitored.

• Be alert for adverse reactions and drug interactions.
• Evaluate patient's and family's knowledge of drug therapy.

Nursing diagnoses
• Altered health maintenance related to presence of leukemia
• Altered protection related to drug-induced myelosuppression
• Knowledge deficit related to drug therapy

▶ **Planning and implementation**
• Know that patients with significant myelosuppression should not receive drug unless benefits outweigh risks.
• Follow institutional policy to minimize risks. Preparation and administration of parenteral form are associated with mutagenic, teratogenic, and carcinogenic risks to personnel.
• Dilute dose (available as aqueous solution of 2 mg/ml in volumes of 10, 12.5, and 15 ml) in at least 50 ml of 0.9% NaCl injection or D₅W injection. Administer drug by direct injection into free-flowing I.V. line of 0.9% NaCl or D₅W injection over at least 3 minutes. Do not mix with other drugs. Heparin is physically incompatible. Do not mix together.
• Although drug is not a vesicant, if drug extravasates, discontinue infusion immediately and notify doctor.
• Be prepared to administer allopurinol, as ordered. Uric acid nephropathy can be avoided by adequately hydrating patient before and during therapy.
• If severe nonhematologic toxicity occurs during first course of therapy, know that second course should be delayed until patient recovers.
• Store undiluted solution at room temperature. Once diluted, mixture is stable for 7 days at room temperature.
Patient teaching
• Inform patient that urine may appear blue-green within 24 hours after administration and that some bluish discoloration

---

of sclera may occur. These effects are not harmful.

• Teach patient infection-control and bleeding precautions. Tell him to watch for and report signs of bleeding and infection.

• Advise female patient of childbearing age to avoid pregnancy during therapy and to consult doctor before becoming pregnant.

☑ **Evaluation**
• Patient responds well to therapy.
• Patient does not develop serious complications as result of drug-induced myelosuppression.
• Patient and family state understanding of drug therapy.

---

mivacurium chloride
(migh-vuh-KYOO-ree-um KLOR-ighd)
Mivacron

Pharmacologic class: nondepolarizing neuromuscular blocker
Therapeutic class: skeletal muscle relaxant
Pregnancy risk category: C

How supplied
Injection: 2 mg/ml in 5-ml and 10-ml vials
Infusion: 0.5 mg/ml in 50 ml of D_5W

Pharmacokinetics
Absorption: not applicable.
Distribution: not extensively distributed to tissues.
Metabolism: rapidly hydrolyzed by plasma pseudocholinesterase to inactive components.
Excretion: metabolites excreted in urine and bile. *Half-life: cis-trans* and *trans-trans* isomers, under 2.3 minutes; *cis-cis* isomer, 55 minutes.

Route	Onset	Peak	Duration
I.V.	1-2 min	2-5 min	20-35 min

Pharmacodynamics
Chemical effect: competes with acetylcholine for receptor sites at motor end plate. Because this action may be antagonized by cholinesterase inhibitors, drug is considered a competitive antagonist. Drug is mixture of three stereoisomers, each possessing neuromuscular blocking activity.
Therapeutic effect: relaxes skeletal muscles.

Indications and dosage
▶ **Adjunct to general anesthesia, to facilitate endotracheal intubation, and to relax skeletal muscles during surgery or mechanical ventilation.** *Adults:* dosage is highly individualized. Usually, 0.15 mg/kg I.V. push over 5 to 15 seconds provides adequate muscle relaxation within 2½ minutes for endotracheal intubation. Supplemental doses of 0.1 mg/kg I.V. q 15 minutes is usually sufficient to maintain muscle relaxation. Alternatively, maintain neuromuscular blockade with continuous infusion of 4 mcg/kg/minute begun simultaneously with initial dose, or 9 to 10 mcg/kg/minute started after evidence of spontaneous recovery caused by initial dose. When used with isoflurane or enflurane anesthesia, dosage is usually reduced about 35% to 40%.
Children ages 2 to 12: 0.20 mg/kg I.V. push given over 5 to 15 seconds. Neuromuscular blockade is usually evident in less than 2 minutes. Maintenance doses are generally required more frequently in children. Alternatively, neuromuscular blockade maintained with continuous I.V. infusion titrated to effect. Most children respond to 5 to 31 mcg/kg/minute (average 14 mcg/kg/minute).

Adverse reactions
CNS: dizziness.
CV: *flushing,* hypotension, tachycardia, bradycardia, *arrhythmias.*

Reactions may be *common,* uncommon, *life-threatening,* or COMMON AND LIFE-THREATENING.

Respiratory: *bronchospasm,* wheezing, *respiratory insufficiency or apnea.*
Skin: rash, urticaria, erythema.
Other: prolonged muscle weakness, phlebitis, muscle spasms.

Interactions

Drug-drug. *Alkaline solutions (such as barbiturate solutions):* physically incompatible; precipitate may form. Do not administer through same I.V. line.
Aminoglycosides (gentamicin, kanamycin, neomycin, streptomycin), bacitracin, colistimethate, colistin, polymyxin B sulfate, tetracycline: potentiated neuromuscular blockade, leading to increased skeletal muscle relaxation and prolongation of effect. Use together cautiously.
Carbamazepine, phenytoin: may prolong time to maximal blockade or shorten duration of blockade with neuromuscular blockers. Monitor patient.
Inhalation anesthetics (especially enflurane, isoflurane), quinidine: may enhance activity (or prolong action) of nondepolarizing neuromuscular blockers. Monitor for excessive weakness.
Magnesium salts: may enhance neuromuscular blockade. Monitor for excessive weakness.

Contraindications and precautions

• Contraindicated in patients with hypersensitivity to drug.
• Use very cautiously, if at all, in patients who are homozygous for atypical plasma pseudocholinesterase gene. Drug is metabolized to inactive compounds by plasma pseudocholinesterase.
• Use cautiously in patients with significant CV disease, in those who may be adversely affected by release of histamine (such as asthmatic patients), and in pregnant or breast-feeding women.
• Also use cautiously, possibly at reduced dosage, in debilitated patients; in patients with metastatic cancer, severe electrolyte disturbances, or neuromuscular diseases; and in those in whom potentiation or difficulty in reversal of neuromuscular

blockade is anticipated. Patients with myasthenia gravis or myasthenic syndrome (Eaton-Lambert syndrome) are particularly sensitive to effects of nondepolarizing relaxants.

NURSING CONSIDERATIONS

⚡ Assessment
• Assess patient's need for drug before therapy and regularly thereafter.
• Monitor respiratory rate closely until patient is fully recovered from neuromuscular blockade, as evidenced by tests of muscle strength (hand grip, head lift, and ability to cough).
• Be alert for adverse reactions and drug interactions.
• Evaluate patient's and family's knowledge of drug therapy.

⊕ Nursing diagnoses
• Ineffective breathing pattern related to drug's effect on respiratory muscle
• Knowledge deficit related to drug therapy

❯ Planning and implementation
• Administer only under direct medical supervision by personnel skilled in use of neuromuscular blockers and techniques for maintaining patent airway. Do not use unless emergency equipment for respiratory support and antagonist are within reach.
• To avoid patient distress, do not administer until patient's consciousness is obtunded by general anesthetic because drug has no effect on consciousness or pain threshold.
• Administer test dose to assess patient's sensitivity to drug. Patients with severe burns develop resistance to nondepolarizing neuromuscular blockers; however, they also may have reduced plasma pseudocholinesterase activity.
• Drug may be given by direct injection over 5 to 15 seconds.
• Prepare drug for I.V. use with D_5W, 0.9% NaCl injection, dextrose 5% in

0.9% NaCl injection, lactated Ringer's injection, or dextrose 5% in lactated Ringer's injection. Diluted solutions are stable for 24 hours at room temperature.
• Remember that when diluted as directed, drug is compatible with alfentanil, fentanyl, sufentanil, droperidol, and midazolam.
• For drug available as premixed infusion in D₅W, remove protective outer wrap, then check container for minor leaks by squeezing bag before administering. Do not add other drugs to container, and do not use container in series connections.
• Nerve stimulator and train-of-four monitoring are recommended to document antagonism of neuromuscular blockade and recovery of muscle strength. Before attempting reversal with neostigmine or edrophonium, some signs of spontaneous recovery should be evident.
• Know that experimental evidence suggests that acid-base and electrolyte balances may influence actions of nondepolarizing neuromuscular blockers. Alkalosis may counteract paralysis; acidosis may enhance it.
• Keep in mind that dosage should be adjusted to ideal body weight in obese patients (patients 30% or more above their ideal weight) to avoid prolonged neuromuscular blockade.
• Duration of effect is increased about 150% in patients with end-stage renal disease and 300% in patients with hepatic dysfunction.
• Be aware that like other neuromuscular blockers, dosage requirements for children are higher on mg/kg basis than those for adults. Onset and recovery of neuromuscular blockade occur more rapidly in children.
Patient teaching
• Describe use of drug to patient and family, and answer their questions.

☑ Evaluation
• Patient maintains adequate ventilation with or without assistance.

• Patient and family state understanding of drug therapy.

---

moexipril hydrochloride
(moh-EKS-eh-pril high-droh-KLOR-ighd)
Univasc

Pharmacologic class: ACE inhibitor
Therapeutic class: antihypertensive
Pregnancy risk category: C (D in second and third trimesters)

How supplied
Tablets: 7.5 mg, 15 mg

Pharmacokinetics
Absorption: incompletely absorbed from GI tract, with bioavailability of about 13%. Food significantly decreases bioavailability.
Distribution: about 50% protein-bound.
Metabolism: metabolized extensively to the active metabolite moexiprilat.
Excretion: excreted primarily in feces, with small amount in urine. *Half-life:* 2 to 9 hours.

Route	Onset	Peak	Duration
P.O.	About 1 hr	3-6 hr	24 hr

Pharmacodynamics
Chemical effect: unknown; thought to result primarily from suppression of renin-angiotensin-aldosterone system. Inhibits ACE, thereby inhibiting production of angiotensin II (a potent vasoconstrictor and stimulator of aldosterone secretion). Other mechanisms also may be involved.
Therapeutic effect: lowers blood pressure.

Indications and dosage
▶ **Hypertension.** *Adults:* 7.5 mg P.O. once daily before meals (3.75 mg for patients receiving diuretics). Inadequate response may lead to increased dose or divided dosing. Recommended dosage is 7.5 to 30 mg daily, in one or two divided dos-

---

Reactions may be *common*, uncommon, *life-threatening*, or COMMON AND LIFE-THREATENING.

es 1 hour before meals. Subsequent adjustments made based on patient response.

Adverse reactions

CNS: *dizziness,* headache, fatigue.
CV: peripheral edema, hypotension, orthostatic hypotension, chest pain, flushing.
EENT: pharyngitis, rhinitis, sinusitis.
GI: diarrhea, dyspepsia, nausea.
GU: urinary frequency.
Hematologic: neutropenia.
Respiratory: *persistent, nonproductive cough,* upper respiratory tract infection.
Skin: rash.
Other: myalgia, *anaphylactoid reactions, angioedema,* hyperkalemia, flu syndrome, pain.

Interactions

Drug-drug. *Antacids:* bioavailability of ACE inhibitors may be decreased. Give drug on an empty stomach.
Capsaicin: capsaicin may cause or exacerbate coughing associated with ACE inhibitor treatment. Avoid concomitant use.
Digoxin: increased plasma digoxin levels. Monitor digoxin levels and patient closely.
Diuretics: risk of excessive hypotension. Monitor blood pressure closely.
Indomethacin: reduced hypotensive effects of ACE inhibitors. Avoid concomitant use.
Lithium: increased serum lithium levels and lithium toxicity. Use together cautiously. Monitor serum lithium levels frequently.
Potassium-sparing diuretics, potassium supplements: risk of hyperkalemia. Monitor serum potassium level closely.
Drug-food. *Salt substitutes containing potassium:* risk of hyperkalemia. Monitor serum potassium level closely.

Contraindications and precautions

• Contraindicated in patients with hypersensitivity to drug or history of angioedema related to previous treatment with ACE inhibitor.

• Drug is not recommended for use in pregnant women.
• Use cautiously in patients with impaired kidney function, heart failure, or renal artery stenosis and in breast-feeding women.
• Safety of drug has not been established in children.

NURSING CONSIDERATIONS

Assessment
• Assess patient's blood pressure before therapy.
• Measure blood pressure at trough (just before dose) to verify adequate control. Drug is less effective in reducing trough blood pressure in blacks than in non-blacks.
• Monitor patient for hypotension.
• Assess kidney function before therapy and periodically thereafter. Monitor serum potassium level, as ordered.
• Know that other ACE inhibitors have been associated with agranulocytosis and neutropenia. Monitor CBC with differential counts before therapy, especially in patient who has collagen-vascular disease with impaired kidney function.
• Be alert for adverse reactions and interactions.
• Evaluate patient's and family's knowledge of drug therapy.

Nursing diagnoses
• Risk for injury related to presence of hypertension
• Sleep pattern disturbance related to cough
• Knowledge deficit related to drug therapy

Planning and implementation
• Excessive hypotension can occur when drug is given with diuretics. If possible, diuretic therapy should be discontinued 2 to 3 days before starting moexipril to decrease potential for excessive hypotensive response. If moexipril does not adequate-

ly control blood pressure, doctor may re-institute diuretic with care.
• Angioedema associated with tongue, glottis, or larynx may be fatal because of airway obstruction. Be prepared with appropriate therapy, such as epinephrine and equipment to ensure a patent airway.
• Notify doctor if drug-induced cough interferes with patient's ability to sleep.

Patient teaching
• Instruct patient to take this drug on an empty stomach; high-fat meals can impair absorption.
• Tell patient to avoid salt substitutes; these products may contain potassium, which can cause hyperkalemia.
• Advise patient to rise slowly to minimize light-headedness. If syncope occurs, tell him to stop drug and call doctor immediately.
• Urge patient to use caution in hot weather and during exercise. Inadequate fluid intake, vomiting, diarrhea, and excessive perspiration can lead to light-headedness and syncope.
• Advise him to report signs of infection, such as fever and sore throat; easy bruising or bleeding; swelling of tongue, lips, face, eyes, mucous membranes, or extremities; difficulty swallowing or breathing; and hoarseness.
• Tell female patient to notify doctor if pregnancy occurs.

☑ **Evaluation**
• Patient's blood pressure is normal.
• Patient states that sleep disturbance does not occur.
• Patient and family state understanding of drug therapy.

---

molindone hydrochloride
(moh-LIN-dohn high-droh-KLOR-ighd)
Moban

Pharmacologic class: dihydroindolone
Therapeutic class: antipsychotic
Pregnancy risk category: NR

How supplied

Tablets: 5 mg, 10 mg, 25 mg, 50 mg, 100 mg
Oral solution: 20 mg/ml

Pharmacokinetics

Absorption: appears to be rapid.
Distribution: distributed widely in body.
Metabolism: metabolized extensively.
Excretion: excreted primarily in urine; some excreted in feces.

Route	Onset	Peak	Duration
P.O.	Unknown	1.5 hr	24-36 hr

Pharmacodynamics

Chemical effect: unknown; probably blocks postsynaptic dopamine receptors in brain.
Therapeutic effect: relieves psychotic signs and symptoms.

Indications and dosage

▶ **Psychotic disorders.** *Adults:* initially, 50 to 75 mg P.O. daily, then increased to 100 to 225 mg/day in 3 or 4 days. Maintenance dosage as follows: mild disease—5 to 15 mg P.O. t.i.d. to q.i.d.; moderate disease—10 to 25 mg P.O. t.i.d. or q.i.d.; acute disease—225 mg/day P.O.

Adverse reactions

CNS: *extrapyramidal reactions* (moderate incidence), *tardive dyskinesia, sedation* (moderate incidence), pseudoparkinsonism, EEG changes, dizziness.
CV: *orthostatic hypotension,* tachycardia, ECG changes.
EENT: *blurred vision.*
GI: *dry mouth, constipation.*
GU: *urine retention,* dark urine, menstrual irregularities, gynecomastia, inhibited ejaculation.
Hematologic: transient leukopenia, hyperprolactinemia.
Hepatic: cholestatic jaundice, abnormal liver function test results.
Skin: *mild photosensitivity,* allergic reactions.

Reactions may be *common,* uncommon, *life-threatening,* or COMMON AND LIFE-THREATENING.

Other: rarely, *neuroleptic malignant syndrome.*

Interactions

Drug-drug. *CNS depressants:* increased CNS depression. Avoid concomitant use.
Drug-lifestyle. *Alcohol use:* increased CNS depression. Avoid concomitant use.

Contraindications and precautions

• Contraindicated in patients with hypersensitivity to drug and in those experiencing coma or severe CNS depression.
• Use cautiously when increased physical activity would be harmful and in patients subject to seizures (may lower seizure threshold). Also use cautiously in pregnant or breast-feeding women.
• Safety of drug has not been established in children.

NURSING CONSIDERATIONS

Assessment
• Assess patient's condition before therapy and regularly thereafter.
• Be alert for adverse reactions and drug interactions.
• Monitor patient for tardive dyskinesia. It may occur after prolonged use. It may not appear until months or years later and may disappear spontaneously or persist for life, despite discontinuation of drug.
• Evaluate patient's and family's knowledge of drug therapy.

Nursing diagnoses
• Altered thought processes related to underlying psychotic disorder
• Risk for injury related to drug-induced adverse CNS reactions
• Knowledge deficit related to drug therapy

Planning and implementation
• Know that drug may be administered in single daily dose.
• Acute dystonic reactions may be treated with diphenhydramine.

Patient teaching
• Warn patient to avoid activities that require alertness or good psychomotor coordination until CNS effects of drug are known.
• Tell patient to avoid alcohol consumption during drug therapy.
• Instruct patient to relieve dry mouth with sugarless gum or hard candy.

Evaluation
• Patient demonstrates decrease in psychotic behavior.
• Patient does not experience injury from adverse CNS reactions.
• Patient and family state understanding of drug therapy.

monoctanoin
(mon-ok-tah-NOH-in)
Moctanin

Pharmacologic class: esterified glycerol
Therapeutic class: cholelitholytic
Pregnancy risk category: C

How supplied

Infusion: 120-ml bottles

Pharmacokinetics

Absorption: not applicable (drug is perfused directly into common bile duct).
Distribution: none.
Metabolism: hydrolyzed by pancreatic and other digestive lipases to produce fatty acids.
Excretion: none.

Route	Onset	Peak	Duration
T tube	≤ 72 hr	Unknown	Unknown

Pharmacodynamics

Chemical effect: dissolves gallstones by rendering them more soluble.
Therapeutic effect: eliminates cholesterol gallstones.

Indications and dosage

▶ **To solubilize cholesterol (radiolu-cent) gallstones that are retained in biliary tract after cholecystectomy.**
Adults: administered as continuous infusion for 2 to 10 days (for elimination or size reduction of stones) through catheter inserted directly into common bile duct by way of T tube at rate of 3 to 5 ml/hour and at pressure of 10 cm H_2O.

Adverse reactions

GI: *pain, discomfort, nausea, vomiting, diarrhea,* anorexia, indigestion.
Other: metabolic acidosis, fever.

Interactions

None significant.

Contraindications and precautions

• Contraindicated in patients with impaired liver function, biliary tract infection, history of recent duodenal ulceration or jejunitis, portosystemic shunting, acute pancreatitis, or active life-threatening problems that would be complicated by perfusion into biliary tract.
• Use cautiously in pregnant or breast-feeding women.
• Safety of drug has not been established in children.

NURSING CONSIDERATIONS

⚡ Assessment
• Assess patient's condition before therapy and regularly thereafter.
• Because impaired liver function may lead to metabolic acidosis during administration, obtain routine liver function tests, as ordered, before perfusion therapy begins.
• Be alert for adverse reactions.
• Monitor patient's hydration status if adverse GI reactions occurs.
• Evaluate patient's and family's knowledge of drug therapy.

🔵 Nursing diagnoses
• Pain related to gallstones

• Risk for fluid volume deficit related to drug-induced adverse GI reactions
• Knowledge deficit related to drug therapy

▶ Planning and implementation
• Monoctanoin treatment should be initiated only by personnel experienced in infusion therapy.
• Do not give parenterally; drug is used for biliary tract infusion only.
• Dilute each vial with sterile water for injection. Diluting drug reduces solution viscosity and enhances bathing of stone.
• Warm solution to 65° to 80° F (18° to 27° C) before perfusion. Temperature of solution should not fall below 65° F (18° C) during administration.
• Use peristaltic infusion pump to regulate infusion. Outpatients may use battery-operated portable pump.
• Keep pressure at 10 cm H_2O to help minimize GI and biliary tract irritation. Pressure must be kept below 15 cm H_2O.
• Reduce GI symptoms by slowing infusion rate or discontinuing infusion during meals, as ordered.
Patient teaching
• Explain to patient and family how drug is administered.
• Instruct patient to promptly report adverse GI reactions.

☑ Evaluation
• Patient's gallstones are dissolved.
• Patient maintains adequate hydration throughout therapy.
• Patient and family state understanding of drug therapy.

montelukast sodium
(mon-tih-LOO-kist SOH-dee-um)
Singulair

Pharmacologic class: leukotriene receptor antagonist
Therapeutic class: antiasthmatic
Pregnancy risk category: B

Reactions may be *common*, uncommon, *life-threatening*, or COMMON AND LIFE-THREATENING.

How supplied

Tablets (film-coated): 10 mg
Tablets (chewable): 5 mg

Pharmacokinetics

Absorption: rapid with an oral bioavailability of 64%.
Distribution: over 99% bound to plasma proteins.
Metabolism: extensively metabolized by cytochrome P-450 isoenzymes.
Excretion: approximately 86% is recovered in the feces, indicating montelukast and its metabolites are excreted almost exclusively via the bile. *Half-life:* 2.7 to 5.5 hours.

Route	Onset	Peak	Duration
P.O. (coated)	Unknown	3-4 hr	Unknown
P.O. (chewable)	Unknown	2-2.5 hr	Unknown

Pharmacodynamics

Chemical effect: causes inhibition of airway cysteinyl leukotriene (CysLT$_1$) receptors. It binds with high affinity and selectivity to the CysLT$_1$ receptor, and inhibits physiologic action of the cysteinyl leukotriene LTD$_4$. This receptor inhibition reduces early- and late-phase bronchoconstriction caused by antigen challenge.
Therapeutic effect: improves breathing.

Indications and dosages

▶ **Prophylaxis and chronic treatment of asthma.** *Adults and children age 15 and older:* 10 mg P.O. once daily in evening. *Children ages 6 to 14:* 5 mg (chewable tablet) P.O. once daily in evening.

Adverse reactions

CNS: *headache,* dizziness, fatigue, asthenia.
EENT: nasal congestion, dental pain.
GI: dyspepsia, infectious gastroenteritis, abdominal pain.
GU: pyuria.

Hepatic: increased ALT and AST levels.
Respiratory: cough.
Skin: rash.
Other: fever, trauma, influenza.

Interactions

Drug-drug. *Phenobarbital, rifampin:* may decrease bioavailability of montelukast due to induction of hepatic metabolism. Monitor closely.

Contraindications and precautions

• Contraindicated in patients with acute asthmatic attacks, status asthmaticus, or hypersensitivity to drug or its components.
• Use cautiously and with appropriate monitoring in patients when systemic corticosteroid medication dosages are reduced.
• Safety and efficacy for patients under age 6 have not been established.

NURSING CONSIDERATIONS

✎ Assessment
• Assess patient's underlying condition and monitor for drug's effectiveness.
• Monitor for adverse reactions and drug interactions.
• Evaluate patient's and family's knowledge of drug therapy.

Nursing diagnoses
• Impaired gas exchange related to asthma
• Activity intolerance related to asthma
• Knowledge deficit related to drug therapy

Planning and implementation
• Do not abruptly substitute drug for inhaled or oral corticosteroids.
• Know that drug is not indicated for use in patients with acute asthmatic attacks, status asthmaticus, or as monotherapy for management of exercise-induced bronchospasm. Appropriate rescue medication should be continued for acute exacerbations.
• Give drug daily and not on as-needed basis.

Patient teaching
• Advise patient to take drug daily, even if asymptomatic, and to contact doctor if asthma is not well controlled.
• Warn patient not to reduce or stop taking other prescribed antiasthma drugs without doctor's approval.
• Warn patient that drug is not beneficial in acute asthma attacks, or in exercise-induced bronchospasm and advise to keep appropriate rescue medications available.
• Advise patient with known aspirin sensitivity to continue to avoid using aspirin and NSAIDs.
• Advise patient with phenylketonuria that chewable tablet contains phenylalanine.

☑ **Evaluation**
• Patient's respiratory signs and symptoms improve.
• Patient is able to perform normal activities of daily living.
• Patient and family state understanding of drug therapy.

---

moricizine hydrochloride
(MOR-ih-sigh-zeen high-droh-KLOR-ighd)
Ethmozine

Pharmacologic class: sodium channel blocker
Therapeutic class: antiarrhythmic
Pregnancy risk category: B

How supplied
Tablets: 200 mg, 250 mg, 300 mg

Pharmacokinetics
Absorption: absorbed from GI tract. Administration within 30 minutes of mealtime delays absorption and lowers peak plasma levels but has no effect on extent of absorption.
Distribution: 95% protein-bound.
Metabolism: undergoes significant first-pass metabolism. At least 26 metabolites have been found; not one represents at least 1% of a dose. Drug induces its own metabolism.
Excretion: 50% excreted in feces; 39% excreted in urine; some recycled through enterohepatic circulation. *Half-life:* 1½ to 3½ hours.

Route	Onset	Peak	Duration
P.O.	≤ 2 hr	0.5-2 hr	10-24 hr

Pharmacodynamics
Chemical effect: class I antiarrhythmic that reduces fast inward current carried by sodium ions across myocardial cell membranes. Moricizine has potent local anesthetic activity and membrane-stabilizing effect.
Therapeutic effect: alleviates ventricular arrhythmias.

Indications and dosage
▶ **Life-threatening ventricular arrhythmias.** *Adults:* individualized dosage is based on clinical response and patient tolerance. Therapy should begin in hospital. Most patients respond to 600 to 900 mg P.O. daily in divided doses q 8 hours. Daily dosage increased within this range q 3 days by 150 mg until desired clinical effect is seen. *In patients with hepatic or renal impairment:* 600 mg or less P.O. daily.

Adverse reactions
CNS: *dizziness, headache, fatigue,* anxiety, hypoesthesia, asthenia, nervousness, paresthesias, sleep disorders.
CV: *proarrhythmic events (ventricular tachycardia, PVCs, supraventricular arrhythmias), ECG abnormalities (including conduction defects, sinus pause, junctional rhythm, or AV block),* **heart failure,** *palpitations,* **cardiac death,** *chest pain.*
EENT: blurred vision.
GI: *nausea, vomiting, abdominal pain, dyspepsia, diarrhea, dry mouth.*
GU: urine retention, urinary frequency, dysuria.
Respiratory: dyspnea.
Skin: rash.

Reactions may be *common,* uncommon, *life-threatening,* or **COMMON AND LIFE-THREATENING.**

Other: drug-induced fever, diaphoresis, musculoskeletal pain.

Interactions

Drug-drug. *Cimetidine:* increased plasma levels and decreased clearance of moricizine. Begin moricizine therapy at low dosage (not more than 600 mg daily) and monitor plasma levels and therapeutic effect closely.
Digoxin, propranolol: additive prolongation of PR interval. Monitor patient closely.
Theophylline: increased clearance and reduced plasma levels of theophylline. Monitor plasma levels and therapeutic response; adjust theophylline dosage as ordered.

Contraindications and precautions

• Contraindicated in patients with hypersensitivity to drug; preexisting second- or third-degree AV block or right bundle-branch heart block when associated with left hemiblock (bifascicular block) unless artificial pacemaker is present; and cardiogenic shock.
• Drug is not recommended for use in breast-feeding women.
• Use with extreme caution in patients with sick sinus syndrome because drug may cause sinus bradycardia or sinus arrest. Also use with extreme caution in patients with coronary artery disease and left ventricular dysfunction because these patients may be at risk for sudden death when treated with drug.
• Administer cautiously to patients with hepatic or renal impairment and to pregnant women.
• Safety of drug has not been established in children.

NURSING CONSIDERATIONS

🔍 **Assessment**
• Assess patient's condition before therapy and regularly thereafter.
• Be alert for adverse reactions and drug interactions.

• Evaluate patient's and family's knowledge of drug therapy.

⊕ **Nursing diagnoses**
• Decreased cardiac output related to presence of ventricular arrhythmia
• Risk for injury related to drug-induced adverse reactions
• Knowledge deficit related to drug therapy

⊠ **Planning and implementation**
• Know that when substituting moricizine for another antiarrhythmic, previous drug should be withdrawn for one or two of drug's half-lives before moricizine is started. Patients with tendency to develop life-threatening arrhythmias after drug withdrawal should be hospitalized during withdrawal of therapy and adjustment to moricizine. Guidelines that doctors use for starting moricizine therapy are as follows:
– disopyramide, 6 to 12 hours after last dose.
– mexiletine, 8 to 12 hours after last dose.
– procainamide, 3 to 6 hours after last dose.
– propafenone, 8 to 12 hours after last dose.
– quinidine, 6 to 12 hours after last dose.
– tocainide, 8 to 12 hours after last dose.
• Determine electrolyte status and correct imbalances before therapy, as ordered. Hypokalemia, hyperkalemia, and hypomagnesemia may alter effects of drug.
Patient teaching
• Tell patient to report adverse reactions promptly.

☑ **Evaluation**
• Patient regains normal cardiac output with alleviation of ventricular arrhythmia.
• Patient does not experience injury from adverse reactions.
• Patient and family state understanding of drug therapy.

morphine hydrochloride
(MOR-feen high-droh-KLOR-ighd)
Morphitec◆, M.O.S.◆, M.O.S.-SR◆

morphine sulfate
Astramorph PF, Duramorph, Duramorph PF, Epimorph◆, Infumorph 200, Infumorph 500, Morphine H.P.◆, MS Contin, MSIR, Oramorph SR, RMS Uniserts, Roxanol, Roxanol 100, Roxanol Rescudose, Roxanol SR, Roxanol UD, Statex◆

morphine tartrate◇
(MOR-feen TAR-trayt)

Pharmacologic class: opioid
Therapeutic class: narcotic analgesic
Controlled substance schedule: II
Pregnancy risk category: C

How supplied

morphine hydrochloride
Tablets: 10 mg◆, 20 mg◆, 40 mg◆, 60 mg◆
Tablets (extended-release): 30 mg◆, 60 mg◆
Oral solution◆: 1 mg/ml, 5 mg/ml, 10 mg/ml, 20 mg/ml, 50 mg/ml
Syrup: 1 mg/ml◆, 5 mg/ml◆, 10 mg/ml◆, 20 mg/ml◆, 50 mg/ml◆
Suppositories: 10 mg◆, 20 mg◆, 30 mg◆
morphine sulfate
Tablets: 15 mg, 30 mg
Tablets (extended-release): 15 mg, 30 mg, 60 mg, 100 mg, 200 mg
Soluble tablets: 10 mg, 15 mg, 30 mg
Oral solution: 10 mg/5 ml, 20 mg/5 ml, 20 mg/ml (concentrate)
Syrup: 1 mg/ml, 5 mg/ml
Injection (with preservative):
500 mcg/ml, 1 mg/ml, 2 mg/ml, 3 mg/ml, 4 mg/ml, 5 mg/ml, 8 mg/ml, 10 mg/ml, 15 mg/ml, 25 mg/ml, 50 mg/ml
Injection (without preservative):
500 mcg/ml, 1 mg/ml, 10 mg/ml, 25 mg/ml

Suppositories: 5 mg, 10 mg, 20 mg, 30 mg
morphine tartrate
Injection: 80 mg/ml◇

Pharmacokinetics

Absorption: absorbed variably from GI tract when administered P.O.; unknown for other routes.
Distribution: distributed widely throughout body.
Metabolism: metabolized primarily in liver.
Excretion: excreted in urine and bile.
Half-life: 2 to 3 hours.

Route	Onset	Peak	Duration
P.O.	≤ 1 hr	1-2 hr	4-12 hr
I.V.	< 5 min	20 min	4-5 hr
I.M.	10-30 min	30-60 min	4-5 hr
S.C.	10-30 min	50-90 min	4-5 hr
P.R.	20-60 min	20-60 min	4-5 hr
Epidural	15-60 min	15-60 min	≤ 24 hr
Intrathecal	15-60 min	Unknown	≤ 24 hr

Pharmacodynamics

Chemical effect: binds with opioid receptors in CNS, altering both perception of and emotional response to pain through unknown mechanism.
Therapeutic effect: relieves pain.

Indications and dosage

▶ **Severe pain.** *Adults:* 10 mg S.C. or I.M. or 2.5 to 15 mg I.V. q 4 hours, p.r.n.; or 10 to 30 mg P.O. or 10 to 20 mg P.R. q 4 hours, p.r.n. When given by continuous I.V. infusion, loading dose of 15 mg I.V. may be followed by continuous infusion of 0.8 to 10 mg/hour. Alternatively, 30 mg controlled-release tablets P.O. q 8 to 12 hours may be administered. As epidural injection, 5 mg by epidural catheter. If adequate pain relief not obtained within 1 hour, additional doses of 1 to 2 mg are given at intervals sufficient to assess efficacy. Maximum total epidural dosage should not exceed 10 mg.
Children: 0.1 to 0.2 mg/kg S.C. q 4 hours. Maximum single dose is 15 mg.

Adverse reactions

CNS: *sedation, somnolence, clouded sensorium, euphoria,* **seizures** (with large doses), dizziness, *nightmares* (with long-acting oral forms).
CV: *hypotension,* **bradycardia, shock, cardiac arrest.**
GI: *nausea, vomiting, constipation,* ileus.
GU: *urine retention.*
Hematologic: *thrombocytopenia.*
Respiratory: *respiratory depression, respiratory arrest.*
Skin: pruritus and flushing (with epidural administration).
Other: *physical dependence.*

Interactions

Drug-drug. *CNS depressants, general anesthetics, hypnotics, MAO inhibitors, other narcotic analgesics, sedatives, tranquilizers, tricyclic antidepressants:* possible respiratory depression, hypotension, profound sedation, or coma. Use together with extreme caution. Reduce morphine dosage and monitor patient response.
Drug-lifestyle. *Alcohol use:* additive effects. Use together cautiously.

Contraindications and precautions

• Contraindicated in patients with hypersensitivity to drug or conditions that preclude I.V. administration of opioids (acute bronchial asthma or upper airway obstruction).
• Use with extreme caution in elderly and debilitated patients and in patients with head injury, increased intracranial pressure, seizures, chronic pulmonary disease, prostatic hyperplasia, severe hepatic or renal disease, acute abdominal conditions, hypothyroidism, Addison's disease, or urethral stricture.
• Use cautiously in pregnant women.
• Breast-feeding women should wait 2 to 3 hours after last dose before breast-feeding to avoid sedation in infant.

NURSING CONSIDERATIONS

⬔ Assessment
• Assess patient's pain before therapy and regularly thereafter.
• Be aware that morphine may worsen or mask gallbladder pain.
• Monitor patient for respiratory depression after administration. When given epidurally, monitor for up to 24 hours after injection. Check respiratory rate and depth every 30 to 60 minutes for 24 hours.
• Be alert for adverse reactions and drug interactions.
• Evaluate patient's and family's knowledge of drug therapy.

⊕ Nursing diagnoses
• Pain related to underlying condition
• Ineffective breathing pattern related to drug's depressive effect on respiratory system
• Knowledge deficit related to drug therapy

▷ Planning and implementation
• Keep narcotic antagonist and resuscitation equipment available.
P.O. use: Oral solutions of various concentrations are available as well as intensified oral solution (20 mg/ml). Carefully note strength administered.
– Do not crush or break extended-release tablets.
– If S.L. administration is ordered, measure oral solution with tuberculin syringe. Administer dose a few drops at a time to allow maximal S.L. absorption and minimize swallowing.
I.V. use: When given by direct injection, 2.5 to 15.0 mg may be diluted in 4 or 5 ml of sterile water for injection and given over 4 to 5 minutes. Alternatively, drug may be mixed with D_5W to concentration of 0.1 to 1.0 mg/ml and administered by continuous-infusion device. Morphine sulfate is compatible with most common I.V. solutions.

---

*Liquid form contains alcohol   **May contain tartrazine   ◆Canada   ◇Australia   †OTC

I.M. and S.C. use: Follow normal protocol.

P.R. use: Be aware that refrigeration of rectal suppository is not necessary. In some patients, P.R. and P.O. absorption may not be equivalent.

Epidural and intrathecal use: Know that preservative-free preparations are available for epidural or intrathecal administration.

• Morphine is drug of choice in relieving pain of MI. It may cause transient decrease in blood pressure.

• An around-the-clock regimen best manages severe, chronic pain.

• Withhold dose and notify doctor if respiratory rate is below 12 breaths/minute.

• Because constipation is often severe with maintenance dosage, ensure that stool softener or other laxative is ordered.

Patient teaching

• Caution ambulatory patient about getting out of bed or walking. Warn outpatient to refrain from driving and performing other potentially hazardous activities that require mental alertness until drug's adverse CNS effects are known.

• Tell patient to report if morphine does not provide pain relief.

• Instruct patient to avoid alcohol consumption during drug therapy.

☑ **Evaluation**

• Patient states that pain is relieved.

• Patient maintains adequate breathing patterns throughout therapy.

• Patient and family state understanding of drug therapy.

---

muromonab-CD3
(myoo-roh-MOH-nab see dee three)
Orthoclone OKT3

Pharmacologic class: monoclonal antibody
Therapeutic class: immunosuppressive
Pregnancy risk category: C

How supplied
Injection: 1 mg/1 ml in 5-ml ampules

Pharmacokinetics
Absorption: not applicable.
Distribution: unknown.
Metabolism: unknown.
Excretion: unknown.

Route	Onset	Peak	Duration
I.V.	Almost immediate	Unknown	1 wk after drug stopped

Pharmacodynamics
Chemical effect: IgG antibody that reacts in T-lymphocyte membrane with a molecule (CD3) needed for antigen recognition. This drug depletes blood of CD3-positive T cells, which leads to restoration of allograft function and reversal of rejection.
Therapeutic effect: halts acute allograft rejection in kidney transplantation.

Indications and dosage

▶ **Acute allograft rejection in kidney transplant patients; steroid-resistant hepatic or cardiac allograft rejection.**
Adults: 5 mg I.V. bolus once daily for 10 to 14 days.

Adverse reactions

CNS: *tremors,* headache, *seizures, encephalopathy, cerebral edema.*
CV: *chest pain,* tachycardia, *cardiac arrest, shock, heart failure.*
GI: *nausea, vomiting,* diarrhea.
Respiratory: *severe pulmonary edema, adult respiratory distress syndrome, dyspnea.*
Other: *fever, chills,* INFECTION*, anaphylaxis, cytokine release syndrome, aseptic meningitis, risk of neoplasia.*

Interactions

Drug-drug. *Immunosuppressants:* increased risk of infection. Monitor closely.
Indomethacin: increased muromonab-CD3 levels with CNS effects.

Reactions may be *common,* uncommon, *life-threatening*, or COMMON AND LIFE-THREATENING.

Encephalopathy has occurred. Monitor patient closely.

Live-virus vaccines: may increase replication and effects of virus vaccine. Postpone vaccination when possible and consult doctor.

Contraindications and precautions

• Contraindicated in pregnant or breastfeeding women and in patients with hypersensitivity to drug or to other products of murine origin. Also contraindicated in patients who have antimouse antibody titers of 1:1,000 or more; who have fluid overload, as evidenced by chest X-ray or weight gain greater than 3% within week before treatment; and who have history of or are predisposed to seizures.

• Safety of drug has not been established in children.

NURSING CONSIDERATIONS

Assessment
• Assess patient's condition before therapy and regularly thereafter.
• Obtain chest X-ray within 24 hours before drug treatment, as ordered.
• Assess patient for signs of fluid overload before treatment.
• Be alert for adverse reactions and drug interactions.
• Monitor patient's hydration status if adverse GI reactions occur.
• Evaluate patient's and family's knowledge of drug therapy.

Nursing diagnoses
• Risk for injury related to presence of acute allograft rejection
• Risk for fluid volume deficit related to drug-induced adverse GI reactions
• Knowledge deficit related to drug therapy

Planning and implementation
• Keep in mind that treatment should begin in facility that is equipped and staffed for cardiopulmonary resuscitation and in which patient can be monitored closely.

• Most adverse reactions develop within 30 minutes to 6 hours after first dose.
• Administer antipyretic, as ordered, before giving drug to help lower incidence of expected pyrexia and chills. Corticosteroids may also be administered, as ordered, before first injection to help decrease incidence of adverse reactions. Methylprednisolone sodium succinate (1 mg/kg) preinjection followed by hydrocortisone sodium succinate (100 mg) 30 minutes postinjection may alleviate severity of first-dose reaction.
• Be aware that muromonab-CD3 is a monoclonal antibody preparation. Patients develop antibodies to this preparation that can lead to loss of effectiveness and more severe adverse reactions if second course of therapy is attempted. Therefore, experts believe that this drug should be used for only single course of treatment.

Patient teaching
• Inform patient of expected adverse reactions, and reassure him that they will lessen as treatment progresses.

Evaluation
• Patient exhibits no signs of organ rejection.
• Patient maintains adequate hydration.
• Patient and family state understanding of drug therapy.

---

mycophenolate mofetil
(migh-koh-FEN-oh-layt MOH-feh-til)
CellCept

mycophenolate mofetil hydrochloride
CellCept Intravenous

Pharmacologic class: mycophenolic acid derivative
Therapeutic class: immunosuppressant
Pregnancy risk category: C

How supplied

mycophenolate mofetil
Capsules: 250 mg
Tablets: 500 mg
mycophenolate mofetil hydrochloride
Injection: 500 mg/vial

Pharmacokinetics

Absorption: absorbed from GI tract.
Distribution: 97% bound to plasma proteins.
Metabolism: undergoes complete presystemic metabolism to mycophenolic acid.
Excretion: excreted primarily in urine, with small amount in feces. *Half-life:* about 17.9 hours.

Route	Onset	Peak	Duration
P.O.	Unknown	Unknown	Unknown
I.V.	Unknown	Unknown	10-17 hr

Pharmacodynamics

Chemical effect: inhibits proliferative responses of T- and B-lymphocytes, suppresses antibody formation by B-lymphocytes, and may inhibit recruitment of leukocytes into sites of inflammation and graft rejection.
Therapeutic effect: prevents organ rejection.

Indications and dosage

► **Prophylaxis of organ rejection in patients receiving allogeneic renal transplant.** Adults: 1 g P.O. or I.V. b.i.d., used with corticosteroids and cyclosporine (begun within 72 hours after transplantation).
► **Prophylaxis of organ rejection in patients receiving allogeneic cardiac transplant.** *Adults:* 1.5 g P.O. or I.V. b.i.d. in combination with cyclosporine and corticosteroids.

Adverse reactions

CNS: *tremor, insomnia, dizziness, headache.*
CV: *chest pain, hypertension, edema.*

GI: *diarrhea, constipation, nausea, dyspepsia, vomiting, oral moniliasis, abdominal pain,* HEMORRHAGE.
GU: urinary tract infection, hematuria, kidney tubular necrosis.
Hematologic: anemia, *leukopenia,* THROMBOCYTOPENIA, hypochromic anemia, leukocytosis.
Metabolic: *hypercholesteremia, hypophosphatemia, hypokalemia,* hyperkalemia, hyperglycemia.
Respiratory: *dyspnea, cough,* pharyngitis, infection, bronchitis, pneumonia.
Skin: *acne, rash.*
Other: *pain, fever, infection, sepsis, asthenia, back pain,* peripheral edema.

Interactions

Drug-drug. *Acyclovir, ganciclovir, other drugs known to undergo tubular secretion:* increased risk of toxicity for both drugs. Monitor patient closely.
Antacids with magnesium and aluminum hydroxides: decreased absorption of mycophenolate mofetil. Separate dosages.
Azathioprine: has not been clinically studied. Avoid concurrent use.
Cholestyramine: may interfere with enterohepatic recirculation, reducing mycophenolate bioavailability. Do not administer concurrently.
Oral contraceptives: may affect efficacy of oral contraceptives. Advise patient to use barrier birth control methods.

Contraindications and precautions

• Contraindicated in patients with hypersensitivity to drug, mycophenolic acid, or other components of product and in pregnant (unless benefits outweigh risks) or breast-feeding women.
• Use cautiously in patients with GI disorders.
• Safety of drug has not been established in children.

NURSING CONSIDERATIONS

𝄪 Assessment
• Obtain history of patient's kidney transplant.
• Monitor CBC regularly, as ordered.
• Be alert for adverse reactions and drug interactions.
• Evaluate patient's and family's knowledge of drug therapy.

⊕ Nursing diagnoses
• Altered health maintenance related to need for kidney transplant
• Altered protection related to drug-induced immunosuppression
• Knowledge deficit related to drug therapy

⟩ Planning and implementation
P.O. use: Administer drug on an empty stomach. Do not crush or open capsules or tablets.
I.V. use: CellCept Intravenous must be reconstituted and diluted to a concentration of 6 mg/ml using 5% dextrose injection.
– Never administer drug by rapid or bolus I.V. injection. Give infusion over at least 2 hours.
• In patients with severe chronic renal impairment (GFR less than 25 ml/minute) outside the immediate post-transplant period, avoid use of doses above 1 g b.i.d.
• Because of potential teratogenic effects, do not open or crush capsules. Avoid inhaling powder in capsules or letting it contact skin or mucous membranes. If contact occurs, wash thoroughly with soap and water; rinse eyes with plain water.
• Notify doctor if neutropenia occurs; he may stop drug or reduce dose, order appropriate diagnostic tests, and provide additional treatment.
Patient teaching
• Warn patient not to open or crush capsule but to swallow it whole on an empty stomach.

• Stress importance of not interrupting therapy without consulting doctor.
• Inform female patient that a pregnancy test should be done 1 week before therapy. Advise her to use effective contraception until at least 6 weeks after discontinuation, even with history of infertility (unless due to hysterectomy). Tell her that two forms of contraception must be used simultaneously, unless abstinence is chosen. If pregnancy occurs despite these measures, have patient contact doctor immediately.

✓ Evaluation
• Patient does not exhibit signs and symptoms of organ rejection.
• Neutropenia does not develop.
• Patient and family state understanding of drug therapy.

nabumetone
(nuh-BYOO-meh-tohn)
Relafen

Pharmacologic class: NSAID
Therapeutic class: antiarthritic
Pregnancy risk category: C

How supplied
Tablets: 500 mg, 750 mg

Pharmacokinetics
Absorption: well absorbed from GI tract. Administration with food increases absorption rate and peak levels of its principal metabolite but doesn't change total drug absorbed.
Distribution: over 99% of metabolite is bound to plasma proteins.
Metabolism: metabolized to inactive metabolites in liver.

Excretion: metabolites excreted primarily in urine; about 9% appears in feces.
Half-life: about 24 hours.

Route	Onset	Peak	Duration
P.O.	Unknown	2-4 hr	Unknown

Pharmacodynamics

Chemical effect: unknown; may inhibit prostaglandin synthesis.
Therapeutic effect: relieves pain.

Indications and dosage

▶ **Rheumatoid arthritis or osteoarthritis.** *Adults:* initially, 1,000 mg P.O. daily as single dose or in divided doses b.i.d. Maximum daily dosage is 2,000 mg.

Adverse reactions

CNS: *dizziness, headache,* fatigue, increased sweating, insomnia, nervousness, somnolence.
CV: vasculitis.
EENT: *tinnitus.*
GI: *diarrhea, dyspepsia, abdominal pain, constipation, flatulence, nausea,* dry mouth, gastritis, stomatitis, vomiting, *bleeding,* ulceration.
Respiratory: dyspnea, pneumonitis.
Skin: *pruritus, rash.*
Other: *edema.*

Interactions

Drug-drug. *Diuretics:* NSAIDs may decrease diuretic effectiveness. Monitor patient closely during therapy.
Drugs highly bound to plasma proteins (such as warfarin): increased risk of adverse effects from displacement of drug by nabumetone. Use cautiously.
Drug-food. *Any food:* increases absorption. Give together.
Drug-lifestyle. *Alcohol use:* associated with increased risk of additive GI toxicity. Avoid concomitant use.

Contraindications and precautions

● Contraindicated in patients with hypersensitivity to drug or history of aspirin- or NSAID-induced asthma, urticaria, or other allergic-type reactions.
● Drug is not recommended for use during third trimester of pregnancy or in breast-feeding women.
● Use cautiously in patients with renal or hepatic impairment; peptic ulcer disease; and heart failure, hypertension, or other conditions that may predispose to fluid retention.
● Safety of drug has not been established in children.

NURSING CONSIDERATIONS

🩺 Assessment
● Assess patient's arthritis before therapy and regularly thereafter.
● During long-term therapy, periodically monitor renal and liver function, CBC, and hematocrit as ordered; assess these patients for signs and symptoms of GI bleeding.
● Be alert for adverse reactions and drug interactions.
● Evaluate patient's and family's knowledge of drug therapy.

Nursing diagnoses
● Pain related to arthritic condition
● Impaired tissue integrity related to adverse drug effect on GI mucosa
● Knowledge deficit related to drug therapy

Planning and implementation
● Administer drug with food to enhance time of absorption.
● Notify doctor of adverse reactions.
Patient teaching
● Instruct patient to take drug with food, milk, or antacids for best absorption.
● Advise patient to limit alcohol intake because of additive GI toxicity.
● Teach patient to recognize and report signs and symptoms of GI bleeding.

✓ Evaluation
● Patient is free from pain.

Reactions may be *common,* uncommon, *life-threatening,* or COMMON AND LIFE-THREATENING.

• Patient's GI tissue integrity is maintained throughout drug therapy.
• Patient and family state understanding of drug therapy.

nadolol
(nay-DOH-lol)
Corgard, Syn-Nadolol ♦

Pharmacologic class: beta blocker
Therapeutic class: antihypertensive, antianginal
Pregnancy risk category: C

How supplied

Tablets: 20 mg, 40 mg, 80 mg, 120 mg, 160 mg

Pharmacokinetics

Absorption: 30% to 40% of dose is absorbed from GI tract.
Distribution: distributed throughout body; about 30% protein-bound.
Metabolism: none.
Excretion: most excreted unchanged in urine; remainder in feces. *Half-life:* about 20 hours.

Route	Onset	Peak	Duration
P.O.	Unknown	2-4 hr	Unknown

Pharmacodynamics

Chemical effect: reduces cardiac oxygen demand by blocking catecholamine-induced increases in heart rate, blood pressure, and myocardial contraction. Depresses renin secretion.
Therapeutic effect: lowers blood pressure and relieves anginal pain.

Indications and dosage

▶ **Angina pectoris.** *Adults:* 40 mg P.O. once daily, initially. Dosage increased in 40- to 80-mg increments until optimum response occurs. Usual maintenance dosage is 40 to 240 mg daily.
▶ **Hypertension.** *Adults:* 20 to 40 mg P.O. once daily, initially. Dosage increased in 40- to 80-mg increments/day until optimum response occurs. Usual maintenance dosage is 40 to 320 mg daily (in rare cases, 640 mg).

Adverse reactions

CNS: fatigue, lethargy, dizziness.
CV: *bradycardia, hypotension,* **heart failure,** peripheral vascular disease.
GI: nausea, vomiting, diarrhea, constipation.
Respiratory: *increased airway resistance.*
Skin: rash.
Other: fever.

Interactions

Drug-drug. *Antihypertensives:* enhanced antihypertensive effect. Monitor patient.
Cardiac glycosides: excessive bradycardia and additive effects on AV conduction. Use together cautiously.
Epinephrine: severe vasoconstriction and reflex bradycardia. Monitor patient closely.
Insulin, oral antidiabetic agents: can alter dosage requirements in diabetic patients. Monitor patient.
NSAIDs: decreased antihypertensive effect. Monitor blood pressure and adjust dosage.

Contraindications and precautions

• Contraindicated in patients with bronchial asthma, sinus bradycardia and greater than first-degree heart block, and cardiogenic shock.
• Drug is not recommended for use in breast-feeding women.
• Use cautiously in patients with heart failure, chronic bronchitis, emphysema, renal or hepatic impairment, or diabetes and in those undergoing major surgery involving general anesthesia.
• Safety of drug has not been established in children.

NURSING CONSIDERATIONS

☜ Assessment
• Assess patient's condition before therapy and regularly thereafter.

• Drug masks common signs of shock and hyperthyroidism.
• Be alert for adverse reactions and drug interactions.
• Evaluate patient's and family's knowledge of drug therapy.

🔁 **Nursing diagnoses**
• Risk for injury related to presence of hypertension
• Pain related to angina
• Knowledge deficit related to drug therapy

▷ **Planning and implementation**
• Always check apical pulse before giving drug. If slower than 60 beats/minute, withhold drug and call doctor.
• If patient develops severe hypotension, give vasopressor, as prescribed.
• Reduce dosage gradually over 1 to 2 weeks. Abrupt discontinuation can exacerbate angina and MI.
Patient teaching
• Explain importance of taking drug as prescribed, even when feeling well. Caution patient not to discontinue drug suddenly.

☑ **Evaluation**
• Patient's blood pressure is normal.
• Patient reports reduced anginal pain.
• Patient and family state understanding of drug therapy.

---

nafarelin acetate
(NAF-ah-rel-in AS-ih-tayt)
Synarel

Pharmacologic class: synthetic decapeptide
Therapeutic class: gonadotropin-releasing hormone (GnRH) analogue
Pregnancy risk category: X

How supplied

Nasal solution: 200 mcg/spray in metered-dose spray bottle (2 mg/ml)

Pharmacokinetics
Absorption: absorbed through nasal mucosa into systemic circulation.
Distribution: 80% of drug is bound to plasma proteins.
Metabolism: degraded by peptidase.
Excretion: unknown. *Half-life:* about 3 hours.

Route	Onset	Peak	Duration
Intranasal	> 4 wk	10-40 min	3-6 mo

Pharmacodynamics
Chemical effect: acts on pituitary to decrease release of follicle-stimulating hormone and luteinizing hormone, thus decreasing ovarian stimulation, lowering circulating estrogens, and improving symptoms of endometriosis.
Therapeutic effect: decreases levels of sex hormones and improves endometriosis.

Indications and dosage
▶ **Management of endometriosis.**
Women age 18 and older: 1 spray in one nostril b.i.d., beginning on day 2, 3, or 4 of menstrual cycle, for up to 6 months.
▶ **Central precocious puberty.**
Children: 2 sprays in each nostril in morning and evening, or 3 sprays (600 mcg) into alternating nostrils t.i.d for total of 9 sprays per day to achieve 1,600 to 1,800 mcg daily.

Adverse reactions
CNS: *headaches, emotional lability, insomnia,* depression.
CV: edema.
EENT: *nasal irritation.*
Skin: *acne,* seborrhea, hirsutism.
Other: *hot flashes, decreased libido, myalgia,* reduced breast size, weight gain or loss, increased libido, decreased bone density, *vaginal dryness.*

Interactions
Drug-drug. *Topical nasal decongestants:* possible interference with drug absorption; Administer at least 30 minutes apart.

Reactions may be *common*, uncommon, *life-threatening*, or COMMON AND LIFE-THREATENING.

Contraindications and precautions

• Contraindicated in patients hypersensitive to GnRH analogues or other components of formulation, in those with undiagnosed vaginal bleeding, and in pregnant or breast-feeding women.
• Studies have confirmed small loss in bone density after 6 months of therapy. Patients with major risk factors for osteoporosis (chronic alcohol or tobacco use, strong family history of osteoporosis, or use of drugs that may reduce bone mass [such as anticonvulsants or corticosteroids]) should not receive additional courses of therapy and should strongly weigh risks and benefits before initial trial of drug.

NURSING CONSIDERATIONS

◪ Assessment
• Assess patient's condition before therapy and regularly thereafter.
• Be alert for adverse reactions.
• Evaluate patient's and family's knowledge of drug therapy.

◉ Nursing diagnoses
• Altered health maintenance related to underlying condition
• Altered thought processes related to drug-induced depression
• Knowledge deficit related to drug therapy

❯ Planning and implementation
• If topical nasal decongestant is required, it should be used at least 30 minutes after nafarelin treatment to reduce possible interference with drug absorption.
Patient teaching
• Instruct patient how to use drug.
• Teach patient that menstruation will stop with regular drug use and to contact doctor if it persists or if breakthrough bleeding occurs.
• Advise patient to use nonhormonal form of contraception (such as barrier contraception). Although drug will usual-

ly inhibit ovulation and stop menstruation, it's not a reliable contraceptive, particularly if patient misses a few doses. Tell patient to stop drug immediately and contact doctor if she believes that she is pregnant.
• Instruct patient to immediately report severe abdominal pain, bloating, swelling of hands or feet, nausea, vomiting, diarrhea, substantial weight gain, or shortness of breath.
• Tell patient who develops a cold or rhinitis during therapy to call doctor.

◪ Evaluation
• Patient responds well to therapy.
• Patient does not exhibit depressive behavior during drug therapy.
• Patient and family state understanding of drug therapy.

nafcillin sodium
(naf-SIL-in SOH-dee-um)
Nafcil, Nallpen, Unipen

Pharmacologic class: penicillinase-resistant penicillin
Therapeutic class: antibiotic
Pregnancy risk category: B

How supplied

Tablets: 500 mg
Capsules: 250 mg
Oral solution: 250 mg/5 ml (after reconstitution)
Injection: 500 mg, 1 g, 2 g
I.V. infusion piggyback: 1 g, 2 g

Pharmacokinetics

Absorption: absorbed erratically and poorly from GI tract after oral administration; unknown after I.M. administration.
Distribution: distributed widely. CSF penetration is poor but enhanced by meningeal inflammation. Drug is 70% to 90% protein-bound.

Metabolism: metabolized primarily in liver; undergoes enterohepatic circulation. *Excretion:* excreted primarily in bile; 25% to 30% is excreted in urine unchanged. *Half-life:* 30 to 90 minutes.

Route	Onset	Peak	Duration
P.O.	Unknown	0.5-2 hr	Unknown
I.V.	Immediate	Immediate	Unknown
I.M.	Unknown	30-60 min	Unknown

Pharmacodynamics

Chemical effect: inhibits cell wall synthesis during microorganism multiplication; bacteria resist penicillins by producing penicillinases—enzymes that hydrolyze penicillins. Nafcillin resists these enzymes.
Therapeutic effect: kills susceptible bacteria, such as penicillinase-producing staphylococci, and some gram-positive aerobic and anaerobic bacilli.

Indications and dosage

▶ **Systemic infections caused by penicillinase-producing staphylococci.**
Adults: 2 to 4 g P.O. daily, divided into doses given q 6 hours; or 2 to 12 g I.M. or I.V. daily in divided doses q 4 to 6 hours.
Children older than age 1 month: 50 mg/kg P.O. daily, divided into doses given q 6 hours; or 50 to 100 mg/kg I.M. or I.V. daily in divided doses q 6 hours for mild to moderate infections. For severe infections, 100 to 200 mg/kg/day I.M. or I.V. in equally divided doses q 4 to 6 hours.

Adverse reactions

GI: *nausea,* vomiting, diarrhea.
Hematologic: transient *leukopenia, neutropenia, granulocytopenia, thrombocytopenia* (with high doses).
Other: hypersensitivity reactions (chills, fever, rash, pruritus, urticaria, *anaphylaxis*), vein irritation, thrombophlebitis.

Interactions

Drug-drug. *Aminoglycosides:* synergistic effect. Monitor closely.

Probenecid: increased blood levels of nafcillin. Probenecid may be used for this purpose.
Rifampin: dose-dependent antagonism. Monitor closely.
Warfarin: increased risk of bleeding when used with I.V. nafcillin. Monitor closely.

Contraindications and precautions

• Contraindicated in patients with hypersensitivity to drug or other penicillins.
• Use cautiously in patients with other drug allergies, especially to cephalosporins, or in those with GI distress. Also use cautiously in pregnant or breast-feeding women.

NURSING CONSIDERATIONS

⚗ Assessment

• Assess patient's infection before therapy and regularly thereafter.
• Before giving, ask patient about allergic reactions to penicillin. However, negative history of penicillin allergy is no guarantee against future allergic reaction.
• Obtain specimen for culture and sensitivity tests before giving first dose. Therapy may begin pending results.
• Be alert for adverse reactions and drug interactions.
• Monitor patient's hydration status if adverse GI reactions occur.
• Evaluate patient's and family's knowledge of drug therapy.

⊞ Nursing diagnoses

• Infection related to susceptible bacteria
• Risk for fluid volume deficit related to drug-induced adverse GI reactions
• Knowledge deficit related to drug therapy

⊳ Planning and implementation

• Give drug at least 1 hour before bacteriostatic antibiotics.
• Drug may falsely elevate or cause false-positive results with certain tests for urine or serum proteins.

Reactions may be *common,* uncommon, *life-threatening,* or COMMON AND LIFE-THREATENING.

P.O. use: Give drug 1 to 2 hours before or 2 to 3 hours after meals. Oral drug may cause GI disturbances. Food may interfere with absorption.
I.V. use: Reconstitute piggyback containers according to manufacturer's instructions. Reconstitute 500-mg, 1-g, or 2-g vials using sterile water for injection, D₅W, or 0.9% NaCl injection. Add 1.7 ml for each 500 mg of drug. Alternatively, dilute with 15 to 30 ml of sterile water for injection or 0.45% or 0.9% NaCl injection, and give by direct injection into vein or into tubing of free-flowing I.V. solution over 5 to 10 minutes. Or, dilute drug to 2 to 40 mg/ml and give by intermittent I.V. infusion over 30 to 60 minutes.
– Avoid continuous I.V. infusions to prevent vein irritation. Change site every 48 hours.
– Aminoglycosides are chemically and physically incompatible with drug; do not mix together in same I.V. solution.
I.M. use: Follow normal protocol.
Patient teaching
• Tell patient to take entire quantity of medication exactly as prescribed, even after he feels better.
• Tell patient to call doctor if rash, fever, or chills develop.

☑ **Evaluation**
• Patient is free from infection.
• Patient maintains adequate hydration throughout drug therapy.
• Patient and family state understanding of drug therapy.

---

nalbuphine hydrochloride
(NAL-byoo-feen high-droh-KLOR-ighd)
Nubain

Pharmacologic class: narcotic agonist-antagonist; opioid partial agonist
Therapeutic class: analgesic; adjunct to anesthesia
Pregnancy risk category: B

How supplied
Injection: 10 mg/ml, 20 mg/ml

Pharmacokinetics
Absorption: unknown for S.C. and I.M. administration.
Distribution: not appreciably bound to plasma proteins.
Metabolism: metabolized in liver.
Excretion: excreted in urine and bile.
Half-life: 5 hours.

Route	Onset	Peak	Duration
I.V.	2-3 min	≤ 30 min	3-4 hr
I.M.	≤ 15 min	≤ 60 min	3-6 hr
S.C.	≤ 15 min	Unknown	3-6 hr

Pharmacodynamics
Chemical effect: binds with opioid receptors in CNS, altering pain perception and response by unknown mechanism.
Therapeutic effect: relieves pain and enhances anesthesia.

Indications and dosage
▶ **Moderate to severe pain.** *Adults:* for average (70 kg; 154-lb) person, give 10 to 20 mg I.V., I.M., or S.C., q 3 to 6 hours, p.r.n. Maximum daily dosage is 160 mg.
▶ **Adjunct to balanced anesthesia.** *Adults:* 0.3 mg/kg to 3 mg/kg I.V. over 10 to 15 minutes, followed by maintenance doses of 0.25 to 0.5 mg/kg in single I.V. doses p.r.n.

Adverse reactions
CNS: *headache, sedation, dizziness, vertigo,* nervousness, depression, restlessness, crying, euphoria, hostility, unusual dreams, confusion, hallucinations, speech difficulty, delusions.
CV: hypertension, hypotension, tachycardia, bradycardia.
EENT: blurred vision, *dry mouth.*
GI: cramps, dyspepsia, bitter taste, *nausea, vomiting,* constipation.
GU: urinary urgency.
Respiratory: *respiratory depression, pulmonary edema.*

Skin: itching; burning; urticaria; *sweaty, clammy feeling.*

Interactions

Drug-drug. *CNS depressants, general anesthetics, hypnotics, MAO inhibitors, sedatives, tranquilizers, tricyclic antidepressants:* possible respiratory depression, hypertension, profound sedation, or coma. Use together with caution. Monitor response.
Narcotic analgesics: possible decreased analgesic effect. Avoid concomitant use.
Drug-lifestyle: *Alcohol use:* possible respiratory depression, hypertension, profound sedation, or coma. Use together with caution. Monitor response.

Contraindications and precautions

• Contraindicated in patients with hypersensitivity to drug.
• Use cautiously in pregnant or breastfeeding women, substance abusers, or in those with emotional instability, head injury, increased intracranial pressure, impaired ventilation, MI accompanied by nausea and vomiting, upcoming biliary surgery, and hepatic or renal disease.

NURSING CONSIDERATIONS

⚎ Assessment
• Assess patient's pain or anesthetic requirement before therapy and regularly thereafter.
• Observe for signs of withdrawal in patient with long-term opioid use.
• Monitor patient closely for respiratory depression.
• Be alert for adverse reactions and drug interactions.
• Evaluate patient's and family's knowledge of drug therapy.

⊕ Nursing diagnoses
• Pain related to condition
• Altered thought processes related to drug's effect on CNS
• Knowledge deficit related to drug therapy

⚎ Planning and implementation
• Be aware that respiratory depression can be reversed with naloxone. Keep resuscitation equipment available, particularly when administering I.V.
• Know that drug acts as narcotic antagonist; may precipitate withdrawal syndrome. For patients with long-term opioid use, administer 25% of usual dose initially, as ordered.
• Withhold dose and notify doctor if respirations are shallow or rate is below 12 breaths/minute.
• Make sure stool softener or other laxative is ordered for severe constipation.
• Know that psychological and physical dependence may occur with prolonged use.
I.V. use: Inject slowly over at least 2 to 3 minutes into vein or into I.V. line containing compatible, free-flowing I.V. solution, such as D_5W, 0.9% NaCl, or lactated Ringer's solution.
I.M. and S.C use: Follow normal protocol.

Patient teaching
• Caution ambulatory patient about getting out of bed or walking. Warn outpatient to avoid hazardous activities until drug's CNS effects are known.

☑ Evaluation
• Patient is free from pain.
• Patient maintains normal thought processes throughout therapy.
• Patient and family state understanding of drug therapy.

nalidixic acid
(nal-uh-DIK-sik AS-id)
NegGram

Pharmacologic class: fluoroquinolone antibiotic
Therapeutic class: urinary tract anti-infective
Pregnancy risk category: B (safe use in first trimester unknown)

How supplied

Tablets: 250 mg, 500 mg, 1 g
Oral suspension: 250 mg/5 ml

Pharmacokinetics

Absorption: well absorbed from GI tract.
Distribution: concentrates in renal tissue and seminal fluid; does not penetrate prostatic tissue and only minimal amounts appear in CSF. Drug is highly protein-bound.
Metabolism: metabolized in liver.
Excretion: 13% of metabolites and 2% to 3% of unchanged drug are excreted by kidneys. *Half-life:* 1 to 2½ hours.

Route	Onset	Peak	Duration
P.O.	Unknown	1-4 hr	Unknown

Pharmacodynamics

Chemical effect: inhibits microbial DNA synthesis by bacterial DNA gyrase.
Therapeutic effect: kills susceptible bacteria, including most gram-negative organisms except *Pseudomonas.*

Indications and dosage

▶ **Acute and chronic urinary tract infections caused by susceptible gram-negative organisms (*Proteus, Klebsiella, Enterobacter,* and *Escherichia coli*).**
Adults: 1 g P.O. q.i.d. for 7 to 14 days; 2 g daily for long-term use. *Children over age 3 months:* 55 mg/kg P.O. daily divided q.i.d. for 7 to 14 days; 33 mg/kg divided q.i.d. for long-term use.

Adverse reactions

CNS: weakness, headache, dizziness, vertigo, *seizures,* malaise, confusion, hallucinations, drowsiness; *increased intracranial pressure and bulging fontanelles* (in infants and children).
EENT: light sensitivity, color perception changes, diplopia, blurred vision.
GI: *abdominal pain, nausea, vomiting,* diarrhea.
Hematologic: eosinophilia, *leukopenia, thrombocytopenia.*
Skin: pruritus, photosensitivity, urticaria, rash.
Other: *angioedema,* fever, chills.

Interactions

Drug-drug. *Oral anticoagulants:* increased anticoagulant effect. Monitor for bleeding.
Drug-lifestyle. *Sun exposure:* photosensitivity reactions may occur. Take precautions.

Contraindications and precautions

• Contraindicated in patients with seizure disorders or hypersensitivity to drug and in infants under age 3 months.
• Use with extreme caution in prepubertal children.
• Use cautiously in pregnant or breast-feeding women and in those with impaired hepatic or renal function, severe cerebral arteriosclerosis, or pulmonary disease (because of increased respiratory depression).

NURSING CONSIDERATIONS

⚖ Assessment
• Assess patient's infection before therapy and regularly thereafter. Resistant bacteria may emerge within first 48 hours of therapy.
• Obtain specimen for culture and sensitivity tests before starting therapy and repeat p.r.n. Therapy may begin pending results.
• Monitor CBC, renal, and liver function studies during long-term therapy, as ordered.
• Be alert for adverse reactions and drug interactions.
• Monitor patient's hydration status if adverse GI reactions occur.
• Evaluate patient's and family's knowledge of drug therapy.

⊕ Nursing diagnoses
• Infection related to susceptible bacteria
• Risk for fluid volume deficit related to drug-induced adverse GI reactions

---

• Knowledge deficit related to drug therapy

❯❯ **Planning and implementation**
• Know that drug may cause false-positive Clinitest reaction. Use Diastix to monitor urine glucose. Also gives false elevations in urine vanillylmandelic acid and 17-ketosteroids. Tests should be repeated after therapy is completed.
Patient teaching
• Tell patient to avoid undue exposure to sunlight because of photosensitivity. The patient may continue to be photosensitive for as long as 3 months after therapy ends.
• Tell patient to report visual disturbances; these usually disappear with reduced dose.

☑ **Evaluation**
• Patient is free from infection.
• Patient maintains adequate hydration throughout drug therapy.
• Patient and family state understanding of drug therapy.

naloxone hydrochloride
(nal-OKS-ohn high-droh-KLOR-ighd)
Narcan

Pharmacologic class: narcotic (opioid) antagonist
Therapeutic class: narcotic antagonist
Pregnancy risk category: B

How supplied
Injection: 0.02 mg/ml, 0.4 mg/ml, 1 mg/ml

Pharmacokinetics
Absorption: unknown after I.M. or S.C. administration.
Distribution: rapidly distributed into body tissues and fluids.
Metabolism: rapidly metabolized in liver.

Excretion: excreted in urine. *Half-life:* 60 to 90 minutes in adults, 3 hours in neonates.

Route	Onset	Peak	Duration
I.V.	1-2 min	Unknown	Varies
I.M., S.C.	2-5 min	Unknown	Varies

Pharmacodynamics
Chemical effect: unknown; may displace narcotic analgesics from their receptors (competitive antagonism). Has no pharmacologic activity of its own.
Therapeutic effect: reverses opioid effects.

Indications and dosage
▶ **Known or suspected narcotic-induced respiratory depression, including that caused by pentazocine and propoxyphene.** *Adults:* 0.4 to 2 mg I.V., I.M, or S.C. Repeated q 2 to 3 minutes, p.r.n. If no response is observed after 10 mg has been administered, diagnosis of narcotic-induced toxicity should be questioned.
▶ **Postoperative narcotic depression.** *Adults:* 0.1 to 0.2 mg I.V. q 2 to 3 minutes, p.r.n. *Children:* 0.005 to 0.01 mg/kg dose I.V. Repeated q 2 to 3 minutes, p.r.n. *Neonates (asphyxia neonatorum):* 0.01 mg/kg I.V. into umbilical vein. May be repeated q 2 to 3 minutes for three doses.

Adverse reactions
CNS: *seizures.*
CV: tachycardia, hypertension (with high doses); *ventricular fibrillation.*
GI: nausea, vomiting (with high doses).
Respiratory: *pulmonary edema.*
Other: tremors, withdrawal symptoms (in narcotic-dependent patients with higher than recommended doses).

Interactions
None significant.

Contraindications and precautions
• Contraindicated in patients with hypersensitivity to drug.

• Use cautiously in pregnant women and in patients with cardiac irritability and opioid addiction. Abrupt reversal of opioid-induced CNS depression may cause nausea, vomiting, diaphoresis, tachycardia, CNS excitement, and increased blood pressure.
• Safety of drug has not been established in breast-feeding women.

NURSING CONSIDERATIONS

Assessment
• Assess patient's opioid use before therapy.
• Assess effectiveness of drug regularly throughout therapy.
• Duration of narcotic may exceed that of naloxone, causing relapse into respiratory depression. Monitor respiratory depth and rate.
• Know that patients who receive naloxone to reverse opioid-induced respiratory depression may exhibit tachypnea.
• Monitor patient's hydration status if adverse GI reactions occur.
• Evaluate patient's and family's knowledge of drug therapy.

Nursing diagnoses
• Altered health maintenance related to opioid use
• Risk for fluid volume deficit related to drug-induced adverse GI reactions
• Knowledge deficit related to drug therapy

Planning and implementation
• Drug is effective only in reversing respiratory depression caused by opioids. Flumazenil should be used to treat respiratory depression caused by diazepam or other benzodiazepines.
• Provide oxygen, ventilation, and other resuscitation measures if severe respiratory depression occurs.
I.V. use: Be prepared to administer continuous I.V. infusion (to control adverse effects of epidural morphine). Adult concentration (0.4 mg) may be diluted by mixing 0.5 ml with 9.5 ml of sterile water or NaCl solution for injection to make neonatal concentration (0.02 mg/ml).
I.M. and S.C. use: Follow normal protocol.
Patient teaching
• Instruct patient to report adverse reactions.

Evaluation
• Patient responds well to drug.
• Patient maintains adequate hydration.
• Patient and family state understanding of drug therapy.

naltrexone hydrochloride
(nal-TREKS-ohn high-droh-KLOR-ighd)
ReVia

Pharmacologic class: narcotic (opioid) antagonist
Therapeutic class: narcotic detoxification adjunct
Pregnancy risk category: C

How supplied
Tablets: 50 mg

Pharmacokinetics
Absorption: well absorbed from GI tract.
Distribution: widely distributed through body but considerable interindividual variation exists. Drug is about 21% to 28% protein-bound.
Metabolism: undergoes extensive first-pass hepatic metabolism. Its major metabolite may be pure antagonist and contribute to its efficacy. Drug and metabolites may undergo enterohepatic recirculation.
Excretion: excreted primarily by kidneys. *Half-life:* about 4 hours.

Route	Onset	Peak	Duration
P.O.	15-30 min	> 12 hr	About 24 hr

Pharmacodynamics

Chemical effect: unknown; may reversibly block subjective effects of I.V. opioids by occupying opioid receptors in brain.
Therapeutic effect: helps prevent opioid dependence and treats alcohol dependence.

Indications and dosage

▶ **Adjunct for maintenance of opioid-free state in detoxified patients.** *Adults:* initially, 25 mg P.O. If no withdrawal signs occur within 1 hour, additional 25 mg is given. Once patient receives 50 mg q 24 hours, flexible maintenance schedule may be used.
▶ **Treatment of alcohol dependence.** *Adults:* 50 mg P.O. once daily.

Adverse reactions

CNS: *insomnia, anxiety, nervousness, headache,* depression, *suicide ideation.*
GI: *nausea, vomiting,* anorexia, *abdominal pain.*
Hepatic: *hepatotoxicity.*
Musculoskeletal: *muscle and joint pain.*

Interactions

Drug-drug. *Thioridazine:* increased somnolence and lethargy. Monitor closely.

Contraindications and precautions

• Contraindicated in patients who are receiving opioid analgesics, are opioid dependent, or have acute opioid withdrawal or a positive urine screen for opioids, and in those with acute hepatitis, liver failure, or hypersensitivity to drug.
• Use cautiously in patients with mild hepatic disease or history of recent hepatic disease and in pregnant women.
• Safety of drug has not been established in breast-feeding women.

NURSING CONSIDERATIONS

▓ **Assessment**
• Assess patient's opioid or alcohol dependence before therapy.

• Monitor effectiveness of drug.
• Evaluate patient's and family's knowledge of drug therapy.

✡ **Nursing diagnoses**
• Health-seeking behavior related to desire to remain free from opioid dependence
• Sleep pattern disturbance related to drug-induced insomnia
• Knowledge deficit related to drug therapy

▶ **Planning and implementation**
• Be aware that treatment for opioid dependency should begin after patient receives naloxone challenge, a provocative test of opioid dependency. If signs of opioid withdrawal persist after challenge, don't administer naltrexone.
• Patient must be completely free from opioids before taking naltrexone or severe withdrawal symptoms may occur. Patient who has been addicted to short-acting opioids, such as heroin and meperidine, must wait at least 7 days after last opioid dose before starting naltrexone. Patient who has been addicted to longer-acting opioids, such as methadone, should wait at least 10 days.
• In emergency, expect patient receiving naltrexone to be given an opioid analgesic, but in a higher dose than usual to surmount naltrexone's effect. Respiratory depression caused by opioid analgesic may be longer and deeper.
• For patient with opioid dependence who is expected to be poor complier, use flexible maintenance regimen: 100 mg on Monday and Wednesday, 150 mg on Friday, as ordered.
• Use naltrexone only as part of comprehensive rehabilitation program.
Patient teaching
• Advise patient to carry medical identification card. Warn him to tell medical personnel that he is taking naltrexone.
• Give patient names of nonopioid drugs he can continue to take for pain, diarrhea, or cough.

Reactions may be *common,* uncommon, *life-threatening,* or COMMON AND LIFE-THREATENING.

⚕ Evaluation

- Patient maintains opioid-free state.
- Patient reports no insomnia.
- Patient and family state understanding of drug therapy.

nandrolone decanoate
(NAN-druh-lohn deh-kuh-NOH-ayt)
Androlone-D, Deca-Durabolin, Hybolin Decanoate, Kabolin, Neo-Durabolic

nandrolone phenpropionate
Durabolin, Hybolin Improved, Nandrobolic

Pharmacologic class: anabolic steroid
Therapeutic class: erythropoietic and anabolic (nandrolone decanoate), antineoplastic (nandrolone phenpropionate)
Controlled substance schedule: III
Pregnancy risk category: X

How supplied

nandrolone decanoate
Injection (in oil): 50 mg/ml, 100 mg/ml, 200 mg/ml
nandrolone phenpropionate
Injection (in oil): 25 mg/ml, 50 mg/ml

Pharmacokinetics

Absorption: nandrolone decanoate is slowly released from I.M. depot. Nandrolone phenpropionate's absorption is unknown.
Distribution: unknown.
Metabolism: nandrolone decanoate is hydrolyzed to free nandrolone by plasma esterase and metabolized in liver. Nandrolone phenpropionate is metabolized in liver.
Excretion: excreted in urine. *Half-life:* 6 to 8 days for nandrolone decanoate; unknown for nandrolone phenpropionate.

Route	Onset	Peak	Duration
I.M.	Unknown	3-6 days (decanoate) 1-2 days (phenpropionate)	Unknown

Pharmacodynamics

Chemical effect: promotes tissue-building processes, reverses catabolism, and stimulates erythropoiesis.
Therapeutic effect: promotes tissue building and RBC growth (decanoate); hinders growth of breast cancer cells (phenpropionate).

Indications and dosage

▶ **Severe debility or disease states, refractory anemias. Nandrolone decanoate.** *Adults:* 50 to 100 mg/week I.M. for females; 100 to 200 mg I.M. at weekly intervals for males. Therapy should be intermittent. *Children ages 2 to 13:* 25 to 50 mg I.M. q 3 to 4 weeks.
▶ **Control of metastatic breast cancer. Nandrolone phenpropionate.** *Adults:* 50 to 100 mg I.M. weekly.

Adverse reactions

CV: edema.
GI: gastroenteritis, nausea, vomiting, diarrhea, change in appetite.
GU: bladder irritability.
Hematologic: thrombocytopenia, elevated serum lipid levels.
Hepatic: reversible jaundice, peliosis hepatis, elevated liver enzyme levels, *liver cell tumors.*
Skin: pain, induration (at injection site).
Other: hypercalcemia, muscle cramps or spasms, androgenic effects in women (acne, edema, *weight gain, hirsutism,* hoarseness, clitoral enlargement, *decrease in breast size,* changes in libido, male-pattern baldness, *oily skin or hair*), hypoestrogenic effects in women (flushing, diaphoresis, vaginitis, vaginal bleeding, nervousness, emotional lability, menstrual irregularities), excessive hormonal effects in men (prepubertal—premature epiphyseal closure, *acne,* priapism, *growth of body and facial hair,* phallic enlargement; postpubertal—testicular atrophy, oligospermia, decreased ejaculatory volume, impotence, gynecomastia, epididymitis).

Interactions

Drug-drug. *Hepatotoxic drugs:* increased risk of hepatotoxicity. Monitor patient closely.
Insulin, oral antidiabetic agents: altered dosage requirements. Monitor blood glucose levels in diabetic patients.
Oral anticoagulants: altered dosage requirements. Monitor PT and INR.

Contraindications and precautions

• Contraindicated in patients with hypersensitivity to anabolic steroids, in males with breast or prostate cancer, in those with nephrosis, in those experiencing nephrotic phase of nephritis, in females with breast cancer and hypercalcemia, and in pregnant or breast-feeding women.
• Use cautiously in patients with diabetes; cardiac, renal, or hepatic disease; epilepsy; or migraine or other conditions that may be aggravated by fluid retention.

NURSING CONSIDERATIONS

Assessment

• Assess patient's condition before therapy and regularly thereafter.
• Ensure that pregnancy test has been performed in female patient of childbearing age and that it is negative before therapy is begun.
• In child, X-rays of wrist bones should be taken before treatment to assess bone maturation. During treatment, bone maturation may proceed rapidly; periodically review X-ray results to monitor it.
• Closely observe boy under age 7 for precocious development of male sexual characteristics.
• Semen evaluation is routinely performed every 3 to 4 months, especially in adolescent male.
• Evaluate hepatic function, as ordered.
• Watch for symptoms of hypoglycemia in diabetic patient. Check blood glucose levels regularly because dosage of antidiabetic agent may need to be adjusted.
• Check quantitative urine and serum calcium levels.

• Be alert for adverse reactions and drug interactions.
• Evaluate patient's and family's knowledge of drug therapy.

Nursing diagnoses

• Altered health maintenance related to underlying condition
• Body image disturbance related to adverse androgenic reactions
• Knowledge deficit related to drug therapy

Planning and implementation

• Inject I.M. drug deeply, preferably into upper outer quadrant of gluteal muscle in adults. Rotate injection sites to prevent muscle atrophy.
• Notify doctor immediately if signs of virilization occur; may be irreversible despite prompt discontinuation of therapy.
• Dosage adjustment may reverse jaundice. If liver function test results are abnormal, therapy should be stopped.
• Drug-induced edema generally can be controlled with sodium restrictions or diuretics.
• When used to promote erythropoiesis, make sure patient has adequate daily iron intake.
• Anabolic steroids may alter results of laboratory studies performed during therapy and for 2 to 3 weeks after therapy ends.
Patient teaching
• Make sure patient understands importance of using effective nonhormonal contraceptive during therapy.
• Advise washing after intercourse to decrease risk of vaginitis. Instruct patient to wear only cotton underwear.
• Tell woman to report menstrual irregularities and to discontinue therapy until the cause has been determined.

Evaluation

• Patient responds well to therapy.
• Patient states acceptance of body image changes.

Reactions may be *common*, uncommon, *life-threatening*, or COMMON AND LIFE-THREATENING.

• Patient and family state understanding of drug therapy.

naphazoline hydrochloride
(naf-AZ-oh-leen high-droh-KLOR-ighd)
Privine†

Pharmacologic class: sympathomimetic
Therapeutic class: decongestant, vaso-constrictor.
Pregnancy risk category: NR

How supplied

Nasal drops: 0.05% solution
Nasal spray: 0.05% solution

Pharmacokinetics

Unknown.

Route	Onset	Peak	Duration
Intranasal	≤ 10 min	Unknown	2-6 hr

Pharmacodynamics

Chemical effect: causes local vasocon-striction of dilated arterioles, reducing blood flow.
Therapeutic effect: relieves nasal con-gestion.

Indications and dosage

▶ **Nasal congestion.** *Adults and children age 12 and older:* 1 or 2 drops or sprays instilled in each nostril q 3 to 4 hours. *Children ages 6 to 12:* 1 to 2 drops or sprays instilled in each nostril q 3 to 6 hours, p.r.n. Not to be used longer than 3 to 5 days.

Adverse reactions

EENT: rebound nasal congestion (with excessive or long-term use), sneezing, stinging, mucosal dryness.
Other: systemic effects (in children after excessive or long-term use), marked sedation.

Interactions

None significant.

Contraindications and precautions

• Contraindicated in patients with hyper-sensitivity to drug.
• Drug use is not recommended in breast-feeding women.
• Use cautiously in pregnant women and in patients with hyperthyroidism, heart disease, hypertension, or diabetes melli-tus.

NURSING CONSIDERATIONS

Assessment

• Assess patient's condition before ther-apy and regularly thereafter.
• Be alert for adverse reactions.
• Evaluate patient's and family's knowl-edge of drug therapy.

Nursing diagnoses

• Altered health maintenance related to nasal congestion
• Altered tissue integrity related to drug's adverse effect on nasal tissue
• Knowledge deficit related to drug therapy

Planning and implementation

• To instill nasal drops, have patient tilt head back as far as possible; instill drops; then have patient lean head forward while inhaling. Repeat procedure for other nos-tril.
• To instill nasal spray, hold spray con-tainer and patient's head upright, then spray. Do not shake container.
Patient teaching
• Teach patient how to use drug.
• Explain that product should be used by only one person to prevent spread of in-fection.
• Warn patient not to exceed recommend-ed dosage.
• Tell patient to contact doctor if nasal congestion persists after 5 days.

Evaluation

• Patient's congestion is relieved.
• Patient's nasal tissue does not dry or crack.

• Patient and family state understanding of drug therapy.

---

naproxen
(nuh-PROK-sin)
Apo-Naproxen♦, Inza◇, Naprosyn, Naprosyn-E♦, Naprosyn SR♦◇, Naxen♦◇, Novo-Naprox♦, Nu-Naprox♦

naproxen sodium
Aleve†, Anaprox, Anaprox DS, Apo-Napro-Na♦, Naprogesic◇, Novo-Naprox Sodium♦, Synflex♦

Pharmacologic class: NSAID
Therapeutic class: nonnarcotic analgesic, antipyretic, anti-inflammatory
Pregnancy risk category: NR

How supplied
naproxen
Tablets: 250 mg, 375 mg, 500 mg
Tablets (extended-release)♦: 750 mg, 1,000 mg
Oral suspension: 125 mg/5 ml
Suppositories: 500 mg◇
naproxen sodium
Tablets (film-coated): 220 mg, 275 mg, 550 mg. *Note:* 275 mg of naproxen sodium = 250 mg of naproxen

Pharmacokinetics
Absorption: absorbed rapidly and completely from GI tract.
Distribution: highly protein-bound.
Metabolism: metabolized in liver.
Excretion: excreted in urine. *Half-life:* 1.3 hours.

Route	Onset	Peak	Duration
P.O.	≤ 1 hr	1-4 hr	About 7 hr
P.R.	Unknown	Unknown	Unknown

Pharmacodynamics
Chemical effect: unknown; produces anti-inflammatory, analgesic, and antipyretic effects, possibly by inhibiting prostaglandin synthesis.

Therapeutic effect: relieves pain, fever, and inflammation.

Indications and dosage
▶ **Rheumatoid arthritis, osteoarthritis, ankylosing spondylitis.** *Adults:* 250 to 500 mg naproxen P.O. b.i.d.; or, 275 to 550 mg naproxen sodium P.O. b.i.d. Alternatively, where suppository is available, give 500 mg P.R. h.s. with oral naproxen during day. Maximum dosage is 1,500 mg daily.
▶ **Juvenile arthritis.** *Children:* 10 mg/kg naproxen P.O. in two divided doses.
▶ **Acute gout.** *Adults:* 750 mg naproxen P.O., followed by 250 mg q 8 hours until attack subsides. Or, 825 mg naproxen sodium initially, then 275 mg q 8 hours until attack subsides.
▶ **Mild to moderate pain, primary dysmenorrhea, acute tendinitis and bursitis.** *Adults:* 500 mg naproxen P.O., followed by 250 mg q 6 to 8 hours p.r.n. Or, 550 mg naproxen sodium P.O. initially, then 275 mg P.O. q 6 to 8 hours p.r.n.

Adverse reactions
CNS: *headache, drowsiness, dizziness,* tinnitus, cognitive dysfunction, aseptic meningitis.
CV: *peripheral edema,* palpitations, digital vasculitis.
EENT: visual disturbances, *tinnitus.*
GI: *epigastric distress, occult blood loss, nausea, **peptic ulceration.***
GU: nephrotoxicity.
Hematologic: prolonged bleeding time, ***agranulocytosis, thrombocytopenia,*** neutropenia.
Hepatic: elevated liver enzymes.
Metabolic: hyperkalemia.
Respiratory: dyspnea.
Skin: *pruritus, rash,* urticaria.

Interactions
Drug-drug. *Antihypertensives, diuretics:* decreased effect of these drugs. Monitor patient.

Reactions may be *common,* uncommon, *life-threatening,* or COMMON AND LIFE-THREATENING.

Aspirin, corticosteroids: increased risk of adverse GI reactions. Use with caution.
Methotrexate: increased risk of toxicity. Monitor closely.
Oral anticoagulants, sulfonylureas, drugs that are highly protein-bound: increased risk of toxicity. Monitor closely.
Probenecid: decreased elimination of naproxen. Monitor for toxicity.
Drug-lifestyle. *Alcohol use:* increased risk of adverse GI reactions. Avoid concomitant use.

Contraindications and precautions

• Contraindicated in patients with asthma, rhinitis, nasal polyps, or hypersensitivity to drug; during last trimester of pregnancy; and in breast-feeding patients.
• Use cautiously in elderly patients and in those with renal disease, CV disease, GI disorders, hepatic disease, or peptic ulcer disease.

NURSING CONSIDERATIONS

Assessment
• Assess patient's condition before therapy and regularly thereafter.
• Monitor CBC and renal and hepatic function every 4 to 6 months or as ordered during long-term therapy.
• NSAIDs may mask signs and symptoms of infection.
• Monitor patient's hydration status if adverse GI reactions occur.
• Evaluate patient's and family's knowledge of drug therapy.

Nursing diagnoses
• Pain related to condition
• Risk for fluid volume deficit related to drug-induced adverse GI reactions
• Knowledge deficit related to drug therapy

Planning and implementation
P.O. use: Give drug with food or milk to minimize GI upset. Tell patient to take a full glass of water or other liquid with each dose.

P.R. use: Not commercially available in the United States. Don't use in patients with inflammatory lesion of the rectum or anus.
• Inform laboratory personnel that patient is taking naproxen. Drug may interfere with urinary assays of 5-hydroxyindoleacetic acid and may falsely elevate urinary 17-ketosteroid concentrations.
Patient teaching
• Tell patient taking prescription doses of naproxen for arthritis that full therapeutic effect may be delayed 2 to 4 weeks.
• Warn patient against taking both naproxen and naproxen sodium at same time.
• Teach patient to recognize and report signs and symptoms of GI bleeding. Serious GI toxicity, including peptic ulceration and bleeding, can occur in patients taking NSAIDs despite absence of GI symptoms.
• Caution patient that concomitant use with aspirin, alcohol, or corticosteroids may increase risk of adverse GI reactions.
• Advise patient to have periodic eye examinations.

Evaluation
• Patient is free from pain.
• Patient maintains adequate hydration.
• Patient and family state understanding of drug therapy.

naratriptan hydrochloride
(nah-rah-TRIP-tin high-droh-KLOR-ighd)
Amerge

Pharmacologic class: selective 5-hydroxytryptamine$_1$ (5HT$_1$) receptor subtype agonist
Therapeutic class: antimigraine
Pregnancy risk category: C

How supplied
Tablets: 1 mg, 2.5 mg

Pharmacokinetics

Absorption: well absorbed with a bioavailability of 70%.
Distribution: Approximately 28% to 31% plasma protein-bound.
Metabolism: metabolized to a number of inactive metabolites by wide range of cytochrome P450 isoenzymes.
Excretion: primarily excreted in urine with 50% of dose recovered unchanged and 30% as metabolites. *Half-life:* 6 hours.

Route	Onset	Peak	Duration
P.O.	Unknown	2-3 hr	Unknown

Pharmacodynamics

Chemical effect: thought to activate receptors located in intracranial blood vessels leading to vasoconstriction and migraine headache relief; also thought that activation of receptors on sensory nerve endings in trigeminal system results in inhibition of proinflammatory neuropeptide release.
Therapeutic effect: relieves migraine pain.

Indications and dosage

▶ **Treatment of acute migraine headache attacks with or without aura.**
Adults: 1 or 2.5 mg P.O. as a single dose. If headache returns or if only partial response occurs, dose may be repeated after 4 hours, for maximum dose of 5 mg within 24 hours.

Adverse reactions

CNS: paresthesias, dizziness, drowsiness, malaise, fatigue, vertigo, syncope.
CV: palpitation, increased blood pressure, *tachyarrhythmias, abnormal ECG changes (PR, QTc prolongation, ST/T wave abnormalities, PVCs, atrial flutter or fibrillation), coronary vasospasm.*
EENT: ear, nose, and throat infections, photophobia.
GI: nausea, hyposalivation, vomiting.
Other: warm or cold temperature sensations, pressure, tightness, heaviness sensations.

Interactions

Drug-drug. *Ergot-containing or ergot-type agents (methysergide, dihydroergotamine), other 5HT$_1$ agonists:* prolonged vasospastic reactions. Do not give within 24 hours of naratriptan.
Oral contraceptives: slightly higher concentrations of naratriptan. Monitor patient.
Selective serotonin reuptake inhibitors (SSRIs) (fluoxetine, fluvoxamine, paroxetine, sertraline): may cause weakness, hyperreflexia, and incoordination. Monitor patient.
Drug-lifestyle. *Smoking:* increased clearance of naratriptan. Discourage concomitant use.

Contraindications and precautions

• Contraindicated in patients with history, symptoms, or signs of cardiac ischemia, cerebrovascular, or peripheral vascular diseases; known hypersensitivity to drug or its components; significant underlying CV diseases; history of uncontrolled hypertension; severe renal impairment (creatinine clearance below 15 ml/minute); severe hepatic impairment (Child-Pugh grade C); in those who have received ergot-containing, ergot-type, or other 5-HT$_1$ agonists within the past 24 hours; and in elderly patients.
• Use cautiously in patients with risk factors for coronary artery disease, such as hypertension, hypercholesterolemia, obesity, diabetes, strong family history of coronary artery disease, women with surgical or physiologic menopause, men over age 40, or smoking unless a CV evaluation has determined patient is free from cardiac disease. For those with cardiac risk factors who have had a satisfactory CV evaluation, give first dose in a medically equipped facility. Consider ECG monitoring.

NURSING CONSIDERATIONS

Assessment
• Assess baseline cardiac function before initiating therapy. Perform periodic car-

---

diac reevaluation in patients who develop risk factors for coronary artery disease.
• Monitor renal and liver function tests before initiating drug therapy and report abnormalities.
• Evaluate patient's and family's knowledge of drug therapy.

🕀 Nursing diagnoses
• Pain related to presence of migraine headache
• Risk of injury related to drug-induced adverse CV reactions
• Knowledge deficit related to drug therapy

❱ Planning and implementation
• Administer drug once a definite diagnosis of migraine has been established. Drug is not intended for prophylactic therapy of migraine headaches or for use in hemiplegic or basilar migraines or for cluster headaches.
• Withhold drug and notify doctor of pain or tightness in chest or throat, arrhythmias, or increases in blood pressure.
• Know that patients with mild to moderate renal or hepatic impairment receive a lower initial dosage. Do not exceed maximum dose of 2.5 mg within a 24-hour period in these patients.
• Do not give to patients with history of known coronary artery disease, hypertension, arrhythmias, or presence of risk factors for coronary artery disease, because drug may cause coronary vasospasm and hypertension.
• For patients with cardiac risk factors who have had a satisfactory cardiac evaluation, administer first dose while monitoring ECG and have emergency equipment readily available.
• Know that safety and effectiveness have not been established for cluster headaches or for treating more than four migraine headaches in a 30-day period.
Patient teaching
• Instruct patient to take drug only as prescribed.

• Tell patient that drug is intended to relieve, not prevent migraine headaches.
• Instruct patient to take dose soon after headache starts. If no response occurs to first tablet, tell patient to seek medical approval before taking second tablet. If physician has approved a second dose, patient may take a second tablet but not sooner than 4 hours after first tablet. Inform patient not to exceed two tablets within 24 hours.
• Instruct patient not to use drug during pregnancy or if it is suspected.
• Teach patient to alert doctor of risk factors for coronary artery disease or if bothersome adverse effects occur.
• Instruct patient to read the accompanying patient leaflet before taking drug.

☑ Evaluation
• Patient has relief of migraine headache.
• Patient does not experience pain or tightness in chest or throat, arrhythmias, or increase in blood pressure.
• Patient and family state understanding of drug therapy.

nedocromil sodium
(nee-DOK-roh-mil SOH-dee-um)
Tilade

Pharmacologic class: pyranoquinoline
Therapeutic class: anti-inflammatory respiratory inhalant
Pregnancy risk category: B

How supplied
Inhalation aerosol: 1.75 mg/activation

Pharmacokinetics
Absorption: 2% to 3% of drug swallowed after inhalation is absorbed. From 6% to 9% of drug deposited in lungs is absorbed.
Distribution: distributed to plasma only. About 89% reversibly bound to plasma proteins when plasma concentrations are 0.5 to 50 mcg/ml.

Metabolism: not metabolized.
Excretion: rapidly excreted unchanged in bile and urine. *Half-life:* about 1.5 to 3.3 hours.

Route	Onset	Peak	Duration
Inhalation	2 days-4 wk	5-90 min	6-12 hr

Pharmacodynamics

Chemical effect: reduces inflammatory changes in airway by blocking release of inflammation mediators from mast cells, eosinophils, monocytes, neutrophils, macrophages, and other immune cells. *Therapeutic effect:* improves gas exchange.

Indications and dosage

▶ **Maintenance in mild-to-moderate reversible obstructive airway disease.** *Adults and children age 12 and over:* 2 inhalations q.i.d., preferably at regular intervals.

Adverse reactions

CNS: headache.
GI: nausea, vomiting.
Respiratory: upper respiratory tract infection, rhinitis, *bronchospasm.*
Other: *unpleasant taste.*

Interactions

None significant.

Contraindications and precautions

• Contraindicated in patients with hypersensitivity to drug or its components and in those experiencing acute asthmatic attack or acute bronchospasm.
• Use cautiously in pregnant or breast-feeding women.
• Safety of drug has not been established in children under age 12.

NURSING CONSIDERATIONS

Assessment
• Assess patient's condition before therapy and regularly thereafter.
• Be alert for adverse reactions.

• Evaluate patient's and family's knowledge of drug therapy.

Nursing diagnoses
• Impaired gas exchange related to respiratory condition
• Pain related to drug-induced headache
• Knowledge deficit related to drug therapy

Planning and implementation
• Dosage may be reduced to two inhalations t.i.d., as ordered, and then b.i.d. after several weeks, when patient's asthma is under control.
• Administer regularly, even during symptom-free periods, to achieve benefit in maintenance therapy.
• Administer mild analgesic, as ordered, for drug-induced headache.
Patient teaching
• Warn patient that drug cannot replace bronchodilators during acute asthmatic attack.
• Tell patient that drug is adjunct to regular bronchodilator regimen and may reduce need for corticosteroids or bronchodilators.
• Explain that regular drug use will help patient feel better. Most patients report benefits after 1 week; some require longer treatment.
• Teach patient how to use inhaler. Instruct him to shake canister and invert it just before use.
• Advise patient to clean inhaler at least twice weekly and to remove canister before rinsing inhaler in hot, running water. Allow inhaler to air dry overnight.

Evaluation
• Patient demonstrates adequate gas exchange with drug therapy.
• Patient is free from drug-induced headache.
• Patient and family state understanding of drug therapy.

Reactions may be *common,* uncommon, *life-threatening,* or COMMON AND LIFE-THREATENING.

nefazodone hydrochloride
(nef-AZ-oh-dohn high-droh-KLOR-ighd)
Serzone

Pharmacologic class: synthetically derived phenylpiperazine
Therapeutic class: antidepressant
Pregnancy risk category: C

How supplied

Tablets: 100 mg, 150 mg, 200 mg, 250 mg

Pharmacokinetics

Absorption: rapidly and completely absorbed with low, variable absolute bioavailability (about 20%).
Distribution: widely distributed in body tissues, including CNS. Drug is extensively bound to plasma proteins.
Metabolism: extensively metabolized.
Excretion: excreted in urine. *Half-life:* 2 to 4 hours.

Route	Onset	Peak	Duration
P.O.	Unknown	About 1 hr	Unknown

Pharmacodynamics

Chemical effect: not precisely defined. Drug inhibits neuronal uptake of serotonin (5-HT-2) and norepinephrine; it also occupies serotonin and alpha$_1$-adrenergic receptors in CNS.
Therapeutic effect: relieves depression.

Indications and dosage

▶ **Depression.** *Adults:* initially, 200 mg/day P.O. in two divided doses. Dosage increased in increments of 100 to 200 mg/day at intervals of no less than 1 week, as indicated. Usual dosage range is 300 to 600 mg/day.

Adverse reactions

CNS: headache, *somnolence, dizziness, asthenia,* insomnia, *light-headedness, confusion,* memory impairment, paresthesia, abnormal dreams, decreased concentration, ataxia, incoordination, taste perversion, psychomotor retardation, tremor, hypertonia.
CV: vasodilation, postural hypotension, hypotension, peripheral edema.
EENT: *blurred vision, abnormal vision,* tinnitus, visual field defect.
GI: *dry mouth, nausea, constipation,* dyspepsia, diarrhea, increased appetite, vomiting.
GU: urinary frequency, urinary tract infection, urine retention.
Respiratory: pharyngitis, cough.
Skin: pruritus, rash.
Other: infection, flu syndrome, chills, fever, neck rigidity, vaginitis, breast pain, thirst, arthralgia.

Interactions

Drug-drug. *Alprazolam, triazolam:* increased effects of these drugs. Do not administer concurrently, or give greatly reduced dosage of alprazolam and triazolam.
Astemizole: may cause decreased metabolism, leading to increased antihistamine levels and cardiotoxicity. Avoid concomitant use.
CNS-active drugs: may alter CNS activity. Use together cautiously.
Digoxin: may increase digoxin level. Use together cautiously and monitor digoxin levels.
MAO inhibitors: may cause severe excitation, hyperpyrexia, seizures, delirium, or coma. Avoid concomitant use.
Other highly bound plasma protein drugs: may increase adverse reactions. Monitor patient closely.
Drug-lifestyle. *Alcohol use:* enhanced CNS depression. Avoid concomitant use.

Contraindications and precautions

• Contraindicated in patients with hypersensitivity to drug or to other phenylpiperazine antidepressants; within 14 days of MAO inhibitor therapy; and in coadministration with astemizole.
• Use cautiously in patients with CV or cerebrovascular disease that could be exacerbated by hypotension (such as history

of MI, angina, or CVA) and conditions that predispose to hypotension (such as dehydration, hypovolemia, and treatment with antihypertensives). Also use cautiously in patients with history of mania and in pregnant or breast-feeding women.
• Safety of drug has not been established in children under age 18.

NURSING CONSIDERATIONS

Ⓩ Assessment
• Assess patient's depression before therapy and regularly thereafter.
• Record mood changes. Monitor patient for suicidal tendencies.
• Be alert for adverse reactions and drug interactions.
• Evaluate patient's and family's knowledge of drug therapy.

⊕ Nursing diagnoses
• Altered thought processes related to depression
• Risk of injury related to drug-induced adverse CNS reactions
• Knowledge deficit related to drug therapy

⧁ Planning and implementation
• At least 1 week should be allowed after stopping drug before patient is started on MAO inhibitor. At least 14 days should be allowed before patient is started on drug after MAO inhibitor therapy has been discontinued.
Patient teaching
• Warn patient not to engage in hazardous activity until drug's CNS effects are known.
• Instruct male patient with prolonged or inappropriate erections to stop drug at once and call doctor.
• Instruct female patient to call doctor if she becomes pregnant or intends to become pregnant during therapy.
• Instruct patient not to take alcoholic beverages during drug therapy.
• Tell patient who develops rash, hives, or related allergic reaction to notify doctor.

• Inform patient that several weeks of therapy may be required to obtain full antidepressant effect. Once improvement is seen, tell patient not to stop drug until directed by doctor.

Ⓥ Evaluation
• Patient exhibits improved behavior.
• Patient experiences no injuries due to drug-induced adverse CNS reactions.
• Patient and family state understanding of drug therapy.

nelfinavir mesylate
(nel-FIN-uh-veer MES-ih-layt)
Viracept

Pharmacologic class: HIV protease inhibitor
Therapeutic class: antiviral
Pregnancy risk category: B

How supplied
Tablets: 250 mg
Powder: 50 mg/g powder

Pharmacokinetics
Absorption: not reported. Higher peak plasma concentrations achieved when taken with food.
Distribution: over 98% bound to plasma protein.
Metabolism: metabolized primarily by cytochrome P-450 3A (CYP3A).
Excretion: excreted primarily in the feces. *Half-life:* 3.5 to 5 hours.

Route	Onset	Peak	Duration
P.O.	Unknown	2-4 hr	Unknown

Pharmacodynamics
Chemical effect: inhibition of the protease enzyme prevents cleavage of the viral polyprotein.
Therapeutic effect: production of immature, noninfectious virus.

Reactions may be *common*, uncommon, *life-threatening*, or COMMON AND LIFE-THREATENING.

Indications and dosage

▶ **Treatment of HIV infection when antiretroviral therapy is warranted.**
Adults: 750 mg P.O. t.i.d. with meals or light snack. *Children ages 2 to 13:* 20 to 30 mg/kg/dose P.O. t.i.d. with meals or light snack; not to exceed 750 mg t.i.d. **Recommended children's dose given t.i.d. is shown below.**

Body weight (kg)	Level 1-g scoops	Level teaspoons	Tablets
7 to < 8.5	4	1	-
8.5 to < 10.5	5	1.25	-
10.5 to < 12	6	1.5	-
12 to < 14	7	1.75	-
14 to < 16	8	2	-
16 to < 18	9	2.25	-
18 to < 23	10	2.5	2
≥ 23	15	3.75	3

Adverse reactions

CNS: asthenia, anxiety, depression, dizziness, emotional lability, hyperkinesia, insomnia, migraine, malaise, headache, paresthesia, *seizures,* sleep disorders, somnolence, *suicidal ideation.*
EENT: iritis, eye disorder, pharyngitis, rhinitis, sinusitis.
GI: abdominal pain, nausea, *diarrhea,* flatulence, anorexia, dyspepsia, epigastric pain, GI bleeding, pancreatitis, mouth ulceration, vomiting.
GU: sexual dysfunction, renal calculus, urine abnormality.
Hematologic: anemia, *leukopenia, thrombocytopenia.*
Hepatic: *hepatitis,* elevated liver function test results.
Metabolic: dehydration, hyperglycemia, hyperlipidemia, hyperuricemia, hypoglycemia, increased amylase and creatinine phosphokinase levels.
Musculoskeletal: back pain, arthralgia, arthritis, cramps, myalgia, myasthenia, myopathy.
Respiratory: dyspnea.
Skin: rash, dermatitis, folliculitis, fungal dermatitis, pruritus, sweating, urticaria.

Other: allergic reactions, fever.

Interactions

Drug-drug. *Amiodarone, astemizole, cisapride, ergot derivatives, midazolam, quinidine, triazolam:* nelfinavir may produce large increases in plasma levels of these drugs, which may increase risk for serious or life-threatening adverse events. Don't administer concurrently.
AntiHIV protease inhibitors (indinavir, ritonavir): may increase nelfinavir plasma levels. Monitor carefully.
Carbamazepine, phenobarbital, phenytoin: may reduce effectiveness of nelfinavir by decreasing nelfinavir plasma concentrations. Monitor patient.
Oral contraceptives (ethinyl estradiol, norethindrone): nelfinavir may decrease plasma levels. Suggest alternate or additional contraceptive measures during nelfinavir therapy.
Rifabutin: increased rifabutin plasma levels. Expect reduced dosage of rifabutin to one-half usual dose.
Rifampin: decreased nelfinavir plasma levels. Don't use together.

Contraindications and precautions

• Contraindicated in patients with hypersensitivity to drug or its components.
• Use cautiously in patients with hepatic dysfunction or hemophilia type A and B.

NURSING CONSIDERATIONS

Assessment
• Obtain baseline assessment of patient's condition and reassess regularly thereafter to monitor drug's effectiveness.
• Monitor liver function tests.
• Assess patient for increased bleeding tendencies, especially if used in patients with hemophilia type A or B.
• Monitor patient for excessive diarrhea and treat as directed by doctor.
• Evaluate patient's and family's knowledge of drug therapy.

⊞ Nursing diagnoses
• Risk of injury related to drug's adverse GI effects
• Potential for impaired skin integrity secondary to drug adverse effects
• Knowledge deficit related to drug therapy

▶ Planning and implementation
• Administer oral powder in children unable to take tablets. May mix oral powder with small amount of water, milk, formula, soy formula, soy milk, or dietary supplements. Tell patient to consume entire contents.
• Don't reconstitute drug with water in its original container.
• Use reconstituted powder within 6 hours.
• Know that mixing with acidic foods or juice is not recommended due to bitter taste.
Patient teaching
• Advise patient not to breast-feed to avoid transmitting virus to infant.
• Advise patient to take drug with food.
• Inform patient that drug is not a cure for HIV infection.
• Tell patient that long-term effects of drug are currently unknown and that there are no data to support assumption that drug reduces risk of HIV transmission to others.
• Advise patient to take drug daily as prescribed and not to alter dose or discontinue drug without medical approval.
• If patient misses a dose, tell him to take it as soon as possible and then return to his normal schedule. If a dose is skipped, advise patient not to double-dose.
• Tell patient that diarrhea is most common adverse effect and it can be controlled with loperamide if necessary.
• Instruct patient taking oral contraceptives to use alternate or additional contraceptive measures while on nelfinavir therapy.
• Warn patient with phenylketonuria that powder contains 11.2 mg phenylalanine per gram.

• Advise patient to report use of other prescribed or OTC drugs because of possible drug interactions.

☑ Evaluation
• Patient does not experience adverse GI reactions.
• Skin integrity remains intact.
• Patient and family state understanding of drug therapy.

neomycin sulfate
(nee-oh-MIGH-sin SUL-fayt)
Mycifradin, Neo-fradin, Neosulf◊, Neo-Tabs

Pharmacologic class: aminoglycoside
Therapeutic class: antibiotic
Pregnancy risk category: NR

How supplied
Tablets: 500 mg
Oral solution: 125 mg/5 ml

Pharmacokinetics
Absorption: absorbed poorly (about 3%), although absorption is enhanced in patients with impaired GI motility or mucosal intestinal ulcerations.
Distribution: distributed locally in GI tract.
Metabolism: not metabolized.
Excretion: excreted primarily unchanged in feces. *Half-life:* 2 to 3 hours.

Route	Onset	Peak	Duration
P.O.	Unknown	1-4 hr	About 8 hr

Pharmacodynamics
Chemical effect: inhibits protein synthesis by binding directly to 30S ribosomal subunit.
Therapeutic effect: kills susceptible bacteria, such as many aerobic gram-negative organisms and some aerobic gram-positive organisms. Inhibits ammonia-forming bacteria in GI tract, reducing am-

---

Reactions may be *common*, uncommon, *life-threatening*, or COMMON AND LIFE-THREATENING.

monia and improving neurologic status of patients with hepatic encephalopathy.

Indications and dosage

▶ **Infectious diarrhea caused by enteropathogenic** *Escherichia coli. Adults:* 50 mg/kg daily P.O. in four divided doses for 2 to 3 days. *Children:* 50 to 100 mg/kg daily P.O. divided q 4 to 6 hours for 2 to 3 days.
▶ **Suppression of intestinal bacteria preoperatively.** *Adults:* 1 g P.O. q hour for four doses, then 1 g q 4 hours for balance of 24 hours. A saline cathartic should precede therapy. *Children:* 40 to 100 mg/kg daily P.O. divided q 4 to 6 hours. First dose should follow saline cathartic.
▶ **Adjunct treatment in hepatic coma.** *Adults:* 1 to 3 g P.O. q.i.d. for 5 to 6 days; or 200 ml of 1% solution or 100 ml of 2% solution as enema retained for 20 to 60 minutes q 6 hours.

Adverse reactions

CNS: headache, lethargy.
EENT: *ototoxicity (tinnitus, vertigo, hearing loss).*
GI: nausea, vomiting.
GU: *nephrotoxicity* (cells or casts in urine, oliguria, proteinuria, decreased creatinine clearance, increased BUN and serum creatinine levels).
Skin: rash, urticaria.
Other: hypersensitivity reactions.

Interactions

Drug-drug. *Acyclovir, amphotericin B, cisplatin, methoxyflurane, other aminoglycosides, vancomycin:* increased nephrotoxicity. Use together cautiously.
Cephalothin: increased nephrotoxicity. Use together cautiously.
Digoxin: decreased digoxin absorption. Monitor closely.
Dimenhydrinate: may mask symptoms of ototoxicity. Use with caution.
I.V. loop diuretics (such as furosemide): increased ototoxicity. Use cautiously.

Oral anticoagulants: inhibited vitamin K-producing bacteria; may potentiate anticoagulant effect.

Contraindications and precautions

• Contraindicated in patients with intestinal obstruction or hypersensitivity to other aminoglycosides.
• Use cautiously in patients with impaired renal function, neuromuscular disorders, or ulcerative bowel lesions and in elderly patients.
• Safety of drug has not been established in breast-feeding women.

NURSING CONSIDERATIONS

✐ Assessment
• Assess patient's condition before therapy and regularly thereafter.
• Evaluate patient's hearing before therapy and regularly thereafter.
• Monitor renal function (output, specific gravity, urinalysis, BUN and creatinine levels, and creatinine clearance).
• Be alert for adverse reactions and drug interactions.
• Monitor patient's hydration status if adverse GI reactions occur.
• Evaluate patient's and family's knowledge of drug therapy.

✐ Nursing diagnoses
• Infection related to organisms
• Risk for fluid volume deficit related to drug-induced adverse GI reactions
• Knowledge deficit related to drug therapy

▶ Planning and implementation
• Drug is nonabsorbable at recommended dosage. More than 4 g/day may be systemically absorbed and lead to nephrotoxicity.
• Ensure that patient is well hydrated while taking drug to minimize chemical irritation of renal tubules.
• For preoperative disinfection, provide low-residue diet and cathartic immedi-

ately before oral administration of drug, as ordered.

• In adjunct treatment of hepatic coma, decrease patient's dietary protein and assess neurologic status frequently during therapy.

• Never administer drug parenterally.

• Know that ototoxic and nephrotoxic properties of neomycin limit its usefulness.

• Drug is available in combination with polymyxin B as urinary bladder irrigant.

• Notify doctor of signs of decreasing renal function or if patient complains of tinnitus, vertigo, or hearing loss. Onset of deafness may occur several weeks after drug is stopped.

Patient teaching

• Instruct patient to report adverse reactions, especially hearing loss or change in urinary elimination.

• Emphasize need to drink 2,000 ml of fluid each day.

• Tell patient to alert doctor if infection worsens or does not improve.

☑ Evaluation

• Patient is free from infection.

• Patient maintains adequate hydration throughout drug therapy.

• Patient and family state understanding of drug therapy.

---

neostigmine bromide
(nee-oh-STIG-meen BROH-mighd)
Prostigmin

neostigmine methylsulfate
Prostigmin

Pharmacologic class: cholinesterase inhibitor
Therapeutic class: muscle stimulant
Pregnancy risk category: C

How supplied

neostigmine bromide
Tablets: 15 mg

neostigmine methylsulfate
Injection: 0.25 mg/ml, 0.5 mg/ml, 1 mg/ml

Pharmacokinetics

Absorption: poorly absorbed (1% to 2%) from GI tract after oral administration. Unknown after S.C. or I.M. administration.
Distribution: about 15% to 25% of dose binds to plasma proteins.
Metabolism: hydrolyzed by cholinesterases and metabolized by microsomal liver enzymes.
Excretion: about 80% of drug excreted in urine.

Route	Onset	Peak	Duration
P.O.	45-75 min	1-2 hr	2-4 hr
I.V.	4-8 min	1-2 hr	2-4 hr
I.M.	20-30 min	1-2 hr	2-4 hr
S.C.	Unknown	1-2 hr	2-4 hr

Pharmacodynamics

Chemical effect: inhibits destruction of acetylcholine released from parasympathetic and somatic efferent nerves. Acetylcholine accumulates, promoting increased stimulation of receptor.
Therapeutic effect: stimulates muscle contraction.

Indications and dosage

▶ **Treatment of myasthenia gravis.**
Adults: 15 to 30 mg P.O. t.i.d. (range is 15 to 375 mg daily); or 0.5 mg S.C. or I.M. *Children:* 7.5 to 15 mg P.O. t.i.d. or q.i.d. Subsequent dosages must be highly individualized, depending on response and tolerance of adverse effects. Therapy may be required day and night.
▶ **Diagnosis of myasthenia gravis.**
Adults: 0.022 mg/kg I.M. 30 minutes after 0.011 mg/kg I.M. of atropine sulfate. *Children:* 0.025 to 0.04 mg/kg. I.M. after 0.011 mg/kg atropine sulfate S.C.
▶ **Postoperative abdominal distention and bladder atony.** *Adults:* 0.25 to 0.5 mg I.M. or S.C. q 4 to 6 hours for 2 to 3 days.

Reactions may be *common*, uncommon, *life-threatening*, or COMMON AND LIFE-THREATENING.

► **Antidote for nondepolarizing neuromuscular blockers.** *Adults:* 0.5 to 2 mg I.V. slowly. Repeat p.r.n. to total of 5 mg. Before antidote dose, 0.6 to 1.2 mg atropine sulfate is given I.V. *Note:* 1:1,000 solution of injectable solution contains 1 mg/ml; 1:2,000 solution contains 0.5 mg/ml.

Adverse reactions

CNS: dizziness, headache, muscle weakness, mental confusion, jitters, sweating.
CV: bradycardia, hypotension, *cardiac arrest.*
EENT: blurred vision, lacrimation, miosis.
GI: *nausea, vomiting, diarrhea, abdominal cramps,* excessive salivation.
GU: urinary frequency.
Musculoskeletal: *muscle cramps,* muscle fasciculations.
Respiratory: *depression, bronchospasm, bronchoconstriction, respiratory arrest.*
Skin: rash (with bromide).
Other: hypersensitivity reactions *(anaphylaxis).*

Interactions

Drug-drug. *Aminoglycosides, anticholinergics, atropine, corticosteroids, magnesium sulfate, procainamide, quinidine:* may reverse cholinergic effects. Observe for lack of drug effect.

Contraindications and precautions

• Contraindicated in patients with hypersensitivity to cholinergics or to bromide and in those with peritonitis or mechanical obstruction of intestine or urinary tract.
• Use cautiously in patients with bronchial asthma, bradycardia, seizure disorders, recent coronary occlusion, vagotonia, hyperthyroidism, arrhythmias, and peptic ulcer.

NURSING CONSIDERATIONS

🔍 **Assessment**
• Assess patient's condition before therapy.

• Monitor patient's response after each dose. Observe closely for improvement in strength, vision, and ptosis 45 to 60 minutes after each dose. Show patient how to record variations in muscle strength.
• Monitor vital signs frequently.
• Evaluate patient's and family's knowledge of drug therapy.

🔄 **Nursing diagnoses**
• Impaired physical mobility related to condition
• Diarrhea related to drug's adverse effect on GI tract
• Knowledge deficit related to drug therapy

▶ **Planning and implementation**
• Stop all other cholinergics before giving drug, as ordered.
• In myasthenia gravis, schedule doses before fatigue. For example, if patient has dysphagia, schedule dose 30 minutes before each meal.
• Be prepared to give atropine injection, as ordered; provide respiratory support as needed.
• Be aware that I.M. neostigmine may be used instead of edrophonium to diagnose myasthenia gravis. May be preferable to edrophonium when limb weakness is only symptom.
• When drug is used to prevent abdominal distention and GI distress, doctor may order rectal tube inserted to help passage of gas.
• Although drug is frequently used to reverse effects of nondepolarizing neuromuscular blockers in patients who have undergone surgery, be aware that it may worsen blockade produced by succinylcholine.
• Know that patient may develop resistance to drug.
P.O. use: Give drug with food or milk. If appropriate, obtain order for hospitalized patient to have bedside supply of tablets. A patient with long-standing disease may insist on self-administration.

I.V. use: Give drug at slow, controlled rate not to exceed 1 mg/minute in adults and 0.5 mg/minute in children.
I.M. and S.C. use: Follow normal protocol.

Patient teaching
• Tell patient to take drug with food or milk to reduce GI distress.
• When using for myasthenia gravis, explain that drug will relieve ptosis, double vision, difficulty in chewing and swallowing, and trunk and limb weakness. Stress need to take drug exactly as ordered. Explain that it may have to be taken for life.
• Advise patient to wear medical identification bracelet indicating myasthenia gravis.

☑ **Evaluation**
• Patient performs activities of daily living without assistance.
• Patient's bowel patterns are normal.
• Patient and family state understanding of drug therapy.

netilmicin sulfate
(net-il-MIGH-sin SUL-fayt)
Netromycin

Pharmacologic class: aminoglycoside
Therapeutic class: antibiotic
Pregnancy risk category: D

How supplied

Injection: 25 mg/ml♦, 50 mg/ml♦, 100 mg/ml

Pharmacokinetics

Absorption: unknown after I.M. administration.
Distribution: distributed widely; CSF penetration is low. Protein binding is minimal.
Metabolism: not metabolized.
Excretion: excreted primarily in urine; small amounts excreted in bile. *Half-life:* 2 to 2½ hours.

Route	Onset	Peak	Duration
I.V.	Immediate	Immediate	8-12 hr
I.M.	Unknown	30-60 min	8-12 hr

Pharmacodynamics

Chemical effect: inhibits protein synthesis by binding directly to 30S ribosomal subunit.
Therapeutic effect: kills susceptible bacteria, such as many aerobic gram-negative organisms (including most strains of *Pseudomonas aeruginosa*) and some aerobic gram-positive organisms.

Indications and dosage

▶ **Serious infections caused by sensitive strains of *P. aeruginosa, Escherichia coli, Proteus, Klebsiella, Serratia, Enterobacter, Citrobacter, Staphylococcus.*** *Adults and children over age 12:* 3 to 6.5 mg/kg/day by I.M. injection or I.V. infusion. May be given q 12 hours to treat serious urinary tract infections (UTI) and q 8 to 12 hours to treat serious systemic infections. *Infants and children ages 6 weeks to 12 years:* 5.5 to 8 mg/kg/day by I.M. injection or I.V. infusion, given either as 1.8 to 2.7 mg/kg q 8 hours or as 2.7 to 4 mg/kg q 12 hours. *Neonates under age 6 weeks:* 4 to 6.5 mg/kg/day by I.M. injection or I.V. infusion given as 2 to 3.25 mg/kg q 12 hours.
▶ **Complicated UTIs.** *Adults with normal renal function:* 3 to 4 mg/kg/day by I.M. injection or I.V. infusion divided into two equal doses given q 12 hours.

Adverse reactions

CNS: headache, lethargy, *neuromuscular blockade, seizures.*
EENT: *ototoxicity (tinnitus, vertigo, hearing loss).*
GU *nephrotoxicity (cells or casts in urine; oliguria; proteinuria; decreased creatinine clearance; increased BUN, nonprotein nitrogen, and serum creatinine levels).*
Other: hypersensitivity reactions *(anaphylaxis).*

Reactions may be *common,* uncommon, *life-threatening,* or **COMMON AND LIFE-THREATENING.**

Interactions

Drug-drug. *Cephalothin:* increased nephrotoxicity. Use together cautiously.
Dimenhydrinate: may mask symptoms of ototoxicity. Use cautiously.
General anesthetics, neuromuscular blocking agents: may potentiate neuromuscular blockade.
I.V. loop diuretics (such as furosemide): increased ototoxicity. Use cautiously.
Other aminoglycosides, acyclovir, amphotericin B, cisplatin, methoxyflurane, vancomycin: increased nephrotoxicity. Use together cautiously.
Parenteral penicillins (such as ticarcillin): netilmicin inactivation. Don't mix together.

Contraindications and precautions

• Contraindicated in patients with hypersensitivity to drug or other aminoglycosides.
• Drug use is not recommended in pregnant or breast-feeding women.
• Use cautiously in patients with impaired renal function or neuromuscular disorders and in neonates, infants, and elderly patients. Drug contains sulfites, which may cause allergic reaction in some patients.

NURSING CONSIDERATIONS

♨ Assessment

• Assess patient's infection before therapy and regularly thereafter.
• Obtain blood for peak drug level 1 hour after I.M. injection and 30 minutes to 1 hour after infusion ends; for trough level, draw blood just before next dose. Don't use heparinized tube because heparin is incompatible with aminoglycosides.
• Blood levels above 16 mcg/ml and trough levels above 4 mcg/ml may be associated with higher incidence of toxicity.
• Obtain specimen for culture and sensitivity tests before giving first dose. Therapy may begin pending results.
• Weigh patient and review renal function studies before therapy begins.

• Evaluate patient's hearing and renal function before beginning therapy. Then monitor hearing and renal function (output, specific gravity, urinalysis, BUN and creatinine levels, and creatinine clearance) as ordered throughout therapy.
• Be alert for adverse reactions and drug interactions.
• Evaluate patient's and family's knowledge of drug therapy.

⊞ Nursing diagnoses

• Infection related to organisms
• Risk for injury related to drug-induced adverse reactions
• Knowledge deficit related to drug therapy

⊠ Planning and implementation

I.V. use: A single dose may be diluted in 50 to 200 ml of 0.9% NaCl or D₅W. Infuse over 30 minutes to 2 hours.
– After completing I.V. infusion, flush line with 0.9% NaCl solution or D₅W.
I.M. use: Follow normal protocol.
• Notify doctor of signs of decreasing renal function or if patient complains of tinnitus, vertigo, or hearing loss.
• Ensure that patient is well hydrated while taking drug to minimize chemical irritation of renal tubules.
• Therapy usually continues for 7 to 10 days. If no response occurs in 3 to 5 days, therapy may be stopped and new specimens obtained for culture and sensitivity testing.

Patient teaching
• Tell patient to drink at least 2,000 ml of fluid daily during therapy.
• Instruct patient to immediately report changes in hearing or voiding.

✓ Evaluation

• Patient is free from infection.
• Patient does not experience injury as result of netilmicin therapy.
• Patient and family state understanding of drug therapy.

---

*Liquid form contains alcohol   **May contain tartrazine   ♦Canada   ◇ Australia   †OTC

nevirapine
(neh-VEER-uh-peen)
Viramune

Pharmacologic class: nonnucleoside reverse transcriptase inhibitor
Therapeutic class: antiviral
Pregnancy risk category: C

How supplied

Tablets: 200 mg

Pharmacokinetics

Absorption: readily absorbed.
Distribution: widely distributed.
Metabolism: metabolized by liver.
Excretion: excreted in urine and feces.

Route	Onset	Peak	Duration
P.O.	Unknown	4 hr	Unknown

Pharmacodynamics

Chemical effect: binds to reverse transcriptase and blocks RNA-dependent and DNA-dependent DNA polymerase activities.
Therapeutic effect: no results available from clinical trials evaluating effect on progression of HIV infection.

Indications and dosage

▶ **Adjunct treatment in patients with HIV-1 infection who have experienced clinical or immunologic deterioration.**
Adults: 200 mg P.O. daily for first 14 days, followed by 200 mg P.O. b.i.d., in combination with nucleoside analogue antiretroviral agents.

Adverse reactions

CNS: *headache,* paresthesia.
GI: *nausea,* diarrhea, abdominal pain, ulcerative stomatitis.
Hematologic: *decreased neutrophil count,* decreased hemoglobin.
Hepatic: hepatitis, increased ALT, AST, gamma-glutamyl transpeptidase (GGT), and total bilirubin levels.

Skin: rash, blistering, *Stevens-Johnson syndrome.*
Other: *fever,* myalgia.

Interactions

Drug-drug. *Drugs extensively metabolized by P-450 CYP3A:* may lower plasma levels of these drugs, requiring dosage adjustment.
Oral contraceptives, other hormonal contraceptives, protease inhibitors: may decrease plasma levels of these drugs. Don't use together.
Rifabutin, rifampin: more data needed to assess whether dosage adjustments are needed. Monitor closely with concomitant use.

Contraindications and precautions

• Contraindicated in patients with hypersensitivity to drug.
• Use cautiously in patients with impaired renal and hepatic function.

NURSING CONSIDERATIONS

✍ Assessment
• Perform clinical chemistry tests, including liver function tests, before and during therapy, as ordered.
• Monitor patient for blistering, oral lesions, conjunctivitis, muscle or joint aches, or general malaise. Be especially alert for severe rash or rash accompanied by fever. Report such signs and symptoms to doctor.

⊕ Nursing diagnoses
• Infection related to presence of virus
• Knowledge deficit related to drug therapy

▷ Planning and implementation
• Know that drug should be used with at least one additional antiretroviral agent.
• Drug is excreted in breast milk.
Patient teaching
• Inform patient that drug is not a cure for HIV and that illnesses associated with advanced HIV-1 infection may occur.

Reactions may be *common,* uncommon, *life-threatening,* or COMMON AND LIFE-THREATENING.

Explain that drug does not reduce risk of HIV-1 transmission.
• Instruct patient to report rash at once and to stop drug.
• Tell patient not to use other drugs unless approved by doctor.
• Advise female patient of childbearing age to avoid use of hormonal contraceptive methods with drug.
• Tell patient to stop breast-feeding during therapy to reduce risk of postnatal HIV transmission.

☑ **Evaluation**
• Patient shows no signs of worsening condition.
• Patient and family state understanding of drug therapy.

niacin
(vitamin B3, nicotinic acid)
(NIGH-uh-sin)
Niac, Niacor, Nico-400, Nicobid†, Nicolar**, Nicotinex, Slo-Niacin, Niacin TR Tablets

niacinamide (nicotinamide)†

Pharmacologic class: B-complex vitamin
Therapeutic class: vitamin B₃, antilipemic, peripheral vasodilator
Pregnancy risk category: C

How supplied
niacin
Tablets: 25 mg†, 50 mg†, 100 mg†, 250 mg†, 500 mg
Tablets (timed-release): 150 mg†, 250 mg†, 500 mg†, 750 mg†
Capsules (timed-release): 125 mg†, 250 mg†, 300 mg†, 400 mg†, 500 mg
Elixir: 50 mg/5 ml†
Injection: 100 mg/ml in 30-ml vials
niacinamide
Tablets: 50 mg†, 100 mg†, 125 mg†, 250 mg†, 500 mg†

Pharmacokinetics
Absorption: absorbed rapidly from GI tract. Absorption unknown after S.C. or I.M. administration.
Distribution: niacin coenzymes are distributed widely in body tissues.
Metabolism: metabolized by liver to active metabolites.
Excretion: excreted in urine. *Half-life:* about 45 minutes.

Route	Onset	Peak	Duration
P.O.	Unknown	45 min	Unknown
I.V., I.M., S.C.	Unknown	Unknown	Unknown

Pharmacodynamics
Chemical effect: niacin and niacinamide stimulate lipid metabolism, tissue respiration, and glycogenolysis; niacin decreases synthesis of low-density lipoproteins and inhibits lipolysis in adipose tissue.
Therapeutic effect: restores normal levels of vitamin B₃, lowers triglyceride and cholesterol levels, and dilates peripheral blood vessels.

Indications and dosage
▶ **RDA.** *Neonates and infants to age 6 months:* 5 mg. *Infants ages 6 months to 1 year:* 6 mg. *Children ages 1 to 3:* 9 mg. *Children ages 4 to 6:* 12 mg. *Children ages 7 to 10:* 13 mg. *Males ages 11 to 14:* 17 mg. *Males ages 15 to 18:* 20 mg. *Males ages 19 to 50:* 19 mg. *Males age 51 and over:* 15 mg. *Females ages 11 to 50:* 15 mg. *Females age 51 and over:* 13 mg. *Pregnant women:* 17 mg. *Breast-feeding women:* 20 mg.
▶ **Pellagra.** *Adults:* 300 to 500 mg P.O., S.C., I.M., or I.V. infusion daily in divided doses, depending on severity of niacin deficiency. *Children:* up to 300 mg P.O. or 100 mg I.V. daily, depending on severity of niacin deficiency. After symptoms subside, advise adequate nutrition and RDA supplements to prevent recurrence.

▶ **Hartnup disease.** *Adults:* 50 to 200 mg P.O. daily.
▶ **Niacin deficiency.** *Adults:* up to 100 mg P.O. daily.
▶ **Hyperlipidemias, especially with hypercholesterolemia.** *Adults:* 1 to 2 g P.O. t.i.d. with meals, increased at intervals to 6 g daily.

Adverse reactions

Most adverse reactions are dose-dependent.
CNS: dizziness, transient headache.
CV: *excessive peripheral vasodilation* (especially niacin), *arrhythmias.*
GI: *nausea, vomiting, diarrhea,* possible activation of peptic ulceration, epigastric or substernal pain.
Hepatic: *hepatic dysfunction.*
Metabolic: hyperglycemia, hyperuricemia.
Skin: *flushing,* pruritus, dryness, tingling.

Interactions

Drug-drug. *Antihypertensive drugs (sympathetic or ganglionic blockers):* potential postural hypotension. Use together cautiously; also warn patient about postural hypotension.

Contraindications and precautions

• Contraindicated in patients with hepatic dysfunction, active peptic ulcers, severe hypotension, arterial hemorrhage, or hypersensitivity to drug.
• Use cautiously in patients with gallbladder disease, diabetes mellitus, or coronary artery disease and in patients with history of liver disease, peptic ulcer, allergy, or gout.

NURSING CONSIDERATIONS

⬛ Assessment
• Assess patient's condition before therapy and regularly thereafter.
• Monitor hepatic function and blood glucose, as ordered.
• Be alert for adverse reactions and drug interactions.

• Monitor patient's hydration status if adverse GI reactions occur.
• Evaluate patient's and family's knowledge of drug therapy.

⬛ Nursing diagnoses
• Altered nutrition: less than body requirements related to decreased intake of vitamin B_3
• Risk for fluid volume deficit related to drug-induced adverse GI reactions
• Knowledge deficit related to drug therapy

⬛ Planning and implementation
• Administer aspirin (325 mg P.O. 30 minutes before niacin dose), as ordered, to possibly reduce flushing.
• Know that timed-release niacin or niacinamide may prevent excessive flushing that occurs with large doses. However, timed-release niacin has been associated with hepatic dysfunction, even at doses as low as 1 g/day.
P.O. use: Give drug with meals to minimize GI adverse effects.
I.V. use: Give drug by slow I.V. (no faster than 2 mg/minute).
I.M. and S.C. use: Follow normal protocol.
Patient teaching
• Explain harmlessness of flushing.
• Stress that drug is a potent medication that may cause serious adverse effects. Explain importance of adhering to therapeutic regimen.
• Advise patient against self-medicating for hyperlipidemia.

⬛ Evaluation
• Patient's vitamin B_3 levels are normal.
• Patient maintains adequate hydration throughout drug therapy.
• Patient and family state understanding of drug therapy.

Reactions may be *common*, uncommon, *life-threatening*, or COMMON AND LIFE-THREATENING.

nicardipine hydrochloride
(nigh-KAR-dih-peen
high-droh-KLOR-ighd)
Cardene, Cardene IV, Cardene SR

Pharmacologic class: calcium channel blocker
Therapeutic class: antianginal, antihypertensive
Pregnancy risk category: C

How supplied

Capsules (immediate-release): 20 mg, 30 mg
Capsules (sustained-release): 30 mg, 45 mg, 60 mg
Injection: 2.5 mg/ml

Pharmacokinetics

Absorption: completely absorbed after oral administration; may be decreased if drug is taken with food.
Distribution: extensively (over 95%) bound to plasma proteins.
Metabolism: absolute bioavailability of about 35%; extensively metabolized in liver.
Excretion: about 60% excreted in urine, 35% in bile. *Half-life:* 2 to 4 hours.

Route	Onset	Peak	Duration
P.O.	≤ 20 min	0.5-4 hr	6-12 hr
I.V.	Immediate	Within min	Rapid decline after infusion ends

Pharmacodynamics

Chemical effect: inhibits calcium ion influx across cardiac and smooth-muscle cells, decreasing myocardial contractility and oxygen demand. Also dilates coronary arteries and arterioles.
Therapeutic effect: lowers blood pressure and relieves anginal pain.

Indications and dosage

▶ **Chronic stable angina (used alone or in combination with other antianginal agents).** *Adults:* initially, 20 mg P.O. t.i.d. (immediate-release only). Dosage titrated based on response q 3 days. Usual dosage range is 20 to 40 mg t.i.d.
▶ **Hypertension.** *Adults:* initially, 20 to 40 mg P.O. t.i.d. (immediate-release) or 30 to 60 mg b.i.d. (sustained-release). Dosage increased based on response. Alternatively, for patients unable to take oral nicardipine, 50 ml/hour (5 mg/hour) I.V. infusion initially; then increased by 25 ml/hour (2.5 mg/hour) q 15 minutes up to 150 ml/hour (15 mg/hour).

Adverse reactions

CNS: *dizziness, light-headedness, headache, paresthesia, drowsiness, asthenia.*
CV: *peripheral edema, palpitations, angina, tachycardia.*
GI: nausea, abdominal discomfort, dry mouth.
Skin: rash, *flushing.*

Interactions

Drug-drug. *Antihypertensives:* enhanced antihypertensive effect. Monitor patient.
Beta blockers: may increase cardiac depressant effects. Monitor patient.
Cimetidine: may decrease metabolism of calcium channel blockers. Monitor patient for toxicity.
Cyclosporine: nicardipine may increase plasma levels of cyclosporine. Monitor closely.
Theophylline: pharmacologic effects of theophylline may be enhanced. Monitor patient.

Contraindications and precautions

• Contraindicated in patients with hypersensitivity to drug and in those with advanced aortic stenosis.
• Drug use is not recommended in breast-feeding women.
• Use cautiously in pregnant women and in patients with cardiac conduction disturbances, hypotension, heart failure, and impaired hepatic or renal function.
• Safety of drug has not been established in children.

NURSING CONSIDERATIONS

⚖ Assessment
• Assess patient's condition before therapy and regularly thereafter.
• Measure blood pressure frequently during initial therapy. Maximum blood pressure response occurs about 1 hour after dosing with immediate-release form and 2 to 4 hours with sustained-release form. Check for potential orthostatic hypotension. Because large swings in blood pressure may occur based on blood level of drug, assess adequacy of antihypertensive effect 8 hours after dosing.
• Be alert for adverse reactions and drug interactions.
• Evaluate patient's and family's knowledge of drug therapy.

Nursing diagnoses
• Risk for injury related to hypertension
• Pain related to angina
• Knowledge deficit related to drug therapy

Planning and implementation
P.O. use: Follow normal protocol.
I.V. use: When switching to oral therapy other than nicardipine, initiate therapy after stopping infusion. If oral nicardipine is to be used, administer first dose of t.i.d. regimen 1 hour before stopping infusion.
– Adjust infusion rate if hypotension or tachycardia occurs, as ordered.
Patient teaching
• Advise patient to report chest pain immediately. Some patients may experience increased frequency, severity, or duration of chest pain at beginning of therapy or during dosage adjustments.
• Stress need to take drug exactly as prescribed even when feeling well.
• Instruct patient how to minimize orthostatic hypotension.

☑ Evaluation
• Patient's blood pressure is normal.
• Patient's anginal attacks are less frequent and severe.

• Patient and family state understanding of drug therapy.

---

nicotine polacrilex (nicotine-polacrilin resin complex)
(NIH-koh-teen poh-luh-KRIGH-leks)
Nicorette, Nicorette DS

Pharmacologic class: nicotinic agonist
Therapeutic class: smoking cessation aid
Pregnancy risk category: X

How supplied
Chewing gum: 2 mg/square, 4 mg/square

Pharmacokinetics
Absorption: nicotine is bound to ion-exchange resin and is released only during chewing. Blood level depends on vigor of gum chewing.
Distribution: not clearly defined.
Metabolism: metabolized by liver and somewhat by kidney and lung.
Excretion: excreted in urine. Excretion increased in acidic urine and by high urine output. *Half-life:* 1 to 2 hours.

Route	Onset	Peak	Duration
P.O.	Unknown	15-30 min	Unknown

Pharmacodynamics
Chemical effect: provides nicotine, which stimulates nicotinic acetylcholine receptors in CNS, neuromuscular junction, autonomic ganglia, and adrenal medulla.
Therapeutic effect: blocks nicotine withdrawal symptoms.

Indications and dosage
▶ **Relief of nicotine withdrawal symptoms in patients undergoing smoking cessation.** *Adults:* initially, one 2-mg square; highly-dependent patients should start treatment with 4-mg squares. Patients should chew one piece of gum slowly and intermittently for 30 minutes whenever urge to smoke occurs. Most patients require 9 to 12 pieces of gum daily

---

during first month. With 4-mg squares, maximum dosage is 20 pieces daily. With 2-mg squares, maximum dosage is 30 pieces daily.

Adverse reactions

CNS: dizziness, light-headedness.
CV: atrial fibrillation.
EENT: throat soreness, jaw muscle ache (from chewing).
GI: nausea, vomiting, indigestion.
Other: hiccups.

Interactions

Drug-drug. *Beta blockers, methylxanthines, propoxyphene, propranolol:* decreased metabolism of these agents, increasing therapeutic effects. Dosages of these agents may be adjusted.
Drug-lifestyle. *Smoking:* reduced effectiveness of drug. Warn patient to avoid smoking while taking drug.

Contraindications and precautions

• Contraindicated in nonsmokers; in patients with recent MI, life-threatening arrhythmias, severe or worsening angina pectoris, or active temporomandibular joint disease, and in pregnant women.
• Drug use is not recommended in breast-feeding women or in children.
• Use cautiously in patients with hyperthyroidism, pheochromocytoma, insulin-dependent diabetes, peptic ulcer disease, history of esophagitis, oral or pharyngeal inflammation, or dental conditions that might be exacerbated by chewing gum.

NURSING CONSIDERATIONS

Assessment
• Assess patient's smoking history before therapy.
• Evaluate effectiveness of drug by assessing for nicotine withdrawal signs and symptoms.
• Be alert for adverse reactions and drug interactions.
• Evaluate patient's and family's knowledge of drug therapy.

Nursing diagnoses
• Altered health maintenance related to smoking
• Risk for injury related to drug-induced adverse CNS reactions
• Knowledge deficit related to drug therapy

Planning and implementation
• Smokers most likely to benefit from nicotine gum are those with high "physical" nicotine dependence—those who smoke more than 15 cigarettes daily, prefer high-nicotine brands, usually inhale smoke, smoke first cigarette within 30 minutes of arising, find first morning cigarette hardest to give up, smoke most frequently during morning, find it difficult to refrain from smoking in places where it's forbidden, or smoke even when ill and confined to bed.
Patient teaching
• Instruct patient to chew gum slowly and intermittently (chew several times, then place between cheek and gums) for about 30 minutes to promote slow, even absorption. Fast chewing tends to produce more adverse reactions.
• Be sure that patient reads and understands patient instruction sheet included in package.
• Emphasize importance of withdrawing gum gradually.
• Tell patient that successful abstainers will begin to gradually withdraw gum usage after 3 months. Use of gum for longer than 6 months is not recommended. For gradual withdrawal, cut gum in halves or quarters and mix with other sugarless gum.

Evaluation
• Patient does not experience nicotine withdrawal symptoms.
• Patient experiences no injuries due to drug-induced CNS reactions.
• Patient and family state understanding of drug therapy.

---

nicotine transdermal system
(NIH-koh-teen trans-DER-mul SIS-tum)
Habitrol, Nicoderm, Nicotrol, ProStep

Pharmacologic class: nicotinic cholinergic agonist
Therapeutic class: smoking cessation aid
Pregnancy risk category: D

How supplied
Habitrol—21 mg/day, 14 mg/day, 7 mg/day
Nicoderm—21 mg/day, 14 mg/day, 7 mg/day
Nicotrol—15 mg/16 hours, 10 mg/16 hours, 5 mg/16 hours
ProStep—22 mg/day, 11 mg/day

Pharmacokinetics
Absorption: rapidly absorbed.
Distribution: plasma protein-binding of drug is below 5%.
Metabolism: metabolized by liver, kidney, and lung.
Excretion: excreted primarily in urine as metabolites; about 10% excreted unchanged. With high urine flow rates or acidified urine, up to 30% can be excreted unchanged. *Half-life:* 1 to 2 hours.

Route	Onset	Peak	Duration
Trans-dermal	Unknown	3-9 hr	Varies

Pharmacodynamics
Chemical effect: provides nicotine, which stimulates nicotinic acetylcholine receptors in CNS, neuromuscular junction, autonomic ganglia, and adrenal medulla.
Therapeutic effect: blocks nicotine withdrawal symptoms.

Indications and dosage
▶ **Relief of nicotine withdrawal symptoms in patients undergoing smoking cessation.** *Adults:* initially, one transdermal system, delivering largest available nicotine dosage in its dosage series, ap-plied once daily in morning to nonhairy part of body and removed before retiring. After 4 to 12 weeks (dependent on brand) dosage tapered to next largest available dosage in series followed in 2 to 4 weeks by lowest dosage in series. Drug is then stopped in 2 to 4 weeks.

Adverse reactions
CNS: somnolence, dizziness, *headache, insomnia.*
EENT: pharyngitis, sinusitis.
GI: abdominal pain, constipation, dyspepsia, nausea.
GU: dysmenorrhea.
Skin: *local or systemic erythema, pruritus, burning* (at application site); cutaneous hypersensitivity, rash.
Other: back pain, myalgia, diaphoresis.

Interactions
Drug-drug. *Acetaminophen, imipramine, oxazepam, pentazocine, propranolol, theophylline:* may decrease induction of hepatic enzymes that help metabolize certain drugs. Dosage may be reduced.
Adrenergic agonists (such as isoproterenol, phenylephrine): may decrease circulating catecholamines. Dosage may be increased.
Adrenergic antagonists (such as labetalol, prazosin): may decrease circulating catecholamines. Dosage may be reduced.
Insulin: may increase amount of subcutaneous insulin absorbed. Insulin dosage may be reduced.
Drug-lifestyle. *Caffeine:* may decrease induction of hepatic enzymes that help metabolize certain drugs. Dosage may be reduced.

Contraindications and precautions
• Contraindicated in patients with recent MI, life-threatening arrhythmias, severe or worsening angina pectoris, or hypersensitivity to nicotine or components of transdermal system and in nonsmokers.

• Drug use is not recommended in pregnant or breast-feeding women and in children.
• Use cautiously in patients with hyperthyroidism, pheochromocytoma, hypertension, insulin-dependent diabetes, or peptic ulcer disease.

NURSING CONSIDERATIONS

Assessment
• Assess patient's smoking history before therapy.
• Evaluate effectiveness of drug by assessing for nicotine withdrawal signs and symptoms.
• Be alert for adverse reactions and drug interactions.
• Evaluate patient's and family's knowledge of drug therapy.

Nursing diagnoses
• Altered health maintenance related to smoking
• Risk for injury related to drug-induced adverse CNS reactions
• Knowledge deficit related to drug therapy

Planning and implementation
• Health care workers' exposure to nicotine in transdermal systems probably is minimal; however, avoid unnecessary contact. Wash hands with water alone because soap can enhance absorption.
Patient teaching
• Discourage use of transdermal system for more than 3 months. Chronic nicotine consumption by any route can be habit-forming.
• Warn patient not to smoke. If he smokes while using system, serious adverse effects may occur because peak serum nicotine levels will be much higher than those achieved by smoking alone.
• Be sure that patient reads and understands patient information that is dispensed with drug.
• Advise patient to apply patch promptly because nicotine can evaporate from

transdermal system once it is removed from its protective packaging. Patch should not be altered in any way (folded or cut) before application. Do not store at temperatures above 86° F (30° C).
• Teach patient proper disposal of transdermal system. After removal, fold patch in half, bringing adhesive sides together. If system comes in protective pouch, place used patch in it. Careful disposal prevents accidental poisoning of children or pets.
• Tell patient who experiences persistent or severe local skin reactions or generalized rash to immediately stop use of patch and contact doctor.
• Explain that patient who cannot stop cigarette smoking during initial 4 weeks of therapy probably will not benefit from continued use of drug. Patient who was unsuccessful may benefit from counseling to identify factors that led to treatment failure. Encourage patient to minimize or eliminate factors contributing to treatment failure and to try again after a while.

Evaluation
• Patient does not experience nicotine withdrawal symptoms.
• Patient experiences no injuries due to drug-induced adverse CNS reactions.
• Patient and family state understanding of drug therapy.

nifedipine
(nigh-FEH-duh-peen)
Adalat, Adalat CC, Adalat P.A.♦, Nu-Nifed♦, Procardia, Procardia XL

Pharmacologic class: calcium channel blocker
Therapeutic class: antianginal
Pregnancy risk category: C

How supplied

Tablets (extended-release): 30 mg, 60 mg, 90 mg
Capsules: 10 mg, 20 mg

Pharmacokinetics

Absorption: about 90% of drug is absorbed rapidly from GI tract; however, only about 65% to 70% of drug reaches systemic circulation because of significant first-pass effect in liver.
Distribution: about 92% to 98% of circulating drug is bound to plasma proteins.
Metabolism: metabolized in liver.
Excretion: excreted in urine and feces as inactive metabolites. *Half-life:* 2 to 5 hours.

Route	Onset	Peak	Duration
P.O.	20 min	0.5-2 hr	4-24 hr

Pharmacodynamics

Chemical effect: unknown; may inhibit calcium ion influx across cardiac and smooth-muscle cells, decreasing myocardial contractility and oxygen demand. Also may dilate coronary arteries and arterioles.
Therapeutic effect: reduces blood pressure and prevents anginal pain.

Indications and dosage

▶ **Vasospastic angina (also called Prinzmetal's [variant] angina) and classic chronic stable angina pectoris.** *Adults:* starting dose is 10 mg P.O. t.i.d. Usual effective dose range is 10 to 20 mg t.i.d. Some patients may require up to 30 mg q.i.d. Maximum daily dosage is 180 mg (capsules).
▶ **Hypertension.** *Adults:* 30 or 60 mg P.O. (extended-release form only) once daily. Titrated over 7- to 14-day period. Maximum daily dosage is 120 mg.

Adverse reactions

CNS: *dizziness, light-headedness, flushing, headache,* weakness, syncope.
CV: peripheral edema, hypotension, palpitations, heart failure, pulmonary edema, **MI.**
EENT: nasal congestion.
GI: nausea, heartburn, diarrhea.
Respiratory: dyspnea.
Skin: rash, pruritus.

Other: muscle cramps, hypokalemia.

Interactions

Drug-drug. *Cimetidine, ranitidine:* decreased nifedipine metabolism. Monitor patient closely.
Propranolol, other beta blockers: may cause hypotension and heart failure. Use together cautiously.
Drug-food. *Grapefruit juice:* increased bioavailability. Give together.

Contraindications and precautions

• Contraindicated in patients with hypersensitivity to drug and in pregnant or breast-feeding women.
• Use cautiously in elderly patients and in those with heart failure or hypotension. Use extended-release tablets cautiously in patients with severe GI narrowing because obstructive symptoms may occur.
• Safety of drug has not been established in children.

NURSING CONSIDERATIONS

☡ Assessment

• Assess patient's condition before therapy and regularly thereafter.
• Monitor blood pressure regularly, especially in patient who also takes beta blockers or antihypertensives.
• Monitor serum potassium level regularly, as ordered.
• Be alert for adverse reactions and drug interactions.
• Evaluate patient's and family's knowledge of drug therapy.

⊕ Nursing diagnoses

• Risk for injury related to presence of hypertension
• Pain related to angina
• Knowledge deficit related to drug therapy

▶ Planning and implementation

• When rapid response to drug is desired, instruct patient to bite and swallow capsule. If he is unable to chew capsules, liq-

---

uid can be withdrawn by puncturing capsule with needle and squeezing contents into mouth. When using these methods, continuous blood pressure and ECG monitoring is recommended.
• Despite widespread S.L. use of nifedipine capsules, avoid this route of administration. Peak serum levels are lower and it takes longer for peak levels to occur than when capsules are bitten and swallowed.
• S.L. nitroglycerin may be taken as needed when anginal symptoms are acute.
• Although rebound effect hasn't been observed when drug is stopped, dosage should still be reduced slowly under doctor's supervision.
Patient teaching
• If patient is kept on nitrate therapy while nifedipine dosage is being titrated, urge continued compliance.
• Warn patient that angina may worsen when beginning drug therapy or when dosage is increased. Reassure him that this is temporary.
• Instruct patient to swallow extended-release tablets without breaking, crushing, or chewing.
• Advise patient who is taking extended-release form of drug that wax-matrix "ghost" from tablet may be passed in stool.
• Warn patient not to switch brands. Procardia XL and Adalat CC are not equivalent because of major differences in their pharmacokinetics.
• Tell patient to protect capsules from direct light and moisture and to store at room temperature.

☑ **Evaluation**
• Patient's blood pressure is normal.
• Patient's anginal attacks are less frequent and severe.
• Patient and family state understanding of drug therapy.

nimodipine
(nigh-MOH-dih-peen)
Nimotop

Pharmacologic class: calcium channel blocker
Therapeutic class: cerebral vasodilator
Pregnancy risk category: C

How supplied
Capsules: 30 mg

Pharmacokinetics
Absorption: well absorbed from GI tract, but bioavailability is 3% to 30%.
Distribution: drug is greater than 95% protein-bound.
Metabolism: extensively metabolized in liver. Drug and metabolites undergo enterohepatic recycling.
Excretion: excreted mainly in feces; less than 1% in urine. *Half-life:* 8 to 9 hours.

Route	Onset	Peak	Duration
P.O.	Unknown	≤ 1 hr	Unknown

Pharmacodynamics
Chemical effect: inhibits calcium ion influx across cardiac and smooth-muscle cells, decreasing myocardial contractility and oxygen demand, and dilates coronary and cerebral arteries and arterioles.
Therapeutic effect: improves neurologic deficits in selected patients.

Indications and dosage
▶ **Improvement of neurologic deficits in patients after subarachnoid hemorrhage from ruptured congenital aneurysms.** *Adults:* 60 mg P.O. q 4 hours for 21 days. Therapy begun within 96 hours after subarachnoid hemorrhage. In patients with hepatic failure, 30 mg P.O. q 4 hours for 21 days.

Adverse reactions
CNS: headache.
CV: decreased blood pressure, flushing, edema.

GI: nausea, diarrhea, abdominal discomfort.
Respiratory: dyspnea.
Skin: dermatitis, rash.
Other: muscle cramps.

Interactions

Drug-drug. *Antihypertensives:* possible enhanced hypotensive effect. Monitor patient.
Calcium channel blockers: possible enhanced CV effects. Monitor patient.

Contraindications and precautions

• No known contraindications.
• Drug use is not recommended in pregnant or breast-feeding women.
• Use cautiously in patients with hepatic failure.
• Safety of drug has not been established in children.

NURSING CONSIDERATIONS

⚗ Assessment
• Assess patient's condition before therapy and regularly thereafter.
• Monitor blood pressure and heart rate, especially at start of therapy.
• Evaluate patient's and family's knowledge of drug therapy.

⊞ Nursing diagnoses
• Altered health maintenance related to underlying condition
• Pain related to drug-induced headache
• Knowledge deficit related to drug therapy

⧩ Planning and implementation
• Nimodipine should be reserved for patients who are in good neurologic condition (for example, Hunt and Hess grades I to II).
Patient teaching
• Inform patient and family that nimodipine therapy is required for 21 days.
• Tell patient to take mild analgesic if headache develops.

• Instruct patient to avoid sudden position changes, which may cause dizziness and orthostatic hypotension.

☑ Evaluation
• Patient responds well to therapy.
• Patient is free from pain.
• Patient and family state understanding of drug therapy.

nisoldipine
(nigh-SOHL-dih-peen)
Sular

Pharmacologic class: calcium channel blocker
Therapeutic class: antihypertensive
Pregnancy risk category: C

How supplied

Extended-release tablets: 10 mg, 20 mg, 30 mg, 40 mg

Pharmacokinetics

Absorption: well absorbed from GI tract; high-fat foods significantly affect release of drug from coat-core formulation.
Distribution: about 99% protein-bound.
Metabolism: extensively metabolized, with five major metabolites identified.
Excretion: excreted in urine. *Half-life:* 7 to 12 hours.

Route	Onset	Peak	Duration
P.O.	Unknown	6-12 hr	Unknown

Pharmacodynamics

Chemical effect: prevents entry of calcium ions into vascular smooth-muscle cells, causing dilation of arterioles, which decreases peripheral vascular resistance.
Therapeutic effect: lowers blood pressure.

Indications and dosage

▶ **Hypertension.** *Adults:* initially, 20 mg (10 mg if patient is over age 65 or has liver dysfunction) P.O. once daily, then increased by 10 mg/week or at longer intervals, as indicated. Usual maintenance dosage is 20 to 40 mg once daily. Dosages above 60 mg daily are not recommended.

Adverse reactions

CNS: *headache,* dizziness.
CV: vasodilation, palpitation, chest pain, *peripheral edema.*
EENT: sinusitis, pharyngitis.
GI: nausea.
Skin: rash.

Interactions

Drug-drug. *Cimetidine:* increases bioavailability and peak concentration of nisoldipine. Monitor patient.
Quinidine: decreases bioavailability, but not peak concentration, of nisoldipine. Monitor patient.
Drug-food. *Grapefruit juice:* increased bioavailability and concentration of drug. Avoid using together.
High-fat meal: increases peak drug concentration. Discourage high-fat meals.

Contraindications and precautions

• Contraindicated in patients with hypersensitivity to dihydropyridine calcium channel blockers.
• Use cautiously in patients with heart failure or compromised ventricular function, particularly those taking beta blockers, or severe hepatic impairment and in pregnant women.
• Drug should not be used in breastfeeding women.

NURSING CONSIDERATIONS

🔧 Assessment
• Assess patient's blood pressure before therapy and monitor regularly thereafter, especially at titration of dosage.
• Monitor patient carefully. Some patients, especially those with severe obstructive coronary artery disease, have developed increased frequency, duration, or severity of angina or acute MI after initiation of calcium channel blocker therapy or at time of dosage increase.
• Be alert for adverse reactions and interactions.
• Evaluate patient's and family's knowledge of drug therapy.

🔧 Nursing diagnoses
• Risk for injury related to hypertension
• Fluid volume excess related to edema
• Knowledge deficit related to drug therapy

🔧 Planning and implementation
• Don't administer drug with a high-fat meal or grapefruit products.
Patient teaching
• Tell patient to take drug as prescribed.
• Instruct patient to swallow tablet whole and not to chew, divide, or crush it.

🔧 Evaluation
• Patient's blood pressure is normal.
• Patient does not exhibit signs of edema.
• Patient and family state understanding of drug therapy.

---

nitrofurantoin macrocrystals
(nigh-troh-fyoo-RAN-toyn MAH-kroh-kris-tuls)
Macrodantin

nitrofurantoin microcrystals
Apo-Nitrofurantoin♦, Furadantin, Furalan, Macrodantin

Pharmacologic class: nitrofuran
Therapeutic class: urinary tract antiinfective
Pregnancy risk category: B

How supplied

nitrofurantoin macrocrystals
Capsules: 25 mg, 50 mg, 100 mg
nitrofurantoin microcrystals
Tablets: 50 mg, 100 mg
Capsules: 50 mg, 100 mg
Oral suspension: 25 mg/5 ml

Pharmacokinetics

Absorption: well absorbed from GI tract. Food aids drug's dissolution and speeds absorption. Macrocrystal form exhibits slower dissolution and absorption.
Distribution: drug crosses into bile; 60% binds to plasma proteins.
Metabolism: metabolized partially in liver.
Excretion: about 30% to 50% of dose is eliminated in urine. *Half-life:* 0.3 to 1 hour.

Route	Onset	Peak	Duration
P.O.	Unknown	Unknown	Unknown

Pharmacodynamics

Chemical effect: unknown; may interfere with bacterial enzyme systems and cell-wall formation.
Therapeutic effect: hinders growth of many common gram-positive and gram-negative urinary pathogens including *Escherichia coli, Staphylococcus aureus,* enterococci, and certain strains of *Klebsiella* and *Enterobacter.*

Indications and dosage

▶ **Urinary tract infection caused by susceptible *E. coli, S. aureus,* enterococci, certain strains of *Klebsiella, Proteus,* and *Enterobacter.*** *Adults and children over age 12:* 50 to 100 mg P.O. q.i.d. with milk or meals. *Children ages 1 month to 12 years:* 5 to 7 mg/kg P.O. daily, divided q.i.d.
▶ **Long-term suppression therapy.** *Adults:* 50 to 100 mg P.O. daily h.s. *Children:* 1 to 2 mg/kg P.O. daily h.s.

Adverse reactions

CNS: *peripheral neuropathy,* headache, dizziness, drowsiness, *ascending polyneuropathy with high doses or renal impairment.*
GI: *anorexia, nausea, vomiting,* abdominal pain, *diarrhea.*
Hematologic: *hemolysis in patients with G6PD deficiency* (reversed after stopping drug), *agranulocytosis, thrombocytopenia.*
Hepatic: *hepatitis, hepatic necrosis.*

Skin: maculopapular, erythematous, or eczematous eruption; pruritus; urticaria; *exfoliative dermatitis; Stevens-Johnson syndrome.*
Other: *asthmatic attacks in patients with history of asthma;* hypersensitivity reactions *(anaphylaxis);* transient alopecia; drug fever; overgrowth of nonsusceptible organisms in urinary tract; pulmonary sensitivity (cough, chest pains, fever, chills, dyspnea).

Interactions

Drug-drug. *Magnesium-containing antacids:* decreased nitrofurantoin absorption. Separate ingestion by 1 hour. *Nalidixic acid, norfloxacin:* possible decreased effectiveness. Avoid using together.
Probenecid, sulfinpyrazone: increased blood levels and decreased urine levels. May result in increased toxicity and lack of therapeutic effect. Don't use together.
Drug-food. *Any food:* increased absorption. Give drug with food.

Contraindications and precautions

● Contraindicated in children age 1 month and under and in patients with moderate to severe renal impairment, anuria, oliguria, or creatinine clearance under 60 ml/minute.
● Use cautiously in pregnant or breast-feeding women and in patients with renal impairment, anemia, diabetes mellitus, electrolyte abnormalities, vitamin B deficiency, debilitating disease, or G6PD deficiency.

NURSING CONSIDERATIONS

� Assessment
● Assess patient's infection before therapy and regularly thereafter.
● Obtain urine specimen for culture and sensitivity tests before starting therapy and repeat p.r.n. Therapy may begin pending results.
● Monitor fluid intake and output. May turn urine brown or darker.

Reactions may be *common,* uncommon, **life-threatening,** or COMMON AND LIFE-THREATENING.

• Monitor CBC and pulmonary status regularly.
• Be alert for adverse reactions and drug interactions.
• Monitor patient's hydration status if adverse GI reactions occur.
• Evaluate patient's and family's knowledge of drug therapy.

🕮 **Nursing diagnoses**
• Infection related to susceptible bacteria
• Risk for fluid volume deficit related to drug-induced adverse GI reactions
• Knowledge deficit related to drug therapy

▷ **Planning and implementation**
• Drug has no effect in blood or tissue outside urinary tract.
• Hypersensitivity may develop during long-term therapy.
• Dual-release capsules (25 mg nitrofurantoin macrocrystals combined with 75 mg nitrofurantoin monohydrate) enable twice-daily dosing.
• Continue treatment for 3 days after urine specimens become sterile.
• Some patients may experience fewer adverse GI effects with nitrofurantoin macrocrystals.
• Store drug in amber container. Keep away from metals other than stainless steel or aluminum to avoid precipitate formation.
• Drug may cause false-positive results with urine glucose test using copper sulfate reduction method (Clinitest) but not with glucose oxidase tests (Diastix).
Patient teaching
• Tell patient to take drug with food or milk to minimize GI distress.
• Teach patient how to measure intake and output. Warn him that drug will turn urine brown or darker.
• Instruct patient how to store drug.

☑ **Evaluation**
• Patient is free from infection.
• Patient maintains adequate hydration throughout drug therapy.

• Patient and family state understanding of drug therapy.

---

nitroglycerin (glyceryl trinitrate)
(nigh-troh-GLIH-suh-rin)
Anginine◇, Deponit, GTN-Pohl◇, Minitran, Nitradisc◇, Nitro-Bid, Nitro-Bid I.V., Nitrocine, Nitrodisc, Nitro-Dur, Nitrogard, Nitroglyn, Nitroject, Nitrol, Nitrolingual, Nitrong, Nitrostat, Transderm-Nitro, Transiderm-Nitro◇, Tridil

Pharmacologic class: nitrate
Therapeutic class: antianginal, vasodilator
Pregnancy risk category: C

How supplied

Tablets (buccal): 1 mg, 2 mg, 3 mg
Tablets (sublingual): 0.15 mg (1/400 gr), 0.3 mg (1/200 gr), 0.4 mg (1/150 gr), 0.6 mg (1/100 gr)
Tablets (sustained-release): 2.6 mg, 6.5 mg, 9 mg
Capsules (sustained-release): 2.5 mg, 6.5 mg, 9 mg, 13 mg
Aerosol (translingual): 0.4 mg metered spray
Topical: 2% ointment
Transdermal: 2.5 mg, 5 mg, 7.5 mg, 10 mg, 15 mg per 24-hour system
I.V.: 0.5 mg/ml, 0.8 mg/ml, 5 mg/ml
I.V. premixed solutions in dextrose: 100 mcg/ml, 200 mcg/ml, 400 mcg/ml

Pharmacokinetics

Absorption: well absorbed from GI tract. However, because it undergoes first-pass metabolism in liver, drug is incompletely absorbed into systemic circulation. S.L. form: absorption from oral mucosa is relatively complete; topical or transdermal form: well absorbed. Data not reported for other forms.
Distribution: distributed widely; about 60% of circulating drug is bound to plasma proteins.
Metabolism: metabolized in liver.

Excretion: metabolites excreted in urine.
Half-life: about 1 to 4 minutes.

Route	Onset	Peak	Duration
P.O.	20-45 min	Unknown	8-12 hr
I.V.	Immediate	Immediate	3-5 min
Buccal	3 min	Unknown	5 hr
Ointment	30 min	Unknown	4-8 hr
S.L.	1-3 min	Unknown	30-60 min
Trans-dermal	30 min	Unknown	≤ 24 hr
Trans-lingual	2-4 min	Unknown	30-60 min

Pharmacodynamics

Chemical effect: reduces cardiac oxygen demand by decreasing left ventricular end-diastolic pressure (preload) and, to a lesser extent, systemic vascular resistance (afterload). Also increases blood flow through collateral coronary vessels.
Therapeutic effect: prevents or relieves acute anginal pain, lowers blood pressure, and helps minimize heart failure caused by MI.

Indications and dosage

▶ **Prophylaxis against chronic anginal attacks.** *Adults:* 2.5 mg or 2.6 mg sustained-release (capsule) q 8 to 12 hours. Alternatively, use of 2% ointment: dosage started with ½″ ointment, increasing by ½″ increments until headache occurs, then decreasing to previous dose. Range of dosage with ointment is ½″ to 5″. Usual dose is 1″ to 2″. Alternatively, transdermal disc or pad (Nitrodisc, Nitro-Dur, or Transderm-Nitro) 0.2 to 0.4 mg/hour once daily.

▶ **Acute angina pectoris, prophylaxis to prevent or minimize anginal attacks when taken immediately before stressful events.** *Adults:* 1 S.L. tablet (gr 1/400, 1/200, 1/150, 1/100) dissolved under tongue or in buccal pouch as soon as angina begins. Repeat q 5 minutes, if needed, for 15 minutes. Or, using Nitrolingual spray, 1 or 2 sprays into mouth, preferably onto or under tongue. Repeat q 3 to 5 minutes if needed, to maximum of three doses within 15-minute period. Alternatively, 1 to 3 mg transmucosally q 3 to 5 hours during waking hours.

▶ **Hypertension associated with surgery; heart failure associated with MI; angina pectoris in acute situations; to produce controlled hypotension during surgery (by I.V. infusion).** *Adults:* initial infusion rate is 5 mcg/minute. Increased as needed, by 5 mcg/minute q 3 to 5 minutes until response is noted. If 20 mcg/minute rate doesn't produce response, dosage is increased by as much as 20 mcg/minute q 3 to 5 minutes. Up to 100 mcg/minute may be needed.

Adverse reactions

CNS: *headache, sometimes with throbbing; dizziness;* weakness.
CV: *orthostatic hypotension, tachycardia, flushing, palpitations,* fainting.
GI: nausea, vomiting.
Skin: cutaneous vasodilation, contact dermatitis (patch), rash.
Other: hypersensitivity reactions, sublingual burning.

Interactions

Drug-drug. *Antihypertensives:* may enhance hypotensive effect. Monitor patient closely.
Drug-lifestyle. *Alcohol use:* may increase hypotension. Advise patient to avoid alcohol consumption during therapy.

Contraindications and precautions

• Contraindicated in patients with hypersensitivity to nitrates and in those with early MI (sublingual nitroglycerin), severe anemia, increased intracranial pressure, angle-closure glaucoma, postural hypotension, and allergy to adhesives (transdermal form).
• I.V. nitroglycerin is contraindicated in patients with cardiac tamponade, restrictive cardiomyopathy, constrictive pericarditis, or hypersensitivity to I.V. form.

Reactions may be *common,* uncommon, *life-threatening*, or COMMON AND LIFE-THREATENING.

• Use cautiously in patients with hypotension or volume depletion and in pregnant or breast-feeding women.
• Safety of drug has not been established in children.

NURSING CONSIDERATIONS

⚖ Assessment
• Assess patient's condition before therapy and regularly thereafter.
• Monitor vital signs and drug response. Be particularly aware of blood pressure. Excessive hypotension may worsen MI.
• Be alert for adverse reactions and drug interactions.
• Evaluate patient's and family's knowledge of drug therapy.

⊞ Nursing diagnoses
• Pain related to angina
• Risk for injury related to drug-induced adverse reactions
• Knowledge deficit related to drug therapy

▷ Planning and implementation
P.O. use: Give oral tablets on empty stomach, either 30 minutes before or 1 to 2 hours after meals; tell patient to swallow oral tablets whole; and not to chew tablets.
I.V. use: Dilute drug with D_5W or 0.9% NaCl injection. Concentration should not exceed 400 mcg/ml. Always administer with infusion control device and titrate to desired response. Also, always mix in glass bottles and avoid I.V. filters because drug binds to plastic. Regular polyvinyl chloride tubing can bind up to 80% of drug, making it necessary to infuse higher dosages. A special nonabsorbent (nonpolyvinyl chloride) tubing is available from manufacturer. Always use same type of infusion set when changing I.V. lines.
– When changing concentration of nitroglycerin infusion, flush I.V. administration set with 15 to 20 ml of new concentration before use. This will clear line of old drug solution.

Buccal use: Tell patient to place transmucosal tablet between lip and gum above incisors, or between cheek and gum. Tablets should be swallowed or chewed.
Topical use: To apply ointment, measure prescribed amount on application paper; then place paper on any nonhairy area. Do not rub in. Cover with plastic film to aid absorption and to protect clothing. If using Tape-Surrounded Appli-Ruler (TSAR) system, keep TSAR on skin to protect patient's clothing and to ensure that ointment remains in place. Remove all excess ointment from previous site before applying next dose. Avoid getting ointment on fingers.
S.L. use: Administer S.L. tablet at first sign of attack. The tablet should be wet with patient's saliva and placed under tongue until completely absorbed, and patient should sit down and rest until pain subsides. Dose may be repeated every 10 to 15 minutes for up to three doses. If drug doesn't provide relief, medical help should be obtained promptly.
– Patient who complains of tingling sensation with drug placed S.L. may try holding tablet in buccal pouch.
Transdermal system use: apply transdermal dosage forms to any nonhairy area except distal parts of arms or legs (absorption will not be maximal from distal sites).
– Be sure to remove transdermal patch before defibrillation. Because of its aluminum backing, electric current may cause patch to explode.
– When stopping transdermal treatment of angina, gradually reduce dose and frequency of application over 4 to 6 weeks, as ordered.
Translingual use: When administering translingual aerosol form, make sure that he does *not* inhale spray. Release it onto or under tongue. Also, have patient wait about 10 seconds or so before swallowing.
• Notify doctor immediately if nitroglycerin is ineffective and keep patient at rest.
• Know that drug may cause headaches, especially at start of therapy. Dosage may

need to be reduced temporarily, but tolerance usually develops. Treat headache with aspirin or acetaminophen.
• Minimize drug tolerance with 10- to 12-hour nitrate-free interval. To achieve this, remove transdermal system in early evening and apply new system next morning or omit last daily dose of buccal, sustained-release, or ointment form. Check with doctor for alterations in dosage regimen if tolerance is suspected.
Patient teaching
• Teach patient how to use form of drug prescribed.
• Caution patient to take drug regularly, as prescribed, and to have it accessible at all times.
• Tell patient that stopping drug abruptly causes coronary vasospasm.
• Inform patient that an additional dose may be taken before anticipated stress or at bedtime if angina is nocturnal.
• Instruct patient to use caution when wearing transdermal patch near microwave oven. Leaking radiation may heat patch's metallic backing and cause burns.
• Advise patient to avoid alcohol during drug therapy.
• Tell patient to change to upright position slowly. Advise him to go up and down stairs carefully and to lie down at first sign of dizziness.
• Inform patient to store drug in cool, dark place in tightly closed container. To ensure freshness, replace supply of S.L. tablets every 3 months. Remove cotton because it absorbs drug.
• Tell patient to store S.L. tablets in original container or other container specifically approved for this use and to carry container in jacket pocket or purse, not in pocket close to body.

☑ **Evaluation**
• Patient reports pain relief.
• Patient does not experience injury from adverse reactions.
• Patient and family state understanding of drug therapy.

nitroprusside sodium
(nigh-troh-PRUS-ighd SOH-dee-um)
Nipride♦, Nitropress

Pharmacologic class: vasodilator
Therapeutic class: antihypertensive
Pregnancy risk category: C

How supplied
Injection: 50 mg/vial in 2-ml, 5-ml vials

Pharmacokinetics
Absorption: not applicable.
Distribution: unknown.
Metabolism: metabolized rapidly in erythrocytes and tissues to cyanide radical and then converted to thiocyanate in liver.
Excretion: excreted primarily as metabolites in urine. *Half-life:* 2 minutes.

Route	Onset	Peak	Duration
I.V.	≤ 1 min	Almost immediate	≤ 10 min

Pharmacodynamics
Chemical effect: relaxes both arteriolar and venous smooth muscle.
Therapeutic effect: lowers blood pressure and reduces preload and afterload.

Indications and dosage
▶ **To lower blood pressure quickly in hypertensive emergencies; to produce controlled hypotension during anesthesia; to reduce preload and afterload in cardiac pump failure or cardiogenic shock (may be used with or without dopamine).** *Adults:* 50-mg vial diluted with 2 to 3 ml of D_5W and then added to 250, 500, or 1,000 ml of D_5W. Infused at 0.3 to 10 mcg/kg/minute. Average dose is 3 mcg/kg/minute. Maximum infusion rate is 10 mcg/kg/minute. Patients taking other antihypertensives are extremely sensitive to nitroprusside. Dosage is adjusted accordingly.

Adverse reactions

The following adverse reactions usually indicate overdose:

CNS: *headache, dizziness,* ataxia, loss of consciousness, *coma, increased intracranial pressure,* weak pulse, absent reflexes, dilated pupils, *restlessness, muscle twitching, diaphoresis.*
CV: distant heart sounds, palpitations, bradycardia, tachycardia, hypotension.
GI: vomiting, nausea, abdominal pain.
Respiratory: dyspnea, shallow breathing.
Skin: pink color.
Other: acidosis, *thiocyanate toxicity, methemoglobinemia, cyanide toxicity.*

Interactions

Drug-drug. *Antihypertensives:* may cause sensitivity to nitroprusside. Adjust dosage as ordered.
Ganglionic blocking agents, general anesthetics, negative inotropic agents, other antihypertensives: additive effects. Monitor blood pressure closely.

Contraindications and precautions

• Contraindicated in patients with compensatory hypertension (such as in arteriovenous shunt or coarctation of aorta), inadequate cerebral circulation, congenital optic atrophy, tobacco-induced amblyopia, or hypersensitivity to drug.
• Use with extreme caution in patients with increased intracranial pressure. Use cautiously in patients with hypothyroidism, hepatic or renal disease, hyponatremia, or low vitamin B_{12} concentration and in pregnant women.
• Safety of drug has not been established in breast-feeding women and in children.

NURSING CONSIDERATIONS

🔲 Assessment
• Assess patient's condition before therapy.
• Obtain baseline vital signs before giving drug, and find out what parameters doctor wants to achieve.

• Excessive doses or rapid infusion greater than 15 mcg/kg/minute can cause cyanide toxicity; therefore, check serum thiocyanate levels every 72 hours. Levels above 100 mcg/ml are associated with toxicity. Watch for signs of toxicity: profound hypotension, metabolic acidosis, dyspnea, headache, loss of consciousness, ataxia, and vomiting.
• Be alert for adverse reactions and drug interactions.
• Evaluate patient's (if appropriate) and family's knowledge of drug therapy.

🔲 Nursing diagnoses
• Risk for injury related to hypertension
• Decreased cardiac output related to heart failure
• Knowledge deficit related to drug therapy

🔲 Planning and implementation
• Keep patient in supine position when initiating or titrating drug.
• Don't use bacteriostatic water for injection or sterile NaCl solution for reconstitution.
• Because drug is sensitive to light, wrap I.V. solution in foil; it's not necessary to wrap tubing. Fresh solution should have faint brownish tint. Discard drug after 24 hours.
• Infuse with infusion pump. Drug is best given by piggyback through peripheral line with no other medication. Don't adjust rate of main I.V. line while drug is being infused. Even small bolus of nitroprusside can cause severe hypotension.
• Check blood pressure every 5 minutes at start of infusion and every 15 minutes thereafter. If severe hypotension occurs, stop infusion—effects of drug quickly reverse. Notify doctor. If possible, start arterial pressure line. Adjust flow to specified level.
• If cyanide toxicity occurs, stop drug immediately and notify doctor.
Patient teaching
• Advise patient, if alert, to report adverse reactions immediately.

☑ **Evaluation**
• Patient's blood pressure is normal.
• Patient has normal cardiac output.
• Patient and family state understanding of drug therapy.

nizatidine
(nigh-ZAT-ih-deen)
Axid, Tazac ◇

Pharmacologic class: H_2-receptor antagonist
Therapeutic class: antiulcer agent
Pregnancy risk category: B

How supplied
Capsules: 75 mg†, 150 mg, 300 mg

Pharmacokinetics
Absorption: well absorbed (greater than 90%) from GI tract. Absorption may be slightly enhanced by food, and slightly impaired by antacids.
Distribution: about 35% of drug is bound to plasma proteins.
Metabolism: unknown, but may undergo hepatic metabolism.
Excretion: more than 90% excreted in urine; less than 6% in feces. *Half-life:* 1 to 2 hours.

Route	Onset	Peak	Duration
P.O.	≤ 30 min	0.5-3 hr	≤ 12 hr

Pharmacodynamics
Chemical effect: competitively inhibits action of H_2 at receptor sites of parietal cells.
Therapeutic effect: decreases gastric acid secretion.

Indications and dosage
▶ **Active duodenal ulcer.** *Adults:* 300 mg P.O. daily h.s. Alternatively, 150 mg P.O. b.i.d.
▶ **Maintenance therapy for duodenal ulcer.** *Adults:* 150 mg P.O. daily h.s.
▶ **Benign gastric ulcer.** *Adults:* 150 mg P.O. b.i.d. or 300 mg h.s. for 8 weeks.

▶ **Gastroesophageal reflux disease.**
Adults: 150 mg P.O. b.i.d. *In patients with impaired renal function:* if clearance is 20 to 50 ml/minute, 150 mg P.O. daily for treatment of active duodenal ulcer or 150 mg every other day for maintenance therapy; if creatinine clearance is below 20 ml/minute, 150 mg P.O. every other day for treatment or 150 mg every third day for maintenance.

Adverse reactions
CNS: *somnolence.*
CV: arrhythmias.
Hematologic: *thrombocytopenia.*
Skin: *diaphoresis,* rash, urticaria, *exfoliative dermatitis.*
Other: liver damage, hyperuricemia, fever.

Interactions
Drug-drug. *Aspirin:* possibly elevated serum salicylate levels (with high doses).
Drug-food. *Tomato-based mixed-vegetable juices:* may decrease drug potency. Monitor diet.

Contraindications and precautions
• Contraindicated in patients hypersensitive to H_2-receptor antagonists.
• Use cautiously in patients with impaired renal function and in pregnant or breast-feeding women.
• Safety of drug has not been established in children.

NURSING CONSIDERATIONS

☑ **Assessment**
• Assess patient's condition before therapy and regularly thereafter.
• Be alert for adverse reactions and drug interactions.
• Evaluate patient's and family's knowledge of drug therapy.

🔁 **Nursing diagnoses**
• Altered tissue integrity related to ulceration of GI mucosa

---

• Decreased cardiac output related to drug-induced arrhythmias
• Knowledge deficit related to drug therapy

≫ **Planning and implementation**
• If necessary, open capsules and mix contents with apple juice. However, drug loses some potency when combined with tomato-based, mixed-vegetable juices.
• Be aware that false-positive test results for urobilinogen may occur.
Patient teaching
• Urge patient to avoid cigarette smoking because it may increase gastric acid secretion and worsen disease.
• Warn patient to take drug as directed, even after pain subsides, to allow for adequate healing.

☑ **Evaluation**
• Patient reports pain relief.
• Patient maintains normal cardiac output throughout drug therapy.
• Patient and family state understanding of drug therapy.

---

norepinephrine bitartrate (levarterenol bitartrate, noradrenaline acid tartrate)
(nor-ep-ih-NEF-rin bigh-TAR-trayt)
Levophed

Pharmacologic class: adrenergic (direct acting)
Therapeutic class: vasopressor
Pregnancy risk category: C

How supplied
Injection: 1 mg/ml

Pharmacokinetics
Absorption: not applicable.
Distribution: drug localizes in sympathetic nerve tissues.
Metabolism: metabolized in liver and other tissues to inactive compounds.

Excretion: excreted in urine. *Half-life:* about 1 minute.

Route	Onset	Peak	Duration
I.V.	Immediate	Immediate	1-2 min

Pharmacodynamics
Chemical effect: stimulates alpha- and beta$_1$-adrenergic receptors within sympathetic nervous system.
Therapeutic effect: raises blood pressure.

Indications and dosage
▶ **To restore blood pressure in acute hypotensive states.** *Adults:* initially, 8 to 12 mcg/minute I.V. infusion, then adjusted to maintain normal blood pressure. Average maintenance dosage is 2 to 4 mcg/minute. *Children:* 2 mcg/m^2/minute I.V. infusion; dosage adjusted based on patient response.
▶ **Severe hypotension during cardiac arrest.** *Children:* initial I.V. infusion rate is 0.1 mcg/kg/minute. Rate adjusted based on patient response.

Adverse reactions
CNS: *headache,* anxiety, weakness, dizziness, tremor, restlessness, insomnia.
CV: bradycardia, *severe hypertension,* marked increase in peripheral resistance, decreased cardiac output, *arrhythmias.*
GU: decreased urine output.
Respiratory: respiratory difficulties, *asthmatic episodes.*
Other: fever, metabolic acidosis, hyperglycemia, increased glycogenolysis, irritation with extravasation, swelling and enlargement of thyroid, *anaphylaxis.*

Interactions
Drug-drug. *Alpha-adrenergic blocking agents:* may antagonize drug effects. Monitor patient.
Antihistamines, ergot alkaloids, guanethidine, methyldopa: use with sympathomimetics may cause severe hypertension. Don't give together.
Inhalation anesthetics: increased risk of arrhythmias. Monitor closely.

MAO inhibitors: increased risk of hypertensive crisis. Monitor patient closely.
Tricyclic antidepressants: increased vasopressor effect. Don't give together.

Contraindications and precautions

• Contraindicated in patients with mesenteric or peripheral vascular thrombosis, profound hypoxia, hypercapnia, or hypotension resulting from blood volume deficits; during cyclopropane and halothane anesthesia; and in pregnant or breast-feeding women.
• Use with extreme caution in patients receiving MAO inhibitors or triptyline or imipramine-type antidepressants. Use cautiously in patients with sulfite sensitivity.

NURSING CONSIDERATIONS

Assessment
• Assess patient's condition before therapy.
• During infusion, frequently monitor ECG, cardiac output, central venous pressure, pulmonary capillary wedge pressure, pulse rate, urine output, and color and temperature of extremities. Also, check blood pressure every 2 minutes until stabilized; then check every 5 minutes.
• Be alert for adverse reactions and drug interactions.
• Monitor vital signs and functions closely when therapy ends. Watch for sudden drop in blood pressure.
• Evaluate patient's and family's knowledge of drug therapy.

Nursing diagnoses
• Decreased cardiac output related to hypotension
• Risk for injury related to drug-induced adverse reactions
• Knowledge deficit related to drug therapy

Planning and implementation
• Know that drug is not a substitute for blood or fluid volume deficit. If deficit

exists, replace fluid before administering vasopressors.
• Use central venous catheter or large vein, such as in antecubital fossa, to minimize risk of extravasation. Administer in dextrose 5% in 0.9% NaCl injection; 0.9% NaCl injection alone is not recommended. Use continuous infusion pump to regulate flow rate and piggyback setup so I.V. line remains open if norepinephrine is stopped.
• Titrate infusion rate according to assessment findings and doctor's guidelines. In previously hypertensive patients, blood pressure should be raised no higher than 40 mm Hg below preexisting systolic pressure.
• Never leave patient unattended during infusion.
• Check site frequently for extravasation. If it occurs, stop infusion immediately and call doctor. He may counteract effect by infiltrating area with 5 to 10 mg phentolamine and 10 to 15 ml of 0.9% NaCl solution. Also check for blanching along course of infused vein; may progress to superficial sloughing.
• If prolonged I.V. therapy is necessary, change injection site frequently.
• Keep emergency drugs on hand to reverse effects of norepinephrine: atropine for reflex bradycardia; phentolamine for vasopressor effects; and propranolol for arrhythmias.
• Report decreased urine output to doctor immediately.
• When stopping drug, gradually slow infusion rate, as ordered, and report sudden drop in blood pressure.
• Be aware that drug solutions deteriorate after 24 hours.
• Protect drug from light. Discard discolored solutions or solutions that contain precipitate.
Patient teaching
• Tell patient to immediately report discomfort at infusion site or difficulty breathing.

Reactions may be *common*, uncommon, *life-threatening*, or COMMON AND LIFE-THREATENING.

☑ Evaluation
• Patient has normal cardiac output.
• Patient experiences no injuries due to drug-induced adverse reactions.
• Patient and family state understanding of drug therapy.

norethindrone
(nor-ETH-in-drohn)
Micronor, Nor-Q.D.

norethindrone acetate
Aygestin, Norlutate

Pharmacologic class: progestin
Therapeutic class: contraceptive
Pregnancy risk category: X

How supplied
norethindrone
Tablets: 0.35 mg, 0.5 mg
norethindrone acetate
Tablets: 5 mg

Pharmacokinetics
Absorption: well absorbed from GI tract.
Distribution: distributed widely; about 80% protein-bound.
Metabolism: metabolized primarily in liver; it undergoes extensive first-pass metabolism.
Excretion: excreted primarily in feces.
Half-life: 5 to 14 hours.

Route	Onset	Peak	Duration
P.O.	Unknown	Unknown	Unknown

Pharmacodynamics
Chemical effect: suppresses ovulation, possibly by inhibiting pituitary gonadotropin secretion, and forms thick cervical mucus.
Therapeutic effect: prevents pregnancy and relieves symptoms of endometriosis, amenorrhea, and abnormal uterine bleeding.

Indications and dosage
▶ **Amenorrhea, abnormal uterine bleeding. Norethindrone acetate.**
Adults: 2.5 to 10 mg P.O. daily on days 5 to 25 of menstrual cycle.
▶ **Endometriosis. Norethindrone acetate.** *Adults:* 5 mg P.O. daily for 14 days; then increased by 2.5 mg daily q 2 weeks up to 15 mg daily.
▶ **Contraception in women. Norethindrone.** *Adults:* initially, 0.35 mg P.O. on first day of menstruation; then 0.35 mg daily.

Adverse reactions
CNS: dizziness, migraine, lethargy, depression.
CV: hypertension, thrombophlebitis, *pulmonary embolism, thromboembolism, CVA,* edema.
GI: nausea, vomiting, abdominal cramps.
GU: breakthrough bleeding, dysmenorrhea, amenorrhea, cervical erosion, abnormal secretions, uterine fibromas, vaginal candidiasis.
Hepatic: cholestatic jaundice.
Skin: melasma, rash.
Other: breast tenderness, enlargement, or secretion; decreased libido; hyperglycemia.

Interactions
Drug-drug. *Barbiturates, carbamazepine, rifampin:* decreased progestin effects. Monitor closely.
Bromocriptine: may possibly cause amenorrhea, thus interfering with bromocriptine effects. Avoid concomitant use.
Drug-food. *Caffeine:* may increase serum caffeine concentrations. Monitor effects.
Drug-lifestyle. *Smoking:* increased risk of CV effects. If smoking continues, may need alternative therapy.

Contraindications and precautions
• Contraindicated in patients with thromboembolic disorders, cerebral apoplexy, or history of these conditions. Also con-

traindicated in those with breast cancer, undiagnosed abnormal vaginal bleeding, severe hepatic disease, missed abortion, or hypersensitivity to drug and in pregnant women.
• Drug use is not recommended in breastfeeding women.
• Use cautiously in patients with diabetes mellitus, seizure disorder, migraine, cardiac or renal disease, asthma, and depression.
• Safety of drug has not been established in children.

NURSING CONSIDERATIONS

⚕ Assessment
• Assess patient's condition before therapy and regularly thereafter.
• Be alert for adverse reactions and drug interactions.
• Evaluate patient's and family's knowledge of drug therapy.

🔟 Nursing diagnoses
• Altered health maintenance related to underlying condition
• Fluid volume excess related to drug-induced edema
• Knowledge deficit related to drug therapy

▷ Planning and implementation
• Norethindrone acetate is twice as potent as norethindrone. It should not be used for contraception.
• Do not use drug as test for pregnancy; norethindrone may cause birth defects and masculinization of female fetus.
• Know that preliminary estrogen treatment is usually needed in patients with menstrual disorders.
• Withhold drug and notify doctor if visual disturbance, migraine, or headache occurs or if pulmonary emboli are suspected; provide supportive care.
Patient teaching
• Ensure that, before receiving first dose, patient reads package insert explaining

adverse effects of progestin. Also provide verbal explanation.
• Instruct patient to report unusual symptoms immediately. Tell her to stop drug and call doctor if visual disturbance or migraine occurs.
• Teach patient how to perform routine monthly breast self-examination.
• Warn patient that edema and weight gain are likely. Advise her to restrict sodium intake.

☑ Evaluation
• Patient responds well to therapy.
• Patient's drug-induced edema is minimized with sodium restriction.
• Patient and family state understanding of drug therapy.

norfloxacin
(nor-FLOKS-uh-sin)
Noroxin

Pharmacologic class: fluoroquinolone
Therapeutic class: broad-spectrum antibiotic
Pregnancy risk category: C

How supplied
Tablets: 400 mg

Pharmacokinetics
Absorption: about 30% to 40% absorbed from GI tract (as dose increases, percentage of absorbed drug decreases). Food may reduce absorption.
Distribution: distributed into renal tissue, liver, gallbladder, prostatic fluid, testicles, seminal fluid, bile, and sputum. From 10% to 15% binds to plasma proteins.
Metabolism: unknown.
Excretion: most systemically absorbed drug is excreted by kidneys, with about 30% appearing in bile. *Half-life:* 3 to 4 hours.

Route	Onset	Peak	Duration
P.O.	Unknown	1-2 hr	Unknown

Pharmacodynamics

Chemical effect: inhibits bacterial DNA synthesis, mainly by blocking DNA gyrase.
Therapeutic effect: kills selected bacteria, such as most aerobic gram-positive and gram-negative urinary pathogens, including *Pseudomonas aeruginosa.*

Indications and dosage

▶ **Complicated or uncomplicated urinary tract infections caused by susceptible strains of *Escherichia coli, Klebsiella, Enterobacter, Proteus, P. aeruginosa, Citrobacter, Staphylococcus aureus, S. epidermidis,* and group D streptococci.** *Adults:* for uncomplicated infections, 400 mg P.O. b.i.d. for 7 to 10 days. For complicated infections, 400 mg b.i.d. for 10 to 21 days.
▶ **Cystitis caused by *E. coli, Klebsiella pneumoniae,* or *Proteus mirabilis.*** *Adults:* 400 mg P.O. b.i.d. for 3 days.
▶ **Acute, uncomplicated gonorrhea.** *Adults:* 800 mg P.O. as single dose, followed by doxycycline therapy to treat any coexisting chlamydial infection. Adults with creatinine clearance of 30 ml/minute or less should receive 400 mg once daily.

Adverse reactions

CNS: fatigue, somnolence, headache, dizziness, *seizures.*
GI: nausea, constipation, flatulence, heartburn, dry mouth.
GU: increased serum creatinine and BUN levels, crystalluria.
Hematologic: eosinophilia.
Musculoskeletal: arthralgia, arthritis, myalgia, joint swelling.
Skin: rash, photosensitivity.
Other: *hypersensitivity reactions (rash, anaphylactoid reactions),* transient elevations of AST and ALT, fever.

Interactions

Drug-drug. *Antacids, iron products, sucralfate:* may hinder absorption. Separate administration times by 2 hours.
Cyclosporine: increased serum concentrations of cyclosporine. Monitor serum levels.
Nitrofurantoin: decreased norfloxacin effectiveness. Don't use together.
Oral anticoagulants: increased anticoagulant effect. Monitor closely.
Probenecid: may increase serum levels of norfloxacin by decreasing its excretion. Monitor for toxicity.
Theophylline: possibly impaired theophylline metabolism, resulting in increased plasma levels and risk of toxicity. Monitor closely.

Contraindications and precautions

• Contraindicated in patients with hypersensitivity to fluoroquinolones and in children.
• Use cautiously in pregnant women and in patients with conditions that may predispose them to seizure disorders, such as cerebral arteriosclerosis.
• Safety of drug has not been established in breast-feeding women.

NURSING CONSIDERATIONS

⚕ Assessment
• Assess patient's infection before therapy and regularly thereafter.
• Obtain culture and sensitivity tests before starting therapy, and repeat as needed throughout therapy.
• Be alert for adverse reactions and drug interactions.
• Evaluate patient's and family's knowledge of drug therapy.

⊞ Nursing diagnoses
• Infection related to bacteria
• Risk for injury related to drug-induced adverse CNS reactions
• Knowledge deficit related to drug therapy

▶ Planning and implementation
• Give drug on empty stomach.

• Make sure patient is well hydrated before and during therapy to avoid crystalluria.

Patient teaching

• Advise patient to take drug 1 hour before or 2 hours after meals to promote absorption.

• Warn patient not to exceed recommended dosage and to drink several glasses of water throughout day to maintain hydration and adequate urine output.

• Caution patient to avoid hazardous activities until CNS effects of drug are known.

☑ **Evaluation**

• Patient is free from infection.

• Patient experiences no injuries due to drug-induced adverse CNS reactions.

• Patient and family state understanding of drug therapy.

---

norgestrel
(nor-JES-trel)
Ovrette**

Pharmacologic class: progestin
Therapeutic class: contraceptive
Pregnancy risk category: X

How supplied

Tablets: 0.075 mg

Pharmacokinetics

Absorption: well absorbed.
Distribution: unknown.
Metabolism: unknown.
Excretion: unknown.

Route	Onset	Peak	Duration
P.O.	Unknown	Unknown	Unknown

Pharmacodynamics

Chemical effect: unknown; may suppress ovulation, possibly by inhibiting pituitary gonadotropin secretion, and forms thick cervical mucus.
Therapeutic effect: prevents pregnancy.

Indications and dosage

▶ **Contraception in women.** *Adults:* 0.075 mg P.O. daily.

Adverse reactions

CNS: cerebral thrombosis or hemorrhage, migraine headache, lethargy, depression.
CV: hypertension, thrombophlebitis, *pulmonary embolism, thromboembolism, CVA,* edema.
GI: nausea, vomiting, abdominal cramps, gallbladder disease.
GU: *breakthrough bleeding, change in menstrual flow,* dysmenorrhea, spotting, amenorrhea, cervical erosion, vaginal candidiasis.
Hepatic: cholestatic jaundice.
Skin: melasma, rash.
Other: breast tenderness, enlargement, or secretion.

Interactions

Drug-drug. *Barbiturates, carbamazepine, rifampin:* decreased progestin effects. Monitor for reduced response.
Bromocriptine: may cause amenorrhea, interfering with bromocriptine's effects. Avoid concomitant use.
Drug-food. *Caffeine:* may increase serum caffeine concentrations. Monitor effects.
Drug-lifestyle. *Smoking.* increased risk of CV effects. If smoking continues, may need alternate therapy.

Contraindications and precautions

• Contraindicated in patients with thromboembolic disorders, cerebral apoplexy, or history of these conditions; hypersensitivity to drug; breast cancer, undiagnosed abnormal vaginal bleeding, severe hepatic disease, or missed abortion and in pregnant or breast-feeding women.

• Use cautiously in patients with diabetes mellitus, seizure disorder, migraine, cardiac or renal disease, asthma, or depression.

• Safety of drug has not been established in children.

Reactions may be *common*, uncommon, *life-threatening*, or COMMON AND LIFE-THREATENING.

NURSING CONSIDERATIONS

🐾 Assessment
• Assess patient's pregnancy status before therapy and regularly thereafter. Failure rate of progestin-only contraceptive is about three times higher than that of combination contraceptives.
• Be alert for adverse reactions and drug interactions.
• Evaluate patient's and family's knowledge of drug therapy.

⊕ Nursing diagnoses
• Health-seeking behavior related to request for contraceptive
• Fluid volume excess related to drug-induced edema
• Knowledge deficit related to drug therapy

⧉ Planning and implementation
• Norgestrel is a progestin-only oral contraceptive known as "minipill."
• Ensure pregnancy test is negative before drug is initiated.
Patient teaching
• Make sure that, before receiving first dose, patient reads package insert explaining adverse effects of progestins. Also provide verbal explanation.
• Tell patient to take pill every day, at same time, even if menstruating.
• Inform patient that risk of pregnancy increases with each tablet missed. Tell patient who misses one tablet to take it as soon as remembered and then take next tablet at regular time. Advise patient who misses two tablets to take one as soon as remembered and then take next regular dose at usual time and to use nonhormonal method of contraception and norgestrel until 14 tablets have been taken. Tell patient who misses three or more tablets to stop drug and use nonhormonal method of contraception until after menses. If menstrual period does not occur within 45 days, test for pregnancy.
• Advise patient using oral contraceptives of increased risk of serious adverse CV

reactions associated with heavy cigarette smoking.
• Instruct patient to immediately report excessive bleeding or bleeding between menstrual cycles, breast pain or tenderness, vaginal discharge, or swelling of hands or feet.
• Tell patient to report unusual symptoms immediately and to stop drug and call doctor if visual disturbance, migraine, or numbness or tingling in limbs occurs.
• Teach patient how to perform routine breast self-examination.

✓ Evaluation
• Patient does not become pregnant.
• Patient develops minimal edema.
• Patient and family state understanding of drug therapy.

nortriptyline hydrochloride
(nor-TRIP-teh-leen high-droh-KLOR-ighd)
Allegron◇, Aventyl*, Pamelor*

Pharmacologic class: tricyclic antidepressant
Therapeutic class: antidepressant
Pregnancy risk category: NR

How supplied
Tablets: 10 mg◇, 25 mg◇
Capsules: 10 mg, 25 mg, 50 mg, 75 mg
Oral solution: 10 mg/5 ml (4% alcohol)

Pharmacokinetics
Absorption: absorbed rapidly.
Distribution: distributed widely into body, including CNS. Drug is 95% protein-bound.
Metabolism: metabolized by liver; significant first-pass effect may account for variability of serum concentrations in different patients taking same dosage.
Excretion: most excreted in urine; some in feces. *Half-life:* 18 to 24 hours.

Route	Onset	Peak	Duration
P.O.	Unknown	7-8.5 hr	Unknown

Pharmacodynamics

Chemical effect: unknown; increases amount of norepinephrine, serotonin, or both in CNS by blocking their reuptake by presynaptic neurons.
Therapeutic effect: relieves depression.

Indications and dosage

▶ **Depression.** *Adults:* 25 mg P.O. t.i.d. or q.i.d., gradually increased to maximum of 150 mg daily. Or, entire dosage may be given h.s.

Adverse reactions

CNS: *drowsiness, dizziness,* excitation, *seizures,* tremor, weakness, confusion, headache, nervousness, EEG changes, extrapyramidal reactions.
CV: *tachycardia,* ECG changes, hypertension, *heart block, stroke, MI.*
EENT: *blurred vision,* tinnitus, mydriasis.
GI: dry mouth, *constipation,* nausea, vomiting, anorexia, paralytic ileus.
GU: *urine retention.*
Hematologic: bone marrow depression, eosinophilia, *agranulocytosis, thrombocytopenia.*
Skin: rash, urticaria, photosensitivity.
Other: diaphoresis, hypersensitivity reaction.
After abrupt withdrawal of long-term therapy: nausea, headache, malaise (does not indicate addiction).

Interactions

Drug-drug. *Barbiturates, CNS depressants:* enhanced CNS depression. Avoid concomitant use.
Cimetidine, methylphenidate: may increase nortriptyline serum levels. Monitor for adverse reactions.
Clonidine, epinephrine, norepinephrine: increased hypertensive effect. Use with caution.
MAO inhibitors: may cause severe excitation, hyperpyrexia, or seizures. Use with caution.
Drug-lifestyle: *Alcohol use:* enhanced CNS depression. Avoid concomitant use.

Smoking: may lower plasma concentrations or nortriptyline. Monitor for lack of clinical effect.
Sun exposure: increased risk of photosensitivity reaction. Take precautions.

Contraindications and precautions

• Contraindicated during acute recovery phase of MI and in patients with hypersensitivity to drug or in those receiving MAO therapy within past 14 days.
• Drug is not recommended for use in pregnant or breast-feeding women or in children.
• Use with extreme caution in patients with glaucoma, suicidal tendency, history of urine retention or seizures, CV disease, or hyperthyroidism and in those receiving thyroid drugs.

NURSING CONSIDERATIONS

✍ Assessment
• Assess patient's depression before therapy and regularly thereafter.
• Be alert for adverse reactions and drug interactions.
• Evaluate patient's and family's knowledge of drug therapy.

⊞ Nursing diagnoses
• Altered thought processes related to depression
• Risk for injury related to drug-induced adverse CNS reactions
• Knowledge deficit related to drug therapy

▷ Planning and implementation
• Dosage should be reduced in elderly or debilitated patient.
• Do not withdraw drug abruptly.
• Because hypertensive episodes have occurred during surgery in patients receiving tricyclic antidepressants, drug should be gradually stopped several days before surgery.
• If signs of psychosis occur or increase, expect to reduce dosage.

Reactions may be *common,* uncommon, *life-threatening*, or COMMON AND LIFE-THREATENING.

Patient teaching
• Whenever possible, advise patient to take full dose at bedtime to reduce risk of orthostatic hypotension.
• Warn patient to avoid hazardous activities until CNS effects of drug are known. Drowsiness and dizziness usually subside after a few weeks.
• Tell patient to avoid alcohol while during drug therapy.
• Warn patient not to stop drug suddenly.
• Advise patient to consult doctor before taking other prescription or OTC drugs.
• Advise patient to use sunblock, wear protective clothing, and avoid prolonged exposure to sunlight.

☑ **Evaluation**
• Patient's depression improves.
• Patient experiences no injuries due to drug-induced adverse CNS reactions.
• Patient and family state understanding of drug therapy.

nystatin
(NIGH-stuh-tin)
Mycostatin*, Nadostine♦, Nilstat, Nystex*

Pharmacologic class: polyene macrolide
Therapeutic class: antifungal
Pregnancy risk category: C

How supplied
Tablets: 500,000 units
Oral suspension: 100,000 units/ml
Vaginal suppositories: 100,000 units

Pharmacokinetics
Absorption: not absorbed from GI tract, intact skin, or mucous membranes.
Distribution: none.
Metabolism: none.
Excretion: oral form excreted almost entirely unchanged in feces.

Route	Onset	Peak	Duration
P.O., topical	Unknown	Unknown	Unknown

Pharmacodynamics
Chemical effect: unknown; probably acts by binding to sterols in fungal cell membrane, altering cell permeability and allowing leakage of intracellular components.
Therapeutic effect: kills susceptible yeasts and fungi.

Indications and dosage
▶ **GI infections.** *Adults:* 500,000 to 1 million units as oral tablets t.i.d.
▶ **Oral, vaginal, and intestinal infections caused by** *Candida albicans* **(Monilia) and other** *Candida* **species.** *Adults:* 500,000 to 1 million units oral suspension t.i.d. for oral candidiasis. *Children and infants over age 3 months:* 250,000 to 500,000 units oral suspension q.i.d. *Neonates and premature infants:* 100,000 units oral suspension q.i.d.
▶ **Vaginal infections.** *Adults:* 100,000 units, as vaginal tablets, inserted high into vagina, daily or b.i.d. for 14 days.

Adverse reactions
GI: transient nausea, vomiting, diarrhea (with large oral dosage).

Interactions
None significant.

Contraindications and precautions
• Contraindicated in patients with hypersensitivity to drug.
• Safety of drug has not been established in breast-feeding women.

NURSING CONSIDERATIONS

☝ **Assessment**
• Assess patient's infection before therapy and regularly thereafter.
• Be alert for adverse reactions.
• Monitor patient's hydration status if adverse GI reactions occur.
• Evaluate patient's and family's knowledge of drug therapy.

◆ Nursing diagnoses

• Infection related to organisms
• Risk for fluid volume deficit related to drug-induced adverse GI reactions
• Knowledge deficit related to drug therapy

◆ Planning and implementation

• Keep in mind that drug is not effective against systemic infections.

P.O. use: For treatment of oral candidiasis (thrush): After mouth is clean of food debris, have patient hold suspension in mouth for several minutes before swallowing. When treating infant, swab medication on oral mucosa. Instruct patient in good oral hygiene techniques.

Mouthwash overuse or poorly fitting dentures, especially in older patients, may alter flora and promote infection.

• For treatment of oral candidiasis, be aware that immunosuppressed patients are sometimes instructed by doctor to suck on vaginal tablets (100,000 units) because this provides prolonged contact with oral mucosa.

Vaginal use: Pregnant patients can use vaginal tablets up to 6 weeks before term to treat infection that may cause thrush in neonates.

Patient teaching

• Advise patient to take drug for at least 2 days after symptoms disappear to prevent reinfection. Consult doctor for duration of therapy.
• Instruct patient to continue therapy during menstruation.
• Explain that predisposing factors of vaginal infection include use of antibiotics, oral contraceptives, and corticosteroids; diabetes; reinfection by sexual partner; and tight-fitting panty hose. Encourage patient to use cotton (not synthetic) underpants.
• Teach patient about hygiene for affected areas, including cleansing perineal area from front to back after defecation.
• Advise patient to report redness, swelling, or irritation.

☑ Evaluation

• Patient is free from infection.
• Patient maintains adequate hydration throughout drug therapy.
• Patient and family state understanding of drug therapy.

octreotide acetate
(ok-TREE-oh-tighd AS-ih-tayt)
Sandostatin

Pharmacologic class: synthetic octapeptide
Therapeutic class: somatotropic hormone
Pregnancy risk category: B

How supplied

Injection: 0.05-mg, 0.1-mg, 0.5-mg ampules; 0.2 mg/ml, 1 mg/ml multidose vials

Pharmacokinetics

Absorption: absorbed rapidly and completely after S.C. injection.
Distribution: distributed to plasma, where it binds to serum lipoprotein and albumin.
Metabolism: not clearly defined.
Excretion: about 35% of drug appears unchanged in urine. *Half-life:* about 1½ hours.

Route	Onset	Peak	Duration
S.C.	≤ 30 min	≤ 30 min	≤ 12 hr

Pharmacodynamics

Chemical effect: mimics action of naturally occurring somatostatin.
Therapeutic effect: relieves flushing and diarrhea caused by selected tumors and treats acromegaly.

Indications and dosage

▶ **Flushing and diarrhea associated with carcinoid tumors.** *Adults:* 0.1 to

0.6 mg daily S.C. in two to four divided doses for first 2 weeks of therapy (usual daily dosage is 0.3 mg). Subsequent dosage based on response.

► **Watery diarrhea associated with vasoactive intestinal polypeptide secreting tumors (VIPomas).** *Adults:* 0.2 to 0.3 mg daily S.C. in two to four divided doses for first 2 weeks of therapy. Subsequent dosage based on individual response; typically, don't exceed 0.45 mg daily.

► **Acromegaly.** *Adults:* initially, 50 mcg S.C. t.i.d., then adjusted according to somatomedin C levels q 2 weeks.

Adverse reactions

CNS: dizziness, light-headedness, fatigue.
CV: *arrhythmias.*
GI: *nausea, diarrhea, abdominal pain or discomfort,* loose stools, vomiting, fat malabsorption, gallbladder abnormalities.
Metabolic: hyperglycemia, hypoglycemia, hypothyroidism.
Skin: flushing, edema, wheal; erythema, pain (at injection site).
Other: pain, burning (at S.C. injection site).

Interactions

Drug-drug. *Cyclosporine:* may decrease plasma levels of cyclosporine. Monitor patient.

Contraindications and precautions

• Contraindicated in patients hypersensitive to drug or its components.
• Use cautiously in pregnant women.
• Safety of drug has not been established in breast-feeding women and in children.

NURSING CONSIDERATIONS

⚕ Assessment
• Assess patient's condition before therapy and regularly thereafter.
• Monitor baseline thyroid function tests as ordered.
• Monitor somatomedin C levels every 2 weeks as ordered. Dosage is adjusted based on this level.

• Monitor laboratory tests periodically, such as thyroid function tests, urine 5-hydroxyindoleacetic acid, plasma serotonin, and plasma substance P (for carcinoid tumors), and plasma vasoactive intestinal peptide (for VIPomas).
• Monitor fluid and electrolyte status.
• Be alert for adverse reactions and drug interactions.
• Evaluate patient's and family's knowledge of drug therapy.

⚕ Nursing diagnoses
• Diarrhea related to condition
• Fatigue related to drug-induced adverse CNS reaction
• Knowledge deficit related to drug therapy

⚕ Planning and implementation
• Administer drug in divided doses for first 2 weeks of therapy; subsequent daily dosage depends on patient's response.
• Read drug labels carefully and check dosage and strength.
• Drug therapy may alter fluid and electrolyte balance and may require adjustment of other drugs.
Patient teaching
• Tell patient to report signs of gallbladder disease such as abdominal discomfort. Drug may be associated with development of cholelithiasis.
• Instruct patient that laboratory tests are needed during therapy.

⚕ Evaluation
• Patient's bowel pattern is normal.
• Patient uses energy-saving measures to combat fatigue.
• Patient and family state understanding of drug therapy.

ofloxacin
(oh-FLOKS-eh-sin)
Floxin

Pharmacologic class: fluoroquinolone

Therapeutic class: antibiotic
Pregnancy risk category: C

How supplied

Tablets: 200 mg, 300 mg, 400 mg
Injection: 20 mg/ml, 40 mg/ml; 4 mg/ml premixed in D_5W

Pharmacokinetics

Absorption: well absorbed after oral administration.
Distribution: widely distributed to body tissues and fluids.
Metabolism: pyridobenzoxazine ring decreases extent of metabolism in liver.
Excretion: 70% to 80% of drug is excreted unchanged in urine; less than 5% in feces.

Route	Onset	Peak	Duration
P.O.	Unknown	1-2 hr	Unknown
I.V.	Almost immediate	Immediate	Unknown

Pharmacodynamics

Chemical effect: unknown; may inhibit bacterial DNA gyrase and prevent DNA replication in susceptible bacteria.
Therapeutic effect: kills susceptible aerobic gram-positive and gram-negative organisms.

Indications and dosage

▶ **Lower respiratory tract infections caused by susceptible strains of** *Haemophilus influenzae* **or** *Streptococcus pneumoniae. Adults:* 400 mg I.V. or P.O. q 12 hours for 10 days.
▶ **Cervicitis or urethritis caused by** *Chlamydia trachomatis* **or** *Neisseria gonorrhoeae. Adults:* 300 mg I.V. or P.O. q 12 hours for 7 days.
▶ **Acute, uncomplicated gonorrhea.** *Adults:* 400 mg I.V. or P.O. as single dose.
▶ **Mild-to-moderate skin and skin structure infections caused by susceptible strains of** *Staphylococcus aureus, S. epidermidis, S. pyogenes,* **or** *Proteus mirabilis. Adults:* 400 mg I.V. or P.O. q 12 hours for 10 days.

▶ **Cystitis caused by** *Escherichia coli* **or** *Klebsiella pneumoniae. Adults:* 200 mg I.V. or P.O. q 12 hours for 3 days.
▶ **Urinary tract infections (UTIs) caused by susceptible strains of** *Citrobacter diversus, Enterobacter aerogenes, E. coli, P. mirabilis,* **or** *Pseudomonas aeruginosa. Adults:* 200 mg I.V. or P.O. q 12 hours for 7 days. Complicated infections may require therapy for 10 days.
▶ **Prostatitis caused by** *E. coli. Adults:* 300 mg I.V. or P.O. q 12 hours for 6 weeks. If creatinine clearance is 10 to 50 ml/minute, decrease dosage interval to once q 24 hours. If clearance is below 10 ml/minute, give half recommended dose q 24 hours.

Adverse reactions

CNS: headache, dizziness, fatigue, lethargy, malaise, drowsiness, sleep disorders, nervousness, light headedness, insomnia, *seizures.*
CV: chest pain.
GI: nausea, anorexia, abdominal pain or discomfort, diarrhea, vomiting, dry mouth, flatulence, dysgeusia.
GU: vaginitis, vaginal discharge, genital pruritus.
Hematologic: eosinophilia.
Hepatic: elevated liver enzymes.
Musculoskeletal: trunk pain, transient arthralgia, myalgia.
Skin: rash, pruritus, photosensitivity.
Other: hypersensitivity reactions *(anaphylactoid reaction),* visual disturbances, fever.

Interactions

Drug-drug. *Antacids containing aluminum or magnesium hydroxide, iron salts, sucralfate, products containing zinc:* may interfere with GI absorption of ofloxacin. Separate administration by at least 2 hours.
Antineoplastic agents: may lower serum levels of fluoroquinolones. Monitor for lack of effect.

Reactions may be *common*, uncommon, *life-threatening*, or COMMON AND LIFE-THREATENING.

Oral anticoagulants: increased effect. Monitor for bleeding and altered PT and INR.
Theophylline: decreased clearance of theophylline with some fluoroquinolones. Monitor theophylline levels.
Drug-food. *Any food:* decreased absorption. Give drug on an empty stomach.
Drug-lifestyle. *Sun exposure:* photosensitivity reactions may occur. Take precautions.

Contraindications and precautions

• Contraindicated in patients with hypersensitivity to drug or other fluoroquinolones.
• Use cautiously in pregnant women and in patients with renal impairment or with history of seizures or other CNS diseases such as cerebral arteriosclerosis.
• Safety of drug has not been established in breast-feeding women and in children.

NURSING CONSIDERATIONS

Assessment
• Assess patient's infection before therapy and regularly thereafter.
• Monitor regular blood studies and hepatic and renal function tests during prolonged therapy, as ordered.
• Patient treated for gonorrhea should have serologic test for syphilis. Drug is not effective against syphilis, and treatment of gonorrhea may mask or delay symptoms of syphilis.
• Be alert for adverse reactions and drug interactions.
• Monitor patient's hydration status if adverse GI reactions occur.
• Evaluate patient's and family's knowledge of drug therapy.

Nursing diagnoses
• Infection related to presence of bacteria
• Risk for fluid volume deficit related to drug-induced adverse GI reactions
• Knowledge deficit related to drug therapy

Planning and implementation
P.O. use: Administer drug on empty stomach.
I.V. use: Dilute concentrate for injection before use. Single-use vials containing 20 or 40 mg/ml must be diluted to maximum concentration of 4 mg/ml using compatible I.V. solution, such as D_5W, 0.9% NaCl injection, D_5W in 0.9% NaCl injection, or sterile water for injection. Infuse over not less than 1 hour.
• Because compatibility with other drugs is not known, don't mix ofloxacin with other drugs. If giving infusion at Y-site, discontinue other solution during infusion.
• If patient experiences restlessness, tremor, confusion, or hallucinations, stop medication and notify doctor. Take seizure precautions.
Patient teaching
• Advise patient to take drug with plenty of fluids, but not with meals, and to avoid antacids, sucralfate, and products with iron or zinc for at least 2 hours before or after each dose.
• Warn patient to avoid hazardous tasks until drug's CNS effects are known.
• Advise patient to use sunblock and protective clothing to avoid photosensitivity reactions.
• Tell patient to stop drug and notify doctor if rash or other signs of hypersensitivity reactions develop.

Evaluation
• Patient is free from infection.
• Patient maintains adequate hydration throughout drug therapy.
• Patient and family state understanding of drug therapy.

olsalazine sodium
(olh-SAL-uh-zeen SOH-dee-um)
Dipentum

Pharmacologic class: salicylate
Therapeutic class: anti-inflammatory
Pregnancy risk category: C

How supplied

Capsules: 250 mg

Pharmacokinetics

Absorption: about 2.4% of single dose is absorbed.
Distribution: liberated mesalamine is absorbed slowly from colon, resulting in very high local concentrations.
Metabolism: 0.1% is metabolized in liver; remainder will reach colon, where it is rapidly converted to mesalamine by colonic bacteria.
Excretion: about 80% excreted in feces; less than 1% excreted in urine. *Half-life:* of two metabolites, 0.9 hours to 7 days.

Route	Onset	Peak	Duration
P.O.	Unknown	1 hr	Unknown

Pharmacodynamics

Chemical effect: unknown; converts to 5-aminosalicylic acid (5-ASA or mesalamine) in colon, where it has local anti-inflammatory effect.
Therapeutic effect: prevents flare-up of ulcerative colitis.

Indications and dosage

▶ **Maintenance of remission of ulcerative colitis in patients intolerant of sulfasalazine.** *Adults:* 500 mg P.O. b.i.d. with meals.

Adverse reactions

CNS: headache, depression, vertigo, dizziness.
GI: *diarrhea,* nausea, abdominal pain, heartburn.
Musculoskeletal: arthralgia.
Skin: rash, itching.

Interactions

Drug-drug. *Anticoagulants, coumarin derivatives:* prolonged PT or INR. Monitor closely.
Drug-food. *Any food:* decreased GI irritation. Administer drug with food.

Contraindications and precautions

• Contraindicated in patients hypersensitive to salicylates.
• Use cautiously in pregnant or breast-feeding women and in patients with pre-existing renal disease. Renal tubular damage may result from absorbed mesalamine or its metabolites.
• Safety of drug has not been established in children.

NURSING CONSIDERATIONS

⬛ Assessment

• Assess patient's condition before therapy and regularly thereafter.
• Monitor BUN and creatinine levels and urinalysis in patient with preexisting renal disease, as ordered.
• Be alert for adverse reactions.
• Evaluate patient's and family's knowledge of drug therapy.

⬛ Nursing diagnoses

• Impaired tissue integrity related to ulcerative colitis
• Diarrhea related to drug's adverse effect on GI tract
• Knowledge deficit related to drug therapy

⬛ Planning and implementation

• Administer drug with food in evenly divided doses.
• Report diarrhea to doctor. Although diarrhea appears dose-related, it is difficult to distinguish from worsening of disease symptoms. Exacerbation of disease has been noted with similar drugs.
Patient teaching
• Teach patient to take drug in evenly divided doses and with food to minimize adverse GI reactions.
• Tell patient to notify doctor of adverse reactions, especially diarrhea or increased pain.

⬛ Evaluation

• Patient is free from signs and symptoms of ulcerative colitis.

Reactions may be *common*, uncommon, *life-threatening*, or COMMON AND LIFE-THREATENING.

• Patient is free from diarrhea.
• Patient and family state understanding of drug therapy.

omeprazole
(oh-MEH-pruh-zohl)
Losec ♦ ◊, Prilosec

Pharmacologic class: substituted benzimidazole
Therapeutic class: gastric acid suppressant.
Pregnancy risk category: C

How supplied

Capsules (delayed-release): 20 mg

Pharmacokinetics

Absorption: absorbed rapidly after drug leaves stomach. However, bioavailability is about 40% because of instability in gastric acid as well as substantial first-pass effect. Bioavailability increases slightly with repeated dosing.
Distribution: protein binding is about 95%.
Metabolism: metabolized primarily in liver.
Excretion: excreted primarily in urine.
Half-life: 30 to 60 minutes.

Route	Onset	Peak	Duration
P.O.	≤ 1 hr	2 hr	≥ 3 days

Pharmacodynamics

Chemical effect: inhibits activity of acid (proton) pump, and binds to hydrogen/potassium adenosine triphosphatase, located at secretory surface of gastric parietal cells to block formation of gastric acid.
Therapeutic effect: relieves symptoms caused by excessive gastric acid.

Indications and dosage

▶ **Erosive esophagitis; symptomatic, poorly responsive gastroesophageal reflux disease (GERD).** *Adults:* 20 mg P.O. daily for 4 to 8 weeks. Patients with GERD should have failed initial therapy with H$_2$ antagonist.
▶ **Pathologic hypersecretory conditions (such as Zollinger-Ellison syndrome).** *Adults:* initially, 60 mg P.O. daily; dosage titrated according to patient response. If daily dosage exceeds 80 mg, administer in divided doses. Dosages up to 120 mg t.i.d. have been given. Continue therapy as long as clinically indicated.
▶ **Duodenal ulcer (short-term treatment).** *Adults:* 20 mg P.O. daily for 4 to 8 weeks.

Adverse reactions

CNS: headache, dizziness.
GI: diarrhea, abdominal pain, nausea, vomiting, constipation, flatulence.
Respiratory: cough.
Skin: rash.
Other: back pain.

Interactions

Drug-drug. *Ampicillin esters, iron derivatives, ketoconazole:* may exhibit poor bioavailability because optimal absorption of these drugs requires low gastric pH. Administer separately.
Diazepam, phenytoin, warfarin: decreased hepatic clearance, possibly leading to increased serum levels. Monitor closely.

Contraindications and precautions

• Contraindicated in patients hypersensitive to drug or its components.
• Use cautiously in pregnant or breast-feeding women.
• Safety of drug has not been established in children.

NURSING CONSIDERATIONS

▨ Assessment
• Assess patient's condition before therapy and regularly thereafter.
• Be alert for adverse reactions and drug interactions.

- Monitor patient's hydration status if adverse GI reactions occur.
- Evaluate patient's and family's knowledge of drug therapy.

🖎 **Nursing diagnoses**
- Altered tissue integrity related to upper gastric disorder
- Risk for fluid volume deficit related to drug-induced adverse GI reactions
- Knowledge deficit related to drug therapy

▶ **Planning and implementation**
- Dosage adjustments are not required for renal or hepatic impairment.
- Administer drug before meals.

Patient teaching
- Explain importance of taking drug exactly as prescribed.
- Tell patient to swallow capsules whole and not to open or crush.

☑ **Evaluation**
- Patient responds well to therapy.
- Patient maintains adequate hydration throughout drug therapy.
- Patient and family state understanding of drug therapy.

---

ondansetron hydrochloride
(on-DAN-seh-tron high-droh-KLOR-ighd)
Zofran

Pharmacologic class: serotonin (5-HT$_3$) receptor antagonist
Therapeutic class: antiemetic
Pregnancy risk category: B

How supplied

Tablets: 4 mg, 8 mg
Injection: 2 mg/ml, 4 mg/ml

Pharmacokinetics

Absorption: absorption is variable with oral administration; bioavailability of 50% to 60%.

Distribution: 70% to 76% is plasma protein-bound.
Metabolism: extensively metabolized.
Excretion: primarily excreted in urine.
Half-life: 4 hours.

Route	Onset	Peak	Duration
P.O., I.V.	Unknown	Unknown	Unknown

Pharmacodynamics

Chemical effect: located in CNS at area postrema (chemoreceptor trigger zone) and in peripheral nervous system on nerve terminals of vagus nerve. Drug's blocking action may occur at both sites.
Therapeutic effect: prevents nausea and vomiting associated with emetogenic chemotherapy or surgery.

Indications and dosage

▶ **Prevention of nausea and vomiting associated with emetogenic chemotherapy.** *Adults and children age 12 and over:* 8 mg P.O. 30 minutes before start of chemotherapy. Follow with 8 mg P.O. 4 and 8 hours after first dose. Then follow with 8 mg q 8 hours for 1 to 2 days. Alternatively, administer single dose of 32 mg by I.V. infusion over 15 minutes beginning 30 minutes before chemotherapy; or three divided doses of 0.15 mg/kg I.V. (first dose given 30 minutes before chemotherapy; subsequent doses given 4 and 8 hours after first dose). Infuse drug over 15 minutes. *Children ages 4 to 12:* 4 mg P.O. 30 minutes before start of chemotherapy. Follow with 4 mg P.O. 4 and 8 hours after first dose. Then follow with 4 mg q 8 hours for 1 to 2 days. Alternatively, three doses of 0.15 mg/kg I.V. Give first dose 30 minutes before chemotherapy; administer subsequent doses 4 and 8 hours after first dose. Infuse drug over 15 minutes.
▶ **Prevention of postoperative nausea and vomiting.** *Adults:* 4 mg I.V. (undiluted) over 2 to 5 minutes.

Adverse reactions

CNS: headache.

GI: diarrhea, constipation.
Hepatic: transient elevations in AST and ALT levels.
Skin: rash.

Interactions

Drug-drug. *Drugs that alter hepatic drug metabolizing enzymes (such as cimetidine phenobarbital):* may alter pharmacokinetics of ondansetron. No dosage adjustment appears necessary.

Contraindications and precautions

• Contraindicated in patients hypersensitive to drug.
• Use cautiously in patients with liver failure and in pregnant or breast-feeding women.

NURSING CONSIDERATIONS

✇ Assessment

• Assess patient's condition before therapy and regularly thereafter.
• Be alert for adverse reactions and drug interactions.
• Evaluate patient's and family's knowledge of drug therapy.

✇ Nursing diagnoses

• Risk for fluid volume deficit related to nausea and vomiting
• Pain related to drug-induced headache
• Knowledge deficit related to drug therapy

✇ Planning and implementation

P.O. use: Follow normal protocol.
I.V. use: Dilute drug in 50 ml of D_5W injection or 0.9% NaCl injection before administration.
– Infuse drug over 15 minutes.
– Drug is also stable for up to 48 hours after dilution in 5% dextrose in 0.9% NaCl injection, 5% dextrose in 0.45% NaCl injection, and 3% NaCl injection.
Patient teaching
• Instruct patient when to take drug.
• Tell patient to report adverse reactions.

✇ Evaluation

• Patient maintains adequate hydration.
• Patient reports no headache.
• Patient and family state understanding of drug therapy.

---

opium tincture*
(OH-pee-um TINK-shur)

opium tincture, camphorated*
(paregoric)

Pharmacologic class: opium
Therapeutic class: antidiarrheal
Controlled substance schedule: II (III for opium tincture, camphorated)
Pregnancy risk category: NR

How supplied

opium tincture
Oral solution: equivalent to morphine 10 mg/ml*
opium tincture, camphorated
Oral solution: each 5 ml contains morphine, 2 mg; anise oil, 0.2 ml; benzoic acid, 20 mg; camphor, 20 mg; glycerin, 0.2 ml; and ethanol to make 5 ml*

Pharmacokinetics

Absorption: absorbed variably.
Distribution: distributed widely in body.
Metabolism: metabolized in liver.
Excretion: excreted in urine.

Route	Onset	Peak	Duration
P.O.	Unknown	Unknown	Unknown

Pharmacodynamics

Chemical effect: increases smooth-muscle tone in GI tract, inhibits motility and propulsion, and diminishes secretions.
Therapeutic effect: relieves diarrhea.

Indications and dosage

▶ **Acute, nonspecific diarrhea. Opium tincture.** *Adults:* 0.6 ml (range 0.3 to 1 ml) P.O. q.i.d. Maximum dosage is 6 ml daily. **Camphorated opium tinc-**

---

ture. *Adults:* 5 to 10 ml once daily, b.i.d., t.i.d., or q.i.d. until diarrhea subsides. *Children:* 0.25 to 0.5 ml/kg P.O. once daily, b.i.d., t.i.d., or q.i.d. until diarrhea subsides.
Note: Do *not* confuse opium tincture with camphorated opium tincture.

Adverse reactions

CNS: dizziness, light-headedness.
GI: nausea, vomiting; physical dependence (after long-term use).

Interactions

None significant.

Contraindications and precautions

• Contraindicated in patients with acute diarrhea resulting from poisoning until toxic material is removed from GI tract or in those with diarrhea caused by organisms that penetrate intestinal mucosa.
• Use cautiously in patients with asthma, prostatic hyperplasia, hepatic disease, or opioid dependence.
• Safety of drug has not been established in pregnant or breast-feeding women.

NURSING CONSIDERATIONS

Assessment
• Assess patient's condition before therapy and regularly thereafter.
• Be alert for adverse reactions.
• Monitor patient's hydration status throughout drug therapy.
• Evaluate patient's and family's knowledge of drug therapy.

Nursing diagnoses
• Diarrhea related to GI disorder
• Risk for fluid volume deficit related to diarrhea and drug-induced adverse GI reactions
• Knowledge deficit related to drug therapy

Planning and implementation
• Read label carefully. *The opium content of opium tincture is 25 times greater than*

camphorated opium tincture. Camphorated opium tincture is more dilute, and teaspoonful doses are easier to measure than dropper quantities of opium tincture.
• Mix drug with water to form a milky fluid.
• Store drug in tightly capped, light-resistant container.
• For overdose, use narcotic antagonist naloxone, as ordered, to reverse respiratory depression.

Patient teaching
• Advise patient against using drug for more than 2 days; risk of dependence increases with long-term use.
• Encourage proper storage to keep drug out of children's hands.

Evaluation
• Patient's diarrhea ceases.
• Patient maintains adequate hydration.
• Patient and family state understanding of drug.

orphenadrine citrate
(or-FEN-uh-dreen SIH-trayt)
Banflex, Flexoject, Flexon, Marflex, Myolin, Norflex, Orphenate

Pharmacologic class: diphenhydramine analogue
Therapeutic class: skeletal muscle relaxant
Pregnancy risk category: NR

How supplied

Tablets: 100 mg
Tablets (extended-release): 100 mg
Injection: 30 mg/ml

Pharmacokinetics

Absorption: rapidly absorbed from GI tract after oral administration. Unknown for I.M. administration.
Distribution: widely distributed throughout body.
Metabolism: biotransformed in liver. Metabolized almost completely to at least

eight metabolites.
Excretion: excreted in urine, mainly as
metabolites. *Half-life:* about 14 hours.

Route	Onset	Peak	Duration
P.O.	≤ 1 hr (regular) 6-8 hr (extended-release)	≤ 2 hr	Unknown
I.V.	Immediate	Immediate	Unknown
I.M.	≤ 5 min	≤ 30 min	Unknown

Pharmacodynamics

Chemical effect: unknown; appears to
modify central perception of pain without
modifying pain reflexes. Blocks interneuronal activity in descending reticular activating system and in spinal cord.
Therapeutic effect: relaxes skeletal muscles.

Indications and dosage

▶ **Adjunct treatment in painful, acute
musculoskeletal conditions.** *Adults:*
100 mg P.O. b.i.d., or 60 mg I.V. or I.M.
q 12 hours, p.r.n. For maintenance therapy, oral therapy begins 12 hours after
last parenteral dose.

Adverse reactions

CNS: disorientation, restlessness, irri-
tability, weakness, *drowsiness,* headache,
dizziness, hallucinations, insomnia.
CV: palpitations, tachycardia.
EENT: dilated pupils, blurred vision, dif-
ficulty swallowing, increased intraocular
pressure.
GI: constipation, *dry mouth,* nausea, vom-
iting, paralytic ileus, epigastric distress.
GU: urinary hesitancy or urine retention.
Hematologic: *aplastic anemia.*
Other: *anaphylaxis.*

Interactions

Drug-drug. *CNS depressants, propoxyphene:* increased CNS depression. Avoid
concomitant use.
Drug-lifestyle. *Alcohol use.* increased
CNS depression. Avoid concomitant use.

Contraindications and precautions

● Contraindicated in patients with glaucoma; prostatic hyperplasia; pyloric, duodenal, or bladder-neck obstruction; myasthenia gravis; peptic ulceration; or hypersensitivity to drug.
● Use cautiously in pregnant women, in
elderly or debilitated patients, and in
those with tachycardia, cardiac disease,
arrhythmias, or sulfite sensitivity.
● Safety of drug has not been established
in children and in breast-feeding women.

NURSING CONSIDERATIONS

🔲 Assessment
● Assess patient's condition before therapy and regularly thereafter.
● When given I.V., assess for paradoxical
initial bradycardia; usually disappears in
2 minutes.
● Monitor CBC, hepatic function, and
urinalysis in patient receiving long-term
therapy as ordered.
● Monitor vital signs carefully.
● Be alert for adverse reactions and drug
interactions.
● Evaluate patient's and family's knowledge of drug therapy.

🔲 Nursing diagnoses
● Pain related to condition
● Risk for injury related to drug-induced
adverse CNS reactions
● Knowledge deficit related to drug
therapy

🔲 Planning and implementation
● Check all dosages; slight overdose can
lead to toxicity. Early signs are excessive
dry mouth, dilated pupils, blurred vision,
skin flushing, and fever.
P.O. and I.M. use: Follow normal protocol.
I.V. use: Inject drug over about 5 minutes
with patient supine. After 5 to 10 minutes, help patient to sit up.

Patient teaching
• Tell patient to report urinary hesitancy and urine retention. Instruct him to void before taking drug.
• Advise patient to relieve dry mouth with sugarless gum or hard candy.
• Warn patient to avoid tasks that require alertness until drug's CNS effects are known.
• Advise patient to avoid alcohol or other CNS depressants during drug therapy.

☑ **Evaluation**
• Patient is free from pain.
• Patient does not experience injury from adverse CNS reactions.
• Patient and family state understanding of drug therapy.

oxacillin sodium
(oks-uh-SIL-in SOH-dee-um)
Bactocill, Prostaphlin

Pharmacologic class: penicillinase-resistant penicillin
Therapeutic class: antibiotic
Pregnancy risk category: B

How supplied
Capsules: 250 mg, 500 mg
Oral solution: 250 mg/5 ml (after reconstitution)
Injection: 250 mg, 500 mg, 1 g, 2 g, 4 g
I.V. infusion: 1 g, 2 g, 4 g

Pharmacokinetics
Absorption: absorbed rapidly but incompletely from GI tract after oral administration; food decreases absorption. Absorption unknown after I.M. administration.
Distribution: distributed widely. CSF penetration is poor but enhanced by meningeal inflammation. Drug is 89% to 94% protein-bound.
Metabolism: metabolized partially.

Excretion: excreted primarily in urine; small amount in bile. *Half-life:* 30 to 60 minutes.

Route	Onset	Peak	Duration
P.O.	Unknown	0.5-2 hr	Unknown
I.V.	Immediate	Immediate	Unknown
I.M.	Unknown	≤ 30 min	Unknown

Pharmacodynamics
Chemical effect: inhibits cell-wall synthesis during microorganism multiplication; bacteria resist penicillins by producing penicillinases—enzymes that convert penicillins to inactive penicilloic acid. Oxacillin resists these enzymes.
Therapeutic effect: kills susceptible bacteria, such as penicillinase-producing staphylococci and a few gram-positive aerobic and anaerobic bacilli.

Indications and dosage
▶ **Systemic infections caused by penicillinase-producing staphylococci.**
Adults and children weighing over 40 kg (88 lb): 500 mg P.O. q 4 to 6 hours; or 1 to 12 g I.M. or I.V. daily, in divided doses q 4 to 6 hours. *Children weighing 40 kg or less:* 50 to 100 mg/kg P.O. daily, in divided doses q 6 hours; or 50 to 200 mg/kg I.M. or I.V. daily, in divided doses q 4 to 6 hours.

Adverse reactions
CNS: neuropathy, neuromuscular irritability, *seizures.*
GI: oral lesions.
GU: interstitial nephritis, transient hematuria, proteinuria.
Hematologic: *agranulocytopenia, thrombocytopenia,* eosinophilia, *hemolytic anemia, transient neutropenia.*
Hepatic: hepatitis, elevated liver enzymes.
Other: hypersensitivity reactions (fever, chills, rash, urticaria, *anaphylaxis*), overgrowth of nonsusceptible organisms, *thrombophlebitis.*

Interactions

Drug-drug. *Aminoglycosides:* possible synergistic effect. Monitor closely.
Probenecid: increased blood levels of oxacillin and other penicillins. Probenecid may be used for this purpose.
Rifampin: possible antagonism. Monitor closely.

Contraindications and precautions

• Contraindicated in patients with hypersensitivity to drug or other penicillins.

• Use cautiously in patients with other drug allergies, especially to cephalosporins; in premature neonates; infants; and in breast-feeding or pregnant women.

NURSING CONSIDERATIONS

⚡ Assessment

• Assess patient's infection before therapy and regularly thereafter.

• Before giving drug, ask about allergic reactions to penicillin. However, negative history of allergy is no guarantee against future allergic reaction.

• Obtain specimen for culture and sensitivity tests before giving first dose. Therapy may begin pending results.

• Monitor CBC and platelet count as ordered.

• Monitor periodic liver function studies; watch for elevated AST and ALT levels.

• Be alert for adverse reactions and drug interactions.

• Evaluate patient's and family's knowledge of drug therapy.

⊞ Nursing diagnoses

• Infection related to presence of bacteria

• Altered protection related to drug-induced adverse hematologic reactions

• Knowledge deficit related to drug therapy

⊵ Planning and implementation

P.O. and I.M. use: Follow normal protocol.

• Give drug 1 to 2 hours before or 2 to 3 hours after meals. When given orally, drug may cause GI disturbances. Food may interfere with absorption.

I.V. use: For direct I.V. injection, reconstitute vials with sterile water for injection or 0.9% NaCl injection. Use 5 ml of diluent for 250- or 500-mg vial, 10 ml of diluent for 1-g vial, 20 ml of diluent for 2-g vial, or 40 ml of diluent for 4-g vial. When solution is clear, withdraw ordered dose and inject slowly over 10 minutes. When giving by piggyback injection, reconstitute 1-g piggyback vial with 20 to 100 ml of diluent; reconstitute 2-g vial with 19 to 99 ml of diluent. For intermittent infusion, further dilute drug to concentration of 5 to 40 mg/ml.

– Know that aminoglycosides are chemically and physically incompatible with drug; do not mix together in same I.V. solution.

– To prevent vein irritation, avoid continuous infusions. Change site every 48 hours.

• Don't give I.V. or I.M. unless ordered and infection is severe or patient can't take oral dose.

• Give drug at least 1 hour before bacteriostatic antibiotics.

• Drug may falsely elevate or cause false-positive results with certain tests for urine or serum proteins.

• Notify doctor of abnormal laboratory test results and be prepared to provide supportive care.

Patient teaching

• Instruct patient to take drug exactly as prescribed, even after he feels better.

• Tell patient to take oral drug on empty stomach.

• Tell patient to call doctor if rash, fever, or chills develop.

✓ Evaluation

• Patient is free from infection.

• Patient does not experience adverse hematologic reactions.

• Patient and family state understanding of drug therapy.

---

*Liquid form contains alcohol   **May contain tartrazine   ◆Canada   ◇Australia   †OTC

oxandrolone
(oks-AN-droh-lohn)
Lonavar◇, Oxandrin

Pharmacologic class: anabolic steroid
Therapeutic class: anticatabolic and tissue-depleting agent
Controlled substance schedule: III
Pregnancy risk category: X

How supplied
Tablets: 2.5 mg

Pharmacokinetics
Absorption: unknown.
Distribution: unknown.
Metabolism: unknown.
Excretion: excreted primarily in urine; small amount excreted in feces. *Half-life:* 0.55 hours during first-phase and 9 hours during second phase.

Route	Onset	Peak	Duration
P.O.	Unknown	Unknown	Unknown

Pharmacodynamics
Chemical effect: reverses catabolism and negative nitrogen balance by promoting protein anabolism and stimulating appetite if calorie and protein intake is sufficient.
Therapeutic effect: promotes tissue-building and reverses catabolism.

Indications and dosage
▶ **To combat catabolic effects of corticosteroid therapy, prevent bone pain associated with osteoporosis, and to promote weight gain following extensive surgery or severe trauma in debilitated patients.** *Adults:* 2.5 mg P.O. b.i.d., t.i.d., or q.i.d., up to 20 mg daily.
Children: 0.1 mg/kg P.O. daily.

Adverse reactions
CV: edema.
GI: gastroenteritis, nausea, vomiting, constipation or diarrhea, change in appetite.
GU: bladder irritability.

Hematologic: thrombocytopenia, elevated serum lipid levels.
Hepatic: reversible jaundice, peliosis hepatis, elevated liver enzyme levels, *liver cell tumors.*
Other: hypercalcemia; muscle cramps or spasms; androgenic effects in women (acne, edema, *weight gain, hirsutism,* hoarseness, clitoral enlargement, *decrease in breast size,* changes in libido, male-pattern baldness, *oily skin or hair*); hypoestrogenic effects in women (flushing; diaphoresis; vaginitis, including itching, dryness, and burning; vaginal bleeding; nervousness; emotional lability; menstrual irregularities); excessive hormonal effects in men (prepubertal—premature epiphyseal closure, *acne,* priapism, *growth of body and facial hair,* phallic enlargement; postpubertal—testicular atrophy, oligospermia, decreased ejaculatory volume, impotence, gynecomastia, epididymitis).

Interactions
Drug-drug. *Hepatotoxic drugs:* increased risk of hepatotoxicity. Monitor closely.
Insulin, oral antidiabetic agents: altered dosage requirements. Monitor blood glucose levels in diabetic patients.
Oral anticoagulants: altered dosage requirements. Monitor PT or INR.

Contraindications and precautions
• Contraindicated in pregnant and breast-feeding women and in patients with nephrosis, nephrotic phase of nephritis, hypersensitivity to anabolic steroids, in males with breast or prostate cancer, and in females with breast cancer and hypercalcemia.
• Use cautiously in patients with diabetes; cardiac, renal, or hepatic disease; epilepsy; or migraine or other conditions that may be aggravated by fluid retention.

NURSING CONSIDERATIONS

☑ Assessment
• Assess patient's condition before therapy and regularly thereafter.

- In child, baseline X-rays of wrist bones should be taken to establish level of bone maturation. During treatment, bones may mature rapidly; ensure intermittent dosage and review X-rays periodically to monitor maturation.
- Watch for signs of virilization, which may be irreversible despite prompt discontinuation of therapy. Doctor must decide if benefits outweigh adverse effects.
- Closely observe boy under age 7 for precocious development of male sexual characteristics.
- Semen evaluation is routinely performed every 3 to 4 months, especially in adolescent male.
- Monitor hepatic function.
- Be alert for adverse reactions and drug interactions.
- Evaluate patient's and family's knowledge of drug therapy.

⊕ Nursing diagnoses
- Altered health maintenance related to condition
- Body image disturbance related to adverse androgenic reactions
- Knowledge deficit related to drug therapy

▷ Planning and implementation
- Avoid use in women of childbearing age until pregnancy is ruled out.
- Control edema with sodium restriction or diuretics, as ordered.
- Unless contraindicated, use with diet high in calories and protein. Give small, frequent feedings.
- Anabolic steroids may alter results of laboratory tests done during and for 2 to 3 weeks after therapy.

Patient teaching
- Tell patient to take drug with food or meals to avoid GI upset.
- Make sure patient understands importance of using effective nonhormonal contraceptive during therapy.
- Advise patient to wash after intercourse to decrease risk of vaginitis. Instruct patient to wear only cotton underwear.

- Tell female patient to report menstrual irregularities and to stop drug until the cause has been determined.

☑ Evaluation
- Patient responds well to therapy.
- Patient accepts body image changes caused by drug.
- Patient and family state understanding of drug therapy.

oxaprozin
(oks-uh-PROH-zin)
Daypro

Pharmacologic class: NSAID
Therapeutic class: nonnarcotic analgesic, antipyretic, anti-inflammatory
Pregnancy risk category: C

How supplied
Caplets: 600 mg

Pharmacokinetics
Absorption: high oral bioavailability (95%); food may reduce rate—but not extent—of absorption.
Distribution: about 99.9% protein-bound.
Metabolism: metabolized in liver.
Excretion: metabolites are excreted in urine (65%) and feces (35%). *Half-life:* 5 hours.

Route	Onset	Peak	Duration
P.O.	Unknown	3-5 hr	Unknown

Pharmacodynamics
Chemical effect: unknown; may inhibit prostaglandin synthesis.
Therapeutic effect: relieves pain, fever, and inflammation.

Indications and dosage

▶ **Osteoarthritis or rheumatoid arthritis.** *Adults:* initially, 1,200 mg P.O. daily. Then, individualized to smallest effective dosage to minimize adverse reactions. Smaller patients or those with mild symptoms may require only 600 mg daily. Maximum is 1,800 mg or 26 mg/kg, whichever is lower, in divided doses.

Adverse reactions

CNS: depression, sedation, somnolence, confusion, sleep disturbances.
EENT: tinnitus, visual disturbances.
GI: *nausea, dyspepsia, diarrhea, constipation,* abdominal pain or distress, anorexia, flatulence, vomiting, *hemorrhage.*
GU: dysuria, urinary frequency.
Hepatic: elevated liver function test results (with chronic use); severe hepatic dysfunction (rare).
Skin: *rash,* photosensitivity.

Interactions

Drug-drug. *Antihypertensives, diuretics:* decreased effect. Monitor closely and adjust dosage as ordered.
Aspirin: oxaprozin displaces salicylates from plasma protein-binding sites, increasing risk of salicylate toxicity. Avoid concomitant use.
Aspirin, corticosteroids: increased risk of adverse GI reactions. Avoid concomitant use.
Methotrexate: increased risk of methotrexate toxicity. Avoid concomitant use.
Oral anticoagulants: increased risk of bleeding. Use together cautiously.
Drug-lifestyle. *Alcohol use:* increased risk of adverse GI reactions. Avoid concomitant use.
Sun exposure: photosensitivity reactions may occur. Take precautions.

Contraindications and precautions

• Contraindicated in patients with syndrome of nasal polyps, angioedema, bronchospastic reactivity to aspirin or other NSAIDs or hypersensitivity to drug.
• Use cautiously in pregnant or breast-feeding women and in those with history of peptic ulcer disease, hepatic or renal dysfunction, hypertension, CV disease, or conditions that predispose to fluid retention.

• Safety of drug has not been established in children.

NURSING CONSIDERATIONS

Assessment
• Assess patient's condition before therapy and regularly thereafter.
• Periodically monitor liver function tests during long-term therapy, and closely monitor patient with abnormal test results. Elevations of liver function tests can occur. These abnormal findings may persist, worsen, or resolve with continued therapy. Rarely, patient may progress to severe hepatic dysfunction.
• Be alert for adverse reactions and drug interactions.
• Evaluate patient's and family's knowledge of drug therapy.

Nursing diagnoses
• Pain related to condition
• Altered tissue integrity related to drug's adverse GI effects
• Knowledge deficit related to drug therapy

Planning and implementation
• Administer drug on empty stomach unless adverse GI reactions occur.
• Notify doctor immediately of adverse reactions, especially GI symptoms.
Patient teaching
• Tell patient to take drug 30 minutes before or 2 hours after meals. If adverse GI reactions occur, patient may take it with milk or meals.
• Explain that full therapeutic effects may be delayed for 2 to 4 weeks.
• Tell patient to report adverse visual or auditory reactions immediately.
• Teach patient to recognize and promptly report signs and symptoms of GI bleeding.
• Advise patient to use sunblock, wear protective clothing, and avoid prolonged exposure to sunlight.

Reactions may be *common*, uncommon, *life-threatening*, or COMMON AND LIFE-THREATENING.

✓ Evaluation
• Patient is free from pain.
• Patient maintains GI tissue integrity.
• Patient and family state understanding of drug therapy.

---

oxazepam
(oks-AZ-ih-pam)
Alepam◇, Apo-Oxazepam♦, Murelax◇, Novoxapam♦, Serax**, Serepax◇

Pharmacologic class: benzodiazepine
Therapeutic class: antianxiety, sedative-hypnotic
Controlled substance schedule: IV
Pregnancy risk category: NR

How supplied
Tablets: 10 mg, 15 mg, 30 mg
Capsules: 10 mg, 15 mg, 30 mg

Pharmacokinetics
Absorption: well absorbed.
Distribution: distributed widely throughout body. Drug is 85% to 95% protein-bound.
Metabolism: metabolized in liver.
Excretion: metabolites are excreted in urine. *Half-life:* 5 to 13 hours.

Route	Onset	Peak	Duration
P.O.	Unknown	About 3 hr	Unknown

Pharmacodynamics
Chemical effect: unknown; believed to stimulate gamma-aminobutyric receptors in ascending reticular activating system.
Therapeutic effect: relieves anxiety and promotes calmness.

Indications and dosage
▶ **Alcohol withdrawal.** *Adults:* 15 to 30 mg P.O. t.i.d. or q.i.d.
▶ **Severe anxiety.** *Adults:* 15 to 30 mg P.O. t.i.d. or q.i.d.
▶ **Mild to moderate anxiety.** *Adults:* 10 to 15 mg P.O. t.i.d. or q.i.d.

Adverse reactions
CNS: drowsiness, lethargy, hangover, fainting.
CV: transient hypotension.
GI: nausea, vomiting, abdominal discomfort.
Hematologic: *leukopenia* (rare).
Hepatic: *hepatic dysfunction.*

Interactions
Drug-drug. *Cimetidine, other CNS depressants:* increased CNS depression. Avoid concomitant use.
Digoxin: may increase serum levels of digoxin, increasing toxicity. Monitor closely.
Drug-lifestyle. *Alcohol use:* increased CNS depression. Avoid concomitant use.
Smoking: increased benzodiazepine clearance. Monitor for lack of effect.

Contraindications and precautions
• Contraindicated in patients hypersensitive to drug.
• Avoid use of drug in pregnant or breast-feeding women.
• Use cautiously in elderly patients and in those with history of drug abuse or in whom drop in blood pressure might lead to cardiac problems.
• Safety of drug has not been established in children.

NURSING CONSIDERATIONS

🗲 Assessment
• Assess patient's condition before therapy and regularly thereafter.
• Monitor liver, renal, and hematopoietic function studies periodically in patient receiving repeated or prolonged therapy, as ordered.
• Be alert for adverse reactions and drug interactions.
• Evaluate patient's and family's knowledge of drug therapy.

⊞ Nursing diagnoses
• Altered thought processes related to condition

- Risk for injury related to drug-induced adverse CNS reactions
- Knowledge deficit related to drug therapy

▶ **Planning and implementation**
- Expect to reduce dosage in elderly or debilitated patient.
- Possibility of abuse and addiction exists. Do not stop drug abruptly; withdrawal symptoms may occur.

Patient teaching
- Warn patient to avoid hazardous activities until CNS effects of drug are known.
- Tell patient to avoid alcohol during drug therapy.

☑ **Evaluation**
- Patient exhibits less anxiety.
- Patient does not experience injury as result of drug therapy.
- Patient and family state understanding of drug therapy.

---

oxybutynin chloride
(oks-ee-BYOO-tih-nin KLOR-ighd)
Ditropan

Pharmacologic class: synthetic tertiary amine
Therapeutic class: antispasmodic
Pregnancy risk category: B

How supplied

Tablets: 5 mg
Syrup: 5 mg/5 ml

Pharmacokinetics

Absorption: absorbed rapidly.
Distribution: unknown.
Metabolism: metabolized by liver.
Excretion: excreted primarily in urine.

Route	Onset	Peak	Duration
P.O.	30-60 min	3-4 hr	6-10 hr

Pharmacodynamics

Chemical effect: produces direct spasmolytic effect and antimuscarinic (atropine-like) effect on urinary tract smooth muscles, increasing bladder capacity and providing some local anesthesia and mild analgesia.
Therapeutic effect: relieves bladder spasms.

Indications and dosage

▶ **Antispasmodic for uninhibited or reflex neurogenic bladder.** *Adults:* 5 mg P.O. b.i.d. to t.i.d., up to 5 mg q.i.d. *Children over age 5:* 5 mg P.O. b.i.d., up to 5 mg t.i.d.

Adverse reactions

CNS: *drowsiness,* dizziness, insomnia, restlessness, impaired alertness.
CV: palpitations, tachycardia.
EENT: *transient blurred vision,* mydriasis, cycloplegia.
GI: nausea, vomiting, *constipation,* bloated feeling, *dry mouth.*
GU: impotence, urinary hesitancy, urine retention.
Skin: rash, urticaria, allergic reactions.
Other: decreased diaphoresis, fever, suppressed lactation, flushing.

Interactions

Drug-drug. *Anticholinergics:* increased anticholinergic effects. Use cautiously.
Atenolol, digoxin: increased levels of these drugs. Monitor closely.
CNS depressants: increased CNS effects. Use cautiously.
Haloperidol, levodopa: decreased levels of these drugs. Monitor closely.
Drug-lifestyle: *Alcohol use:* increased CNS effects. Use cautiously.
Exercise, hot weather: may precipitate heat stroke. Use cautiously.

Contraindications and precautions

- Contraindicated in patients with myasthenia gravis, GI obstruction, glaucoma, adynamic ileus, megacolon, severe colitis, ulcerative colitis when megacolon is

---

present, obstructive uropathy, or hypersensitivity to drug; in elderly or debilitated patients with intestinal atony; and in hemorrhaging patients with unstable CV status.

• Use cautiously in pregnant or breastfeeding women, in elderly patients, and in those with autonomic neuropathy, reflux esophagitis, or hepatic or renal disease.

NURSING CONSIDERATIONS

⚞ Assessment
• Assess patient's bladder condition before therapy.
• Before giving drug, anticipate confirmation of neurogenic bladder by cystometry and rule out partial intestinal obstruction in patients with diarrhea, especially those with colostomy or ileostomy.
• Prepare patient for periodic cystometry to evaluate response to therapy.
• Be alert for adverse reactions.
• Drug may aggravate symptoms of hyperthyroidism, coronary artery disease, heart failure, arrhythmias, tachycardia, hypertension, or prostatic hyperplasia.
• Evaluate patient's and family's knowledge of drug therapy.

⚟ Nursing diagnoses
• Pain related to bladder spasms
• Risk for injury related to drug-induced adverse CNS reactions
• Knowledge deficit related to drug therapy

⚟ Planning and implementation
• If urinary tract infection is present, administer antibiotics, as ordered.
• To minimize tendency toward tolerance, be prepared to stop therapy periodically to determine whether patient can get along without it.
Patient teaching
• Warn patient to avoid hazardous activities until CNS effects are known.
• Caution patient that using drug in hot weather may precipitate fever or heatstroke.

• Advise patient to store drug in tightly closed containers at 59° to 86° F (15° to 30° C).

☑ Evaluation
• Patient is free from bladder pain.
• Patient sustains no injuries due to drug-induced adverse CNS reactions.
• Patient and family state understanding of drug therapy.

oxycodone hydrochloride
(oks-ee-KOH-dohn high-droh-KLOR-ighd)
Endone◇, Roxicodone, Roxicodone Intensol, Supeudol◆

oxycodone pectinate
Proladone◇

Pharmacologic class: opioid
Therapeutic class: analgesic
Controlled substance schedule: II
Pregnancy risk category: NR

How supplied

oxycodone hydrochloride
Tablets: 5 mg
Oral solution: 5 mg/5 ml, 20 mg/ml (concentrate)
Suppositories: 10 mg, 20 mg
oxycodone pectinate
Suppositories: 30 mg◇

Pharmacokinetics

Absorption: unknown.
Distribution: unknown.
Metabolism: metabolized in liver.
Excretion: excreted primarily in urine.
Half-life: 2 to 3 hours.

Route	Onset	Peak	Duration
P.O.	10-15 min	≤ 1 hr	3-6 hr
P.R.	Unknown	Unknown	Unknown

Pharmacodynamics

Chemical effect: binds with opioid receptors in CNS, altering response to pain via unknown mechanism.

Therapeutic effect: relieves pain.

Indications and dosage

▶ **Moderate to severe pain.** *Adults:*
5 mg P.O. q 6 hours, p.r.n. Alternatively,
10 to 40 mg P.R., p.r.n., t.i.d. or q.i.d.
Children ages 6 to 12: 0.61 mg of combined salts P.O. q 6 hours, p.r.n. *Children
age 12 and older:* 1.22 mg of combined
salts P.O. q 6 hours, p.r.n.

Adverse reactions

CNS: *sedation, somnolence, clouded
sensorium, euphoria,* dizziness.
CV: *hypotension,* bradycardia.
GI: nausea, vomiting, constipation, ileus.
GU: urine retention.
Respiratory: *respiratory depression.*
Other: physical dependence.

Interactions

Drug-drug. *Anticoagulants:* oxycodone
products containing aspirin may increase
anticoagulant effect. Monitor clotting
times. Use together cautiously.
*CNS depressants, general anesthetics,
hypnotics, MAO inhibitors, other narcotic analgesics, sedatives, tranquilizers, tricyclic antidepressants:* additive effects.
Use together with extreme caution.
Reduce oxycodone dose and monitor patient response.
Drug-lifestyle. *Alcohol use:* increased
CNS depression. Avoid concomitant use.

Contraindications and precautions

• Contraindicated in patients with hypersensitivity to drug
• Use with extreme caution in elderly or
debilitated patients and in those with
head injury, increased intracranial pressure, seizures, asthma, COPD, prostatic
hypertrophy, severe hepatic or renal disease, acute abdominal conditions, urethral stricture, hypothyroidism, Addison's
disease, or arrhythmias.
• Use cautiously in pregnant or breast-
feeding women.

NURSING CONSIDERATIONS

⬛ Assessment
• Assess patient's pain before and after
drug administration.
• Monitor circulatory and respiratory status.
• Be alert for adverse reactions and drug
interactions.
• Evaluate patient's and family's knowledge of drug therapy.

⬛ Nursing diagnoses
• Pain related to condition
• Ineffective breathing pattern related to
drug-induced respiratory depression
• Knowledge deficit related to drug
therapy

⬛ Planning and implementation
P.O. use: Give drug with food or milk to
avoid GI upset.
P.R. use: Not commercially available in
the United States.
• Administer drug before patient has intense pain for best results.
• Know that single-agent oxycodone solution or tablets are especially good for
patient who shouldn't take aspirin or acetaminophen.
• Withhold dose and notify doctor if respirations are shallow or if rate falls below
12 breaths/minute.
Patient teaching
• Instruct patient to take drug with food
or milk to minimize adverse GI upset.
Also tell patient to ask for drug before intense pain occurs.
• Caution ambulatory patient about getting out of bed or walking. Warn outpatient to avoid hazardous activities until
drug's CNS effects are known.

⬛ Evaluation
• Patient is free from pain.
• Patient's respiratory rate and pattern re-
main within normal limits.
• Patient and family state understanding
of drug therapy.

Reactions may be *common,* uncommon, *life-threatening,* or COMMON AND LIFE-THREATENING.

oxymetazoline hydrochloride
(oks-ee-met-AHZ-oh-leen high-droh-KLOR-ighd)

Afrin†, Afrin Children's Strength Nose Drops†, Allerest 12-Hour Nasal†, Chlorphed-LA†, Dristan Long Lasting†, Drixine Nasal◇, Duramist Plus†, Duration†, 4-Way Long-Acting Nasal, Genasal Spray†, Neo-Synephrine 12 Hour†, Nostrilla†, NTZ Long Acting Nasal†, Sinarest 12-Hour†, Sinex Long-Acting†, Twice-A-Day Nasal†

Pharmacologic class: sympathomimetic
Therapeutic class: decongestant, vaso-constrictor
Pregnancy risk category: NR

How supplied

Nasal solution: 0.025% , 0.05%

Pharmacokinetics

Unknown.

Route	Onset	Peak	Duration
Intranasal	5-10 min	≤ 6 hr	< 12 hr

Pharmacodynamics

Chemical effect: may cause local vaso-constriction of dilated arterioles, reducing blood flow and nasal congestion.
Therapeutic effect: relieves nasal congestion.

Indications and dosage

▶ **Nasal congestion.** *Adults and children age 6 and older:* 2 to 3 drops or sprays of 0.05% solution in each nostril b.i.d. *Children ages 2 to 6:* 2 to 3 drops of 0.025% solution in each nostril b.i.d. Do not use for more than 5 days.

Adverse reactions

CNS: headache, drowsiness, dizziness, insomnia, possible sedation.
CV: palpitations, *CV collapse,* hypertension.
EENT: rebound nasal congestion or irritation (with excessive or long-term use),
dryness of nose and throat, increased nasal discharge, stinging, sneezing.
Other: systemic effects in children (with excessive or long-term use).

Interactions

None significant.

Contraindications and precautions

• Contraindicated in patients with hypersensitivity to drug.
• Use cautiously in pregnant or breast-feeding women and in patients with hyperthyroidism, cardiac disease, hypertension, or diabetes mellitus.

NURSING CONSIDERATIONS

Assessment
• Assess patient's congestion before therapy and regularly thereafter.
• Be alert for adverse reactions.
• Evaluate patient's and family's knowledge of drug therapy.

Nursing diagnoses
• Altered health maintenance related to nasal congestion
• Risk for injury related to drug-induced adverse CNS reactions
• Knowledge deficit related to drug therapy

Planning and implementation
• When administering drug, have patient hold head upright, insert nozzle, and sniff spray briskly.
Patient teaching
• Teach patient how to use drug.
• Inform patient that product should be used by only one person to prevent spread of infection.
• Tell patient not to exceed recommended dosage and to use only when needed.
• Warn patient that excessive use may cause bradycardia, hypotension, dizziness, and weakness.

Evaluation
• Patient's nasal congestion is relieved.

• Patient sustains no injuries due to drug-induced adverse CNS reactions.
• Patient and family state understanding of drug therapy.

oxymorphone hydrochloride
(oks-ee-MOR-fohn high-droh-KLOR-ighd)
Numorphan, Numorphan H.P.

Pharmacologic class: opioid
Therapeutic class: analgesic
Controlled substance schedule: II
Pregnancy risk category: C

How supplied

Injection: 1 mg/ml, 1.5 mg/ml
Suppositories: 5 mg

Pharmacokinetics

Absorption: well absorbed.
Distribution: widely distributed.
Metabolism: metabolized primarily in liver.
Excretion: excreted primarily in urine.

Route	Onset	Peak	Duration
I.V.	5-10 min	15-30 min	3-4 hr
I.M.	10-15 min	30-90 min	3-6 hr
S.C.	10-20 min	60-90 min	3-6 hr
P.R.	15-30 min	About 2 hr	3-6 hr

Pharmacodynamics

Chemical effect: binds with opioid receptors in CNS, altering response to pain via unknown mechanism.
Therapeutic effect: relieves pain.

Indications and dosage

▶ **Moderate to severe pain.** *Adults:* 1 to 1.5 mg I.M. or S.C. q 4 to 6 hours, p.r.n.; or 0.5 mg I.V. q 4 to 6 hours, p.r.n.; or 5 mg P.R. q 4 to 6 hours, p.r.n.

Adverse reactions

CNS: *sedation, somnolence, clouded sensorium, euphoria,* dizziness, *seizures* (with large doses).
CV: *hypotension,* bradycardia.

GI: nausea, vomiting, constipation, ileus.
GU: urine retention.
Respiratory: *respiratory depression.*
Other: physical dependence.

Interactions

Drug-drug. *CNS depressants, general anesthetics, MAO inhibitors, tricyclic antidepressants:* additive effects. Use together with extreme caution.
Drug-lifestyle. *Alcohol use:* additive effects. Avoid concomitant use.

Contraindications and precautions

• Contraindicated in patients with hypersensitivity to drug.
• Use with extreme caution in elderly or debilitated patients and in those with head injury, increased intracranial pressure, seizures, asthma, COPD, acute abdominal conditions, prostatic hyperplasia, severe hepatic or renal disease, urethral stricture, respiratory depression, hypothyroidism, Addison's disease, or arrhythmias.
• Use with caution in pregnant or breast-feeding women.

NURSING CONSIDERATIONS

⚡ Assessment
• Assess patient's pain before and after drug administration.
• Be alert for adverse reactions and drug interactions.
• Evaluate patient's and family's knowledge of drug therapy.

Nursing diagnoses
• Pain related to condition
• Ineffective breathing pattern related to drug-induced respiratory depression
• Knowledge deficit related to drug therapy

Planning and implementation
• Keep narcotic antagonist (naloxone) and resuscitation equipment available.
• Do not give drug for mild to moderate pain. May worsen gallbladder pain.

Reactions may be *common*, uncommon, *life-threatening*, or COMMON AND LIFE-THREATENING.

• Give drug before patient has intense pain.

• Withhold dose and notify doctor if respirations decrease or rate is below 12 breaths/minute.

• Dependence can develop with long-term use.

I.V. use: Give drug by direct I.V. injection. If needed, dilute drug in 0.9% NaCl. Keep patient supine during administration to minimize hypotension.

I.M., S.C., and P.R. use: Follow normal protocol.

Patient teaching

• Instruct patient to take drug before pain becomes intense.

• Caution ambulatory patient about getting out of bed or walking. Warn outpatient to avoid hazardous activities until drug's CNS effects are known.

• Tell patient or family to report if patient's respiratory rate decreases.

☑ Evaluation

• Patient is free from pain.

• Patient's respiratory status is within normal limits.

• Patient and family state understanding of drug therapy.

oxytetracycline hydrochloride
(oks-ih-teh-truh-SIGH-kleen high-droh-KLOR-ighd)
Terramycin, Tija

Pharmacologic class: tetracycline
Therapeutic class: antibiotic
Pregnancy risk category: D

How supplied

Capsules: 250 mg
Injection: 50 mg/ml, 125 mg/ml (with lidocaine 2%)

Pharmacokinetics

Absorption: 60% absorbed from GI tract after oral administration in fasting patients. Absorption is significantly reduced by food or milk and other dairy products. I.M. absorption is erratic and incomplete. *Distribution:* distributed widely into body tissues and fluids, including synovial, pleural prostatic, and seminal fluids; bronchial secretions; saliva; and aqueous humor. CSF penetration is poor. Drug is 10% to 40% protein-bound. *Metabolism:* not metabolized. *Excretion:* excreted primarily unchanged in urine. *Half-life:* 6 to 10 hours.

Route	Onset	Peak	Duration
P.O.	Unknown	2-4 hr	Unknown
I.M.	Unknown	Unknown	Unknown

Pharmacodynamics

Chemical effect: unknown; may bind to 30S ribosomal subunit of microorganisms, thus inhibiting protein synthesis. *Therapeutic effect:* hinders bacterial growth of many gram-negative and gram-positive organisms, *Mycoplasma, Rickettsia, Chlamydia,* and spirochetes.

Indications and dosage

▶ **Infections caused by sensitive gram-negative and gram-positive organisms, trachoma, rickettsiae.** *Adults:* 250 to 500 mg P.O. q 6 hours, 100 mg I.M. q 8 to 12 hours, or 250 mg I.M. as single dose. *Children over age 8:* 25 to 50 mg/kg P.O. daily, in divided doses q 6 hours; 15 to 25 mg/kg I.M. daily, in divided doses q 8 to 12 hours.

▶ **Brucellosis.** *Adults:* 500 mg P.O. q.i.d. for 3 weeks combined with 1 g of streptomycin I.M. q 12 hours first week, once daily second week.

▶ **Syphilis in patients sensitive to penicillin.** *Adults:* 30 to 40 g total dosage P.O., divided equally over 15 days.

▶ **Gonorrhea in patients sensitive to penicillin.** *Adults:* initially, 1.5 g P.O., followed by 0.5 g q.i.d., for total of 9 g.

Adverse reactions

CNS: *intracranial hypertension* (pseudotumor cerebri).
CV: pericarditis.

EENT: dysphagia, glossitis; permanent discoloration of teeth and enamel defects (in children under age 8).
GI: *anorexia, nausea,* vomiting, *diarrhea,* oral candidiasis, enterocolitis, anogenital inflammation.
GU: increased BUN levels.
Hematologic: neutropenia, eosinophilia.
Hepatic: elevated liver enzymes.
Musculoskeletal: bone growth retardation (in children under age 8).
Skin: maculopapular and erythematous rashes, urticaria, photosensitivity, increased pigmentation.
Other: hypersensitivity reactions *(anaphylaxis),* superinfection, *thrombophlebitis, irritation* (after I.M. injection).

Interactions

Drug-drug. *Antacids (including sodium bicarbonate) and laxatives containing aluminum, magnesium, calcium; antidiarrheals:* decreased antibiotic absorption. Give antibiotic 1 hour before or 2 hours after any of above agents.
Ferrous sulfate, other iron products, zinc: decreased antibiotic absorption. Give antibiotic 3 hours after or 2 hours before iron.
Methoxyflurane: may cause nephrotoxicity with tetracyclines. Monitor carefully.
Oral anticoagulants: increased anticoagulant effect. Monitor PT and INR and adjust dosage as ordered.
Oral contraceptives: decreased contraceptive effectiveness and increased risk of breakthrough bleeding. Use nonhormonal form of birth control.
Penicillins: may interfere with bactericidal action of penicillins. Avoid use together.
Drug-food. *Food, milk, or other dairy products:* decreased antibiotic absorption. Give antibiotic 1 hour before or 2 hours after any of above agents.

Contraindications and precautions

• Contraindicated in patients with hypersensitivity to drug or other tetracyclines.
• Use cautiously in patients with impaired renal or hepatic function. Use dur-

ing last half of pregnancy and in children under age 8 may cause permanent discoloration of teeth, enamel defects, and bone growth retardation.

NURSING CONSIDERATIONS

⚠ Assessment
• Assess patient's infection before therapy and regularly thereafter.
• Obtain specimen for culture and sensitivity tests. Therapy may begin pending results.
• Ask patient about hypersensitivity reactions to local anesthetics when administering I.M. preparations.
• Be alert for adverse reactions and drug interactions.
• Monitor patient's hydration status if adverse GI reactions occur.
• Evaluate patient's and family's knowledge of drug therapy.

⊕ Nursing diagnoses
• Infection related to presence of bacteria
• Risk for fluid volume deficit related to drug-induced adverse GI reactions
• Knowledge deficit related to drug therapy

❯ Planning and implementation
• Check expiration date. Outdated or deteriorated oxytetracyclines have been associated with reversible nephrotoxicity (Fanconi's syndrome).
• Don't expose drug to light or heat.
P.O. use: Administer drug on empty stomach. Give last dose of day at least 1 hour before bedtime.
I.M. use: Inject drug deeply into large muscle mass. Rotate sites. I.M. preparations contain local anesthetic.
• Parenteral form may cause false-positive reading of copper sulfate tests (Clinitest). All forms may cause false-negative reading of glucose enzymatic tests (Diastix).
Patient teaching
• Warn patient that I.M. injection may be painful.

- Explain to patient that oral drug's effectiveness is reduced when taken with milk or other dairy products, food, antacids, or iron products. Tell him to take each dose with full glass of water at least 1 hour before or 2 hours after meals. Advise him to take last dose at least 1 hour before bedtime to prevent esophagitis.
- Tell patient to take drug exactly as prescribed, even after he feels better.
- Warn patient to avoid direct sunlight and ultraviolet light and to use a sunscreen. Photosensitivity persists for some time after therapy ends.

☑ **Evaluation**
- Patient is free from infection.
- Patient maintains adequate hydration throughout drug therapy.
- Patient and family state understanding of drug therapy.

---

oxytocin, synthetic injection
(oks-ih-TOH-sin, sin-THET-ik in-JEK-shun)
Oxytocin, Pitocin

Pharmacologic class: exogenous hormone
Therapeutic class: oxytocic, lactation stimulant
Pregnancy risk category: C

How supplied
Injection: 10 units/ml ampule or vial

Pharmacokinetics
Absorption: unknown after I.M. administration.
Distribution: distributed through extracellular fluid.
Metabolism: metabolized rapidly in kidneys and liver. In early pregnancy, a circulating enzyme, oxytocinase, can inactivate drug.
Excretion: small amounts excreted in urine. *Half-life:* 3 to 5 minutes.

Route	Onset	Peak	Duration
I.V.	Immediate	Unknown	1 hr
I.M.	3-5 min	Unknown	2-3 hr

Pharmacodynamics
Chemical effect: causes potent and selective stimulation of uterine and mammary gland smooth muscle.
Therapeutic effect: induces labor and milk ejection and reduces postpartum bleeding.

Indications and dosage
▶ **Induction or stimulation of labor.**
Adults: initially, 1 ml (10 units) ampule in 1,000 ml of dextrose 5% injection or 0.9% NaCl solution I.V. infused at 1 to 2 milliunits/minute. Rate increased in increments of no more than 1 to 2 milliunits/minute at 15- to 30-minute intervals until normal contraction pattern is established. Rate decreased when labor is firmly established.
▶ **Reduction of postpartum bleeding after expulsion of placenta.** *Adults:* 10 to 40 units added to 1,000 ml of D_5W or 0.9% NaCl solution infused at rate necessary to control bleeding, usually 20 to 40 milliunits/minute. Also, 1 ml (10 units) can be given I.M. after delivery of placenta.
▶ **Incomplete or inevitable abortion.**
Adults: 10 units of oxytocin I.V. in 500 ml of 0.9% NaCl solution or dextrose 5% in 0.9% NaCl solution. Infuse at rate of 20 to 40 drops/minute.

Adverse reactions
Maternal
CNS: *subarachnoid hemorrhage* (from hypertension); *seizures, coma* (from water intoxication).
CV: *hypertension;* increased heart rate, systemic venous return, and cardiac output; *arrhythmias.*
GI: nausea, vomiting.
Hematologic: afibrinogenemia (may be related to postpartum bleeding).
Other: hypersensitivity reactions *(anaphylaxis),* tetanic uterine contractions,

---

abruptio placentae, impaired uterine blood flow, pelvic hematoma, *increased uterine motility.*
Fetal
CV: bradycardia, tachycardia, *PVCs.*
Hematologic: hyperbilirubinemia.
Respiratory: *anoxia, asphyxia.*

Interactions

Drug-drug. *Cyclopropane anesthetics:* less pronounced bradycardia and hypotension. Use together cautiously.
Thiopental anesthetics: possible delayed induction. Use together cautiously.
Vasoconstrictors: severe hypertension if oxytocin is given within 3 to 4 hours of vasoconstrictor in patients receiving caudal block anesthetic. Avoid concomitant use.

Contraindications and precautions

• Contraindicated in cephalopelvic disproportion or delivery that requires conversion, as in transverse lie; in fetal distress when delivery isn't imminent, prematurity, and other obstetric emergencies; and in patients with severe toxemia, hypertonic uterine patterns, drug hypersensitivity, total placenta previa, or vasoprevia.
• Use with extreme caution during first and second stages of labor because cervical laceration, uterine rupture, and maternal and fetal death have been reported.
• Use with extreme caution, if at all, in patients with history of cervical or uterine surgery, grand multiparity, uterine sepsis, traumatic delivery, or overdistended uterus and in invasive cervical carcinoma.

NURSING CONSIDERATIONS

Assessment
• Assess patient's condition before therapy and regularly thereafter.
• Monitor and record uterine contractions, heart rate, blood pressure, intrauterine pressure, fetal heart rate, and blood loss every 15 minutes.
• Be alert for adverse reactions and drug interactions.

• Monitor fluid intake and output. Antidiuretic effect may lead to fluid overload, seizures, and coma.
• Evaluate patient's and family's knowledge of drug therapy.

Nursing diagnoses
• Risk for fluid volume deficit related to postpartum bleeding
• Fluid volume excess related to drug-induced antidiuretic effect
• Knowledge deficit related to drug therapy

Planning and implementation
• Drug is used to induce or reinforce labor only when pelvis is known to be adequate, vaginal delivery is indicated, fetal maturity is assured, and fetal position is favorable. Should be used only in hospital where critical care facilities and doctor are immediately available.
I.V. use: Don't give drug by I.V. bolus injection. Administer by infusion only; give by piggyback infusion so drug may be discontinued without interrupting I.V. line. Use infusion pump.
I.M. use: Drug is not recommended for routine I.M. use. However, 10 units may be given I.M. after delivery of placenta to control postpartum uterine bleeding.
• Never give oxytocin simultaneously by more than one route.
• Have magnesium sulfate (20% solution) available for relaxation of myometrium.
• If contractions occur less than 2 minutes apart and if contractions above 50 mm Hg are recorded, or if contractions last 90 seconds or longer, stop infusion, turn patient on her side, and notify doctor.
Patient teaching
• Instruct patient to report unusual feelings or adverse effects at once.

Evaluation
• Patient maintains adequate fluid balance with drug therapy.
• Patient shows no signs of edema.
• Patient and family state understanding of drug therapy.

Reactions may be *common,* uncommon, *life-threatening*, or COMMON AND LIFE-THREATENING.

paclitaxel
(pak-lih-TAK-sil)
Taxol

Pharmacologic class: novel anti-
microtubule
Therapeutic class: antineoplastic
Pregnancy risk category: D

How supplied

Injection: 30 mg/5 ml

Pharmacokinetics

Absorption: not applicable.
Distribution: about 89% to 98% of drug
is bound to serum proteins.
Metabolism: may be metabolized in liver.
Excretion: unknown.

Route	Onset	Peak	Duration
I.V.	Unknown	Unknown	Unknown

Pharmacodynamics

Chemical effect: prevents depolymerization of cellular microtubules, thus inhibiting normal reorganization of microtubule
network necessary for mitosis and other
vital cellular functions.
Therapeutic effect: hinders ovarian and
breast cancer cell activity.

Indications and dosage

▶ **Metastatic ovarian cancer after failure of first-line or subsequent chemotherapy.** *Adults:* 135 mg/m² or 175 mg/
m² I.V. over 3 hours q 3 weeks.
▶ **Breast cancer after failure of combination chemotherapy for metastatic
disease or relapse within 6 months of
adjuvant chemotherapy.** *Adults:*
175 mg/m² I.V. over 3 hours q 3 weeks.

Adverse reactions

CNS: *peripheral neuropathy.*

CV: *bradycardia, hypotension, abnormal
ECG.*
GI: *nausea, vomiting, diarrhea, mucosi-
tis.*
Hematologic: NEUTROPENIA, LEUKOPE-
NIA, THROMBOCYTOPENIA, *anemia,
bleeding.*
Hepatic: elevated liver enzymes.
Musculoskeletal: *myalgia, arthralgia,*
Other: hypersensitivity reactions *(ana-
phylaxis),* alopecia, phlebitis; cellulitis
(at injection site).

Interactions

Drug-drug. *Cisplatin:* possible additive
myelosuppressive effects. Use together
cautiously.
Ketoconazole: inhibited paclitaxel metabolism. Use together cautiously.

Contraindications and precautions

• Contraindicated in patients who are hypersensitive to drug or to polyoxyethylated castor oil, a vehicle used in drug solution, and in patients with baseline neutrophil counts below 1,500/mm³.
• Drug use is not recommended in pregnant or breast-feeding women.
• Use cautiously in patients who have received prior radiation therapy; they may
display more frequent or severe myelosuppression.
• Safety of drug has not been established
in children.

NURSING CONSIDERATIONS

Assessment
• Assess patient's condition before therapy and regularly thereafter.
• Continuously monitor patient for first
30 minutes of infusion. Monitor closely
throughout infusion.
• Monitor blood counts frequently during
therapy.
• Be alert for adverse reactions and drug
interactions.
• Evaluate patient's and family's knowledge of drug therapy.

🔁 Nursing diagnoses
• Altered health maintenance related to neoplastic disease
• Altered protection related to drug-induced adverse hematologic reactions
• Knowledge deficit related to drug therapy

⟩ Planning and implementation
• To reduce severe hypersensitivity, expect to pretreat patient with corticosteroids, such as dexamethasone, and antihistamines, as ordered. H_1-receptor antagonists, such as diphenhydramine, and H_2-receptor antagonists, such as cimetidine or ranitidine, may be used.
• Follow institutional protocol for safe handling, preparation, and use of chemotherapeutic drugs. Preparation and administration of parenteral form are associated with carcinogenic, mutagenic, and teratogenic risks for personnel. Mark all waste materials with "CHEMOTHERAPY HAZARD" labels.
• Dilute concentrate to 0.3 to 1.2 mg/ml before infusion. Compatible solutions include 0.9% NaCl injection, D_5W, 5% dextrose in 0.9% NaCl injection, and 5% dextrose in Ringer's lactate injection. Diluted solutions are stable for 27 hours at room temperature.
• Prepare and store infusion solutions in glass containers. The undiluted concentrate shouldn't come in contact with polyvinylchloride I.V. bags or tubing. Store diluted solution in glass or polypropylene bottles, or use polypropylene or polyolefin bags. Administer through polyethylene-lined administration sets, and use in-line 0.22-micron filter.
• Take care to avoid extravasation.
Patient teaching
• Warn patient to watch for signs of bleeding and infection.
• Teach patient symptoms of peripheral neuropathy, such as tingling or burning sensation or numbness in extremities, and advise her to report them immediately. Although mild symptoms are common,

severe symptoms occur infrequently. Dosage reduction may be necessary.
• Warn patient that alopecia is common (up to 82% of patients).
• Advise female patient of childbearing age to avoid pregnancy during therapy. Also recommend consulting with doctor before becoming pregnant.

☑ Evaluation
• Patient responds well to therapy.
• Patient develops no serious complications as result of drug-induced adverse hematological reactions.
• Patient and family state understanding of drug therapy.

---

pamidronate disodium
(pam-ih-DROH-nayt digh-SOH-dee-um)
Aredia

Pharmacologic class: bisphosphonate; pyrophosphate analogue
Therapeutic class: antihypercalcemic
Pregnancy risk category: C

How supplied
Injection: 30 mg/vial, 60 mg/vial, 90 mg/vial

Pharmacokinetics
Absorption: not applicable.
Distribution: about 50% to 60% of dose is rapidly taken up by bone; drug is also taken up by kidneys, liver, spleen, teeth, and tracheal cartilage.
Metabolism: none.
Excretion: excreted by kidneys. *Half-life:* alpha, 1.6 hours; beta, 27.2 hours.

Route	Onset	Peak	Duration
I.V.	Unknown	Unknown	Unknown

Pharmacodynamics
Chemical effect: inhibits bone resorption. Adsorbs to hydroxyapatite crystals in bone and may directly block calcium phosphate dissolution.

Therapeutic effect: lowers blood calcium levels.

Indications and dosage

► **Moderate to severe hypercalcemia associated with cancer (with or without bone metastases).** *Adults:* dosage depends on severity of hypercalcemia. Serum calcium levels are corrected for serum albumin as follows:

Corrected serum   serum   0.8 (4 - serum
calcium (CCa) = calcium + albumin)
(in mg/dl)   (in mg/dl)   (in g/dl)

Patients with moderate hypercalcemia (CCa levels of 12 to 13.5 mg/dl) may receive 60 to 90 mg by I.V. infusion; 60-mg dose given over at least 4 hours, 90-mg dose infused over 24 hours. Those with severe hypercalcemia (CCa levels over 13.5 mg/dl) may receive 90 mg by I.V. infusion over 24 hours. At least 7 days should elapse before retreatment to allow full response to initial dose.

► **Moderate to severe Paget's disease.** *Adults:* 30 mg I.V. as 4-hour infusion on 3 consecutive days for total dose of 90 mg. Cycle repeated, p.r.n.

Adverse reactions

CNS: *seizures.*
CV: *fluid overload, hypertension, atrial fibrillation.*
GI: *abdominal pain, anorexia, constipation, nausea, vomiting, GI hemorrhage.*
GU: *urinary tract infection.*
Hematologic: *leukopenia, thrombocytopenia,* anemia.
Metabolism: hypophosphatemia, hypokalemia, hypomagnesemia, hypocalcemia.
Other: bone pain, fever, redness, swelling, pain.

Interactions

None significant.

Contraindications and precautions

• Contraindicated in patients hypersensitive to drug or to other biphosphonates, such as etidronate.

• Use with extreme caution in patients with renal impairment.
• Use cautiously in pregnant or breast-feeding women.
• Safety of drug has not been established in children.

NURSING CONSIDERATIONS

Assessment
• Assess patient's condition before therapy and regularly thereafter.
• Assess hydration before treatment.
• Closely monitor serum electrolytes, creatinine level, CBC and differential, hematocrit, and hemoglobin, as ordered.
• Carefully monitor patient with preexisting anemia, leukopenia, or thrombocytopenia during first 2 weeks of therapy.
• Monitor patient's temperature. Fever is most likely 24 to 48 hours after therapy.
• Be alert for adverse reactions and drug interactions.
• Evaluate patient's and family's knowledge of drug therapy.

Nursing diagnoses
• Altered health maintenance related to hypercalcemia
• Risk for injury related to drug-induced hypocalcemia
• Knowledge deficit related to drug therapy

Planning and implementation
• Use drug only after patient has been vigorously hydrated with NaCl solution. In patients with mild to moderate hypercalcemia, hydration alone may be sufficient.
• Reconstitute vial with 10 ml of sterile water for injection. After drug is dissolved, add to 1,000 ml of 0.45% or 0.9% NaCl injection or D₅W. Do not mix with infusion solutions that contain calcium, such as Ringer's injection or lactated Ringer's injection. Inspect for precipitate before administering.
• Give drug only by I.V. infusion. Animals have developed nephropathy when drug is given as bolus.

• Know that short-term administration of calcium may be necessary in patient with severe hypocalcemia.
• Solution is stable for 24 hours at room temperature.

Patient teaching
• Instruct patient to report unusual signs or symptoms at once.
• Inform patient of need for frequent tests to monitor effectiveness of drug and detect adverse reactions.

☑ **Evaluation**
• Patient's blood calcium level returns to normal.
• Patient does not develop hypocalcemia during drug therapy.
• Patient and family state understanding of drug therapy.

---

pancreatin

(pan-kree-AH-tin)
Dizymes Tablets†, Donnazyme, 8X Pancreatin 900 mg†, Entozyme, 4X Pancreatin 600 mg†, Hi-Vegi-Lip Tablets†, Pancrezyme 4X Tablets†

Pharmacologic class: pancreatic enzyme
Therapeutic class: digestant
Pregnancy risk category: C

How supplied

Bioglan Panazyme†
Tablets: 468 mg pancreatin, 7,200 units lipase, 656 units protease, and 9,200 units amylase
Dizymes
Tablets (enteric-coated): 250 mg pancreatin, 6,750 units lipase, 41,250 units protease, and 43,750 units amylase†
Donnazyme
Tablets: 500 mg pancreatin, 1,000 units lipase, 12,500 units protease, and 12,500 units amylase
8X Pancreatin 900 mg
Tablets (enteric-coated): 7,200 mg pancreatin, 22,500 units lipase, 180,000 units protease, and 180,000 units amylase†

Entozyme
Tablets: 500 mg pancreatin, 600 units lipase, 7,500 units protease, and 7,500 units amylase
4X Pancreatin 600 mg
Tablets (enteric-coated): 2,400 mg pancreatin, 12,000 units lipase, 60,000 units protease, and 60,000 units amylase†
Hi-Vegi-Lip
Tablets (enteric-coated): 2,400 mg pancreatin, 4,800 units lipase, 60,000 units protease, and 60,000 units amylase†
Pancrezyme 4X
Tablets (enteric-coated): 2,400 mg pancreatin, 12,000 units lipase, 60,000 units protease, and 60,000 units amylase†

Pharmacokinetics

Absorption: not absorbed; it acts locally in GI tract.
Distribution: none.
Metabolism: none.
Excretion: excreted in feces.

Route	Onset	Peak	Duration
P.O.	Unknown	1-2 hr	Unknown

Pharmacodynamics

Chemical effect: replaces endogenous exocrine pancreatic enzymes.
Therapeutic effect: aids digestion of starches, fats, and proteins.

Indications and dosage

▶ **Exocrine pancreatic secretion insufficiency; digestive aid in diseases associated with deficiency of pancreatic enzymes, such as cystic fibrosis.** *Adults and children:* dosage varies with condition being treated. Usual initial dosage is 8,000 to 24,000 units of lipase activity before or with each meal or snack. Total daily dose also may be given in divided doses at 1- to 2-hour intervals throughout day.

Adverse reactions

GI: nausea, diarrhea (with high doses).
Metabolic: hyperuricuria (with high doses).

Reactions may be *common*, uncommon, *life-threatening*, or COMMON AND LIFE-THREATENING.

Interactions

Drug-drug. *Antacids:* may negate pancreatin's effect. Avoid concomitant use.

Contraindications and precautions

• Contraindicated in patients with acute pancreatitis, acute exacerbations of chronic pancreatitis, and hypersensitivity to drug or to pork protein or enzymes.
• Use with caution in pregnant or breast-feeding women.

NURSING CONSIDERATIONS

Assessment

• Assess patient's condition before therapy and regularly thereafter. Decreased number of bowel movements and improved stool consistency indicate effective therapy.
• Monitor patient's diet to ensure proper balance of fat, protein, and starch intake to avoid indigestion. Dosage varies according to degree of maldigestion and malabsorption, amount of fat in diet, and enzyme activity of drug.
• Evaluate patient's and family's knowledge of drug therapy.

Nursing diagnoses

• Altered nutrition: less than body requirements related to condition
• Noncompliance related to long-term therapy
• Knowledge deficit related to drug therapy

Planning and implementation

• USP standards dictate that each milligram of bovine or porcine pancreatin contain lipase 2 units, protease 25 units, and amylase 25 units.
• Drug is not effective in GI disorders unrelated to pancreatic enzyme deficiency.
• Enteric coating on some products may reduce availability of enzyme in upper portion of jejunum.
Patient teaching
• Tell patient not to crush or chew enteric-coated dosage forms. However, capsules containing enteric-coated microspheres may be opened and contents sprinkled on small quantity of soft food or applesauce.
• Tell patient to store in airtight containers at room temperature.

Evaluation

• Patient maintains normal digestion of fats, carbohydrates, and proteins.
• Patient complies with prescribed drug regimen.
• Patient and family state understanding of drug therapy.

pancrelipase

(pan-krih-LIGH-pays)
Cotazym Capsules, Cotazym-S Capsules, Creon 5 Delayed-Release Minimicrospheres Capsules, Creon 10 Delayed-Release Minimicrospheres Capsules, Creon 20 Delayed-Release Minimicrospheres Capsules, Ilozyme Tablets, Ku-Zyme HP Capsules, Pancrease Capsules, Pancrease MT 4, Pancrease MT 10, Pancrease MT 16, Pancrelipase Capsules, Protilase Capsules, Ultrase MT 12, Ultrase MT 20, Viokase Powder, Viokase Tablets, Zymase Capsules

Pharmacologic class: pancreatic enzyme
Therapeutic class: digestant
Pregnancy risk category: C

How supplied

Cotazym
Capsules: 8,000 units lipase, 30,000 units protease, 30,000 units amylase, and 25 mg calcium carbonate
Cotazym-S
Capsules (enteric-coated spheres): 5,000 units lipase, 20,000 units protease, and 20,000 units amylase
Creon 5
Capsules (delayed-release minimicrospheres): 5,000 units lipase, 18,750 units protease, 16,600 units amylase

Creon 10
Capsules (delayed-release minimicrospheres): 10,000 units lipase, 37,500 units protease, 33,200 units amylase
Creon 20
Capsules (delayed-release minimicrospheres): 20,000 units lipase, 75,000 units protease, 66,400 units amylase
Ilozyme
Tablets: 11,000 units lipase, 30,000 units protease, and 30,000 units amylase
Ku-Zyme HP
Capsules: 8,000 units lipase, 30,000 units protease, and 30,000 units amylase
Pancrease
Capsules (enteric-coated microspheres): 4,000 units lipase, 25,000 units protease, and 20,000 units amylase
Pancrease MT 4
Capsules (enteric-coated microtablets): 4,000 units lipase, 12,000 units protease, and 12,000 units amylase
Pancrease MT 10
Capsules (enteric-coated microtablets): 10,000 units lipase, 30,000 units protease, and 30,000 units amylase
Pancrease MT 16
Capsules (enteric-coated microtablets): 16,000 units lipase, 48,000 units protease, and 48,000 units amylase
Pancrelipase
Capsules (enteric-coated pellets): 4,000 units lipase, 25,000 units protease, and 20,000 units amylase
Protilase
Capsules (enteric-coated spheres): 4,000 units lipase, 25,000 units protease, and 20,000 units amylase
Ultrase MT 12
Capsules (delayed-release): 12,000 units lipase, 39,000 units protease, and 39,000 units amylase
Ultrase MT 20
Capsules: 20,000 units lipase, 65,000 units protease, and 65,000 units amylase
Viokase
Tablets: 8,000 units lipase, 30,000 units protease, 30,000 units amylase

Powder: 16,800 units lipase, 70,000 units protease, and 70,000 units amylase per 0.7 g powder
Zymase
Capsules (enteric-coated spheres): 12,000 units lipase, 24,000 units protease, and 24,000 units amylase

Pharmacokinetics
Absorption: not absorbed; it acts locally in GI tract.
Distribution: none.
Metabolism: none.
Excretion: excreted in feces.

Route	Onset	Peak	Duration
P.O.	Varies	Varies	Varies

Pharmacodynamics
Chemical effect: replaces endogenous exocrine pancreatic enzymes.
Therapeutic effect: aids digestion of starches, fats, and proteins.

Indications and dosage
▶ Exocrine pancreatic secretion insufficiency, cystic fibrosis in adults and children, steatorrhea and other disorders of fat metabolism secondary to insufficient pancreatic enzymes. *Adults and children:* dosage titrated to patient's response. Usual initial dosage is 4,000 to 33,000 units of lipase activity with each meal or snack.

Adverse reactions
GI: *nausea,* cramping, diarrhea (high doses).

Interactions
Drug-drug. *Antacids:* may destroy enteric coating and enhance degradation of pancrelipase. Avoid concomitant use.

Contraindications and precautions
• Contraindicated in patients with acute pancreatitis, acute exacerbations of chronic pancreatitis, and hypersensitivity to drug or to pork protein or enzymes.

Reactions may be *common,* uncommon, *life-threatening,* or COMMON AND LIFE-THREATENING.

• Use with caution in pregnant or breast-feeding women.

NURSING CONSIDERATIONS

Assessment
• Assess patient's condition before therapy and regularly thereafter. Decreased number of bowel movements and improved stool consistency indicate effective therapy.
• Monitor patient's diet to ensure proper balance of fat, protein, and starch intake to avoid indigestion. Dosage varies according to degree of maldigestion and malabsorption, amount of fat in diet, and enzyme activity of drug.
• Be alert for adverse reactions and drug interactions.
• Evaluate patient's and family's knowledge of drug therapy.

Nursing diagnoses
• Altered nutrition: less than body requirements related to condition
• Noncompliance related to long-term therapy
• Knowledge deficit related to drug therapy

Planning and implementation
• For infant, mix powder with applesauce and give with meals. Avoid contact with or inhalation of powder; it may be irritating. Older child may take capsules with food.
• USP standards dictate that each mg of pancrelipase contain 24 units lipase, 100 units protease, and 100 units amylase.
• Know that enteric coating on some products may reduce availability of enzyme in upper portion of jejunum.
• Drug is not effective in GI disorders unrelated to pancreatic enzyme deficiency.
Patient teaching
• Advise patient not to crush or chew enteric-coated dosage forms.
• Tell patient to store in airtight containers at room temperature.

Evaluation
• Patient maintains normal digestion of fats, carbohydrates, and proteins.
• Patient complies with prescribed drug regimen.
• Patient and family state understanding of drug therapy.

pancuronium bromide
(pan-kyoo-ROH-nee-um BROH-mighd)
Pavulon

Pharmacologic class: nondepolarizing neuromuscular blocker
Therapeutic class: skeletal muscle relaxant
Pregnancy risk category: C

How supplied
Injection: 1 mg/ml, 2 mg/ml

Pharmacokinetics
Absorption: not applicable.
Distribution: drug has very low protein binding regardless of dose.
Metabolism: unknown.
Excretion: excreted mainly in urine; some biliary excretion. *Half-life:* 114 to 116 minutes.

Route	Onset	Peak	Duration
I.V.	30-45 sec	3-4.5 min	35-45 min

Pharmacodynamics
Chemical effect: prevents acetylcholine from binding to receptors on muscle end plate, thus blocking depolarization.
Therapeutic effect: relaxes skeletal muscles.

Indications and dosage
▶ **Adjunct to anesthesia to induce skeletal muscle relaxation; to facilitate intubation; to lessen muscle contractions in pharmacologically or electrically induced seizures; to assist with mechanical ventilation.** Dosage depends on anesthetic used, individual needs, and

response. Dosages are representative and must be adjusted. *Adults and children age 1 month and over:* initially, 0.04 to 0.1 mg/kg I.V.; then 0.01 mg/kg q 25 to 60 minutes. *Neonates up to age 1 month:* individualized.

Adverse reactions

CV: tachycardia, increased blood pressure.
Musculoskeletal: residual muscle weakness.
Respiratory: prolonged, *dose-related respiratory insufficiency or apnea;* wheezing.
Skin: transient rashes.
Other: burning sensation, excessive sweating and salivation, allergic or idiosyncratic hypersensitivity reactions.

Interactions

Drug-drug. *Aminoglycoside antibiotics, including amikacin, gentamicin, kanamycin, neomycin, streptomycin; clindamycin; general anesthetics; polymyxin antibiotics (such as polymyxin B sulfate, colistin, polymyxin B sulfate); quinidine:* potentiated neuromuscular blockade, leading to increased skeletal muscle relaxation and prolongation of effect. Use cautiously during surgical and postoperative periods.
Lithium, opioid analgesics: potentiated neuromuscular blockade, leading to increased skeletal muscle relaxation and possible respiratory paralysis. Use with extreme caution, and reduce dose of pancuronium.
Succinylcholine: increased intensity and duration of blockade. Allow succinylcholine effects to subside before giving pancuronium.

Contraindications and precautions

• Contraindicated in patients with hypersensitivity to bromides or preexisting tachycardia and in those for whom even minor increase in heart rate is undesirable.

• Use cautiously in elderly or debilitated patients and in those with renal, hepatic, or pulmonary impairment; respiratory depression; myasthenia gravis; myasthenic syndrome of lung cancer or bronchogenic carcinoma; dehydration; thyroid disorders; collagen diseases; porphyria; electrolyte disturbances; hyperthermia; or toxemic states. Use large doses cautiously in pregnant women undergoing cesarean section and in breast-feeding women.

NURSING CONSIDERATIONS

Assessment
• Assess patient's condition before therapy and regularly thereafter.
• Monitor baseline electrolyte determinations (electrolyte imbalance can potentiate neuromuscular effects) and vital signs.
• Measure fluid intake and output; renal dysfunction may prolong duration of action because 25% of drug is unchanged before excretion.
• Nerve stimulator and train-of-four monitoring are recommended to confirm antagonism of neuromuscular blockade and recovery of muscle strength. Before attempting pharmacologic reversal with neostigmine, one should see some evidence of spontaneous recovery.
• Monitor respirations closely until patient fully recovers from neuromuscular blockade, as evidenced by tests of muscle strength (hand grip, head lift, and ability to cough).
• Be alert for adverse reactions and drug interactions.
• Evaluate patient's and family's knowledge of drug therapy.

Nursing diagnoses
• Altered health maintenance related to condition
• Ineffective breathing pattern related to drug's effect on respiratory muscles
• Knowledge deficit related to drug therapy

Reactions may be *common*, uncommon, *life-threatening*, or COMMON AND LIFE-THREATENING.

▶ Planning and implementation
• Administer sedatives or general anesthetics before neuromuscular blockers, as ordered. Neuromuscular blockers do not obtund consciousness or alter pain threshold.
• Pancuronium should be used only by personnel skilled in airway management.
• Do not mix drug with alkaline solutions, such as barbiturate solutions, because precipitate will form; use only fresh solutions.
• Allow succinylcholine effects to subside before giving pancuronium, as ordered.
• Store drug in refrigerator. Do not store in plastic containers or syringes, although plastic syringes may be used for administration.
• Give analgesics, as ordered, for pain. Remember, patient will not be able to indicate that pain is present.
• Have emergency respiratory support equipment (endotracheal equipment, ventilator, oxygen, atropine, edrophonium, epinephrine, and neostigmine) immediately available.
• Once spontaneous recovery starts, drug-induced neuromuscular blockade may be reversed with anticholinesterase agent (such as neostigmine or edrophonium). Usually administered with anticholinergic (such as atropine).
Patient teaching
• Explain all events and happenings to patient because he can still hear.
• Reassure patient that he is being monitored at all times and that pain medication will be provided, if appropriate.
• Tell patient that he may feel burning sensation at injection site.

☑ Evaluation
• Patient's condition improves.
• Patient maintains adequate ventilation with mechanical assistance.
• Patient and family state understanding of drug therapy.

papaverine hydrochloride
(puh-PAV-eh-reen high-droh-KLOR-ighd)
Cerespan, Genabid, Pavabid, Pavabid HP, Pavabid Plateau, Pavacels, Pavagen, Pavarine, Pavased, Pavatym, Paverolan

Pharmacologic class: benzylisoquinoline derivative, opioid alkaloid
Therapeutic class: peripheral vasodilator
Pregnancy risk category: C

How supplied
Tablets: 60 mg, 100 mg, 200 mg, 300 mg
Tablets (timed-release): 200 mg
Capsules (timed-release): 150 mg
Injection: 30 mg/ml, 32.5 mg/ml ♦

Pharmacokinetics
Absorption: 54% of oral drug is bioavailable; sustained-release forms are sometimes absorbed poorly and erratically. Absorption unknown after I.M. administration.
Distribution: drug tends to localize in adipose tissue and in liver; remainder is distributed throughout body. About 90% of drug is protein-bound.
Metabolism: metabolized by liver.
Excretion: excreted in urine as metabolites.

Route	Onset	Peak	Duration
P.O.	Rapid	1-2 hr	12 hr (timed-release); Unknown (regular)
I.V.	Unknown	Unknown	Unknown
I.M.	Unknown	Unknown	Unknown

Pharmacodynamics
Chemical effect: has direct, nonspecific relaxant effect on vascular, cardiac, and other smooth muscle.
Therapeutic effect: relieves vascular spasms.

Indications and dosage
▶ **Relief of cerebral and peripheral ischemia associated with arterial spasm**

and myocardial ischemia; treatment of coronary occlusion and certain cerebral angiospastic states. *Adults:* 100 to 300 mg P.O. three to five times daily, or 150- to 300-mg timed-release preparations q 8 to 12 hours; 30 to 120 mg I.M. or I.V. slowly over 1 to 2 minutes q 3 hours, as indicated.

Adverse reactions

CNS: *headache,* depression, malaise.
CV: *increased heart rate, increased blood pressure* (parenteral use), depressed AV and intraventricular conduction, hypotension, *arrhythmias.*
GI: constipation, dry mouth, *nausea.*
Hepatic: *hepatitis (jaundice, eosinophilia, abnormal liver function tests), cirrhosis.*
Respiratory: increased depth of respiration, *apnea.*
Other: *diaphoresis, flushing.*

Interactions

Drug-drug. *Levodopa:* papaverine may interfere with levodopa's therapeutic effects in patients with Parkinson's disease. Monitor patient closely.

Contraindications and precautions

• I.V. use is contraindicated in patients with Parkinson's disease or complete AV block.
• Use cautiously in patients with glaucoma and in pregnant women.
• Safety of drug has not been established in breast-feeding women and in children.

NURSING CONSIDERATIONS

✎ Assessment
• Assess patient's condition before therapy and regularly thereafter.
• Monitor blood pressure and heart rate and rhythm, especially in patient with cardiac disease.
• Be alert for adverse reactions and drug interactions.
• Monitor for adverse hepatic reactions during long-term therapy.

• Evaluate patient's and family's knowledge of drug therapy.

⊕ Nursing diagnoses
• Altered tissue perfusion (cerebral, cardiopulmonary, peripheral, gastrointestinal) related to vascular spasms
• Constipation related to drug's effect on GI tract
• Knowledge deficit related to drug therapy

⊠ Planning and implementation
P.O. and I.M. use: Follow normal protocol.
I.V. use: Give drug by direct injection over 1 to 2 minutes to minimize risk of serious adverse reactions. Do not add to lactated Ringer's injection, because precipitate forms.
• Drug is most effective when given early in course of disorder.
• FDA has announced this drug may not be effective for diseases indicated.
• Hold dose and notify doctor at once if vital signs change.
Patient teaching
• Tell patient to take drug regularly; long-term therapy is required.
• Advise patient to avoid hazardous activities until drug's CNS effects are known.
• Instruct patient to avoid sudden position changes.

☑ Evaluation
• Patient maintains adequate tissue perfusion.
• Patient states measures used to prevent constipation.
• Patient and family state understanding of drug therapy.

paromomycin sulfate
(PAR-oh-moh-migh-sin SUL-fayt)
Humatin

Pharmacologic class: aminoglycoside
Therapeutic class: amebicide

Pregnancy risk category: C

How supplied

Capsules: 250 mg

Pharmacokinetics

Absorption: very small amounts absorbed in GI tract; however, larger amounts may be absorbed in patients with ulcerative intestinal disorders or renal insufficiency.
Distribution: unknown.
Metabolism: no metabolites have been detected.
Excretion: almost 100% excreted unchanged in feces; systemically absorbed drug excreted in urine.

Route	Onset	Peak	Duration
P.O.	Unknown	Unknown	Unknown

Pharmacodynamics

Chemical effect: unknown, but may inhibit protein synthesis in susceptible bacteria at 30S segment of ribosome.
Therapeutic effect: kills intestinal amoebae, such as trophozoite and encysted forms of *Entamoeba histolytica* and against *Diphyllobothrium latum* (fish tapeworm), *Dipylidium caninum* (dog and cat tapeworm), *Hymenolepis nana* (dwarf tapeworm), *Taenia saginata* (beef tapeworm), and *Taenia solium* (pork tapeworm).

Indications and dosage

▶ **Intestinal amebiasis, acute and chronic.** *Adults and children:* 25 to 35 mg/kg daily P.O. in three doses with meals for 5 to 10 days.
▶ **Tapeworms (fish, beef, pork, dog).** *Adults:* 1 g P.O. q 15 minutes for four doses. *Children:* 11 mg/kg P.O. q 15 minutes for four doses.

Adverse reactions

CNS: headache, vertigo.
EENT: ototoxicity.
GI: anorexia, *nausea, vomiting, epigastric pain and burning, abdominal cramps,* diarrhea, constipation, increased motility, steatorrhea, pruritus ani, malabsorption syndrome.
GU: hematuria, *nephrotoxicity.*
Hematologic: eosinophilia.
Skin: rash, exanthema, pruritus.
Other: overgrowth of nonsusceptible organisms.

Interactions

None significant.

Contraindications and precautions

• Contraindicated in patients with impaired renal function, intestinal obstruction, or hypersensitivity to drug.
• Use cautiously in pregnant women and in patients with ulcerative lesions of bowel.
• Safety of drug has not been established in breast-feeding women.

NURSING CONSIDERATIONS

▨ **Assessment**
• Assess patient's infection before therapy and regularly thereafter.
• Ask about history of sensitivity to drug before giving first dose.
• Criterion of cure is absence of amoebae in stools examined weekly for 6 weeks after treatment and thereafter at monthly intervals for 2 years. Examine feces of family members or suspected contacts.
• Be alert for adverse reactions.
• Monitor patient's hydration status if adverse GI reactions occur.
• Evaluate patient's and family's knowledge of drug therapy.

▧ **Nursing diagnoses**
• Infection related to presence of amoebae
• Risk for fluid volume deficit related to drug-induced adverse GI reactions
• Knowledge deficit related to drug therapy

⊠ Planning and implementation
• Patient should avoid high doses or prolonged therapy.
• Notify doctor if patient reports ringing in ears, hearing impairment, or dizziness.
Patient teaching
• Teach patient about need for personal hygiene, especially good hand-washing technique. Instruct him to refrain from preparing food for others until stools are negative.
• Tell patient to take drug with meals.
• Instruct patient to notify doctor if adverse reactions occur.

☑ Evaluation
• Patient is free from amoebae infection.
• Patient maintains adequate hydration throughout drug therapy.
• Patient and family state understanding of drug therapy.

---

paroxetine hydrochloride
(par-OKS-eh-teen high-droh-KLOR-ighd)
Paxil

Pharmacologic class: selective serotonin reuptake inhibitor
Therapeutic class: antidepressant
Pregnancy risk category: B

How supplied
Tablets: 20 mg, 30 mg

Pharmacokinetics
Absorption: completely absorbed.
Distribution: distributed throughout body, including CNS; only 1% remains in plasma. About 93% to 95% bound to plasma protein.
Metabolism: about 36% metabolized in liver.
Excretion: about 64% excreted in urine.
Half-life: about 24 hours.

Route	Onset	Peak	Duration
P.O.	1-4 wk	2-8 hr	Unknown

Pharmacodynamics
Chemical effect: unknown; presumed to be linked to its inhibition of CNS neuronal uptake of serotonin.
Therapeutic effect: relieves depression.

Indications and dosage
▶ **Depression.** *Adults:* initially, 20 mg P.O. daily, preferably in morning as indicated. If patient does not respond after full antidepressant effect has occurred, dosage increased in 10-mg/day increments at weekly intervals, to maximum of 50 mg daily. *Elderly or debilitated patients; patients with severe hepatic or renal disease:* initially, 10 mg P.O. daily, preferably in morning as indicated. If patient does not respond after full antidepressant effect has occurred, dosage increased in 10-mg/day increments at weekly intervals, to maximum of 40 mg daily.

Adverse reactions
CNS: *asthenia,* blurred vision, *somnolence, dizziness, insomnia, tremor, nervousness,* anxiety, paresthesia, confusion.
CV: palpitations, vasodilation, orthostatic hypotension.
EENT: lump or tightness in throat, taste perversion, dysgeusia.
GI: *dry mouth, nausea, constipation, diarrhea, decreased appetite* or increased appetite, flatulence, vomiting, dyspepsia, increased appetite.
GU: ejaculatory disturbances, male genital disorders (including anorgasmy, erectile difficulties, delayed ejaculation or orgasm, impotence, and sexual dysfunction), urinary frequency, other urinary disorder, female genital disorder (including anorgasmy, difficulty with orgasm).
Metabolic: hyponatremia.
Musculoskeletal: myopathy, myalgia, myasthenia.
Skin: rash.
Other: *diaphoresis,* decreased libido, yawning.

Reactions may be *common*, uncommon, *life-threatening*, or COMMON AND LIFE-THREATENING.

Interactions

Drug-drug. *Cimetidine:* decreased hepatic metabolism of paroxetine, leading to risk of toxicity. Dosage adjustments may be necessary.
Digoxin: may decrease digoxin levels. Monitor closely.
MAO inhibitors: may increase risk of serious, sometimes fatal, adverse reactions. Avoid concomitant use.
Phenobarbital, phenytoin: may alter pharmacokinetics of both drugs. Dosage adjustments may be needed.
Procyclidine: may increase procyclidine levels. Monitor for excessive anticholinergic effects.
Tryptophan: may increase incidence of adverse reactions, such as nausea and dizziness. Avoid concomitant use.
Warfarin: increased risk of bleeding. Use concomitantly with caution.
Drug-lifestyle. *Alcohol use:* may alter psychomotor function. Limit intake.

Contraindications and precautions

• Contraindicated in patients taking MAO inhibitors.
• Use cautiously in pregnant or breast-feeding women and in patients with history of seizures or mania; in those with severe, concomitant systemic illness; and in patients at risk for volume depletion.
• Safety of drug has not been established in children.

NURSING CONSIDERATIONS

Assessment
• Assess patient's depression before therapy and regularly thereafter.
• Be alert for adverse reactions and drug interactions.
• Evaluate patient's and family's knowledge of drug therapy.

Nursing diagnoses
• Altered thought processes related to depression
• Risk for injury related to drug-induced adverse CNS reactions

• Knowledge deficit related to drug therapy

Planning and implementation
• Don't administer drug with, or within 14 days of discontinuing, MAO inhibitor therapy. Allow at least 2 weeks after discontinuing paroxetine before starting treatment with MAO inhibitor, as ordered.
• If signs of psychosis occur or increase, expect to reduce dosage.
Patient teaching
• Warn patient to avoid hazardous activities until CNS effects of drug are known.
• Tell patient that he may notice improvement in 1 to 4 weeks but that he must continue with prescribed regimen to obtain continued benefits.
• Tell patient to abstain from alcohol during drug therapy.

Evaluation
• Patient's depression improves.
• Patient sustains no injuries due to drug-induced adverse CNS reactions.
• Patient and family state understanding of drug therapy.

pegaspargase
(PEG-L-asparaginase)
(peg-AHS-per-jays)
Oncaspar

Pharmacologic class: modified version of enzyme L-asparaginase
Therapeutic class: antineoplastic
Pregnancy risk category: C

How supplied

Injection: 750 IU/ml

Pharmacokinetics

Unknown.

Route	Onset	Peak	Duration
I.V., I.M.	Unknown	Unknown	Unknown

Pharmacodynamics

Chemical effect: exerts its cytotoxic activity by inactivating amino acid asparagine. Asparagine is required by tumor cells to synthesize proteins. Because tumor cells cannot synthesize their own asparagine, protein synthesis and, eventually, synthesis of DNA and RNA are inhibited.
Therapeutic effect: kills selected leukemic cells.

Indications and dosage

▶ **Acute lymphoblastic leukemia (ALL) in patients who require L-asparaginase but have developed hypersensitivity to native forms of L-asparaginase.** *Adults and children with body surface area of at least 0.6 m²:* 2,500 IU/m² I.M. or I.V. q 14 days.
Children with body surface area less than 0.6 m²: 82.5 IU/kg I.M. or I.V. q 14 days.

Adverse reactions

CNS: *seizures,* headache, paresthesia, *status epilepticus,* somnolence, coma, mental status changes, dizziness, emotional lability, mood changes, parkinsonism, confusion, disorientation, fatigue. Malaise.
CV: hypotension, tachycardia, chest pain, subacute bacterial endocarditis, hypertension.
EENT: epistaxis.
GI: nausea, vomiting, abdominal pain, anorexia, diarrhea, constipation, indigestion, flatulence, GI pain, mucositis, *pancreatitis (sometimes fulminant and fatal),* increased serum amylase and lipase levels, colitis.
GU: increased BUN level, increased creatinine level, increased urinary frequency, hematuria, severe hemorrhagic cystitis, renal dysfunction, *renal failure.*
Hematologic: *thrombosis, leukopenia, pancytopenia, agranulocytosis, thrombocytopenia,* prolonged PT and PTT, decreased antithrombin III, disseminated intravascular coagulation, decreased fibrinogen, hemolytic anemia, increased thromboplastin, easily bruised, ecchymosis, *hemorrhage* (may be fatal).

Hepatic: jaundice, bilirubinemia, increased ALT and AST, ascites, hypoalbuminemia, fatty changes in liver, *liver failure.*
Metabolic: hyperuricemia, hyponatremia, uric acid nephropathy, hypoproteinemia, proteinuria, weight loss, metabolic acidosis, increased blood ammonia level, hyperglycemia, hypoglycemia.
Musculoskeletal: arthralgia, myalgia, musculoskeletal pain, joint stiffness, cramps.
Respiratory: cough, *severe bronchospasm,* upper respiratory tract infection.
Skin: itching, alopecia, fever blister, purpura, hand whiteness, fungal changes, nail whiteness and ridging, erythema simplex, petechial rash.
Other: *hypersensitivity reactions, including anaphylaxis,* rash, erythema, edema, pain, fever, chills, urticaria, dyspnea, or bronchospasm; pain in extremities; peripheral edema; nighttime sweating; mouth tenderness; infection; *sepsis; septic shock,* injection pain or reaction, localized edema.

Interactions

Drug-drug. *Aspirin, dipyridamole, heparin, NSAIDs, warfarin:* imbalances in coagulation factors may occur, predisposing patient to bleeding or thrombosis. Use together cautiously.
Methotrexate: may interfere with action of methotrexate, which requires cell replication for its lethal effect. Monitor for decreased effectiveness.
Protein-bound drugs: serum protein depletion may increase toxicity of other drugs that bind to proteins. Monitor for toxicity. May interfere with enzymatic detoxification of other drugs, particularly in liver. Administer concomitantly with caution.

Contraindications and precautions

• Contraindicated in patients with pancreatitis or history of pancreatitis; in those who have had significant hemorrhagic events associated with prior L-asparaginase therapy; and in those with

---

Reactions may be *common,* uncommon, *life-threatening,* or COMMON AND LIFE-THREATENING.

previous serious allergic reactions, such as generalized urticaria, bronchospasm, laryngeal edema, hypotension, or other unacceptable adverse reactions to pegaspargase.
• Drug use is not recommended in pregnant or breast-feeding women.
• Use cautiously in patients with liver dysfunction.

NURSING CONSIDERATIONS

Assessment
• Assess patient's condition before therapy and regularly thereafter.
• Monitor patient closely for hypersensitivity reactions, including life-threatening anaphylaxis, which may occur during therapy, especially in patient with hypersensitivity to other forms of L-asparaginase.
• Monitor patient's peripheral blood count and bone marrow, as ordered. A fall in circulating lymphoblasts is often noted after initiating therapy. This may be accompanied by marked rise in serum uric acid levels.
• Monitor serum amylase levels, as ordered, to detect early evidence of pancreatitis. Monitor patient's blood sugar during therapy because hyperglycemia may occur.
• Monitor for liver dysfunction when pegaspargase is used with hepatotoxic chemotherapeutic agents.
• Drug may affect number of plasma proteins; therefore, monitor fibrinogen, PT, and PTT. Question doctor if not ordered.
• Be alert for adverse reactions and drug interactions.
• Evaluate patient's and family's knowledge of drug therapy.

Nursing diagnoses
• Altered health maintenance related to leukemia
• Altered protection related to drug-induced adverse hematologic reactions
• Knowledge deficit related to drug therapy

Planning and implementation
• Drug should be used as sole induction agent only in unusual situation when combined regimen that uses other chemotherapeutic agents is inappropriate because of toxicity or other specific patient-related factors, or in patients refractory to other therapy.
• I.M. route is preferred over I.V. route because of its lower incidence of hepatotoxicity, coagulopathy, and GI and renal disorders.
• Don't use if there is indication that it has been frozen. Although drug may not look different, its activity is destroyed after freezing. Obtain new dose from pharmacist.
• Avoid excessive agitation; do *not* shake. Keep refrigerated at 36° to 46° F (2° to 8° C). Do not use if cloudy, if precipitate is present, or if stored at room temperature for more than 48 hours. Do not freeze. Discard unused portions. Use only one dose per vial; do not reenter vial. Do not save unused drug for later use.
I.V. use: Give drug over 1 to 2 hours in 100 ml of 0.9% NaCl or dextrose 5% injection through infusion that is already running.
I.M. use: Limit volume administered at single injection site to 2 ml. If volume to be administered is greater than 2 ml, use multiple injection sites.
• Keep patient under observation for 1 hour and have resuscitation equipment and other agents necessary to treat anaphylaxis (such as epinephrine, oxygen, and I.V. steroids) readily available. Moderate to life-threatening hypersensitivity reactions require discontinuation of drug.
• Handle and administer solution with care. Gloves are recommended. Avoid inhalation of vapors and contact with skin or mucous membranes, especially those of eyes. If contact occurs, wash with copious amounts of water for at least 15 minutes.
Patient teaching
• Inform patient about hypersensitivity reactions and importance of alerting staff at once if they occur.

• Instruct patient not to take other drugs, including OTC preparations, until approved by doctor. Concomitant use may increase risk of bleeding or may increase toxicity of other drugs.
• Instruct patient to report signs and symptoms of infection (fever, chills, and malaise) to doctor because drug may suppress immune system.

☑ **Evaluation**
• Patient responds well to therapy.
• Patient develops no serious complications caused by drug-induced adverse hematologic reactions.
• Patient and family state understanding of drug therapy.

pemoline
(PEH-moh-leen)
Cylert, Cylert Chewable

Pharmacologic class: oxazolidinedione derivative
Therapeutic class: analeptic
Controlled substance schedule: IV
Pregnancy risk category: B

How supplied

Tablets: 18.75 mg, 37.5 mg, 75 mg
Tablets (chewable): 37.5 mg

Pharmacokinetics

Absorption: well absorbed.
Distribution: distribution is unknown. Drug is 50% protein-bound.
Metabolism: metabolized in liver.
Excretion: excreted in urine. *Half-life:* 12 hours.

Route	Onset	Peak	Duration
P.O.	Unknown	2-4 hr	Unknown

Pharmacodynamics

Chemical effect: may promote nerve impulse transmission by releasing stored norepinephrine from nerve terminals in brain, mainly in cerebral cortex and reticular activating system.
Therapeutic effect: promotes calmness in children with attention deficit.

Indications and dosage

▶ **Attention deficit hyperactivity disorder.** *Children age 6 and older:* initially, 37.5 mg P.O. in a.m. Daily dosage raised by 18.75 mg weekly, as necessary. Effective dosage range is 56.25 to 75 mg daily; maximum dosage is 112.5 mg daily.

Adverse reactions

CNS: *insomnia,* malaise, dyskinetic movements, irritability, fatigue, mild depression, dizziness, headache, drowsiness, hallucinations, nervousness (with large doses), *seizures, Tourette syndrome,* psychosis.
CV: *tachycardia* (with large doses).
GI: anorexia, abdominal pain, nausea, diarrhea.
Hematologic: *aplastic anemia.*
Hepatic: elevated liver enzymes, hepatitis, jaundice, *hepatic failure.*
Skin: rash.

Interactions

Drug-drug. *Insulin, oral antidiabetic agents:* may decrease antidiabetic agent requirements. Monitor blood glucose levels.

Contraindications and precautions

• Contraindicated in patients with hepatic dysfunction and hypersensitivity or idiosyncrasy to drug.
• Because of risk of hepatic failure, drug should not be considered as first-line therapy.
• Use cautiously in patients with impaired renal function.

NURSING CONSIDERATIONS

☑ **Assessment**
• Assess patient's condition, including liver function tests, before and during therapy.

• May precipitate Tourette syndrome in child. Monitor especially at start of therapy.

• Monitor for blood or hepatic function changes and growth suppression.

• Know that drug should be stopped if significant hepatic dysfunction occurs.

• Drug may produce similar adverse reactions to amphetamines or methylphenidate, including lowered seizure threshold. Has potential for abuse and dependence.

• Evaluate patient's and family's knowledge of drug therapy.

Nursing diagnoses

• Risk for injury related to attention deficit hyperactivity disorder

• Sleep pattern disturbance related to drug-induced insomnia

• Knowledge deficit related to drug therapy

Planning and implementation

• Give drug at least 6 hours before bedtime.

Patient teaching

• Warn patient to avoid hazardous activities until effects of drug are known.

• Tell patient to report insomnia and other adverse effects.

Evaluation

• Patient exhibits less hyperactivity.

• Patient is able to sleep without difficulty throughout drug therapy.

• Patient and family state understanding of drug therapy.

---

penbutolol sulfate
(pen-BYOO-toh-lol SUL-fayt)
Levatol

Pharmacologic class: beta blocker
Therapeutic class: antihypertensive
Pregnancy risk category: C

How supplied

Tablets: 20 mg

Pharmacokinetics

Absorption: almost completely absorbed from GI tract.
Distribution: 80% to 98% of drug is bound to plasma proteins.
Metabolism: metabolized by liver.
Excretion: most metabolites excreted in urine. *Half-life:* 5 hours.

Route	Onset	Peak	Duration
P.O.	≤ 1 hr	1.5-3 hr	≤ 24 hr

Pharmacodynamics

Chemical effect: unknown.
Therapeutic effect: lowers blood pressure.

Indications and dosage

▶ **Mild to moderate hypertension.**
Adults: 20 mg P.O. once daily. Usually given with other antihypertensives, such as thiazide diuretics.

Adverse reactions

CNS: *dizziness,* vertigo, headache, fatigue, sleep disturbances.
CV: *bradycardia,* chest pain, **heart failure.**
GI: gastric pain, flatulence, nausea, constipation, heartburn, vomiting, taste alteration, dry mouth.
GU: impotence, nocturia, urine retention.
Metabolic: hyperglycemia, hypoglycemia.
Respiratory: respiratory distress, shortness of breath.
Skin: pallor, flushing, rash.
Other: hypersensitivity reactions, decreased libido.

Interactions

Drug-drug. *Clonidine:* may cause paradoxical hypertension. May enhance rebound hypertension when clonidine is withdrawn.
Digoxin, diltiazem, verapamil: may cause additive depression of AV node conduction. Monitor closely.

Insulin, oral antidiabetic agents: hypoglycemic response to these drugs may be altered. Monitor patient closely.
NSAIDs: may decrease antihypertensive effects. Monitor patient.
Prazosin, terazosin: "first-dose" orthostatic hypotension may be enhanced. Monitor patient closely.
Sympathomimetics, including dobutamine, dopamine, isoproterenol, norepinephrine: decreased hypotensive response. Monitor patient.
Theophylline: may decrease bronchodilator effect. Monitor patient.

Contraindications and precautions

• Contraindicated in patients with sinus bradycardia, cardiogenic shock, overt cardiac failure, greater than first-degree heart block, chronic bronchitis, and hypersensitivity to it or other beta blockers.
• Use cautiously in pregnant or breastfeeding women and in patients with heart failure controlled by drug therapy or history of bronchospastic disease. Also use cautiously in diabetic patients because drug may mask signs and symptoms of hypoglycemia.
• Safety of drug has not been established in children.

NURSING CONSIDERATIONS

✎ Assessment
• Assess patient's condition before therapy and regularly thereafter.
• Monitor ECG and heart rate and rhythm frequently.
• Be alert for adverse reactions and drug interactions.
• Evaluate patient's and family's knowledge of drug therapy.

✦ Nursing diagnoses
• Risk for injury related to hypertension
• Altered tissue perfusion (cerebral, cardiopulmonary, peripheral) related to drug-induced adverse reactions
• Knowledge deficit related to drug therapy

➤ Planning and implementation
• Always check patient's apical pulse before giving drug. If you detect extremes in pulse rates, withhold drug and call doctor immediately.
• Do not stop therapy abruptly; sudden withdrawal of other beta blockers has precipitated angina and MI.
• To slowly discontinue drug, taper dosage over 1 to 2 weeks, especially in patient with ischemic heart disease. If symptoms of angina develop, notify doctor immediately because drug should be immediately reinstituted, at least temporarily, and supportive care may be needed to control patient's unstable angina.
Patient teaching
• Tell patient to avoid abrupt discontinuation of therapy.
• Teach patient signs and symptoms of heart failure (edema and pulmonary congestion). Advise him to contact doctor if these symptoms occur.
• Teach patient how to take his pulse and tell him to contact doctor if pulse is slower than usual. Also tell him to report other adverse reactions.

✔ Evaluation
• Patient's blood pressure is normal.
• Patient maintains adequate tissue perfusion.
• Patient and family state understanding of drug therapy.

---

penicillamine
(pen-ih-SIL-uh-meen)
Cuprimine, Depen, D-Penamine◇

Pharmacologic class: chelating agent
Therapeutic class: heavy metal antagonist, antirheumatic
Pregnancy risk category: NR

How supplied
Tablets: 125 mg◇, 250 mg
Capsules: 125 mg, 250 mg

Reactions may be *common*, uncommon, *life-threatening*, or COMMON AND LIFE-THREATENING.

Pharmacokinetics

Absorption: well absorbed from GI tract.
Distribution: only limited data available.
Metabolism: uncomplexed penicillamine is metabolized in liver to inactive disulfides.
Excretion: only small amount of penicillamine excreted unchanged; after 24 hours, 50% of drug excreted in urine, 20% in feces, and 30% is unaccounted for.

Route	Onset	Peak	Duration
P.O.	Unknown	1 hr	Unknown

Pharmacodynamics

Chemical effect: chelates heavy metals and may inhibit collagen formation; unknown for rheumatoid arthritis.
Therapeutic effect: chelates copper in Wilson's disease, combines with cystine to form complex more soluble than cystine alone, and relieves symptoms of rheumatoid arthritis.

Indications and dosage

▶ **Wilson's disease.** *Adults and children:* 250 mg P.O. q.i.d. 30 to 60 minutes before meals. Dosage adjusted to achieve urinary copper excretion of 0.5 to 1 mg daily.
▶ **Cystinuria.** *Adults:* 250 mg to 1 g P.O. q.i.d. before meals. Dosage adjusted to achieve urinary cystine excretion of less than 100 mg daily when renal calculi are present or 100 to 200 mg daily when no calculi are present. Maximum dosage is 4 g daily. *Children:* 30 mg/kg P.O. daily divided q.i.d. before meals. Dosage adjusted to achieve urinary cystine excretion of less than 100 mg daily when renal calculi are present or 100 to 200 mg daily when no calculi are present.
▶ **Rheumatoid arthritis.** *Adults:* initially, 125 to 250 mg P.O. daily, with increases of 125 to 250 mg q 1 to 3 months, if necessary. Maximum dosage is 1.5 g daily.

Adverse reactions

EENT: tinnitus, *optic neuritis.*
GI: *anorexia, epigastric pain, nausea, vomiting, diarrhea, loss of or altered taste perception, stomatitis.*
GU: nephrotic syndrome, glomerulonephritis, proteinuria, hematuria.
Hematologic: *leukopenia, eosinophilia, thrombocytopenia, monocytosis, agranulocytopenia, aplastic anemia,* elevated sedimentation rate, lupuslike syndrome.
Hepatic: *hepatotoxicity.*
Skin: alopecia, friability, especially at pressure spots; wrinkling; erythema; urticaria; ecchymoses.
Other: myasthenia gravis syndrome with long-term use; *allergic reactions (rash, pruritus, fever), arthralgia, lymphadenopathy,* or *pneumonitis.*

Interactions

Drug-drug. *Antacids, oral iron:* decreased effectiveness of D-penicillamine. Give at least 2 hours apart.
Drug-food. *Any food:* delayed absorption of drug. Administer drug 1 hour before or 3 hours after meals.

Contraindications and precautions

• Contraindicated in pregnancy except for the treatment of Wilson's disease or certain cases of cystinuria, in patients with previous penicillamine-related aplastic anemia or granulocytosis, and in rheumatoid arthritis patients with renal insufficiency.
• Use with extreme caution, if at all, in patients with hypersensitivity to penicillin.
• Safety of drug has not been established in breast-feeding women.

NURSING CONSIDERATIONS

⚕ Assessment
• Obtain history of patient's underlying condition before therapy.
• Monitor effectiveness by evaluating patient's urinary copper or cysteine excre-

tion or improvement in rheumatoid arthritis condition.
• Monitor CBC and kidney and liver function every 2 weeks for first 6 months, then monthly, as ordered.
• Monitor urinalysis regularly for protein loss.
• Check patient's range of motion and joint mobility.
• Be alert for adverse reactions and drug interactions.
• Evaluate patient's and family's knowledge of drug therapy.

Nursing diagnoses
• Impaired physical mobility related to Wilson's disease
• Altered urinary elimination related to drug-induced renal dysfunction
• Knowledge deficit related to drug therapy

Planning and implementation
• Give dose on empty stomach to facilitate absorption, preferably 1 hour before or 3 hours after meals.
• Keep in mind that patient should receive supplemental pyridoxine daily.
• If patient has a skin reaction, give antihistamines, as prescribed. Handle patient carefully to avoid skin damage.
• Report rash and fever (important signs of toxicity) to doctor immediately.
• Withhold drug and notify doctor if WBC count falls below 3,500/mm³ or platelet count falls below 100,000/mm³. A progressive decline in platelet or WBC count in three successive blood tests may necessitate temporary cessation of therapy, even if such counts are within normal limits.
Patient teaching
• Tell patient that therapeutic effect may be delayed up to 3 months in treatment of rheumatoid arthritis.
• Tell patient to maintain adequate fluid intake, especially at night.
• Advise patient to report early signs of granulocytopenia: fever, sore throat, chills, bruising, and prolonged bleeding time.

• Reassure patient that taste impairment usually resolves in 6 weeks without change in dosage.

Evaluation
• Patient reports increase in physical mobility.
• Patient maintains normal urinary elimination pattern.
• Patient and family state understanding of drug therapy.

---

penicillin G benzathine (benzylpenicillin benzathine)
(pen-ih-SIL-in gee BENZ-uh-theen)
Bicillin L-A, Permapen

Pharmacologic class: natural penicillin
Therapeutic class: antibiotic
Pregnancy risk category: B

How supplied
Injection: 300,000 units/ml, 600,000 units/ml

Pharmacokinetics
Absorption: absorbed slowly from I.M. injection site.
Distribution: distributed widely into synovial, pleural, pericardial, and ascitic fluids and bile, and into liver, skin, lungs, kidneys, muscle, intestines, tonsils, maxillary sinuses, saliva, and erythrocytes. CSF penetration is poor but is enhanced in patients with inflamed meninges. Drug is 45% to 68% protein-bound.
Metabolism: between 16% and 30% of drug is metabolized to inactive compounds.
Excretion: excreted primarily in urine.
Half-life: 30 to 60 minutes.

Route	Onset	Peak	Duration
I.M.	Unknown	13-24 hr	1-4 wk

Pharmacodynamics
Chemical effect: inhibits cell-wall synthesis during microorganism multiplica-

---

tion; bacteria resist penicillins by producing penicillinases—enzymes that convert penicillins to inactive penicilloic acid. *Therapeutic effect:* kills susceptible bacteria, such as most nonpenicillinase-producing strains of gram-positive and gram-negative aerobic cocci; spirochetes; and some gram-positive aerobic and anaerobic bacilli.

Indications and dosage

▶ **Congenital syphilis.** *Children under age 2:* 50,000 units/kg I.M. as single dose.

▶ **Group A streptococcal upper respiratory tract infections.** *Adults:* 1.2 million units I.M. as single injection. *Children over 27 kg:* 900,000 units I.M. as single injection. *Children weighing under 27 kg (59 lb):* 300,000 to 600,000 units I.M. as single injection.

▶ **Prophylaxis of poststreptococcal rheumatic fever.** *Adults and children:* 1.2 million units I.M. once monthly or 600,000 units twice monthly.

▶ **Syphilis of less than 1 year's duration.** *Adults:* 2.4 million units I.M. as single dose.

▶ **Syphilis of more than 1 year's duration.** *Adults:* 2.4 million units I.M. weekly for 3 successive weeks.

Adverse reactions

CNS: neuropathy; *seizures* (with high doses).
Hematologic: eosinophilia, hemolytic anemia, *thrombocytopenia, leukopenia.*
Other: hypersensitivity reactions (maculopapular and *exfoliative dermatitis,* chills, fever, edema, *anaphylaxis*); pain, sterile abscess (at injection site).

Interactions

Drug-drug. *Colestipol:* decreased serum concentrations of penicillin G benzathine. Give penicillin 1 hour before or 4 hours after colestipol.
Probenecid: increased blood levels of penicillin. Probenecid may be used for this purpose.

Contraindications and precautions

• Contraindicated in patients with hypersensitivity to drug or other penicillins.
• Use cautiously in pregnant women and in patients with other drug allergies, especially to cephalosporins.
• Drug is excreted in breast milk; use in breast-feeding women may sensitize infant to penicillin and cause some adverse effects.

NURSING CONSIDERATIONS

⚇ Assessment
• Assess patient's infection before therapy and regularly thereafter.
• Before giving drug, ask patient about allergic reactions to penicillin. However, negative history of penicillin allergy is no guarantee against future allergic reaction.
• Obtain specimen for culture and sensitivity tests before giving first dose. Therapy may begin pending results.
• Be alert for adverse reactions and drug interactions.
• Observe closely. With large doses and prolonged therapy, bacterial or fungal superinfection may occur, especially in elderly, debilitated, or immunosuppressed patient.
• Evaluate patient's and family's knowledge of drug therapy.

⚇ Nursing diagnoses
• Infection related to presence of bacteria
• Altered protection related to risk of hypersensitivity reactions to drug
• Knowledge deficit related to drug therapy

⚇ Planning and implementation
• Shake drug well before injection.
• Never give drug I.V.—inadvertent I.V. administration has caused cardiac arrest and death.
• Inject deeply into upper outer quadrant of buttocks in adult; in midlateral thigh in infant and young child. Avoid injection into or near major nerves or blood vessels to prevent neurovascular damage.

• Give drug at least 1 hour before bacteriostatic antibiotics.
• Drug's extremely slow absorption makes allergic reactions difficult to treat. Stop drug immediately if patient develops signs of anaphylactic shock (rapidly developing dyspnea and hypotension). Notify doctor and prepare for immediate treatment with epinephrine, corticosteroids, antihistamines, and other resuscitative measures as indicated.
Patient teaching
• Tell patient to call doctor if rash, fever, or chills develop.
• Warn patient that injection may be painful but that ice applied to site may ease discomfort.

☑ **Evaluation**
• Patient is free from infection.
• Patient shows no signs of allergy.
• Patient and family state understanding of drug therapy.

---

penicillin G potassium (benzylpenicillin potassium)
(pen-ih-SIL-in gee poh-TAH-see-um)
Megacillin♦, Pfizerpen

Pharmacologic class: natural penicillin
Therapeutic class: antibiotic
Pregnancy risk category: B

How supplied

Tablets: 500,000 units♦
Oral suspension: 250,000 units♦, 500,000 units♦
Injection: 1 million units, 5 million units, 10 million units, 20 million units

Pharmacokinetics

Absorption: only 15% to 30% of oral dose is absorbed; remainder is hydrolyzed by gastric secretions. Food in stomach reduces rate and extent of absorption. Absorbed rapidly from I.M. injection site.

Distribution: distributed widely into synovial, pleural, pericardial, and ascitic fluids and bile, and into liver, skin, lungs, kidneys, muscle, intestines, tonsils, maxillary sinuses, saliva, and erythrocytes. CSF penetration is poor but is enhanced in patients with inflamed meninges. Drug is 45% to 68% protein-bound.
Metabolism: hepatic metabolism accounts for less than 30% of biotransformation of penicillin.
Excretion: excreted primarily in urine.
Half-life: 30 to 60 minutes.

Route	Onset	Peak	Duration
P.O.	Unknown	0.5-1 hr	Unknown
I.V.	Immediate	Immediate	Unknown
I.M.	Unknown	15-30 min	Unknown

Pharmacodynamics

Chemical effect: inhibits cell-wall synthesis during microorganism multiplication; bacteria resist penicillins by producing penicillinases—enzymes that convert penicillins to inactive penicilloic acid.
Therapeutic effect: kills susceptible bacteria, such as most nonpenicillinase-producing strains of gram-positive and gram-negative aerobic cocci; spirochetes; and certain gram-positive aerobic and anaerobic bacilli.

Indications and dosage

▶ **Moderate to severe systemic infections.** *Adults:* 500,000 units P.O. q 6 to 8 hours; 12 to 24 million units I.M. or I.V. daily in divided doses q 4 hours. *Children:* 25,000 to 90,000 units/kg/day P.O. in three to six divided doses; or 25,000 to 300,000 units/kg I.M. or I.V. daily in divided doses q 4 hours.

Adverse reactions

CNS: neuropathy; *seizures* (with high doses).
Hematologic: *hemolytic anemia, thrombocytopenia,* leukopenia.
Other: hypersensitivity reactions (rash, urticaria, maculopapular eruptions, *exfoliative dermatitis,* chills, fever, edema,

---

Reactions may be *common*, uncommon, *life-threatening*, or COMMON AND LIFE-THREATENING.

anaphylaxis), overgrowth of nonsusceptible organisms, possible severe potassium poisoning with high doses (hyper-reflexia, *seizures, coma*), thrombophlebitis; pain (at injection site).

Interactions

Drug-drug. *Colestipol:* decreased serum concentrations of penicillin G potassium. Give penicillin 1 hour before or 4 hours after colestipol.
Potassium-sparing diuretics: possible increased risk of hyperkalemia. Do not use together.
Probenecid: increased blood levels of penicillin. Probenecid may be used for this purpose.

Contraindications and precautions

• Contraindicated in patients with hypersensitivity to drug or other penicillins.
• Use cautiously in pregnant women and in patients with other drug allergies, especially to cephalosporins.
• Drug is excreted in breast milk; use in breast-feeding women may sensitize infant to penicillin and cause some adverse effects.

NURSING CONSIDERATIONS

🔧 Assessment
• Assess patient's infection before therapy and regularly thereafter.
• Before giving, ask patient about any allergic reactions to penicillin. However, negative history of penicillin allergy is no guarantee against future allergic reaction.
• Obtain specimen for culture and sensitivity tests before first dose. Therapy may begin pending results.
• Be alert for adverse reactions and drug interactions.
• Observe closely. With large doses and prolonged therapy, bacterial or fungal superinfection may occur, especially in elderly, debilitated, or immunosuppressed patient.
• Evaluate patient's and family's knowledge of drug therapy.

🔧 Nursing diagnoses
• Infection related to presence of bacteria
• Altered protection related to risk of hypersensitivity reactions to drug
• Knowledge deficit related to drug therapy

▶ Planning and implementation
• Reconstitute vials with sterile water for injection, D_5W, or 0.9% NaCl injection. Volume of diluent varies with manufacturer.
• Give drug at least 1 hour before bacteriostatic antibiotics.
P.O. use: Give drug 1 to 2 hours before or 2 to 3 hours after meals. Drug may cause GI disturbances. Food may interfere with absorption.
I.V. use: Use continuous I.V. infusion when large doses are required (10 million units or more). Otherwise, give via intermittent I.V. infusion over 1 to 2 hours.
– Aminoglycosides are physically and chemically incompatible with drug. Administer separately.
I.M. use: Administer drug deeply into large muscle; may be painful.
Patient teaching
• Tell patient to take drug exactly as prescribed, even after he feels better.
• Warn patient never to use leftover penicillin for new illness or to share penicillin with family and friends.
• Tell patient to call doctor if rash, fever, or chills develop.
• Warn patient that I.M. injection may be painful but that ice applied to site may ease discomfort.

🗹 Evaluation
• Patient is free from infection.
• Patient shows no signs of allergy.
• Patient and family state understanding of drug therapy.

---

penicillin G procaine
(benzylpenicillin procaine)
(pen-ih-SIL-in gee PROH-kayn)
Ayercillin♦, Crysticillin-300 A.S., Pfizerpen-AS, Wycillin

Pharmacologic class: natural penicillin
Therapeutic class: antibiotic
Pregnancy risk category: B

How supplied

Injection: 300,000 units/ml, 500,000 units/ml, 600,000 units/ml

Pharmacokinetics

Absorption: absorbed slowly.
Distribution: distributed widely into synovial, pleural, pericardial, and ascitic fluids and bile, and into liver, skin, lungs, kidneys, muscle, intestines, tonsils, maxillary sinuses, saliva, and erythrocytes. CSF penetration usually poor, but enhanced in patients with inflamed meninges. Drug is 45% to 68% protein-bound.
Metabolism: from 16% to 30% metabolized to inactive compounds.
Excretion: excreted primarily in urine.
Half-life: 30 to 60 minutes.

Route	Onset	Peak	Duration
I.M.	Unknown	1-4 hr	1-2 days

Pharmacodynamics

Chemical effect: inhibits cell-wall synthesis during microorganism multiplication; bacteria resist penicillins by producing penicillinases—enzymes that convert penicillins to inactive penicilloic acid.
Therapeutic effect: kills susceptible bacteria, such as most nonpenicillinase-producing strains of gram-positive and gram-negative aerobic cocci, spirochetes, and some gram-positive aerobic and anaerobic bacilli.

Indications and dosage

▶ **Moderate to severe systemic infections.** *Adults:* 600,000 to 1.2 million units I.M. daily in single dose.

Children over age 1 month: 25,000 to 50,000 units/kg I.M. daily in single dose.
▶ **Uncomplicated gonorrhea.** *Adults and children over age 12:* 1 g probenecid; after 30 minutes, 4.8 million units of penicillin G procaine I.M., divided between two injection sites.
▶ **Pneumococcal pneumonia.** *Adults and children over age 12:* 600,000 units to 1.2 million units I.M. daily for 7 to 10 days.

Adverse reactions

CNS: *seizures.*
Hematologic: *thrombocytopenia,* hemolytic anemia, *leukopenia.*
Other: arthralgia, hypersensitivity reactions (rash, urticaria, chills, fever, edema, prostration, *anaphylaxis*), overgrowth of nonsusceptible organisms.

Interactions

Drug-drug. *Colestipol:* decreased serum concentrations of penicillin G procaine. Give penicillin 1 hour before or 4 hours after colestipol.
Probenecid: increased blood levels of penicillin. Probenecid may be used for this purpose.

Contraindications and precautions

• Contraindicated in patients with hypersensitivity to drug or other penicillins.
• Use cautiously in pregnant women and in patients with other drug allergies, especially to cephalosporins.
• Drug is excreted in breast milk; use in breast-feeding women may sensitize infant to penicillin and cause some adverse effects.

NURSING CONSIDERATIONS

⚱ Assessment
• Assess patient's infection before therapy and regularly thereafter.
• Before giving, ask patient about allergic reactions to penicillin. However, negative history of penicillin allergy is no guarantee against future allergic reaction.

• Obtain specimen for culture and sensitivity tests before giving first dose. Therapy may begin pending results.
• Be alert for adverse reactions and drug interactions.
• Observe closely. With large doses and prolonged therapy, bacterial or fungal superinfection may occur, especially in elderly, debilitated, or immunosuppressed patient.
• Evaluate patient's and family's knowledge of drug therapy.

🔟 **Nursing diagnoses**
• Infection related to presence of bacteria
• Altered protection related to risk of hypersensitivity reactions to drug
• Knowledge deficit related to drug therapy

⧉ **Planning and implementation**
• Shake drug well before injection.
• Never give I.V.—inadvertent I.V. administration has caused cardiac arrest and death.
• Inject deeply into upper outer quadrant of buttocks in adults; in midlateral thigh in infants and small children. Avoid injection into or near major nerves or blood vessels to prevent neurovascular damage.
• Give penicillin G procaine at least 1 hour before bacteriostatic antibiotics.
• Drug's extremely slow absorption makes allergic reactions difficult to treat. Stop drug immediately if patient develops signs of anaphylactic shock (rapidly developing dyspnea and hypotension). Notify doctor and prepare for immediate treatment with epinephrine, corticosteroids, antihistamines, and other resuscitative measures as indicated.
Patient teaching
• Tell patient to call doctor if rash, fever, or chills develop.
• Warn patient that injection may be painful but that ice applied to site may ease discomfort.

☑ **Evaluation**
• Patient is free from infection.

• Patient shows no signs of allergy.
• Patient and family state understanding of drug therapy.

penicillin G sodium (benzylpenicillin sodium)
(pen-ih-SIL-in gee SOH-dee-um)
Crystapen◆

Pharmacologic class: natural penicillin
Therapeutic class: antibiotic
Pregnancy risk category: B

How supplied
Injection: 5 million-units vial

Pharmacokinetics
Absorption: absorbed rapidly from I.M. injection site.
Distribution: distributed widely into synovial, pleural, pericardial, and ascitic fluids and bile, and into liver, skin, lungs, kidneys, muscle, intestines, tonsils, maxillary sinuses, saliva, and erythrocytes. CSF penetration is poor but is enhanced in patients with inflamed meninges. Drug is 45% to 68% protein-bound.
Metabolism: between 16% and 30% of drug is metabolized to inactive compounds.
Excretion: excreted primarily in urine.
Half-life: 30 to 60 minutes.

Route	Onset	Peak	Duration
I.V.	Immediate	Immediate	Unknown
I.M.	Unknown	15-30 min	Unknown

Pharmacodynamics
Chemical effect: inhibits cell-wall synthesis during microorganism multiplication; bacteria resist penicillins by producing penicillinases—enzymes that convert penicillins to inactive penicilloic acid.
Therapeutic effect: kills susceptible bacteria, such as most non-penicillinase-producing strains of gram-positive and gram-negative aerobic cocci, spirochetes,

---

and some gram-positive aerobic and anaerobic bacilli.

Indications and dosage

▶ **Moderate to severe systemic infections.** *Adults:* 12 to 24 million units daily I.M. or I.V. in divided doses q 4 to 6 hours. *Children:* 25,000 to 300,000 units/kg daily I.M. or I.V. in divided doses q 4 to 6 hours.
▶ **Endocarditis prophylaxis for dental surgery.** *Adults and children weighing over 27 kg (59 lb):* 2 million units I.V. or I.M. 30 to 60 minutes before procedure; then 1 million units 6 hours later.

Adverse reactions

CNS: neuropathy, *seizures.*
Hematologic: hemolytic anemia, *leukopenia, thrombocytopenia.*
Other: arthralgia, hypersensitivity reactions *(exfoliative dermatitis,* urticaria, *anaphylaxis),* overgrowth of nonsusceptible organisms, vein irritation, thrombophlebitis, pain (at injection site).

Interactions

Drug-drug. *Colestipol:* decreased serum concentrations of penicillin G sodium. Give penicillin 1 hour before or 4 hours after colestipol.
Probenecid: increased blood levels of penicillin. Probenecid may be used for this purpose.

Contraindications and precautions

• Contraindicated in patients with hypersensitivity to drug or other penicillins.
• Use cautiously in pregnant women and in patients with other drug allergies, especially to cephalosporins.
• Drug is excreted in breast milk; use in breast-feeding women may sensitize infant to penicillin and cause some adverse effects.

NURSING CONSIDERATIONS

⚕ Assessment
• Assess patient's infection before therapy and regularly thereafter.

• Before giving, ask patient about allergic reactions to penicillin. However, negative history of penicillin allergy is no guarantee against future allergic reaction.
• Obtain specimen for culture and sensitivity tests before first dose. Therapy may begin pending results.
• Be alert for adverse reactions and drug interactions.
• Observe closely. With large doses and prolonged therapy, bacterial or fungal superinfection may occur, especially in elderly, debilitated, or immunosuppressed patient.
• Evaluate patient's and family's knowledge of drug therapy.

⚌ Nursing diagnoses
• Infection related to presence of bacteria
• Altered protection related to risk of hypersensitivity reactions to drug
• Knowledge deficit related to drug therapy

⟩ Planning and implementation
I.V. use: Reconstitute vials with sterile water for injection, 0.9% NaCl injection, or D_5W. Volume of diluent varies with manufacturer and concentration needed.
– For patient receiving 10 million units of drug or more daily, dilute in 1 to 2 liters of compatible solution and administer over 24 hours. Otherwise, give by intermittent I.V. infusion: Dilute drug in 50 to 100 ml and give over 1 to 2 hours q 4 to 6 hours.
– In neonate or child, give divided doses usually over 15 to 30 minutes.
– Aminoglycosides are physically and chemically incompatible with drug. Administer separately.
I.M. use: Give drug deeply in upper outer quadrant of buttocks in adult; in midlateral thigh in young child. Don't massage injection site. Avoid injection near major nerves or blood vessels to prevent neurovascular damage.
• Do not give S.C.
• Give penicillin G sodium at least 1 hour before bacteriostatic antibiotics.

Patient teaching
• Tell patient to alert nurse if discomfort is felt at I.V. site
• Warn patient that I.M. injection may be painful but that ice applied to site may ease discomfort.

☑ Evaluation
• Patient is free from infection.
• Patient shows no signs of allergy.
• Patient and family state understanding of drug therapy.

penicillin V
(phenoxymethyl penicillin)
(pen-ih-SIL-in VEE)

penicillin V potassium
(phenoxymethylpenicillin potassium)
Abbocillin VK◇, Apo-Pen-VK◇, Beepen-VK, Betapen-VK, Cilicaine VK◇, Ledercillin VK, Nadopen-V-200♦, Nadopen-V-400♦, Nadopen-VK♦, NovoPen-VK♦, Nu-Pen VK♦, Pen Vee, Pen Vee K, PVF K♦, PVK◇, Robicillin VK, V-Cillin K, Veetids**

Pharmacologic class: natural penicillin
Therapeutic class: antibiotic
Pregnancy risk category: B

How supplied
penicillin V
Tablets: 250 mg, 500 mg
Oral suspension: 125 mg/5 ml, 250 mg/5 ml (after reconstitution)
penicillin V potassium
Tablets: 125 mg, 250 mg, 500 mg
Tablets (film-coated): 250 mg, 500 mg
Capsules: 250 mg◇
Oral suspension: 125 mg/5 ml, 250 mg/5 ml (after reconstitution)

Pharmacokinetics
Absorption: about 60% to 75% absorbed from GI tract.

Distribution: distributed widely into synovial, pleural, pericardial, and ascitic fluids and bile, and into liver, skin, lungs, kidneys, muscle, intestines, tonsils, maxillary sinuses, saliva, and erythrocytes. CSF penetration is poor but is enhanced in patients with inflamed meninges. It is 75% to 89% protein-bound.
Metabolism: between 35% and 70% metabolized to inactive compounds.
Excretion: excreted primarily in urine.
Half-life: 30 minutes.

Route	Onset	Peak	Duration
P.O.	Unknown	30-60 min	Unknown

Pharmacodynamics
Chemical effect: inhibits cell-wall synthesis during microorganism multiplication; bacteria resist penicillins by producing penicillinases.
Therapeutic effect: kills susceptible bacteria, such as most nonpenicillinase-producing strains of gram-positive and gram-negative aerobic cocci, spirochetes, and some gram-positive aerobic and anaerobic bacilli.

Indications and dosage
▶ **Mild to moderate systemic infections.** *Adults:* 125 to 500 mg (200,000 to 800,000 units) P.O. q 6 hours. *Children:* 15 to 50 mg/kg (25,000 to 90,000 units/kg) P.O. daily, in divided doses q 6 to 8 hours.
▶ **Endocarditis prophylaxis for dental surgery.** *Adults:* 2 g P.O. 30 to 60 minutes before procedure; then 500 mg P.O. q 6 hours for eight doses. *Children weighing under 30 kg (66 lb):* half of adult dose.

Adverse reactions
CNS: neuropathy.
GI: *epigastric distress,* vomiting, diarrhea, *nausea.*
Hematologic: eosinophilia, hemolytic anemia, *leukopenia, thrombocytopenia.*
Other: hypersensitivity reactions (rash, urticaria, chills, fever, edema, *anaphy-*

---

laxis), overgrowth of nonsusceptible organisms.

Interactions

Drug-drug. *Oral contraceptives containing estrogen:* decreased effectiveness of oral contraceptive. Monitor for breakthrough bleeding.
Probenecid: increased blood levels of penicillin. Probenecid may be used for this purpose.

Contraindications and precautions

• Contraindicated in patients with hypersensitivity to drug or other penicillins.
• Use cautiously in pregnant women and in patients with other drug allergies, especially to cephalosporins.
• Drug is excreted in breast milk; use in breast-feeding women may sensitize infant to penicillin and cause some adverse effects.

NURSING CONSIDERATIONS

Assessment
• Assess patient's infection before therapy and regularly thereafter.
• Before giving drug, ask patient about any allergic reactions to penicillin. However, negative history of penicillin allergy is no guarantee against future allergic reaction.
• Obtain specimen for culture and sensitivity tests before giving first dose. Therapy may begin pending results.
• As ordered, periodically assess renal and hematopoietic function in patient receiving long-term therapy.
• Be alert for adverse reactions and drug interactions.
• Observe closely. With large doses and prolonged therapy, bacterial or fungal superinfection may occur, especially in elderly, debilitated, or immunosuppressed patient.
• Evaluate patient's and family's knowledge of drug therapy.

Nursing diagnoses
• Infection related to presence of bacteria
• Altered protection related to risk of hypersensitivity reactions to drug
• Knowledge deficit related to drug therapy

Planning and implementation
• Give drug at least 1 hour before bacteriostatic antibiotics.
• American Heart Association considers amoxicillin the preferred agent for endocarditis prophylaxis because GI absorption is better and serum levels are sustained longer. Penicillin V is considered an alternative agent.
Patient teaching
• Tell patient to take drug exactly as prescribed, even after he feels better.
• Tell patient that drug may be taken without regard to meals. However, if GI disturbances occur, drug may be taken with meals.
• Warn patient never to use leftover penicillin V for new illness or to share penicillin with family and friends.
• Tell patient to call doctor if rash, fever, or chills develop.

Evaluation
• Patient is free from infection.
• Patient shows no signs of allergy.
• Patient and family state understanding of drug therapy.

pentamidine isethionate
(pen-TAM-eh-deen
ighs-eh-THIGH-oh-nayt)
NebuPent, Pentacarinat, Pentam 300, Pneumopent

Pharmacologic class: diamidine derivative
Therapeutic class: antiprotozoal
Pregnancy risk category: C

How supplied

Injection: 300-mg vial

Aerosol: 300-mg vial

Pharmacokinetics

Absorption: absorption is limited after aerosol administration. Unknown after I.M. administration.
Distribution: drug appears to be extensively tissue-bound. CNS penetration is poor. Extent of plasma protein-binding is unknown.
Metabolism: unknown.
Excretion: excreted unchanged in urine.
Half-life: varies according to route of administration: 9.1 to 13.2 hours for I.M., about 6.5 hours for I.V., and unknown for aerosol.

Route	Onset	Peak	Duration
I.V.	Unknown	Immediate	Unknown
I.M.	Unknown	0.5-1 hr	Unknown
Aerosol	Unknown	Unknown	Unknown

Pharmacodynamics

Chemical effect: interferes with organism's biosynthesis of DNA, RNA, phospholipids, and proteins.
Therapeutic effect: hinders growth of susceptible organisms, such as *Pneumocystis carinii* and *Trypanosoma.*

Indications and dosage

▶ *P. carinii* **pneumonia.** *Adults and children:* 4 mg/kg I.V. or I.M. once daily for 14 to 21 days.
▶ **Prevention of** *P. carinii* **pneumonia in high-risk patients.** *Adults:* 300 mg by inhalation (using Respirgard II nebulizer) once q 4 weeks.

Adverse reactions

CNS: confusion, hallucinations.
CV: *hypotension,* tachycardia.
GI: nausea, anorexia, metallic taste.
GU: *elevated serum creatinine,* renal toxicity, *acute renal failure.*
Hematologic: *leukopenia, thrombocytopenia,* anemia.
Hepatic: elevated liver enzymes.
Metabolic: *hypoglycemia,* hyperglycemia, hypocalcemia.

Respiratory: cough, bronchospasm.
Skin: rash, facial flushing, pruritus, *Stevens-Johnson syndrome.*
Other: fever, *sterile abscess; pain, induration* (at injection site).

Interactions

Drug-drug. *Aminoglycosides, amphotericin B, capreomycin, cisplatin, colistin, methoxyflurane, polymyxin B, vancomycin:* increased risk of nephrotoxicity. Monitor patient closely.

Contraindications and precautions

• Contraindicated in patients with history of anaphylactic reaction to drug.
• Drug use is not recommended in breast-feeding women.
• Use cautiously in pregnant women and in patients with hypertension, hypotension, hypoglycemia, hypocalcemia, leukopenia, thrombocytopenia, anemia, or hepatic or renal dysfunction.

NURSING CONSIDERATIONS

☞ Assessment
• Assess patient's infection before therapy and regularly thereafter.
• Monitor blood glucose, serum calcium, serum creatinine, and BUN levels daily. After parenteral administration, blood glucose level may decrease initially; hypoglycemia may be severe in 5% to 10% of patients. This may be followed by hyperglycemia and insulin-dependent diabetes mellitus, which may be permanent.
• Closely monitor blood pressure during I.V. administration.
• Be alert for adverse reactions and drug interactions.
• Evaluate patient's and family's knowledge of drug therapy.

☷ Nursing diagnoses
• Infection related to presence of organisms
• Risk for injury related to drug-induced adverse CNS reactions

---

• Knowledge deficit related to drug therapy

▷ **Planning and implementation**
I.V. use: Reconstitute drug with 3 ml of sterile water for injection, then dilute in 50 to 250 ml of D_5W. Inject over at least 1 hour.
– To minimize hypotension, infuse drug slowly with patient lying down.
I.M. use: Reconstitute drug with 3 ml of sterile water for solution containing 100 mg/ml; administer deeply. Expect pain and induration to occur.
• In patient with AIDS, pentamidine may produce less severe adverse reactions than co-trimoxazole, the alternative treatment, and may be treatment of choice.
Aerosol use: Administer aerosol form only by Respirgard II nebulizer manufactured by Marquest. Dosage recommendations are based on particle size and delivery rate of this device. To use aerosol, mix contents of one vial in 6 ml of sterile water for injection. *Do not* use 0.9% NaCl solution; it will cause precipitation. Do not mix with other drugs.
– Do not use low-pressure (below 20 psi) compressors. The flow rate should be 5 to 7 liters/minute from 40- to 50-psi air or oxygen source.
Patient teaching
• Instruct patient to use aerosol device until chamber is empty, which may take up to 45 minutes.
• Warn patient that I.M. injection causes pain at administration site. However, application of warm soaks is helpful.
• Stress need to report light-headedness or signs and symptoms of hypoglycemia immediately.

☑ **Evaluation**
• Patient is free from infection.
• Patient sustains no injuries due to drug-induced adverse CNS reactions.
• Patient and family state understanding of drug therapy.

pentazocine hydrochloride
(pen-TAZ-oh-seen high-droh-KLOR-ighd)
Fortral♦◊, Talwin

pentazocine hydrochloride and naloxone hydrochloride
Talwin Nx

pentazocine lactate
Fortral◊, Talwin

Pharmacologic class: narcotic agonist-antagonist, opioid partial agonist
Therapeutic class: analgesic, adjunct to anesthesia
Controlled substance schedule: IV
Pregnancy risk category: NR

How supplied

pentazocine hydrochloride
Tablets: 25 mg◊, 50 mg♦◊
pentazocine hydrochloride and naloxone hydrochloride
Tablets: 50 mg pentazocine hydrochloride and 500 mcg naloxone hydrochloride
pentazocine lactate
Injection: 30 mg/ml

Pharmacokinetics

Absorption: well absorbed after oral or parenteral administration, although oral form undergoes first-pass metabolism in liver and less than 20% of dose reaches systemic circulation unchanged. Bioavailability is increased in patients with hepatic dysfunction; patients with cirrhosis absorb 60% to 70% of drug.
Distribution: appears to be widely distributed throughout body.
Metabolism: metabolized in liver. Metabolism may be prolonged in patients with impaired hepatic function.
Excretion: excreted primarily in urine, with very small amounts excreted in feces. *Half-life:* 2 to 3 hours.

Route	Onset	Peak	Duration
P.O.	15-30 min	60-90 min	2-3 hr
I.V.	2-3 min	15-30 min	2-3 hr
I.M., S.C.	15-20 min	30-60 min	2-3 hr

Pharmacodynamics

Chemical effect: binds with opioid receptors at many sites in CNS, altering pain response by unknown mechanism. **Therapeutic effect:** relieves pain.

Indications and dosage

▶ **Moderate to severe pain.** *Adults:* 50 to 100 mg P.O. q 3 to 4 hours, p.r.n. Maximum oral dosage is 600 mg/day. Alternatively, 30 mg I.M., I.V., or S.C. q 3 to 4 hours, p.r.n. Maximum parenteral dosage is 360 mg/day. Single doses above 30 mg I.V. or 60 mg I.M. or S.C. are not recommended.
▶ **Labor.** *Adults:* 30 mg I.M. or 20 mg I.V. q 2 to 3 hours when contractions become regular.

Adverse reactions

CNS: *sedation,* visual disturbances, hallucinations, drowsiness, *dizziness, lightheadedness,* confusion, *euphoria,* headache, psychotomimetic effects.
CV: hypotension, *shock.*
EENT: dry mouth, dysgeusia.
GI: *nausea, vomiting,* constipation.
GU: urine retention.
Respiratory: *respiratory depression.*
Skin: induration, nodules, sloughing, and sclerosis of injection site.
Other: hypersensitivity reactions *(anaphylaxis),* physical and psychological dependence.

Interactions

Drug-drug. *CNS depressants:* additive effects. Use together cautiously.
Narcotic analgesics: possible decreased analgesic effect. Avoid concomitant use.
Drug-lifestyle. *Alcohol use:* additive effects. Use together cautiously.
Smoking: may increase requirements for pentazocine. Monitor drug's effectiveness.

Contraindications and precautions

● Contraindicated in patients with hypersensitivity to drug or its components.
● Drug is not recommended for children under age 12.
● Use cautiously in pregnant or breastfeeding women and in patients with hepatic or renal disease, acute MI, head injury, increased intracranial pressure, or respiratory depression.

NURSING CONSIDERATIONS

⚙ Assessment

● Assess patient's pain before and after drug administration.
● Monitor vital signs closely, especially respirations.
● Be alert for adverse reactions and drug interactions.
● Evaluate patient's and family's knowledge of drug therapy.

⊕ Nursing diagnoses

● Pain related to condition
● Ineffective breathing patterns related to drug-induced respiratory depression
● Knowledge deficit related to drug therapy

▶ Planning and implementation

P.O. use: Talwin Nx, the oral pentazocine available in the U.S., contains the narcotic antagonist naloxone. This prevents illicit I.V. use.
I.V. use: Give drug by direct I.V. injection. Administer slowly. Do not mix in same syringe with aminophylline, barbiturates, or other alkaline substances.
I.M. and S.C. use: Rotate injection sites to minimize tissue irritation. If possible, avoid giving by S.C. route.
● Drug possesses narcotic antagonist properties. May precipitate withdrawal syndrome in narcotic-dependent patient.
● Dependence may occur with prolonged use.
● Hold drug and notify doctor if respiratory rate drops significantly. Have nalox-

---

one readily available to reverse respiratory depression.
• Drug may interfere with certain laboratory tests for urinary 17-hydroxycorticosteroids.

Patient teaching
• Caution ambulatory patient about getting out of bed or walking. Warn outpatient to avoid hazardous activities until drug's CNS effects are known.
• Warn patient about drug's potential for causing dependence.

☑ Evaluation
• Patient is free from pain.
• Patient maintains respiratory rate and pattern within normal limits.
• Patient and family state understanding of drug therapy.

pentobarbital (pentobarbitone)
(pen-toh-BAR-beh-tol)
Nembutal* **

pentobarbital sodium
Carbrital◇, Nembutal Sodium*,
Nova Rectal♦, Novopentobarb♦

Pharmacologic class: barbiturate
Therapeutic class: anticonvulsant, sedative-hypnotic
Controlled substance schedule: II
Pregnancy risk category: D

How supplied
pentobarbital
Elixir: 18.2 mg/5 ml
pentobarbital sodium
Capsules: 50 mg, 100 mg
Injection: 50 mg/ml
Suppositories: 30 mg, 60 mg, 120 mg, 200 mg

Pharmacokinetics
Absorption: absorbed rapidly after oral or rectal administration. Unknown after I.M. administration.

Distribution: distributed widely throughout body. About 35% to 45% of drug is protein-bound.
Metabolism: metabolized in liver.
Excretion: 99% of drug is excreted in urine. **Half-life:** 35 to 50 hours.

Route	Onset	Peak	Duration
P.O.	≤ 15 min	30-60 min	1-4 hr
I.V.	Immediate	Immediate	15 min
I.M.	10-25 min	Unknown	Unknown
P.R.	≤ 15 min	Unknown	1-4 hr

Pharmacodynamics
Chemical effect: unknown; may interfere with transmission of impulses from thalamus to cortex of brain.
Therapeutic effect: promotes sleep and calmness.

Indications and dosage
► **Sedation.** *Adults:* 20 to 40 mg P.O. b.i.d., t.i.d., or q.i.d. *Children:* 2 to 6 mg/kg daily P.O. in three divided doses. Maximum daily dosage is 100 mg.
► **Insomnia.** *Adults:* 100 mg P.O. h.s. or 150 to 200 mg I.M.; initially, 100 mg I.V., then additional doses up to 500 mg; 120 or 200 mg P.R. *Children:* 2 to 6 mg/kg I.M. Maximum dosage is 100 mg. P.R. doses are: ages 2 months to 1 year, 30 mg; ages 1 to 4, 30 or 60 mg; ages 5 to 12, 60 mg; ages 12 to 14, 60 or 120 mg.
► **Preoperative sedation.** *Adults:* 150 to 200 mg I.M. *Children:* 5 mg/kg P.O. or I.M. if age 10 or older; 5 mg/kg I.M. or P.R. if younger than age 10.

Adverse reactions
CNS: *drowsiness, lethargy, hangover;* paradoxical excitement (in elderly patients).
GI: nausea, vomiting.
Hematologic: exacerbation of porphyria.
Skin: rash, *urticaria, Stevens-Johnson syndrome.*
Other: *angioedema, respiratory depression.*

Reactions may be *common*, uncommon, *life-threatening*, or COMMON AND LIFE-THREATENING.

Interactions

Drug-drug. *Corticosteroids, doxycycline, estrogens and oral contraceptives, oral anticoagulants:* pentobarbital may enhance metabolism of these drugs. Monitor for decreased effect.
CNS depressants, including narcotic analgesics: excessive CNS and respiratory depression. Use together cautiously.
Griseofulvin: decreased absorption of griseofulvin.
MAO inhibitors: inhibited metabolism of barbiturates; may cause prolonged CNS depression. Reduce barbiturate dosage.
Rifampin: may decrease barbiturate levels. Monitor for decreased effect.
Drug-lifestyle. *Alcohol use:* excessive CNS and respiratory depression. Avoid concomitant use.

Contraindications and precautions

• Contraindicated in patients with porphyria or hypersensitivity to barbiturates.
• Drug use is not recommended in pregnant or breast-feeding women.
• Use cautiously in elderly or debilitated patients and in those with acute or chronic pain, depression, suicidal tendencies, history of drug abuse, or hepatic impairment.

NURSING CONSIDERATIONS

Assessment
• Assess patient's condition before therapy and regularly thereafter.
• Assess mental status before therapy and use reduced doses, as ordered. Elderly patients are more sensitive to drug's adverse CNS effects.
• Inspect patient's skin. Skin eruptions may precede potentially fatal reactions to barbiturate therapy.
• Be alert for adverse reactions and drug interactions.
• Evaluate patient's and family's knowledge of drug therapy.

Nursing diagnoses
• Sleep pattern disturbance related to condition

• High risk for injury related to drug-induced adverse CNS reactions
• Knowledge deficit related to drug therapy

Planning and implementation
P.O. use: Follow normal protocol.
I.V. use: I.V. use of barbiturates may cause severe respiratory depression, laryngospasm, or hypotension. Have emergency resuscitation equipment available.
– To minimize deterioration, use I.V injection solution within 30 minutes after opening container. Don't use cloudy solution.
– Reserve I.V. injection for emergency treatment, which should be given under close supervision. Give slowly (50 mg/minute or less).
– Parenteral solution is alkaline. Local tissue reactions and injection site pain have followed I.V. use. Avoid extravasation. Assess patency of I.V. site before and during administration.
– Do not mix in syringe or in I.V. solutions or lines with other drugs.
I.M. use: Give I.M. injection deeply. Superficial injection may cause pain, sterile abscess, and sloughing.
P.R. use: To ensure accurate dosage, don't divide suppositories.
• Stop drug if skin reactions occur and call doctor. In some patients, high fever, stomatitis, headache, or rhinitis may precede skin reactions.
• Pentobarbital has no analgesic effect and may cause restlessness or delirium in patient with pain.
• Long-term use is not recommended; drug loses its efficacy in promoting sleep after 14 days of continued use. Long-term high dosage may cause drug dependence, and may lead to withdrawal symptoms if drug is suddenly discontinued. Withdraw barbiturates gradually.
Patient teaching
• Warn patient about performing activities that require alertness or physical coordination. For inpatient, supervise walk-

ing and raise bed rails, particularly for elderly patient.

• Inform patient that morning hangover is common after hypnotic dose, which suppresses REM sleep. Patient may experience increased dreaming after drug is discontinued.

• Tell patient who uses oral contraceptives that she should consider alternate birth control methods because drug may enhance contraceptive hormone metabolism and decrease its effect.

☑ **Evaluation**
• Patient reports satisfactory sleep.
• Patient sustains no injuries due to drug-induced adverse CNS reactions.
• Patient and family state understanding of drug therapy.

---

pentostatin (2'-deoxycoformycin)
(pen-toh-STAH-tin)
Nipent

Pharmacologic class: antimetabolite (adenosine deaminase [ADA] inhibitor)
Therapeutic class: antineoplastic agent
Pregnancy risk category: D

How supplied

Powder for injection: 10 mg/vial

Pharmacokinetics

Absorption: not applicable.
Distribution: plasma protein–binding is low (about 4%).
Metabolism: unknown.
Excretion: over 90% excreted in urine.
Half-life: about 6 hours.

Route	Onset	Peak	Duration
I.V.	Unknown	Unknown	Unknown

Pharmacodynamics

Chemical effect: inhibits ADA, causing increase in intracellular levels of deoxyadenosine triphosphate. This leads to cell damage and death. Greatest activity

of ADA is in cells of lymphoid system (especially malignant T cells).
Therapeutic effect: kills selected leukemic cells.

Indications and dosage

▶ **Alpha-interferon–refractory hairy-cell leukemia.** *Adults:* 4 mg/m^2 I.V. every other week.

Adverse reactions

CNS: asthenia, malaise, *headache, neurologic symptoms, anxiety, confusion, depression, dizziness, insomnia, nervousness, paresthesia, somnolence, abnormal thinking, fatigue.*
CV: chest pain, *arrhythmias,* abnormal ECG, thrombophlebitis, peripheral edema, *hemorrhage.*
EENT: abnormal vision, conjunctivitis, ear pain, eye pain, epistaxis, pharyngitis, rhinitis, sinusitis.
GI: abdominal pain, nausea, vomiting, anorexia, diarrhea, constipation, flatulence, stomatitis.
GU: *hematuria, dysuria, increased BUN and creatinine levels.*
Hematologic: *myelosuppression,* LEUKOPENIA, anemia, THROMBOCYTOPENIA, *lymphocytopenia,* lymphadenopathy.
Hepatic: *elevated liver enzyme levels.*
Musculoskeletal: back pain, myalgia, arthralgia.
Respiratory: *cough, bronchitis, dyspnea, pulmonary edema, pneumonia.*
Skin: photosensitivity, contact dermatitis, ecchymosis, petechiae, rash, eczema, dry skin, herpes simplex or zoster, maculopapular rash, vesiculobullous rash, pruritus, seborrhea, discoloration.
Other: fever, diaphoresis, INFECTION, pain, HYPERSENSITIVITY REACTIONS, *death, neoplasm,* chills, sepsis, flulike syndrome, weight loss, increased LD level.

Interactions

Drug-drug. *Cytarabine, vidarabine:* increased adverse reactions to either drug. Avoid concomitant use.

Reactions may be *common,* uncommon, *life-threatening*, or COMMON AND LIFE-THREATENING.

Fludarabine: risk of fatal pulmonary toxicity. Don't use together.

Contraindications and precautions

• Contraindicated in patients hypersensitive to drug.
• Drug use is not recommended in pregnant or breast-feeding women.
• Safety of drug has not been established in children.

NURSING CONSIDERATIONS

Assessment
• Assess patient's condition before therapy and regularly thereafter.
• Be alert for adverse reactions and drug interactions.
• Evaluate patient's and family's knowledge of drug therapy.

Nursing diagnoses
• Altered health maintenance related to leukemia
• Altered protection related to drug-induced adverse hematologic reactions
• Knowledge deficit related to drug therapy

Planning and implementation
• Use drug only under supervision of doctor qualified and experienced in use of chemotherapeutic agents. Adverse reactions after therapy are common.
• Make sure patient is well hydrated before therapy. Administer 500 to 1,000 ml of D_5W in 0.45% NaCl injection, as ordered, for hydration.
• Follow institutional policy to reduce risks. Preparation and administration of parenteral form are associated with mutagenic, teratogenic, and carcinogenic risks to personnel.
• Add 5 ml of sterile water for injection to vial containing pentostatin powder for injection. Mix thoroughly to make solution of 5 mg/ml. Drug may be administered by I.V. bolus injection or diluted further in 25 or 50 ml of D_5W or 0.9%

NaCl injection and infused over 20 to 30 minutes.
• Use reconstituted solution within 8 hours; it contains no preservatives.
• Treat all spills and waste products with 5% sodium hypochlorite (household bleach).
• Give additional 500 ml of D_5W, as ordered, for hydration after drug is administered.
• Optimal duration of therapy is unknown. Current recommendations suggest two additional courses of therapy after complete response. If partial response is not evident after 6 months, drug will be discontinued. If partial response is evident, drug will be continued for another 6 months or for two courses of therapy after complete response.
• Withhold drug in patients with CNS toxicity, severe rash, or active infection and notify doctor. Drug may be resumed when infection clears. Avoid use in patients with renal damage (creatinine clearance of 60 ml/minute or less).
• Temporarily withhold drug and notify doctor if absolute neutrophil count falls below 200/mm³ and pretreatment level was over 500/mm³. No recommendations exist for dosage adjustments in patients with anemia, neutropenia, or thrombocytopenia.
• Use drug only in patients with hairy-cell leukemia refractory to alpha-interferon (disease that progresses after minimum of 3 months of treatment with alpha-interferon or disease that does not exhibit response after 6 months of therapy).
Patient teaching
• Teach patient how to take infection-control and bleeding precautions.
• Tell patient to notify doctor of adverse reactions.

Evaluation
• Patient responds well to therapy.
• Patient does not develop serious complications from adverse reactions.
• Patient and family state understanding of drug therapy.

pentoxifylline
(pen-tok-SIH-fi-lin)
Trental

Pharmacologic class: xanthine derivative
Therapeutic class: hemorrheologic
Pregnancy risk category: C

How supplied
Tablets (extended-release): 400 mg

Pharmacokinetics
Absorption: absorbed almost completely but slowed by food. Undergoes first-pass hepatic metabolism.
Distribution: bound by erythrocyte membrane.
Metabolism: metabolized extensively by erythrocytes and liver.
Excretion: excreted primarily in urine; less than 4% of drug is excreted in feces.
Half-life: about 30 to 45 minutes.

Route	Onset	Peak	Duration
P.O.	Unknown	2-4 hr	Unknown

Pharmacodynamics
Chemical effect: unknown; thought to increase RBC flexibility and lower blood viscosity.
Therapeutic effect: improves capillary blood flow.

Indications and dosage
▶ **Intermittent claudication caused by chronic occlusive vascular disease.**
Adults: 400 mg P.O. t.i.d. with meals.

Adverse reactions
CNS: headache, dizziness.
GI: dyspepsia, nausea, vomiting.

Interactions
Drug-drug. *Anticoagulants:* increased anticoagulant effect. Adjust anticoagulant dosage as ordered.
Antihypertensives: increased hypotensive effect. Dosage adjustments may be necessary.

Drug-lifestyle. *Smoking:* vasoconstriction may result. Advise patient to avoid smoking, it may worsen his condition.

Contraindications and precautions
• Contraindicated in patients who are intolerant to methylxanthines, such as caffeine and theophylline, and in those with recent cerebral or retinal hemorrhage.
• Drug is not recommended for use in breast-feeding women.
• Use cautiously in pregnant women.
• Safety of drug has not been established in children.

NURSING CONSIDERATIONS

Assessment
• Assess patient's condition before therapy and regularly thereafter.
• Be alert for adverse reactions and drug interactions.
• Be aware that elderly patients may be more sensitive to drug's effects.
• Monitor patient's hydration status if adverse GI reactions.
• Evaluate patient's and family's knowledge of drug therapy.

Nursing diagnoses
• Altered peripheral tissue perfusion related to condition
• Risk for fluid volume deficit related to drug-induced adverse GI reactions
• Knowledge deficit related to drug therapy

Planning and implementation
• Know that drug is useful in patients who are not good surgical candidates.
• Report adverse reactions to doctor; dosage may need to be reduced.
Patient teaching
• Advise patient to take with meals to minimize GI upset.
• Instruct patient to swallow drug whole, without breaking, crushing, or chewing.
• Tell patient to report adverse GI or CNS reactions.

Reactions may be *common*, uncommon, **life-threatening**, or COMMON AND LIFE-THREATENING.

• Advise patient to avoid smoking because nicotine causes vasoconstriction that can worsen his condition.
• Tell patient not to discontinue drug during first 8 weeks of therapy unless directed by doctor.

☑ **Evaluation**
• Patient exhibits adequate peripheral tissue perfusion.
• Patient maintains adequate hydration throughout therapy.
• Patient and family state understanding of drug therapy.

pergolide mesylate
(PER-goh-lighd MES-ih-layt)
Permax

Pharmacologic class: dopaminergic agonist
Therapeutic class: antiparkinsonian agent
Pregnancy risk category: B

How supplied

Tablets: 0.05 mg, 0.25 mg, 1 mg

Pharmacokinetics

Absorption: well absorbed.
Distribution: drug is about 90% protein-bound.
Metabolism: metabolized to at least 10 different compounds, some of which retain pharmacologic activity.
Excretion: excreted mainly by kidneys.

Route	Onset	Peak	Duration
P.O.	Unknown	Unknown	Unknown

Pharmacodynamics

Chemical effect: directly stimulates dopamine receptors in nigrostriatal system.
Therapeutic effect: helps to relieve signs and symptoms of Parkinson's disease.

Indications and dosage

▶ **Adjunct treatment with carbidopa-levodopa in management of symptoms associated with Parkinson's disease.** *Adults:* initially, 0.05 mg P.O. daily for first 2 days followed by increased dosage of 0.1 to 0.15 mg every third day over 12 days. Subsequent dosage increased by 0.25 mg every third day until optimum response is seen if needed. Drug usually is administered in divided doses t.i.d. Gradual reductions in carbidopa-levodopa dosage could be made during dosage titration.

Adverse reactions

CNS: headache, asthenia, *dyskinesia, dizziness, hallucinations,* dystonia, confusion, *somnolence,* insomnia, anxiety, depression, tremor, abnormal dreams, personality disorder, psychosis, abnormal gait, akathisia, extrapyramidal syndrome, incoordination, akinesia, hypertonia, neuralgia, speech disorder, twitching paresthesia.
CV: chest pain, *orthostatic hypotension,* vasodilation, palpitations, hypotension, syncope, hypertension, *arrhythmias, MI.*
EENT: *rhinitis,* epistaxis, abnormal vision, diplopia, eye disorder.
GI: dry mouth, dysgeusia, abdominal pain, *nausea, constipation,* diarrhea, dyspepsia, anorexia, vomiting.
GU: urinary frequency, urinary tract infection, hematuria.
Musculoskeletal: neck, and back pain, arthralgia; bursitis; myalgia.
Skin: rash.
Other: diaphoresis, flulike syndrome, chills; infection; facial, peripheral, or generalized edema; weight gain.

Interactions

Drug-drug. *Butyrophenones, metoclopramide, other dopamine antagonists, phenothiazines, thioxanthenes:* may antagonize effects of pergolide. Avoid concomitant use.

Contraindications and precautions

• Contraindicated in patients hypersensitive to drug or ergot alkaloids.

• Use cautiously in pregnant women and in patients prone to arrhythmias.
• Safety of drug has not been established in children and in breast-feeding women.

NURSING CONSIDERATIONS

⚖ Assessment
• Assess patient's condition before therapy. Monitor drug's effectiveness by regularly checking patient's body movements for improvement.
• Monitor blood pressure and heart rate and rhythm. Symptomatic orthostatic or sustained hypotension may occur in some patients, especially at start of therapy, and arrhythmias may be induced by drug.
• Be alert for adverse reactions and drug interactions.
• Evaluate patient's and family's knowledge of drug therapy.

🔁 Nursing diagnoses
• Impaired physical mobility related to Parkinson's disease
• Decreased cardiac output related to drug-induced adverse CV reactions
• Knowledge deficit related to drug therapy

❯ Planning and implementation
• Know that dosage is gradually increased according to patient's response and tolerance.
• Notify doctor if significant changes in vital signs or mental status occur.
Patient teaching
• Inform patient of potential adverse reactions, especially hallucinations and confusion (27% incidence).
• Warn patient to avoid activities that could result in injury from orthostatic hypotension and syncope.

☑ Evaluation
• Patient exhibits improved mobility.
• Patient maintains cardiac output.
• Patient and family state understanding of drug therapy.

perphenazine
(per-FEN-uh-zeen)
Apo-Perphenazine♦, PMS-Perphenazine♦, Trilafon, Trilafon Concentrate

Pharmacologic class: phenothiazine (piperazine derivative)
Therapeutic class: antipsychotic, antiemetic
Pregnancy risk category: NR

How supplied
Tablets: 2 mg, 4 mg, 8 mg, 16 mg
Oral concentrate: 16 mg/5 ml
Syrup: 2 mg/5 ml♦
Injection: 5 mg/ml

Pharmacokinetics
Absorption: rate and extent vary: oral tablet absorption is erratic and variable; oral concentrate absorption is much more predicable; I.M. drug is rapidly absorbed from injection site.
Distribution: distributed widely in body; 91% to 99% of drug is protein-bound.
Metabolism: metabolized extensively by liver.
Excretion: most of drug excreted in urine; some in feces.

Route	Onset	Peak	Duration
P.O., I.M.	Varies	Unknown	Unknown

Pharmacodynamics
Chemical effect: unknown; probably blocks postsynaptic dopamine receptors in brain and inhibits medullary chemoreceptor trigger zone.
Therapeutic effect: relieves signs and symptoms of psychosis as well as nausea and vomiting.

Indications and dosage
▶ **Psychosis in nonhospitalized patients.** *Adults:* initially, 4 to 8 mg P.O. t.i.d., reduced as soon as possible to minimum effective dosage. *Children over age 12:* lowest adult dose.

▶ **Psychosis in hospitalized patients.**
Adults: initially, 8 to 16 mg P.O. b.i.d.,
t.i.d., or q.i.d., increased to 64 mg daily
as needed. Alternatively, 5 to 10 mg I.M.
q 6 hours p.r.n. Maximum dosage is
30 mg. *Children over age 12:* lowest limit of adult dosage.
▶ **Severe nausea and vomiting.** *Adults:*
5 to 10 mg I.M. p.r.n.

Adverse reactions

CNS: *extrapyramidal reactions* (high in-
cidence), *tardive dyskinesia,* sedation
(low incidence), pseudoparkinsonism,
EEG changes, dizziness, *seizures.*
CV: *orthostatic hypotension,* tachycardia,
ECG changes, *cardiac arrest.*
EENT: ocular changes, blurred vision.
GI: dry mouth, constipation.
GU: *urine retention,* dark urine, menstrual irregularities, gynecomastia, inhibited
ejaculation.
Hematologic: transient leukopenia, hyperprolactinemia, *agranulocytosis, hemolytic anemia, thrombocytopenia.*
Hepatic: cholestatic jaundice, abnormal
liver function test results.
Skin: *mild photosensitivity,* allergic reactions, pain at I.M. injection site, sterile
abscess.
Other: weight gain; increased appetite;
rarely, *neuroleptic malignant syndrome.*
**After abrupt withdrawal of long-term
therapy:** gastritis, nausea, vomiting,
dizziness, tremors, feeling of warmth or
cold, diaphoresis, tachycardia, headache,
insomnia.

Interactions

Drug-drug. *Antacids:* inhibited oral phenothiazine absorption. Administer separately.
Barbiturates: may decrease phenothiazine effect. Observe patient closely.
Other CNS depressants: increased CNS
depression. Avoid concomitant use.
Drug-lifestyle. *Alcohol use:* increased
CNS depression. Avoid concomitant use.
Sun exposure: increased photosensitivity
reaction; take precautions.

Contraindications and precautions

• Contraindicated in patients with hypersensitivity to drug; in patients experiencing coma; in those with CNS depression,
blood dyscrasia, bone marrow depression, liver damage, or subcortical damage; and in those receiving large doses of
CNS depressants.
• Use cautiously with other CNS depressants or anticholinergics, and in elderly
or debilitated patients or in pregnant or
breast-feeding women.
• Also use cautiously in patients with alcohol withdrawal, psychic depression,
suicidal tendency, severe adverse reactions to other phenothiazines, impaired
renal function, and respiratory disorders.
• Safety of drug has not been established
in children age 12 and under.

NURSING CONSIDERATIONS

Assessment
• Assess patient's condition before therapy and regularly thereafter.
• Obtain baseline blood pressure before
therapy and monitor regularly. Watch for
orthostatic hypotension, especially with
I.M. administration.
• Monitor weekly bilirubin tests during
first month; periodic blood tests (CBC
and liver function); and ophthalmic tests
(long-term use) as ordered.
• Be alert for adverse reactions and drug
interactions.
• Monitor patient for tardive dyskinesia.
It may occur after prolonged use. It may
not appear until months or years later and
may disappear spontaneously or persist
for life despite discontinuation of drug.
• Monitor patient's hydration status if
drug is used for nausea and vomiting.
• Evaluate patient's and family's knowledge of drug therapy.

Nursing diagnoses
• Altered thought processes related to
psychosis
• Risk for fluid volume deficit related to
nausea or vomiting

● Knowledge deficit related to drug therapy

▶ **Planning and implementation**
P.O. use: Dilute liquid concentrate with fruit juice, milk, carbonated beverage, or semisolid food just before giving. Exceptions: oral concentrate causes turbidity or precipitation in colas, black coffee, grape or apple juice, or tea. Do not mix with them.
I.M. use: Inject drug deeply only in upper outer quadrant of buttocks. Massage slowly afterward to prevent sterile abscess. Injection may sting. Keep patient supine for 1 hour after injection because of risk of hypotension.
● Prevent contact dermatitis by keeping drug away from skin and clothes. Wear gloves when preparing liquid forms.
● Protect drug from light. Slight yellowing of injection or concentrate does not affect potency. Discard markedly discolored solutions.
● Do not stop drug abruptly unless required by severe adverse reactions.
● Withhold dose and notify doctor if patient develops jaundice, symptoms of blood dyscrasia (fever, sore throat, infection, cellulitis, weakness), or persistent extrapyramidal reactions (longer than a few hours).
● Acute dystonic reactions may be treated with diphenhydramine.
Patient teaching
● Advise patient to change positions slowly to minimize effects of orthostatic hypotension.
● Warn patient to avoid hazardous activities until CNS effects of drug are known. Drowsiness and dizziness usually subside after a few weeks.
● Tell patient to avoid alcohol during drug therapy.
● Advise patient to report urine retention or constipation.
● Tell patient to use sunblock and to wear protective clothing to avoid photosensitivity reactions.

● Tell patient to relieve dry mouth with sugarless gum or hard candy.

☑ **Evaluation**
● Patient's thought processes are normal.
● Patient maintains adequate hydration throughout drug therapy.
● Patient and family state understanding of drug therapy.

phenazopyridine hydrochloride (phenylazo diamino pyridine hydrochloride)
(fen-eh-soh-PEER-eh-deen high-droh-KLOR-ighd)
Azo-Standard†, Baridium†, Eridium†, Geridium†, Phenazo♦, Phenazodine†, Prodium†, Pyridiate†, Pyridium, Urodine†, Urogesic†, Viridium†

Pharmacologic class: azo dye
Therapeutic class: urinary analgesic
Pregnancy risk category: B

How supplied
Tablets: 95 mg†, 100 mg†, 200 mg

Pharmacokinetics
Absorption: unknown.
Distribution: unknown.
Metabolism: metabolized in liver.
Excretion: excreted in urine.

Route	Onset	Peak	Duration
P.O.	Unknown	Unknown	Unknown

Pharmacodynamics
Chemical effect: unknown; exerts local anesthetic action on urinary mucosa.
Therapeutic effect: relieves urinary tract pain.

Indications and dosage
▶ **Pain with urinary tract irritation or infection.** *Adults:* 200 mg P.O. t.i.d. *Children:* 12 mg/kg P.O. daily in three equally divided doses.

Reactions may be *common*, uncommon, *life-threatening*, or COMMON AND LIFE-THREATENING.

Adverse reactions
CNS: headache, vertigo.
GI: nausea.
Skin: rash.

Interactions
None significant.

Contraindications and precautions
• Contraindicated in patients with glomerulonephritis, severe hepatitis, uremia, pyelonephritis during pregnancy, or renal insufficiency.
• Use cautiously in children.
• Safety of drug has not been established in breast-feeding women.

NURSING CONSIDERATIONS

⚕ Assessment
• Assess patient's pain before and after drug administration.
• Be alert for adverse reactions.
• Monitor patient's hydration status if nausea occurs.
• Evaluate patient's and family's knowledge of drug therapy.

⊕ Nursing diagnoses
• Pain related to underlying urinary tract condition
• Risk for fluid volume deficit related to drug-induced nausea
• Knowledge deficit related to drug therapy

▶ Planning and implementation
• Administer drug with food to minimize nausea.
• Drug may alter Diastix results but does not affect Chemstrip uG used to test urine glucose.
Patient teaching
• Advise patient that taking drug with meals may minimize nausea.
• Caution patient to stop taking drug and to notify doctor if skin or sclera becomes yellow-tinged.
• Alert patient that drug colors urine red or orange. It may stain fabrics.

☑ Evaluation
• Patient is free from pain.
• Patient maintains adequate hydration.
• Patient and family state understanding of drug therapy.

---

phenobarbital (phenobarbitone)
(feen-oh-BAR-bih-tol)
Ancalixir♦, Barbita, Solfoton

phenobarbital sodium (phenobarbitone sodium)
Luminal Sodium

Pharmacologic class: barbiturate
Therapeutic class: anticonvulsant, sedative-hypnotic
Controlled substance schedule: IV
Pregnancy risk category: D

How supplied
Tablets: 15 mg, 16 mg, 30 mg, 32 mg, 60 mg, 65 mg, 100 mg
Capsules: 16 mg
Elixir:* 15 mg/5 ml, 20 mg/5 ml
Injection: 30 mg/ml, 60 mg/ml, 65 mg/ml, 130 mg/ml

Pharmacokinetics
Absorption: absorbed well after oral administration. Absorption from I.M. injection site is 100%.
Distribution: distributed widely throughout body. Drug is about 25% to 30% protein-bound.
Metabolism: metabolized in liver.
Excretion: excreted in urine. *Half-life:* 5 to 7 days.

Route	Onset	Peak	Duration
P.O.	20-60 min	Unknown	10-12 hr
I.V.	5 min	≥ 15 min	10-12 hr
I.M.	> 60 min	Unknown	10-12 hr

Pharmacodynamics
Chemical effect: unknown; may depress CNS synaptic transmission and increase seizure activity threshold in motor cortex.

As sedative, may interfere with transmission of impulses from thalamus to brain cortex.
Therapeutic effect: prevents and stops seizure activity; promotes calmness and sleep.

Indications and dosage

▶ **All forms of epilepsy except absent seizures, febrile seizures in children.**
Adults: 60 to 250 mg P.O. daily, in divided doses t.i.d. or as single dose h.s.
Children: 1 to 6 mg/kg P.O. daily, divided q 12 hours for total of 100 mg; can be given once daily, usually h.s.
▶ **Status epilepticus.** *Adults:* 10 to 20 mg/kg I.V.; repeat if necessary.
Children: 15 to 20 mg/kg I.V. Do not exceed 50 mg/minute.
▶ **Sedation.** *Adults:* 30 to 120 mg P.O. daily in two or three divided doses.
Children: 3 to 5 mg/kg P.O. daily in divided doses t.i.d.
▶ **Insomnia.** *Adults:* 100 to 200 mg P.O. or I.M. h.s.
▶ **Preoperative sedation.** *Adults:* 100 to 200 mg I.M. 60 to 90 minutes before surgery. *Children:* 1 to 3 mg/kg I.V. or I.M. 60 to 90 minutes before surgery.

Adverse reactions

CNS: drowsiness, lethargy, hangover; paradoxical excitement (in elderly).
CV: bradycardia, hypotension.
GI: nausea, vomiting.
Hematologic: exacerbation of porphyria.
Respiratory: *respiratory depression, apnea.*
Skin: rash, *erythema multiforme, Stevens-Johnson syndrome,* urticaria; pain, swelling, thrombophlebitis, necrosis; nerve injury (at injection site).
Other: *angioedema.*

Interactions

Drug-drug. *Chloramphenicol, MAO inhibitors, valproic acid:* potentiated barbiturate effect. Monitor for increased CNS and respiratory depression.

CNS depressants, including narcotic analgesics: excessive CNS depression. Use cautiously.
Corticosteroids, digitoxin, doxycycline, estrogens and oral contraceptives, oral anticoagulants, tricyclic antidepressants: phenobarbital may enhance metabolism of these drugs. Monitor for decreased effect.
Diazepam: increased effects of both drugs. Use together cautiously.
Griseofulvin: decreased absorption of griseofulvin. Administer separately.
Mephobarbital, primidone: excessive phenobarbital blood levels; monitor closely.
Rifampin: may decrease barbiturate levels. Monitor for decreased effect.
Valproic acid: increased phenobarbital levels. Monitor for toxicity.
Drug-lifestyle. *Alcohol use:* excessive CNS depression. Use cautiously.

Contraindications and precautions

• Contraindicated in patients with barbiturate hypersensitivity, history of manifest or latent porphyria, hepatic dysfunction, respiratory disease with dyspnea or obstruction, and nephritis.
• Drug use is not recommended in pregnant or breast-feeding women.
• Use cautiously in patients with acute or chronic pain, depression, suicidal tendencies, history of drug abuse, blood pressure alterations, CV disease, shock, uremia, and in elderly or debilitated patients.

NURSING CONSIDERATIONS

⚕ **Assessment**
• Assess patient's condition before therapy and regularly thereafter.
• Monitor blood levels closely. Therapeutic level is 15 to 40 mcg/ml.
• Be alert for adverse reactions and drug interactions.
• Evaluate patient's and family's knowledge of drug therapy.

⊕ Nursing diagnoses

• Risk for trauma related to seizures
• Risk for injury related to drug-induced adverse CNS reactions
• Knowledge deficit related to drug therapy

⊠ Planning and implementation

P.O. use: Follow normal protocol.
I.V. use: Know that I.V. injection is reserved for emergency treatment. Monitor respirations closely. When administering, do not give more than 60 mg/minute. Have resuscitation equipment available.
I.M. use: Give drug by deep I.M. injection. Superficial injection may cause pain, sterile abscess, and tissue sloughing.
• Do not mix parenteral form with acidic solutions.
• Do not use injectable solution if it contains precipitate.
• Don't stop drug abruptly; seizures may worsen. Call doctor immediately if adverse reactions occur.
Patient teaching
• Make sure patient knows that phenobarbital is available in different strengths and sizes. Advise him to check prescription and refills closely.
• Inform him that full effects are not seen for 2 to 3 weeks, except when loading dose is used.
• Advise him to avoid hazardous activities until drug's CNS effects are known.
• Warn patient and parents not to discontinue drug abruptly.
• Advise patient using oral contraceptives to consider alternate birth control methods.

☑ Evaluation

• Patient is free from seizure activity.
• Patient does not experience injury from drug-induced adverse CNS reactions.
• Patient and family state understanding of drug therapy.

phensuximide
(fen-SUK-sih-mighd)
Milontin

Pharmacologic class: succinimide derivative
Therapeutic class: anticonvulsant
Pregnancy risk category: NR

How supplied

Capsules: 500 mg

Pharmacokinetics

Absorption: absorbed from GI tract.
Distribution: distributed widely throughout body.
Metabolism: unknown.
Excretion: partially excreted in urine.
Half-life: 5 to 12 hours.

Route	Onset	Peak	Duration
P.O.	Unknown	1-4 hr	Unknown

Pharmacodynamics

Chemical effect: unknown; probably increases seizure threshold. Reduces paroxysmal spike-and-wave pattern of absence seizures by depressing nerve transmission in motor cortex.
Therapeutic effect: prevents seizure activity.

Indications and dosage

▶ **Absence seizures.** *Adults and children:* 500 mg to 1 g P.O. b.i.d. or t.i.d.

Adverse reactions

CNS: muscular weakness, *drowsiness,* dizziness, ataxia, headache.
GI: *nausea, vomiting,* anorexia.
GU: urinary frequency, renal damage, hematuria.
Hematologic: transient leukopenia, *pancytopenia, agranulocytosis, fatal blood dyscrasias.*
Skin: pruritus, eruptions, erythema, *Stevens-Johnson syndrome.*
Other: lupuslike syndrome.

Interactions

None significant.

Contraindications and precautions

• Contraindicated in patients with hypersensitivity to succinimide derivatives.
• Drug use is not recommended in pregnant or breast-feeding women.
• Use with extreme caution in patients with hepatic or renal disease.

NURSING CONSIDERATIONS

⚡ Assessment
• Assess patient's disorder before therapy and regularly thereafter.
• Monitor blood levels as ordered. Therapeutic level is 40 to 80 mcg/ml.
• Check CBC every 3 to 4 months and urinalysis and liver function tests every 6 months, as ordered.
• Be alert for adverse reactions.
• Monitor patient's hydration status if adverse GI reactions occur.
• Evaluate patient's and family's knowledge of drug therapy.

⊞ Nursing diagnoses
• Risk for trauma related to seizures
• Risk for fluid volume deficit related to adverse GI reactions
• Knowledge deficit related to drug therapy

⊠ Planning and implementation
• Abrupt withdrawal may precipitate absence seizures. Call doctor immediately if adverse reactions develop.
Patient teaching
• Advise patient to avoid hazardous activities until drug's CNS effects are known.
• Warn patient and parents not to stop drug therapy suddenly.
• Tell patient to report lupuslike symptoms immediately.
• Caution patient that drug may color urine pink, red, or red brown.

☑ Evaluation
• Patient is free from seizure activity.

• Patient maintains adequate hydration.
• Patient and family state understanding of drug therapy.

---

phentermine hydrochloride
(FEN-ter-meen high-droh-KLOR-ighd)
Adipex-P, Duromine♦, Fastin, Obe-Cap, Obe-Nix, Obephen, Panshape M, Phentercot, Phentride, Phentride Caplets, Phentrol, Phentrol-2, Phentrol-4, Phentrol-5, T-Diet, Teramine, Zantryl

Pharmacologic class: amphetamine congener
Therapeutic class: short-term adjunct anorexigenic
Controlled substance schedule: IV
Pregnancy risk category: NR

How supplied

Tablets: 8 mg, 30 mg, 37.5 mg
Capsules: 15 mg, 18.75 mg, 30 mg, 37.5 mg
Capsules (resin complex, sustained-release): 15 mg, 30 mg

Pharmacokinetics

Absorption: absorbed readily from GI tract.
Distribution: distributed throughout body.
Metabolism: unknown.
Excretion: excreted in urine. *Half-life:* 19 to 24 hours.

Route	Onset	Peak	Duration
P.O.	Unknown	Unknown	12-14 hr

Pharmacodynamics

Chemical effect: unknown; probably promotes nerve impulse transmission by releasing stored norepinephrine from nerve terminals in brain. Main sites appear to be cerebral cortex and reticular activating system.
Therapeutic effect: depresses appetite.

Indications and dosage

▶ **Short-term adjunct in exogenous obesity.** *Adults:* 8 mg P.O. t.i.d. ½ hour before meals; or 15 to 30 mg (resin complex) daily 2 hours before breakfast (or 1 to 2 hours after breakfast).

Adverse reactions

CNS: overstimulation, headache, euphoria, dysphoria, dizziness, *insomnia.*
CV: palpitations, tachycardia, increased blood pressure.
EENT: mydriasis, eye irritation, blurred vision.
GI: dry mouth, dysgeusia, constipation, diarrhea, other GI disturbances.
GU: impotence.
Skin: urticaria.
Other: altered libido.

Interactions

Drug-drug. *Acetazolamide, antacids, sodium bicarbonate:* increased renal reabsorption.
Ammonium chloride, ascorbic acid: decreased plasma levels and increased renal excretion of phentermine. Monitor for decreased effects.
Guanethidine: may decrease hypotensive effect. Monitor closely.
Haloperidol, phenothiazines, tricyclic antidepressants: increased CNS effects. Avoid concomitant use.
Insulin, oral antidiabetic agents: may alter antidiabetic agent requirements. Monitor blood glucose levels.
MAO inhibitors: severe hypertension; possible hypertensive crisis. Don't use together or within 14 days of MAO inhibitor discontinuation.
Drug-food. *Caffeine:* may increase CNS stimulation.

Contraindications and precautions

• Contraindicated in patients with hyperthyroidism, moderate to severe hypertension, advanced arteriosclerosis, symptomatic CV disease, glaucoma, or hypersensitivity or idiosyncrasy to sympatho-mimetic amines; within 14 days of MAO inhibitor therapy; and in agitated patients.
• Drug use is not recommended in pregnant or breast-feeding women.
• Use cautiously in patients with mild hypertension.
• Safety of drug has not been established in children.

NURSING CONSIDERATIONS

Assessment
• Weigh patient before therapy and regularly thereafter.
• Be alert for adverse reactions and drug interactions.
• Monitor patient for habituation and tolerance.
• Evaluate patient's and family's knowledge of drug therapy.

Nursing diagnoses
• Altered nutrition: more than body requirements related to food intake
• Sleep pattern disturbance related to drug-induced insomnia
• Knowledge deficit related to drug therapy

Planning and implementation
• Give drug at least 6 hours before bedtime to avoid insomnia.
• Make sure patient also is on weight-reduction program.
Patient teaching
• Instruct patient to take drug at least 6 hours before bedtime to avoid sleep interference.
• Warn patient to avoid hazardous activities until CNS effects of drug are known.
• Tell patient to avoid drinks containing caffeine, which increase effects of amphetamines and related amines.
• Tell patient to report signs of excessive stimulation.
• Inform patient that fatigue may result as drug effects wear off.

Evaluation
• Patient loses weight.

- Patient does not have insomnia.
- Patient and family state understanding of drug therapy.

phentolamine mesylate
(fen-TOH-luh-meen MES-ih-layt)
Regitine, Rogitine ◆

Pharmacologic class: alpha-adrenergic blocker
Therapeutic class: antihypertensive agent for pheochromocytoma; cutaneous vasodilator
Pregnancy risk category: C

How supplied

Injection: 5 mg/ml in 1-ml vials, 10 mg/ml ◆

Pharmacokinetics

Absorption: unknown.
Distribution: unknown.
Metabolism: unknown.
Excretion: about 10% of drug is excreted unchanged in urine; excretion of remainder is unknown. *Half-life:* 19 minutes after I.V. administration; unknown for I.M. administration.

Route	Onset	Peak	Duration
I.V., I.M.	Unknown	Unknown	Unknown

Pharmacodynamics

Chemical effect: competitively blocks effects of catecholamines on alpha-adrenergic receptors.
Therapeutic effect: lowers blood pressure; minimizes dermal damage from norepinephrine infiltration.

Indications and dosage

▶ **To aid in diagnosis of pheochromocytoma; to control or prevent hypertension before or during pheochromocytomectomy.** *Adults:* I.V. diagnostic dose is 5 mg, with close monitoring of blood pressure. Before surgical removal of tumor, 5 mg I.M. or I.V. During surgery, pa-

tient may need 5 mg I.V. *Children:* I.V. diagnostic dose is 1 mg with close monitoring of blood pressure. Before surgical removal of tumor, 1 mg, 0.1 mg/kg, or 3 mg/m² I.V. or I.M. During surgery, patient may need 1 mg I.V.
▶ **Dermal necrosis and sloughing following I.V. extravasation of norepinephrine.** *Adults and children:* infiltrate area with 5 to 10 mg phentolamine in 10 ml 0.9% NaCl solution or give half dosage through infiltrated I.V. and other half around site. Must be done within 12 hours.

Adverse reactions

CNS: dizziness, weakness, flushing, *cerebrovascular occlusion.*
CV: hypotension, *shock,* arrhythmias, palpitations, tachycardia, angina pectoris, *MI.*
EENT: nasal congestion.
GI: *diarrhea,* abdominal pain, *nausea, vomiting,* hyperperistalsis.
Metabolic: hypoglycemia.

Interactions

Drug-drug. *Epinephrine:* excessive hypotension. Use cautiously and monitor patient closely.
Narcotics, rauwolfia alkaloids, sedatives: false-positive test results for pheochromocytoma. Don't give 24 hours before phentolamine is given as diagnostic test. Withdraw rauwolfia alkaloids at least 4 weeks before such testing.

Contraindications and precautions

- Contraindicated in patients with angina, coronary artery disease, MI, history of MI, or hypersensitivity to drug.
- Drug use is not recommended in breast-feeding women.
- Use cautiously in patients with gastritis or peptic ulcer and in pregnant women.

NURSING CONSIDERATIONS

Assessment
- Assess patient's condition before therapy and regularly thereafter.

• Before drug is given as diagnostic test for pheochromocytoma, check blood pressure, and monitor frequently during administration.
• Know that test is positive for pheochromocytoma if I.V. test dose causes severe hypotension.
• Be alert for adverse reactions and drug interactions.
• Evaluate patient's and family's knowledge of drug therapy.

⊞ **Nursing diagnoses**
• Altered health maintenance related to underlying condition
• Decreased cardiac output related to adverse CV reactions
• Knowledge deficit related to drug therapy

▷ **Planning and implementation**
• Drug is supplied as powder. Use it immediately after reconstitution.
I.V. use: Dilute 5 to 10 mg of drug in 500 ml of 0.9% NaCl, and use infusion pump to control rate.
I.M. use: Follow normal protocol.
Local use: Infiltrate area with 5 to 10 mg of drug in 10 ml normal saline solution or give half dosage through infiltrated I.V. and other half around site. Must be done within 12 hours of infiltration.
• Don't administer epinephrine to treat phentolamine-induced hypotension because it may cause additional fall in blood pressure ("epinephrine reversal"). Use norepinephrine instead.
Patient teaching
• Explain if drug will be used as diagnostic test.
• Tell patient to report adverse reactions immediately.

☑ **Evaluation**
• Patient responds well to therapy.
• Patient maintains adequate cardiac output.
• Patient and family state understanding of drug therapy.

phenylephrine hydrochloride
(fen-il-EF-rin high-droh-KLOR-ighd)
Neo-Synephrine

Pharmacologic class: adrenergic
Therapeutic class: vasoconstrictor
Pregnancy risk category: C

How supplied
Injection: 10 mg/ml

Pharmacokinetics
Absorption: unknown after I.M. and S.C. administration.
Distribution: unknown.
Metabolism: metabolized in liver and intestine.
Excretion: unknown.

Route	Onset	Peak	Duration
I.V.	Immediate	Unknown	15-20 min
I.M.	10-15 min	Unknown	0.5-2 hr
S.C.	10-15 min	Unknown	50-60 min

Pharmacodynamics
Chemical effect: predominantly stimulates alpha-adrenergic receptors in sympathetic nervous system.
Therapeutic effect: raises blood pressure and abolishes paroxysmal supraventricular tachycardia.

Indications and dosage
▶ **Hypotensive emergencies during spinal anesthesia.** *Adults:* initially, 0.1 to 0.2 mg I.V., then subsequent doses of 0.1 to 0.2 mg, p.r.n.
▶ **Maintenance of blood pressure during spinal or inhalation anesthesia.**
Adults: 2 to 3 mg S.C. or I.M. 3 or 4 minutes before anesthesia. *Children:* 0.044 to 0.088 mg/kg S.C. or I.M.
▶ **Prolongation of spinal anesthesia.**
Adults: 2 to 5 mg added to anesthetic solution.
▶ **Vasoconstrictor for regional anesthesia.** *Adults:* 1 mg phenylephrine added to 20 ml local anesthetic.

▶ **Mild to moderate hypotension.**
Adults: 2 to 5 mg S.C. or I.M.; repeated
in 1 to 2 hours as needed and tolerated.
Initial dose should not exceed 5 mg.
Alternatively, 0.1 to 0.5 mg slow I.V., not
to be repeated more often than 10 to 15
minutes. *Children:* 0.1 mg/kg I.M. or
S.C.; repeated in 1 to 2 hours as needed
and tolerated.
▶ **Severe hypotension and shock (including drug-induced).** *Adults:* 10 mg in
250 to 500 ml of D₅W or 0.9% NaCl injection. I.V. infusion started at 100 to
180 mcg/minute, then decreased to maintenance infusion of 40 to 60 mcg/minute
when blood pressure stabilizes.
▶ **Paroxysmal supraventricular tachycardia.** *Adults:* initially, 0.5 mg rapid
I.V.; subsequent doses should not exceed
preceding dose by more than 0.1 to
0.2 mg and should not exceed 1 mg.

Adverse reactions

CNS: *headache, restlessness, lightheadedness, weakness.*
CV: palpitations, bradycardia, *arrhythmias,* hypertension, anginal pain, decreased cardiac output.
EENT: blurred vision.
GI: vomiting.
Skin: pilomotor response, feeling of
coolness.
Other: tachyphylaxis (may occur with
continued use), decreased organ perfusion (with prolonged use), tissue sloughing (with extravasation), *anaphylaxis,
asthmatic episodes.*

Interactions

Drug-drug. *Alpha-adrenergic blockers,
phenothiazines:* decreased vasopressor
response. Monitor closely.
Beta blockers: block cardiostimulatory
effects. Monitor closely.
MAO inhibitors: may cause severe hypertension (hypertensive crisis). Monitor patient and blood pressure closely.
Oxytocics, tricyclic antidepressants: increased pressor response. Monitor patient.

Contraindications and precautions

• Contraindicated in patients with severe
hypertension, ventricular tachycardia, or
hypersensitivity to drug.
• Use with extreme caution in patients
with heart disease, hyperthyroidism, severe atherosclerosis, bradycardia, partial
heart block, myocardial disease, or sulfite
sensitivity and in elderly patients.
• Use cautiously in pregnant or breastfeeding women.

NURSING CONSIDERATIONS

🔍 Assessment
• Assess patient's condition before therapy and regularly thereafter.
• Monitor blood pressure frequently;
avoid severe increase. Maintain blood
pressure slightly below patient's normal
level, as ordered. In previously normotensive patient, maintain systolic pressure at
80 to 100 mm Hg; in previously hypertensive patient, maintain systolic pressure
at 30 to 40 mm Hg below usual level.
• Monitor ECG throughout therapy.
• Be alert for adverse reactions and drug
interactions.
• Evaluate patient's and family's knowledge of drug therapy.

🔄 Nursing diagnoses
• Altered tissue perfusion (cerebral, cardiopulmonary, peripheral, GI, renal) related to underlying condition
• Decreased cardiac output related to
drug-induced adverse reaction
• Knowledge deficit related to drug
therapy

➤ Planning and implementation
I.V. use: For direct injection, dilute
10 mg (1 ml) with 9 ml sterile water for
injection to provide solution containing
1 mg/ml. I.V. infusions are usually prepared by adding 10 mg of drug to 500 ml
of D₅W or 0.9% NaCl injection. Initial
infusion rate is usually 100 to 180 mcg/
minute; maintenance rate is usually 40 to
60 mcg/minute.

Reactions may be *common,* uncommon, *life-threatening,* or COMMON AND LIFE-THREATENING.

– With prolonged I.V. infusions, avoid abrupt withdrawal. During infusion, frequently monitor ECG, blood pressure, cardiac output, central venous pressure, pulmonary capillary wedge pressure, pulse rate, urine output, and color and temperature of extremities. Titrate infusion rate according to findings and doctor's guidelines. Use continuous infusion pump to regulate flow rate.

– Use central venous catheter or large vein, as in antecubital fossa, to minimize risk of extravasation. Use continuous infusion pump to regulate infusion flow rate.

– To treat extravasation, infiltrate site promptly with 10 to 15 ml of 0.9% NaCl injection containing 5 to 10 mg phentolamine. Use fine needle.

– Keep in mind that drug is incompatible with butacaine sulfate, alkalis, ferric salts, and oxidizing agents.

I.M. and S.C. use: Follow normal protocol.

Patient teaching

• Tell patient to report discomfort at infusion site immediately.

☑ Evaluation

• Patient maintains tissue perfusion and cellular oxygenation.

• Patient maintains adequate cardiac output.

• Patient and family state understanding of drug therapy.

---

phenylephrine hydrochloride
(fen-il-EF-rin high-droh-KLOR-ighd)
Alconefrin 12†, Alconefrin 25†, Alconefrin 50†, Duration†, Neo-Synephrine†, Nōstril†, Rhinall†, Rhinall-10†, Sinex†, St. Joseph Measured-Dose Nasal Decongestant†

Pharmacologic class: adrenergic
Therapeutic class: vasoconstrictor
Pregnancy risk category: NR

How supplied

Nasal solution: 0.125%, 0.16%, 0.25%, 0.5%, 1%

Pharmacokinetics

Absorption: small amounts may be absorbed.
Distribution: distributed locally to nasal tissue.
Metabolism: metabolized in liver.
Excretion: excreted in urine.

Route	Onset	Peak	Duration
Intranasal	Rapid	Unknown	0.5-4 hr

Pharmacodynamics

Chemical effect: causes local vasoconstriction of dilated arterioles, reducing blood flow.
Therapeutic effect: relieves nasal congestion.

Indications and dosage

▶ **Nasal congestion.** *Adults and children age 12 and older:* 2 to 3 drops or 1 to 2 sprays instilled in each nostril, p.r.n. *Children ages 6 to 12:* 2 to 3 drops or 1 to 2 sprays of 0.25% solution instilled in each nostril q 3 to 4 hours, p.r.n. *Children under age 6:* 2 to 3 drops of 0.125% solution q 4 hours, p.r.n.

Adverse reactions

CNS: headache, tremor, dizziness, nervousness.
CV: *palpitations, tachycardia, PVCs,* hypertension, pallor.
EENT: transient burning or stinging, dryness of nasal mucosa; rebound nasal congestion (with continued use).
GI: nausea.

Interactions

None significant.

Contraindications and precautions

• Contraindicated in patients with hypersensitivity to drug.
• Use cautiously in patients with hyperthyroidism, marked hypertension, type 1

---

diabetes mellitus, cardiac disease, or advanced arteriosclerotic changes; in children of low body weight; in elderly patients; and in pregnant or breast-feeding women.

NURSING CONSIDERATIONS

☒ Assessment
• Assess patient's condition before therapy and regularly thereafter.
• Be alert for adverse reactions.
• Evaluate patient's and family's knowledge of drug therapy.

☒ Nursing diagnoses
• Altered health maintenance related to nasal congestion
• Altered tissue integrity related to adverse effect on nasal tissue
• Knowledge deficit related to drug therapy

☒ Planning and implementation
• To administer drug, have patient hold head upright, insert nozzle and then have patient sniff spray briskly.
Patient teaching
• Teach patient how to administer drug.
• Tell patient not to share drug to prevent spread of infection.
• Warn patient not to exceed recommended dosage.
• Advise patient to contact doctor if symptoms persist beyond 3 days.

☒ Evaluation
• Patient's nasal congestion is relieved with phenylephrine therapy.
• Patient maintains normal nasal tissue integrity.
• Patient and family state understanding of drug therapy.

phenytoin (diphenylhydantoin)
(FEN-uh-toyn)
Dilantin, Dilantin-30 Pediatric,
Dilantin-125, Dilantin Infatabs

phenytoin sodium
Dilantin, Phenytex

phenytoin sodium (extended)
Dilantin Kapseals

Pharmacologic class: hydantoin derivative
Therapeutic class: anticonvulsant
Pregnancy risk category: NR

How supplied

phenytoin
Tablets (chewable): 50 mg
Oral suspension: 30 mg/5 ml,
125 mg/5 ml
phenytoin sodium
Capsules: 30 mg (27.6-mg base), 100 mg (92-mg base)
Injection: 50 mg/ml (46-mg base)
phenytoin sodium (extended)
Capsules: 30 mg (27.6-mg base), 100 mg (92-mg base)

Pharmacokinetics

Absorption: absorbed slowly from small intestine after oral administration. Absorption is formulation-dependent and bioavailability may differ among products. Absorbed erratically from I.M. absorption site.
Distribution: distributed widely throughout body. Drug is about 90% protein-bound.
Metabolism: metabolized by liver.
Excretion: excreted in urine; exhibits dose-dependent (zero-order) elimination kinetics; above certain dosage level, small increases in dosage disproportionately increase serum levels. *Half-life:* varies with dose and serum concentration changes.

Route	Onset	Peak	Duration
P.O.	Unknown	1.5-12 hr	Unknown
I.V.	Immediate	1-2 hr	Unknown
I.M.	Unknown	Unknown	Unknown

Pharmacodynamics

Chemical effect: unknown; probably stabilizes neuronal membranes and limits seizure activity by either increasing efflux or decreasing influx of sodium ions across cell membranes in motor cortex during generation of nerve impulses. *Therapeutic effect:* prevents and abolishes seizure activity.

Indications and dosage

▶ **Control of tonic-clonic (grand mal) and complex partial (temporal lobe) seizures, post-head trauma, Reye's syndrome.** *Adults:* highly individualized. Initially, 100 mg P.O. t.i.d., increased in increments of 100 mg P.O. q 2 to 4 weeks until desired response is obtained. Usual range is 300 to 600 mg daily. If stabilized with extended-release capsules, once-daily dosing with 300-mg extended-release capsules possible as alternative. *Children:* 5 mg/kg or 250 mg/m² P.O. daily b.i.d. or t.i.d. Maximum daily dosage is 300 mg.
▶ **For patient requiring loading dose.** *Adults:* initially, 1 g P.O. daily divided into three doses and administered at 2-hour intervals. Alternatively, 10 to 15 mg/kg I.V. at rate not exceeding 50 mg/minute. Normal maintenance dosage instituted 24 hours later. *Children:* 5 mg/kg/day P.O. in two or three equally divided doses with subsequent dosage individualized to maximum of 300 mg daily.
▶ **Prevention and treatment of seizures occurring during neurosurgery.** *Adults:* 100 to 200 mg I.M. q 4 hours during surgery and continued during postoperative period.
▶ **Status epilepticus.** *Adults:* loading dose of 10 to 15 mg/kg I.V. (1 to 1.5 g may be needed) at rate not exceeding 50 mg/minute followed by maintenance dosage (once controlled) of 300 mg P.O. daily. *Children:* loading dose of 15 to 20 mg/kg I.V., at rate not exceeding 1 to 3 mg/kg/minute followed by highly individualized maintenance dosages.

Adverse reactions

CNS: *ataxia, slurred speech, confusion,* dizziness, insomnia, nervousness, twitching, headache.
CV: hypotension.
EENT: nystagmus, diplopia, blurred vision, gingival hyperplasia (especially in children).
GI: nausea, vomiting.
Hematologic: *thrombocytopenia, leukopenia, agranulocytosis, pancytopenia,* macrocythemia, megaloblastic anemia.
Hepatic: *toxic hepatitis.*
Skin: scarlatiniform or morbilliform rash; bullous, *exfoliative,* or purpuric dermatitis; *Stevens-Johnson syndrome;* lupus erythematosus; *hirsutism; toxic epidermal necrolysis;* photosensitivity; pain, necrosis, inflammation (at injection site); discoloration ("purple glove syndrome") if given by I.V. push in back of hand.
Other: periarteritis nodosa, lymphadenopathy, hyperglycemia, osteomalacia, hypertrichosis.

Interactions

Drug-drug. *Amiodarone, antihistamines, chloramphenicol, cimetidine, cycloserine, diazepam, disulfiram, influenza vaccine, isoniazid, phenylbutazone, salicylates, sulfamethizole, valproate:* increased therapeutic effects of phenytoin. Monitor for toxicity.
Dexamethasone, diazoxide, folic acid: decreased phenytoin activity. Monitor closely.
Drug-food. *Oral tube feedings with Osmolite or Isocal:* may interfere with absorption of oral phenytoin. Schedule feedings as far as possible from drug administration.
Drug-lifestyle. *Alcohol use:* decreased phenytoin activity. Avoid concomitant use.

Contraindications and precautions

• Contraindicated in patients with hydantoin hypersensitivity, sinus bradycardia, SA block, second- or third-degree AV block, or Adams-Stokes syndrome.
• Drug use is not recommended in pregnant or breast-feeding women.
• Use cautiously in patients with hepatic dysfunction, hypotension, myocardial insufficiency, diabetes, or respiratory depression; in elderly or debilitated patients; and in patients receiving other hydantoin derivatives.

NURSING CONSIDERATIONS

☰ Assessment

• Assess patient's condition before therapy and regularly thereafter.
• Monitor blood levels as ordered. Therapeutic level is 10 to 20 mcg/ml.
• Monitor CBC and serum calcium level every 6 months, and periodically monitor hepatic function as ordered.
• Check vital signs, blood pressure, and ECG during I.V. administration.
• Be alert for adverse reactions and drug interactions.
• Mononucleosis may decrease phenytoin levels. Monitor for increased seizure activity.
• Evaluate patient's and family's knowledge of drug therapy.

⊕ Nursing diagnoses

• Risk for trauma related to seizures
• Altered oral mucous membrane related to gingival hyperplasia
• Knowledge deficit related to drug therapy

⊅ Planning and implementation

• Elderly patients tend to metabolize phenytoin slowly and may require lower dosages.
• Use only clear solution for injection. A slight yellow color is acceptable. Don't refrigerate.

P.O. use: Divided doses given with or after meals may decrease adverse GI reactions.
– Suspension available as 30 mg/5 ml or 125 mg/5 ml. Read label carefully. Shake suspension well before use.
– Dilantin capsule is only oral form that can be given once daily. Toxic levels may result if any other brand or form is given once daily. Dilantin brand tablets and oral suspension should not be taken once daily.
I.V. use: Administer drug slowly (50 mg/minute) as I.V. bolus. If giving as infusion, don't mix drug with D_5W because it will precipitate. Clear I.V. tubing first with 0.9% NaCl solution. Never use cloudy solution. May mix with 0.9% NaCl solution if necessary and infuse over 30 to 60 minutes when possible. Infusion must begin within 1 hour after preparation and should run through in-line filter. Discard 4 hours after preparation.
– Check patency of I.V. catheter before administering. Extravasation has caused severe local tissue damage.
– Avoid giving phenytoin by I.V. push into veins on back of hand to avoid discoloration known as purple glove syndrome. Inject into larger veins or central venous catheter if available.
I.M. use: Don't give drug I.M. unless dosage adjustments are made. Drug may precipitate at site, cause pain, and be erratically absorbed.
• Discontinue drug if rash appears. If rash is scarlatiniform or morbilliform, drug may be resumed after rash clears. If rash reappears, therapy should be discontinued. If rash is exfoliative, purpuric, or bullous, drug will not be resumed.
• Don't withdraw drug suddenly; seizures may worsen. Call doctor at once if adverse reactions develop.
• Know that phenytoin may cause altered laboratory test results, including reduced serum protein-bound iodine and free thyroxine levels without clinical signs of hypothyroidism; slight decrease in urinary 17-hydroxysteroid and 17-ketosteroid

---

Reactions may be *common,* uncommon, *life-threatening,* or COMMON AND LIFE-THREATENING.

levels; increased urine 6-hydroxycortisol excretion and serum levels of alkaline phosphatase or μ-glutamyltransferase; and decreased values for dexamethasone suppression or metyrapone tests.
• If megaloblastic anemia is evident, doctor may order folic acid and vitamin B_{12}.
Patient teaching
• Advise patient to avoid hazardous activities until drug's CNS effects are known.
• Advise patient not to change brands or dosage forms.
• Warn patient and parents not to stop drug abruptly.
• Promote oral hygiene and regular dental examinations. Gingivectomy may be necessary periodically if dental hygiene is poor.
• Caution patient that drug may color urine pink, red, or red-brown.
• Inform patient that heavy alcohol use may diminish drug's benefits.

☑ **Evaluation**
• Patient is free from seizure activity.
• Patient expresses importance of good oral hygiene and regular dental examinations.
• Patient and family state understanding of drug therapy.

physostigmine salicylate (eserine salicylate)
(fiz-oh-STIG-meen SAL-i-sil-ayt)
Antilirium

Pharmacologic class: cholinesterase inhibitor
Therapeutic class: antimuscarinic antidote
Pregnancy risk category: NR

How supplied

Injection: 1 mg/ml

Pharmacokinetics

Absorption: absorbed well from injection site when administered I.M.

Distribution: distributed widely and crosses blood-brain barrier.
Metabolism: cholinesterase hydrolyzes physostigmine relatively quickly.
Excretion: primary mode of excretion unknown; small amount excreted in urine.

Route	Onset	Peak	Duration
I.V.	3-5 min	≤ 5 min	30-60 min
I.M.	3-5 min	20-30 min	30-60 min

Pharmacodynamics

Chemical effect: inhibits destruction of acetylcholine released from parasympathetic and somatic efferent nerves. Acetylcholine accumulates, promoting increased stimulation of receptor.
Therapeutic effect: reverses anticholinergic signs and symptoms.

Indications and dosage

▶ **To reverse CNS toxicity associated with clinical or toxic dosages of drugs capable of producing anticholinergic syndrome.** *Adults:* 0.5 to 2 mg I.M. or I.V. (1 mg/minute I.V.) repeated q 10 minutes as necessary if life-threatening signs recur (coma, seizures, arrhythmias). *Children:* reserved for life-threatening situations only. 0.02 mg/kg I.M. or slow I.V. repeated q 5 to 10 minutes until response is obtained. Maximum dosage is 2 mg.

Adverse reactions

CNS: *seizures,* hallucinations, muscle twitching, muscle weakness, ataxia, *restlessness, excitability, sweating.*
CV: irregular pulse, palpitations, bradycardia, hypotension.
EENT: miosis.
GI: nausea, vomiting, epigastric pain, *diarrhea, excessive salivation.*
GU: urinary urgency.
Respiratory: *bronchospasm,* bronchial constriction, dyspnea.

Interactions

Drug-drug. *Anticholinergic agents, atropine, procainamide, quinidine:* may re-

verse cholinergic effects. Observe for lack of drug effect.
Ganglionic blockers: may decrease blood pressure. Avoid concomitant use.

Contraindications and precautions

• Contraindicated in patients with mechanical obstruction of intestine or urogenital tract, asthma, gangrene, diabetes, CV disease, or vagotonia and in those receiving choline esters or depolarizing neuromuscular blocking agents.
• Use cautiously in patients with sensitivity or allergy to sulfites.
• Use cautiously in pregnant women.
• Safety of drug has not been established in breast-feeding women.

NURSING CONSIDERATIONS

🏥 Assessment

• Assess patient's condition before therapy and regularly thereafter. Effectiveness is often immediate and dramatic, but may be transient and require repeated doses.
• Monitor vital signs frequently, especially respirations.
• Be alert for adverse reactions and drug interactions.
• Evaluate patient's and family's knowledge of drug therapy.

🔖 Nursing diagnoses

• Altered health maintenance related to underlying condition
• Risk for injury related to drug-induced adverse CNS reactions
• Knowledge deficit related to drug therapy

➤ Planning and implementation

I.V. use: Give drug I.V. at controlled rate; use direct injection at no more than 1 mg/minute.
I.M. use: Follow normal protocol.
• Use only clear solution. Darkening of solution may indicate loss of potency.
• Position patient to ease breathing. Have atropine injection available and be pre-

pared to give 0.5 mg S.C. or slow I.V. push as ordered. Provide respiratory support as needed. Best administered in presence of doctor.
• Put up side rails of bed if patient becomes restless or hallucinates. Adverse reactions may indicate drug toxicity. Notify doctor.
Patient teaching
• Tell patient to report adverse reactions.

☑ Evaluation

• Patient responds well to therapy.
• Patient does not experience injury from adverse CNS reactions.
• Patient and family state understanding of drug therapy.

phytonadione (vitamin K₁)
(figh-toh-neh-DIGH-ohn)
AquaMEPHYTON, Konakion, Mephyton

Pharmacologic class: vitamin K
Therapeutic class: blood coagulation modifier
Pregnancy risk category: C

How supplied

Tablets: 5 mg
Injection (aqueous colloidal solution): 2 mg/ml, 10 mg/ml
Injection (aqueous dispersion): 2 mg/ml, 10 mg/ml

Pharmacokinetics

Absorption: drug requires presence of bile salts for GI tract absorption after oral administration. Absorption unknown after I.M. or S.C. administration.
Distribution: concentrates in liver for short time.
Metabolism: metabolized rapidly by liver.
Excretion: not clearly defined.

Route	Onset	Peak	Duration
P.O.	6-12 hr	Unknown	12-14 hr
I.V., I.M., S.C.	1-2 hr	Unknown	12-14 hr

Pharmacodynamics

Chemical effect: an antihemorrhagic factor that promotes hepatic formation of active prothrombin.
Therapeutic effect: controls abnormal bleeding.

Indications and dosage

► **RDA.** *Neonates and infants to age 6 months:* 5 mcg. *Infants age 6 months to 1 year:* 10 mcg. *Children ages 1 to 3:* 15 mcg. *Children ages 4 to 6:* 20 mcg. *Children ages 7 to 10:* 30 mcg. *Children ages 11 to 14:* 45 mcg. *Males ages 15 to 18:* 65 mcg. *Males ages 19 to 24:* 70 mcg. *Males age 25 and over:* 80 mcg. *Females ages 15 to 18:* 55 mcg. *Females ages 19 to 24:* 60 mcg. *Females age 25 and over; pregnant or breast-feeding women:* 65 mcg.

► **Hypoprothrombinemia secondary to vitamin K malabsorption, drug therapy, or excessive vitamin A dosage.**
Adults: depending on severity, 2 to 25 mg P.O., S.C., or I.M. repeated and increased up to 50 mg if necessary. *Children:* 5 to 10 mg P.O. or parenterally. I.V. injection rate for infants and children should not exceed 3 mg/m²/minute or total of 5 mg. *Infants:* 2 mg P.O. or parenterally.

► **Hypoprothrombinemia secondary to effect of oral anticoagulants.** *Adults:* 2.5 to 10 mg P.O., S.C., or I.M. based on PT, repeated if necessary within 12 to 48 hours after oral dose or within 6 to 8 hours after parenteral dose. In emergency, 10 to 50 mg slow I.V., rate not to exceed 1 mg/minute, repeated q 4 hours, p.r.n.

► **Prevention of hemorrhagic disease of newborn.** *Neonates:* 0.5 to 1 mg I.M. or S.C. within 1 hour after birth.

► **Treatment of hemorrhagic disease of newborn.** *Neonates:* 1 mg S.C. or I.M. based on laboratory tests. Higher doses may be necessary if mother has been receiving oral anticoagulants.

► **To differentiate between hepatocellular disease or biliary obstruction as source of hypoprothrombinemia.**
Adults and children: 10 mg I.M. or S.C.

► **Prevention of hypoprothrombinemia related to vitamin K deficiency in long-term parenteral nutrition.** *Adults:* 5 to 10 mg I.M. weekly. *Children:* 2 to 5 mg I.M. weekly.

► **Prevention of hypoprothrombinemia in infants receiving less than 0.1 mg/L vitamin K in breast milk or milk substitutes.** *Infants:* 1 mg I.M. monthly.

Adverse reactions

CNS: dizziness, seizure-like movements.
CV: transient hypotension (after I.V. administration), rapid and weak pulse, cardiac irregularities.
Skin: diaphoresis, flushing, erythema.
Other: cramp-like pain, *anaphylaxis and anaphylactoid reactions* (usually after rapid I.V. administration); pain, swelling, hematoma (at injection site).

Interactions

Drug-drug. *Anticoagulants:* temporary resistance to prothrombin-depressing anticoagulants may result, especially when larger doses of phytonadione are used. Monitor closely.
Cholestyramine resin, mineral oil: inhibited GI absorption of oral vitamin K. Administer separately.

Contraindications and precautions

• Contraindicated in patients with hypersensitivity to drug.
• Use cautiously in pregnant or breast-feeding women.

NURSING CONSIDERATIONS

⚙ Assessment
• Assess patient's condition before therapy and regularly thereafter.
• Monitor PT to determine dosage effectiveness, as ordered.
• Failure to respond to vitamin K may indicate coagulation defects.
• Be alert for adverse reactions and drug interactions.
• Be aware that phytonadione therapy for hemorrhagic disease in infants causes

---

fewer adverse reactions than do other vitamin K analogues.
• Monitor patient's hydration status if adverse GI reactions occur.
• Evaluate patient's and family's knowledge of drug therapy.

🖏 **Nursing diagnoses**
• Altered protection related to underlying vitamin K deficiency
• Risk for fluid volume deficit related to adverse GI reactions
• Knowledge deficit related to drug therapy

▨ **Planning and implementation**
• Check brand name labels for administration route restrictions.
P.O. and S.C. use: Follow normal protocol.
I.V. use: Dilute drug with 0.9% NaCl injection, D_5W, or D_5W in 0.9% NaCl injection. Give I.V. by slow infusion over 2 to 3 hours. Infusion rate shouldn't exceed 1 mg/minute in adult or 3 mg/m²/minute in child.
– Protect parenteral products from light. Wrap infusion container with aluminum foil.
– Anticipate order of weekly addition of 5 to 10 mg of phytonadione to total parenteral nutrition solutions.
I.M. use: Administer drug in upper outer quadrant of buttocks in adult or older child; inject in anterolateral aspect of thigh or deltoid region in infant.
• If severe bleeding occurs, don't delay other measures, such as fresh frozen plasma or whole blood.
Patient teaching
• Explain drug's purpose.
• Instruct patient to report adverse reactions.

✅ **Evaluation**
• Patient achieves normal PT levels with drug therapy.
• Patient maintains adequate hydration throughout drug therapy.

• Patient and family state understanding of drug therapy.

---

pimozide
(PIH-mih-zighd)
Orap

Pharmacologic class: diphenylbutylpiperidine
Therapeutic class: antipsychotic
Pregnancy risk category: C

How supplied
Tablets: 2 mg, 4 mg♦, 10 mg♦

Pharmacokinetics
Absorption: absorbed slowly and incompletely from GI tract.
Distribution: distributed widely into body.
Metabolism: metabolized by liver; significant first-pass effect exists.
Excretion: about 40% of drug is excreted in urine as parent drug and metabolites; about 15% is excreted in feces. *Half-life:* about 29 hours.

Route	Onset	Peak	Duration
P.O.	Unknown	4-12 hr	Unknown

Pharmacodynamics
Chemical effect: may block dopamine nonselectively at pre- and postsynaptic receptors on neurons in CNS.
Therapeutic effect: abolishes tics associated with Tourette syndrome.

Indications and dosage
▶ **Suppression of motor and phonic tics in patients with Tourette syndrome refractory to first line therapy.** *Adults and children over age 12:* initially, 1 to 2 mg P.O. daily in divided doses. Then increased every other day, as needed. Maximum dosage is 20 mg daily.

Adverse reactions
CNS: *parkinsonian-like symptoms,* other extrapyramidal symptoms (dystonia, aka-

thisia, hyperreflexia, opisthotonos, oculogyric crisis), *tardive dyskinesia, sedation.*
CV: *ECG changes (prolonged QT interval),* hypotension.
EENT: visual disturbances.
GI: dry mouth, constipation.
GU: impotence.
Musculoskeletal: muscle rigidity; *neuroleptic malignant syndrome* (rare).

Interactions

Drug-drug. *Antiarrhythmics, phenothiazines, tricyclic antidepressants:* increased incidence of ECG abnormalities. Monitor patient closely.
CNS depressants: increased CNS depression. Avoid concomitant use.
Drug-lifestyle. *Alcohol use:* increased CNS depression. Avoid concomitant use.

Contraindications and precautions

• Contraindicated in patients with hypersensitivity to drug, in treatment of simple tics or tics other than those associated with Tourette syndrome, concurrent drug therapy known to cause motor and phonic tics, congenital long QT syndrome or history of arrhythmias, patients with severe toxic CNS depression, and patients experiencing coma.
• Use cautiously in patients with hepatic or renal dysfunction, glaucoma, prostatic hyperplasia, seizure disorder, or EEG abnormalities.
• Safety of drug has not been established in breast-feeding women.

NURSING CONSIDERATIONS

🕮 Assessment
• Assess patient's tics before therapy and regularly thereafter.
• Perform ECG before therapy and periodically thereafter as ordered. Monitor for prolonged QT interval.
• Monitor patient for tardive dyskinesia. It may occur after prolonged use. It may not appear until months or years later and may disappear spontaneously or persist for life despite discontinuation of drug.

• Monitor patient who also is taking anticonvulsants for increased seizure activity. Pimozide may lower seizure threshold.
• Be alert for adverse reactions and drug interactions.
• Evaluate patient's and family's knowledge of drug therapy.

🕮 Nursing diagnoses
• Body image disturbance related to presence of tics
• Impaired physical mobility related to adverse reactions
• Knowledge deficit related to drug therapy

🕮 Planning and implementation
• Acute dystonic reactions may be treated with diphenhydramine.
• Avoid concurrent administration of other drugs that prolong QT interval, such as antiarrhythmics.
Patient teaching
• Warn patient not to stop taking drug abruptly and not to exceed prescribed dosage.
• Tell patient to avoid alcohol during drug therapy.
• Tell patient to use sugarless hard candy, gum, and liquids to relieve dry mouth.

🕮 Evaluation
• Patient states positive feelings about self with absence of tics.
• Patient is able to perform activities of daily living.
• Patient and family state understanding of drug therapy.

pindolol
(PIN-duh-lol)
Barbloc♦, Novo-Pindol♦, Syn-Pindolol♦, Visken

Pharmacologic class: beta blocker
Therapeutic class: antihypertensive
Pregnancy risk category: B

How supplied

Tablets: 5 mg, 10 mg, 15 mg ♦

Pharmacokinetics

Absorption: absorbed rapidly from GI tract. Food does not reduce bioavailability but may increase rate of GI absorption.
Distribution: distributed widely throughout body and is 40% to 60% protein-bound.
Metabolism: about 60% to 65% of drug is metabolized in liver.
Excretion: 35% to 50% of dose excreted unchanged in urine. *Half-life:* about 3 to 4 hours.

Route	Onset	Peak	Duration
P.O.	Unknown	1-2 hr	24 hr

Pharmacodynamics

Chemical effect: unknown; possible mechanisms include reduced cardiac output, decreased sympathetic outflow to peripheral vasculature, and inhibition of renin release by kidneys.
Therapeutic effect: lowers blood pressure.

Indications and dosage

▶ **Hypertension.** *Adults:* initially, 5 mg P.O. b.i.d. Increased as needed and tolerated to maximum of 60 mg daily.

Adverse reactions

CNS: insomnia, fatigue, dizziness, nervousness, vivid dreams, hallucinations, lethargy.
CV: *edema,* bradycardia, **heart failure,** peripheral vascular disease, hypotension.
EENT: visual disturbances.
GI: *nausea,* vomiting, diarrhea.
Metabolic: hypoglycemia without tachycardia.
Musculoskeletal: *muscle pain, joint pain.*
Respiratory: increased airway resistance.
Skin: rash.

Interactions

Drug-drug. *Cardiac glycosides, diltiazem, verapamil:* excessive bradycardia and additive depression of AV node. Use together cautiously.
Epinephrine: severe vasoconstriction. Monitor blood pressure and observe patient carefully.
Indomethacin: decreased antihypertensive effect. Monitor blood pressure and adjust dosage.
Insulin, oral antidiabetic agents: can alter requirements for these drugs in previously stabilized diabetic patients. Monitor patient for hypoglycemia.

Contraindications and precautions

• Contraindicated in patients with bronchial asthma, severe bradycardia, heart block greater than first degree, cardiogenic shock, overt cardiac failure, or hypersensitivity to drug.
• Drug use is not recommended in breast-feeding women.
• Use cautiously in patients with heart failure, nonallergic bronchospastic disease, diabetes, hyperthyroidism, or impaired renal or hepatic function and in pregnant women.
• Safe use of drug has not been established in children.

NURSING CONSIDERATIONS

Assessment
• Assess patient's blood pressure before therapy and regularly thereafter.
• Always check patient's apical pulse rate before giving drug.
• Be alert for adverse reactions and drug interactions.
• Evaluate patient's and family's knowledge of drug therapy.

Nursing diagnoses
• Risk for injury related to presence of hypertension
• Fatigue related to drug's adverse effect
• Knowledge deficit related to drug therapy

⟫ Planning and implementation

• If you detect extremes in pulse rates, withhold medication and call doctor immediately.

• Notify doctor if severe hypotension occurs.

• Abrupt discontinuation can exacerbate angina and precipitate MI. Withdraw over 1 to 2 weeks after long-term administration, as ordered.

Patient teaching

• Teach patient how to take his pulse and tell him to take his pulse before taking each dose of pindolol. Tell patient to notify doctor before taking any more doses if his pulse rate varies significantly from its usual level.

• Tell patient not to discontinue this drug suddenly even if unpleasant adverse reactions occur, but to discuss problem with doctor. Explain that abrupt discontinuation can exacerbate angina and MI.

• Instruct patient to check with doctor before taking OTC medications.

• Teach patient and family caregiver to take blood pressure measurements. Tell them to notify doctor of any significant change.

⚞ Evaluation

• Patient's blood pressure is normal.

• Patient states energy-conserving measures to combat fatigue.

• Patient and family state understanding of drug therapy.

---

pipecuronium bromide
(pigh-peh-kyoor-OH-nee-um BROH-mighd)
Arduan

Pharmacologic class: nondepolarizing neuromuscular blocker
Therapeutic class: skeletal muscle relaxant
Pregnancy risk category: C

How supplied
Powder for injection: 10 mg/vial

Pharmacokinetics
Absorption: not applicable.
Distribution: volume of distribution is about 0.25 L/kg and increases in patients with renal failure. Other conditions associated with increased volume distribution (including edema, old age, and CV disease) may delay onset.
Metabolism: about 20% to 40% of drug is metabolized, probably in liver.
Excretion: excreted primarily in urine.
Half-life: about 1.7 hours.

Route	Onset	Peak	Duration
I.V.	1-2 min	≤ 5 min	About 24 min

Pharmacodynamics
Chemical effect: competes with acetylcholine for receptor sites at motor end plate. Because this action may be antagonized by cholinesterase inhibitors, drug is considered a competitive antagonist.
Therapeutic effect: relaxes skeletal muscles.

Indications and dosage

▶ **To provide skeletal muscle relaxation during surgery as adjunct to general anesthesia.** Dosage is highly individualized. The following doses may serve as a guide for use in nonobese patients with normal renal function. *Adults and children:* initially, 70 to 85 mcg/kg I.V. provides conditions considered ideal for endotracheal intubation and maintains paralysis for 1 to 2 hours. If succinylcholine is used for endotracheal intubation, initial dose of 50 mcg/kg I.V. provides good relaxation for 45 minutes or more. Maintenance dose of 10 to 15 mcg/kg provides relaxation for about 50 minutes.

Adverse reactions
CV: hypotension, bradycardia, hypertension, myocardial ischemia, *CVA,* throm-

---

bosis, atrial fibrillation, *ventricular extrasystole*.
GU: anuria.
Respiratory: dyspnea, respiratory depression, *respiratory insufficiency or apnea*.
Other: prolonged muscle weakness, increased creatinine levels.

Interactions

Drug-drug. *Aminoglycosides (gentamicin, kanamycin, neomycin, streptomycin), bacitracin, colistimethate, colistin, polymyxin B sulfate, tetracyclines:* potentiated neuromuscular blockade, leading to increased skeletal muscle relaxation and prolongation of effect. Use together cautiously.
Inhalation anesthetics, quinidine: enhanced activity (or prolonged action) of nondepolarizing neuromuscular blocking agents.
Magnesium salts: may enhance neuromuscular blockade. Monitor for excessive weakness.

Contraindications and precautions

• Contraindicated in patients with hypersensitivity to drug.
• Use cautiously and with dosage adjustments in patients with renal failure because drug is excreted by kidneys. No information is available regarding use of drug in patients with hepatic disease. Also use cautiously in pregnant or breast-feeding women.
• Drug is not recommended for use in neonates and infants younger than 3 months. Limited evidence suggests that infants and children (ages 1 to 14) under balanced anesthesia or halothane anesthesia may be less sensitive than adults.

NURSING CONSIDERATIONS

⚕ Assessment

• Assess patient's condition before therapy and regularly thereafter.
• Monitor respirations closely until patient is fully recovered from neuromuscular blockade, as evidenced by tests of

muscle strength (hand grip, head lift, and ability to cough).
• Monitor for bradycardia during anesthesia due to drug's minimal vagolytic action.
• Nerve stimulator and train-of-four monitoring are recommended to document antagonism of neuromuscular blockade and recovery of muscle strength. Before attempting pharmacologic reversal with neostigmine, some evidence of spontaneous recovery should be evident.
• Be alert for adverse reactions and drug interactions.
• Evaluate patient's and family's knowledge of drug therapy.

🔟 Nursing diagnoses

• Altered health maintenance related to underlying condition
• Ineffective breathing pattern related to drug's effect on respiratory muscles
• Knowledge deficit related to drug therapy

⬎ Planning and implementation

• Use drug under direct medical supervision by personnel skilled in use of neuromuscular blockers and techniques for maintaining patent airway. Do not use drug unless facilities and equipment for artificial respiration, mechanical ventilation, oxygen therapy, and intubation and antagonist are within reach.
• Give pipecuronium after succinylcholine when latter is used to facilitate intubation. However, no evidence exists to support safe use of pipecuronium before succinylcholine to decrease adverse effects of latter drug.
• Give patient sedatives or general anesthetics before neuromuscular blockers are administered, as ordered. Neuromuscular blockers do not obtund consciousness or alter pain threshold.
• Reconstitute drug with 10 ml solution before use to yield solution of 1 mg/ml. Large volumes of diluent or addition of drug to hanging I.V. solution is not recommended.

Reactions may be *common*, uncommon, *life-threatening*, or COMMON AND LIFE-THREATENING.

• After reconstitution with sterile water for injection or other compatible I.V. solutions (such as 0.9% NaCl injection, D_5W, lactated Ringer's injection, dextrose 5% in 0.9% NaCl), know that drug is stable for 24 hours if refrigerated.
• After reconstitution with solutions other than bacteriostatic water for injection, discard unused drug.
• After reconstitution with bacteriostatic water for injection, drug is stable for 5 days at room temperature or in refrigerator. Bacteriostatic water contains benzyl alcohol and is not intended for use in neonates.
• Store powder at room temperature or in refrigerator (36° to 86° F [2° to 30° C]).
• Drug is not recommended for use in patients requiring prolonged mechanical ventilation in intensive care unit, before or after administration of other nondepolarizing neuromuscular blockers, or during cesarean section.
• Patients with myasthenia gravis or myasthenic syndrome (Eaton-Lambert syndrome) are particularly sensitive to nondepolarizing relaxants. Shorter-acting agents are recommended.
• Know that dosage should be adjusted to ideal body weight in obese patients (30% or more over their ideal weight) to avoid prolonged neuromuscular blockade.
• Experimental evidence suggests that acid-base and electrolyte balances may influence actions of nondepolarizing neuromuscular blocking agents. Alkalosis may counteract paralysis and acidosis may enhance it.
Patient teaching
• Inform patient and family that drug will be given as part of anesthesia.
• Reassure patient that he will be monitored continuously.

☑ Evaluation
• Patient responds well to therapy.
• Patient maintains adequate breathing pattern with mechanical assistance.
• Patient and family state understanding of drug therapy.

piperacillin sodium
(pigh-PER-uh-sil-in SOH-dee-um)
Pipracil, Pipril♦

Pharmacologic class: extended-spectrum penicillin, acyclaminopenicillin
Therapeutic class: antibiotic
Pregnancy risk category: B

How supplied
Injection: 2 g, 3 g, 4 g

Pharmacokinetics
Absorption: unknown after I.M. administration.
Distribution: distributed widely in body. It penetrates minimally into uninflamed meninges and slightly into bone and sputum. Drug is 16% to 22% protein-bound.
Metabolism: unknown.
Excretion: excreted mainly in urine (42% to 90%); some excreted in bile.
Half-life: 30 to 90 minutes.

Route	Onset	Peak	Duration
I.V.	Immediate	Immediate	Unknown
I.M.	Unknown	30-50 min	Unknown

Pharmacodynamics
Chemical effect: inhibits cell-wall synthesis during microorganism multiplication; bacteria resist penicillins by producing penicillinases—enzymes that convert penicillins to inactive penicilloic acid.
Therapeutic effect: kills susceptible bacteria. Spectrum of activity includes many gram-negative aerobic and anaerobic bacilli, many gram-positive and gram-negative cocci, and some gram-positive aerobic and anaerobic bacilli. Drug may be effective against some strains of carbenicillin-resistant and ticarcillin-resistant gram-negative bacilli.

Indications and dosage
▶ **Systemic infections caused by susceptible strains of gram-positive and especially gram-negative organisms**

(including *Proteus* and *Pseudomonas aeruginosa*). *Adults and children over age 12:* 12 to 18 g/day in divided doses q 4 to 6 hours I.V. Dosage for children under age 12 has not been established.
▶ **Prophylaxis of surgical infections.** *Adults:* 2 g I.V., given 30 to 60 minutes before surgery. Dose may be repeated during surgery and once or twice more after surgery.

Adverse reactions

CNS: neuromuscular irritability, *seizures,* headache, dizziness.
GI: nausea, diarrhea.
Hematologic: bleeding with high doses, *neutropenia,* eosinophilia, *leukopenia, thrombocytopenia.*
Other: *hypokalemia,* hypersensitivity reactions (edema, fever, chills, rash, pruritus, urticaria, *anaphylaxis*), overgrowth of nonsusceptible organisms, pain at injection site, vein irritation, phlebitis.

Interactions

Drug-drug. *Probenecid:* increased blood levels of piperacillin. Probenecid may be used for this purpose.

Contraindications and precautions

● Contraindicated in patients with hypersensitivity to drug or other penicillins.
● Use cautiously in patients with other drug allergies, especially to cephalosporins (possible cross-sensitivity); in those with bleeding tendencies, uremia, or hypokalemia; and in pregnant or breast-feeding women.
● Safety of drug has not been established in children under age 12.

NURSING CONSIDERATIONS

✎ Assessment
● Assess patient's infection before therapy and regularly thereafter.
● Before giving, ask patient about any allergic reactions to penicillin. However, negative history is no guarantee against future reaction.

● Obtain specimen for culture and sensitivity tests before first dose. Therapy may begin pending results.
● Check CBC and platelet counts frequently, as ordered. Drug may cause thrombocytopenia.
● Monitor serum potassium level.
● Be alert for adverse reactions and drug interactions.
● Cystic fibrosis patients tend to be most susceptible to fever or rash.
● Monitor patient's hydration status if adverse GI reactions occur.
● Evaluate patient's and family's knowledge of drug therapy.

⊞ Nursing diagnoses
● Infection related to presence of susceptible bacteria
● Risk for fluid volume deficit related to adverse GI reactions
● Knowledge deficit related to drug therapy

▷ Planning and implementation
● Dosage should be altered in patient with impaired renal function.
● Keep in mind that drug is typically used with another antibiotic, such as gentamicin.
I.V. use: Reconstitute each gram of drug with 5 ml of diluent, such as sterile or bacteriostatic water for injection, 0.9% NaCl injection (with or without preservative), D_5W, or dextrose 5% in 0.9% NaCl injection. Shake until dissolved. Inject reconstituted solution directly into vein or into I.V. line of free-flowing solution over 3 to 5 minutes. Alternatively, dilute with at least 50 ml of compatible I.V. solution and give by intermittent infusion over 30 minutes.
– Avoid continuous infusions to prevent vein irritation. Change site every 48 hours.
– Aminoglycoside antibiotics (such as gentamicin and tobramycin) are chemically incompatible with drug. Don't mix in same I.V. container.

Reactions may be *common,* uncommon, *life-threatening,* or COMMON AND LIFE-THREATENING.

I.M. use: Reconstitute drug with sterile or bacteriostatic water for injection, 0.9% NaCl injection (with or without preservative), or 0.5% to 1% lidocaine hydrochloride. Add 2 ml of diluent for each gram of drug. Final solution will contain 1 g/2.5 ml.

• Give drug at least 1 hour before bacteriostatic antibiotics.

• Institute seizure precautions. Patients with high serum levels of this drug may have seizures.

Patient teaching

• Tell patient to inform nurse of pain or discomfort at I.V. site.

• Instruct patient to limit salt intake while taking piperacillin because drug contains 1.98 mEq sodium per gram.

• Tell patient to report adverse reactions.

☑ Evaluation

• Patient is free from infection.

• Patient maintains adequate hydration throughout drug therapy.

• Patient and family state understanding of drug therapy.

---

piperacillin sodium and tazobactam sodium
(pigh-PER-uh-sil-in SOH-dee-um and taz-oh-BAK-tem SOH-dee-um)
Zosyn

Pharmacologic class: extended-spectrum penicillin/beta-lactamase inhibitor.
Therapeutic class: antibiotic
Pregnancy risk category: B

How supplied

Powder for injection: 2 g piperacillin and 0.25 g tazobactam per vial, 3 g piperacillin and 0.375 g tazobactam per vial, 4 g piperacillin and 0.5 g tazobactam per vial
Pharmacy bulk package: 40.5 g

Pharmacokinetics

Absorption: not applicable.

Distribution: both drugs are about 30% protein-bound.
Metabolism: piperacillin is metabolized to a minor, microbiologically active desethyl metabolite. Tazobactam is metabolized to a single metabolite that lacks pharmacologic and antibacterial activities.
Excretion: excreted in urine and bile.
Half-life: piperacillin, 0.7 hour; tazobactam, 1.2 hours.

Route	Onset	Peak	Duration
I.V.	Immediate	Immediate	Unknown

Pharmacodynamics

Chemical effect: piperacillin inhibits cell-wall synthesis during microorganism multiplication; tazobactam increases piperacillin effectiveness by inactivating beta lactamases, which destroy penicillins.
Therapeutic effect: kills susceptible bacteria. Spectrum of activity includes *Escherichia coli, Bacteroides fragilis, Bacteroides ovatus, Bacteroides thetaiotaomicron, Bacteroides vulgatus, Staphylococcus aureus,* and *Haemophilus influenzae.*

Indications and dosage

▶ **Appendicitis (complicated by rupture or abscess) and peritonitis caused by *E. coli, B. fragilis, B. ovatus, B. thetaiotaomicron,* or *B. vulgatus;* skin and skin-structure infections caused by *S. aureus;* postpartum endometritis or pelvic inflammatory disease caused by *E. coli;* moderately severe community-acquired pneumonia caused by *H. influenzae.*** *Adults:* 3 g piperacillin and 0.375 g tazobactam I.V. q 6 hours. *In adult patients with renal impairment:* if creatinine clearance is 20 to 40 ml/minute, 2 g piperacillin and 0.25 g tazobactam I.V. q 6 hours. If creatinine clearance is below 20 ml/minute, 2 g piperacillin and 0.25 g tazobactam I.V. q 8 hours.

Adverse reactions

CNS: *headache, insomnia,* agitation, dizziness, anxiety.
CV: hypertension, tachycardia, chest pain, edema.
EENT: rhinitis.
GI: *diarrhea, nausea, constipation,* vomiting, dyspepsia, stool changes, abdominal pain.
Respiratory: dyspnea.
Skin: rash (including maculopapular, bullous, urticarial, and eczematoid), pruritus.
Other: fever; pain, *thrombocytopenia, anaphylaxis,* candidiasis; inflammation, phlebitis (at I.V. site).

Interactions

Drug-drug. *Probenecid:* increased blood levels of piperacillin. Probenecid may be used for this purpose.
Vecuronium: prolongation of neuromuscular blockage. Monitor closely.

Contraindications and precautions

● Contraindicated in patients with hypersensitivity to drug or other penicillins.
● Use cautiously in patients with other drug allergies, especially to cephalosporins (possible cross-sensitivity); in those with bleeding tendencies, uremia, or hypokalemia; and in pregnant or breast-feeding women.
● Safety of drug has not been established in children under age 12.

NURSING CONSIDERATIONS

⚕ Assessment

● Before giving drug, ask patient about previous allergic reactions to this drug or other penicillins. However, negative history of penicillin allergy does not guarantee future safety.
● Assess patient's infection before therapy and regularly thereafter.
● Obtain specimen for culture and sensitivity tests before first dose. Therapy may begin pending results.

● Be alert for adverse reactions and drug interactions.
● Monitor patient's hydration status if adverse GI reactions occur.
● Evaluate patient's and family's knowledge of drug therapy.

⚙ Nursing diagnoses

● Infection related to presence of bacteria
● Risk of fluid volume deficit related to adverse GI reactions
● Knowledge deficit related to drug therapy

⬚ Planning and implementation

● Reconstitute each gram of piperacillin with 5 ml of diluent, such as sterile or bacteriostatic water for injection, 0.9% NaCl injection, bacteriostatic 0.9% NaCl injection, D_5W, dextrose 5% in 0.9% NaCl injection, or dextran 6% in 0.9% NaCl injection. Don't use lactated Ringer's injection. Shake until dissolved. Further dilute to final volume of 50 ml before infusion.
● Infuse drug over at least 30 minutes. Discontinue other primary infusions during administration if possible. Aminoglycoside antibiotics (such as gentamicin and tobramycin) are chemically incompatible with drug. Don't mix in same I.V. container.
● Don't mix with other drugs.
● Use drug immediately after reconstitution. Discard unused drug after 24 hours if held at room temperature; 48 hours if refrigerated. Once diluted, drug is stable in I.V. bags for 24 hours at room temperature or 1 week if refrigerated.
● Change I.V. site every 48 hours.
● Because hemodialysis removes 6% of piperacillin dose and 21% of tazobactam dose, be aware that supplemental doses may be needed after hemodialysis.
Patient teaching
● Tell patient to inform nurse if pain or discomfort occurs at I.V. site.
● Advise patient to limit salt intake while taking drug because piperacillin contains 1.98 mEq Na/g.

Reactions may be *common,* uncommon, *life-threatening*, or COMMON AND LIFE-THREATENING.

• Tell patient to report adverse reactions.

☑ **Evaluation**

• Patient is free from infection.
• Patient maintains adequate hydration.
• Patient and family state understanding of drug therapy.

---

pirbuterol acetate
(pir-BYOO-teh-rol AS-ih-tayt)
Maxair

Pharmacologic class: beta-adrenergic agonist
Therapeutic class: bronchodilator
Pregnancy risk category: C

How supplied
Inhaler: 0.2 mg/metered dose

Pharmacokinetics
Absorption: negligible serum levels are achieved after inhalation.
Distribution: distributed locally.
Metabolism: metabolized in liver.
Excretion: about 50% of inhaled dose is excreted in urine as parent drug and metabolites.

Route	Onset	Peak	Duration
Inhalation	≤ 5 min	30-60 min	5 hr

Pharmacodynamics
Chemical effect: relaxes bronchial smooth muscle by acting on beta$_2$-adrenergic receptors.
Therapeutic effect: improves breathing ability.

Indications and dosage
▶ **Prevention and reversal of bronchospasm, asthma.** *Adults and children age 12 and over:* 1 or 2 inhalations (0.2 to 0.4 mg) repeated q 4 to 6 hours. Not to exceed 12 inhalations daily.

Adverse reactions
CNS: tremor, nervousness, dizziness, insomnia, headache.
CV: tachycardia, palpitations, increased blood pressure.
EENT: dryness or irritation of throat.

Interactions
Drug-drug. *MAO inhibitors, tricyclic antidepressants:* may potentiate action of beta-adrenergic agonist on vascular system. Use together cautiously.
Propranolol, other beta blockers: decreased bronchodilating effects. Avoid concomitant use.

Contraindications and precautions
• Contraindicated in patients with hypersensitivity to drug.
• Use cautiously in pregnant or breastfeeding women and in patients with CV disorders, hyperthyroidism, diabetes, and seizure disorders or in those who are unusually responsive to sympathomimetic amines.
• Safety of drug has not been established in children under age 12.

NURSING CONSIDERATIONS

☜ **Assessment**
• Assess patient's condition before therapy.
• Monitor effectiveness by checking respiratory rate and auscultating lung fields frequently and following laboratory studies such as arterial blood gases as ordered.
• Be alert for adverse reactions and drug interactions.
• Evaluate patient's and family's knowledge of drug therapy.

⊕ **Nursing diagnoses**
• Impaired gas exchange related to presence of bronchospasms
• Sleep pattern disturbance related to drug-induced insomnia
• Knowledge deficit related to drug therapy

⟩ Planning and implementation
- Shake canister well before each use.
- Store drug away from heat and direct sunlight.
- If patient is also to receive steroid inhaler, always administer pirbuterol first, then wait about 5 minutes before administering steroid inhaler.
- Notify doctor if patient's condition does not improve or worsens.

Patient teaching
- Give these instructions for using metered-dose inhaler: Clear nasal passages and throat. Breathe out, expelling as much air from lungs as possible. Place mouthpiece well into mouth as dose from inhaler is released, and inhale deeply. Hold breath for several seconds, remove mouthpiece, and exhale slowly.
- If more than one inhalation is ordered, tell patient to wait at least 2 minutes before repeating procedure.
- Tell patient also using steroid inhaler to use bronchodilator first, then wait about 5 minutes before using steroid. This allows bronchodilator to open air passages for maximum effectiveness.
- Tell patient to notify doctor if increased bronchospasm occurs after using drug.
- Advise patient to seek medical attention if previously effective dosage does not control symptoms; this may signify worsening of disease.

☑ Evaluation
- Patient exhibits improved gas exchange, as demonstrated by improved lung sounds and arterial blood gas measurements.
- Patient does not experience insomnia.
- Patient and family state understanding of drug therapy.

---

piroxicam
(peer-OK-sih-cam)
Apo-Piroxicam♦, Feldene,
Novo-Pirocam♦

Pharmacologic class: NSAID

Therapeutic class: nonnarcotic analgesic, antipyretic, anti-inflammatory
Pregnancy risk category: NR

How supplied
Capsules: 10 mg, 20 mg

Pharmacokinetics
Absorption: absorbed rapidly from GI tract. Food delays absorption.
Distribution: drug is highly protein-bound.
Metabolism: metabolized in liver.
Excretion: excreted in urine. *Half-life:* about 50 hours.

Route	Onset	Peak	Duration
P.O.	15-30 min	3-5 hr	About 24 hr

Pharmacodynamics
Chemical effect: unknown; produces anti-inflammatory, analgesic, and antipyretic effects, possibly by inhibiting prostaglandin synthesis.
Therapeutic effect: relieves pain, fever, and inflammation.

Indications and dosage
▶ **Osteoarthritis and rheumatoid arthritis.** *Adults:* 20 mg P.O. daily. If desired, dosage may be divided b.i.d.

Adverse reactions
CNS: headache, drowsiness, dizziness, paresthesia, somnolence.
CV: peripheral edema.
EENT: auditory disturbances.
GI: *epigastric distress, nausea, occult blood loss,* **peptic ulceration, severe GI bleeding.**
GU: *nephrotoxicity,* elevated BUN level.
Hematologic: prolonged bleeding time, anemia, leukopenia, *aplastic anemia, agranulocytosis, thrombocytopenia.*
Hepatic: elevated liver enzymes.
Metabolism: hyperkalemia, acidosis, dilutional hypernatremia.
Respiratory: *bronchospasm.*
Skin: pruritus, rash, urticaria, *photosensitivity.*

Reactions may be *common*, uncommon, *life-threatening*, or COMMON AND LIFE-THREATENING.

Interactions

Drug-drug. *Aspirin, corticosteroids:* increased risk of GI toxicity. Decreased plasma levels of piroxicam.
Lithium: increased plasma lithium levels. Monitor for toxicity.
Oral anticoagulants: enhanced risk of bleeding. Monitor patient closely.
Oral antidiabetic agents: enhanced antidiabetic effects. Monitor patient.
Drug-lifestyle. *Alcohol use:* increased risk of GI toxicity. Decreased plasma levels of piroxicam. Avoid concomitant use.
Sun exposure: risk of photosensitivity reaction. Take precautions.

Contraindications and precautions

• Contraindicated in patients with bronchospasm, angioedema precipitated by aspirin or NSAIDs, or hypersensitivity to drug and in pregnant or breast-feeding women.
• Use cautiously in elderly patients and in those with GI disorders, history of renal or peptic ulcer disease, cardiac disease, hypertension, or conditions predisposing to fluid retention.
• Safety of drug has not been established in children.

NURSING CONSIDERATIONS

⚕ Assessment
• Assess patient's condition before therapy and regularly thereafter. Effectiveness is not seen for at least 2 weeks after therapy begins. Evaluate response to drug by assessing for reduced symptoms.
• Check renal, hepatic, and auditory function and CBC periodically during prolonged therapy.
• Be alert for adverse reactions and drug interactions.
• Evaluate patient's and family's knowledge of drug therapy.

Nursing diagnoses
• Pain related to arthritis
• Altered tissue integrity related to adverse effect on GI mucosa

• Knowledge deficit related to drug therapy

Planning and implementation
• Give drug with milk, antacids, or food if GI adverse reactions occur.
• Stop drug and notify doctor if laboratory abnormalities occur.
Patient teaching
• Tell patient that full therapeutic effects may be delayed for 2 to 4 weeks.
• Teach patient to recognize and report signs and symptoms of GI bleeding.
• Advise patient to use sunblock, wear protective clothing, and avoid prolonged exposure to sunlight.

☑ Evaluation
• Patient is free from pain.
• Patient maintains normal GI tissue integrity.
• Patient and family state understanding of drug therapy.

plasma protein fraction
(PLAZ-muh PROH-teen FRAK-shun)
Plasmanate, Plasma-Plex, Plasmatein, Protenate

Pharmacologic class: blood derivative
Therapeutic class: plasma volume expander
Pregnancy risk category: C

How supplied

Injection: 5% solution in 50-ml, 250-ml, 500-ml vials

Pharmacokinetics

Absorption: not applicable.
Distribution: distributed into intravascular space and extravascular sites, including skin, muscle, and lungs.
Metabolism: unknown.
Excretion: unknown.

Route	Onset	Peak	Duration
I.V.	Immediate	Immediate	Unknown

Pharmacodynamics

Chemical effect: supplies colloid to blood and expands plasma volume.
Therapeutic effect: raises serum protein levels and expands plasma volume.

Indications and dosage

▶ **Shock.** *Adults:* varies with patient's condition and response, but usual dose is 250 to 500 ml I.V. (12.5 to 25 g protein), usually no faster than 10 ml/minute.
Infants and young children: 6.6 to 33 ml/kg (0.33 to 1.65 g/kg of protein) I.V., 5 to 10 ml/minute.
▶ **Hypoproteinemia.** *Adults:* 1,000 to 1,500 ml I.V. daily. Maximum infusion rate is 8 ml/minute.

Adverse reactions

CNS: headache.
CV: various effects on blood pressure (after rapid infusion or intra-arterial administration); *vascular overload* (after rapid infusion).
GI: nausea, vomiting, hypersalivation.
Respiratory: dyspnea, *pulmonary edema*.
Skin: erythema, urticaria.
Other: flushing, chills, fever, back pain.

Interactions

None significant.

Contraindications and precautions

• Contraindicated in patients with severe anemia or heart failure and in those having undergone cardiac bypass surgery.
• Use cautiously in patients with hepatic or renal failure, low cardiac reserve, and restricted sodium intake.
• Also use cautiously in pregnant or breast-feeding women.

NURSING CONSIDERATIONS

☒ Assessment
• Assess patient's condition before therapy and regularly thereafter.
• Monitor vital signs at least hourly.
• Be alert for adverse reactions.

• Evaluate patient's and family's knowledge of drug therapy.

⊞ Nursing diagnoses
• Decreased cardiac output related to underlying condition
• Pain related to headache
• Knowledge deficit related to drug therapy

▧ Planning and implementation
• Check expiration date before using. Don't use solutions that are cloudy, contain sediment, or have been frozen. Discard solutions in containers opened for more than 4 hours because it contains no preservatives.
• If patient is dehydrated, give additional fluids P.O. or I.V., as ordered.
• Do not give more than 250 g or 5,000 ml in 48 hours.
• Be prepared to slow or stop infusion if hypotension occurs. Vital signs should return to normal gradually.
• Keep in mind that drug contains 130 to 160 mEq sodium/L.
• Administer mild analgesic as ordered for drug-induced headache.
Patient teaching
• Tell patient and family purpose of plasma protein fraction and keep them informed of drug effectiveness.
• Instruct patient to report adverse reactions.

☑ Evaluation
• Patient regains normal cardiac output.
• Patient is free from pain.
• Patient and family state understanding of drug therapy.

plicamycin (mithramycin)
(pligh-keh-MIGH-sin)
Mithracin

Pharmacologic class: antibiotic antineoplastic (cell cycle–phase nonspecific)

Therapeutic class: antineoplastic, hypocalcemic agent
Pregnancy risk category: X

How supplied

Injection: 2.5-mg vials

Pharmacokinetics

Absorption: not applicable.
Distribution: distributes mainly into Kupffer's cells of liver, into renal tubular cells, and along formed bone surfaces. Also crosses blood-brain barrier and achieves appreciable concentrations in CSF.
Metabolism: unknown.
Excretion: excreted primarily in urine.

Route	Onset	Peak	Duration
I.V.	1-2 days	3 days	7-10 days

Pharmacodynamics

Chemical effect: unknown; may form a complex with DNA, thus inhibiting RNA synthesis. Also inhibits osteocytic activity, blocking calcium and phosphorus resorption from bone.
Therapeutic effect: hinders growth of testicular cancer cells and lowers blood calcium levels.

Indications and dosage

Dosage and indications may vary. Check protocol with doctor.
▶ **Hypercalcemia associated with advanced malignancy.** *Adults:* 15 to 25 mcg/kg/day I.V. for 3 to 4 days. Dosage repeated at weekly intervals until desired response is obtained.
▶ **Testicular cancer.** *Adults:* 25 to 30 mcg/kg/day I.V. for 8 to 10 days or until toxicity occurs.

Adverse reactions

CNS: drowsiness, weakness, lethargy, headache, dizziness, nervousness, depression.
GI: *nausea, vomiting,* anorexia, diarrhea, stomatitis, metallic taste.

GU: proteinuria; increased BUN and serum creatinine levels.
Hematologic: *leukopenia, thrombocytopenia; bleeding syndrome from epistaxis to generalized hemorrhage; facial flushing.*
Hepatic: elevated liver enzymes levels, *hepatotoxicity.*
Metabolic: *decreased serum calcium,* potassium, and phosphorus levels.
Other: irritation, cellulitis with extravasation, *death.*

Interactions

None significant.

Contraindications and precautions

● Contraindicated in patients with thrombocytopenia, bone marrow suppression, or coagulation and bleeding disorder; in women who are or may become pregnant; and in breast-feeding patients.
● Use with extreme caution in patients with significant renal or hepatic impairment.
● Safety of drug has not been established in children.

NURSING CONSIDERATIONS

Assessment
● Assess patient's condition before therapy and regularly thereafter.
● Obtain baseline platelet count and PT before therapy, and monitor during therapy, as ordered.
● Know that facial flushing is early indicator of bleeding.
● Monitor LD, AST, ALT, alkaline phosphatase, BUN, creatinine, potassium, calcium, and phosphorus levels, as ordered.
● Monitor patient for tetany, carpopedal spasm, Chvostek's sign, and muscle cramps; check serum calcium level. Precipitous drop is possible.
● Be alert for adverse reactions.
● Evaluate patient's and family's knowledge of drug therapy.

🖑 **Nursing diagnoses**
• Altered health maintenance related to underlying condition
• Altered protection related to adverse hematologic reactions
• Knowledge deficit related to drug therapy

▶ **Planning and implementation**
• Give antiemetic before administering drug, as ordered.
• Follow institutional policy to reduce risks. Preparation and administration of parenteral form are associated with carcinogenic, mutagenic, and teratogenic risks for personnel.
• To prepare solution, add 4.9 ml of sterile water for injection to vial and shake to dissolve. Then dilute for I.V infusion in 1,000 ml of D_5W or 0.9% NaCl. Infuse over 4 to 6 hours. Discard unused drug.
• Be aware that slow infusion reduces nausea that develops with I.V. push.
• Avoid extravasation. Drug is a vesicant. If I.V. solution infiltrates, stop immediately, notify doctor, and use ice packs. Restart I.V. line.
• Avoid contact with skin or mucous membranes.
• Discontinue drug if WBC count is less than 4,000/mm³, platelet count falls to less than 150,000/mm³, or if PT is prolonged more than 4 seconds longer than control and notify doctor.
• Store lyophilized powder in refrigerator and protect from light.
Patient teaching
• Warn patient to watch for signs of infection (fever, sore throat, fatigue) and bleeding (easy bruising, nosebleeds, bleeding gums, melena). Have patient take temperature daily. Instruct patient and family on infection-control and bleeding precautions.
• Tell patient to use salicylate-free medication for pain or fever.

☑ **Evaluation**
• Patient responds well to therapy.

• Patient does not develop serious complications from adverse hematologic reactions.
• Patient and family state understanding of drug therapy.

---

polyethylene glycol and electrolyte solution
(pol-ee-ETH-ih-leen GLIGH-kohl and ee-LEK-troh-light soh-LOO-shun)
Colovage, CoLyte, Glycoprep♦, GoLYTELY, NuLYTELY, OCL

Pharmacologic class: polyethylene glycol 3350 nonabsorbable solution
Therapeutic class: laxative and bowel evacuant
Pregnancy risk category: C

How supplied

Powder for oral solution: polyethylene glycol (PEG) 3350 (6 g), anhydrous sodium sulfate (568 mg), NaCl (146 mg), potassium chloride (74.5 mg) per 100 ml (Colovage); PEG 3350 (120 g), sodium sulfate (3.36 g), NaCl (2.92 g), potassium chloride (1.49 g) per 2 L (CoLyte); PEG 3350 (60 g), NaCl (1.46 g), potassium chloride (745 mg), sodium bicarbonate (1.68 g), sodium sulfate (5.68 g) per liter (Glycoprep♦); PEG 3350 (236 g), sodium sulfate (22.74 g), sodium bicarbonate (6.74 g), NaCl (5.86 g), potassium chloride (2.97 g) per 4.8 L (GoLYTELY); PEG 3350 (420 g), sodium bicarbonate (5.72 g), NaCl (11.2 g), potassium chloride (1.48 g) per 4 L (NuLYTELY); PEG 3350 (6 g), sodium sulfate decahydrate (1.29 g), NaCl (146 mg), potassium chloride (75 mg), polysorbate-80 (30 mg) per 100 ml (OCL)

Pharmacokinetics

Absorption: not absorbed.
Distribution: not applicable because drug is not absorbed.
Metabolism: not applicable because drug is not absorbed.

Excretion: excreted via GI tract.

Route	Onset	Peak	Duration
P.O.	≤ 1 hr	Varies	Varies

Pharmacodynamics
Chemical effect: PEG 3350, a nonabsorbable solution, acts as osmotic agent. Sodium sulfate greatly reduces sodium absorption. The electrolyte concentration causes virtually no net absorption or secretion of ions.
Therapeutic effect: cleanses bowel.

Indications and dosage

▶ **Bowel preparation before GI examination.** *Adults:* 240 ml P.O. q 10 minutes until 4 L are consumed. Typically, give 4 hours before examination, allowing 3 hours for drinking and 1 hour for bowel evacuation.

Adverse reactions
GI: nausea, bloating, cramps, vomiting.

Interactions
Drug-drug. *Orally administered drugs:* decreased absorption if given within 1 hour of starting therapy. Don't give with other oral drugs.

Contraindications and precautions
• Contraindicated in patients with GI obstruction or perforation, gastric retention, toxic colitis, or megacolon.
• Use cautiously in pregnant or breast-feeding women.

NURSING CONSIDERATIONS

☲ Assessment
• Assess patient's condition before therapy and regularly thereafter.
• Be alert for adverse reactions and drug interactions.
• Evaluate patient's and family's knowledge of drug therapy.

⊕ Nursing diagnoses
• Health-seeking behavior (testing) related to need to determine cause of underlying GI problem
• Risk for fluid volume deficit related to adverse GI reactions
• Knowledge deficit related to drug therapy

▷ Planning and implementation
• Use tap water to reconstitute powder. Shake vigorously to ensure that all powder is dissolved. Refrigerate solution but use within 48 hours.
• Do not add flavoring or additional ingredients to solution or administer chilled solution. Hypothermia has been reported after ingestion of large amounts of chilled solution.
• Administer solution early in morning if patient is scheduled for midmorning examination. Orally administered solution induces diarrhea (onset 30 to 60 minutes) that rapidly cleans bowel, usually within 4 hours.
• When used as preparation for barium enema, administer solution the evening before examination, to avoid interfering with barium coating of colonic mucosa.
• If given to semiconscious patient or to patient with impaired gag reflex, take care to prevent aspiration.
• No major shifts in fluid or electrolyte balance have been reported.
Patient teaching
• Tell patient to fast for 4 hours before taking solution and to ingest only clear fluids until examination is complete.
• Warn patient about adverse GI reactions to drug.

☑ Evaluation
• Patient is able to have examination performed.
• Patient maintains adequate fluid volume.
• Patient and family state understanding of drug therapy.

polysaccharide iron complex
(pol-ee-SAK-uh-righd IGH-ern KOM-pleks)
Hytinic, Niferex, Niferex-150, Nu-Iron, Nu-Iron 150

Pharmacologic class: oral iron supplement
Therapeutic class: hematinic
Pregnancy risk category: NR

How supplied
Capsules: 150 mg
Solution: 100 mg/5 ml
Tablets (film-coated): 50 mg

Pharmacokinetics
Absorption: iron is absorbed from entire length of GI tract, but primary absorption sites are duodenum and proximal jejunum. Up to 10% of iron is absorbed by healthy individuals; patients with iron-deficiency anemia may absorb up to 60%.
Distribution: iron is transported through GI mucosal cells directly into blood, where it is immediately bound to carrier protein, transferrin, and transported to bone marrow for incorporation into hemoglobin. Iron is highly protein-bound.
Metabolism: iron is liberated by destruction of hemoglobin, but is conserved and reused by body.
Excretion: men and postmenopausal women lose about 1 mg/day; premenopausal women, about 1.5 mg/day. Loss usually occurs in nails, hair, feces, and urine; trace amounts lost in bile and sweat.

Route	Onset	Peak	Duration
P.O.	≤ 3 days	5-30 days	2 months

Pharmacodynamics
Chemical effect: provides elemental iron, an essential component in formation of hemoglobin.
Therapeutic effect: restores normal iron levels in body.

Indications and dosage
▶ **Treatment of uncomplicated iron deficiency anemia.** *Adults and children age 12 and over:* 150 to 300 mg P.O. as capsules or tablets daily or 1 to 2 teaspoonsful of elixir P.O. daily. *Children ages 6 to 12:* 150 mg to 300 mg P.O. as tablets or 1 teaspoonful of elixir P.O. daily. *Children ages 2 to 6:* ½ teaspoonful P.O. daily.

Adverse reactions
Although nausea, constipation, black stools, and epigastric pain are common adverse reactions associated with iron therapy, few, if any, occur with polysaccharide iron complex.

Interactions
Drug-drug. *Antacids, cholestyramine resin, cimetidine, tetracycline, vitamin E:* decreased iron absorption. Separate doses by 2 to 4 hours.
Chloramphenicol: delayed response to iron therapy. Monitor patient.
Fluoroquinolones, levodopa, methyldopa, penicillamine: decreased GI absorption, possibly resulting in decreased serum levels or efficacy. Administer separately.
Vitamin C: may increase iron absorption. Can be used for this effect.
Drug-food. *Cereals, cheese, coffee, eggs, milk, teas, whole-grain breads, yogurt:* may impair iron absorption. Don't administer together.

Contraindications and precautions
• Contraindicated in patients with hemochromatosis, hemosiderosis, and hypersensitivity to drug or its components.

NURSING CONSIDERATIONS

🔁 Assessment
• Assess patient's condition before therapy and regularly thereafter.
• Be alert for adverse reactions and drug interactions.
• Evaluate patient's and family's knowledge of drug therapy.

Reactions may be *common,* uncommon, *life-threatening,* or COMMON AND LIFE-THREATENING.

⊕ Nursing diagnoses
• Fatigue related to anemia
• Knowledge deficit related to drug therapy

▶ Planning and implementation
• Give drug with juice (preferably orange juice) or water but not with milk or antacids.
Patient teaching
• Inform patient that drug may turn stools black.
• Inform parents that as few as three tablets can cause iron poisoning in children. Store out of reach of children.
• If patient misses dose, tell him to take it as soon as he remembers but not to double-dose.
• Advise patient to avoid foods that may impair absorption, including yogurt, cheese, eggs, milk, whole-grain breads and cereals, tea, and coffee. Tell him to take drug with juice or water.

☑ Evaluation
• Patient states that fatigue is relieved as hemoglobin and reticulocyte count return to normal.
• Patient and family state understanding of drug therapy.

---

potassium acetate
(puh-TAS-ee-um AS-ih-tayt)
Pharmacologic class: potassium supplement
Therapeutic class: therapeutic agent for electrolyte balance
Pregnancy risk category: C

How supplied

Injection: 2 mEq/ml in 20-ml, 30-ml vials

Pharmacokinetics

Absorption: not applicable.
Distribution: distributed throughout body.
Metabolism: none significant.

Excretion: excreted largely by kidneys; small amounts may be excreted via skin and intestinal tract, but intestinal potassium is usually reabsorbed.

Route	Onset	Peak	Duration
I.V.	Immediate	Immediate	Unknown

Pharmacodynamics

Chemical effect: aids in transmitting nerve impulses; contracting cardiac and skeletal muscle; and maintaining intracellular tonicity, cellular metabolism, acid-base balance, and normal renal function.
Therapeutic effect: replaces and maintains potassium level.

Indications and dosage

▶ **Treatment of hypokalemia.** *Adults:* no more than 20 mEq hourly in concentration of 40 mEq/L or less. Total 24-hour dosage should not exceed 150 mEq (3 mEq/kg in children). Potassium replacement should be done with ECG monitoring and frequent serum potassium determinations. I.V. should be used only for life-threatening hypokalemia or when oral replacement not feasible.
▶ **Prevention of hypokalemia.** *Adults:* dosage is individualized to patient's needs, not to exceed 150 mEq/day. Given as additive to I.V. infusions. Usual dose is 40 mEq/L infused at rate not to exceed 20 mEq/hour. *Children:* individualized dosage not to exceed 3 mEq/kg/day. Given as additive to I.V. infusions.

Adverse reactions

CNS: paresthesia of extremities, listlessness, mental confusion, weakness or heaviness of legs, flaccid paralysis.
CV: *arrhythmias, possible cardiac arrest, heart block,* ECG changes.
GI: nausea, vomiting, abdominal pain, diarrhea, bowel ulceration.
GU: oliguria.
Skin: cold skin, gray pallor.
Other: pain, redness (at infusion site); *respiratory paralysis.*

Interactions

Drug-drug. *ACE inhibitors, potassium-sparing diuretics:* increased risk of hyperkalemia. Use with extreme caution.

Contraindications and precautions

• Contraindicated in patients with severe renal impairment with oliguria, anuria, or azotemia; in those with untreated Addison's disease; and in those with acute dehydration, heat cramps, hyperkalemia, hyperkalemic form of familial periodic paralysis, and conditions associated with extensive tissue breakdown.
• Use cautiously in patients with cardiac disease or renal impairment and in pregnant or breast-feeding women.

NURSING CONSIDERATIONS

⚕ Assessment
• Assess patient's condition before therapy and regularly thereafter.
• During therapy, monitor ECG, renal function, fluid intake and output, and serum potassium, serum creatinine, and BUN levels.
• Be alert for adverse reactions and drug interactions.
• Evaluate patient's and family's knowledge of drug therapy.

⊞ Nursing diagnoses
• Altered health maintenance related to presence of hypokalemia
• Risk for injury related to drug-induced hyperkalemia
• Knowledge deficit related to drug therapy

⧁ Planning and implementation
• Give drug by I.V. infusion only; never I.V. push or I.M. Observe for pain and redness at infusion site. Large-bore needle reduces local irritation.
• Administer drug slowly as diluted solution; potentially fatal hyperkalemia may result from too-rapid infusion.
• Reconstitute potassium acetate powder with liquids; give after meals with full

glass of water or fruit juice to minimize GI irritation.
• Never give potassium postoperatively until urine flow is established.

Patient teaching
• Inform patient of need for potassium supplementation.
• Tell patient that drug will be administered through I.V. line.
• Instruct patient to report adverse reactions.

☑ Evaluation
• Patient's potassium level returns to normal with drug therapy.
• Patient does not develop hyperkalemia as result of drug therapy.
• Patient and family state understanding of drug therapy.

---

potassium bicarbonate
(puh-TAS-ee-um bigh-KAR-buh-nayt)
K+Care ET, K-Ide, Klor-Con/EF, K-Lyte

Pharmacologic class: potassium supplement
Therapeutic class: therapeutic agent for electrolyte balance
Pregnancy risk category: NR

How supplied

Effervescent tablets: 6.5 mEq, 25 mEq

Pharmacokinetics

Absorption: well absorbed from GI tract.
Distribution: distributed throughout body.
Metabolism: none significant.
Excretion: excreted largely by kidneys; small amounts may be excreted via skin and intestinal tract, but intestinal potassium is usually reabsorbed.

Route	Onset	Peak	Duration
P.O.	Unknown	≤ 4 hr	Unknown

Pharmacodynamics

Chemical effect: aids in transmitting nerve impulses; contracting cardiac and

---

skeletal muscle; and maintaining intracellular tonicity, cellular metabolism, acid-base balance, and normal renal function. *Therapeutic effect:* replaces and maintains potassium level.

Indications and dosage

▶ **Hypokalemia.** *Adults:* 25 to 50 mEq dissolved in 4 to 8 oz of water (120 to 240 ml) once daily to b.i.d.

Adverse reactions

CNS: paresthesia of extremities, listlessness, mental confusion, weakness or heaviness of legs, flaccid paralysis.
CV: *arrhythmias, cardiac arrest, heart block,* ECG changes (prolonged PR interval; widened QRS complex; ST-segment depression; tall, tented T waves).
GI: *nausea, vomiting, abdominal pain,* diarrhea, ulcerations, hemorrhage, obstruction, perforation.

Interactions

Drug-drug. *ACE inhibitors, potassium-sparing diuretics:* risk of hyperkalemia.

Contraindications and precautions

• Contraindicated in patients with untreated Addison's disease, acute dehydration, heat cramps, hyperkalemia, hyperkalemic form of familial periodic paralysis, other conditions associated with extensive tissue breakdown, and severe renal impairment with oliguria, anuria, or azotemia.
• Use cautiously in patients with cardiac disease or renal impairment and in pregnant or breast-feeding women.
• Safety of drug has not been established in children.

NURSING CONSIDERATIONS

Assessment
• Assess patient's condition before therapy and regularly thereafter.
• During therapy, monitor ECG, renal function, fluid intake and output, and serum potassium, serum creatinine, and BUN levels.
• Be alert for adverse reactions and drug interactions.
• Evaluate patient's and family's knowledge of drug therapy.

Nursing diagnoses
• Altered health maintenance related to presence of hypokalemia
• Risk for injury related to potassium-induced hyperkalemia
• Knowledge deficit related to drug therapy

Planning and implementation
• Dissolve potassium bicarbonate tablets completely in 6 to 8 oz of cold water to minimize GI irritation.
• Ask patient's flavor preference. Available in lime and orange flavors.
• Have patient take with meals and sip slowly over 5 to 10 minutes.
• Don't administer potassium supplements postoperatively until urine flow has been established.
• Never switch potassium products without doctor's order. Potassium bicarbonate cannot be given instead of potassium chloride.
Patient teaching
• Inform patient of need for potassium supplementation.
• Teach patient how to prepare and take drug.
• Instruct patient to report adverse reactions.

Evaluation
• Patient's potassium level returns to normal.
• Patient does develop hyperkalemia as result of drug therapy.
• Patient and family state understanding of drug therapy.

---

*Liquid form contains alcohol   **May contain tartrazine   ◆Canada   ◇ Australia   †OTC

potassium chloride

(puh-TAS-ee-um KLOR-ighd)
Cena-K, K+10, Kaochlor 10%*, Kaochlor S-F 10%*, Kaon-Cl, Kaon-Cl 20%*, Kato Powder, Kay Ciel*, K+Care, K-Dur, K-Lease, K-Lor, Klor-Con, Klor-Con 10, Klorvess, Klotrix, K-Lyte/Cl, K-Norm, K-Tab, Micro-K Extencaps, Rum-K, Slow-K, Ten-K

Pharmacologic class: potassium supplement
Therapeutic class: therapeutic agent for electrolyte balance
Pregnancy risk category: C.

How supplied

Tablets: 1.22 mEq (99 mg), 8 mEq (600 mg), 10 mEq (750 mg), 20 mEq (1,500 mg), 25 mEq (1,875 mg)
Tablets (controlled-release): 6.7 mEq (500 mg), 8 mEq (600 mg), 10 mEq (750 mg), 20 mEq (1,500 mg)
Tablets (enteric-coated): 4 mEq (300 mg), 13.4 mEq (1,000 mg)
Capsules (controlled-release): 8 mEq (600 mg), 10 mEq (750 mg)
Oral liquid: 5% (10 mEq/15 ml), 7.5% (15 mEq/15 ml), 10% (20 mEq/15 ml), 15% (30 mEq/15 ml), 20% (40 mEq/ 15 ml)
Powder for oral use: 15 mEq/packet, 20 mEq/packet, 25 mEq/packet, 25 mEq/ dose
Injection: 20 mEq, 40 mEq ampules; additive syringes containing 30 mEq or 40 mEq; 10 mEq, 20 mEq, 30 mEq, 40 mEq, 45 mEq, 60 mEq, 100 mEq, 200 mEq, 400 mEq, or 1,000 mEq vials

Pharmacokinetics

Absorption: well absorbed from GI tract when administered orally.
Distribution: distributed throughout body.
Metabolism: none significant.
Excretion: excreted largely by kidneys; small amounts may be excreted via skin and intestinal tract, but intestinal potassium is usually reabsorbed.

Route	Onset	Peak	Duration
P.O.	Unknown	≤ 4 hr	Unknown
I.V.	Immediate	Immediate	Unknown

Pharmacodynamics

Chemical effect: aids in transmitting nerve impulses; contracting cardiac and skeletal muscle; and maintaining intracellular tonicity, cellular metabolism, acid-base balance, and normal renal function.
Therapeutic effect: replaces and maintains potassium level.

Indications and dosage

▶ **Hypokalemia.** *Adults:* 40 to 100 mEq P.O. daily in three or four divided doses for treatment; 20 mEq for prevention. Further dosage based on serum potassium level. *Children:* 3 mEq/kg daily. Total dosage not to exceed 150 mEq daily or 40 mEq/m². Use I.V. route only when oral replacement is not feasible or when hypokalemia is life-threatening. If serum potassium is less than 2 mEq/ml, maximum infusion rate is 40 mEq/hour; maximum infusion concentration is 80 mEq/L; and maximum 24-hour dose is 400 mEq. If serum potassium level is greater than 2 mEq/ml, maximum infusion rate is 10 mEq/hour; maximum infusion concentration is 40 mEq/L; and maximum 24-hour dose is 200 mEq. For routine supplementation, usual dose 20 mEq hourly in concentration of 40 mEq/L or less.

Adverse reactions

CNS: paresthesia of extremities, listlessness, mental confusion, weakness or heaviness of limbs, flaccid paralysis.
CV: *arrhythmias, heart block, possible cardiac arrest,* ECG changes (prolonged PR interval; widened QRS complex; ST-segment depression; tall, tented T waves).
GI: *nausea, vomiting, abdominal pain,* diarrhea, GI ulcerations (possible stenosis, hemorrhage, obstruction, perforation).

Reactions may be *common*, uncommon, *life-threatening*, or COMMON AND LIFE-THREATENING.

GU: oliguria.
Skin: cold skin, gray pallor.
Other: postinfusion phlebitis, *respiratory paralysis.*

Interactions

Drug-drug. *ACE inhibitors, potassium-sparing diuretics:* risk of hyperkalemia. Use with extreme caution.

Contraindications and precautions

• Contraindicated in patients with in those with untreated Addison's disease, acute dehydration, heat cramps, hyperkalemia, hyperkalemic form of familial periodic paralysis, other conditions associated with extensive tissue breakdown, and severe renal impairment with oliguria, anuria, or azotemia.
• Use cautiously in patients with cardiac disease or renal impairment and in pregnant or breast-feeding women.

NURSING CONSIDERATIONS

Assessment
• Assess patient's condition before therapy and regularly thereafter.
• During therapy, monitor ECG, renal function, fluid intake and output, and serum potassium, serum creatinine, and BUN levels.
• Be alert for adverse reactions and drug interactions.
• Evaluate patient's and family's knowledge of drug therapy.

Nursing diagnoses
• Altered health maintenance related to presence of hypokalemia
• Risk for injury related to drug-induced hyperkalemia
• Knowledge deficit related to drug therapy

Planning and implementation
P.O. use: Give oral potassium supplements with extreme caution because its many forms deliver varying amounts of potassium. Never switch products without doctor's order.
– Make sure powders are completely dissolved before administering.
– Don't crush sustained-release potassium products.
– Give potassium with or after meals with full glass of water or fruit juice to lessen GI distress.
• Use sugar-free liquid (Kaochlor S-F 10%) if tablet or capsule passage is likely to be delayed, such as in GI obstruction. Have patient sip slowly to minimize GI irritation.
• Know that enteric-coated tablets are not recommended because of increased potential for GI bleeding and small-bowel ulcerations.
• Tablets in wax matrix sometimes lodge in esophagus and cause ulceration in cardiac patients who have esophageal compression from enlarged left atrium. Use liquid form in such patients and in those with esophageal stasis or obstruction.
• Know that drug is often used orally with potassium-wasting diuretics to maintain potassium levels.
• Never give potassium postoperatively until urine flow is established.
I.V. use: Give drug by infusion only; never I.V. push or I.M. Give slowly as dilute solution; potentially fatal hyperkalemia may result from too-rapid infusion.
Patient teaching
• Inform patient of need for potassium supplementation.
• Teach patient how to prepare and take supplement.
• Instruct patient to report adverse reactions.

Evaluation
• Patient's potassium level returns to normal.
• Patient does not develop hyperkalemia.
• Patient and family state understanding of drug therapy.

potassium gluconate
(puh-TAS-ee-um GLOO-kuh-nayt)
Glu-K, Kaon Liquid*, Kaon Tablets,
Kaylixir*, K-G Elixir*, Potassium-
Rougier♦

Pharmacologic class: potassium
supplement
Therapeutic class: therapeutic agent for
electrolyte balance
Pregnancy risk category: C

How supplied

Tablets: 500 mg (2 mEq K⁺), 1,170 mg
(5 mEq K⁺)
Elixir♦: 4.68 g (20 mEq K⁺)/15 ml*

Pharmacokinetics

Absorption: well absorbed from GI tract.
Distribution: distributed throughout body.
Metabolism: none significant.
Excretion: excreted largely by kidneys;
small amounts may be excreted via skin
and intestinal tract, but intestinal potassium is usually reabsorbed.

Route	Onset	Peak	Duration
P.O.	Unknown	≤ 4 hr	Unknown

Pharmacodynamics

Chemical effect: aids in transmitting
nerve impulses; contracting cardiac and
skeletal muscle; and maintaining intracellular tonicity, cellular metabolism, acid-
base balance, and normal renal function.
Therapeutic effect: replaces and maintains potassium level.

Indications and dosage

▶ **Hypokalemia.** *Adults:* 40 to 100 mEq
P.O. daily in three or four divided doses
for treatment; 20 mEq P.O. daily for prevention. Further dosage based on serum
potassium determinations.

Adverse reactions

CNS: paresthesia of extremities, listlessness, mental confusion, weakness or
heaviness of legs, flaccid paralysis.

CV: *arrhythmias,* ECG changes (prolonged PR interval; widened QRS complex; ST-segment depression; tall, tented
T waves).
GI: *nausea, vomiting, abdominal pain,*
diarrhea; GI ulcerations that may be accompanied by stenosis, hemorrhage, obstruction, perforation (with oral products,
especially enteric-coated tablets).

Interactions

Drug-drug. *ACE inhibitors, potassium-
sparing diuretics:* risk of hyperkalemia.
Use with extreme caution.

Contraindications and precautions

• Contraindicated in patients with untreated Addison's disease, acute dehydration,
heat cramps, hyperkalemia, hyperkalemic
form of familial periodic paralysis, other
conditions associated with extensive tissue
breakdown, and severe renal impairment
with oliguria, anuria, or azotemia.
• Use cautiously in patients with cardiac
disease or renal impairment and in pregnant or breast-feeding women.
• Safety of drug has not been established
in children.

NURSING CONSIDERATIONS

⬛ Assessment
• Assess patient's condition before therapy and regularly thereafter.
• During therapy, monitor ECG, renal
function, fluid intake and output, and
serum potassium, serum creatinine, and
BUN levels.
• Be alert for adverse reactions and drug
interactions.
• Evaluate patient's and family's knowledge of drug therapy.

⬛ Nursing diagnoses
• Altered health maintenance related to
presence of hypokalemia
• Risk for injury related to potassium-
induced hyperkalemia
• Knowledge deficit related to drug
therapy

Reactions may be *common,* uncommon, *life-threatening,* or COMMON AND LIFE-THREATENING.

⧁ Planning and implementation
• Give oral potassium supplements with extreme caution because their many forms deliver varying amounts of potassium. Never switch products without doctor's order.
• Give drug with or after meals with glass of water or fruit juice.
• Have patient sip liquid potassium slowly to minimize GI irritation.
• Know that enteric-coated tablets are not recommended because of increased potential for GI bleeding and small-bowel ulcerations.
• Don't administer potassium supplements postoperatively until urine flow has been established.
Patient teaching
• Inform patient of need for potassium supplementation.
• Teach patient how to take drug.
• Instruct patient to report adverse reactions.

☑ Evaluation
• Patient's potassium level returns to normal.
• Patient does develop hyperkalemia as result of drug therapy.
• Patient and family state understanding of drug therapy.

---

potassium iodide
(puh-TAS-ee-um IGH-uh-dighd)
Iosat, Pima, Thyro-Block

potassium iodide, saturated solution SSKI)

strong iodine solution (Lugol's solution)

Pharmacologic class: electrolyte
Therapeutic class: antihyperthyroid agent, expectorant
Pregnancy risk category: D

How supplied
potassium iodide
Tablets: 130 mg
Oral solution: 500 mg/15 ml
Syrup: 325 mg/5 ml
potassium iodide, saturated solution
Oral solution: 1 g/ml
strong iodine solution
Oral solution: iodine 50 mg/ml and potassium iodide 100 mg/ml

Pharmacokinetics
Unknown.

Route	Onset	Peak	Duration
P.O.	≤ 24 hr	10-15 days	Unknown

Pharmacodynamics
Chemical effect: inhibits thyroid hormone formation by blocking iodotyrosine and iodothyronine synthesis, limits iodide transport into thyroid gland, and blocks thyroid hormone release.
Therapeutic effect: lowers thyroid hormone levels.

Indications and dosage
▶ **Preparation for thyroidectomy.**
Strong iodine solution, USP. *Adults and children:* 0.1 to 0.3 ml P.O. t.i.d. **SSKI.** *Adults and children:* 1 to 5 drops in water P.O. t.i.d., after meals for 10 to 14 days before surgery.
▶ **Thyrotoxic crisis.** *Adults and children:* 500 mg P.O. q 4 hours (about 10 drops of SSKI).
▶ **Radiation protectant for thyroid gland.** *Adults:* 130 mg P.O. immediately before and for 3 to 14 days after radiation exposure.

Adverse reactions
CNS: frontal headache.
EENT: acute rhinitis, inflammation of salivary glands, tooth discoloration, periorbital edema, conjunctivitis, hyperemia.
GI: burning, irritation, *nausea,* vomiting, diarrhea (sometimes bloody), *metallic taste.*

Skin: acneiform rash, mucous membrane ulceration.
Other: fever; *hypersensitivity reactions, potassium toxicity* (confusion, irregular heart beat, numbness, tingling, pain or weakness of hands and feet, tiredness).

Interactions

Drug-drug. *ACE inhibitors, potassium-sparing diuretics:* risk of hyperkalemia. Avoid concomitant use.
Antithyroid medications: potassium iodide may potentiate hypothyroid or goitrogenic effects. Monitor closely.
Lithium carbonate: hypothyroidism may occur. Use with caution.

Contraindications and precautions

• Contraindicated in patients with tuberculosis, acute bronchitis, iodide hypersensitivity, or hyperkalemia. Some forms contain sulfites, which may precipitate allergic reactions in hypersensitive individuals.
• Drug use is not recommended for pregnant or breast-feeding women.
• Use cautiously in patients with hypocomplementemic vasculitis, presence of goiter, or autoimmune thyroid disease.

NURSING CONSIDERATIONS

⚄ Assessment
• Assess patient's condition before therapy and regularly thereafter.
• Be alert for adverse reactions and drug interactions.
• Earliest signs of delayed hypersensitivity reactions caused by iodides are irritation and swelling of eyelids.
• Evaluate patient's and family's knowledge of drug therapy.

⊞ Nursing diagnoses
• Altered health maintenance related to underlying thyroid condition
• Altered protection related to hypersensitivity reactions
• Knowledge deficit related to drug therapy

⧁ Planning and implementation
• Potassium iodide is usually given with other antithyroid drugs.
• Know that doctor may avoid prescribing enteric-coated tablets, which have been associated with small bowel lesions and can lead to serious complications, including perforation, hemorrhage, or obstruction.
• Dilute oral doses in water, milk, or fruit juice, and give after meals to prevent gastric irritation, to hydrate patient, and to mask very salty taste.
• Give iodides through straw to avoid tooth discoloration.
• Store drug in light-resistant container.
Patient teaching
• Teach patient how to administer drug.
• Warn patient that sudden withdrawal may precipitate thyroid crisis.
• Tell patient to ask doctor about using iodized salt and eating shellfish.
• Tell him to report adverse reactions.

☑ Evaluation
• Patient's thyroid hormone level is lower with potassium iodide therapy.
• Patient does not experience hypersensitivity reactions.
• Patient and family state understanding of drug therapy.

pralidoxime chloride (pyridine-2-aldoxime methochloride; 2-PAM chloride)
(pral-ih-DOKS-eem KLOR-ighd)
Protopam Chloride

Pharmacologic class: quaternary ammonium oxime
Therapeutic class: antidote
Pregnancy risk category: C

How supplied

Injection: 1 g/20 ml in 20-ml vial without diluent or syringe; 1 g/20 ml in 20-ml vial with diluent, syringe, needle, and alcohol swab (emergency kit); 600 mg/2 ml auto-injector, parenteral

---

Pharmacokinetics

Absorption: absorption unknown after I.M. or S.C. administration.
Distribution: distributed throughout extracellular water; it is not appreciably bound to plasma protein. It does not readily pass into CNS.
Metabolism: unknown but hepatic metabolism is considered likely.
Excretion: excreted rapidly in urine.

Route	Onset	Peak	Duration
I.V.	Unknown	5-15 min	Unknown
I.M.	Unknown	10-20 min	Unknown
S.C.	Unknown	Unknown	Unknown

Pharmacodynamics

Chemical effect: reactivates cholinesterase that has been inactivated by organophosphorus pesticides and related compounds, permitting degradation of accumulated acetylcholine and facilitating normal functioning of neuromuscular junctions.
Therapeutic effect: alleviates signs and symptoms of organophosphate poisoning and cholinergic crisis in myasthenia gravis.

Indications and dosage

▶ **Antidote for organophosphate poisoning.** *Adults:* 1 to 2 g in 100 ml of NaCl solution by I.V. infusion over 15 to 30 minutes. If pulmonary edema is present, give by slow I.V. push over at least 5 minutes. Repeat in 1 hour if muscle weakness persists; may give further doses cautiously. I.M. or S.C. injection may be used if I.V. is not feasible. *Children:* 20 to 40 mg/kg I.V. administered as for adults.
▶ **Anticholinesterase overdose.** *Adults:* 1 to 2 g I.V., followed by 250 mg I.V. q 5 minutes, p.r.n.

Adverse reactions

CNS: dizziness, headache, drowsiness, excitement, manic behavior after recovery of consciousness.
CV: tachycardia.

EENT: blurred vision, diplopia, impaired accommodation, laryngospasm.
GI: nausea.
Musculoskeletal: muscular weakness, muscle rigidity.
Respiratory: hyperventilation.

Interactions

None significant.

Contraindications and precautions

• No known contraindications.
• Use with extreme caution in patients with myasthenia gravis (overdosage may precipitate myasthenic crisis).
• Use cautiously in pregnant women.
• Safety of drug has not been established in breast-feeding women.

NURSING CONSIDERATIONS

⚕ Assessment
• Assess patient's condition before therapy and regularly thereafter. Drug relieves paralysis of respiratory muscles but is less effective in relieving depression of respiratory center.
• Drug is not effective against poisoning due to phosphorus, inorganic phosphates, or organophosphates with no anticholinesterase activity.
• Observe patient for 48 to 72 hours if poison was ingested. Delayed absorption may occur from lower bowel. It is difficult to distinguish between toxic effects produced by atropine or by organophosphate compounds and those resulting from pralidoxime.
• Observe patient with myasthenia gravis treated for overdose of cholinergic drugs closely for signs of rapid weakening. This patient can pass quickly from cholinergic crisis to myasthenic crisis, and requires more cholinergic drugs to treat myasthenia. Keep edrophonium (Tensilon) available in such situations for establishing differential diagnosis.
• Be alert for adverse reactions.
• Evaluate patient's and family's knowledge of drug therapy.

🔲 **Nursing diagnoses**
• Altered health maintenance related to underlying condition
• Risk for injury related to adverse CNS reactions
• Knowledge deficit related to drug therapy

▶ **Planning and implementation**
• Initially, remove secretions, maintain patent airway, and institute artificial ventilation if needed. After dermal exposure to organophosphate, remove patient's clothing and wash his skin and hair with sodium bicarbonate, soap, water, and alcohol as soon as possible. A second washing may be necessary. When washing patient, wear protective gloves and clothes to avoid exposure.
• Draw blood for cholinesterase levels before giving drug.
• Drug should be used in hospitalized patient only; have respiratory and other supportive measures available. If possible, obtain accurate medical history and chronology of poisoning. Drug should be given as soon as possible after poisoning; treatment is most effective if initiated within 24 hours after exposure.
I.V. use: Give I.V. preparation slowly as diluted solution. Dilute with sterile water without preservatives.
• To ameliorate muscarinic effects and block accumulation of acetylcholine associated with organophosphate poisoning, give atropine 2 to 6 mg I.V. along with pralidoxime if cyanosis is not present, as ordered. (If cyanosis is present, atropine should be given I.M.) Give atropine every 5 to 60 minutes in adults, as ordered, until muscarinic signs and symptoms disappear; if they reappear, repeat the dose. Know that atropinization should be maintained for at least 48 hours.
I.M. and S.C. use: Follow normal protocol.
Patient teaching
• Tell patient to report adverse reactions immediately.

• Caution patient treated for organophosphate poisoning to avoid contact with insecticides for several weeks.

🔲 **Evaluation**
• Patient responds well to therapy.
• Patient does not experience injury from adverse CNS reactions.
• Patient and family state understanding of drug therapy.

---

pramipexole dihydrochloride
(pram-ih-PEKS-ohl digh-high-droh-KLOR-ighd)
Mirapex

Pharmacologic class: dopamine agonist
Therapeutic class: antiparkinsonian agent
Pregnancy risk category: C

How supplied
Tablets: 0.125 mg, 0.25 mg, 1 mg, 1.5 mg

Pharmacokinetics
Absorption: rapid. Absolute bioavailability exceeds 90%.
Distribution: extensively distributed throughout the body.
Metabolism: 90% of dose is excreted unchanged in urine.
Excretion: primary route of elimination is urinary excretion. *Half-life:* 8 to 12 hours.

Route	Onset	Peak	Duration
P.O.	Rapid	2 hr	8-12 hr

Pharmacodynamics
Chemical effect: precise mechanism is unknown, but thought to stimulate dopamine receptors in striatum.
Therapeutic effect: relieves symptoms of idiopathic Parkinson's disease.

Reactions may be *common*, uncommon, *life-threatening*, or COMMON AND LIFE-THREATENING.

Indications and dosages

▶ **Treatment of signs and symptoms of idiopathic Parkinson's disease.** *Adults:* initially, 0.375 mg P.O. daily given in three divided doses; do not increase more frequently than q 5 to 7 days. Maintenance dosage range is 1.5 to 4.5 mg/day in three divided doses.

Adverse reactions

CNS: malaise, akathisia, amnesia, *asthenia, confusion,* delusions, *dizziness, dream abnormalities, dyskinesia,* dystonia, *extrapyramidal syndrome,* gait abnormalities, *hallucinations,* hypoesthesia, hypertonia, *insomnia,* myoclonus, paranoid reaction, *somnolence,* sleep disorders, thought abnormalities.
CV: chest pain, peripheral edema, *orthostatic hypotension.*
EENT: accommodation abnormalities, diplopia, dry mouth, rhinitis, vision abnormalities.
GI: anorexia, *constipation,* dysphagia, *nausea.*
GU: decreased libido, impotence, urinary frequency, urinary tract infection, urinary incontinence.
Musculoskeletal: arthritis, bursitis, twitching, myasthenia.
Respiratory: dyspnea, pneumonia.
Skin: skin disorders.
Other: *accidental injury,* fever, general edema, weight loss.

Interactions

Drug-drug. *Butyrophenones, metoclopramide, phenothiazines, thiothixenes:* may diminish effectiveness of pramipexole. Monitor closely.
Cimetidine, diltiazem, quinidine, quinine, ranitidine, triamterene, verapamil: decreased clearance of pramipexole. Adjust dose as needed.
Levodopa: increased adverse effects of levodopa. Adjust levodopa dose as needed.

Contraindications and precautions

• Contraindicated in patients with hypersensitivity to drug or its components.

• Use with caution in patients who have renal impairment and the elderly, because dosing may need to be adjusted.
• Use with caution in breast-feeding women because it is not known if drug is excreted in breast milk.

NURSING CONSIDERATIONS

🗠 Assessment
• Monitor vital signs carefully because drug may cause orthostatic hypotension, especially during dose escalation.
• Assess patient's risk for physical injury due to drug's CNS adverse effects (dyskinesia, dizziness, hallucinations, and somnolence).
• Assess patient's response to drug therapy and adjust dose, as ordered by doctor.
• Evaluate patient's and family's knowledge of drug therapy.

🗠 Nursing diagnoses
• Impaired physical mobility related to underlying Parkinson's disease
• Altered thought processes related to drug-induced CNS adverse reactions
• Knowledge deficit related to drug therapy

🗠 Planning and implementation
• Institute safety precautions.
• Adjust dose in renal impairment as follows: in patients with normal to mild renal impairment (creatinine clearance over 60 ml/minute), initial dose 0.125 mg P.O. t.i.d., up to 1.5 mg t.i.d.; in those with moderate impairment (creatinine clearance between 35 and 59 ml/minute), initial dose 0.125 mg P.O. b.i.d. up to 1.5 mg b.i.d.; and in those with severe impairment (creatinine clearance of 15 to 34 ml/minute), initial dose 0.125 mg P.O. daily, up to 1.5 mg daily.
• Do not withdraw drug abruptly. Titrate dosage gradually, as ordered, according to patient's response and tolerance.
• Provide ice chips, drinks, or hard, sugarless candy to relieve dry mouth, and in-

crease fluid and fiber intake to prevent constipation as appropriate.

Patient teaching

• Instruct patient not to rise rapidly after sitting or lying down because of risk of orthostatic hypotension.

• Caution patient not to drive a car or operate complex machinery until response to drug is known.

• Tell patient to use caution before taking drug with other CNS depressants.

• Tell patient that hallucinations may occur, especially if he is elderly.

• Advise patient to take drug with food if nausea develops.

• Tell female patient to notify doctor if she is breast-feeding or intends to do so.

☑ **Evaluation**

• Patient exhibits improved mobility with reduction of muscular rigidity and tremor.

• Patient remains mentally alert.

• Patient and family state understanding of drug therapy.

---

pravastatin sodium (eptastatin)
(PRAH-vuh-stat-in SOH-dee-um)
Pravachol

Pharmacologic class: HMG-CoA reductase inhibitor
Therapeutic class: antilipemic
Pregnancy risk category: X

How supplied

Tablets: 10 mg, 20 mg, 40 mg

Pharmacokinetics

Absorption: rapidly absorbed. Although food reduces bioavailability, drug effects are same if drug is taken with or 1 hour before meals.
Distribution: about 50% bound to plasma proteins. Drug experiences extensive first-pass extraction, possibly because of active transport system into hepatocytes.

Metabolism: metabolized in liver; at least six metabolites have been identified. Some are active.
Excretion: excreted by liver and kidneys.
Half-life: 1.3 to 2.4 hours.

Route	Onset	Peak	Duration
P.O.	Unknown	1 hr	Unknown

Pharmacodynamics

Chemical effect: inhibits 3-hydroxy-3-methylglutaryl coenzyme A reductase. This enzyme is early (and rate-limiting) step in synthetic pathway of cholesterol.
Therapeutic effect: lowers low-density lipoprotein (LDL) and total cholesterol levels in some patients.

Indications and dosage

▶ **Reduction of LDL and total cholesterol levels in patients with primary hypercholesterolemia (types IIa and IIb).** *Adults:* initially, 10 or 20 mg P.O. daily h.s. Dosage adjusted q 4 weeks based on patient tolerance and response; maximum daily dosage is 40 mg. Most elderly patients respond to daily dosage of 20 mg or less.

Adverse reactions

CNS: headache, fatigue, dizziness.
CV: chest pain.
EENT: rhinitis.
GI: vomiting, diarrhea, heartburn, nausea.
Musculoskeletal: myositis, myopathy, localized muscle pain, myalgia, *rhabdomyolysis*.
Respiratory: cough.
Skin: rash.
Other: flulike symptoms, renal failure secondary to myoglobinuria.

Interactions

Drug-drug. *Cholestyramine, colestipol:* decreased plasma levels of pravastatin. Administer pravastatin 1 hour before or 4 hours after these drugs.
Drugs that decrease levels or activity of endogenous steroids (such as cimetidine,

---

ketoconazole, spironolactone): may increase risk of developing endocrine dysfunction. No intervention appears necessary. Take complete drug history in patients who develop endocrine dysfunction.

Erythromycin, fibric acid derivatives (such as clofibrate, gemfibrozil), high doses of niacin (nicotinic acid; 1 g or more daily), immunosuppressants (such as cyclosporine): may increase risk of rhabdomyolysis. Monitor patient closely if concomitant use cannot be avoided.

Gemfibrozil: decreases protein-binding and urinary clearance of pravastatin. Avoid concomitant use.

Hepatotoxic drugs: increased risk of hepatotoxicity. Avoid concomitant use.

Drug-lifestyle. *Alcohol use:* increased risk of hepatotoxicity. Avoid concomitant use.

Contraindications and precautions

• Contraindicated in patients with hypersensitivity to drug, active liver disease, or unexplained persistent elevations of serum transaminase levels; in pregnant and breast-feeding women; and in women of childbearing age unless there is no risk of pregnancy.

• Use cautiously in patients who consume large quantities of alcohol or have history of liver disease.

• Safety of drug has not been established in children.

NURSING CONSIDERATIONS

Assessment

• Assess patient's condition before therapy and regularly thereafter.

• Liver function tests should be performed at start of therapy and periodically thereafter. A liver biopsy may be performed if elevations persist.

• Be alert for adverse reactions and drug interactions.

• Monitor patient's hydration status if adverse GI reactions occur.

• Evaluate patient's and family's knowledge of drug therapy.

Nursing diagnoses

• Risk for injury related to elevated cholesterol levels

• Risk for fluid volume deficit related to adverse GI reactions

• Knowledge deficit related to drug therapy

Planning and implementation

• Know that drug therapy should be initiated only after diet and other nonpharmacologic therapies have proved ineffective. Patients should be on standard low-cholesterol diet during therapy.

• Be aware that dosage is adjusted about every 4 weeks. If cholesterol level falls below target range, dosage may be reduced.

Patient teaching

• Instruct patient to take recommended dosage in evening, preferably at bedtime.

• Teach patient about proper dietary management of serum lipids (restricting total fat and cholesterol intake), as well as measures to control other cardiac disease risk factors. When appropriate, recommend weight control, exercise, and smoking cessation programs.

• Inform female patient that drug is contraindicated during pregnancy. Advise her to notify doctor immediately if pregnancy occurs.

Evaluation

• Patient's LDL and total cholesterol levels are within normal range.

• Patient maintains adequate hydration.

• Patient and family state understanding of drug therapy.

prazosin hydrochloride
(PRAH-zoh-sin high-droh-KLOR-ighd)
Minipress

Pharmacologic class: alpha-adrenergic blocker

Therapeutic class: antihypertensive
Pregnancy risk category: C

How supplied

Capsules: 1 mg, 2 mg, 5 mg

Pharmacokinetics

Absorption: variable.
Distribution: distributed throughout body and is highly protein-bound (about 97%).
Metabolism: metabolized extensively in liver.
Excretion: over 90% excreted in feces via bile; remainder excreted in urine.
Half-life: 2 to 4 hours.

Route	Onset	Peak	Duration
P.O.	30-90 min	2-4 hr	7-10 hr

Pharmacodynamics

Chemical effect: unknown; its alpha-adrenergic blocking activity probably accounts for its effects.
Therapeutic effect: lowers blood pressure.

Indications and dosage

▶ **Mild to moderate hypertension, alone or in combination with diuretic or other antihypertensive.** *Adults:* initial dose is 1 mg P.O. t.i.d. Dosage increased slowly. Maximum daily dosage is 20 mg. Maintenance dosage is 6 to 15 mg daily in three divided doses. Some patients require larger dosages (up to 40 mg daily). If other antihypertensives or diuretics are added to this drug, prazosin is decreased to 1 to 2 mg t.i.d. and retitrated.

Adverse reactions

CNS: *dizziness,* headache, drowsiness, weakness, *"first-dose syncope,"* depression.
CV: orthostatic hypotension, *palpitations.*
EENT: blurred vision.
GI: vomiting, diarrhea, abdominal cramps, constipation, *nausea,* dry mouth.
GU: priapism, impotence.

Interactions

Drug-drug. *Diuretics, propranolol and other beta blockers:* increased frequency of syncope with loss of consciousness. Advise patient to sit or lie down if dizziness occurs.

Contraindications and precautions

• No known contraindications.
• Drug use in breast-feeding women is not recommended.
• Use cautiously in patients receiving other antihypertensives and in pregnant women.
• Safety of drug has not been established in children.

NURSING CONSIDERATIONS

◩ Assessment

• Assess patient's condition before therapy and regularly thereafter.
• Monitor patient's blood pressure and pulse rate frequently.
• Elderly patients may be more sensitive to drug's hypotensive effects.
• Be alert for adverse reactions and drug interactions.
• Evaluate patient's and family's knowledge of drug therapy.

◫ Nursing diagnoses

• Risk for injury related to presence of hypertension
• Sexual dysfunction related to drug-induced impotence
• Knowledge deficit related to drug therapy

▶ Planning and implementation

• If initial dose is greater than 1 mg, severe syncope with loss of consciousness may occur ("first-dose syncope").
• Do not stop therapy abruptly.
• Compliance *may* be improved with twice-daily dosing. Suggest this dosing change with doctor if you suspect compliance problems.

Reactions may be *common,* uncommon, *life-threatening*, or COMMON AND LIFE-THREATENING.

Patient teaching
- Tell patient not to suddenly stop taking drug, but to call doctor, if unpleasant adverse reactions occur.
- Advise patient to minimize orthostatic hypotension by rising slowly and avoiding sudden position changes. Dry mouth can be relieved with chewing gum, sour hard candy, or ice chips.

☑ Evaluation
- Patient's blood pressure is normal.
- Patient seeks counseling for alternative methods of sexual gratification because of drug-induced impotence.
- Patient and family state understanding of drug therapy.

---

prednisolone
(pred-NIS-uh-lohn)
Delta-Cortef, Deltasolone♦, Panafcortelone♦, Prelone, Solone♦

prednisolone acetate
Articulose-50, Key-Pred 25, Key-Pred 50, Predaject-50, Predalone 50, Predate 50, Predcor-25, Predcor-50, Predicort-50

prednisolone sodium phosphate
Hydeltrasol, Key-Pred-SP, Pediapred, Predate S, Predicort-RP, Predsol Retention Enema♦, Predsol Suppositories♦

prednisolone steaglate
Sintisone♦

prednisolone tebutate
Hydeltra-TBA, Nor-Pred TBA, Predalone TBA, Predate TBA, Predcor TBA

Pharmacologic class: glucocorticoid, mineralocorticoid
Therapeutic class: anti-inflammatory, immunosuppressant
Pregnancy risk category: NR

How supplied

prednisolone
Tablets: 1 mg♦, 5 mg, 25 mg♦
Syrup: 15 mg/5 ml
prednisolone acetate
Injection (suspension): 25 mg/ml, 50 mg/ml, 100 mg/ml
prednisolone acetate and prednisolone sodium phosphate
Injection (suspension): 80 mg acetate and 20 mg sodium phosphate/ml
prednisolone sodium phosphate
Oral solution: 5 mg/5 ml
Injection: 20 mg/ml
Retention enema: 20 mg/100 ml♦
Suppositories: 5 mg♦
prednisolone steaglate
Tablets: 6.65 mg (equal to 3.5 mg prednisolone)♦
prednisolone tebutate
Injection (suspension): 20 mg/ml

Pharmacokinetics

Absorption: absorbed readily after oral administration; variable with other routes.
Distribution: distributed to muscle, liver, skin, intestines, and kidneys. Drug is extensively bound to plasma proteins. Only unbound portion is active.
Metabolism: metabolized in liver.
Excretion: inactive metabolites and small amounts of unmetabolized drug are excreted in urine; insignificant quantities excreted in feces. *Half-life:* 18 to 36 hours.

Route	Onset	Peak	Duration
P.O.	Rapid	1-2 hr	30-36 hr
I.V.	Rapid	≤ 1 hr	Unknown
I.M.	Rapid	≤ 1 hr	≤ 4 wk
P.R.	Unknown	Unknown	Unknown
Intra-lesional, intra-articular	1-2 days	Unknown	3 days-4 wk

Pharmacodynamics

Chemical effect: not clearly defined; decreases inflammation, mainly by stabilizing leukocyte lysosomal membranes;

suppresses immune response; stimulates bone marrow; and influences protein, fat, and carbohydrate metabolism. *Therapeutic effect:* relieves inflammation and induces immunosuppression.

Indications and dosage

▶ **Severe inflammation or immunosuppression.** *Adults:* 2.5 to 15 mg P.O. b.i.d., t.i.d., or q.i.d.; 2 to 30 mg I.M. (acetate, phosphate) or I.V. (phosphate) q 12 hours; or 2 to 30 mg (phosphate) into joints, lesions, or soft tissue; or 4 to 40 mg (tebutate) into joints and lesions; or 0.25 to 1 ml (sodium phosphate-acetate suspension) into joints weekly, p.r.n.
▶ **Proctitis**◊. *Adults:* 1 suppository b.i.d., preferably in morning and h.s.
▶ **Ulcerative colitis**◊. *Adults:* 1 retention enema h.s. nightly for 2 to 4 weeks. The contents of enema should be retained overnight.

Adverse reactions

Most reactions to corticosteroids are dose- or duration-dependent.
CNS: *euphoria, insomnia,* psychotic behavior, pseudotumor cerebri, *seizures*.
CV: *heart failure, thromboembolism,* hypertension, edema.
EENT: cataracts, glaucoma.
GI: *peptic ulceration,* GI irritation, increased appetite, pancreatitis.
Metabolic: hypokalemia, hyperglycemia, and carbohydrate intolerance.
Musculoskeletal: muscle weakness, osteoporosis, growth suppression in children.
Skin: hirsutism, delayed wound healing, acne, various skin eruptions.
Other: susceptibility to infections; *acute adrenal insufficiency may occur with increased stress (infection, surgery, or trauma) or abrupt withdrawal after long-term therapy.*
After abrupt withdrawal: rebound inflammation, fatigue, weakness, arthralgia, fever, dizziness, lethargy, depression, fainting, orthostatic hypotension, dysp-

nea, anorexia, hypoglycemia. *After prolonged use, sudden withdrawal may be fatal.*

Interactions

Drug-drug. *Aspirin, indomethacin, other NSAIDs:* increased risk of GI distress and bleeding. Avoid concomitant use.
Barbiturates, phenytoin, rifampin: decreased corticosteroid effect. Increase corticosteroid dosage, as ordered.
Oral anticoagulants: altered dosage requirements. Monitor PT and INR closely.
Potassium-depleting drugs (such as thiazide diuretics): enhanced potassium-wasting effects of prednisolone. Monitor serum potassium levels.
Skin-test antigens: decreased response. Defer skin testing until therapy is completed.
Toxoids, vaccines: decreased antibody response and increased risk of neurologic complications. Check with doctor regarding when to reschedule vaccine if possible.

Contraindications and precautions

• Contraindicated in patients with fungal infections and hypersensitivity to drug or its ingredients.
• Use of high doses is not recommended in breast-feeding women.
• Use with extreme caution in patient with recent MI and in pregnant women.
• Use cautiously in patients with GI ulcer, renal disease, hypertension, osteoporosis, diabetes mellitus, hypothyroidism, cirrhosis, diverticulitis, nonspecific ulcerative colitis, recent intestinal anastomoses, thromboembolic disorders, seizures, myasthenia gravis, heart failure, tuberculosis, ocular herpes simplex, emotional instability, and psychotic tendencies.

NURSING CONSIDERATIONS

⚕ Assessment
• Assess patient's condition before therapy and regularly thereafter.

• Monitor patients' weight, blood pressure, and serum electrolyte levels.
• Watch for depression or psychotic episodes, especially with high doses.
• Diabetic patient may need increased insulin; monitor blood glucose levels.
• Monitor patient's stress level; dosage adjustment may be needed.
• Be alert for adverse reactions and drug interactions.
• Evaluate patient's and family's knowledge of drug therapy.

⊞ **Nursing diagnoses**
• Altered health maintenance related to underlying condition
• Altered protection related to drug-induced adverse reactions
• Knowledge deficit related to drug therapy

▶ **Planning and implementation**
• Don't confuse drug with prednisone.
• Always titrate to lowest effective dose, as ordered. However, expect to increase dose as ordered during times of physiologic stress (surgery, trauma, or infection).
• Prednisolone salts (acetate, sodium phosphate, and tebutate) are used parenterally less often than other corticosteroids that have more potent anti-inflammatory action.
• Know that drug may be used for alternate-day therapy.
P.O. use: Give oral dose with food when possible to reduce GI irritation.
I.V. use: Use only prednisolone sodium phosphate; never give acetate form I.V. When administering as direct injection, inject undiluted over at least 1 minute. When administering as intermittent or continuous infusion, dilute solution according to manufacturer's instructions and give over prescribed duration. D_5W or 0.9% NaCl are recommended as diluents for I.V. infusions.
I.M. use: Inject drug deeply into gluteal muscle. Rotate injection sites to prevent muscle atrophy.

P.R. use: Follow normal protocol.
Intralesional and intra-articular use: Assist doctor with administration as directed.
• Avoid S.C. injection because atrophy and sterile abscesses may occur.
• Gradually reduce drug dosage after long-term therapy as ordered.
• Unless contraindicated, give low-sodium diet high in potassium and protein. Administer potassium supplements as needed.
• Notify doctor immediately if serious adverse reactions occur and be prepared to give supportive care.
Patient teaching
• Tell patient not to discontinue drug without doctor's consent.
• Tell patient to take drug as ordered. Give patient instructions on what to do if dose is inadvertently missed.
• Advise patient to take oral form with meals to minimize GI reactions.
• Teach signs of early adrenal insufficiency: fatigue, muscular weakness, joint pain, fever, anorexia, nausea, dyspnea, dizziness, and fainting.
• Instruct patient to carry card identifying need for systemic glucocorticoids during stress.
• Warn patient on long-term therapy about cushingoid symptoms.
• Tell patient to report sudden weight gain, swelling, or slow healing.
• Advise patient on long-term therapy to consider exercise or physical therapy and to ask doctor about vitamin D or calcium supplements.

☑ **Evaluation**
• Patient responds well to therapy.
• Patient does not experience serious adverse reactions.
• Patient and family state understanding of drug therapy.

---

prednisone
(PRED-nih-sohn)
Apo-Prednisone♦, Deltasone, Liquid
Pred*, Meticorten, Novo-prednisone♦,
Orasone, Panafcort♦, Panasol-S,
Prednicen-M, Prednisone Intensol*,
Sone♦, Sterapred, Winpred♦

Pharmacologic class: adrenocorticoid
Therapeutic class: anti-inflammatory,
immunosuppressant
Pregnancy risk category: NR

How supplied
Tablets: 1 mg, 2.5 mg, 5 mg, 10 mg,
20 mg, 25 mg, 50 mg
Oral solution: 5 mg/5 ml*, 5 mg/ml
(concentrate)*
Syrup: 5 mg/5 ml*

Pharmacokinetics
Absorption: absorbed readily after oral
administration.
Distribution: distributed to muscle, liver,
skin, intestines, and kidneys. Drug is extensively bound to plasma proteins. Only
unbound portion is active.
Metabolism: metabolized in liver.
Excretion: inactive metabolites and small
amounts of unmetabolized drug are excreted in urine; insignificant quantities excreted in feces. *Half-life:* 18 to 36 hours.

Route	Onset	Peak	Duration
P.O.	Varies	Varies	Varies

Pharmacodynamics
Chemical effect: not clearly defined; decreases inflammation; suppresses immune response; stimulates bone marrow;
and influences protein, fat, and carbohydrate metabolism.
Therapeutic effect: relieves inflammation
and induces immunosuppression.

Indications and dosage
▶ **Severe inflammation or immunosuppression.** *Adults:* 5 to 60 mg/day P.O. in
single or divided doses. Maximum dose

is 250 mg/day. Maintenance dosage giv-
en once daily or every other day. Dosage
must be individualized.
▶ **Acute exacerbations of multiple sclerosis.** *Adults:* 200 mg P.O. daily for 1
week; then 80 mg P.O. every other day
for 1 month.

Adverse reactions
Most reactions to corticosteroids are
dose- or duration-dependent.
CNS: *euphoria, insomnia,* psychotic behavior, pseudotumor cerebri, *seizures.*
CV: *heart failure, thromboembolism,*
hypertension, edema.
EENT: cataracts, glaucoma.
GI: *peptic ulceration,* GI irritation, increased appetite, pancreatitis.
Metabolic: hypokalemia, hyperglycemia,
and carbohydrate intolerance.
Musculoskeletal: muscle weakness, osteoporosis, growth suppression in children.
Skin: hirsutism, delayed wound healing,
acne, various skin eruptions.
Other: susceptibility to infections, *acute
adrenal insufficiency may occur with increased stress or abrupt withdrawal after long-term therapy.*
After abrupt withdrawal: rebound inflammation, fatigue, weakness, arthralgia, fever, dizziness, lethargy, depression,
fainting, orthostatic hypotension, dyspnea, anorexia, hypoglycemia. *After prolonged use, sudden withdrawal may be
fatal.*

Interactions
Drug-drug. *Aspirin, indomethacin, other
NSAIDs:* increased risk of GI distress and
bleeding. Give together cautiously.
Barbiturates, phenytoin, rifampin: decreased corticosteroid effect. Increase
corticosteroid dosage, as ordered.
Oral anticoagulants: altered dosage requirements. Monitor PT and INR closely.
*Potassium-depleting drugs (such as thi-
azide diuretics):* enhanced potassium-
wasting effects of prednisone. Monitor
serum potassium levels.

Reactions may be *common*, uncommon, *life-threatening*, or COMMON AND LIFE-THREATENING.

Skin-test antigens: decreased response. Defer skin testing until therapy is completed.
Toxoids, vaccines: decreased antibody response and increased risk of neurologic complications. Avoid concomitant use.

Contraindications and precautions

• Contraindicated in patients with systemic fungal infections or hypersensitivity to drug.
• Use of high doses is not recommended in breast-feeding women.
• Use with extreme caution in pregnant women.
• Use cautiously in patients with GI ulcer, renal disease, hypertension, osteoporosis, diabetes mellitus, hypothyroidism, cirrhosis, diverticulitis, nonspecific ulcerative colitis, recent intestinal anastomoses, thromboembolic disorders, seizures, myasthenia gravis, heart failure, tuberculosis, ocular herpes simplex, emotional instability, and psychotic tendencies.

NURSING CONSIDERATIONS

Assessment
• Assess patient's condition before therapy and regularly thereafter.
• Monitor patient's weight, blood pressure, and serum electrolyte levels.
• Watch for depression or psychotic episodes, especially with high doses.
• Diabetic patient may need increased insulin; monitor blood glucose levels.
• Monitor patient's stress level; dosage adjustment may be needed.
• Be alert for adverse reactions and drug interactions.
• Evaluate patient's and family's knowledge of drug therapy.

Nursing diagnoses
• Altered health maintenance related to underlying condition
• Altered protection related to drug-induced adverse reactions
• Knowledge deficit related to drug therapy

Planning and implementation
• Don't confuse drug with prednisolone.
• Always titrate to lowest effective dose, as ordered. However, expect to increase dose as ordered during times of physiologic stress (surgery, trauma, or infection).
• Know that drug may be used for alternate-day therapy.
• For better results and less toxicity, give once-daily dose in morning.
• Give oral dose with food when possible to reduce GI irritation.
• Gradually reduce drug dosage after long-term therapy as ordered.
• Unless contraindicated, give low-sodium diet high in potassium and protein. Administer potassium supplements as needed.
• Notify doctor immediately if serious adverse reactions occur and be prepared to give supportive care.
Patient teaching
• Tell patient not to discontinue drug without doctor's consent.
• Tell patient to take drug as ordered. Give patient instructions on what to do if dose is inadvertently missed.
• Advise patient to take oral form with meals to minimize GI reactions.
• Teach signs of early adrenal insufficiency: fatigue, muscular weakness, joint pain, fever, anorexia, nausea, dyspnea, dizziness, and fainting.
• Instruct patient to carry card identifying need for systemic glucocorticoids during stress.
• Warn patient on long-term therapy about cushingoid symptoms.
• Tell patient to report sudden weight gain, swelling, or slow healing.
• Advise patient receiving long-term therapy to consider exercise or physical therapy, to ask doctor about vitamin D or calcium supplements, and to have periodic eye examinations.

Evaluation
• Patient responds well to therapy.

• Patient does not experience serious adverse reactions.
• Patient and family state understanding of drug therapy.

primaquine phosphate
(PRIH-muh-kwin FOS-fayt)

Pharmacologic class: 8-aminoquinoline
Therapeutic class: antimalarial
Pregnancy risk category: NR

How supplied
Tablets: 7.5 mg (base)♦, 15 mg (base)

Pharmacokinetics
Absorption: well absorbed from GI tract.
Distribution: distributed widely into liver, lungs, heart, brain, skeletal muscle, and other tissues.
Metabolism: metabolized in liver.
Excretion: small amount excreted unchanged in urine. *Half-life:* 4 to 10 hours.

Route	Onset	Peak	Duration
P.O.	Unknown	2-3 hr	Unknown

Pharmacodynamics
Chemical effect: unknown; it may be effective because it can bind to and alter properties of DNA.
Therapeutic effect: prevents or treats relapsing *Plasmodium vivax* malaria.

Indications and dosage
▶ Radical cure of relapsing *P. vivax* malaria, eliminating symptoms and infection completely; prevention of relapse.
Adults: 15 mg (base) P.O. daily for 14 days. (26.3-mg tablet = 15 mg of base.)

Adverse reactions
GI: nausea, vomiting, epigastric distress, abdominal cramps.
Hematologic: *leukopenia, hemolytic anemia in G6PD deficiency,* methemoglobinemia in NADH methemoglobin reductase deficiency.

Interactions
Drug-drug. *Magnesium and aluminum salts:* decreased GI absorption. Separate administration times.
Quinacrine: enhanced toxicity of primaquine. Don't use together.

Contraindications and precautions
• Contraindicated in patients with systemic diseases in which granulocytopenia may develop (such as lupus erythematosus or rheumatoid arthritis) and in those taking bone marrow suppressants and potentially hemolytic drugs.
• Use cautiously in patients with previous idiosyncratic reaction (manifested by hemolytic anemia, methemoglobinemia, or leukopenia); in those with family or personal history of favism; and in those with erythrocytic G6PD deficiency or NADH methemoglobin reductase deficiency. Also use cautiously in pregnant women.
• Safety of drug has not been established in children and in breast-feeding women.

NURSING CONSIDERATIONS

▣ Assessment
• Assess patient's condition before therapy and regularly thereafter.
• Obtain frequent blood studies and urine examinations as ordered in light-skinned patient taking more than 30 mg (base) daily, dark-skinned patient taking more than 15 mg (base) daily, and patient with severe anemia or suspected sensitivity.
• Monitor patient for sudden fall in hemoglobin concentration, erythrocyte or leukocyte count, or marked darkening of urine, which suggests impending hemolytic reactions.
• Be alert for adverse reactions and drug interactions.
• Evaluate patient's and family's knowledge of drug therapy.

▣ Nursing diagnoses
• Infection related to malaria
• Altered protection related to adverse hematologic reactions

---

• Knowledge deficit related to drug therapy

❯ Planning and implementation
• Administer drug with meals.
• A fast-acting antimalarial (such as chloroquine) is usually given with primaquine to reduce possibility of drug-resistant strains.
• Stop drug immediately and notify doctor of abnormal CBC results or pronounced darkening of urine.
Patient teaching
• Instruct patient to take drug with meals.
• Tell patient to notify doctor if adverse reactions occur, especially a marked darkening of urine.
• Tell patient to avoid hazardous activities if visual disturbances occur.

✔ Evaluation
• Patient is free from malaria.
• Patient does not develop serious adverse hematologic reactions.
• Patient and family state understanding of drug therapy.

---

primidone
(PRIH-mih-dohn)
Apo-Primidone♦, Mysoline,
PMS Primidone♦, Sertan♦

Pharmacologic class: barbiturate analogue
Therapeutic class: anticonvulsant
Pregnancy risk category: NR

How supplied
Tablets: 50 mg, 250 mg
Oral suspension: 250 mg/5 ml

Pharmacokinetics
Absorption: absorbed readily from GI tract.
Distribution: distributed widely throughout body.
Metabolism: metabolized slowly by liver to phenylethylmalonamide (PEMA) and

phenobarbital; PEMA is the major metabolite.
Excretion: excreted in urine.

Route	Onset	Peak	Duration
P.O.	Unknown	3-4 hr	Unknown

Pharmacodynamics
Chemical effect: unknown; some activity may be caused by PEMA and phenobarbital.
Therapeutic effect: prevents seizure activity.

Indications and dosage
▶ **Generalized tonic-clonic, focal, and complex-partial (psychomotor) seizures.** *Adults and children age 8 and over:* initially, 100 to 125 mg P.O. h.s. on days 1 to 3; then 100 to 125 mg P.O. b.i.d. on days 4 to 6; then 100 to 125 mg P.O. t.i.d. on days 7 to 9; followed by maintenance dosage of 250 mg P.O. t.i.d. Maintenance dosage increased to 250 mg q.i.d. if needed. *Children under age 8:* initially, 50 mg P.O. h.s. for 3 days, then 50 mg P.O. b.i.d. for 4-6 days, then 100 mg P.O. b.i.d. for 7-9 days followed by maintenance dosage of 125 to 250 mg P.O. t.i.d.
▶ **Benign familial tremor (essential tremor).** *Adults:* 750 mg P.O. daily.

Adverse reactions
CNS: *drowsiness, ataxia,* emotional disturbances, vertigo, hyperirritability, fatigue.
EENT: *diplopia,* nystagmus, edema of eyelids.
GI: anorexia, nausea, vomiting, thirst.
GU: impotence, polyuria.
Hematologic: leukopenia, eosinophilia, *thrombocytopenia.*
Skin: morbilliform rash, alopecia.
Other: edema.

Interactions
Drug-drug. *Carbamazepine:* increased primidone levels. Observe for toxicity.

Phenytoin: stimulated conversion of primidone to phenobarbital. Observe for increased phenobarbital effect.

Contraindications and precautions

• Contraindicated in patients with phenobarbital hypersensitivity or porphyria and in pregnant or breast-feeding women.

NURSING CONSIDERATIONS

Assessment
• Assess patient's condition before therapy and regularly thereafter.
• Monitor blood levels as ordered. Therapeutic level of primidone is 5 to 12 mcg/ml. Therapeutic level of phenobarbital is 15 to 40 mcg/ml.
• Monitor CBC and routine blood chemistry every 6 months, as ordered.
• Monitor patient's hydration status throughout drug therapy.
• Evaluate patient's and family's knowledge of drug therapy.

Nursing diagnoses
• Risk for trauma related to seizures
• Risk for fluid volume deficit related to adverse reactions
• Knowledge deficit related to drug therapy

Planning and implementation
• Shake liquid suspension well.
• Don't withdraw drug suddenly because seizures may worsen.
• Call doctor immediately if adverse reactions develop.
Patient teaching
• Advise patient to avoid hazardous activities until drug's CNS effects are known.
• Warn patient and parents not to stop drug therapy suddenly.
• Tell patient that full therapeutic response may take 2 weeks or more.

Evaluation
• Patient is free from seizure activity.
• Patient maintains adequate hydration throughout drug therapy.

• Patient and family state understanding of drug therapy.

---

probenecid
(proh-BEN-uh-sid)
Benemid, Benuryl♦, Probalan

Pharmacologic class: sulfonamide-derivative
Therapeutic class: uricosuric agent
Pregnancy risk category: NR

How supplied
Tablets: 500 mg

Pharmacokinetics
Absorption: completely absorbed.
Distribution: distributed throughout body; about 75% protein-bound.
Metabolism: metabolized in liver to active metabolites, with some uricosuric effect.
Excretion: drug and metabolites excreted in urine; probenecid (but not metabolites) is actively reabsorbed. *Half-life:* 3 to 8 hours after 500-mg dose, 6 to 12 hours after larger doses.

Route	Onset	Peak	Duration
P.O.	Unknown	2-4 hr	About 8 hr

Pharmacodynamics
Chemical effect: blocks renal tubular reabsorption of uric acid, increasing excretion, and inhibits active renal tubular secretion of many weak organic acids, such as penicillins and cephalosporins.
Therapeutic effect: lowers uric acid and prolongs penicillin action.

Indications and dosage
▶ **Adjunct to penicillin therapy.** *Adults and children over age 14 or weighing over 50 kg (110 lb):* 500 mg P.O. q.i.d. *Children ages 2 to 14 or weighing 50 kg or less:* initially, 25 mg/kg P.O., then 40 mg/kg in divided doses q.i.d.
▶ **Gonorrhea.** *Adults:* 3.5 g ampicillin P.O. with 1 g probenecid P.O. given to-

---

gether; or 1 g probenecid P.O. 30 minutes before dose of 4.8 million units of aqueous penicillin G procaine I.M., injected at two different sites.
► **Hyperuricemia of gout, gouty arthritis.** *Adults:* 250 mg P.O. b.i.d. for first week, then 500 mg b.i.d., to maximum of 2 to 3 g daily. Maintenance dosage should be reviewed q 6 months and reduced by increments of 500 mg if indicated.

Adverse reactions

CNS: *headache,* dizziness.
CV: hypotension.
GI: anorexia, nausea, vomiting, sore gums, *gastric distress.*
GU: urinary frequency, renal colic.
Hematologic: *hemolytic anemia, aplastic anemia.*
Skin: dermatitis, pruritus.
Other: flushing, fever, alopecia, *hypersensitivity reaction, hepatic necrosis, anaphylaxis.*

Interactions

Drug-drug. *Indomethacin:* decreased indomethacin excretion. Lower indomethacin dosages may be required.
Methotrexate: decreased methotrexate excretion. Lower methotrexate dosage may be required. Serum levels should be determined.
Oral antidiabetic agents: enhanced hypoglycemic effect. Monitor blood glucose levels closely. Dosage adjustment may be required.
Salicylates: inhibited uricosuric effect of probenecid, causing urate retention. Don't use together.
Drug-lifestyle. *Alcohol use:* increased urate levels. Avoid concomitant use.

Contraindications and precautions

• Contraindicated in patients with uric acid kidney stones, blood dyscrasias, or hypersensitivity to drug; in acute gout attack; and in children under age 2.
• Use cautiously in patients with peptic ulcer or renal impairment and in pregnant or breast-feeding women.

NURSING CONSIDERATIONS

☝ Assessment

• Assess patient's condition before therapy and regularly thereafter.
• Monitor periodic BUN and renal function tests in long-term therapy, as ordered.
• Know that drug is ineffective in patients with chronic renal insufficiency (glomerular filtration rate less than 30 ml/minute).
• Be alert for adverse reactions and drug interactions.
• Monitor patient's hydration status if adverse GI reactions occur.
• Evaluate patient's and family's knowledge of drug therapy.

⊞ Nursing diagnoses

• Altered health maintenance related to underlying condition
• Risk for fluid volume deficit related to adverse GI reactions
• Knowledge deficit related to drug therapy

≫ Planning and implementation

• Give with milk, food, or antacids to minimize GI distress. Continued disturbances might indicate need to lower dosage.
• Force fluids to maintain minimum daily output of 2 to 3 L. Alkalinize urine with sodium bicarbonate or potassium citrate, as ordered. These measures will prevent hematuria, renal colic, urate stone development, and costovertebral pain.
• Keep in mind that therapy is not initiated until acute attack subsides. Drug contains no analgesic or anti-inflammatory agent and is not useful during acute gout attacks.
• Drug may increase frequency, severity, and duration of acute gout attacks during first 6 to 12 months of therapy. Prophylactic colchicine or another anti-inflammatory agent is given during first 3 to 6 months.
• Be aware that drug may produce false-positive glucose tests with Benedict's so-

lution or Clinitest, but not with glucose oxidase method (Diastix).

• Know that drug decreases urinary excretion of 17-ketosteroids, Bromsulphalein (BSP), aminohippuric acid, and iodine-related organic acids, interfering with laboratory procedures.

Patient teaching

• Instruct patient to take drug with food or milk to minimize GI distress.

• Advise patient with gout to avoid all medications that contain aspirin, which may precipitate gout. Acetaminophen may be used for pain.

• Tell patient with gout to avoid alcohol during drug therapy; it increases urate level.

• Tell patient with gout to limit intake of foods high in purine: anchovies, liver, sardines, kidneys, sweetbreads, peas, and lentils.

• Instruct patient and family that drug must be taken regularly as ordered or gout attacks may result. Tell him to visit doctor regularly so uric acid can be monitored and dosage adjusted, if necessary. Lifelong therapy may be required in patients with hyperuricemia.

☑ Evaluation

• Patient responds positively to therapy.

• Patient maintains adequate hydration.

• Patient and family state understanding of drug therapy.

---

procainamide hydrochloride
(proh-KAYN-uh-mighd high-droh-KLOR-ighd)
Procainamide Durules♦, Procan SR, Promine, Pronestyl**, Pronestyl-SR

Pharmacologic class: procaine derivative
Therapeutic class: ventricular antiarrhythmic, supraventricular antiarrhythmic.
Pregnancy risk category: C

How supplied

Tablets: 250 mg, 375 mg, 500 mg

Tablets (sustained-release): 250 mg, 500 mg, 750 mg
Capsules: 250 mg, 375 mg, 500 mg
Injection: 100 mg/ml, 500 mg/ml

Pharmacokinetics

Absorption: rate and extent of drug's absorption from intestines vary; usually 75% to 95% of orally administered dose is absorbed. Unknown after I.M. administration.

Distribution: distributed widely in most body tissues, including cerebrospinal fluid, liver, spleen, kidneys, lungs, muscles, brain, and heart. About 15% binds to plasma proteins.

Metabolism: metabolized in liver.

Excretion: excreted in urine. *Half-life:* about 2½ to 4¾ hours.

Route	Onset	Peak	Duration
P.O.	2 hr	1-1.5 hr	Unknown
I.V.	Immediate	Immediate	Unknown
I.M.	10-30 min	15-60 min	Unknown

Pharmacodynamics

Chemical effect: class Ia antiarrhythmic that decreases excitability, conduction velocity, automaticity, and membrane responsiveness with prolonged refractory period. Larger doses may induce AV block.

Therapeutic effect: restores normal sinus rhythm.

Indications and dosage

▶ **Life-threatening ventricular arrhythmias.** *Adults:* 50 to 100 mg by slow I.V. push q 5 minutes, no faster than 25 to 50 mg/minute until arrhythmias disappear, adverse reactions develop, or 500 mg has been given. Usual effective dose is 500 to 600 mg. When arrhythmias disappear, give continuous infusion of 2 to 6 mg/minute. If arrhythmias recur, repeat bolus as above and increase infusion rate. Alternatively, 50 mg/kg I.M. given in divided doses q 3 to 6 hours until oral therapy begins. *For oral therapy:* 50 mg/kg daily q 3 hours; average is 250 to 500 mg q 3 hours. *In patients with renal or hepatic dysfunction:* decreased dosages or longer dosing intervals may be needed.

Adverse reactions

CNS: hallucinations, confusion, depression, dizziness.
CV: hypotension, *ventricular asystole, bradycardia,* AV block, *ventricular fibrillation* (after parenteral use), *heart failure, cardiac death.*
GI: nausea, vomiting, anorexia, diarrhea, bitter taste (with high doses).
Hematologic: *thrombocytopenia, neutropenia* (especially with sustained-release forms), *agranulocytosis, hemolytic anemia,* increased antinuclear antibody (ANA) titer.
Skin: maculopapular rash.
Other: *fever, lupuslike syndrome* (especially after prolonged administration), *myalgia.*

Interactions

Drug-drug. *Amiodarone:* increased procainamide levels and toxicity; additive effects on QT interval and QRS complex. Avoid concomitant use.
Anticholinergics: additive anticholinergic effects. Monitor patient closely.
Anticholinesterase agents: may decrease effect of anticholinesterase. Dosage of anticholinesterase may need to be increased.
Cimetidine: may increase procainamide blood levels. Monitor closely.
Neuromuscular blockers: increased skeletal muscle relaxant effects. Monitor patient.

Contraindications and precautions

● Contraindicated in patients with hypersensitivity to procaine and related drugs; in those with complete, second-, or third-degree heart block in absence of artificial pacemaker; and in patients with myasthenia gravis or systemic lupus erythematosus. Also contraindicated in patients with atypical ventricular tachycardia (torsades de pointes) because procainamide may aggravate this condition.

● Drug is not recommended for use in breast-feeding women.
● Use with extreme caution when treating ventricular tachycardia during coronary occlusion.
● Use cautiously in pregnant women and in patients with heart failure or other conduction disturbances, such as bundle-branch heart block, sinus bradycardia, or cardiac glycoside intoxication; hepatic or renal insufficiency; preexisting blood dyscrasias; or bone marrow suppression.
● Safety of drug has not been established in children.

NURSING CONSIDERATIONS

Assessment

● Assess patient's condition before therapy and regularly thereafter.
● Monitor plasma levels of procainamide and its active metabolite NAPA. To suppress ventricular arrhythmias, therapeutic serum concentrations of procainamide are 4 to 8 mcg/ml; therapeutic levels of NAPA are 10 to 30 mcg/ml.
● Monitor QT interval closely in patient with renal failure.
● Hypokalemia predisposes patient to arrhythmias; monitor serum electrolytes, especially potassium level.
● Monitor blood pressure and ECG continuously during I.V. administration. Watch for prolonged QT intervals and QRS complexes, heart block, or increased arrhythmias.
● Monitor CBC frequently during first 3 months, particularly in patient taking sustained-release form.
● Be alert for adverse reactions and drug interactions.
● Evaluate patient's and family's knowledge of drug therapy.

Nursing diagnoses

● Decreased cardiac output related to presence of arrhythmia
● Altered protection related to adverse hematologic reactions

---

• Knowledge deficit related to drug therapy

▷ **Planning and implementation**

P.O. and I.M. use: Follow normal protocol.

I.V. use: Patient receiving infusions must be attended *at all times.* Use infusion control device to administer infusion precisely.

– Note that vials for I.V. injection contain 1 g of drug: 100 mg/ml (10 ml) or 500 mg/ml (2 ml).

– Keep patient in supine position during I.V. administration. If drug is given too rapidly, hypotension can occur. Watch closely for adverse reactions during infusion and notify doctor if they occur.

– If procainamide solution becomes discolored, check with pharmacy and prepare to discard.

• If blood pressure changes significantly or ECG changes occur, withhold drug, obtain rhythm strip, and notify doctor immediately.

• Be aware that positive ANA titer is common in about 60% of patients who don't have symptoms of lupuslike syndrome. This response seems to be related to prolonged use, not dosage. May progress to systemic lupus erythematosus if drug is not discontinued.

Patient teaching

• Instruct patient to report fever, rash, muscle pain, diarrhea, bleeding, bruises, or pleuritic chest pain.

• Stress importance of taking drug exactly as prescribed. This may require use of alarm clock for nighttime doses.

• Reassure patient taking extended-release form that wax-matrix "ghost" from tablet may be passed in stool. Drug is completely absorbed before this occurs.

☑ **Evaluation**

• Patient regains normal cardiac output after drug abolishes abnormal heart rhythm.

• Patient maintains normal CBC.

• Patient and family state understanding of drug therapy.

procarbazine hydrochloride
(proh-KAR-buh-zeen high-droh-KLOR-ighd)
Matulane, Natulan

Pharmacologic class: antibiotic antineoplastic (cell cycle–phase specific, S phase)
Therapeutic class: antineoplastic
Pregnancy risk category: D

How supplied

Capsules: 50 mg

Pharmacokinetics

Absorption: rapidly and completely absorbed.
Distribution: distributes widely into body tissues, with highest concentrations found in liver, kidneys, intestinal wall, and skin. Drug crosses blood-brain barrier.
Metabolism: extensively metabolized in liver; some metabolites have cytotoxic activity.
Excretion: drug and metabolites excreted primarily in urine. *Half-life:* about 10 minutes.

Route	Onset	Peak	Duration
P.O.	Unknown	Unknown	Unknown

Pharmacodynamics

Chemical effect: unknown; thought to inhibit DNA, RNA, and protein synthesis.
Therapeutic effect: kills selected cancer cells.

Indications and dosage

Dosage and indications may differ. Check with doctor for treatment protocol.

▶ **Hodgkin's disease; lymphomas; brain and lung cancer.** *Adults:* 2 to 4 mg/kg P.O. daily in single dose or divided doses for first week. Then, 4 to 6 mg/kg/day until WBC count decreases to below 4,000/mm³ or platelet count decreases to below 100,000/mm³. After bone marrow recovers, maintenance dosage of 1 to 2 mg/kg/day resumed. *Children:* 50 mg/

Reactions may be *common*, uncommon, *life-threatening*, or COMMON AND LIFE-THREATENING.

m² P.O. daily for first week; then 100 mg/m² until response or toxicity occurs. Maintenance dosage is 50 mg/m² P.O. daily after bone marrow recovery.

Adverse reactions

CNS: nervousness, depression, insomnia, nightmares, paresthesia, neuropathy, *hallucinations,* confusion, *seizures, coma.*
EENT: retinal hemorrhage, nystagmus, photophobia.
GI: *nausea, vomiting,* anorexia, stomatitis, dry mouth, dysphagia, diarrhea, constipation.
Hematologic: *bleeding tendency, thrombocytopenia, leukopenia, anemia.*
Respiratory: *pleural effusion,* pneumonitis.
Skin: dermatitis.
Other: reversible alopecia, *hepatotoxicity.*

Interactions

Drug-drug. *CNS depressants:* additive depressant effects. Avoid concomitant use.
Digoxin: may decrease serum digoxin levels. Monitor closely.
Local anesthetics, sympathomimetics, tricyclic antidepressants: possible tremors, palpitations, increased blood pressure. Monitor closely.
Meperidine: may cause severe hypotension and possible death. Don't give together.
Drug-food. *Caffeine:* concurrent use may result in arrhythmias, severe hypertension. Discourage caffeine intake.
Foods high in tyramine (cheese, Chianti wine): possible tremors, palpitations, increased blood pressure. Monitor closely.
Drug-lifestyle. *Alcohol use:* mild disulfiram-like reaction. Warn patient to avoid alcohol.

Contraindications and precautions

• Contraindicated in patients hypersensitive to drug and in those with inadequate bone marrow reserve as shown by bone marrow aspiration.
• Drug is not recommended in pregnant or breast-feeding women.

• Use cautiously in patients with impaired hepatic or renal function.

NURSING CONSIDERATIONS

☲ Assessment
• Assess patient's condition before therapy and regularly thereafter.
• Monitor CBC and platelet counts.
• Be alert for adverse reactions and drug interactions.
• Evaluate patient's and family's knowledge of drug therapy.

⊞ Nursing diagnoses
• Altered health maintenance related to presence of neoplastic disease
• Altered protection related to adverse hematologic reactions
• Knowledge deficit related to drug therapy

▷ Planning and implementation
• Give drug at bedtime to lessen nausea.
• Be prepared to discontinue drug if patient becomes confused, or if paresthesia or other neuropathies develop. Notify doctor.
Patient teaching
• Advise patient to take drug at bedtime and in divided doses.
• Warn patient to watch for signs of infection (fever, sore throat, fatigue) and bleeding (easy bruising, nosebleeds, bleeding gums, melena). Take temperature daily.
• Warn patient to avoid alcohol during drug therapy. Tell him to stop drug and check with doctor immediately if disulfiram-like reaction (chest pains, rapid or irregular heartbeat, severe headache, stiff neck) occurs.
• Warn patient to avoid hazardous activities until CNS effects are known.
• Advise female patient of childbearing age to avoid becoming pregnant during therapy and to consult with doctor before becoming pregnant.

✓ **Evaluation**
• Patient responds well to therapy.
• Patient does not develop serious adverse hematologic reactions.
• Patient and family state understanding of drug therapy.

prochlorperazine
(proh-klor-PER-ah-zeen)
Compazine, PMS Prochlorperazine♦,
Prorazin♦, Stemetil

prochlorperazine edisylate
Compa-Z, Compazine Syrup, Cotranzine,
Ultrazine-10

prochlorperazine maleate
Anti-Naus♦, Compazine Spansule, PMS
Prochlorperazine♦, Prorazin♦, Stemetil

Pharmacologic class: phenothiazine
(piperazine derivative)
Therapeutic class: antipsychotic,
antiemetic, antianxiety agent
Pregnancy risk category: NR

How supplied
prochlorperazine
Tablets: 5 mg, 10 mg
Injection: 5 mg/ml
Suppositories: 2.5 mg, 5 mg, 25 mg
prochlorperazine edisylate
Syrup: 1 mg/ml
prochlorperazine maleate
Tablets: 5 mg, 10 mg, 25 mg
Capsules (sustained-release): 10 mg,
15 mg, 30 mg

Pharmacokinetics
Absorption: erratic and variable with oral
tablet, more predictable with oral concentrate, unknown for P.R. administration,
rapid absorption with I.M. administration.
Distribution: distributed widely into
body; 91% to 99% protein-bound.
Metabolism: metabolized extensively by
liver, but no active metabolites are formed.

Excretion: excreted primarily in urine;
some excreted in feces.

Route	Onset	Peak	Duration
P.O.	30-40 min	Unknown	3-12 hr
I.V.	Immediate	Immediate	Unknown
I.M.	10-20 min	Unknown	3-4 hr
P.R.	60 min	Unknown	3-4 hr

Pharmacodynamics
Chemical effect: acts on chemoreceptor
trigger zone to inhibit nausea and vomiting; in larger doses, partially depresses
vomiting center.
Therapeutic effect: relieves nausea and
vomiting, signs and symptoms of psychosis, and anxiety.

Indications and dosage
▶ **Preoperative nausea control.** *Adults:* 5
to 10 mg I.M. 1 to 2 hours before induction of anesthesia; repeat once in 30 minutes, if necessary. Alternatively, 5 to
10 mg I.V. 15 to 30 minutes before induction of anesthesia; repeat once if necessary; or 20 mg/L D_5W or 0.9% NaCl solution by I.V. infusion, added to infusion 15
to 30 minutes before induction. Maximum
parenteral dosage is 40 mg daily.
▶ **Severe nausea and vomiting.** *Adults:*
5 to 10 mg P.O., t.i.d. or q.i.d.; 15 mg
sustained-release form P.O. on arising;
10 mg sustained-release form P.O. q 12
hours; 25 mg P.R., b.i.d.; or 5 to 10 mg
I.M. repeated q 3 to 4 hours, p.r.n.
Alternatively, 5 to 10 mg may be given
I.V. Maximum I.M. dosage is 40 mg daily. *Children weighing 9 to 13 kg (20 to
29 lb):* 2.5 mg P.O. or P.R. once daily or
b.i.d. Maximum dosage is 7.5 mg daily.
Or give 0.132 mg/kg by deep I.M. injection. Control usually is obtained with one
dose. *Children weighing 14 to 17 kg (30
to 38 lb):* 2.5 mg P.O. or P.R., b.i.d. or
t.i.d. Maximum dosage is 10 mg daily. Or
give 0.132 mg/kg by deep I.M. injection.
Control usually is obtained with one dose.
*Children weighing 18 to 39 kg (40 to
86 lb):* 2.5 mg P.O. or P.R., t.i.d.; or 5 mg
P.O. or P.R., b.i.d. Maximum dosage is

Reactions may be *common,* uncommon, *life-threatening,* or COMMON AND LIFE-THREATENING.

15 mg daily. Or, give 0.132 mg/kg by deep I.M. injection. Control usually is obtained with one dose.

▶ **To manage symptoms of psychotic disorders.** *Adults:* 5 to 10 mg P.O., t.i.d. or q.i.d. *Children ages 2 to 12:* 2.5 mg P.O. or P.R., b.i.d. or t.i.d. Do not exceed 10 mg on day 1. Increase dosage gradually to recommended maximum (if necessary). In children ages 2 to 5, maximum daily dosage is 20 mg. In children ages 6 to 10, maximum daily dosage is 25 mg.

▶ **To manage symptoms of severe psychoses.** *Adults:* 10 to 20 mg I.M. repeated in 1 to 4 hours, if needed. Rarely, patients may receive 10 to 20 mg q 4 to 6 hours. Institute oral therapy after symptoms are controlled. *Children ages 2 to 12:* 0.13 mg/kg I.M.

▶ **Nonpsychotic anxiety.** *Adults:* 5 to 10 mg by deep I.M. injection q 3 to 4 hours, not to exceed 40 mg daily; or 5 to 10 mg P.O., t.i.d. or q.i.d. Alternatively, give 15 mg extended-release capsule once daily or 10 mg extended-release capsule q 12 hours.

Adverse reactions

CNS: *extrapyramidal reactions,* sedation, pseudoparkinsonism, EEG changes, dizziness.
CV: *orthostatic hypotension,* tachycardia, ECG changes.
EENT: *ocular changes, blurred vision.*
GI: *dry mouth, constipation.*
GU: *urine retention,* dark urine, menstrual irregularities, inhibited ejaculation.
Hematologic: *transient leukopenia, agranulocytosis.*
Hepatic: cholestatic jaundice.
Skin: *mild photosensitivity,* allergic reactions, *exfoliative dermatitis.*
Other: hyperprolactinemia, gynecomastia, weight gain, increased appetite.

Interactions

Drug-drug. *Antacids:* inhibited absorption of oral phenothiazines. Separate doses by at least 2 hours.

Anticholinergics, including antidepressants and antiparkinsonian agents: increased anticholinergic activity and aggravated parkinsonian symptoms. Use together cautiously.
Barbiturates: may decrease phenothiazine effect.
Drug-lifestyle. *Sun exposure:* potential photosensitivity reaction. Take precautions.

Contraindications and precautions

• Contraindicated in patients with hypersensitivity to phenothiazines; CNS depression including coma; during pediatric surgery; when using spinal or epidural anesthetic, adrenergic blockers, or alcohol; and in children under age 2.
• Use cautiously in patients with impaired CV function, glaucoma, seizure disorders; in those who have been exposed to extreme heat; and in children with acute illness. Also use cautiously in breast-feeding women.
• Safety of drug has not been established in pregnant women.

NURSING CONSIDERATIONS

⚕ Assessment
• Assess patient's condition before therapy and regularly thereafter.
• Watch for orthostatic hypotension, especially when giving drug I.V.
• Monitor CBC and liver function studies during prolonged therapy.
• Be alert for adverse reactions and drug interactions.
• Evaluate patient's and family's knowledge of drug therapy.

Nursing diagnoses
• Risk for fluid volume deficit related to nausea and vomiting
• Altered thought processes related to presence of psychosis
• Knowledge deficit related to drug therapy

⚡ Planning and implementation

P.O. use: Dilute oral solution with tomato or fruit juice, milk, coffee, carbonated beverage, tea, water or soup, or mix with pudding.

I.V. use: Drug may be given undiluted or diluted in an isotonic solution. Rate of administration should not exceed 5 mg per minute. Don't give by bolus injection.

I.M. use: Inject deeply into upper outer quadrant of gluteal region.

P.R. use: Follow normal protocol.

• Do not give S.C. or mix in syringe with another drug.

• Avoid getting concentrate or injection solution on hands or clothing.

• Know that drug is used only if vomiting can't be otherwise controlled or if only few doses are required. If more than four doses are needed in 24 hours, notify doctor.

• Store drug in light-resistant container. Slight yellowing does not affect potency; discard extremely discolored solutions.

Patient teaching

• Tell patient to mix oral solution with flavored liquid to mask taste.

• Advise patient to wear protective clothing when exposed to sunlight.

• Tell patient to notify doctor of adverse reactions.

☑ Evaluation

• Patient's nausea and vomiting are relieved.

• Patient behavior and communication show better thought processes.

• Patient and family state understanding of drug therapy.

---

progesterone
(proh-JES-teh-rohn)
Gesterol 50, PMS-Progesterone♦,
Progestasert

Pharmacologic class: progestin
Therapeutic class: hormonal agent
Pregnancy risk category: X

How supplied
Injection (in oil): 50 mg/ml
Intrauterine device (IUD): 38 mg (with barium sulfate, dispersed in silicone fluid)

Pharmacokinetics
Absorption: unknown.
Distribution: unknown.
Metabolism: metabolized in liver.
Excretion: excreted in urine. *Half-life:* several minutes.

Route	Onset	Peak	Duration
I.M.	Unknown	Unknown	Unknown

Pharmacodynamics
Chemical effect: suppresses ovulation and forms thick cervical mucus.
Therapeutic effect: alleviates amenorrhea and dysfunctional uterine bleeding.

Indications and dosage
▶ **Amenorrhea.** *Adults:* 5 to 10 mg I.M. daily for 6 to 8 days usually beginning 8 to 10 days before anticipated start of menstruation.

▶ **Dysfunctional uterine bleeding.** *Adults:* 5 to 10 mg I.M. daily for six doses.

▶ **Contraception (as an IUD).** *Adults:* Progestasert system inserted into uterine cavity; replaced annually.

Adverse reactions
CNS: dizziness, migraine, lethargy, depression.
CV: hypertension, thrombophlebitis, *thromboembolism, pulmonary embolism, CVA,* edema.
GI: nausea, vomiting, abdominal cramps.
GU: breakthrough bleeding, dysmenorrhea, amenorrhea, cervical erosion, abnormal secretions, uterine fibromas, vaginal candidiasis.
Hepatic: cholestatic jaundice.
Skin: melasma, rash.
Other: breast tenderness, enlargement, or secretion; decreased libido; hyperglycemia, pain (at injection site).

Reactions may be *common*, uncommon, *life-threatening*, or COMMON AND LIFE-THREATENING.

Interactions

Drug-drug. *Barbiturates, carbamazepine, rifampin:* decreased progestin effects. Avoid concomitant use.
Bromocriptine: may cause amenorrhea. Monitor patient.

Contraindications and precautions

• Contraindicated in patients with thromboembolic disorders, cerebral apoplexy, or history of these conditions; hypersensitivity to drug; breast cancer, undiagnosed abnormal vaginal bleeding, severe hepatic disease, missed abortion; and in pregnant or breast-feeding women.
• Use cautiously in patients with diabetes mellitus, seizure disorder, migraine, cardiac or renal disease, asthma, and depression.
• Safety of drug has not been established in children.

NURSING CONSIDERATIONS

Assessment
• Assess patient's condition before therapy and regularly thereafter.
• Be alert for adverse reactions and drug interactions.
• Evaluate patient's and family's knowledge of drug therapy.

Nursing diagnoses
• Risk for fluid volume deficit related to excessive uterine bleeding
• Risk for injury related to dizziness
• Knowledge deficit related to drug therapy

Planning and implementation
• Know that preliminary estrogen treatment is usually needed in menstrual disorders.
• Give oil solutions (peanut oil or sesame oil) by deep I.M. injection. Check sites frequently for irritation. Rotate injection sites.
Patient teaching
• Ensure patient reads package insert explaining possible adverse effects of pro-

gestins before taking first dose. Also provide verbal explanation.
• Tell patient not to perform hazardous activities if dizziness occurs.
• Tell patient to report any unusual symptoms immediately and to stop drug and call doctor if visual disturbances or migraine occurs.
• Teach patient how to perform routine breast self-examination.

Evaluation
• Patient's uterine bleeding ceases.
• Patient does not experience injury from drug-induced dizziness.
• Patient and family state understanding of drug therapy.

---

promazine hydrochloride
(PROH-muh-zeen high-droh-KLOR-ighd)
Primazine, Prozine-50, Sparine**

Pharmacologic class: aliphatic phenothiazine
Therapeutic class: antipsychotic, antiemetic
Pregnancy risk category: NR

How supplied

Tablets: 25 mg, 50 mg, 100 mg
Injection: 25 mg/ml, 50 mg/ml

Pharmacokinetics

Absorption: usually absorbed well from GI tract and rapidly following I.M. injection.
Distribution: distributed widely into body; 91% to 99% protein-bound.
Metabolism: metabolized extensively by liver, but no active metabolites are formed.
Excretion: excreted primarily as metabolites in urine; some excreted in feces.

Route	Onset	Peak	Duration
P.O., I.V., I.M.	Varies	Unknown	Unknown

Pharmacodynamics

Chemical effect: unknown; probably blocks postsynaptic dopamine receptors in brain.
Therapeutic effect: relieves signs and symptoms of psychosis.

Indications and dosage

▶ **Psychosis.** *Adults:* 10 to 200 mg P.O. or I.M. q 4 to 6 hours, up to 1 g daily, p.r.n. In acutely agitated patients, 50 to 150 mg initially I.M. or I.V.; repeated within 5 to 10 minutes, p.r.n. Give I.V. dose in concentrations of 25 mg/ml or less. *Children over age 12:* 10 to 25 mg P.O. or I.M. q 4 to 6 hours.

Adverse reactions

CNS: *extrapyramidal reactions* (moderate incidence), *tardive dyskinesia, sedation* (high incidence), pseudoparkinsonism, EEG changes, dizziness, *seizures.*
CV: orthostatic hypotension, tachycardia, ECG changes.
EENT: ocular changes, blurred vision.
GI: dry mouth, constipation.
GU: *urine retention,* dark urine, menstrual irregularities, gynecomastia, inhibited ejaculation.
Hematologic: transient leukopenia, *agranulocytosis, thrombocytopenia, hemolytic anemia,* hyperprolactinemia.
Hepatic: cholestatic jaundice, abnormal liver function test results.
Skin: *mild photosensitivity,* allergic reactions, sterile abscess; pain (at I.M. injection site).
Other: weight gain; increased appetite; *neuroleptic malignant syndrome* (rare).
After abrupt withdrawal of long-term therapy: gastritis, nausea, vomiting, dizziness, tremors, feeling of warmth or cold, diaphoresis, tachycardia, headache, insomnia.

Interactions

Drug-drug. *Antacids:* inhibited absorption of oral phenothiazines. Use together cautiously. Separate antacid and phenothiazine doses by at least 2 hours.

Anticholinergics, including antidepressants and antiparkinsonian agents: increased anticholinergic activity, aggravated parkinsonian symptoms. Use together cautiously.
Barbiturates, lithium: may decrease phenothiazine effect. Observe patient.
Centrally acting antihypertensives: decreased antihypertensive effect. Monitor blood pressure.
Other CNS depressants: increased CNS depression. Use together cautiously.
Drug-lifestyle. *Alcohol use:* increased CNS depression. Avoid concomitant use.

Contraindications and precautions

• Contraindicated in patients with hypersensitivity to drug or in those experiencing coma or CNS depression, bone marrow suppression, or subcortical damage.
• Drug use not recommended in breastfeeding women.
• Use cautiously in elderly or debilitated patients and in patients with hepatic or renal disease, severe CV disease (may cause sudden drop in blood pressure); exposure to extreme heat or cold (including antipyretic therapy) or to organophosphate insecticides; respiratory disorder; hypocalcemia; seizure disorder (may lower seizure threshold); severe reactions to insulin or electroconvulsive therapy; glaucoma; or prostatic hyperplasia.
• Safety of drug has not been established in children age 12 and under or in pregnant women.

NURSING CONSIDERATIONS

🔅 Assessment

• Assess patient's condition before therapy and regularly thereafter.
• Monitor blood pressure with patient lying and standing before starting therapy, and routinely throughout course of treatment.
• Monitor patient for tardive dyskinesia. It may occur after prolonged use. It may not appear until months or years later and may disappear spontaneously or persist for life despite discontinuation of drug.

• Monitor therapy with weekly bilirubin tests during first month; periodic blood tests (CBC and liver function); and ophthalmic tests (long-term use) as ordered.
• Be alert for adverse reactions and drug interactions.
• Evaluate patient's and family's knowledge of drug therapy.

Nursing diagnoses
• Altered thought processes related to presence of psychosis
• Risk of injury related to adverse CNS reactions
• Knowledge deficit related to drug therapy

Planning and implementation
• Prevent contact dermatitis by keeping drug away from skin and clothes. Wear gloves when preparing liquid forms.
P.O. use: Dilute liquid concentrate with fruit juice, milk, semisolid food, or chocolate-flavored drinks just before giving. For best taste, use at least 10 ml diluent per 25 mg drug.
I.V. use: Give drug by direct injection; not recommended for intermittent or continuous infusion. Administer I.V. only to hospitalized patient. Drug should be changed to oral therapy as soon as possible.
I.M. use: Inject drug deeply only in upper outer quadrant of buttocks. Massage slowly afterward to prevent sterile abscess. Injection may sting.
• Protect drug from light. Slight yellowing of injection or concentrate is common; does not affect potency. Discard markedly discolored solutions.
• Keep patient supine for 1 hour afterward and have patient change positions slowly.
• Do not stop drug abruptly unless required by severe adverse reactions.
• Withhold dose and notify doctor if patient develops jaundice, symptoms of blood dyscrasia (fever, sore throat, infection, cellulitis, weakness), persistent extrapyramidal reactions (longer than a few hours).

• Acute dystonic reactions may be treated with diphenhydramine.
Patient teaching
• Warn patient to avoid hazardous activities until CNS effects of drug are known.
• Tell patient to avoid alcohol during drug therapy.
• Instruct patient to report urine retention or constipation.
• Tell patient to use sunblock and to wear protective clothing to avoid photosensitivity reactions.
• Tell patient to relieve dry mouth with sugarless gum or hard candy.

Evaluation
• Patient behavior and communication reveal improved thought processes with drug therapy.
• Patient does not experience injury from CNS reactions.
• Patient and family state understanding of drug therapy.

promethazine hydrochloride
(proh-METH-uh-zeen high-droh-KLOR-ighd)
Anergan 25, Anergan 50, Histantil◆, Pentazine, Phenameth, Phenazine 25, Phenazine 50, Phencen-50, Phenergan*, Phenergan Fortis*, Phenergan Plain*, Phenoject-50, PMS-Promethazine◆, Pro-50, Prometh-25, Prometh-50, Promethegan, Prorex-25, Prorex-50, Prothazine*, Prothazine Plain, V-Gan-25, V-Gan-50

promethazine theoclate
Avomine◆

Pharmacologic class: phenothiazine derivative
Therapeutic class: antiemetic, antivertigo agent, antihistamine (H_1-receptor antagonist), sedative
Pregnancy risk category: NR

How supplied

promethazine hydrochloride
Tablets: 12.5 mg, 25 mg, 50 mg
Syrup: 5 mg/5 ml†*, 6.25 mg/5 ml*,
10 mg/5 ml*, 25 mg/5 ml*
Injection: 25 mg/ml, 50 mg/ml
Suppositories: 12.5 mg, 25 mg, 50 mg
promethazine theoclate
Tablets: 25 mg†

Pharmacokinetics

Absorption: well absorbed from GI tract
after P.O. use; absorbed fairly rapidly after P.R. or I.M. use.
Distribution: distributed widely throughout body.
Metabolism: metabolized in liver.
Excretion: excreted in urine and feces.

Route	Onset	Peak	Duration
P.O.	15-60 min	Unknown	≤ 12 hr
I.V.	3-5 min	Unknown	≤ 12 hr
I.M., P.R.	20 min	Unknown	≤ 12 hr

Pharmacodynamics

Chemical effect: competes with histamine for H_1-receptor sites on effector
cells. Prevents, but does not reverse,
histamine-mediated responses.
Therapeutic effect: prevents motion sickness and relieves nausea, nasal congestion, and allergy symptoms. Also promotes calmness.

Indications and dosage

► **Motion sickness.** *Adults:* 25 mg P.O.
b.i.d. *Children:* 12.5 to 25 mg P.O., I.M.,
or P.R. b.i.d.
► **Nausea.** *Adults:* 12.5 to 25 mg P.O.,
I.M., or P.R. q 4 to 6 hours, p.r.n.
Children: 0.25 to 0.5 mg/kg I.M. or P.R.
q 4 to 6 hours, p.r.n.
► **Rhinitis, allergy symptoms.** *Adults:*
12.5 to 25 mg P.O. q.i.d.; or 25 mg P.O.
h.s. *Children:* 6.25 to 12.5 mg P.O. t.i.d.
or 25 mg P.O. or P.R. h.s.
► **Sedation.** *Adults:* 25 to 50 mg P.O. or
I.M. h.s. or p.r.n. *Children:* 12.5 to 25 mg
P.O., I.M., or P.R. h.s.

► **Routine preoperative or postopera-
tive sedation or adjunct to analgesics.**
Adults: 25 to 50 mg I.M., I.V., or P.O.
Children: 12.5 to 25 mg I.M., I.V., or P.O.

Adverse reactions

CNS: *sedation,* confusion, restlessness,
tremors, *drowsiness* (especially elderly
patients).
CV: hypotension.
EENT: transient myopia, nasal conges-
tion.
GI: anorexia, nausea, vomiting, constipa-
tion, *dry mouth.*
GU: urine retention.
Hematologic: leukopenia, *agranulocyto-
sis, thrombocytopenia.*
Other: photosensitivity.

Interactions

Drug-drug. *Anticholinergics, phenothiazines, tricyclic antidepressants:* increased effects. Don't give together.
CNS depressants: increased sedation.
Use together cautiously.
Epinephrine: promethazine may block or
reverse effects of epinephrine. Other vasopressor agents should be used.
Levodopa: promethazine may decrease
levodopa's antiparkinsonian action.
Avoid concomitant use.
Lithium: promethazine may reduce GI
absorption or enhance renal elimination
of lithium. Avoid concomitant use.
MAO inhibitors: increased extrapyramidal effects. Don't use together.
Drug-lifestyle. *Alcohol use:* increased
sedation. Avoid concomitant use.
Sun exposure: possible photosensitivity
reaction; take precautions.

Contraindications and precautions

• Contraindicated in patients with intestinal obstruction, prostatic hyperplasia,
bladder-neck obstruction, seizure disorders, coma, CNS depression, stenosing
peptic ulcerations, or hypersensitivity to
drug; in newborns and premature neonates; in breast-feeding women; and in
acutely ill or dehydrated children.

Reactions may be *common,* uncommon, *life-threatening,* or COMMON AND LIFE-THREATENING.

• Use cautiously in patients with pulmonary, hepatic, or CV disease or asthma.
• Safety of drug has not been established in pregnant women.

NURSING CONSIDERATIONS

⚖ Assessment
• Assess patient's condition before therapy and regularly thereafter.
• Be alert for adverse reactions and drug interactions.
• Evaluate patient's and family's knowledge of drug therapy.

⊕ Nursing diagnoses
• Altered health maintenance related to underlying condition
• Risk for injury related to drug's sedating effects
• Knowledge deficit related to drug therapy

⧁ Planning and implementation
• Pronounced sedative effect limits use in many ambulatory patients.
• Drug is used as adjunct to analgesics (usually to increase sedation); it has no analgesic activity.
P.O. use: Give drug with food or milk to reduce GI distress.
I.V. use: Don't give in concentration greater than 25 mg/ml or at rate exceeding 25 mg/minute. Shield I.V. infusion from direct light.
I.M. use: Inject deeply into large muscle mass. Rotate injection sites.
P.R. use: Follow normal protocol.
• Do not administer S.C.
• Be aware that drug may be safely mixed with meperidine (Demerol) in same syringe.
• In patient scheduled for myelogram, discontinue drug 48 hours before procedure and do not resume drug until 24 hours after procedure, as ordered, because of risk of seizures.
• Know that drug may cause false-positive immunologic urine pregnancy test using Gravindex and false-negative using Prepurex or Dap tests. Also may interfere with blood typing of ABO group.

Patient teaching
• When treating for motion sickness, tell patient to take first dose 30 to 60 minutes before travel. On succeeding days of travel, he should take dose upon rising and with evening meal.
• Warn patient to avoid alcohol and hazardous activities until drug's CNS effects are known.
• Tell patient that coffee or tea may reduce drowsiness. Sugarless gum, sugarless sour hard candy, or ice chips may relieve dry mouth.
• Warn patient about possible photosensitivity and precautions to avoid it.
• Advise patient to stop drug 4 days before allergy skin tests.

☑ Evaluation
• Patient responds well to therapy.
• Patient does not experience injury from adverse reactions.
• Patient and family state understanding of drug therapy.

---

propafenone hydrochloride
(proh-puh-FEE-nohn high-droh-KLOR-Ighd)
Rythmol

Pharmacologic class: sodium channel antagonist
Therapeutic class: antiarrhythmic (class IC)
Pregnancy risk category: C

How supplied
Tablets: 150 mg, 300 mg

Pharmacokinetics
Absorption: well absorbed from GI tract. Because of significant first-pass effect, bioavailability is limited; however, it increases with dosage.
Distribution: 97% protein-bound.

Metabolism: metabolized in liver.
Excretion: excreted mainly in feces; some in urine. *Half-life:* 2 to 32 hours.

Route	Onset	Peak	Duration
P.O.	Unknown	≤ 3.5 hr	Unknown

Pharmacodynamics

Chemical effect: reduces inward sodium current in Purkinje and myocardial cells. Decreases excitability, conduction velocity, and automaticity in AV nodal, His-Purkinje, and intraventricular tissue; causes slight but significant prolongation of refractory period in AV nodal tissue. *Therapeutic effect:* restores normal sinus rhythm.

Indications and dosage

▶ **Suppression of life-threatening ventricular arrhythmias, such as sustained ventricular tachycardia.** *Adults:* initially, 150 mg P.O. q 8 hours. Dosage may be increased at 3- to 4-day intervals to 225 mg q 8 hours, if necessary, increase dosage to 300 mg q 8 hours. Maximum daily dosage is 900 mg. Manufacturer recommends dosage reduction of 20% to 30% in patients with hepatic failure.

Adverse reactions

CNS: anxiety, ataxia, dizziness, drowsiness, fatigue, headache, insomnia, syncope, tremor, weakness.
CV: atrial fibrillation, bradycardia, bundle branch block, *heart failure,* chest pain, edema, first-degree AV block, hypotension, increased QRS duration, intraventricular conduction delay, palpitations, *proarrhythmic events (ventricular tachycardia, PVCs).*
EENT: blurred vision.
GI: abdominal pain or cramps, constipation, diarrhea, dyspepsia, flatulence, nausea, vomiting, dry mouth, unusual taste, anorexia.
Respiratory: dyspnea.
Skin: rash.
Other: diaphoresis, joint pain.

Interactions

Drug-drug. *Antiarrhythmics:* increased risk of heart failure. Monitor patient closely.
Cardiac glycosides, oral anticoagulants: propafenone may increase serum levels of these agents by about 35% to 85%, resulting in toxicity. Monitor patient closely.
Cimetidine: decreased metabolism of propafenone. Monitor patient closely.
Local anesthetics: increased risk of CNS toxicity. Monitor patient closely.
Metoprolol, propranolol: propafenone slows metabolism of these agents. Monitor for toxicity.
Quinidine: slowed metabolism of propafenone. Avoid concomitant use.
Rifampin: increased clearance of propafenone. Monitor closely.

Contraindications and precautions

• Contraindicated in patients hypersensitive to drug and in those with severe or uncontrolled heart failure, cardiogenic shock; SA, AV, or intraventricular disorders of impulse conduction in absence of pacemaker; bradycardia; marked hypotension; bronchospastic disorders; and electrolyte imbalance.
• Drug is not recommended in breast-feeding women.
• Use cautiously in patients with heart failure because propafenone can exert negative inotropic effect on heart. Also use cautiously in patients taking other cardiac depressant drugs and in those with hepatic or renal failure.
• Safety of drug has not been established in children and in pregnant women.

NURSING CONSIDERATIONS

⚥ Assessment

• Assess patient's condition before therapy and regularly thereafter.
• Continuous cardiac monitoring is recommended during initiation of therapy and dosage adjustments.

Reactions may be *common,* uncommon, *life-threatening,* or COMMON AND LIFE-THREATENING.

• Be alert for adverse reactions and drug interactions.
• Evaluate patient's and family's knowledge of drug therapy.

⊞ **Nursing diagnoses**
• Decreased cardiac output related to presence of arrhythmia
• Altered protection related to drug-induced proarrhythmias
• Knowledge deficit related to drug therapy

⊠ **Planning and implementation**
• Administer drug with food to minimize adverse GI reactions.
• If PR interval or QRS complex increases by more than 25%, notify doctor because reduction in dosage may be necessary.
• During concomitant use with digoxin, frequently monitor ECG and serum digoxin levels.
Patient teaching
• Tell patient to take drug with food.
• Stress importance of taking drug exactly as ordered.
• Warn patient to avoid hazardous activities if adverse CNS disturbances occur.

☑ **Evaluation**
• Patient regains adequate cardiac output when arrhythmia is corrected.
• Patient does not develop any proarrhythmic events.
• Patient and family state understanding of drug therapy.

---

propantheline bromide
(proh-PAN-thuh-leen BROH-mighd)
Pro-Banthine, Propanthel♦

Pharmacologic class: anticholinergic
Therapeutic class: antimuscarinic, GI antispasmodic
Pregnancy risk category: C

How supplied
Tablets: 7.5 mg, 15 mg

Pharmacokinetics
Absorption: about 10% to 25% absorbed (varies among patients).
Distribution: unknown.
Metabolism: appears to undergo considerable metabolism in upper small intestine and liver.
Excretion: absorbed drug is excreted in urine. *Half-life:* 1.6 hours.

Route	Onset	Peak	Duration
P.O.	Unknown	2 hr	6 hr

Pharmacodynamics
Chemical effect: blocks acetylcholine, which decreases GI motility and inhibits gastric acid secretion.
Therapeutic effect: relieves peptic ulcer pain.

Indications and dosage
▶ **Adjunct treatment of peptic ulcer, irritable bowel syndrome, and other GI disorders; reduce duodenal motility during diagnostic radiologic procedures.** *Adults:* 15 mg P.O. t.i.d. before meals, and 30 mg h.s. *Elderly patients:* 7.5 mg P.O. t.i.d. before meals.

Adverse reactions
CNS: headache, insomnia, drowsiness, dizziness, *confusion or excitement in elderly patients,* nervousness, weakness.
CV: palpitations, tachycardia.
EENT: *blurred vision,* mydriasis, increased intraocular pressure, cycloplegia, photophobia.
GI: *dry mouth,* dysphagia, constipation, heartburn, loss of taste, nausea, vomiting, paralytic ileus.
GU: urinary hesitancy, urine retention, impotence.
Skin: urticaria, decreased sweating or possible anhidrosis, other dermal manifestations.
Other: fever, allergic reactions, *anaphylaxis.*

---

*Liquid form contains alcohol   **May contain tartrazine   ♦Canada   ◊ Australia   †OTC

Note: Overdose may cause curare-like effects, such as respiratory paralysis.

Interactions

Drug-drug. *Amantadine, antihistamines, antiparkinsonian agents, disopyramide, glutethimide, meperidine, phenothiazines, procainamide, quinidine, tricyclic antidepressants:* additive adverse effects. Avoid concomitant use.
Antacids: decreased absorption of oral anticholinergics. Separate administration times by 2 to 3 hours.
Digoxin: increased serum digoxin levels. Monitor for cardiac toxicity.
Ketoconazole: anticholinergics may interfere with ketoconazole absorption. Avoid concomitant use.
Methotrimeprazine: anticholinergics may enhance risk of extrapyramidal reactions. Monitor patient closely.

Contraindications and precautions

• Contraindicated in patients with angle-closure glaucoma, obstructive uropathy, obstructive disease of GI tract, severe ulcerative colitis, myasthenia gravis, hypersensitivity to anticholinergics, paralytic ileus, intestinal atony, unstable CV status in acute hemorrhage, or toxic megacolon.
• Use cautiously in patients with autonomic neuropathy, hyperthyroidism, coronary artery disease, arrhythmias, heart failure, hypertension, hiatal hernia associated with reflux esophagitis, hepatic or renal disease, or ulcerative colitis; in patients in hot or humid environments (drug-induced heatstroke can develop); and in pregnant or breast-feeding women.
• Safety of drug has not been established in children.

NURSING CONSIDERATIONS

⚕ Assessment
• Assess patient's condition before therapy and regularly thereafter.
• Monitor patient's vital signs and urine output carefully.

• Evaluate patient's and family's knowledge of drug therapy.

⊞ Nursing diagnoses
• Pain related to peptic ulcer
• Constipation related to drug's adverse effect on GI tract
• Knowledge deficit related to drug therapy

⊡ Planning and implementation
• Give 30 minutes to 1 hour before meals and h.s. Bedtime doses can be larger; give at least 2 hours after last meal of day.
Patient teaching
• Tell patient when drug should be taken throughout day and at h.s.
• Instruct patient to avoid driving and other hazardous activities if he is drowsy, dizzy, or has blurred vision; to drink plenty of fluids to help prevent constipation; and to report any rash or skin eruption.
• Advise him to use sugarless gum or hard candy to relieve dry mouth.

☑ Evaluation
• Patient is free from pain.
• Patient states measures used to prevent constipation.
• Patient and family state understanding of drug therapy.

---

propoxyphene hydrochloride (dextropropoxyphene hydrochloride)
(proh-POK-sih-feen high-droh-KLOR-ighd)
Darvon, Dolene, 642♦

propoxyphene napsylate (dextropropoxyphene napsylate)
Darvon-N, Doloxene♦

Pharmacologic class: opioid
Therapeutic class: analgesic
Controlled substance schedule: IV
Pregnancy risk category: C

How supplied

propoxyphene hydrochloride
Capsules: 32 mg, 65 mg
propoxyphene napsylate
Tablets: 100 mg
Oral suspension: 10 mg/ml

Pharmacokinetics

Absorption: absorbed primarily in upper small intestine.
Distribution: drug enters CSF.
Metabolism: metabolized in liver; about one-quarter of dose is metabolized to norpropoxyphene, an active metabolite.
Excretion: excreted in urine. *Half-life:* 6 to 12 hours.

Route	Onset	Peak	Duration
P.O.	15-60 min	2-2.5 hr	4-6 hr

Pharmacodynamics

Chemical effect: binds with opioid receptors in CNS, altering both perception of and emotional response to pain through unknown mechanism.
Therapeutic effect: relieves pain.

Indications and dosage

▶ **Mild to moderate pain.**
Propoxyphene hydrochloride. *Adults:* 65 mg P.O. q 4 hours p.r.n. Maximum dosage is 390 mg/day. **Propoxyphene napsylate.** *Adults:* 100 mg P.O. q 4 hours p.r.n. Maximum dosage is 600 mg/day.

Adverse reactions

CNS: *dizziness,* headache, *sedation,* euphoria, paradoxical excitement, insomnia.
GI: nausea, vomiting, constipation.
Respiratory: *respiratory depression.*
Other: psychological and physical dependence.

Interactions

Drug-drug. *Barbiturate anesthetics:* may increase respiratory and CNS depression. Use together cautiously.
Carbamazepine: may increase carbamazepine levels. Monitor closely.

CNS depressants: additive effects. Use together cautiously.
Warfarin: increased anticoagulant effect. Monitor PT and INR.
Drug-lifestyle. *Alcohol use:* additive effects. Avoid concomitant use.

Contraindications and precautions

• Contraindicated in patients with hypersensitivity to drug.
• Use cautiously in patients with hepatic or renal disease, emotional instability, or history of drug or alcohol abuse and in pregnant or breast-feeding women.
• Safety of drug has not been established in children.

NURSING CONSIDERATIONS

⚖ Assessment
• Assess patient's pain before and after drug administration.
• Be alert for adverse reactions and drug interactions.
• Monitor patient's hydration status if adverse GI reactions occur.
• Evaluate patient's and family's knowledge of drug therapy.

⊞ Nursing diagnoses
• Pain related to underlying condition
• Risk for fluid volume deficit related to GI reactions
• Knowledge deficit related to drug therapy

▷ Planning and implementation
• Administer with food to minimize adverse GI reactions.
• Remember that 65 mg of propoxyphene hydrochloride equals 100 mg of propoxyphene napsylate.
• Know that drug can be considered a mild narcotic analgesic, but pain relief is equivalent to that provided by aspirin. Tolerance and physical dependence have been observed. Typically used with aspirin or acetaminophen to maximize analgesia.
• Drug may cause false decreases in urinary steroid excretion tests.

---

*Liquid form contains alcohol   **May contain tartrazine   ◆ Canada   ◇ Australia   †OTC

Patient teaching
- Advise patient to take drug with food or milk to minimize GI upset.
- Warn patient not to exceed recommended dosage. Respiratory depression, hypotension, profound sedation, and coma may result if used in excessive doses or with other CNS depressants. Propoxyphene-containing products alone or in combination with other drugs are major cause of drug-related overdose and death.
- Advise patient to avoid alcohol during drug therapy.
- Caution ambulatory patient about getting out of bed or walking. Warn outpatient to avoid driving and other hazardous activities until drug's CNS effects are known.

☑ **Evaluation**
- Patient is free from pain.
- Patient maintains adequate hydration.
- Patient and family state understanding of drug therapy.

---

propranolol hydrochloride
(proh-PRAH-nuh-lohl high-droh-KLOR-ighd)
Apo-Propranolol♦, Deralin♦, Detensol♦, Inderal, Inderal LA, Novopranol♦, pms Propranolol♦

Pharmacologic class: beta blocker
Therapeutic class: antihypertensive, antianginal, antiarrhythmic, adjunct therapy for migraine, adjunct therapy for MI
Pregnancy risk category: C

How supplied
Tablets: 10 mg, 20 mg, 40 mg, 60 mg, 80 mg, 90 mg
Capsules (extended-release): 60 mg, 80 mg, 120 mg, 160 mg
Oral solution: 4 mg/ml, 8 mg/ml, 80 mg/ml (concentrate)
Injection: 1 mg/ml

Pharmacokinetics
Absorption: absorbed almost completely from GI tract after oral administration. Absorption is enhanced when given with food.
Distribution: distributed widely throughout body. Drug is more than 90% protein-bound.
Metabolism: metabolized almost totally in liver. Oral form undergoes extensive first-pass metabolism.
Excretion: about 96% to 99% excreted in urine as metabolites; remainder excreted in feces as unchanged drug and metabolites. *Half-life:* about 4 hours.

Route	Onset	Peak	Duration
P.O.	30 min	60-90 min	About 12 hr
I.V.	≤ 1 min	≤ 1 min	< 5 min

Pharmacodynamics
Chemical effect: reduces cardiac oxygen demand by blocking catecholamine-induced increases in heart rate, blood pressure, and force of myocardial contraction. Depresses renin secretion and prevents vasodilation of cerebral arteries.
Therapeutic effect: relieves anginal and migraine pain, lowers blood pressure, restores normal sinus rhythm, and helps limit MI damage.

Indications and dosage
▶ **Angina pectoris.** *Adults:* total daily doses of 80-320 mg P.O. when given b.i.d, t.i.d. or q.i.d. Or one 80-mg extended-release capsule daily. Dosage increased at 7- to 10-day intervals.
▶ **Mortality reduction after MI.** *Adults:* 180 to 240 mg P.O. daily in divided doses beginning 5 to 21 days after MI has occurred. Usually administered t.i.d. or q.i.d.
▶ **Supraventricular, ventricular, and atrial arrhythmias; tachyarrhythmias caused by excessive catecholamine action during anesthesia, hyperthyroidism, or pheochromocytoma.** *Adults:* 0.5 to 3 mg by slow I.V. push, not to exceed 1 mg/minute. After 3 mg have been giv-

en, another dose may be given in 2 minutes; subsequent doses, no sooner than q 4 hours. May be diluted and infused slowly. Usual maintenance dosage is 10 to 30 mg P.O. t.i.d. or q.i.d.

▶ **Hypertension.** *Adults:* initially, 80 mg P.O. daily in two to four divided doses or extended-release form once daily. Increased at 3- to 7-day intervals to maximum daily dosage of 640 mg. Usual maintenance dosage is 160 to 480 mg daily.

▶ **Prevention of frequent, severe, uncontrollable, or disabling migraine or vascular headache.** *Adults:* initially, 80 mg P.O. daily in divided doses or one extended-release capsule daily. Usual maintenance dosage is 160 to 240 mg daily, t.i.d. or q.i.d.

▶ **Essential tremor.** *Adults:* 40 mg (tablets, oral solution) P.O. b.i.d. Usual maintenance dosage is 120 to 320 mg daily in three divided doses.

▶ **Hypertrophic subaortic stenosis.** *Adults:* 10 to 20 mg P.O. t.i.d. or q.i.d. before meals and h.s.

▶ **Adjunct therapy in pheochromocytoma.** *Adults:* 60 mg P.O. daily in divided doses with alpha-adrenergic blocker 3 days before surgery.

Adverse reactions

CNS: *fatigue, lethargy,* vivid dreams, hallucinations, mental depression.
CV: *bradycardia, hypotension, heart failure,* intermittent claudication.
GI: nausea, vomiting, diarrhea.
Hematologic: *agranulocytosis.*
Musculoskeletal: arthralgia.
Respiratory: increased airway resistance.
Skin: rash.
Other: fever.

Interactions

Drug-drug. *Aminophylline:* antagonized beta-blocking effects of propranolol. Use together cautiously.
Cardiac glycosides, diltiazem, verapamil: hypotension, bradycardia, and increased depressant effect on myocardium. Use together cautiously.
Cimetidine: inhibits propranolol's metabolism. Monitor for increased beta-blocking effect.
Epinephrine: severe vasoconstriction. Monitor blood pressure and observe patient carefully.
Glucagon, isoproterenol: antagonized propranolol effect. May be used therapeutically and in emergencies.
Insulin, oral antidiabetic agents: can alter requirements for these drugs in previously stabilized diabetics. Monitor for hypoglycemia.
Drug-lifestyle. *Cocaine use:* increases angina-inducing potential of cocaine. Do not use together.

Contraindications and precautions

• Contraindicated in patients with bronchial asthma, sinus bradycardia, heart block greater than first-degree, cardiogenic shock, and heart failure (unless failure is secondary to tachyarrhythmia that can be treated with propranolol).
• Drug use is not recommended in breast-feeding women.
• Use cautiously in patients taking other antihypertensives; in those with renal impairment, nonallergic bronchospastic diseases, hepatic disease, diabetes mellitus (drug blocks some symptoms of hypoglycemia), or thyrotoxicosis (drug may mask some signs of that disorder); and in pregnant women.
• Safety of drug has not been established in children.

NURSING CONSIDERATIONS

Assessment
• Assess patient's condition before therapy and regularly thereafter.
• Monitor blood pressure, ECG, and heart rate and rhythm frequently, especially during I.V. administration.
• Be alert for adverse reactions and drug interactions.

• Evaluate patient's and family's knowledge of drug therapy.

⊞ Nursing diagnoses
• Altered health maintenance related to underlying condition
• Impaired gas exchange related to airway resistance
• Knowledge deficit related to drug therapy

⊠ Planning and implementation
• Always check patient's apical pulse before giving drug. If extremes in pulse rates occur, withhold drug and call doctor immediately.
• Double-check dose and route. I.V. doses are much smaller than oral doses.
P.O. use: Give drug consistently with meals. Food may increase absorption of propranolol.
I.V. use: Give drug by direct injection into large vessel or into I.V. line containing free-flowing, compatible solution; continuous I.V. infusion generally is not recommended. Alternatively, dilute drug with 0.9% NaCl and give by intermittent infusion over 10 to 15 minutes in 0.1- to 0.2-mg increments. Drug is compatible with D_5W, 0.45% and 0.9% NaCl, and lactated Ringer's solution.
• Don't discontinue drug before surgery for pheochromocytoma. Before any surgical procedure, notify anesthesiologist that patient is receiving propranolol.
• Notify doctor if patient develops severe hypotension; vasopressor may be prescribed.
• Know that elderly patient may experience enhanced adverse reactions and may need dosage adjustment.
• Do not discontinue drug abruptly.
• For overdose, give I.V. isoproterenol, I.V. atropine, or glucagon; refractory cases may require pacemaker.
Patient teaching
• Teach patient how to check pulse rate and to do so before each dose. Tell him to notify doctor if significant change occurs in pulse rate.

• Tell patient that taking drug twice daily or as extended-release capsule may improve compliance. Check with doctor.
• Advise patient to continue taking drug as prescribed, even when he's feeling well. Tell him not to discontinue drug suddenly because this can exacerbate angina and MI.

⊠ Evaluation
• Patient responds well to therapy.
• Patient maintains adequate gas exchange.
• Patient and family state understanding of drug therapy.

---

propylthiouracil (PTU)
(proh-pil-thigh-oh-YOOR-uh-sil)
Propyl-Thyracil♦

Pharmacologic class: thyroid hormone antagonist
Therapeutic class: antihyperthyroid agent
Pregnancy risk category: D

How supplied
Tablets: 50 mg, 100 mg♦

Pharmacokinetics
Absorption: about 80% of drug is absorbed rapidly and readily from GI tract.
Distribution: drug appears to be concentrated in thyroid gland. About 75% to 80% of drug is protein-bound.
Metabolism: metabolized rapidly in the liver.
Excretion: about 35% excreted in urine.
Half-life: 1 to 2 hours.

Route	Onset	Peak	Duration
P.O.	Unknown	1-1.5 hr	Unknown

Pharmacodynamics
Chemical effect: inhibits oxidation of iodine in thyroid gland, blocking iodine's ability to combine with tyrosine to form T_4, and may prevent coupling of mono-

---

iodotyrosine and diiodotyrosine to form T_4 and T_3.
Therapeutic effect: lowers thyroid hormone level.

Indications and dosage

▶ **Hyperthyroidism.** *Adults:* 100 to 150 mg P.O. t.i.d.; up to 1,200 mg daily have been used in severe cases. Maintenance dosage is 100 to 150 mg once daily in divided doses t.i.d. *Children over age 10:* 150 to 300 mg P.O. daily in divided doses t.i.d. Maintenance dosage is determined by patient response. *Children ages 6 to 10:* 50 to 150 mg P.O. daily in divided doses t.i.d. Maintenance dosage is determined by patient response.
▶ **Thyrotoxic crisis.** *Adults and children:* 200 to 400 mg P.O. q 4 to 6 hours on first day; after symptoms are under control, dosage is gradually reduced to usual maintenance levels.

Adverse reactions

CNS: headache, drowsiness, vertigo.
CV: vasculitis.
EENT: visual disturbances.
GI: diarrhea, *nausea, vomiting* (may be dose-related), salivary gland enlargement, loss of taste.
Hematologic: *agranulocytosis, thrombocytopenia, aplastic anemia,* leukopenia.
Hepatic: jaundice, *hepatotoxicity.*
Musculoskeletal: arthralgia, myalgia.
Skin: rash, urticaria, skin discoloration, pruritus.
Other: drug-induced fever, lymphadenopathy; dose-related hypothyroidism (mental depression; cold intolerance; hard, nonpitting edema).

Interactions

Drug-drug. *Aminophylline, oxtriphylline, theophylline:* decreased clearance. Dosage may need adjusted.
Anticoagulants: anticoagulants may be increased. Monitor PT, PTT, or INR.

Cardiac glycosides: increased serum levels of glycosides. May need to decrease dose.
Potassium iodide: may decrease response to drug. May need to increase dose of antithyroid drug.

Contraindications and precautions

• Contraindicated in patients hypersensitive to drug or in breast-feeding women.
• Use cautiously in pregnant women.

NURSING CONSIDERATIONS

✎ Assessment
• Assess patient's condition before therapy and regularly thereafter.
• Watch for signs of hypothyroidism (depression; cold intolerance; hard, nonpitting edema); adjust dosage as ordered.
• Monitor CBC as ordered to detect impending leukopenia, thrombocytopenia, and agranulocytosis.
• Be alert for adverse reactions.
• Monitor patient's hydration status if adverse GI reactions occur.
• Evaluate patient's and family's knowledge of drug therapy.

⊕ Nursing diagnoses
• Altered health maintenance related to thyroid condition
• Risk for fluid volume deficit related to adverse GI reactions
• Knowledge deficit related to drug therapy

❯ Planning and implementation
• Give drug with meals to reduce adverse GI reactions.
• Know that pregnant woman may require less drug as pregnancy progresses. Monitor thyroid function studies closely. Thyroid may be added to regimen. Drug may be stopped during last few weeks of pregnancy.
• Discontinue drug if severe rash or enlarged cervical lymph nodes develop and notify doctor.
• Store drug in light-resistant container.

Patient teaching
• Warn patient to report skin eruptions (sign of hypersensitivity) and fever, sore throat, or mouth sores (early signs of agranulocytosis).
• Tell patient to ask doctor about using iodized salt and eating shellfish.
• Warn patient against OTC cough medicines; many contain iodine.

☑ **Evaluation**
• Patient's thyroid hormone level is normal.
• Patient maintains adequate hydration.
• Patient and family state understanding of drug therapy.

protamine sulfate
(PROH-tuh-meen SUL-fayt)

Pharmacologic class: antidote
Therapeutic class: heparin antagonist
Pregnancy risk category: C

How supplied
Injection: 10 mg/ml

Pharmacokinetics
Absorption: not applicable.
Distribution: unknown.
Metabolism: unknown, although it appears to be partially degraded, with release of some heparin.
Excretion: unknown.

Route	Onset	Peak	Duration
I.V.	30-60 sec	Unknown	2 hr

Pharmacodynamics
Chemical effect: forms inert complex with heparin sodium.
Therapeutic effect: blocks heparin's effects.

Indications and dosage
▶ **Heparin overdose.** *Adults:* dosage based on venous blood coagulation studies, usually 1 mg for each 90 to 115 units

of heparin. Give by slow I.V. injection over 1 to 3 minutes, not to exceed 50 mg in any 10-minute period.

Adverse reactions
CV: fall in blood pressure, bradycardia, *circulatory collapse.*
Respiratory: dyspnea, *pulmonary edema, acute pulmonary hypertension.*
Other: transitory flushing, feeling of warmth, *anaphylaxis, anaphylactoid reactions.*

Interactions
None significant.

Contraindications and precautions
• Contraindicated in patients with hypersensitivity to drug.
• Use cautiously after cardiac surgery and in pregnant or breast-feeding women.
• Safety of drug has not been established in children.

NURSING CONSIDERATIONS

🝔 **Assessment**
• Obtain assessment of patient's heparin overdose before therapy.
• Monitor patient continually. Check vital signs frequently.
• Watch for spontaneous bleeding (heparin "rebound"), especially in patients undergoing dialysis and in those who have undergone cardiac surgery. Protamine sulfate may act as anticoagulant in very high doses.
• Evaluate patient's and family's knowledge of drug therapy.

🝔 **Nursing diagnoses**
• Altered protection related to heparin overdose
• Risk for injury related to anaphylaxis
• Knowledge deficit related to drug therapy

🝔 **Planning and implementation**
• Calculate dosage carefully. One mg of protamine neutralizes 90 to 115 units of

heparin depending on salt (heparin calcium or heparin sodium) and source of heparin (beef or pork).
• Give drug slowly by direct injection. Be prepared to treat shock.
Patient teaching
• Instruct patient to report adverse reactions immediately.

☑ **Evaluation**
• Patient does not experience injury.
• Patient and family state understanding of drug therapy.

---

pseudoephedrine hydrochloride
(soo-doh-eh-FED-rin high-droh-KLOR-ighd)
Cenafed†, Children's Sudafed Liquid†, Deco-fed†, De Fed-60†, Dorcol Children's Decongestant†, Drixoral Non-Drowsy Formula†, Efidac/24†, Eltor 120♦†, Genaphed†, Halofed†, Halofed Adult Strength†, Maxenal♦†, Myfedrine†, Novafed†, PediaCare Infants' Oral Decongestant Drops†, Pseudo†, Pseudo-frin♦, Pseudogest†, Robidrine♦†, Sudafed†, Sudafed 12 Hour†, Sudafed-60†, Sufedrin†

pseudoephedrine sulfate
Afrin†, Drixoral♦

Pharmacologic class: adrenergic
Therapeutic class: decongestant
Pregnancy risk category: C

How supplied

pseudoephedrine hydrochloride
Tablets: 30 mg†, 60 mg†
Tablets (extended-release): 120 mg†, 240 mg†
Capsules: 60 mg
Capsules (extended-release): 20 mg
Oral solution: 15 mg/5 ml , 30 mg/5 ml , 7.5 mg/0.8 ml
Syrup: 30 mg/5 ml

pseudoephedrine sulfate
Tablets (extended-release): 120 mg (60 mg immediate-release, 60 mg delayed-release)

Pharmacokinetics

Absorption: unknown.
Distribution: widely distributed throughout body.
Metabolism: incompletely metabolized in liver to inactive compounds.
Excretion: excreted in urine; rate is accelerated with acidic urine.

Route	Onset	Peak	Duration
P.O.	15-30 min	30-60 min	3-12 hr

Pharmacodynamics

Chemical effect: stimulates alpha-adrenergic receptors in respiratory tract, resulting in vasoconstriction.
Therapeutic effect: acts to relieve congestion of nasal and eustachian tube.

Indications and dosage

▶ **Nasal and eustachian tube decongestion.** *Adults and children age 12 and older:* 60 mg P.O. q 4 to 6 hours. Maximum dosage is 240 mg daily. Or, 120 mg extended-release tablet P.O. q 12 hours or 240 mg extended-release (Efidac/24) once daily. *Children ages 6 to 11:* 30 mg P.O. regular-release form q 4 to 6 hours. Maximum dosage is 120 mg daily. *Children ages 2 to 5:* 15 mg P.O. regular-release form q 4 to 6 hours. Maximum dosage is 60 mg/day.

Adverse reactions

CNS: *anxiety,* transient stimulation, tremor, dizziness, headache, insomnia, *nervousness.*
CV: arrhythmias, *palpitations,* tachycardia.
GI: anorexia, nausea, vomiting, dry mouth.
GU: difficulty urinating.
Respiratory: respiratory difficulty.
Skin: pallor.

Interactions

Drug-drug. *Antihypertensives:* may attenuate hypotensive effect. Monitor closely.
MAO inhibitors: may cause severe hypertension (hypertensive crisis). Avoid concomitant use.

Contraindications and precautions

• Contraindicated in patients with severe hypertension or severe coronary artery disease, in those receiving MAO inhibitors, and in breast-feeding women. Extended-release preparations are contraindicated in children under age 12.
• Use cautiously in patients with hypertension, cardiac disease, diabetes, glaucoma, hyperthyroidism, and prostatic hyperplasia.

NURSING CONSIDERATIONS

⚐ Assessment
• Assess patient's condition before therapy and regularly thereafter.
• Be alert for adverse reactions and drug interactions.
• Be aware that elderly patients are more sensitive to drug's effects.
• Evaluate patient's and family's knowledge of drug therapy.

⊞ Nursing diagnoses
• Altered health maintenance related to congestion
• Sleep pattern disturbance related to drug-induced insomnia
• Knowledge deficit related to drug therapy

⊠ Planning and implementation
• Do not crush or break extended-release forms.
• Give last dose at least 2 hours before bedtime to minimize insomnia.
Patient teaching
• Warn patient against using OTC products containing other sympathomimetics.

• Tell patient not to take drug within 2 hours of bedtime because it can cause insomnia.
• Tell patient to relieve dry mouth with sugarless gum or hard candy.
• Tell patient to stop drug if he becomes unusually restless and to notify doctor promptly.

☑ Evaluation
• Patient's congestion is relieved.
• Patient and family state understanding of drug therapy.

---

psyllium
(SIL-ee-um)
Alramucil†, Cillium†, Fiberall†, Hydrocil Instant†, Konsyl†, Metamucil†, Metamucil Instant Mix†, Metamucil Sugar-Free†, Modane Bulk†, Naturacil†, Perdiem, Prodiem Plain♦†, Pro-Lax†, Reguloid†, Serutan†, Siblin†, Syllact†, V-Lax†

Pharmacologic class: adsorbent
Therapeutic class: bulk laxative
Pregnancy risk category: NR

How supplied

Chewable pieces: 1.7 g/piece†
Effervescent powder: 3.4 g/packet†, 3.7 g/packet†
Granules: 2.5 g/tsp†, 4.03 g/tsp†
Powder: 3.3 g/tsp†, 3.4 g/tsp†, 3.5 g/tsp†, 4.94 g/tsp†
Wafers: 3.4 g/wafer†

Pharmacokinetics

Absorption: none.
Distribution: distributed locally in GI tract.
Metabolism none.
Excretion: excreted in feces.

Route	Onset	Peak	Duration
P.O.	12-24 hr	≤ 3 days	Varies

Pharmacodynamics

Chemical effect: absorbs water and expands to increase bulk and moisture content of stool, thus encouraging peristalsis and bowel movement.
Therapeutic effect: relieves constipation.

Indications and dosage

▶ **Constipation, bowel management, irritable bowel syndrome.** *Adults:* 1 to 2 rounded teaspoonfuls P.O. in full glass of liquid once daily, b.i.d., or t.i.d., followed by second glass of liquid; 1 packet dissolved in water once daily, b.i.d., or t.i.d.; or 2 wafers b.i.d. or t.i.d. *Children over age 6:* 1 level teaspoonful P.O. in half a glass of liquid h.s.

Adverse reactions

GI: nausea, vomiting, diarrhea (with excessive use); esophageal, gastric, small intestinal, or colonic strictures (with dry form); abdominal cramps (in severe constipation).

Interactions

None significant.

Contraindications and precautions

• Contraindicated in patients with intestinal obstruction or ulceration, disabling adhesions, or difficulty swallowing, hypersensitivity to drug, or abdominal pain, nausea, vomiting, or other symptoms of appendicitis.
• Use cautiously in pregnant or breast-feeding women.

NURSING CONSIDERATIONS

⚖ Assessment
• Assess patient's condition before therapy and regularly thereafter.
• Before giving for constipation, determine if patient has adequate fluid intake, exercise, and diet.
• Be alert for adverse reactions.
• Evaluate patient's and family's knowledge of drug therapy.

⊞ Nursing diagnoses
• Constipation related to underlying condition
• Pain related to abdominal cramps
• Knowledge deficit related to drug therapy

❯ Planning and implementation
• Mix drug with at least 8 oz (240 ml) of cold, pleasant-tasting liquid, such as orange juice, to mask grittiness, and stir only a few seconds. Have patient drink mixture immediately so it does not congeal. Follow with additional glass of liquid.
• For dosages in children under age 6, consult doctor.
• Know that drug may reduce appetite if taken before meals.
• Drug is not absorbed systemically and is nontoxic. It is especially useful in debilitated patients and those with postpartum constipation, irritable bowel syndrome, and diverticular disease. Also useful to treat chronic laxative abuse and with other laxatives to empty colon before barium enema examinations.
Patient teaching
• Teach patient how to properly mix drug. To enhance effect and prevent intestinal obstruction, tell him to take drug with plenty of water. Advise him that inhaling powder may cause allergic reactions.
• Tell patient that laxative effect usually occurs in 12 to 24 hours, but may be delayed up to 3 days.
• Advise diabetic patient to check label and use brand of drug that does not contain sugar.
• Teach patient about dietary sources of bulk, including bran and other cereals, fresh fruit, and vegetables.

☑ Evaluation
• Patient's constipation is relieved.
• Patient's abdominal cramping is minimal and tolerable.
• Patient and family state understanding of drug therapy.

---

*Liquid form contains alcohol   **May contain tartrazine   ◆Canada   ◇Australia   †OTC

pyrantel embonate
(peer-AN-tul EM-boh-nayt)
Anthel♦, Combantrin♦, Early Bird♦

pyrantel pamoate
Antiminth, Combantrin♦, Pin-Rid†,
Reese's Pinworm Medicine

Pharmacologic class: pyrimidine derivative
Therapeutic class: anthelmintic
Pregnancy risk category: NR

How supplied

pyrantel embonate
Tablets: 125 mg♦, 250 mg♦
Oral suspension: 50 mg/ml♦
Granules: 100 mg/g♦
Squares (chocolate-flavored): 100 mg♦
pyrantel pamoate
Tablets: 125 mg♦
Capsules: 180 mg†
Oral suspension: 50 mg/ml

Pharmacokinetics

Absorption: poorly absorbed.
Distribution: unknown.
Metabolism: small amount partially metabolized in liver.
Excretion: over 50% excreted in feces; about 7% excreted in urine.

Route	Onset	Peak	Duration
P.O.	Varies	1-3 hr	Varies

Pharmacodynamics

Chemical effect: blocks neuromuscular action, paralyzing worm and causing its expulsion by normal peristalsis.
Therapeutic effect: relieves roundworm and pinworm infestation. Spectrum of activity includes *Enterobius vermicularis, Ascaris lumbricoides, Ancylostoma duodenale, Necator americanus,* and *Trichostrongylus orientalis.*

Indications and dosage

► **Roundworm and pinworm.** *Adults and children over age 2:* 11 mg/kg P.O.
given as single dose. Maximum dosage is 1 g. For pinworm, dosage should be repeated in 2 weeks.

Adverse reactions

CNS: headache, dizziness, drowsiness, insomnia, weakness.
GI: anorexia, nausea, vomiting, gastralgia, cramps, diarrhea, tenesmus.
Hepatic: transient elevation of AST.
Skin: rash.
Other: fever.

Interactions

Drug-drug. *Piperazine salts:* possible antagonism. Don't give together.

Contraindications and precautions

• Contraindicated in patients with hypersensitivity to drug.
• Use cautiously in patients with hepatic dysfunction or severe malnutrition or anemia and in pregnant women.
• Safety of drug has not been established in breast-feeding women.

NURSING CONSIDERATIONS

⚱ Assessment
• Assess patient's condition before therapy and regularly thereafter.
• Be alert for adverse reactions and drug interactions.
• Monitor patient's hydration status if adverse GI reactions occur.
• Evaluate patient's and family's knowledge of drug therapy.

⊕ Nursing diagnoses
• Infection related to worm infestation
• Risk for fluid volume deficit related to adverse GI reactions
• Knowledge deficit related to drug therapy

▷ Planning and implementation
• Be aware that no dietary restrictions, laxatives, or enemas are needed.

Reactions may be *common,* uncommon, *life-threatening,* or COMMON AND LIFE-THREATENING.

• Drug should be administered to all family members, as prescribed, to prevent risk of spreading infection.
• Drug may be taken with food, milk, or fruit juices. Shake suspension well.

Patient teaching
• Tell patient to shake suspension form well before administration. Inform patient that drug may be taken with food or beverages.
• Teach patient about personal hygiene, especially good hand-washing technique. To avoid reinfection, teach him to wash perianal area daily, to change undergarments and bedclothes daily, and to wash hands and clean fingernails before meals and after bowel movements. Advise patient to refrain from preparing food for others during infestation.

☑ Evaluation
• Patient is free from infestation.
• Patient maintains adequate hydration.
• Patient and family state understanding of drug therapy.

---

pyrazinamide
(peer-uh-ZIN-uh-mighd)
pms-Pyrazinamide♦, Tebrazid♦, Zinamide♦

Pharmacologic class: synthetic pyrazine analogue of nicotinamide
Therapeutic class: antituberculosis agent
Pregnancy risk category: C

How supplied

Tablets: 500 mg

Pharmacokinetics

Absorption: absorbed well.
Distributed: distributed widely into body tissues and fluids, including lungs, liver, and CSF. Drug is 50% protein-bound.
Metabolism: hydrolyzed in liver and in stomach.
Excretion: excreted almost completely in urine. *Half-life:* 9 to 10 hours.

Route	Onset	Peak	Duration
P.O.	Unknown	1-2 hr	Unknown

Pharmacodynamics

Chemical effect: unknown.
Therapeutic effect: helps eradicate tuberculosis. Spectrum of activity is only *Mycobacterium tuberculosis.*

Indications and dosage

▶ **Adjunct treatment of tuberculosis (when primary and secondary antitubercular drugs cannot be used or have failed).** *Adults:* 15 to 30 mg/kg P.O. once daily, not to exceed 3 g/day. Or, twice-weekly dose of 50 to 70 mg/kg (based on lean body weight) to promote compliance. Dosage adjustment recommended in renal failure.

Adverse reactions

CNS: malaise
GI: anorexia, nausea, vomiting, diarrhea.
GU: dysuria.
Hematologic: sideroblastic anemia, *thrombocytopenia.*
Hepatic: *hepatitis.*
Metabolic: interference with control in diabetes mellitus, *hyperuricemia.*
Other: fever, arthralgia.

Interactions

None significant.

Contraindications and precautions

• Contraindicated in patients with severe hepatic disease or hypersensitivity to drug.
• Use cautiously in patients with diabetes mellitus, renal failure, or gout, and in pregnant women.
• Safety not established in children and in breast-feeding women.

NURSING CONSIDERATIONS

☲ Assessment
• Assess patient's condition before therapy and regularly thereafter.

• Monitor hematopoietic studies and serum uric acid levels, as ordered.

• Monitor liver function studies; examine for jaundice and liver tenderness or enlargement before and frequently during therapy.

• Watch closely for signs of gout and of liver impairment.

• Monitor patient's hydration status if adverse GI reactions occur.

• Evaluate patient's and family's knowledge of drug therapy.

🔯 **Nursing diagnoses**

• Infection related to tuberculosis

• Risk for fluid volume deficit related to adverse GI reactions

• Knowledge deficit related to drug therapy

▶ **Planning and implementation**

• Be aware that drug should always be administered with other antitubercular agents to prevent development of resistant organisms.

• Keep in mind that reduced dosage is needed in patients with renal impairment because nearly 100% of drug is excreted in urine.

• Question doses that exceed 35 mg/kg; they may cause liver damage.

• Notify doctor at once if liver dysfunction is suspected.

• Be aware that when drug is used with surgical management of tuberculosis, it is started 1 to 2 weeks before surgery and continued for 4 to 6 weeks after.

• Know that patients with concomitant HIV infection may require longer course.

Patient teaching

• Stress importance of taking drug exactly as prescribed; warn patient against discontinuing drug without doctor's approval.

• Teach patient to watch for and immediately report signs of gout and hepatic impairment.

✅ **Evaluation**

• Patient is free from infection.

• Patient maintains adequate hydration.

• Patient and family state understanding of drug therapy.

pyridostigmine bromide
(peer-ih-doh-STIG-meen BROH-mighd)
Mestinon*, Mestinon-SR♦, Mestinon Timespans, Regonol

Pharmacologic class: cholinesterase inhibitor
Therapeutic class: muscle stimulant
Pregnancy risk category: NR

How supplied

Tablets: 60 mg
Tablets (extended-release): 180 mg
Syrup: 60 mg/5 ml
Injection: 5 mg/ml in 2-ml ampules or 5-ml vials

Pharmacokinetics

Absorption: poorly absorbed from GI tract.
Distribution: unknown.
Metabolism: unknown.
Excretion: excreted in urine.

Route	Onset	Peak	Duration
P.O.	20-60 min	1-2 hr	3-12 hr
I.V.	2-5 min	Unknown	2-3 hr
I.M.	15 min	Unknown	2-3 hr

Pharmacodynamics

Chemical effect: inhibits destruction of acetylcholine released from parasympathetic and somatic efferent nerves. Acetylcholine accumulates, promoting increased stimulation of receptor.
Therapeutic effect: reverses effect of nondepolarizing neuromuscular blocking agents and myasthenia gravis.

Indications and dosage

▶ **Antidote for nondepolarizing neuromuscular blocking agents.** *Adults:* 10 to 20 mg I.V. preceded by atropine sulfate 0.6 to 1.2 mg I.V.

Reactions may be *common*, uncommon, *life-threatening*, or COMMON AND LIFE-THREATENING.

► **Myasthenia gravis.** *Adults:* 60 to 120 mg P.O. t.i.d. Usual dosage is 600 mg daily but higher dosage may be needed (up to 1,500 mg daily). For I.M. or I.V. use, 1/30 of oral dosage is given. Dosage must be adjusted for each patient, depending on response and tolerance. Alternatively, 180 to 540 mg timed-release tablets (1 to 3 tablets) P.O. b.i.d., with at least 6 hours between doses. *Children:* 7 mg/kg or 200 mg/m² daily in five or six divided doses.

► **Supportive treatment of neonates born to myasthenic mothers.** *Neonates:* 0.05 to 0.15 mg/kg I.M. q 4 to 6 hours. Dosage decreased daily until drug can be withdrawn.

Adverse reactions

CNS: headache (with high doses), weakness, sweating, *seizures.*
CV: bradycardia, hypotension, thrombophlebitis.
EENT: miosis.
GI: abdominal cramps, nausea, vomiting, diarrhea, excessive salivation.
Musculoskeletal: muscle cramps, muscle fasciculations.
Respiratory: *bronchospasm, bronchoconstriction,* increased bronchial secretions.
Skin: rash.

Interactions

Drug-drug. *Aminoglycosides, anesthetics:* may decrease response to drug. Use together cautiously.
Anticholinergic agents, atropine, corticosteroids, magnesium, procainamide, quinidine: may antagonize cholinergic effects. Observe for lack of drug effect.
Ganglionic blockers: increased risk of hypotension. Monitor closely.

Contraindications and precautions

• Contraindicated in patients hypersensitive to anticholinesterase agents and in those with mechanical obstruction of intestine or urinary tract.

• Use cautiously in patients with bronchial asthma, bradycardia, and arrhythmias.
• Safety of drug has not been established in pregnant or breast-feeding women.

NURSING CONSIDERATIONS

⬚ Assessment
• Assess patient's condition before therapy and regularly thereafter.
• Monitor and document patient's response after each dose. Optimum dosage is difficult to judge.
• Monitor patient's vital signs, especially respirations.
• Be alert for adverse reactions and drug interactions.
• Evaluate patient's and family's knowledge of drug therapy.

⬚ Nursing diagnoses
• Impaired physical mobility related to underlying condition
• Ineffective breathing pattern related to adverse respiratory reactions
• Knowledge deficit related to drug therapy

⬚ Planning and implementation
• Stop all other cholinergics before giving drug, as ordered.
P.O. use: Don't crush timed-release tablets.
• When using sweet syrup for patient who has difficulty swallowing, give over ice chips if he can't tolerate flavor.
I.V. use: Administer I.V. injection no faster than 1 mg/minute. If I.V. administration is too rapid, bradycardia and seizures may result.
I.M. use: Follow normal protocol.
• Position patient to ease breathing. Have atropine injection readily available; provide respiratory support as needed.
• If patient's muscle weakness is severe, keep in mind that doctor determines if it is caused by drug-induced toxicity or exacerbation of myasthenia gravis. Test dose of edrophonium I.V. will aggravate drug-

induced weakness, but will temporarily relieve weakness caused by disease.
• The United States formulation of Regonol contains benzyl ethanol preservative that may cause toxicity in neonates if administered in high doses. The Canadian formulation of this drug does not contain benzyl ethanol.
• If appropriate, obtain doctor's order for hospitalized patient to have bedside supply of tablets. Patients with long-standing disease often insist on self-administration.
Patient teaching
• When using for myasthenia gravis, stress importance of taking drug exactly as ordered, on time, in evenly spaced doses. If doctor has ordered extended-release tablets, explain that patient must take tablets at same time each day, at least 6 hours apart. Tell him that he may have to take drug for life.
• Advise patient to carry medical identification at all times.

☑ Evaluation
• Patient exhibits improved physical mobility.
• Patient maintains adequate respiratory pattern.
• Patient and family state understanding of drug therapy.

pyridoxine hydrochloride (vitamin B₆)
(peer-ih-DOKS-een high-droh-KLOR-ighd)
Beesix, Nestrex†, Rodex

Pharmacologic class: water-soluble vitamin
Therapeutic class: nutritional supplement
Pregnancy risk category: A

How supplied

Tablets: 10 mg†, 25 mg†, 50 mg†, 100 mg†, 200 mg†, 250 mg†, 500 mg†
Tablets (timed-release): 100 mg
Capsules: 500 mg
Capsules (timed-release): 100 mg
Injection: 100 mg/ml

Pharmacokinetics

Absorption: drug and its substituents are absorbed readily from GI tract. Absorption may be diminished in patients with malabsorption syndromes or following gastric resection.
Distribution: drug is stored mainly in liver.
Metabolism: metabolized in liver.
Excretion: in erythrocytes, pyridoxine is converted to pyridoxal phosphate, and pyridoxamine is converted to pyridoxamine phosphate. The phosphorylated form of pyridoxine is transaminated to pyridoxal and pyridoxamine, which is phosphorylated rapidly. The conversion of pyridoxine phosphate to pyridoxal phosphate requires riboflavin. *Half-life:* 15 to 20 days.

Route	Onset	Peak	Duration
P.O, I.V., I.M.	Unknown	Unknown	Unknown

Pharmacodynamics

Chemical effect: acts as coenzyme that stimulates various metabolic functions, including amino acid metabolism.
Therapeutic effect: raises pyridoxine levels, prevents and relieves seizure activity related to pyridoxine deficiency or dependency, and blocks effects of isoniazid poisoning.

Indications and dosage

▶ **RDA.** *Neonates and infants up to 6 months:* 0.3 mg. *Infants ages 6 months to 1 year:* 0.6 mg. *Children ages 1 to 3:* 1 mg. *Children ages 4 to 6:* 1.1 mg. *Children ages 7 to 10:* 1.4 mg. *Males ages 11 to 14:* 1.7 mg. *Males age 15 and over:* 2 mg. *Females ages 11 to 14:* 1.4 mg. *Females ages 15 to 18:* 1.5 mg. *Females age 19 and over:* 1.6 mg. *Pregnant women:* 2.2 mg. *Breast-feeding women:* 2.1 mg.
▶ **Dietary vitamin B₆ deficiency.** *Adults:* 2.5 to 10 mg P.O., I.M., or I.V.

daily for 3 weeks, then 2 to 5 mg daily as supplement to proper diet.
▶ **Seizures related to vitamin B₆ deficiency or dependency.** *Adults and children:* 10 to 100 mg I.M. or I.V. in single dose.
▶ **Vitamin B₆-responsive anemias or dependency syndrome (inborn errors of metabolism).** *Adults:* up to 600 mg/day I.M., P.O., or I.V. until symptoms subside, then 30 mg/day for life.
▶ **Prevention of vitamin B₆ deficiency during drug therapy.** *Adults:* 6 to 100 mg P.O. daily for isoniazid therapy.
▶ **Drug-induced vitamin B₆ deficiency.** *Adults:* 100 to 200 mg P.O. daily for 3 weeks, followed by 25 to 100 mg P.O. daily to prevent relapse.
▶ **Antidote for isoniazid poisoning.** *Adults:* 4 g I.V., followed by 1 g I.M. q 30 minutes until amount of pyridoxine administered equals amount of isoniazid ingested.

Adverse reactions

CNS: drowsiness, paresthesia, unstable gait.

Interactions

Drug-drug. *Levodopa:* decreased levodopa effect. Avoid concomitant use.
Phenobarbital, phenytoin: decreased anticonvulsant serum levels, increasing risk of seizures.
Drug-lifestyle. *Alcohol use:* risk of possible delirium and lactic acidosis. Avoid concomitant use.

Contraindications and precautions

• Contraindicated in patients hypersensitive to pyridoxine.

NURSING CONSIDERATIONS

⬛ Assessment
• Assess patient's condition before therapy and regularly thereafter.
• Be alert for adverse CNS reactions and drug interactions. Patient taking high doses (2 to 6 g/day) may experience diffi-

culty walking because of diminished proprioceptive and sensory function.
• Monitor patient's diet and snacking habits. Excessive protein intake increases daily drug requirements.
• Evaluate patient's and family's knowledge of drug therapy.

⬛ Nursing diagnoses
• Altered health maintenance related to underlying condition
• Risk for injury related to drug-induced adverse CNS reactions
• Knowledge deficit related to drug therapy

⬛ Planning and implementation
P.O. and I.M. use: Follow normal protocol.
I.V. use: Inject undiluted drug into I.V. line containing free-flowing compatible solution. Alternatively, infuse diluted drug over prescribed duration for intermittent infusions. Do not use for continuous infusion.
• Protect drug from light. Do not use solution if it contains precipitate, although slight darkening is acceptable.
• When using drug to treat isoniazid toxicity, expect to administer anticonvulsants.
• If sodium bicarbonate is required to control acidosis in isoniazid toxicity, do not mix in same syringe with pyridoxine.
Patient teaching
• Advise patient taking levodopa alone to avoid multivitamins containing pyridoxine because of decreased levodopa effect.
• Stress importance of compliance and of good nutrition if prescribed for maintenance therapy to prevent recurrence of deficiency. Explain that pyridoxine in combination therapy with isoniazid has specific therapeutic purpose and is not just a vitamin.

⬛ Evaluation
• Patient responds well to therapy.
• Patient does not experience injury from adverse CNS reactions.

• Patient and family state understanding of drug therapy.

---

pyrimethamine
(peer-ih-METH-uh-meen)
Daraprim

pyrimethamine with sulfadoxine
Fansidar

Pharmacologic class: aminopyrimidine derivative (folic acid antagonist)
Therapeutic class: antimalarial
Pregnancy risk category: C

How supplied
pyrimethamine
Tablets: 25 mg
pyrimethamine with sulfadoxine
Tablets: pyrimethamine 25 mg, sulfadoxine 500 mg

Pharmacokinetics
Absorption: well absorbed from intestinal tract.
Distribution: distributed to kidneys, liver, spleen, and lungs. It is about 80% bound to plasma proteins.
Metabolism: metabolized to several unidentified compounds.
Excretion: excreted in urine. *Half-life:* 2 to 6 hours.

Route	Onset	Peak	Duration
P.O.	Unknown	1.5-8 hr	Unknown

Pharmacodynamics
Chemical effect: inhibits enzyme dihydrofolate reductase, thereby impeding reduction of dihydrofolic acid to tetrahydrofolic acid. Sulfadoxine competitively inhibits use of PABA.
Therapeutic effect: prevents malaria and treats malaria and toxoplasmosis infections. Spectrum of activity includes asexual erythrocytic forms of susceptible plasmodia and *Toxoplasma gondii.*

Indications and dosage
► **Malaria prophylaxis and transmission control. Pyrimethamine.** *Adults and children over age 10:* 25 mg P.O. weekly. *Children ages 4 to 10:* 12.5 mg P.O. weekly. *Children under age 4:* 6.25 mg P.O. weekly. Needs to be continued in all age groups at least 10 weeks after leaving endemic areas.
► **Acute attacks of malaria. Fansidar.** *Adults:* 2 to 3 tablets as single dose, either alone or in sequence with quinine. *Children ages 9 to 14:* 2 tablets. *Children ages 4 to 8:* 1 tablet. *Children under age 4:* ½ tablet.
► **Malaria prophylaxis. Fansidar.** *Adults:* 1 tablet weekly, or 2 tablets q 2 weeks. *Children ages 9 to 14:* ¾ tablet weekly, or 1½ tablets q 2 weeks. *Children ages 4 to 8:* ½ tablet weekly, or 1 tablet q 2 weeks. *Children under age 4:* ¼ tablet weekly, or ½ tablet q 2 weeks.
► **Acute attacks of malaria. Pyrimethamine.** *Adults and children over age 10:* 25 mg P.O. daily for 2 days when used with faster-acting antimalarials; when used alone, 50 mg P.O. daily for 2 days. *Children ages 4 to 10:* 25 mg P.O. daily for 2 days.
► **Toxoplasmosis. Pyrimethamine.** *Adults:* initially, 50 to 75 mg P.O. daily for 1 to 3 weeks, then 25 mg P.O. daily for 4 to 5 weeks; at same time, 1 g sulfadiazine is given P.O. q 6 hours. *Children:* initially, 1 mg/kg P.O. (not to exceed 100 mg) in two equally divided doses for 2 to 4 days, then 0.5 mg/kg daily for 4 weeks, along with 100 mg sulfadiazine/kg P.O. daily, divided q 6 hours.

Adverse reactions
CNS: stimulation and seizures (acute toxicity).
GI: anorexia, vomiting, diarrhea, atrophic glossitis.
Hematologic: *agranulocytosis, aplastic anemia,* megaloblastic anemia, *bone marrow suppression, leukopenia, thrombocytopenia, pancytopenia.*

Reactions may be *common,* uncommon, *life-threatening,* or COMMON AND LIFE-THREATENING.

Skin: rash, *erythema multiforme (Stevens-Johnson syndrome), toxic epidermal necrolysis.*

Interactions

Drug-drug. *Co-trimoxazole, methotrexate, sulfonamides:* increased risk of bone marrow suppression. Don't use together. *Folic acid, PABA:* decreased antitoxoplasmic effects. May require dosage adjustment.

Contraindications and precautions

• Contraindicated in patients with hypersensitivity to drug and in those with megaloblastic anemia caused by folic acid deficiency. Fansidar is contraindicated in patients with porphyria because it contains sulfadoxine, a sulfonamide.
• Repeated use of Fansidar is contraindicated in patients with severe renal insufficiency, marked liver parenchymal damage or blood dyscrasias, known hypersensitivity to pyrimethamine or sulfonamides, or documented megaloblastic anemia due to folate deficiency; in infants under age 2 months; in pregnancy at term; and in breast-feeding women.
• Use cautiously in patients with impaired hepatic or renal function, severe allergy or bronchial asthma, or G6PD deficiency; in those with seizure disorders (smaller doses may be needed); and after treatment with chloroquine.

NURSING CONSIDERATIONS

📛 Assessment
• Assess patient's condition before therapy and regularly thereafter.
• Obtain twice-weekly blood counts, including platelets, as ordered, for patients with toxoplasmosis because dosages used approach toxic levels.
• Be alert for adverse reactions and drug interactions.
• Evaluate patient's and family's knowledge of drug therapy.

📋 Nursing diagnoses
• Infection related to presence of susceptible organism
• Altered protection related to adverse hematologic reactions
• Knowledge deficit related to drug therapy

▶ Planning and implementation
• Give drug with meals to minimize GI distress.
• If signs of folic acid or folinic acid deficiency develop, dosage should be reduced or discontinued while patient receives parenteral folinic acid (leucovorin) until blood counts become normal.
• When used to treat toxoplasmosis in patients with AIDS, therapy may last for several months. Chronic suppressive therapy for patient's lifetime may also be necessary.
• Because of possibility of severe skin reactions, Fansidar should be used only in regions where chloroquine-resistant malaria is prevalent and only when traveler plans to stay in region longer than 3 weeks.

Patient teaching
• Advise patient to take drug with food.
• Teach patient to watch for and immediately report signs of folic or folinic acid deficiency and acute toxicity.
• Warn patient taking Fansidar to stop drug and notify doctor at first sign of rash.
• Instruct patient to take first prophylactic dose of Fansidar 1 to 2 days before traveling to endemic area.

✔ Evaluation
• Patient is free from infection.
• Patient maintains normal hematologic parameters.
• Patient and family state understanding of drug therapy.

quazepam
(KWAZ-uh-pam)
Doral

Pharmacologic class: benzodiazepine
Therapeutic class: hypnotic
Controlled substance schedule: IV
Pregnancy risk category: X

How supplied
Tablets: 7.5 mg, 15 mg

Pharmacokinetics
Absorption: well absorbed from GI tract.
Distribution: more than 95% bound to plasma proteins.
Metabolism: metabolized in liver.
Excretion: excreted in urine and feces.
Half-life: 39 hours for parent drug and active metabolite 2-oxoquazepam; 733 hours for active metabolite *N*-desalkyl-2-oxoquazepam.

Route	Onset	Peak	Duration
P.O.	Unknown	About 2 hr	Unknown

Pharmacodynamics
Chemical effect: unknown, although drug acts on limbic system and thalamus of CNS by binding to specific benzodiazepine receptors.
Therapeutic effect: induces sleep.

Indications and dosage
▶ **Insomnia.** *Adults:* 15 mg P.O. h.s. Patient may respond to lower dosage. Dosage decreased in elderly patients after 2 days of therapy, if possible.

Adverse reactions
CNS: fatigue, dizziness, daytime drowsiness, headache.
CV: palpitations, chest pain.
GI: dry mouth, dyspepsia.

Other: physical and psychological dependence.

Interactions
Drug-drug. *Anticonvulsants, antihistamines, psychotropic drugs, other drugs that produce CNS depression:* additive CNS depressant effects. Avoid concomitant use.
Drug-lifestyle. *Alcohol use:* additive CNS depressant effects. Avoid concomitant use.

Contraindications and precautions
• Contraindicated in patients with hypersensitivity to drug or other benzodiazepines, in those with suspected or established sleep apnea; and in pregnant women.
• Drug is not recommended for use in breast-feeding women.
• Use cautiously in patients with hepatic, renal, or respiratory disease or depression and in elderly patients.
• Safety of drug has not been established in children.

NURSING CONSIDERATIONS

Assessment
• Assess patient's insomnia before therapy and regularly thereafter.
• Be alert for adverse CNS reactions and drug interactions.
• Evaluate patient's and family's knowledge of drug therapy.

Nursing diagnoses
• Sleep pattern disturbance related to presence of insomnia
• Fatigue related to drug-induced adverse CNS reactions
• Knowledge deficit related to drug therapy

Planning and implementation
• Before leaving bedside, make sure patient has swallowed drug.
• Prevent hoarding or self-overdosing by patient who is depressed, suicidal, or

drug-dependent or who has a history of drug abuse.
• Patient on long-term therapy may experience withdrawal symptoms if drug is suddenly withdrawn (possibly after 6 weeks of continuous therapy).
Patient teaching
• Warn patient to avoid tasks that require mental alertness or physical coordination.
• Caution patient not to increase dosage but to tell doctor if drug isn't effective.
• Warn patient that additive depression can occur if alcohol is consumed within 24 hours of drug.

☑ **Evaluation**
• Patient states that drug is effective in inducing sleep.
• Patient shows ways to conserve energy to cope with fatigue.
• Patient and family state understanding of drug therapy.

quetiapine fumarate
(KWET-ee-uh-peen FYOO-muh-rayt)
Seroquel

Pharmacologic class: dibenzothiazepine derivative
Therapeutic class: antipsychotic
Pregnancy risk category: C

How supplied
Tablets: 25 mg, 100 mg, 200 mg

Pharmacokinetics
Absorption: rapid following oral administration; 100% bioavailable.
Distribution: widely distributed throughout body; 83% bound to plasma protein.
Metabolism: extensively metabolized by liver to inactive metabolites.
Excretion: about 73% is recovered in urine; 20% is recovered in feces. *Half-life:* 6 hours.

Route	Onset	Peak	Duration
P.O.	Unknown	1.5 hr	Unknown

Pharmacodynamics
Chemical effect: exact mechanism of action is unknown, but drug is thought to exert antipsychotic activity through blocking dopamine D-2 receptors and serotonin 5-HT$_2$ receptors in the brain and may also act at histamine H$_1$ receptors and adrenergic alpha$_1$ receptors.
Therapeutic effect: improves symptoms associated with psychotic disorders.

Indications and dosages
▶ **Management of the manifestations of psychotic disorders.** *Adults:* initially, 25 mg b.i.d., with increases in increments of 25 to 50 mg b.i.d. or t.i.d. on days 2 and 3, as tolerated. Target dose range of 300 to 400 mg daily, divided into two or three doses, by day 4. Further dosage adjustments, if indicated, should generally occur at intervals of not less than 2 days. Dosages can be increased or decreased by 25 to 50 mg b.i.d. Antipsychotic efficacy is generally in dose range of 150 to 750 mg/day. Safety of doses above 800 mg/day has not been evaluated.

Adverse reactions
CNS: asthenia, *dizziness, headache, somnolence,* hypertonia, dysarthria.
CV: postural hypotension, tachycardia, palpitations, peripheral edema.
EENT: pharyngitis, rhinitis, ear pain.
GI: dry mouth, dyspepsia, abdominal pain, constipation, anorexia.
Hematologic: *leukopenia.*
Metabolic: *weight gain.*
Respiratory: increased cough, dyspnea.
Skin: rash, sweating.
Other: back pain, fever, flulike syndrome.

Interactions
Drug-drug. *Antihypertensive agents:* increased effects. Monitor blood pressure. *Carbamazepine, glucocorticoids, phenobarbital, phenytoin, rifampin:* increased quetiapine clearance. Adjust dose as needed.

CNS depressants: increased CNS effects. Use cautiously.

Erythromycin, fluconazole, itraconazole, ketoconazole: decreased quetiapine clearance. Use cautiously.

Lorazepam: reduced clearance of lorazepam. Monitor patient.

Drug-lifestyle. *Alcohol use:* increased CNS effects. Use cautiously.

Contraindications and precautions

• Contraindicated in patients hypersensitive to drug or its ingredients.

• Use with caution in patients with CV or cerebrovascular disease or conditions that predispose them to hypotension; in those with history of seizures or conditions that lower seizure threshold; and in those who will be experiencing conditions in which core body temperature may be elevated.

NURSING CONSIDERATIONS

Assessment

• Monitor patient for tardive dyskinesia. Condition may not appear until months or years after starting drug and may disappear spontaneously or persist for life, despite discontinuation of drug.

• Monitor patient's vital signs carefully, especially during the 3- to 5-day period of initial dose titration, when re-initiating treatment, or when increasing dosages.

• Assess patient's risk for physical injury due to drug's CNS side effects.

• Be alert for adverse reactions and drug interactions.

• Evaluate patient's and family's knowledge of drug therapy.

Nursing diagnoses

• Risk for altered body temperature related to drug-induced hyperpyrexia

• Impaired physical mobility related to drug-induced CNS side effects

• Knowledge deficit related to drug therapy

Planning and implementation

• Know that elderly or debilitated patients or patients with hepatic impairment or predisposition to hypotensive reactions usually require lower initial doses and more gradual dosage titration.

• Withhold drug and notify doctor if symptoms of neuroleptic malignant syndrome occur (hyperpyrexia, muscular rigidity, altered mental status, and autonomic instability).

• Provide ice chips, drinks, or sugarless hard candy to help relieve dry mouth.

Patient teaching

• Advise patient of risk of orthostatic hypotension. Risk is greatest during 3- to 5-day period of initial dose titration, when re-initiating treatment, or when increasing dosages.

• Tell patient to avoid becoming overheated or dehydrated during therapy.

• Warn patient to avoid activities that require mental alertness such as driving a car or operating hazardous machinery until CNS effects of drug are known.

• Remind patient to have initial eye examination before starting drug therapy and every 6 months during therapy to monitor for possibility of cataract formation.

• Tell patient to notify doctor of other medications (prescription or OTC) he is taking or plans to take.

• Tell female patient to notify doctor if she becomes pregnant or intends to become pregnant during drug therapy. Advise her not to breast-feed during therapy.

• Advise patient to avoid alcohol during therapy.

Evaluation

• Patient maintains normal body temperature.

• Patient maintains physical mobility and does not experience extrapyramidal side effects of drug.

• Patient and family state understanding of drug therapy.

Reactions may be *common,* uncommon, *life-threatening,* or COMMON AND LIFE-THREATENING.

quinapril hydrochloride
(KWIN-eh-pril high-droh-KLOR-ighd)
Accupril, Asig◇

Pharmacologic class: ACE inhibitor
Therapeutic class: antihypertensive
Pregnancy risk category: C (D second and third trimesters)

How supplied
Tablets: 5 mg, 10 mg, 20 mg, 40 mg

Pharmacokinetics
Absorption: at least 60% absorbed; rate and extent drop by 25% to 30% when given with high-fat meals.
Distribution: about 97% of drug and active metabolite are bound to plasma proteins.
Metabolism: 38% of dose de-esterified in liver to active metabolite.
Excretion: excreted primarily in urine.
Half-life: about 25 hours.

Route	Onset	Peak	Duration
P.O.	≤ 1 hr	1-2 hr	About 24 hr

Pharmacodynamics
Chemical effect: unknown; may be related to inhibition of angiotensin I to angiotensin II, which lowers peripheral arterial resistance and decreases aldosterone secretion.
Therapeutic effect: lowers blood pressure.

Indications and dosage
▶ **Hypertension.** *Adults:* initially, 10 mg P.O. daily. Dosage adjusted based on patient response at intervals of about 2 weeks. Most patients are controlled at 20, 40, or 80 mg daily as single dose or in two divided doses.
▶ **Heart failure.** *Adults:* initially, 5 mg P.O. b.i.d. if patient is receiving a diuretic and 10 mg P.O. b.i.d. if patient is not receiving a diuretic. Dosage increased at weekly intervals. Usual effective dose is 20 to 40 mg b.i.d. in equally divided doses.
▶ **Initial dose in renal patients.** *Adults:* 10 mg P.O. if creatinine clearance is over 60 ml/minute, 5 mg if it is 30 to 60 ml/minute, and 2.5 mg if it is 10 to 30 ml/minute; no dose recommendations available for level below 10 ml/minute.

Adverse reactions
CNS: somnolence, vertigo, lightheadedness, syncope, malaise, nervousness, depression.
CV: palpitations, vasodilation, tachycardia, hypertensive crisis, angina, orthostatic hypotension, *rhythm disturbances.*
EENT: dry throat.
GI: dry mouth, abdominal pain, constipation, hemorrhage.
Hepatic: elevated liver enzyme levels.
Metabolic: hyperkalemia.
Musculoskeletal: back pain.
Respiratory: dry, persistent, tickling, nonproductive cough.
Skin: pruritus, *exfoliative dermatitis, photosensitivity.*
Other: *angioedema,* diaphoresis.

Interactions
Drug-drug. *Diuretics, other antihypertensives:* risk of excessive hypotension. Expect to stop diuretic or lower dose of drug.
Lithium: increased serum lithium levels and lithium toxicity. Avoid concomitant use.
Potassium-sparing diuretics: risk of hyperkalemia. Monitor during concomitant use.
Drug-food. *Sodium substitutes containing potassium:* risk of hyperkalemia. Monitor during concomitant use.

Contraindications and precautions
● Contraindicated in patients with hypersensitivity to ACE inhibitors or with history of angioedema related to previous treatment with ACE inhibitor.
● Drug is not recommended for use in pregnant women in their second or third trimester.
● Use cautiously in patients with impaired kidney function and in breastfeeding women.

• Safety of drug has not been established in children.

NURSING CONSIDERATIONS

≋ Assessment

• Assess patient's blood pressure before therapy and regularly thereafter. Take blood pressure when drug levels are at their peak (2 to 6 hours after dosing) and at their trough (just before dosing) to verify adequate blood pressure control.

• Assess kidney and liver function before and throughout therapy.

• Monitor serum potassium levels. Risk factors for development of hyperkalemia include renal insufficiency, diabetes, and concomitant use of drugs that raise potassium level.

• Other ACE inhibitors have been associated with agranulocytosis and neutropenia. Monitor CBC with differential counts before therapy, every 2 weeks for first 3 months of therapy, and periodically thereafter.

• Be alert for adverse reactions and drug interactions.

• Evaluate patient's and family's knowledge of drug therapy.

⬚ Nursing diagnoses

• Risk for injury related to presence of hypertension

• Sleep pattern disturbance related to drug-induced cough

• Knowledge deficit related to drug therapy

⬙ Planning and implementation

• Dosage adjustment is necessary for patient with renal impairment.

• Give drug on empty stomach; high-fat meals can impair absorption.

Patient teaching

• Advise patient to report signs of infection, such as fever and sore throat.

• Tell patient to report signs such as swelling of face, eyes, lips, or tongue or breathing difficulty; angioedema (includ-

ing laryngeal edema) may occur, especially after first dose.

• Warn patient that light-headedness can occur, especially at first. Tell him to rise slowly and report symptoms. Patient who experiences syncope should stop drug and call doctor.

• Inadequate fluid intake, vomiting, diarrhea, and excessive perspiration can lead to light-headedness and syncope. Tell patient to use caution in hot weather and during exercise.

• Warn patient to avoid sodium substitutes during therapy.

• Tell female patient to notify doctor if pregnancy occurs or is suspected. Drug will need to be stopped.

☑ Evaluation

• Patient's blood pressure is normal.

• Patient's sleep patterns are undisturbed throughout therapy.

• Patient and family state understanding of drug therapy.

---

quinidine bisulfate
(KWIN-eh-deen bigh-SUL-fayt)
(66.4% quinidine base)
Biquin Durules◆, Kinidin Durules◇

quinidine gluconate
(62% quinidine base)
Quinaglute Dura-tabs, Quinalan, Quinate◆

quinidine polygalacturonate
(60.5% quinidine base)
Cardioquin

quinidine sulfate
(83% quinidine base)
Apo-Quinidine◆, Cin-Quin, Novoquinidin◆, Quinidex Extentabs, Quinora

---

Pharmacologic class: cinchona alkaloid
Therapeutic class: antiarrhythmic
Pregnancy risk category: C

How supplied

quinidine bisulfate
Tablets (extended-release): 250 mg♦◊
quinidine gluconate
Tablets (extended-release): 324 mg,
325 mg♦, 330 mg
Injection: 80 mg/ml
quinidine polygalacturonate
Tablets: 275 mg
quinidine sulfate
Tablets: 200 mg, 300 mg
Tablets (extended-release): 300 mg
Capsules: 200 mg, 300 mg
Injection: 200 mg/ml

Pharmacokinetics

Absorption: although all quinidine salts
are well absorbed from GI tract after P.O.
administration, serum drug levels vary
greatly among individuals.
Distribution: well distributed in all tissues except brain; about 80% bound to
plasma proteins.
Metabolism: about 60% to 80% metabolized in liver to two metabolites that may
have some pharmacologic activity.
Excretion: 10% to 30% excreted in
urine. Urine acidification increases excretion; alkalinization decreases it. *Half-life:*
5 to 12 hours.

Route	Onset	Peak	Duration
P.O.	1-3 hr	1-2 hr	6-8 hr
I.V.	Immediate	Immediate	Unknown
I.M.	Unknown	Unknown	Unknown

Pharmacodynamics

Chemical effect: class Ia antiarrhythmic
that has both direct and indirect (anticholinergic) effects on cardiac tissue.
Automaticity, conduction velocity, and
membrane responsiveness are decreased.
The effective refractory period is prolonged. Anticholinergic action reduces
vagal tone.
Therapeutic effect: restores normal sinus
rhythm and relieves signs and symptoms
of malaria infection.

Indications and dosage

▶ **Atrial flutter or fibrillation.** *Adults:*
200 mg of quinidine sulfate or equivalent
base P.O. q 2 to 3 hours for five to eight
doses, with subsequent daily increases
until sinus rhythm is restored or toxic effects develop. Quinidine is given only after digitalization to avoid increasing AV
conduction. Maximum dosage is 3 to 4 g
daily.
▶ **Paroxysmal supraventricular tachycardia.** *Adults:* 400 to 600 mg of quinidine sulfate P.O. q 2 to 3 hours until toxic
adverse reactions develop or arrhythmia
subsides.
▶ **Premature atrial and ventricular
contractions; paroxysmal AV junctional
rhythm; paroxysmal atrial tachycardia;
paroxysmal ventricular tachycardia;
maintenance after cardioversion of atrial fibrillation or flutter.** *Adults:* quinidine
sulfate or equivalent base 200 to 400 mg
P.O. q 4 to 6 hours; or quinidine gluconate
400 mg I.M. q 2 hours, adjusting each
dose by the effect of the previous; or
quinidine gluconate infused I.V. at up to
0.25 mg/kg/minute (1 ml/kg/hour).
Children: test dose is 2 mg/kg; then
30 mg/kg/day P.O. or 900 mg/m^2/day P.O.
in five divided doses.
▶ **Severe** *Plasmodium falciparum*
malaria. *Adults:* 10 mg/kg quinidine gluconate I.V. diluted in 250 ml of 0.9%
NaCl and infused over 1 to 2 hours, then
continuous maintenance infusion of
0.02 mg/kg/minute for 72 hours or until
parasitemia is reduced to less than 1%.
Patients with impaired liver function or
heart failure require reduced dosage.

Adverse reactions

CNS: *vertigo, headache, light-
headedness,* confusion, restlessness, cold
sweats, pallor, fainting, dementia.
CV: *PVCs; ventricular tachycardia;
atypical ventricular tachycardia (torsades de pointes); severe hypotension;
SA and AV block; ventricular fibrillation,* tachycardia; *aggravated heart failure,* ECG changes (widening of QRS

---

complex, notched P waves, widened QT interval, ST-segment depression).
EENT: *tinnitus,* blurred vision.
GI: *diarrhea, nausea, vomiting,* excessive salivation, anorexia, abdominal pain.
Hematologic: *hemolytic anemia, thrombocytopenia, agranulocytosis.*
Hepatic: *hepatotoxicity.*
Respiratory: acute asthma attack, *respiratory arrest.*
Skin: rash, petechial hemorrhage of buccal mucosa, pruritus.
Other: *angioedema,* fever, cinchonism.

Interactions

Drug-drug. *Acetazolamide, antacids, sodium bicarbonate, thiazide diuretics:* may increase quinidine blood levels because of alkaline urine. Monitor for increased effect.
Amiodarone, cimetidine: increased serum quinidine levels. Monitor for increased effect.
Barbiturates, phenytoin, rifampin: may lower blood levels of quinidine. Monitor for decreased quinidine effect.
Digoxin: increased serum digoxin levels after initiating quinidine therapy. Monitor patient closely.
Nifedipine: may decrease quinidine blood levels. Monitor patient carefully.
Other antiarrhythmics (such as lidocaine, phenytoin, procainamide, propranolol): increased risk of toxicity. Use together cautiously.
Verapamil: may result in hypotension, bradycardia, or AV block. Monitor blood pressure and heart rate.
Warfarin: increased anticoagulant effect. Monitor patient closely.

Contraindications and precautions

• Contraindicated in patients with idiosyncrasy or hypersensitivity to quinidine or related cinchona derivatives, intraventricular conduction defects, digitalis toxicity when AV conduction is grossly impaired, or abnormal rhythms due to escape mechanisms.

• Drug is not recommended for use in breast-feeding women.
• Use cautiously in patients with asthma, muscle weakness, or infection with fever (hypersensitivity reactions to drug may be masked); in patients with hepatic or renal impairment; and in pregnant women.

NURSING CONSIDERATIONS

Assessment
• Assess patient's arrhythmia before therapy and regularly thereafter.
• Monitor serum quinidine levels. Therapeutic plasma levels for antiarrhythmic effects are 2 to 5 mcg/ml.
• Check apical pulse rate and blood pressure before starting therapy.
• Monitor liver function tests during first 4 to 8 weeks of therapy.
• Be alert for adverse reactions and drug interactions.
• Evaluate patient's and family's knowledge of drug therapy.

Nursing diagnoses
• Decreased cardiac output related to presence of arrhythmia
• Risk for fluid volume deficit related to drug-induced adverse GI reactions
• Knowledge deficit related to drug therapy

Planning and implementation
• Anticoagulant therapy is commonly advised before quinidine therapy in long-standing atrial fibrillation because restoration of normal sinus rhythm may dislodge thrombi from atrial wall, causing thromboembolism.
P.O. use: Do not crush extended-release tablets.
I.V. use: I.V. route should only be used to treat acute arrhythmias. Mix 10 ml of quinidine gluconate with 40 ml of D_5W and infuse at an initial rate of up to 0.25 mg/minute (1ml/kg/hr). Never use discolored (brownish) quinidine solution.
I.M. use: Follow normal protocol.

• When used to treat severe malaria, patient should be hospitalized in intensive-care setting and continuously monitored. Decrease infusion rate if plasma quinidine level exceeds 6 mcg/ml, uncorrected QT interval exceeds 0.6 second, or QRS complex widening exceeds 25% of baseline.
• Store drug away from heat and direct light.
• If extremes in pulse rate occur, stop drug and tell doctor at once.
• When changing route of administration, be aware that dosage needs to be altered to compensate for variations in quinidine base content.
• Report adverse GI reactions, especially diarrhea; these are signs of toxicity. Blood levels above 8 mcg/ml are toxic.
Patient teaching
• Tell patient to take drug with meals.
• Teach patient signs of toxicity, and tell him to report them at once.
• Stress importance of close follow-up care and frequent diagnostic studies to monitor effectiveness of quinidine and detect adverse reactions.

☑ **Evaluation**
• Patient regains normal cardiac output with resolution of arrhythmia.
• Patient maintains adequate hydration throughout therapy.
• Patient and family state understanding of drug therapy.

rabies immune globulin, human
(RAY-bees ih-MYOON GLOH-byoo-lin, HYOO-mun)
Hyperab, Imogam

Pharmacologic class: immune serum
Therapeutic class: rabies prophylaxis agent

Pregnancy risk category: C

How supplied
Injection: 150 IU/ml in 2-ml, 10-ml vials

Pharmacokinetics
Absorption: absorption is slow after I.M. administration.
Distribution: unknown.
Metabolism: unknown.
Excretion: unknown. *Half-life:* about 24 days.

Route	Onset	Peak	Duration
I.M.	Unknown	24 hr	Unknown

Pharmacodynamics
Chemical effect: provides passive immunity to rabies.
Therapeutic effect: prevents rabies.

Indications and dosage
▶ **Rabies exposure.** *Adults and children:* 20 IU/kg I.M. at time of first dose of rabies vaccine. Half of dose used to infiltrate wound area. Remainder given I.M.

Adverse reactions
Skin: *rash,* pain, redness, induration (at injection site).
Other: slight fever, *anaphylaxis, angioedema, nephrotic syndrome.*

Interactions
Drug-drug. *Corticosteroids, immunosuppressive agents:* interfere with response. Avoid during postexposure immunization period.
Live-virus vaccines (measles, mumps, polio, rubella): interferes with response to vaccine. Delay immunization if possible.

Contraindications and precautions
• No known contraindications.
• Use with caution in pregnant women, in patients with history of systemic allergic reactions after administration of human immunoglobulin preparations, and in those with immunoglobulin A deficiency or hypersensitivity to thimerosal.

• Safety of drug has not been established in breast-feeding women.

NURSING CONSIDERATIONS

⚕ Assessment
• Obtain history of animal bites, allergies, and immunization reactions.
• Ask patient when last tetanus immunization was received; doctor may order booster at this time.
• Be alert for adverse reactions and drug interactions.
• Evaluate patient's and family's knowledge of drug therapy.

⊞ Nursing diagnoses
• Risk for injury related to rabies exposure
• Altered protection related to drug-induced hypersensitivity reaction
• Knowledge deficit related to drug therapy

⧉ Planning and implementation
• Use only with rabies vaccine and immediate local treatment of wound. Don't give in same syringe or at same site with rabies vaccine. Give drug regardless of interval between exposure and initiation of therapy.
• Don't administer live-virus vaccines within 3 months of rabies immune globulin.
• Drug provides passive immunity. Don't confuse with rabies vaccine, which is suspension of attenuated or killed microorganisms used to confer active immunity. The two drugs are often given together prophylactically after exposure to known or suspected rabid animals.
• Have epinephrine 1:1,000 available to treat anaphylaxis.
• Don't give more than 5 ml I.M. at one injection site; divide I.M. doses greater than 5 ml, and give at different sites.
Patient teaching
• Explain that slight fever, pain, and redness at injection site may occur.
• Advise patient that tetanus booster may be necessary at this time.

• Instruct patient to report immediately signs of hypersensitivity.

☑ Evaluation
• Patient exhibits passive immunity to rabies.
• Patient does not exhibit signs of hypersensitivity after receiving drug.
• Patient and family state understanding of drug therapy.

radioactive iodine (sodium iodide)¹³¹I
(ray-dee-oh-AK-tiv IGH-oh-dighn)
Iodotope, Sodium Iodide ¹³¹I Therapeutic

Pharmacologic class: thyroid hormone antagonist
Therapeutic class: antihyperthyroid agent
Pregnancy risk category: X

How supplied
All radioactivity concentrations are determined at time of calibration.
Iodotope
Capsules: radioactivity range is 8 to 100 millicuries (mCi)/capsule
Oral solution: radioactivity concentration is 7.05 mCi/ml; in vials containing approximately 7, 14, 28, 70, or 106 mCi
Sodium Iodide ¹³¹I Therapeutic
Capsules: radioactivity range is 0.8 to 100 mCi/capsule
Oral solution: radioactivity range is 3.5 to 150 mCi/vial

Pharmacokinetics
Absorption: readily absorbed from GI tract.
Distribution: distributed in extracellular fluid. It is selectively concentrated and bound to tyrosyl residues of thyroglobulin in thyroid gland. It is also concentrated in stomach, choroid plexus, and salivary glands.
Metabolism: converted readily to protein-bound iodine by thyroid.

Reactions may be *common*, uncommon, *life-threatening*, or COMMON AND LIFE-THREATENING.

Excretion: excreted by kidneys. *Half-life:* 138 days; effective radioactive half-life is 7.6 days.

Route	Onset	Peak	Duration
P.O.	2-4 wk	2-4 mo	Unknown

Pharmacodynamics

Chemical effect: limits thyroid hormone secretion by destroying thyroid tissue. The affinity of thyroid tissue for radioactive iodine facilitates uptake of drug by cancerous thyroid tissue that has metastasized to other sites in body.
Therapeutic effect: decreases thyroid function.

Indications and dosage

▶ **Hyperthyroidism.** *Adults:* usual dosage is 4 to 10 mCi P.O. Dosage based on estimated weight of thyroid gland and thyroid uptake. Treatment repeated after 6 weeks, according to serum T_4 level.
▶ **Thyroid cancer.** *Adults:* 50 to 150 mCi P.O. Dosage based on estimated malignant thyroid tissue and metastatic tissue as determined by total body scan. Treatment repeated according to clinical status.

Adverse reactions

CV: chest pain, tachycardia.
EENT: *fullness in neck,* pain on swallowing, sore throat, cough.
Hematologic: anemia; blood dyscrasia; *leukopenia; thrombocytopenia;* possible increased risk of developing *leukemia* later in life after sufficient ^{131}I dosage for thyroid ablation after cancer surgery.
Other: hypothyroidism; radiation-induced thyroiditis; radiation sickness (nausea, vomiting); temporary thinning of hair; allergic-type reactions; possible increased risk of birth defects in offspring after sufficient ^{131}I dosage for thyroid ablation after cancer surgery, **death.**

Interactions

Drug-drug. *Lithium carbonate:* hypothyroidism may occur. Use with caution.

The following drugs can interfere with action of ^{131}I and should be withheld for specified time before administering ^{131}I dose:
Adrenocorticoids: 1 week.
Benzodiazepines: 1 month.
Cholecystographic agents: 6 to 9 months.
Contrast media containing iodine: 1 to 2 months.
Iodine-containing products, including antitussives, expectorants, topical agents, and vitamins: 2 weeks.
Salicylates: 1 to 2 weeks.

Contraindications and precautions

• Contraindicated in pregnant women, except to treat thyroid cancer, and in breast-feeding women.
• Drug is not recommended for use in patients under age 30, unless other treatments are precluded.

NURSING CONSIDERATIONS

⬚ Assessment
• Assess patient's thyroid condition before therapy and regularly thereafter.
• Monitor thyroid function by way of serum T_4 levels, as ordered.
• Be alert for adverse reactions and drug interactions.
• Evaluate patient's and family's knowledge of drug therapy.

⬚ Nursing diagnoses
• Altered health maintenance related to presence of thyroid dysfunction
• Risk for injury related to drug's possible long-term effects
• Knowledge deficit related to drug therapy

⬚ Planning and implementation
• All antithyroid medications and thyroid preparations need to be stopped 1 week before ^{131}I dose. If they're not stopped, patient may receive thyroid-stimulating hormone for 3 days before ^{131}I dose. When treating female patient of child-

---

bearing age, give dose during menstruation or within 7 days after menstruation.
• Institute full radiation precautions. Have patient use appropriate disposal methods when coughing and expectorating. After dose for hyperthyroidism, urine and saliva are slightly radioactive for 24 hours; vomitus is highly radioactive for 6 to 8 hours.
• After dose for thyroid cancer, urine, saliva, and perspiration are radioactive for 3 days. Isolate patient. Do not allow pregnant personnel to care for patient, use disposable eating utensils and linens, and instruct patient to save all urine in lead containers for 24 to 48 hours so amount of radioactive material excreted can be determined. Tell patient to drink as much fluid as possible for 48 hours after drug dose to facilitate excretion. Limit patient contact to 30 minutes per shift per person first day and increase time, as needed, to 1 hour second day and longer on third day.
Patient teaching
• Tell patient to fast overnight before dose. Food may delay absorption.
• Inform patient that after therapy for hyperthyroidism, he should not resume antithyroid drugs but should continue propranolol or other drugs used to treat symptoms of hyperthyroidism until onset of full ^{131}I effect occurs (usually 6 weeks).
• Review safety precautions to take after radioactive iodine dose. Warn patient who is discharged less than 7 days after ^{131}I dose for thyroid cancer to avoid close, prolonged contact with young children and not to sleep in same room with spouse for 7 days after treatment. Tell patient he can use same bathroom as rest of family.

☑ **Evaluation**
• Patient's thyroid function returns to normal.
• Patient does not develop complications as result of therapy.
• Patient and family state understanding of drug therapy.

raloxifene hydrochloride
(rah-LOKS-ih-feen
high-droh-KLOR-ighd)
Evista

Pharmacologic class: selective estrogen receptor modulator (SERM) of the benzothiophene class
Therapeutic class: antiosteoporotic
Pregnancy risk category: X

How supplied

Tablets: 60 mg

Pharmacokinetics

Absorption: rapid, with about 60% of the dose absorbed after oral administration.
Distribution: widely distributed and highly bound to plasma proteins.
Metabolism: extensive first-pass metabolism to glucuronide conjugates.
Excretion: primarily excreted in the feces, with less than 0.2% excreted unchanged in the urine. *Half-life:* 27.7 hours.

Route	Onset	Peak	Duration
P.O.	Unknown	Unknown	24 hr

Pharmacodynamics

Chemical effect: SERM that reduces resorption of bone and decreases overall bone turnover. These effects on bone are manifested as reductions in serum and urine levels of bone turnover markers and increases in bone mineral density
Therapeutic effect: prevents bone breakdown in postmenopausal women.

Indications and dosage

▶ **Prevention of osteoporosis in postmenopausal women.** *Adults:* 60 mg P.O. once daily.

Adverse reactions

CNS: depression, insomnia, migraine.
CV: *hot flashes,* chest pain.
EENT: *sinusitis,* pharyngitis, laryngitis.

Reactions may be *common,* uncommon, *life-threatening*, or COMMON AND LIFE-THREATENING.

GI: nausea, dyspepsia, vomiting, flatulence, GI disorder, gastroenteritis, abdominal pain.
GU: vaginitis, urinary tract infection, cystitis, leukorrhea, endometrial disorder, vaginal bleeding.
Metabolic: weight gain, fever.
Musculoskeletal: *arthralgia,* myalgia, arthritis, leg cramps, breast pain.
Respiratory: increased cough, pneumonia.
Skin: rash, sweating.
Other: *infection, flu syndrome,* peripheral edema.

Interactions

Drug-drug. *Cholestyramine:* causes a significant reduction in absorption of raloxifene. Don't coadminister these drugs.
Highly protein-bound drugs (such as clofibrate, diazepam, diazoxide, ibuprofen, indomethacin, naproxen): may interfere with binding sites. Use with caution.
Warfarin: may cause a decrease in PT. Monitor PT and INR closely.

Contraindications and precautions

• Contraindicated in pregnant women or those planning pregnancy or breast-feeding and in children.
• Also contraindicated in women hypersensitive to drug or its constituents; or in women with past history of, or currently active, venous thromboembolic events, including deep vein thrombosis (DVT), pulmonary embolism, and retinal vein thrombosis.
• Use cautiously in patients with severe hepatic impairment.

NURSING CONSIDERATIONS

Assessment
• Obtain history of patient's condition and reassess during therapy.
• Monitor for signs of blood clots. The greatest risk for thromboembolic events occurs during first 4 months of treatment.

• Monitor for breast abnormalities that occur during treatment.
• Monitor serum lipid levels, blood pressure, body weight, and liver function, as ordered.
• Evaluate patient's and family's knowledge of drug therapy.

Nursing diagnoses
• Altered peripheral tissue perfusion related to potential DVT formation
• Altered nutrition: Less than body requirements related to drug-induced adverse GI reactions
• Knowledge deficit related to drug therapy

Planning and implementation
• Know that drug should be discontinued at least 72 hours before prolonged immobilization and resumed only after patient is fully mobilized.
• Withhold drug and notify doctor if thromboembolic event is suspected.
• Know that unexplained uterine bleeding should be reported to doctor.
• Safety and efficacy have not been evaluated in men.
• Be aware that effect on bone mineral density beyond 2 years of drug treatment is not known.
• Know that concomitant use of drug with hormone replacement therapy or systemic estrogen is not recommended.
Patient teaching
• Advise patient to avoid long periods of restricted movement (such as during traveling) because of increased risk of venous thromboembolic events.
• Inform patient that hot flashes or flushing may occur and that drug does not aid in reducing them.
• Instruct patient to take other bone-loss prevention measures, including supplemental calcium and vitamin D if dietary intake is inadequate, performing weight-bearing exercises, and stopping alcohol consumption and smoking.
• Tell patient that drug may be taken without regard for food.

• Advise patient to report any unexplained uterine bleeding or breast abnormalities that occur during treatment.
• Explain side effects and instruct patient to read package insert before starting therapy and to re-read each time prescription is renewed.

☑ **Evaluation**
• Patient does not develop pain, redness, or swelling in lower extremities.
• Patient maintains normal dietary intake.
• Patient and family state understanding of drug therapy.

ramipril
(reh-MIH-pril)
Altace, Ramace◇, Tritace◇

Pharmacologic class: ACE inhibitor
Therapeutic class: antihypertensive
Pregnancy risk category: C (D in second and third trimesters)

How supplied
Capsules: 1.25 mg, 2.5 mg, 5 mg, 10 mg

Pharmacokinetics
Absorption: 50% to 60% absorbed from GI tract.
Distribution: 73% serum protein-bound; ramiprilat (metabolite), 58%.
Metabolism: almost completely converted to ramiprilat, which is six times more potent than parent drug.
Excretion: 60% in urine; 40% in feces.
Half-life: ramipril, 5.1 hours; ramiprilat, 13 to 17 hours.

Route	Onset	Peak	Duration
P.O.	1-2 hr	≤ 1 hr (ramipril) 3 hr (ramiprilat)	About 24 hr

Pharmacodynamics
Chemical effect: unknown; thought to be related to inhibition of angiotensin I to angiotensin II, a potent vasoconstrictor. This decreases peripheral arterial resistance, thus decreasing aldosterone secretion.
Therapeutic effect: lowers blood pressure.

Indications and dosage
▶ **Hypertension.** *Adults:* initially, 2.5 mg P.O. once daily for patients not receiving diuretic, and 1.25 mg P.O. once daily for patients receiving diuretic. Dosage increased as needed based on patient response. Maintenance dosage is 2.5 to 20 mg daily as single dose or in divided doses. *In patients with renal insufficiency:* if creatinine clearance is less than 40 ml/minute, 1.25 mg P.O. daily. Dosage is titrated gradually based on response. Maximum daily dosage is 5 mg.
▶ **Heart failure post-MI.** *Adults:* 2.5 mg P.O. b.i.d. Titrate to target dose of 5 mg P.O. b.i.d.

Adverse reactions
CNS: headache, dizziness, fatigue, asthenia, malaise, light-headedness, anxiety, amnesia, *seizures,* depression, insomnia, nervousness, neuralgia, neuropathy, paresthesia, somnolence, tremors, vertigo.
CV: orthostatic hypotension, syncope, angina, *arrhythmias,* chest pain, palpitations, *MI.*
EENT: epistaxis, tinnitus.
GI: nausea, vomiting, abdominal pain, anorexia, constipation, diarrhea, dyspepsia, dry mouth, gastroenteritis.
GU: impotence.
Musculoskeletal: arthralgia, arthritis, myalgia.
Respiratory: *dry, persistent, tickling, nonproductive cough;* dyspnea.
Skin: hypersensitivity reactions, rash, dermatitis, pruritus, photosensitivity.
Other: *angioedema,* edema, hyperkalemia, increased diaphoresis, weight gain.

Interactions
Drug-drug. *Diuretics:* excessive hypotension, especially at start of therapy.

Discontinue diuretic at least 3 days before therapy begins, increase sodium intake, or reduce starting dose of ramipril.
Insulin, oral antidiabetic agents: risk of hypoglycemia, especially at initiation of ramipril therapy. Monitor patient closely.
Lithium: increased serum lithium levels. Use together cautiously and monitor serum lithium levels.
Potassium-sparing diuretics, potassium supplements: increased risk of hyperkalemia because ramipril attenuates potassium loss. Monitor plasma potassium levels closely.
Drug-food. *Salt substitutes containing potassium:* increased risk of hyperkalemia because ramipril attenuates potassium loss. Monitor plasma potassium levels closely.

Contraindications and precautions

• Contraindicated in patients with hypersensitivity to ACE inhibitors or history of angioedema related to previous treatment with ACE inhibitor.
• Drug is not recommended for use in pregnant or breast-feeding women.
• Use cautiously in patients with renal impairment.
• Safety of drug in children has not been established.

NURSING CONSIDERATIONS

Assessment

• Assess patient's blood pressure before therapy and regularly thereafter.
• Closely assess kidney function during first few weeks of therapy. Regular assessment (serum creatinine and BUN levels) is advisable. Patients with severe heart failure whose kidney function depends on angiotensin-aldosterone system have experienced acute renal failure during ACE inhibitor therapy. Hypertensive patient with renal artery stenosis also may show signs of worsening kidney function at start of therapy.
• Monitor CBC with differential counts before therapy, every 2 weeks for first 3 months of therapy, and periodically thereafter. These effects may occur especially in patient with impaired kidney function or collagen vascular disease (systemic lupus erythematosus or scleroderma).
• Monitor serum potassium levels. Risk factors for development of hyperkalemia include renal insufficiency, diabetes, and concomitant use of agents that raise potassium levels.
• Be alert for adverse reactions and drug interactions.
• Evaluate patient's and family's knowledge of drug therapy.

Nursing diagnoses

• Risk for injury related to presence of hypertension
• Sleep pattern disturbance related to drug-induced cough
• Knowledge deficit related to drug therapy

Planning and implementation

• Diuretic therapy should be stopped 2 to 3 days before start of ramipril therapy, if possible.
Patient teaching
• Tell patient to avoid abrupt discontinuation of therapy.
• Advise patient to report signs of angioedema, which may occur after first dose.
• To avoid initial light-headedness, tell patient to rise slowly and to report symptoms. If syncope occurs, he should stop drug and call doctor.
• Tell patient to report signs of infection.
• Warn patient to avoid sodium substitutes during therapy.
• Tell female patient to report pregnancy. Drug will need to be stopped.

Evaluation

• Patient's blood pressure is normal.
• Patient's sleep patterns are undisturbed throughout therapy.
• Patient and family state understanding of drug therapy.

ranitidine hydrochloride

(ruh-NIH-tuh-deen high-droh-KLOR-ighd)
Zantac*, Zantac-C♦, Zantac EFFERdose,
Zantac 75†

Pharmacologic class: H$_2$-receptor
antagonist
Therapeutic class: antiulcer agent
Pregnancy risk category: B

How supplied

Tablets: 75 mg†, 150 mg, 300 mg
Tablets (dispersible): 150 mg†
Tablets (effervescent): 150 mg
Granules (effervescent): 150 mg
Syrup: 15 mg/ml*
Injection: 25 mg/ml
Infusion: 0.5 mg/ml in 100-ml containers

Pharmacokinetics

Absorption: about 50% to 60% of P.O.
dose absorbed; absorbed rapidly from
parenteral sites after I.M. dose.
Distribution: distributed to many body
tissues and appears in CSF; about 10% to
19% protein-bound.
Metabolism: metabolized in liver.
Excretion: excreted in urine and feces.
Half-life: 2 to 3 hours.

Route	Onset	Peak	Duration
P.O.	≤ 1 hr	1-3 hr	≤ 13 hr
I.V., I.M.	Unknown	Unknown	≤ 13 hr

Pharmacodynamics

Chemical effect: competitively inhibits
action of H$_2$ at receptor sites of parietal
cells, decreasing gastric acid secretion.
Therapeutic effect: relieves GI discomfort.

Indications and dosage

▶ **Duodenal and gastric ulcer (short-
term treatment); pathological hypersecretory conditions, such as Zollinger-
Ellison syndrome.** *Adults:* 150 mg P.O.
b.i.d. or 300 mg daily h.s. Alternatively,
50 mg I.V. or I.M. q 6 to 8 hours. Patients
with Zollinger-Ellison syndrome may require dosages up to 6 g P.O. daily.

▶ **Maintenance therapy for duodenal
ulcer.** *Adults:* 150 mg P.O. h.s.
▶ **Gastroesophageal reflux disease.**
Adults: 150 mg P.O. b.i.d.
▶ **Erosive esophagitis.** *Adults:* 150 mg
P.O. q.i.d.
▶ **Self-medication for relief of occasional heartburn, acid indigestion, and
sour stomach.** *Adults and children age
12 and older:* 75 mg once or twice daily;
maximum daily dosage is 150 mg.

Adverse reactions

CNS: vertigo, malaise.
EENT: *blurred vision.*
Hematologic: reversible leukopenia,
pancytopenia.
Hepatic: elevated liver enzyme levels,
jaundice.
Other: burning and itching at injection
site, *anaphylaxis,* angioneurotic edema.

Interactions

Drug-drug. *Antacids:* may interfere with
ranitidine absorption. Stagger doses if
possible.
Diazepam: decreased absorption of diazepam. Monitor for decreased effectiveness.
Glipizide: possible increased hypoglycemic effect. Adjust glipizide dosage
as necessary.
Procainamide: possible decreased renal
clearance of procainamide. Monitor for
procainamide toxicity.
Warfarin: possible interference with warfarin clearance. Monitor closely.

Contraindications and precautions

• Contraindicated in patients hypersensitive to drug.
• Use cautiously in patients with hepatic
dysfunction and in pregnant or breast-
feeding women. Adjust dosage in patients
with impaired kidney function, as ordered.

NURSING CONSIDERATIONS

⚕ Assessment
• Assess patient's GI condition before
therapy and regularly thereafter.

Reactions may be *common,* uncommon, *life-threatening*, or COMMON AND LIFE-THREATENING.

• Be alert for adverse reactions and drug interactions.
• Evaluate patient's and family's knowledge of drug therapy.

⊞ Nursing diagnoses
• Altered tissue integrity related to underlying GI condition
• Risk for injury related to drug-induced adverse CNS reactions
• Knowledge deficit related to drug therapy

⧁ Planning and implementation
• Don't use aluminum-based needles or equipment when mixing or giving drug parenterally. Drug is incompatible with aluminum.
P.O. use: Administer once-daily dosage at bedtime.
I.V. use: When administering by I.V. push, dilute to total volume of 20 ml and inject over period of 5 minutes.
– When giving by intermittent I.V. infusion, dilute 50 mg ranitidine in 100 ml of D$_5$W and infuse over 15 to 20 minutes. Or, give by continuous I.V. infusion: 150 mg in 250 ml of compatible solution. Administer at 6.25 mg/hour using infusion pump.
– For premixed I.V. infusion, give by slow I.V. drip (over 15 to 20 minutes). Don't add other drugs to solution. If used with primary I.V. fluid system, stop primary solution during infusion.
I.M. use: Follow normal protocol. No dilution is needed when giving drug I.M.
Patient teaching
• Remind patient taking drug once daily to take it at bedtime.
• Instruct patient to take without regard to meals.
• Urge patient to avoid cigarette smoking because it may increase gastric acid secretion and worsen disease.

☑ Evaluation
• Patient states that GI discomfort is relieved.

• Patient does not experience injury as result of drug-induced adverse CNS reactions.
• Patient and family state understanding of drug therapy.

---

repaglinide
(reh-PAG-lih-nighd)
Prandin

Pharmacologic class: meglitinide
Therapeutic class: antidiabetic
Pregnancy risk category: C

How supplied
Tablets: 0.5 mg, 1 mg, 2 mg

Pharmacokinetics
Absorption: rapidly and completely absorbed from the gastrointestinal tract. Absolute bioavailability is 56%.
Distribution: more than 98% bound to plasma proteins.
Metabolism: completely metabolized by oxidative biotransformation and direct conjugation with glucuronic acid.
Excretion: about 90% is recovered in feces and 8% in urine. *Half-life:* 1 hour.

Route	Onset	Peak	Duration
P.O.	Unknown	1 hr	Unknown

Pharmacodynamics
Chemical effect: stimulates the release of insulin from the beta cells in the pancreas to lower the blood glucose level.
Therapeutic effect: lowers blood glucose levels.

Indications and dosage
▶ **Adjunct to diet and exercise in lowering blood glucose in patient with type 2 (non-insulin-dependent) diabetes mellitus whose hyperglycemia cannot be controlled by diet and exercise alone.**
Adults: for patients not previously treated or whose glycosylated hemoglobin (HbA$_{1c}$) is below 8%, starting dose is

---

0.5 mg P.O. taken immediately to 30 minutes before each meal; for those previously treated with glucose-lowering drugs and whose HbA$_{1c}$ is 8% or more, initial dose is 1 to 2 mg P.O. taken immediately to 30 minutes before each meal. Recommended dosage range is 0.5 to 4 mg with meals preprandially divided b.i.d., t.i.d., or q.i.d. Maximum daily dosage is 16 mg.

Adverse reactions

CNS: *headache,* paresthesia.
CV: angina, chest pain.
EENT: rhinitis, sinusitis, tooth disorder.
GI: constipation, diarrhea, dyspepsia, nausea, vomiting.
GU: urinary tract infection.
Metabolic: HYPOGLYCEMIA, hyperglycemia.
Musculoskeletal: arthralgia, back pain.
Respiratory: bronchitis, *upper respiratory infection.*

Interactions

Drug-drug. *Barbiturates, carbamazepine, rifampin, troglitazone:* may increase metabolism of repaglinide. Monitor glucose level.
Beta-adrenergic blocking agents, chloramphenicol, coumarins, MAO inhibitors, NSAIDs, other drugs that are highly protein-bound, probenecid, salicylates, sulfonamides: may potentiate hypoglycemic action of repaglinide. Monitor glucose level.
Calcium channel blocking drugs, corticosteroids, estrogens, isoniazid, nicotinic acid, oral contraceptives, phenothiazines, phenytoin, sympathomimetics, thiazides and other diuretics, thyroid products: may produce hyperglycemia resulting in a loss of glycemic control. Monitor glucose level.
Erythromycin, inhibitors of P-450 cytochrome system 3A4, ketoconazole, miconazole: may inhibit metabolism of repaglinide. Monitor glucose levels.

Contraindications and precautions

● Contraindicated in patients with hypersensitivity to drug or its inactive ingredients and in those with insulin-dependent diabetes mellitus or diabetic ketoacidosis.
● Use cautiously in patients with hepatic insufficiency in whom reduced metabolism could cause elevated blood levels of repaglinide and hypoglycemia.
● Use cautiously in elderly, debilitated, or malnourished patients and those with adrenal or pituitary insufficiency because they are more susceptible to the hypoglycemic effect of glucose-lowering drugs.

NURSING CONSIDERATIONS

⚕ Assessment
● Monitor blood glucose level before therapy and regularly thereafter.
● Be alert for adverse reactions and drug interactions.
● Monitor elderly patients and patients taking beta-adrenergic blocking agents carefully because hypoglycemia may be difficult to recognize in these populations.
● Evaluate patient's and family's knowledge of drug therapy.

⊕ Nursing diagnoses
● Altered nutrition: More than body requirements related to patient's underlying condition
● Risk for injury related to drug-induced hypoglycemic episode
● Knowledge deficit related to drug therapy

▶ Planning and implementation
● Make increases in drug dosage carefully in patients with impaired renal function or renal failure requiring dialysis.
● Know that metformin may be added if repaglinide monotherapy is inadequate.
● Be aware that loss of glycemic control can occur during stress, such as fever, trauma, infection, or surgery. Discontinue drug as ordered and administer insulin.
● Know that administration of oral antidiabetic drugs has been reported to be associated with increased CV mortality compared with diet treatment alone.

Reactions may be *common,* uncommon, *life-threatening*, or COMMON AND LIFE-THREATENING.

• Give drug immediately to 30 minutes before meals.
Patient teaching
• Teach patient about importance of diet and exercise in combination with drug therapy.
• Discuss symptoms of hypoglycemia with patient and family.
• Advise patient to monitor blood glucose periodically to determine minimum effective dose.
• Encourage patient to keep regular appointments and have glucose levels checked as ordered to determine long-term glucose control.
• Tell patient to take drug before meals, usually 15 minutes before start of meal; however, time can vary from immediately preceding meal to up to 30 minutes before meal.
• Tell patient that if a meal is skipped or an extra meal added, he should skip the dose or add an extra dose of drug for that meal.
• Teach patient how to monitor blood glucose carefully and what to do when he is ill, undergoing surgery, or under added stress.

☑ **Evaluation**
• Patient's blood glucose is controlled and an adequate nutritional balance is maintained.
• Patient does not experience severe decreases in blood glucose levels.
• Patient and family state understanding of drug therapy.

reserpine
(re-SER-peen)
Novoreserpine♦, Serpalan, Serpasil♦*

Pharmacologic class: rauwolfia alkaloid, peripherally acting adrenergic blocker
Therapeutic class: antihypertensive
Pregnancy risk category: C

How supplied
Tablets: 0.1 mg, 0.25 mg, 1 mg

Pharmacokinetics
Absorption: appears to be absorbed rapidly.
Distribution: appears to be distributed widely in body; high concentrations are found in adipose tissue.
Metabolism: metabolized extensively to inactive compounds.
Excretion: excreted slowly in urine and feces. *Half-life:* 33 hours.

Route	Onset	Peak	Duration
P.O	3 days-3 wk	3-6 wk	1-6 wk

Pharmacodynamics
Chemical effect: unknown; thought to be due to reduced cardiac output and, possibly, decreased peripheral resistance.
Therapeutic effect: lowers blood pressure.

Indications and dosage
▶ **Mild to moderate essential hypertension.** *Adults:* initially, 0.5 mg P.O. in single daily dose or divided into two doses daily. Maintenance dosage is 0.25 mg/day.

Adverse reactions
CNS: confusion, drowsiness, sedation, nervousness, paradoxical anxiety, nightmares, depression, extrapyramidal symptoms.
CV: orthostatic hypotension, *bradycardia,* syncope.
EENT: nasal congestion, glaucoma.
GI: hyperacidity, nausea, vomiting, dry mouth, bleeding.
GU: impotence.
Skin: pruritus, rash.
Other: weight gain, *thrombocytopenic purpura.*

Interactions
Drug-drug. *Cardiac glycosides, quinidine:* arrhythmias may occur. Monitor patient closely.
CNS depressants: additive CNS effects. Avoid concomitant use.
MAO inhibitors: may cause excitability and hypertension. Use together cautiously.
Tricyclic antidepressants: decreased antihypertensive effect. Monitor closely.

Drug-lifestyle. *Alcohol use:* additive CNS effects. Avoid concomitant use.

Contraindications and precautions

• Contraindicated in patients with hypersensitivity to drug, depression, ulcerative colitis, or peptic ulcer disease and in those receiving electroconvulsive therapy.
• Drug is not recommended for use in breast-feeding women.
• Use cautiously in patients with history of peptic ulcer, ulcerative colitis, or gallstones and in pregnant women.

NURSING CONSIDERATIONS

Assessment
• Obtain history of patient's blood pressure and pulse rate before therapy and reassess regularly thereafter.
• Be alert for adverse reactions and drug interactions.
• Monitor patient's hydration status if adverse GI reactions occur.
• Evaluate patient's and family's knowledge of drug therapy.

Nursing diagnoses
• Risk for injury related to presence of hypertension
• Risk for fluid volume deficit related to drug-induced adverse GI reactions
• Knowledge deficit related to drug therapy

Planning and implementation
• Administer drug with meals.
• Do not discontinue drug abruptly.
Patient teaching
• Warn patient to avoid activities that require alertness until drug's CNS effects are known.
• Tell patient to rise slowly and avoid sudden position changes to lessen orthostatic hypotension.
• Tell patient that dry mouth can be relieved with ice chips or sugarless chewing gum or sour hard candy.
• Tell patient to contact doctor if relief is needed for nasal congestion.

• Tell patient to weigh himself daily and report weight gain over 2.27 kg (5 lb).
• Suggest periodic eye examinations.
• Tell family to watch patient for signs of depression. Warn patient to promptly report nightmares.

Evaluation
• Patient's blood pressure is normal.
• Patient states that mild analgesic relieves drug-induced headache.
• Patient and family state understanding of drug therapy.

reteplase, recombinant
(REE-teh-plays, ree-KUHM-buh-nent)
Retavase

Pharmacologic class: recombinant plasminogen activator; enzyme
Therapeutic class: thrombolytic enzyme
Pregnancy risk category: C

How supplied
Injection: 10.8 units (18.8 mg)/vial. Supplied in kit with components for reconstitution for 2 single-use vials.

Pharmacokinetics
Absorption: not applicable with I.V. administration.
Distribution: rapid distribution.
Metabolism: unknown.
Excretion: in urine and feces.

Route	Onset	Peak	Duration
I.V.	Unknown	Unknown	Unknown

Pharmacodynamics
Chemical effect: enhances cleavage of plasminogen to generate plasmin.
Therapeutic effect: fibrinolysis and thrombolytic action.

Indications and dosage
▶ **Management of acute MI.** *Adults:* administered as double-bolus injection of 10 + 10 U. Give each bolus I.V. over 2

minutes. If complications don't occur after first bolus, give second bolus 30 minutes after start of first.

Adverse reactions

CNS: *intracranial hemorrhage.*
CV: *arrhythmias, cholesterol embolization, hemorrhage.*
GI: *hemorrhage.*
GU: hematuria.
Hematologic: anemia, *bleeding tendency.*
Other: bleeding at puncture sites.

Interactions

Drug-drug. *Heparin, oral anticoagulants, platelet inhibitors (abciximab, aspirin, dipyridamole):* may increase risk of bleeding. Use together cautiously.

Contraindications and precautions

• Contraindicated in patients with active internal bleeding, known bleeding diathesis, history of cerebrovascular accident, recent intracranial or intraspinal surgery or trauma, severe uncontrolled hypertension, intracranial neoplasm, arteriovenous malformation, or aneurysm.
• Use cautiously in patients with recent (within 10 days) major surgery, obstetric delivery, organ biopsy, or trauma; previous puncture of noncompressible vessel; cerebrovascular disease; recent GI or GU bleeding; heart disease.

NURSING CONSIDERATIONS

☞ Assessment
• Monitor ECG during treatment.
• Monitor patient for bleeding. Avoid I.M. injections, invasive procedures, and nonessential handling of patient.
• Evaluate patient's and family's knowledge of drug therapy.

⊕ Nursing diagnoses
• Altered cardiopulmonary tissue perfusion related to underlying condition
• Risk for injury related to adverse effects of drug

• Knowledge deficit related to drug therapy

⊠ Planning and implementation
• Know that reteplase is administered I.V. as double-bolus injection. If bleeding or anaphylactoid reaction occurs after first bolus, notify doctor.
• Reconstitute drug according to manufacturer's instructions.
• Do not administer drug with other I.V. medications through the same line. Note that heparin and reteplase are incompatible in solution.
• Avoid noncompressible pressure sites during therapy. If an arterial puncture is needed, an upper extremity vessel that can be compressed manually should be used. Apply pressure for at least 30 minutes; then apply a pressure dressing. Check site frequently for bleeding.
Patient teaching
• Tell patient and family about drug.
• Tell patient to report adverse reactions immediately.

☑ Evaluation
• Patient's cardiopulmonary assessment findings show improved perfusion.
• Patient is free from serious adverse reactions associated with therapy.
• Patient and family state understanding of drug therapy.

Rh₀(D) immune globulin, human
(R H O D ih-MYOON GLOH-byoo-lin, HYOO-mun)
Gamulin Rh, HypRho-D, MICRhoGAM, Mini-Gamulin Rh, Rhesonativ, RhoGAM

Pharmacologic class: immune serum
Therapeutic class: anti-Rh₀(D)-positive prophylaxis agent
Pregnancy risk category: C

How supplied

Injection: 300 mcg of Rh₀(D) immune globulin/vial (standard dose); 50 mcg of

Rh$_o$(D) immune globulin/vial (micro-dose)

Pharmacokinetics

Unknown.

Route	Onset	Peak	Duration
I.M.	Unknown	Unknown	Unknown

Pharmacodynamics

Chemical effect: suppresses active antibody response and formation of anti-Rh$_o$(D) in Rh$_o$(D)-negative, D^u-negative individuals exposed to Rh-positive blood. *Therapeutic effect:* blocks adverse effects of Rh-positive exposure.

Indications and dosage

▶ **Rh exposure.** *Adults (postabortion, postmiscarriage, ectopic pregnancy, postpartum, or threatened abortion 13 weeks or beyond):* transfusion unit or blood bank determines fetal packed RBC volume entering patient's blood; then give one vial I.M. if fetal packed RBC volume is below 15 ml. More than one vial I.M. may be required if large fetomaternal hemorrhage occurs. Must be given within 72 hours after delivery or miscarriage.

▶ **Transfusion accident.** *Adults and children:* consult blood bank or transfusion unit at once. Must be given within 72 hours.

▶ **Postabortion or postmiscarriage to prevent Rh antibody formation up to and including 12 weeks' gestation.** *Adults:* consult transfusion unit or blood bank. One microdose vial suppresses immune reaction to 2.5 ml Rh$_o$(D)-positive RBCs. Should be given within 3 hours but may be given up to 72 hours after abortion or miscarriage.

▶ **Amniocentesis or abdominal trauma during pregnancy.** *Women:* dose based on extent of fetomaternal hemorrhage.

Adverse reactions

Skin: discomfort (at injection site).
Other: slight fever, *anaphylaxis.*

Interactions

Drug-drug. *Live-virus vaccines:* may interfere with response. Delay immunization for 3 months if possible.

Contraindications and precautions

• Contraindicated in Rh$_o$(D)-positive or D^u-positive patients, in those previously immunized to Rh$_o$(D) blood factor, and in those with anaphylactic or severe systemic reaction to human globulin.
• Use cautiously in pregnant or breast-feeding women.

NURSING CONSIDERATIONS

☣ Assessment

• Obtain history of Rh-negative patient's Rh-positive exposure and allergies and reaction to immunization.
• Evaluate patient's and family's knowledge of drug therapy.

⚕ Nursing diagnoses

• Risk for injury related to Rh-positive exposure
• Altered protection related to drug-induced anaphylaxis
• Knowledge deficit related to drug therapy

⟫ Planning and implementation

• Make sure epinephrine 1:1,000 is available in case of anaphylaxis.
• After delivery, have neonate's cord blood typed and crossmatched; confirm if mother is Rh$_o$(D)-negative and D^u-negative. Administer to mother, as ordered, only if infant is Rh$_o$(D)-positive or D^u-positive.
• Drug gives passive immunity to patient exposed to Rh$_o$(D)-positive fetal blood during pregnancy; prevents formation of maternal antibodies, which would endanger future Rh$_o$(D)-positive pregnancies.
• Defer vaccination with live-virus vaccines for 3 months after administration of drug.
• MICRhoGAM is recommended for every patient undergoing abortion or miscarriage up to 12 weeks' gestation unless

she is $Rh_o(D)$-positive or D^u-positive or has Rh antibodies, or father or fetus is Rh-negative.
• Refrigerate drug at 36° to 46° F (2° to 8° C).

Patient teaching
• Explain to patient how drug protects future $Rh_o(D)$-positive fetuses.

☑ **Evaluation**
• Patient exhibits evidence of passive immunity to exposure to $Rh_o(D)$-positive blood.
• Patient does not develop anaphylaxis after drug administration.
• Patient and family state understanding of drug therapy.

ribavirin
(righ-bəh-VIGH-rin)
Virazole

Pharmacologic class: synthetic nucleoside
Therapeutic class: antiviral
Pregnancy risk category: X

How supplied

Powder to be reconstituted for inhalation: 6 g in 100-ml glass vial

Pharmacokinetics

Absorption: some ribavirin is absorbed systemically.
Distribution: ribavirin concentrates in bronchial secretions.
Metabolism: metabolized to 1,2,4-triazole-3-carboxamide (deribosylated ribavirin).
Excretion: most of drug excreted in urine. *Half-life:* first phase, 9½ hours; second phase, 40 hours.

Route	Onset	Peak	Duration
Inhalation	Immediate	Immediate	Unknown

Pharmacodynamics

Chemical effect: inhibits viral activity by unknown mechanism, possibly by inhibiting RNA and DNA synthesis by depleting intracellular nucleotide pools.
Therapeutic effect: inhibits activity of respiratory syncytial virus (RSV).

Indications and dosage

▶ **Hospitalized infants and young children infected by RSV.** *Infants and young children:* solution in concentration of 20 mg/ml delivered by Viratek Small Particle Aerosol Generator (SPAG-2) and mechanical ventilator or oxygen hood, face mask, or oxygen tent at rate of about 12.5 L of mist per minute. Treatment lasts for 12 to 18 hours/day for 3 to 7 days.

Adverse reactions

CV: *cardiac arrest,* hypotension.
EENT: conjunctivitis, rash or erythema of eyelids.
Hematologic: reticulocytosis.
Hepatic: elevated bilirubin, AST, ALT levels.
Respiratory: worsening of respiratory state, apnea, bacterial pneumonia, pneumothorax.

Interactions

Drug-drug. *Acetaminophen, aspirin, cimetidine:* may affect plasma concentrations of drug. Monitor patient.

Contraindications and precautions

• Contraindicated in patients with hypersensitivity to drug and in women who are or may become pregnant during treatment.
• Drug is not indicated for use in breast-feeding women.

NURSING CONSIDERATIONS

☒ **Assessment**
• Assess patient's respiratory infection before therapy and regularly thereafter.
• Monitor ventilator function. Drug may precipitate in ventilator apparatus, causing equipment malfunction with serious consequences.
• Watch for anemia in patient receiving drug longer than 1 to 2 weeks.

• Be alert for adverse reactions.
• Evaluate patient's and family's knowledge of drug therapy.

🖉 Nursing diagnoses
• Infection related to presence of RSV
• Risk for injury related to drug-induced adverse CV reactions
• Knowledge deficit related to drug therapy

⯈ Planning and implementation
• Ribavirin aerosol is indicated only for severe lower respiratory tract infection caused by RSV. Treatment may start pending test results, but existence of RSV infection must eventually be documented.
• Most infants and children with RSV infection don't require treatment. Infants with underlying conditions, such as prematurity or cardiopulmonary disease, benefit most from treatment with ribavirin aerosol.
• Give drug by SPAG-2 only. Don't use any other device.
• Use sterile USP water for injection, *not* bacteriostatic water, for reconstitution. Water used to reconstitute this drug must not contain an antimicrobial agent.
• Discard solutions placed in SPAG-2 unit at least every 24 hours before adding newly reconstituted solution.
• Avoid unnecessary occupational exposure to drug. Adverse effects reported in health care personnel exposed to aerosolized ribavirin include eye irritation and headache.
• Store reconstituted solutions at room temperature for 24 hours.
• Continue providing supportive respiratory and fluid management.
Patient teaching
• Inform parents of need for drug therapy and answer questions.

☑ Evaluation
• Patient is free from infection.
• Patient does not develop adverse CV reactions after drug administration.

• Parents state understanding of drug therapy.

riboflavin (vitamin B$_2$)†
(righ-boh-FLAY-vin)

Pharmacologic class: water-soluble vitamin
Therapeutic class: vitamin B complex vitamin
Pregnancy risk category: NR

How supplied
Tablets: 10 mg†, 25 mg†, 50 mg†, 100 mg†
Tablets (sugar-free): 50 mg†, 100 mg†

Pharmacokinetics
Absorption: absorbed readily from GI tract, although extent of absorption is limited. Absorption occurs at specialized segment of mucosa; riboflavin absorption is limited by duration of drug's contact with this area. Before being absorbed, riboflavin 5-phosphate is rapidly dephosphorylated in GI lumen. GI absorption increases when drug is given with food and decreases when hepatitis, cirrhosis, biliary obstruction, or probenecid administration is present.
Distribution: riboflavin, a coenzyme, functions in forms of flavin adenine dinucleotide (FAD) and flavin mononucleotide (FMN). FAD and FMN are distributed widely to body tissues. Riboflavin is stored in limited amounts in liver, spleen, kidneys, and heart, mainly in form of FAD. FAD and FMN are about 60% protein-bound in blood.
Metabolism: riboflavin is metabolized to FMN in erythrocytes, GI mucosal cells, and liver. FMN is converted to FAD in liver.
Excretion: excreted in urine. *Half-life:* 66 to 84 minutes.

Route	Onset	Peak	Duration
P.O.	Unknown	Unknown	Unknown

Pharmacodynamics

Chemical effect: converts to two other coenzymes that are necessary for normal tissue respiration.
Therapeutic effect: relieves riboflavin deficiency.

Indications and dosage

▶ **RDA.** *Males age 51 and over:* 1.4 mg. *Males ages 19 to 50:* 1.7 mg. *Males ages 15 to 18:* 1.8 mg. *Males ages 11 to 14:* 1.5 mg. *Females age 51 and over:* 1.2 mg. *Females ages 11 to 50:* 1.3 mg. *Pregnant women:* 1.6 mg. *Breast-feeding women (first 6 months):* 1.8 mg. *Breast-feeding women (second 6 months):* 1.7 mg. *Children ages 7 to 10:* 1.2 mg. *Children ages 4 to 6:* 1.1 mg. *Children ages 1 to 3:* 0.8 mg. *Infants age 6 months to 1 year:* 0.5 mg. *Neonates and infants to age 6 months:* 0.4 mg.

▶ **Riboflavin deficiency or adjunct to thiamine treatment for polyneuritis or cheilosis secondary to pellagra.** *Adults and children age 12 and over:* 5 to 30 mg P.O. daily, depending on severity. *Children under age 12:* 3 to 10 mg P.O. daily, depending on severity. For maintenance, increase nutritional intake and supplement with vitamin B complex.

▶ **Microcytic anemia associated with splenomegaly and glutathione reductase deficiency.** *Adults:* 10 mg P.O. daily for 10 days.

Adverse reactions

GU: bright yellow urine.

Interactions

Drug-drug. *Probenecid:* reduced urinary excretion of riboflavin. Use together cautiously.
Propantheline, other anticholinergics: decreased rate and extent of absorption. Avoid concomitant use.

Contraindications and precautions

• No known contraindications.

NURSING CONSIDERATIONS

⚕ Assessment
• Assess patient's riboflavin deficiency before and during therapy.
• Be alert for change in urine color.
• Evaluate patient's and family's knowledge of drug therapy.

⊞ Nursing diagnoses
• Altered nutrition: Less than body's needs related to drug deficiency
• Knowledge deficit related to drug therapy

▷ Planning and implementation
• Drug may be given I.M. or I.V. as component of multiple vitamins.
• Know that riboflavin deficiency usually accompanies other vitamin B complex deficiencies and may require multivitamin therapy.
• Protect drug from air and light.
Patient teaching
• Encourage patient to take with meals to increase absorption.
• Stress proper nutritional habits to prevent recurrence of deficiency.

☑ Evaluation
• Patient's drug deficiency is resolved.
• Patient and family state understanding of drug therapy.

rifabutin
(rif-uh-BYOO-tin)
Mycobutin

Pharmacologic class: semisynthetic ansamycin
Therapeutic class: antibiotic
Pregnancy risk category: B

How supplied

Capsules: 150 mg

Pharmacokinetics

Absorption: readily absorbed from GI tract.
Distribution: because of its high lipophilicity, rifabutin demonstrates high propensity for distribution and intracellular tissue uptake. About 85% of drug is bound in concentration-independent manner to plasma proteins.
Metabolism: metabolized in liver.
Excretion: excreted primarily in urine; about 30% excreted in feces. *Half-life:* 45 hours.

Route	Onset	Peak	Duration
P.O.	Unknown	1.5-4 hr	Unknown

Pharmacodynamics

Chemical effect: inhibits DNA-dependent RNA polymerase in susceptible bacteria, blocking bacterial protein synthesis.
Therapeutic effect: prevents disseminated *Mycobacterium avium* complex (MAC) in patients with advanced HIV infection.

Indications and dosage

▶ **Prevention of disseminated MAC in patients with advanced HIV infection.**
Adults: 300 mg P.O. daily as single dose or divided b.i.d. taken with food.

Adverse reactions

GI: dyspepsia, eructation, flatulence, diarrhea, nausea, vomiting, abdominal pain.
GU: discolored urine.
Hematologic: eosinophilia, LEUKOPENIA, NEUTROPENIA, *thrombocytopenia.*
Skin: rash.
Other: fever, headache, myalgia.

Interactions

Drug-drug: *Drugs metabolized by liver, zidovudine:* decreased serum levels of zidovudine. Because rifabutin, like rifampin, induces liver enzymes, it may lower serum levels of many other drugs as well. Although dosage adjustments may be necessary, further study is needed.

Oral contraceptives: decreased effectiveness. Instruct patient to use nonhormonal forms of birth control.
Drug-food. *High-fat foods:* slows absorption of drug. Avoid taking drug with high-fat meals.

Contraindications and precautions

• Contraindicated in patients with hypersensitivity to drug or other rifamycin derivatives (such as rifampin) and in those with active tuberculosis because single-agent therapy with rifabutin increases risk of inducing bacterial resistance to both rifabutin and rifampin.
• Drug is not recommended for use in breast-feeding women.
• Use cautiously in patients with preexisting neutropenia and thrombocytopenia.
• Safety of drug has not been established in children.

NURSING CONSIDERATIONS

⚕ Assessment
• Assess patient's condition before therapy and regularly thereafter.
• Perform baseline hematologic studies and repeat periodically, as ordered.
• Be alert for adverse reactions and drug interactions.
• Evaluate patient's and family's knowledge of drug therapy.

⊞ Nursing diagnoses
• Infection related to presence of advanced HIV infection
• Altered protection related to drug-induced adverse hematologic reactions
• Knowledge deficit related to drug therapy

⊠ Planning and implementation
• Know that high-fat meals slow rate but not extent of absorption.
• Mix with soft foods for patient who has difficulty swallowing.
• No evidence exists that drug will provide effective prophylaxis against *Mycobacterium tuberculosis.* Patients re-

quiring prophylaxis against both *M. tuberculosis* and MAC may require rifampin and rifabutin.

Patient teaching
• Tell patient that drug may turn urine, feces, sputum, saliva, tears, and skin brownish-orange. Tell him not to wear soft contacts because they may be permanently stained.
• Instruct patient to report photophobia, excessive lacrimation, or eye pain. Drug may rarely cause uveitis.

✓ Evaluation
• Patient does not develop disseminated MAC.
• Patient maintains normal hematologic values throughout therapy.
• Patient and family state understanding of drug therapy.

rifampin (rifampicin)

(rih-FAM-pin)
Rifadin, Rifadin IV, Rimactane, Rimycin◇, Rofact♦

Pharmacologic class: semisynthetic rifamycin B derivative (macrocytic antibiotic)
Therapeutic class: antitubercular agent
Pregnancy risk category: C

How supplied

Capsules: 150 mg, 300 mg
Injection: 600 mg

Pharmacokinetics

Absorption: absorbed completely from GI tract after P.O. administration. Food delays absorption.
Distribution: distributed widely in body tissues and fluids, including CSF, ascitic, pleural, and seminal fluids as well as tears and saliva and in liver, prostate, lungs, and bone. It is 84% to 91% protein-bound.
Metabolism: metabolized extensively in liver. Drug undergoes enterohepatic circulation.

Excretion: drug and metabolite excreted primarily in bile; drug, but not metabolite, is reabsorbed. Some of drug and its metabolite are excreted in urine. *Half-life:* 1½ to 5 hours.

Route	Onset	Peak	Duration
P.O.	Unknown	2-4 hr	Unknown
I.V.	Unknown	Unknown	Unknown

Pharmacodynamics

Chemical effect: inhibits DNA-dependent RNA polymerase, thus impairing RNA synthesis (bactericidal).
Therapeutic effect: kills susceptible bacteria. Spectrum of activity includes *Mycobacterium bovis, M. kansasii, M. marinum, M. tuberculosis* and some strains of *M. avium-intracellulare* and *M. fortuitum* as well as many gram-positive and some gram-negative bacteria.

Indications and dosage

▶ **Pulmonary tuberculosis.** *Adults:* 600 mg P.O. or I.V. daily in single dose. *Children over age 5:* 10 to 20 mg/kg P.O. or I.V. daily in single dose. Maximum dosage is 600 mg daily. Concomitant use with other antitubercular agents is recommended.
▶ **Meningococcal carriers.** *Adults:* 600 mg P.O. or I.V. b.i.d. for 2 days. *Children ages 1 month to 12 years:* 10 mg/kg P.O. or I.V. b.i.d. for 2 days, not to exceed 600 mg/day. *Neonates:* 5 mg/kg P.O. or I.V. b.i.d. for 2 days.
▶ **Prophylaxis of *Haemophilus influenzae* type b.** *Adults and children:* 20 mg/kg P.O. daily for 4 days, not to exceed 600 mg/day.
Note: Reduce dosage in patients with liver dysfunction.

Adverse reactions

CNS: ataxia, behavioral changes, confusion, dizziness, fatigue, headache, drowsiness, generalized numbness.
EENT: visual disturbances, exudative conjunctivitis.

GI: epigastric distress, anorexia, nausea, vomiting, abdominal pain, diarrhea, flatulence, sore mouth and tongue, pseudomembranous colitis, *pancreatitis*.
GU: hemoglobinuria, hematuria, *acute renal failure,* menstrual disturbances.
Hematologic: eosinophilia, transient leukopenia, *thrombocytopenia,* hemolytic anemia.
Hepatic: *hepatotoxicity, transient abnormalities in liver function tests*, porphyria exacerbation.
Skin: pruritus, urticaria, rash.
Other: flulike syndrome, discoloration of body fluids, hyperuricemia, shortness of breath, wheezing, *shock,* osteomalacia.

Interactions

Drug-drug. *Analgesics, anticoagulants, anticonvulsants, barbiturates, beta blockers, cardiac glycosides, chloramphenicol, clofibrate, corticosteroids, cyclosporine, dapsone, diazepam, disopyramide, methadone, mexiletine, narcotics, oral contraceptives, progestins, quinidine, sulfonylureas, theophylline, verapamil:* reduced effectiveness of these drugs. Avoid concomitant use.
Halothane: may increase risk of hepatotoxicity in both drugs. Monitor liver function closely.
Ketoconazole, para-aminosalicylate sodium: may interfere with absorption of rifampin. Give these drugs 8 to 12 hours apart.
Probenecid: may increase rifampin levels. Use cautiously.
Drug-lifestyle. *Alcohol use:* may increase risk of hepatotoxicity. Avoid concomitant use.

Contraindications and precautions

• Contraindicated in patients with hypersensitivity to drug.
• Use cautiously in patients with liver disease and in pregnant or breast-feeding women.

NURSING CONSIDERATIONS

⬆ Assessment
• Assess patient's infection before therapy and regularly thereafter.
• Monitor liver function, hematopoiesis, and serum uric acid levels.
• Be alert for adverse reactions and drug interactions.
• Know that drug may cause hemorrhage in neonates of rifampin-treated mothers.
• Watch closely for signs of hepatic impairment.
• Monitor patient's hydration status if adverse GI reactions occur.
• Evaluate patient's and family's knowledge of drug therapy.

⬚ Nursing diagnoses
• Infection related to presence of susceptible bacteria
• Risk for fluid volume deficit related to drug-induced adverse reactions
• Knowledge deficit related to drug therapy

⬚ Planning and implementation
• Be aware that concomitant treatment with at least one other antitubercular agent is recommended.
P.O. use: Give drug 1 hour before or 2 hours after meals for optimal absorption; if GI irritation occurs, patient may take rifampin with meals.
I.V. use: Reconstitute vial with 10 ml of sterile water for injection to make solution containing 60 mg/ml. Add to 100 ml of D₅W and infuse over 30 minutes, or add to 500 ml of D₅W and infuse over 3 hours. When dextrose is contraindicated, drug may be diluted with 0.9% NaCl injection. Do not use other I.V. solutions.
• Report hepatic impairment.
Patient teaching
• Warn patient about drowsiness and possible red-orange discoloration of urine, feces, saliva, sweat, sputum, and tears. Soft contact lenses may be permanently stained.

Reactions may be *common*, uncommon, *life-threatening*, or COMMON AND LIFE-THREATENING.

• Advise patient to avoid alcoholic beverages while taking this drug.

☑ **Evaluation**
• Patient is free from infection.
• Patient maintains adequate hydration throughout therapy.
• Patient and family state understanding of drug therapy.

---

rifapentine
(rif-ah-PEN-tin)
Priftin

Pharmacologic class: rifamycin derivative antibiotic
Therapeutic class: antituberculosis agent
Pregnancy risk category: C

How supplied:
Tablets (film-coated): 150 mg

Pharmacokinetics
Absorption: relative bioavailability is 70%.
Distribution: about 98% bound to plasma proteins.
Metabolism: hydrolyzed by an esterase enzyme to the microbiologically active 25-desacetyl rifapentine. Rifapentine contributes 62% to drug's activity and 25-desacetyle contributes 38%.
Excretion: about 17% is excreted in urine and 70% in feces. *Half-life:* 13 hours.

Route	Onset	Peak	Duration
P.O.	Unknown	5-6 hr	Unknown

Pharmacodynamics
Chemical effect: inhibits DNA-dependent RNA polymerase in susceptible strains of *Mycobacterium tuberculosis*. It has bactericidal activity against the organism both intra- and extracellularly. Rifapentine and rifampin share similar antimicrobial action.
Therapeutic effect: kills susceptible bacteria.

Indications and dosage
▶ **Pulmonary tuberculosis, in conjunction with at least one other antitubercular agent to which the isolate is susceptible.** *Adults:* during intensive phase of short-course therapy, 600 mg P.O. twice weekly for 2 months, with an interval between doses of not less than 3 days (72 hours). During the continuation phase of short-course therapy, 600 mg P.O. once weekly for 4 months in combination with isoniazid or another agent to which the isolate is susceptible.

Adverse reactions
CNS: headache, dizziness.
CV: hypertension.
GI: anorexia, nausea, vomiting, dyspepsia, diarrhea.
GU: pyuria, proteinuria, hematuria, urinary casts.
Hematologic: *neutropenia,* lymphopenia, anemia, *leukopenia,* thrombocytosis.
Hepatic: elevated AST and ALT.
Respiratory: hemoptysis.
Skin: rash, pruritus, acne, maculopapular rash.
Other: *hyperuricemia,* arthralgia, pain.

Interactions
Drug-drug. *Antiarrhythmics (disopyramide, mexiletine, quinidine, tocainide), antibiotics (chloramphenicol, clarithromycin, dapsone, doxycycline, fluoroquinolones), anticonvulsants (phenytoin), antifungals (fluconazole, itraconazole, ketoconazole), barbiturates, benzodiazepines (diazepam), beta blockers, calcium channel blockers (diltiazem, nifedipine, verapamil), cardiac glycosides, clofibrate, corticosteroids, haloperidol, HIV protease inhibitors (indinavir, nelfinavir, ritonavir, saquinavir), immunosuppressants (cyclosporine, tacrolimus), levothyroxine, narcotic analgesics (methadone), oral anticoagulants (warfarin), oral hypoglycemics (sulfonylureas), oral or other systemic hormonal contraceptives, progestins, quinine, reverse transcriptase inhibitors (delavir-*

---

dine, zidovudine), sildenafil, theophylline, tricyclic antidepressants (amitriptyline, nortriptyline): induces metabolism of hepatic cytochrome P-450 enzyme system, decreasing the activity of these medications. Dosage adjustments may be required.

Contraindications and precautions

• Contraindicated in patients with history of hypersensitivity to a rifamycin (rifapentine, rifampin, or rifabutin).
• Use drug cautiously and with frequent monitoring in patients with liver disease.

NURSING CONSIDERATIONS

⚗ Assessment
• Assess patient's condition before therapy and regularly thereafter.
• Assess patient's understanding of disease and stress importance of strict compliance with drug and daily companion medications, as well as necessary follow-up visits and laboratory tests.
• Monitor liver function, CBC, and serum uric acid levels.
• Monitor patient for persistent or severe diarrhea and notify doctor if it occurs.
• Evaluate patient's and family's knowledge of drug therapy.

⊞ Nursing diagnoses
• Infection related to patient's underlying condition
• Noncompliance related to long-term therapeutic regimen
• Knowledge deficit related to drug therapy

❯ Planning and implementation
• Know that concomitant administration of pyridoxine (vitamin B_6) is recommended in malnourished patients, in those predisposed to neuropathy (alcoholics, diabetics), and in adolescents.
• Know that drug must be given with appropriate daily companion drugs. Compliance with all medications, especially with daily companion drugs on the days

when rifapentine is not given, is crucial for early sputum conversion and protection from relapse of tuberculosis.
• Administration of drug during last 2 weeks of pregnancy may lead to postnatal hemorrhage in mother or infant. Monitor clotting parameters closely.
Patient teaching
• Stress importance of strict compliance with drug and daily companion medications, as well as necessary follow-up visits and laboratory tests.
• Advise patient to use nonhormonal methods of birth control.
• Tell patient to take drug with food if nausea, vomiting, or GI upset occurs.
• Instruct patient to notify doctor if the following occur: fever, loss of appetite, malaise, nausea, vomiting, darkened urine, yellowish discoloration of skin and eyes, pain or swelling of joints, and excessive loose stools or diarrhea.
• Instruct patient to protect pills from excessive heat.
• Tell patient that drug can turn body fluids red-orange. If patient wears contact lenses, these can become permanently stained.

☑ Evaluation
• Patient experiences sputum conversion and recovers from tuberculosis.
• Patient is compliant with therapeutic regimen.
• Patient and family state understanding of drug therapy.

---

riluzole
(RIGH-loo-zohl)
Rilutek

Pharmacologic class: benzothiazole
Therapeutic class: neuroprotector
Pregnancy risk category: C

How supplied

Tablets: 50 mg

Pharmacokinetics

Absorption: well absorbed from GI tract, with average absolute oral bioavailability of about 60%. High-fat meal decreases absorption.
Distribution: 96% protein-bound.
Metabolism: extensively metabolized in liver.
Excretion: excreted primarily in urine, with small amount excreted in feces.
Half-life: 12 hours with repeated doses.

Route	Onset	Peak	Duration
P.O.	Unknown	Unknown	Unknown

Pharmacodynamics

Chemical effect: unknown.
Therapeutic effect: improves signs and symptoms associated with amyotrophic lateral sclerosis (ALS).

Indications and dosage

▶ **ALS.** *Adults:* 50 mg P.O. q 12 hours on empty stomach.

Adverse reactions

CNS: headache, aggravation reaction, *asthenia,* hypertonia, depression, dizziness, insomnia, malaise, somnolence, vertigo, circumoral paresthesia.
CV: hypertension, tachycardia, palpitation, orthostatic hypotension.
EENT: *rhinitis, sinusitis.*
GI: abdominal pain, *nausea,* vomiting, dyspepsia, anorexia, diarrhea, flatulence, stomatitis, tooth disorder, dry mouth, oral moniliasis.
GU: urinary tract infection, dysuria.
Respiratory: *decreased lung function,* increased cough.
Skin: pruritus, eczema, alopecia, exfoliative dermatitis.
Other: back pain, phlebitis, weight loss, peripheral edema, arthralgia.

Interactions

Drug-drug. *Allopurinol, methyldopa, sulfasalazine:* increased risk of hepatotoxicity. Monitor patient closely.
Inducers of CVP 1AZ (omeprazole, rifampicin): may increase riluzole elimination. Monitor closely.
Potential inhibitors of CYP 1A2 (amitriptyline, phenacetin, quinolones, theophylline): may decrease riluzole elimination. Monitor closely.
Drug-food. *Any food:* decreased bioavailability. Administer 1 hour before or 2 hours after meals.
Caffeine: may decrease riluzole elimination. Monitor closely.
Charbroiled foods: may increase riluzole elimination. Avoid taking together.
Drug-lifestyle. *Alcohol use:* may increase risk of hepatotoxicity. Avoid excessive use.
Smoking: may increase riluzole elimination. Advise patient to refrain from smoking.

Contraindications and precautions

• Contraindicated in patients with history of severe hypersensitivity reaction to drug or components of the tablets.
• Drug is not recommended for use in breast-feeding women.
• Use cautiously in patients with hepatic or renal dysfunction, in elderly patients, and in females and Japanese patients (who may have a lower metabolic capacity to eliminate riluzole compared to males and white subjects, respectively).
• Safety of drug has not been established in children.

NURSING CONSIDERATIONS

⚏ Assessment
• Obtain history of patient's ALS.
• Obtain liver function studies before and during therapy.
• Evaluate patient's and family's knowledge of drug therapy.

⚏ Nursing diagnoses
• Impaired physical mobility related to ALS
• Risk for fluid volume deficit related to adverse GI reactions

---

• Knowledge deficit related to drug therapy

▶ **Planning and implementation**
• Baseline elevations in liver function studies (especially elevated bilirubin level) should preclude use of riluzole. In many patients, drug may cause serum aminotransferase level elevations. If level exceeds 10 times upper limit of normal range, or if clinical jaundice develops, notify doctor.
• Give drug at least 1 hour before or 2 hours after a meal to avoid a food-related decrease in bioavailability.
Patient teaching
• Tell patient to take drug at same time each day. If he misses a dose, tell him to take the next tablet as planned.
• Instruct patient to report febrile illness; his WBC count should be checked.
• Warn patient to avoid hazardous activities until drug's CNS effects are known.
• Advise patient to limit alcohol intake during therapy.
• Tell patient to store drug at room temperature, protected from bright light and out of children's reach.

☑ **Evaluation**
• Patient responds well to therapy.
• Patient maintains adequate hydration.
• Patient and family state understanding of drug therapy.

rimantadine hydrochloride
(righ-MAN-tuh-deen high-droh-KLOR-ighd)
Flumadine

Pharmacologic class: adamantine
Therapeutic class: antiviral
Pregnancy risk category: C

How supplied
Tablets: 100 mg
Syrup: 50 mg/5 ml

Pharmacokinetics
Absorption: well absorbed from GI tract.
Distribution: plasma protein–binding is about 40%.
Metabolism: metabolized extensively in liver.
Excretion: excreted in urine. *Half-life:* 25.4 to 32 hours.

Route	Onset	Peak	Duration
P.O.	Unknown	1-4 hr	Unknown

Pharmacodynamics
Chemical effect: unknown; appears to prevent viral uncoating, an early step in virus reproductive cycle.
Therapeutic effect: inhibits viral reproduction. Spectrum of activity is influenza A virus.

Indications and dosage
▶ **Prophylaxis against influenza A virus.** *Adults and children age 10 and over:* 100 mg P.O. b.i.d. *Elderly patients, patients with severe hepatic or renal dysfunction:* 100 mg P.O. daily. *Children under age 10:* 5 mg/kg (not to exceed 150 mg/day) P.O. once daily.
▶ **Treatment of influenza A virus infections.** *Adults:* 100 mg P.O. b.i.d. for 7 days from onset of symptoms. *Elderly patients, patients with severe hepatic or renal dysfunction:* 100 mg P.O. daily.

Adverse reactions
CNS: insomnia, headache, dizziness, nervousness, fatigue, asthenia.
GI: nausea, vomiting, anorexia, dry mouth, abdominal pain.

Interactions
Drug-drug. *Acetaminophen, aspirin:* reduced concentration of rimantadine. Monitor for decreased effectiveness of rimantadine.
Cimetidine: may decrease clearance of rimantadine. Monitor for adverse reactions.

Reactions may be *common*, uncommon, *life-threatening*, or COMMON AND LIFE-THREATENING.

Contraindications and precautions

• Contraindicated in patients hypersensitive to drug or amantadine and in breastfeeding women.
• Use cautiously in patients with renal or hepatic impairment or history of seizures and in pregnant women.

NURSING CONSIDERATIONS

⏣ Assessment

• Obtain history of patient's exposure to influenza A virus before therapy and reassess regularly thereafter.
• Monitor patient's hydration status throughout rimantadine therapy.
• Evaluate patient's and family's knowledge of drug therapy.

⏣ Nursing diagnoses

• Infection related to exposure to influenza A virus
• Risk for fluid volume deficit related to drug-induced adverse GI reactions
• Knowledge deficit related to drug therapy

⏵ Planning and implementation

• For influenza infections, give within 48 hours of onset of symptoms and continue for 7 days after initial signs and symptoms occurred.
• Consider risk to contacts of treated patients who may be subject to morbidity from influenza A. Influenza A–resistant strains can emerge during therapy. Patients taking drug may still be able to spread disease.
Patient teaching
• Instruct patient to take drug several hours before bedtime to prevent insomnia.

⏣ Evaluation

• Patient is free from infection.
• Patient maintains adequate hydration throughout therapy.
• Patient and family state understanding of drug therapy.

Ringer's injection
(RING-erz in-JEK-shun)

Pharmacologic class: electrolyte solution
Therapeutic class: electrolyte and fluid replenishment
Pregnancy risk category: NR

How supplied

Injection: 250 ml, 500 ml, 1,000 ml

Pharmacokinetics

Absorption: not applicable with I.V. administration.
Distribution: widely distributed.
Metabolism: not significant.
Excretion: excreted primarily in urine and minimally in feces.

Route	Onset	Peak	Duration
I.V.	Immediate	Immediate	Unknown

Pharmacodynamics

Chemical effect: replaces fluids and electrolytes.
Therapeutic effect: restores normal fluid and electrolyte balance.

Indications and dosage

▶ **Fluid and electrolyte replacement.**
Adults and children: dose highly individualized but usually 1.5 to 3 L (2% to 6% body weight) infused I.V. over 18 to 24 hours.

Adverse reactions

CV: fluid overload.
Metabolic: electrolyte imbalance.

Interactions

None significant.

Contraindications and precautions

• Contraindicated in patients with renal failure, except as emergency volume expander.
• Use cautiously in patients with heart failure, circulatory insufficiency, renal

dysfunction, hypoproteinemia, or pulmonary edema and in pregnant women.

NURSING CONSIDERATIONS

⚕ Assessment
• Obtain history of patient's fluid and electrolyte status before therapy and reassess regularly thereafter.
• Be alert for fluid overload.
• Evaluate patient's and family's knowledge of drug therapy.

⊞ Nursing diagnoses
• Fluid volume deficit related to underlying condition
• Knowledge deficit related to drug therapy

▶ Planning and implementation
• Know that drug contains sodium, 147 mEq/L; potassium, 4 mEq/L; calcium, 4.5 mEq/L; and chloride, 155.5 mEq/L.
• Electrolyte content is not enough to treat severe electrolyte deficiencies, but it does provide electrolytes in levels approximating those of blood.
Patient teaching
• Inform patient of need for drug, and instruct him to report signs of fluid overload, such as difficulty breathing.

▣ Evaluation
• Patient regains normal fluid and electrolyte balance.
• Patient and family state understanding of drug therapy.

Ringer's injection, lactated (Hartmann's solution, Ringer's lactate solution)
(RING-erz in-JEK-shun, LAK-tayt-ed)

Pharmacologic class: electrolyte-carbohydrate solution
Therapeutic class: electrolyte and fluid replenishment
Pregnancy risk category: NR

How supplied
Injection: 150 ml, 250 ml, 500 ml, 1,000 ml

Pharmacokinetics
Absorption: not applicable with I.V. administration.
Distribution: widely distributed.
Metabolism: not significant for electrolytes. Lactate is oxidized to bicarbonate.
Excretion: excreted primarily in urine and minimally in feces.

Route	Onset	Peak	Duration
I.V.	Immediate	Immediate	Unknown

Pharmacodynamics
Chemical effect: replaces fluids and electrolytes.
Therapeutic effect: restores normal fluid and electrolyte balance.

Indications and dosage
▶ **Fluid and electrolyte replacement.**
Adults and children: dosage highly individualized according to patient's size and clinical condition.

Adverse reactions
CV: fluid overload.
Metabolic: electrolyte imbalance.

Interactions
None significant.

Contraindications and precautions
• Contraindicated in patients with renal failure, except as emergency volume expander.
• Use cautiously in patients with heart failure, circulatory insufficiency, renal dysfunction, hypoproteinemia, or pulmonary edema and in pregnant women.

NURSING CONSIDERATIONS

⚕ Assessment
• Obtain history of patient's fluid and electrolyte status before therapy and reassess regularly thereafter.

• Be alert for fluid overload.
• Evaluate patient's knowledge of drug therapy.

🖼 **Nursing diagnoses**
• Fluid volume deficit related to underlying condition
• Knowledge deficit related to drug therapy

▷ **Planning and implementation**
• Know that drug contains sodium, 130 mEq/L; potassium, 4 mEq/L; calcium, 3 mEq/L; chloride, 109.7 mEq/L; and lactate, 28 mEq/L.
• Lactated Ringer's injection more closely approximates electrolyte concentration in blood plasma.
Patient teaching
• Inform patient of need for drug. Instruct him to report signs of fluid overload, such as difficulty breathing.

☑ **Evaluation**
• Patient regains normal fluid and electrolyte balance.
• Patient and family state understanding of drug therapy.

---

risperidone
(ris-PER-ih-dohn)
Risperdal

Pharmacologic class: benzisoxazole derivative
Therapeutic class: antipsychotic
Pregnancy risk category: C

How supplied
Tablets: 1 mg, 2 mg, 3 mg, 4 mg

Pharmacokinetics
Absorption: well absorbed; absolute oral bioavailability is 70%.
Distribution: plasma protein binding is about 90% for risperidone and 77% for its major active metabolite.

Metabolism: extensively metabolized in liver.
Excretion: metabolite excreted in urine.

Route	Onset	Peak	Duration
P.O.	Unknown	About 1 hr	Unknown

Pharmacodynamics
Chemical effect: blocks dopamine and serotonin receptors as well as alpha$_1$, alpha$_2$, and H$_1$ receptors in CNS.
Therapeutic effect: relieves signs and symptoms of psychosis.

Indications and dosage
▶ **Psychosis.** *Adults:* initially, 1 mg P.O. b.i.d. Increased in increments of 1 mg b.i.d. on days 2 and 3 of treatment to target dose of 3 mg b.i.d. At least 1 week must pass before dosage is adjusted further. *Elderly or debilitated patients, hypotensive patients, or patients with severe renal or hepatic impairment:* initially, 0.5 mg P.O. b.i.d. Increased in increments of 0.5 mg b.i.d. on days 2 and 3 of treatment to target dosage of 1.5 mg P.O. b.i.d. At least 1 week must pass before dosage is increased further.

Adverse reactions
CNS: *somnolence, extrapyramidal symptoms,* headache, *insomnia, agitation, anxiety,* tardive dyskinesia, aggressiveness.
CV: tachycardia, chest pain, orthostatic hypotension, *prolonged QT interval.*
EENT: *rhinitis,* coughing, upper respiratory tract infection, sinusitis, pharyngitis, abnormal vision.
GI: *constipation, nausea, vomiting, dyspepsia.*
Musculoskeletal: arthralgia, back pain.
Skin: rash, dry skin, photosensitivity.
Other: fever; *neuroleptic malignant syndrome* (rare).

Interactions
Drug-drug. *Carbamazepine:* increased clearance of risperidone, leading to decreased effectiveness. Monitor patient closely.

Clozapine: decreased clearance of risperidone, increasing toxicity. Monitor patient closely.
CNS depressants: additive CNS depression. Avoid concomitant use.
Levodopa: antagonized effects. Don't use together.
Drug-lifestyle. *Alcohol use:* additive CNS depression. Avoid concomitant use.
Sun exposure: increased photosensitivity reactions. Avoid prolonged or unprotected sun exposure.

Contraindications and precautions

• Contraindicated in patients hypersensitive to drug and in breast-feeding women.
• Use with extreme caution in pregnant women.
• Use cautiously in patients with prolonged QT interval, CV disease, cerebrovascular disease, dehydration, hypovolemia, history of seizures, exposure to extreme heat, or conditions that could affect metabolism or hemodynamic responses.
• Safety of drug has not been established in children.

NURSING CONSIDERATIONS

Assessment
• Assess patient's psychosis before therapy and regularly thereafter.
• Assess blood pressure before therapy and monitor regularly. Watch for orthostatic hypotension, especially during initial dosage titration.
• Be alert for adverse reactions and drug interactions.
• Watch for tardive dyskinesia. It may occur after prolonged use. It may not appear until months or years later and may disappear spontaneously or persist for life despite stopping drug.
• Evaluate patient's and family's knowledge of drug therapy.

Nursing diagnoses
• Altered thought processes related to presence of psychosis

• Risk for injury related to drug-induced adverse CNS reactions
• Knowledge deficit related to drug therapy

Planning and implementation
• When restarting therapy for patient who has been off drug, follow 3-day dose initiation schedule.
• When switching patient to drug from another antipsychotic agent, immediate discontinuation of the other agent on initiation of risperidone therapy is recommended when medically appropriate.
Patient teaching
• Warn patient to rise slowly, avoid hot showers, and use extra caution during first few days of therapy to avoid fainting.
• Warn patient to avoid activities that require alertness until CNS effects of drug are known. Drowsiness and dizziness usually subside after a few days.
• Tell patient to avoid alcohol during therapy.
• Advise patient to use caution in hot weather to prevent heatstroke; drug may affect thermoregulation.
• Tell patient to use sunblock and to wear protective clothing.
• Tell female patient to notify doctor if she is or plans to become pregnant.

Evaluation
• Patient behavior and communication indicate improved thought processes.
• Patient does not experience injury as result of drug-induced adverse CNS reactions.
• Patient and family state understanding of drug therapy.

---

ritodrine hydrochloride
(RIGH-toh-dreen high-droh-KLOR-ighd)
Yutopar

Pharmacologic class: beta-receptor agonist

Therapeutic class: adjunct agent in suppression of preterm labor
Pregnancy risk category: B

How supplied

Tablets: 10 mg
Injection: 10 mg/ml, 15 mg/ml

Pharmacokinetics

Absorption: 30% absorbed after P.O. dose. Food may inhibit absorption and effectiveness of oral drug.
Distribution: distributed to tissues; protein binding is low.
Metabolism: metabolized in liver.
Excretion: about 70% to 90% excreted in urine.

Route	Onset	Peak	Duration
P.O.	30-60 min	Unknown	Unknown
I.V.	5 min	Unknown	Unknown

Pharmacodynamics

Chemical effect: stimulates beta$_2$-adrenergic receptors in uterine smooth muscle, inhibiting contractility.
Therapeutic effect: stops uterine contractions.

Indications and dosage

▶ **Preterm labor.** *Adults:* Usual initial dose is 0.05 mg/minute I.V., gradually increased by 0.05 mg/minute q 10 minutes until desired result is obtained or maternal heart rate is 130 beats/minute. Effective dosage is usually 0.15 to 0.35 mg/minute. Oral maintenance: 10 mg P.O. about 30 minutes before I.V. therapy stopped. Usual dosage for first 24 hours of maintenance is 10 mg P.O. q 2 hours. Then, 10 to 20 mg P.O. q 4 to 6 hours. Maximum daily dosage is 120 mg.

Adverse reactions

CNS: nervousness, anxiety, *headache, tremors,* emotional upset, malaise.
CV: dose-related alterations in blood pressure, palpitations, *pulmonary edema, tachycardia.*
GI: *nausea, vomiting.*
Hematologic: *leukopenia, agranulocytosis.*
Metabolic: *hyperglycemia,* hypokalemia.
Other: *erythema, anaphylactic shock.*

Interactions

Drug-drug. *Atropine:* may potentiate systemic hypertension. Monitor blood pressure.
Beta blockers: may inhibit ritodrine's action. Avoid concurrent use.
Corticosteroids: may produce pulmonary edema in mother. Monitor patient closely.
Inhalation anesthetics: potentiated adverse cardiac effects, arrhythmias, and hypotension. Monitor patient.
Sympathomimetics: additive sympathomimetic effects. Use together cautiously.

Contraindications and precautions

● Contraindicated in pregnant women before 20th week of gestation and in women with antepartum hemorrhage, eclampsia, intrauterine fetal death, chorioamnionitis, maternal cardiac disease, pulmonary hypertension, maternal hyperthyroidism, or uncontrolled maternal diabetes mellitus as well as in patients who are hypersensitive to drug or with preexisting maternal medical conditions that would be seriously affected by known pharmacologic properties of drug, such as hypovolemia, pheochromocytoma, or uncontrolled hypertension.
● Use cautiously in patients with sulfite sensitivity.

NURSING CONSIDERATIONS

⚗ Assessment
● Assess patient's uterine contractions before therapy and regularly thereafter.
● Because CV responses are common and more pronounced during I.V. administration, monitor CV effects, including maternal pulse rate and blood pressure and fetal heart rate. Maternal tachycardia of over 140 beats/minute or persistent respi-

ratory rate of over 20 breaths/minute may signal impending pulmonary edema.
• Monitor blood glucose concentrations during infusion, especially in diabetic mother.
• Monitor amount of fluids given I.V. to prevent circulatory overload.
• Be alert for adverse reactions and drug interactions.
• Evaluate patient's and family's knowledge of drug therapy.

⊞ **Nursing diagnoses**
• Pain related to uterine contractions
• Risk for fluid volume deficit related to drug-induced adverse GI reactions
• Knowledge deficit related to drug therapy

▶ **Planning and implementation**
P.O. use: Follow normal protocol. Start oral therapy about 30 minutes before I.V. therapy stopped.
I.V. use: Dilute 150 mg (3 ampules) in 500 ml of fluid (final concentration is 0.3 mg/ml).
– Continue I.V. infusion for 12 hours after contractions have stopped.
– Don't use ritodrine I.V. if solution is discolored or contains precipitate.
– Use solution within 48 hours of preparation.
• Discontinue drug if pulmonary edema develops and notify doctor.
Patient teaching
• Caution patient not to stop taking oral drug without medical approval.
• Advise patient to keep scheduled follow-up appointments and to report adverse reactions promptly.

☑ **Evaluation**
• Patient's uterine contractions cease.
• Patient maintains adequate fluid balance throughout therapy.
• Patient and family state understanding of drug therapy.

ritonavir
(rih-TOH-nuh-veer)
Norvir

Pharmacologic class: protease inhibitor
Therapeutic class: antiviral
Pregnancy risk category: B

How supplied
Capsules: 100 mg
Oral solution: 80 mg/ml

Pharmacokinetics
Absorption: food enhances absorption.
Distribution: absolute bioavailability unknown; 98% to 100% bound to serum albumin.
Metabolism: in liver and kidneys.
Excretion: in urine and feces.

Route	Onset	Peak	Duration
P.O.	Unknown	2-4 hr	Unknown

Pharmacodynamics
Chemical effect: HIV protease inhibitor with activity against HIV-1 and HIV-2 proteases; binds to protease-active site and inhibits enzyme activity.
Therapeutic effect: prevents cleavage of viral polyproteins, resulting in formation of immature noninfectious viral particles.

Indications and dosage
▶ **Treatment of HIV infection in combination with nucleoside analogues or as monotherapy when antiretroviral therapy is warranted.** *Adults:* 600 mg P.O. b.i.d with meals. If nausea occurs, escalation of dosage may provide relief: 300 mg b.i.d. for 1 day, 400 mg b.i.d. for 2 days, 500 mg b.i.d. for 1 day, and then 600 mg b.i.d. thereafter.

Adverse reactions
CNS: *asthenia,* headache, malaise, circumoral paresthesia, dizziness, insomnia, paresthesia, peripheral paresthesia, somnolence, thinking abnormality, migraine headache.

Reactions may be *common,* uncommon, *life-threatening*, or COMMON AND LIFE-THREATENING.

CV: vasodilation.
EENT: local throat irritation, diplopia, pharyngitis, photophobia, *taste perversion.*
GI: abdominal pain, anorexia, constipation, *diarrhea, nausea, vomiting,* dyspepsia, flatulence.
Hematologic: decreased hemoglobin and hematocrit levels, *leukopenia, thrombocytopenia.*
Musculoskeletal: myalgia.
Skin: rash, sweating.
Other: fever, increased CK level, hyperlipidemia, blepharitis, elevated transaminases.

Interactions

Drug-drug. *Agents that increase CYP3A activity (carbamazepine, dexamethasone, phenobarbital, phenytoin, rifabutin, rifampin):* may increase clearance of ritonavir, resulting in decreased ritonavir plasma concentrations. Monitor patient closely.
Alprazolam, clorazepate, diazepam, estazolam, flurazepam, midazolam, triazolam, zolpidem: significantly increased levels of these drugs. Because of potential for extreme sedation and respiratory depression, don't administer these agents concurrently with ritonavir.
Amiodarone, astemizole, bepridil, bupropion, cisapride, clozapine, encainide, flecainide, meperidine, piroxicam, propafenone, propoxyphene, quinidine, rifabutin: significantly increases plasma levels of these drugs, which increases patient's risk of arrhythmias, hematologic abnormalities, seizures, or other potentially serious adverse effects. Don't administer drugs concurrently.
Clarithromycin: reduces creatinine clearance. Patients with impaired renal function receiving drug with ritonavir require reduction in clarithromycin dose of 50% if creatinine clearance is 30 to 60 ml/minute and a 75% reduction if it is below 30 ml/minute.
Desipramine: increases serum levels of desipramine. Monitor patient.
Disulfiram or other drugs that produce disulfiram-like reactions (metronidazole): increases risk of disulfiram-like reactions (alcohol in ritonavir formulation). Monitor patient closely.
Glucuronosyltransferases: may increase activity of these drugs with loss of therapeutic effects. If used concomitantly, monitor therapeutic drug levels. Dosage reduction greater than 50% may be required for agents extensively metabolized by CYP3A.
Oral contraceptives containing ethinyl estradiol: decreases serum levels of contraceptive. Concomitant therapy may require higher oral contraceptive dosage or alternative method.
Saquinavir: inhibits metabolism of saquinavir, resulting in increased plasma levels. Monitor for toxicity.
Theophylline: decreases serum levels of theophylline. Monitor level.
Drug-food. *Any food:* increased absorption. Give drug with food.
Drug-lifestyle. *Smoking:* decreased serum levels of drug. Advise against tobacco use.

Contraindications and precautions

• Contraindicated in patients with hypersensitivity to drug.

NURSING CONSIDERATIONS

⚕ Assessment
• Use cautiously in patients with hepatic insufficiency.
• Evaluate patient's and family's understanding of drug therapy.

⊕ Nursing diagnoses
• Infection related to presence of virus
• Knowledge deficit related to drug therapy

⊵ Planning and implementation
• Know that it is unclear if drug is excreted in breast milk.
Patient teaching
• Inform patient that drug is not a cure for HIV infection and that illnesses associated with HIV infection may occur.

Drug does not reduce risk of HIV transmission.
- Tell patient that the taste of oral drug solution may be improved by mixing it with flavored milk within 1 hour of dose.
- Tell patient to take drug with meal.
- If a dose is missed, instruct patient to take next dose at once; he should not double doses.
- Advise patient to report use of other drugs, including OTCs.
- Tell patient to stop breast-feeding to prevent transmission of HIV.

☑ **Evaluation**
- Patient's infection is eradicated.
- Patient and family state understanding of drug therapy.

---

rizatriptan benzoate
(rih-zah-TRIP-tin BEN-zoh-ayt)
Maxalt, Maxalt-MLT

Pharmacologic class: selective 5-hydroxytryptamine receptor agonist
Therapeutic class: antimigraine
Pregnancy risk category: C

How supplied

Tablets: 5 mg, 10 mg
Tablets (orally disintegrating): 5 mg, 10 mg

Pharmacokinetics

Absorption: completely absorbed with an absolute bioavailability of 45%.
Distribution: widely distributed, 14 % bound to plasma proteins.
Metabolism: primarily by oxidative deamination by monoamine oxidase-A.
Excretion: excreted primarily in the urine (82%). *Half-life:* 2 to 3 hours.

Route	Onset	Peak	Duration
P.O.	Unknown	1-1.5 hr	Unknown

Pharmacodynamics

Chemical effect: believed to exert its effect by acting as an agonist at serotonin receptors on the extracerebral intracranial blood vessels, which results in vasoconstriction of the affected vessels, inhibition of neuropeptide release, and reduction of pain transmission in the trigeminal pathways.
Therapeutic effect: relieves migraine pain.

Indications and dosage

▶ **Treatment of acute migraine headaches with or without aura.**
Adults: initially, 5 to 10 mg P.O. If first dose is ineffective, another dose can be given at least 2 hours after first dose. Maximum daily dosage is 30 mg. For patients receiving propranolol, 5 mg P.O., up to maximum of three doses (15 mg total) in 24 hours.

Adverse reactions

CNS: dizziness, headache, somnolence, paresthesia, asthenia, fatigue, hypesthesia, decreased mental acuity, euphoria, tremor.
CV: chest pain, pressure or heaviness, palpitations, *coronary artery vasospasm.*
EENT: neck, throat and jaw pain, pressure or heaviness.
GI: dry mouth, nausea, diarrhea, vomiting.
Respiratory: dyspnea.
Skin: flushing.
Other: pain, warm or cold sensations, hot flashes.

Interactions

Drug-drug. *Ergot-containing or ergot-type drugs (dihydroergotamine, methysergide), other 5-HT$_1$ agonists:* prolonged vasospastic reactions. Do not use within 24 hours of rizatriptan.
MAO inhibitors (moclobemide), nonselective MAO inhibitors (types A and B; isocarboxazid, pargyline, phenelzine, tranylcypromine): increased plasma con-

---

Reactions may be *common,* uncommon, *life-threatening,* or COMMON AND LIFE-THREATENING.

centrations of rizatriptan. Avoid concurrent use and allow at least 14 days to elapse between discontinuation of an MAO inhibitor and taking rizatriptan. *Propranolol:* increased rizatriptan levels. Reduce rizatriptan dose to 5 mg. *Selective serotonin reuptake inhibitors (fluoxetine, fluvoxamine, paroxetine, sertraline):* weakness, hyperreflexia, incoordination may occur. Monitor patient.

Contraindications and precautions

• Contraindicated in patients with ischemic heart disease (angina pectoris, history of MI, or documented silent ischemia) or those with symptoms or findings consistent with ischemic heart disease, coronary artery vasospasm (Prinzmetal's variant angina), or other significant underlying CV disease. Also contraindicated in patients with uncontrolled hypertension and within 24 hours of treatment with another 5-HT$_1$ agonist, or an ergotamine-containing or ergottype medication like dihydroergotamine or methysergide. Do not use within 2 weeks of discontinuation of MAO inhibitor. Also contraindicated in patients hypersensitive to drug or its inactive ingredients.
• Use cautiously in patients with hepatic or renal impairment.
• Use with caution in patients with risk factors for coronary artery disease (hypertension, hypercholesterolemia, smoking, obesity, diabetes, strong family history of coronary artery disease, women with surgical or physiological menopause, or men over age 40), unless a cardiac evaluation provides evidence that patient is free from cardiac disease.

NURSING CONSIDERATIONS

Assessment
• Use drug only after a definite diagnosis of migraine is established.
• Assess patient for history of coronary artery disease, hypertension, arrhythmias,
or presence of risk factors for coronary artery disease.
• Perform baseline and periodic CV evaluation in patients who develop risk factors for coronary artery disease during treatment.
• Monitor renal and liver function tests prior to initiating drug therapy and report abnormalities.
• Evaluate patient's and family's knowledge of drug therapy.

Nursing diagnoses
• Pain related to presence of migraine headache
• Risk for activity intolerance related to adverse drug reactions
• Knowledge deficit related to drug therapy

Planning and implementation
• Don't administer to patients with hemiplegic or basilar migraine or cluster headaches.
• Don't administer drug within 24 hours of an ergot-containing medication or 5-HT$_1$ agonists or within 2 weeks of discontinuing MAO inhibitor therapy.
• For patients with cardiac risk factors who have had a satisfactory cardiac evaluation, administer first dose while monitoring ECG and have emergency equipment readily available.
• Withhold drug and notify doctor for neck, throat, and jaw pain, pressure, or heaviness and palpitations and report abnormalities to doctor.
• Know that safety of treating, on average, more than four headaches in a 30-day period has not been established.
• Safety and effectiveness have not been evaluated in children under age 18.
• Know that drug contains phenylalanine.
Patient teaching
• Inform patient that drug does not prevent headache from occurring.
• For Maxalt-MLT, tell patient to remove blister pack from sachet, then remove drug from blister pack immediately before use. Tablet should not be popped out

of blister pack, but pack should be carefully peeled away with dry hands, and tablet placed on tongue and allowed to dissolve. Tablet is then swallowed with the saliva. No water is necessary or recommended. Tell patient that orally dissolving tablet does not provide more rapid headache relief.

• Advise patient that if headache returns after initial dose, a second dose may be taken with medical approval at least 2 hours after the first dose. Do not take more than 30 mg in a 24-hour period.

• Tell patient that food may delay drug's onset of action.

• Advise patient to notify doctor if pregnancy occurs or is suspected.

• Instruct patient not to breast-feed because the effects on the infant are unknown.

🗹 **Evaluation**
• Patient has relief from migraine headache.
• Patient maintains baseline activity level.
• Patient and family state understanding of drug therapy.

rocuronium bromide
(roh-kyoo-ROH-nee-um BROH-mighd)
Zemuron

Pharmacologic class: nondepolarizing neuromuscular blocker
Therapeutic class: skeletal muscle relaxant
Pregnancy risk category: B

How supplied
Injection: 10 mg/ml

Pharmacokinetics
Absorption: not applicable with I.V. administration.
Distribution: about 30% bound to human plasma proteins.
Metabolism: unknown, although hepatic clearance is possibly significant.

Excretion: about 33% excreted in urine.

Route	Onset	Peak	Duration
I.V.	≤ 1 min	≤ 2 min	Dose-dependent

Pharmacodynamics
Chemical effect: prevents acetylcholine from binding to receptors on muscle end plate, thus blocking depolarization.
Therapeutic effect: relaxes skeletal muscles.

Indications and dosage
▶ **Adjunct to general anesthesia, to facilitate endotracheal intubation, and to provide skeletal muscle relaxation during surgery or mechanical ventilation.**
Dosage depends on anesthetic used, individual needs, and response. Dosages are representative and must be adjusted.
Adults and children age 3 months or older: initially, 0.6 mg/kg (adults, up to 1.2 mg/kg) I.V. bolus. In most patients, tracheal intubation may be performed within 2 minutes; muscle paralysis should last about 31 minutes. A maintenance dosage of 0.1 mg/kg should provide additional 12 minutes of muscle relaxation, 0.15 mg/kg will add 17 minutes, and 0.2 mg/kg will add 24 minutes to duration of effect.

Adverse reactions
CV: tachycardia, abnormal ECG, *arrhythmias* (rare), transient hypotension, hypertension.
GI: nausea, vomiting.
Respiratory: asthma, *respiratory insufficiency, apnea.*
Skin: rash, edema, pruritus.
Other: hiccups.

Interactions
Drug-drug. *Aminoglycoside antibiotics (including amikacin, gentamicin, kanamycin, neomycin, streptomycin); anticonvulsants; clindamycin; general anesthetics (such as enflurane, halothane, isoflurane); opioid analgesics;*

Reactions may be *common*, uncommon, **life-threatening**, or COMMON AND LIFE-THREATENING.

polymyxin antibiotics (colistin, polymyxin B sulfate); quinidine; succinylcholine; tetracyclines: potentiated neuromuscular blockade, leading to increased skeletal muscle relaxation and potentiation of effect. Use cautiously during surgical and postoperative periods.

Contraindications and precautions

• Contraindicated in patients with hypersensitivity to bromides.
• Use cautiously in pregnant women and in patients with altered circulation time caused by CV disease, old age, and edematous states; hepatic disease; severe obesity; bronchogenic carcinoma; electrolyte disturbances; and neuromuscular disease.
• Safety of drug has not been established in breast-feeding women.

NURSING CONSIDERATIONS

⚕ Assessment
• Assess patient's condition before therapy and regularly thereafter.
• Be alert for adverse reactions and drug interactions.
• Monitor patients with liver disease; they may need higher doses to achieve adequate muscle relaxation and may exhibit prolonged effects from drug.
• Monitor respirations closely until patient is fully recovered from neuromuscular blockade, as evidenced by tests of muscle strength (hand grip, head lift, and ability to cough).
• Evaluate patient's and family's knowledge of drug therapy.

✋ Nursing diagnoses
• Altered health maintenance related to underlying condition
• Ineffective breathing pattern related to drug's effect on respiratory muscles
• Knowledge deficit related to drug therapy

➤ Planning and implementation
• Know that drug should be used only by personnel skilled in airway management.

• Administer sedatives or general anesthetics before neuromuscular blockers, as ordered. Neuromuscular blockers do not obtund consciousness or alter pain threshold.
• Give analgesics, as ordered, for pain.
• Keep airway clear. Have emergency respiratory support equipment (endotracheal equipment, ventilator, oxygen, atropine, edrophonium, epinephrine, and neostigmine) on hand.
• Give drug by rapid I.V. injection; or give by continuous I.V. infusion. Infusion rates are highly individualized but have ranged from 0.004 to 0.16 mg/kg/minute. Compatible solutions include D_5W, 0.9% NaCl injection, dextrose 5% in 0.9% NaCl injection, sterile water for injection, and lactated Ringer's injection.
• Store reconstituted solution in refrigerator. Discard after 24 hours.
• Nerve stimulator and train-of-four monitoring are recommended to confirm antagonism of neuromuscular blockade and recovery of muscle strength. Before attempting pharmacologic reversal with neostigmine, some evidence of spontaneous recovery should be evident.
• Keep in mind that prior administration of succinylcholine may enhance neuromuscular blocking effect and duration of action.
Patient teaching
• Explain all events and happenings to patient because he can still hear.
• Reassure patient that he is being monitored and that muscle use will return when drug has worn off.

☑ Evaluation
• Patient exhibits positive response to drug therapy.
• Patient maintains adequate breathing pattern with mechanical assistance throughout therapy.
• Patient and family state understanding of drug therapy.

ropinirole hydrochloride

(roh-PIN-er-ohl high-droh-KLOR-ighd)
Requip

Pharmacologic class: nonergoline
dopamine agonist
Therapeutic class: antiparkinsonian agent
Pregnancy risk category: C

How supplied

Tablets: 0.25 mg, 0.5 mg, 1 mg, 2 mg,
5 mg

Pharmacokinetics

Absorption: rapid with an absolute
bioavailability of 55%.
Distribution: widely distributed with
about 40% bound to plasma protein.
Metabolism: extensively metabolized by
the liver to inactive metabolites.
Excretion: less than 10% excreted unchanged in urine. *Half-life:* 6 hours.

Route	Onset	Peak	Duration
P.O.	Unknown	1-2 hr	6 hr

Pharmacodynamics

Chemical effect: unknown. A nonergoline dopamine agonist thought to stimulate postsynaptic dopamine D_2 receptors
within the caudate-putamen in the brain.
Therapeutic effect: improves physical
mobility in patients with parkinsonism.

Indications and dosage

▶ **Idiopathic Parkinson's disease.** *Adults:*
initially, 0.25 mg P.O. t.i.d. Dosages can be
titrated on weekly basis. After week 4,
dosage may be increased weekly by
1.5 mg/day on a weekly basis up to dosage
of 9 mg/day and then increased weekly by
up to 3 mg/day to maximum of 24 mg/day.

Adverse reactions

**Early Parkinson's disease (without lev-
odopa)—**
CNS: asthenia, *fatigue,* malaise, hallucinations, *dizziness,* aggravated Parkinson's
disease, *somnolence,* headache, confusion, hyperkinesia, hypesthesia, vertigo,
amnesia, impaired concentration.
CV: hypotension, orthostatic symptoms,
hypertension, *syncope,* edema, chest
pain, extrasystoles, *atrial fibrillation,*
palpitation, tachycardia.
EENT: pharyngitis, dry mouth, abnormal
vision, eye abnormality, xerophthalmia,
rhinitis, sinusitis.
GI: *nausea, vomiting, dyspepsia,* flatulence, abdominal pain, anorexia, constipation, abdominal pain.
GU: urinary tract infection, impotence
(male).
Respiratory: bronchitis, dyspnea.
Skin: flushing.
Other: *viral infection,* pain, increased
sweating, yawning, peripheral ischemia.
**Advanced Parkinson's disease (with
levodopa)—**
CNS: *dizziness,* aggravated parkinsonism,
somnolence, headache, insomnia, *halluci-
nations,* abnormal dreaming, confusion,
tremor, anxiety, nervousness, amnesia.
CV: hypotension, syncope, paresthesia.
EENT: diplopia.
GI: *nausea,* abdominal pain, dry mouth,
vomiting, constipation, diarrhea, dyspha-
gia, flatulence.
GU: urinary tract infection, pyuria, uri-
nary incontinence.
Hematologic: anemia.
Metabolic: weight decrease.
Musculoskeletal: *dyskinesia,* hypokine-
sia, paresis, arthralgia, arthritis.
Respiratory: upper respiratory infection,
dyspnea.
Skin: increased sweating.
Other: injury, *falls,* viral infection, in-
creased drug level, increased saliva, pain.

Interactions

Drug-drug. *CNS depressants:* increased
CNS effects. Use cautiously.
*Dopamine antagonists (bretyrophenones,
metoclopramide, phenothiazines, thioxanthenes):* may decrease the effectiveness of ropinirole. Monitor closely.
Estrogens: reduced clearance of ropinirole. Adjust ropinirole dose if estrogens

---

Reactions may be *common,* uncommon, *life-threatening*, or COMMON AND LIFE-THREATENING.

are started or stopped during treatment with ropinirole.
Inhibitors or substrates of cytochrome P-450: altered clearance. Adjust ropinirole dose if drugs are started or stopped during treatment with ropinirole.
Drug-lifestyle. *Alcohol use:* increased sedative effects. Use cautiously.
Smoking: may increase clearance of drug. Advise patient against tobacco use.

Contraindications and precautions

• Contraindicated in patients with known hypersensitivity to drug.
• Use cautiously in patients with severe hepatic or renal impairment.

NURSING CONSIDERATIONS

Assessment
• Assess patient before and during therapy to evaluate effectiveness.
• Monitor patient carefully for orthostatic hypotension, especially during dose escalation.
• Assess patient for adequate nutritional intake.
• Evaluate patient's and family's knowledge of drug therapy.

Nursing diagnoses
• Impaired physical mobility related to underlying Parkinson's disease
• Altered thought processes related to drug-induced CNS adverse reactions
• Knowledge deficit related to drug therapy

Planning and implementation
• Give drug with food to decrease the occurrence of nausea.
• Know that clearance is reduced in patients above age 65, however, doses are individually titrated to clinical response.
• Know that BUN and alkaline phosphatase levels may be increased during therapy.
• Be aware that drug can potentiate the dopaminergic adverse effects of levodopa and may cause or exacerbate existing

dyskinesia. It may be necessary to decrease levodopa dose.
• Do not abruptly discontinue drug. Withdraw gradually over 7 days to avoid hyperpyrexia and confusion.
Patient teaching
• Advise patient to take drug with food if nausea is a problem.
• Advise patient that hallucinations can occur, particularly in the elderly.
• Instruct patient not to rise rapidly after sitting or lying down because of risk of orthostatic hypotension, which may occur more frequently during initial therapy or with an increase in dose.
• Advise patient to use caution in driving a car or operating machinery until CNS effects are known.
• Tell patient to avoid alcohol during drug therapy.
• Tell female patient to notify doctor if pregnancy is suspected or is being planned; also tell her to inform doctor if she is breast-feeding.

Evaluation
• Patient exhibits improved mobility with reduction of muscular rigidity and tremor.
• Patient remains mentally alert.
• Patient and family state understanding of drug therapy.

salmeterol xinafoate
(sal-MEE-ter-ohl zee-neh-FOH-ayt)
Serevent

Pharmacologic class: selective beta$_2$-adrenergic stimulating agonist
Therapeutic class: bronchodilator
Pregnancy risk category: C

How supplied

Inhalation aerosol: 21 mcg per metered spray

Pharmacokinetics

Absorption: because of low therapeutic dose, systemic levels of drug are low or undetectable after inhalation of recommended doses.
Distribution: distributed locally to lungs; 94% to 99% bound to plasma proteins.
Metabolism: extensively metabolized by hydroxylation.
Excretion: excreted primarily in feces.

Route	Onset	Peak	Duration
Inhalation	10-20 min	About 3 hr	About 12 hr

Pharmacodynamics

Chemical effect: not clearly defined; selectively activates beta$_2$-adrenergic receptors, which results in bronchodilation. Drug also blocks release of allergic mediators from mast cells lining the respiratory tract.
Therapeutic effect: improves breathing ability.

Indications and dosage

▶ **Long-term maintenance treatment of asthma; prevention of bronchospasm in patients with nocturnal asthma or reversible obstructive airway disease who require regular treatment with short-acting beta agonists.** *Adults and children over age 12:* 2 inhalations b.i.d., 1 in morning and 1 in evening. Drug should not be used to treat acute symptoms.
▶ **Prevention of exercise-induced bronchospasm.** *Adults and children age 12 and over:* 2 inhalations at least 30 to 60 minutes before exercise.

Adverse reactions

CNS: *headache,* sinus headache, tremors, nervousness, dizziness.
CV: tachycardia, palpitations, *ventricular arrhythmias.*

EENT: *upper respiratory tract infection, nasopharyngitis,* nasal cavity or sinus disorder.
GI: nausea, vomiting, diarrhea, heartburn.
Musculoskeletal: joint and back pain, myalgia.
Respiratory: cough, lower respiratory tract infection, **bronchospasm.**
Other: hypersensitivity reactions (rash, urticaria).

Interactions

Drug-drug. *Beta-adrenergic agonists, other methylxanthines, theophylline:* possible adverse cardiac effects with excessive use. Monitor patient closely.
MAO inhibitors: risk of severe adverse CV effects. Avoid use within 14 days of MAO therapy.
Tricyclic antidepressants: risk of moderate to severe adverse CV effects. Use with extreme caution.

Contraindications and precautions

• Contraindicated in patients with hypersensitivity to drug or its components.
• Use cautiously in patients with coronary insufficiency, arrhythmias, hypertension or other CV disorders, thyrotoxicosis, or seizure disorders and in patients who are unusually responsive to sympathomimetics. Also use cautiously in pregnant women.
• Safety of drug has not been established in breast-feeding women and in children age 12 or less.

NURSING CONSIDERATIONS

Assessment
• Assess patient's respiratory condition before therapy and regularly thereafter.
• Be alert for adverse reactions and drug interactions.
• Evaluate patient's and family's knowledge of drug therapy.

⊞ Nursing diagnoses
• Ineffective breathing pattern related to respiratory condition
• Pain related to drug-induced headache
• Knowledge deficit related to drug therapy

⯈ Planning and implementation
• Don't give drug for acute broncho-spasm.
• Report insufficient relief or worsening condition.
• Obtain order for mild analgesic if drug-induced headache occurs.
Patient teaching
• Tell patient to take drug at about 12-hour intervals and to take even when feeling better.
• Tell patient taking drug to prevent exercise-induced bronchospasm to take it 30 to 60 minutes before exercise.
• Instruct patient not to take drug to treat acute bronchospasm. Patient must be provided with short-acting beta agonist (such as albuterol) to treat such exacerbations.
• Tell patient to contact doctor if short-acting agonist no longer provides sufficient relief or if more than four inhalations are needed per day. This may be a sign that asthma symptoms are worsening. Tell patient not to increase dosage of drug.
• If patient is taking inhaled corticosteroid, he should continue to use it. Warn him not to take other drugs without doctor's consent.

☑ Evaluation
• Patient exhibits normal breathing pattern.
• Patient states that drug-induced headache is relieved after analgesic administration.
• Patient and family state understanding of drug therapy.

salsalate (disalicylic acid, salicylsalicylic acid)
(SAL-sah-layt)
Amigesic, Argesic-SA, Arthra-G, Disalcid, Mono-Gesic, Salflex, Salsitab

Pharmacologic class: salicylate
Therapeutic class: nonnarcotic analgesic, antipyretic, anti-inflammatory
Pregnancy risk category: C

How supplied
Tablets: 500 mg, 750 mg
Caplets: 750 mg
Capsules: 500 mg

Pharmacokinetics
Absorption: absorbed rapidly and completely from GI tract, mainly in small intestine.
Distribution: distributed widely to most body fluids and tissues. Protein-binding varies from 75% to 90%; it is concentration-dependent and decreases as serum concentrations increase.
Metabolism: hydrolyzed in liver, plasma, blood, and GI mucosa to salicylic acid.
Excretion: metabolite and parent drug excreted in urine.

Route	Onset	Peak	Duration
P.O.	Unknown	1.5-4 hr	Unknown

Pharmacodynamics
Chemical effect: salicylic ester of salicylic acid. Each molecule of salsalate is hydrolyzed to two molecules of salicylate in vivo. Drug produces analgesia by blocking prostaglandin synthesis (peripheral action). Salicylates prevent lowering of pain threshold that occurs when prostaglandins sensitize pain receptors to mechanical and chemical stimulation. Salsalate also has ill-defined effect on hypothalamus. Exact mechanism of anti-inflammatory action unknown.
Therapeutic effect: relieves pain, fever, and inflammation.

Indications and dosage

► **Arthritis.** *Adults:* 3 g P.O. daily in divided doses b.i.d. or t.i.d.

Adverse reactions

EENT: tinnitus, hearing loss.
GI: nausea, vomiting, GI distress, occult bleeding (rare).
Hepatic: abnormal liver function studies, *hepatitis.*
Skin: *rash,* bruising.
Other: hypersensitivity reactions (*anaphylaxis,* asthma), *Reye's syndrome.*

Interactions

Drug-drug. *Ammonium chloride and other urine acidifiers:* increased blood levels of salicylates. Monitor for salicylate toxicity.
Antacids in high doses, other urine alkalinizers: decreased levels of salicylates. Monitor for decreased salicylate effect.
Corticosteroids: enhanced salicylate excretion. Monitor for decreased salicylate effect.
Methotrexate: increased risk of methotrexate toxicity. Avoid concomitant use.
NSAIDs, steroids: increased risk of GI bleeding. Avoid concomitant use.
Oral anticoagulants: possible increased risk of bleeding. Avoid using together if possible.
Drug-lifestyle. *Alcohol use:* increased risk of GI bleeding. Avoid concomitant use.

Contraindications and precautions

• Contraindicated in patients with salsalate hypersensitivity.
• Use cautiously in patients with bleeding disorders, peptic ulcer disease, renal insufficiency, hypoprothrombinemia, vitamin K deficiency, thrombocytopenia, thrombotic thrombocytopenic purpura, or severe hepatic impairment and in pregnant women.
• Because of epidemiologic association with Reye's syndrome, the Centers for Disease Control and Prevention recommends not giving salicylates to children or teenagers with chickenpox or influenza-like illness.

• Safety of drug has not been established in breast-feeding women.

NURSING CONSIDERATIONS

▨ Assessment

• Assess patient's arthritis before therapy and regularly thereafter.
• Monitor serum salicylate level. Therapeutic blood level in arthritis is 10 to 30 mg/dl. Tinnitus may occur at plasma levels of 30 mg/dl and above, but this is not a reliable indicator of toxicity, especially in very young patients and those over age 60. With long-term therapy, mild toxicity may occur at plasma levels of 20 mg/dl.
• Obtain hemoglobin and PT tests periodically in patients on long-term therapy.
• Be alert for adverse reactions and drug interactions.
• Evaluate patient's and family's knowledge of drug therapy.

▨ Nursing diagnoses

• Pain related to arthritis
• Sensory or perceptual alterations (auditory) related to drug-induced hearing loss
• Knowledge deficit related to drug therapy

▧ Planning and implementation

• Store drug in tightly closed container in cool, dry place away from light.
Patient teaching
• Tell patient to take this drug with food, milk, antacid, or large glass of water.
• Advise patient receiving long-term treatment with large doses to watch for petechiae, bleeding gums, and signs of GI bleeding and to maintain adequate fluid intake. Encourage use of soft-bristled toothbrush.

▨ Evaluation

• Patient is free from pain.
• Patient does not experience hearing loss.
• Patient and family state understanding of drug therapy.

Reactions may be *common,* uncommon, *life-threatening,* or COMMON AND LIFE-THREATENING.

saquinavir mesylate
(sah-KWIN-ah-veer MES-eh-layt)
Invirase

Pharmacologic class: HIV-1 and HIV-2
proteinase inhibitor
Therapeutic class: antiviral
Pregnancy risk category: B

How supplied

Capsules: 200 mg

Pharmacokinetics

Absorption: poorly absorbed from GI
tract.
Distribution: more than 98% bound to
plasma proteins.
Metabolism: rapidly metabolized.
Excretion: excreted mainly in feces.
Half-life: 1 to 2 hours.

Route	Onset	Peak	Duration
P.O.	Unknown	Unknown	Unknown

Pharmacodynamics

Chemical effect: inhibits activity of HIV
protease and prevents cleavage of HIV
polyproteins, which are essential for HIV
maturation.
Therapeutic effect: hinders HIV activity.

Indications and dosage

▶ **Adjunct treatment of advanced HIV
infection in selected patients.** *Adults:*
600-mg capsule P.O. t.i.d. within 2 hours
after full meal and in combination with a
nucleoside analogue, such as zalcitabine
(at dosage of 0.75 mg P.O. t.i.d.) or zidovudine (at dosage of 200 mg P.O.
t.i.d.).

Adverse reactions

CNS: asthenia, paresthesia, headache,
dizziness.
CV: chest pain.
GI: diarrhea, ulcerated buccal mucosa,
abdominal pain, nausea, pancreatitis.
Hematologic: *pancytopenia, thrombocytopenia.*

Musculoskeletal: musculoskeletal pain.
Respiratory: bronchitis, cough.
Skin: rash.

Interactions

Drug-drug. *Astemizole:* increased serum
level of this drug, increased risk of arrhythmias, and sudden death. Avoid concomitant use.
Ketoconazole, ritonavir: increased serum
saquinavir concentrations. Monitor patient closely.
*Phenobarbital, phenytoin, rifabutin, ri-
fampin:* reduces steady-state concentration
of saquinavir. Use together cautiously.
Drug-food. *Any food:* increased absorption. Give drug with food.

Contraindications and precautions

• Contraindicated in patients with hypersensitivity to drug or components of capsule.
• Safety of drug has not been established
in pregnant or breast-feeding women and
in children under age 16.

NURSING CONSIDERATIONS

Assessment
• Obtain history of patient's HIV infection.
• Evaluate CBC, platelet count, and electrolyte, uric acid, liver enzyme, and
bilirubin levels before therapy and at appropriate intervals during therapy, as ordered.
• Be alert for adverse reactions and interactions, including those associated with
adjunct therapy (zidovudine or zalcitabine).
• Monitor patient's hydration status if adverse GI reactions occur.
• Evaluate patient's and family's knowledge of drug therapy.

Nursing diagnoses
• Infection related to presence of HIV
• Risk for fluid volume deficit related to
adverse GI reactions

---

*Liquid form contains alcohol   **May contain tartrazine   ◆Canada   ◇Australia   †OTC

• Knowledge deficit related to drug therapy

⊠ Planning and implementation
• If severe toxicity occurs during treatment, drug should be discontinued until cause is identified or toxicity resolves. Therapy may resume with no dosage modifications.
• Notify doctor of adverse reactions, and obtain an order for a mild analgesic, antiemetic, or antidiarrheal agent, if necessary.
Patient teaching
• Tell patient to take drug within 2 hours after a full meal.
• Urge patient to notify doctor of adverse reactions.
• Inform patient that drug is usually administered with other AIDS-related antiviral agents.

☑ Evaluation
• Patient responds well to therapy.
• Patient maintains adequate hydration.
• Patient and family state understanding of drug therapy.

---

sargramostim (granulocyte macrophage colony–stimulating factor, GM-CSF)
(sar-GRAH-moh-stim)
Leukine

Pharmacologic class: biological response modifier
Therapeutic class: colony-stimulating factor
Pregnancy risk category: C

How supplied
Powder for injection: 250 mcg, 500 mcg

Pharmacokinetics
Absorption: not applicable with I.V. administration.
Distribution: bound to specific receptors on target cells.
Metabolism: unknown.

Excretion: unknown. *Half-life:* about 2 hours.

Route	Onset	Peak	Duration
I.V.	≤ 30 min	2 hr	Unknown

Pharmacodynamics
Chemical effect: glycoprotein manufactured by recombinant DNA technology in yeast expression system; differs from natural human GM-CSF. Drug induces cellular responses by binding to specific receptors on cell surfaces of target cells.
Therapeutic effect: stimulates formation of granulocytes (neutrophils, eosinophils) and macrophages.

Indications and dosage
▶ **Acceleration of hematopoietic reconstitution after autologous bone marrow transplantation in patients with malignant lymphoma or acute lymphoblastic leukemia or during autologous bone marrow transplantation in patients with Hodgkin's disease.** *Adults:* 250 mcg/m² daily for 21 consecutive days given as 2-hour I.V. infusion beginning 2 to 4 hours after bone marrow transplantation.
▶ **Bone marrow transplantation failure or engraftment delay.** *Adults:* 250 mcg/m²/day for 14 days as 2-hour I.V. infusion. Dose may be repeated after 7 days off of therapy. If engraftment still has not occurred, a third course of 500 mcg/m²/day I.V. for 14 days may be tried after another 7 days off therapy.
▶ **Acute myelogenous leukemia.** *Adults:* 250 mcg/m²/day I.V. infusion over 4 hours. Start therapy about day 11 or 4 days after end of induction therapy.

Adverse reactions
CNS: *malaise, CNS disorders, asthenia.*
CV: *blood dyscrasias, edema, **hemorrhage, supraventricular arrhythmia,*** pericardial effusion.
GI: *nausea, vomiting, diarrhea, anorexia, **hemorrhage**, GI disorder, stomatitis.*
GU: *urinary tract disorder,* abnormal kidney function.

Reactions may be *common,* uncommon, *life-threatening*, or COMMON AND LIFE-THREATENING.

Hepatic: *liver damage.*
Respiratory: *dyspnea, lung disorders,* pleural effusion.
Skin: *alopecia, rash.*
Other: *fever, mucous membrane disorder, peripheral edema,* SEPSIS.

Interactions

Drug-drug. *Corticosteroids, lithium:* may potentiate myeloproliferative effects of sargramostim. Use together cautiously.

Contraindications and precautions

• Contraindicated in patients with excessive leukemic myeloid blasts in bone marrow or peripheral blood and in those with hypersensitivity to drug or its components or to yeast-derived products.
• Use cautiously in patients with preexisting cardiac disease, hypoxia, preexisting fluid retention, pulmonary infiltrates, heart failure, or impaired kidney or liver function and in pregnant or breast-feeding women.
• Safety of drug has not been established in children.

NURSING CONSIDERATIONS

Assessment
• Assess patient's condition before therapy and regularly thereafter.
• Know that drug effect may be limited in patient who has received extensive radiotherapy to hematopoietic sites for treatment of primary disease in abdomen or chest or who has been exposed to multiple agents (alkylating, anthracycline antibiotics, antimetabolites) before autologous bone marrow transplantation.
• Be aware that drug is effective in accelerating myeloid recovery in patients receiving bone marrow purged from monoclonal antibodies.
• Drug can act as growth factor for tumors, particularly myeloid cancers.
• Blood counts return to normal or baseline levels within 3 to 7 days after stopping treatment.

• Monitor CBC with differential, including examination for presence of blast cells, biweekly, as ordered.
• Be alert for adverse reactions and drug interactions.
• Monitor patient's hydration status throughout drug therapy.
• Evaluate patient's and family's knowledge of drug therapy.

Nursing diagnoses
• Altered health maintenance related to underlying condition
• Risk for fluid volume deficit related to drug-induced adverse effects
• Knowledge deficit related to drug therapy

Planning and implementation
• Reconstitute drug with 1 ml of sterile water for injection. Direct stream of sterile water against side of vial and *gently swirl* contents to minimize foaming. Avoid excessive or vigorous agitation or shaking. Dilute in 0.9% NaCl solution. If final concentration is below 10 mcg/ml, add human albumin at final concentration of 0.1% to NaCl solution *before* adding sargramostim to prevent adsorption to components of delivery system. For final concentration of 0.1% human albumin, add 1 mg human albumin/1 ml NaCl. Administer as soon as possible after mixing and no later than 6 hours after reconstituting.
• Discard unused portion. Vials are for single-dose use and contain no preservatives. Do not reenter vial.
• Don't add other drugs to infusion solution because no data exist on solution compatibility and stability.
• Anticipate reducing dose by half or temporarily discontinue if severe adverse reactions occur, and notify doctor. Therapy may be resumed when reactions abate. Transient rashes and local reactions at injection site may occur; no serious allergic or anaphylactic reactions have been reported.

• Don't give drug within 24 hours of last dose of chemotherapy or within 12 hours of last dose of radiotherapy; rapidly dividing progenitor cells may be sensitive to these cytotoxic therapies and drug would be ineffective.
• Stimulation of marrow precursors may result in rapid rise of WBC count. If blast cells appear or increase to 10% or more of WBC count or if progression of underlying disease occurs, therapy should be discontinued. If absolute neutrophil count is above 20,000/mm³ or if platelet count is above 50,000/mm³, drug is temporarily discontinued or dose is reduced by half.
• Refrigerate sterile powder, reconstituted solution, and diluted solution for injection. Don't freeze or shake.

Patient teaching
• Inform patient and family about need for therapy.
• Advise patient to report adverse reactions immediately.

☑ **Evaluation**
• Patient exhibits positive response to sargramostim therapy.
• Patient maintains adequate hydration throughout therapy.
• Patient and family state understanding of drug therapy.

scopolamine (hyoscine)
(skoh-POL-uh-meen)
Scop◇, Transderm Scōp, Transderm-V♦

scopolamine butylbromide (hyoscine butylbromide)
Buscopan♦ ◇

scopolamine hydrobromide (hyoscine hydrobromide)

Pharmacologic class: anticholinergic
Therapeutic class: antimuscarinic, antiemetic, antivertigo, antiparkinsonian agent
Pregnancy risk category: C

How supplied

scopolamine
Transdermal patch: 1.5 mg
scopolamine butylbromide
Capsules: 0.25 mg
Suppositories: 10 mg♦
Tablets: 10 mg♦
scopolamine hydrobromide
Injection: 0.3, 0.4, 0.5, 0.6, and 1 mg/ml in 1-ml vials and ampules; 0.86 mg/ml in 0.5-ml ampules

Pharmacokinetics

Absorption: well absorbed percutaneously from behind ear with transdermal patch application. Well absorbed from GI tract when given P.O. or P.R. Absorbed rapidly when given I.M. or S.C.
Distribution: distributed widely throughout body tissues; probably crosses blood-brain barrier.
Metabolism: thought to be metabolized completely in liver.
Excretion: may be excreted in urine as metabolites. *Half-life:* 8 hours.

Route	Onset	Peak	Duration
P.O.	30-60 min	Unknown	4-6 hr
I.V., I.M., S.C.	30 min	Unknown	4 hr
P.R.	Unknown	Unknown	Unknown
Trans-dermal	Unknown	Unknown	≤ 72 hr

Pharmacodynamics

Chemical effect: inhibits muscarinic actions of acetylcholine on autonomic effectors innervated by postganglionic cholinergic neurons. Scopolamine also may affect neural pathways originating in labyrinth (inner ear) to inhibit nausea and vomiting.
Therapeutic effect: relieves spasticity, nausea, and vomiting; reduces secretions; and blocks cardiac vagal reflexes.

Indications and dosage

▶ **Spastic states.** *Adults:* 10 to 20 mg P.O. t.i.d. or q.i.d. Dosage adjusted, p.r.n.

Reactions may be *common*, uncommon, **life-threatening**, or COMMON AND LIFE-THREATENING.

Or, 10 to 20 mg (butylbromide) S.C., I.M., or I.V. t.i.d. or q.i.d.
► **Preoperatively to reduce secretions.** **Scopolamine hydrobromide.** *Adults:* 0.2 to 0.6 mg I.M. 30 to 60 minutes before induction of anesthesia. *Children ages 8 to 12:* 300 mcg I.M. 45 minutes before induction of anesthesia. *Children ages 3 to 8:* 200 mcg I.M. 45 minutes before induction of anesthesia. *Children ages 7 months to 3 years:* 150 mcg I.M. 45 minutes before induction of anesthesia. *Infants ages 4 to 7 months:* 100 mcg I.M. 45 minutes before induction of anesthesia.
► **Prevention of nausea and vomiting associated with motion sickness.** **Scopolamine.** *Adults:* one Transderm Scōp or Transderm-V patch (a circular flat unit) programmed to deliver 0.5 mg daily over 3 days (72 hours), applied to skin behind ear several hours before antiemetic is required. **Scopolamine hydrobromide.** *Adults:* 300 to 600 mcg S.C., I.M., or I.V. *Children:* 6 mcg/kg or 200 mcg/m² of body surface S.C., I.M., or I.V.

Adverse reactions

Adverse reactions may be caused by pending atropine-like toxicity and are dose-related. Individual tolerance varies greatly. Many adverse reactions (such as dry mouth, constipation) are expected extension of drug's pharmacologic activity.
CNS: disorientation, restlessness, irritability, dizziness, drowsiness, headache, confusion, hallucinations, delirium.
CV: palpitations, tachycardia, *paradoxical bradycardia.*
EENT: dilated pupils, blurred vision, photophobia, increased intraocular pressure, difficulty swallowing.
GI: *constipation, dry mouth, nausea, vomiting, epigastric distress.*
GU: urinary hesitancy, urine retention.
Respiratory: bronchial plugging, depressed respirations.
Skin: rash, flushing, dryness, contact dermatitis (with transdermal patch).
Other: fever.

Interactions

Drug-drug. *Centrally acting anticholinergics (antihistamines, phenothiazines, tricyclic antidepressants):* increased incidence of adverse CNS reactions. Monitor patient closely.
CNS depressants: increased incidence of CNS depression. Monitor patient closely.
Digoxin: increased digoxin levels. Monitor patient for cardiac toxicity.
Drug-lifestyle. *Alcohol use:* increased incidence of CNS depression. Monitor patient closely.

Contraindications and precautions

• Contraindicated in patients with angle-closure glaucoma, obstructive uropathy, obstructive disease of GI tract, asthma, chronic pulmonary disease, myasthenia gravis, paralytic ileus, intestinal atony, unstable CV status in acute hemorrhage, or toxic megacolon.
• Drug should not be used in breast-feeding women.
• Use cautiously in patients with autonomic neuropathy, hyperthyroidism, coronary artery disease, arrhythmias, heart failure, hypertension, hiatal hernia associated with reflux esophagitis, hepatic or renal disease, or ulcerative colitis; in pregnant women; in children under age 6; and in patients in hot or humid environments (drug-induced heatstroke is possible).

NURSING CONSIDERATIONS

⚕ Assessment
• Assess patient's condition before therapy and regularly thereafter.
• Be alert for adverse reactions and drug interactions.
• Evaluate patient's and family's knowledge of drug therapy.

⊕ Nursing diagnoses
• Risk for fluid volume deficit related to nausea and vomiting
• Risk for injury related to drug-induced adverse CNS reactions

● Knowledge deficit related to drug therapy

▶ **Planning and implementation**
P.O., I.M., S.C., and P.R. use: Follow normal protocol.
I.V. use: Intermittent and continuous infusions are not recommended. For direct injection, dilute with sterile water and inject diluted drug at ordered rate through patent I.V. line.
– Protect I.V. solutions from freezing and light, and store at room temperature.
Transdermal patch use: Apply patch night before patient's expected travel.
● Raise bed's side rails as precaution because some patients become temporarily excited or disoriented. Symptoms disappear when sedative effect is complete.
● Know that in therapeutic doses, scopolamine may produce amnesia, drowsiness, and euphoria; patient may need to be reoriented.
● Tolerance may develop when scopolamine is given over a long time.
Patient teaching
● Advise patient to apply patch the night before planned trip. Transdermal method releases controlled therapeutic amount of drug. Transderm Scōp is effective if applied 2 to 3 hours before experiencing motion but is more effective if applied 12 hours before.
● Advise patient to wash and dry hands thoroughly before and after applying transdermal patch on dry skin behind ear and before touching eye because pupil may dilate. After removing system, he should discard it and wash hands and application site thoroughly.
● Tell patient that if patch becomes displaced, he should remove it and replace it with another patch on fresh skin site behind ear.
● Alert patient about risk of withdrawal symptoms (nausea, vomiting, headache, dizziness) if transdermal system is used longer than 72 hours.
● Have patient ask pharmacist for brochure that comes with transdermal product.

● Instruct patient about P.O. or P.R. administration, if applicable.
● Advise patient to refrain from activities that require alertness until drug's CNS effects are known.
● Instruct patient to report signs of urinary hesitancy or urine retention.
● Recommend use of sugarless gum or hard candy to help minimize dry mouth.

☑ **Evaluation**
● Patient responds well to therapy.
● Patient does not experience injury from adverse CNS reactions.
● Patient and family state understanding of drug therapy.

secobarbital sodium
(sek-oh-BAR-bih-tohl SOH-dee-um)
Novosecobarb♦, Seconal Sodium

Pharmacologic class: barbiturate
Therapeutic class: sedative-hypnotic, anticonvulsant
Controlled substance schedule: II
Pregnancy risk category: D

How supplied
Capsules: 50 mg, 100 mg
Injection: 50 mg/ml

Pharmacokinetics
Absorption: 90% of drug absorbed rapidly after P.O. administration; unknown after I.M. administration.
Distribution: distributed rapidly throughout body tissues and fluids; about 30% to 45% protein-bound.
Metabolism: oxidized in liver to inactive metabolites.
Excretion: excreted in urine. *Half-life:* about 30 hours.

Route	Onset	Peak	Duration
P.O.	≤ 15 min	5-30 min	1-4 hr
I.V.	Almost immediate	1-3 min	15 min
I.M.	Unknown	7-10 min	Unknown

Pharmacodynamics

Chemical effect: unknown; probably interferes with transmission of impulses from thalamus to cortex of brain.
Therapeutic effect: promotes pain relief and calmness and relieves acute seizures.

Indications and dosage

▶ **Preoperative sedation.** *Adults:* 100 to 300 mg P.O. 1 to 2 hours before surgery. *Children:* 50 to 100 mg P.O. 1 to 2 hours before surgery. Maximum single dose is 100 mg.
▶ **Insomnia.** *Adults:* 100 mg P.O., 100 to 200 mg I.M., or 50 to 250 mg I.V.
▶ **Acute tetanus seizure.** *Adults:* 5.5 mg/kg I.M. or slow I.V., repeated q 3 to 4 hours, if needed; I.V. injection rate not to exceed 50 mg/15 seconds.
▶ **Status epilepticus.** *Children:* 15 to 20 mg/kg I.V. over 15 minutes.

Adverse reactions

CNS: *drowsiness, lethargy, hangover,* paradoxical excitement in elderly patients, somnolence.
CV: hypotension (with I.V. use).
GI: nausea, vomiting.
Hematologic: exacerbation of porphyria.
Respiratory: *respiratory depression.*
Skin: rash, urticaria, *Stevens-Johnson syndrome,* tissue reactions and injection-site pain.
Other: *angioedema,* physical and psychological dependence.

Interactions

Drug-drug. *Acidic solutions, lactated Ringer's solution:* incompatible with I.V. form of drug. Don't mix together.
Chloramphenicol, MAO inhibitors, valproic acid: inhibited metabolism of barbiturates; may cause prolonged CNS depression. Reduce barbiturate dosage.
CNS depressants, including narcotic analgesics: excessive CNS and respiratory depression. Use together cautiously.
Corticosteroids, digitoxin, doxycycline, estrogens and oral contraceptives, oral anticoagulants, theophylline, tricyclic an-

tidepressants, verapamil: secobarbital may enhance metabolism of these drugs. Monitor for decreased effect.
Griseofulvin: decreased absorption of griseofulvin. Monitor for decreased griseofulvin effectiveness.
Rifampin: may decrease barbiturate levels. Monitor for decreased effect.
Drug-lifestyle. *Alcohol use:* excessive CNS and respiratory depression. Use together cautiously.

Contraindications and precautions

• Contraindicated in patients with marked liver impairment, respiratory disease in which dyspnea or obstruction is evident, porphyria, or hypersensitivity to barbiturates.
• Drug not recommended for use in pregnant or breast-feeding women.
• Use cautiously in patients with acute or chronic pain, depression, suicidal tendencies, history of drug abuse, or hepatic impairment.

NURSING CONSIDERATIONS

☞ Assessment

• Assess patient's condition before therapy and regularly thereafter.
• Assess mental status before therapy. Elderly patients are more sensitive to drug's adverse CNS effects.
• Be alert for adverse reactions and drug interactions.
• Evaluate patient's and family's knowledge of drug therapy.

Nursing diagnoses

• Sleep pattern disturbance related to underlying condition
• Risk for injury related to drug-induced adverse CNS reactions
• Knowledge deficit related to drug therapy

Planning and implementation
P.O. use: Prevent hoarding or self-overdosing by patient who is depressed,

suicidal, or drug-dependent or who has history of drug abuse.

I.V. use: I.V. injection is reserved for emergency treatment and given under close supervision by direct injection. It is administered slowly at rate not exceeding 50 mg/15 seconds. Drug may be given as supplied or diluted.

– Local tissue reactions and injection-site pain have been noted with I.V. use. Assess patency of I.V. site before and during administration.

– Know that I.V. administration of barbiturates may cause severe respiratory depression, laryngospasm, or hypotension. Have emergency resuscitation equipment readily available.

– Know that secobarbital sodium injection is not compatible with lactated Ringer's solution but is compatible with Ringer's solution, sterile water for injection, and 0.9% NaCl. Don't mix with acidic solutions.

• Use injection solution within 30 minutes after opening container to minimize deterioration. Don't use cloudy solution.

I.M. use: Give I.M. injection deeply. Superficial injection may cause pain, sterile abscess, and sloughing.

• Be aware that skin eruptions may precede potentially fatal reactions to barbiturate therapy. Discontinue drug when skin reactions occur and notify physician. In some patients, high fever, stomatitis, headache, or rhinitis may precede skin reactions.

• Long-term use is not recommended; drug loses its efficacy in promoting sleep after 14 days of continued use.

Patient teaching

• Caution patient to avoid activities that require mental alertness or physical coordination. For inpatient, supervise walking and raise bed rails, particularly for elderly patient.

• Inform patient that morning hangover is common after hypnotic dose, which suppresses REM sleep. Patient may experience increased dreaming after drug is discontinued.

• Advise patient who uses oral contraceptives to consider alternate birth control methods; drug may enhance contraceptive hormone metabolism and decrease its effect.

☑ Evaluation

• Patient states that drug effectively induces sleep.

• Patient does not experience injury from adverse CNS reactions.

• Patient and family state understanding of drug therapy.

---

selegiline hydrochloride (L-deprenyl hydrochloride)
(see-LEJ-eh-leen high-droh-KLOR-ighd)
Eldepryl

Pharmacologic class: MAO inhibitor
Therapeutic class: antiparkinsonian agent
Pregnancy risk category: C

How supplied
Tablets: 5 mg

Pharmacokinetics
Absorption: unknown.
Distribution: unknown.
Metabolism: three metabolites have been detected in serum and urine: N-desmethyldeprenyl, L-amphetamine, and L-methamphetamine.
Excretion: 45% excreted in urine as metabolite. *Half-life:* selegiline, 2 to 10 hours; N-desmethyldeprenyl, 2 hours; L-amphetamine, 17.7 hours; L-methamphetamine, 20.5 hours.

Route	Onset	Peak	Duration
P.O.	Unknown	0.5-2 hr	Unknown

Pharmacodynamics
Chemical effect: unknown; probably acts by selectively inhibiting MAO type B (found mostly in brain). At higher-than-recommended doses, it is nonselective inhibitor of MAO, including MAO type A

(found in GI tract). It also may directly increase dopaminergic activity by decreasing reuptake of dopamine into nerve cells. Its active metabolites, amphetamine and methamphetamine, may contribute to this effect.
Therapeutic effect: improves physical mobility.

Indications and dosage

▶ **Adjunct treatment with carbidopa-levodopa in management of symptoms associated with Parkinson's disease.**
Adults: 10 mg P.O. daily, taken as 5 mg at breakfast and 5 mg at lunch. After 2 or 3 days of therapy, gradual decrease of carbidopa-levodopa dosage is attempted.

Adverse reactions

CNS: *dizziness,* increased tremors, chorea, loss of balance, restlessness, increased bradykinesia, facial grimacing, stiff neck, dyskinesia, involuntary movements, twitching, increased apraxia, behavioral changes, fatigue, headache, confusion, hallucinations, vivid dreams, malaise.
CV: orthostatic hypotension, hypertension, hypotension, *arrhythmias,* palpitations, new or increased anginal pain, tachycardia, peripheral edema, syncope.
EENT: blepharospasm.
GI: dry mouth, *nausea,* vomiting, constipation, weight loss, abdominal pain, anorexia or poor appetite, dysphagia, diarrhea, heartburn.
GU: slow urination, transient nocturia, prostatic hyperplasia, urinary hesitancy, urinary frequency, urine retention, sexual dysfunction.
Skin: rash, hair loss.
Other: diaphoresis.

Interactions

Drug-drug. *Adrenergic agents:* possible increased pressor response, particularly in patients who have taken overdose of selegiline. Use together cautiously.
Meperidine: may cause stupor, muscle rigidity, severe agitation, and elevated temperature. Avoid concomitant use.

Drug-food. *Foods high in tyramine:* possible hypertensive crisis. Monitor blood pressure.

Contraindications and precautions

• Contraindicated in patients with hypersensitivity to drug and in those receiving meperidine.
• Use cautiously in pregnant women.
• Safety of drug has not been established in children and in breast-feeding women.

NURSING CONSIDERATIONS

⚗ Assessment
• Assess patient's condition before therapy and regularly thereafter.
• Be alert for adverse reactions and drug interactions.
• Evaluate patient's and family's knowledge of drug therapy.

⊞ Nursing diagnoses
• Impaired physical mobility related to underlying condition
• Risk for injury related to drug-induced adverse CNS reactions
• Knowledge deficit related to drug therapy

❱ Planning and implementation
• Be aware that some patients experience increased adverse reactions associated with levodopa and require a 10% to 30% reduction of carbidopa-levodopa dosage.
Patient teaching
• Warn patient to move cautiously at start of therapy because dizziness may occur.
• Advise patient not to take more than 10 mg daily because greater amount of drug will not improve efficacy and may increase adverse reactions.

✔ Evaluation
• Patient exhibits improved physical mobility.
• Patient does not experience injury from adverse CNS reactions.
• Patient and family state understanding of drug therapy.

---

senna
(SEN-uh)
Black-Draught†, Fletcher's Castoria†,
Senexon†, Senokot†, Senolax†,
X-Prep Liquid*†

Pharmacologic class: anthraquinone
derivative
Therapeutic class: stimulant laxative
Pregnancy risk category: C

How supplied
Tablets: 187 mg†, 217 mg†, 600 mg†
Granules: 326 mg/tsp†, 1.65 g/½ tsp†
Suppositories: 652 mg†
Syrup: 218 mg/5 ml†

Pharmacokinetics
Absorption: absorbed minimally from GI
tract after P.O. or P.R. use.
Distribution: distributed in bile, saliva,
colonic mucosa.
Metabolism: absorbed portion metabolized in liver.
Excretion: unabsorbed senna excreted
mainly in feces; absorbed drug excreted
in urine and feces.

Route	Onset	Peak	Duration
P.O.	6-10 hr	Varies	Varies
P.R.	30 min-2 hr	Varies	Varies

Pharmacodynamics
Chemical effect: unknown; increases peristalsis probably by direct effect on smooth
muscle of intestine. Senna may either irritate musculature or stimulate colonic intramural plexus. It also promotes fluid accumulation in colon and small intestine.
Therapeutic effect: relieves constipation
and cleanses bowel.

Indications and dosage
▶ **Acute constipation; preparation for
bowel or rectal examination.** *Adults and
children age 12 and over:* usual dose is 2
tablets, 1 teaspoonful of granules dissolved in water, 1 suppository, or 10 to
15 ml syrup h.s. Maximum dosage varies

with preparation used. Dosage for Black-
Draught is 2 tablets or ¼ to ½ level teaspoonfuls of granules mixed with water.
X-Prep Liquid used solely as single dose
for preradiographic bowel evacuation.
Children weighing over 27 kg (59 lb): ½
adult dose of tablets, granules, or syrup
(except Black-Draught tablets and granules—not recommended for children).
Children ages 1 month to 1 year: 1.25 to
2.5 ml Senokot syrup P.O. h.s.

Adverse reactions
GI: *nausea,* vomiting, diarrhea, malabsorption of nutrients, yellow or yellow-
green cast to feces; *abdominal cramps,*
(especially in severe constipation);
"cathartic colon" (syndrome resembling
ulcerative colitis radiologically; with
chronic misuse); possible constipation after catharsis; diarrhea (in breast-feeding
infants of mothers receiving senna); darkened pigmentation of rectal mucosa (with
long-term use; usually reversible within 4
to 12 months after stopping drug); laxative dependence; loss of normal bowel
function (with excessive use).
GU: red-pink discoloration in alkaline
urine; yellow-brown color to acidic urine.
Other: protein-losing enteropathy, electrolyte imbalance (such as hypokalemia).

Interactions
None significant.

Contraindications and precautions
• Contraindicated in patients with ulcerative bowel lesions; nausea, vomiting, abdominal pain, or other symptoms of appendicitis or acute surgical abdomen; fecal impaction; or intestinal obstruction or
perforation.
• Use cautiously in pregnant or breast-
feeding women.

NURSING CONSIDERATIONS

☢ Assessment
• Assess patient's condition before therapy and regularly thereafter.

- Before giving for constipation, determine if patient has adequate fluid intake, exercise, and diet.
- Be alert for adverse reactions.
- Evaluate patient's and family's knowledge of drug therapy.

⊞ **Nursing diagnoses**
- Constipation related to underlying condition
- Diarrhea related to drug-induced adverse GI reactions
- Knowledge deficit related to drug therapy

⊠ **Planning and implementation**
P.O. use: Limit diet to clear liquids after X-Prep Liquid is taken.
P.R. use: Follow normal protocol.
- Avoid exposing drug to excessive heat or light.
- Know that drug is used for short-term treatment.
- Be aware that senna is one of the most effective laxatives for counteracting constipation caused by narcotic analgesics.
Patient teaching
- Teach patient about dietary sources of bulk, which include bran and other cereals, fresh fruit, and vegetables.

☑ **Evaluation**
- Patient's constipation is relieved.
- Patient states that diarrhea does not occur.
- Patient and family state understanding of drug therapy.

---

sertraline hydrochloride
(SER-truh-leen high-droh-KLOR-ighd)
Zoloft

Pharmacologic class: serotonin uptake inhibitor
Therapeutic class: antidepressant
Pregnancy risk category: B

How supplied
Tablets: 25 mg, 50 mg, 100 mg

Pharmacokinetics
Absorption: well absorbed from GI tract. Absorption rate and extent are enhanced when taken with food.
Distribution: highly protein-bound (greater than 98%).
Metabolism: metabolism is probably hepatic.
Excretion: excreted mostly as metabolites in urine and feces. *Half-life:* 26 hours.

Route	Onset	Peak	Duration
P.O.	2-4 wk	4.5-8.5 hr	Unknown

Pharmacodynamics
Chemical effect: unknown; may be linked to its inhibition of neuronal uptake of serotonin in CNS.
Therapeutic effect: relieves depression.

Indications and dosage
▶ **Depression.** *Adults:* 50 mg P.O. daily. Dosage adjusted as tolerated and needed; clinical trials involved dosage of 50 to 200 mg daily. Dosage adjustments should be made at intervals of no less than 1 week.

Adverse reactions
CNS: *headache, tremors, dizziness, insomnia, somnolence,* paresthesias, hypoesthesia, hyperesthesia, *fatigue,* twitching, hypertonia, nervousness, anxiety, confusion.
CV: palpitations, chest pain, hot flashes.
GI: *dry mouth, nausea, diarrhea, loose stools, dyspepsia,* vomiting, constipation, thirst, flatulence, anorexia, abdominal pain, increased appetite.
GU: *male sexual dysfunction,* decreased libido.
Musculoskeletal: myalgia.
Skin: rash, pruritus.
Other: *diaphoresis,* flushing.

Interactions

Drug-drug. *Benzodiazepines (except lorazepam and oxazepam), tolbutamide:* decreased clearance of these drugs. Clinical significance unknown; monitor patient for increased drug effects.
Cimetidine: decreased clearance of sertraline. Monitor closely.
MAO inhibitors: may cause serious, sometimes fatal, reactions including myoclonus rigidity, mental status changes, hyperthermia, autonomic nervous system instability, rapid fluctuations of vital signs, delirium, coma, and death. Avoid concomitant use.
Warfarin, other highly protein-bound drugs: may increase plasma levels of sertraline or other highly bound drug. Small (8%) increases in PT and INR have been noted with concomitant use of warfarin. Monitor patient closely.

Contraindications and precautions

- No known contraindications.
- Use cautiously in patients at risk for suicide and in those with seizure disorder, major affective disorder, or diseases or conditions that affect metabolism or hemodynamic responses. Also use cautiously in pregnant or breast-feeding women.
- Safety of drug has not been established in children.

NURSING CONSIDERATIONS

Assessment

- Assess patient's depression before therapy and reassess regularly thereafter.
- Be alert for adverse reactions and drug interactions.
- Evaluate patient's and family's knowledge of drug therapy.

Nursing diagnoses

- Altered thought processes related to presence of depression
- Risk for injury related to drug-induced adverse CNS reactions
- Knowledge deficit related to drug therapy

Planning and implementation

- Administer drug once daily, either in morning or evening. Drug may be given with or without food.
- Know that drug should not be administered with or within 14 days of discontinuing MAO inhibitor therapy. Allow 14 days after discontinuing drug before starting treatment with MAO inhibitor, as ordered.
- Know that drug may change several laboratory values—increases in serum cholesterol and triglyceride levels, decreases in uric acid concentrations, and elevations in AST and ALT (usually within first 9 weeks of therapy). AST and ALT values return to normal after discontinuing drug; clinical significance is unknown.

Patient teaching

- Advise patient to use caution when performing hazardous tasks that require alertness and to avoid alcohol while taking this drug. Drugs that influence CNS may impair judgment.
- Caution patient to check with doctor or pharmacist before taking OTC medications.

Evaluation

- Patient behavior and communication indicate improved thought processes.
- Patient does not experience injury from adverse CNS reactions.
- Patient and family state understanding of drug therapy.

sibutramine hydrochloride monohydrate

(sigh-BYOO-truh-meen high-droh-KLOR-ighd muh-noh-HIGH-drayt)
Meridia

Pharmacologic class: serotonin, norepinephrine, and dopamine reuptake inhibitor
Therapeutic class: antiobesity
Controlled substance schedule: IV
Pregnancy risk category: C

How supplied

Capsules: 5 mg, 10 mg, 15 mg

Pharmacokinetics

Absorption: rapid; about 77% of administered dose is absorbed.
Distribution: rapid and extensive. Active metabolites are extensively bound to plasma proteins.
Metabolism: extensive first-pass metabolism by the liver to two active metabolites, M_1 and M_2.
Excretion: about 77% is excreted in urine. *Half-life:* M_1 is 14 hours and M_2 is 16 hours.

Route	Onset	Peak	Duration
P.O.	Unknown	3-4 hr	Unknown

Pharmacodynamics

Chemical effect: inhibits reuptake of norepinephrine, serotonin, and dopamine.
Therapeutic effect: assists patient with weight loss.

Indications and dosages

▶ **Management of obesity.** *Adults:*
10 mg P.O. once daily with or without food. May increase dose to 15 mg P.O. daily after 4 weeks if there is inadequate weight loss. Patients who do not tolerate the 10-mg dose may receive 5 mg P.O. daily. Doses above 15 daily are not recommended.

Adverse reactions

CNS: asthenia, *headache, insomnia,* dizziness, nervousness, anxiety, depression, paresthesia, somnolence, CNS stimulation, emotional lability, migraine.
CV: tachycardia, vasodilation, hypertension, palpitation, chest pain.
EENT: thirst, *dry mouth, rhinitis, pharyngitis,* sinusitis, taste perversion, ear disorder, ear pain.
GI: *anorexia, constipation,* increased appetite, nausea, dyspepsia, gastritis, vomiting, abdominal pain, rectal disorder.
GU: dysmenorrhea, urinary tract infection, vaginal candidiasis, metrorrhagia.

Musculoskeletal: arthralgia, myalgia, tenosynovitis, joint disorder, neck or back pain.
Respiratory: cough increase, laryngitis.
Skin: rash, sweating, herpes simplex, acne.
Other: flu syndrome, injury, accident, *allergic reaction,* generalized edema.

Interactions

Drug-drug. *CNS depressants:* may enhance CNS depression. Use with caution. *Dextromethorphan, dihydroergotamine, fentanyl, fluoxetine, fluvoxamine, lithium, MAO inhibitors, meperidine, paroxetine, pentazocine, sertraline, sumatriptan, tryptophan, venlafaxine:* may cause hyperthermia, tachycardia, loss of consciousness. Avoid concomitant use. *Ephedrine, phenylpropanolamine, pseudoephedrine:* may increase blood pressure or heart rate. Use with caution.
Drug-lifestyle. *Alcohol use:* enhanced CNS depression. Avoid concomitant use.

Contraindications and precautions

● Contraindicated in patients taking MAO inhibitors or other centrally acting appetite suppressant drugs, and in those with anorexia nervosa or hypersensitivity to drug or its active ingredients.
● Do not use drug in patients with severe renal or hepatic dysfunction, history of hypertension, seizures, coronary artery disease, heart failure, arrhythmias, or stroke.
● Use cautiously in patients with narrow-angle glaucoma.

NURSING CONSIDERATIONS

⚠ Assessment
● Monitor for adverse reactions and drug interactions.
● Assess patient for organic causes of obesity before starting therapy.
● Measure blood pressure and pulse before starting therapy, with dosage changes, and at regular intervals during therapy.

• Evaluate patient's and family's knowledge of drug therapy.

⊞ Nursing diagnoses
• Altered nutrition: More than body requirements related to increased caloric intake
• Sleep pattern disturbance related to drug-induced insomnia
• Knowledge deficit related to drug therapy

❯ Planning and implementation
• Be aware drug may cause elevated liver function tests.
• Know that at least 2 weeks should elapse between stopping an MAO inhibitor and starting drug therapy, and vice versa.
• Give patient ice chips or sugarless hard candy to relieve dry mouth.
• Safety and effectiveness in children under age 16 have not been established.
Patient teaching
• Advise patient to report rash, hives, or other allergic reactions immediately.
• Instruct patient to inform doctor if he is taking or plans to take prescription or OTC drugs.
• Advise patient to have blood pressure and pulse monitored at regular intervals. Stress importance of regular follow-up visits with doctor.
• Advise patient to use drug with reduced calorie diet.
• Tell patient that weight loss can precipitate gallstone formation. Teach patient signs and symptoms and to report them to doctor promptly.

☑ Evaluation
• Patient achieves nutritional balance with the use of medication and a reduced calorie diet.
• Patient experiences normal sleep patterns.
• Patient and family state understanding of drug therapy.

sildenafil citrate
(sil-DEN-ah-fil SIGH-trayt)
Viagra

Pharmacologic class: selective inhibitor of cyclic guanosine monophosphate-specific phosphodiesterase type 5
Therapeutic class: therapy for erectile dysfunction
Pregnancy risk category: B

How supplied
Tablets: 25 mg, 50 mg 100 mg

Pharmacokinetics
Absorption: rapidly absorbed following oral administration. Absolute bioavailability is 40%.
Distribution: extensively into body tissues. About 96% bound to plasma proteins.
Metabolism: primarily metabolized in the liver to an active metabolite with properties similar to those of parent drug.
Excretion: following oral administration, about 80% is excreted in feces and 13% in urine. *Half-life:* 4 hours.

Route	Onset	Peak	Duration
P.O.	Unknown	0.5-2 hr	4 hr

Pharmacodynamics
Chemical effect: drug has no direct relaxant effect on isolated human corpus cavernosum, but enhances the effect of nitric oxide (NO) by inhibiting phosphodiesterase type 5 (PDE5), which is responsible for degradation of cyclic guanosine monophosphate (cGMP) in the corpus cavernosum. When sexual stimulation causes local release of NO, inhibition of PDE5 by sildenafil causes increased levels of cGMP in the corpus cavernosum, resulting in smooth muscle relaxation and inflow of blood to the corpus cavernosum.
Therapeutic effect: patient achieves an erection.

Reactions may be *common*, uncommon, *life-threatening*, or COMMON AND LIFE-THREATENING.

Indications and dosages

▶ **Treatment of erectile dysfunction.**
Adults under age 65: 50 mg P.O., p.r.n., about 1 hour before sexual activity. Dosage range is 25 mg to 100 mg based on effectiveness and toleration. Maximum of 1 dose per day. *Elderly (age 65 and older):* 25 mg P.O., p.r.n. about 1 hour before sexual activity. Dose may be adjusted based on patient response. Maximum of 1 dose per day.

Adverse reactions

CNS: anxiety, *headache,* dizziness, *seizures,* somnolence, vertigo.
CV: *MI, sudden cardiac death, ventricular arrhythmia, cerebrovascular hemorrhage,* transient ischemic attack, hypertension, *flushing.*
EENT: diplopia, temporary vision loss, decreased vision, ocular redness or bloodshot appearance, increased intraocular pressure, retinal vascular disease, retinal bleeding, vitreous detachment or traction, paramacular edema, abnormal vision (photophobia, color tinged vision, blurred vision); ocular burning, swelling, or pressure.
GI: dyspepsia, diarrhea.
GU: hematuria, prolonged erection, priapism, urinary tract infection.
Musculoskeletal: arthralgia, back pain.
Respiratory: respiratory tract infection.
Skin: rash.
Other: flu syndrome.

Interactions

Drug-drug. *Beta blockers, loop and potassium-sparing diuretics:* increased blood levels of major metabolite of sildenafil, N-desmethyl sildenafil. Clinical significance of this interaction not known.
CYP3A4 inducers, rifampin: reduced sildenafil plasma levels. Monitor effect.
Hepatic isoenzyme inhibitors (such as cimetidine, erythromycin, itraconazole, ketoconazole): may reduce clearance of sildenafil. Avoid concomitant use.
Nitrates: sildenafil enhances hypotensive effects. Don't use together.

Drug-food. *High-fat meals:* reduced rate of absorption and decreased peak serum concentrations. Separate administration time from meals.

Contraindications and precautions

• Contraindicated with concomitant use of organic nitrates at any frequency and in any form, and in patients with underlying CV disease or known hypersensitivity to drug or its components.
• Use cautiously in patients age 65 or older; in those with hepatic or severe renal impairment, anatomic deformation of the penis or conditions that may predispose them to priapism (such as sickle-cell anemia, multiple myeloma, leukemia), retinitis pigmentosa, bleeding disorders, or active peptic ulcer disease; in patients who have suffered an MI, stroke, or life-threatening arrhythmia within last 6 months; and in those with history of cardiac failure, coronary artery disease, uncontrolled high or low blood pressure.

NURSING CONSIDERATIONS

Assessment
• Discuss patient's history of erectile dysfunction to establish need for drug versus other therapies.
• Discuss with patient his response to drug and if he is experiencing adverse effects.
• Assess patient for preexisting CV risk factors because serious events have been reported with drug use, and report risk factors to doctor.
• Evaluate patient's and family's knowledge of drug therapy.

Nursing diagnoses
• Sexual dysfunction related to patient's underlying condition
• Altered cardiopulmonary tissue perfusion related to drug-induced effects on blood pressure and cardiac output
• Knowledge deficit related to drug therapy

⫸ Planning and implementation

• Know that dosage for adults with hepatic or severe renal impairment is 25 mg P.O. about 1 hour before sexual activity. Dose may be adjusted based on patient response. Maximum of 1 dose per day.

• Know that drug's systemic vasodilatory properties cause transient decreases in supine blood pressure and cardiac output (about 2 hours postingestion). Together with the potential cardiac risk of sexual activity, the risk for patients with underlying CV disease is increased.

• Know that serious CV events, including MI, sudden cardiac death, ventricular arrhythmia, cerebrovascular hemorrhage, transient ischemic attack, and hypertension, have occurred in patients during or shortly after sexual activity.

Patient teaching

• Advise patient that drug is contraindicated with regular or intermittent use of nitrates.

• Advise patient of potential cardiac risk of sexual activity especially in presence of preexisting CV risk factors. Instruct him that if symptoms occur (such as angina pectoris, dizziness, nausea) on initiation of sexual activity, to refrain from further activity and to notify doctor.

• Warn patient that erections lasting more than 4 hours and priapism (painful erections more than 6 hours) can occur and should be reported immediately. Penile tissue damage and permanent loss of potency may result if priapism is not treated immediately.

• Inform patient that drug does not offer protection against sexually transmitted diseases and that protective measures such as condoms should be used.

• Instruct patient to take drug 30 minutes to 4 hours before sexual activity; maximum benefit can be expected less than 2 hours after ingesting drug.

• Advise patient that drug is most rapidly absorbed if taken on an empty stomach.

• Inform patient to avoid potentially hazardous activities that rely on color dis-crimination because impairment of blue/green discrimination may occur.

• Instruct patient to notify doctor if visual changes occur.

• Advise patient that drug is effective only in the presence of sexual stimulation.

• Caution patient to take drug only as prescribed.

✓ Evaluation

• Sexual activity improves with drug therapy.

• Patient does not experience adverse CV events.

• Patient and family state understanding of drug therapy.

---

simethicone
(sigh-METH-ih-kohn)
Extra Strength Gas-X†, Gas Relief†, Gas-X†, Maximum Strength Gas Relief†, Maximum Strength Phazyme†, Mylanta Gas†, Mylanta Gas, Maximum Strength†, Mylanta Gas Regular Strength†, Mylicon-80†, Mylicon-125†, Ovol♦, Ovol-40♦, Ovol-80♦, Phazyme†, Phazyme 95†, Phazyme 125†

Pharmacologic class: dispersant
Therapeutic class: antiflatulent
Pregnancy risk category: NR

How supplied

Tablets: 40 mg†, 50 mg†, 60 mg†, 80 mg†, 95 mg†, 125 mg†
Capsules: 125 mg
Drops: 40 mg/0.6 ml†

Pharmacokinetics

Absorption: none.
Distribution: none.
Metabolism: none.
Excretion: excreted in feces.

Route	Onset	Peak	Duration
P.O.	Immediate	Immediate	Unknown

Pharmacodynamics

Chemical effect: by its defoaming action, disperses or prevents formation of mucus-surrounded gas pockets in GI tract.
Therapeutic effect: relieves gas.

Indications and dosage

▶ **Flatulence, functional gastric bloating.** *Adults and children over age 12:* 40 to 125 mg P.O. after each meal and h.s.

Adverse reactions

GI: expulsion of excessive liberated gas as belching, rectal flatus.

Interactions

None significant.

Contraindications and precautions

• Contraindicated in patients hypersensitive to drug.
• Use cautiously in pregnant or breast-feeding women.
• Safety of drug has not been established in children age 12 and younger.

NURSING CONSIDERATIONS

☑ Assessment
• Assess patient's condition before therapy and regularly thereafter.
• Be alert for adverse GI reactions.
• Evaluate patient's and family's knowledge of drug therapy.

⊞ Nursing diagnoses
• Pain related to gas in GI tract
• Knowledge deficit related to drug therapy

▷ Planning and implementation
• Make sure patient chews tablet before swallowing.
Patient teaching
• Advise patient that medication does not prevent formation of gas.
• Encourage patient to change position frequently and ambulate to aid in passing flatus.

☑ Evaluation
• Patient's gas pain is relieved.
• Patient and family state understanding of drug therapy.

---

simvastatin (synvinolin)
(sim-vuh-STAT-in)
Lipex◊, Zocor

Pharmacologic class: HMG-CoA reductase inhibitor
Therapeutic class: antilipemic, cholesterol-lowering agent
Pregnancy risk category: X

How supplied

Tablets: 5 mg, 10 mg, 20 mg, 40 mg

Pharmacokinetics

Absorption: readily absorbed; however, extensive hepatic extraction limits plasma availability of active inhibitors to 5% of dose or less. Individual absorption varies considerably.
Distribution: parent drug and active metabolites are more than 95% bound to plasma proteins.
Metabolism: hydrolysis occurs in plasma; at least three major metabolites have been identified.
Excretion: excreted primarily in bile.
Half-life: 3 hours.

Route	Onset	Peak	Duration
P.O.	Unknown	1.3-2.4 hr	Unknown

Pharmacodynamics

Chemical effect: inhibits 3-hydroxy-3-methylglutaryl coenzyme A reductase. This enzyme is early (and rate-limiting) step in synthetic pathway of cholesterol.
Therapeutic effect: lowers low-density lipoprotein (LDL) and total cholesterol levels.

Indications and dosage

▶ **Reduction of LDL and total cholesterol levels in patients with primary hy-**

---

percholesterolemia (types IIa and IIb). *Adults:* 5 to 10 mg P.O. daily in evening. Dosage adjusted q 4 weeks based on patient tolerance and response; maximum daily dosage is 40 mg. Maximum daily dosage in elderly is 20 mg. *Patients receiving immunosuppressants:* 5 mg/day initially; maximum daily dosage is 10 mg. *Patients with severe renal impairment:* initially, 5 mg P.O. daily.

Adverse reactions

CNS: headache, asthenia.
GI: abdominal pain, constipation, diarrhea, dyspepsia, flatulence, nausea.
Hepatic: elevated liver enzyme levels.
Respiratory: upper respiratory tract infection.

Interactions

Drug-drug. *Digoxin:* simvastatin may elevate digoxin levels slightly. Closely monitor plasma digoxin levels at initiation of simvastatin therapy.
Drugs that decrease levels or activity of endogenous steroids (such as cimetidine, ketoconazole, spironolactone): may increase risk of developing endocrine dysfunction. *Erythromycin, fibric acid derivatives (such as clofibrate, gemfibrozil), high doses of niacin (nicotinic acid; 1 g or more daily), immunosuppressants (such as cyclosporine):* may increase risk of rhabdomyolysis. Monitor patient closely if concomitant use cannot be avoided. Limit daily dosage of simvastatin to 10 mg if patient must take cyclosporine. *Hepatotoxic drugs:* increased risk of hepatotoxicity. Avoid concomitant use. *Warfarin:* anticoagulant effect may be slightly enhanced. Monitor PT at start of therapy and during dosage adjustments.
Drug-lifestyle. *Alcohol use:* increased risk of hepatotoxicity. Avoid concomitant use.

Contraindications and precautions

• Contraindicated in patients with hypersensitivity to drug and in those with active liver disease or conditions that have unexplained persistent elevations of serum transaminase levels; in pregnant or breast-feeding women; and in women of childbearing age unless there is no risk of pregnancy.
• Use cautiously in patients who consume substantial quantities of alcohol or have history of liver disease.
• Safety of drug has not been established in children.

NURSING CONSIDERATIONS

⚕ Assessment

• Obtain history of patient's LDL and total cholesterol levels before therapy and reassess regularly thereafter.
• Know that liver function tests should be performed at start of therapy and periodically thereafter. A liver biopsy may be performed if enzyme level elevations persist.
• Be alert for adverse reactions and drug interactions.
• Evaluate patient's and family's knowledge of drug therapy.

⊕ Nursing diagnoses

• Risk for injury related to presence of elevated cholesterol levels
• Constipation related to drug-induced adverse GI reactions
• Knowledge deficit related to drug therapy

⊠ Planning and implementation

• Know that drug is initiated only after diet and other nonpharmacologic therapies have proved ineffective. The patient should be on standard low-cholesterol diet during therapy.
• Administer drug with evening meal for enhanced effectiveness.
• If cholesterol level falls below target range, dosage may be reduced.
Patient teaching
• Tell patient to take drug with evening meal; absorption is enhanced and cholesterol biosynthesis is greater.
• Teach patient dietary management of serum lipids (restricting total fat and cholesterol intake) and measures to control

---

Reactions may be *common*, uncommon, *life-threatening*, or COMMON AND LIFE-THREATENING.

other cardiac disease risk factors. If appropriate, suggest weight control, exercise, and smoking cessation programs.

• Tell patient to inform doctor if adverse reactions occur, particularly muscle aches and pains.

• Inform female patient that drug is contraindicated during pregnancy. Advise her to notify doctor immediately if pregnancy occurs.

☑ **Evaluation**
• Patient's LDL and total cholesterol levels are within normal limits.
• Patient regains and maintains normal bowel pattern throughout therapy.
• Patient and family state understanding of drug therapy.

sodium bicarbonate†
(SOH-dee-um bigh-KAR-buh-nayt)
Arm and Hammer Pure Baking Soda, Bell/ans, Citrocarbonate, Soda Mint

Pharmacologic class: alkalinizing agent
Therapeutic class: systemic and urinary alkalinizer, systemic hydrogen ion buffer, oral antacid
Pregnancy risk category: NR

How supplied

Tablets†: 300 mg, 325 mg, 520 mg, 600 mg, 650 mg
Injection: 4% (2.4 mEq/5 ml), 4.2% (5 mEq/10 ml), 5% (297.5 mEq/500 ml), 7.5% (8.92 mEq/10 ml and 44.6 mEq/50 ml), 8.4% (10 mEq/10 ml and 50 mEq/50 ml)

Pharmacokinetics

Absorption: well absorbed after P.O. administration.
Distribution: bicarbonate is confined to systemic circulation.
Metabolism: none.
Excretion: bicarbonate is filtered and reabsorbed by kidneys; less than 1% of filtered bicarbonate is excreted.

Route	Onset	Peak	Duration
P.O.	Unknown	Unknown	Unknown
I.V.	Immediate	Immediate	Unknown

Pharmacodynamics

Chemical effect: restores body's buffering capacity and neutralizes excess acid.
Therapeutic effect: restores normal acid-base balance and relieves acid indigestion.

Indications and dosage

▶ **Cardiac arrest.** *Adults and children:* 1 mEq/kg I.V. of 7.5% or 8.4% solution, followed by 0.5 mEq/kg I.V. every 10 minutes, depending on blood gases. Further dosages based on results of blood gas analysis. If blood gas analysis is unavailable, use 0.5 mEq/kg I.V. every 10 minutes until spontaneous circulation returns. *Infants up to age 2:* not to exceed 8 mEq/kg I.V. daily of 4.2% solution.
▶ **Metabolic acidosis.** *Adults and children:* dosage depends on blood CO_2 content, pH, and patient's clinical condition. Generally, 2 to 5 mEq/kg I.V. infused over 4- to 8-hour period.
▶ **Systemic or urinary alkalinization.** *Adults:* initially, 4 g P.O., followed by 1 to 2 g q 4 hours. *Children:* 84 to 840 mg/kg P.O. daily.
▶ **Antacid.** *Adults:* 300 mg to 2 g P.O. up to q.i.d. taken with glass of water.

Adverse reactions

GI: gastric distention, belching, flatulence.
Other: *metabolic alkalosis,* hypernatremia, hypokalemia, hyperosmolarity (with overdose); local pain and irritation (at injection site).

Interactions

Drug-drug. *Anorexiants, flecainide, mecamylamine, quinidine, sympathomimetics:* increased urine alkalinization causes increased renal clearance of these drugs and reduced effectiveness. Monitor patient closely.
Chlorpropamide, lithium, methotrexate, salicylates, tetracycline: urine alkaliniza-

tion causes decreased renal clearance of these drugs and increased risk of toxicity. Monitor patient closely.
Enteric-coated drugs: may be released prematurely in stomach. Avoid concomitant use.
Ketoconazole: concurrent use may decrease absorption. Use with caution.

Contraindications and precautions

• Contraindicated in patients with metabolic or respiratory alkalosis; in patients who are losing chlorides by vomiting or from continuous GI suction; in those receiving diuretics known to produce hypochloremic alkalosis; and in those with hypocalcemia in which alkalosis may produce tetany, hypertension, seizures, or heart failure. Oral sodium bicarbonate is contraindicated in patients with acute ingestion of strong mineral acids.
• Use with extreme caution in patients with heart failure or other edematous or sodium-retaining conditions or renal insufficiency.
• Use cautiously in pregnant or breast-feeding women.

NURSING CONSIDERATIONS

⚕ Assessment
• Assess patient's condition before therapy and regularly thereafter.
• To avoid risk of alkalosis, obtain blood pH, PaO_2, $PaCO_2$, and serum electrolyte levels.
• If sodium bicarbonate is being used to produce alkaline urine, monitor urine pH every 4 to 6 hours (should be greater than 7).
• Be alert for adverse reactions and drug interactions.
• Evaluate patient's and family's knowledge of drug therapy.

⊞ Nursing diagnoses
• Altered health maintenance related to underlying condition
• Risk for injury related to drug-induced adverse reactions

• Knowledge deficit related to drug therapy

▶ Planning and implementation
• Be aware that drug is not routinely recommended for use in cardiac arrest because it may produce paradoxical acidosis from CO_2 production. It should not be routinely administered during early stages of resuscitation unless preexisting acidosis is clearly present. Drug may be used at team leader's discretion after such interventions as defibrillation, cardiac compression, and administration of first-line drugs.
P.O. use: Administer drug with water, not milk.
I.V. use: Drug is usually administered by I.V. infusion. When immediate treatment is necessary, drug may be given by direct, rapid I.V. injection. However, in neonates and children younger than age 2, slow I.V. administration is preferred to avoid hypernatremia, decreased CSF pressure, and possible intracranial hemorrhage.
– Be aware that sodium bicarbonate inactivates such catecholamines as norepinephrine and dopamine and forms precipitate with calcium. Do not mix sodium bicarbonate with I.V. solutions of these agents, and flush I.V. line adequately.
• Keep doctor informed of serum laboratory results.
Patient teaching
• Tell patient not to take with milk. Drug may cause hypercalcemia, alkalosis or, possibly, renal calculi.
• Discourage use as antacid. Offer nonabsorbable alternate antacid if it is to be used repeatedly.

☑ Evaluation
• Patient regains normal acid-base balance in body.
• Patient does not experience injury from drug-induced adverse reactions.
• Patient and family state understanding of drug therapy.

sodium chloride
(SOH-dee-um KLOR-ighd)

Pharmacologic class: electrolyte
Therapeutic class: sodium and chloride replacement
Pregnancy risk category: NR

How supplied

Tablets (enteric-coated): 650 mg, 1 g, 2.25 g
Tablets (slow-release): 600 mg
Injection: 0.45% NaCl solution 500 ml, 1,000 ml; 0.9% NaCl solution 50 ml, 100 ml, 150 ml, 250 ml, 500 ml, 1,000 ml; 3% NaCl solution 500 ml; 5% NaCl solution 500 ml; 14.6% NaCl solution 20 ml, 40 ml, 200 ml; 23.4% NaCl solution 30 ml, 50 ml, and 200 ml.

Pharmacokinetics

Absorption: absorbed readily from GI tract after P.O. administration.
Distribution: distributed widely in body.
Metabolism: none significant.
Excretion: excreted primarily in urine; some excreted in sweat, tears, and saliva.

Route	Onset	Peak	Duration
P.O.	Unknown	Unknown	Unknown
I.V.	Immediate	Immediate	Unknown

Pharmacodynamics

Chemical effect: replaces and maintains sodium and chloride levels.
Therapeutic effect: restores normal sodium and chloride levels.

Indications and dosage

▶ **Fluid and electrolyte replacement in hyponatremia caused by electrolyte loss, severe salt depletion.** *Adults:* dosage is highly individualized. The 3% and 5% solutions are used only with frequent electrolyte determination and given only slow I.V. With 0.45% solution: 3% to 8% of body weight, according to deficiencies, over 18 to 24 hours; with 0.9% solution: 2% to 6% of body weight, ac-cording to deficiencies, over 18 to 24 hours.
▶ **Management of heat cramp caused by excessive perspiration.** *Adults:* 1 g P.O. with every glass of water.

Adverse reactions

CV: aggravation of heart failure; edema (if given too rapidly or in excess).
Metabolic: hypernatremia, aggravation of existing metabolic acidosis (with excessive infusion); serious electrolyte disturbances, loss of potassium.
Respiratory: *pulmonary edema* (if given too rapidly or in excess).
Other: local tenderness, abscess, tissue necrosis (at injection site), thrombophlebitis.

Interactions

None significant.

Contraindications and precautions

• Contraindicated in patients with conditions in which sodium and chloride administration is detrimental. NaCl 3% and 5% injections are contraindicated in patients with increased, normal, or only slightly decreased serum electrolyte levels.
• Use cautiously in patients with heart failure, circulatory insufficiency, renal dysfunction, or hypoproteinemia; in elderly or postoperative patients; and in pregnant or breast-feeding women.

NURSING CONSIDERATIONS

☑ Assessment
• Obtain history of patient's sodium and chloride levels before therapy and reassess regularly thereafter.
• Monitor other serum electrolyte levels.
• Be alert for adverse reactions.
• Evaluate patient's and family's knowledge of drug therapy.

☷ Nursing diagnoses
• Altered nutrition: Less than body requirements related to subnormal levels of sodium and chloride

- Fluid volume excess related to NaCl's water-drawing power
- Knowledge deficit related to drug therapy

➤ **Planning and implementation**
P.O. use: Administer tablet with glass of water.
I.V. use: Infuse 3% and 5% solutions very slowly and cautiously to avoid pulmonary edema. Use only for critical situations, and observe patient continually.
– Don't confuse concentrates (14.6%, 23.4%) available to add to parenteral nutrient solutions with 0.9% NaCl injection, and never give without diluting. Read label carefully.
Patient teaching
- Tell patient to report adverse reactions promptly.

☑ **Evaluation**
- Patient's sodium and chloride levels are normal.
- Patient does not exhibit signs and symptoms of fluid retention.
- Patient and family state understanding of drug therapy.

---

sodium fluoride
(SOH-dee-um FLOR-ighd)
Fluor-A-Day◆, Fluoritab, Fluorodex, Fluotic◆, Flura, Flura-Drops, Flura-Loz, Karidium, Luride, Luride Lozi-Tabs, Luride-SF, Luride-SF Lozi-Tabs, Pediaflor, Pedi-Dent◆, Pharmaflur, Pharmaflur df, Pharmaflur 1.1, Phos-Flur, Solu-Flur◆

sodium fluoride, topical
ACT†, Fluorigard†, Fluorinse, Gel-Kam, Gel-Tin†, Karigel, Karigel-N, Listermint with Fluoride, MInute-Gel, Point-Two, Prevident, Thera-Flur, Thera-Flur-N

Pharmacologic class: trace mineral
Therapeutic class: dental caries prophylactic
Pregnancy risk category: NR

How supplied
sodium fluoride
Tablets: 1 mg
Tablets (chewable): 0.5 mg, 1 mg
Drops: 0.125 mg/drop, 0.25 mg/drop, 0.2 mg/ml, 0.5 mg/ml
Lozenges: 1 mg
sodium fluoride, topical
Gel: 0.1%, 0.5%, 1.23%
Gel drops: 0.5%
Rinse: 0.01%†, 0.02%†, 0.09%

Pharmacokinetics
Absorption: absorbed readily and almost completely from GI tract. A large amount may be absorbed in stomach, and rate of absorption may depend on gastric pH. Oral fluoride absorption may be decreased by simultaneous ingestion of aluminum or magnesium hydroxide. Simultaneous ingestion of calcium also may decrease absorption of large doses.
Distribution: stored in bones and developing teeth after absorption. Skeletal tissue also has high storage capacity for fluoride ions. Because of storage-mobilization mechanism in skeletal tissue, constant fluoride supply may be provided. Although teeth have small mass, they also serve as storage sites. Fluoride deposited in teeth is not released readily. Fluoride has been found in all organs and tissues with low accumulation in noncalcified tissues. Fluoride is distributed into sweat, tears, hair, and saliva.
Metabolism: none.
Excretion: excreted rapidly, mainly in urine.

Route	Onset	Peak	Duration
P.O.	Unknown	30-60 min	Unknown

Pharmacodynamics
Chemical effect: stabilizes apatite crystal of bone and teeth.
Therapeutic effect: prevents dental caries.

Indications and dosage
▶ **Prevention of dental caries.** *Adults and children over age 12:* 10 ml of rinse

---

or thin ribbon of gel applied to teeth with toothbrush or mouth trays for at least 1 minute h.s. *Children ages 6 to 12:* 5 ml of rinse or thin ribbon of gel applied to teeth with toothbrush or mouth trays for at least 1 minute h.s. *Children ages 6 to 16:* 1 mg P.O. (tablet or lozenge) daily. *Children ages 3 to 6:* 0.5 mg P.O. (tablet or drops) daily. *Children ages 6 months to 3 years:* 0.25 mg P.O. (tablet or drops) daily.

Adverse reactions

CNS: headache, weakness.
GI: gastric distress.
Skin: hypersensitivity reactions (atopic dermatitis, eczema, urticaria).
Other: staining of teeth.

Interactions

Drug-drug. *Aluminum hydroxide, calcium, iron, magnesium:* may decrease absorption. Administer separately.
Drug-food. *Dairy products:* incompatibility may occur due to formation of calcium fluoride, which is poorly absorbed. Avoid ingestion during sodium fluoride therapy.

Contraindications and precautions

• Contraindicated in patients hypersensitive to fluoride or when fluoride intake from drinking water exceeds 0.7 ppm.
• Use cautiously in pregnant or breast-feeding women.

NURSING CONSIDERATIONS

⚖ Assessment
• Obtain history of patient's dental history and fluoride intake before therapy and reassess regularly thereafter.
• Be alert for adverse reactions and drug interactions.
• Know that chronic toxicity (fluorosis) may result from prolonged use of higher-than-recommended doses.
• Evaluate patient's and family's knowledge of drug therapy.

⊕ Nursing diagnoses
• Health-seeking behavior related to desire for good dental care
• Risk for fluid volume deficit related to drug-induced adverse GI reactions
• Knowledge deficit related to drug therapy

❯ Planning and implementation
• Administer oral drops undiluted or mixed with fluids or food.
• Fluoride in prenatal vitamins has produced healthier teeth in infants.
Patient teaching
• Tell patient that tablets may be dissolved in mouth, chewed, or swallowed whole.
• Advise parents that topical rinses and gels should not be swallowed by children under age 3 or used if water supply is fluorinated.
• Tell patient that sodium fluoride is most effective when used immediately after brushing teeth. Tell patient to rinse around and between teeth for 1 minute, then spit out.
• Tell patient to dilute drops or rinses in plastic rather than glass containers.
• Advise patient to notify dentist of tooth mottling.

☑ Evaluation
• Patient is free from dental caries.
• Patient maintains adequate hydration throughout therapy.
• Patient and family state understanding of drug therapy.

sodium lactate
(SOH-dee-um LAK-tayt)
Pharmacologic class: alkalinizing agent
Therapeutic class: systemic alkalizer
Pregnancy risk category: NR

How supplied

Injection: 1/6 molar solution (167 mEq/L)
Injection: 5 mEq/ml

Pharmacokinetics

Absorption: not applicable.
Distribution: lactate ion occurs naturally throughout body.
Metabolism: metabolized in liver.
Excretion: none.

Route	Onset	Peak	Duration
I.V.	Immediate	Immediate	Unknown

Pharmacodynamics

Chemical effect: metabolized to sodium bicarbonate, producing buffering effect.
Therapeutic effect: restores normal acid-base balance.

Indications and dosage

▶ **Urine alkalinization.** *Adults:* 30 ml of 1/6 molar solution per kilogram of body weight P.O. given in divided doses over 24 hours.
▶ **Metabolic acidosis.** *Adults:* 1/6 molar injection (167 mEq lactate/L) I.V.; dosage depends on degree of bicarbonate deficit.

Adverse reactions

Metabolic: *metabolic alkalosis,* hypernatremia, hyperosmolarity (with overdose).
Other: fever; infection, thrombophlebitis (at injection site).

Interactions

None significant.

Contraindications and precautions

• Contraindicated in patients with hypernatremia, lactic acidosis, or conditions in which sodium administration is detrimental.
• Use with extreme caution in patients with metabolic or respiratory alkalosis, severe hepatic or renal disease, shock, hypoxia, or beriberi.
• Use cautiously in pregnant or breast-feeding women.

NURSING CONSIDERATIONS

Assessment
• Obtain history of patient's underlying acid-base imbalance before therapy and reassess regularly thereafter.
• Monitor serum electrolyte levels.
• Evaluate patient's and family's knowledge of drug therapy.

Nursing diagnoses
• Altered health maintenance related to underlying condition
• Altered protection related to drug-induced adverse reactions
• Knowledge deficit related to drug therapy

Planning and implementation
• Add drug to other I.V. solutions or give as isotonic 1/6 molar solution. Drug is compatible with most common I.V. solutions.
• Do not mix with sodium bicarbonate because drugs are physically incompatible.
Patient teaching
• Instruct patient to report discomfort at I.V. site immediately.

Evaluation
• Patient regains normal acid-base balance.
• Patient does not experience serious adverse reactions.
• Patient and family state understanding of drug therapy.

sodium phosphates
(SOH-dee-um FOS-fayts)
Fleet Phospho-soda†

Pharmacologic class: acid salt
Therapeutic class: saline laxative
Pregnancy risk category: NR

How supplied

Liquid: 2.4 g/5 ml sodium phosphate and 900 mg sodium biphosphate/5 ml

---

Reactions may be *common,* uncommon, *life-threatening,* or COMMON AND LIFE-THREATENING.

Enema: 160 mg/ml sodium phosphate and 60 mg/ml sodium biphosphate

Pharmacokinetics

Absorption: about 1% to 20% of P.O. dose absorbed; unknown after P.R. administration.
Distribution: unknown.
Metabolism: unknown.
Excretion: unknown.

Route	Onset	Peak	Duration
P.O.	0.5-3 hr	Varies	Varies
P.R.	5-10 min	Varies	Ceases with evacuation

Pharmacodynamics

Chemical effect: produces osmotic effect in small intestine by drawing water into intestinal lumen.
Therapeutic effect: relieves constipation.

Indications and dosage

▶ **Constipation.** *Adults:* 20 to 30 ml of solution mixed with 120 ml of cold water P.O.; or 120 ml P.R. (as enema). *Children:* 5 to 10 ml of solution mixed with 120 ml of cold water P.O.; or 60 ml P.R. in children over age 2.
▶ **Purgative action.** *Adults:* 45 ml solution mixed with 120 ml cold water.

Adverse reactions

GI: *abdominal cramping.*
Metabolic: fluid and electrolyte disturbances (such as hypernatremia, hyperphosphatemia; with daily use).
Other: laxative dependence (with long-term or excessive use).

Interactions

None significant.

Contraindications and precautions

• Contraindicated in patients with abdominal pain, nausea, vomiting, or other symptoms of appendicitis or acute surgical abdomen; intestinal obstruction or perforation; edema; heart failure; mega-colon; or impaired renal function and in patients on sodium-restricted diets.
• Use cautiously in patients with large hemorrhoids or anal excoriations and in pregnant or breast-feeding women.

NURSING CONSIDERATIONS

Assessment
• Assess patient's condition before therapy and regularly thereafter.
• Before giving for constipation, determine if patient has adequate fluid intake, exercise, and diet.
• Be alert for adverse reactions.
• Be aware that up to 10% of sodium content of drug may be absorbed.
• Evaluate patient's and family's knowledge of drug therapy.

Nursing diagnoses
• Constipation related to underlying condition
• Pain related to drug-induced abdominal cramping
• Knowledge deficit related to drug therapy

Planning and implementation
P.O. use: Dilute drug with water before giving orally (add 30 ml of drug to 120 ml of cold water). Follow administration with full glass of water.
P.R. use: Follow normal protocol.
Patient teaching
• Teach patient about dietary sources of bulk, which include bran and other cereals, fresh fruit, and vegetables.

Evaluation
• Patient's constipation is relieved.
• Patient's abdominal cramping ceases.
• Patient and family state understanding of drug therapy.

sodium polystyrene sulfonate
(SOH-dee-um pol-ee-STIGH-reen SUL-fuh-nayt)
Kayexalate, SPS

Pharmacologic class: cation-exchange resin
Therapeutic class: potassium-removing resin
Pregnancy risk category: C

How supplied

Powder: 1-lb jar (3.5 g/teaspoon)
Suspension: 60 ml*, 120 ml*, 200 ml*, 480 ml*, 500 ml*

Pharmacokinetics

Absorption: not absorbed.
Distribution: none.
Metabolism: none.
Excretion: excreted unchanged in feces.

Route	Onset	Peak	Duration
P.O., P.R.	Unknown	Unknown	Unknown

Pharmacodynamics

Chemical effect: exchanges sodium ions for potassium ions in intestine: 1 g of sodium polystyrene sulfonate is exchanged for 0.5 to 1.0 mEq of potassium. The resin is then eliminated. Much of exchange capacity is used for cations other than potassium (calcium and magnesium) and, possibly, fats and proteins.
Therapeutic effect: lowers serum potassium level.

Indications and dosage

▶ **Hyperkalemia.** *Adults:* 15 g P.O. daily to q.i.d. in water or sorbitol (3 to 4 ml/g of resin). Alternatively, mix powder with appropriate medium—aqueous suspension or diet appropriate for renal failure—and instill in nasogastric (NG) tube. Or 30 to 50 g q 6 hours as warm emulsion deep into sigmoid colon (20 cm). In persistent vomiting or paralytic ileus, high-retention enema of sodium polystyrene sulfonate (30 g) suspended in 200 ml of 10% methylcellulose, 10% dextrose, or 25% sorbitol solution may be given. *Children:* 1 g of resin P.O. or P.R. for each milliequivalent of potassium to be removed. P.O. administration preferred because drug should remain in intestine for at least 6 hours.

Adverse reactions

GI: *constipation,* fecal impaction (in elderly patients), anorexia, gastric irritation, nausea, vomiting, *diarrhea* (with sorbitol emulsions).
Metabolic: hypokalemia, hypocalcemia, sodium retention.

Interactions

Drug-drug. *Antacids and laxatives (non-absorbable cation-donating types, including magnesium hydroxide):* systemic alkalosis and reduced potassium exchange capability. Don't use together.

Contraindications and precautions

• Contraindicated in patients with hypokalemia or hypersensitivity to drug.
• Use cautiously in patients with severe heart failure, severe hypertension, or marked edema and in pregnant or breast-feeding women.

NURSING CONSIDERATIONS

Assessment
• Obtain history of patient's serum potassium level before therapy.
• Monitor serum potassium level at least once daily, as ordered. Treatment may result in potassium deficiency. Treatment is usually stopped when potassium level is reduced to 4 or 5 mEq/L.
• Watch for other signs of hypokalemia: irritability, confusion, arrhythmias, ECG changes, severe muscle weakness and paralysis, and cardiac toxicity in digitalized patients.
• Monitor for symptoms of other electrolyte deficiencies (magnesium, calcium) because drug is nonselective. Monitor serum calcium level in patient

receiving sodium polystyrene therapy for more than 3 days. Supplementary calcium may be needed.
• Watch for sodium overload. Drug contains about 100 mg of sodium/g. About one third of resin's sodium is retained.
• Be alert for adverse reactions and drug interactions.
• Watch for constipation with P.O. or NG administration.
• Evaluate patient's and family's knowledge of drug therapy.

🔲 **Nursing diagnoses**
• Altered health maintenance related to presence of hyperkalemia
• Constipation related to drug-induced adverse GI reactions
• Knowledge deficit related to drug therapy

▶ **Planning and implementation**
• Don't heat resin; this impairs drug's effectiveness.
P.O. use: Mix resin only with water or sorbitol for P.O. administration. *Never* mix with orange juice (high potassium content) to disguise taste.
– Chill oral suspension for greater palatability.
– If sorbitol is given, mix with resin suspension.
– Consider solid form. Resin cookie and candy recipes are available; ask pharmacist or dietitian to supply.
– To prevent constipation with oral drug, use sorbitol (10 to 20 ml of 70% syrup every 2 hours, as needed) to produce one or two watery stools daily.
P.R. use: Know that premixed forms are available (SPS and others).
– If preparing manually, mix polystyrene resin only with water and sorbitol for P.R. use. Do not use mineral oil for P.R. administration to prevent impaction; ion exchange requires aqueous medium. Sorbitol content prevents impaction.
– Prepare rectal dose at room temperature. Stir emulsion gently during administration.

– Use #28 French rubber tube for rectal dose. Insert tube 20 cm into sigmoid colon and tape in place. Alternatively, consider Foley catheter with 30-ml balloon inflated distal to anal sphincter to aid in retention. This is especially helpful for patients with poor sphincter control (for example, after CVA). Use gravity flow. Drain returns constantly through Y-tube connection. Place patient in knee-chest position or with hips on pillow for a while if back leakage occurs.
– After P.R. administration, flush tubing with 50 to 100 ml of nonsodium fluid to ensure delivery of all medication. Flush rectum to remove resin.
– Prevent fecal impaction in elderly patient by administering resin P.R., as ordered. Give cleansing enema before P.R. administration. Explain to patient the need to retain enema—for 6 to 10 hours is ideal, but 30 to 60 minutes is acceptable.
• If hyperkalemia is severe, know that doctor does not depend solely on polystyrene resin to lower serum potassium level. Dextrose 50% with regular insulin I.V. push may be given.
Patient teaching
• Explain importance of following prescribed low-potassium diet.
• Explain necessity of retaining enema (6 to 10 hours is ideal, but 30 to 60 minutes is acceptable).
• Tell patient to report adverse reactions.

🔲 **Evaluation**
• Patient's serum potassium level is normal.
• Patient does not develop constipation.
• Patient and family state understanding of drug therapy.

---

somatrem
(SOH-muh-trem)
Protropin

Pharmacologic class: anterior pituitary hormone

Therapeutic class: human growth hormone (GH)
Pregnancy risk category: C

How supplied

Injectable lyophilized powder: 5 mg (10 IU)/vial

Pharmacokinetics

Absorption: unknown.
Distribution: unknown.
Metabolism: about 90% metabolized in liver.
Excretion: about 0.1% excreted unchanged in urine. *Half-life:* 20 to 30 minutes.

Route	Onset	Peak	Duration
I.M., S.C.	Unknown	Unknown	12-48 hr

Pharmacodynamics

Chemical effect: purified GH of recombinant DNA origin that stimulates linear, skeletal muscle, and organ growth.
Therapeutic effect: stimulates growth in children.

Indications and dosage

▶ **Long-term treatment of children who have growth failure because of lack of adequate endogenous GH secretion.** *Children (prepuberty):* highly individualized; up to 0.1 mg/kg I.M. or S.C. three times weekly.

Adverse reactions

Metabolic: hypothyroidism, hyperglycemia.
Other: antibodies to GH.

Interactions

Drug-drug. *Glucocorticoids:* may inhibit growth-promoting action of somatrem. Adjust glucocorticoid dosage as necessary.

Contraindications and precautions

• Contraindicated in patients with epiphyseal closure, active neoplasia, or hypersensitivity to benzyl alcohol.

• Use cautiously in patients with hypothyroidism and in those whose GH deficiency results from an intracranial lesion.

• Drug is not indicated for use in pregnant or breast-feeding women.

NURSING CONSIDERATIONS

⚕ Assessment

• Assess child's growth before therapy and regularly thereafter.
• Be alert for adverse reactions and drug interactions.
• Know that toxicity in neonates has occurred from exposure to benzyl alcohol used in drug as preservative.
• Monitor height and blood with regular checkups; radiologic studies are also necessary.
• Observe patient for signs of glucose intolerance and hyperglycemia.
• Monitor periodic thyroid function tests for hypothyroidism, as ordered, which may require treatment with thyroid hormone.
• Evaluate patient's and family's knowledge of drug therapy.

Nursing diagnoses

• Altered growth and development related to lack of adequate endogenous GH
• Altered health maintenance related to adverse metabolic reactions
• Knowledge deficit related to drug therapy

Planning and implementation

• Check drug's expiration date.
• To prepare solution, inject supplied bacteriostatic water for injection into vial containing drug. Then swirl vial with gentle rotary motion until contents are dissolved. *Don't shake vial.*
• After reconstitution, vial solution should be clear. Don't inject if solution is cloudy or contains particles.
• If drug is administered to neonate, reconstitute immediately before use with

---

Reactions may be *common,* uncommon, *life-threatening,* or COMMON AND LIFE-THREATENING.

sterile water for injection (without bacteriostat). Use vial once, then discard.
• Store reconstituted vial in refrigerator; use within 7 days.
I.M. and S.C. use: Follow normal protocol.
Patient teaching
• Reassure patient and family members that somatrem is *pure* and *safe*. Drug replaces pituitary-derived human GH, which was removed from market in 1985 because of an association with rare but fatal viral infection (Jakob-Creutzfeldt disease).

☑ **Evaluation**
• Patient exhibits growth.
• Patient's thyroid function studies and blood glucose level are normal.
• Patient and family state understanding of drug therapy.

somatropin
(soh-muh-TROH-pin)
Genotropin, Humatrope, Norditropin, Nutropin, Saizen, Serostim

Pharmacologic class: anterior pituitary hormone
Therapeutic class: human growth hormone (GH)
Pregnancy risk category: C

How supplied

Injection: 1.5 mg/ml; 5 mg/5 ml; 4-mg, 5-mg, 8-mg, 10-mg vials

Pharmacokinetics

Absorption: unknown.
Distribution: unknown.
Metabolism: about 90% metabolized in liver.
Excretion: about 0.1% excreted unchanged in urine. *Half-life:* 20 to 30 minutes.

Route	Onset	Peak	Duration
I.M, S.C.	Unknown	7.5 hr	12-48 hr

Pharmacodynamics

Chemical effect: purified GH of recombinant DNA origin that stimulates linear, skeletal muscle, and organ growth.
Therapeutic effect: stimulates growth.

Indications and dosage

▶ **Long-term treatment of growth failure in children with inadequate secretion of endogenous GH.** *Children:* 0.18 mg/kg body weight S.C. weekly divided equally and given on 3 alternate days, six times weekly or daily using Humatrope; or 0.30 mg/kg body weight S.C. weekly in daily divided doses using Nutropin; or 0.06 mg/kg S.C. or I.M. three times weekly using Saizen; or 0.024 to 0.034 mg/kg S.C. six or seven times weekly using Norditropin; or 0.16 to 0.24 mg/kg/week divided into six or seven S.C. injections using Genotropin; or about 1 mg/kg S.C. daily h.s. using Serostim. See manufacturer's dosing chart.
▶ **Growth failure in children associated with chronic renal insufficiency up to time of renal transplantation (Nutropin).** *Children:* 0.35 mg/kg body weight S.C. weekly in daily divided doses.

Adverse reactions

CNS: headache, weakness.
CV: mild, transient edema.
Hematologic: *leukemia.*
Metabolic: mild hyperglycemia, hypothyroidism.
Other: injection site pain, localized muscle pain, antibodies to GH.

Interactions

Drug-drug. *Corticosteroids, corticotropin:* long-term use inhibits growth response to GH. Monitor patient.

Contraindications and precautions

• Contraindicated in patients with closed epiphyses or an active underlying intracranial lesion. Humatrope should not be reconstituted with supplied diluent for patients with known sensitivity to either *m*-cresol or glycerin.

• Use cautiously in children with hypothyroidism and in those whose GH deficiency is caused by an intracranial lesion. Be aware that these children should be examined frequently for progression or recurrence of underlying disease.

• Drug is not indicated for use in pregnant or breast-feeding women.

NURSING CONSIDERATIONS

⊠ Assessment
• Assess child's growth before therapy and regularly thereafter.

• Be alert for adverse reactions.

• Know that toxicity in neonates has occurred from exposure to benzyl alcohol used in drug as preservative.

• Know that regular checkups with monitoring of height and of blood and radiologic studies are necessary.

• Observe patient for signs of glucose intolerance and hyperglycemia.

• Monitor periodic thyroid function tests for hypothyroidism, as ordered, which may require treatment with thyroid hormone.

• Evaluate patient's and family's knowledge of drug therapy.

⊞ Nursing diagnoses
• Altered growth and development related to lack of adequate endogenous GH

• Altered health maintenance related to adverse metabolic reactions

• Knowledge deficit related to drug therapy

≥ Planning and implementation
• To prepare solution, inject supplied diluent into vial containing drug by aiming stream of liquid against glass wall of vial. Then swirl vial with gentle rotary motion until contents are completely dissolved. *Don't shake vial.*

• After reconstitution, vial solution should be clear. Don't inject solution if it is cloudy or contains particles.

• Store reconstituted vial in refrigerator; use within 14 days.

• If sensitivity to diluent should occur, vials may be reconstituted with sterile water for injection. When drug is reconstituted in this manner, use only one reconstituted dose per vial, refrigerate solution if it is not used immediately after reconstitution, use reconstituted dose within 24 hours, and discard unused portion.

I.M. and S.C. use: Follow normal protocol.

• Know that excessive glucocorticoid therapy inhibits growth-promoting effect of somatropin. Patient with coexisting corticotropin deficiency should have glucocorticoid replacement dosage carefully adjusted to avoid an inhibitory effect on growth.

Patient teaching
• Inform parents that child with endocrine disorders (including GH deficiency) may develop slipped capital epiphyses more frequently. Tell them that if they notice limp in their child, they should notify doctor.

☑ Evaluation
• Patient exhibits growth.

• Patient's thyroid function studies and blood glucose level are normal.

• Patient and family state understanding of drug therapy.

sotalol hydrochloride
(SOH-tuh-lol high-droh-KLOR-ighd)
Betapace, Sotacor♦ ◊

Pharmacologic class: beta blocker
Therapeutic class: antiarrhythmic, antihypertensive, antianginal
Pregnancy risk category: B

How supplied
Tablets: 80 mg, 160 mg, 240 mg

Pharmacokinetics

Absorption: well absorbed with bioavailability of 90% to 100%. Food may interfere with absorption.
Distribution: unknown; does not bind to plasma proteins and crosses blood-brain barrier poorly.
Metabolism: not metabolized.
Excretion: excreted primarily in urine in unchanged form. *Half-life:* 12 hours.

Route	Onset	Peak	Duration
P.O.	Unknown	2.5-4 hr	Unknown

Pharmacodynamics

Chemical effect: depresses sinus heart rate, slows AV conduction, decreases cardiac output, and lowers systolic and diastolic blood pressure.
Therapeutic effect: restores normal sinus rhythm, lowers blood pressure, and relieves anginal pain.

Indications and dosage

▶ **Documented, life-threatening ventricular arrhythmias.** *Adults:* initially, 80 mg P.O. b.i.d. Dosage is increased q 2 to 3 days as needed and tolerated; most patients respond to daily dosage of 160 to 320 mg. A few patients with refractory arrhythmias have received as much as 640 mg daily. *In patients with renal failure:* if creatinine clearance is over 60 ml/minute, dosage adjustment is not necessary. If creatinine clearance is 30 to 60 ml/minute, interval is increased to q 24 hours; 10 to 30 ml/minute, q 36 to 48 hours; less than 10 ml/minute, individualized dosage.

Adverse reactions

CNS: *asthenia, headache, dizziness, weakness, fatigue,* sleep problems, *lightheadedness.*
CV: *bradycardia, **arrhythmias, heart failure, AV block, proarrhythmic events (ventricular tachycardia, PVCs, ventricular fibrillation),** edema, palpitations, chest pain,* ECG abnormalities, hypotension.

GI: *nausea,* vomiting, diarrhea, dyspepsia.
Respiratory: *dyspnea, **bronchospasm.***

Interactions

Drug-drug. *Antiarrhythmics:* additive effects. Avoid concomitant use.
Antihypertensives, catecholamine-depleting drugs (such as guanethidine, haloperidol, and reserpine): enhanced hypotensive effects. Monitor patient closely.
Calcium channel blockers: enhanced myocardial depression. Monitor patient carefully.
Clonidine: beta blockers may enhance rebound effect seen after withdrawal of clonidine. Discontinue sotalol several days before withdrawing clonidine.
General anesthetics: may cause additional myocardial depression. Monitor patient closely.
Insulin, oral antidiabetic agents: may cause hyperglycemia. Adjust dose. May mask symptoms of hyperglycemia.
Drug-food. *Any food:* increased absorption. Give drug on an empty stomach.

Contraindications and precautions

• Contraindicated in patients with severe sinus node dysfunction, sinus bradycardia, second- or third-degree AV block in absence of an artificial pacemaker, congenital or acquired long QT syndrome, cardiogenic shock, uncontrolled heart failure, bronchial asthma, or hypersensitivity to drug.
• Use cautiously in patients with renal impairment or diabetes mellitus and in pregnant women.
• Safety of drug has not been established in children and in breast-feeding women.

NURSING CONSIDERATIONS

Assessment
• Assess patient's condition before therapy and regularly thereafter.
• Monitor serum electrolyte levels and ECG regularly, especially if patient is receiving diuretics. Electrolyte imbalances, such as hypokalemia and hypomagne-

semia, may enhance QT-interval prolongation and increase risk of serious arrhythmias such as torsades de pointes.
• Be alert for adverse reactions and drug interactions.
• Evaluate patient's and family's knowledge of drug therapy.

🖫 **Nursing diagnoses**
• Altered health maintenance related to underlying condition
• Fatigue related to adverse reactions
• Knowledge deficit related to drug therapy

▶ **Planning and implementation**
• Because proarrhythmic events may occur at start of therapy and during dosage adjustments, be aware that patient should be hospitalized. Facilities and personnel should be available for cardiac rhythm monitoring and interpretation of ECG.
• Note that although patients receiving I.V. lidocaine have started sotalol therapy without ill effect, other antiarrhythmic drugs should be withdrawn before therapy with sotalol. Sotalol therapy typically is delayed until two or three half-lives of withdrawn drug have elapsed. After withdrawal of amiodarone, sotalol shouldn't be administered until QT interval normalizes.
• Be aware that dosage should be adjusted slowly, allowing 2 to 3 days between dosage increments for adequate monitoring of QT intervals and for plasma levels of drug to reach steady-state level.
Patient teaching
• Explain importance of taking drug as prescribed, even when feeling well. Caution patient not to discontinue drug suddenly.
• Tell patient to take drug 1 hour before or 2 hours after meals.

☑ **Evaluation**
• Patient responds well to therapy.
• Patient states energy-conserving measures to combat fatigue.
• Patient and family state understanding of drug therapy.

spectinomycin hydrochloride
(spek-tih-noh-MIGH-sin high-droh-KLOR-ighd)
Trobicin

Pharmacologic class: aminocyclitol
Therapeutic class: antibiotic
Pregnancy risk category: B

How supplied

Injection: 2-g vial with 3.2-ml diluent; 4-g vial with 6.2-ml diluent
Powder for injection: 2 g, 4 g

Pharmacokinetics

Absorption: absorbed rapidly after I.M. injection.
Distribution: unknown.
Metabolism: unknown.
Excretion: most excreted unchanged in urine. *Half-life:* 1 to 3 hours.

Route	Onset	Peak	Duration
I.M.	Unknown	1-2 hr	Unknown

Pharmacodynamics

Chemical effect: inhibits protein synthesis by binding to 30S subunit of ribosome.
Therapeutic effect: hinders bacterial growth. Drug is bactericidal; its spectrum of activity includes many gram-positive and gram-negative organisms. However, spectinomycin hydrochloride is used mostly against penicillin-resistant *Neisseria gonorrhoeae.*

Indications and dosage

▶ **Gonorrhea.** *Adults:* 2 to 4 g I.M. as single dose injected deeply into upper outer quadrant of buttock.

Adverse reactions

CNS: insomnia, dizziness.
GI: nausea.
GU: decreased urine output, decrease in creatinine clearance, increase in BUN level.
Hematologic: decrease in hemoglobin and hematocrit values.

Reactions may be *common,* uncommon, *life-threatening,* or COMMON AND LIFE-THREATENING.

Hepatic: transient increases in liver enzyme levels.
Skin: urticaria.
Other: *anaphylaxis,* fever, chills (may mask or delay symptoms of incubating syphilis), pain at injection site.

Interactions

None significant.

Contraindications and precautions

• Contraindicated in patients with hypersensitivity to drug.
• Use cautiously in pregnant women.
• Safety of drug has not been established in children and in breast-feeding women.

NURSING CONSIDERATIONS

🕮 Assessment
• Assess patient's infection before therapy and regularly thereafter.
• Drug is not effective in treatment of syphilis. Serologic test for syphilis should be done before treatment dose and 3 months afterward.
• Be alert for adverse reactions and drug interactions.
• Monitor patient's hydration status if adverse GI reactions occur.
• Evaluate patient's and family's knowledge of drug therapy.

◎ Nursing diagnoses
• Infection related to presence of susceptible bacteria
• Risk for fluid volume deficit related to drug-induced adverse GI reactions
• Knowledge deficit related to drug therapy

▶ Planning and implementation
• Shake vial vigorously after reconstitution and before withdrawing dose. Store at room temperature after reconstitution, and use within 24 hours.
• Use 20G needle to administer drug. Divide 4-g dose (10 ml) into two 5-ml injections—give one in each buttock.

Patient teaching
• Inform patient that sexual partners must be treated.

☑ Evaluation
• Patient is free from infection.
• Patient maintains adequate hydration throughout therapy.
• Patient and family state understanding of drug therapy.

---

spironolactone
(spih-ron-uh-LAK-tohn)
Aldactone, Novo-Spiroton♦, Spiractin◊

Pharmacologic class: potassium-sparing diuretic
Therapeutic class: management of edema; antihypertensive; diagnosis of primary hyperaldosteronism; treatment of diuretic-induced hypokalemia
Pregnancy risk category: NR

How supplied

Tablets: 25 mg, 50 mg, 100 mg

Pharmacokinetics

Absorption: about 90% absorbed from GI tract.
Distribution: more than 90% plasma protein–bound.
Metabolism: metabolized rapidly and extensively to canrenone, its major active metabolite.
Excretion: canrenone and other metabolites excreted primarily in urine, minimally in feces. *Half-life:* 13 to 24 hours.

Route	Onset	Peak	Duration
P.O.	1-2 days	2-3 days	2-3 days

Pharmacodynamics

Chemical effect: antagonizes aldosterone in distal tubule.
Therapeutic effect: promotes water and sodium excretion and hinders potassium excretion, lowers blood pressure, and helps to diagnose primary hyperaldosteronism.

---

*Liquid form contains alcohol   **May contain tartrazine   ♦Canada   ◊Australia   †OTC

Indications and dosage

▶ **Edema.** *Adults:* 25 to 200 mg P.O. daily or in divided doses. *Children:* 3.3 mg/kg P.O. daily or in divided doses.
▶ **Hypertension.** *Adults:* 50 to 100 mg P.O. daily or in divided doses.
▶ **Diuretic-induced hypokalemia.** *Adults:* 25 to 100 mg P.O. daily when oral potassium supplements are contraindicated.
▶ **Detection of primary hyperaldosteronism.** *Adults:* 400 mg P.O. daily for 4 days (short test) or 3 to 4 weeks (long test). If hypokalemia and hypertension are corrected, presumptive diagnosis of primary hyperaldosteronism is made.
▶ **Management of primary hyperaldosteronism.** *Adults:* 100 to 400 mg P.O. daily.

Adverse reactions

CNS: headache, drowsiness, lethargy, confusion, ataxia.
GI: diarrhea, gastric bleeding, ulceration, cramping, gastritis, vomiting.
GU: transient elevation in BUN level, inability to maintain an erection, menstrual disturbances in women.
Metabolic: *hyperkalemia,* hyponatremia, mild acidosis.
Skin: urticaria, hirsutism, maculopapular eruptions.
Other: *agranulocytosis,* dehydration, gynecomastia, breast soreness, drug fever, *anaphylaxis.*

Interactions

Drug-drug. *ACE inhibitors, indomethacin, other potassium sparing diuretics, potassium supplements:* increased risk of hyperkalemia. Don't use together, especially in patients with renal impairment.
Aspirin: possible blocked diuretic effect of spironolactone. Watch for diminished spironolactone response.
Digoxin: may alter digoxin clearance, increasing risk of digoxin toxicity. Monitor digoxin levels.

Warfarin: decreased anticoagulant effect. Monitor PT and INR.
Drug-food. *Potassium-containing salt substitutes, potassium-rich foods (such as citrus fruits, tomatoes):* increased risk of hyperkalemia. Use low-potassium salt substitutes. Ingest high-potassium foods cautiously.

Contraindications and precautions

• Contraindicated in patients with anuria, acute or progressive renal insufficiency, or hyperkalemia.
• Use cautiously in patients with fluid or electrolyte imbalances, impaired kidney function, or hepatic disease, and in pregnant women.
• Safety of drug has not been established in breast-feeding women.

NURSING CONSIDERATIONS

Assessment
• Assess patient's condition before therapy and regularly thereafter. Maximum antihypertensive response may be delayed up to 2 weeks.
• Monitor serum electrolyte levels, fluid intake and output, weight, and blood pressure.
• Be alert for adverse reactions and drug interactions.
• Evaluate patient's and family's knowledge of drug therapy.

Nursing diagnoses
• Fluid volume excess related to presence of edema
• Altered urinary elimination related to diuretic therapy
• Knowledge deficit related to drug therapy

Planning and implementation
• Give drug with meals to enhance absorption.
• Protect drug from light.
• Inform laboratory that patient is taking spironolactone because it may interfere

with some laboratory tests that measure digoxin levels.

Patient teaching
• Warn patient to avoid excessive ingestion of potassium-rich foods, potassium-containing salt substitutes, and potassium supplements to prevent serious hyperkalemia.
• Tell patient to take drug with meals and, if possible, early in day to avoid interruption of sleep due to nocturia.

☑ **Evaluation**
• Patient shows no signs of edema.
• Patient demonstrates adjustment of lifestyle to deal with altered patterns of urinary elimination.
• Patient and family state understanding of drug therapy.

---

stanozolol
(STAN-oh-zoh-lol)
Winstrol

Pharmacologic class: anabolic steroid
Therapeutic class: angioedema prophylactic
Controlled substance schedule: III
Pregnancy risk category: X

How supplied
Tablets: 2 mg

Pharmacokinetics
Absorption: unknown.
Distribution: unknown.
Metabolism: metabolized in liver.
Excretion: unknown.

Route	Onset	Peak	Duration
P.O.	Unknown	Unknown	Unknown

Pharmacodynamics
Chemical effect: promotes tissue-building processes, reverses catabolism, and stimulates erythropoiesis.
Therapeutic effect: prevents or relieves angioedema.

Indications and dosage
▶ **Prevention of hereditary angioedema.** *Adults:* initially, 2 mg P.O. t.i.d. Dosage gradually reduced at 1- to 3-month intervals to dosage of 2 mg P.O. daily. *Children ages 6 to 12:* up to 2 mg P.O. daily. *Children under age 6:* 1 mg P.O. daily.
Note: Drug is used in children only during an acute attack.

Adverse reactions
CNS: excitation, insomnia, habituation, depression.
CV: edema.
GI: nausea, vomiting, constipation, diarrhea.
GU: bladder irritability, hypoestrogenic effects in women (flushing; diaphoresis; vaginitis, including itching, dryness, and burning; vaginal bleeding; nervousness; emotional lability; menstrual irregularities); excessive hormonal effects in men (prepubertal—premature epiphyseal closure, *acne,* priapism, *growth of body and facial hair,* phallic enlargement; postpubertal—testicular atrophy, oligospermia, decreased ejaculatory volume, impotence, gynecomastia, epididymitis).
Hematologic: elevated serum lipid levels, suppression of clotting factors.
Hepatic: reversible jaundice, peliosis hepatis, elevated liver enzyme levels, liver cell tumors, **hepatic necrosis.**
Other: androgenic effects in women (acne, edema, *weight gain, hirsutism,* hoarseness, clitoral enlargement, *decrease in breast size,* changes in libido, male-pattern baldness, *oily skin or hair*).

Interactions
Drug-drug. *Hepatotoxic drugs:* increased risk of hepatotoxicity. Monitor patient closely.
Insulin, oral antidiabetic agents: altered dosage requirements. Monitor blood glucose level in diabetic patients.
Oral anticoagulants: altered dosage requirements. Monitor PT and INR.

---

*Liquid form contains alcohol   **May contain tartrazine   ◆Canada   ◇ Australia   †OTC

Contraindications and precautions

• Contraindicated in patients with hypersensitivity to anabolic steroids; in males with breast cancer or prostate cancer; in nephrosis or nephrotic phase of nephritis; in females with carcinoma of breast and with hypercalcemia; and in pregnant or breast-feeding women.

• Use cautiously in patients with diabetes; cardiac, renal, or hepatic disease; epilepsy; or migraine or other conditions that may be aggravated by fluid retention.

Ⓐ Assessment

• Assess patient's condition before therapy and regularly thereafter.

• In children, X-rays of wrist bones should be taken before therapy to establish level of bone maturation. During treatment, bone maturation may proceed more rapidly than linear growth; ensure intermittent dosage and review X-ray results periodically to monitor bone maturation.

• Closely observe boys under age 7 for precocious development of male sexual characteristics.

• Know that semen evaluation is routinely performed every 3 to 4 months, especially in adolescent males.

• Periodically evaluate liver function. Watch for symptoms of jaundice; dosage adjustment may reverse it.

• Be alert for adverse reactions and drug interactions.

• Evaluate patient's and family's knowledge of drug therapy.

Ⓝ Nursing diagnoses

• Risk for injury related to potential for angioedema

• Body image disturbance related to adverse androgenic reactions

• Knowledge deficit related to drug therapy

Ⓟ Planning and implementation

• Avoid use in female patient of childbearing age until pregnancy is ruled out.

• Lower dosage in young women (2 mg b.i.d.) is recommended to avoid virilization. Watch for signs of virilization, which may be irreversible despite prompt discontinuation. Doctor must decide if benefits of therapy outweigh adverse effects.

• Administer drug before or with meals to minimize GI distress.

• Unless contraindicated, use with diet high in calories and protein. Give small, frequent feedings.

• Edema is generally controllable with sodium restriction or diuretics.

• Notify doctor if liver function test results are abnormal; therapy should be discontinued.

• Know that anabolic steroids may alter results of laboratory studies performed during therapy and for 2 to 3 weeks after therapy ends.

Patient teaching

• Instruct patient to take drug with food.

• Make sure patient understands importance of using an effective nonhormonal contraceptive during therapy.

• Advise female patient to wash after intercourse to decrease risk of vaginitis. Instruct her to wear cotton underwear.

• Tell female patient to report menstrual irregularities and to discontinue therapy until the cause has been determined.

Ⓔ Evaluation

• Patient does not develop angioedema.

• Patient states acceptance of body image changes caused by drug.

• Patient and family state understanding of drug therapy.

---

stavudine (2,3-didehydro-3-deoxythymidine, d4T)
(stay-VYOO-deen)
Zerit

Pharmacologic class: synthetic thymidine nucleoside analogue
Therapeutic class: antiviral
Pregnancy risk category: C

How supplied

Capsules: 15 mg, 20 mg, 30 mg, 40 mg
Powder for oral solution: 1 mg/ml

Pharmacokinetics

Absorption: rapidly absorbed with mean absolute bioavailability of 86.4%.
Distribution: distributed equally between RBCs and plasma; binds poorly to plasma proteins.
Metabolism: not extensively metabolized.
Excretion: renal elimination accounts for about 40% of overall clearance. *Half-life:* 1 to 2 hours.

Route	Onset	Peak	Duration
P.O.	Unknown	≤ 1hr	Unknown

Pharmacodynamics

Chemical effect: prevents replication of HIV by inhibiting enzyme reverse transcriptase.
Therapeutic effect: inhibits HIV growth.

Indications and dosage

▶ **Patients with advanced HIV infection who are intolerant or unresponsive to other antiviral therapies.** *Adults weighing 60 kg (132 lb) or more:* 40 mg P.O. q 12 hours. *Adults weighing below 60 kg:* 30 mg P.O. q 12 hours.

Adverse reactions

CNS: *asthenia, peripheral neuropathy, headache, malaise, insomnia, anxiety, depression, nervousness,* dizziness.
CV: chest pain.
EENT: conjunctivitis.
GI: *abdominal pain, diarrhea, nausea, vomiting, anorexia,* dyspepsia, constipation, weight loss.
Hematologic: *neutropenia, thrombocytopenia,* anemia.
Musculoskeletal: myalgia, *back pain, arthralgia.*
Respiratory: *dyspnea.*
Skin: *rash, diaphoresis, pruritus,* maculopapular rash.
Other: *hepatotoxicity, chills, fever.*

Interactions

Drug-drug. *Ketoconazole, ritonavir:* increased stavudine level. Monitor closely.
Myelosuppressants: additive myelosuppression. Avoid concomitant use.

Contraindications and precautions

• Contraindicated in patients with hypersensitivity to drug.
• Use cautiously in patients with renal impairment or history of peripheral neuropathy and in pregnant women.
• Safety of drug has not been established in children and in breast-feeding women.

NURSING CONSIDERATIONS

⚚ Assessment
• Assess patient's condition before therapy and regularly thereafter.
• Periodically monitor CBC and serum levels of creatinine, AST, ALT, and alkaline phosphatase, as ordered.
• Be alert for adverse reactions and drug interactions.
• Evaluate patient's and family's knowledge of drug therapy.

⚙ Nursing diagnoses
• Infection related to presence of HIV
• Sensory or perceptual alteration (peripheral) related to drug-induced peripheral neuropathy
• Knowledge deficit related to drug therapy

❯ Planning and implementation
• Know that peripheral neuropathy appears to be major dose-limiting adverse effect, that may or may not resolve after drug is discontinued.
• Be aware that dosage is calculated based on patient's weight.
Patient teaching
• Tell patient that drug may be taken without regard to meals.
• Advise patient that he cannot receive drug if he experienced peripheral neuropathy while receiving other nucleoside

analogues or if his treatment plan includes cytotoxic antineoplastic agents.
• Warn patient not to take any other drugs for HIV or AIDS (especially street drugs) unless doctor has approved them.
• Teach patient signs and symptoms of peripheral neuropathy—pain, burning, aching, weakness, or pins and needles in extremities—and tell him to report these immediately.

☑ **Evaluation**
• Patient's infection is controlled.
• Patient maintains normal peripheral neurologic function.
• Patient and family state understanding of drug therapy.

streptokinase
(strep-toh-KIGH-nayz)
Kabikinase, Streptase

Pharmacologic class: plasminogen activator
Therapeutic class: thrombolytic enzyme
Pregnancy risk category: C

How supplied

Injection: 100,000 IU, 250,000 IU, 600,000 IU, 750,000 IU, 1.5 million IU in vials for reconstitution

Pharmacokinetics

Absorption: not applicable.
Distribution: unknown.
Metabolism: insignificant.
Excretion: removed from circulation by antibodies and reticuloendothelial system. *Half-life:* first phase, 18 minutes; second phase, 83 minutes.

Route	Onset	Peak	Duration
I.V.	Immediate	20 min-2 hr	About 4 hr

Pharmacodynamics

Chemical effect: activates plasminogen in two steps: plasminogen and streptokinase form a complex that exposes plasminogen-activating site; plasminogen is then converted to plasmin by cleavage of peptide bond.
Therapeutic effect: dissolves blood clots.

Indications and dosage

▶ **Arteriovenous cannula occlusion.** *Adults:* 250,000 IU in 2 ml I.V. solution by I.V. pump infusion into each occluded limb of cannula over 25 to 35 minutes. Clamp off cannula for 2 hours. Then aspirate contents of cannula; flush with saline solution and reconnect.
▶ **Venous thrombosis, pulmonary embolism, arterial thrombosis and embolism.** *Adults:* loading dose is 250,000 IU I.V. infusion over 30 minutes. Sustaining dose is 100,000 IU/hour I.V. infusion for 72 hours for deep vein thrombosis and 100,000 IU/hour over 24 hours by I.V. infusion pump for pulmonary embolism.
▶ **Lysis of coronary artery thrombi after acute MI.** *Adults:* 140,000 units administered as loading dose, followed by maintenance infusion. Loading dose is 20,000 IU by coronary catheter, followed by infusion of maintenance dose of 2,000 IU/minute for 60 minutes. Alternatively, may be administered as an I.V. infusion. Usual adult dose is 1.5 million units infused over 60 minutes.

Adverse reactions

CNS: polyradiculoneuropathy, headache.
CV: *hypotension,* vasculitis, *reperfusion arrhythmias.*
EENT: periorbital edema.
GI: nausea.
Hematologic: *bleeding.*
Respiratory: minor breathing difficulty, *bronchospasm, pulmonary edema.*
Skin: urticaria, pruritus, flushing.
Other: phlebitis at injection site, hypersensitivity reactions *(anaphylaxis), delayed hypersensitivity reactions* (interstitial nephritis, vasculitis, serum sickness–like reactions), musculoskeletal pain, *angioedema,* fever.

Interactions

Drug-drug. *Anticoagulants:* increased risk of bleeding. Monitor patient closely.
Antifibrinolytic agents: streptokinase activity is inhibited and reversed by antifibrinolytic agents such as aminocaproic acid. Use only when indicated during streptokinase therapy.
Aspirin, dipyridamole, drugs affecting platelet activity, indomethacin, phenylbutazone: increased risk of bleeding. Monitor patients closely. Combined therapy with low-dose aspirin (162.5 mg) or dipyridamole has improved acute and long-term results.

Contraindications and precautions

• Contraindicated in patients with ulcerative wounds, active internal bleeding, recent CVA, recent trauma with possible internal injuries, visceral or intracranial malignant neoplasms, ulcerative colitis, diverticulitis, severe hypertension, acute or chronic hepatic or renal insufficiency, uncontrolled hypocoagulation, chronic pulmonary disease with cavitation, subacute bacterial endocarditis or rheumatic valvular disease, or recent cerebral embolism, thrombosis, or hemorrhage.
• Also contraindicated within 10 days after intra-arterial diagnostic procedure or any surgery, including liver or kidney biopsy, lumbar puncture, thoracentesis, paracentesis, or extensive or multiple cutdowns.
• I.M. injections and other invasive procedures are contraindicated during streptokinase therapy.
• Use cautiously when treating arterial embolism that originates from left side of heart because of danger of cerebral infarction. Also use cautiously in pregnant women.
• Safety of drug has not been established in children and in breast-feeding women.

NURSING CONSIDERATIONS

⏚ Assessment

• Assess patient's condition before therapy and regularly thereafter.
• Before initiating therapy, draw blood to determine PTT and PT. Rate of I.V. infusion depends on thrombin time and streptokinase resistance. Then repeat studies often, as ordered, and keep laboratory flow sheet on patient's chart to monitor PTT, PT, and hemoglobin and hematocrit levels.
• Monitor patient for excessive bleeding every 15 minutes for first hour, every 30 minutes for second through eighth hours, then once every shift.
• Monitor pulse rates, color, and sensation of extremities every hour.
• Be alert for adverse reactions and drug interactions.
• Evaluate patient's and family's knowledge of drug therapy.

⊞ Nursing diagnoses

• Altered cardiopulmonary tissue perfusion related to condition
• Risk for fluid volume deficit related to potential for bleeding
• Knowledge deficit related to drug therapy

❯ Planning and implementation

• Know that only doctors with wide experience in thrombotic disease management where clinical and laboratory monitoring can be performed should use streptokinase.
• Before using streptokinase to clear an occluded arteriovenous cannula, try flushing with heparinized NaCl solution, as ordered.
• To check for hypersensitivity reactions, give 100 IU intradermally, as ordered; wheal and flare response within 20 minutes means patient is probably allergic. Monitor vital signs frequently.
• Be aware that if patient has had either recent streptococcal infection or recent

---

treatment with streptokinase, higher loading dose may be necessary.
● Reconstitute each vial with 5 ml of 0.9% NaCl solution for injection. Further dilute to 45 ml. Don't shake; roll gently to mix. Some flocculation may be present; discard if large amounts appear. Filter solution with 0.8-micron or larger filter. Use within 24 hours. Store powder at room temperature and refrigerate after reconstitution.
● If bleeding occurs, stop therapy and notify doctor. Pretreatment with heparin or drugs affecting platelets causes high risk of bleeding but may improve long-term results.
● Keep aminocaproic acid available to treat bleeding, and corticosteroids to treat allergic reactions.
● Have typed and crossmatched packed RBCs and whole blood ready to treat possible hemorrhage.
● Maintain involved extremity in straight alignment to prevent bleeding from infusion site.
● Avoid unnecessary handling of patient; pad side rails. Bruising is more likely during therapy.
● Keep venipuncture sites to minimum; use pressure dressing on puncture sites for at least 15 minutes.
● Notify doctor immediately if hypersensitivity occurs. Antihistamines or corticosteroids may be used to treat mild reactions. If severe reaction occurs, infusion should be stopped immediately and doctor notified.
● Heparin by continuous infusion is usually started within 1 hour after stopping streptokinase. Use infusion pump to administer heparin.
● Keep in mind that thrombolytic therapy in patient with acute MI may decrease infarct size, improve ventricular function, and decrease incidence of heart failure. Drug must be administered within 6 hours of onset of symptoms for optimal effect.
Patient teaching
● Tell patient to report oozing, bleeding, or signs of hypersensitivity immediately.

☑ **Evaluation**
● Patient responds well to therapy.
● Patient maintains adequate fluid balance.
● Patient and family state understanding of drug therapy.

streptomycin sulfate
(strep-toh-MIGH-sin SUL-fayt)

Pharmacologic class: aminoglycoside
Therapeutic class: antibiotic
Pregnancy risk category: D

How supplied
Injection: 400 mg/ml, 1-g/2.5 ml ampules

Pharmacokinetics
Absorption: unknown after I.M. administration.
Distribution: wide distribution although CSF penetration is low; 36% protein-bound.
Metabolism: none.
Excretion: mainly in urine; less so in bile. *Half-life:* 2 to 3 hours.

Route	Onset	Peak	Duration
I.M.	Unknown	1-2 hr	Unknown

Pharmacodynamics
Chemical effect: inhibits protein synthesis by binding directly to 30S ribosomal subunit. Drug is generally bactericidal.
Therapeutic effect: kills bacteria. Spectrum of activity includes many aerobic gram-negative organisms and some aerobic gram-positive organisms. Drug is also active against *Brucella* and *Mycobacterium.*

Indications and dosage
▶ **Streptococcal endocarditis.** *Adults:* 1 g I.M. q 12 hours for 1 week, then 500 mg q 12 hours for 1 week, given with penicillin. Patients over age 60

Reactions may be *common*, uncommon, *life-threatening*, or COMMON AND LIFE-THREATENING.

should receive 500 mg I.M. q 12 hours
for entire 2 weeks.
▶ **Primary and adjunct treatment in
tuberculosis.** *Adults:* 1 g or 15 mg/kg
I.M. daily for 2 to 3 months, then 1 g two
or three times weekly. *Children:* 20 to
40 mg/kg I.M. daily in divided doses injected deeply into large muscle mass.
Given concurrently with other antitubercular agents but *not* with capreomycin.
Continued until sputum specimen becomes negative.
▶ **Enterococcal endocarditis.** *Adults:*
1 g I.M. q 12 hours for 2 weeks, then
500 mg q 12 hours for 4 weeks, given
with penicillin.
▶ **Tularemia.** *Adults:* 1 to 2 g I.M. daily
in divided doses injected deep into upper
outer quadrant of buttocks. Continued
until patient is afebrile for 5 to 7 days.
▶ **Dosage in renal failure.** *Adults and
children:* initial dosage same for normal
renal function. Subsequent doses and frequency determined by renal function
study results and blood serum concentrations.

Adverse reactions

CNS: *neuromuscular blockade.*
EENT: *ototoxicity (tinnitus, vertigo,
hearing loss).*
GI: vomiting, nausea.
GU: some nephrotoxicity (not as much
as other aminoglycosides).
Hematologic: eosinophilia, *leukopenia,
thrombocytopenia.*
Respiratory: *apnea.*
Skin: *exfoliative dermatitis.*
Other: *hypersensitivity reactions* (rash,
fever, urticaria, angioedema); *anaphy-
laxis.*

Interactions

Drug-drug. *Cephalosporins:* increased
nephrotoxicity. Use together cautiously.
Dimenhydrinate: may mask symptoms of
streptomycin-induced ototoxicity. Use together cautiously.

*General anesthetics, neuromuscular
blockers:* may potentiate neuromuscular
blockade. Monitor patient.
I.V. loop diuretics (such as furosemide):
increased ototoxicity. Use with caution.
*Other aminoglycosides, acyclovir, am-
photericin B, cisplatin, methoxyflurane,
vancomycin:* increased nephrotoxicity.
Monitor patient.

Contraindications and precautions

• Contraindicated in patients with
labyrinthine disease or hypersensitivity to
drug or other aminoglycosides and in
pregnant women. Never give I.V.
• Use cautiously in patients with impaired kidney function or neuromuscular
disorders, in elderly patients, and in
breast-feeding women.

NURSING CONSIDERATIONS

⚕ Assessment
• Assess patient's infection before therapy and regularly thereafter.
• Obtain specimen for culture and sensitivity tests before first dose except when
treating tuberculosis. Therapy may begin
pending results.
• Obtain blood for peak streptomycin level 1 to 2 hours after I.M. injection; for
trough levels, draw blood just before next
dose. Don't use heparinized tube because
heparin is incompatible with aminoglycosides.
• Evaluate patient's hearing before beginning therapy, during therapy, and 6
months after therapy.
• Be alert for adverse reactions and drug
interactions.
• Evaluate patient's and family's knowledge of drug therapy.

⊞ Nursing diagnoses
• Infection related to presence of susceptible bacteria
• Sensory or perceptual alterations (auditory) related to drug-induced adverse reactions

• Knowledge deficit related to drug therapy

❯ Planning and implementation
• Protect hands when preparing because drug is irritating.
• Inject drug deeply into upper outer quadrant of buttocks. Rotate injection sites.
• Encourage adequate fluid intake; patient should be well hydrated while taking drug to minimize chemical irritation of renal tubules.
• In primary treatment of tuberculosis, drug is discontinued when sputum becomes negative.
Patient teaching
• Warn patient that injection may be painful.
• Emphasize need to drink at least 2,000 ml per day (if not contraindicated) during therapy.
• Instruct patient to report hearing loss, roaring noises, or fullness in ears immediately.

☑ Evaluation
• Patient is free from infection.
• Patient's auditory function remains normal.
• Patient and family state understanding of drug therapy.

---

streptozocin
(strep-tuh-ZOH-sin)
Zanosar

Pharmacologic class: antibiotic antineoplastic nitrosourea (cell cycle–phase nonspecific)
Therapeutic class: antineoplastic
Pregnancy risk category: C

How supplied
Injection: 1-g vials

Pharmacokinetics
Absorption: not applicable.

Distribution: distributed mainly in liver, kidneys, intestines, and pancreas. Drug does not cross blood-brain barrier; however, its metabolites achieve concentrations in CSF equivalent to concentration in plasma.
Metabolism: extensively metabolized in liver and kidneys.
Excretion: excreted primarily in urine, minimally in expired air. *Half-life:* first phase, 5 minutes; second phase, 35 to 40 minutes.

Route	Onset	Peak	Duration
I.V.	Unknown	Unknown	Unknown

Pharmacodynamics
Chemical effect: unknown; probably cross-links strands of cellular DNA and interferes with RNA transcription, causing an imbalance of growth that leads to cell death.
Therapeutic effect: kills selected cancer cells.

Indications and dosage
▶ **Metastatic islet cell carcinoma of pancreas.** *Adults and children:* 500 mg/ m^2 I.V. for 5 consecutive days q 6 weeks until maximum benefit or toxicity is observed. Alternatively, 1,000 mg/m^2 at weekly intervals for first 2 weeks. Not to exceed single dose of 1,500 mg/m^2. Because of renal toxicity, drug should only be used in patients with symptomatic or progressive metastatic disease.

Adverse reactions
CNS: confusion, lethargy, depression.
GI: *nausea, vomiting,* diarrhea.
GU: *renal toxicity* (evidenced by azotemia, glycosuria, and renal tubular acidosis), mild proteinuria.
Hematologic: *anemia, leukopenia, thrombocytopenia.*
Hepatic: *elevated liver enzyme levels, liver dysfunction.*
Metabolic: hyperglycemia, hypoglycemia, diabetes mellitus.

Reactions may be *common,* uncommon, *life-threatening,* or COMMON AND LIFE-THREATENING.

Interactions

Drug-drug. *Doxorubicin:* prolonged elimination half-life of doxorubicin. Dose of doxorubicin should be reduced. *Other potentially nephrotoxic drugs (such as aminoglycosides):* increased risk of nephrotoxicity. Use cautiously. *Phenytoin:* may decrease effectiveness of streptozocin in patients with pancreatic cancer. Monitor patient.

Contraindications and precautions

• No known contraindications.
• Drug is not recommended for use in pregnant or breast-feeding women.
• Use cautiously in patients with renal disease.

NURSING CONSIDERATIONS

⚡ Assessment
• Assess patient's condition before therapy and regularly thereafter.
• Obtain kidney function tests before therapy, and monitor after each course of therapy, as ordered. Nephrotoxicity resulting from streptozocin therapy is dose-related and cumulative. Urinalysis; BUN, creatinine, and serum electrolyte levels; and creatinine clearance should be obtained at least weekly during drug administration. Weekly monitoring should continue for 4 weeks after each course.
• Monitor CBC and liver function studies at least weekly, as ordered.
• Be alert for adverse reactions and drug interactions.
• Evaluate patient's and family's knowledge of drug therapy.

⊞ Nursing diagnoses
• Altered health maintenance related to presence of neoplastic disease
• Altered protection related to adverse nephrotoxic reactions
• Knowledge deficit related to drug therapy

⊠ Planning and implementation
• Follow institutional policy to reduce risks. Preparation and administration of parenteral form are associated with carcinogenic, mutagenic, and teratogenic risks for personnel.
• Reconstitute streptozocin powder with 9.5 ml of D_5W or 0.9% NaCl injection. This produces pale gold solution. Drug may be further diluted with D_5W or 0.9% NaCl injection. Infuse over at least 15 minutes to minimize risk of phlebitis.
• If extravasation occurs, stop infusion immediately and notify doctor.
• Use within 12 hours of reconstitution. Product lacks preservatives and is not intended as multiple-dose vial.
• To minimize risk of nephrotoxicity, ensure adequate hydration using oral or parenteral fluids, as ordered.
• Monitor urine protein and glucose levels each shift. Mild proteinuria is one of first signs of nephrotoxicity; notify doctor if this occurs. Dosage reduction may be necessary.
• Make sure patient is being treated with an antiemetic. Nausea and vomiting occur in most patients.
• Store unopened and unreconstituted vials in refrigerator.
Patient teaching
• Warn patient to watch for signs of infection (fever, sore throat, fatigue) and bleeding (easy bruising, nosebleeds, bleeding gums, melena). Have patient take temperature daily.
• Review other potential adverse reactions and explain how to prevent or decrease their severity and when to notify doctor.

☑ Evaluation
• Patient responds well to therapy.
• Patient maintains adequate kidney function.
• Patient and family state understanding of drug therapy.

---

strontium-89 chloride
(STRON-tee-um 89 KLOR-ighd)
Metastron

Pharmacologic class: radioisotope
Therapeutic class: radioisotope for
metastatic bone pain
Pregnancy risk category: D

How supplied

Injection: 4 millicuries (mCi)/10 ml

Pharmacokinetics

Absorption: not applicable.
Distribution: rapidly cleared from blood
and selectively localized in bone mineral.
Uptake of strontium-89 by bone occurs
preferentially in sites of active osteogenesis; thus, primary bone tumors and areas
of metastatic involvement (blastic lesions) can accumulate significantly
greater concentrations of strontium-89
than surrounding normal bone.
Metabolism: decays by beta emission
with physical half-life of 50½ days.
Excretion: about 66% excreted in urine
and 33% in feces in patients with bone
metastases. Urine excretion, which is
higher in patients without bone lesions, is
greatest in first 2 days after injection.

Route	Onset	Peak	Duration
I.V.	Within hr	7-20 days	4-12 mo

Pharmacodynamics

Chemical effect: acts as calcium analogue that is actively taken up by bone,
particularly in areas of active osteogenesis
such as metastatic bone tumors. Drug locally irradiates tissue with beta radiation.
Therapeutic effect: relief from bone pain.

Indications and dosage

▶ **Relief from bone pain in patients with
painful metastatic lesions.** *Adults:* 4 mCi
by slow I.V. injection over 1 to 2 minutes.

Adverse reactions

CV: cutaneous flushing (with rapid injection).
Hematologic: *bone marrow suppression.*
Musculoskeletal: transient increase in
bone pain ("flare" reaction).

Interactions

Drug-drug. *Calcium supplements:* decreased effectiveness of strontium-89.
Discontinue calcium supplements about 2
weeks before strontium-89 therapy.
Cytotoxic agents: additive bone marrow
suppression. Monitor patient closely.

Contraindications and precautions

• No known contraindications.
• Drug is not recommended for use in
pregnant or breast-feeding women.
• Use cautiously in patients with platelet
counts below 60,000/mm^3 or WBC
counts below 2,400/mm^3.
• Safety of drug has not been established
in children.

NURSING CONSIDERATIONS

⚐ Assessment
• Obtain history of patient's bone pain
before therapy.
• Frequently assess degree of pain relief
after administration. Pain relief usually
occurs after 2 to 3 weeks. In clinical trials, more than 75% of patients received
substantial relief, allowing reduction or
elimination of opioid analgesics.
• Monitor CBC, as ordered.
• Be alert for adverse reactions and drug
interactions.
• Evaluate patient's and family's knowledge of drug therapy.

⚐ Nursing diagnoses
• Pain related to underlying condition
• Altered protection related to drug-
induced immunosuppression
• Knowledge deficit related to drug
therapy

⟩⟩ Planning and implementation
• Follow institutional safety measures to minimize radiation exposure. Urinary excretion of radiation is greatest during first 2 days after administration.
• Consider placing an indwelling urinary catheter in incontinent patient to minimize contamination of environment with radiation.
• Because drug is potential carcinogen, know that use should be restricted to patients with documented metastatic bone cancer.
• Because of delayed onset of pain relief, drug should not be used in patient with short life expectancy.
• Be aware that during first week, transient increase in pain may necessitate dosage increase in concomitantly administered analgesics.
Patient teaching
• Teach patient proper radiation precautions; during first few days of treatment, patient should flush toilet twice, wipe spilled urine with tissue that is subsequently flushed, and immediately launder linens soiled with blood or urine. Make sure patient understands that drug has low level of radioactivity and that he will pose no risk to family members.
• Advise female patient of childbearing age to avoid becoming pregnant.

☑ Evaluation
• Patient is free from pain.
• Patient does not develop serious complications from drug-induced immunosuppression.
• Patient and family state understanding of drug therapy.

succimer
(SUK-sih-mer)
Chemet

Pharmacologic class: heavy metal
Therapeutic class: chelating agent
Pregnancy risk category: C

How supplied
Capsules: 100 mg

Pharmacokinetics
Absorption: rapid but variable.
Distribution: unknown.
Metabolism: rapid and extensive.
Excretion: 39% excreted in feces as nonabsorbed drug; remainder is excreted primarily in urine. *Half-life:* 48 hours.

Route	Onset	Peak	Duration
P.O.	Unknown	1-2 hr	Unknown

Pharmacodynamics
Chemical effect: forms water-soluble complexes with lead and increases its excretion in urine.
Therapeutic effect: relieves signs and symptoms of lead poisoning.

Indications and dosage
▶ **Lead poisoning in children with blood lead levels above 45 mcg/dl.**
Children: 10 mg/kg or 350 mg/m^2 q 8 hours for 5 days. Dosage rounded to nearest 100 mg (see chart). Then, frequency is decreased to q 12 hours for an additional 2 weeks.

Weight (kg)	Dose (mg)
8 to 15	100
16 to 23	200
24 to 34	300
35 to 44	400
> 45	500

Adverse reactions
CNS: *drowsiness, dizziness, sensory motor neuropathy, sleepiness, paresthesias, headache.*
CV: *arrhythmias.*
EENT: plugged ears, cloudy film in eyes, otitis media, watery eyes, sore throat, rhinorrhea, nasal congestion.
GI: *nausea, vomiting, diarrhea, loss of appetite, abdominal cramps, hemorrhoidal symptoms, metallic taste in mouth, loose stools.*

GU: decreased urination, difficult urination, proteinuria.
Hematologic: increased platelet count, intermittent eosinophilia.
Hepatic: *elevated serum AST, ALT, alkaline phosphatase, or cholesterol level.*
Musculoskeletal: *leg, kneecap, back, stomach, rib, or flank pain.*
Respiratory: cough, head cold.
Skin: papular rash, herpetic rash, mucocutaneous eruptions, pruritus.
Other: *flulike symptoms;* candidiasis.

Interactions

None reported.

Contraindications and precautions

• Contraindicated in patients with hypersensitivity to drug.
• Use cautiously in patients with compromised kidney function.
• Drug is not indicated for use in pregnant or breast-feeding women.

NURSING CONSIDERATIONS

Assessment
• Assess child's condition before therapy and regularly thereafter.
• Measure severity by initial blood lead level and by rate and degree of rebound of blood lead level. Severity should be used as guide for more frequent blood lead monitoring.
• Monitor serum transaminase level before and at least weekly during therapy, as ordered. Transient, mild elevations of serum transaminase level have been observed. Patient with history of hepatic disease should be monitored more closely.
• Monitor patient at least once weekly for rebound blood lead levels, as ordered. Elevated blood lead levels and associated symptoms may return rapidly after drug is discontinued because of redistribution of lead from bone to soft tissues and blood.
• Be alert for adverse reactions.
• Monitor patient's hydration status if adverse GI reactions occur.

• Evaluate parents' knowledge of drug therapy.

Nursing diagnoses
• Altered health maintenance related to presence of lead poisoning
• Risk for fluid volume deficit related to drug-induced adverse GI reactions
• Knowledge deficit related to drug therapy

Planning and implementation
• Be aware that course of treatment lasts 19 days. Repeated courses may be necessary if indicated by weekly monitoring of blood lead levels.
• Know that a minimum of 2 weeks between courses is recommended unless high blood lead level indicates need for immediate therapy.
• Know that false-positive results for ketones in urine using nitroprusside reagents (Ketostix) and falsely decreased levels of serum uric acid and CK have been reported.
• Know that concurrent administration of succimer with other chelating agents is not recommended. Patient who has received edetate calcium disodium with or without dimercaprol may use succimer as subsequent therapy after 4-week interval.
Patient teaching
• Tell parents of child who cannot swallow capsules to open it and sprinkle contents on small amount of soft food. Alternatively, medicated beads from capsule may be poured on spoon; follow with flavored beverage such as a fruit drink.
• Assist parents with identifying and removing sources of lead in child's environment. Chelation therapy is not a substitute for preventing further exposure.
• Tell parents to consult doctor if rash occurs. Consider possibility of allergic or other mucocutaneous reactions each time drug is used.

Evaluation
• Patient responds well to therapy.

Reactions may be *common*, uncommon, *life-threatening*, or COMMON AND LIFE-THREATENING.

• Patient maintains adequate hydration.
• Parents state understanding of drug therapy.

succinylcholine chloride (suxamethonium chloride)

(SUK-seh-nil-KOH-leen KLOR-ighd)

Anectine, Anectine Flo-Pack, Quelicin, Scoline◇, Sucostrin

Pharmacologic class: depolarizing neuromuscular blocker
Therapeutic class: skeletal muscle relaxant
Pregnancy risk category: C

How supplied

Injection: 20 mg/ml, 50 mg/ml, 100 mg/ml; 100 mg/vial, 500 mg/vial, 1 g/vial

Pharmacokinetics

Absorption: unknown after I.M. administration.
Distribution: distributed in extracellular fluid and rapidly reaches its site of action.
Metabolism: occurs rapidly by plasma pseudocholinesterase.
Excretion: about 10% excreted unchanged in urine.

Route	Onset	Peak	Duration
I.M.	2-3 min	Unknown	10-30 min
I.V.	0.5-1 min	1-2 min	4-10 min

Pharmacodynamics

Chemical effect: prolongs depolarization of muscle end plate.
Therapeutic effect: relaxes skeletal muscles.

Indications and dosage

▶ **Adjunct to anesthesia to induce skeletal muscle relaxation; to facilitate intubation and assist with mechanical ventilation or orthopedic manipulations (drug of choice); to lessen muscle contractions in pharmacologically or** **electrically induced seizures.** Dosage depends on anesthetic used, individual needs, and response. *Adults:* 0.6 mg/kg I.V., then 2.5 mg/minute, p.r.n., or 2.5 mg/kg I.M. up to maximum of 150 mg I.M. in deltoid muscle. *Children:* 1 to 2 mg/kg I.M. or I.V. Maximum I.M. dosage is 150 mg. (Children may be less sensitive to succinylcholine than adults.)

Adverse reactions

CV: *bradycardia,* tachycardia, hypertension, hypotension, *arrhythmias,* flushing, *cardiac arrest.*
EENT: increased intraocular pressure.
Musculoskeletal: muscle fasciculation, *postoperative muscle pain,* myoglobinemia.
Respiratory: *prolonged respiratory depression, apnea, bronchoconstriction.*
Other: *malignant hyperthermia,* excessive salivation, allergic or idiosyncratic hypersensitivity reactions *(anaphylaxis).*

Interactions

Drug-drug. *Aminoglycoside antibiotics (including amikacin, gentamicin, kanamycin, neomycin, streptomycin); cholinesterase inhibitors (such as echothiophate, edrophonium, neostigmine, physostigmine, or pyridostigmine); general anesthetics (such as enflurane, halothane, isoflurane); polymyxin antibiotics (colistin, polymyxin B sulfate):* potentiated neuromuscular blockade, leading to increased skeletal muscle relaxation and potentiation of effect. Use cautiously during surgical and postoperative periods.
Cardiac glycosides: may cause arrhythmias. Use together cautiously.
Cyclophosphamide, lithium, MAO inhibitors: prolonged apnea. Monitor patient closely.
Methotrimeprazine, opioid analgesics: potentiated neuromuscular blockade, leading to increased skeletal muscle relaxation and, possibly, respiratory paralysis. Use with extreme caution.
Parenteral magnesium sulfate: potentiated neuromuscular blockade, increased

skeletal muscle relaxation and, possibly, respiratory paralysis. Use with caution, preferably with reduced doses.

Contraindications and precautions

• Contraindicated in patients with abnormally low plasma pseudocholinesterase level, angle-closure glaucoma, malignant hyperthermia, penetrating eye injuries, or hypersensitivity to drug.
• Use cautiously in elderly or debilitated patients; in patients receiving quinidine or cardiac glycoside therapy; in those with severe burns or trauma, electrolyte imbalances, hyperkalemia, paraplegia, spinal neuraxis injury, CVA, degenerative or dystrophic neuromuscular disease, myasthenia gravis, myasthenic syndrome of lung cancer or bronchogenic carcinoma, dehydration, thyroid disorders, collagen diseases, porphyria, fractures, muscle spasms, eye surgery, pheochromocytoma, respiratory depression, or hepatic, renal, or pulmonary impairment. Also, use large doses cautiously in women undergoing cesarean delivery and in breast-feeding women.

NURSING CONSIDERATIONS

⬛ Assessment

• Assess patient's condition before therapy and regularly thereafter.
• Monitor baseline electrolyte determinations and vital signs (check respiratory rate every 5 to 10 minutes during infusion).
• Monitor respiratory rate closely until patient is fully recovered from neuromuscular blockade, as evidenced by tests of muscle strength (hand grip, head lift, and ability to cough).
• Be alert for adverse reactions and drug interactions.
• Evaluate patient's and family's knowledge of drug therapy.

⬛ Nursing diagnoses

• Altered health maintenance related to underlying condition

• Ineffective breathing pattern related to drug's effect on respiratory muscles
• Knowledge deficit related to drug therapy

⬛ Planning and implementation

• Be aware that drug should be used only by personnel skilled in airway management.
• Know that succinylcholine is drug of choice for short procedures (less than 3 minutes) and for orthopedic manipulations; use caution in fractures or dislocations.
• Administer sedatives or general anesthetics before neuromuscular blockers, as ordered. Neuromuscular blockers do not obtund consciousness or alter pain threshold.
• Keep airway clear. Have emergency respiratory support equipment immediately available.
I.V. use: To evaluate patient's ability to metabolize succinylcholine, give test dose (10 mg I.M. or I.V.) after patient has been anesthetized. Normal response (no respiratory depression or transient depression for up to 5 minutes) indicates drug may be given. Do not give subsequent doses if patient develops respiratory paralysis sufficient to permit endotracheal intubation. (Recovery within 30 to 60 minutes.)
I.M. use: Give deep I.M., preferably high into deltoid muscle.
• Store injectable form in refrigerator. Store powder form at room temperature in tightly closed container. Use immediately after reconstitution. Do not mix with alkaline solutions (thiopental sodium, sodium bicarbonate, or barbiturates).
• Administer analgesics, as ordered.
• Know that reversing agents should not be used. Unlike nondepolarizing agents, neostigmine or edrophonium may worsen neuromuscular blockade.
• Know that repeated or continuous infusions of succinylcholine are not advised; they may reduce response or prolong muscle relaxation and apnea.

Reactions may be *common*, uncommon, *life-threatening*, or COMMON AND LIFE-THREATENING.

Patient teaching
• Explain all events and happenings to patient because he can still hear.
• Reassure patient that he is being monitored at all times.
• Inform him that postoperative stiffness is normal and will soon subside.

☑ **Evaluation**
• Patient responds well to therapy.
• Patient maintains adequate respiratory patterns with mechanical assistance.
• Patient and family state understanding of drug therapy.

sucralfate
(SOO-krahl-fayt)
Carafate, SCF◇, Sulcrate♦

Pharmacologic class: pepsin inhibitor
Therapeutic class: antiulcer agent
Pregnancy risk category: B

How supplied
Tablets: 1 g
Suspension: 500 mg/5 ml

Pharmacokinetics
Absorption: only about 3% to 5% absorbed from GI tract.
Distribution: sucralfate acts locally, at ulcer site. Absorbed drug is distributed to many body tissues.
Metabolism: none.
Excretion: about 90% excreted in feces; absorbed drug excreted unchanged in urine.

Route	Onset	Peak	Duration
P.O.	Unknown	≤6 hr	Unknown

Pharmacodynamics
Chemical effect: unknown; probably adheres to and protects ulcer's surface by forming barrier.
Therapeutic effect: aids in duodenal ulcer healing.

Indications and dosage
▶ **Short-term (up to 8 weeks) treatment of duodenal ulcer.** *Adults:* 1 g P.O. q.i.d. 1 hour before meals and h.s.
▶ **Maintenance therapy for duodenal ulcer.** *Adults:* 1 g P.O. b.i.d.

Adverse reactions
CNS: dizziness, sleepiness, headache, vertigo.
GI: constipation, nausea, gastric discomfort, diarrhea, bezoar formation, vomiting, flatulence, dry mouth, indigestion.
Musculoskeletal: back pain.
Skin: rash, pruritus.

Interactions
Drug-drug. *Antacids:* may decrease binding of drug to gastroduodenal mucosa, impairing effectiveness. Don't administer within 30 minutes of each other. *Cimetidine, digoxin, norfloxacin, phenytoin, ranitidine, tetracycline, theophylline, quinolones:* decreased absorption. Separate administration times by at least 2 hours.

Contraindications and precautions
• No known contraindications.
• Use with caution in patients with chronic renal failure and in pregnant or breast-feeding women.
• Safety of drug has not been established in children.

NURSING CONSIDERATIONS
☑ **Assessment**
• Assess patient's ulcer before therapy and regularly thereafter.
• Be alert for adverse reactions and drug interactions.
• Monitor for severe, persistent constipation.
• Evaluate patient's and family's knowledge of drug therapy.

⊕ **Nursing diagnoses**
• Altered tissue integrity related to presence of duodenal ulcer

• Constipation related to drug-induced adverse GI reactions
• Knowledge deficit related to drug therapy

⟩ **Planning and implementation**
• Administer drug on an empty stomach for best results.
Patient teaching
• Instruct patient to take drug 1 hour before each meal and at bedtime.
• Tell patient to continue on prescribed regimen to ensure complete healing. Pain and ulcerative symptoms may subside within first few weeks of therapy.
• Urge patient to avoid cigarette smoking because it may increase gastric acid secretion and worsen disease.

☑ **Evaluation**
• Patient's ulcer pain is gone.
• Patient maintains normal bowel elimination patterns.
• Patient and family state understanding of drug therapy.

---

sufentanil citrate
(soo-FEN-tih-nil SIGH-trayt)
Sufenta

Pharmacologic class: opioid
Therapeutic class: analgesic, adjunct to anesthesia, anesthetic
Controlled substance schedule: II
Pregnancy risk category: C

How supplied
Injection: 50 mcg/ml

Pharmacokinetics
Absorption: not applicable.
Distribution: highly protein-bound and redistributed rapidly.
Metabolism: unknown, although appears to be metabolized mainly in liver and small intestine.

Excretion: drug and its metabolites excreted primarily in urine. *Half-life:* about 2½ hours.

Route	Onset	Peak	Duration
I.V.	1-2 min	1-2 min	0.7-5 min

Pharmacodynamics
Chemical effect: binds with opioid receptors in CNS, altering perception of and emotional response to pain through unknown mechanism.
Therapeutic effect: relieves pain and promotes loss of consciousness.

Indications and dosage
▶ **Adjunct to general anesthetic.**
Adults: 1 to 8 mcg/kg I.V. administered with nitrous oxide and oxygen.
▶ **As primary anesthetic.** *Adults:* 8 to 30 mcg/kg I.V. administered with 100% oxygen and muscle relaxant.

Adverse reactions
CNS: chills, somnolence.
CV: *hypotension,* hypertension, ***bradycardia,*** tachycardia, ***arrhythmias.***
GI: nausea, vomiting.
Musculoskeletal: intraoperative muscle movement.
Respiratory: *chest wall rigidity, apnea, bronchospasm.*
Skin: *pruritus,* erythema.

Interactions
Drug-drug. *CNS depressants:* additive effects. Use together cautiously.
Drug-lifestyle. *Alcohol use:* additive effects. Use together cautiously.

Contraindications and precautions
• Contraindicated in patients with hypersensitivity to drug.
• Drug is not recommended for prolonged use or use of high doses at term in pregnant women.
• Use with extreme caution in patients with head injury; pulmonary, hepatic, or renal disease; or decreased respiratory reserve and in elderly or debilitated patients.

• Safety of drug has not been established in breast-feeding women and in children.

NURSING CONSIDERATIONS

⚗ Assessment
• Assess patient's condition before therapy and regularly thereafter.
• Because drug decreases rate and depth of respirations, monitoring arterial oxygen saturation may aid in assessing respiratory depression.
• Monitor respiratory rate of neonates exposed to drug during labor.
• Monitor postoperative vital signs.
• Be alert for adverse reactions and drug interactions.
• Evaluate patient's and family's knowledge of drug therapy.

⊞ Nursing diagnoses
• Altered health maintenance related to underlying condition
• Ineffective breathing pattern related to respiratory depression
• Knowledge deficit related to drug therapy

⊠ Planning and implementation
• Know that drug should be administered only by personnel specifically trained in use of I.V. anesthetics.
• Reduced dosage is required for elderly and debilitated patients.
• Know that for obese patient who exceeds 20% of his ideal body weight, dosage calculations should be based on an estimate of ideal weight.
• Give drug by direct I.V. injection. Although drug has been given by intermittent I.V. infusion, its compatibility and stability in I.V. solutions have not been fully investigated.
• When used at doses over 8 mcg/kg, postoperative mechanical ventilation and observation are essential because of prolonged respiratory depression.
• Keep narcotic antagonist (naloxone) and resuscitation equipment available.

• Notify doctor if respiratory rate falls below 12 breaths/minute.
• Know that high doses can produce muscle rigidity reversible by neuromuscular blockers; however, patient must be artificially ventilated.
Patient teaching
• Inform patient and family that sufentanil will be used as part of patient's anesthesia. Answer questions patient or family may have.

☑ Evaluation
• Patient responds well to therapy.
• Patient maintains adequate ventilation with mechanical support.
• Patient and family state understanding of drug therapy.

sulfadiazine
(sul-fuh-DIGH-uh-zeen)

Pharmacologic class: sulfonamide
Therapeutic class: antibiotic
Pregnancy risk category: C (contraindicated at term)

How supplied
Tablets: 500 mg

Pharmacokinetics
Absorption: absorbed from GI tract.
Distribution: distributed widely in most body tissues and fluids; 32% to 56% protein-bound.
Metabolism: metabolized partially in liver.
Excretion: excreted unchanged mainly in urine. Urine solubility of unchanged drug increases as urine pH increases. *Half-life:* about 10 hours.

Route	Onset	Peak	Duration
P.O.	Unknown	≤ 6 hr	Unknown

Pharmacodynamics
Chemical effect: inhibits formation of dihydrofolic acid from PABA, decreasing bacterial folic acid synthesis.

Therapeutic effect: hinders bacterial activity. Spectrum of activity includes many gram-positive bacteria, *Chlamydia trachomatis,* many enterobacteriaceae, and some strains of *Plasmodium falciparum* and *Toxoplasma gondii.*

Indications and dosage

▶ **Urinary tract infection.** *Adults:* initially, 2 to 4 g P.O., then 2 to 4 g daily in three to six divided doses. *Children age 2 months and older:* initially, 75 mg/kg or 2 g/m² P.O., then 150 mg/kg or 4 g/m² P.O. in four to six divided doses daily. Maximum daily dosage 6 g.
▶ **Rheumatic fever prophylaxis, as an alternative to penicillin.** *Children weighing 30 kg (66 lb) and over:* 1 g P.O. daily. *Children weighing under 30 kg:* 500 mg P.O. daily.
▶ **Adjunct treatment in toxoplasmosis.** *Adults:* 2 to 8 g P.O. daily in divided doses q 6 hours. Usually given with pyrimethamine. *Children:* 100 to 200 mg/kg P.O. daily. Usually given with pyrimethamine.

Adverse reactions

CNS: headache, mental depression, *seizures,* hallucinations.
GI: *nausea, vomiting, diarrhea,* abdominal pain, anorexia, stomatitis.
GU: *toxic nephrosis with oliguria and anuria,* crystalluria, hematuria.
Hematologic: *agranulocytosis, aplastic anemia,* megaloblastic anemia, *leukopenia, hemolytic anemia, thrombocytopenia.*
Skin: *erythema multiforme (Stevens-Johnson syndrome), generalized skin eruption, epidermal necrolysis, exfoliative dermatitis,* photosensitivity, urticaria, pruritus.
Other: hypersensitivity *(serum sickness, drug fever, anaphylaxis),* jaundice, local irritation, extravasation.

Interactions

Drug-drug. *Methotrexate:* may increase methotrexate levels. Use together cautiously.
Oral anticoagulants: increased anticoagulant effect. Monitor for bleeding.
Oral antidiabetic agents: increased hypoglycemic effect. Monitor blood glucose level.
Oral contraceptives: decreased contraceptive effectiveness and increased risk of breakthrough bleeding. Suggest nonhormonal contraceptive.
Drug-lifestyle. *Sun exposure:* photosensitivity reactions may occur. Take precautions.

Contraindications and precautions

• Contraindicated in patients with hypersensitivity to sulfonamides, in patients with porphyria, in infants under age 2 months (except in congenital toxoplasmosis), in pregnant women at term, and in breast-feeding women.
• Use cautiously and in reduced doses in patients with impaired liver or kidney function, bronchial asthma, history of multiple allergies, G6PD deficiency, or blood dyscrasia.

NURSING CONSIDERATIONS

⚕ Assessment
• Assess patient's condition before therapy and regularly thereafter.
• Obtain specimen for culture and sensitivity tests before first dose. Therapy may begin pending results.
• Monitor urine cultures, CBCs, and urinalyses before and during therapy.
• Monitor urine pH daily.
• Be alert for adverse reactions and drug interactions.
• Monitor patient's hydration if adverse GI reactions occur.
• Evaluate patient's and family's knowledge of drug therapy.

⊞ Nursing diagnoses
- Infection related to presence of susceptible bacteria
- Risk for fluid volume deficit related to drug-induced adverse GI reactions
- Knowledge deficit related to drug therapy

▷ Planning and implementation
- Give drug on schedule to maintain constant blood level.
- Folic or folinic acid may be used during rest periods in toxoplasmosis therapy to reverse hematopoietic depression or anemia associated with pyrimethamine and sulfadiazine.
- Have patient drink between 3,000 and 4,000 ml daily (for adults) to prevent crystalluria. Know that sodium bicarbonate may be administered to alkalinize urine.

Patient teaching
- Tell patient to drink full glass of water with each dose and plenty of water throughout day.
- Tell patient to take entire amount of medication exactly as prescribed, even if he feels better.
- Warn patient to avoid direct sunlight and ultraviolet light to prevent photosensitivity reaction.

☑ Evaluation
- Patient is free from infection.
- Patient maintains adequate hydration.
- Patient and family state understanding of drug therapy.

---

sulfamethoxazole (sulphamethoxazole)
(sul-fuh-meth-OKS-uh-zohl)
Apo-Sulfamethoxazole♦, Gantanol

Pharmacologic class: sulfonamide
Therapeutic class: antibiotic
Pregnancy risk category: C (contraindicated at term)

How supplied
Tablets: 500 mg
Oral suspension: 500 mg/5 ml

Pharmacokinetics
Absorption: absorbed from GI tract.
Distribution: distributed widely in most body tissues and fluids; 50% to 70% protein-bound.
Metabolism: metabolized partially in liver.
Excretion: unchanged drug and metabolites excreted primarily in urine. Urine solubility of unchanged drug increases as urine pH increases. *Half-life:* 7 to 12 hours.

Route	Onset	Peak	Duration
P.O.	Unknown	≤ 2 hr	Unknown

Pharmacodynamics
Chemical effect: inhibits formation of dihydrofolic acid from PABA, decreasing bacterial folic acid synthesis.
Therapeutic effect: hinders bacterial activity. Spectrum of activity includes many gram-positive bacteria, *Chlamydia trachomatis*, many enterobacteriaceae, and some strains of *Plasmodium falciparum* and *Toxoplasma gondii*.

Indications and dosage
▶ **Urinary tract and systemic infections.** *Adults:* initially, 2 g P.O., then 1 g P.O. b.i.d. up to t.i.d. for severe infections. *Children and infants over age 2 months:* initially, 50 to 60 mg/kg P.O., then 25 to 30 mg/kg b.i.d. Maximum dosage should not exceed 75 mg/kg daily.

Adverse reactions
CNS: headache, mental depression, *seizures,* hallucinations, aseptic meningitis, tinnitus, apathy.
GI: *nausea, vomiting, diarrhea,* abdominal pain, anorexia, stomatitis, *pancreatitis,* pseudomembranous colitis.
GU: *toxic nephrosis with oliguria and anuria,* crystalluria, hematuria, interstitial nephritis.

Hematologic: *agranulocytosis, aplastic anemia,* megaloblastic anemia, *thrombocytopenia, leukopenia, hemolytic anemia.*
Skin: *erythema multiforme (Stevens-Johnson syndrome), generalized skin eruption,* **epidermal necrolysis, exfoliative dermatitis,** photosensitivity, urticaria, pruritus.
Other: hypersensitivity reactions *(serum sickness, drug fever,* **anaphylaxis***), jaundice.*

Interactions

Drug-drug. *Methotrexate:* may increase methotrexate levels. Use together cautiously.
Oral anticoagulants: increased anticoagulant effect. Monitor for bleeding.
Oral antidiabetic agents: increased hypoglycemic effect. Monitor blood glucose level.
Oral contraceptives: decreased contraceptive effectiveness and increased risk of breakthrough bleeding. Suggest nonhormonal form of contraception.
Phenytoin: may increase phenytoin effect. Monitor patient closely.
Drug-lifestyle. *Sun exposure:* may cause photosensitivity reactions. Take precautions.

Contraindications and precautions

• Contraindicated in patients with hypersensitivity to sulfonamides, in those with porphyria, in infants under age 2 months (except in congenital toxoplasmosis), in pregnant women at term, and in breast-feeding women.
• Use cautiously and in reduced dosages in patients with impaired liver or kidney function, severe allergy or bronchial asthma, G6PD deficiency, or blood dyscrasia.

NURSING CONSIDERATIONS

📖 Assessment
• Assess patient's condition before therapy and regularly thereafter.

• Obtain specimen for culture and sensitivity tests before first dose. Therapy may begin pending results.
• Monitor urine cultures, CBCs, and urinalyses before and during therapy, as ordered.
• Monitor urine pH daily.
• Be alert for adverse reactions and drug interactions.
• Monitor patient's hydration if adverse GI reactions occur.
• Evaluate patient's and family's knowledge of drug therapy.

🔧 Nursing diagnoses
• Infection related to presence of susceptible bacteria
• Risk for fluid volume deficit related to drug-induced adverse GI reactions
• Knowledge deficit related to drug therapy

▷ Planning and implementation
• Give drug on schedule to maintain constant blood level.
• Be aware that folic or folinic acid may be used during rest periods in toxoplasmosis therapy to reverse hematopoietic depression or anemia associated with pyrimethamine and sulfamethoxazole.
• Have patient drink between 3,000 and 4,000 ml daily (for adults) to prevent crystalluria. Know that sodium bicarbonate may be administered to alkalinize urine.
Patient teaching
• Tell patient to drink full glass of water with each dose and to drink plenty of water throughout day to prevent crystalluria. Teach patient how to monitor fluid intake and output. Intake should be sufficient to produce output of 1,500 ml daily for children and between 3,000 and 4,000 ml daily for adults.
• Tell patient to take entire amount of drug exactly as prescribed.
• Warn patient to avoid direct sunlight and ultraviolet light to prevent photosensitivity reaction.

☑ Evaluation
• Patient is free from infection.
• Patient maintains adequate hydration.
• Patient and family state understanding of drug therapy.

---

sulfasalazine
(salazosulfapyridine, sulphasalazine)
(sul-fuh-SAL-uh-zeen)
Azulfidine, Azulfidine EN-tabs, PMS Sulfasalazine E.C.♦, Salazopyrin♦◇, Salazopyrin EN-Tabs♦◇, S.A.S.-500♦, S.A.S. Enteric-500♦

Pharmacologic class: sulfonamide
Therapeutic class: anti-inflammatory agent
Pregnancy risk category: B

How supplied
Tablets (with or without enteric coating): 500 mg
Oral suspension: 250 mg/5 ml

Pharmacokinetics
Absorption: absorbed poorly from GI tract; 70% to 90% transported to colon, where intestinal flora metabolize drug to its active ingredients, which exert their effects locally. One metabolite, sulfapyridine, is absorbed from colon, but only small portion of metabolite 5-aminosalicytic acid is absorbed.
Distribution: distributed locally in colon. Distribution of absorbed metabolites is unknown.
Metabolism: cleaved by intestinal flora in colon.
Excretion: systemically absorbed sulfasalazine is excreted chiefly in urine.
Half-life: 6 to 8 hours.

Route	Onset	Peak	Duration
P.O.	Unknown (parent drug) 12-24 hr (metabolites)	1.5-6 hr	Unknown

Pharmacodynamics
Chemical effect: unknown.
Therapeutic effect: relieves inflammation in GI tract.

Indications and dosage
▶ **Mild to moderate ulcerative colitis, adjunct therapy in severe ulcerative colitis, Crohn's disease.** *Adults:* initially, 3 to 4 g P.O. daily in evenly divided doses; usual maintenance dosage is 2 g P.O. daily in divided doses q 6 hours. Dosage may be started with 1 to 2 g, with gradual increase in dosage to minimize adverse effects. *Children over age 2:* initially, 40 to 60 mg/kg P.O. daily, divided into three to six doses; then 30 mg/kg daily in four doses. Dosage may be started at lower dose if GI intolerance occurs.
▶ **Rheumatoid arthritis in patients who have responded inadequately to salicylates or NSAIDs.** *Adults:* 2 g P.O. daily b.i.d. in evenly divided doses. Dosage may be started at 0.5 to 1 g daily and gradually increased over 3 weeks to reduce possible GI intolerance.

Adverse reactions
CNS: headache, depression, *seizures,* hallucinations.
GI: *nausea, vomiting, diarrhea,* abdominal pain, anorexia, stomatitis.
GU: *toxic nephrosis with oliguria and anuria,* crystalluria, hematuria, oligospermia, infertility.
Hematologic: *agranulocytosis, aplastic anemia,* megaloblastic anemia, *thrombocytopenia, leukopenia,* hemolytic anemia.
Hepatic: jaundice, *hepatotoxicity.*
Skin: *erythema multiforme (Stevens-Johnson syndrome), generalized skin eruption, epidermal necrolysis, exfoliative dermatitis,* photosensitivity, urticaria, pruritus.
Other: *hypersensitivity reactions (serum sickness, drug fever, anaphylaxis).*

Interactions

Drug-drug. *Antibiotics:* may alter action of sulfasalazine by altering internal flora. Monitor patient closely.
Digoxin: may reduce absorption of digoxin. Monitor patient closely.
Folic acid: absorption may be decreased. No intervention necessary.
Iron: lowered blood concentrations of sulfasalazine caused by iron chelation. Monitor patient closely.
Oral anticoagulants: increased anticoagulant effect. Monitor for bleeding.
Oral antidiabetic agents: increased hypoglycemic effect. Monitor blood glucose level.
Oral contraceptives: decreased contraceptive effectiveness and increased risk of breakthrough bleeding. Suggest nonhormonal contraceptive.

Contraindications and precautions

• Contraindicated in patients with porphyria, intestinal and urinary obstruction, or hypersensitivity to drug or its metabolites and in infants under age 2.
• Use cautiously and in reduced dosages in patients with impaired liver or kidney function, severe allergy, bronchial asthma, or G6PD deficiency. Also use cautiously in pregnant or breast-feeding women.

NURSING CONSIDERATIONS

Assessment
• Assess patient's condition before therapy and regularly thereafter.
• Be alert for adverse reactions and drug interactions.
• Monitor patient's hydration status throughout drug therapy.
• Evaluate patient's and family's knowledge of drug therapy.

Nursing diagnoses
• Pain related to inflammation of GI tract
• Risk for fluid volume deficit related to drug-induced adverse GI reactions

• Knowledge deficit related to drug therapy

Planning and implementation
• Minimize adverse GI symptoms by spacing doses evenly and administering after food intake.
• Be aware that drug colors alkaline urine orange-yellow.
• Discontinue immediately if patient shows signs and symptoms of hypersensitivity, and notify doctor.
Patient teaching
• Instruct patient to take drug after meals and to space doses evenly.
• Warn patient that drug may cause urine to turn orange-yellow as well as skin and that drug may permanently stain soft contact lenses yellow.
• Warn patient to avoid direct sunlight and ultraviolet light to prevent photosensitivity reaction.

Evaluation
• Patient is free from pain.
• Patient maintains adequate hydration.
• Patient and family state understanding of drug therapy.

sulfinpyrazone
(sul-fin-PEER-uh-zohn)
Anturan♦, Anturane

Pharmacologic class: uricosuric agent
Therapeutic class: renal tubular-blocking agent, platelet aggregation inhibitor
Pregnancy risk category: NR

How supplied
Tablets: 100 mg
Capsules: 200 mg

Pharmacokinetics
Absorption: absorbed completely from GI tract.
Distribution: 98% to 99% protein-bound.
Metabolism: metabolized rapidly in liver.

Excretion: excreted in urine; about 50% excreted unchanged. *Half-life:* 4 to 6 hours.

Route	Onset	Peak	Duration
P.O.	Unknown	1-2 hr	4-6 hr

Pharmacodynamics

Chemical effect: blocks renal tubular reabsorption of uric acid, increasing excretion, and inhibits platelet aggregation.
Therapeutic effect: relieves signs and symptoms of gouty arthritis.

Indications and dosage

▶ **Intermittent or chronic gouty arthritis.** *Adults:* 200 to 400 mg P.O. b.i.d. first week, then 400 mg P.O. b.i.d. Maximum dosage is 800 mg daily.

Adverse reactions

GI: *nausea, dyspepsia,* epigastric pain, reactivation of peptic ulcerations.
Hematologic: *blood dyscrasias* (such as anemia, *leukopenia, agranulocytosis, thrombocytopenia, aplastic anemia*).
Respiratory: *bronchoconstriction* (in patients with aspirin-induced asthma).
Skin: rash.

Interactions

Drug-drug. *Aspirin, niacin, salicylates:* inhibited uricosuric effect of sulfinpyrazone. Do not use together.
Oral anticoagulants: increased anticoagulant effect and risk of bleeding. Use together cautiously.
Oral antidiabetic agents: increased effects. Monitor patient closely.
Probenecid: inhibited renal excretion of sulfinpyrazone. Use together cautiously.
Theophylline, verapamil: increased clearance. Use cautiously.
Drug-lifestyle. *Alcohol use:* decreased effectiveness. Avoid concomitant use.

Contraindications and precautions

• Contraindicated in patients with active peptic ulcer, symptoms of GI inflammation or ulceration, blood dyscrasias, or hypersensitivity to pyrazole derivatives (including oxyphenbutazone and phenylbutazone).
• Use cautiously in patients with healed peptic ulcer and in pregnant women.
• Safety of drug has not been established in breast-feeding women and in children.

NURSING CONSIDERATIONS

🗷 Assessment
• Assess patient's condition before therapy and regularly thereafter.
• Monitor BUN level, CBC, and kidney function studies periodically during long-term use, as ordered.
• Monitor fluid intake and output. Therapy may lead to renal colic and formation of uric acid stones until acid levels are normal (about 6 mg/dl).
• Be alert for adverse reactions and drug interactions.
• Evaluate patient's and family's knowledge of drug therapy.

🖽 Nursing diagnoses
• Altered health maintenance related to presence of gouty arthritis
• Risk for injury related to drug-induced adverse CNS reactions
• Knowledge deficit related to drug therapy

▷ Planning and implementation
• Give drug with milk, food, or antacids to minimize GI disturbances.
• Force fluids to maintain minimum daily output of 2 to 3 L. Alkalinize urine with sodium bicarbonate or other agent, as ordered. Keep in mind that alkalinizing agents are used therapeutically to increase drug activity, preventing urolithiasis.
• Know that drug is recommended for patients unresponsive to probenecid. Suitable for long-term use; neither cumulative effects nor tolerance develops.
• Drug contains no analgesic or anti-inflammatory agent and is of no value during acute gout attacks.

• Be aware that drug may increase frequency, severity, and length of acute gout attacks during first 6 to 12 months of therapy. Prophylactic colchicine or another anti-inflammatory agent is given during first 3 to 6 months.
• Lifelong therapy may be required in patient with hyperuricemia.
• Drug decreases urinary excretion of aminohippuric acid, interfering with laboratory test results.

Patient teaching
• Warn patient with gout not to take aspirin-containing medications because they may precipitate gout. Acetaminophen may be used for pain.
• Tell patient to take drug with food, milk, or antacid. Also instruct him to drink plenty of water.
• Instruct patient with gout to avoid foods high in purine: anchovies, liver, sardines, kidneys, sweetbreads, peas, and lentils.
• Instruct patient and family that drug must be taken regularly, as ordered, or gout attacks may result. Tell him to visit doctor regularly so blood levels can be monitored and dosage adjusted if necessary.

☑ **Evaluation**
• Patient regains and maintains normal uric acid levels.
• Patient does not experience injury from adverse CNS reactions.
• Patient and family state understanding of drug therapy.

sulfisoxazole (sulfafurazole, sulphafurazole)
(sul-fih-SOKS-uh-zohl)
Azo-Sulfisoxazole, Gantrisin, Novo-Soxazole ♦

Pharmacologic class: sulfonamide
Therapeutic class: antibiotic
Pregnancy risk category: C (contraindicated at term)

How supplied
Tablets: 500 mg
Liquid: 500 mg/5 ml

Pharmacokinetics
Absorption: absorbed readily from GI tract.
Distribution: distributed widely in most body tissues and fluids; 85% protein-bound.
Metabolism: metabolized partially in liver.
Excretion: unchanged drug and metabolites excreted primarily in urine. Urine solubility of unchanged drug increases as urine pH increases. *Half-life:* 4½ to 8 hours.

Route	Onset	Peak	Duration
P.O.	Unknown	2-4 hr	Unknown

Pharmacodynamics
Chemical effect: decreases bacterial folic acid synthesis.
Therapeutic effect: hinders activity of some gram-positive bacteria, *Chlamydia trachomatis,* many enterobacteriaceae, and some strains of *Plasmodium falciparum* and *Toxoplasma gondii.*

Indications and dosage
▶ **Urinary tract and systemic infections.** *Adults:* initially, 2 to 4 g P.O., then 4 to 8 g daily divided in four to six doses. *Children over age 2 months:* initially, 75 mg/kg P.O. daily or 2 g/m² P.O. daily in divided doses q 6 hours, then 150 mg/kg or 4 g/m² P.O. daily in divided doses q 6 hours.

Adverse reactions
CNS: headache, mental depression, *seizures,* hallucinations.
CV: tachycardia, palpitations, syncope, cyanosis.
GI: *nausea, vomiting, diarrhea,* abdominal pain, anorexia, stomatitis, pseudomembranous colitis, *hepatitis.*
GU: *toxic nephrosis with oliguria and anuria, acute renal failure,* crystalluria, hematuria, *acute renal failure.*

Reactions may be *common,* uncommon, *life-threatening,* or COMMON AND LIFE-THREATENING.

Hematologic: *agranulocytosis, aplastic anemia,* megaloblastic anemia, *thrombocytopenia, leukopenia, hemolytic anemia.* **Skin:** *erythema multiforme, generalized skin eruption, epidermal necrolysis, exfoliative dermatitis,* photosensitivity, urticaria, pruritus.
Other: hypersensitivity reactions *(serum sickness, drug fever, anaphylaxis),* jaundice.

Interactions

Drug-drug. *Methotrexate:* may increase methotrexate levels. Use together cautiously.
Oral anticoagulants: increased anticoagulant effect. Monitor for bleeding.
Oral antidiabetic agents: increased hypoglycemic effect. Monitor blood glucose levels.
Oral contraceptives: decreased contraceptive effectiveness, increased risk of breakthrough bleeding. Suggest nonhormonal form of contraception.
Drug-lifestyle. *Sun exposure:* photosensitivity reactions may occur. Use precautions.

Contraindications and precautions

• Contraindicated in patients with hypersensitivity to sulfonamides, in infants under age 2 months (except in congenital toxoplasmosis), in pregnant women at term, and in breast-feeding women.
• Use cautiously in patients with impaired liver or kidney function, severe allergy or bronchial asthma, or G6PD deficiency.

NURSING CONSIDERATIONS

⚕ Assessment
• Assess patient's condition before therapy and regularly thereafter.
• Obtain specimen for culture and sensitivity tests before giving first dose. Therapy may begin pending results.
• Monitor urine cultures, CBCs, and urinalyses before and during therapy.
• Monitor urine pH daily.

• Be alert for adverse reactions and drug interactions.
• Monitor patient's hydration if adverse GI reactions occur.
• Evaluate patient's and family's knowledge of drug therapy.

⚕ Nursing diagnoses
• Infection related to presence of susceptible bacteria
• Risk for fluid volume deficit related to drug-induced adverse GI reactions
• Knowledge deficit related to drug therapy

▷ Planning and implementation
• Give drug on schedule to maintain constant blood level.
• Have patient drink between 3,000 and 4,000 ml daily (for adults) to prevent crystalluria. Know that sodium bicarbonate may be administered to alkalinize urine.
Patient teaching
• Teach patient how to monitor fluid intake and output.
• Tell patient to take entire amount of drug exactly as prescribed.
• Warn patient to avoid direct sunlight and ultraviolet light to prevent photosensitivity reaction.

☑ Evaluation
• Patient is free from infection.
• Patient maintains adequate hydration.
• Patient and family state understanding of drug therapy.

sulindac
(SUL-in-dak)
Aclin◇, Apo-Sulin♦, Clinoril, Novo-Sundac♦

Pharmacologic class: NSAID
Therapeutic class: nonnarcotic analgesic, antipyretic, anti-inflammatory
Pregnancy risk category: NR

How supplied

Tablets: 100 mg◊, 150 mg, 200 mg

Pharmacokinetics

Absorption: absorbed rapidly and completely from GI tract.
Distribution: highly protein-bound.
Metabolism: drug is inactive and metabolized in liver to an active sulfide metabolite.
Excretion: excreted in urine. *Half-life:* parent drug, 8 hours; active metabolite, about 16 hours.

Route	Onset	Peak	Duration
P.O.	Unknown	2-4 hr	Unknown

Pharmacodynamics

Chemical effect: unknown; produces anti-inflammatory, analgesic, and antipyretic effects, possibly by inhibiting prostaglandin synthesis.
Therapeutic effect: relieves pain, fever, and inflammation.

Indications and dosage

▶ **Osteoarthritis, rheumatoid arthritis, ankylosing spondylitis.** *Adults:* initially, 150 mg P.O. b.i.d.; increased to 200 mg b.i.d., as necessary.
▶ **Acute subacromial bursitis or supraspinatus tendinitis, acute gouty arthritis.** *Adults:* 200 mg P.O. b.i.d. for 7 to 14 days. Dose reduced as symptoms subside.

Adverse reactions

CNS: dizziness, headache, nervousness, psychosis.
CV: hypertension, *heart failure,* palpitations.
EENT: tinnitus, transient visual disturbances.
GI: *epigastric distress, peptic ulceration, pancreatitis, GI bleeding,* occult blood loss, nausea, constipation, dyspepsia, flatulence, anorexia.
GU: interstitial nephritis, *nephrotic syndrome, renal failure.*
Hematologic: prolonged bleeding time, *aplastic anemia, thrombocytopenia,*

neutropenia, agranulocytosis, hemolytic anemia.
Hepatic: elevated liver enzyme levels.
Skin: *rash,* pruritus.
Other: edema, drug fever, *anaphylaxis, hypersensitivity syndrome, angioedema.*

Interactions

Drug-drug. *Anticoagulants:* increased risk of bleeding. Monitor PT closely.
Aspirin: decreased sulindac plasma concentration and increased risk of adverse GI reactions. Avoid concomitant use.
Cyclosporine: increased nephrotoxicity of cyclosporine. Monitor patient.
Diflunisal, dimethyl sulfoxide: decreased metabolism of sulindac to its active metabolite, reducing its effectiveness. Don't use together.
Methotrexate: increased methotrexate toxicity. Avoid concomitant use.
Probenecid: increased plasma levels of sulindac and its active metabolite. Monitor for toxicity.
Sulfonamides, sulfonylureas, other highly protein-bound drugs: possible displacement of these drugs from plasma protein-binding sites, leading to increased toxicity. Monitor patient closely.

Contraindications and precautions

• Contraindicated in patients with hypersensitivity to drug or in whom acute asthmatic attacks, urticaria, or rhinitis is precipitated by aspirin or NSAIDs.
• Drug is not recommended for use in pregnant women.
• Use cautiously in patients with history of ulcers and GI bleeding, renal dysfunction, compromised cardiac function or hypertension, or conditions predisposing to fluid retention.
• Safety of drug has not been established in breast-feeding women and in children.

NURSING CONSIDERATIONS

Assessment
• Assess patient's condition before therapy and regularly thereafter.

• Periodically monitor liver and kidney function and CBC in patient receiving long-term therapy, as ordered.
• Be alert for adverse reactions and drug interactions.
• Evaluate patient's and family's knowledge of drug therapy.

⊞ **Nursing diagnoses**
• Pain related to presence of arthritis
• Impaired tissue integrity related to drug's adverse effect on GI mucosa
• Knowledge deficit related to drug therapy

▶ **Planning and implementation**
• Notify doctor of adverse reactions.
Patient teaching
• Tell patient to take drug with food, milk, or antacids to reduce adverse GI reactions.
• Advise patient to refrain from driving or performing other hazardous activities that require mental alertness until CNS effects are known.
• Teach patient signs and symptoms of GI bleeding, and tell him to contact doctor immediately if they occur. Serious GI toxicity, including peptic ulceration and bleeding, can occur in patient taking NSAIDs despite absence of GI symptoms.
• Tell patient to notify doctor immediately if easy bruising or prolonged bleeding occurs.
• Instruct patient to report edema and have blood pressure checked monthly. Drug causes sodium retention but is thought to have less effect on kidneys than other NSAIDs.
• Tell patient to notify doctor and undergo complete eye examination if visual disturbances occur.

☑ **Evaluation**
• Patient is free from pain.
• Patient does not experience adverse GI reactions.
• Patient and family state understanding of drug therapy.

sumatriptan succinate
(soo-muh-TRIP-ten SEK-seh-nayt)
Imitrex

Pharmacologic class: selective 5-hydroxytryptamine (5-HT₁) receptor agonist
Therapeutic class: antimigraine
Pregnancy risk category: C

How supplied

Tablets: 25 mg, 50 mg, 100 mg (base) ♦
Injection: 6 mg/0.5 ml (12 mg/ml) in 0.5-ml prefilled syringes and vials
Nasal spray: 5 mg/spray; 20 mg/spray

Pharmacokinetics

Absorption: rapidly absorbed after P.O. administration but with low absolute bioavailability (about 15%); absorbed well from injection site after S.C. administration.
Distribution: drug has low protein-binding of about 14% to 21%.
Metabolism: about 80% metabolized in liver.
Excretion: excreted primarily in urine.
Half-life: about 2 hours.

Route	Onset	Peak	Duration
P.O.	30 min	2-4 hr	Unknown
S.C.	10-20 min	1-2 hr	Unknown
Intranasal	Rapid	1 to 2 hr	Unknown

Pharmacodynamics

Chemical effect: unknown; thought to selectively activate vascular serotonin (5-HT) receptors. Stimulation of specific receptor subtype 5-HT₁, present on cranial arteries and the dura mater, causes vasoconstriction of cerebral vessels but has minimal effects on systemic vessels, tissue perfusion, and blood pressure.
Therapeutic effect: relieves acute migraine pain.

Indications and dosage

▶ **Acute migraine attacks (with or without aura).** *Adults:* 6 mg S.C. Maximum recommended dosage is two

6-mg injections in 24 hours, separated by at least 1 hour. Alternatively, 25 to 100 mg P.O. If headache returns or only partial response has occurred, dose may be repeated after 2 hours. Maximum daily dosage is 300 mg P.O. Intranasally, 5 mg, 10 mg, or 20 mg in one nostril (for 10 mg dose—one spray of 5 mg concentration into each nostril); if headache returns, may repeat once after 2 hours. Maximum daily dosage is 40 mg.

Adverse reactions

CNS: *dizziness, vertigo,* drowsiness, headache, anxiety, malaise, fatigue.
CV: *atrial fibrillation, ventricular fibrillation, ventricular tachycardia, MI,* ECG changes such as ischemic ST-segment elevation (rare).
EENT: discomfort of throat, nasal cavity or sinus, mouth, jaw, or tongue; altered vision.
GI: abdominal discomfort, dysphagia.
Skin: flushing.
Other: *tingling; warm or hot sensation; burning sensation; heaviness, pressure, or tightness;* feeling of strangeness; tight feeling in head; cold sensation; pressure or tightness in chest; neck pain; myalgia; muscle cramps; diaphoresis; *injection site reaction.*

Interactions

Drug-drug. *Ergot, ergot derivatives:* prolonged vasospastic effects. Don't use these drugs and sumatriptan within 24 hours of sumatriptan dosage.
MAO inhibitors: increased effects of sumatriptan. Avoid concomitant use or within 2 weeks of discontinuing MAO inhibitor therapy.

Contraindications and precautions

• Contraindicated in patients with uncontrolled hypertension or ischemic heart disease (such as angina pectoris, Prinzmetal's angina, history of MI, or documented silent ischemia), hemiplegic or basilar migraine, or hypersensitivity to drug and in those taking ergotamine or within 14 days of MAO therapy.

• Use cautiously in women who are pregnant or intend to become pregnant. Also use cautiously in patients who may have unrecognized coronary artery disease (CAD), such as postmenopausal women, men over age 40, and patients with risk factors such as hypertension, hypercholesterolemia, obesity, diabetes, smoking, or family history of CAD.
• Safety of drug has not been established in children and in breast-feeding women.

NURSING CONSIDERATIONS

⚕ Assessment
• Assess patient's condition before therapy and regularly thereafter.
• Be alert for adverse reactions and drug interactions.
• Evaluate patient's and family's knowledge of drug therapy.

⚕ Nursing diagnoses
• Pain related to presence of acute migraine attack
• Risk for injury related to drug-induced adverse reactions
• Knowledge deficit related to drug therapy

⚕ Planning and implementation
• Consider administering first dose in doctor's office to patient at risk for unrecognized CAD.
P.O. use: Administer single tablet whole with fluids as soon as patient complains of symptoms of migraine headache. Administer second tablet if symptoms come back, but do not administer sooner than 2 hours after first tablet.
S.C. use: Maximum recommended dosage given in one 24-hour period is no more than two 6-mg injections separated by at least 1 hour. Notify doctor if patient does not obtain relief.
– Serious adverse cardiac effects can follow S.C. administration of this drug, but such events are rare.
– Most patients experience relief within 1 to 2 hours.

Reactions may be *common,* uncommon, *life-threatening,* or COMMON AND LIFE-THREATENING.

– Be aware that redness or pain at injection site should subside within 1 hour after injection.
Intranasal use: Follow normal protocol.
• Know that no more than 300 mg should be administered in any 24 hours. Notify doctor if patient does not obtain relief.
Patient teaching
• Be sure patient understands that drug is intended only to treat migraine attack, not to prevent or reduce number of attacks.
• Tell patient that drug may be given at any time during migraine attack but should be given as soon as symptoms appear.
• Drug is available in spring-loaded injector system that facilitates self-administration. Review detailed information with patient. Be sure patient understands how to load injector, administer injection, and dispose of used syringes.
• Instruct patient taking oral form when and how often to take drug. Warn patient that no more than 300 mg should be taken within 24 hours.
• Instruct patient to use intranasal spray in one nostril (if 10 mg dose is ordered— 1 spray into each nostril). A second spray may be administered if headache returns, but not before 2 hours has elapsed from the first use.
• Tell patient who experiences persistent or severe chest pain to call doctor immediately. Patient who experiences pain or tightness in throat, wheezing, heart throbbing, rash, lumps, hives, or swollen eyelids, face, or lips should stop using drug and call doctor.
• Tell female patient who is pregnant or intends to become pregnant not to take this drug. Advise her to discuss with doctor the risks and benefits of using drug during pregnancy.

☑ **Evaluation**
• Patient is free from pain.
• Patient does not experience injury from adverse CV reactions.
• Patient and family state understanding of drug therapy.

tacrine hydrochloride
(TAK-reen high-droh-KLOR-ighd)
Cognex

Pharmacologic class: centrally acting reversible cholinesterase inhibitor
Therapeutic class: psychotherapeutic agent for Alzheimer's disease
Pregnancy risk category: C

How supplied
Capsules: 10 mg, 20 mg, 30 mg, 40 mg

Pharmacokinetics
Absorption: rapidly absorbed with absolute bioavailability being about 17%. Food reduces tacrine bioavailability by 30% to 40%.
Distribution: about 55% bound to plasma proteins.
Metabolism: undergoes first-pass metabolism, which is dose-dependent; extensively metabolized.
Excretion: excreted in urine. *Half-life:* 2 to 4 hours.

Route	Onset	Peak	Duration
P.O.	Unknown	0.5-3 hr	Unknown

Pharmacodynamics
Chemical effect: reversibly inhibits enzyme cholinesterase in CNS, allowing buildup of acetylcholine.
Therapeutic effect: improves thinking ability in patients with Alzheimer's disease.

Indications and dosage
▶ **Mild to moderate dementia of Alzheimer's type.** *Adults:* initially, 10 mg P.O. q.i.d. After 6 weeks and if patient tolerates treatment and transaminase levels are not elevated, dosage increased to 20 mg q.i.d. After 6 weeks, dosage

titrated upward to 30 mg q.i.d. If still tolerated, increased to 40 mg q.i.d. after another 6 weeks.

Adverse reactions

CNS: agitation, ataxia, insomnia, abnormal thinking, somnolence, depression, anxiety, *headache,* fatigue, *dizziness,* confusion.
CV: chest pain.
GI: *nausea, vomiting,* anorexia, *diarrhea,* dyspepsia, loose stools, changes in stool color, constipation.
Musculoskeletal: myalgia.
Respiratory: rhinitis, upper respiratory tract infection, cough.
Skin: rash, jaundice, facial flushing.
Other: weight loss.

Interactions

Drug-drug. *Anticholinergics:* may decrease effectiveness of anticholinergics. Monitor patient closely.
Cholinergics (such as bethanechol), cholinesterase inhibitors: additive effects. Monitor for toxicity.
Succinylcholine: enhanced neuromuscular blockade and prolonged duration of action. Monitor patient.
Theophylline: increased theophylline serum levels and prolonged theophylline half-life. Carefully monitor theophylline plasma levels, and adjust dosage, as ordered.
Drug-food. *Any food:* decreased absorption of tacrine if taken concomitantly. Take drug 1 hour before a meal.
Drug-lifestyle. *Smoking:* decreased plasma concentrations of drug. Monitor response.

Contraindications and precautions

• Contraindicated in patients hypersensitive to drug or acridine derivatives and in those who have previously developed tacrine-related jaundice, which has been confirmed with elevated total bilirubin level of more than 3 mg/dl.
• Drug is not recommended for use in pregnant or breast-feeding women.

• Use cautiously in patients with sick sinus syndrome or bradycardia; in those at risk for peptic ulceration (including patients taking NSAIDs or those with history of peptic ulcer); in those with history of hepatic disease; and in those with renal disease, asthma, prostatic hyperplasia, or other urinary outflow impairment.
• Drug is not indicated for use in children.

NURSING CONSIDERATIONS

⚕ Assessment
• Assess patient's cognitive ability before therapy and regularly thereafter.
• Monitor serum ALT levels weekly during first 18 weeks of therapy. If ALT is modestly elevated after first 18 weeks (twice upper limit of normal range), continue weekly monitoring. If no problems occur, determinations decreased to every 3 months. Whenever dosage is increased, resume weekly monitoring for at least 6 weeks.
• Be alert for adverse reactions and drug interactions.
• Evaluate patient's and family's knowledge of drug therapy.

⚕ Nursing diagnoses
• Altered thought processes related to Alzheimer's disease
• Diarrhea related to drug-induced adverse GI reactions
• Knowledge deficit related to drug therapy

⚕ Planning and implementation
• Give drug between meals. If GI upset becomes a problem, give drug with meals, although plasma levels may drop by 30% to 40%.
• If drug is discontinued for 4 weeks or more, full dosage titration and monitoring schedule must be restarted.
• Obtain order for antidiarrheal agent, if indicated.
Patient teaching
• Help patient and family members understand that drug only alleviates symp-

toms. Effect of therapy depends on drug administration at regular intervals.
• Instruct caregivers when to give drug. Explain that dosage titration is integral part of safe use. Abrupt discontinuation or large reduction in daily dosage (80 mg or more per day) may trigger behavioral disturbances and decline in cognitive function.
• Advise patient and caregivers to report immediately significant adverse effects or changes in status.

☑ **Evaluation**
• Patient exhibits improved cognitive ability.
• Patient or caregiver states that drug-induced diarrhea has not occurred.
• Patient and family state understanding of drug therapy.

tacrolimus
(tek-roh-LEE-mus)
Prograf

Pharmacologic class: bacteria-derived macrolide
Therapeutic class: immunosuppressant
Pregnancy risk category: C

How supplied

Capsules: 1 mg, 5 mg
Injection: 5 mg/ml

Pharmacokinetics

Absorption: absorption of oral tacrolimus from GI tract varies. The presence of food reduces absorption and bioavailability of drug.
Distribution: distribution between whole blood and plasma depends on several factors, such as hematocrit, temperature of separation of plasma, drug concentration, and plasma protein concentration. Drug is 75% to 99% protein-bound.
Metabolism: extensively metabolized.
Excretion: excreted primarily in bile; less than 1% excreted unchanged in urine.

Route	Onset	Peak	Duration
P.O., I.V.	Unknown	1.5-3.5 hr	Unknown

Pharmacodynamics

Chemical effect: precise mechanism unknown; inhibits T-lymphocyte activation, which results in immunosuppression.
Therapeutic effect: prevents organ rejection.

Indications and dosage

▶ **Prophylaxis of organ rejection in allogenic liver transplantation.** *Adults:* 0.05 to 0.1 mg/kg/day I.V. as continuous infusion administered no sooner than 6 hours after transplantation. Oral therapy should be substituted as soon as possible, with first dose given 8 to 12 hours after discontinuing I.V. infusion. Recommended initial oral dosage is 0.15 to 0.3 mg/kg/day in two divided doses q 12 hours. Dosage should be titrated according to clinical response. *Children:* initially, 0.1 mg/kg/day I.V., followed by 0.3 mg/kg/day P.O. on schedule similar to that for adults, adjusted as needed.

Adverse reactions

CNS: *asthenia, headache, tremors, insomnia, paresthesias, delirium,* **coma.**
CV: *hypertension, peripheral edema.*
GI: *diarrhea, nausea, constipation, abnormal liver function test results, anorexia, vomiting, abdominal pain.*
GU: *abnormal kidney function,* increased creatinine or BUN level, urinary tract infection, oliguria.
Hematologic: *anemia,* leukocytosis, THROMBOCYTOPENIA.
Metabolic: *hyperkalemia, hypokalemia, hyperglycemia, hypomagnesemia.*
Respiratory: *pleural effusion, atelectasis, dyspnea.*
Skin: *photosensitivity.*
Other: *pain, fever, back pain, ascites,* **anaphylaxis.**

Interactions

Drug-drug. *Bromocriptine, cimetidine, clarithromycin, clotrimazole, cyclosporine,*

danazol, diltiazem, erythromycin, fluconazole, itraconazole, ketoconazole, methylprednisolone, metoclopramide, nicardipine, verapamil: may increase tacrolimus level. Monitor for adverse effects.
Carbamazepine, phenobarbital, phenytoin, rifabutin, rifampin: may decrease tacrolimus level. Monitor effectiveness of tacrolimus.
Cyclosporine: increased risk of excess nephrotoxicity. Do not administer together.
Immunosuppressants (except adrenocorticosteroids): may oversuppress immune system. Monitor patient closely, especially during times of stress.
Inducers of cytochrome P-450 enzyme system: may increase tacrolimus metabolism and decrease plasma level. Dosage adjustment may be needed.
Inhibitors of cytochrome P-450 enzyme system: may decrease tacrolimus metabolism and increase plasma level. Dosage adjustment may be needed.
Nephrotoxic drugs (such as aminoglycosides, amphotericin B, cisplatin, cyclosporine): may cause additive or synergistic effects. Monitor patient closely.
Viral vaccines: tacrolimus may interfere with immune response to live virus vaccines.
Drug-food. *Any food:* inhibited drug absorption. Take drug on an empty stomach.
Grapefruit juice: increased drug blood levels in liver transplant patients. Avoid concomitant use.

Contraindications and precautions

• Contraindicated in patients with hypersensitivity to drug; I.V. form is contraindicated in patients hypersensitive to castor oil derivatives.
• Drug is not recommended for use in pregnant or breast-feeding women.

NURSING CONSIDERATIONS

Assessment
• Obtain history of patient's organ transplant before therapy, and reassess regularly thereafter.

• Monitor continuously during first 30 minutes of infusion; then monitor frequently for anaphylaxis.
• Monitor patient for signs of neurotoxicity and nephrotoxicity, especially in patients receiving high dosage or with renal dysfunction.
• Obtain serum potassium and blood glucose levels regularly. Monitor patient for hyperglycemia.
• Know that drug increases risk for infections, lymphomas, and other cancers.
• Be alert for adverse reactions and drug interactions.
• Evaluate patient's and family's knowledge of drug therapy.

Nursing diagnoses
• Risk for injury related to potential organ transplant rejection
• Altered protection related to drug-induced immunosuppression
• Knowledge deficit related to drug therapy

Planning and implementation
• Because of risk of anaphylaxis, injection should be used only in patient who cannot take oral form.
• Keep epinephrine 1:1,000 readily available to treat anaphylaxis.
• Be aware that child with normal kidney and liver function may require higher dosage than adult.
• Patient with hepatic or renal dysfunction needs lowest dosage possible.
• Expect to give adrenocorticosteroids concomitantly with this drug.
P.O. use: Give drug on empty stomach.
I.V. use: Dilute drug with 0.9% NaCl injection or 5% dextrose injection to concentration between 0.004 mg/ml and 0.02 mg/ml before use. Store diluted solution for no more than 24 hours in glass or polyethylene containers. Don't store drug in polyvinyl chloride container. Each required daily dose of diluted drug is infused continuously over 24 hours.

Reactions may be *common,* uncommon, *life-threatening,* or COMMON AND LIFE-THREATENING.

• Other immunosuppressants (except for adrenocorticosteroids) should not be used during therapy.
• Avoid use of potassium-sparing diuretics during therapy.
Patient teaching
• Instruct patient to take oral drug on empty stomach and not to take it with grapefruit juice.
• Explain need for repeated tests during therapy to monitor for adverse reactions and drug effectiveness.
• Advise female patient of childbearing age to notify doctor if she becomes pregnant or plans to do so.
• Instruct patient to check with doctor before taking other medications.

☑ Evaluation
• Patient does not exhibit signs and symptoms of organ rejection.
• Patient does not develop serious complications as result of drug-induced adverse reactions.
• Patient and family state understanding of drug therapy.

tamoxifen citrate
(teh-MOKS-uh-fen SIGH-trayt)
Apo-Tamox♦, Nolvadex, Nolvadex-D♦◇, Novo-Tamoxifen♦, Tamofen♦, Tamone♦, Tamoplex♦

Pharmacologic class: nonsteroidal antiestrogen
Therapeutic class: antineoplastic
Pregnancy risk category: D

How supplied

Tablets: 10 mg, 20 mg
Tablets (enteric-coated)♦: 10 mg, 20 mg

Pharmacokinetics

Absorption: appears to be well absorbed across GI tract.
Distribution: distributed widely in total body water.

Metabolism: metabolized extensively in liver to several metabolites.
Excretion: drug and metabolites excreted mainly in feces, mostly as metabolites.
Half-life: over 7 days.

Route	Onset	Peak	Duration
P.O.	4-10 wk	Unknown	Several wk

Pharmacodynamics

Chemical effect: exact antineoplastic action is unknown; acts as estrogen antagonist.
Therapeutic effect: hinders function of breast cancer cells.

Indications and dosage

▶ **Advanced postmenopausal breast cancer.** *Adults:* 10 to 20 mg P.O. b.i.d.
▶ **Adjunct treatment for breast cancer.** *Adults:* 10 mg P.O. b.i.d. to t.i.d. for no more than 2 years.
▶ **Reduction of breast cancer in high-risk women.** *Adults:* 20 mg P.O. daily for 5 years.

Adverse reactions

CNS: confusion, weakness, headache, sleepiness.
EENT: corneal changes, cataracts, retinopathy.
GI: *nausea, vomiting, diarrhea.*
GU: *vaginal discharge* and bleeding, *irregular menses,* increased BUN, *amenorrhea.*
Hematologic: transient fall in WBC or platelet count, *leukopenia, thrombocytopenia.*
Hepatic: changes in liver enzymes, fatty liver, cholestasis, *hepatic necrosis.*
Skin: *skin changes,* rash.
Other: *hypercalcemia,* temporary bone or tumor pain, *hot flashes,* brief exacerbation of pain from osseous metastases, *weight gain or loss, fluid retention.*

Interactions

Drug-drug. *Antacids:* may affect absorption of enteric-coated tablet. Do not use within 2 hours of tamoxifen dose.

Bromocriptine: may elevate tamoxifen levels. Monitor closely.
Coumadin-type anticoagulants: may cause significant increase in anticoagulant effect. Monitor patient, PT, and INR closely.

Contraindications and precautions

• Contraindicated in patients hypersensitive to drug.
• Contraindicated in women receiving coumarin-type anticoagulants or with history of deep vein thrombosis or pulmonary emboli.
• Drug is not recommended for use in pregnant or breast-feeding women.
• Use cautiously in patients with existing leukopenia or thrombocytopenia.
• Safety of drug has not been established in children.

NURSING CONSIDERATIONS

Assessment
• Assess patient's breast cancer before therapy and regularly thereafter.
• Monitor CBC closely in patient with existing leukopenia or thrombocytopenia, as ordered.
• Monitor serum lipid levels during long-term therapy in patients with preexisting hyperlipidemia.
• Monitor serum calcium level, as ordered. Drug may compound hypercalcemia related to bone metastases during initiation of therapy.
• Be alert for adverse reactions. Such reactions are usually minor.
• Monitor patient's hydration status if adverse GI reactions occur.
• Evaluate patient's and family's knowledge of drug therapy.

Nursing diagnoses
• Altered health maintenance related to presence of breast cancer
• Risk for fluid volume deficit related to drug-induced adverse GI reactions
• Knowledge deficit related to drug therapy

Planning and implementation
• Drug acts as antiestrogen. Best results have been reported in patients with positive estrogen receptors.
• Make sure patient swallows enteric-coated tablets whole. Don't give antacids within 2 hours of dose.
Patient teaching
• Reassure patient that acute bone pain during drug therapy usually means that drug will produce good response. Tell her to take an analgesic for pain.
• Encourage female patient who is taking or has taken drug to have regular gynecologic examinations because of increased risk of uterine cancer.
• Advise patient to use barrier form of contraception because short-term therapy induces ovulation in premenopausal women.
• Advise female patient of childbearing age to avoid becoming pregnant during therapy and to consult with doctor before becoming pregnant.

Evaluation
• Patient responds well to drug.
• Patient maintains adequate hydration.
• Patient and family state understanding of drug therapy.

---

tamsulosin hydrochloride
(tam-soo-LOH-sin high-droh-KLOR-ighd)
Flomax

Pharmacologic class: alpha$_1$-adrenoceptor antagonist
Therapeutic class: BPH agent
Pregnancy risk category: B

How supplied
Capsules: 0.4 mg

Pharmacokinetics
Absorption: almost complete with over 90% absorbed following oral administration. Food increases bioavailability by 30%.

Distribution: distributed into extracellular fluids. Extensively bound to protein (94% to 99%).
Metabolism: primarily by cytochrome P-450 enzymes in the liver.
Excretion: 76% of drug eliminated in urine; 21% in feces. *Half-life:* 9 to 13 hours.

Route	Onset	Peak	Duration
P.O.	Unknown	4-5 hr	9-15 hr

Pharmacodynamics

Chemical effect: selectively blocks alpha receptors in the prostate, leading to relaxation of smooth muscles in the bladder neck and prostate, improving urine flow and reduction in symptoms of BPH.
Therapeutic effect: improves urine flow.

Indications and dosage

▶ **Treatment of BPH.** *Adults:* 0.4 mg P.O. once daily, administered 30 minutes after same meal each day. If no response after 2 to 4 weeks, dose may be increased to 0.8 mg P.O. once daily.

Adverse reactions

CNS: asthenia, *dizziness, headache,* insomnia, somnolence, syncope, vertigo.
CV: chest pain, orthostatic hypotension.
EENT: amblyopia, pharyngitis, *rhinitis,* sinusitis.
GI: diarrhea, nausea, tooth disorder.
GU: abnormal ejaculation, decreased libido.
Respiratory: increased cough.
Other: back pain, *infection.*

Interactions

Drug-drug. *Alpha-adrenergic blocking agents:* may interact with tamsulosin. Avoid concomitant use.
Cimetidine: decreased clearance of tamsulosin. Use with caution.

Contraindications and precautions

• Contraindicated in patients with hypersensitivity to drug or its components.

NURSING CONSIDERATIONS

✍ Assessment

• Assess patient for signs of prostatic hypertrophy including frequency of urination, nocturnal urination, and incidence of urinary hesitancy.
• Monitor patient for decreases in blood pressure and notify doctor.
• Evaluate patient's and family's knowledge of drug therapy.

✇ Nursing diagnoses

• Risk for injury related to decreased blood pressure and resulting syncope
• Altered urinary elimination related to underlying prostatic hypertrophy
• Knowledge deficit related to drug therapy

❯ Planning and implementation

• Know that symptoms of BPH and carcinoma of the prostate are similar; carcinoma should be ruled out before therapy starts.
• If treatment is interrupted for several days or more, restart therapy at one capsule daily as ordered.
• Know that drug may cause a sudden drop in blood pressure, especially after the first dose or when changing doses.
Patient teaching
• Instruct patient not to crush, chew, or open capsules.
• Tell patient to get up slowly from chair or bed during initiation of therapy and to avoid situations where injury could occur due to syncope. Advise him that drug may cause a sudden drop in blood pressure, especially after the first dose or when changing doses.
• Instruct patient not to drive or perform hazardous tasks for 12 hours following the initial dose or changes in dose until response can be monitored.
• Tell patient to take drug about 30 minutes following same meal each day.

✓ Evaluation

• Patient does not experience sudden decreases in blood pressure.

• Patient experiences normal urinary elimination patterns.
• Patient and family state understanding of drug therapy.

telmisartan
(tel-mih-SAR-tan)
Micardis

Pharmacologic class: angiotensin II receptor antagonist
Therapeutic class: antihypertensive
Pregnancy risk category: C (D in second and third trimesters)

How supplied
Tablets: 40 mg, 80 mg

Pharmacokinetics
Absorption: readily absorbed after oral administration.
Distribution: highly protein-bound; volume of distribution is about 500 L.
Metabolism: metabolized by conjugation to an inactive metabolite.
Elimination: mainly excreted unchanged in feces.

Route	Onset	Peak	Duration
P.O.	Unknown	0.5-1 hr	24 hr

Pharmacodynamics
Chemical effect: blocks the vasoconstricting and aldosterone-secreting effects of angiotensin II by selectively blocking the binding of angiotensin II to the AT_1 receptor in many tissues, such as vascular smooth muscle and the adrenal gland.
Therapeutic effect: lowers blood pressure.

Indications and dosage
Treatment of hypertension (used alone or in combination with other antihypertensive agents). *Adults:* 40 mg P.O. daily. Blood pressure response is dose-related over the range of 20 to 80 mg daily.

Adverse reactions
CNS: dizziness, pain, fatigue, headache.
CV: chest pain, hypertension, peripheral edema.
EENT: pharyngitis, sinusitis.
GI: abdominal pain, diarrhea, dyspepsia, nausea.
GU: urinary tract infection.
Hepatic: elevated liver enzymes.
Musculoskeletal: back pain, myalgia.
Respiratory: cough, upper respiratory tract infection.
Other: flulike symptoms.

Interactions
Drug-drug. *Digoxin:* increased digoxin plasma concentrations. Monitor digoxin levels closely.
Warfarin: slightly decreased warfarin plasma concentrations. Monitor INR.

Contraindications and precautions
• Contraindicated in patients hypersensitive to drug or its components. Safety and effectiveness have not been studied in patients age 18 or less.
• Use cautiously in patients with renal and hepatic insufficiency and in those with an activated renin-angiotensin system, such as volume- or salt-depleted patients (such as those being treated with high doses of diuretics).
• Know that drugs, such as telmisartan, that act directly on the renin-angiotensin system can cause fetal and neonatal morbidity and death when given to pregnant women. These problems have not been detected when exposure has been limited to the first trimester. If pregnancy is suspected, notify doctor because drug should be discontinued.

NURSING CONSIDERATIONS

Assessment
• Monitor for hypotension following initiation of drug. Place patient in supine position if hypotension occurs and administer I.V. of normal saline if necessary.

• Know that in patients whose renal function may depend on the activity of the renin-angiotensin-aldosterone system (such as those with severe heart failure), treatment with ACE inhibitors and angiotensin receptor antagonists has been associated with oliguria or progressive azotemia and (rarely) with acute renal failure or death.
• Be aware drug levels may be increased in patients with biliary obstruction because of inability to excrete drug.
• Drug is not removed by hemodialysis. Patients undergoing dialysis may develop orthostatic hypotension. Closely monitor blood pressure.
• Evaluate patient's and family's knowledge of drug therapy.

❖ **Nursing diagnoses**
• Risk for injury related to presence of hypertension
• Altered cerebral and cardiopulmonary tissue perfusion related to drug-induced hypotension
• Knowledge deficit related to drug therapy

▶ **Planning and implementation**
• Most of the antihypertensive effect is present within 2 weeks. Maximal blood pressure reduction is generally attained after 4 weeks. Diuretic may be added if blood pressure is not controlled by drug alone.
Patient teaching
• Inform female patient of childbearing age of consequences of second and third trimester exposure to drug. Instruct patient to report suspected pregnancy to doctor immediately.
• Advise breast-feeding patient about risk for adverse effects on infant and need to stop breast-feeding or discontinue drug, taking into account importance of drug to patient.
• Tell patient that transient hypotension may occur. Instruct him to lie down if feeling dizzy and to rise slowly from a lying to standing position or when climbing stairs.

• Instruct patient with heart failure to notify doctor about decreased urine output.
• Tell patient that drug may be taken without regard to meals.
• Inform patient that drug should not be removed from blister-sealed packet until immediately before use.

☑ **Evaluation**
• Patient does not experience injury from underlying disease.
• Patient does not experience hypotension and maintains adequate tissue perfusion.
• Patient and family state understanding of drug therapy.

temazepam
(teh-MAZ-ih-pam)
Euhypnos 10◇, Euhypnos 20◇, Normison◇, Restoril, Temaze◇

Pharmacologic class: benzodiazepine
Therapeutic class: sedative-hypnotic
Controlled substance schedule: IV
Pregnancy risk category: X

How supplied
Capsules: 7.5 mg, 15 mg, 20 mg◇, 30 mg

Pharmacokinetics
Absorption: well absorbed through GI tract.
Distribution: distributed widely throughout body; 98% protein-bound.
Metabolism: metabolized in liver to primarily inactive metabolites.
Excretion: metabolites excreted in urine.
Half-life: 10 to 17 hours.

Route	Onset	Peak	Duration
P.O.	Unknown	1-2 hr	Unknown

Pharmacodynamics
Chemical effect: unknown; probably acts on limbic system, thalamus, and hypothalamus of CNS to produce hypnotic effects.
Therapeutic effect: promotes sleep.

---

*Liquid form contains alcohol   **May contain tartrazine   ◆Canada   ◇ Australia   †OTC

Indications and dosage

► **Insomnia.** *Adults age 65 or less:* 7.5 to 30 mg P.O. 30 minutes before bedtime. *Adults over age 65:* 7.5 mg P.O. h.s.

Adverse reactions

CNS: *drowsiness, dizziness, lethargy,* disturbed coordination, daytime sedation, confusion, nightmares, vertigo, euphoria, weakness, headache, fatigue, nervousness, anxiety, depression.
EENT: blurred vision.
GI: diarrhea, nausea, dry mouth.
Other: physical and psychological dependence.

Interactions

Drug-drug. *CNS depressants, including narcotic analgesics:* increased CNS depression. Use together cautiously.
Drug-lifestyle. *Alcohol use:* increased CNS depression. Avoid concomitant use.

Contraindications and precautions

• Contraindicated in patients with hypersensitivity to benzodiazepines and in pregnant women.
• Drug is not recommended for use in breast-feeding women.
• Use cautiously in patients with chronic pulmonary insufficiency, impaired liver or kidney function, severe or latent depression, suicidal tendencies, or history of drug abuse.
• Safety of drug has not been established in children.

NURSING CONSIDERATIONS

⚕ Assessment
• Assess patient's sleeping disorder before therapy and regularly thereafter.
• Assess mental status before therapy. Elderly patients are more sensitive to drug's adverse CNS effects.
• Be alert for adverse reactions and drug interactions.
• Evaluate patient's and family's knowledge of drug therapy.

⊞ Nursing diagnoses
• Sleep pattern disturbance related to presence of insomnia
• Risk for injury related to drug-induced adverse CNS reactions
• Knowledge deficit related to drug therapy

⊠ Planning and implementation
• Prevent hoarding or self-overdosing by patient who is depressed, suicidal, or drug-dependent or who has history of drug abuse.
• Make sure patient has swallowed capsule before leaving bedside.
• Supervise walking and raise bed rails, particularly for elderly patient.
Patient teaching
• Warn patient to avoid activities that require mental alertness or physical coordination.

☑ Evaluation
• Patient states that drug induces sleep.
• Patient does not experience injury from adverse CNS reactions.
• Patient and family state understanding of drug therapy.

teniposide (VM-26)
(teh-NIP-uh-sighd)
Vumon

Pharmacologic class: podophyllotoxin (cell-cycle–phase-specific, G_2 and late S phase)
Therapeutic class: antineoplastic
Pregnancy risk category: D

How supplied

Injection: 50 mg/5 ml

Pharmacokinetics

Absorption: not applicable.
Distribution: distributed mainly in liver, kidneys, small intestine, and adrenals. Drug crosses blood-brain barrier to limited extent; highly bound to plasma proteins.

Reactions may be *common,* uncommon, *life-threatening,* or COMMON AND LIFE-THREATENING.

Metabolism: metabolized extensively in liver.
Excretion: about 40% eliminated through kidneys as unchanged drug or metabolites. *Half-life:* 5 hours.

Route	Onset	Peak	Duration
I.V.	Unknown	Unknown	Unknown

Pharmacodynamics

Chemical effect: acts in late S or early G_2 phase of cell cycle, thus preventing cells from entering mitosis.
Therapeutic effect: prevents reproduction of leukemic cells.

Indications and dosage

▶ **Refractory childhood acute lymphoblastic leukemia.** *Children:* optimum dosage hasn't been established. One protocol reported by manufacturer is 165 mg/m^2 I.V. twice weekly for eight or nine doses. Usually used in combination with other agents.

Adverse reactions

CV: hypotension from rapid infusion.
GI: *nausea, vomiting, mucositis, diarrhea.*
Hematologic: MYELOSUPPRESSION (dose-limiting), LEUKOPENIA, NEUTROPENIA, THROMBOCYTOPENIA, anemia.
Other: alopecia, *anaphylaxis* (rare), *hypersensitivity reactions* (chills, fever, urticaria, tachycardia, *bronchospasm,* dyspnea, hypotension, flushing); *phlebitis at injection site with extravasation.*

Interactions

Drug-drug. *Methotrexate:* may increase clearance and intracellular levels of methotrexate. Monitor closely.
Sodium salicylate, sulfamethizole, tolbutamide: may displace teniposide from protein-binding sites and increase toxicity. Monitor closely.

Contraindications and precautions

• Contraindicated in patients hypersensitive to drug or polyoxyethylated castor oil, an injection vehicle.

• Drug is not recommended for use in pregnant or breast-feeding women.

NURSING CONSIDERATIONS

✍ Assessment
• Assess patient's condition before therapy and regularly thereafter.
• Obtain baseline blood counts and kidney and liver function tests, as ordered, and then monitor periodically.
• Monitor blood pressure before therapy and at 30-minute intervals during infusion.
• Be alert for adverse reactions and drug interactions.
• Evaluate patient's and family's knowledge of drug therapy.

✠ Nursing diagnoses
• Altered health maintenance related to presence of leukemia
• Altered protection related to drug-induced immunosuppression
• Knowledge deficit related to drug therapy

▶ Planning and implementation
• Some doctors may decide to use drug despite patient's history of hypersensitivity because therapeutic benefits may outweigh risks. Such patients should be treated with antihistamines and corticosteroids before infusion begins and be closely watched during drug administration.
• Have diphenhydramine, hydrocortisone, epinephrine, and appropriate emergency equipment available to establish airway in case of anaphylaxis.
• Follow institutional policy to reduce risks. Preparation and administration of parenteral form are associated with carcinogenic, mutagenic, and teratogenic risks for personnel.
• Dilute drug in D_5W or 0.9% NaCl injection to concentration of 0.1, 0.2, 0.4, or 1 mg/ml. Don't agitate vigorously; precipitation may occur. Discard cloudy solutions. Prepare and store in glass con-

---

*Liquid form contains alcohol   **May contain tartrazine   ◆Canada   ◇Australia   †OTC

tainers. Infuse over 45 to 90 minutes to prevent hypotension.
• Don't mix with other drugs or solutions.
• Heparin is physically incompatible with drug. Don't mix together.
• Ensure careful placement of I.V. catheter. Extravasation can result in local tissue necrosis or sloughing.
• Don't administer drug through membrane-type in-line filter because diluent may dissolve filter.
• Know that solutions containing 0.5 to 1 mg/ml are stable for 4 hours; those containing 0.1 to 0.2 mg/ml are stable for 6 hours at room temperature.
• Report systolic blood pressure below 90 mm Hg and stop infusion.

Patient teaching
• Tell patient to report discomfort at I.V. site immediately.
• Encourage adequate fluid intake to increase urine output and facilitate excretion of uric acid.
• Review infection-control and bleeding precautions to take during therapy.
• Reassure patient that hair growth should return after treatment stops.
• Instruct patient and parents to notify doctor if adverse reactions occur.

☑ **Evaluation**
• Patient responds well to drug.
• Patient does not develop serious complications from immunosuppression.
• Patient and family state understanding of drug therapy.

---

terazosin hydrochloride
(ter-uh-ZOH-sin high-droh-KLOR-ighd)
Hytrin

Pharmacologic class: selective alpha$_1$-adrenergic blocker
Therapeutic class: antihypertensive
Pregnancy risk category: C

How supplied
Capsules: 1 mg, 2 mg, 5 mg, 10 mg

Pharmacokinetics
Absorption: absorbed rapidly with about 90% of dose being bioavailable.
Distribution: about 90% to 94% plasma protein-bound.
Metabolism: metabolized in liver.
Excretion: about 40% excreted in urine, 60% in feces, mostly as metabolites. Up to 30% may be excreted unchanged.
Half-life: about 12 hours.

Route	Onset	Peak	Duration
P.O.	≤ 15 min	2-3 hr	24 hr

Pharmacodynamics
Chemical effect: decreases blood pressure by vasodilation produced in response to blockade of alpha$_1$-adrenergic receptors. Improves urine flow in patients with BPH by blocking alpha$_1$-adrenergic receptors in smooth muscle of bladder neck and prostate, thus relieving urethral pressure and reestablishing urine flow.
Therapeutic effect: lowers blood pressure and relieves symptoms of BPH.

Indications and dosage
▶ **Hypertension.** *Adults:* initially, 1 mg P.O. h.s., increased gradually based on response. Usual dosage range is 1 to 5 mg daily. Maximum recommended dosage is 20 mg/day.
▶ **Symptomatic BPH.** *Adults:* initially, 1 mg P.O. h.s. Dosage increased in stepwise manner to 2 mg, 5 mg, and 10 mg once daily to achieve optimal response. Most patients require 10 mg daily for optimal response.

Adverse reactions
CNS: *asthenia, dizziness, headache,* nervousness, paresthesias, somnolence.
CV: palpitation*s,* postural hypotension, tachycardia, *peripheral edema.*
EENT: nasal congestion, sinusitis, blurred vision.
GI: nausea.
GU: impotence, decreased libido.
Musculoskeletal: back pain, muscle pain.
Respiratory: dyspnea.

Reactions may be *common,* uncommon, *life-threatening,* or COMMON AND LIFE-THREATENING.

Interactions

Drug-drug. *Antihypertensives:* excessive hypotension. Use together cautiously. *Clonidine:* clonidine's antihypertensive effect may be decreased. Monitor patient.

Contraindications and precautions

• Contraindicated in patients with hypersensitivity to drug.
• Use cautiously in pregnant or breast-feeding women.
• Safety of drug has not been established in children.

NURSING CONSIDERATIONS

⬛ Assessment
• Assess patient's condition before therapy and regularly thereafter.
• Monitor blood pressure frequently.
• Be alert for adverse reactions and drug interactions.
• Evaluate patient's and family's knowledge of drug therapy.

⬕ Nursing diagnoses
• Risk for injury related to presence of hypertension
• Sexual dysfunction related to drug-induced impotence
• Knowledge deficit related to drug therapy

⬲ Planning and implementation
• If drug is stopped for several days, patient will need to be retitrated using initial dosing regimen.
Patient teaching
• Tell patient not to stop drug but to call doctor if adverse reactions occur.
• Tell patient to take the first dose at bedtime and go to sleep. If he must get up, he should do so slowly to prevent syncope.
• Warn patient to avoid activities that require mental alertness for 12 hours after first dose.

⬛ Evaluation
• Patient's blood pressure is normal.

• Patient develops and maintains positive attitude toward his sexuality despite impotence.
• Patient and family state understanding of drug therapy.

terbutaline sulfate

(ter-BYOO-tuh-leen SUL-fayt)
Brethaire, Brethine, Bricanyl

Pharmacologic class: beta$_2$-adrenergic agonist
Therapeutic class: bronchodilator
Pregnancy risk category: B

How supplied

Tablets: 2.5 mg, 5 mg
Aerosol inhaler: 200 mcg/metered spray
Injection: 1 mg/ml

Pharmacokinetics

Absorption: 33% to 50% of oral dose absorbed through GI tract; unknown after inhalation or S.C. administration.
Distribution: widely distributed throughout body.
Metabolism: partially metabolized in liver to inactive compounds.
Excretion: excreted primarily in urine.

Route	Onset	Peak	Duration
P.O.	30 min	2-3 hr	4-8 hr
S.C.	≤ 15 min	30-60 min	1.5-4 hr
Inhalation	5-30 min	1-2 hr	3-6 hr

Pharmacodynamics

Chemical effect: relaxes bronchial smooth muscle by acting on beta$_2$-adrenergic receptors.
Therapeutic effect: improves breathing ability.

Indications and dosage

▶ **Bronchospasm in patients with reversible obstructive airway disease.**
Adults and children age 15 and older: 5 mg P.O. t.i.d. at 6-hour intervals. Alternatively, 0.25 mg S.C. may be re-

peated in 15 to 30 minutes; maximum 0.5 mg q 4 hours. Or, 2 inhalations q 4 to 6 hours, with 1 minute elapsing between inhalations. *Children ages 12 to 15:* 2.5 mg P.O. t.i.d. Alternatively, 2 inhalations q 4 to 6 hours with 1 minute elapsing between inhalations.

Adverse reactions

CNS: *nervousness, tremors, headache, drowsiness, dizziness,* weakness.
CV: *palpitations,* tachycardia, *arrhythmias,* flushing.
EENT: dryness and irritation of nose and throat (with inhaled form).
GI: *vomiting, nausea,* heartburn.
Respiratory: *paradoxical bronchospasm* (with prolonged use), dyspnea.
Other: hypokalemia (with high doses), diaphoresis.

Interactions

Drug-drug. *Cardiac glycosides, cyclopropane, halogenated inhalation anesthetics, levodopa:* increased risk of arrhythmias. Monitor patient closely.
CNS stimulants: increased CNS stimulation. Avoid concomitant use.
MAO inhibitors: when given with sympathomimetics, may cause severe hypertension (hypertensive crisis). Avoid concomitant use.
Propranolol, other beta blockers: blocked bronchodilating effects of terbutaline. Avoid concomitant use.

Contraindications and precautions

• Contraindicated in patients with hypersensitivity to drug or sympathomimetic amines.
• Use cautiously in patient with CV disorders, hyperthyroidism, diabetes, or seizure disorders and in pregnant or breast-feeding women.
• Safety of drug has not been established in children age 11 and younger.

NURSING CONSIDERATIONS

Assessment
• Assess patient's respiratory condition before therapy and regularly thereafter.
• Monitor closely for toxicity, especially if patient is using tablets and aerosol concomitantly.
• Evaluate patient's and family's knowledge of drug therapy.

Nursing diagnoses
• Ineffective breathing pattern related to underlying respiratory condition
• Pain related to drug-induced headache
• Knowledge deficit related to drug therapy

Planning and implementation
P.O. use: Follow normal protocol.
S.C. use: Inject in lateral deltoid area.
– Protect injection from light. Do not use if discolored.
Inhalation use: Follow normal protocol. If patient is also to receive steroid by inhalation, administer terbutaline first, wait 5 minutes, and then administer steroid inhaler.
• Know that patient may use tablets and aerosol concomitantly.
• Notify doctor immediately if bronchospasms develop during therapy.
• Obtain order for mild analgesic to treat drug-induced headache.
Patient teaching
• Ensure that patient and family understand why drug is needed.
• Teach patient to use metered-dose inhaler: Clear nasal passages and throat. Breathe out, expelling as much air from lungs as possible. Place mouthpiece well into mouth as dose from inhaler is released, and inhale deeply. Hold breath for several seconds, remove mouthpiece, and exhale slowly.
• If more than one inhalation is ordered, tell patient to wait at least 2 minutes before repeating procedure.
• Tell patient who also is using steroid inhaler to use bronchodilator first, then

---

Reactions may be *common,* uncommon, *life-threatening,* or COMMON AND LIFE-THREATENING.

wait about 5 minutes before using steroid.
• Warn patient to report paradoxical bronchospasm and stop drug.
• Warn patient that tolerance may develop with prolonged use.

🗹 **Evaluation**
• Patient's breathing is improved.
• Patient's headache is relieved with mild analgesic.
• Patient and family state understanding of drug therapy.

terconazole
(ter-KON-uh-zohl)
Terazol 3 Vaginal Cream, Terazol 3 Vaginal Suppositories, Terazol 7 Vaginal Cream

Pharmacologic class: triazole derivative
Therapeutic class: antifungal
Pregnancy risk category: C

How supplied
Vaginal cream: 0.4%, 0.8%
Vaginal suppositories: 80 mg

Pharmacokinetics
Absorption: minimal absorption may range from 5% to 16%.
Distribution: mainly local.
Metabolism: unknown.
Excretion: unknown.

Route	Onset	Peak	Duration
Vaginal	Unknown	Unknown	Unknown

Pharmacodynamics
Chemical effect: unknown; may increase fungal cell membrane permeability (*Candida* species only).
Therapeutic effect: impairs fungus function. Spectrum of activity is *Candida* species only.

Indications and dosage
▶ **Vulvovaginal candidiasis.** *Adults:* 1 applicatorful of cream or 1 suppository

inserted into vagina h.s.; 0.4% cream used for 7 consecutive days; 0.8% cream or 80-mg suppository used for 3 consecutive days. Course repeated, if necessary, after reconfirmation by smear or culture.

Adverse reactions
CNS: *headache.*
GI: abdominal pain.
GU: dysmenorrhea, pain of the female genitalia, vulvovaginal burning.
Skin: irritation, photosensitivity, *pruritus.*
Other: fever, chills, body aches.

Interactions
None significant.

Contraindications and precautions
• Contraindicated in patients with known hypersensitivity to drug or inactive ingredients in formulation.
• Drug is not recommended for use in breast-feeding women.
• Use cautiously in pregnant women.

NURSING CONSIDERATIONS
Assessment
• Assess patient's infection before therapy and regularly thereafter.
• Be alert for adverse reactions.
• Evaluate patient's and family's knowledge of drug therapy.

Nursing diagnoses
• Infection related to presence of susceptible fungi
• Pain related to drug-induced burning
• Knowledge deficit related to drug therapy

Planning and implementation
• Insert cream using applicator supplied.
• If vaginal suppository is used, have patient remain supine for about 30 minutes after insertion.
• Report fever, chills, other flulike symptoms, or sensitivity, and stop drug.

Patient teaching
• Instruct patient how to insert cream or suppository.
• Advise patient to continue treatment during menstrual period. Tell her not to use tampons.
• Tell patient to use for full treatment period prescribed. Explain how to prevent reinfection.

☑ **Evaluation**
• Patient is free from infection.
• Patient states that drug-induced burning is tolerable.
• Patient and family state understanding of drug therapy.

testolactone
(tes-tuh-LAK-tohn)
Teslac

Pharmacologic class: androgen
Therapeutic class: antineoplastic
Controlled substance schedule: III
Pregnancy risk category: C

How supplied

Tablets: 50 mg

Pharmacokinetics

Absorption: absorbed well across GI tract.
Distribution: widely distributed in total body water.
Metabolism: extensively metabolized in liver.
Excretion: testolactone and its metabolites excreted primarily in urine.

Route	Onset	Peak	Duration
P.O.	6-12 wk	Unknown	Unknown

Pharmacodynamics

Chemical effect: exact antineoplastic action unknown; probably changes tumor's hormonal environment and alters neoplastic process.
Therapeutic effect: hinders breast cancer cell activity.

Indications and dosage

▶ **Advanced postmenopausal breast cancer.** *Women:* 250 mg P.O. q.i.d.

Adverse reactions

CNS: paresthesias, peripheral neuropathy.
CV: increased blood pressure, edema.
GI: nausea, vomiting, diarrhea, anorexia, glossitis.
Skin: erythema, nail changes, alopecia.

Interactions

Drug-drug. *Oral anticoagulants:* increased pharmacologic effects. Monitor patient carefully.

Contraindications and precautions

• Contraindicated in patients hypersensitive to drug and in men with breast cancer.
• Drug is not recommended for use in breast-feeding women.
• Use cautiously in pregnant women.
• Drug is not indicated for use in children.

NURSING CONSIDERATIONS

☢ **Assessment**
• Assess patient's breast cancer before therapy and regularly thereafter.
• Monitor fluid and electrolyte levels, especially calcium level.
• Be alert for adverse reactions and drug interactions.
• Evaluate patient's and family's knowledge of drug therapy.

⊞ **Nursing diagnoses**
• Altered health maintenance related to presence of breast cancer
• Sensory or perceptual alterations (tactile) related to drug-induced paresthesia and peripheral neuropathy
• Knowledge deficit related to drug therapy

▷ **Planning and implementation**
• Force fluids to aid calcium excretion, and encourage exercise to prevent hyper-

calcemia. Immobilized patients are prone to hypercalcemia.
• Higher-than-recommended doses do not promote remission.
Patient teaching
• Inform patient that therapeutic response isn't immediate; it may take up to 3 months for benefit to be noted.
• Encourage patient to perform exercises and to drink plenty of fluids to help prevent hypercalcemia.
• Tell patient to report adverse effects.

☑ **Evaluation**
• Patient responds well to drug.
• Patient lists ways to protect against risk of injury caused by diminished tactile sensation.
• Patient and family state understanding of drug therapy.

---

testosterone
(tes-TOS-teh-rohn)
Andronaq-50, Histerone-50, Histerone 100, Testamone 100, Testaqua, Testoject-50

testosterone cypionate
Andronate 100, Andronate 200, depAndro 100, depAndro 200, Depotest, Depo-Testosterone, Duratest-100, Duratest-200, T-Cypionate, Testred Cypionate 200, Virilon IM

testosterone enanthate
Andro L.A. 200, Andropository 200, Andryl 200, Delatest, Delatestryl, Durathate-200, Everone 200, Testrin-P.A.

testosterone propionate
Malogen in Oil♦, Testex

Pharmacologic class: androgen
Therapeutic class: androgen replacement, antineoplastic
Controlled substance schedule: III
Pregnancy risk category: X

How supplied
testosterone
Injection (aqueous suspension):
25 mg/ml, 50 mg/ml, 100 mg/ml
testosterone cypionate
Injection (in oil): 100 mg/ml, 200 mg/ml
testosterone enanthate
Injection (in oil): 100 mg/ml, 200 mg/ml
testosterone propionate
Injection (in oil): 100 mg/ml

Pharmacokinetics
Absorption: unknown.
Distribution: 98% to 99% plasma protein–bound, primarily to testosterone-estradiol–binding globulin.
Metabolism: metabolized in liver.
Excretion: excreted in urine. *Half-life:* 10 to 100 minutes.

Route	Onset	Peak	Duration
I.M.	Unknown	Unknown	Unknown

Pharmacodynamics
Chemical effect: stimulates target tissues to develop normally in androgen-deficient men. Drug may have some antiestrogen properties, making it useful to treat certain estrogen-dependent breast cancers. Its action in postpartum breast engorgement is not known because drug does not suppress lactation.
Therapeutic effect: increases testosterone levels, inhibits some estrogen activity, and relieves postpartum breast pain and engorgement.

Indications and dosage
▶ **Male hypogonadism. Testosterone.**
Adults: 10 to 25 mg I.M. two to three times weekly. **Testosterone cypionate, testosterone enanthate.** *Adults:* 50 to 400 mg I.M. q 2 to 4 weeks.
Testosterone propionate. *Adults:* 10 to 25 mg I.M. two to three times weekly.
▶ **Delayed puberty in males. Testosterone, testosterone propionate.** *Children:* 25 to 50 mg I.M. two or three times weekly for up to 6 months.

▶ **Metastatic breast cancer in women 1 to 5 years postmenopausal. Testosterone.** *Adults:* 100 mg I.M. three times weekly. **Testosterone propionate.** *Adults:* 50 to 100 mg I.M. three times weekly. **Testosterone cypionate, testosterone enanthate.** *Adults:* 200 to 400 mg I.M. q 2 to 4 weeks.
▶ **Postpartum breast pain and engorgement. Testosterone, testosterone propionate.** *Adults:* 25 to 50 mg I.M. daily for 3 to 4 days.

Adverse reactions

CNS: headache, anxiety, depression, paresthesia, sleep apnea syndrome.
GI: nausea.
GU: hypoestrogenic effects in women (*acne, edema, oily skin, hirsutism, hoarseness weight gain,* clitoral enlargement, decreased or increased libido); hypoestrogenic effects in women (flushing; diaphoresis; vaginitis, including itching, drying, and burning; vaginal bleeding; menstrual irregularities); excessive hormonal effects in men (prepubertal—premature epiphyseal closure, *acne,* priapism, *growth of body and facial hair,* phallic enlargement; postpubertal—testicular atrophy, oligospermia, decreased ejaculatory volume, impotence, gynecomastia, epididymitis); bladder irritability.
Hematologic: polycythemia, suppression of clotting factors.
Hepatic: reversible jaundice, cholestatic hepatitis, abnormal liver enzyme levels.
Metabolic: hypercalcemia.
Skin: pain and induration at injection site, local edema, hypersensitivity skin manifestations.
Other: edema, androgenic effects in women.

Interactions

Drug-drug. *Hepatotoxic drugs:* increased risk of hepatotoxicity. Monitor patient closely.
Insulin, oral antidiabetic agents: altered dosage requirements. Monitor blood glucose level in diabetic patients.

Oral anticoagulants: altered dosage requirements. Monitor PT and INR.

Contraindications and precautions

• Contraindicated in men with breast or prostate cancer; in patients with hypercalcemia; in those with cardiac, hepatic, or renal decompensation; and in pregnant or breast-feeding women.
• Use cautiously in elderly patients.

NURSING CONSIDERATIONS

⚏ Assessment
• Assess patient's condition before therapy and regularly thereafter.
• Periodically monitor calcium level and liver function test results.
• Monitor prepubertal boys by X-ray for rate of bone maturation.
• Be alert for adverse reactions and drug interactions.
• Evaluate patient's and family's knowledge of drug therapy.

⊞ Nursing diagnoses
• Altered health maintenance related to underlying condition
• Body image disturbance related to drug-induced adverse androgenic reactions
• Knowledge deficit related to drug therapy

⊠ Planning and implementation
• Avoid use in female patient of childbearing age until pregnancy is ruled out.
• Administer daily dosage requirement in divided doses for best results.
• Store preparations at room temperature. If crystals appear, warm and shake bottle to disperse them.
• Inject deep into upper outer quadrant of gluteal muscle. Rotate sites to prevent muscle atrophy. Report soreness at site because of possibility of postinfection furunculosis.
• Unless contraindicated, use with diet high in calories and protein. Give small, frequent feedings.

Reactions may be *common,* uncommon, *life-threatening,* or COMMON AND LIFE-THREATENING.

• Report signs of virilization in female patient.

• Know that edema generally can be controlled with sodium restriction or diuretics.

• Therapeutic response in breast cancer usually appears within 3 months. Therapy should be stopped if signs of disease progression appear. In metastatic breast cancer, hypercalcemia usually signals progression of bone metastases. Report signs of hypercalcemia.

• Androgens may alter results of laboratory studies during therapy and for 2 to 3 weeks after therapy ends.

Patient teaching

• Make sure patient understands importance of using effective nonhormonal contraceptive during therapy.

• Instruct male patient to report priapism, reduced ejaculatory volume, and gynecomastia. Drug may need to be discontinued.

• Inform female patient that virilization may occur. Tell her to report androgenic effects immediately. Stopping drug will prevent further androgenic changes but will probably not reverse those already present.

• Teach patient to recognize and report signs of hypoglycemia.

• Instruct patient to follow dietary measures to combat drug-induced adverse reactions.

☑ **Evaluation**

• Patient responds well to drug.

• Patient states acceptance of altered body image.

• Patient and family state understanding of drug therapy.

---

testosterone transdermal system
(tes-TOS-teh-rohn tranz-DER-mal SIHS-tum)
Androderm, Testoderm

Pharmacologic class: androgen
Therapeutic class: androgen replacement

Controlled substance schedule: III
Pregnancy risk category: X

How supplied
Transdermal system: 2.5 mg/day, 4 mg/day, 5 mg/day, 6 mg/day

Pharmacokinetics
Absorption: absorbed from scrotal skin after application.
Distribution: chiefly bound in serum to sex hormone–binding globulin.
Metabolism: metabolized in liver.
Excretion: excreted in urine. *Half-life:* 10 to 100 minutes.

Route	Onset	Peak	Duration
Trans-dermal	Unknown	2-4 hr	2 hr after removal

Pharmacodynamics
Chemical effect: stimulates target tissues to develop normally in androgen-deficient men.
Therapeutic effect: increases testosterone in androgen-deficient men.

Indications and dosage
▶ **Primary or hypogonadotropic hypogonadism in men age 18 and older.**
Testoderm. *Adults:* one 6-mg/day patch applied to scrotal area daily. If scrotal area is inadequate for 6-mg/day patch, therapy started with 4-mg/day patch. Patch worn for 22 to 24 hours daily.
Androderm. *Adults:* 5 mg/day either as two 2.5 mg/day systems or one 5 mg/day system applied h.s. to clean, dry skin on back, abdomen, upper arms, or thighs.

Adverse reactions
CV: *CVA,* headache, depression.
GU: gynecomastia, prostatitis, prostate abnormalities, urinary tract infection, breast tenderness.
Skin: acne, *pruritus,* irritation, *blister under system,* allergic contact dermatitis; burning, induration (at application site).
Other: GI bleeding.

Interactions

Drug-drug. *Antidiabetic agents:* altered antidiabetic agent dosage requirements. Monitor blood glucose level.
Oral anticoagulants: altered anticoagulant dosage requirements. Monitor PT and INR.
Oxyphenbutazone: may elevate serum level of oxyphenbutazone. Monitor patient for adverse reactions.

Contraindications and precautions

• Contraindicated in patients hypersensitive to drug, in women, and in men with known or suspected breast or prostate cancer.
• Use cautiously in elderly men because they may be at greater risk for prostatic hyperplasia or prostate cancer and in patients with preexisting renal, hepatic, or cardiac disease.
• Drug is not indicated for use in children.

NURSING CONSIDERATIONS

🖎 Assessment
• Assess patient's condition before therapy and regularly thereafter.
• Because chronic use of systemic androgens is associated with polycythemia, monitor hematocrit and hemoglobin values periodically in patient on long-term therapy, as ordered.
• Periodically assess liver function tests, serum lipid profiles, and prostatic acid phosphatase and prostate-specific antigen levels, as ordered.
• Be alert for adverse reactions and drug interactions.
• Evaluate patient's and family's knowledge of drug therapy.

🖎 Nursing diagnoses
• Sexual dysfunction related to androgen deficiency
• Risk for impaired skin integrity related to drug-induced irritation at application site
• Knowledge deficit related to drug therapy

🖎 Planning and implementation
• Apply Testoderm system on clean, dry scrotal skin. Dry shave scrotal hair (don't use chemical depilatories).
• Apply Androderm to clean, dry skin on back, abdomen, upper arms, or thighs.
Patient teaching
• Teach patient how to apply transdermal system.
• Tell patient that topical testosterone preparations can cause virilization in female partners. These women should report acne or changes in body hair distribution.
• Advise patient to report persistent erections, nausea, vomiting, changes in skin color, or ankle edema to doctor.

🖎 Evaluation
• Patient states that he can resume normal sexual activity.
• Patient maintains normal skin integrity.
• Patient and family state understanding of drug therapy.

---

tetanus immune globulin, human
(TET-uh-nus ih-MYOON GLOH-byoo-lin, HYOO-mun)
Homo-Tet, Hu-Tet, Hyper-Tet

Pharmacologic class: immune serum
Therapeutic class: tetanus prophylaxis
Pregnancy risk category: C

How supplied

Injection: 250 units per vial or syringe

Pharmacokinetics

Absorption: absorbed slowly.
Distribution: unknown.
Metabolism: unknown.
Excretion: unknown. *Half-life:* about 28 days.

Route	Onset	Peak	Duration
I.M.	Unknown	2-3 days	About 4 wk

Pharmacodynamics

Chemical effect: provides passive immunity to tetanus.
Therapeutic effect: prevents tetanus.

Indications and dosage

▶ **Tetanus exposure.** *Adults and children over age 7:* 250 units I.M. *Children under age 7:* 4 units/kg I.M.
▶ **Tetanus treatment.** *Adults and children:* single doses of 3,000 to 6,000 units I.M. have been used. Optimal dosage has not been established.

Adverse reactions

Skin: pain, stiffness, erythema at injection site.
Other: slight fever, *hypersensitivity reactions, anaphylaxis, angioedema,* nephrotic syndrome.

Interactions

Drug-drug. *Live-virus vaccines:* may interfere with response. Defer administration of live-virus vaccines for 3 months after administration of tetanus immune globulin.

Contraindications and precautions

• Contraindicated in patients with thrombocytopenia or coagulation disorders that would contraindicate I.M. injection unless potential benefits outweigh risks.
• Use cautiously in pregnant or breast-feeding women.

NURSING CONSIDERATIONS

Assessment
• Obtain history of injury, tetanus immunizations, last tetanus toxoid injection, allergies, and reaction to immunizations.
• Antibodies remain at effective level for about 4 weeks (several times the duration of antitoxin-induced antibodies), which protects patient for incubation period of most tetanus cases.
• Be alert for adverse reactions and drug interactions.

• Evaluate patient's and family's knowledge of drug therapy.

Nursing diagnoses
• Risk for injury related to potential for tetanus to occur
• Knowledge deficit related to drug therapy

Planning and implementation
• Have epinephrine 1:1,000 available to treat hypersensitivity reactions.
• Drug is used only if wound is more than 24 hours old or if patient has had fewer than two tetanus toxoid injections.
• Thoroughly clean wound and remove all foreign matter.
• Inject drug into deltoid muscle for adult and child age 3 and older and into anterolateral aspect of thigh in neonate and child under age 3.
• Do not confuse drug with tetanus toxoid. Tetanus immune globulin is not a substitute for tetanus toxoid, which should be given at same time to produce active immunization. Don't give at same site as toxoid.
Patient teaching
• Warn patient that pain and tenderness at injection site may occur. Suggest use of mild analgesic for pain relief.

Evaluation
• Patient does not develop tetanus.
• Patient and family state understanding of drug therapy.

tetracycline hydrochloride
(tet-ruh-SIGH-kleen high-droh-KLOR-ighd)
Achromycin V, Apo-Tetra♦, Mysteclin 250◊, Nor-Tet, Novo-Tetra♦, Panmycin**, Panmycin P◊, Robitet, Sumycin, Tetracap, Tetralan, Tetrex◊

Pharmacologic class: tetracycline
Therapeutic class: antibiotic
Pregnancy risk category: NR

How supplied

Tablets: 250 mg, 500 mg
Capsules: 100 mg, 250 mg, 500 mg
Oral suspension: 125 mg/5 ml

Pharmacokinetics

Absorption: 75% to 80% absorbed. Food or milk products significantly reduce oral absorption.
Distribution: distributed widely in body tissues and fluids. CSF penetration is poor. Drug is 20% to 67% protein-bound.
Metabolism: not metabolized.
Excretion: excreted primarily unchanged in urine. *Half-life:* 6 to 11 hours.

Route	Onset	Peak	Duration
P.O.	Unknown	2-4 hr	Unknown

Pharmacodynamics

Chemical effect: unknown; thought to exert bacteriostatic effect by binding to 30S ribosomal subunit of microorganisms, thus inhibiting protein synthesis.
Therapeutic effect: hinders bacterial activity. Spectrum of activity includes such gram-negative and gram-positive organisms as *Chlamydia, Mycoplasma, Rickettsia,* and spirochetes.

Indications and dosage

▶ **Infections caused by sensitive gram-negative and gram-positive organisms, including *Chlamydia, Mycoplasma, Rickettsia,* and organisms that cause trachoma.** *Adults:* 1 to 2 g P.O. divided into two to four doses. *Children over age 8:* 25 to 50 mg/kg P.O. daily divided into four doses.
▶ **Uncomplicated urethral, endocervical, or rectal infection caused by *Chlamydia trachomatis.*** *Adults:* 500 mg P.O. q.i.d. for at least 7 days.
▶ **Brucellosis.** *Adults:* 500 mg P.O. q 6 hours for 3 weeks combined with 1 g of streptomycin I.M. q 12 hours first week and daily the second week.
▶ **Gonorrhea in patients sensitive to penicillin.** *Adults:* initially, 1.5 g P.O.; then 500 mg q 6 hours for 4 days.

▶ **Syphilis in nonpregnant patients sensitive to penicillin.** *Adults:* 500 mg P.O. q.i.d. for 15 days.
▶ **Acne.** *Adults and adolescents:* initially, 125 to 250 mg P.O. q 6 hours; then 125 to 500 mg daily or every other day.

Adverse reactions

CNS: dizziness, headache, *intracranial hypertension (pseudotumor cerebri).*
CV: pericarditis.
EENT: sore throat, glossitis, dysphagia.
GI: anorexia, *epigastric distress, nausea,* vomiting, *diarrhea,* esophagitis, oral candidiasis, stomatitis, enterocolitis, inflammatory lesions in anogenital region.
GU: *increased BUN level.*
Hematologic: *neutropenia, thrombocytopenia,* eosinophilia.
Hepatic: elevated liver enzyme levels.
Musculoskeletal: *permanent discoloration of teeth, enamel defects, and retardation of bone growth if used in children under age 9.*
Skin: candidal superinfection, maculopapular and erythematous rashes, urticaria, photosensitivity, increased pigmentation.
Other: hypersensitivity reactions.

Interactions

Drug-drug. *Antacids (including sodium bicarbonate); antidiarrheals containing kaolin, pectin, or bismuth subsalicylate; laxatives containing aluminum, magnesium, or calcium:* decreased antibiotic absorption. Give antibiotic 1 hour before or 2 hours after any of the above.
Ferrous sulfate, other iron products, zinc: decreased antibiotic absorption. Give tetracyclines 3 hours after or 2 hours before iron.
Lithium carbonate: may alter serum lithium level. Monitor patient.
Methoxyflurane: may cause severe nephrotoxicity with tetracyclines. Monitor patient carefully.
Oral anticoagulants: potentiated anticoagulant effects. Monitor PT and adjust anticoagulant dosage.

Reactions may be *common*, uncommon, *life-threatening*, or COMMON AND LIFE-THREATENING.

Oral contraceptives: decreased contraceptive effectiveness and increased risk of breakthrough bleeding. Use nonhormonal form of birth control.
Penicillins: may interfere with bactericidal action of penicillins. Avoid using together.
Drug-food. *Milk, dairy products, other foods:* decreased antibiotic absorption. Give antibiotic 1 hour before or 2 hours after any of the above.
Drug-lifestyle. *Sun exposure:* photosensitivity reactions may occur. Take precautions.

Contraindications and precautions

• Contraindicated in patients with hypersensitivity to tetracyclines.
• Drug is not recommended for use in breast-feeding women.
• Use with extreme caution in patients with impaired kidney or liver function. Also use with extreme caution (if at all) during last half of pregnancy and in children under age 8 because drug may cause permanent discoloration of teeth, enamel defects, and bone growth retardation.

NURSING CONSIDERATIONS

Assessment
• Assess patient's infection before therapy and regularly thereafter.
• Obtain specimen for culture and sensitivity tests before first dose. Therapy may begin pending results.
• Monitor patient's hydration status if adverse GI reactions occur.
• Be alert for adverse reactions and drug interactions.
• Evaluate patient's and family's knowledge of drug therapy.

Nursing diagnoses
• Infection related to presence of susceptible bacteria
• Risk for fluid volume deficit related to drug-induced adverse GI reactions
• Knowledge deficit related to drug therapy

Planning and implementation
• Check expiration date. Outdated or deteriorated tetracyclines have been associated with reversible nephrotoxicity (Fanconi's syndrome).
• Administer drug on empty stomach.
• Don't expose drug to light or heat.
• Know that drug may cause false-negative reading with glucose enzymatic tests (Diastix).
Patient teaching
• Explain that effectiveness of drug is reduced when taken with milk or other dairy products, food, antacids, or iron products. Tell patient to take drug with full glass of water on empty stomach, at least 1 hour before or 2 hours after meals. Also, tell him to take drug at least 1 hour before bedtime to prevent esophagitis.
• Tell patient to take drug exactly as prescribed, even after he feels better, and to take entire amount prescribed.
• Warn patient to avoid direct sunlight and ultraviolet light. Recommend use of sunscreen to help prevent photosensitivity reactions. Tell him that photosensitivity persists after drug is stopped.

Evaluation
• Patient is free from infection.
• Patient maintains adequate hydration.
• Patient and family state understanding of drug therapy.

theophylline
(thee-OF-ih-lin)
Immediate-release liquids
Accurbron*, Aquaphyllin, Asmalix*, Bronkodyl*, Elixomin*, Elixophyllin*, Lanophyllin*, Slo-Phyllin, Theolair Liquid
Immediate-release tablets and capsules
Bronkodyl, Elixophyllin, Nuelin◊, Slo-Phyllin
Timed-release tablets
Constant-T, Quibron-T/SR Dividose, Respbid, Sustaire, Theo-Dur, Theolair-SR, Theo-Time, Theo-X, Uniphyl

---

Timed-release capsules
Aerolate, Elixophyllin SR, Nuelin-SR◊,
Slo-bid Gyrocaps, Slo-Phyllin, Theo-24,
Theobid Duracaps, Theobid Jr.
Duracaps, Theochron, Theo-Dur Sprinkle,
Theospan-SR, Theovent Long-Acting

theophylline sodium glycinate

Pharmacologic class: xanthine derivative
Therapeutic class: bronchodilator
Pregnancy risk category: C

How supplied

theophylline
Tablets: 100 mg, 125 mg, 200 mg,
250 mg, 300 mg
Tablets (chewable): 100 mg
Tablets (extended-release): 100 mg,
200 mg, 250 mg, 300 mg, 400 mg,
450 mg, 500 mg
Capsules: 100 mg, 200 mg
Capsules (extended-release): 50 mg,
60 mg, 65 mg, 75 mg, 100 mg, 125 mg,
130 mg, 200 mg, 250 mg, 260 mg,
300 mg
Elixir: 27 mg/5 ml, 50 mg/5 ml*
Oral solution: 27 mg/5 ml, 50 mg/5 ml
Syrup: 27 mg/5 ml, 50 mg/5 ml
Dextrose 5% injection: 200 mg in 50 ml
or 100 ml; 400 mg in 100 ml, 250 ml,
500 ml, or 1,000 ml; 800 mg in 500 ml or
1,000 ml
theophylline sodium glycinate
Elixir: 110 mg/5 ml (equivalent to 55 mg
of anhydrous theophylline/5 ml)

Pharmacokinetics

Absorption: well absorbed after oral administration. Food may further alter rate of
absorption, especially of some extended-
release preparations.
Distribution: distributed throughout extracellular fluids; equilibrium between
fluid and tissues occurs within 1 hour of
I.V. loading dose.
Metabolism: metabolized in liver to inactive compounds.
Excretion: about 10% excreted unchanged in urine. *Half-life:* adults, 7 to 9

hours; smokers, 4 to 5 hours; children, 3
to 5 hours; premature infants, 20 to 30
hours.

Route	Onset	Peak	Duration
P.O.	15-60 min	1-2 hr (regular) 5 hr (enteric-coated) 4-7 hr (extended-release)	Unknown
I.V.	15 min	15-30 min	Unknown

Pharmacodynamics

Chemical effect: inhibits phosphodiesterase, the enzyme that degrades
cAMP, and relaxes smooth muscle of
bronchial airways and pulmonary blood
vessels.
Therapeutic effect: improves breathing
ability.

Indications and dosage

▶ **Oral theophylline for acute bronchospasm in patients not receiving
theophylline.** *Loading dose:* 6 mg/kg
P.O., then—*Adults (nonsmokers):* 3 mg/
kg q 6 hours for two doses. Maintenance
dosage is 3 mg/kg q 8 hours. *Children
ages 9 to 16 and young adult smokers:*
3 mg/kg q 4 hours for three doses, then
3 mg/kg q 6 hours. *Children ages 6
months to 9 years:* 4 mg/kg q 4 hours for
three doses, then 4 mg/kg q 6 hours.
*Older adults or those with cor pul-
monale:* 2 mg/kg q 6 hours for two doses,
then 2 mg/kg q 8 hours. *Adults with heart
failure or liver disease:* 2 mg/kg q 8
hours for two doses, then 1 to 2 mg/kg q
12 hours.
Note: Extended-release preparations
should not be used for treatment of acute
bronchospasm.
▶ **Parenteral theophylline for patients
not receiving theophylline.** *Loading
dose:* 4.7 mg/kg I.V. slowly; then maintenance infusion. *Adults (nonsmokers):*
0.55 mg/kg/hour I.V. for 12 hours, then
0.39 mg/kg/hour. *Older adults or those*

with cor pulmonale: 0.47 mg/kg/hour I.V. for 12 hours, then 0.24 mg/kg/hour. *Adults with heart failure or liver disease:* 0.39 mg/kg/hour I.V. for 12 hours, then 0.08 to 0.16 mg/kg/hour. *Children ages 9 to 16:* 0.79 mg/kg/hour I.V. for 12 hours, then 0.63 mg/kg/hour. *Children ages 6 months to 9 years:* 0.95 mg/kg/hour I.V. for 12 hours, then 0.79 mg/kg/hour.

▶ **Oral and parenteral theophylline for acute bronchospasm in patients receiving theophylline.** *Adults and children:* each 0.5 mg/kg I.V. or P.O. (loading dose) increases plasma level by 1 mcg/ml. Ideally, dose is based on current theophylline level. In emergencies, some clinicians recommend 2.5 mg/kg P.O. dose of rapidly absorbed form if no obvious signs of theophylline toxicity are present.

▶ **Chronic bronchospasm.** *Adults and children:* 16 mg/kg or 400 mg P.O. daily (whichever is less) given in three or four divided doses at 6- to 8-hour intervals. Alternatively, 12 mg/kg or 400 mg P.O. daily (whichever is less) using extended-release preparation given in two or three divided doses at 8- or 12-hour intervals. Dosage increased as tolerated at 2- to 3-day intervals to maximum dosage as follows: *Adults and children age 16 and over:* 13 mg/kg or 900 mg P.O. daily (whichever is less) in divided doses. *Children ages 12 to 16:* 18 mg/kg P.O. daily in divided doses. *Children ages 9 to 12:* 20 mg/kg P.O. daily in divided doses. *Children under age 9:* 24 mg/kg P.O. daily in divided doses.

Adverse reactions

CNS: *restlessness, dizziness,* headache, *insomnia,* irritability, *seizures,* muscle twitching.
CV: *palpitations, sinus tachycardia,* extrasystoles, flushing, marked hypotension, *arrhythmias.*
GI: *nausea, vomiting,* diarrhea, epigastric pain.
Respiratory: increased respiratory rate, *respiratory arrest.*

Interactions

Drug-drug. *Adenosine:* decreased antiarrhythmic effectiveness. Higher doses of adenosine may be necessary.
Barbiturates, carbamazepine, phenytoin, rifampin: enhanced metabolism and decreased theophylline blood level. Monitor for decreased effect.
Beta blockers: antagonism. Propranolol and nadolol, especially, may cause bronchospasm in sensitive patients. Use together cautiously.
Cimetidine, fluoroquinolone antibiotics (such as ciprofloxacin), influenza virus vaccine, macrolide antibiotics (such as erythromycin), oral contraceptives: decreased hepatic clearance of theophylline; elevated theophylline level. Monitor for toxicity.
Drug-food. *Any food:* accelerated absorption. Give Theo-24 to patient on an empty stomach.
Caffeine: decreased hepatic clearance of theophylline; elevated theophylline level. Monitor for toxicity.
Drug-lifestyle. *Smoking:* increased elimination of theophylline, increasing dosage requirements. Monitor theophylline response and serum concentration.

Contraindications and precautions

• Contraindicated in patients with active peptic ulcer, seizure disorders, or hypersensitivity to xanthine compounds (caffeine, theobromine).
• Use cautiously in young children, infants, and neonates; in elderly patients; in pregnant women; and in those with COPD, cardiac failure, cor pulmonale, renal or hepatic disease, peptic ulceration, hyperthyroidism, diabetes mellitus, glaucoma, severe hypoxemia, hypertension, compromised cardiac or circulatory function, angina, acute MI, or sulfite sensitivity.
• Drug is excreted in breast milk and may cause irritability, insomnia, or fretfulness in breast-fed infant.

NURSING CONSIDERATIONS

✒ Assessment
• Assess patient's condition before therapy and regularly thereafter.
• Monitor vital signs; measure fluid intake and output. Expected clinical effects include improvement in quality of pulse and respirations.
• Xanthine metabolism rate varies among individuals; dosage is determined by monitoring response, tolerance, pulmonary function, and serum theophylline level. Serum theophylline concentration should range from 10 to 20 mcg/ml in adults and 5 to 15 mcg/ml in children.
• Be alert for adverse reactions and drug interactions.
• Monitor patient's hydration status if adverse GI reactions occur.
• Evaluate patient's and family's knowledge of drug therapy.

🖐 Nursing diagnoses
• Impaired gas exchange related to presence of bronchospasms
• Risk for fluid volume deficit related to drug-induced adverse GI reactions
• Knowledge deficit related to drug therapy

▶ Planning and implementation
P.O. use: Don't confuse sustained-release forms with standard-release forms.
– Give drug around-the-clock, using sustained-release product at bedtime.
I.V. use: Use commercially available infusion solution, or mix drug in D_5W. Use infusion pump for continuous infusion.
• Dosage may need to be increased in cigarette smokers and in habitual marijuana smokers; smoking causes drug to be metabolized faster.
• Be aware that daily dosage may need to be decreased in patients with heart failure or hepatic disease and in elderly patients because metabolism and excretion may be decreased.

Patient teaching
• Warn patient not to dissolve, crush, or chew slow-release products. For children unable to swallow, contents of capsules may be sprinkled over soft food and ingested (without chewing).
• Supply instructions for home care and dosage schedule.
• Tell patient to relieve GI symptoms by taking oral drug with full glass of water after meals, although food in stomach delays absorption.
• Warn patient to take drug regularly, as directed. Patients tend to want to take extra "breathing pills."
• Warn elderly patient that dizziness, a common adverse reaction at start of therapy, may occur.
• Caution patient to check with doctor about other drugs used. OTC drugs may contain ephedrine in combination with theophylline salts; excessive CNS stimulation may result.

☑ Evaluation
• Patient demonstrates improved gas exchange, exhibited in arterial blood gas values and respiratory status.
• Patient maintains adequate hydration.
• Patient and family state understanding of drug therapy.

---

thiabendazole
(thigh-uh-BEN-duh-zohl)
Mintezol

Pharmacologic class: benzimidazole
Therapeutic class: anthelmintic
Pregnancy risk category: C

How supplied
Tablets (chewable): 500 mg
Oral suspension: 500 mg/5 ml

Pharmacokinetics
Absorption: absorbed readily from GI tract.
Distribution: unknown.

Reactions may be *common*, uncommon, *life-threatening*, or COMMON AND LIFE-THREATENING.

Metabolism: metabolized almost completely by hydroxylation and conjugation. *Excretion:* excreted primarily in urine as metabolites; about 5% excreted in feces. *Half-life:* about 1.2 hours.

Route	Onset	Peak	Duration
P.O.	Unknown	1-2 hr	Unknown

Pharmacodynamics

Chemical effect: unknown; appears to inhibit helminth-specific enzyme fumarate reductase.
Therapeutic effect: eliminates helminthic infestation.

Indications and dosage

▶ **Cutaneous infestations with larva migrans (creeping eruption).** *Adults and children:* 25 mg/kg P.O. b.i.d. for 2 to 5 days. Maximum dosage is 3 g daily. If lesions persist after 2 days, course is repeated.
▶ **Systemic infections with pinworm, roundworm, threadworm, whipworm, visceral larva migrans, and trichinosis.** *Adults and children weighing between 13.6 and 70 kg (30 and 154 lb):* 25 mg/kg P.O. q 12 hours for 2 successive days. *Adults and children weighing over 70 kg (154 lb):* 1.5 g q 12 hours for 2 successive days. Maximum dosage is 3 g daily. *Trichinosis:* two doses daily for 2 to 4 successive days. *Visceral larva migrans:* two doses daily for 7 successive days.

Adverse reactions

CNS: impaired mental alertness, impaired coordination, numbness, *seizures, drowsiness, fatigue,* giddiness, *headache,* dizziness.
CV: *hypotension.*
EENT: tinnitus, blurry vision, dry mouth and eyes, xanthopsia.
GI: *anorexia, nausea, vomiting,* diarrhea, epigastric distress, cholestasis.
GU: hematuria, enuresis, crystalluria, malodorous urine.
Hematologic: *leukopenia.*

Hepatic: jaundice, *parenchymal liver damage.*
Skin: *rash, pruritus, erythema multiforme, Stevens-Johnson syndrome.*
Other: lymphadenopathy, fever, flushing, chills, *angioedema, anaphylaxis.*

Interactions

Drug-drug. *Theophylline:* may impair hepatic metabolism of theophylline, increasing risk of toxicity. Monitor patient closely.

Contraindications and precautions

• Contraindicated in patients with hypersensitivity to drug.
• Use cautiously in patients with hepatic or renal dysfunction, severe malnutrition, or anemia and in those who are vomiting. Also use cautiously in pregnant women.
• Safety of drug has not been established in breast-feeding women.

NURSING CONSIDERATIONS

⚙ Assessment
• Assess patient's infection before therapy and regularly thereafter.
• Be alert for adverse reactions and drug interactions.
• Monitor patient's hydration status if adverse GI reactions occur.
• Evaluate patient's and family's knowledge of drug therapy.

⊞ Nursing diagnoses
• Infection related to presence of helminthic infestation
• Risk for fluid volume deficit related to drug-induced adverse reactions
• Knowledge deficit related to drug therapy

▷ Planning and implementation
• Drug should be given to all family members, as prescribed, to prevent risk of spreading infection.
• Know that dietary restrictions, laxatives, or enemas are not needed. Provide

supportive therapy for anemic, dehydrated, or malnourished patients.

Patient teaching

• Teach patient to take drug after meals, to shake oral suspension before measuring, and to chew tablets.

• Advise patient to avoid hazardous activities, such as driving, because drug may cause drowsiness.

• Teach patient about personal hygiene, especially good hand-washing technique. To avoid reinfection, teach him to wash perianal area daily, change undergarments and bedclothes daily, and wash hands and clean fingernails before meals and after bowel movements. Tell him not to prepare food for others during infestation.

☑ **Evaluation**

• Patient is free from infection.

• Patient maintains adequate hydration.

• Patient and family state understanding of drug therapy.

thiamine hydrochloride (vitamin B₁)

(THIGH-eh-min high-droh-KLOR-ighd)
Betamin◇, Beta-Sol◇, Biamine, Thiamilate

Pharmacologic class: water-soluble vitamin
Therapeutic class: nutritional supplement
Pregnancy risk category: A

How supplied

Tablets: 5 mg†, 10 mg†, 25 mg†, 50 mg†, 100 mg†, 250 mg†, 500 mg†
Tablet (enteric-coated): 20 mg
Elixir♦: 250 mcg/5 ml
Injection: 100 mg/ml, 200 mg/ml

Pharmacokinetics

Absorption: absorbed readily after small oral doses; after large oral dose, total amount absorbed is limited. In alcoholics and in patients with cirrhosis or malabsorption, GI absorption of thiamine is de-

creased. When given with meals, drug's GI rate of absorption decreases, but total absorption remains same. After I.M. dose, drug is absorbed rapidly and completely.

Distribution: distributed widely in body tissues. When intake exceeds minimal requirements, tissue stores become saturated.

Metabolism: metabolized in liver.

Excretion: excess thiamine excreted in urine.

Route	Onset	Peak	Duration
P.O., I.V., I.M.	Unknown	Unknown	Unknown

Pharmacodynamics

Chemical effect: combines with adenosine triphosphate to form coenzyme necessary for carbohydrate metabolism.

Therapeutic effect: restores normal thiamine level.

Indications and dosage

▶ **RDA.** *Males age 51 and over:* 1.2 mg. *Males ages 15 to 50:* 1.5 mg. *Males ages 11 to 14:* 1.3 mg. *Females age 51 and over:* 1 mg. *Females ages 11 to 50:* 1.1 mg. *Pregnant women:* 1.5 mg. *Breast-feeding women:* 1.6 mg. *Children ages 7 to 10:* 1 mg. *Children ages 4 to 6:* 0.9 mg. *Children ages 1 to 3:* 0.7 mg. *Infants age 6 months to 1 year:* 0.4 mg. *Neonates and infants under age 6 months:* 0.3 mg.

▶ **Beriberi.** *Adults:* depending on severity, 10 to 20 mg I.M. t.i.d. for 2 weeks, followed by dietary correction and multivitamin supplement containing 5 to 10 mg of thiamine daily for 1 month. *Children:* depending on severity, 10 to 50 mg I.M. daily for several weeks with adequate diet.

▶ **Wet beriberi with myocardial failure.** *Adults and children:* 10 to 30 mg I.V. for emergency treatment.

▶ **Wernicke's encephalopathy.** *Adults:* initially, 100 mg I.V., then 50 to 100 mg I.V. or I.M. daily until patient is consuming regular balanced diet.

Adverse reactions

CNS: restlessness.
CV: *CV collapse, angioedema,* cyanosis.
EENT: tightness of throat (allergic reaction).
GI: nausea, *hemorrhage.*
Respiratory: *pulmonary edema.*
Skin: feeling of warmth, pruritus, urticaria, diaphoresis.
Other: weakness; tenderness, induration (after I.M. administration).

Interactions

None significant.

Contraindications and precautions

• Contraindicated in patients hypersensitive to thiamine products.
• Use cautiously in pregnant women if dose exceeds RDA.

NURSING CONSIDERATIONS

🔍 Assessment
• Assess patient's condition before therapy and regularly thereafter.
• Be alert for adverse reactions.
• Evaluate patient's and family's knowledge of drug therapy.

Nursing diagnoses
• Altered nutrition: Less than body requirements related to presence of thiamine deficiency
• Diarrhea related to drug-induced adverse GI reactions
• Knowledge deficit related to drug therapy

Planning and implementation
• Parenteral route should be used only when P.O. route is not feasible.
P.O. and I.M. use: Follow normal protocol.
I.V. use: Dilute drug before administration.
– Give large I.V. doses cautiously; administer patient skin test on patient before starting therapy if he has history of hyper-

sensitivity reactions. Have epinephrine on hand to treat anaphylaxis if it occurs.
• For treating alcoholic patient, give thiamine before dextrose infusions to prevent encephalopathy.
• Do not use with materials that yield alkaline solutions. Unstable in alkaline solutions.
• Know that drug malabsorption is most likely in alcoholism, cirrhosis, and GI disease.
• Clinically significant deficiency can occur in about 3 weeks of thiamine-free diet. Thiamine deficiency usually requires concurrent treatment for multiple deficiencies.
• Keep in mind that doses larger than 30 mg t.i.d. may not be fully utilized. Tissues may become saturated with thiamine and drug is excreted in urine as pyrimidine.
• Be aware that if beriberi occurs in breast-fed infant, both mother and child should be treated with thiamine.
Patient teaching
• Stress proper nutritional habits to prevent recurrence of deficiency.

✓ Evaluation
• Patient regains normal thiamine level.
• Patient maintains normal bowel pattern.
• Patient and family state understanding of drug therapy.

thioguanine
(6-thioguanine, 6-TG)
(thigh-oh-GWAH-neen)
Lanvis ◆

Pharmacologic class: antimetabolite (cell cycle–phase specific, S phase)
Therapeutic class: antineoplastic
Pregnancy risk category: D

How supplied

Tablets (scored): 40 mg

Pharmacokinetics

Absorption: incomplete and variable; average bioavailability is 30%.
Distribution: distributed well in bone marrow cells.
Metabolism: extensively metabolized to less active form in liver and other tissues.
Excretion: excreted in urine, mainly as metabolites. *Half-life:* initial phase, 15 minutes; terminal phase, 11 hours.

Route	Onset	Peak	Duration
P.O.	Unknown	Unknown	Unknown

Pharmacodynamics

Chemical effect: inhibits purine synthesis.
Therapeutic effect: inhibits selected leukemic cell reproduction.

Indications and dosage

▶ **Acute nonlymphocytic leukemia, chronic myelogenous leukemia.** *Adults and children:* initially, 2 mg/kg P.O. daily (usually calculated to nearest 20 mg). If necessary, dose is then increased gradually to 3 mg/kg/day, as tolerated.

Adverse reactions

GI: nausea, vomiting, stomatitis, diarrhea, anorexia.
Hematologic: *leukopenia, anemia, thrombocytopenia* (occurs slowly over 2 to 4 weeks).
Hepatic: *hepatotoxicity,* jaundice, hepatic fibrosis, toxic hepatitis.
Other: hyperuricemia.

Interactions

Drug-drug. *Myelosuppressant drugs:* increased risk of toxicity, especially myelosuppression, hepatotoxicity, and bleeding. Use together cautiously.

Contraindications and precautions

• Contraindicated in patients whose disease has shown resistance to drug.
• Drug is not recommended for use in pregnant or breast-feeding women.
• Use cautiously in patients with renal or hepatic dysfunction.

NURSING CONSIDERATIONS

⚕ Assessment
• Assess patient's condition before therapy and regularly thereafter.
• Monitor CBC daily during induction and then weekly during maintenance therapy, as ordered.
• Monitor serum uric acid level.
• Watch for jaundice.
• Be alert for adverse reactions and drug interactions.
• Evaluate patient's and family's knowledge of drug therapy.

⊕ Nursing diagnoses
• Altered health maintenance related to presence of leukemia
• Altered protection related to drug-induced immunosuppression
• Knowledge deficit related to drug therapy

▶ Planning and implementation
• Dosage modification may be required in renal or hepatic dysfunction.
• Drug may be ordered as 6-thioguanine. The numeral 6 is part of drug name and does not signify dosage units.
• Report jaundice; it may be reversible if drug is stopped promptly. Also, drug must be stopped if hepatotoxicity or hepatic tenderness occurs.
• Force fluids to prevent hyperuricemia.
Patient teaching
• Warn patient to watch for signs of infection and bleeding, and instruct him on infection-control and bleeding precautions to use in daily living.
• Tell patient to increase fluid intake.
• Advise female patient of childbearing age to avoid becoming pregnant during therapy. Also recommend that she consult with doctor before becoming pregnant.

☑ Evaluation
• Patient responds well to drug.
• Patient does not develop serious complications from drug-induced immunosuppression.

Reactions may be *common*, uncommon, *life-threatening*, or COMMON AND LIFE-THREATENING.

• Patient and family state understanding of drug therapy.

thioridazine hydrochloride
(thigh-oh-RIGH-duh-zeen high-droh-KLOR-ighd)
AldazineL, Apo-Thioridazinel, Mellaril*, Mellaril Concentrate, Novo-Ridazinel, PMS Thioridazinel

Pharmacologic class: phenothiazine (piperidine derivative)
Therapeutic class: antipsychotic
Pregnancy risk category: NR

How supplied

Tablets: 10 mg, 15 mg, 25 mg, 50 mg, 100 mg, 150 mg, 200 mg
Oral suspension: 25 mg/5 ml, 100 mg/5 ml
Oral concentrate: 30 mg/ml, 100 mg/ml (3% to 4.2% alcohol)

Pharmacokinetics

Absorption: erratic and variable, although oral concentrates and syrups are more predictable than tablets.
Distribution: distributed widely in body; 91% to 99% protein-bound.
Metabolism: extensively by liver.
Excretion: most as metabolites in urine; some, in feces.

Route	Onset	Peak	Duration
P.O.	Varies	Unknown	Unknown

Pharmacodynamics

Chemical effect: unknown; probably blocks postsynaptic dopamine receptors in brain.
Therapeutic effect: relieves signs of psychosis, depression, anxiety, stress, fears, and sleep disturbances.

Indications and dosage

▶ **Psychosis.** *Adults:* initially, 50 to 100 mg P.O. t.i.d., with gradual, incre-

mental increases up to 800 mg daily in divided doses, if needed. Dosage varies.
▶ **Short-term treatment of moderate to marked depression with variable degrees of anxiety; dementia in elderly patients; behavioral problems in children.** *Adults:* initially, 25 mg P.O. t.i.d. Maximum daily dosage is 200 mg. *Children ages 2 to 12:* 0.5 to 3 mg/kg P.O. daily in divided doses. Give 10 mg b.i.d. to t.i.d. to children with moderate disorders and 25 mg b.i.d. to t.i.d. to hospitalized, severely disturbed, or psychotic children.

Adverse reactions

CNS: extrapyramidal reactions (low incidence), *tardive dyskinesia, sedation* (high incidence), EEG changes, dizziness.
CV: *orthostatic hypotension,* tachycardia, ECG changes.
EENT: *ocular changes, blurred vision,* retinitis pigmentosa.
GI: *dry mouth, constipation.*
GU: *urine retention,* dark urine, menstrual irregularities, gynecomastia, inhibited ejaculation.
Hematologic: transient leukopenia, *agranulocytosis,* hyperprolactinemia.
Hepatic: cholestatic jaundice.
Skin: *mild photosensitivity,* allergic reactions.
Other: weight gain; increased appetite; rarely, *neuroleptic malignant syndrome.*
After abrupt withdrawal of long-term therapy: gastritis, nausea, vomiting, dizziness, tremors, feeling of warmth or cold, diaphoresis, tachycardia, headache, insomnia.

Interactions

Drug-drug. *Antacids:* inhibited absorption of oral phenothiazines. Separate doses by at least 2 hours.
Barbiturates, lithium: may decrease phenothiazine effect. Monitor patient.
Centrally acting antihypertensives: decreased antihypertensive effect. Monitor blood pressure.

Other CNS depressants: increased CNS depression. Use together cautiously.
Drug-lifestyle. *Alcohol use:* increased CNS depression. Avoid concomitant use.
Sun exposure: increased photosensitivity reactions. Avoid prolonged or unprotected sun exposure.

Contraindications and precautions

• Contraindicated in patients with CNS depression, severe hypertensive or hypotensive cardiac disease, coma, or hypersensitivity to drug.
• Use cautiously in elderly or debilitated patients; in pregnant or breast-feeding women; and in patients with hepatic disease, CV disease, exposure to extreme heat or cold (including antipyretic therapy) or to organophosphate insecticides, respiratory disorder, hypocalcemia, seizure disorder, or severe reactions to insulin or electroconvulsive therapy.

NURSING CONSIDERATIONS

⚅ Assessment
• Assess patient's condition before therapy and regularly thereafter.
• Monitor patient for tardive dyskinesia. It may occur after prolonged use, or may not appear until months or years later. It may disappear spontaneously or persist for life, despite discontinuation of drug.
• Monitor therapy with weekly bilirubin tests during first month, periodic blood tests (CBC and liver function), and ophthalmologic tests (long-term therapy), as ordered.
• Be alert for adverse reactions and drug interactions.
• Evaluate patient's and family's knowledge of drug therapy.

⊞ Nursing diagnoses
• Altered thought processes related to underlying condition
• Risk for injury related to drug-induced adverse CNS reactions
• Knowledge deficit related to drug therapy

⊠ Planning and implementation
• Different liquid formulations have different concentrations. Check dosage.
• Prevent contact dermatitis by keeping drug away from skin and clothes. Wear gloves when preparing liquid forms.
• Dilute liquid concentrate with water or fruit juice just before giving.
• Shake suspension well before using.
• Do not withdraw abruptly unless required by severe adverse reactions.
• Report jaundice, symptoms of blood dyscrasia (fever, sore throat, infection, cellulitis, weakness), or persistent extrapyramidal reactions (longer than a few hours), especially in pregnant woman or in child, and withhold drug.
• Acute dystonic reactions may be treated with diphenhydramine.

Patient teaching
• Warn patient to avoid activities that require alertness until drug's CNS effects are known. Drowsiness and dizziness usually subside after a few weeks.
• Tell patient to watch for orthostatic hypotension, especially with parenteral administration. Advise patient to change position slowly.
• Tell patient to avoid alcohol while taking drug.
• Instruct patient to report urine retention or constipation.
• Inform patient that drug may discolor urine.
• Tell patient to watch for and notify doctor of blurred vision.
• Advise patient to relieve dry mouth with sugarless gum or hard candy.
• Tell patient to use sunblock and to wear protective clothing to avoid photosensitivity reactions.

☑ Evaluation
• Patient's behavior and communication exhibit improved thought processes.
• Patient does not experience injury from adverse CNS reactions.
• Patient and family state understanding of drug therapy.

Reactions may be *common*, uncommon, *life-threatening*, or COMMON AND LIFE-THREATENING.

thiotepa
(thigh-oh-TEE-puh)
Thioplex

Pharmacologic class: alkylating agent
(cell cycle–phase nonspecific)
Therapeutic class: antineoplastic
Pregnancy risk category: D

How supplied

Injection: 15-mg vials

Pharmacokinetics

Absorption: absorption from bladder after instillation ranges from 10% to 100% of instilled dose; also variable after intracavitary administration; increased by certain pathologic conditions.
Distribution: crosses blood-brain barrier.
Metabolism: metabolized extensively in liver.
Excretion: thiotepa and its metabolites excreted in urine.

Route	Onset	Peak	Duration
I.V., bladder instillation, intracavitary	Unknown	Unknown	Unknown

Pharmacodynamics

Chemical effect: cross-links strands of cellular DNA and interferes with RNA transcription, causing growth imbalance that leads to cell death.
Therapeutic effect: kills selected cancer cells.

Indications and dosage

▶ **Breast and ovarian cancers, lymphoma, Hodgkin's disease.** *Adults and children over age 12:* 0.3 to 0.4 mg/kg I.V. q 1 to 4 weeks or 0.2 mg/kg 4 to 5 days at intervals of 2 to 4 weeks.
▶ **Bladder tumor.** *Adults and children over age 12:* 60 mg in 30 to 60 ml of 0.9% NaCl solution instilled in bladder for 2 hours once weekly for 4 weeks.

▶ **Neoplastic effusions.** *Adults and children over age 12:* 0.6 to 0.8 mg/kg intracavitarily or intratumor q 1 to 4 weeks.

Adverse reactions

CNS: headache, dizziness, fatigue, weakness.
EENT: blurred vision, laryngeal edema, conjunctivitis.
GI: *nausea, vomiting,* abdominal pain, anorexia, stomatitis.
GU: amenorrhea, decreased spermatogenesis, dysuria, urine retention, hemorrhagic cystitis.
Hematologic: *leukopenia* (begins within 5 to 10 days), *thrombocytopenia; neutropenia; anemia.*
Respiratory: asthma.
Skin: urticaria, rash, dermatitis, alopecia, pain at injection site.
Other: fever, *hypersensitivity, anaphylaxis.*

Interactions

Drug-drug. *Anticoagulants, aspirin:* increased bleeding risk. Avoid concomitant use.
Neuromuscular blocking agents: may prolong muscular paralysis. Monitor closely.
Other alkylating agents, irradiation therapy: may intensify toxicity rather than enhance therapeutic response. Avoid concurrent use.
Succinylcholine: increased apnea with concomitant use. Monitor patient closely.

Contraindications and precautions

● Contraindicated in patients hypersensitive to drug and in those with severe bone marrow, hepatic, or renal dysfunction.
● Drug is not recommended for use in pregnant or breast-feeding women.
● Use cautiously in patients with mild bone marrow suppression or renal or hepatic dysfunction.
● Safety of drug has not been established in children age 12 and younger.

NURSING CONSIDERATIONS

⚕ Assessment
• Assess patient's condition before therapy and regularly thereafter.
• Adverse genitourinary reactions are reversible in 6 to 8 months.
• Monitor CBC weekly for at least 3 weeks after last dose, as ordered.
• Monitor serum uric acid levels.
• Be alert for adverse reactions and drug interactions.
• Evaluate patient's and family's knowledge of drug therapy.

⊞ Nursing diagnoses
• Altered health maintenance related to presence of neoplastic disease
• Altered protection related to drug-induced immunosuppression
• Knowledge deficit related to drug therapy

⧁ Planning and implementation
• Follow institutional policy to minimize risks. Preparation and administration of parenteral form are associated with mutagenic, teratogenic, and carcinogenic risks to personnel.
I.V. use: Reconstitute drug with 1.5 ml of sterile water for injection. Do not reconstitute with other solutions. Further dilute solution with 0.9% NaCl injection, D_5W, dextrose 5% in 0.9% NaCl injection, Ringer's injection, or lactated Ringer's injection. Drug may be given by rapid I.V. administration in doses of 0.3 to 0.4 mg/kg at intervals of 1 to 4 weeks. Solutions are stable for up to 5 days if refrigerated.
– Use local anesthetic at injection site, as ordered, if intense pain occurs.
– If pain occurs at insertion site, dilute further or use local anesthetic. Make sure drug does not infiltrate.
– Discard if solution appears grossly opaque or has precipitate. Solutions should be clear to slightly opaque.
Intracavitary use: For neoplastic effusions, mix drug with 2% procaine hy-

drochloride or epinephrine hydrochloride 1:1,000, as ordered.
Bladder instillation use: Dehydrate patient 8 to 10 hours before therapy. Instill drug into bladder by catheter; ask patient to retain solution for 2 hours. Volume may be reduced to 30 ml if discomfort is too great with 60 ml. Reposition patient every 15 minutes for maximum area contact.
• Be aware that drug can be given by all parenteral routes, including direct injection into tumor.
• Refrigerate and protect dry powder from direct sunlight.
• Report WBC count below 3,000/mm³ or platelet count below 150,000/mm³ and stop drug, as ordered.
• To prevent hyperuricemia with resulting uric acid nephropathy, know that allopurinol may be used with adequate hydration.
Patient teaching
• Warn patient to watch for signs of infection (fever, sore throat, fatigue) and bleeding (easy bruising, nosebleeds, bleeding gums, melena). Tell patient to take temperature daily and to report even mild infections.
• Instruct patient to avoid OTC products containing aspirin.
• Advise breast-feeding woman to stop breast-feeding during therapy because of possible infant toxicity.
• Advise female patient of childbearing age to avoid becoming pregnant during therapy and to consult with doctor before becoming pregnant.

☑ Evaluation
• Patient responds well to drug.
• Patient does not develop serious complications from drug-induced immunosuppression.
• Patient and family state understanding of drug therapy.

Reactions may be *common*, uncommon, *life-threatening*, or COMMON AND LIFE-THREATENING.

thiothixene
(thigh-oh-THIKS-een)
Navane

thiothixene hydrochloride
Navane*

Pharmacologic class: thioxanthene
Therapeutic class: antipsychotic
Pregnancy risk category: C

How supplied

thiothixene
Capsules: 1 mg, 2 mg, 5 mg, 10 mg,
20 mg
thiothixene hydrochloride
Oral concentrate: 5 mg/ml (7% alcohol)
Injection: 2 mg/ml, 5 mg/ml

Pharmacokinetics

Absorption: rapid after P.O. and I.M. administration.
Distribution: distributed widely in body;
91% to 99% protein-bound.
Metabolism: minimal.
Excretion: most of drug excreted as parent drug in feces.

Route	Onset	Peak	Duration
P.O., I.M.	Several wk	Unknown	Unknown

Pharmacodynamics

Chemical effect: unknown; probably blocks postsynaptic dopamine receptors in brain.
Therapeutic effect: relieves signs and symptoms of psychosis.

Indications and dosage

▶ **Mild to moderate psychosis.** *Adults:*
initially, 2 mg P.O. t.i.d. Increased gradually to 15 mg daily.
▶ **Severe psychosis.** *Adults:* initially, 5 mg
P.O. b.i.d. Increased gradually to 20 to
30 mg daily. Maximum recommended dosage is 60 mg daily. Alternatively, 4 mg
I.M. b.i.d. or q.i.d. Maximum dosage is
30 mg I.M. daily. An oral form should supplant injectable form as soon as possible.

Adverse reactions

CNS: *extrapyramidal reactions, tardive dyskinesia,* sedation, pseudoparkinsonism, EEG changes, dizziness, restlessness, agitation, insomnia.
CV: *orthostatic hypotension,* tachycardia, ECG changes.
EENT: ocular changes, *blurred vision,* nasal congestion.
GI: *dry mouth, constipation.*
GU: *urine retention,* menstrual irregularities, gynecomastia, inhibited ejaculation.
Hematologic: transient leukopenia, leukocytosis, *agranulocytosis.*
Hepatic: jaundice.
Skin: *mild photosensitivity,* allergic reactions, pain at I.M. injection site, sterile abscess.
Other: weight gain; rarely, *neuroleptic malignant syndrome.*
After abrupt withdrawal of long-term therapy: gastritis, nausea, vomiting, dizziness, tremors, feeling of warmth or cold, diaphoresis, tachycardia, headache, insomnia.

Interactions

Drug-drug. *Other CNS depressants:* increased CNS depression. Avoid concomitant use.
Drug-lifestyle. *Alcohol use:* increased CNS depression. Avoid concomitant use.
Sun exposure: increased photosensitivity reactions. Avoid prolonged or unprotected sun exposure.

Contraindications and precautions

● Contraindicated in patients with circulatory collapse, coma, CNS depression, blood dyscrasia, or hypersensitivity to drug.
● Use with extreme caution in patients with history of seizure disorder or during alcohol withdrawal.
● Use cautiously in elderly or debilitated patients; in patients with CV disease (may cause sudden drop in blood pressure), exposure to extreme heat, glaucoma, or prostatic hyperplasia; and in pregnant or breast-feeding women.

NURSING CONSIDERATIONS

Assessment
• Assess patient's psychosis before therapy and regularly thereafter.
• Watch for orthostatic hypotension, especially with parenteral route.
• Monitor for tardive dyskinesia. It may occur after prolonged use or may not appear until months or years later. It may disappear spontaneously or persist for life, despite stopping drug.
• Monitor therapy with weekly bilirubin tests during first month, periodic blood tests (CBC and liver function), and ophthalmologic tests (long-term therapy), as ordered.
• Be alert for adverse reactions and drug interactions.
• Evaluate patient's and family's knowledge of drug therapy.

Nursing diagnoses
• Altered thought processes related to presence of psychosis
• Risk for injury related to drug-induced adverse CNS reactions
• Knowledge deficit related to drug therapy

Planning and implementation
P.O. use: Prevent contact dermatitis by keeping drug away from skin and clothes. Wear gloves when preparing liquid forms.
– Dilute liquid concentrate with water or fruit juice just before giving.
I.M. use: Give I.M. only in upper outer quadrant of buttocks or midlateral thigh. Massage slowly afterward to prevent sterile abscess. Injection may sting.
– Keep patient in supine position for 1 hour after drug administration.
• Know that slight yellowing of injection or concentrate is common and does not affect potency. Discard markedly discolored solutions.
• Do not withdraw drug abruptly unless required by severe adverse reactions.
• Report jaundice, symptoms of blood dyscrasia (fever, sore throat, infection,

cellulitis, weakness), or persistent extrapyramidal reactions (longer than a few hours), especially in pregnant woman or in child, and withhold dose.
• Know that acute dystonic reactions may be treated with diphenhydramine.
Patient teaching
• Warn patient to avoid activities that require alertness until drug's CNS effects are known. Drowsiness and dizziness usually subside after a few weeks.
• Tell patient to avoid alcohol while taking drug.
• Instruct patient to notify doctor if urine retention or constipation occurs.
• Tell patient to relieve dry mouth with sugarless gum or hard candy.
• Tell patient to use sunblock and to wear protective clothing to avoid photosensitivity reactions.
• Tell patient to watch for orthostatic hypotension, especially with parenteral administration. Advise patient to change position slowly.

Evaluation
• Patient's behavior and communication exhibit improved thought processes.
• Patient does not experience injury from adverse CNS reactions.
• Patient and family state understanding of drug therapy.

thyroid
(THIGH-royd)
Armour Thyroid, S-P-T, Thyrar, Thyroid Strong, Thyroid USP, Westhroid

Pharmacologic class: thyroid hormone
Therapeutic class: thyroid agent
Pregnancy risk category: A

How supplied
Tablets: 15 mg, 30 mg, 60 mg, 65 mg, 90 mg, 120 mg, 130 mg, 180 mg, 240 mg, 300 mg
Tablets (bovine origin): 30 mg, 60 mg, 120 mg

Tablets (porcine origin): 15 mg, 30 mg, 60 mg, 120 mg, 200 mg, 250 mg, 300 mg
Tablets (enteric-coated): 60 mg, 120 mg
Strong tablets (50% stronger than thyroid USP, and containing 0.3% iodine): 32.5 mg, 65 mg, 130 mg, 200 mg
Capsules (porcine origin): 60 mg, 120 mg, 180 mg, 300 mg

Pharmacokinetics

Absorption: absorbed from GI tract.
Distribution: highly protein-bound.
Metabolism: not fully understood.
Excretion: not fully understood. *Half-life:* T_4, 7 days; T_3, 2 days.

Route	Onset	Peak	Duration
P.O.	Unknown	Unknown	Unknown

Pharmacodynamics

Chemical effect: not clearly defined; stimulates metabolism of body tissues by accelerating cellular oxidation.
Therapeutic effect: raises thyroid hormone level in body.

Indications and dosage

▶ **Adult hypothyroidism.** Initially, 30 mg P.O. daily, increased by 15 mg q 14 to 30 days, depending on disease severity until desired response is achieved. Usual maintenance dosage is 60 to 180 mg P.O. daily as a single dose.
▶ **Congenital hypothyroidism.** *Children over age 12:* may approach adult dosage (60 to 180 mg daily), depending on response. *Children ages 6 to 12:* 60 to 90 mg P.O. daily. *Children ages 1 to 5:* 45 to 60 mg P.O. daily. *Children ages 6 to 12 months:* 30 to 45 mg P.O. daily. *Children up to age 6 months:* 15 to 30 mg P.O. daily.
Note: Thyroid Strong is 50% stronger than Thyroid USP. Each grain is equivalent to 1½ grains of Thyroid USP.

Adverse reactions

Adverse reactions to thyroid hormones are extensions of their pharmacologic properties and reflect patient sensitivity to them.
CNS: *nervousness, insomnia,* tremors, headache.
CV: *tachycardia, arrhythmias,* angina pectoris, increased blood pressure, *cardiac decompensation and collapse.*
GI: diarrhea, vomiting.
Musculoskeletal: accelerated rate of bone maturation in infants and children.
Other: weight loss, heat intolerance, diaphoresis, menstrual irregularities, allergic reactions.

Interactions

Drug-drug. *Cholestyramine:* impaired thyroid absorption. Separate doses by 4 to 5 hours.
Insulin, oral antidiabetic agents: altered blood glucose level. Monitor level; adjust dosage as needed.
I.V. phenytoin: free thyroid released. Monitor for tachycardia.
Oral anticoagulants: altered PT. Monitor PT and INR; adjust dosage as needed.
Sympathomimetics (such as epinephrine): increased risk of coronary insufficiency. Monitor patient closely.

Contraindications and precautions

• Contraindicated in patients with hypersensitivity to drug, acute MI uncomplicated by hypothyroidism, untreated thyrotoxicosis, or uncorrected adrenal insufficiency.
• Use with extreme caution in patients with angina pectoris, hypertension, or other CV disorders; renal insufficiency; ischemic states; and in elderly patients.
• Use cautiously in patients with myxedema, diabetes mellitus, or diabetes insipidus and in breast-feeding women.

NURSING CONSIDERATIONS

⚗ Assessment
• Assess patient's thyroid condition before therapy and regularly thereafter.
• Monitor pulse rate and blood pressure.

• Be aware that sleeping pulse rate and basal morning temperature in children guide treatment.
• In patient with coronary artery disease who must receive drug, watch for possible coronary insufficiency.
• Be alert for adverse reactions and drug interactions.
• Evaluate patient's and family's knowledge of drug therapy.

▣ Nursing diagnoses
• Altered health maintenance related to presence of hypothyroidism
• Sleep pattern disturbance related to drug-induced insomnia
• Knowledge deficit related to drug therapy

▷ Planning and implementation
• Drug requirements are about 25% lower in patients over age 60 than in young adults.
• Thyroid hormones alter thyroid function test results.
• Know that patient taking drug usually requires decreased anticoagulant dosage.
Patient teaching
• Tell patient to take drug at same time each day, preferably before breakfast, to maintain constant levels.
• Suggest patient take dosage in the morning to prevent insomnia.
• Advise patient who has achieved stable response not to change brands.
• Warn patient (especially elderly patient) to notify doctor promptly if chest pain, palpitations, sweating, nervousness, or other signs of overdose occur or if chest pain, dyspnea, and tachycardia develop.
• Tell patient to report unusual bleeding and bruising.

▨ Evaluation
• Patient regains normal thyroid function.
• Patient expresses importance of taking thyroid in morning if insomnia occurs.
• Patient and family state understanding of drug therapy.

thyrotropin (thyroid-stimulating hormone, or TSH)
(thigh-ROH-troh-pin)
Thytropar

Pharmacologic class: anterior pituitary hormone
Therapeutic class: thyrotropic hormone
Pregnancy risk category: C

How supplied
Powder for injection: 10 IU/vial

Pharmacokinetics
Absorption: occurs within minutes from I.M. or S.C. injection site.
Distribution: concentrated primarily in thyroid gland.
Metabolism: not fully understood.
Excretion: not fully understood.

Route	Onset	Peak	Duration
I.M., S.C.	Min	≤ 24 hr	Effects rapidly reverse after withdrawal

Pharmacodynamics
Chemical effect: stimulates uptake of radioactive iodine (^{131}I) in patients with thyroid carcinoma and promotes thyroid hormone production by anterior pituitary gland.
Therapeutic effect: evaluates thyroid function and inhibits thyroid cancer cell activity.

Indications and dosage
▶ **Diagnosis of thyroid cancer remnant with ^{131}I after surgery.** *Adults:* 10 IU I.M. or S.C. for 3 to 7 days.
▶ **Differential diagnosis of primary and secondary hypothyroidism.** *Adults:* 10 IU I.M. or S.C. for 1 to 3 days.
▶ **In protein-bound iodine or ^{131}I uptake determinations for differential diagnosis of subclinical hypothyroidism or low thyroid reserve.** *Adults:* 10 IU I.M. or S.C.

▶ **Therapy for thyroid carcinoma (local or metastatic) with** ^{131}**I.** *Adults:* 10 IU I.M. or S.C. for 3 to 8 days.
▶ **To determine thyroid status of patient receiving thyroid hormone.** *Adults:* 10 IU I.M. or S.C. for 1 to 3 days.

Adverse reactions

CNS: headache.
CV: *tachycardia,* atrial fibrillation, angina pectoris, *heart failure,* hypotension.
GI: nausea, vomiting.
Other: thyroid hyperplasia (with large doses), fever, hypersensitivity reactions (postinjection flare, urticaria, *anaphylaxis*), menstrual irregularities.

Interactions

Drug-drug. *Insulin, oral antidiabetic agents:* altered blood glucose level. Monitor level. Dosage may need adjustment.
Oral anticoagulants: altered PT. Monitor PT and INR. Dosage adjustment may be necessary.
Sympathomimetics (such as epinephrine): increased risk of coronary insufficiency. Monitor patient closely.

Contraindications and precautions

• Contraindicated in patients with coronary thrombosis, untreated Addison's disease, or hypersensitivity to drug.
• Use cautiously in patients with angina pectoris, heart failure, hypopituitarism, adrenocortical suppression and in pregnant or breast-feeding women.

NURSING CONSIDERATIONS

Assessment
• Assess patient's condition before therapy and regularly thereafter.
• Be alert for adverse reactions and drug interactions.
• Evaluate patient's and family's knowledge of drug therapy.

Nursing diagnoses
• Health-seeking behavior (desire to have thyroid problem diagnosed) related to thyroid dysfunction
• Altered protected related to drug-induced hypersensitivity reaction
• Knowledge deficit related to drug therapy

Planning and implementation
I.M. and S.C. use: Folow normal protocol.
• Know that 3-day dosage schedule may be used in long-standing pituitary myxedema or with prolonged use of thyroid medication.
Patient teaching
• Warn patient to report immediately itching, redness, or swelling at injection site; rash; tightness of throat or wheezing chest pain; irritability; nervousness; rapid heartbeat; shortness of breath; or unusual sweating.

Evaluation
• Patient's thyroid dysfunction is diagnosed.
• Patient does not experience drug-induced hypersensitivity reaction.
• Patient and family state understanding of drug therapy.

tiagabine hydrochloride
(tigh-AG-ah-been high-droh-KLOR-ighd)
Gabitril

Pharmacologic class: gamma aminobutyric acid (GABA) uptake inhibitor
Therapeutic class: anticonvulsant
Pregnancy risk category: C

How supplied

Tablets: 4 mg, 12 mg, 16 mg, 20 mg

Pharmacokinetics

Absorption: drug is rapidly and nearly completely absorbed (more than 95%). Absolute bioavailability is 90%.

Distribution: about 96% bound to plasma protein.
Metabolism: likely to be metabolized by cytochrome P-450 3A isoenzymes.
Excretion: about 25% is excreted in urine (2% unchanged); 63% in feces.
Half-life: 7 to 9 hours.

Route	Onset	Peak	Duration
P.O.	Rapid	45 min	7-9 hr

Pharmacodynamics

Chemical effect: unknown, but tiagabine may act by enhancing the activity of GABA, the major inhibitory neurotransmitter in the central nervous system. It binds to recognition sites associated with the GABA uptake carrier and may thus permit more GABA to be available for binding to receptors on postsynaptic cells. *Therapeutic effect:* prevents partial seizures.

Indications and dosage

▶ **Adjunctive therapy in the treatment of partial seizures.** *Adults:* initially, 4 mg P.O. once daily. Total daily dosage may be increased by 4 to 8 mg at weekly intervals until clinical response or up to 56 mg/day. Total daily dosage should be given in divided doses b.i.d. to q.i.d. *Adolescents ages 12 to 18:* initially, 4 mg P.O. once daily. Total daily dosage may be increased by 4 mg at the beginning of week 2 and thereafter by 4 to 8 mg/week until clinical response or up to 32 mg/day. Total daily dosage should be given in divided doses b.i.d. to q.i.d.

Adverse reactions

CNS: generalized weakness, *dizziness, asthenia, somnolence, nervousness,* tremor, difficulty with concentration and attention, insomnia, ataxia, confusion, speech disorder, difficulty with memory, paresthesia, depression, emotional lability, abnormal gait, hostility, language problems, agitation.
CV: vasodilation.
EENT: nystagmus, pharyngitis.

GI: abdominal pain, *nausea,* diarrhea, vomiting, increased appetite, mouth ulceration.
Musculoskeletal: myasthenia.
Respiratory: increased cough.
Skin: rash, pruritus.
Other: pain.

Interactions

Drug-drug. *Carbamazepine, phenobarbital, phenytoin:* increased tiagabine clearance. Monitor closely.
CNS depressants: enhanced CNS effects. Use cautiously.
Drug-lifestyle. *Alcohol use:* enhanced CNS effects. Use cautiously.

Contraindications and precautions

• Contraindicated in patients with hypersensitivity to drug or its ingredients.
• Use cautiously in breast-feeding patients.

NURSING CONSIDERATIONS

⚎ Assessment
• Assess patient's seizure disorder before therapy and regularly thereafter.
• Assess patient's compliance with therapy at each follow-up visit.
• Monitor patient carefully for status epilepticus because sudden unexpected death has occurred in patients receiving antiepilepsy drugs, including tiagabine.
• Assess for adverse reactions and drug interactions.
• Evaluate patient's and family's knowledge of drug therapy.

⊕ Nursing diagnoses
• Risk for injury related to seizure disorder
• Impaired physical mobility related to drug-induced generalized weakness
• Knowledge deficit related to drug therapy

▷ Planning and implementation
• Reduced initial and maintenance doses or longer dosing intervals may be re-

quired in patients with impaired liver function.

• Never withdraw drug suddenly because seizure frequency may increase. Withdraw gradually unless safety concerns require a more rapid withdrawal.

• Know that patients who are *not* receiving at least one concomitant enzyme-inducing antiepilepsy drug at the time of tiagabine initiation may require lower doses or a slower dose titration.

• Report breakthrough seizure activity to doctor.

Patient teaching
• Advise patient to take drug only as prescribed.

• Advise patient to take tiagabine with food.

• Warn patient that drug may cause dizziness, somnolence, and other symptoms and signs of CNS depression. Advise patient to avoid driving and other potentially hazardous activities that require mental alertness until drug's CNS effects are known.

• Tell female patient to call doctor if she becomes pregnant or plans to become pregnant during therapy.

• Tell female patient to notify doctor if planning to breast-feed because drug may be excreted in breast milk.

☑ **Evaluation**
• Patient is free from seizure activity.

• Patient receives therapeutic medication dose and does not experience muscle weakness.

• Patient and family state understanding of drug therapy.

---

ticarcillin disodium
(tigh-kar-SIL-in digh-SOH-dee-um)
Ticar, Ticillin◊

Pharmacologic class: extended-spectrum penicillin, alpha-carboxypenicillin
Therapeutic class: antibiotic
Pregnancy risk category: B

How supplied
Injection: 1 g, 3 g, 6 g
I V. infusion: 3 g

Pharmacokinetics
Absorption: unknown after I.M. administration.
Distribution: distributed widely. Drug penetrates minimally into CSF with uninflamed meninges; 45% to 65% protein-bound.
Metabolism: about 13% metabolized by hydrolysis to inactive compounds.
Excretion: excreted mostly in urine; also in bile. *Half-life:* about 1 hour.

Route	Onset	Peak	Duration
I.V.	Immediate	Immediate	Unknown
I.M.	Unknown	30-75 min	Unknown

Pharmacodynamics
Chemical effect: inhibits cell-wall synthesis during microorganism multiplication; bacteria resist penicillins by producing penicillinases—enzymes that convert penicillins to inactive penicilloic acid.
Therapeutic effect: kills bacteria. Activity includes many gram-negative aerobic and anaerobic bacilli, many gram-positive and gram-negative aerobic cocci, some gram-positive aerobic and anaerobic bacilli. May be effective against some carbenicillin-resistant gram-negative bacilli.

Indications and dosage
▶ **Severe systemic infections caused by susceptible strains of gram-positive and especially gram-negative organisms (including *Pseudomonas* and *Proteus*).** *Adults:* 200 to 300 mg/kg I.V. daily in divided doses q 4 to 6 hours.
Children over age 1 month and weighing under 40 kg (88 lb): 200 to 300 mg/kg I.V. daily in divided doses q 4 to 6 hours.

Adverse reactions
CNS: *seizures,* neuromuscular excitability.
CV: vein irritation, phlebitis.

GI: nausea, diarrhea, vomiting.
Hematologic: *leukopenia, neutropenia,* eosinophilia, *thrombocytopenia,* hemolytic anemia.
Other: hypersensitivity reactions (rash, pruritus, urticaria, chills, fever, edema, *anaphylaxis*), overgrowth of nonsusceptible organisms, hypokalemia, pain at injection site.

Interactions

Drug-drug. *Lithium:* altered renal elimination of lithium. Monitor serum lithium level closely.
Oral contraceptives: efficacy of oral contraceptives may be decreased. Additional form of contraception recommended during penicillin therapy.
Probenecid: increased blood levels of ticarcillin and other penicillins. Probenecid may be used for this purpose.

Contraindications and precautions

• Contraindicated in patients with hypersensitivity to penicillins.
• Use cautiously in patients with other drug allergies, especially to cephalosporins (possible cross-sensitivity); in those with impaired kidney function, hemorrhagic conditions, hypokalemia, or sodium restrictions (contains 5.2 to 6.5 mEq sodium/g); and in pregnant or breast-feeding women.

NURSING CONSIDERATIONS

Assessment
• Assess patient's infection before therapy and regularly thereafter.
• Before giving, ask patient if he is allergic to penicillin. Negative history of penicillin allergy is no guarantee against future allergic reaction.
• Obtain specimen for culture and sensitivity tests before giving first dose. Therapy may begin pending results.
• Monitor serum potassium level.
• Monitor CBC and platelet count.
• Be alert for adverse reactions and drug interactions.

• Monitor patient's hydration status if adverse GI reactions occur.
• Evaluate patient's and family's knowledge of drug therapy.

Nursing diagnoses
• Infection related to presence of susceptible bacteria
• Risk for fluid volume deficit related to drug-induced adverse GI reactions
• Knowledge deficit related to drug therapy

Planning and implementation
• Dosage should be decreased in patient with impaired kidney function.
I.V. use: Reconstitute vials using D_5W, 0.9% NaCl injection, sterile water for injection, or other compatible solution. Add 4 ml of diluent for each gram of drug. Further dilute to maximum concentration of 50 mg/ml, and inject slowly directly into vein or I.V. line containing free-flowing solution. Or, dilute to concentration of 10 to 100 mg/ml, and intermittently infuse over 30 minutes to 2 hours in adults or 10 to 20 minutes in neonates.
– Know that aminoglycoside antibiotics (such as gentamicin and tobramycin) are chemically incompatible. Don't mix in same I.V. container.
– Continuous infusion may cause vein irritation. Change site every 48 hours.
I.M. use: Reconstitute vials with sterile water for injection, 0.9% NaCl injection, or lidocaine 1% (without epinephrine). Use 2 ml of diluent per gram of drug. Inject deeply into large muscle. Don't exceed 2 g per injection.
• Give drug at least 1 hour before bacteriostatic antibiotics.
• Institute seizure precautions. Patient with high blood level of ticarcillin may develop seizures.
• Drug is typically used with another antibiotic, such as gentamicin.
Patient teaching
• Instruct patient to report adverse reactions.

Reactions may be *common*, uncommon, *life-threatening*, or COMMON AND LIFE-THREATENING.

☑ **Evaluation**
• Patient is free from infection.
• Patient maintains adequate hydration.
• Patient and family state understanding of drug therapy.

---

ticarcillin disodium/clavulanate potassium
(tigh-kar-SIL-in digh-SOH-dee-um/ KLAV-yoo-lan-nayt poh-TAH-see-um)
Timentin

Pharmacologic class: extended-spectrum penicillin, beta-lactamase inhibitor
Therapeutic class: antibiotic
Pregnancy risk category: B

How supplied

Injection: 3 g ticarcillin and 100 mg clavulanic acid

Pharmacokinetics

Absorption: not applicable with I.V. administration.
Distribution: ticarcillin disodium distributed widely; penetrates minimally into CSF with uninflamed meninges. Clavulanic acid penetrates into pleural fluid, lungs, and peritoneal fluid.
Metabolism: about 13% of ticarcillin dose metabolized by hydrolysis to inactive compounds; clavulanic acid is thought to undergo extensive metabolism but its fate is unknown.
Excretion: ticarcillin excreted primarily in urine; also excreted in bile. Clavulanate's metabolites are excreted in urine.
Half-life: about 1 hour.

Route	Onset	Peak	Duration
I.V.	Immediate	Immediate	Unknown

Pharmacodynamics

Chemical effect: ticarcillin is an extended-spectrum penicillin that inhibits cell-wall synthesis during microorganism replication; clavulanic acid increases ticarcillin's effectiveness by inactivating beta lactamases, which destroy ticarcillin.
Therapeutic effect: kills susceptible bacteria. Spectrum of activity for ticarcillin includes many gram-negative aerobic and anaerobic bacilli, many gram-positive and gram-negative aerobic cocci, and some gram-positive aerobic and anaerobic bacilli. The combination of ticarcillin and clavulanate potassium is also effective against many beta-lactamase– producing strains, including *Bacteroides fragilis, Escherichia coli, Haemophilus influenzae, Klebsiella, Neisseria gonorrhoeae, Providencia,* and *Staphylococcus aureus.*

Indications and dosage

▶ **Lower respiratory tract, urinary tract, bone and joint, skin, and skin-structure infections and septicemia when caused by beta-lactamase– producing strains of bacteria or by ticarcillin-susceptible organisms.**
Adults: 3.1 g (3 g ticarcillin and 100 mg clavulanate acid) administered by I.V. infusion q 4 to 6 hours.

Adverse reactions

CNS: *seizures,* neuromuscular excitability, headache, giddiness.
CV: vein irritation, phlebitis.
GI: nausea, diarrhea, stomatitis, vomiting, epigastric pain, flatulence, pseudomembranous colitis, taste and smell disturbances.
Hematologic: *leukopenia, neutropenia,* eosinophilia, *thrombocytopenia,* hemolytic anemia, anemia.
Other: hypersensitivity reactions (rash, pruritus, urticaria, chills, fever, edema, *anaphylaxis*), overgrowth of nonsusceptible organisms, hypokalemia, pain at injection site.

Interactions

Drug-drug. *Oral contraceptives:* efficacy of oral contraceptives may be decreased. Recommend an additional form of contraception during penicillin therapy.

Probenecid: increased blood levels of ticarcillin. Probenecid may be used for this purpose.

Contraindications and precautions

• Contraindicated in patients with hypersensitivity to penicillins.

• Use cautiously in patients with other drug allergies, especially to cephalosporins (possible cross-sensitivity); in those with impaired kidney function, hemorrhagic condition, hypokalemia, or sodium restrictions (contains 4.5 mEq sodium/g); and in pregnant or breast-feeding women.

NURSING CONSIDERATIONS

Assessment

• Assess patient's infection before therapy and regularly thereafter.

• Before giving drug, ask patient if he's allergic to penicillin. Negative history of penicillin allergy is no guarantee against future allergic reaction.

• Obtain specimen for culture and sensitivity tests before giving first dose. Therapy may begin pending results.

• Monitor CBC and platelet count.

• Be alert for adverse reactions and drug interactions.

• Monitor patient's hydration status if adverse GI reactions occur.

• Evaluate patient's and family's knowledge of drug therapy.

Nursing diagnoses

• Infection related to presence of susceptible bacteria

• Risk for fluid volume deficit related to drug-induced adverse GI reactions

• Knowledge deficit related to drug therapy

Planning and implementation

• Dosage should be decreased in patient with impaired kidney function.

• Reconstitute drug with 13 ml of sterile water for injection or 0.9% NaCl injection. Further dilute to maximum of 10 to 100 mg/ml (based on ticarcillin component) and infuse over 30 minutes. In fluid-restricted patient, dilute to maximum of 48 mg/ml if using D_5W, 43 mg/ml if using 0.9% NaCl injection, or 86 mg/ml if using sterile water for injection.

• Aminoglycoside antibiotics (such as gentamicin and tobramycin) are chemically incompatible. Don't mix in same I.V. container.

• Give drug at least 1 hour before bacteriostatic antibiotics.

Patient teaching

• Instruct patient to report adverse reactions immediately.

Evaluation

• Patient is free from infection.

• Patient maintains adequate hydration.

• Patient and family state understanding of drug therapy.

ticlopidine hydrochloride
(tigh-KLOH-peh-deen high-droh-KLOR-ighd)
Ticlid

Pharmacologic class: platelet aggregation inhibitor
Therapeutic class: antithrombotic agent
Pregnancy risk category: B

How supplied

Tablets: 250 mg

Pharmacokinetics

Absorption: rapidly and extensively absorbed; enhanced by food.
Distribution: 98% bound to serum proteins and lipoproteins.
Metabolism: extensively metabolized by liver. More than 20 metabolites have been identified; it is unknown if parent drug or active metabolites are responsible for pharmacologic activity.
Excretion: 60% excreted in urine and 23% in feces.

Route	Onset	Peak	Duration
P.O.	≤ 2 days	About 2 hr	1-2 wk

Pharmacodynamics

Chemical effect: unknown; probably blocks adenosine diphosphate–induced platelet-fibrinogen and platelet-platelet binding.
Therapeutic effect: prevents blood clots from forming.

Indications and dosage

▶ **To reduce risk of thrombotic stroke in patients with history of stroke or who have experienced stroke precursors.**
Adults: 250 mg P.O. b.i.d. with meals.

Adverse reactions

CNS: dizziness, *intracerebral bleeding.*
CV: vasculitis.
EENT: epistaxis, conjunctival hemorrhage.
GI: *diarrhea,* nausea, dyspepsia, vomiting, flatulence, anorexia, *abdominal pain,* bleeding.
GU: hematuria, *nephrotic syndrome,* dark-colored urine.
Hematologic: *neutropenia, agranulocytosis, pancytopenia, immune thrombocytopenia.*
Hepatic: hepatitis, cholestatic jaundice, abnormal liver function tests.
Metabolic: *hyponatremia.*
Musculoskeletal: arthropathy, myositis.
Respiratory: *allergic pneumonitis.*
Skin: *rash,* purpura, pruritus, ecchymosis, urticaria, *thrombocytopenic purpura.*
Other: hypersensitivity reactions, postoperative bleeding, systemic lupus erythematosus, *serum sickness.*

Interactions

Drug-drug. *Antacids:* decreased plasma ticlopidine level. Separate administration times by at least 2 hours.
Aspirin: aspirin effects on platelets potentiated. Don't use together.
Cimetidine: decreased clearance of ticlopidine and increased risk of toxicity. Avoid concomitant use.

Digoxin: slight decrease in serum digoxin level. Monitor level.
Theophylline: decreased theophylline clearance and risk of toxicity. Monitor patient closely and adjust theophylline dosage, as ordered.

Contraindications and precautions

● Contraindicated in patients with hematopoietic disorders (such as neutropenia, thrombocytopenia, or disorders of hemostasis), active pathologic bleeding (such as peptic ulceration or active intracranial bleeding), severe hepatic impairment, or hypersensitivity to drug.
● Drug is reserved for patients intolerant to aspirin.
● Drug is not recommended for use in breast-feeding women.
● Use cautiously in pregnant women.
● Safety of drug has not been established in children.

NURSING CONSIDERATIONS

≈ Assessment
● Assess patient's condition before therapy and regularly thereafter.
● Obtain baseline liver function tests before therapy. Monitor closely, especially during first 4 months of treatment, and repeat when liver dysfunction is suspected.
● Determine baseline CBC and WBC differentials and then repeat at second week of therapy and every 2 weeks until end of third month. Frequency of tests increased if patient shows signs of declining neutrophil count or if count falls 30% below baseline. After first 3 months, CBC and WBC differential determinations should be performed only in patient showing signs of infection.
● Be alert for adverse reactions and drug interactions.
● Evaluate patient's and family's knowledge of drug therapy.

▩ Nursing diagnoses
● Impaired cerebral tissue perfusion related to stroke potential or history

---

• Altered protection related to drug-induced adverse hematologic reactions
• Knowledge deficit related to drug therapy

> ⬧ **Planning and implementation**
• Thrombocytopenia has occurred rarely. Report platelet count of 80,000/mm³ or less, and stop drug. If ordered, give 20 mg of methylprednisolone I.V. to normalize bleeding time within 2 hours. Platelet transfusions may also be used.
• When used preoperatively, drug may decrease incidence of graft occlusion in patient receiving coronary artery bypass grafts and reduce severity of drop in platelet count in patient receiving extracorporeal hemoperfusion during open heart surgery.
Patient teaching
• Tell patient to take drug with meals; this substantially increases bioavailability and improves GI tolerance.
• Tell patient to avoid aspirin-containing products and to check with doctor before taking OTC drugs.
• Explain that drug prolongs bleeding time but to report unusual or prolonged bleeding. Advise him to tell dentist and other doctors that he is taking this drug.
• Stress importance of regular blood tests. Because neutropenia can increase risk of infection, tell patient to promptly report such signs as fever, chills, and sore throat.
• If drug is substituted for fibrinolytic or anticoagulant, tell patient to discontinue those drugs before starting ticlopidine therapy, as ordered.
• Advise patient to stop drug 10 to 14 days before elective surgery.
• Tell patient to report yellow skin or sclera, severe or persistent diarrhea, rashes, subcutaneous bleeding, light-colored stools, and dark urine.

☑ **Evaluation**
• Patient maintains adequate cerebral perfusion.

• Patient does not develop serious complications.
• Patient and family state understanding of drug therapy.

timolol maleate
(TIH-moh-lol MAL-ee-ayt)
Apo-Timol♦, Blocadren

Pharmacologic class: beta blocker
Therapeutic class: antihypertensive, adjunct in MI, antimigraine
Pregnancy risk category: C

How supplied
Tablets: 5 mg, 10 mg, 20 mg

Pharmacokinetics
Absorption: about 90% absorbed from GI tract.
Distribution: distributed throughout body; depending on assay method, drug is 10% to 60% protein-bound.
Metabolism: about 80% metabolized in liver to inactive metabolites.
Excretion: drug and its metabolites excreted primarily in urine. *Half-life:* about 4 hours.

Route	Onset	Peak	Duration
P.O.	15-30 min	1-2 hr	6-12 hr

Pharmacodynamics
Chemical effect: mechanism of antihypertensive action unknown. In MI, drug may decrease myocardial oxygen requirements. It also prevents arterial dilation through beta blockade for migraine headache prophylaxis.
Therapeutic effect: lowers blood pressure and helps to prevent MI and migraine headaches.

Indications and dosage
▶ **Hypertension.** *Adults:* initially, 10 mg P.O. b.i.d. Usual daily maintenance dosage is 20 to 40 mg. Maximum daily

dosage is 60 mg. Allow at least 7 days to elapse between increases in dosage.
► **MI (long-term prophylaxis in patients who have survived acute phase).**
Adults: 10 mg P.O. b.i.d.
► **Prevention of migraine headache.**
Adults: usual dose is 10 mg P.O. b.i.d. During maintenance therapy, 20-mg daily dose may be given once daily. Maximum daily dosage is 30 mg in divided doses (10 mg in morning, and 20 mg in evening). If maximum dosage for 6 to 8 weeks does not achieve an adequate response, another therapy should be instituted.

Adverse reactions

CNS: fatigue, lethargy, dizziness.
CV: bradycardia, hypotension, peripheral vascular disease, *arrhythmias, heart failure.*
GI: nausea, vomiting, diarrhea.
Respiratory: dyspnea, *bronchospasm, increased airway resistance.*
Skin: pruritus.

Interactions

Drug-drug. *Cardiac glycosides, diltiazem, verapamil:* excessive bradycardia and increased depressant effect on myocardium. Use together cautiously.
Catecholamine-depleting drugs (such as reserpine): may have additive effects when given with beta blockers. Monitor for hypotension and bradycardia.
Indomethacin: decreased antihypertensive effect. Monitor blood pressure and adjust dosage.
Insulin, oral antidiabetic agents: can alter requirements for these drugs in previously stabilized diabetic patients. Monitor patient for hypoglycemia.

Contraindications and precautions

• Contraindicated in patients with bronchial asthma, severe COPD, sinus bradycardia and heart block greater than first-degree, cardiogenic shock, overt heart failure, or hypersensitivity to drug.

• Drug is not recommended for use in breast-feeding women.
• Use cautiously in patients with compensated heart failure; hepatic, renal, or respiratory disease; diabetes; or hyperthyroidism and in pregnant women.
• Safety of drug has not been established in children.

NURSING CONSIDERATIONS

Assessment
• Assess patient's condition before therapy and regularly thereafter.
• Monitor blood pressure frequently.
• Be alert for adverse reactions and drug interactions.
• Evaluate patient's and family's knowledge of drug therapy.

Nursing diagnoses
• Risk for injury related to history of hypertension or MI
• Pain related to migraine headache
• Knowledge deficit related to drug therapy

Planning and implementation
• Check patient's apical pulse rate before giving drug. Report extreme pulse rate, and withhold drug.
• Don't stop drug abruptly; this can exacerbate angina and precipitate MI. Dosage should be reduced gradually over 1 to 2 weeks.
Patient teaching
• Explain importance of taking drug exactly as prescribed.
• Tell patient not to discontinue drug abruptly because serious complications can occur. Instead, tell him to report adverse reactions.

Evaluation
• Patient does not experience injury from underlying disease.
• Patient does not develop migraine headaches.
• Patient and family state understanding of drug therapy.

tioconazole
(tigh-uh-KON-uh-zohl)
Vagistat-1

Pharmacologic class: imidazole
derivative
Therapeutic class: antifungal
Pregnancy risk category: C

How supplied
Vaginal ointment: 6.5%

Pharmacokinetics
Absorption: negligible.
Distribution: unknown.
Metabolism: unknown.
Excretion: unknown.

Route	Onset	Peak	Duration
Vaginal	Unknown	Unknown	Unknown

Pharmacodynamics
Chemical effect: alters cell-wall permeability.
Therapeutic effect: kills fungi causing
vulvovaginal candidiasis.

Indications and dosage
▶ **Vulvovaginal candidiasis.** *Adults:* one
applicatorful (about 4.6 g) inserted intravaginally h.s. as a single dose.

Adverse reactions
GU: burning, pruritus, discharge, vaginal
pain, dysuria, dyspareunia, vulvar edema,
irritation.

Interactions
None significant.

Contraindications and precautions
● Contraindicated in patients hypersensitive to drug or other imidazole antifungal
agents (miconazole, ketoconazole).
● Drug is not recommended for use in
breast-feeding women.
● Use cautiously in pregnant women.
● Safety of drug has not been established
in children.

NURSING CONSIDERATIONS

⚖ Assessment
● Assess patient's infection before therapy and regularly thereafter.
● Be alert for adverse reactions.
● Evaluate patient's and family's knowledge of drug therapy.

⊞ Nursing diagnoses
● Infection related to presence of susceptible fungi
● Knowledge deficit related to drug
therapy

▷ Planning and implementation
● Insert one applicatorful into vagina.
● To avoid contamination of ointment,
open applicator just before use.
Patient teaching
● Review proper use of drug with patient.
Written instructions for patient are available with product. Tell patient to insert
drug high into vagina.
● Suggest that patient use sanitary napkin
to avoid staining her clothing.
● Advise patient to avoid sexual intercourse during therapy, or suggest condom
to prevent reinfection.
● Tell patient to report adverse reaction to
doctor.

☑ Evaluation
● Patient is free from infection.
● Patient and family state understanding
of drug therapy.

tizanidine hydrochloride
(tigh-ZAN-eh-deen high-droh-KLOR-ighd)
Zanaflex

Pharmacologic class: alpha$_2$-adrenergic
agonist
Therapeutic class: antispasticity agent
Pregnancy risk category: C

How supplied
Tablets: 4 mg

Reactions may be *common*, uncommon, *life-threatening*, or COMMON AND LIFE-THREATENING.

Pharmacokinetics

Absorption: almost completely absorbed.
Distribution: throughout body.
Metabolism: in liver.
Excretion: in urine and feces. *Half-life:* 2.5 hours.

Route	Onset	Peak	Duration
P.O.	Unknown	1-2 hr	3-6 hr

Pharmacodynamics

Chemical effect: agonist at alpha$_2$-adrenergic receptor sites.
Therapeutic effect: reduces spasticity; reduces facilitation of spinal motor neurons.

Indications and dosage

▶ **Acute and intermittent management of increased muscle tone associated with spasticity.** *Adults:* initially, 4 mg P.O. q 6 to 8 hours p.r.n. to maximum of three doses in 24 hours. Dosage can be increased gradually in 2- to 4-mg increments. Maximum daily dosage is 36 mg.

Adverse reactions

CNS: *somnolence, sedation, asthenia, dizziness,* speech disorder, dyskinesia, nervousness, hallucinations.
CV: *hypotension,* **bradycardia.**
EENT: amblyopia, pharyngitis, rhinitis.
GI: *dry mouth,* constipation, vomiting.
GU: *urinary tract infection,* urinary frequency.
Hepatic: elevations of liver function tests, hepatic injury.
Other: infection, flulike syndrome.

Interactions

Drug-drug. *Antihypertensives, other alpha$_2$-adrenergic agonists:* may cause hypotension. Monitor patient closely. Do not use with other alpha$_2$-adrenergic agonists.
Baclofen, benzodiazepines, other CNS depressants: additive CNS depressant effects. Avoid concomitant use.
Oral contraceptives: decreased clearance of tizanidine. Dosage may be reduced.

Drug-lifestyle. *Alcohol use:* additive CNS depressant effects. Avoid concomitant use.

Contraindications and precautions

• Contraindicated in patients with known hypersensitivity to drug.

NURSING CONSIDERATIONS

Assessment
• Use cautiously in patients who are taking antihypertensives, in those with renal or hepatic impairment, and in the elderly.
• Obtain baseline liver function tests as ordered before treatment; during treatment at 1, 3, and 6 months; and then periodically thereafter.
• Evaluate patient's and family's knowledge of drug therapy.

Nursing diagnoses
• Risk for injury related to drug-induced adverse CNS reactions
• Knowledge deficit related to drug therapy

Planning and implementation
• Know that dosage is reduced in patient with renal impairment. If higher dosage is needed, individual dose rather than frequency is increased.
Patient teaching
• Inform patient of limited clinical experience with drug.
• Warn patient that drug-induced drowsiness may occur and to avoid alcohol and activities that require alertness.
• Inform patient to rise slowly and avoid sudden position changes.

Evaluation
• Patient does not experience injury from adverse CNS reactions.
• Patient and family state understanding of drug therapy.

---

*Liquid form contains alcohol   **May contain tartrazine   ◆ Canada   ◇ Australia   †OTC

tobramycin sulfate
(toh-breh-MIGH-sin SUL-fayt)
Nebcin

Pharmacologic class: aminoglycoside
Therapeutic class: antibiotic
Pregnancy risk category: D

How supplied

Injection: 40 mg/ml, 10 mg/ml (pediatric)
Powder for injection: 30 mg/ml after reconstitution
Premixed parenteral injection for I.V. infusion: 60 mg or 80 mg in 0.9% NaCl

Pharmacokinetics

Absorption: unknown after I.M. administration.
Distribution: distributed widely, although CSF penetration is low, even in patients with inflamed meninges. Protein-binding is minimal.
Metabolism: not metabolized.
Excretion: excreted primarily in urine; small amount may be excreted in bile.
Half-life: 2 to 3 hours.

Route	Onset	Peak	Duration
I.V.	Immediate	Immediate	About 8 hr
I.M.	Unknown	30-90 min	About 8 hr

Pharmacodynamics

Chemical effect: inhibits protein synthesis by binding directly to 30S ribosomal subunit. Drug is generally bactericidal.
Therapeutic effect: kills susceptible bacteria. Spectrum of activity includes many aerobic gram-negative organisms, including most strains of *Pseudomonas aeruginosa* and some aerobic gram-positive organisms.

Indications and dosage

▶ **Serious infections caused by sensitive strains of** *Citrobacter, Enterobacter, Escherichia coli, Klebsiella, Proteus, Providencia, Pseudomonas, Serratia, Staphylococcus aureus.* Adults and chil-

dren with normal renal function: 3 mg/kg I.M. or I.V. daily divided q 8 hours. Up to 5 mg/kg daily divided q 6 to 8 hours for life-threatening infections. *Neonates under age 1 week or premature infants:* up to 4 mg/kg I.V. or I.M. daily in two equal doses q 12 hours.

Adverse reactions

CNS: headache, lethargy, confusion, disorientation.
EENT: *ototoxicity.*
GI: nausea, vomiting, diarrhea.
GU: *nephrotoxicity.*
Hematologic: anemia, eosinophilia, *leukopenia, thrombocytopenia, agranulocytosis.*
Other: hypersensitivity reactions *(anaphylaxis).*

Interactions

Drug-drug. *Acyclovir, amphotericin B, cisplatin, methoxyflurane, other aminoglycosides, vancomycin:* increased nephrotoxicity. Use together cautiously.
Cephalothin: increased nephrotoxicity. Use together cautiously.
Dimenhydrinate: may mask symptoms of ototoxicity. Use with caution.
General anesthetics, neuromuscular blockers: may potentiate neuromuscular blockade. Monitor patient closely.
I.V. loop diuretics (such as furosemide): increased ototoxicity. Use together cautiously.
Parenteral penicillins (such as ticarcillin): tobramycin inactivation in vitro. Don't mix together.

Contraindications and precautions

• Contraindicated in patients with hypersensitivity to aminoglycosides.
• Drug is not recommended for use in pregnant or breast-feeding women.
• Use cautiously in patients with impaired kidney function or neuromuscular disorders and in elderly patients.

NURSING CONSIDERATIONS

📝 Assessment
• Assess patient's infection before therapy and regularly thereafter.
• Obtain specimen for culture and sensitivity tests before giving first dose. Therapy may begin pending results.
• Draw blood for peak tobramycin level 1 hour after I.M. injection and 30 minutes to 1 hour after infusion ends; draw blood for trough level just before next dose. Don't collect blood in heparinized tube because heparin is incompatible with drug.
• Weigh patient and review baseline kidney function studies before therapy.
• Evaluate patient's hearing before and during therapy. Report tinnitus, vertigo, or hearing loss.
• Be aware that blood levels over 12 mcg/ml and trough levels over 2 mcg/ml may be associated with increased incidence of toxicity.
• Monitor kidney function (output, specific gravity, urinalysis, BUN and creatinine levels, and creatinine clearance).
• Be alert for adverse reactions and drug interactions.
• Evaluate patient's and family's knowledge of drug therapy.

🔲 Nursing diagnoses
• Infection related to susceptible bacteria
• Risk for injury related to potential for drug-induced nephrotoxicity
• Knowledge deficit related to drug therapy

▶ Planning and implementation
I.M. use: Follow normal protocol.
I.V. use: Dilute in 50 to 100 ml of 0.9% NaCl solution or D_5W for adults and in less volume for children. Infuse over 20 to 60 minutes. After I.V. infusion, flush line with 0.9% NaCl solution or D_5W.
• Notify doctor of signs of decreasing kidney function.
• Patient should be well hydrated while taking drug to minimize chemical irritation of renal tubules.

• Be aware that if no response occurs in 3 to 5 days, therapy may be stopped and new specimens obtained for culture and sensitivity testing.
Patient teaching
• Emphasize need to drink 2,000 ml of fluid each day.
• Instruct patient to report adverse reactions.

🔲 Evaluation
• Patient is free from infection.
• Patient maintains normal kidney function.
• Patient and family state understanding of drug therapy.

tocainide hydrochloride
(TOH-kay-nighd high-droh-KLOR-ighd)
Tonocard

Pharmacologic class: local anesthetic
Therapeutic class: ventricular antiarrhythmic
Pregnancy risk category: C

How supplied
Tablets: 400 mg, 600 mg

Pharmacokinetics
Absorption: rapidly and completely absorbed from GI tract.
Distribution: not clearly defined, although drug appears to be widely distributed and apparently crosses blood-brain barrier. Only about 10% to 20% bound to plasma protein.
Metabolism: metabolized apparently in liver to inactive metabolites.
Excretion: excreted in urine. *Half-life:* about 11 to 23 hours.

Route	Onset	Peak	Duration
P.O.	Unknown	0.5-2 hr	8 hr

Pharmacodynamics
Chemical effect: class Ib antiarrhythmic that blocks fast sodium channel in car-

diac tissues, especially Purkinje network, without involvement of autonomic nervous system. It reduces rate of rise and amplitude of action potential and decreases automaticity in Purkinje fibers. It shortens duration of action potential and, to lesser extent, decreases effective refractory period in Purkinje fibers.
Therapeutic effect: restores normal sinus rhythm.

Indications and dosage

▶ **Suppression of symptomatic life-threatening ventricular arrhythmias, such as sustained ventricular tachycardia.** *Adults:* initially, 400 mg P.O. q 8 hours. Usual dosage is between 1,200 and 1,800 mg daily in three divided doses.

Adverse reactions

CNS: *light-headedness, tremors,* restlessness, paresthesias, confusion, *dizziness, vertigo,* drowsiness, fatigue, confusion, headache.
CV: hypotension, *new or worsened arrhythmias, heart failure, bradycardia,* palpitations.
EENT: blurred vision, tinnitus.
GI: *nausea,* vomiting, diarrhea, anorexia.
Hematologic: *blood dyscrasia.*
Hepatic: hepatitis.
Respiratory: *respiratory arrest,* pulmonary fibrosis, pneumonitis, *pulmonary edema.*
Skin: rash, diaphoresis.

Interactions

Drug-drug. *Beta blockers:* decreased myocardial contractility; increased CNS toxicity. Avoid concomitant use.
Cimetidine: may decrease tocainide peak concentration. Monitor closely.
Disopyramide, lidocaine, mexiletine, phenytoin, procainamide, quinidine: additive pharmacologic effect and CNS toxicity. Monitor closely.
Rifampin: increased clearance of tocainide. Monitor efficacy of tocainide.

Contraindications and precautions

• Contraindicated in patients with hypersensitivity to lidocaine or other amide-type local anesthetics and in those with second- or third-degree AV block in absence of artificial pacemaker.
• Use cautiously in patients with heart failure or diminished cardiac reserve and in those with hepatic or renal impairment. These patients often may be treated effectively with lower dose.
• Safety of drug has not been established in breast-feeding women and in children.

NURSING CONSIDERATIONS

Assessment
• Assess patient's condition before therapy and regularly thereafter.
• Monitor therapeutic blood level. Therapeutic blood levels range from 4 to 10 mcg/ml. Report deviations.
• Monitor patient for tremors, which may indicate that maximum dosage has been reached.
• Monitor patient during transition from lidocaine to tocainide.
• Be alert for adverse reactions and drug interactions.
• Evaluate patient's and family's knowledge of drug therapy.

Nursing diagnoses
• Decreased cardiac output related to presence of cardiac arrhythmia
• Risk for injury related to drug-induced adverse reactions
• Knowledge deficit related to drug therapy

Planning and implementation
• Be aware that drug is considered by cardiologists as "oral lidocaine." It may ease transition from I.V. lidocaine to oral antiarrhythmic therapy.
Patient teaching
• Instruct patient to take drug with food.
• Tell patient to report unusual bruising or bleeding or signs of infection. Agranulocytosis and bone marrow sup-

---

Reactions may be *common,* uncommon, *life-threatening,* or COMMON AND LIFE-THREATENING.

pression have been reported in patients taking usual doses of drug. Most cases have been reported within first 12 weeks of therapy.
• Tell patient to report sudden onset of pulmonary symptoms, such as coughing, wheezing, and exertional dyspnea. Drug has been associated with serious pulmonary toxicity.
• Dizziness and falling are more likely to occur in elderly patient. Tell patient to take safety precautions.

☑ **Evaluation**
• Patient exhibits normal cardiac output with abolishment of arrhythmia.
• Patient does not experience injury from adverse reactions.
• Patient and family state understanding of drug therapy.

tolazamide
(tohl-AZ-ah-mighd)
Tolinase

Pharmacologic class: sulfonylurea
Therapeutic class: antidiabetic
Pregnancy risk category: C

How supplied
Tablets: 100 mg, 250 mg, 500 mg

Pharmacokinetics
Absorption: absorbed slowly but well from GI tract.
Distribution: probably distributed in extracellular fluid.
Metabolism: metabolized to several mildly active metabolites.
Excretion: excreted in urine. *Half-life:* 7 hours.

Route	Onset	Peak	Duration
P.O.	4-6 hr	4-6 hr	12-24 hr

Pharmacodynamics
Chemical effect: unknown; probably stimulates insulin release from pancreatic beta cells and reduces glucose output by liver. An extrapancreatic effect increases peripheral sensitivity to insulin.
Therapeutic effect: lowers blood glucose levels.

Indications and dosage
► **Adjunct to diet to lower blood glucose levels in patients with type 2 (non-insulin-dependent) diabetes mellitus.** *Adults:* initially, 100 mg P.O. daily with breakfast if fasting blood sugar (FBS) is under 200 mg/dl, or 250 mg P.O. if FBS is over 200 mg/dl. Dosage adjusted at weekly intervals by 100 to 250 mg, as necessary. To avoid hypoglycemia in underweight, undernourished or elderly patients, increase dosage by 50 to 125 mg daily at weekly intervals, as needed. Maximum daily dosage is 500 mg b.i.d. before meals.
► **To change from insulin to oral therapy.** *Adults:* if insulin dosage is under 20 units daily, insulin may be stopped and oral therapy started at 100 mg P.O. daily with breakfast. If insulin dosage is 20 to 40 units daily, insulin may be stopped and oral therapy started at 250 mg P.O. daily with breakfast. If insulin dosage is over 40 units daily, insulin may be decreased by 50% and oral therapy started at 250 mg P.O. daily with breakfast. Dosage may be adjusted by 100 to 250 mg.

Adverse reactions
GI: nausea, vomiting.
Hematologic: *thrombocytopenia, aplastic anemia, agranulocytosis.*
Skin: rash, urticaria, facial flushing.
Other: *hypersensitivity reactions, hypoglycemia.*

Interactions
Drug-drug. *Anabolic steroids, chloramphenicol, clofibrate, guanethidine, MAO inhibitors, phenylbutazone, salicylates, sulfonamides:* increased hypoglycemic activity. Monitor blood glucose levels carefully.

Beta blockers, clonidine: prolonged hypoglycemic effect and masked symptoms of hypoglycemia. Monitor patient closely.

Corticosteroids, glucagon, rifampin, thiazide diuretics: decreased hypoglycemic response. Monitor blood glucose level.

Hydantoins: increased blood level of hydantoins. Monitor blood level.

Oral anticoagulants: increased hypoglycemic activity or enhanced anticoagulant effect. Monitor blood glucose levels and PT and INR.

Drug-lifestyle. *Alcohol use:* possible disulfiram-like reaction. Don't use with moderate to large amounts of alcohol.

Contraindications and precautions

• Contraindicated for treating type 1 diabetes (insulin-dependent) or diabetes that can be adequately controlled by diet. Also contraindicated in patients with type 2 diabetes complicated by ketosis, acidosis, coma, or other acute complications such as major surgery, severe infection, and severe trauma; in patients with uremia or hypersensitivity to sulfonylureas, and in pregnant or breast-feeding women.

• Use cautiously in elderly, debilitated, or malnourished patients or in those with impaired liver or kidney function or porphyria.

• Safety of drug has not been established in children.

NURSING CONSIDERATIONS

Assessment

• Assess patient's blood glucose before therapy and regularly thereafter.

• Patient transferring from insulin therapy to oral antidiabetic agent requires blood glucose level testing at least three times a day before meals.

• Be alert for adverse reactions and drug interactions.

• Elderly patient may be more sensitive to drug's adverse effects.

• Evaluate patient's and family's knowledge of drug therapy.

Nursing diagnoses

• Altered health maintenance related to presence of hyperglycemia

• Risk for injury related to drug-induced hypoglycemia

• Knowledge deficit related to drug therapy

Planning and implementation

• Be aware that patient transferring from another oral antidiabetic agent usually needs no transition period.

• Administer drug with food if adverse GI reactions occur.

• Tablets may be crushed to ease administration.

Patient teaching

• Make sure patient knows that therapy relieves symptoms only.

• Teach patient about the disease. Stress importance of adhering to therapeutic regimen and diet, weight reduction, exercise, and personal hygiene programs. Emphasize need to avoid infection. Explain how and when to perform self-monitoring of blood glucose level, and teach recognition of and intervention for hypoglycemia and hyperglycemia.

• Tell patient not to change drug dosage without doctor's consent and to report abnormal blood or urine glucose test results.

• Teach patient to carry candy or other simple sugars to treat mild hypoglycemic episodes. Severe episodes may require hospital treatment.

• Advise patient not to take other medications, including OTC drugs, without first checking with doctor.

• Advise patient to avoid moderate to large intake of alcohol because of possible disulfiram-like reaction.

• Advise patient to carry medical identification at all times.

Evaluation

• Patient's blood glucose level is normal.

• Patient does not experience hypoglycemia.

• Patient and family state understanding of drug therapy.

tolazoline hydrochloride
(toh-LAHZ-oh-leen
high-droh-KLOR-ighd)
Priscoline

Pharmacologic class: peripheral
vasodilatory, alpha-adrenergic blocker
Therapeutic class: antihypertensive
Pregnancy risk category: C

How supplied
Injection: 25 mg/ml

Pharmacokinetics
Absorption: not applicable.
Distribution: concentrates primarily in
kidneys and liver.
Metabolism: none.
Excretion: excreted in urine. *Half-life:*
1½ to 41 hours (inversely related to urine
output).

Route	Onset	Peak	Duration
I.V.	≤ 30 min	Unknown	Unknown

Pharmacodynamics
Chemical effect: direct-acting vasodilator; may have some alpha-receptor blocking effects.
Therapeutic effect: reduces pulmonary
hypertension in neonate.

Indications and dosage
► **Persistent pulmonary hypertension
of neonate.** *Neonates:* initially, 1 to
2 mg/kg I.V. over 10 minutes, followed
by infusion of 1 to 2 mg/kg/hour.

Adverse reactions
CV: *arrhythmias,* anginal pain, *hyperten-
sion, flushing,* tachycardia, *hypotension.*
GI: nausea, vomiting, diarrhea, *GI hem-
orrhage.*
GU: hematuria, oliguria, edema.
Hematologic: *leukopenia, thrombocy-
topenia.*
Respiratory: *pulmonary hemorrhage.*
Skin: increased pilomotor activity with
tingling and chilliness, rash.

Interactions
Drug-drug. *Vasopressors (epinephrine,
norepinephrine):* may cause paradoxical
fall in blood pressure. Monitor closely.

Contraindications and precautions
● Contraindicated in neonates with hypersensitivity to drug.
● Use cautiously in patients with known
or suspected mitral stenosis.
● Drug is not indicated for use in pregnant or breast-feeding women.

NURSING CONSIDERATIONS

▨ Assessment
● Assess patient's condition before therapy and regularly thereafter.
● Know that response to treatment of persistent pulmonary hypertension of
neonate should be evident within 30 minutes. Little information exists regarding
infusions lasting longer than 48 hours.
● Be alert for adverse reactions and drug
interactions.
● Monitor vital signs and ECG. Watch especially for blood pressure changes and
arrhythmias.
● Evaluate patient's and family's knowledge of drug therapy.

▥ Nursing diagnoses
● Altered health maintenance related to
presence of pulmonary hypertension
● Decreased cardiac output related to
drug-induced arrhythmias
● Knowledge deficit related to drug
therapy

▧ Planning and implementation
● Place patient in supine position during
infusion.
● To increase response, keep patient
warm during administration.
● Appearance of flushing usually indi-
cates maximum tolerable dose.
Patient teaching
● Tell parents about need for drug.

---

*Liquid form contains alcohol **May contain tartrazine   ◆ Canada   ◊ Australia   †OTC

☑ Evaluation
• Patient exhibits positive response to drug.
• Patient does not develop drug-induced arrhythmias.
• Parents state understanding of drug therapy.

---

tolbutamide
(tole-BYOO-tah-mide)
Apo-Tolbutamide, Mobenol♦,
Novo-Butamide♦, Orinase

Pharmacologic class: sulfonylurea
Therapeutic class: antidiabetic
Pregnancy risk category: C

How supplied

Tablets: 250 mg, 500 mg

Pharmacokinetics

Absorption: absorbed well from GI tract.
Distribution: probably distributed in extracellular fluid.
Metabolism: metabolized in liver to inactive metabolites.
Excretion: excreted in urine and feces.
Half-life: 4 to 5 hours.

Route	Onset	Peak	Duration
P.O.	≤ 1 hr	3-5 hr	6-12 hr

Pharmacodynamics

Chemical effect: unknown; probably stimulates insulin release from pancreatic beta cells and reduces glucose output by liver. An extrapancreatic effect increases peripheral sensitivity to insulin.
Therapeutic effect: lowers blood glucose levels.

Indications and dosage

▶ **Adjunct to diet to lower blood glucose levels in patients with type 2 diabetes mellitus (non-insulin-dependent).**
Adults: initially, 1 to 2 g P.O. daily as single dose or in divided doses b.i.d. to t.i.d. Dosage adjusted, if necessary, to maximum of 3 g daily; manufacturer states that little benefit occurs with dosages greater than 2 g daily.
▶ **To change from insulin to oral therapy.** *Adults:* if insulin dosage is under 20 units daily, insulin stopped and oral therapy started at 1 to 2 g P.O. daily. If insulin dosage is 20 to 40 units daily, insulin reduced by 30% to 50% and oral therapy started as above. If insulin dosage is over 40 units daily, insulin reduced by 20% and oral therapy started as above. Further reductions in insulin are based on patient's response to oral therapy.

Adverse reactions

GI: nausea, heartburn.
Hematologic: *thrombocytopenia, aplastic anemia, agranulocytosis.*
Skin: rash, pruritus, facial flushing.
Other: *hypersensitivity reactions, hypoglycemia, dilutional hyponatremia.*

Interactions

Drug-drug. *Anabolic steroids, chloramphenicol, clofibrate, guanethidine, MAO inhibitors, phenylbutazone, salicylates, sulfonamides:* increased hypoglycemic activity. Monitor blood glucose level.
Beta blockers, clonidine: prolonged hypoglycemic effect and masked symptoms of hypoglycemia. Use together cautiously.
Corticosteroids, glucagon, rifampin, thiazide diuretics: decreased hypoglycemic response. Monitor blood glucose level.
Hydantoins: increased blood levels of hydantoins. Monitor blood levels.
Oral anticoagulants: increased hypoglycemic activity or enhanced anticoagulant effect. Monitor blood glucose level, PT, and INR.
Drug-lifestyle. *Alcohol use:* possible disulfiram-like reaction. Avoid concomitant use of moderate to large amount of alcohol.

Contraindications and precautions

• Contraindicated for treating type 1 diabetes mellitus (insulin-dependent) or diabetes that can be adequately controlled

---

by diet. Also contraindicated in patients with type 2 diabetes mellitus complicated by fever, ketosis, acidosis, coma, or other acute complications such as major surgery, severe infection, or severe trauma; in patients with hypersensitivity to sulfonylureas or severe renal insufficiency; and in pregnant or breast-feeding women.

• Use cautiously in elderly, debilitated, or malnourished patients or patients with impaired liver or kidney function or porphyria.

• Safety of drug has not been established in children.

NURSING CONSIDERATIONS

⚘ Assessment
• Assess patient's blood glucose level before therapy and regularly thereafter.
• Patient transferring from insulin therapy to oral antidiabetic agent requires blood glucose level testing at least three times daily before meals.
• Be alert for adverse reactions and drug interactions.
• Elderly patient may be more sensitive to drug's adverse effects.
• Evaluate patient's and family's knowledge of drug therapy.

⊞ Nursing diagnoses
• Altered health maintenance related to presence of hyperglycemia
• Risk for injury related to drug-induced hypoglycemia
• Knowledge deficit related to drug therapy

⊠ Planning and implementation
• Be aware that patient transferring from another oral antidiabetic agent usually needs no transition period.
• To avoid GI intolerance for patient on large doses and to improve control of hyperglycemia, give divided doses before morning and evening meals.
• Be aware that tablets may be crushed to ease administration.

Patient teaching
• Make sure patient knows that therapy relieves symptoms only.
• Teach patient about the disease. Stress the importance of adhering to therapeutic regimen and diet, weight reduction, exercise, and personal hygiene programs. Emphasize the need to avoid infection. Explain how and when to perform self-monitoring of blood glucose level and teach recognition of and intervention for hypoglycemia and hyperglycemia.
• Tell patient not to change drug dosage without doctor's consent and to report abnormal blood or urine glucose test results.
• Teach patient to carry candy or other simple sugars to treat mild hypoglycemic episodes. Severe episodes may require hospital treatment.
• Advise patient not to take other medication, including OTC drugs, without first checking with doctor.
• Advise patient to avoid moderate to large intake of alcohol because of possible disulfiram-like reaction.
• Advise patient to carry medical identification at all times.

☑ Evaluation
• Patient's blood glucose level is normal.
• Patient does not experience hypoglycemia.
• Patient and family state understanding of drug therapy.

tolcapone
(TOHL-cah-pohn)
Tasmar

Pharmacologic class: catechol-O-methyltransferase (COMT) inhibitor
Therapeutic class: antiparkinsonian agent
Pregnancy risk category: C

How supplied
Tablets: 100 mg, 200 mg

Pharmacokinetics

Absorption: rapid. Absolute bioavailability is 65% following oral administration.
Distribution: not widely distributed into tissues; over 99.9% is bound to plasma proteins.
Metabolism: almost completely metabolized before excretion mainly by glucuronidation.
Excretion: following oral administration, 60% excreted in urine and 40% in feces.
Half-life: 2 to 3 hours.

Route	Onset	Peak	Duration
P.O.	Unknown	2 hr	Unknown

Pharmacodynamics

Chemical effect: exact mechanism unknown. Thought to reversibly inhibit human erythrocyte COMT when given in combination with levodopa/carbidopa, resulting in a decrease in levodopa clearance and a twofold increase in levodopa bioavailability. Decreased clearance of levodopa prolongs elimination half-life of levodopa from 2 to 3.5 hours.
Therapeutic effect: improves physical mobility in patients with parkinsonism.

Indications and dosages

▶ **Adjunct to levodopa and carbidopa for treatment of signs and symptoms of idiopathic Parkinson's disease.** *Adults:* initially, 100 mg P.O. t.i.d. (in combination with levodopa/carbidopa). Recommended daily dosage is 100 mg P.O. t.i.d. although 200 mg P.O. t.i.d. can also be given if the anticipated clinical benefit is justified. If initiating treatment with 200 mg t.i.d. and dyskinesia occurs, reduced dosage of levodopa may be necessary. Maximum daily dosage is 600 mg.

Adverse reactions

CNS: *dyskinesia, sleep disorder, dystonia, excessive dreaming, somnolence,* dizziness, *confusion, headache, hallucinations,* hyperkinesia, hypertonia, fatigue, falling, syncope, balance loss, depression, tremor, speech disorder, pares-
thesia, agitation, irritability, mental deficiency, hyperactivity, hypokinesia.
CV: *orthostatic complaints,* chest pain, chest discomfort, palpitation, hypotension.
EENT: pharyngitis, tinnitus, sinus congestion.
GI: *nausea, anorexia, diarrhea,* flatulence, *vomiting,* constipation, abdominal pain, dyspepsia, dry mouth.
GU: urinary tract infection, urine discoloration, hematuria, micturition disorder, urinary incontinence, impotence.
Musculoskeletal: *muscle cramps,* stiffness, arthritis, neck pain.
Respiratory: bronchitis, dyspnea, upper respiratory infections.
Skin: increased sweating, rash.
Other: bleeding, burning, fever, influenza.

Interactions

Drug-drug. *CNS depressants:* enhanced sedative effects. Use cautiously.
Desipramine: increased incidence of adverse effects. Use cautiously.
Nonselective MAO inhibitors (phenelzine, tranylcypromine): possible hypertensive crisis. Avoid concomitant use.

Contraindications and precautions

• Contraindicated in patients with liver disease, elevated ALT or AST values, or known or demonstrated hypersensitivity to drug or its components; in those who were withdrawn from tolcapone because of evidence of drug-induced hepatocellular injury; or in patients with history of nontraumatic rhabdomyolysis or hyperpyrexia and confusion possibly related to drug.
• Use cautiously in patients with severe renal impairment and in breast-feeding women.

NURSING CONSIDERATIONS

☒ Assessment
• Assess patient's history of Parkinson's disease and reassess during therapy.
• Monitor liver enzymes before therapy, then every 2 weeks during first 3 years of therapy, then every 2 weeks for the next 6

Reactions may be *common,* uncommon, *life-threatening*, or COMMON AND LIFE-THREATENING.

months, then every 8 weeks thereafter because of risk of liver toxicity. Stop drug if results are elevated or if patient appears jaundiced. Assess patient's risk for physical injury due to drug's CNS adverse effects.
• Monitor for orthostatic hypotension and syncope.
• Evaluate patient's and family's knowledge of drug therapy.

⊞ **Nursing diagnoses**
• Impaired physical mobility related to underlying Parkinson's disease
• Altered thought processes related to drug-induced CNS adverse reactions
• Knowledge deficit related to drug therapy

❯ **Planning and implementation**
• Know that patient should provide a written informed consent before drug is used. Use drug only in patients on levodopa and carbidopa who do not respond to or who are not appropriate candidates for other adjunctive therapies because of risk of liver toxicity.
• Administer first dose of day with first daily dose of levodopa/carbidopa.
• Know that patients with severe renal dysfunction may require a reduced dose.
• Withhold drug and notify doctor if hepatic transaminases are elevated or if patient appears jaundiced.
• Because of risk of liver toxicity, stop treatment if patient shows no benefit within 3 weeks, as ordered.
• Know that because of highly protein-bound nature of tolcapone, drug is not expected to be removed significantly during dialysis.
• Notify doctor if severe diarrhea occurs that is associated with drug therapy.
Patient teaching
• Advise patient to take drug exactly as prescribed.
• Teach patient signs of liver injury (jaundice, fatigue, loss of appetite, persistent nausea, pruritus, dark urine or right upper

quadrant tenderness) and instruct him to report them immediately.
• Warn patient about risk of orthostatic hypotension; tell him to use caution when rising from a seated or recumbent position.
• Caution patient to avoid hazardous activities until CNS effects of drug are known.
• Tell patient that nausea may occur at the start of therapy.
• Inform patient about risk of increased dyskinesia or dystonia.
• Tell patient to report if pregnancy is being planned or suspected during therapy.
• Instruct patient to report adverse effects, including diarrhea and hallucinations, to doctor.
• Inform patient that drug may be taken without regard to meals.

☑ **Evaluation**
• Patient exhibits improved mobility with reduction of muscular rigidity and tremor.
• Patient remains mentally alert.
• Patient and family state understanding of drug therapy.

tolmetin sodium
(TOHL-meh-tin SOH-dee-um)
Tolectin 200, Tolectin 600, Tolectin DS

Pharmacologic class: NSAID
Therapeutic class: nonnarcotic analgesic, antipyretic, anti-inflammatory
Pregnancy risk category: C

How supplied
Tablets: 200 mg, 600 mg
Capsules: 400 mg

Pharmacokinetics
Absorption: absorbed rapidly from GI tract.
Distribution: highly protein-bound.
Metabolism: metabolized in liver.

Excretion: excreted in urine. *Half-life:* 1 to 2 hours.

Route	Onset	Peak	Duration
P.O.	Unknown	30-60 min	Unknown

Pharmacodynamics

Chemical effect: unknown; produces anti-inflammatory, analgesic, and antipyretic effects, possibly by inhibiting prostaglandin synthesis.
Therapeutic effect: relieves pain, fever, and inflammation.

Indications and dosage

▶ **Rheumatoid arthritis, osteoarthritis, juvenile rheumatoid arthritis.** *Adults:* 400 mg P.O. t.i.d. Maximum daily dosage is 1.8 g. *Children age 2 and over:* 15 to 30 mg/kg P.O. daily in three or four divided doses.

Adverse reactions

CNS: headache, dizziness, drowsiness.
EENT: tinnitus, visual disturbances.
GI: *epigastric distress, peptic ulceration,* occult blood loss, *nausea, GI bleeding.*
GU: *nephrotoxicity,* pseudoproteinuria, *renal failure.*
Hematologic: prolonged bleeding time, granulocytopenia, *thrombocytopenia, agranulocytosis.*
Skin: rash, urticaria, pruritus.
Other: sodium retention, edema, *anaphylaxis,* weight gain.

Interactions

Drug-drug. *Aspirin:* decreased tolmetin levels. Avoid concurrent use.
Methotrexate: increased risk of methotrexate toxicity. Monitor patient closely.
Oral anticoagulants: increased risk of bleeding. Monitor patient closely.
Drug-lifestyle. *Alcohol use:* increased risk of GI toxicity. Avoid concomitant use.

Contraindications and precautions

• Contraindicated in patients with hypersensitivity to drug; in those whose acute asthmatic attacks, urticaria, or rhinitis is precipitated by aspirin or NSAIDs; and in breast-feeding women.
• Drug is not recommended for use during second half of pregnancy.
• Use cautiously in patients with cardiac or renal disease, GI bleeding, history of peptic ulcer disease, hypertension, or conditions predisposing to fluid retention.

NURSING CONSIDERATIONS

⚏ Assessment
• Assess patient's arthritis before therapy and regularly thereafter.
• During prolonged therapy, patient should have regular eye examinations, hearing tests, CBCs, and kidney function tests to monitor for toxicity.
• Be alert for adverse reactions and drug interactions.
• Evaluate patient's and family's knowledge of drug therapy.

⊞ Nursing diagnoses
• Pain related to presence of arthritis
• Impaired tissue integrity related to drug's adverse effect on GI mucosa
• Knowledge deficit related to drug therapy

❯ Planning and implementation
• Be aware that drug may interfere with certain tests for urinary proteins; it does not interfere with dye-impregnated reagent strips.
• Report signs of serious GI toxicity.
Patient teaching
• Tell patient to take drug with food, milk, or antacids.
• Tell patient that therapeutic effect begins within 1 week but that full effect may be delayed 2 to 4 weeks.
• Advise patient to avoid activities that require alertness until drug's CNS effects are known.
• Teach patient signs of GI bleeding and tell him to report them promptly.
• Instruct patient to report immediately changes in vision or hearing.

☑ Evaluation

- Patient has relief from pain.
- Patient does not exhibit signs of GI toxicity.
- Patient and family state understanding of drug therapy.

---

topiramate
(toh-PEER-uh-mayt)
Topamax

Pharmacologic class: sulfamate-substituted monosaccharide
Therapeutic class: antiepileptic
Pregnancy risk category: C

How supplied

Tablets: 25 mg, 100 mg, 200 mg

Pharmacokinetics

Absorption: rapid absorption following oral dose.
Distribution: up to 17% bound to plasma proteins.
Metabolism: not extensively metabolized.
Excretion: primarily eliminated unchanged in urine. *Half-life:* 21 hours.

Route	Onset	Peak	Duration
P.O.	Unknown	2 hr	Unknown

Pharmacodynamics

Chemical effect: precise mechanism of action unknown. Thought to block action potential, suggestive of a sodium channel blocking action. Drug may also potentiate activity of gamma-aminobutyrate (GABA) and antagonize ability of kainate to activate the kainate/alpha-amino-3-hydroxy-5-methylisoxazole-4-proprionic acid subtype of excitatory amino acid (glutamate) receptor. Drug also has weak carbonic anhydrase inhibitor activity, which is unrelated to its antiepileptic properties.
Therapeutic effect: prevents partial-onset seizures.

Indications and dosages

▶ **Adjunctive therapy of partial-onset seizures.** *Adults:* titrate up to maximum daily dosage of 400 mg P.O. in divided doses b.i.d. Titration schedule is as follows: Week 1, 50 mg P.O. in evening; week 2, 50 mg P.O. b.i.d.; week 3, 50 mg P.O. in morning and 100 mg P.O. in evening; week 4, 100 mg P.O. b.i.d.; week 5, 100 mg P.O. in morning and 150 mg P.O. in evening; week 6, 150 mg P.O. b.i.d.; week 7, 150 mg P.O. in morning and 200 mg P.O. in evening; week 8, 200 mg P.O. b.i.d.

Adverse reactions

CNS: *fatigue,* abnormal coordination, aggressive reaction, agitation, apathy, asthenia, *ataxia, confusion,* depression, depersonalization, *dizziness,* emotional lability, euphoria, **grand mal seizures,** hallucination, hyperkinesia, hypertonia, hypoesthesia, hypokinesia, insomnia, *nervousness, nystagmus, paresthesia,* personality disorder, *psychomotor slowing,* psychosis, *somnolence, speech disorders,* stupor, **suicide attempts,** *tremor,* vertigo; malaise, mood problems; difficulty with concentration, attention, language, or *memory.*
CV: chest pain, palpitations.
EENT: *abnormal vision,* conjunctivitis, *diplopia,* eye pain, hearing problems, pharyngitis, sinusitis, taste perversion, tinnitus.
GI: abdominal pain, anorexia, constipation, diarrhea, dry mouth, dyspepsia, flatulence, gastroenteritis, gingivitis, *nausea,* vomiting.
GU: amenorrhea, decreased libido, dysuria, dysmenorrhea, hematuria, impotence, intermenstrual bleeding, menstrual disorder, menorrhagia, micturition frequency, renal calculus, urinary incontinence, urinary tract infection, vaginitis.
Hematologic: anemia, epistaxis, *leukopenia.*
Metabolic: increased or decreased weight.
Musculoskeletal: arthralgia, back or leg pain, muscle weakness, myalgia, rigors.

---

*Liquid form contains alcohol   **May contain tartrazine   ♦Canada   ◊ Australia   †OTC

Respiratory: bronchitis, coughing, dyspnea, *upper respiratory infection.*
Skin: acne, alopecia, increased sweating, pruritus, rash.
Other: breast pain, body odor, edema, fever, flulike symptoms, hot flashes, leukorrhea.

Interactions

Drug-drug. *Carbamazepine:* decreased topiramate concentrations. Monitor patient.
Carbonic anhydrase inhibitors (acetazolamide, dichlorphenamide): increased risk of renal calculus formation. Avoid concomitant use.
CNS depressants: possible topiramate-induced CNS depression, as well as other adverse cognitive and neuropsychiatric events. Use with caution.
Oral contraceptives: decreased efficacy. Report changes in bleeding patterns.
Phenytoin: decreased topiramate concentrations and increased phenytoin concentrations. Monitor levels.
Valproic acid: decrease in valproic acid and topiramate levels. Monitor patient.
Drug-lifestyle. *Alcohol use:* possible topiramate-induced CNS depression, as well as other adverse cognitive and neuropsychiatric events. Avoid concomitant use.

Contraindications and precautions

• Contraindicated in patients with hypersensitivity to drug or its components.
• Use with caution in patients with hepatic impairment and in breast-feeding or pregnant women.

NURSING CONSIDERATIONS

⚕ Assessment
• Assess patient's seizure disorder before therapy and regularly thereafter.
• Carefully monitor patients taking topiramate in conjunction with other antiepileptic drugs; dosage adjustments may be needed to achieve optimal response.
• Assess patient's compliance with therapy at each follow-up visit.

• Evaluate patient's and family's knowledge of drug therapy.

⚕ Nursing diagnoses
• Risk for injury related to seizure disorder
• Pain related to increased risk of renal calculi formation
• Knowledge deficit related to drug therapy

⚕ Planning and implementation
• Know that renal insufficiency requires a reduced dose. For hemodialysis patients, supplemental doses may be required to avoid rapid drops in drug levels during prolonged dialysis treatment.
• Expect to adjust dosage according to patient's response.
• Initiate safety precautions as indicated.
Patient teaching
• Tell patient to maintain adequate fluid intake during therapy to minimize risk of forming renal calculi.
• Advise patient not to drive or operate hazardous machinery until CNS effects of drug are known.
• Tell patient that drug may decrease effectiveness of oral contraceptives and to use a barrier form of birth control.
• Tell patient to avoid crushing or breaking tablets because of bitter taste.
• Tell patient that drug can be taken without regard to food.

☑ Evaluation
• Patient is free from seizure activity.
• Patient maintains adequate fluid hydration to prevent renal calculus formation.
• Patient and family state understanding of drug therapy.

---

topotecan hydrochloride
(toh-poh-TEE-ken high-droh-KLOR-ighd)
Hycamtin

Pharmacologic class: antitumor
Therapeutic class: antineoplastic
Pregnancy risk category: NR

How supplied

Injection: 4-mg single-dose vial

Pharmacokinetics

Absorption: proportional to dose.
Distribution: about 35% bound to plasma proteins.
Metabolism: by liver.
Excretion: 30% excreted in urine.

Route	Onset	Peak	Duration
I.V.	Unknown	Unknown	Unknown

Pharmacodynamics

Chemical effect: relieves torsional strain in DNA and prevents relegation of single-strand breaks.
Therapeutic effect: cytotoxicity is thought to be due to double-strand DNA damage produced during DNA synthesis when replication enzymes interact with the complex formed.

Indications and dosage

▶ **Metastatic carcinoma of ovary after failure of initial or subsequent chemotherapy.** *Adults:* 1.5 mg/m^2 by I.V. daily for 5 consecutive days, starting on day 1 of a 21-day cycle, for minimum of four cycles. For patients with creatinine clearance of 20 to 39 ml/minute, decrease dosage to 0.75 mg/m^2. If severe neutropenia occurs, reduce dosage by 0.25 mg/m^2 for subsequent courses. Alternatively, in severe neutropenia, give granulocyte-colony stimulating factor (GSF) after subsequent course (before resorting to dosage reduction) starting from day 6 of the course (24 hours after topotecan administration).

Adverse reactions

CNS: *fatigue, asthenia, headache,* paresthesia.
GI: *nausea, vomiting, diarrhea, constipation, abdominal pain, stomatitis, anorexia.*
Hematologic: NEUTROPENIA, LEUKOPENIA, THROMBOCYTOPENIA, *anemia.*
Hepatic: transient elevation of AST, ALT, and bilirubin levels.

Respiratory: *dyspnea.*
Skin: *alopecia.*
Other: *sepsis, fever.*

Interactions

Drug-drug. *Cisplatin:* increases severity of myelosuppression. Use both drugs very cautiously.
GSF: prolongs duration of neutropenia. If GSF is used, don't start it until day 6 of course, 24 hours after completion of topotecan treatment.

Contraindications and precautions

• Contraindicated in patients with severe bone marrow depression or hypersensitivity to drug or its components and in pregnant or breast-feeding women.

NURSING CONSIDERATIONS

⧆ Assessment
• Patient must have a baseline neutrophil count above 1,500 cells/mm^3 and platelet count above 100,000 cells/mm^3 before initiating therapy.
• Frequent monitoring of peripheral blood cell count is critical. Don't give repeated doses until neutrophil count is over 1,000 cells/mm^3, platelet count is over 100,000 cells/mm^3, and hemoglobin level over 9 mg/dl.
• Evaluate patient's and family's understanding of drug therapy.

⧆ Nursing diagnoses
• Altered health maintenance related to neoplastic disease
• Knowledge deficit related to drug therapy

⧆ Planning and implementation
• Prepare drug under a vertical laminar flow hood while wearing gloves and protective clothing. If drug contacts skin, wash immediately and thoroughly with soap and water. If mucous membranes are affected, flush with water.
• Reconstitute each 4-mg vial with 4 ml sterile water for injection. Dilute appro-

priate volume of reconstituted solution in 0.9% NaCl solution or D₅W before use. Infuse over 30 minutes.

• Protect unopened vials of drug from light. Reconstituted vials stored at 68° to 77° F (20° to 25° C) and exposed to ambient lighting are stable for 24 hours.

Patient teaching

• Instruct patient to report promptly sore throat, fever, chills, or unusual bleeding or bruising.

• Advise female patient of childbearing age to avoid pregnancy and breast-feeding during treatment.

• Tell patient and family about need for close monitoring of blood counts.

☑ **Evaluation**

• Patient shows positive response to drug.

• Patient and family state understanding of drug therapy.

---

torsemide
(TOR-seh-mighd)
Demadex

Pharmacologic class: loop diuretic
Therapeutic class: diuretic, antihypertensive
Pregnancy risk category: B

How supplied

Injection: 10 mg/ml
Tablets: 5 mg, 10 mg, 20 mg, 100 mg

Pharmacokinetics

Absorption: absorbed with little first-pass metabolism after oral administration.
Distribution: extensively bound to plasma protein.
Metabolism: metabolized in liver.
Excretion: 22% to 34% excreted unchanged in urine.

Route	Onset	Peak	Duration
P.O.	1 hr	1-2 hr	6-8 hr
I.V.	≤ 10 min	≤ 1 hr	6-8 hr

Pharmacodynamics

Chemical effect: enhances excretion of sodium, chloride, and water by acting on ascending portion of loop of Henle.
Therapeutic effect: promotes water and sodium excretion and lowers blood pressure.

Indications and dosage

▶ **Diuresis in patients with heart failure.** *Adults:* initially, 10 to 20 mg P.O. or I.V. once daily. If response is inadequate, dose is doubled until response is obtained. Maximum dosage is 200 mg daily.

▶ **Diuresis in patients with chronic renal failure.** *Adults:* initially, 20 mg P.O. or I.V. once daily. If response is inadequate, dose is doubled until response is obtained. Maximum dosage is 200 mg daily.

▶ **Diuresis in patients with hepatic cirrhosis.** *Adults:* initially, 5 to 10 mg P.O. or I.V. once daily with aldosterone antagonist or potassium-sparing diuretic. If response is inadequate, dose is doubled until response is obtained. Maximum dosage is 40 mg daily.

▶ **Hypertension.** *Adults:* initially, 5 mg P.O. daily. Increased to 10 mg in 4 to 6 weeks if needed and tolerated. If response is still inadequate, another antihypertensive agent should be added.

Adverse reactions

CNS: asthenia; dizziness, headache, nervousness, insomnia, syncope.
CV: ECG abnormalities, chest pain, edema, increased cholesterol level, *dehydration,* orthostatic hypertension.
EENT: rhinitis, cough, sore throat.
GI: *excessive thirst,* diarrhea, constipation, nausea, dyspepsia, *hemorrhage.*
GU: *excessive urination,* impotence.
Metabolic: electrolyte imbalances including *hypokalemia, hypomagnesemia,* hypocalcemia, hyperuricemia, gout, hyperglycemia; increased uric acid, hypochloremic alkalosis.
Musculoskeletal: arthralgia; myalgia.

Reactions may be *common,* uncommon, *life-threatening,* or COMMON AND LIFE-THREATENING.

Interactions

Drug-drug. *Cholestyramine:* decreased absorption of torsemide. Separate administration times by at least 3 hours.
Digoxin: decreased torsemide clearance. Dosage adjustments not needed.
Indomethacin: decreased diuretic effectiveness in sodium-restricted patients. Avoid concomitant use.
Lithium, ototoxic drugs (such as aminoglycosides, ethacrynic acid): possible increased toxicity of these agents. Avoid concomitant use.
NSAIDs: may potentiate nephrotoxicity of NSAIDs. Use together cautiously.
Probenecid: decreased diuretic effectiveness. Avoid concomitant use.
Salicylates: decreased excretion, possibly leading to salicylate toxicity. Avoid concomitant use.
Spironolactone: decreased renal clearance of spironolactone. Dosage adjustments not necessary.

Contraindications and precautions

• Contraindicated in patients with anuria or hypersensitivity to drug or other sulfonylurea derivatives.
• Use cautiously in patients with hepatic disease and associated cirrhosis and ascites; sudden changes in fluid and electrolyte balance may precipitate hepatic coma in these patients. Also use cautiously in pregnant or breast-feeding women.
• Safety of drug has not been established in children.

NURSING CONSIDERATIONS

Assessment

• Assess patient's condition before therapy and regularly thereafter.
• Monitor elderly patients, who are especially susceptible to excessive diuresis, with potential for circulatory collapse and thromboembolic complications.
• Monitor fluid intake and output, serum electrolyte levels, blood pressure, weight, and pulse rate during rapid diuresis and routinely with chronic use. Drug can cause profound diuresis and water and electrolyte depletion.
• Watch for signs of hypokalemia, such as muscle weakness and cramps.
• Be alert for adverse reactions and drug interactions.
• Evaluate patient's and family's knowledge of drug therapy.

Nursing diagnoses

• Fluid volume excess related to presence of edema
• Risk for injury related to presence of hypertension
• Knowledge deficit related to drug therapy

Planning and implementation

P.O. use: Give drug in morning to prevent nocturia.
I.V. use: Inspect ampules for precipitate or discoloration before use. Drug may be given by direct injection over at least 2 minutes. Rapid injection may cause ototoxicity. Don't give more than 200 mg at a time.
• Consult doctor and dietitian to provide high-potassium diet. Foods rich in potassium include citrus fruits, tomatoes, bananas, dates, and apricots.
Patient teaching
• Tell patient to take drug in morning to prevent sleep interruption.
• Advise patient to change position slowly to prevent dizziness and to limit alcohol intake and strenuous exercise in hot weather to prevent orthostatic hypotension.
• Advise patient to immediately report ringing in ears because it may indicate toxicity.
• Tell patient to check with doctor or pharmacist before taking other OTC medications.

Evaluation

• Patient shows no signs of edema.
• Patient's blood pressure is normal.
• Patient and family state understanding of drug therapy.

---

*Liquid form contains alcohol   **May contain tartrazine   ♦Canada   ◊ Australia   †OTC

trace elements
(trays EL-uh-ments)

chromium (chromic chloride)
(KROH-mee-um)
Chroma-Pak, Chromic Chloride

copper (cupric sulfate)
(KAH-per)
Cupric Sulfate

iodine (sodium iodide)
(IGH-oh-dighn)
Iodopen

manganese (manganese chloride, manganese sulfate)
(MAN-geh-nees)

selenium (selenious acid)
(seh-LEHN-ee-um)
Sele-Pak, Selepen

zinc (zinc chloride, zinc sulfate)
(zink)
Zinca-Pak

Pharmacologic class: trace elements
Therapeutic class: nutritional agents
Pregnancy risk category: C

How supplied
chromium
Injection: 4 mcg/ml, 20 mcg/ml
copper
Injection: 0.4 mg/ml, 2 mg/ml
iodine
Injection: 100 mcg/ml
manganese
Injection: 0.1 mg/ml
selenium
Injection: 40 mcg/ml
zinc
Injection: 1 mg/ml, 5 mg/ml

Pharmacokinetics
Absorption: not applicable.
Distribution: not reported.

Metabolism: not reported.
Excretion: not reported.

Route	Onset	Peak	Duration
I.V.	Immediate	Immediate	Unknown

Pharmacodynamics
Chemical effect: participates in synthesis and stabilization of proteins and nucleic acids in subcellular and membrane transport systems.
Therapeutic effect: restores normal body levels of trace elements.

Indications and dosage
▶ **Prevention of individual trace element deficiencies in patients receiving long-term total parenteral nutrition (TPN). Chromium.** *Adults:* 10 to 15 mcg I.V. daily. *Children:* 0.14 to 0.20 mcg/kg I.V. daily. **Copper.** *Adults:* 0.5 to 1.5 mg I.V. daily. *Children:* 20 mcg/kg I.V. daily. **Iodine.** *Adults:* 1 to 2 mcg/kg I.V. daily. *Children:* 2 to 3 mcg/kg I.V. daily. **Manganese.** *Adults:* 0.15 to 0.8 mg I.V. daily. *Children:* 2 to 10 mcg/kg I.V. daily. **Selenium.** *Adults:* 20 to 40 mcg I.V. daily. *Children:* 3 mcg/kg I.V. daily. **Zinc.** *Adults:* 2.5 to 4 mg I.V. daily. *Children age 5 or younger:* 100 mcg/kg I.V. daily. *Neonates:* 300 mcg/kg/I.V. daily.

Adverse reactions
None reported with suggested dosages except for hypersensitivity to iodides.

Interactions
None significant at suggested dosages.

Contraindications and precautions
• No known contraindications.

NURSING CONSIDERATIONS

❧ Assessment
• Obtain history of patient's underlying trace element deficiency before therapy and reassess regularly thereafter. Keep in mind that normal serum levels are

0.85 ng/ml chromium; 0.07 to 0.15 mg/ml copper; 4 to 20 mcg/dl manganese; 0.1 to 0.19 mcg/ml selenium; and 0.05 to 0.15 mg/dl zinc.
• Check serum levels of trace elements in patients who have received TPN for 2 months or longer, as ordered. Call doctor's attention to low serum levels of these elements because supplement may be needed.
• Evaluate patient's and family's knowledge of drug therapy.

⊞ Nursing diagnoses
• Altered nutrition: Less than body requirements related to presence of deficiency of trace elements
• Knowledge deficit related to drug therapy

⊠ Planning and implementation
• Cautiously infuse diluted solution through patent I.V. line over ordered duration.
• Don't administer undiluted due to potential for phlebitis.
• Be aware that solutions of trace elements are compounded by pharmacy for addition to TPN solutions according to various formulas. One common trace element solution is Shil's solution, which contains copper 1 mg/ml, iodide 0.06 mg ml, manganese 0.4 mg/ml, and zinc 2 mg/ml.
Patient teaching
• Inform patient and family of need for trace elements.

☑ Evaluation
• Patient regains normal serum levels of trace elements.
• Patient and family state understanding of drug therapy.

---

tramadol hydrochloride
(TRAM-uh-dohl high-droh-KLOR-ighd)
Ultram

Pharmacologic class: synthetic analgesic

Therapeutic class: analgesic
Pregnancy risk category: C

How supplied

Tablets: 50 mg

Pharmacokinetics

Absorption: rapidly and almost completely absorbed from GI tract.
Distribution: about 20% bound to plasma proteins.
Metabolism: extensively metabolized.
Excretion: 30% excreted in urine as unchanged drug and 60% as metabolites.
Half-life: 6 to 7 hours.

Route	Onset	Peak	Duration
P.O.	Unknown	About 2 hr	Unknown

Pharmacodynamics

Chemical effect: unknown; centrally acting synthetic analgesic compound not chemically related to opioids that is thought to bind to opioid receptors and inhibit reuptake of norepinephrine and serotonin.
Therapeutic effect: relieves pain.

Indications and dosage

▶ **Moderate to moderately severe pain.**
Adults: 50 to 100 mg P.O. q 4 to 6 hours, p.r.n. Maximum dosage is 400 mg daily.

Adverse reactions

CNS: *dizziness, vertigo, headache, somnolence, CNS stimulation, asthenia,* anxiety, confusion, coordination disturbance, euphoria, nervousness, sleep disorder, *seizures.*
CV: vasodilation.
EENT: visual disturbances.
GI: *nausea, constipation, vomiting,* dyspepsia, dry mouth, diarrhea, abdominal pain, anorexia, flatulence.
GU: urine retention, urinary frequency, menopausal symptoms.
Musculoskeletal: malaise, hypertonia.
Respiratory: *respiratory depression.*
Skin: *pruritus,* sweating, rash.

Interactions

Drug-drug. *Carbamazepine:* increased tramadol metabolism. Patients receiving chronic carbamazepine therapy at dosage of up to 800 mg daily may require up to twice recommended dose of tramadol. *CNS depressants:* additive effects. Use together with caution. Dosage of tramadol may need to be reduced.
MAO inhibitors, neuroleptics: increased risk of seizures. Monitor patient closely.

Contraindications and precautions

• Contraindicated in patients with hypersensitivity to drug or with acute intoxication from alcohol, hypnotics, centrally acting analgesics, opioids, or psychotropic drugs.
• Drug is not recommended for use in breast-feeding women.
• Use cautiously in patients at risk for seizures or respiratory depression; in patients with increased intracranial pressure or head injury, acute abdominal conditions, or renal or hepatic impairment; and in patients physically dependent on opioids.
• Safety has not been established in children or pregnant women.

NURSING CONSIDERATIONS

⏱ Assessment

• Assess patient's pain before therapy and regularly thereafter.
• Monitor CV and respiratory status.
• Closely monitor patient at risk for seizures. Drug has been reported to reduce seizure threshold.
• Monitor patient for drug dependence. Tramadol can produce dependence similar to that of codeine or dextropropoxyphene and thus has potential to be abused.
• Be alert for adverse reactions and drug interactions.
• Evaluate patient's and family's knowledge of drug therapy.

⊞ Nursing diagnoses

• Pain related to underlying condition
• Constipation related to drug-induced adverse GI reactions
• Knowledge deficit related to drug therapy

⟩ Planning and implementation

• Be aware that for better analgesic effect, drug should be given before onset of intense pain.
• Withhold dose and notify doctor if respiratory rate decreases or falls below 12 breaths/minute.
• Because constipation is a common adverse effect, anticipate need for laxative therapy.
Patient teaching
• Instruct patient to take drug only as prescribed and not to increase dosage or dosage interval unless instructed by doctor.
• Caution ambulatory patient to be careful when getting out of bed and walking. Warn outpatient to refrain from driving and performing other potentially hazardous activities that require mental alertness until drug's CNS effects are known.
• Advise patient to check with doctor before taking OTC medications; drug interactions can occur.

☑ Evaluation

• Patient is free from pain.
• Patient regains normal bowel pattern.
• Patient and family state understanding of drug therapy.

trandolapril
(tran-DOH-luh-pril)
Mavik

Pharmacologic class: ACE inhibitor
Therapeutic class: antihypertensive
Pregnancy risk category: C (D in second and third trimesters)

How supplied

Tablets: 1 mg, 2 mg, 4 mg

Pharmacokinetics

Absorption: food slows absorption.
Distribution: unknown.
Metabolism: in liver.
Excretion: in urine and feces.

Route	Onset	Peak	Duration
P.O.	Unknown	1 hr (drug); 4-10 hr (metabolite)	Unknown

Pharmacodynamics

Chemical effect: inhibits circulating and tissue ACE activity, thus reducing angiotensin II formation, decreasing vasoconstriction, decreasing aldosterone secretion, and increasing plasma renin.
Therapeutic effect: decreases aldosterone secretion leading to diuresis, natriuresis, and small increase in serum potassium.

Indications and dosage

▶ **Hypertension.** *Adults:* for patient not receiving a diuretic, initially 1 mg for a nonblack patient and 2 mg for a black patient P.O. once daily. If response isn't adequate, dosage may be increased at intervals of at least 1 week. Maintenance dosage range is 2 to 4 mg daily for most patients. Some patients receiving 4-mg once-daily doses may need b.i.d. doses. For patient also receiving diuretic, initial dose is 0.5 mg P.O. once daily. Subsequent dosages adjusted based on blood pressure response.

Adverse reactions

CNS: dizziness, headache, fatigue, drowsiness, insomnia, paresthesia, vertigo, anxiety.
CV: chest pain, first-degree AV block, *bradycardia,* edema, flushing, hypotension, palpitations.
EENT: epistaxis, throat irritation, upper respiratory tract infection.
GI: diarrhea, dyspepsia, abdominal distention, abdominal pain or cramps, constipation, vomiting, pancreatitis.

GU: urinary frequency, impotence, decreased libido.
Hematologic: *neutropenia, leukopenia.*
Metabolic: hyperkalemia, hyponatremia.
Respiratory: dry, persistent, tickling, nonproductive cough; dyspnea.
Skin: rash, pruritus, pemphigus.
Other: *anaphylactic reactions, angioedema.*

Interactions

Drug-drug. *Diuretics:* increased risk of excessive hypotension. Monitor blood pressure closely.
Lithium: increased serum lithium levels and lithium toxicity. Avoid use together; monitor serum lithium levels.
Potassium-sparing diuretics, potassium supplements: increased risk of hyperkalemia. Monitor serum potassium closely.
Drug-food. *Salt substitutes containing potassium:* increased risk of hyperkalemia. Monitor serum potassium closely.

Contraindications and precautions

• Contraindicated in patients with hypersensitivity to drug or history of angioedema related to previous treatment with ACE inhibitor and in pregnant women.
• Use cautiously in patients with impaired renal function, heart failure, or renal artery stenosis.

NURSING CONSIDERATIONS

⚖ Assessment
• Monitor patient's blood pressure and serum potassium levels before and during drug therapy.
• Monitor for hypotension. If possible, stop diuretic therapy 2 to 3 days before starting drug.
• Monitor patient's compliance with treatment.
• Evaluate patient's and family's knowledge of drug therapy.

▦ Nursing diagnoses
• Risk for injury related to hypertension

• Knowledge deficit related to drug therapy

▶ Planning and implementation
• Take steps to prevent or minimize orthostatic hypotension
• Maintain patient's nonpharmacologic therapies, such as sodium restriction, stress management, and exercise program.
Patient teaching
• Advise patient to report infection and other adverse reactions.
• Tell patient to avoid salt substitutes.
• Tell patient to use caution in hot weather and during exercise.
• Tell female patient to report suspected pregnancy immediately.
• Advise patient about to undergo surgery or anesthesia to inform doctor about use of this drug.

✓ Evaluation
• Patient's blood pressure is normal.
• Patient and family state understanding of drug therapy.

---

tranylcypromine sulfate
(tran-il-SIGH-proh-meen SUL-fayt)
Parnate

Pharmacologic class: MAO inhibitor
Therapeutic class: antidepressant
Pregnancy risk category: NR

How supplied
Tablets: 10 mg

Pharmacokinetics
Absorption: absorbed rapidly and completely from GI tract.
Distribution: unknown.
Metabolism: metabolized in liver.
Excretion: excreted primarily in urine; some excreted in feces. *Half-life:* 2½ hours.

Route	Onset	Peak	Duration
P.O.	2-21 days	1-3.5 hr	≤ 10 days after drug stopped

Pharmacodynamics
Chemical effect: unknown; probably promotes accumulation of neurotransmitters by inhibiting MAO.
Therapeutic effect: relieves depression.

Indications and dosage
▶ **Depression.** *Adults:* 10 mg P.O. t.i.d. Increased by 10 mg daily at 1- to 3-week intervals to maximum of 60 mg daily, if necessary, after 2 weeks of initial therapy.

Adverse reactions
CNS: *dizziness, vertigo, headache,* anxiety, agitation, drowsiness, weakness, numbness, paresthesias, tremors, jitters, confusion.
CV: *orthostatic hypotension, tachycardia,* paradoxical hypertension, palpitations.
EENT: blurred vision, tinnitus.
GI: dry mouth, *anorexia,* nausea, diarrhea, constipation, abdominal pain.
GU: impotence, SIADH, urinary retention, impaired ejaculation.
Hematologic: anemia, *leukopenia, agranulocytosis, thrombocytopenia.*
Skin: rash.
Other: *edema,* hepatitis, muscle spasm, myoclonic jerks, chills.

Interactions
Drug-drug. *Amphetamines, antihistamines, ephedrine, levodopa, meperidine, metaraminol, methylphenidate, phenylephrine, phenylpropanolamine, sympathomimetics:* enhanced pressor effects of these drugs. Avoid concomitant use.
Antiparkinsonian drugs, barbiturates, dextromethorphan, methotrimeprazine, narcotics, other sedatives, selective serotonin reuptake inhibitors, tricyclic antidepressants: enhanced adverse CNS effects. Use with caution and in reduced dosage.
Buspirone: may elevate blood pressure. Monitor patient closely.

Insulin, oral antidiabetic agents: increased risk of hypoglycemia. Use with caution and in reduced dosages.
Drug-food. *Foods high in tryptophan, tyramine, caffeine:* may cause hypertensive crisis. Avoid concomitant use.
Drug-lifestyle. *Alcohol use:* enhanced adverse CNS effects. Avoid concomitant use.

Contraindications and precautions

• Contraindicated in patients receiving MAO inhibitors or dibenzazepine derivatives; sympathomimetics (including amphetamines); some CNS depressants (including alcohol); some serotonin reuptake inhibitors; antihypertensive, diuretic, antihistaminic, sedative, or anesthetic drugs; bupropion hydrochloride, buspirone hydrochloride, dextromethorphan, meperidine; foods high in tyramine or tryptophan; or excessive quantities of caffeine.
• Also contraindicated in patients with confirmed or suspected cerebrovascular defect, CV disease, hypertension, or history of headache and in those undergoing elective surgery.
• Drug is not recommended for use in pregnant women.
• Use cautiously with antiparkinsonian drugs or spinal anesthetics; in patients with renal disease, diabetes, seizure disorder, Parkinson's disease, or hyperthyroidism; and in patients at risk for suicide.
• Safety of drug has not been established in breast-feeding women and in children.

NURSING CONSIDERATIONS

Assessment
• Assess patient's condition before therapy and regularly thereafter.
• Obtain baseline blood pressure, heart rate, CBC, and liver function test results before beginning therapy; monitor throughout treatment.
• Be alert for adverse reactions and drug interactions.
• Evaluate patient's and family's knowledge of drug therapy.

Nursing diagnoses
• Altered thought processes related to presence of depression
• Risk for injury related to drug-induced adverse CNS reactions
• Knowledge deficit related to drug therapy

Planning and implementation
• Dosage usually is reduced to maintenance level as soon as possible.
• Do not withdraw drug abruptly.
• In most patients, discontinue MAO inhibitors 14 days before elective surgery, as ordered, to avoid drug interactions that may occur during anesthetic procedure.
• If patient develops symptoms of overdose (palpitations, severe hypotension, or frequent headaches), withhold dose and notify doctor.
• Have phentolamine available to combat severe hypertension.
• Continue precautions for 10 days after stopping drug because it has long-lasting effects.
Patient teaching
• Warn patient to avoid foods high in tyramine or tryptophan and large amounts of caffeine. Tranylcypromine is the MAO inhibitor most often reported to cause hypertensive crisis with ingestion of foods high in tyramine, including aged cheese, Chianti wine, beer, avocados, chicken livers, chocolate, bananas, soy sauce, meat tenderizers, salami, and bologna.
• Tell patient to avoid alcohol during drug therapy.
• Instruct patient to sit up for 1 minute before getting out of bed to avoid dizziness.
• Warn patient to avoid overexertion because MAO inhibitors may suppress anginal pain.
• Advise patient to consult doctor before taking other prescription or OTC medications. Severe adverse effects can occur if MAO inhibitors are taken with OTC cold, hay fever, or diet preparations.
• Warn patient not to stop drug suddenly.

☑ Evaluation
● Patient's behavior and communication exhibit improved thought processes.
● Patient does not experience injury from adverse CNS reactions.
● Patient and family state understanding of drug therapy.

---

trastuzumab
(trahs-TOO-zuh-mab)
Herceptin

Pharmacologic class: monoclonal antibody
Therapeutic class: antineoplastic
Pregnancy risk category: B

How supplied
Injection: Lyophilized sterile powder containing 440 mg per vial

Pharmacokinetics
Absorption: no information available.
Distribution: drug's volume of distribution was 44 ml/kg.
Metabolism: no information available.
Excretion: no information available.
Half-life: 5.8 days (range 1 to 32 days).

Route	Onset	Peak	Duration
I.V.	Unknown	Unknown	Unknown

Pharmacodynamics
Chemical effect: trastuzumab is a recombinant DNA-derived monoclonal antibody that selectively binds to human epidermal growth factor receptor 2 protein (HER2). Trastuzumab has been shown to inhibit the proliferation of human tumor cells that overexpress HER2.
Therapeutic effect: hinders function of specific breast cancer tumor cells that overexpress HER2.

Indications and dosage
▶ **Single-agent treatment of patients with metastatic breast cancer whose tumors overexpress the HER2 protein** and who have received one or more chemotherapy regimens for their metastatic disease; or in combination with paclitaxel for metastatic breast cancer in patients whose tumors overexpress the HER2 protein and who have not received chemotherapy for their metastatic disease. *Adults:* initial loading dose of 4 mg/kg I.V. over 90 minutes. Maintenance dose is 2 mg/kg I.V. weekly as a 30-minute I.V. infusion if the initial loading dose was well tolerated.

Adverse reactions
CNS: *headache, asthenia, insomnia, dizziness,* paresthesia, depression, peripheral neuritis, neuropathy.
CV: tachycardia, **heart failure,** *peripheral edema.*
EENT: *rhinitis, pharyngitis,* sinusitis.
GI: *nausea, diarrhea, vomiting, anorexia, abdominal pain.*
GU: urinary tract infection.
Hematologic: anemia, **leukopenia.**
Musculoskeletal: bone pain, arthralgia, *back pain.*
Respiratory: *increased cough, dyspnea.*
Skin: *rash,* herpes simplex, acne.
Other: *pain, fever, chills, infection, flu syndrome,* **allergic reaction,** edema.

Interactions
None reported.

Effects on diagnostic tests
None reported.

Contraindications and precautions
● Use cautiously in patients with preexisting cardiac dysfunction, the elderly, and in patients with known hypersensitivity to drug or its components.
● Safety and effectiveness in children have not been established.

NURSING CONSIDERATIONS

☑ Assessment
● Before beginning therapy, patient should undergo thorough baseline cardiac

---

assessment including history and physical examination and appropriate evaluation methods to identify those at risk of developing cardiotoxicity.
• Know that drug should only be used in patients with metastatic breast cancer whose tumors have HER2 protein overexpression.
• Assess patient for chills and fever especially during the first infusion.
• Monitor patient closely for signs and symptoms of cardiac dysfunction especially if receiving concurrent anthracyclines and cyclophosphamide.
• Monitor for dyspnea, increased cough, paroxysmal nocturnal dyspnea, peripheral edema, and S_3 gallop. Patients also receiving chemotherapy concurrently should be monitored closely for cardiac dysfunction or failure, anemia, and leukopenia, diarrhea, and infection.
• Evaluate patient's and family's understanding of drug therapy.

▦ **Nursing diagnoses**
• Altered nutrition: Less than body requirements related to drug-induced GI adverse effects
• Decreased cardiac output related to drug-induced decreased left ventricular function
• Knowledge deficit related to drug therapy

▧ **Planning and implementation**
• Treat first infusion-associated symptoms with acetaminophen, diphenhydramine, and meperidine (with or without reducing the rate of infusion) as ordered.
• Notify doctor if patient develops a clinically significant decrease in cardiac function.
• Reconstitute each vial with 20 ml of bacteriostatic water for injection, USP, 1.1% benzyl alcohol preserved, as supplied, to yield a multidose solution containing 21 mg/ml. Immediately upon reconstitution, label vial for drug expiration 28 days from date of reconstitution.

• Know that if patient has known hypersensitivity to benzyl alcohol, drug must be reconstituted with sterile water for injection. Drug reconstituted with sterile water for injection must be used immediately; unused portion must be discarded. Avoid use of other reconstitution diluents.
• Don't administer as an I.V. push or bolus.
• Determine dose (mg) of trastuzumab needed, based on loading dose of 4 mg/kg or maintenance dose of 2 mg/kg. Calculate volume of 21 mg/ml solution and withdraw amount from vial; add it to an infusion bag containing 250 ml of 0.9% NaCl. Dextrose 5% solution should not be used.
• Don't mix or dilute trastuzumab with other drugs.
• Know that vials of drug are stable at 36° to 46° F (2° to 8° C) before reconstitution. Discard reconstituted solution after 28 days. Store trastuzumab solution diluted in 0.9% NaCl for injection at 36° to 46° F before use; it is stable for up to 24 hours.
Patient teaching
• Tell patient about possibility of first-dose, infusion-associated adverse effects.
• Instruct patient to notify doctor immediately if signs and symptoms of cardiac dysfunction develop, such as shortness of breath, increased cough, or peripheral edema.
• Instruct patient to report adverse effects to doctor.
• Advise breast-feeding women to discontinue breast-feeding during drug therapy and for 6 months after last dose.

▨ **Evaluation**
• Patient does not experience adverse GI effects (nausea, vomiting, diarrhea).
• Patient does not exhibit dyspnea, increased cough, paroxysmal nocturnal dyspnea, peripheral edema, or S_3 gallop as result of drug-induced cardiac dysfunction.
• Patient and family state understanding of drug therapy.

---

*Liquid form contains alcohol   **May contain tartrazine   ◆ Canada   ◊ Australia   †OTC

trazodone hydrochloride
(TRAYZ-oh-dohn high-droh-KLOR-ighd)
Desyrel, Trazon, Trialodine

Pharmacologic class: triazolopyridine
derivative
Therapeutic class: antidepressant
Pregnancy risk category: C

How supplied
Tablets: 50 mg, 100 mg, 150 mg, 300 mg

Pharmacokinetics
Absorption: well absorbed from GI tract.
Concomitant ingestion of food delays absorption but increases amount of drug absorbed by 20%.
Distribution: distributed widely in body;
does not concentrate in any particular tissue.
Metabolism: metabolized by liver.
Excretion: about 75% excreted in urine;
remainder excreted in feces. *Half-life:*
first phase, 3 to 6 hours; second phase, 5
to 9 hours.

Route	Onset	Peak	Duration
P.O.	2-4 wk	1-2 hr	Unknown

Pharmacodynamics
Chemical effect: unknown, although it
inhibits serotonin uptake in brain. Not a
tricyclic derivative.
Therapeutic effect: relieves depression.

Indications and dosage
▶ **Depression.** *Adults:* initial dosage,
150 mg P.O. daily in divided doses.
Increased by 50 mg daily q 3 to 4 days,
p.r.n. Average dosage ranges from 150 to
400 mg daily. Maximum daily dosage is
600 mg.

Adverse reactions
CNS: *drowsiness, dizziness,* nervousness,
fatigue, confusion, tremors, weakness,
hostility, anger, nightmares, vivid
dreams, headache, insomnia.

CV: orthostatic hypotension, tachycardia,
hypertension, syncope, shortness of breath.
EENT: blurred vision, tinnitus, nasal
congestion.
GI: dry mouth, dysgeusia, constipation,
nausea, vomiting, anorexia.
GU: urine retention; priapism, possibly
leading to impotence; decreased libido;
hematuria.
Hematologic: anemia.
Skin: rash, urticaria.
Other: diaphoresis.

Interactions
Drug-drug. *Antihypertensives:* increased
hypotensive effect of trazodone. Monitor
blood pressure; antihypertensive dosage
may have to be decreased.
Clonidine, CNS depressants: enhanced
CNS depression. Avoid concomitant use.
Digoxin, phenytoin: may increase serum
levels of these drugs. Monitor for toxicity.
MAO inhibitors: no clinical experience.
Use together with extreme caution.
Drug-lifestyle. *Alcohol use:* enhanced
CNS depression. Avoid concomitant use.

Contraindications and precautions
● Contraindicated during initial recovery
phase of MI and in patients with hypersensitivity to drug.
● Use cautiously in patients with cardiac
disease and in those at risk for suicide.
● Safety of drug has not been established
in pregnant or breast-feeding women and
in children.

NURSING CONSIDERATIONS

⬚ Assessment
● Assess patient's condition before therapy and regularly thereafter.
● Be alert for adverse reactions and drug
interactions.
● Evaluate patient's and family's knowledge of drug therapy.

⬚ Nursing diagnoses
● Altered thought processes related to
presence of depression

Reactions may be *common*, uncommon, *life-threatening*, or COMMON AND LIFE-THREATENING.

• Risk for injury related to drug-induced adverse CNS reactions
• Knowledge deficit related to drug therapy

❯ **Planning and implementation**
• Administer after meals or light snack for optimal absorption and to decrease incidence of dizziness.
• Don't discontinue drug abruptly. However, it should be discontinued at least 48 hours before surgery.
• Notify doctor if adverse reactions occur.
Patient teaching
• Instruct patient to take drug after meals or light snack.
• Inform male patient that priapism is potential problem in men taking trazodone. Advise him to notify doctor immediately if it occurs; it may require surgical intervention.
• Warn patient to avoid activities that require alertness and good psychomotor coordination until CNS effects of drug are known. Drowsiness and dizziness usually subside after first few weeks.
• Teach patient's family how to recognize signs of suicidal tendency or suicidal ideation.

☑ **Evaluation**
• Patient's behavior and communication exhibit improved thought processes.
• Patient does not experience adverse CNS reactions.
• Patient and family state understanding of drug therapy.

tretinoin
(TRET-ih-noyn)
Vesanoid

Pharmacologic class: retinoid
Therapeutic class: antineoplastic
Pregnancy risk category: D

How supplied
Capsules: 10 mg

Pharmacokinetics
Absorption: absorbed from GI tract.
Distribution: about 95% protein-bound.
Metabolism: drug induces its own metabolism.
Excretion: in urine and feces.

Route	Onset	Peak	Duration
P.O.	Unknown	1-2 hr	Unknown

Pharmacodynamics
Chemical effect: unknown.
Therapeutic effect: induces remission in selected patients with certain types of leukemia.

Indications and dosage
▶ **Induction of remission in patients with acute promyelocytic leukemia (APL), French-American-British (FAB) classification M3 (including M3 variant), characterized by presence of the t(15,17) translocation or the PML/RAR alpha gene, who are refractory to or have relapsed from anthracycline chemotherapy or for whom anthracycline-based chemotherapy is contraindicated.** *Adults and children age 1 and older:* 45 mg/m² P.O. daily administered as two evenly divided doses until complete remission is documented. Therapy should be discontinued 30 days after achievement of complete remission or after 90 days of treatment, whichever occurs first.

Adverse reactions
CNS: hypothermia, weakness, fatigue, *malaise, headache,* dizziness, *paresthesias, anxiety, insomnia, depression, confusion,* **cerebral hemorrhage, CVA,** intracranial hypertension, agitation, hallucinations, abnormal gait, agnosia, aphasia, asterixis, cerebellar edema, cerebellar disorders, *seizures, coma,* CNS depression, dysarthria, encephalopathy, facial paralysis, hemiplegia, hyporeflexia, hypotaxia, no light reflex, neurologic reaction, spinal cord disorder, tremors, leg weakness, unconsciousness, dementia, forgetfulness, somnolence, slow speech.

CV: *chest discomfort,* ARRHYTHMIAS, *hypotension, hypertension, phlebitis, edema,* HEART FAILURE, **MI,** enlarged heart, heart murmur, ischemia, myocarditis, pericarditis, secondary cardiomyopathy, *pericardial effusions,* impaired myocardial contractility, progressive hypoxemia.
EENT: *earache, ear fullness,* changed visual acuity, visual field defects, hearing loss, *visual disturbances, ocular disorders.*
GI: *GI hemorrhage, nausea, vomiting, anorexia, abdominal pain, GI disorders, diarrhea, constipation, dyspepsia, abdominal distention,* hepatosplenomegaly, ulcer.
GU: *renal insufficiency,* dysuria, *acute renal failure,* urinary frequency, renal tubular necrosis, enlarged prostate.
Hematologic: *leukocytosis,* HEMORRHAGE, DIC.
Hepatic: hepatitis, unspecified liver disorder, *hypercholesterolemia, hypertriglyceridemia, abnormal liver function test results.*
Musculoskeletal: *myalgia, bone pain,* flank pain, bone inflammation.
Respiratory: *pneumonia, upper respiratory tract disorders, dyspnea, respiratory insufficiency, pleural effusion, crackles, expiratory wheezing,* lower respiratory tract disorders, pulmonary infiltrates, bronchial asthma, pulmonary edema, laryngeal edema, unspecified pulmonary disease, pulmonary hypertension.
Skin: *flushing, skin and mucous membrane dryness, pruritus, increased sweating, alopecia, skin changes, rash.*
Other: *retinoic acid-APL syndrome, fever, infections, shivering, peripheral edema, pain, weight gain or loss, injection site reactions, mucositis, septicemia, multiorgan failure,* cellulitis, facial edema, fluid imbalance, pallor, lymph disorder, acidosis, ascites.

Interactions

None reported.

Contraindications and precautions

- Contraindicated in patients with known hypersensitivity to retinoids or to parabens, which are used as preservatives in the gelatin capsule.
- Drug is not recommended for use in pregnant or breast-feeding women.

NURSING CONSIDERATIONS

Assessment
- Assess patient's condition before therapy.
- Monitor CBC and platelet count regularly. Patients with elevated WBC counts at diagnosis have an increased risk of further rapid increase in WBC counts. Rapidly evolving leukocytosis is associated with a higher risk of life-threatening complications.
- Monitor patient, especially a child, for signs and symptoms of pseudotumor cerebri. Early signs and symptoms include papilledema, headache, nausea, vomiting, and visual disturbances.
- Monitor cholesterol and triglyceride levels, coagulation profile, and liver function studies for abnormalities.
- Be alert for adverse reactions.
- Evaluate patient's knowledge of drug therapy.

Nursing diagnoses
- Altered health maintenance related to leukemia
- Risk for injury related to adverse reactions
- Knowledge deficit related to drug therapy

Planning and implementation
- Because patients with APL are at high risk in general and can have severe adverse reactions, drug should be given under supervision of a doctor experienced in managing such patients and in a facility with laboratory and supportive services sufficient to monitor drug tolerance and to protect and maintain a patient compromised by toxicity.

Reactions may be *common,* uncommon, *life-threatening,* or COMMON AND LIFE-THREATENING.

• About 25% of patients treated during clinical studies have experienced a syndrome called retinoic acid-APL syndrome, which is characterized by fever, dyspnea, weight gain, radiographic pulmonary infiltrates, and pleural or pericardial effusion. Notify doctor immediately if these signs and symptoms appear; this syndrome may be accompanied by impaired myocardial contractility and episodic hypotension with or without leukocytosis. Some patients have died of progressive hypoxemia and multiorgan failure. The syndrome generally occurs during the first month of therapy. Prompt treatment with high-dose steroids may reduce morbidity and mortality.

• Notify doctor immediately if signs and symptoms of pseudotumor cerebri occur.

• Ensure that pregnancy testing and contraception counseling are repeated monthly throughout therapy and for 1 month after therapy.

Patient teaching

• Inform female patient that a pregnancy test is required within 1 week before therapy. When possible, therapy is delayed until a negative result is obtained. Also advise her to use effective contraception during therapy and for 1 month after discontinuation, even with a history of infertility or menopause (unless hysterectomy has been performed). Urge her to use two forms of contraception simultaneously, unless abstinence is the chosen method. Tell her to alert doctor immediately of suspected pregnancy.

• Instruct patient on infection-control and bleeding precautions. Tell her to notify doctor of signs of infection (fever, sore throat, fatigue) or bleeding (easy bruising, nosebleeds, bleeding gums, melena) and to take temperature daily.

☑ **Evaluation**

• Patient responds well to therapy.

• Patient does not experience injury from adverse reactions.

• Patient and family state understanding of drug therapy.

triamcinolone
(trigh-am-SIN-oh-lohn)
Aristocort, Atolone, Kenacort**

triamcinolone acetonide
Cenocort A-40, Cinonide 40, Kenaject-40, Kenalog-10, Kenalog-40, Tac-3, Tac-40, Triam-A, Triamonide 40, Tri-Kort, Trilog

triamcinolone diacetate
Amcort, Aristocort, Aristocort Forte, Aristocort Intralesional, Articulose-L.A., Cenocort Forte, Cinalone 40, Kenacort Diacetate, Triam Forte, Triamolone 40, Trilone, Tristoject

triamcinolone hexacetonide
Aristospan Intra-Articular, Aristospan Intralesional

Pharmacologic class: glucocorticoid
Therapeutic class: anti-inflammatory, immunosuppressant
Pregnancy risk category: C

How supplied

triamcinolone
Tablets: 1 mg, 2 mg, 4 mg, 8 mg
Syrup: 2 mg/ml, 4 mg/ml
triamcinolone acetonide
Injection (suspension): 3 mg/ml, 10 mg/ml, 40 mg/ml
triamcinolone diacetate
Injection (suspension): 25 mg/ml, 40 mg/ml
triamcinolone hexacetonide
Injection (suspension): 5 mg/ml, 20 mg/ml

Pharmacokinetics

Absorption: absorbed readily after oral administration. Absorption is variable after other routes of administration, depending on whether drug is injected into intra-articular space or muscle and on blood supply to that muscle.
Distribution: distributed to muscle, liver, skin, intestines, and kidneys. Drug is ex-

---

tensively bound to plasma proteins. Only unbound portion is active.
Metabolism: metabolized in liver.
Excretion: excreted in urine; insignificant quantities also excreted in feces.
Half-life: 18 to 36 hours.

Route	Onset	Peak	Duration
P.O., I.M., intralesional, intra-articular, intrasynovial	Varies	Varies	Varies

Pharmacodynamics

Chemical effect: not clearly defined; decreases inflammation, mainly by stabilizing leukocyte lysosomal membranes; suppresses immune response; stimulates bone marrow; and influences protein, fat, and carbohydrate metabolism.
Therapeutic effect: relieves inflammation and suppresses immune system function.

Indications and dosage

▶ **Severe inflammation or immunosuppression. Triamcinolone.** *Adults:* 8 to 16 mg P.O. daily, in a single or divided dose. **Triamcinolone diacetate.** *Adults:* 40 mg I.M. weekly or 2 to 40 mg into lesions, joints or soft tissue, or 4 to 48 mg P.O. divided q.i.d. **Triamcinolone hexacetonide.** *Adults:* up to 0.5 mg per square inch of affected skin intralesionally, or 2 to 20 mg intra-articularly q 3 to 4 weeks, p.r.n. **Triamcinolone acetonide.** *Adults:* initially, 2.5 to 60 mg I.M. Additional doses of 20 to 100 mg may be given p.r.n. at 6-week intervals. Alternatively, 2.5 to 15 mg intra-articularly, or up to 1 mg intralesionally, p.r.n.

Adverse reactions

Most adverse reactions to corticosteroids are dose- or duration-dependent.
CNS: *euphoria, insomnia,* psychotic behavior, pseudotumor cerebri, vertigo, headache, paresthesia, *seizures.*
CV: *heart failure,* hypertension, edema, *arrhythmias,* thrombophlebitis, *thromboembolism.*

EENT: cataracts, glaucoma.
Endocrine: menstrual irregularities, cushingoid state (moonface, buffalo hump, central obesity).
GI: *peptic ulceration,* GI irritation, increased appetite, *pancreatitis,* nausea, vomiting.
Metabolic: hypokalemia, hyperglycemia, carbohydrate intolerance.
Musculoskeletal: muscle weakness, osteoporosis, growth suppression in children.
Skin: hirsutism, delayed wound healing, acne, various skin eruptions.
Other: susceptibility to infections; *acute adrenal insufficiency may occur with increased stress (infection, surgery, or trauma) or abrupt withdrawal.*
After abrupt withdrawal: rebound inflammation, fatigue, weakness, arthralgia, fever, dizziness, lethargy, depression, fainting, orthostatic hypotension, dyspnea, anorexia, hypoglycemia. *After prolonged use, sudden withdrawal may be fatal.*

Interactions

Drug-drug. *Aspirin, indomethacin, other NSAIDs:* increased risk of GI distress and bleeding. Give together cautiously.
Barbiturates, phenytoin, rifampin: decreased corticosteroid effect. Increase corticosteroid, as ordered.
Oral anticoagulants: altered dosage requirements. Monitor PT closely.
Potassium-depleting drugs (such as thiazide diuretics): enhanced potassium-wasting effects of triamcinolone. Monitor serum potassium level.
Skin-test antigens: decreased response. Defer skin testing.
Toxoids, vaccines: decreased antibody response and increased risk of neurologic complications. Avoid concomitant use.

Contraindications and precautions

• Contraindicated in patients with systemic fungal infections or hypersensitivity to drug or its components.
• Use cautiously in pregnant or breast-feeding women and in patients with GI ulcer, renal disease, hypertension, osteo-

porosis, diabetes mellitus, hypothyroidism, cirrhosis, diverticulitis, nonspecific ulcerative colitis, recent intestinal anastomoses, thromboembolic disorders, seizures, myasthenia gravis, heart failure, tuberculosis, ocular herpes simplex, emotional instability, or psychotic tendencies.

NURSING CONSIDERATIONS

☢ Assessment
• Assess patient before and after therapy; monitor weight, blood pressure, and serum electrolyte levels.
• Watch for adverse reactions, drug interactions, depression, or psychotic episodes, especially with high doses.
• Evaluate patient's and family's knowledge of drug therapy.

⊞ Nursing diagnoses
• Altered health maintenance related to underlying condition
• Risk for injury related to drug-induced adverse reactions
• Knowledge deficit related to drug therapy

⧉ Planning and implementation
• Know that drug is not used for alternate-day therapy.
• Always titrate to lowest effective dose, as ordered.
• For better results and less toxicity, give once-daily dose in morning.
P.O. use: Give dose with food when possible to reduce GI irritation.
I.M. use: Give I.M. injection deeply into gluteal muscle. Rotate injection sites to prevent muscle atrophy.
Intralesional, intra-articular, intrasynovial use: Assist doctor with administration, as directed.
• Parenteral form is *not* for I.V. use.
• Don't use diluents that contain preservatives; flocculation may occur.
• Unless contraindicated, give low-sodium diet high in potassium and protein. Administer potassium supplements, as needed.

• Gradually reduce drug dosage after long-term therapy, as ordered.
Patient teaching
• Tell patient not to discontinue drug abruptly or without doctor's consent.
• Instruct patient to take oral drug with food.
• Teach patient signs of early adrenal insufficiency: fatigue, muscle weakness, joint pain, fever, anorexia, nausea, dyspnea, dizziness, and fainting.
• Instruct patient to carry medical identification at all times.
• Warn patient on long-term therapy about cushingoid symptoms and to report sudden weight gain and swelling to doctor.
• Tell patient to report slow healing.
• Advise patient receiving long-term therapy to consider exercise or physical therapy. Also tell patient to ask doctor about vitamin D or calcium supplements.

☑ Evaluation
• Patient responds well to drug.
• Patient does not experience injury from adverse reactions.
• Patient and family state understanding of drug therapy.

triamcinolone acetonide
(trigh-am-SIN-oh-lohn as-EE-tuh-nighd)
Azmacort

Pharmacologic class: glucocorticoid
Therapeutic class: anti-inflammatory, immunosuppressant
Pregnancy risk category: C

How supplied
Inhalation aerosol: 100 mcg/metered spray

Pharmacokinetics
Absorption: absorbed slowly from lungs and GI tract.
Distribution: without use of spacer, about 10% to 25% of inhaled dose is de-

posited in airways; remainder is deposited in mouth and throat and swallowed. A greater percentage of inhaled dose may reach lungs with use of spacer device. *Metabolism:* metabolized in liver. Some drug that reaches lungs may be metabolized locally. *Excretion:* excreted in urine and feces. *Half-life:* 18 to 36 hours.

Route	Onset	Peak	Duration
Inhalation	1-4 wk	Unknown	Unknown

Pharmacodynamics

Chemical effect: unknown; probably decreases inflammation, mainly by stabilizing leukocyte lysosomal membranes. *Therapeutic effect:* improves breathing ability.

Indications and dosage

▶ **Steroid-dependent asthma.** *Adults:* 2 inhalations t.i.d. to q.i.d. Maximum dosage is 16 inhalations daily. In some patients, maintenance can be accomplished when total daily dosage is given b.i.d. *Children ages 6 to 12:* 1 or 2 inhalations t.i.d. to q.i.d. Maximum dosage is 12 inhalations daily.

Adverse reactions

Most adverse reactions to corticosteroids are dose- or duration-dependent.
EENT: dry or irritated nose or throat, hoarseness.
GI: *oral candidiasis,* dry or irritated tongue or mouth.
Respiratory: cough, wheezing.
Other: facial edema, *hypothalamic-pituitary-adrenal function suppression,* adrenal insufficiency.

Interactions

None significant.

Contraindications and precautions

• Contraindicated in patients with status asthmaticus or hypersensitivity to drug or its components.

• Drug is not recommended for use in breast-feeding women.
• Use with extreme caution, if at all, in patients with tuberculosis of respiratory tract; untreated fungal, bacterial, or systemic viral infections; or ocular herpes simplex.
• Use cautiously in patients receiving systemic corticosteroids and in pregnant women.

NURSING CONSIDERATIONS

⚕ Assessment
• Assess patient's asthma before therapy and regularly thereafter.
• Be alert for adverse reactions.
• Evaluate patient's and family's knowledge of drug therapy.

⚙ Nursing diagnoses
• Ineffective breathing pattern related to presence of asthma
• Impaired tissue integrity related to drug's adverse effect on oral mucosa
• Knowledge deficit related to drug therapy

▶ Planning and implementation
• Know that patient who has recently been transferred to oral inhaled steroids from systemic administration of steroids may need to be placed back on systemic steroids during periods of stress or severe asthma attacks.
• Taper oral therapy slowly, as ordered.
• If patient is also to receive bronchodilator by inhalation, administer bronchodilator first, wait several minutes, then administer triamcinolone.
• If more than one inhalation of triamcinolone is ordered for each dose, allow 1 minute to elapse before repeat inhalations.
• Store drug between 36° and 86° F (2° and 30° C).
Patient teaching
• Inform patient that inhaled corticosteroids don't provide relief for emergency asthma attacks.

Reactions may be *common*, uncommon, *life-threatening*, or COMMON AND LIFE-THREATENING.

• Advise patient to ensure delivery of proper dose of medication by gently warming canister to room temperature before using. Some patients carry canister in pocket to keep it warm.
• Instruct patient requiring bronchodilator to use it several minutes before triamcinolone. Tell him to allow 1 minute to elapse before repeat inhalations and to hold breath for a few seconds to enhance drug action.
• Teach patient to check mucous membranes frequently for signs of fungal infection.
• Tell patient to prevent oral fungal infections by gargling or rinsing mouth with water after each use of inhaler but not to swallow water.
• Inform patient to keep inhaler clean and unobstructed by washing it with warm water and drying it thoroughly after use.
• Instruct patient to contact the doctor if response to therapy decreases; doctor may need to adjust dosage. Tell patient not to exceed recommended dosage on his own.
• Instruct patient to carry medical identification at all times.

☑ **Evaluation**
• Patient exhibits improved breathing ability.
• Patient maintains normal oral mucosa integrity.
• Patient and family state understanding of drug therapy.

---

triamcinolone acetonide
(trigh-am-SIN-oh-lohn as-EE-tuh-nighd)
Nasacort

Pharmacologic class: glucocorticoid
Therapeutic class: anti-inflammatory
Pregnancy risk category: C

How supplied
Nasal aerosol: 55 mcg/metered spray

Pharmacokinetics
Absorption: minimally absorbed.
Distribution: locally.
Metabolism: metabolized in liver.
Excretion: excreted primarily in feces.
Half-life: 4 hours.

Route	Onset	Peak	Duration
Intranasal	≤ 12 hr	3-4 days	Several days after drug is stopped

Pharmacodynamics
Chemical effect: unknown.
Therapeutic effect: relieves signs and symptoms of nasal inflammation.

Indications and dosage
▶ **Relief of symptoms of seasonal or perennial allergic rhinitis.** *Adults and children age 12 and over:* initially, 2 sprays (110 mcg) in each nostril once daily. Increased as needed up to 220 mcg daily either as once-daily dosage or in divided doses up to four times daily. After desired effect is obtained, dosage decreased, if possible, to as little as 1 spray (55 mcg) in each nostril daily.

Adverse reactions
CNS: *headache.*
EENT: *nasal irritation,* dry mucous membranes, nasal and sinus congestion, irritation, burning, stinging, throat discomfort, sneezing, epistaxis.

Interactions
None known.

Contraindications and precautions
• Contraindicated in patients hypersensitive to drug or its components.
• Use with extreme caution, if at all, in patients with active or quiescent tuberculosis infection of respiratory tract and in patients with untreated fungal, bacterial, or systemic viral infection or ocular herpes simplex.

• Use cautiously in patients already receiving systemic corticosteroids because of increased likelihood of hypothalamic-pituitary-adrenal suppression compared with therapeutic dosage of either one alone. Also use cautiously in patients with recent nasal septal ulcers, nasal surgery, or trauma because of inhibitory effect on wound healing. Also use with caution in pregnant or breast-feeding women.

• Safety of drug has not been established in children under age 12.

NURSING CONSIDERATIONS

🔏 Assessment
• Assess patient's condition before therapy and regularly thereafter.
• Be alert for adverse reactions.
• Evaluate patient's and family's knowledge of drug therapy.

⊕ Nursing diagnoses
• Altered health maintenance related to presence of allergic rhinitis
• Impaired tissue integrity related to drug's adverse effect on nasal mucosa
• Knowledge deficit related to drug therapy

▷ Planning and implementation
• Be aware that when excessive doses are used, signs and symptoms of hyperadrenocorticism and adrenal suppression may occur; drug should be discontinued slowly.
• To administer drug, shake canister before each use and have patient blow his nose. To instill drug, tilt patient's head forward slightly and insert nozzle into nostril, pointing it away from septum. Have patient hold other nostril closed and then inspire gently when drug is sprayed. Repeat procedure for other nostril after shaking canister.
Patient teaching
• Urge patient to read instruction sheet in package before using drug for first time.
• To instill, instruct patient to shake canister before using; to blow nose to clear nasal passages; and to tilt head slightly

forward and insert nozzle into nostril, pointing away from septum. Tell him to hold other nostril closed and then to inspire gently and spray. Next, have patient shake canister again and repeat this procedure in other nostril.
• Tell patient to discard canister after 100 actuations.
• Stress importance of using drug on regular schedule because its effectiveness depends on regular use. Caution patient not to exceed dosage prescribed because serious adverse reactions may occur.
• Tell patient to notify doctor if symptoms don't improve within 2 to 3 weeks or if condition worsens.
• Warn patient to avoid exposure to chickenpox or measles and, if exposed to either, to obtain medical advice.
• Instruct patient to watch for signs and symptoms of nasal infection. If symptoms occur, tell patient to notify doctor because drug may need to be discontinued and appropriate local therapy given.
• Advise patient not to break or incinerate canister or store it in extreme heat; contents are under pressure and may explode.

☑ Evaluation
• Patient's allergic rhinitis is visibly improved.
• Patient maintains normal tissue integrity in nasal passages.
• Patient and family state understanding of drug therapy.

triamterene
(trigh-AM-tuh-reen)
Dyrenium

Pharmacologic class: potassium-sparing diuretic
Therapeutic class: diuretic
Pregnancy risk category: B

How supplied
Tablets ◆: 50 mg, 100 mg
Capsules: 50 mg, 100 mg

Pharmacokinetics

Absorption: absorbed rapidly from GI tract but extent varies.
Distribution: about 67% protein-bound.
Metabolism: metabolized by hydroxylation and sulfation.
Excretion: excreted in urine. *Half-life:* 100 to 150 minutes.

Route	Onset	Peak	Duration
P.O.	2-4 hr	6-8 hr	7-9 hr

Pharmacodynamics

Chemical effect: inhibits sodium reabsorption and potassium and hydrogen excretion by direct action on distal tubule.
Therapeutic effect: promotes water and sodium excretion.

Indications and dosage

▶ **Diuresis.** *Adults:* initially, 100 mg P.O. b.i.d. after meals. Total dosage should not exceed 300 mg daily.

Adverse reactions

CNS: dizziness, weakness, fatigue, headache.
CV: hypotension.
GI: dry mouth, nausea, vomiting, diarrhea.
GU: interstitial nephritis, nephrolithiasis, transient elevation in BUN or creatinine level.
Hematologic: megaloblastic anemia related to low folic acid levels, *thrombocytopenia, agranulocytosis.*
Hepatic: jaundice, increased liver enzyme abnormalities.
Metabolic: *hyperkalemia,* acidosis, hypokalemia, hyponatremia, hyperglycemia, azotemia.
Musculoskeletal: muscle cramps.
Skin: photosensitivity, rash.
Other: *anaphylaxis.*

Interactions

Drug-drug. *ACE inhibitors, potassium supplements:* increased risk of hyperkalemia. Don't use together.

Amantadine: increased risk of amantadine toxicity. Don't use together.
Lithium: decreased lithium clearance, increasing risk of lithium toxicity. Monitor lithium level.
NSAIDs: may enhance risk of nephrotoxicity. Avoid concomitant use.
Quinidine: may interfere with some laboratory tests that measure quinidine levels. Inform laboratory that patient is taking triamterene.
Drug-food. *Potassium-containing salt substitutes, potassium-rich foods:* increased risk of hyperkalemia. Don't use together.
Drug-lifestyle. *Sun exposure:* photosensitivity reactions may occur. Take precautions.

Contraindications and precautions

• Contraindicated in patients with anuria, severe or progressive renal disease or dysfunction, severe hepatic disease, hyperkalemia, or hypersensitivity to drug.
• Use cautiously in patients with impaired liver function or diabetes mellitus; in elderly or debilitated patients; and in pregnant women.
• Safe use of drug has not been established in breast-feeding women.

NURSING CONSIDERATIONS

Assessment
• Obtain history of patient's edema before therapy and reassess regularly thereafter. Full effect of triamterene delayed 2 to 3 days when used alone.
• Monitor blood pressure and BUN and serum electrolyte levels.
• Watch for blood dyscrasia.
• Be alert for adverse reactions and drug interactions.
• Evaluate patient's and family's knowledge of drug therapy.

Nursing diagnoses
• Fluid volume excess related to underlying condition

• Altered health maintenance related to drug-induced hyperkalemia
• Knowledge deficit related to drug therapy

» **Planning and implementation**
• Give drug after meals to minimize nausea.
• Withdraw drug gradually, as ordered, to minimize excessive rebound potassium excretion.
• Be aware that drug is less potent than thiazides and loop diuretics and is useful as adjunct to other diuretic therapy. Triamterene is usually used with potassium-wasting diuretics.
Patient teaching
• Tell patient to take drug after meals.
• Warn patient to avoid excessive ingestion of potassium-rich foods, potassium-containing salt substitutes, and potassium supplements to prevent serious hyperkalemia.
• Teach patient to avoid direct sunlight, wear protective clothing, and use sunblock to prevent photosensitivity reactions.

☑ **Evaluation**
• Patient exhibits no signs of edema.
• Patient's serum potassium level is normal.
• Patient and family state understanding of drug therapy.

---

triazolam
(trigh-AH-zoh-lam)
Alti-Triazolam♦, Apo-Triazo♦, Halcion, Novo-Triolam♦

Pharmacologic class: benzodiazepine
Therapeutic class: sedative-hypnotic
Controlled substance schedule: IV
Pregnancy risk category: X

How supplied
Tablets: 0.125 mg, 0.25 mg

Pharmacokinetics
Absorption: well absorbed through GI tract.
Distribution: distributed widely throughout body; 90% protein-bound.
Metabolism: metabolized in liver.
Excretion: excreted in urine. *Half-life:* 1½ to 5½ hours.

Route	Onset	Peak	Duration
P.O.	Unknown	1-2 hr	Unknown

Pharmacodynamics
Chemical effect: unknown; probably acts on limbic system, thalamus, and hypothalamus of CNS to produce hypnotic effects.
Therapeutic effect: promotes sleep.

Indications and dosage
▶ **Insomnia.** *Adults:* 0.125 to 0.5 mg P.O. h.s. *Adults over age 65:* 0.125 mg P.O. h.s.; increased, p.r.n., to 0.25 mg P.O. h.s.

Adverse reactions
CNS: *drowsiness, dizziness, headache,* rebound insomnia, amnesia, lightheadedness, lack of coordination, confusion, depression, nervousness, ataxia.
GI: nausea, vomiting.
Other: physical or psychological abuse.

Interactions
Drug-drug. *Cimetidine, erythromycin:* may cause prolonged triazolam blood levels. Monitor for increased sedation.
Other CNS depressants, including narcotic analgesics: excessive CNS depression. Use together cautiously.
Drug-lifestyle. *Alcohol use:* excessive CNS depression. Use together cautiously.

Contraindications and precautions
• Contraindicated in patients with hypersensitivity to benzodiazepines and in pregnant women.
• Drug is not recommended for use in breast-feeding women.

• Use cautiously in patients with impaired liver or kidney function, chronic pulmonary insufficiency, sleep apnea, depression, suicidal tendencies, or history of drug abuse.
• Safe use of drug has not been established in children.

NURSING CONSIDERATIONS

Assessment
• Assess patient's condition before therapy and regularly thereafter.
• Assess mental status before initiating therapy. Elderly patients are more sensitive to drug's CNS effects.
• Be alert for adverse reactions and drug interactions.
• Evaluate patient's and family's knowledge of drug therapy.

Nursing diagnoses
• Sleep pattern disturbance related to underlying disorder
• Risk for injury related to drug-induced adverse CNS reactions
• Knowledge deficit related to drug therapy

Planning and implementation
• Store drug in cool, dry place away from light.
• Institute safety precautions once drug has been administered.
Patient teaching
• Warn patient not to take more than prescribed amount because overdose can occur at total daily dosage of 2 mg (or four times the highest recommended amount).
• Caution patient about performing activities that require mental alertness or physical coordination. For inpatient, supervise walking and raise bed rails, particularly for elderly patient.
• Inform patient that drug is very short-acting and therefore has less tendency to cause morning drowsiness.
• Tell patient that rebound insomnia may develop for 1 or 2 nights after stopping therapy.

Evaluation
• Patient states that drug produces sleep.
• Patient does not experience injury from adverse CNS reactions.
• Patient and family state understanding of drug therapy.

trifluoperazine hydrochloride
(trigh-floo-oh-PER-eh-zeen
high-droh-KLOR-ighd)
Apo-Trifluoperazine♦, Novo-Flurazine♦, PMS Trifluoperazine♦, Solazine♦, Stelazine, Stelazine Concentrate, Terfluzine♦, Terfluzine Concentrate♦

Pharmacologic class: phenothiazine (piperazine derivative)
Therapeutic class: antipsychotic, antiemetic
Pregnancy risk category: C

How supplied
Tablets (regular and film-coated): 1 mg, 2 mg, 5 mg, 10 mg
Oral concentrate: 10 mg/ml
Injection: 2 mg/ml

Pharmacokinetics
Absorption: variable with P.O. administration; rapid after I.M. use.
Distribution: distributed widely in body; 91% to 99% protein-bound.
Metabolism: metabolized extensively by liver.
Excretion: excreted primarily in urine; some excreted in feces.

Route	Onset	Peak	Duration
P.O., I.M.	Up to several wk	Unknown	Unknown

Pharmacodynamics
Chemical effect: unknown; probably blocks postsynaptic dopamine receptors in brain.
Therapeutic effect: relieves anxiety and signs and symptoms of psychotic disorders.

Indications and dosage

▶ **Anxiety.** *Adults:* 1 to 2 mg P.O. b.i.d. Maximum dosage is 6 mg/day. Drug should not be used longer than 12 weeks for anxiety.

▶ **Schizophrenia and other psychotic disorders.** *Adult outpatients:* 1 to 2 mg P.O. b.i.d., increased as needed. Or 1 to 2 mg deep I.M. q 4 to 6 hours, p.r.n. *Hospitalized adults:* 2 to 5 mg P.O. b.i.d.; may increase gradually to 40 mg daily. *Children ages 6 to 12 (hospitalized or under close supervision):* 1 mg P.O. daily or b.i.d.; may increase gradually to 15 mg daily, if needed.

Adverse reactions

CNS: *extrapyramidal reactions, tardive dyskinesia,* pseudoparkinsonism, dizziness, drowsiness, insomnia, fatigue, headache.
CV: *orthostatic hypotension,* tachycardia, ECG changes.
EENT: ocular changes, *blurred vision.*
GI: *dry mouth, constipation,* nausea.
GU: *urine retention.*
Hematologic: transient leukopenia, *agranulocytosis.*
Hepatic: cholestatic jaundice.
Skin: *photosensitivity,* allergic reactions, pain at I.M. injection site, sterile abscess, rash.
Other: weight gain; rarely, *neuroleptic malignant syndrome* (fever, tachycardia, tachypnea, profuse diaphoresis); menstrual irregularities; gynecomastia; inhibited lactation.
After abrupt withdrawal of long-term therapy: gastritis, nausea, vomiting, dizziness, tremors, feeling of warmth or cold, diaphoresis, tachycardia, headache, insomnia, anorexia, muscle rigidity, altered mental status, evidence of autonomic instability.

Interactions

Drug-drug. *Antacids:* inhibited absorption of oral phenothiazines. Separate doses by at least 2 hours.
Barbiturates, lithium: may decrease phenothiazine effect. Monitor patient.

Centrally acting antihypertensives: decreased antihypertensive effect. Monitor blood pressure.
CNS depressants: increased CNS depression. Use together cautiously.
Propranolol: increased levels of both propranolol and trifluoperazine. Monitor patient closely.
Warfarin: decreased effect of oral anticoagulants. Monitor PT and INR.
Drug-lifestyle. *Alcohol use:* increased CNS depression. Avoid concomitant use.

Contraindications and precautions

● Contraindicated in patients with hypersensitivity to phenothiazines or in patients experiencing coma, CNS depression, bone marrow suppression, or liver damage.
● Use cautiously in patients with CV disease (may cause drop in blood pressure), exposure to extreme heat, seizure disorder, glaucoma, or prostatic hyperplasia and in elderly or debilitated patients.
● Safety of drug has not been established in pregnant or breast-feeding women and in children under age 6.

NURSING CONSIDERATIONS

Assessment

● Assess patient's condition before therapy and regularly thereafter.
● Watch for orthostatic hypotension, especially with parenteral use.
● Monitor patient for tardive dyskinesia. It may occur after prolonged use. It may not appear until months or years later and may disappear spontaneously or persist for life, despite discontinuation of drug.
● Monitor therapy with weekly bilirubin tests during first month; periodic blood tests (CBC and liver function); and ophthalmologic tests (long-term use), as ordered.
● Be alert for adverse reactions and drug interactions.
● Evaluate patient's and family's knowledge of drug therapy.

Reactions may be *common,* uncommon, *life-threatening,* or COMMON AND LIFE-THREATENING.

⊞ Nursing diagnoses
• Anxiety related to underlying condition
• Altered thought processes related to underlying psychotic disorder
• Knowledge deficit related to drug therapy

⟩ Planning and implementation
• Although there is little likelihood of contact dermatitis, people with known sensitivity to phenothiazine drugs should avoid direct contact. Wear gloves when preparing liquid forms.
P.O. use: Dilute liquid concentrate with 60 ml of tomato or fruit juice, carbonated beverages, coffee, tea, milk, water, or semisolid food.
I.M. use: Give deeply I.M. only in upper outer quadrant of buttocks. Massage slowly afterward to prevent sterile abscess. Injection may sting.
– Protect drug from light. Slight yellowing of injection or concentrate is common; it does not affect potency. Discard markedly discolored solutions.
• Keep patient supine for 1 hour after drug administration, and advise him to change position slowly.
• Do not withdraw drug abruptly unless severe adverse reactions occur.
• Withhold dose and notify doctor if patient develops jaundice, symptoms of blood dyscrasia (fever, sore throat, infection, cellulitis, weakness), or persistent extrapyramidal reactions (longer than a few hours), especially in pregnant woman or in child.
• Know that acute dystonic reactions may be treated with diphenhydramine.
Patient teaching
• Teach patient or caregiver how to prepare oral form of drug.
• Warn patient to avoid activities that require alertness or good psychomotor coordination until CNS effects of drug are known. Drowsiness and dizziness usually subside after a few weeks.
• Tell patient to avoid alcohol during drug therapy.

• Instruct patient to report urine retention or constipation.
• Tell patient to use sunblock and to wear protective clothing to avoid photosensitivity reactions.
• Tell patient to relieve dry mouth with sugarless gum or hard candy.

☑ Evaluation
• Patient's anxiety is reduced.
• Patient's behavior and communication exhibit improved thought processes.
• Patient and family state understanding of drug therapy.

---

trihexyphenidyl hydrochloride
(trigh-heks-eh-FEEN-ih-dil high-droh-KLOR-ighd)
Apo-Trihex♦, Artane*, Artane Sequels, PMS Trihexyphenidyl, Trihexane, Trihexy-2, Trihexy-5

Pharmacologic class: anticholinergic
Therapeutic class: antiparkinsonian agent
Pregnancy risk category: C

How supplied
Tablets: 2 mg, 5 mg
Capsules (sustained-release): 5 mg
Elixir: 2 mg/5 ml

Pharmacokinetics
Absorption: readily absorbed from GI tract.
Distribution: unknown; crosses blood-brain barrier.
Metabolism: unknown.
Excretion: excreted in urine.

Route	Onset	Peak	Duration
P.O.	≤ 1 hr	2-3 hr	6-12 hr

Pharmacodynamics
Chemical effect: unknown; blocks central cholinergic receptors, helping to balance cholinergic activity in basal ganglia.

Therapeutic effect: improves physical mobility in patients with parkinsonism.

Indications and dosage

▶ **All forms of parkinsonism and adjunct treatment to levodopa in management of parkinsonism.** *Adults:* 1 mg P.O. first day, 2 mg second day, then increased by 2 mg q 3 to 5 days until total of 6 to 10 mg is given daily. Usually given t.i.d. with meals. Sometimes given q.i.d. (last dose h.s.). Postencephalitic parkinsonism may require total daily dosage of 12 to 15 mg.
▶ **Drug-induced parkinsonism.** *Adults:* 5 to 15 mg P.O. daily.

Adverse reactions

CNS: nervousness, dizziness, headache, hallucinations, drowsiness, weakness.
CV: tachycardia.
EENT: blurred vision, mydriasis, increased intraocular pressure.
GI: *dry mouth,* constipation, *nausea, vomiting.*
GU: urinary hesitancy, urine retention.

Interactions

Drug-drug. *Amantadine:* additive anticholinergic reactions, such as confusion and hallucinations. Reduce dosage of trihexyphenidyl before administering.
Levodopa: increased effect when used concomitantly with levodopa. May require lower doses of both agents.
Drug-lifestyle. *Alcohol use:* increased sedative effects. Avoid concomitant use.

Contraindications and precautions

• Contraindicated in patients hypersensitive to drug.
• Drug is not recommended for use in breast-feeding women.
• Use cautiously in patients with glaucoma; cardiac, hepatic, or renal disorders; obstructive disease of GI and GU tracts; or prostatic hyperplasia.
• Safety of drug has not been established in pregnant women and in children.

NURSING CONSIDERATIONS

⚗ Assessment
• Assess patient's condition before therapy and regularly thereafter.
• Gonioscopic evaluation and monitoring of intraocular pressure are needed, especially in patient over age 40.
• Be alert for adverse reactions and drug interactions. Adverse reactions are dose-related and usually transient.
• Monitor the elderly for mental confusion or disorientation.
• Evaluate patient's and family's knowledge of drug therapy.

⊞ Nursing diagnoses
• Impaired physical mobility related to presence of parkinsonism
• Risk for injury related to drug-induced adverse CNS reactions
• Knowledge deficit related to drug therapy

▷ Planning and implementation
• Be aware that dosage may need to be gradually increased in patient who develops tolerance to drug.
• Administer drug with meals.
Patient teaching
• Alert patient that drug may cause nausea if taken before meals.
• Tell patient to avoid activities that require alertness until CNS effects of drug are known.
• Advise patient to report urinary hesitancy or urine retention.
• Tell patient to relieve dry mouth with cool drinks, ice chips, or sugarless gum or hard candy.

☑ Evaluation
• Patient exhibits improved physical mobility.
• Patient does not experience injury from adverse reactions.
• Patient and family state understanding of drug therapy.

trimethobenzamide hydrochloride
(trigh-meth-oh-BEN-zuh-mighd high-droh-KLOR-ighd)
Arrestin, Bio-Gan, Stemetic, Tebamide, Tegamide, T-Gen, Ticon, Tigan, Triban, Tribenzagan

Pharmacologic class: ethanolamine-related antihistamine
Therapeutic class: antiemetic
Pregnancy risk category: NR

How supplied
Capsules: 100 mg, 250 mg
Injection: 100 mg/ml
Suppositories: 100 mg, 200 mg

Pharmacokinetics
Absorption: about 60% absorbed after P.O. administration; unknown after P.R. or I.M. administration.
Distribution: unknown.
Metabolism: about 50% to 70% metabolized, probably in liver.
Excretion: excreted in urine and feces.

Route	Onset	Peak	Duration
P.O.	10-20 min	Unknown	3-4 hr
I.M.	15-30 min	Unknown	2-3 hr
P.R.	Unknown	Unknown	Unknown

Pharmacodynamics
Chemical effect: unknown; probably acts on chemoreceptor trigger zone to inhibit nausea and vomiting.
Therapeutic effect: prevents or relieves nausea and vomiting.

Indications and dosage
▶ **Nausea, vomiting.** *Adults:* 250 mg P.O. t.i.d. or q.i.d.; or 200 mg I.M. or P.R. t.i.d. or q.i.d.
▶ **Prevention of postoperative nausea and vomiting.** *Adults:* 200 mg I.M. or P.R. as single dose before or during surgery; if needed, repeat 3 hours after termination of anesthesia. Limit use to prolonged vomiting from known cause.

Children weighing 13 to 40 kg (28 to 88 lb): 100 to 200 mg P.O. or P.R. t.i.d. or q.i.d. *Children weighing under 13 kg:* 100 mg P.R. t.i.d. or q.i.d.

Adverse reactions
CNS: *drowsiness,* dizziness (in large doses), headache, disorientation, depression, parkinsonian-like symptoms, *coma, seizures.*
CV: hypotension.
GI: diarrhea.
Hepatic: jaundice.
Skin: hypersensitivity reaction (pain, stinging, burning, redness, swelling at I.M. injection site); blurred vision; muscle cramps.

Interactions
Drug-drug. *CNS depressants:* additive CNS depression. Avoid concomitant use.
Drug-lifestyle. *Alcohol use:* additive CNS depression. Avoid concomitant use.

Contraindications and precautions
• Contraindicated in patients with hypersensitivity to drug. Suppositories are contraindicated in patients hypersensitive to benzocaine hydrochloride or similar local anesthetics.
• Use cautiously in children. Drug is not recommended for use in children with viral illness because it may contribute to development of Reye's syndrome.
• Safety of drug has not been established in pregnant or breast-feeding women.

NURSING CONSIDERATIONS

≋ Assessment
• Assess patient's condition before therapy and regularly thereafter.
• Be alert for adverse reactions and drug interactions.
• Evaluate patient's and family's knowledge of drug therapy.

▦ Nursing diagnoses
• Risk for fluid volume deficit related to potential for or presence of nausea and vomiting

• Diarrhea related to drug-induced adverse GI reactions
• Knowledge deficit related to drug therapy

▷ **Planning and implementation**
P.O. use: Follow normal protocol.
I.M. use: Inject deeply into upper outer quadrant of gluteal region to reduce pain and local irritation.
P.R. use: Refrigerate suppositories.
• Withhold drug if skin hypersensitivity reaction occurs.
Patient teaching
• Advise patient of possibility of drowsiness and dizziness, and caution against driving or performing other activities requiring alertness until CNS effects of drug are known.
• Warn patient that I.M. administration of drug may be painful.
• If patient will be self-administering suppositories, instruct him to remove foil and, if necessary, moisten suppository with water for 10 to 30 seconds before inserting. Tell him to store suppositories in refrigerator.

☑ **Evaluation**
• Patient maintains adequate hydration with cessation of nausea and vomiting.
• Patient maintains normal bowel pattern.
• Patient and family state understanding of drug therapy.

trimethoprim
(trigh-METH-uh-prim)
Alprim◇, Proloprim, Trimpex, Triprim◇

Pharmacologic class: synthetic folate antagonist
Therapeutic class: antibiotic
Pregnancy risk category: C

How supplied
Tablets: 100 mg, 200 mg

Pharmacokinetics
Absorption: absorbed quickly and completely.
Distribution: distributed widely; about 42% to 46% protein-bound.
Metabolism: less than 20% metabolized in liver.
Excretion: mostly excreted in urine.
Half-life: 8 to 11 hours.

Route	Onset	Peak	Duration
P.O.	Unknown	1-4 hr	Unknown

Pharmacodynamics
Chemical effect: interferes with action of dihydrofolate reductase, inhibiting bacterial synthesis of folic acid.
Therapeutic effect: inhibits selected bacteria activity. Spectrum of activity includes many gram-positive and gram-negative organisms, including most enterobacteriaceae organisms (except *Pseudomonas*), *Escherichia coli, Klebsiella,* and *Proteus mirabilis.*

Indications and dosage
▶ **Uncomplicated urinary tract infections caused by susceptible strains of *Enterobacter, E. coli, Klebsiella,* and *P. mirabilis.*** *Adults:* 200 mg P.O. daily as single dose or in divided doses q 12 hours for 10 days.

Adverse reactions
GI: epigastric distress, nausea, vomiting, glossitis.
Hematologic: *thrombocytopenia, leukopenia,* megaloblastic anemia, methemoglobinemia.
Skin: *rash, pruritus, exfoliative dermatitis.*
Other: fever.

Interactions
Drug-drug. *Phenytoin:* may decrease phenytoin metabolism and increase its serum level. Monitor for toxicity.

Contraindications and precautions
• Contraindicated in patients with hypersensitivity to drug and in those with doc-

---

Reactions may be *common,* uncommon, *life-threatening,* or COMMON AND LIFE-THREATENING.

umented megaloblastic anemia caused by folate deficiency.
• Drug is not recommended for use in breast-feeding women.
• Use cautiously in patients with impaired liver function. Dosage should be decreased in patients with severely impaired kidney function. Also use cautiously in pregnant women.
• Safety of drug has not been established in children under age 12.

NURSING CONSIDERATIONS

☲ Assessment
• Assess patient's infection before therapy and regularly thereafter.
• Obtain urine specimen for culture and sensitivity tests before giving first dose. Therapy may begin pending results.
• Monitor CBC routinely. Clinical signs such as sore throat, fever, pallor, or purpura may be early indications of serious blood disorders. Prolonged use of trimethoprim at high doses may cause bone marrow suppression.
• Be alert for adverse reactions and drug interactions.
• Monitor patient's hydration status if adverse GI reactions occur.
• Evaluate patient's and family's knowledge of drug therapy.

⊕ Nursing diagnoses
• Infection related to presence of susceptible bacteria
• Risk for fluid volume deficit related to drug-induced adverse GI reactions
• Knowledge deficit related to drug therapy

⊳ Planning and implementation
• Because resistance to trimethoprim develops rapidly when administered alone, it is usually given in combination with other drugs.
• Be aware that drug is not recommended for use in patient with creatinine clearance less than 15 ml/minute.

Patient teaching
• Instruct patient to take drug as prescribed, even if he feels better.

✓ Evaluation
• Patient is free from infection.
• Patient maintains adequate hydration.
• Patient and family state understanding of drug therapy.

---

trimipramine maleate
(trigh-MIH-pruh-meen MAL-ee-ayt)
Apo-Trimip♦, Novo-Tripramine♦, Rhotrimine♦, Surmontil

Pharmacologic class: tricyclic antidepressant (TCA)
Therapeutic class: antidepressant
Pregnancy risk category: C

How supplied
Tablets: 25 mg◊
Capsules: 25 mg, 50 mg, 100 mg

Pharmacokinetics
Absorption: absorbed rapidly from GI tract.
Distribution: distributed widely in body; 90% protein-bound.
Metabolism: metabolized in liver; significant first-pass effect may explain variability of serum level in different patients taking same dosage.
Excretion: most of drug excreted in urine; some excreted in feces. *Half-life:* 9 hours.

Route	Onset	Peak	Duration
P.O.	Unknown	2 hr	Unknown

Pharmacodynamics
Chemical effect: unknown; increases amount of norepinephrine, serotonin, or both in CNS by blocking their reuptake by presynaptic neurons.
Therapeutic effect: relieves depression.

Indications and dosage

▶ **Depression.** *Adults:* 75 to 100 mg P.O. daily in divided doses, increased to 200 to 300 mg daily. Dosages over 300 mg daily not recommended in hospitalized patients; dosages over 200 mg not recommended in outpatients.

Adverse reactions

CNS: *drowsiness, dizziness,* paresthesia, ataxia, hallucinations, delusions, anxiety, agitation, insomnia, tremors, weakness, confusion, headache, nervousness, EEG changes, *seizures,* extrapyramidal reactions.
CV: *orthostatic hypotension, tachycardia,* hypertension, *arrhythmias, heart block, MI, stroke.*
EENT: *blurred vision,* tinnitus, mydriasis.
GI: *dry mouth, constipation,* nausea, vomiting, anorexia, paralytic ileus.
GU: *urine retention.*
Skin: rash, urticaria, photosensitivity.
Other: *diaphoresis, hypersensitivity reaction.*
After abrupt withdrawal of long-term therapy: nausea, headache, malaise (does not indicate addiction).

Interactions

Drug-drug. *Barbiturates:* decreased TCA blood level. Monitor for decreased antidepressant effect.
Cimetidine, methylphenidate: may increase drug serum level. Monitor for increased adverse reactions.
Clonidine, epinephrine, norepinephrine: increased hypertensive effect. Use with caution.
CNS depressants: enhanced CNS depression. Avoid concomitant use.
MAO inhibitors: may cause severe excitation, hyperpyrexia, or seizures, usually with high dosage. Use with caution.
Drug-lifestyle. *Alcohol use:* enhanced CNS depression. Avoid concomitant use.
Sun exposure: increased risk of photosensitivity reactions. Avoid unprotected or prolonged sun exposure.

Contraindications and precautions

• Contraindicated during acute recovery phase of MI; in patients with hypersensitivity to drug; and in those receiving MAO inhibitor within 14 days.
• Use with extreme caution in patients with CV disease, increased intraocular pressure, hyperthyroidism, impaired liver function, or history of urine retention, angle-closure glaucoma, or seizures and in those receiving thyroid medications, guanethidine, or similar agents.
• Use cautiously in pregnant women.
• Safety of drug has not been established in children and in breast-feeding women.

NURSING CONSIDERATIONS

⚗ Assessment
• Assess patient's depression before therapy and regularly thereafter.
• Be alert for adverse reactions and drug interactions.
• Evaluate patient's and family's knowledge of drug therapy.

⊞ Nursing diagnoses
• Altered thought processes related to presence of depression
• Risk for injury related to drug-induced adverse CNS reactions
• Knowledge deficit related to drug therapy

▷ Planning and implementation
• Administer full dose at bedtime if patient exhibits daytime sedation.
• Know that dosage should be reduced in elderly or debilitated patient.
• Do not withdraw drug abruptly.
• Because hypertensive episodes have occurred during surgery in patients receiving TCAs, be aware that dosage should be discontinued gradually several days before surgery.
• If signs of psychosis occur or increase, expect doctor to reduce dosage.
Patient teaching
• Tell patient to take full dosage at bedtime to avoid daytime sedation. Warn him

about possible morning orthostatic hypotension.
• Warn patient to avoid hazardous activities that require alertness and good psychomotor coordination until CNS effects of drug are known. Drowsiness and dizziness usually subside after a few weeks.
• Tell patient to avoid alcohol during drug therapy.
• Warn patient not to stop taking drug suddenly. Advise him to consult doctor before taking other prescription or OTC medications.
• Advise patient to use sunblock, wear protective clothing, and avoid prolonged exposure to sunlight to prevent photosensitivity reactions.

☑ **Evaluation**
• Patient's behavior and communication exhibit improved thought processes.
• Patient does not experience injury from adverse CNS reactions.
• Patient and family state understanding of drug therapy.

---

tripelennamine citrate
(trigh-peh-LEN-uh-meen SIH-trayt)
PBZ*

tripelennamine hydrochloride
PBZ, PBZ-SR, Pelamine, Pyribenzamine

Pharmacologic class: ethylenediamine-derivative antihistamine
Therapeutic class: antihistamine
(H_1-receptor antagonist)
Pregnancy risk category: NR

How supplied

tripelennamine citrate
Elixir: 37.5 mg/5 ml (equivalent to 25 mg/5 ml of tripelennamine hydrochloride)*
tripelennamine hydrochloride
Tablets: 25 mg, 50 mg
Tablets (extended-release): 100 mg

Pharmacokinetics
Absorption: well absorbed from GI tract.
Distribution: distributed in high concentrations in liver.
Metabolism: appears to be almost completely metabolized.
Excretion: excreted almost entirely in urine.

Route	Onset	Peak	Duration
P.O.	15-60 min	Unknown	4-6 hr

Pharmacodynamics
Chemical effect: competes with histamine for H_1-receptor sites on effector cells. Drug prevents but does not reverse histamine-mediated responses.
Therapeutic effect: relieves allergy symptoms.

Indications and dosage
▶ **Rhinitis, allergy symptoms.** *Adults:* 25 to 50 mg P.O. q 4 to 6 hours (maximum dosage 600 mg daily); or 50 to 100 mg extended-release b.i.d. or t.i.d. *Children:* 5 mg/kg P.O. daily in four to six divided doses. Maximum dosage is 300 mg daily. Do not use extended-release tablets in children.

Adverse reactions
CNS: (especially in elderly patients) *drowsiness,* dizziness, confusion, restlessness, tremors, irritability, insomnia.
CV: palpitations.
GI: anorexia, diarrhea, constipation, *nausea, vomiting, dry mouth.*
GU: urinary frequency, urine retention.
Respiratory: thick bronchial secretions.
Skin: urticaria, rash.

Interactions
Drug-drug. *CNS depressants:* increased sedation. Use together cautiously.
MAO inhibitors: increased anticholinergic effects. Don't use together.

Contraindications and precautions
• Contraindicated in patients with hypersensitivity to drug or related compounds;

---

in those with angle-closure glaucoma, stenosing peptic ulcer, symptomatic prostatic hypertrophy, pyloroduodenal or bladder-neck obstruction, or lower respiratory tract symptoms, including asthma; and in premature infants, neonates, or breast-feeding women.

• Use cautiously in elderly patients and in patients with increased intraocular pressure, hyperthyroidism, CV disease, hypertension, or history of bronchial asthma.

• Safety of drug has not been established in pregnant women.

NURSING CONSIDERATIONS

Assessment
• Assess patient before and after therapy. Be alert for adverse reactions and drug interactions.
• Evaluate patient's and family's knowledge of drug therapy.

Nursing diagnoses
• Altered health maintenance related to allergies
• Risk for injury related to drug-induced adverse CNS reactions
• Knowledge deficit related to drug therapy

Planning and implementation
• Know that extended-release preparations should not be used in children.
• Give drug with food or milk to reduce likelihood of GI distress.
Patient teaching
• Tell patient to take drug with food or milk and to use ice chips, sugarless gum or hard candy to relieve dry mouth.
• Warn patient to avoid alcohol, driving, and other activities that require alertness until CNS effects are known; coffee or tea may reduce drowsiness.
• Advise patient to stop drug 4 days before allergy skin tests.
• Tell patient to notify doctor if tolerance develops.
• Tell patient that extended-release tablets should not be crushed or chewed.

Evaluation
• Patient responds well to drug.
• Patient does not experience injury from adverse CNS reactions.
• Patient and family state understanding of drug therapy.

triprolidine hydrochloride
(trigh-PROH-lih-deen high-droh-KLOR-ighd)
Actifed Cold and Allergy†, Active†, Allerfrim†, Aprodine†, Triposed†, Unifed†

Pharmacologic class: propylamine antihistamine derivative
Therapeutic class: antihistamine (H₁-receptor antagonist)
Pregnancy risk category: C

How supplied
Tablets: 2.5 mg† and pseudoephedrine hydrochloride 60 mg
Syrup: 1.25 mg/5 ml*† and pseudoephedrine hydrochloride 30 mg/5 ml

Pharmacokinetics
Absorption: well absorbed from GI tract.
Distribution: unknown.
Metabolism: metabolized in liver.
Excretion: excreted in urine. *Half-life:* 2 to 6 hours.

Route	Onset	Peak	Duration
P.O.	15-60 min	2 hr	4-8 hr

Pharmacodynamics
Chemical effect: competes with histamine for H₁-receptor sites on effector cells. Drug prevents but does not reverse histamine-mediated responses.
Therapeutic effect: relieves allergy symptoms.

Indications and dosage
▶ **Colds and allergy symptoms.** *Adults and children age 12 and over:* 2.5 mg P.O. q 4 to 6 hours. Maximum dosage is 10 mg/day. *Children ages 6 to 11:*

1.25 mg P.O. q 4 to 6 hours. Maximum dosage is 5 mg/day. *Children ages 4 to 5:* 0.9 mg P.O. q 4 to 6 hours. Maximum dosage is 3.75 mg/day. *Children ages 2 to 3:* 0.6 mg P.O. q 4 to 6 hours. Maximum dosage is 2.5 mg/day. *Children ages 4 months to 2 years:* 0.3 mg P.O. q 4 to 6 hours. Maximum dosage is 1.25 mg/day.

Adverse reactions

CNS: *drowsiness,* dizziness, confusion, restlessness, insomnia, headache, *sedation, sleepiness, incoordination,* fatigue, anxiety, nervousness, tremor, *seizures, stimulation* (especially in elderly patients).
CV: hypotension, palpitations, tachycardia.
EENT: *dry nose and throat.*
GI: anorexia, diarrhea, constipation, nausea, vomiting, *dry mouth,* epigastric distress.
GU: urinary frequency, urine retention.
Hematologic: hemolytic anemia, *thrombocytopenia, agranulocytosis.*
Skin: urticaria, rash, photosensitivity, diaphoresis.
Other: *anaphylactic shock,* chills, thickening of bronchial secretions.

Interactions

Drug-drug. *CNS depressants:* increased sedation. Avoid concomitant use.
MAO inhibitors: increased anticholinergic effects. Don't use together.
Drug-lifestyle. *Sun exposure:* photosensitivity reactions may occur. Take precautions.

Contraindications and precautions

• Contraindicated in patients with acute asthma attacks or hypersensitivity to drug and in neonates, premature infants, or breast-feeding women.
• Use with extreme caution in patients with increased intraocular pressure, angle-closure glaucoma, hyperthyroidism, CV disease, hypertension, bronchial asthma, prostatic hyperplasia, bladder-neck obstruction, or stenosing peptic ulcerations.
• Use cautiously in pregnant women.
• Use drug in children under age 12 only as directed by doctor.

NURSING CONSIDERATIONS

☯ Assessment
• Assess patient's condition before therapy and regularly thereafter.
• Be alert for adverse reactions and drug interactions.
• Evaluate patient's and family's knowledge of drug therapy.

⊞ Nursing diagnoses
• Altered health maintenance related to allergies
• Risk for injury related to drug-induced adverse CNS reactions
• Knowledge deficit related to drug therapy

▷ Planning and implementation
• Reduce GI distress by giving drug with food or milk.
Patient teaching
• Advise patient to take drug with food or milk.
• Warn patient to avoid alcohol as well as driving or other activities that require alertness until drug's CNS effects are known.
• Tell patient that coffee or tea may reduce drowsiness.
• Tell patient that ice chips or sugarless gum or hard candy may relieve dry mouth.
• Advise patient to stop drug 4 days before allergy skin tests to preserve accuracy of tests.

☑ Evaluation
• Patient responds well to drug.
• Patient does not experience injury from adverse CNS reactions.
• Patient and family state understanding of drug therapy.

---

*Liquid form contains alcohol   **May contain tartrazine   ♦Canada   ◇Australia   †OTC

troglitazone
(troh-GLIH-tuh-zohn)
Rezulin

Pharmacologic class: thiazolidinedione
antihyperglycemic
Therapeutic class: antidiabetic
Pregnancy risk category: B

How supplied

Tablets: 200 mg, 300 mg, 400 mg

Pharmacokinetics

Absorption: rapidly absorbed.
Distribution: 99% bound to serum albumin.
Metabolism: in liver.
Excretion: 88% in feces; 3% in urine.
Half-life: 16-34 hours.

Route	Onset	Peak	Duration
P.O.	Rapid	2-3 hr	Unknown

Pharmacodynamics

Chemical effect: decreases hepatic glucose
output and increases insulin-dependent
glucose disposal in skeletal muscle.
Therapeutic effect: enhances insulin's
effects.

Indications and dosage

▶ **Adjunct to diet and insulin therapy
in patients with type 2 diabetes mellitus (non-insulin-dependent) whose hyperglycemia is inadequately controlled
with insulin therapy over 30 units/daily given as multiple injections.** *Adults:*
initially, for patients on insulin therapy,
continue with current insulin dose and
begin therapy with 200 mg P.O. once daily with a meal. Dosage may be increased
after 2 to 4 weeks if needed. Usual daily
dose is 400 mg; maximum is 600 mg.
Insulin dose may be decreased by 10% to
25% when fasting glucose levels are below 120 mg/dl in patients receiving both
troglitazone and insulin.

Adverse reactions

CNS: *headache,* asthenia, dizziness.
CV: peripheral edema.
EENT: rhinitis, pharyngitis.
GI: nausea, diarrhea.
GU: urinary tract infection.
Hepatic: *hepatotoxicity.*
Musculoskeletal: back pain.
Other: *infection, pain,* accidental injury.

Interactions

Drug-drug. *Cholestyramine:* reduced absorption of troglitazone. Avoid concomitant use.
Oral contraceptives: may reduce plasma
hormone levels, resulting in contraceptive
effect. Suggest other form of contraception.
Drug-food. *Any food:* increased absorption. Take drug with food.

Contraindications and precautions

• Contraindicated in patients with known
hypersensitivity to drug.

NURSING CONSIDERATIONS

⚖ Assessment
• Use cautiously in patients with hepatic
disease or class III or IV heart failure.
• When used with insulin, watch for hypoglycemia.
• Monitor glucose levels, especially during times of increased stress, such as infection, fever, surgery, and trauma.
• Evaluate patient's and family's knowledge of drug therapy.

⊕ Nursing diagnoses
• Altered health maintenance related to
hyperglycemia
• Risk for injury related to drug-induced
hypoglycemia
• Knowledge deficit related to drug
therapy

≥ Planning and implementation
• Don't use for treating type 1 diabetes
mellitus (insulin-dependent) or ketoacidosis.

• Before starting drug therapy, investigate and address secondary causes of poor glycemic control (including infection and poor injection technique).

Patient teaching
• Instruct patient and family about diabetes and importance of following treatment, avoiding infection, and adhering to diet, weight-reduction, exercise, and personal-hygiene programs. Teach him to self-monitor blood glucose level, signs of hypoglycemia and hyperglycemia, and what to do if those conditions occur.
• Tell patient to take drug with meals. For missed dose, tell him to take it with next meal.
• Tell a premenopausal anovulatory patient that drug may cause resumption of ovulation.
• Instruct patient to carry medical identification at all times.

☑ **Evaluation**
• Patient's blood glucose is normal.
• Patient treats hypoglycemia early before injury occurs.
• Patient and family state understanding of drug therapy.

---

tromethamine
(troh-METH-eh-meen)
Tham

Pharmacologic class: sodium-free organic amine
Therapeutic class: systemic alkalinizer
Pregnancy risk category: C

How supplied
Injection: 18 g/500 ml

Pharmacokinetics
Absorption: not applicable.
Distribution: at pH of 7.4 about 25% of drug is unionized; this portion may enter cells to neutralize acidic ions of intracellular fluid.
Metabolism: none.

Excretion: rapidly excreted in urine as bicarbonate salt. *Half-life:* 7 to 40 minutes.

Route	Onset	Peak	Duration
I.V.	Immediate	Immediate	Unknown

Pharmacodynamics
Chemical effect: combines with hydrogen ions and associated acid anions; resulting salts are excreted. Drug also has osmotic diuretic effect.
Therapeutic effect: restores normal acid-base balance in body.

Indications and dosage
▶ **Metabolic acidosis associated with cardiac bypass surgery or cardiac arrest.** *Adults:* dosage depends on bicarbonate deficit. Calculate as follows: each milliliter of 0.3 M tromethamine solution required = weight in kg × base deficit (mEq/L).

Adverse reactions
CV: venospasm; I.V. thrombosis.
Hepatic: hemorrhagic hepatic necrosis.
Metabolic: hypoglycemia, *hyperkalemia* (with decreased urine output).
Respiratory: *respiratory depression.*
Other: inflammation, necrosis, sloughing (if extravasation occurs); fever.

Interactions
None significant.

Contraindications and precautions
• Contraindicated in patients with anuria, uremia, or chronic respiratory acidosis and in pregnant women (except in acute, life-threatening situations).
• Use cautiously in patients with renal disease and poor urine output.

NURSING CONSIDERATIONS

☜ **Assessment**
• Assess patient's condition before therapy and regularly thereafter.

• Monitor ECG and serum potassium level in patient with renal disease and poor urine output.
• Make the following determinations before, during, and after therapy: blood pH; carbon dioxide tension; bicarbonate, glucose, and electrolyte levels.
• Be alert for adverse reactions.
• Evaluate patient's and family's knowledge of drug therapy.

🔲 **Nursing diagnoses**
• Altered health maintenance related to presence of acid-base imbalance
• Altered tissue integrity related to tromethamine extravasation
• Knowledge deficit related to drug therapy

▷ **Planning and implementation**
• Give slowly through 18G to 20G needle into largest antecubital vein or by indwelling I.V. catheter.
• Total dosage should be administered over at least 1 hour and should not exceed 500 mg/kg. Additional therapy based on serial determinations of existing bicarbonate deficit.
• Be aware that drug should not be used longer than 1 day except in life-threatening situations.
• Have mechanical ventilation available for patients with associated respiratory acidosis.
• To prevent blood pH from rising above normal, be prepared to adjust dosage carefully, as ordered.
• If extravasation occurs, infiltrate area with 1% procaine and 150 units hyaluronidase, as ordered; this may reduce vasospasm and dilute remaining drug locally.
Patient teaching
• Inform patient and family of need for drug and be prepared to answer their questions.

☑ **Evaluation**
• Patient regains normal acid-base balance.

• Patient does not exhibit signs and symptoms of extravasation.
• Patient and family state understanding of drug therapy.

---

trovafloxacin mesylate (alatrofloxacin mesylate)
(troh-vah-FLOKS-ah-sin MES-eh-layt)
Trovan, Trovan I.V.

Pharmacologic class: fluoroquinolone
Therapeutic class: antibiotic
Pregnancy risk category: C

How supplied
Trovan
Tablets (trovafloxacin): 100 mg, 200 mg
Trovan I.V.
Injection (alatrofloxacin): 5 mg/ml in 40-ml (200 mg) and 60-ml (300 mg) vials

Pharmacokinetics
Absorption: well absorbed following oral administration. Absolute bioavailability is about 88%.
Distribution: widely and rapidly throughout body with about 76% bound to plasma proteins.
Metabolism: metabolized by conjugation.
Excretion: about 43% of drug excreted unchanged in feces and 6% unchanged in urine following oral administration. *Half-life:* 9 to 12 hours.

Route	Onset	Peak	Duration
P.O., I.V.	Unknown	1 hr	Unknown

Pharmacodynamics
Chemical effect: trovafloxacin is related to the fluoroquinolones with in vitro activity against a wide range of gram-positive and gram-negative aerobic and anaerobic microorganisms. Bactericidal action results from inhibition of DNA gyrase and topoisomerase IV, two enzymes involved in bacterial replication.

Therapeutic effect: hinders a wide range of gram-positive and gram-negative bacterial activity.

Indications and dosages

▶ **Nosocomial pneumonia caused by** *Escherichia coli, Pseudomonas aeruginosa, Haemophilus influenzae,* **or** *Staphylococcus aureus;* **gynecologic and pelvic infections caused by** *E. coli, Bacteroides fragilis,* **viridans group streptococci,** *Enterococcus faecalis, Streptococcus agalactiae, Peptostreptococcus* **species,** *Prevotella* **species, or** *Gardnerella vaginalis;* **complicated intra-abdominal infections including postsurgical infections caused by** *E. coli, B. fragilis,* **viridans group streptococci,** *P. aeruginosa, Klebsiella pneumoniae, Peptostreptococcus* **species,** *or Prevotella* **species.** *Adults:* 300 mg I.V. daily followed by 200 mg P.O. daily for 7 to 14 days. (10 to 14 days for pneumonia.)

▶ **Community-acquired pneumonia caused by** *Streptococcus pneumoniae, H. influenzae, K. pneumoniae, S. aureus, Mycoplasma pneumoniae, Moraxella catarrhalis, Legionella pneumophila,* **or** *Chlamydia pneumoniae;* **complicated skin and skin-structure infections including diabetic foot infections caused by** *S. aureus, S. agalactiae, P. aeruginosa, E. faecalis, E. coli,* **or** *Proteus mirabilis* **(not for treatment of osteomyelitis).** *Adults:* 200 mg P.O. or I.V. daily followed by 200 mg P.O. daily for 7 to 14 days (10 to 14 days for complicated skin and skin-structure infections).

▶ **Prophylaxis of infection associated with elective colorectal surgery or vaginal and abdominal hysterectomy.** *Adults:* 200 mg P.O. or I.V as a single dose 30 minutes to 4 hours before surgery.

▶ **Acute sinusitis caused by** *H. influenzae, M. catarrhalis,* **or** *S. pneumoniae;* **chronic prostatitis caused by** *E. coli, E. faecalis,* **or** *Staphylococcus epidermis;*

cervicitis caused by *Chlamydia trachomatis;* **and pelvic inflammatory disease (mild to moderate) caused by** *Neisseria gonorrhoeae* **or** *C. trachomatis.* *Adults:* 200 mg P.O. daily for 5 days (cervicitis), 10 days (acute sinusitis), 14 days (pelvic inflammatory disease), or 28 days (chronic prostatitis).

▶ **Uncomplicated urinary tract infections caused by** *E. coli;* **uncomplicated skin and skin-structure infections caused by** *S. aureus, Streptococcus pyogenes,* **or** *S. agalactiae;* **acute bacterial exacerbation of chronic bronchitis caused by** *H. influenzae, M. catarrhalis, S. pneumoniae, S. aureus,* **or** *Haemophilus parainfluenzae;* **and uncomplicated gonorrhea caused by** *N. gonorrhoeae.* *Adults:* 100 mg P.O. daily for 3 days (urinary tract infections), 7 to 10 days (skin and skin structure infections, bronchitis) or single dose for treatment of gonorrhea.

Adverse reactions

CNS: *dizziness,* light-headedness, headache, *seizures,* psychosis.
GI: diarrhea, nausea, vomiting, abdominal pain, pseudomembranous colitis.
GU: vaginitis, increased BUN and creatinine.
Hematologic: bone marrow aplasia (anemia, *thrombocytopenia, leukopenia*), decreased hemoglobin and hematocrit, increased platelets.
Hepatic: increased ALT and AST.
Musculoskeletal: arthralgia, arthropathy, myalgia.
Skin: pruritus, rash, injection-site reaction (I.V.), photosensitivity.

Interactions

Drug-drug. *Antacids containing aluminum, magnesium, or citric acid buffered with sodium citrate (Bicitra), sucralfate, iron-containing preparations, and I.V. morphine:* bioavailability of trovafloxacin is significantly reduced following concomitant use with these agents. Give these agents 2 hours before

---

*Liquid form contains alcohol   **May contain tartrazine   ◆Canada   ◇Australia   †OTC

or 2 hours after trovafloxacin. Avoid morphine I.V. for 4 hours if trovafloxacin is taken with food.
Drug-lifestyle. *Sun exposure:* photosensitivity reactions may occur. Take precautions.

Contraindications and precautions

• Contraindicated in patients with hypersensitivity to drug, alatrofloxacin, other quinolone antimicrobials, or other components of these products.
• Use cautiously in patients with CNS disorders (such as cerebral atherosclerosis or epilepsy) and in those at increased risk for seizures. As with other quinolones, drug may cause neurologic complications such as seizures, psychosis, or increased intracranial pressure may occur. Monitor patient with preexisting condition closely.

NURSING CONSIDERATIONS

Assessment
• Assess patient's infection before therapy and regularly thereafter.
• Obtain specimen for culture and sensitivity tests before giving first dose, as ordered. Therapy may begin pending test results.
• Assess patient for history of CNS disorders or increased risk for seizures and monitor patient with preexisting condition closely.
• Perform periodic assessment of liver function due to potential for increases in ALT, AST, and alkaline phosphatase levels and report abnormalities to doctor.
• Be aware that patients with mild to moderate cirrhosis will require reduced dosages.
• Evaluate patient and family's knowledge of drug therapy.

Nursing diagnoses
• Infection related to bacteria susceptible to drug
• Risk for injury related to drug-induced neurologic complications

• Knowledge deficit related to drug therapy

Planning and implementation
P.O. use: Be aware that no dosage adjustment is necessary when switching from I.V. to oral form. Give drug with meals or at bedtime if patient experiences dizziness.
I.V. use: Alatrofloxacin mesylate is supplied in single-use vials which must be further diluted with an appropriate solution (D_5W, 0.45% NaCl) before administration. Don't dilute drug with 0.9% NaCl or lactated Ringer's solution. Follow package insert for specific instructions regarding preparation of desired dosage.
– After dilution, administer by I.V. infusion over 60 minutes. Avoid rapid bolus or infusion. Do not administer drug with solutions containing multivalent cations (such as magnesium) through same I.V. line.
• Know that if *P. aeruginosa* is the known or presumed pathogen, combination therapy with either an aminoglycoside or aztreonam may be indicated.
Patient teaching
• Inform patient that drug may be taken without regard to meals; however, advise patient to take drug with meals or at bedtime if light-headedness or dizziness occurs.
• Warn patient to avoid excessive sunlight or artificial ultraviolet light and to use an effective sunscreen to prevent burn.
• Instruct patient to discontinue treatment, refrain from exercise, and seek medical advice if pain, inflammation, or rupture of a tendon occurs.
• Advise patient to discontinue treatment at first sign of rash, hives, difficulty swallowing or breathing, or other symptoms suggesting an allergic reaction and to seek medical help immediately.
• Instruct patient to notify doctor if severe diarrhea occurs.

Reactions may be *common*, uncommon, *life-threatening*, or COMMON AND LIFE-THREATENING.

☑ Evaluation
• Patient is free from infection.
• Patient does not experience neurologic complications such as seizures or psychosis.
• Patient and family state understanding of drug therapy.

---

tubocurarine chloride
(too-boh-kyoo-RAH-reen KLOR-ighd)
Tubarine ♦

Pharmacologic class: nondepolarizing neuromuscular blocker
Therapeutic class: skeletal muscle relaxant
Pregnancy risk category: C

How supplied
Injection: 3 mg (20 units)/ml; 10 mg/ml

Pharmacokinetics
Absorption: not applicable.
Distribution: distributed in extracellular fluid and rapidly reaches its site of action; 40% to 45% bound to plasma proteins, mainly globulins.
Metabolism: undergoes *N*-demethylation in liver.
Excretion: about 33% to 75% excreted unchanged in urine in 24 hours; up to 11% excreted in bile.

Route	Onset	Peak	Duration
I.V., I.M.	≤ 1 min	2-5 min	20-40 min

Pharmacodynamics
Chemical effect: prevents acetylcholine from binding to receptors on muscle end plate, thus blocking depolarization.
Therapeutic effect: relaxes skeletal muscles; diagnostic aid for myasthenia gravis.

Indications and dosage
▶ **Adjunct to anesthesia to induce skeletal muscle relaxation; to facilitate intubation, orthopedic manipulations.**
Dosage depends on anesthetic used, individual needs, and response. Dosages listed are representative and must be adjusted. *Adults:* 1 unit/kg or 0.165 mg/kg I.V. slowly over 60 to 90 seconds. Average dose is initially 6 to 9 mg I.V. or I.M., followed by 3 to 4.5 mg in 3 to 5 minutes, if needed. Additional doses of 3 mg may be given if needed during prolonged anesthesia. *Children:* 0.6 mg/kg I.V or I.M.
▶ **To assist with mechanical ventilation.** *Adults and children:* initially, 0.0165 mg/kg I.V. (average 1 mg), then adjust subsequent doses to patient response.
▶ **To lessen muscle contractions in pharmacologically or electrically induced seizures.** *Adults and children:* 1 unit/kg or 0.165 mg/kg over 60 to 90 seconds. Initial dose is 3 mg less than calculated dose.
▶ **Diagnosis of myasthenia gravis.** *Adults:* 0.004 to 0.033 mg/kg as single I.V. or I.M. dose.

Adverse reactions
CV: hypotension, *arrhythmias, bradycardia, cardiac arrest.*
Respiratory: *respiratory depression or apnea, bronchospasm.*
Other: profound and prolonged muscle relaxation, hypersensitivity reactions, idiosyncrasy, residual muscle weakness, increased salivation.

Interactions
Drug-drug. *Aminoglycoside antibiotics (including amikacin, gentamicin, kanamycin, neomycin, streptomycin), general anesthetics (such as enflurane, halothane, isoflurane), polymyxin antibiotics (colistin, polymyxin B sulfate):* potentiated neuromuscular blockade, leading to increased skeletal muscle relaxation and potentiation of effect. Use cautiously during surgical and postoperative periods.
Amphotericin B, ethacrynic acid, furosemide, methotrimeprazine, opioid analgesics, propranolol, thiazide diuret-

---

*Liquid form contains alcohol   **May contain tartrazine   ♦Canada   ◊ Australia   †OTC

ics: potentiated neuromuscular blockade, leading to increased skeletal muscle relaxation and, possibly, respiratory paralysis. Use with extreme caution during surgical and postoperative periods.
Quinidine: prolonged neuromuscular blockade. Use together with caution. Monitor patient closely.

Contraindications and precautions

• Contraindicated in patients with hypersensitivity to drug and in those for whom histamine release is hazardous (such as asthmatic patients).
• Use cautiously in elderly or debilitated patients and in those with hepatic or pulmonary impairment, hypothermia, respiratory depression, myasthenia gravis, myasthenic syndrome of lung cancer or bronchogenic carcinoma, dehydration, thyroid disorders, collagen diseases, porphyria, electrolyte disturbances, fractures, or muscle spasms. Also use large doses cautiously in women undergoing cesarean delivery and in breast-feeding women.

NURSING CONSIDERATIONS

Assessment
• Assess patient's condition before therapy and regularly thereafter.
• Monitor baseline electrolyte determinations (imbalance can potentiate neuromuscular blocking effects).
• Check vital signs every 15 minutes.
• Measure fluid intake and output; renal dysfunction prolongs duration of action because much of drug is unchanged before excretion.
• Monitor respiratory rate closely until patient is fully recovered from neuromuscular blockade, as evidenced by tests of muscle strength (hand grip, head lift, and ability to cough).
• Be alert for adverse reactions and drug interactions.
• Evaluate patient's and family's knowledge of drug therapy.

Nursing diagnoses
• Altered health maintenance related to underlying condition
• Ineffective breathing pattern related to drug-induced respiratory depression
• Knowledge deficit related to drug therapy

Planning and implementation
• Allow succinylcholine effects to subside before giving tubocurarine.
• Administer sedatives or general anesthetics before neuromuscular blockers, as ordered. Neuromuscular blockers do not obtund consciousness or alter pain threshold.
• Know that only personnel skilled in airway management should administer tubocurarine.
• Keep airway clear. Have emergency respiratory support equipment immediately available.
I.V. use: Give drug I.V. over 60 to 90 seconds.
– Do not mix drug with barbiturates (precipitate will form). Use only fresh solutions and discard if discolored.
I.M. use: Follow normal protocol.
• Notify doctor at once if changes in vital signs occur.
• Nerve stimulator and train-of-four monitoring are recommended to confirm antagonism of neuromuscular blockade and recovery of muscle strength. Before attempting pharmacologic reversal with neostigmine, some evidence of spontaneous recovery should be evident.
• Administer analgesics, as ordered.
Patient teaching
• Explain all events and happenings to patient because he still can hear.
• Reassure patient that he is being monitored at all times.

Evaluation
• Patient responds well to drug.
• Patient maintains adequate breathing patterns with or without mechanical assistance.
• Patient and family state understanding of drug therapy.

urea (carbamide)
(yoo-REE-eh)
Ureaphil

Pharmacologic class: carbonic acid salt
Therapeutic class: osmotic diuretic
Pregnancy risk category: C

How supplied
Injection: 40 g/150 ml

Pharmacokinetics
Absorption: not applicable.
Distribution: distributed in intracellular and extracellular fluid, including lymph, bile, and CSF.
Metabolism: hydrolyzed in GI tract by bacterial uridase.
Excretion: excreted by kidneys.

Route	Onset	Peak	Duration
I.V.	30-45 min	1-2 hr	3-10 hr

Pharmacodynamics
Chemical effect: increases osmotic pressure of glomerular filtrate, inhibiting tubular reabsorption of water and electrolytes. Drug also elevates blood plasma osmolality, resulting in enhanced water flow into extracellular fluid.
Therapeutic effect: promotes water excretion, which in turn reduces intracranial and intraocular pressure.

Indications and dosage
▶ **Elevated intracranial or intraocular pressure.** *Adults:* 1 to 1.5 g/kg as 30% solution by slow I.V. infusion over 1 to 2½ hours. Maximum dosage is 120 g daily. *Children:* 0.5 to 1.5 g/kg slow I.V. infusion or 35 g/m² in 24 hours. Children under age 2 may receive as little as 0.1 g/kg slow I.V. infusion.

Adverse reactions
CNS: *headache,* syncope, disorientation.
CV: hypotension, tachycardia, dizziness, ECG changes.
GI: *nausea, vomiting.*
Other: *hyponatremia,* hypokalemia, fluid overload; irritation, necrotic sloughing (with extravasation) hemolysis (with rapid administration).

Interactions
Drug-drug. *Lithium:* increased lithium clearance and decreased lithium effectiveness. Monitor lithium level.

Contraindications and precautions
• Contraindicated in patients with severely impaired kidney function, marked dehydration, frank hepatic failure, active intracranial bleeding, or sickle cell disease with CNS involvement.
• Use cautiously in patients with cardiac disease or hepatic or renal impairment and in pregnant or breast-feeding women.

NURSING CONSIDERATIONS

Assessment
• Assess patient's condition before therapy and regularly thereafter.
• Assess breath sounds for crackles, indicating pulmonary edema.
• Watch for signs of hyponatremia (nausea, vomiting, tachycardia) or hypokalemia (muscle weakness, lethargy); they may indicate electrolyte depletion before serum levels are reduced.
• Monitor blood pressure, fluid intake and output, and serum electrolyte levels.
• In patient with renal disease, monitor BUN level.
• Be alert for adverse reactions and drug interactions.
• Evaluate patient's and family's knowledge of drug therapy.

Nursing diagnoses
• Fluid volume excess related to presence of water retention
• Pain related to drug-induced headache

• Knowledge deficit related to drug therapy

▶ **Planning and implementation**
• To prepare 135 ml of 30% solution, mix contents of 40-g vial of urea with 105 ml of D_5W or dextrose 10% in water or 10% invert sugar in water. Each milliliter of 30% solution provides 300 mg of urea.
• Use freshly reconstituted urea only for I.V. infusion; solution becomes ammonia on standing. Use within minutes of reconstitution and discard within 24 hours.
• Avoid rapid I.V. infusion; it may cause hemolysis or increased capillary bleeding. Maximum infusion rate is 4 ml/minute. Avoid extravasation; it may cause reactions ranging from mild irritation to necrosis.
• Don't give drug through same infusion set as blood or blood derivatives.
• Don't infuse drug into leg veins; this may cause phlebitis or thrombosis, especially in elderly patients.
• Maintain adequate hydration.
• To ensure bladder emptying in comatose patient, use indwelling urinary catheter. Use hourly urometer collection bag for accurate evaluation of diuresis.
• If satisfactory diuresis does not occur in 6 to 12 hours, know that urea should be discontinued and kidney function reevaluated.
• Administer mild analgesic if drug-induced headache occurs.
Patient teaching
• Inform patient and family of need for urea therapy, and answer any questions.

▨ **Evaluation**
• Patient exhibits decreased intracranial or intraocular pressure.
• Patient states that drug-induced headache is relieved with mild analgesic.
• Patient and family state understanding of drug therapy.

urokinase
(yoo-roh-KIGH-nays)
Abbokinase Open-Cath, Ukidan◇

Pharmacologic class: thrombolytic enzyme
Therapeutic class: thrombolytic enzyme
Pregnancy risk category: B

How supplied
Injection: 5,000 units (IU) per unit-dose vial; 9,000 units (IU) per unit-dose vial; 250,000-IU vial

Pharmacokinetics
Absorption: not applicable.
Distribution: rapidly cleared from circulation; most of drug accumulates in kidneys and liver.
Metabolism: rapidly metabolized in liver.
Excretion: small amount excreted in urine and bile. *Half-life:* 10 to 20 minutes.

Route	Onset	Peak	Duration
I.V.	Immediate	20 min-2 hr	About 4 hr

Pharmacodynamics
Chemical effect: activates plasminogen by directly cleaving peptide bonds at two sites.
Therapeutic effect: dissolves blood clots in lungs, coronary arteries, and venous catheters.

Indications and dosage
▶ **Lysis of acute massive pulmonary embolism or of pulmonary embolism accompanied by unstable hemodynamics.** *Adults:* priming dose: 4,400 IU/kg I.V. given over 10 minutes, followed by 4,400 IU/kg hourly for 12 hours. Total volume should not exceed 200 ml. Therapy followed with continuous I.V. infusion of heparin, then oral anticoagulants.
▶ **Coronary artery thrombosis.** *Adults:* after bolus dose of heparin ranging from 2,500 to 10,000 units, 6,000 IU/minute of urokinase is infused into occluded artery

for up to 2 hours. Average total dosage is 500,000 IU.
▶ **Venous catheter occlusion.** *Adults:* 5,000 IU instilled into occluded line and aspirated after 5-minute wait. Aspiration attempts repeated q 5 minutes for 30 minutes. If not patent after 30 minutes, line is capped and urokinase left to work for 30 to 60 minutes before aspirating again. May require second instillation.

Adverse reactions

CV: *reperfusion arrhythmias,* hypotension.
Hematologic: *bleeding.*
Respiratory: *bronchospasm,* minor breathing difficulties.
Other: phlebitis at injection site, hypersensitivity reactions *(anaphylaxis),* fever, chills, nausea, vomiting.

Interactions

Drug-drug. *Anticoagulants:* increased risk of bleeding. Monitor patient closely. *Aspirin, dipyridamole, indomethacin, phenylbutazone, other drugs affecting platelet activity:* increased risk of bleeding. Monitor patient closely.

Contraindications and precautions

• Contraindicated in patients with active internal bleeding; history of CVA; aneurysm; arteriovenous malformation; known bleeding diathesis; recent trauma with possible internal injuries; visceral or intracranial cancer; ulcerative colitis; diverticulitis; severe hypertension; hemostatic defects, including those secondary to severe hepatic or renal insufficiency; uncontrolled hypocoagulation; chronic pulmonary disease with cavitation; subacute bacterial endocarditis or rheumatic valvular disease; or recent cerebral embolism, thrombosis, or hemorrhage.
• Also contraindicated in pregnant women and during the first 10 days postpartum and within 10 days after intraarterial diagnostic procedure or surgery (liver or kidney biopsy, lumbar puncture, thoracentesis, paracentesis, or extensive

or multiple cutdowns) or within 2 months after intracranial or intraspinal surgery.
• I.M. injections and other invasive procedures are contraindicated during urokinase therapy.
• Safety of drug has not been established in children.

NURSING CONSIDERATIONS

⚕ Assessment
• Assess patient's condition before therapy and regularly thereafter.
• Monitor patient for excessive bleeding every 15 minutes for first hour; every 30 minutes for second through eighth hours; then once every shift. Pretreatment with drugs affecting platelets places patient at high risk for bleeding.
• Monitor pulse rates, color, and sensation of extremities every hour.
• Although incidence of hypersensitivity is low, watch for signs of this reaction.
• Keep laboratory flowsheet on patient's chart to monitor PTT, PT, INR, and hemoglobin and hematocrit levels.
• Monitor vital signs.
• Be alert for adverse reactions and drug interactions.
• Evaluate patient's and family's knowledge of drug therapy.

🔟 Nursing diagnoses
• Altered tissue perfusion (cardiopulmonary, peripheral) related to presence of blood clot(s)
• Altered protection related to drug-induced bleeding
• Knowledge deficit related to drug therapy

❯ Planning and implementation
• Have typed and crossmatched RBCs, whole blood, and aminocaproic acid available to treat bleeding and corticosteroids to treat allergic reactions.
• Add 5 ml of sterile water for injection to vial. Dilute further with 0.9% NaCl solution or D_5W solution before infusion. Total volume of fluid administered

---

should not exceed 200 ml. Don't use bacteriostatic water for injection to reconstitute; it contains preservatives. Urokinase solutions may be filtered through 0.45-mcg or smaller cellulose membrane filter before administration. Administer by infusion pump only.
• Keep venipuncture sites to a minimum; use pressure dressing on puncture sites for at least 15 minutes.
• Maintain involved extremity in straight alignment to prevent bleeding from infusion site.
• Avoid unnecessary handling of patient; pad side rails. Bruising is more likely during therapy.
• Be aware that heparin by continuous infusion should be initiated when patient's thrombin time has decreased to less than twice the normal control value after urokinase has been stopped to prevent recurrent thrombosis.
Patient teaching
• Instruct patient to report symptoms of bleeding and other adverse reactions.

☑ **Evaluation**
• Patient regains normal tissue perfusion with dissolution of blood clots.
• Patient does not experience serious complications from drug-induced bleeding.
• Patient and family state understanding of drug therapy.

ursodiol
(ur-sih-DIGH-al)
Actigall

Pharmacologic class: bile acid
Therapeutic class: gallstone solubilizing agent
Pregnancy risk category: B

How supplied
Capsules: 300 mg

Pharmacokinetics
Absorption: about 90% of therapeutic dose absorbed in small bowel after administration.
Distribution: after absorption, ursodiol enters portal vein and is extracted from portal blood by liver (first-pass effect), where it is conjugated and then secreted into hepatic bile ducts. Ursodiol in bile is concentrated in gallbladder and expelled into duodenum in gallbladder bile. A small amount appears in systemic circulation.
Metabolism: metabolized in liver. A small amount undergoes bacterial degradation with each cycle of enterohepatic circulation.
Excretion: excreted primarily in feces. Very small amount excreted in urine. Reabsorbed free ursodiol reconjugated by liver.

Route	Onset	Peak	Duration
P.O.	Unknown	1-3 hr	Unknown

Pharmacodynamics
Chemical effect: unknown; probably suppresses hepatic synthesis and secretion of cholesterol as well as intestinal cholesterol absorption. After long-term administration, ursodiol can solubilize cholesterol from gallstones.
Therapeutic effect: dissolves cholesterol gallstones.

Indications and dosage
▶ **Dissolution of gallstones less than 20 mm in diameter in patients who are poor candidates for surgery or who refuse surgery.** *Adults:* 8 to 10 mg/kg P.O. daily in two or three divided doses.

Adverse reactions
CNS: *headache,* fatigue, anxiety, depression, *dizziness,* sleep disorders.
EENT: rhinitis.
GI: *nausea, vomiting, dyspepsia,* metallic taste, *abdominal pain,* biliary pain, cholecystitis, *diarrhea, constipation,* stomatitis, flatulence.
GU: urinary tract infection.

Reactions may be *common,* uncommon, *life-threatening,* or COMMON AND LIFE-THREATENING.

Musculoskeletal: arthralgia, myalgia, back pain.
Respiratory: cough.
Skin: pruritus, rash, dry skin, urticaria, hair thinning, diaphoresis.

Interactions

Drug-drug. *Aluminum-containing antacids, cholestyramine, colestipol:* bind ursodiol and prevent its absorption. Avoid concomitant use.
Clofibrate, estrogens, oral contraceptives: increased hepatic cholesterol secretion; may counteract effects of ursodiol. Avoid concomitant use.

Contraindications and precautions

• Contraindicated in patients hypersensitive to ursodiol or other bile acids.
• Also contraindicated in patients with chronic hepatic disease, unremitting acute cholecystitis, cholangitis, biliary obstruction, gallstone-induced pancreatitis, or biliary fistula.
• Use cautiously in pregnant or breast-feeding women.
• Safety of drug has not been established in children.

NURSING CONSIDERATIONS

Assessment
• Assess patient's condition before therapy and regularly thereafter.
• Know that usually therapy is long term and requires ultrasound images of gallbladder taken at 6-month intervals. If partial stone dissolution does not occur within 12 months, eventual success is unlikely. Safety of use for longer than 24 months has not been established.
• Monitor liver function test results, including AST and ALT, at beginning of therapy and after 1 month, 3 months, and then every 6 months during ursodiol therapy, as ordered. Abnormal test results may indicate worsening of disease. A theoretical risk exists that hepatotoxic metabolite of ursodiol may be formed in some patients.

• Be alert for adverse reactions and drug interactions.
• Monitor patient's hydration status if adverse GI reactions occur.
• Evaluate patient's and family's knowledge of drug therapy.

Nursing diagnoses
• Risk for injury related to presence of gallstones
• Risk for fluid volume deficit related to drug-induced adverse GI reactions
• Knowledge deficit related to drug therapy

Planning and implementation
• Be aware that drug will not dissolve calcified cholesterol stones, radiolucent bile pigment stones, or radiopaque stones.
Patient teaching
• Tell patient about alternative therapies, including "watchful waiting" (no intervention) and cholecystectomy because relapse rate after bile acid therapy may be as high as 50% after 5 years.

Evaluation
• Patient is free from gallstones.
• Patient maintains adequate hydration.
• Patient and family state understanding of drug therapy.

valacyclovir hydrochloride
(val-ay-SIGH-kloh-veer
high-droh-KLOR-ighd)
Valtrex

Pharmacologic class: synthetic purine nucleoside
Therapeutic class: antiviral
Pregnancy risk category: B

How supplied
Caplets: 500 mg

Pharmacokinetics

Absorption: rapidly absorbed from GI tract; absolute bioavailability of about 54.5%.
Distribution: protein binding ranges from 13.5% to 17.9%.
Metabolism: rapidly and nearly completely converted to acyclovir and L-valine by first-pass intestinal or hepatic metabolism.
Excretion: excreted in urine and feces.
Half-life: averages 2.5 to 3.3 hours.

Route	Onset	Peak	Duration
P.O.	About 30 min	Unknown	Unknown

Pharmacodynamics

Chemical effect: rapidly converted to acyclovir, which becomes incorporated into viral DNA and inhibits viral DNA polymerase, thereby inhibiting viral replication.
Therapeutic effect: inhibits susceptible viral growth of herpes zoster.

Indications and dosage

▶ **Treatment of herpes zoster (shingles) in immunocompetent patients.**
Adults: 1 g P.O. t.i.d. daily for 7 days. Dosage is adjusted for patients with impaired kidney function, based on creatinine clearance levels.

Adverse reactions

CNS: *headache,* dizziness, asthenia.
GI: *nausea,* vomiting, diarrhea, constipation, abdominal pain, anorexia.

Interactions

Drug-drug. *Cimetidine, probenecid:* reduces rate (but not extent) of conversion from valacyclovir to acyclovir and reduces renal clearance of acyclovir, thereby increasing acyclovir blood levels. Monitor for possible toxicity.

Contraindications and precautions

• Contraindicated in patients with hypersensitivity or intolerance to valacyclovir, acyclovir, or components of their formulations.
• Drug is not recommended for use in immunocompromised patients. Thrombotic thrombocytopenic purpura and hemolytic uremic syndrome have resulted in death in some patients with advanced HIV disease and in bone marrow transplant and renal transplant recipients.
• Use cautiously in patients with renal impairment and in those receiving other nephrotoxic drugs.
• Safety and efficacy have not been established in children and in breast-feeding women. Drug should be used in pregnancy only if potential benefits outweigh potential risk to the fetus.

NURSING CONSIDERATIONS

Assessment
• Assess patient's infection before therapy.
• Evaluate patient's and family's knowledge of drug therapy.

Nursing diagnoses
• Infection related to herpes zoster
• Risk for fluid volume deficit related to adverse GI reactions
• Knowledge deficit related to drug therapy

Planning and implementation
• Follow-up studies have not shown an increased risk for birth defects for infants born to patients exposed to the drug during pregnancy.
• Dosage adjustment may be necessary in elderly patient, depending on underlying renal status.
• Although overdosage has not been reported, precipitation of acyclovir in renal tubules may occur when solubility (2.5 mg/ml) is exceeded in the intratubular fluid. In the event of acute renal failure and anuria, the patient may benefit from hemodialysis until kidney function is restored.

Reactions may be *common,* uncommon, **life-threatening**, or COMMON AND LIFE-THREATENING.

Patient teaching

• Inform patient that drug may be taken without regard to meals.

• Review signs and symptoms of herpes infection (rash, tingling, itching, and pain), and advise patient to notify doctor immediately if they occur. Treatment should begin as soon as possible after symptoms appear, preferably within 48 hours.

☑ **Evaluation**

• Patient is free from infection.

• Patient maintains adequate hydration.

• Patient and family state understanding of drug therapy.

valproate sodium
(val-PROH-ayt SOH-dee-um)
Depacon, Depakene Syrup, Epilim◊

valproic acid
Depakene, Myproic Acid

divalproex sodium
Depakote, Depakote Sprinkle, Epival◆

Pharmacologic class: carboxylic acid derivative
Therapeutic class: anticonvulsant
Pregnancy risk category: D

How supplied

valproate sodium
Syrup: 250 mg/ml
Injection: 100 mg/ml
valproic acid
Tablets (enteric-coated): 200 mg◊, 500 mg◊
Crushable tablets: 100 mg◊
Capsules: 250 mg
Syrup: 200 mg/5 ml◊
divalproex sodium
Capsules (delayed-release): 125 mg
Tablets (enteric-coated): 125 mg, 250 mg, 500 mg

Pharmacokinetics

Absorption: valproate sodium and divalproex sodium quickly convert to valproic acid after administration.
Distribution: distributed rapidly throughout body; 80% to 95% protein-bound.
Metabolism: metabolized by liver.
Excretion: excreted primarily in urine; some excreted in feces and exhaled air.
Half-life: 6 to 16 hours (may be considerably longer in patient with liver function impairment, in elderly patient, and in child up to age 18 months; may be considerably shorter in patient receiving hepatic enzyme-inducing anticonvulsants).

Route	Onset	Peak	Duration
P.O.	Unknown	1-4 hr	Unknown
I.V.	Unknown	Unknown	Unknown

Pharmacodynamics

Chemical effect: unknown; probably increases brain levels of gamma-aminobutyric acid, which transmits inhibitory nerve impulses in CNS.
Therapeutic effect: prevents and treats certain types of seizure activity.

Indications and dosage

▶ **Simple and complex absence seizures, mixed seizure types (including absence seizures).** *Adults and children:* initially, 15 mg/kg P.O. daily; then increased by 5 to 10 mg/kg daily at weekly intervals up to maximum of 60 mg/kg daily. When dosage exceeds 250 mg daily, drug should be equally divided into two or more doses. Alternatively, 10 to 15 mg/kg/day I.V., increased by 5 to 10 mg/kg/week to clinical response. Maximum dosage is 60 mg/kg/day I.V.

Adverse reactions

Because drug typically is used in combination with other anticonvulsants, adverse reactions reported may not be caused by valproic acid alone.

CNS: *sedation,* emotional upset, depression, psychosis, aggressiveness, hyperactivity, behavioral deterioration, muscle weakness, tremors, ataxia, headache, dizziness, incoordination.
EENT: nystagmus, diplopia.
GI: *nausea, vomiting, indigestion,* diarrhea, abdominal cramps, constipation, increased appetite and weight gain, anorexia, *pancreatitis. (Note*: Lower incidence of GI effects occur with divalproex sodium.)
Hematologic: petechiae, bruising, eosinophilia, *hemorrhage, leukopenia, bone marrow suppression, thrombocytopenia,* increased bleeding time.
Hepatic: *elevated liver enzyme levels, toxic hepatitis.*
Skin: rash, alopecia, pruritus, photosensitivity, *erythema multiforme.*

Interactions

Drug-drug. *Aspirin, chlorpromazine, cimetidine, felbamate:* may cause valproic acid toxicity. Use together cautiously and monitor blood levels.
Benzodiazepines, other CNS depressants: excessive CNS depression. Avoid concomitant use.
Erythromycin: increased serum valproate concentrations. Monitor for toxicity.
Lamotrigine: increased lamotrigine levels, decreased valproate levels. Monitor levels closely.
Phenobarbital: increased phenobarbital level. Monitor patient closely.
Phenytoin: increased or decreased phenytoin level. Monitor patient closely.
Rifampin: may decrease valproate levels. Monitor levels.
Warfarin: valproic acid may displace warfarin from binding sites. Monitor PT and INR.
Drug-lifestyle. *Alcohol use:* excessive CNS depression. Avoid concomitant use.

Contraindications and precautions

• Contraindicated in patients with hypersensitivity to drug.
• Drug is not recommended for use in pregnant or breast-feeding women.

• Use with extreme caution in patients with history of hepatic dysfunction.

NURSING CONSIDERATIONS

⊠ Assessment
• Assess patient's condition before therapy and regularly thereafter.
• Monitor blood levels, as ordered. Therapeutic blood level is 50 to 100 mcg/ml.
• Monitor liver function studies, platelet counts, and PT before starting drug and periodically thereafter, as ordered.
• Be alert for adverse reactions and drug interactions.
• Evaluate patient's and family's knowledge of drug therapy.

⊞ Nursing diagnoses
• Risk for trauma related to seizure activity
• Altered thought processes related to drug-induced adverse CNS reactions
• Knowledge deficit related to drug therapy

⊠ Planning and implementation
P.O. use: Don't administer syrup to patient who requires sodium restriction. Check with doctor.
– Administer drug with food or milk to minimize adverse GI reactions.
I.V. use: Dilute with at least 50 ml with a compatible diluent (dextrose 5%, NaCl, lactated Ringer's injection) and administer I.V. over 1 hour. Do not exceed 20 mg/minute.
• Know that sudden withdrawal may worsen seizures. Call doctor at once if adverse reactions develop.
• Be aware that serious or fatal hepatotoxicity may follow nonspecific symptoms, such as malaise, fever, and lethargy. Notify doctor at once because drug will need to be discontinued in presence of suspected or apparent substantial hepatic dysfunction.
• Know that patients at high risk for developing hepatotoxicity include those

---

Reactions may be *common,* uncommon, **life-threatening**, or COMMON AND LIFE-THREATENING.

with congenital metabolic disorders, mental retardation, or organic brain disease; those taking multiple anticonvulsants; and children under age 2.
• Notify doctor if tremors occur. Dosage may need to be reduced.
• Know that drug may produce false-positive test results for ketones in urine.
Patient teaching
• Tell patient that drug may be taken with food or milk to reduce adverse GI effects.
• Advise patient not to chew capsules.
• Tell patient and parents that syrup shouldn't be mixed with carbonated beverages.
• Tell patient and parents to keep drug out of children's reach.
• Warn patient and parents not to stop drug therapy abruptly.
• Advise patient to refrain from driving or performing other potentially hazardous activities that require mental alertness until drug's CNS effects are known.

☑ **Evaluation**
• Patient is free from seizure activity.
• Patient maintains normal thought processes.
• Patient and family state understanding of drug therapy.

valsartan
(val-SAR-tin)
Diovan

Pharmacologic class: angiotensin II receptor blocker
Therapeutic class: antihypertensive
Pregnancy risk category: C (D in second and third trimesters)

How supplied

Capsules: 80 mg, 160 mg

Pharmacokinetics

Absorption: bioavailability about 25%; food decreases absorption.

Distribution: does not distribute into tissues extensively; 95% bound to serum proteins.
Metabolism: in liver and kidneys.
Excretion: in urine and feces.

Route	Onset	Peak	Duration
P.O.	Within 2 hr	2-4 hr	24 hr

Pharmacodynamics

Chemical effect: blocks binding of angiotensin II to receptor sites in vascular smooth muscle and adrenal gland.
Therapeutic effect: inhibits pressor effects of renin-angiotensin system.

Indications and dosage

▶ **Hypertension, used alone or in combination with other antihypertensives.**
Adults: initially, 80 mg P.O. once daily. Expect a reduction in blood pressure in 2 to 4 weeks. If additional antihypertensive effect is needed, dosage may be increased to 160 or 320 mg daily, or a diuretic may be added. (Addition of a diuretic has a greater effect than dosage increases beyond 80 mg.) Usual dosage range is 80 to 320 mg daily.

Adverse reactions

CNS: headache, dizziness, fatigue.
CV: hyperkalemia, edema.
GI: abdominal pain, diarrhea, nausea.
Hematologic: *neutropenia.*
Musculoskeletal: arthralgia.
Respiratory: upper respiratory infection, cough, rhinitis, sinusitis, pharyngitis.
Other: viral infection.

Interactions

Drug-drug. *Diuretics:* risk of hypotension. Assess fluid status before starting concomitant therapy. Monitor closely.
Drug-food. *Any food:* decreased peak levels. Give drug on an empty stomach.

Contraindications and precautions

• Contraindicated in patients with known hypersensitivity to drug.

NURSING CONSIDERATIONS

⚖ Assessment
- Use cautiously in patients with severe renal or hepatic disease.
- Monitor for hypotension. Correct volume and salt depletions as ordered before starting drug therapy.

🔁 Nursing diagnoses
- Risk for injury related to presence of hypertension
- Knowledge deficit related to drug therapy

➢ Planning and implementation
- Don't use drug in second or third trimester of pregnancy or in breast-feeding women.
- Safety and effectiveness in children have not been established.

Patient teaching
- Tell female patient to notify doctor if pregnancy occurs.

☑ Evaluation
- Patient's blood pressure becomes normal.
- Patient and family state understanding of drug therapy.

---

vancomycin hydrochloride
(van-koh-MIGH-sin high-droh-KLOR-ighd)
Vancocin, Vancoled

Pharmacologic class: glycopeptide
Therapeutic class: antibiotic
Pregnancy risk category: C

How supplied
Capsules: 125 mg, 250 mg
Powder for oral solution: 1-g, 10-g bottles
Powder for injection: 500-mg, 1-g vials
Pharmacy bulk package: 5 g, 10 g

Pharmacokinetics
Absorption: minimal systemic absorption with oral administration. (Drug may ac-

cumulate in patients with colitis or renal failure.)
Distribution: distributed in body fluids; achieves therapeutic levels in CSF if meninges inflamed.
Metabolism: unknown.
Excretion: excreted in urine with parenteral administration; excreted in feces with P.O. administration. *Half-life:* 6 hours.

Route	Onset	Peak	Duration
P.O.	Unknown	Unknown	Unknown
I.V.	Immediate	Immediate	Unknown

Pharmacodynamics
Chemical effect: hinders bacterial cell-wall synthesis, damaging bacterial plasma membrane and making cell more vulnerable to osmotic pressure.
Therapeutic effect: kills susceptible bacteria. Spectrum of activity includes many gram-positive organisms, including those resistant to other antibiotics. It is useful for *Staphylococcus epidermidis,* methicillin-resistant *Staphylococcus aureus,* and penicillin-resistant *Streptococcus pneumoniae.*

Indications and dosage
▶ **Severe staphylococcal infections when other antibiotics are ineffective or contraindicated.** *Adults:* 500 mg I.V. q 6 hours, or 1 g q 12 hours. *Children:* 40 mg/kg I.V. daily in divided doses q 6 hours. *Neonates:* initially, 15 mg/kg; then 10 mg/kg I.V. daily, divided q 12 hours for first week of life; then q 8 hours up to age 1 month.
▶ **Antibiotic-associated pseudomembranous and staphylococcal enterocolitis.** *Adults:* 125 to 500 mg P.O. q 6 hours for 7 to 10 days. *Children:* 40 mg/kg P.O. daily in divided doses q 6 to 8 hours for 7 to 10 days. Maximum daily dosage is 2 g.
▶ **Endocarditis prophylaxis for dental procedures.** *Adults:* 1 g I.V. slowly over 1 hour, starting 1 hour before procedure. *Children:* 20 mg/kg I.V. over 1 hour, starting 1 hour before procedure.

Reactions may be *common,* uncommon, *life-threatening*, or COMMON AND LIFE-THREATENING.

Adverse reactions

EENT: tinnitus, ototoxicity.
GI: nausea.
GU: *nephrotoxicity,* pseudomembranous colitis.
Hematologic: eosinophilia, *leukopenia.*
Skin: "red-neck" or "red-man" syndrome (maculopapular rash on face, neck, trunk, and extremities [with rapid I.V. infusion]; pruritus, hypotension [with histamine release]).
Other: chills, fever, *anaphylaxis,* superinfection, hypotension, wheezing, dyspnea; pain, thrombophlebitis (at injection site).

Interactions

Drug-drug. *Aminoglycosides, amphotericin B, cisplatin, pentamidine:* increased risk of nephrotoxicity and ototoxicity. Monitor patient closely.

Contraindications and precautions

• Contraindicated in patients with hypersensitivity to drug.
• Use cautiously in patients receiving other neurotoxic, nephrotoxic, or ototoxic drugs; in patients over age 60; in those with impaired liver or kidney function, preexisting hearing loss, or allergies to other antibiotics; and in pregnant women.
• Safety of drug has not been established in breast-feeding women.

NURSING CONSIDERATIONS

⚚ Assessment
• Assess patient's infection before therapy and regularly thereafter.
• Obtain urine specimen for culture and sensitivity tests before giving first dose. Therapy may begin pending test results.
• Obtain hearing evaluation and kidney function studies before therapy and repeat, as ordered, during therapy.
• Check serum levels regularly, especially in the elderly, premature infants, and those with decreased renal function.
• Be alert for adverse reactions and drug interactions.

• Evaluate patient's and family's knowledge of drug therapy.

⊞ Nursing diagnoses
• Infection related to presence of susceptible bacteria
• Risk for injury related to drug-induced adverse reactions
• Knowledge deficit related to drug therapy

▶ Planning and implementation
• Know that patient with renal dysfunction requires dosage adjustment.
P.O. use: Know that oral preparation is stable for 2 weeks if refrigerated.
I.V. use: For I.V. infusion, dilute in 200 ml of NaCl injection or D_5W and infuse over 60 minutes. Check site daily for phlebitis and irritation. Report pain at infusion site. Avoid extravasation; severe irritation and necrosis can result.
– If red-neck or red-man syndrome occurs because drug is infused too rapidly, stop infusion and report to doctor.
– Refrigerate I.V. solution after reconstitution and use within 96 hours.
• Do not give drug I.M.
• Be aware that when using drug to treat staphylococcal endocarditis, it is given for at least 4 weeks.
Patient teaching
• Tell patient to take entire amount of drug exactly as directed, even after he feels better.
• Tell patient to stop drug immediately and report adverse reactions, especially fullness or ringing in ears.

☑ Evaluation
• Patient is free from infection.
• Patient does not experience injury from adverse reactions.
• Patient and family state understanding of drug therapy.

vasopressin (ADH)
(VAY-soh-preh-sin)
Pitressin

Pharmacologic class: posterior pituitary hormone
Therapeutic class: ADH, peristaltic stimulant
Pregnancy risk category: C

How supplied
Injection: 0.5-ml and 1-ml ampules, 20 units/ml

Pharmacokinetics
Absorption: unknown.
Distribution: distributed throughout extracellular fluid, without evidence of protein-binding.
Metabolism: most of drug is destroyed rapidly in liver and kidneys.
Excretion: excreted in urine. *Half-life:* 10 to 20 minutes.

Route	Onset	Peak	Duration
S.C., I.M, intranasal	Unknown	Unknown	2-8 hr

Pharmacodynamics
Chemical effect: increases permeability of renal tubular epithelium to adenosine monophosphate and water; epithelium promotes reabsorption of water and produces concentrated urine (ADH effect).
Therapeutic effect: promotes water reabsorption and stimulates GI motility.

Indications and dosage
▶ **Nonnephrogenic, nonpsychogenic diabetes insipidus.** *Adults:* 5 to 10 units I.M. or S.C. b.i.d. to q.i.d., p.r.n.; or intranasally (aqueous solution used as spray or applied to cotton balls) in individualized dosages, based on response. *Children:* 2.5 to 10.0 units I.M. or S.C. b.i.d. to q.i.d., p.r.n.; or intranasally (aqueous solution used as spray or applied to cotton balls) in individualized doses.

▶ **Postoperative abdominal distention.** *Adults:* initially, 5 units (aqueous) I.M.; then q 3 to 4 hours, dose increased to 10 units, if needed. Dosage reduced proportionately for children.
▶ **To expel gas before abdominal X-ray.** *Adults:* 5 to 15 units S.C. at 2 hours; then again at 30 minutes before X-ray.

Adverse reactions
CNS: tremors, vertigo, headache.
CV: angina in patients with vascular disease; vasoconstriction, *arrhythmias, cardiac arrest,* myocardial ischemia, circumoral pallor, decreased cardiac output.
GI: abdominal cramps, nausea, vomiting, flatulence.
Skin: cutaneous gangrene.
Other: water intoxication (drowsiness, listlessness, headache, confusion, weight gain, *seizures, coma*), hypersensitivity reactions (urticaria, *angioedema, bronchoconstriction, anaphylaxis*), diaphoresis.

Interactions
Drug-drug. *Carbamazepine, chlorpropamide, clofibrate, fludrocortisone, tricyclic antidepressants:* increased antidiuretic response. Use together cautiously. *Demeclocycline, heparin, lithium, norepinephrine:* reduced antidiuretic activity. Use together cautiously.
Drug-lifestyle. *Alcohol use:* reduced antidiuretic activity. Avoid use.

Contraindications and precautions
• Contraindicated in patients with chronic nephritis accompanied by nitrogen retention.
• Use cautiously in children, elderly patients, pregnant or breast-feeding women, preoperative and postoperative polyuric patients, and those with seizure disorders, migraine headache, asthma, CV disease, heart failure, renal disease, goiter with cardiac complications, arteriosclerosis, or fluid overload.

Reactions may be *common*, uncommon, *life-threatening*, or COMMON AND LIFE-THREATENING.

NURSING CONSIDERATIONS

Assessment
• Assess patient's condition before therapy and regularly thereafter.
• Monitor specific gravity of urine and fluid intake and output to aid evaluation of drug effectiveness.
• To prevent possible seizures, coma, and death, observe patient closely for early signs of water intoxication.
• Monitor blood pressure of patient on vasopressin twice daily. Watch for excessively elevated blood pressure or lack of response to drug, which may be indicated by hypotension. Also monitor daily weight.
• Be alert for adverse reactions and drug interactions.
• Evaluate patient's and family's knowledge of drug therapy.

Nursing diagnoses
• Risk for fluid volume deficit related to polyuria from diabetes insipidus
• Diarrhea related to drug-induced increased GI motility
• Knowledge deficit related to drug therapy

Planning and implementation
• Know that drug may be used for transient polyuria resulting from ADH deficiency related to neurosurgery or head injury.
• Never inject during first stage of labor; this may cause uterus to rupture.
• Know that minimum effective dosage should be used to reduce adverse reactions.
• Give drug with one to two glasses of water to reduce adverse reactions and to improve therapeutic response.
• Know that a rectal tube facilitates gas expulsion after vasopressin injection.
I.M. and S.C. use: Follow normal protocol.
Intranasal use: Aqueous solution can be used as a spray or applied to cotton balls.

Follow manufacturer's guidelines for intranasal use.
Patient teaching
• Instruct patient how to administer drug. Tell patient taking drug S.C. to rotate injection sites to prevent tissue damage.
• Stress importance of monitoring fluid intake and output.
• Tell patient to notify doctor immediately if adverse reactions occur.

Evaluation
• Patient maintains adequate hydration.
• Patient does not experience diarrhea.
• Patient and family state understanding of drug therapy.

vecuronium bromide
(veh-kyoo-ROH-nee-um BROH-mighd)
Norcuron

Pharmacologic class: nondepolarizing neuromuscular blocker
Therapeutic class: skeletal muscle relaxant
Pregnancy risk category: C

How supplied
Injection: 10 mg/vial; 20 mg/vial

Pharmacokinetics
Absorption: not applicable.
Distribution: distributed in extracellular fluid and rapidly reaches its site of action (skeletal muscles); 60% to 90% plasma protein–bound.
Metabolism: undergoes rapid and extensive hepatic metabolism.
Excretion: excreted in feces and urine.
Half-life: 20 minutes.

Route	Onset	Peak	Duration
I.V.	≤ 1 min	3-5 min	25-30 min

Pharmacodynamics
Chemical effect: prevents acetylcholine from binding to receptors on muscle end plate, thus blocking depolarization.

Therapeutic effect: relaxes skeletal muscle.

Indications and dosage

► **Adjunct to general anesthesia; to facilitate endotracheal intubation and to provide skeletal muscle relaxation during surgery or mechanical ventilation.** Dosage depends on anesthetic used, individual needs, and response. Dosages are representative and must be adjusted.
Adults and children over age 9: initially, 0.08 to 0.1 mg/kg I.V. bolus. Maintenance doses of 0.01 to 0.015 mg/kg within 25 to 40 minutes of initial dose should be administered during prolonged surgical procedures. Maintenance doses may be given q 12 to 15 minutes in patients receiving balanced anesthesia. *Children under age 9:* may require slightly higher initial dose as well as supplementation slightly more often than adults. Alternatively, drug may be given by continuous I.V. infusion of 1 mcg/kg/minute initially, then 0.8 to 1.2 mcg/kg/minute.

Adverse reactions

Musculoskeletal: skeletal muscle weakness.
Respiratory: *prolonged, dose-related respiratory insufficiency or apnea.*

Interactions

Drug-drug. *Aminoglycoside antibiotics, including amikacin, gentamicin, kanamycin, neomycin, streptomycin; bacitracin; clindamycin; general anesthetics (such as enflurane, halothane, isoflurane); other skeletal muscle relaxants, polymyxin antibiotics (colistin, polymyxin B sulfate); quinidine; tetracyclines:* potentiated neuromuscular blockade, leading to increased skeletal muscle relaxation and potentiation of effect. Use cautiously during surgical and postoperative periods.
Opioid analgesics: potentiated neuromuscular blockade, leading to increased skeletal muscle relaxation and, possibly, respiratory paralysis. Use with extreme caution, and reduce dose of vecuronium.

Contraindications and precautions

• Contraindicated in patients with hypersensitivity to bromides.
• Use cautiously in elderly patients; in patients with altered circulation caused by CV disease and edematous states; and in those with hepatic disease, severe obesity, bronchogenic carcinoma, electrolyte disturbances, or neuromuscular disease.
• Also use cautiously in pregnant or breast-feeding women.

NURSING CONSIDERATIONS

⚕ Assessment

• Assess patient's condition before therapy and regularly thereafter.
• Monitor respiratory rate closely until patient is fully recovered from neuromuscular blockade as evidenced by tests of muscle strength (hand grip, head lift, and ability to cough).
• Be alert for adverse reactions and drug interactions.
• Evaluate patient's and family's knowledge of drug therapy.

⊞ Nursing diagnoses

• Altered health maintenance related to underlying condition
• Ineffective breathing pattern related to drug's effect on respiratory muscles
• Knowledge deficit related to drug therapy

▶ Planning and implementation

• Keep airway clear. Have emergency respiratory support equipment available immediately.
• Know that drug should be used only by personnel skilled in airway management.
• Keep in mind that prior administration of succinylcholine may enhance neuromuscular blocking effect and duration of action.
• Administer sedatives or general anesthetics before neuromuscular blockers, as ordered. Neuromuscular blockers do not obtund consciousness or alter pain threshold.

Reactions may be *common*, uncommon, *life-threatening*, or COMMON AND LIFE-THREATENING.

• Administer drug by rapid I.V. injection. Alternatively, 10 to 20 mg may be added to 100 ml of compatible solution and given by I.V. infusion. Compatible solutions include D₅W, 0.9% NaCl injection, dextrose 5% in 0.9% NaCl injection, and lactated Ringer's injection.

• Do not mix drug with alkaline solutions.

• Store reconstituted solution in refrigerator. Discard after 24 hours.

• Administer analgesics, as ordered, for pain.

• Know that nerve stimulator and train-of-four monitoring are recommended to confirm antagonism of neuromuscular blockade and recovery of muscle strength. Before attempting pharmacologic reversal with neostigmine, some evidence of spontaneous recovery should be seen.

Patient teaching
• Explain all events and happenings to patient because he can still hear.
• Reassure patient that he is being monitored at all times.

☑ **Evaluation**
• Patient responds well to drug.
• Patient maintains effective breathing pattern with mechanical assistance.
• Patient and family state understanding of drug therapy.

---

venlafaxine hydrochloride
(ven-leh-FAKS-een high-droh-KLOR-ighd)
Effexor

Pharmacologic class: neuronal serotonin, norepinephrine, and dopamine reuptake inhibitor
Therapeutic class: antidepressant
Pregnancy risk category: C

How supplied

Tablets: 25 mg, 37.5 mg, 50 mg, 75 mg, 100 mg

Pharmacokinetics
Absorption: about 92% absorbed after oral administration.
Distribution: about 25% to 29% protein-bound in plasma.
Metabolism: extensively metabolized in liver.
Excretion: excreted in urine.

Route	Onset	Peak	Duration
P.O.	Unknown	Unknown	Unknown

Pharmacodynamics
Chemical effect: blocks reuptake of norepinephrine and serotonin into neurons in CNS.
Therapeutic effect: relieves depression.

Indications and dosage

▶ **Depression.** *Adults:* initially, 75 mg P.O. daily in two or three divided doses with food. Dosage increased as tolerated and needed in increments of 75 mg/day at intervals of no less than 4 days. For moderately depressed outpatients, usual maximum dosage is 225 mg/day; in certain severely depressed patients, dosage may be as high as 350 mg/day.

Adverse reactions

CNS: *asthenia, headache, somnolence, dizziness, nervousness, insomnia,* anxiety, tremors, abnormal dreams, paresthesia, agitation.
CV: hypertension.
EENT: blurred vision.
GI: *nausea, constipation,* vomiting, *dry mouth, anorexia,* diarrhea, dyspepsia, flatulence.
GU: *abnormal ejaculation,* impotence, urinary frequency, impaired urination.
Other: *diaphoresis,* weight loss, rash, yawning, chills, infection.

Interactions

Drug-drug. *MAO inhibitors:* may precipitate syndrome similar to neuroleptic malignant syndrome (myoclonus, hyperthermia, seizures, and death). Do not start venlafaxine within 14 days of discontinu-

---

ing therapy with MAO inhibitor, and don't start MAO inhibitor therapy within 7 days of stopping venlafaxine.

Contraindications and precautions

• Contraindicated in patients hypersensitive to drug and in those within 14 days of MAO inhibitor therapy.
• Use cautiously in patients with renal impairment or diseases or conditions that could affect hemodynamic responses or metabolism and in those with history of mania or seizures.
• Also use cautiously in pregnant or breast-feeding women.
• Safety of drug has not been established in children.

NURSING CONSIDERATIONS

🔏 Assessment
• Assess patient's depression before therapy and regularly thereafter.
• Carefully monitor blood pressure. Venlafaxine therapy is associated with sustained, dose-dependent increases in blood pressure. Greatest increases (averaging about 7 mm Hg above baseline) occur in patients taking 375 mg daily.
• Be alert for adverse reactions and drug interactions.
• Evaluate patient's and family's knowledge of drug therapy.

🔄 Nursing diagnoses
• Altered thought processes related to presence of depression
• Risk for injury related to drug-induced adverse CNS reactions
• Knowledge deficit related to drug therapy

▶ Planning and implementation
• Know that total daily dosage should be reduced by 50% in patient with hepatic impairment. In patient with moderate renal impairment (GFR of 10 to 70 ml/minute), total daily dosage should be reduced by 25%. In patient undergoing hemodialysis, know that dose should be withheld until dialysis session is completed and daily dosage reduced by 50%.
• Administer drug with food.
• Do not discontinue drug abruptly if administered for 6 weeks or more. Discontinue drug by tapering dosage over 2-week period, as instructed by doctor.
Patient teaching
• Instruct patient to take with food.
• Caution patient not to operate hazardous machinery, including motor vehicle, until reasonably certain that venlafaxine does not adversely affect ability to engage in such activities.
• Tell patient it may take several weeks before the full antidepressant effect is seen.
• Tell patient to avoid alcohol while taking drug and to notify doctor before taking other medication, including OTC preparations, because of potential interactions.
• Instruct patient to notify doctor if adverse reactions occur.

☑ Evaluation
• Patient's behavior and communication exhibit improved thought processes.
• Patient does not experience injury from adverse CNS reactions.
• Patient and family state understanding of drug therapy.

---

verapamil
(veh-RAP-uh-mil)
Apo-Verap♦, Calan, Isoptin, Novo-Veramil♦, Nu-Verap♦

verapamil hydrochloride
Anpec◇, Calan, Calan SR, Cordilox◇, Cordilox SR◇, Covera-HS, Isoptin, Isoptin SR, Veracaps SR◇, Verelan

Pharmacologic class: calcium channel blocker
Therapeutic class: antianginal, antihypertensive, antiarrhythmic
Pregnancy risk category: C

How supplied

verapamil
Tablets: 40 mg, 80 mg, 120 mg
verapamil hydrochloride
Tablets: 40 mg◊, 80 mg◊, 120 mg◊,
160 mg◊
Tablets (extended-release): 120 mg,
180 mg, 240 mg
Capsules (extended-release): 120 mg,
160 mg◊, 180 mg, 240 mg, 360 mg
Injection: 2.5 mg/ml

Pharmacokinetics

Absorption: absorbed rapidly and completely from GI tract after P.O. administration; only about 20% to 35% reaches systemic circulation.
Distribution: about 90% of circulating drug is bound to plasma proteins.
Metabolism: metabolized in liver.
Excretion: excreted in urine as unchanged drug and active metabolites.
Half-life: 6 to 12 hours.

Route	Onset	Peak	Duration
P.O.	1-2 hr	1-9 hr	8-24 hr
I.V.	1-5 min	Immediate	1-6 hr

Pharmacodynamics

Chemical effect: not clearly defined; inhibits calcium ion influx across cardiac and smooth-muscle cells, thus decreasing myocardial contractility and oxygen demand. Drug also dilates coronary arteries and arterioles.
Therapeutic effect: relieves anginal pain, lowers blood pressure, and restores normal sinus rhythm.

Indications and dosage

▶ **Vasospastic angina and classic chronic, stable angina pectoris; chronic atrial fibrillation.** *Adults:* starting dose is 80 to 120 mg P.O. t.i.d. Dosage increased at weekly intervals as needed. Some patients may require up to 480 mg daily.
▶ **Supraventricular arrhythmias.**
Adults: 0.075 to 0.15 mg/kg (5 to 10 mg) by I.V. push over 2 minutes with ECG

and blood pressure monitoring. If no response occurs, give a second dose of 10 mg (0.15 mg/kg) 15 to 30 minutes after the initial dose. *Children ages 1 to 15:* 0.1 to 0.3 mg/kg as I.V. bolus over 2 minutes. *Children under age 1:* 0.1 to 0.2 mg/kg as I.V. bolus over 2 minutes with continuous ECG monitoring. Repeat in 30 minutes if no response.
▶ **Hypertension.** *Adults:* initiate therapy with sustained-release capsules at 180 mg (240 mg for Verelan) P.O. daily in the morning. Adjust dosage based on clinical effectiveness 24 hours after dosing. Increase in increments of 120 mg daily to a maximum daily dosage of 480 mg.

Adverse reactions

CNS: dizziness, headache, asthenia.
CV: transient hypotension, *heart failure, bradycardia,* pulmonary edema, AV block, *ventricular asystole, ventricular fibrillation,* peripheral edema.
GI: constipation, nausea.
Hepatic: elevated liver enzyme levels.
Skin: rash.

Interactions

Drug-drug. *Antihypertensives, quinidine:* may cause hypotension. Monitor blood pressure.
Carbamazepine, cardiac glycosides: may increase serum levels of these drugs. Monitor patient for toxicity.
Cyclosporine: may increase cyclosporine serum level. Monitor cyclosporine level.
Disopyramide, flecainide, propranolol, other beta blockers: may cause heart failure. Use together cautiously.
Lithium: may decrease serum lithium level. Monitor patient closely.
Rifampin: may decrease oral bioavailability of verapamil. Monitor patient for lack of effect.
Drug-food. *Any food:* increased absorption. Take drug with food.
Drug-lifestyle. *Alcohol use:* may enhance effects of alcohol. Avoid use together.

---

*Liquid form contains alcohol   **May contain tartrazine   ◆Canada   ◊Australia   †OTC

Contraindications and precautions

• Contraindicated in patients with hypersensitivity to drug; severe left ventricular dysfunction; cardiogenic shock; second- or third-degree AV block or sick sinus syndrome, except in presence of functioning pacemaker; atrial flutter or fibrillation and accessory bypass tract syndrome; severe heart failure (unless secondary to verapamil therapy); or severe hypotension. I.V. verapamil contraindicated in patients with ventricular tachycardia and in those receiving I.V. beta blockers.

• Drug is not recommended for use in breast-feeding women.

• Use cautiously in elderly patients, in pregnant women, and in patients with increased intracranial pressure or hepatic or renal disease.

NURSING CONSIDERATIONS

⚕ Assessment

• Assess patient's condition before therapy and regularly thereafter.

• Be aware that all patients receiving I.V. verapamil should be on cardiac monitor. Monitor R-R interval.

• Monitor blood pressure at start of therapy and during dosage adjustments.

• Monitor liver function studies during prolonged treatment, as ordered.

• Be alert for adverse reactions and drug interactions.

• Evaluate patient's and family's knowledge of drug therapy.

⚕ Nursing diagnoses

• Pain related to presence of angina

• Decreased cardiac output related to presence of arrhythmia

• Knowledge deficit related to drug therapy

⚕ Planning and implementation

• Know that patient with severely compromised cardiac function or patient taking beta blockers should receive lower doses of verapamil.

P.O. use: Although drug should be taken with food, be aware that taking extended-release tablets with food may decrease rate and extent of absorption but allows smaller fluctuations of peak and trough blood levels.

I.V. use: Give drug by direct injection into vein or into tubing of free-flowing, compatible I.V. solution. Compatible solutions include D_5W, 0.45% and 0.9% NaCl, and Ringer's and lactated Ringer's solutions. Administer I.V. doses slowly over period of no less than 2 minutes, or for elderly patients no less than 3 minutes to minimize risk of adverse reactions. Perform continuous ECG and blood pressure monitoring during administration.

• Be aware that if verapamil is being used to terminate supraventricular tachycardia, doctor may have patient perform vagal maneuvers after receiving drug.

• Assist patient with ambulation because dizziness may occur.

• Notify doctor if signs of heart failure, such as swelling of hands and feet or shortness of breath, occur.

Patient teaching

• Instruct patient to take drug with food.

• If patient is kept on nitrate therapy during titration of oral verapamil dosage, urge continued compliance. S.L. nitroglycerin, especially, may be taken as needed when anginal symptoms are acute.

• Encourage patient to increase fluid and fiber intake to combat constipation. Administer stool softener, as ordered.

• Instruct patient to report adverse reactions, especially swelling of hands and feet and shortness of breath.

⚕ Evaluation

• Patient has reduced severity or frequency of anginal pain.

• Patient regains normal cardiac output with restoration of normal sinus rhythm.

• Patient and family state understanding of drug therapy.

vinblastine sulfate (VLB)
(vin-BLAH-steen SUL-fayt)
Velban, Velbe♦◊

Pharmacologic class: vinca alkaloid
(cell cycle–phase specific, M phase)
Therapeutic class: antineoplastic
Pregnancy risk category: D

How supplied

Injection: 10-mg vials (lyophilized powder), 1 mg/ml in 10-ml vials

Pharmacokinetics

Absorption: not applicable.
Distribution: distributed widely in body tissues; crosses blood-brain barrier but does not achieve therapeutic concentrations in CSF.
Metabolism: metabolized partially in liver to active metabolite.
Excretion: excreted primarily in bile as unchanged drug; smaller portion excreted in urine. *Half-life:* alpha phase, 3.7 minutes; beta phase, 1.6 hours; terminal phase, 24.8 hours.

Route	Onset	Peak	Duration
I.V.	Unknown	Unknown	Unknown

Pharmacodynamics

Chemical effect: arrests mitosis in metaphase, blocking cell division.
Therapeutic effect: inhibits replication of selected cancer cells.

Indications and dosage

▶ **Breast or testicular cancer, Hodgkin's and non-Hodgkin's lymphoma, choriocarcinoma, lymphosarcoma, mycosis fungoides, Kaposi's sarcoma, histiocytosis.** *Adults:* 0.1 mg/kg or 3.7 mg/m² I.V. weekly or q 2 weeks. May be increased to maximum dosage of 0.5 mg/kg or 18.5 mg/m² weekly according to response. Dosage should not be repeated if WBC count is less than 4,000/mm³. *Children:* 2.5 mg/m² I.V. as a single dose every week, increased weekly in increments of 1.25 mg/m² to a maximum of 7.5 mg/m².

Adverse reactions

CNS: depression, *paresthesias, peripheral neuropathy and neuritis, numbness, loss of deep tendon reflexes, muscle pain and weakness, seizures, CVA,* headache.
CV: hypertension, *MI, phlebitis.*
EENT: pharyngitis.
GI: *nausea, vomiting,* ulcer, bleeding, *constipation, ileus, anorexia,* diarrhea, abdominal pain, *stomatitis.*
GU: oligospermia, aspermia, urine retention.
Hematologic: anemia, *leukopenia* (nadir, days 4 to 10; lasts another 7 to 14 days), *thrombocytopenia.*
Respiratory: *acute bronchospasm,* shortness of breath.
Skin: reversible alopecia, vesiculation, cellulitis, necrosis with extravasation.
Other: hyperuricemia, uric acid nephropathy, *weight loss, irritation.*

Interactions

Drug-drug. *Erythromycin, other drugs that inhibit cytochrome P-450 pathway:* may increase toxicity of vinblastine. Monitor patient closely.
Mitomycin: increased risk of bronchospasm and shortness of breath. Monitor patient closely.
Phenytoin: decreased plasma phenytoin level. Monitor patient closely.

Contraindications and precautions

• Contraindicated in patients with severe leukopenia or bacterial infection.
• Drug is not recommended for use in pregnant or breast-feeding women.
• Use cautiously in patients with hepatic dysfunction.

NURSING CONSIDERATIONS

⚗ Assessment
• Assess patient's condition before therapy and regularly thereafter.

• After administering, monitor for development of life-threatening acute bronchospasm. Reaction is most likely to occur in patient also receiving mitomycin.
• Be alert for adverse reactions and drug interactions.
• Assess for numbness and tingling in hands and feet. Assess gait for early evidence of footdrop. Know that drug is less neurotoxic than vincristine.
• Evaluate patient's and family's knowledge of drug therapy.

🔷 **Nursing diagnoses**
• Altered health maintenance related to presence of neoplastic disease
• Altered protection related to drug-induced adverse hematologic reactions
• Knowledge deficit related to drug therapy

▶ **Planning and implementation**
• Give antiemetic before administering drug, as ordered.
• Follow institutional policy to reduce risks. Preparation and administration of parenteral form are associated with carcinogenic, mutagenic, and teratogenic risks for personnel.
• Reconstitute 10-mg vial with 10 ml of NaCl injection or sterile water. This yields 1 mg/ml. Refrigerate reconstituted solution. Discard after 30 days.
• Inject drug directly into vein or running I.V. line over 1 minute. Drug may also be given in 50 ml of D₅W or 0.9% NaCl solution infused over 15 minutes. If extravasation occurs, stop infusion immediately and notify doctor. The manufacturer recommends that moderate heat be applied to area of leakage. Local injection of hyaluronidase may help disperse drug, as ordered. Some clinicians prefer to apply ice packs on and off every 2 hours for 24 hours, with local injection of hydrocortisone or 0.9% NaCl.
• Don't administer drug into limb with compromised circulation.
• If acute bronchospasm occurs after administration, notify doctor immediately.

• Ensure that patient maintains adequate fluid intake to facilitate excretion of uric acid.
• Be prepared to stop drug if stomatitis occurs, and notify doctor.
• Know that dosage should not be repeated more frequently than every 7 days or severe leukopenia will develop.
• Take care to avoid confusing vinblastine with vincristine or vindesine.
• Anticipate decrease in dosage by 50% if bilirubin level is greater than 3 mg/dl.
Patient teaching
• Teach patient about infection-control and bleeding precautions to take in everyday living.
• Warn patient that alopecia may occur, but that it's usually reversible.
• Tell patient to report promptly adverse reactions.
• Encourage adequate fluid intake to increase urine output and facilitate excretion of uric acid.

☑ **Evaluation**
• Patient responds well to drug.
• Patient does not develop serious complications from adverse hematologic reactions.
• Patient and family state understanding of drug therapy.

---

vincristine sulfate
(vin-KRIH-steen SUL-fayt)
Oncovin, Vincasar PFS

Pharmacologic class: vinca alkaloid (cell cycle–phase specific, M phase)
Therapeutic class: antineoplastic
Pregnancy risk category: D

How supplied

Injection: 1 mg/ml in 1-ml, 2-ml, 5-ml multiple-dose vials; 1 mg/ml in 1-ml, 2-ml preservative-free vials

Pharmacokinetics

Absorption: not applicable.

Distribution: distributed widely in body tissues and bound to erythrocytes and platelets; crosses blood-brain barrier but does not achieve therapeutic concentrations in CSF.
Metabolism: metabolized extensively in liver.
Excretion: excreted primarily in bile; smaller portion excreted in urine. *Half-life:* first phase, 4 minutes; second phase, 2.25 hours; terminal phase, 85 hours.

Route	Onset	Peak	Duration
I.V.	Unknown	Unknown	Unknown

Pharmacodynamics

Chemical effect: arrests mitosis in metaphase, blocking cell division.
Therapeutic effect: inhibits replication of selected cancer cells.

Indications and dosage

► **Acute lymphoblastic and other leukemias, Hodgkin's disease, non-Hodgkin's lymphoma, neuroblastoma, rhabdomyosarcoma, Wilms' tumor.**
Adults: 1.4 mg/m^2 I.V. weekly. Maximum weekly dosage is 2 mg. *Children weighing over 10 kg (22 lb):* 2 mg/m^2 I.V. weekly. Maximum single dose is 2 mg. *Children weighing 10 kg and less:* 0.05 mg/kg I.V. once weekly.

Adverse reactions

CNS: *peripheral neuropathy,* sensory loss, *loss of deep tendon reflexes, paresthesia, wristdrop and footdrop,* headache, ataxia, cranial nerve palsies, *jaw pain,* hoarseness, vocal cord paralysis, *muscle weakness and cramps, seizures, coma;* some neurotoxicities may be permanent.
CV: hypotension, hypertension, *phlebitis.*
EENT: visual disturbances, diplopia, optic and extraocular neuropathy, ptosis.
GI: diarrhea, *constipation, cramps,* ileus that mimics surgical abdomen, *nausea, vomiting,* anorexia, dysphagia, *intestinal necrosis, stomatitis.*
GU: urine retention, SIADH, dysuria, acute uric acid neuropathy, polyuria.

Hematologic: anemia, *leukopenia, thrombocytopenia.*
Metabolic: hyponatremia, hyperuricemia.
Respiratory: *acute bronchospasm.*
Skin: rash, *reversible alopecia,* cellulitis at injection site, severe local reaction with extravasation.
Other: fever, weight loss.

Interactions

Drug-drug. *Asparaginase:* decreased hepatic clearance of vincristine. Monitor patient closely for toxicity.
Calcium channel blockers: enhanced vincristine accumulation. Monitor for toxicity.
Digoxin: decreased digoxin effects. Monitor serum digoxin level.
Mitomycin: possible increased frequency of bronchospasm and acute pulmonary reactions. Monitor patient closely.
Phenytoin: may reduce phenytoin levels. Monitor closely.

Contraindications and precautions

• Contraindicated in patients hypersensitive to drug or who have demyelinating form of Charcot-Marie-Tooth syndrome. Don't administer to patients who are concurrently receiving radiation therapy through ports that include liver.
• Drug is not recommended for use in pregnant or breast-feeding women.
• Use cautiously in patients with hepatic dysfunction, neuromuscular disease, or infection.

NURSING CONSIDERATIONS

Assessment
• Assess patient's condition before therapy and regularly thereafter.
• After administering, monitor for development of life-threatening acute bronchospasm.
• Monitor for hyperuricemia, especially in patient with leukemia or lymphoma.
• Be alert for adverse reactions and drug interactions.
• Check for depression of Achilles tendon reflex, numbness, tingling, footdrop

or wristdrop, difficulty in walking, ataxia, and slapping gait. Also check ability to walk on heels.
• Monitor bowel function. Constipation may be early sign of neurotoxicity.
• Evaluate patient's and family's knowledge of drug therapy.

⊕ Nursing diagnoses
• Altered health maintenance related to presence of neoplastic disease
• Altered protection related to drug-induced adverse hematologic reactions
• Knowledge deficit related to drug therapy

❯ Planning and implementation
• Give antiemetic before administering drug, as ordered.
• Follow institutional policy to reduce risks. Preparation and administration of parenteral form are associated with carcinogenic, mutagenic, and teratogenic risks for personnel.
• Inject drug directly into vein or running I.V. line slowly over 1 minute. Drug may also be given in 50 ml of D₅W or 0.9% NaCl solution infused over 15 minutes. If drug extravasates, stop infusion immediately and notify doctor. Apply heat on and off every 2 hours for 24 hours. Administer 150 units of hyaluronidase, as ordered, to area of infiltrate.
• Don't administer to one patient as single dose. The 5-mg vials are for multiple-dose use only.
• Take care to avoid confusing vincristine with vinblastine or vindesine.
• Know that all vials (1-mg, 2-mg, 5-mg) contain 1 mg/ml solution and should be refrigerated.
• Because of risk of neurotoxicity, know that drug should not be given more than once a week. Children are more resistant to neurotoxicity than adults. Neurotoxicity is dose-related and usually reversible.
• If acute bronchospasm occurs after administration, notify doctor immediately.

• Maintain good hydration, and administer allopurinol, as ordered, to prevent uric acid nephropathy.
• Be aware that fluid restriction may be necessary if SIADH develops.
• Give stool softener or laxative, as ordered, or water before dosing to help prevent constipation.
Patient teaching
• Instruct patient on infection-control and bleeding precautions to take in everyday living.
• Warn patient that alopecia may occur, but that it's usually reversible.
• Tell patient to report promptly adverse reactions.
• Encourage fluid intake to facilitate excretion of uric acid.
• Advise female patient of childbearing age to avoid becoming pregnant during therapy. Also recommend that she consult with doctor before becoming pregnant.

☑ Evaluation
• Patient responds well to drug.
• Patient does not develop serious complications from adverse hematologic reactions.
• Patient and family state understanding of drug therapy.

---

vinorelbine
(vin-oh-REL-been)
Navelbine

Pharmacologic class: semisynthetic vinca alkaloid
Therapeutic class: antineoplastic
Pregnancy risk category: D

How supplied
Injection: 10 mg/ml, 50 mg/5 ml

Pharmacokinetics
Absorption: not applicable.
Distribution: distributed widely in body tissues and bound to lymphocytes and platelets.

Metabolism: metabolized extensively in liver.
Excretion: excreted primarily in bile; smaller portion excreted in urine. *Half-life:* 27.7 to 43.6 hours.

Route	Onset	Peak	Duration
I.V.	Unknown	Unknown	Unknown

Pharmacodynamics

Chemical effect: arrests mitosis in metaphase, blocking cell division.
Therapeutic effect: inhibits replication of selected cancer cells.

Indications and dosage

▶ **Alone or as adjunct therapy with cisplatin for first-line treatment of ambulatory patients with nonresectable advanced non-small-cell lung cancer (NSCLC); alone or with cisplatin in stage IV of NSCLC; with cisplatin in stage III of NSCLC.** *Adults:* 30 mg/m^2 I.V. weekly. In combination treatment, same dosage used along with 120 mg/m^2 of cisplatin, given on days 1 and 29, then every 6 weeks.

Adverse reactions

CNS: *peripheral neuropathy, asthenia, fatigue.*
GI: *nausea, vomiting, anorexia, diarrhea, constipation, stomatitis.*
Hematologic: **bone marrow suppression** *(agranulocytosis,* LEUKOPENIA, *thrombocytopenia,* anemia*).*
Hepatic: *abnormal liver function test results, bilirubinemia.*
Musculoskeletal: jaw pain, chest pain, myalgia, arthralgia, loss of deep tendon reflexes.
Respiratory: dyspnea.
Skin: *alopecia,* rash, *injection pain or reaction.*
Other: SIADH.

Interactions

Drug-drug. *Cisplatin:* increased risk of bone marrow suppression when used concomitantly with cisplatin. Monitor patient's hematologic status closely.
Mitomycin: may cause pulmonary reactions. Monitor patient's respiratory status closely.

Contraindications and precautions

• Contraindicated in patients with pretreatment granulocyte counts below 1,000 cells/mm^3.
• Drug is not recommended for use in pregnant or breast-feeding women.
• Use with extreme caution in patients whose bone marrow may have been compromised by previous exposure to radiation therapy or chemotherapy or whose bone marrow is still recovering from previous chemotherapy.
• Use cautiously in patients with hepatic impairment.
• Safety of drug has not been established in children.

NURSING CONSIDERATIONS

Assessment
• Assess patient's condition before therapy and regularly thereafter.
• Monitor patient closely for hypersensitivity reactions.
• As a guide to effects of therapy, monitor patient's peripheral blood count and bone marrow, as ordered.
• Be alert for adverse reactions and drug interactions.
• Assess for numbness and tingling in hands and feet. Assess gait for early evidence of footdrop.
• Evaluate patient's and family's knowledge of drug therapy.

Nursing diagnoses
• Altered health maintenance related to presence of neoplastic disease
• Altered protection related to drug-induced adverse hematologic reactions
• Knowledge deficit related to drug therapy

▶ **Planning and implementation**
• Give antiemetic before administering drug, as ordered.
• Check patient's granulocyte count before administration. The count should be 1,000 cells/mm³ or more for drug to be administered. Withhold drug and notify doctor if count is less.
• Know that drug must be diluted before administration. Administer drug I.V. over 6 to 10 minutes into side port of free-flowing I.V. line that is closest to I.V. bag, followed by flushing with 75 to 125 ml of D₅W or 0.9% NaCl solution.
• Take great care to avoid extravasation during administration because drug can cause considerable irritation, localized tissue necrosis, and thrombophlebitis. If extravasation occurs, drug administration should be stopped immediately and remaining dosage portion injected into different vein.
• Be aware that dosage adjustments are made according to hematologic toxicity or hepatic insufficiency, whichever results in lower dosage. Expect dosage to be halved if patient's granulocyte count falls below 1,500 cells/mm³ but is greater than 1,000 cells/mm³. If three consecutive doses are skipped because of agranulocytosis, know that further vinorelbine therapy should not be given.
• Know that drug may be a contact irritant, and solution must be handled and administered with care. Gloves are recommended. Inhalation of vapors and contact with skin or mucous membranes, especially those of eyes, must be avoided. In case of contact, wash with copious amounts of water for at least 15 minutes.
Patient teaching
• Instruct patient on infection-control and bleeding precautions to take in everyday living.
• Warn patient that alopecia may occur, but that it's usually reversible.
• Instruct patient not to take other drugs, including OTC preparations, until approved by doctor.

• Instruct patient to report signs and symptoms of infection (fever, chills, malaise) to doctor because drug may have immunosuppressant activity.

☑ **Evaluation**
• Patient responds well to drug.
• Patient does not develop serious complications from adverse hematologic reactions.
• Patient and family state understanding of drug therapy.

vitamin A (retinol)
(VIGH-tuh-min ay)
Aquasol A, Del-Vi-A

Pharmacologic class: fat-soluble vitamin
Therapeutic class: vitamin
Pregnancy risk category: A (X if used in doses exceeding RDA)

How supplied

Tablets: 5,000 IU, 10,000 IU
Capsules: 10,000 IU, 25,000 IU, 50,000 IU
Drops: 30 ml with dropper (50,000 IU/0.1 ml)
Injection: 2-ml vials (50,000 IU/ml with 0.5% chlorobutanol, polysorbate 80, butylated hydroxyanisol, and butylated hydroxytoluene)

Pharmacokinetics

Absorption: in normal doses, absorbed readily and completely if fat absorption is normal; larger doses or regular dose in patients with fat malabsorption, low protein intake, or hepatic or pancreatic disease may be absorbed incompletely. Because vitamin A is fat-soluble, absorption requires bile salts, pancreatic lipase, and dietary fat.
Distribution: stored (primarily as palmitate) in Kupffer's cells of liver. Normal adult liver stores are sufficient to provide vitamin A requirements for 2 years. Lesser amounts of retinyl palmitate are

stored in kidneys, lungs, adrenal glands, retinas, and intraperitoneal fat. Vitamin A circulates bound to specific alpha, protein, retinol-binding protein (RBP). *Metabolism:* metabolized in liver. *Excretion:* retinol (fat-soluble) combines with glucuronic acid and is metabolized to retinal and retinoic acid. Retinoic acid undergoes biliary excretion in feces. Retinal, retinoic acid, and other water-soluble metabolites are excreted in urine and feces.

Route	Onset	Peak	Duration
P.O., I.M.	Unknown	3-5 hr	Unknown

Pharmacodynamics

Chemical effect: stimulates retinal function, bone growth, reproduction, and integrity of epithelial and mucosal tissues. *Therapeutic effect:* raises vitamin A levels in body.

Indications and dosage

▶ **RDA**. *Note:* RDAs have been converted to retinol equivalents (RE). One RE has activity of 1 mcg of all-*trans* retinol, 6 mcg of beta carotene, or 12 mcg of carotenoid provitamins. *Males over age 11:* 1,000 mcg RE or 5,000 IU. *Females over age 11:* 800 mcg RE or 4,000 IU. *Pregnant women:* 800 mcg RE or 4,000 IU. *Breast-feeding women (first 6 months):* 1,300 mcg RE or 6,500 IU. *Breast-feeding women (second 6 months):* 1,200 mcg RE or 6,000 IU. *Children ages 7 to 10:* 700 mcg RE or 3,500 IU. *Children ages 4 to 6:* 500 mcg RE or 2,500 IU. *Children ages 1 to 3:* 400 mcg RE or 2,000 IU. *Neonates and infants to age 1:* 375 mcg RE or 1,875 IU.
▶ **Severe vitamin A deficiency.** *Adults and children over age 8:* 100,000 IU I.M. or P.O. daily for 3 days, followed by 50,000 IU I.M. or P.O. daily for 2 weeks; then 10,000 to 20,000 IU P.O. daily for 2 months. Follow with adequate dietary nutrition and RDA vitamin A supplements. *Children ages 1 to 8:* 17,500 to 35,000 IU I.M. daily for 10 days. *Infants under age 1:* 7,500 to 15,000 IU I.M. daily for 10 days.
▶ **Maintenance dosage to prevent recurrence of vitamin A deficiency.** *Children ages 1 to 8:* 5,000 to 10,000 IU P.O. daily for 2 months, then adequate dietary nutrition and RDA vitamin A supplements.

Adverse reactions

Adverse reactions are usually seen only with toxicity.
CNS: irritability, headache, *increased intracranial pressure,* fatigue, lethargy, malaise.
EENT: papilledema, exophthalmos.
GI: anorexia, epigastric pain, vomiting, polydipsia.
GU: hypomenorrhea, polyuria.
Hepatic: jaundice, hepatomegaly, *cirrhosis,* elevated liver enzyme levels.
Metabolic: slow growth, decalcification of bone, hypercalcemia, periostitis, premature closure of epiphyses, migratory arthralgia, cortical thickening over radius and tibia.
Skin: alopecia; drying, cracking, scaling of skin; pruritus; lip fissures; erythema; inflamed tongue, lips, and gums; massive desquamation; increased pigmentation; night sweating.
Other: splenomegaly, *anaphylactic shock.*

Interactions

Drug-drug. *Cholestyramine resin, mineral oil:* reduced GI absorption of fat-soluble vitamins. If needed, give mineral oil at bedtime.
Isotretinoin, multivitamins containing vitamin A: increased risk of toxicity. Avoid concomitant use.
Neomycin (oral): decreased vitamin A absorption. Avoid concomitant use.
Oral contraceptives: may increase plasma vitamin A levels. Monitor closely.
Warfarin: increased risk of bleeding. Monitor PT and INR closely.

Contraindications and precautions

• Contraindicated for oral administration in patients with malabsorption syndrome; if malabsorption is from inadequate bile secretion, oral route may be used with concurrent administration of bile salts (dehydrocholic acid). Also contraindicated in patients with hypervitaminosis A or hypersensitivity to other ingredients in product.

• I.V. administration contraindicated except for special water-miscible forms intended for infusion with large parenteral volumes. I.V. push of vitamin A of any type is also contraindicated (anaphylaxis or anaphylactoid reactions and death have resulted).

• Use cautiously in pregnant or breast-feeding women, avoiding doses exceeding RDA.

NURSING CONSIDERATIONS

⚕ Assessment

• Assess patient's vitamin A intake from fortified foods, dietary supplements, self-administered drugs, and prescription drug sources before therapy and reassess regularly thereafter.

• Be alert for adverse reactions (if dose is high). Be aware that acute toxicity has resulted from single doses of 25,000 IU/kg of body weight; 350,000 IU in infants and over 2 million IU in adults have also proved acutely toxic. Doses that do not exceed RDA are usually nontoxic.

• Be aware that chronic toxicity in infants (3 to 6 months) has resulted from doses of 18,500 IU daily for 1 to 3 months. In adults, chronic toxicity has resulted from doses of 50,000 IU daily for more than 18 months; 500,000 IU daily for 2 months, and 1 million IU daily for 3 days.

• Be alert for drug interactions.

• Evaluate patient's and family's knowledge of drug therapy.

⊕ Nursing diagnoses

• Altered nutrition: Less than body requirements related to inadequate intake

• Altered health maintenance related to vitamin A toxicity caused by excessive intake

• Knowledge deficit related to drug therapy

⊠ Planning and implementation

P.O. use: Follow normal protocol.
– Liquid preparations available if nasogastric administration is necessary. They may be mixed with cereal or fruit juice.

• Know that adequate vitamin A absorption requires suitable protein, vitamin E, and zinc intake and bile secretion; give supplemental salts, if necessary and ordered. Zinc supplements may be necessary in patient receiving long-term total parenteral nutrition.

I.M. use: Keep in mind that absorption is fastest and most complete with water-miscible preparations, intermediate with emulsions, and slowest with oil suspensions.

• Protect drug from light.

Patient teaching

• Warn patient against self-administration of megadoses of vitamins without specific indications. Also stress that he not share prescribed vitamins with others.

• Explain importance of avoiding prolonged use of mineral oil while taking this drug because mineral oil reduces vitamin A absorption.

• Instruct patient on signs and symptoms of vitamin A toxicity, and tell him to report such occurrences immediately.

• Advise patient to consume adequate protein, vitamin E, and zinc, which, along with bile, are necessary for vitamin A absorption.

• Instruct patient to store vitamin A in tight, light-resistant container.

☑ Evaluation

• Patient regains normal vitamin A levels.

• Patient does not exhibit signs and symptoms of vitamin A toxicity.

• Patient and family state understanding of drug therapy.

---

vitamin C (ascorbic acid)
(VIGH-tuh-min see)
Ascorbicap†, Cebid Timecelles†, Cecon†, Cenolate†, Cetane†, Cevalin†, Cevi-Bid, Ce-Vi-Sol*, Dull-C†, Flavorcee†, N'ice w/Vitamin C Drops†, Penta-Vite◇, Redoxon♦, Vita-C Crystals†

Pharmacologic class: water-soluble vitamin
Therapeutic class: vitamin
Pregnancy risk category: A (C if used in doses exceeding RDA)

How supplied
Tablets: 25 mg†, 50 mg†, 100 mg†, 250 mg†, 500 mg†, 1,000 mg†
Tablets (chewable): 50 mg, 100 mg†, 250 mg†, 500 mg†, 1,000 mg†
Tablets (effervescent): 1,000 mg sugar-free†
Tablets (timed-release): 500 mg†, 1,000 mg†, 1,500 mg
Capsules (timed-release): 500 mg†
Crystals: 100 g (4 g/tsp)†, 500 g (4 g/tsp)†
Lozenges: 60 mg†
Oral liquid: 50 ml (35 mg/0.6 ml)*†
Oral solution: 60 mg/ml†, 100 mg/ml†
Powder: 100 g (4 g/tsp)†, 500 g (4 g/tsp)†
Syrup: 20 mg/ml in 120 ml, 480 ml†; 500 mg/5 ml in 5 ml†, 120 ml†, 480 ml†
Injection: 100 mg/ml; 250 mg/ml; 500 mg/ml

Pharmacokinetics
Absorption: after oral administration, ascorbic acid is absorbed readily from GI tract. After very large doses, absorption may be limited because absorption is an active process. Absorption also may be reduced in patients with diarrhea or GI diseases. Degree of absorption unknown after I.M. or S.C. administration.
Distribution: distributed widely in body with large concentrations found in liver, leukocytes, platelets, glandular tissues, and lens of eye. Protein binding is low.
Metabolism: metabolized in liver.

Excretion: excreted in urine. Renal excretion is directly proportional to blood concentrations.

Route	Onset	Peak	Duration
All routes	Unknown	Unknown	Unknown

Pharmacodynamics
Chemical effect: stimulates collagen formation and tissue repair; involved in oxidation-reduction reactions throughout body.
Therapeutic effect: raises vitamin C levels in body.

Indications and dosage
▶ **RDA.** *Adults and children age 15 and over:* 60 mg. Pregnant women: 70 mg. *Breast-feeding women (first 6 months):* 95 mg. *Breast-feeding women (second 6 months):* 90 mg. *Children ages 11 to 14:* 50 mg. *Children ages 4 to 10:* 45 mg. *Children ages 1 to 3:* 40 mg. *Infants ages 6 months to 1 year:* 35 mg. *Neonates and infants to age 6 months:* 30 mg.
▶ **Frank and subclinical scurvy.** *Adults:* depending on severity, 300 mg to 1 g P.O., S.C., I.M., or I.V. daily, then at least 50 mg daily for maintenance. *Children:* depending on severity, 100 to 300 mg P.O., S.C., I.M., or I.V. daily, then at least 30 mg daily for maintenance. *Premature infants:* 75 to 100 mg P.O., I.M., I.V., or S.C. daily.
▶ **Extensive burns, delayed fracture or wound healing, postoperative wound healing, severe febrile or chronic disease states.** *Adults:* 300 to 500 mg P.O., S.C., I.M., or I.V. daily for 7 to 10 days. For extensive burns, 1 to 2 g daily. *Children:* 100 to 200 mg P.O., S.C., I.M., or I.V. daily.
▶ **Prevention of vitamin C deficiency in patients with poor nutritional habits or increased requirements.** *Adults:* 70 to 150 mg P.O., S.C., I.M., or I.V. daily. *Pregnant or breast-feeding women:* at least 70 to 150 mg P.O., S.C., I.M., or I.V. daily. *Children:* at least 40 mg P.O.,

S.C., I.M., or I.V. daily. *Infants:* at least 35 mg P.O., S.C., I.M., or I.V. daily.
▶ **Potentiation of methenamine in urine acidification.** *Adults:* 4 to 12 g P.O. daily in divided doses.

Adverse reactions

CNS: faintness, dizziness (with too-fast I.V. administration).
GI: diarrhea.
GU: acid urine, oxaluria, renal calculi.
Other: discomfort (at injection site).

Interactions

Drug-drug. *Aspirin (high doses):* increased risk of ascorbic acid deficiency. Monitor patient closely.
Contraceptives, estrogen: increased serum levels of estrogen. Monitor patient.
Oral iron supplements: increased iron absorption. A beneficial drug interaction.
Warfarin: decreased anticoagulant effect. Monitor patient closely.

Contraindications and precautions

No known contraindications.

NURSING CONSIDERATIONS

❧ Assessment
• Assess patient's condition before therapy and regularly thereafter.
• When administering for urine acidification, check urine pH to ensure efficacy.
• Be alert for adverse reactions and drug interactions.
• Monitor patient's hydration status if adverse GI reactions occur.
• Evaluate patient's and family's knowledge of drug therapy.

⊞ Nursing diagnoses
• Altered nutrition: Less than body requirements related to inadequate intake
• Risk for fluid volume deficit related to drug-induced adverse GI reactions
• Knowledge deficit related to drug therapy

⊠ Planning and implementation
P.O. use: Administer oral solutions directly into mouth or mix with food. Effervescent tablets should be dissolved in glass of water immediately before ingestion.
I.V. use: Administer I.V. infusion cautiously in patients with renal insufficiency. – Avoid rapid I.V. administration.
I.M. use: Know that utilization of vitamin may be better with I.M. route, the preferred parenteral route.
S.C. use: Follow normal protocol.
• Protect solution from light, and refrigerate ampules.
Patient teaching
• Stress proper nutritional habits to prevent recurrence of deficiency.
• Advise patient with vitamin C deficiency to decrease or stop smoking.

☑ Evaluation
• Patient regains normal vitamin C levels.
• Patient maintains adequate hydration.
• Patient and family state understanding of drug therapy.

vitamin D

cholecalciferol (vitamin D₃)
(koh-lih-kal-SIF-eh-rol)
Delta-D†, Vitamin D₃†

ergocalciferol (vitamin D₂)
(er-goh-kal-SIF-er-ohl)
Calciferol, Deltalin Gelseals, Drisdol, Radiostol Forte♦, Vitamin D

Pharmacologic class: fat-soluble vitamin
Therapeutic class: vitamin
Pregnancy risk category: C

How supplied

Tablets: 1.25 mg (50,000 IU)
Capsules: 1.25 mg (50,000 IU)
Oral liquid: 8,000 IU/ml in 60-ml dropper bottle†
Injection: 12.5 mg (500,000 IU)/ml

Pharmacokinetics

Absorption: absorbed from small intestine with P.O. administration; unknown for I.M. administration.
Distribution: widely distributed throughout body; bound to proteins stored in liver.
Metabolism: metabolized in liver and kidneys.
Excretion: excreted primarily in bile; small amount excreted in urine. *Half-life:* 24 hours.

Route	Onset	Peak	Duration
P.O., I.M.	2-24 hr	3-12 hr	Varies

Pharmacodynamics

Chemical effect: promotes absorption and utilization of calcium and phosphate, helping to regulate calcium homeostasis.
Therapeutic effect: helps to maintain normal calcium and phosphate levels in body.

Indications and dosage

▶ **RDA for cholecalciferol.** *Adults age 25 and over:* 200 IU. *Pregnant or breastfeeding women:* 400 IU. *Adults under age 25 and children age 6 months and over:* 400 IU. *Neonates and infants to age 6 months:* 300 IU.
▶ **Rickets and other vitamin D deficiency diseases.** *Adults:* initially, 12,000 IU P.O. or I.M. daily, usually increased as indicated by response up to 500,000 IU daily. After correction of deficiency, maintenance includes adequate diet and RDA supplements.
▶ **Hypoparathyroidism.** *Adults and children:* 50,000 to 200,000 IU P.O. or I.M. daily with calcium supplement.
▶ **Familial hypophosphatemia.** *Adults:* 10,000 to 80,000 IU P.O. or I.M. daily with phosphorus supplement.

Adverse reactions

Adverse reactions listed are usually seen only in vitamin D toxicity.
CNS: headache, weakness, somnolence, decreased libido, overt psychosis, irritability, hyperthermia.
CV: *calcifications of soft tissues including, heart, arrhythmias,* hypertension, *arrhythmias.*
EENT: rhinorrhea, conjunctivitis (calcific), photophobia.
GI: anorexia, nausea, vomiting, constipation, dry mouth, metallic taste, polydipsia.
GU: polyuria, albuminuria, hypercalciuria, nocturia, *impaired kidney function,* reversible azotemia.
Metabolic: *hypercalcemia.*
Musculoskeletal: bone and muscle pain, bone demineralization, weight loss.
Skin: pruritus.

Interactions

Drug-drug. *Cardiac glycosides:* increased risk of arrhythmias. Monitor serum calcium level.
Cholestyramine resin, mineral oil: inhibited GI absorption of oral vitamin D. Space doses. Use together cautiously.
Corticosteroids: antagonized effect of vitamin D. Monitor vitamin D level closely.
Phenobarbital, phenytoin: increased vitamin D metabolism, which decreases half-life as well as drug's effectiveness. Monitor patient closely.
Thiazide diuretics: may cause hypercalcemia in patients with hypoparathyroidism. Monitor patient closely.
Verapamil: atrial fibrillation has occurred due to increased calcium. Monitor closely.

Contraindications and precautions

• Contraindicated in patients with hypercalcemia, hypervitaminosis A, or renal osteodystrophy with hyperphosphatemia.
• Administer ergocalciferol with extreme caution, if at all, to patients with impaired kidney function, heart disease, renal stones, or arteriosclerosis.
• Use cautiously in cardiac patients, especially those receiving cardiac glycosides; in patients with increased sensitivity to these drugs; and in pregnant or breastfeeding women.

---

*Liquid form contains alcohol   **May contain tartrazine   ◆Canada   ◇Australia   †OTC

NURSING CONSIDERATIONS

Assessment
- Assess patient's condition before therapy and regularly thereafter.
- Monitor patient's eating and bowel habits; dry mouth, nausea, vomiting, metallic taste, and constipation may be early signs and symptoms of toxicity.
- Monitor serum and urine calcium, potassium, and urea levels when high therapeutic dosages are used.
- Be alert for adverse reactions and drug interactions.
- Evaluate patient's and family's knowledge of drug therapy.

Nursing diagnoses
- Altered nutrition: Less than body requirements related to inadequate intake
- Altered health maintenance related to vitamin D toxicity
- Knowledge deficit related to drug therapy

Planning and implementation
P.O. use: Follow normal protocol.
I.M. use: Use I.M. injection of vitamin D dispersed in oil for patient unable to absorb oral form, as ordered.
- Keep in mind that dosages of 60,000 IU/day can cause hypercalcemia.
- Be aware that malabsorption from inadequate bile or hepatic dysfunction may require addition of exogenous bile salts with oral form.
- Know that patient with hyperphosphatemia requires dietary phosphate restrictions and binding agents to avoid metastatic calcifications and renal calculus formation.
Patient teaching
- Warn patient of dangers of increasing dosage without consulting doctor. Vitamin D is fat-soluble.
- Tell patient taking vitamin D to restrict his intake of magnesium-containing antacids.

Evaluation
- Patient regains normal vitamin D level.
- Patient does not develop vitamin D toxicity.
- Patient and family state understanding of drug therapy.

vitamin E (tocopherol)
(VIGH-tuh-min ee)
Amino-Opti-E†, Aquasol E†, E-Complex-600†, E-200 I.U. Softgels†, E-400 I.U. Softgels†, E-Vitamin Succinate†, Vita-Plus E Softgels†

Pharmacologic class: fat-soluble vitamin
Therapeutic class: vitamin
Pregnancy risk category: NR

How supplied
Tablets (chewable): 200 IU†, 400 IU†
Capsules: 200 IU†, 400 IU†, 500 IU†, 600 IU†, 1,000 IU†, 73.5 mg, 147 mg, 330 mg
Oral solution: 50 mg/ml†

Pharmacokinetics
Absorption: GI absorption depends on presence of bile. Only 20% to 60% of vitamin obtained from dietary sources is absorbed. As dosage increases, fraction of vitamin E absorbed decreases.
Distribution: distributed to all tissues and stored in adipose tissues.
Metabolism: metabolized in liver.
Excretion: excreted primarily in bile; small amount excreted in urine.

Route	Onset	Peak	Duration
P.O.	Unknown	Unknown	Unknown

Pharmacodynamics
Chemical effect: unknown; thought to act as an antioxidant and protect RBC membranes against hemolysis.
Therapeutic effect: raises vitamin E level in body.

Indications and dosage

▶ **RDA.** *Note:* RDAs for vitamin E have been converted to alpha-tocopherol equivalents (alpha-TE). One alpha-TE equals 1 mg of D-alpha tocopherol or 1.49 IU. *Males age 11 and over:* 10 alpha-TE or 15 IU. *Females age 11 and over:* 8 alpha-TE or 12 IU. *Pregnant women:* 10 alpha-TE or 15 IU. *Breast-feeding women (first 6 months):* 12 alpha-TE or 18 IU. *Breast-feeding women (second 6 months):* 11 alpha-TE or 16 IU. *Children ages 4 to 10:* 7 alpha-TE or 10 IU. *Children over age 1 to age 3:* 6 alpha-TE or 9 IU. *Infants ages 6 months to 1 year:* 4 alpha-TE or 6 IU. *Neonates and infants to age 6 months:* 3 alpha-TE or 4 IU.
▶ **Vitamin E deficiency in adults and in children with malabsorption syndrome.** *Adults:* depending on severity, 60 to 75 IU P.O. daily. *Children:* 1 IU/kg P.O. daily.

Adverse reactions

None reported with recommended dosages.

Interactions

Drug-drug. *Cholestyramine resin, mineral oil:* inhibited GI absorption of oral vitamin E. Space doses. Use together cautiously.
Iron: may catalyze oxidation and increase daily requirements. Administer separately.
Oral anticoagulants: hypoprothrombinemic effects may be increased, possibly causing bleeding. Monitor patient closely.
Vitamin K: antagonized effects of vitamin K possible with large doses of vitamin E. Avoid concurrent use.

Contraindications and precautions

No known contraindications.

NURSING CONSIDERATIONS

🔍 **Assessment**
• Assess patient's condition before therapy and regularly thereafter.

• Monitor patient with liver or gallbladder disease for response to therapy. Adequate bile is essential for vitamin E absorption.
• Be alert for drug interactions.
• Evaluate patient's and family's knowledge of drug therapy.

🔟 **Nursing diagnoses**
• Altered nutrition: Less than body requirements related to inadequate intake
• Knowledge deficit related to drug therapy

❯ **Planning and implementation**
• Know that requirements increase with rise in dietary polyunsaturated acids.
• Ensure that patient swallows tablets or capsules whole.
• Store drug in tightly closed light-resistant container.
• Know that vitamin E should be given concurrently with bile salts if patient has malabsorption caused by lack of bile.
Patient teaching
• Tell patient not to crush tablets or open capsules. An oral solution and chewable tablets are commercially available.
• Discourage patient from self-medication with megadoses, which can cause thrombophlebitis. Vitamin E is fat-soluble.

🔲 **Evaluation**
• Patient regains normal vitamin E level.
• Patient and family state understanding of drug therapy.

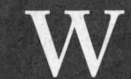

warfarin sodium
(WAR-feh-rin SOH-dee-um)
Coumadin, Sofarin, Warfilone♦

Pharmacologic class: coumarin derivative

Therapeutic class: anticoagulant
Pregnancy risk category: X

How supplied

Tablets: 1 mg, 2 mg, 2.5 mg, 4 mg, 5 mg, 7.5 mg, 10 mg

Pharmacokinetics

Absorption: rapidly and completely absorbed from GI tract.
Distribution: highly bound to plasma proteins, especially albumin.
Metabolism: metabolized in liver.
Excretion: metabolites reabsorbed from bile and excreted in urine. *Half-life:* 1 to 3 days.

Route	Onset	Peak	Duration
P.O.	0.5-3 days	4 hr	2-5 days

Pharmacodynamics

Chemical effect: inhibits vitamin K–dependent activation of clotting factors II, VII, IX, and X, formed in liver.
Therapeutic effect: reduces blood's ability to clot.

Indications and dosage

▶ **Pulmonary embolism associated with deep vein thrombosis, MI, rheumatic heart disease with heart valve damage, prosthetic heart valves, chronic atrial fibrillation.** *Adults:* initially, 2 to 5 mg P.O.; then daily PT and INR are used to establish optimal dose. Usual maintenance dosage is 2 to 10 mg daily.

Adverse reactions

GI: anorexia, nausea, vomiting, cramps, *diarrhea,* mouth ulcerations, sore mouth, melena.
GU: hematuria, excessive menstrual bleeding.
Hematologic: *hemorrhage* (with excessive dosage).
Hepatic: hepatitis, elevated liver function tests, jaundice.
Skin: dermatitis, urticaria, necrosis, gangrene, alopecia, *rash.*
Other: *fever,* headache.

Interactions

Drug-drug. *Acetaminophen:* may increase bleeding with chronic (over 2 weeks) therapy with high doses (over 2 g/day) of acetaminophen. Monitor patient very carefully.
Allopurinol, amiodarone, anabolic steroids, cephalosporins, chloramphenicol, cimetidine, ciprofloxacin, clofibrate, danazol, diazoxide, diflunisal, disulfiram, erythromycin, ethacrynic acid, fenoprofen calcium, fluoroquinolones, glucagon, heparin, ibuprofen, influenza virus vaccine, isoniazid, ketoprofen, lovastatin, meclofenamate, methimazole, methylthiouracil, metronidazole, miconazole, nalidixic acid, neomycin (oral), pentoxifylline, propafenone, propoxyphene, propylthiouracil, quinidine, streptokinase, sulfinpyrazone, sulfonamides, sulindac, tamoxifen, tetracyclines, thiazides, thyroid drugs, tricyclic antidepressants, urokinase, vitamin E: increased PT. Monitor for bleeding. Consider anticoagulant dosage reduction.
Anticonvulsants: increased serum levels of phenytoin and phenobarbital. Monitor closely.
Barbiturates, carbamazepine, corticosteroids, corticotropin, ethchlorvynol, griseofulvin, mercaptopurine, methaqualone, nafcillin, oral contraceptives containing estrogen, rifampin, spironolactone, sucralfate, trazodone: decreased PT with reduced anticoagulant effect. Monitor patient carefully.
Chloral hydrate, glutethimide, propylthiouracil, sulfinpyrazone: increased or decreased PT. Avoid use, if possible. Monitor patient carefully.
Cholestyramine: decreased response when administered too close together. Administer 6 hours after oral anticoagulants.
NSAIDs, salicylates: increased PT; ulcerogenic effects. Don't use together.
Sulfonylureas (oral antidiabetic agents): increased hypoglycemic response. Monitor blood glucose level.
Drug-food. *Foods or enteral products containing vitamin K:* may impair antico-

agulation. Tell patient to maintain consistent daily intake of leafy green vegetables.
Drug-lifestyle. *Alcohol use:* enhanced anticoagulant effects. Tell patient receiving oral anticoagulants to avoid excessive alcohol intake; however, one or two drinks daily are unlikely to affect warfarin response.

Contraindications and precautions

• Contraindicated in pregnant women; in patients with bleeding or hemorrhagic tendencies, GI ulcerations, severe hepatic or renal disease, severe uncontrolled hypertension, subacute bacterial endocarditis, polycythemia vera, or vitamin K deficiency; and after recent eye, brain, or spinal cord surgery.
• Use cautiously in patients with diverticulitis, colitis, mild or moderate hypertension, mild or moderate hepatic or renal disease, drainage tubes in any orifice, or regional or lumbar block anesthesia; in any condition increasing risk of hemorrhage; and in breast-feeding women.
• Infants, especially neonates, may be more susceptible to anticoagulants because of vitamin K deficiency.

NURSING CONSIDERATIONS

⚕ Assessment
• Assess patient's condition before therapy and regularly thereafter.
• Draw blood to establish baseline coagulation parameters before therapy.
• Know that INR determinations are essential for proper control. Clinicians typically try to maintain INR at two to three times normal; high incidence of bleeding when INR exceeds six times normal.
• Be alert for adverse reactions and drug interactions. Be aware that elderly patients and patients with renal or hepatic failure are especially sensitive to warfarin effect.
• Regularly inspect patient for bleeding gums, bruises on arms or legs, petechiae, nosebleeds, melena, tarry stools, hematuria, and hematemesis.

• Observe breast-feeding infant of patient on drug for unexpected bleeding.
• Evaluate patient's and family's knowledge of drug therapy.

⚕ Nursing diagnoses
• Risk for injury related to potential for blood clot formation from underlying condition
• Altered protection related to increased risk of bleeding
• Knowledge deficit related to drug therapy

⚕ Planning and implementation
• Give drug at same time daily.
• Be aware that I.V. form may be obtained from manufacturer in rare instances that oral therapy cannot be given. Follow manufacturer guidelines carefully regarding preparation and administration.
• Because onset of action is delayed, keep in mind that heparin sodium is often given during first few days of treatment. When heparin is being given simultaneously, blood for PT should not be drawn within 5 hours of intermittent I.V. heparin administration. However, blood for PT may be drawn at any time during continuous heparin infusion.
• Know that the elderly are more prone to bleeding so lower doses are usually used.
• Withhold drug and call doctor immediately if fever and rash (signal severe adverse reactions) occur.
• Be aware that drug's anticoagulant effect can be neutralized by vitamin K injections.
• Be aware that drug is best oral anticoagulant for patient taking antacids or phenytoin.
Patient teaching
• Stress importance of compliance with prescribed dosage and follow-up appointments. Patient should carry a medical identification card that identifies him as potential bleeder.
• Instruct patient and family to watch for signs of bleeding and to notify doctor immediately if they occur.

• Warn patient to avoid OTC products containing aspirin, other salicylates, or drugs that may interact with warfarin.
• Tell patient to notify doctor if menses is heavier than usual; dosage adjustment may be necessary.
• Tell patient to use electric razor when shaving to avoid scratching skin and to use soft toothbrush.
• Caution patient to read food labels. Food and enteral feedings that contain vitamin K may impair anticoagulation.
• Tell patient to eat a daily, consistent amount of leafy green vegetables that contain vitamin K. Eating different amounts daily may alter anticoagulant effects.

✓ **Evaluation**
• Patient does not develop blood clots.
• Patient states appropriate bleeding precautions to take.
• Patient and family state understanding of drug therapy.

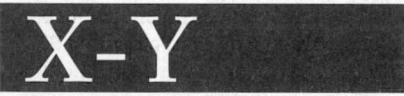

xylometazoline hydrochloride
(zigh-loh-met-uh-ZOH-leen high-droh-KLOR-ighd)
Otrivin

Pharmacologic class: sympathomimetic
Therapeutic class: decongestant, vaso-constrictor
Pregnancy risk category: NR

How supplied
Nasal solution: 0.05%, 0.1%

Pharmacokinetics
Unknown.

Route	Onset	Peak	Duration
Intranasal	5-10 min	Unknown	5-6 hr

Pharmacodynamics
Chemical effect: unknown; thought to cause local vasoconstriction of dilated arterioles, reducing blood flow and nasal congestion.
Therapeutic effect: relieves nasal congestion.

Indications and dosage
▶ **Nasal congestion.** *Adults and children age 12 and over:* 2 to 3 drops or sprays of 0.1% solution in each nostril q 8 to 10 hours. *Children ages 6 months to 12 years:* 2 to 3 drops of 0.05% solution in each nostril q 8 to 10 hours. *Children under 6 months:* 1 drop of 0.05% in each nostril q 6 hours, p.r.n.

Adverse reactions
EENT: transient burning, stinging; dryness or ulceration of nasal mucosa; sneezing; rebound nasal congestion or irritation (with excessive or long-term use).

Interactions
None significant.

Contraindications and precautions
• Contraindicated in patients with angle-closure glaucoma or hypersensitivity to drug.
• Use cautiously in patients with hyperthyroidism, cardiac disease, hypertension, diabetes mellitus, or advanced arteriosclerosis.
• Safety of drug has not been established in pregnant or breast-feeding women.

NURSING CONSIDERATIONS

✓ **Assessment**
• Assess patient's condition before therapy and regularly thereafter.
• Be alert for adverse reactions.
• Evaluate patient's and family's knowledge of drug therapy.

⊞ **Nursing diagnoses**
• Altered health maintenance related to presence of nasal congestion

• Altered tissue integrity related to drug's adverse effect on nasal mucosa
• Knowledge deficit related to drug therapy

▶ Planning and implementation
• When administering more than one spray, be aware that drug is more effective if 3 to 5 minutes elapse between sprays and nose is cleared before each spray.
Patient teaching
• Teach patient how to use drug. Have patient hold head upright to minimize swallowing of medication, then sniff spray briskly. Instruct him to wait 3 to 5 minutes between sprays and to clear nose before each spray.
• Instruct patient that product should be used by only one person to prevent spread of infection.
• Tell patient not to exceed recommended dose and to use only as needed for 3 to 5 days.

☑ Evaluation
• Patient's nasal congestion is eliminated.
• Patient maintains normal intranasal mucosa.
• Patient and family state understanding of drug therapy.

zafirlukast
(zay-FEER-loo-kast)
Accolate

Pharmacologic class: synthetic, selective peptide leukotriene receptor antagonist
Therapeutic class: antiasthma, bronchodilator
Pregnancy risk category: B

How supplied
Tablets: 20 mg

Pharmacokinetics
Absorption: rapidly absorbed.
Distribution: unknown.
Metabolism: extensively metabolized.
Excretion: in feces; 10% in urine.

Route	Onset	Peak	Duration
P.O.	Unknown	3 hr	Unknown

Pharmacodynamics
Chemical effect: selectively competes for leukotriene receptor sites.
Therapeutic effect: blocks inflammatory action, inhibits bronchoconstriction, improves breathing.

Indications and dosage
▶ **Prophylaxis and chronic treatment of asthma.** *Adults and children age 12 and older:* 20 mg P.O. b.i.d. taken 1 hour before or 2 hours after meals.

Adverse reactions
CNS: *headache,* asthenia, dizziness.
GI: nausea, diarrhea, abdominal pain, vomiting, dyspepsia.
Hepatic: elevated liver enzymes.
Musculoskeletal: myalgia, back pain.
Other: infection, pain, accidental injury, fever.

Interactions
Drug-drug. *Aspirin:* increased plasma levels of zafirlukast. Monitor patient.
Erythromycin, theophylline: decreased plasma levels of zafirlukast. Monitor patient.
Warfarin: increased PT. Monitor PT and INR levels, and adjust dosage of anticoagulant, as ordered.
Drug-food. *Any food:* reduced rate and extent of drug absorption. Give drug 1 hour before or 2 hours after meals.

Contraindications and precautions
• Contraindicated in patients with known hypersensitivity to drug.

NURSING CONSIDERATIONS

Assessment
• Use cautiously in patients with hepatic impairment and in the elderly.
• Evaluate patient's and family's understanding of drug therapy.

Nursing diagnoses
• Impaired gas exchange related to bronchospasm
• Knowledge deficit related to drug therapy

Planning and implementation
• Do not use drug for reversing bronchospasm in acute asthma attack.
• Safety and effectiveness in patients under age 12 have not been established.
Patient teaching
• Tell patient to keep taking drug even if symptoms disappear.
• Advise patient to continue taking other antiasthma drugs as ordered.
• Instruct patient to take drug 1 hour before or 2 hours after meals.

Evaluation
• Patient demonstrates improved gas exchange.
• Patient and family state understanding of drug therapy.

---

zalcitabine (ddC, dideoxycytidine)
(zal-SIGH-tuh-been)
Hivid

Pharmacologic class: nucleoside analogue
Therapeutic class: antiviral
Pregnancy risk category: C

How supplied
Tablets: 0.375 mg, 0.75 mg

Pharmacokinetics
Absorption: mean absolute bioavailability is above 80%. Administering drug with food decreases rate and extent of absorption.
Distribution: enters CNS.
Metabolism: doesn't appear to undergo significant hepatic metabolism; phosphorylation to active form occurs within cells.
Excretion: excreted primarily in urine.
Half-life: 2 hours.

Route	Onset	Peak	Duration
P.O.	Unknown	1-2 hr	Unknown

Pharmacodynamics
Chemical effect: inhibits replication of HIV by blocking viral DNA synthesis.
Therapeutic effect: reduces symptoms associated with advanced HIV infection.

Indications and dosage
▶ **Advanced HIV infection (CD4+ T-cell count below 300 cells/mm³) in patients who have demonstrated significant clinical or immunologic deterioration.** *Adults and children age 13 or older weighing at least 30 kg (66 lb):* 0.75 mg P.O. q 8 hours. Drug must be taken with zidovudine 200 mg P.O. q 8 hours.

Adverse reactions
CNS: *peripheral neuropathy, headache, fatigue,* dizziness, confusion, *seizures,* impaired concentration, amnesia, insomnia, depression, tremors, hypertonia, asthenia, agitation, abnormal thinking, anxiety.
CV: cardiomyopathy, *heart failure,* chest pain.
EENT: pharyngitis, cough, ocular pain, abnormal vision, ototoxicity, nasal discharge.
GI: nausea, vomiting, diarrhea, abdominal pain, anorexia, constipation, stomatitis, esophageal ulcer, glossitis, *pancreatitis.*
Hematologic: anemia, *neutropenia, leukopenia, thrombocytopenia.*
Hepatic: increased liver function tests.

Metabolic: hypoglycemia.
Musculoskeletal: myalgia, arthralgia.
Skin: pruritus; night sweats; *erythematous, maculopapular, or follicular rash;* urticaria.
Other: *fever.*

Interactions

Drug-drug. *Aminoglycosides, amphotericin B, foscarnet, other drugs that may impair kidney function:* increased risk of nephrotoxicity. Avoid concomitant use.
Antacids: decreased zalcitabine absorption. Administer separately.
Antacids containing aluminum or magnesium: decreased bioavailability of zalcitabine. Do not use together.
Chloramphenicol, cisplatin, dapsone, disulfiram, ethionamide, glutethimide, gold salts, hydralazine, iodoquinol, isoniazid, metronidazole, nitrofurantoin, phenytoin, ribavirin, and vincristine as well as other drugs that can cause peripheral neuropathy: increased risk of peripheral neuropathy. Avoid concomitant use.
Cimetidine, probenecid: increased serum zalcitabine levels. Monitor patient carefully.
Pentamidine: increased risk of pancreatitis. Avoid concomitant use.
Drug-food. *Any food:* decreased rate of absorption. Give drug on empty stomach.

Contraindications and precautions

• Contraindicated in patients with hypersensitivity to drug or its components.
• Use with extreme caution in patients with preexisting peripheral neuropathy.
• Use cautiously in patients with renal impairment (creatinine clearance below 55 ml/minute) because they may be at increased risk for toxicity to drug.
• Also use cautiously in patients with hepatic failure. In clinical trials, drug regimen (zalcitabine plus zidovudine) exacerbated hepatic dysfunction in patients with preexisting hepatic impairment.
• Additionally, use cautiously in patients with history of pancreatitis. Rarely, pan-creatitis has been fatal in patients receiving zalcitabine. In patients receiving zalcitabine as only treatment, pancreatitis was rare (less than 1%).
• Use cautiously in patients with baseline cardiomyopathy or history of heart failure.
• Safety of drug in children under age 13 and in pregnant women has not been established.

NURSING CONSIDERATIONS

🔍 Assessment
• Assess patient's condition before therapy and regularly thereafter.
• Assess for signs of peripheral neuropathy, characterized by numbness and burning in extremities, the major toxicity resulting from drug.
• Be alert for adverse reactions and drug interactions.
• Evaluate patient's and family's knowledge of drug therapy.

🔩 Nursing diagnoses
• Infection related to presence of HIV
• Sensory or perceptual alterations (tactile) related to drug-induced peripheral neuropathy
• Knowledge deficit related to drug therapy

▷ Planning and implementation
• Know that dosage adjustments are necessary in patient with moderate to severe renal failure.
• Don't administer drug with food because it decreases rate and extent of absorption.
• Notify doctor if signs and symptoms of peripheral neuropathy occur. If drug isn't withdrawn, peripheral neuropathy can progress to sharp, shooting pain or severe continuous burning pain requiring opioid analgesics. It may or may not be reversible.
• If patient experiences symptoms that resemble peripheral neuropathy, prepare to withdraw drug. Drug should be discon-

tinued if symptoms are bilateral and persist beyond 72 hours. If symptoms persist or worsen beyond 1 week, drug should be permanently discontinued. If all findings relevant to peripheral neuropathy have resolved to minor symptoms, drug may be reintroduced at 0.375 mg P.O. q 8 hours, as ordered.

• If zalcitabine is discontinued because of toxicity, be aware that patient should resume recommended dose for zidovudine (100 mg q 4 hours).

Patient teaching
• Make sure patient understands that drug doesn't cure HIV infection and that opportunistic infections may occur despite continued use. Review safe sex practices with patient.
• Inform patient that peripheral neuropathy is the major toxicity associated with this drug and that pancreatitis is the major life-threatening toxicity. Review signs and symptoms of these adverse reactions, and instruct patient to call doctor promptly if they appear.
• Instruct female patient of childbearing age to use effective contraceptive during drug therapy.

☑ **Evaluation**
• Patient responds well to drug.
• Patient does not develop peripheral neuropathy.
• Patient and family state understanding of drug therapy.

zidovudine (azidothymidine, AZT)
(zigh-DOH-vyoo-deen)
Apo-Zidovudine♦, Novo-AZT♦, Retrovir

Pharmacologic class: thymidine analogue
Therapeutic class: antiviral
Pregnancy risk category: C

How supplied
Capsules: 100 mg
Syrup: 50 mg/5 ml

Injection: 10 mg/ml

Pharmacokinetics
Absorption: absorbed rapidly from GI tract.
Distribution: preliminary data reveal good CSF penetration; about 36% plasma protein-bound.
Metabolism: metabolized rapidly to inactive compound.
Excretion: excreted in urine. *Half-life:* 1 hour.

Route	Onset	Peak	Duration
P.O.	Unknown	0.5-1.5 hr	Unknown
I.V.	Immediate	0.5-1.5 hr	Unknown

Pharmacodynamics
Chemical effect: prevents replication of HIV by inhibiting the enzyme reverse transcriptase.
Therapeutic effect: reduces symptoms of HIV infection.

Indications and dosage
▶ **Symptomatic HIV infection, including AIDS.** *Adults and children age 12 and older:* 100 mg P.O. q 4 hours. *Children ages 3 months to 12 years:* 180 mg/m^2 P.O. q 6 hours (720 mg/m^2/day), not to exceed 200 mg q 6 hours.
▶ **Selected patients with AIDS or advanced AIDS-related complex (ARC) who have history of *Pneumocystis carinii* pneumonia or CD4+ lymphocyte count below 200 cells/mm^3.** *Adults:* 1 to 2 mg/kg I.V. infused over 1 hour q 4 hours around the clock, followed by 200 mg P.O. q 4 hours around the clock when P.O. administration can replace parenteral administration.
▶ **Asymptomatic HIV infection.** *Adults and children age 12 and older:* 100 mg P.O. q 4 hours while awake (500 mg daily). *Children ages 3 months to 12 years:* 180 mg/m^2 P.O. q 6 hours (720 mg/m^2/day), not to exceed 200 mg q 6 hours.
▶ **To reduce risk of transmission of HIV from infected mother with baseline CD4+ lymphocyte counts greater**

than 200 cells/mm³ to neonate. *Adults:*
100 mg P.O. q 4 hours while awake (total
of five doses daily) given initially between 14 and 34 weeks' gestation and
continued throughout pregnancy. During
labor, give loading dose of 2 mg/kg, followed by infusion of 1 mg/kg/hour until
delivery. *Infants:* 2 mg/kg P.O. (syrup) q
6 hours for 6 weeks starting 12 hours after birth.

Adverse reactions

CNS: *asthenia, headache, seizures,*
paresthesias, *malaise,* insomnia, *dizzi-
ness,* somnolence.
EENT: taste perversion.
GI: *nausea, anorexia, abdominal pain,
vomiting,* constipation, *diarrhea,* dyspep-
sia.
Hematologic: *severe bone marrow sup-
pression (resulting in anemia), agranu-
locytosis, thrombocytopenia.*
Hepatic: increased liver enzymes.
Metabolic: lactic acidosis.
Musculoskeletal: myalgia.
Skin: *rash.*
Other: diaphoresis, *fever.*

Interactions

Drug-drug. *Acetaminophen, aspirin, indomethacin:* may impair hepatic metabolism of zidovudine, increasing drug's toxicity. Avoid concomitant use.
Acyclovir: possible seizures, lethargy,
and fatigue. Use together cautiously.
*Amphotericin B, dapsone, flucytosine,
pentamidine:* increased risk of nephrotoxicity and bone marrow suppression.
Monitor patient closely.
Fluconazole, methadone, valproic acid:
increased zidovudine concentration.
Monitor for toxicity.
Ganciclovir: increased risk and hematologic toxicity. Monitor patient.
Other cytotoxic drugs: additive adverse
effects on bone marrow. Avoid concomitant use.
Probenecid: may decrease renal clearance of zidovudine. Avoid concomitant
use.

Ribavirin: antagonizes antiviral activity of
zidovudine against HIV. Use cautiously.

Contraindications and precautions

• Contraindicated in patients with hypersensitivity to drug.
• Use cautiously and with close monitoring in patients with advanced symptomatic HIV infection and in those with severe bone marrow depression.
• Use with caution in patients with hepatomegaly, hepatitis, or other known
risk factors for hepatic disease.

NURSING CONSIDERATIONS

⚗ Assessment
• Assess patient's condition before therapy and regularly thereafter.
• Monitor blood studies every 2 weeks,
as ordered, to detect anemia or agranulocytosis.
• Be alert for adverse reactions and drug
interactions.
• Evaluate patient's and family's knowledge of drug therapy.

⊕ Nursing diagnoses
• Infection related to presence of HIV
• Altered protection related to drug-
induced adverse hematologic reactions
• Knowledge deficit related to drug
therapy

▶ Planning and implementation
• Be aware that zidovudine has been
shown to temporarily decrease morbidity
and mortality in certain patients with
AIDS or ARC.
• Know that optimum duration of treatment as well as dosage for optimum effectiveness and minimum toxicity are not
yet known.
P.O. use: Follow normal protocol.
I.V. use: Dilute drug before use. Remove
calculated dose from vial; add to D₅W to
achieve concentration that does not exceed 4 mg/ml.

–Infuse drug over 1 hour at constant rate; give every 4 hours around the clock. Avoid rapid infusion or bolus injection.
– Adding mixture to biological or colloidal fluids (for example, blood products, protein solutions) is not recommended.
– After drug is diluted, solution is physically and chemically stable for 24 hours at room temperature and for 48 hours if refrigerated at 35.6° to 46. 4° F (2° to 8° C) to minimize risk of microbial contamination. Store undiluted vials at 59° to 77° F (15° to 25° C) and protect them from light.
• Notify doctor of abnormal hematologic study results. Patient may require dosage reduction or temporary discontinuation of drug.
Patient teaching
• Advise patient that blood transfusions may be needed during treatment. Drug often causes low RBC count.
• Stress importance of compliance with every-4-hour dosage schedule. Suggest ways to avoid missing doses, perhaps by using an alarm clock.
• Warn patient not to take other drugs for AIDS (especially those available on street) unless approved by doctor. Some purported AIDS cures may interfere with drug's effectiveness.
• Advise pregnant, HIV-infected women that drug therapy only *reduces* risk of HIV transmission to neonates. Long-term risks to infants are unknown.
• Advise health care worker who considers zidovudine prophylaxis after occupational exposure (for example, after needle-stick injury) that drug's safety and efficacy haven't been proven.

☑ **Evaluation**
• Patient exhibits reduced severity and frequency of symptoms associated with HIV infection.
• Patient does not develop complications from therapy.
• Patient and family state understanding of drug therapy.

zileuton
(zigh-LOO-tun)
Zyflo

Pharmacologic class: leukotriene inhibitor
Therapeutic class: antiasthma agent, bronchodilator
Pregnancy risk category: C

How supplied
Tablets: 600 mg

Pharmacokinetics
Absorption: rapidly absorbed.
Distribution: unknown; plasma protein-bound; well absorbed into systemic circulation.
Metabolism: by liver.
Excretion: in feces and urine. *Half-life:* mean terminal half-life is 2½ hours.

Route	Onset	Peak	Duration
P.O.	Unknown	2 hr	Unknown

Pharmacodynamics
Chemical effect: inhibits enzyme which forms leukotrienes.
Therapeutic effect: reduces inflammatory response.

Indications and dosage
▶ **Prophylaxis and chronic treatment of asthma.** *Adults and children age 12 and older:* 600 mg P.O. q.i.d.

Adverse reactions
CNS: *headache,* asthenia, dizziness, insomnia, nervousness, somnolence, malaise.
CV: chest pain.
EENT: conjunctivitis.
GI: dyspepsia, nausea, abdominal pain, constipation, flatulence, vomiting.
GU: urinary tract infection, vaginitis.
Hematologic: *leukopenia.*
Hepatic: elevated liver enzymes.
Musculoskeletal: myalgia, arthralgia, hypertonia, neck pain and rigidity.
Skin: pruritus.

Reactions may be *common*, uncommon, **life-threatening**, or COMMON AND LIFE-THREATENING.

Other: pain, accidental injury, fever, lymphadenopathy.

Interactions

Drug-drug. *Propranolol, other beta blockers:* increased beta blocker effect. Monitor and reduce dosage as needed. *Theophylline:* lowers theophylline clearance. Reduce theophylline dose, as ordered, and monitor serum levels. *Warfarin:* increased PT. Monitor PT and INR, and adjust dosage of anticoagulant, as ordered.

Contraindications and precautions

• Contraindicated in patients with active liver disease, transaminase levels at least three times upper normal limit, or known hypersensitivity to drug.
• Use cautiously in patients with hepatic impairment or history of heavy alcohol use.

NURSING CONSIDERATIONS

Assessment
• Obtain baseline and periodic liver enzyme levels, as ordered.
• Evaluate patient's and family's understanding of drug therapy.

Nursing diagnoses
• Altered health maintenance related to underlying condition
• Knowledge deficit related to drug therapy

Planning and implementation
• Know that drug is not indicated for reversing bronchospasm in acute asthma attack.
• Safety and effectiveness in children under age 12 not established.
Patient teaching
• Tell patient to keep taking drug even if symptoms disappear.
• Warn patient not to use drug for an acute asthma attack.
• Advise patient to continue taking other antiasthma drugs, as ordered.

• Instruct patient to notify doctor if a short-acting bronchodilator doesn't relieve symptoms.
• Tell patient of need to regularly check liver enzyme levels.
• Tell patient to notify doctor at once if signs of liver dysfunction occur.
• Tell patient to avoid alcohol during therapy and to consult doctor before taking OTC or new prescription drugs.

Evaluation
• Patient exhibits improvement in underlying condition.
• Patient and family state understanding of drug therapy.

zolmitriptan
(zohl-muh-TRIP-tan)
Zomig

Pharmacologic class: selective 5-hydroxytryptamine receptor agonist
Therapeutic class: antimigraine
Pregnancy risk category: C

How supplied
Tablets: 2.5 mg, 5 mg

Pharmacokinetics
Absorption: well absorbed following oral administration with an absolute bioavailability of 40%.
Distribution: 25% bound to plasma protein.
Metabolism: converted to active N-desmethyl metabolite.
Excretion: about 65% of dose is recovered in the urine (8% unchanged) and 30% in feces. *Half-life:* 3 hours.

Route	Onset	Peak	Duration
P.O.	Unknown	2 hr	3 hr

Pharmacodynamics
Chemical effect: selective serotonin receptor agonist that can abort migraine headaches by causing constriction of cra-

nial blood vessels and inhibition of pro-inflammatory neuropeptide release. *Therapeutic effect:* relieves migraine headache pain.

Indications and dosage

▶ **Treatment of acute migraine headaches.** *Adults:* initially, 2.5 mg or lower P.O. increased to 5 mg per dose p.r.n. If headache returns after initial dose, second dose may be administered after 2 hours. Maximum dosage is 10 mg in 24-hour period.

Adverse reactions

CNS: somnolence, vertigo, *dizziness,* syncope, hyperesthesias, paresthesia, warm or cold sensations, asthenia, sweating.
CV: pain or heaviness in chest, *arrhythmias,* hypertension, *pain, tightness, or pressure in the neck, throat, or jaw.*
GI: dry mouth, dyspepsia, dysphagia, nausea.
Musculoskeletal: myalgia.

Interactions

Drug-drug. *Cimetidine:* doubles half-life of zolmitriptan. Monitor patient.
Ergot-type or ergot-containing drugs 5HT₁ agonists: may cause additive vasospastic reactions. Avoid concomitant use.
Fluoxetine, fluvoxamine, paroxetine, sertraline: may cause weakness, hyperreflexia, and incoordination. Use cautiously.
MAO inhibitors: increased effects of drug. Avoid concomitant use.

Contraindications and precautions

• Contraindicated in patients with ischemic heart disease or other significant heart disease (including Wolff-Parkinson-White syndrome), uncontrolled hypertension, or hypersensitivity to drug. Don't give drug within 24 hours of 5HT₁ agonists, ergot- containing or ergot-type drugs. Concurrent administration of MAO inhibitor therapy or use of zolmitriptan within 2 weeks of discontinuing MAO inhibitor is also contraindicated.
• Use cautiously in patients with liver disease.
• Drug is not intended for prophylactic therapy of migraine headaches or for use in hemiplegic or basilar migraines.
• Safety has not been established for cluster headaches.
• Don't administer to female patient who is or may be pregnant or one who is breast-feeding.

NURSING CONSIDERATIONS

Assessment
• Assess patient's history of migraine headaches and drug's effectiveness.
• Assess patient for history of known coronary artery disease, hypertension, arrhythmias, or presence of risk factors for coronary artery disease.
• Monitor liver function tests prior to initiating drug therapy and report abnormalities.
• Know that drug should only be used when a clear diagnosis of migraine has been established.
• Evaluate patient's and family's knowledge of drug therapy.

Nursing diagnoses
• Pain related to presence of migraine headache
• Altered cardiopulmonary tissue perfusion related to drug-induced adverse cardiac events
• Knowledge deficit related to drug therapy

Planning and implementation
• Know that a lower dose is indicated in patients with moderate to severe hepatic impairment as ordered.
• Don't give drug for prophylactic therapy of migraine headaches or for use in hemiplegic or basilar migraines or for cluster headaches.

Reactions may be *common,* uncommon, *life-threatening,* or COMMON AND LIFE-THREATENING.

• Don't administer drug within 24 hours of ergot-containing drugs or within 2 weeks of discontinuing MAO inhibitor therapy.

Patient teaching
• Tell patient that drug is intended to relieve the symptoms of migraines, not to prevent them.
• Advise patient to take drug as prescribed. Do not take a second dose unless instructed by doctor. Tell patient that if a second dose is indicated and permitted, to only take it 2 hours after initial dose.
• Advise patient to report pain or tightness in chest or throat, heart throbbing, rash, skin lumps, or swelling of face, lips or eyelids immediately.
• Tell female patient not to take drug if pregnancy is being planned or is suspected.

☑ **Evaluation**
• Patient has relief from migraine headache.
• Patient does not experience pain or tightness in the chest or throat, arrhythmias, increases in blood pressure, or MI.
• Patient and family state understanding of drug therapy.

---

zolpidem tartrate
(ZOHL-peh-dim TAR-trayt)
Ambien

Pharmacologic class: imidazopyridine
Therapeutic class: hypnotic
Controlled substance schedule: IV
Pregnancy risk category: B

How supplied
Tablets: 5 mg, 10 mg

Pharmacokinetics
Absorption: absorbed rapidly from GI tract. Food delays drug absorption.
Distribution: protein-binding about 92.5%.
Metabolism: metabolized in liver.

Excretion: excreted primarily in urine.
Half-life: 2.6 hours.

Route	Onset	Peak	Duration
P.O.	Rapid	0.5-2 hr	Unknown

Pharmacodynamics
Chemical effect: interacts with one of three identified GABA-benzodiazepine (gamma-aminobutyric acid benzodiazepine) receptor complexes but isn't a benzodiazepine. It exhibits hypnotic activity, but no muscle relaxant or anticonvulsant properties.
Therapeutic effect: promotes sleep.

Indications and dosage
► **Short-term management of insomnia.** *Adults:* 10 mg P.O. h.s. *In elderly or debilitated patients and in patients with hepatic insufficiency:* 5 mg P.O. h.s. Maximum daily dosage is 10 mg.

Adverse reactions
CNS: daytime drowsiness, lightheadedness, abnormal dreams, amnesia, dizziness, *headache,* hangover effect, sleep disorder, lethargy, depression.
CV: palpitations.
EENT: sinusitis, pharyngitis, dry mouth.
GI: nausea, vomiting, diarrhea, dyspepsia, constipation, abdominal pain.
Musculoskeletal: back or chest pain, myalgia, arthralgia.
Skin: rash.
Other: flulike symptoms, hypersensitivity reactions.

Interactions
Drug-drug. *CNS depressants:* enhanced CNS depression. Use together cautiously.
Drug-food. *Any food:* decreased rate and extent of absorption. Take drug on an empty stomach.
Drug-lifestyle. *Alcohol use:* excessive CNS depression. Avoid concomitant use.

Contraindications and precautions
• No known contraindications.

• Drug is not recommended for use in breast-feeding women.
• Use cautiously in patients with diseases or conditions that could affect metabolism or hemodynamic responses and in those with compromised respiratory status because hypnotics may depress respiratory drive. Also use cautiously in patients with depression or history of alcohol or drug abuse and in pregnant women.
• Safety of drug has not been established in children.

NURSING CONSIDERATIONS

⊠ Assessment
• Assess patient's condition before therapy and regularly thereafter.
• Be alert for adverse reactions and drug interactions.
• Evaluate patient's and family's knowledge of drug therapy.

⊞ Nursing diagnoses
• Sleep pattern disturbance related to presence of insomnia
• Risk for injury related to drug-induced adverse CNS reactions
• Knowledge deficit related to drug therapy

▶ Planning and implementation
• Drug has a rapid onset of action and should be given when patient is ready to go to bed.
• Be aware that hypnotics should be used only for short-term management of insomnia, usually 7 to 10 days. Persistent insomnia may indicate primary psychiatric or medical disorder.
• Know that because most adverse reactions are dose-related, smallest effective dose should be used in all patients, especially elderly or debilitated patient.
• Administer at least 1 hour before meals or 2 hours after meals.
Patient teaching
• Tell patient to take drug immediately before going to bed.

• For faster sleep onset, instruct patient not to take drug with or immediately after meals. Food decreases drug's absorption.
• Caution patient about performing activities that require mental alertness or physical coordination. For inpatient, supervise walking and raise bed rails, particularly for elderly patient.

☑ Evaluation
• Patient states that drug effectively promotes sleep.
• Patient does not experience injury from adverse CNS reactions.
• Patient and family state understanding of drug therapy.

Herbal
Medicines

HERBAL MEDICINES

aloe
(AH-loh)
aloe vera, Barbados aloe, Cape aloe, Curacao aloe, lily of the desert

Common forms

In capsules or as cream, hair conditioner, jelly, juice, liniment, lotion, ointment, shampoo, skin cream, soap, sunscreen, and in facial tissues. Also as an ingredient in Benzoin Compound Tincture.
Capsules: 75 mg, 100 mg, 200 mg aloe vera extract or aloe vera powder
Gel: 98%, 99.5%, 99.6% aloe vera gel
Juice: 99.6%, 99.7% aloe vera juice

Actions

When taken internally, aloin produces a metabolite that irritates the large intestines and stimulates colonic activity. It also causes active secretion of fluids and electrolytes and inhibits reabsorption of fluids from the colon, resulting in a feeling of distention and increased peristalsis. The cathartic effect occurs 8 to 12 hours after ingestion.

When taken externally, besides acting as a moisturizer on burns and other wounds, aloe reduces inflammation. Its antipruritic effect may result from blockage of the conversion of histidine to histamine. Wound healing may result from increased blood flow to the wound area.

Reported uses

Used externally as a topical gel for minor burns, sunburn, cuts, frostbite, skin irritation, and other wounds and abrasions.

Used internally as a stimulant laxative. Also to treat amenorrhea, asthma, colds, seizures, bleeding, and ulcers.

Aloe preparations also used to treat acne, AIDS, arthritis, asthma, blindness, bursitis, cancer, colitis, depression, diabetes, glaucoma, hemorrhoids, multiple sclerosis, peptic ulcers, and varicose veins.

Dosages

► **For pruritus, skin irritation, burns, and other wounds (external forms).** Applied liberally, p.r.n. Although internal use is not recommended, some sources suggest 100 to 200 mg aloe or 50 to 100 mg aloe extract P.O., taken in the evening. Information about dosages for aloe juice is lacking.

Adverse reactions

GI: painful intestinal spasms, damage to intestinal mucosa (may be irreversible), harmless brown discoloration of intestinal mucous membranes, severe hemorrhagic diarrhea.
GU: kidney damage, red discoloration of urine (with frequent use), reflex stimulation of uterine musculature (may cause spontaneous abortion or premature birth during late pregnancy).
Metabolic: fluid and electrolyte loss (with frequent use); loss of potassium from intestine, leading to reduced serum potassium.
Skin: contact dermatitis, delayed healing of deep wounds (with topical use).
Other: accumulation of blood in the pelvic region (with large doses), death (from overdose).

Interactions

Antiarrhythmics, cardiac glycosides, loop diuretics, other potassium-wasting drugs, steroids, thiazides: increased effects when aloe used internally. Avoid internal use of aloe when taking these drugs.

Contraindications and precautions

● External aloe preparations contraindicated in patients known to be hypersensitive to aloe or in those with history of allergic

This section on herbal medicines is adapted from Fetrow, C.W., and Avila, J.R. *Professional's Handbook of Complementary & Alternative Medicines.* Springhouse, Pa.: Springhouse Corporation, 1999.

reactions to plants in the Liliaceae family (such as garlic, onions, and tulips).
• Internal use contraindicated in menstruating, pregnant, or breast-feeding women, in children, and in patients with cardiac or kidney disease (because of risk of hypokalemia and disturbance of cardiac rhythm).

NURSING CONSIDERATIONS

• Know that oral use can cause severe abdominal discomfort and serious hypokalemia and electrolyte imbalance.
• Be aware that unapproved use of aloe vera injections for cancer has been associated with death.
• Know that use of injectable aloe vera preparations or chemical constituents of aloe vera is not recommended.
Patient teaching
• Caution patient against use of aloe vera gel or aloe vera juice for internal use.

angelica
(an-JEL-ih-kah)
angelica root, angelique, dong quai, garden angelica, tang-kuei, wild angelica

Common forms

Fluid extract, tincture, essential oil, or cut, dried, or powdered root.

Actions

Root extracts may have antitumor properties in animals; may also have anti-inflammatory and analgesic actions.

Isolated substances extracted from the root inhibit platelet aggregation, exert antimicrobial action, and decrease myocardial injury and the incidence of PVCs and arrhythmias induced by myocardial reperfusion.

Improved pulmonary function and decreased mean arterial pulmonary pressures occurred when compounds were used with nifedipine in patients with chronic obstructive pulmonary disease and pulmonary hypertension.

Reported uses

Used to treat gynecologic disorders, postmenopausal symptoms, menstrual discomfort, regulation of the menstrual cycle, and anemia. Also used to treat headaches and backaches, improve circulation in the extremities, and relieve osteoporosis, hay fever, asthma, and eczema.

Dosages

No consensus exists.

Adverse reactions

CV: hypotension.
Skin: photodermatitis, phototoxicity.
Other: increased risk of bleeding (when used with drugs such as heparin or warfarin).

Interactions

Warfarin: significantly prolonged PT when administered with warfarin. Avoid concomitant use.

Contraindications and precautions

• Contraindicated in pregnant or breast-feeding women because of potential stimulant effects on the uterus.
• Use cautiously in diabetic patients because various species of this plant contain polysaccharides that may disrupt blood glucose control.

NURSING CONSIDERATIONS

• Monitor patients taking angelica for signs of bleeding—especially those already receiving anticoagulants.
Patient teaching
• Advise patient that using angelica poses a cancer risk.
• Warn patient to watch for signs of allergic reactions to this plant and to report such reactions promptly to doctor.
• Advise patient to take precautions against direct sun exposure while taking angelica preparations.

bilberry
(BIL-beh-ree)
bilberries, bog bilberries, European
blueberries, huckleberries, whortleberries

Common forms

Capsules: 60 mg, 80 mg, 120 mg,
450 mg
Also available in liquid, tincture, fluid extract, and dried root, leaves, and berries.

Actions

May reduce vascular permeability and tissue edema. Also may aid blood flow. Exerts potent antioxidant effects and a protective effect on low-density lipoproteins.

Chemical components of bilberry may exert changes in the retina, allowing better adaptation to darkness and light, decrease excessive platelet aggregation, and exert preventative and curative antiulcer actions.

Reported uses

Used to treat visual and circulatory problems, glaucoma, cataracts, diabetic retinopathy, macular degeneration, varicose veins, and hemorrhoids. Also used to improve night vision.

Dosages

Suggested dosages vary considerably. Most herbalists recommend using standardized products consisting of 25% anthocyanoside content.
▶ **To improve night vision.** 60 to 120 mg of bilberry extract P.O. daily.
▶ **For visual and circulatory problems.** 240 to 480 mg P.O. daily in two or three divided doses.

Adverse reactions

Other: toxic reactions. (Long-term consumption of large doses of bilberry leaves can be poisonous. Dosages of 1.5 g/kg/day or higher may be fatal.)

Interactions

Anticoagulants, other antiplatelet agents: inhibition of platelet aggregation, potentially enhancing the risk of bleeding if used concurrently. Monitor patient.
Disulfiram: disulfiram reaction if patient takes form containing alcohol. Avoid concurrent use.

Contraindications and precautions

• Contraindicated in pregnant and breast-feeding women.
• Use cautiously in patients taking anticoagulants.

NURSING CONSIDERATIONS

• Monitor for signs and symptoms of bleeding if patient is taking an anticoagulant.
Patient teaching
• Warn patient taking disulfiram not to take bilberry product containing alcohol.

capsicum
(KAP-sih-kem)
bell pepper, capsaicin, cayenne pepper,
chili pepper, hot pepper, paprika,
red pepper, tabasco pepper

Common forms

Cream: 0.025%, 0.075%, 0.25%
Gel: 0.025%
Lotion: 0.025%, 0.075%
Roll-on: 0.075%
Self-defense spray: 5%, 10%
Also available as the vegetable, pepper.

Actions

Topical capsicum produces an extremely intense irritation at the contact point. Initial dose causes profound pain; however, repeated applications cause desensitization, with analgesic and anti-inflammatory effects.

Juices from the fruits may have antibacterial properties in vitro.

Reported uses

Used to treat bowel disorders, chronic laryngitis, and peripheral vascular disease. Various preparations of capsicum are applied topically as counterirritants and external analgesics. Topical preparations also used to treat pain associated with postherpetic neuralgia, rheumatoid arthritis, osteoarthritis, diabetic neuropathy, postsurgical pain (including postmastectomy and postamputation pain), and other neuropathic pain and complex pain syndromes. Also used to treat refractory pruritus and pruritus associated with renal failure and as a nonlethal self-defense spray.

Dosages

Concentrations of topical preparations range from 0.025% to 0.25%. Preparations are most effective when applied t.i.d. or q.i.d. and have a duration of action of about 4 to 6 hours. Applications given less frequently typically result in incomplete analgesia.

Adverse reactions

Intensity of adverse reactions is dose- and concentration-dependent.
EENT: blepharospasm, extreme burning pain, lacrimation, conjunctival edema, hyperemia, burning pain in nose, sneezing, serous discharge. (Ocular complications rare; usually because of eye rubbing.)
GI: discomfort (minimized if seeds are removed before ingestion).
Respiratory: transient bronchoconstriction, cough, retrosternal discomfort.
Skin: transient skin irritation, itching, stinging, erythema without vesicular eruption (diminishes with repeated use).

Interactions

Centrally acting adrenergic agents: may reduce effectiveness of antihypertensives such as clonidine or methyldopa. Avoid concomitant use.
MAO inhibitors: may promote toxicity (hypertensive crisis) when used together. Avoid concomitant use.

Contraindications and precautions

• Contraindicated in patients hypersensitive to capsicum or chili pepper products.
• Also contraindicated in pregnant women because of possible uterine stimulant effects.

NURSING CONSIDERATIONS

• Know that, after topical application, relief occurs as early as 3 days, but may take as long as 14 to 28 days, depending on the condition requiring analgesia.
• Know that here is no evidence that topical application causes permanent neurologic injury.
Patient teaching
• Tell patient to avoid contact with eyes, mucous membranes, and broken skin.
• If incidental contact occurs, inform patient to flush exposed area with cool running water for as long as necessary.
• Caution patient taking MAO inhibitors or centrally acting adrenergics against use of this herb.
• Advise female patient to avoid use of herb during pregnancy or when breastfeeding.

cat's-claw
(KATS-klaw)
life-giving vine of Peru, samento, una de gato

Common forms

In tablets and capsules; also as teas or tinctures and the cut, dried, or powdered bark, roots, and leaves.
Tablets, capsules: 25 mg, 150 mg, 175 mg, 300 mg, 350 mg (standard extract); 400 mg, 500 mg, 800 mg, 1 g, 5 g (raw herb)

Actions

Some chemical components stimulate immune system function and exert antitumor activity. Other components may inhibit platelet aggregation and the sympathetic nervous system, reduce the heart rate, decrease peripheral vascular resistance, and lower blood pressure. They also may exhibit antiviral activity and antioxidant properties in vitro. One component has weak diuretic properties.

Reported uses

Used to treat systemic inflammatory diseases (such as arthritis and rheumatism) and inflammatory GI disorders (such as diverticulitis, gastritis, Crohn's disease, dysentery, and ulcerations). Also used as a contraceptive.

Dosages

No consensus exists. Herbal literature suggests 500 to 1,000 mg P.O. t.i.d.

Adverse reactions

CV: potential hypotension.

Interactions

Antihypertensives: may potentiate effects. Avoid concomitant use.

Contraindications and precautions

• Contraindicated in patients undergoing skin grafts and organ transplants and in those with coagulation disorders or receiving anticoagulants.
• Avoid use in pregnant or breast-feeding women; effects are unknown.

NURSING CONSIDERATIONS

• Monitor patient for signs of bleeding, such as petechiae or epistaxis, and for unusual bruising or bleeding gums.
Patient teaching
• Recommend another method of contraception if herb is being used for this purpose.
• Tell patient to rise slowly from a sitting or lying position to avoid dizziness from possible hypotension.
• Advise patient to watch for signs of bleeding, especially if anticoagulants are also being taken.

• Advise female patient to avoid use of herb during pregnancy or when breast-feeding.

chamomile
(KAH-meh-mighl)
common chamomile, English chamomile, German chamomile, Hungarian chamomile, sweet false chamomile

Common forms

As capsules, liquid, tea, and in many cosmetic products.
Capsules: 354 mg, 360 mg

Actions

Exhibits anti-inflammatory, antiallergenic, antidiuretic, sedative, antibacterial, and antifungal properties. May lower serum urea concentrations. Some compounds may stimulate liver regeneration following oral administration; others exhibit in vitro antitumor activity. One component may have antiulcer effects.

Reported uses

Used to treat stomach disorders, such as GI spasms, other GI inflammatory conditions, and insomnia because of chamomile's sedative properties. Also used to treat menstrual disorders, migraine, epidermolysis bullosa, eczema, eye irritation, throat discomfort, and hemorrhoids, and as a topical bacteriostat, sleep inducer, and mouthwash.

Dosages

Usually taken as a tea, prepared by adding 1 tablespoon (3 g) of the flower head to hot water and steeping for 10 to 15 minutes; it is then taken up to q.i.d.

Adverse reactions

EENT: allergic conjunctivitis.
GI: emesis.
Skin: contact dermatitis.
Other: anaphylaxis.

Interactions

Anticoagulants: may potentiate effects. Avoid concomitant use.
Other medications taken concurrently: potential for decreased absorption of these agents secondary to chamomile's antispasmodic activity in the GI tract. Avoid concomitant use.

Contraindications and precautions

• Avoid use in pregnant or breast-feeding women. Chamomile is believed to be an abortifacient, and some of its components have shown teratogenic effects in animals.
• Use cautiously in patients with hypersensitivity to components of volatile oils or in those at risk for contact dermatitis.

NURSING CONSIDERATIONS

• Monitor patient for allergic reactions.
Patient teaching
• Caution patient with history of allergies against use of this herb.
• Advise female patient to avoid use of herb during pregnancy or when breast-feeding.

echinacea
(eh-kih-NAY-zyah)
American cone flower, black sampson, black susans, coneflower, echinacea care liquid, Indian head

Common forms

In capsules and tablets; also as hydroalcoholic extracts, fresh-pressed juice, glycerite, lozenges, and tinctures.
Capsules: 125 mg, 355 mg (85 mg herbal extract powder), 500 mg
Tablets: 335 mg

Actions

Extract stimulates the immune system and reduces growth of bacteria responsible for vaginal infections. Components may exert local anesthetic effects and anti-inflammatory activities. Essential oil components produce a tingling sensation on the tongue. Some compounds also exhibit direct antitumor activity and insecticidal activity. Conjugates in the plant activate adrenal cortex activity. The fresh-pressed juice of the aerial portion and the extract of the roots may inhibit influenza, herpes infections, and vesicular stomatitis virus.

Reported uses

Used as a wound-healing agent for abscesses, burns, eczema, varicose ulcers of the leg and other skin wounds, and as a nonspecific immunostimulant for the supportive treatment of upper respiratory tract infections and urinary tract infections.

Dosages

Expressed juice: 6 to 9 ml P.O. daily.
Capsules containing powdered herb: equivalent to 900 mg to 1 g P.O. t.i.d.; doses can vary. *Tincture:* 0.75 to 1.5 ml (15 to 30 gtt) P.O. two to five times daily. The tincture has been given as 60 gtt P.O. t.i.d. *Tea:* 2 teaspoons (4 g) of coarsely powdered herb simmered in 1 cup of boiling water for 10 minutes. Avoid this method of administration because some active compounds are water-insoluble.

Adverse reactions

Adverse effects are uncommon. Allergic reactions may occur in patients allergic to plants belonging to the daisy family.

Interactions

None reported.

Contraindications and precautions

• Contraindicated in patients with severe illnesses such as HIV infection, collagen disease, leukosis, multiple sclerosis, and tuberculosis or other autoimmune diseases.
• Avoid use of herb in pregnant or breast-feeding women; effects are unknown.

• Know that many tinctures contain significant concentrations of alcohol (ranging from 15% to 90%) and may not be suitable for children, alcoholic patients, those with liver disease, or those taking disulfiram or metronidazole.
• Monitor for immune suppression in cases of excessive use.

Patient teaching
• Advise patient taking herb for prolonged time that overstimulation of the immune system and possible immune suppression may occur. Echinacea should not be used longer than 8 weeks; therapy lasting 10 to 14 days is probably sufficient.
• Advise patient not to delay treatment for an illness that does not resolve after taking herb.
• Advise female patient to avoid use of herb during pregnancy or when breast-feeding.

eucalyptus
(yoo-kah-LIP-tes)
fevertree, gum tree, Tasmanian blue gum

Common forms

As an oil and a lotion.

Actions

Produces a stimulant effect on nasal cold receptors. Acts as a counterirritant and causes an increase in cutaneous blood flow. Also exhibits antimicrobial, antifungal, and anti-inflammatory effects.

Reported uses

Used to relieve nasal congestion.

Dosages

▶ **For various uses.** Typical oral dosages include 0.05 to 0.2 ml (eucalyptol), 0.05 to 0.2 ml (eucalyptus oil), or 2 to 4 g (fluid extract).

▶ **For topical use.** 30 ml oil mixed with 500 ml water.

Adverse reactions

CNS, GI, and respiratory reactions may occur even with low dosages.
CNS: delirium, dizziness, seizures.
EENT: miosis.
GI: epigastric burning, nausea, vomiting.
Musculoskeletal: muscular weakness.
Respiratory: cyanosis.

Interactions

None reported.

Contraindications and precautions

• Eucalyptus oil is contraindicated in patients receiving hypoglycemic therapy and in pregnant or breast-feeding women.

• Monitor for adverse reactions, and institute seizure precautions where appropriate.

Patient teaching
• Advise patient that herb should be diluted before internal or external use.
• Advise patient to keep this agent away from children and pets.
• Advise female patient to avoid use of herb during pregnancy or when breast-feeding.

fennel
(FEN-el)
bitter fennel, carosella, common fennel, fenchel, fenouil, fenouille, sweet fennel

Common forms

Volatile oil in water: 2% (sweet fennel), 4% (bitter fennel)

Actions

May exhibit stimulant and antiflatulent properties. Fennel oil with methylparaben inhibits the growth of

Salmonella enteritidis and, to a lesser extent, *Listeria monocytogenes.*

Reported uses

Used to increase milk secretion, promote menses, facilitate birth, and increase libido.

Dosages

▶ **For GI complaints.** Herbalists recommend 0.1 to 0.6 ml P.O. of the oil daily; or 5 to 7 g of the fruit daily.

Adverse reactions

CNS: seizures.
GI: nausea, vomiting.
Respiratory: pulmonary edema (rare).
Skin: contact dermatitis, photodermatitis.
Other: tumors. (An essential oil component, estragole, caused tumors in animals.)

Interactions

None reported.

Contraindications and precautions

• Use cautiously in patients allergic to other members of the Umbelliferae family, such as celery, carrots, or mugwort.
• Avoid use in pregnant women.

NURSING CONSIDERATIONS

• Monitor patient for allergic reactions.
Patient teaching
• Inform patient that herb cannot be recommended for any use because of insufficient evidence.
• Remind patient that long-term risks of herb's use are not known.
• Advise patient to avoid sun exposure if photodermatitis occurs.
• Advise female patient to avoid use of herb during pregnancy or when breast-feeding.

feverfew
(FEE-ver-fyoo)
altamisa, bachelors' button, chamomile grande, featherfew, featherfoil, midsummer daisy

Common forms

As capsules, liquid, and tablets. The leaves are commonly used to make infusions or teas.
Capsules: 250 mg (leaf extract), 380 mg (pure leaf)

Actions

Main active ingredients may inhibit serotonin release by human platelets. Extracts of feverfew contain chemicals that inhibit activation of leukocytes and the synthesis of leukotrienes and prostaglandins.

Reported uses

Used as an antipyretic and to treat psoriasis, toothache, insect bites, rheumatism, asthma, stomachache, menstrual problems, and threatened miscarriage. Also used for migraine prophylaxis.

Dosages

▶ **For migraine treatment.** Average dosage of 543 mcg P.O. parthenolide (a component of feverfew) daily.
▶ **For migraine prophylaxis.** 25 mg of freeze-dried leaf extract P.O. daily, or 50 mg of leaf P.O. daily with food, or 50 to 200 mg of aerial parts of plant P.O. daily.

Adverse reactions

GI: mouth ulcerations (commonly with crude drug).
Other: hypersensitivity reactions, post–feverfew syndrome (withdrawal syndrome characterized by moderate to severe pain and joint and muscle stiffness).

Interactions

None reported.

Contraindications and precautions

• Contraindicated in pregnant or breast-feeding women.

NURSING CONSIDERATIONS

• Monitor patient for allergic reaction.
• Monitor for mouth ulcerations. Encourage proper oral hygiene.
• Know that feverfew potency is often based on the parthenolide content in the preparation, which is variable.
Patient teaching
• Instruct patient not to withdraw herb abruptly, but to taper its use gradually because of risk of post-feverfew syndrome.
• Assure patient that several other strategies for migraine treatment and prophylaxis exist and that these should be attempted before taking products with unknown benefits and risks.
• Remind patient to promptly report unusual signs and symptoms, such as mouth sores or skin ulcerations.

flax
(flaks)
flaxseed, linseed, lint bells, linum

Common forms

As a powder, capsules, softgel capsules, and an oil.
Softgel capsules: 1,000 mg

Actions

Decreases total cholesterol and low-density lipoprotein levels. May decrease thrombin-mediated platelet aggregation. Flax contains lignans, which may have weak estrogenic, antiestrogenic, and steroidlike activity. Diets high in flax may lower the risk of breast and other hormone-dependent cancers. Linolenic acid supplement, derived from flax, arginine, and yeast RNA, may improve weight gain in some patients with HIV.

Reported uses

Used to treat constipation, functional disorders of the colon resulting from laxative abuse, irritable bowel syndrome, and diverticulitis. Also used as a supplement to decrease the risk of hypercholesterolemia and atherosclerosis. Externally, flax has been made into a poultice and used to treat areas of local inflammation.

Dosages

▶ **For all systemic uses.** 1 to 2 tablespoons of oil or mature seeds daily in two or three divided doses. Average dosage is 1 oz of oil or mature seeds daily.
▶ **For topical use.** 30 to 50 g of flax meal applied as a hot, moist poultice or compress as needed.

Adverse reactions

Immature seedpods are especially poisonous. Overdose symptoms include, but are not limited to, shortness of breath, tachypnea, weakness, and unstable gait, progressing to paralysis and seizures.
GI: diarrhea, flatulence, nausea.

Interactions

Laxatives, stool softeners: possible increase in laxative actions of flax. Avoid concurrent use.
Oral medications taken concurrently with herb: possible diminished absorption of oral medications. Avoid taking flax and other drugs concurrently.

Contraindications and precautions

• Contraindicated in pregnant and breast-feeding women because herb's hormonal effects may cause teratogenicity or spontaneous abortion.
• Avoid use in suspected or actual ileus and in prostate cancer.

NURSING CONSIDERATIONS

• Monitor patient for potential toxicity related to oral ingestion of herb; cyanosis is a symptom of flax toxicity.

Patient teaching
• Encourage patient to drink plenty of fluids to minimize risk of flatulence.
• Instruct patient to refrigerate flaxseed oil to prevent breakdown of essential fatty acids.
• Remind patient that other cholesterol-lowering therapies exist that have been proven to improve survival and lower the risk of cardiac disease; flax has no such clinical support.
• Instruct patient never to ingest immature seeds and to keep flax away from children and pets.
• Remind patient that long-term risks of flax use are unknown.
• Tell patient to report decreased effects of other drugs being taken.

garlic
(GAR-lik)
allium, camphor of the poor, da-suan, la-suan, nectar of the gods, poor man's treacle, stinking rose

Common forms

In tablets; also as fresh bulb, antiseptic oil, fresh extract, powdered, freeze-dried garlic powder, and garlic oil (essential oil).
Tablets (garlic extract): 100 mg, 320 mg, 400 mg, 600 mg
Tablets (allicin total potential): 2 to 5 mg
Dried powder: 400 to 1,200 mg
Fresh bulb: 2 to 5 g

Actions

May exhibit antithrombotic, lipid-lowering, cholesterol-lowering, anti-tumor, and antimicrobial effects. May have hypoglycemic activity and hypotensive properties, as well as antibacterial, antifungal, larvicidal, insecticidal, amebicidal, and antiviral activities. A component in garlic oil may inhibit adenosine diphosphate–induced platelet aggrega-

tion. Also may decrease a type of carcinogen and nitrite accumulation.

Reported uses

Used to treat asthma, diabetes, inflammation, heavy metal poisoning, constipation, and athlete's foot. Also used as an antimicrobial and to improve serum lipid profiles in some patients and reduce morbidity in patients with AIDS.

Dosages

▶ **For lipid-lowering action.** 600 to 900 mg daily; or average of 4 g (fresh garlic) or 8 mg (garlic oil) daily.

Adverse reactions

CNS: dizziness.
GI: irritation of mouth, esophagus, and stomach; nausea; vomiting.
Hematologic: decreased hemoglobin production and lysis of RBCs (with chronic use or excessive dosages).
Skin: contact dermatitis, diaphoresis, hypothyroidism.
Other: allergic reactions (asthma, rash, anaphylaxis [rare]), "garlic odor."

Interactions

Anticoagulants: may increase risk of bleeding when used concomitantly. Monitor patient.
Antiplatelets: may enhance effects of antiplatelet therapy. Monitor patient.

Contraindications and precautions

• Contraindicated in patients sensitive to garlic or other members of the Lilaceae family and in those with GI disorders, such as peptic ulcer or reflux disease.
• Also contraindicated in pregnant women because of its oxytocic effects.

NURSING CONSIDERATIONS

• Perform periodic CBCs on patients taking high-dose or long-term garlic.
Patient teaching
• Advise patient that cholesterol-lowering agents are commonly used for hypercho-

lesterolemia because of their proven survival data and ability to lower cholesterol levels more effectively than garlic.

• Instruct patient to watch for signs of bleeding (bleeding gums, easy bruising, tarry stools, petechiae) if garlic supplements are taken with hemostatic agents.

• Remind patient to report such symptoms as burning of the mouth or gums, recurring heartburn, chest pain or stomach ulcer–like pain.

ginger
(JIN-jer)
zingiber

Common forms

As root, extract, liquid, powder, capsules, tablets, and teas.
Root: 530 mg
Extract: 250 mg
Liquid, powder, capsules: 100 mg, 465 mg
Tablets (chewable): 67.5 mg

Actions

Inhibits platelet aggregation induced by adenosine diphosphate and epinephrine. May exhibit anti-inflammatory and positive inotropic effects. Specific components of ginger produce varying CV effects.

Reported uses

Used as an antiemetic, GI protectant, anti-inflammatory agent useful for arthritis treatment, CV stimulant, antitumor agent, antioxidant, and as a therapy for microbial and parasitic infestations. Also used to treat morning, motion, or sea sickness; postoperative nausea and vomiting; and to provide relief from pain and swelling caused by rheumatoid arthritis, osteoarthritis, or muscular discomfort.

Dosages

Dosage forms and strengths vary with each disease state.

▶ **As an antiemetic.** 500 to 1,000 mg powdered ginger P.O., or 1,000 mg fresh ginger root P.O.

Adverse reactions

CNS: CNS depression (with overdose).
CV: arrhythmias (with overdose).

Interactions

Anticoagulants: may enhance risk of bleeding. Monitor patient.

Contraindications and precautions

• Contraindicated in pregnant women; effects are unknown.

NURSING CONSIDERATIONS

• Use only under medical supervision in patients receiving anticoagulants because ginger may affect bleeding time by inhibiting platelet function.

• Monitor patient for bleeding.

Patient teaching

• Advise female patient to avoid use of ginger during pregnancy.

• Instruct patient to watch for signs of bleeding when taking ginger.

• Explain that no consensus exists with respect to dosing and monitoring.

ginkgo
(GIN-koh)
EGB 761, GBE, GBE 24, GBX, ginkgo biloba, ginkogink, LI 1370, rokan, sophium, tanakan, tebonin

Common forms

As ginkgo biloba extract in capsules, tablets, and sublingual sprays (standardized to contain 24% flavone glycosides and 6% terpenes) and as concentrated alcoholic extract of fresh leaf.

Tablets, capsules: 30 mg, 40 mg, 60 mg, 120 mg, 260 mg, 420 mg
Capsules (ginkgo biloba extract [24% standardized extract] bound to phosphatidylcholine): 80 mg
Sublingual sprays: 15 mg/spray, 40 mg/spray

Actions

Produces arterial and venous vasoactive changes that increase tissue perfusion and cerebral blood flow. Also produces arterial vasodilation, inhibits arterial spasms, decreases capillary permeability, reduces capillary fragility, decreases blood viscosity, and reduces erythrocyte aggregation. Ginkgo biloba extract acts as an antioxidant, and ginkgolide B (a component of gingko) may be a potent inhibitor of platelet activating factor.

Reported uses

Used to treat cerebrovascular disease, peripheral vascular insufficiency, arrhythmias, asthma, impotence secondary to serotonin reuptake inhibitors, premenstrual syndrome, senile macular degeneration, hearing loss, and vestibular disorders. Also used to improve mental alertness and overall brain function.

Dosages

▶ **For dementia syndromes.** 120 to 240 mg P.O. daily in two or three divided doses.
▶ **For peripheral arterial disease, vertigo, and tinnitus.** 120 to 160 mg P.O. daily in two or three divided doses.

Adverse reactions

CNS: headache, seizures (with excessive ingestion of ginkgo seeds by children [more than 50 seeds]).
GI: diarrhea, flatulence, nausea, vomiting.
Skin: contact hypersensitivity reactions, dermatitis (if contact with fruit occurs).
Other: bleeding (subdural hematoma, hyphema [rare]).

Interactions

Anticoagulants, antiplatelets: because of its effect on platelet activating factor, use ginkgo biloba extract with careful monitoring in patients taking anticoagulant or antiplatelet medications.

Contraindications and precautions

• Contraindicated in patients with history of allergy to ginkgo preparations.
• Also contraindicated in children and pregnant women.
• Use cautiously in patients taking anticoagulant medications.

NURSING CONSIDERATIONS

• Monitor patient for bleeding or unusual bruising.
• Know that the fruit pulp and seed coats contain ginkgolic acid and bilobin, which are structurally related to the urushiols found in poison ivy, mango fruit rind, and cashew nut shells.
Patient teaching
• Advise patient to report unusual bleeding or bruising.
• Instruct patient to keep seeds out of reach of children because of potential risk of seizures with ingestion.
• Advise patient to avoid contact with the fruit pulp or seed coats because of the risk of contact dermatitis. More potent preparations may cause irritation or blistering of skin or mucous membranes if applied externally.

ginseng
(JIN-sehng)
American ginseng, Asiatic ginseng, Chinese ginseng, G115, Japanese ginseng, jintsam, Korean ginseng

Common forms

As capsules, teas, extract, root powder, whole root (by the pound), and oil.
Capsules: 100 mg, 250 mg, 500 mg

Tea bags: 1,500 mg ginseng root
Extract: 2 oz root extract (in alcohol base)
Root powder: 1 oz, 4 oz

Actions

Ginseng compounds may exert opposing effects. For example, one compound has CNS-depressant, anticonvulsant, analgesic, and antipsychotic effects and stress-ulcer preventing action. Another compound has CNS-stimulating, antifatigue, hypertensive, and stress-ulcer aggravating effects. Some components enhance cardiac performance, whereas others depress cardiac function.

Oral ginseng may reduce cholesterol and triglycerides, decrease platelet adhesiveness, impair coagulation, and increase fibrinolysis. It may also reduce stress by acting on the adrenal gland.

Extracts of ginseng may exhibit antioxidant activity.

Reported uses

Used to minimize or reduce the activity of the thymus gland. Also used as a sedative, demulcent (soothes irritated or inflamed internal tissues or organs), aphrodisiac, antidepressant, sleep aid, and diuretic. May be used to improve stamina, concentration, healing, stress-resistance, vigilance, and work efficiency and to improve "well-being" in elderly patients with debilitated or degenerative conditions.

Also used to decrease fasting blood glucose and hemoglobin A_{1c} in diabetic and nondiabetic patients, and to treat hyperlipidemia, hepatic dysfunction, and impaired cognitive function.

Dosages

Dosages vary with the disease state; usually, 0.5 to 2 g dry ginseng root daily or 200 to 600 mg ginseng extract daily, in one or two equal doses.
▶ **For improved well-being in debilitated elderly patients.** 0.4 to 0.8 g root P.O. daily on a continual basis.

Adverse reactions

Ginseng abuse syndrome occurs when large doses of the herb are taken concomitantly with other psychomotor stimulants, such as tea and coffee; symptoms include diarrhea, hypertension, restlessness, insomnia, skin eruptions, depression, appetite suppression, euphoria, and edema.
CNS: headache, insomnia, nervousness.
CV: chest pain, palpitations, hypertension.
EENT: epistaxis.
GI: diarrhea, nausea, vomiting.
GU: impotence, vaginal bleeding.
Skin: pruritus, skin eruptions (with ginseng abuse).
Other: breast pain.

Interactions

Antidiabetic agents, insulin: use cautiously because of ginseng's hypoglycemic effect.
MAO inhibitors (hypericin, parnate, phenelzine, selegiline, tranylcypromine): adverse reactions including headache, tremors, mania. Avoid concomitant use.

Contraindications and precautions

● Use cautiously in patients with CV disease, hypertension, hypotension, or diabetes, and in those also receiving steroid therapy.
● Avoid use in pregnant or breast-feeding women; effects are unknown.

NURSING CONSIDERATIONS

● Monitor patient for signs and symptoms of ginseng abuse syndrome.
● Monitor diabetic patient for signs and symptoms of hypoglycemia.
Patient teaching
● Advise patient not to take ginseng for a prolonged time.
● Tell patient with preexisting medical conditions to check with doctor before taking ginseng.

• Advise diabetic patient to check glucose levels closely until effects on serum glucose are known.

• Instruct patient to watch for unusual symptoms (nervousness, insomnia, palpitations, diarrhea) because of risk of ginseng toxicity.

• Advise pregnant or breast-feeding patient to consult doctor before taking ginseng because safety has not been established.

goldenseal
(GOHL-den-seel)
eye balm, eye root, goldsiegel, ground raspberry, Indian dye, Indian turmeric, jaundice root

Common forms

In capsules and tablets; also as ethanol and water extracts, dried ground root powder, tinctures, and teas.
Capsules, tablets: 250 mg, 350 mg, 400 mg, 404 mg, 470 mg, 500 mg, 535 mg, 540 mg

Actions

May have astringent, anti-inflammatory, oxytocic, antihemorrhagic, and laxative properties. Inhibits muscular contractions.

Decreases the anticoagulant effect of heparin and acts as a cardiac stimulant (at lower dosages), increases coronary perfusion, and inhibits cardiac activity (at higher dosages). May exhibit antipyretic activity (greater than aspirin) and antimuscarinic, antihistaminic, antitumor, antimicrobial, antiparasitic, and hypotensive effects.

Causes vasoconstriction and produces significant changes in blood pressure.

Reported uses

Used to treat GI disorders, gastritis, peptic ulceration, anorexia, postpartum hemorrhage, dysmenorrhea, eczema, pruritus, tuberculosis, cancer, mouth ulcerations, otorrhea, tinnitus, and conjunctivitis; also used as a wound antiseptic, diuretic, laxative, and anti-inflammatory agent.

Used to shorten the duration of acute *Vibrio cholera* diarrhea and diarrhea caused by some species of *Giardia, Salmonella, Shigella,* and some Enterobacteriaceae. May be used to improve biliary secretion and function in patients with hepatic cirrhosis.

Dosages

Ethanol and water extract: 250 mg P.O. t.i.d. *Dried rhizome:* 0.5 to 1 g t.i.d.

Adverse reactions

CNS: CNS depression, paralysis (with higher dosages), paresthesia, seizures.
CV: asystole, bradycardia, heart block.
GI: diarrhea, GI cramping and pain, mouth ulceration, nausea, vomiting.
Hematologic: leukocytosis.
Respiratory: respiratory depression (with high dosages).
Skin: contact dermatitis.
Other: death may be caused by large alkaloid doses. Symptoms of overdose include GI upset, nervousness, depression, exaggerated reflexes, and seizures that progress to respiratory paralysis and CV collapse.

Interactions

Alcohol, benzodiazepines, other CNS depressants: may enhance sedative effects when taken with goldenseal. Avoid use with goldenseal.
Anticoagulants: may offset the beneficial effects of therapeutic anticoagulants. Avoid concomitant use.
Antihypertensive agents: may interfere or enhance hypotensive effects when taken with goldenseal or its extracts. Don't use together.
Beta blockers, calcium channel blockers, digoxin: may enhance or interfere with the cardiac effects of these drugs. Don't use together.

Contraindications and precautions

• Contraindicated in patients with CV disease, particularly hypertension, heart failure, or arrhythmia, and in pregnant women.

NURSING CONSIDERATIONS

• Monitor patient for unusual symptoms.
• Monitor patient for signs of vitamin B deficiencies (megaloblastic anemia, peripheral neuropathy, seizures, cheilosis, glossitis, angular stomatitis, seborrheic dermatitis, and infertility).
Patient teaching
• Tell patient to avoid hazardous activities until CNS effects of the herb are known.
• Instruct patient to avoid consumption of herb because of risk of serious adverse reactions.

grapeseed; pinebark
(GRAYP-seed; PIGHN-bahrk)
muskat, Pinus maritima, Pinus nigra, Vitis coignetiae, Vitis vinifera

Common forms

Tablets, capsules: 25 mg to 300 mg

Actions

Demonstrates antilipoperoxidant activity and xanthine oxidase inhibition. Inhibits enzymes responsible for skin turnover. Extract exhibits therapeutic effects in Ehrlich ascites carcinoma and inhibits growth of *Streptococcus mutans*.

Reported uses

Used as an antioxidant to treat circulatory disorders (hypoxia from atherosclerosis, inflammation, and cardiac or cerebral infarction). Also used to treat pain, limb heaviness, and swelling in patients with peripheral circulatory disorders and to treat inflammatory conditions, varicose veins, and cancer.

Dosages

Tablets, capsules: 25 to 300 mg P.O. daily for up to 3 weeks; then, a maintenance dosage of 40 to 80 mg P.O. once daily.

Adverse reactions

None reported.

Interactions

None reported.

Contraindications and precautions

No known contraindications.

NURSING CONSIDERATIONS

• Evaluate underlying condition for which patient claims to be using herb to self-treat.
Patient teaching
• Instruct patient with a circulatory disorder not to delay seeking medical attention if signs and symptoms worsen (changes in sensation, color, or temperature of extremity).

kava
(KAH-veh)
ava, awa, kava-kava, kawa, kew, sakau, tonga, yagona

Common forms

Prepared as a drink from pulverized roots, tablets, capsules, or extract.

Actions

Components of the root may cause local anesthetic activity that is similar to cocaine but lasts longer than benzocaine. Some components show fungistatic properties against several fungi.
Induces muscular relaxation and inhibits the limbic system, an effect associated with suppression of emotional excitability and mood enhancement. Produces mild euphoria with no effect on thoughts and memory during the intoxi-

cation. Other effects include analgesia, sedation, hyporeflexia, impaired gait, and pupil dilation.

Reported uses

Used in attenuating spinal seizures and as an antipsychotic. Also used for seizure control in epileptic patients. Used to treat anxiety disorders, depression, insomnia, asthma, pain, rheumatism, venereal disease, and muscle spasms and to promote wound healing.

Dosages

▶ **For anxiety.** 90 to 110 mg dried kava extract t.i.d. *Freshly prepared kava beverages:* 400 to 900 g weekly.

Adverse reactions

CNS: changes in motor reflexes and judgment.
EENT: visual disturbances.
With chronic, heavy use:
EENT: reddened eyes.
GI: weight loss.
Hematologic: decreased platelet and lymphocyte count.
Respiratory: shortness of breath, pulmonary hypertension.
Skin: dry, flaking discolored skin.
Other: dopamine antagonism, increased patellar reflexes, reduced plasma protein, urea, and bilirubin levels.

Interactions

Alcohol use: increased kava toxicity. Avoid concomitant use.
Alprazolam: may cause coma. Avoid concomitant use.
Benzodiazepines, other CNS depressants: additive sedative effects. Avoid concomitant use.
Levodopa: increased parkinsonian symptoms. Avoid concomitant use.
Pentobarbital: may cause additive effects. Avoid concomitant use.

Contraindications and precautions

• Avoid use of herb in pregnant or breast-feeding women and in children under age 12; effects are unknown.
• Use cautiously in patients with renal disease, thrombocytopenia, or neutropenia.

NURSING CONSIDERATIONS

• Avoid concomitant use with psychotropic agents.
• Monitor patient for adverse effects with long-term use.
Patient teaching
• Inform patient that significant adverse reactions may occur with long-term use of kava.
• Tell patient to avoid alcohol and other CNS depressants while taking kava because they enhance herb's sedative and toxic effects.
• Inform patient that absorption of kava may be enhanced if taken with food.
• Advise female patient to avoid taking herb during pregnancy or when breast-feeding.

milk thistle
(MILK THIH-sel)
Carduus marianus L., Cnicus marianus, holy thistle, Lady's thistle, Marian thistle, Mary thistle, St. Mary thistle

Common forms

In capsules, tablets, and as an extract.
Capsules: 50 mg, 100 mg, 175 mg, 200 mg, 505 mg
Tablets: 85 mg (standardized to contain 80% silymarin with the flavonoid silibinin)

Actions

Exerts hepatoprotective and antihepatotoxic actions over liver toxins by altering the outer liver membrane cell structure so that toxins cannot enter the cell. Also leads to activation of the regenerative capacity of the liver through cell development.

Reported uses

Used as a liver-cleansing agent; also, extracts have been used as an antidote after the accidental ingestion of *Amanita phalloides* and other poisonous mushrooms.

Used to improve liver function test results and blunt hepatotoxicity in patients with psychotic drug–induced hepatic damage. Extracts used to treat acute and chronic liver disease and hepatitis C.

Dosages

420 to 800 mg P.O. daily as a single dose, or divided into two to three doses; or 200 to 400 mg of silymarin component P.O. daily, calculated as the silibinin component.

Adverse reactions

GI: mild laxative effect (with standardized extracts).
GU: uterine stimulant effect.

Interactions

None reported.

Contraindications and precautions

• Contraindicated in pregnant or breast-feeding women.
• Use cautiously in patients with hypersensitivity to plants belonging to the Asteraceae family.

NURSING CONSIDERATIONS

• Monitor liver function test results during therapy with milk thistle.
Patient teaching
• Advise patient to consult a medical professional specialized in liver disease before pursuing this therapy.
• Advise female patient to report planned or suspected pregnancy.
• Instruct patient to report unusual symptoms immediately.

nettle
(NEH-tel)
common nettle, greater nettle, stinging nettle

Common forms

Available as capsules and dried leaf and root extract or tincture.
Capsules: 150 mg, 300 mg

Actions

Acts primarily as a diuretic by increasing urine volume and decreasing systolic blood pressure. May stimulate uterine contractions. Extract reduces urine flow, nocturia, and residual urine.

Reported uses

Used as an antispasmodic and expectorant and to treat rheumatism, asthma, cough, and tuberculosis. Juice may be applied to the scalp to stimulate hair growth. Also used to treat nosebleeds, uterine bleeding, diabetes, gout, cancer, and eczema, and for wound healing.

Used to treat hypertension, heart failure, and urinary, bladder, and kidney disorders. Used for bladder irrigation in the treatment of prostatic adenoma and to reduce postoperative blood loss, bacteriuria, and inflammation. Used for the early treatment of BPH and for treating allergic rhinitis.

Dosages

▶ **For allergic rhinitis.** 150 to 300 mg capsules P.O. *Tea:* mix 1 to 2 teaspoons dried herb in 1 cup boiling water; take up to 2 cups daily. *Tincture:* ½ to 1 teaspoon up to b.i.d.

Adverse reactions

Skin: contact urticaria (leaves).
With internal use:
GI: diarrhea, gastric irritation, stomach irritation.
GU: decreased urine volume, oliguria.
Other: edema.

Interactions

Diuretics: may potentiate effects. Avoid concomitant use.

Contraindications and precautions

• Contraindicated in pregnant and breast-feeding women because of its diuretic and uterine stimulation properties.
• Also contraindicated in children under age 2.
• Use cautiously, and in reduced dosages, in older children and adults over age 65.

NURSING CONSIDERATIONS

• Monitor patient's urine output.
• Monitor for adverse skin reactions if leaves contact skin.
Patient teaching
• Advise patient to eat foods high in potassium, such as bananas and fresh vegetables, to replenish electrolytes lost through diuresis.
• Caution patient against self-medicating with nettle for BPH or to relieve fluid accumulation associated with heart failure without medical approval and supervision.
• Tell patient to wash thoroughly with soap and water, use antihistamines and steroid creams, and to wear heavy gloves if plant is to be handled. If rubbed against the skin, nettles can cause intense burning for up to 12 hours or more.

passion flower
(PAH-shen flow-er)
apricot vine, granadilla, Jamaican honeysuckle, maypop, passion fruit, water lemon

Common forms

As liquid extract, crude extract, tincture, dried herb, and in several homeopathic remedies.
Liquid extract: 1:1 in 25% alcohol

Tincture: 1:8 in 45% alcohol, or containing 0.7% flavonoids

Actions

Exerts both stimulatory and depressant CNS effects. May have anticonvulsant effects and may reduce spontaneous motor activity.

Reported uses

Used as a sedative and to treat nervousness.

Dosages

▶ **For Parkinson's disease.** 10 to 30 drops P.O. (0.7% flavonoids) t.i.d. *Dried herb:* 0.25 to 1 g P.O. t.i.d. *Liquid extract:* 0.5 to 1 ml P.O. t.i.d. *Tea:* 4 to 8 g (3 to 6 teaspoons) daily in divided doses. *Tincture:* 0.5 to 2 ml P.O. t.i.d.

Adverse reactions

CNS: CNS depression (with large doses).

Interactions

MAO inhibitors: may potentiate action. Monitor patient.
Other CNS depressants: possible additive effects. Use cautiously.

Contraindications and precautions

• Contraindicated in pregnant and breast-feeding women; harman alkaloids may act as a uterine stimulant.

NURSING CONSIDERATIONS

• Monitor patient for possible adverse CNS effects.
Patient teaching
• Advise female patient to report planned or suspected pregnancy.
• Advise female patient to avoid use of herb during pregnancy or when breast-feeding.
• Warn patient of potential untoward effects on alertness (sedation) if considering consumption of herb.

primrose, evening
(PRIHM-rohz, EEV-ning)
king's-cure-all

Common forms

Capsules: 50 mg, 500 mg, 1,300 mg
Gelcaps: 500 mg, 1,300 mg

Actions

Aids prostaglandin synthesis.

Reported uses

Infusion used for sedative and astringent properties. Used to treat asthmatic coughs, GI disorders, whooping cough, psoriasis, multiple sclerosis, asthma, Raynaud's disease, and Sjögren's syndrome. Poultices made with evening primrose oil may be used to speed wound healing.

Used to treat pruritic symptoms of atopic dermatitis and eczema, breast pain and tenderness associated with premenstrual syndrome, benign breast disease, and diabetic neuropathy.

Used in rheumatoid arthritis to improve patients' symptoms and reduce the need for pain medication; also to lower serum cholesterol, improve hypertension, and decrease platelet aggregation.

Also may be used to calm hyperactive children and to reduce mammary tumors from baseline size.

Dosages

The following dosages are based on a standardized gamma linoleic acid content of 8%.
▶ **For eczema.** *Adults:* 320 mg to 8 g P.O. daily. *Children ages 1 to 12:* 160 mg to 4 g P.O. daily; continue for 3 months.
▶ **For breast pain.** 3 to 4 g P.O. daily. No consensus exists for all other disorders.

Adverse reactions

CNS: headache, temporal lobe epilepsy (most common in schizophrenic patients or those taking drugs such as phenothiazines).
GI: nausea.
Skin: rash.
Other: inflammation, thrombosis, immunosuppression (may occur after use for over 1 year).

Interactions

Phenothiazines: may increase risk of seizures. Avoid concomitant use.

Contraindications and precautions

• Avoid use of herb in pregnant women; effects are unknown.
• Use cautiously, if at all, in schizophrenic patients or in those taking seizure drugs.

NURSING CONSIDERATIONS

• Monitor patient for adverse effects, especially with long-term use.
Patient teaching
• Instruct patient with seizure disorders to reconsider need to use herb.
• Caution parents to use herb for a hyperactive child only under medical supervision.

Saint John's wort
(SAYNT JAHNS WART)
amber, devil's scourge, goatweed, grace of God, Hypericum, klamath weed, St. John's wort

Common forms

As capsules, sublingual capsules, and liquid tinctures.
Capsules: 100 mg, 300 mg, 500 mg (standardized to 0.3% hypericin); 250 mg (standardized to 0.14% hypericin)

Actions

Inhibits stress-induced increase in corticotropin-releasing hormone, corticotropin, and cortisol. Also has antiviral activity, including action against retroviruses.

Reported uses

Used to treat depression, bronchial inflammation, burns, cancer, enuresis, gastritis, hemorrhoids, hypothyroidism, insect bites and stings, insomnia, kidney disorders, and scabies, and has been used as a wound-healing agent. Saint John's wort can be used to treat HIV infection; also can be used topically for phototherapy of skin diseases, including psoriasis, cutaneous T-cell lymphoma, warts, and Kaposi's sarcoma.

Dosages

▶ **For depression.** 300 mg standardized extract preparations (standardized to 0.3% hypericin) P.O. t.i.d. for 4 to 6 weeks; or 2 to 4 g tea that has been steeped in 1 to 2 cups of water for about 10 minutes and taken P.O. daily for 4 to 6 weeks.
▶ **For burns and skin lesions.** Cream applied topically; strength is not standardized.

Adverse reactions

Adverse effects are uncommon.
CNS: dizziness, restlessness, sleep disturbances.
GI: constipation, dry mouth, GI distress.
Other: allergic hypersensitivity, phototoxicity (rare).

Interactions

Alcohol use, MAO inhibitors, narcotics, OTC cold and flu medications, sympathomimetics, tyramine-containing foods: may enhance MAO inhibition activity. Avoid concurrent use.
Paroxetine: may result in sedative-hypnotic intoxication with concurrent ingestion of the herb.
Serotonergic drugs (amphetamines, serotonin reuptake inhibitors, trazodone, tricyclic antidepressants): serotonin syndrome may occur when used in combination with these agents. Use cautiously together.

Contraindications and precautions

• Contraindicated in patients with history of allergy to St. John's wort or its components.
• Avoid use in children and in pregnant or breast-feeding women; effects are unknown.

NURSING CONSIDERATIONS

• Patient's depression should be medically evaluated. Conventional therapy may be prudent for a more moderate to severe disorder.
Patient teaching
• Tell patient to purchase herbs only from a reputable source, and that products and their contents may vary among different manufacturers.
• Caution patient against using herb with alcohol and OTC cold and flu medications.
• Advise patient to take precautions against sun exposure.

saw palmetto
(SAW pal-MEH-toh)
American dwarf palm tree, cabbage palm, IDS 89, LSESR, sabal

Common forms

As tablets, capsules, teas, berries (fresh or dried), and liquid extract.

Actions

Has an anti-inflammatory effect and inhibits prolactin and growth factor–induced prostatic cell proliferation. May inhibit hormonally induced prostate enlargement.

Reported uses

Used as a mild diuretic; also used to treat genitourinary problems such as BPH and to increase sperm production, breast size, and sexual vigor.

Dosages

▶ **For BPH.** 320 mg P.O. daily in two divided doses for 3 months. Other recommendations include 1 to 2 g fresh saw palmetto berries or 0.5 to 1 g dried berry in decoction P.O. t.i.d.

Adverse reactions

CNS: headache.
CV: hypertension.
GI: abdominal pain, constipation, diarrhea, nausea.
GU: dysuria, impotence, urine retention.
Musculoskeletal: back pain.
Other: decreased libido.

Interactions

None reported.

Contraindications and precautions

• Contraindicated during pregnancy and in women of childbearing age because of herb's potential hormonal effects.
• Use cautiously in conditions other than BPH because of lack of data regarding its effects.

NURSING CONSIDERATIONS

• Obtain a baseline prostate-specific antigen (PSA) before starting treatment because of the concern that the herb causes a false-negative PSA result. However, saw palmetto probably does not alter the size of the prostate.
• Know that herb should be taken with the morning and evening meal to minimize GI effects.
Patient teaching
• Inform patient wishing to use herb for BPH symptoms to do so only after a diagnosis has been made, and on doctor's advice.
• Advise female patient to avoid use of herb during pregnancy or when breastfeeding.

• Advise patient to take herb with meals to minimize GI upset.

valerian
(veh-LEHR-ee-ehn)
all heal, amantilla, herba benedicta, katzenwurzel, phu germanicum, phu parvum

Common forms

As standardized capsules, tablets, and tinctures; also as tinctures and teas containing crude dried herb and in combination with other dietary supplements.
Standardized capsules, tablets (0.8% valerenic acid): 250 mg, 400 mg, 450 mg, 493 mg, 530 mg, 550 mg
Standardized tinctures: 2% essential oil

Actions

May exhibit a sedative effect and weak anticonvulsant and antidepressant properties. Also has antispasmodic effects on GI smooth muscle, produces coronary dilation, and has antiarrhythmic activity.

Reported uses

Used as a sedative and antispasmodic and as a daytime sedative for restlessness and tension. Also used to treat restlessness and nervous disturbances of sleep.

Dosages

The composition and purity of valerian preparations vary greatly.
▶ **For sleep disorders.** 400 to 900 mg standardized valerian extract ½ to 1 hour before bedtime. *Tea:* 2 to 3 g (1 teaspoon) of crude dried herb several times daily. *Tincture:* 3 to 5 ml (½ to 1 teaspoon) several times daily.

Adverse reactions

With acute overdose or chronic use:
CNS: excitability, headache, insomnia.
CV: cardiac disturbance.
EENT: blurred vision.

GI: nausea.
Other: hypersensitivity reactions, hepatotoxicity (from combination products containing valerian, and from overdosage averaging 2.5 g).

Interactions

Alcohol use, CNS depressants: potential additive effects. Avoid concomitant use.
Disulfiram: disulfiram reaction may occur if herbal extract or tincture contains alcohol. Avoid concomitant use.

Contraindications and precautions

• Contraindicated in patients with history of allergy to valerian.
• Avoid use in patients with hepatic impairment because of risk of hepatotoxicity.
• Avoid use in pregnant or breast-feeding women; effects are unknown.

NURSING CONSIDERATIONS

• Monitor periodic liver function tests in patients with preexisting hepatic disease or with prolonged use.
Patient teaching
• Inform patient that many extract products contain 40% to 60% alcohol and may not be appropriate for all patients.
• Warn patient taking disulfiram not to take herbal form containing alcohol.
• Counsel patient about herb's sedative effects and to avoid hazardous activities until CNS effects of herb are known.
• Advise female patient to avoid use of herb during pregnancy or when breast-feeding.
• Inform patient that safety and efficacy have not been established in children.

Appendices
and Index

Selected topical drugs

Drug	Indications and dosages	Special considerations
Antibacterial drugs		
bacitracin	▶ Topical infections, impetigo, abrasions, cuts, and minor burns or wounds. *Adults and children:* apply thin film b.i.d., t.i.d., or p.r.n., depending on severity.	● Pregnancy risk categories for antibacterial topical agents are as follows: − NR (gentamicin, neomycin) − B (clindamycin, erythromycin, metronidazole, mupirocin, silver sulfadiazine, tetracycline)
chloramphenicol	▶ Superficial skin infections. *Adults and children:* after thoroughly cleaning the skin, rub into infected area b.i.d. or t.i.d.	− C (bacitracin, chloramphenicol, mafenide, nitrofurazone) − D (tetracycline) ● Antibacterial topical agents are contraindicated in patients hypersensitive to the drugs.
clindamycin phosphate	▶ Acne vulgaris. *Adults and adolescents:* apply b.i.d., morning and evening. ▶ Bacterial vaginosis. *Adults:* 100 mg intravaginally h.s. for 7 consecutive days.	● Mafenide requires cautious use in patients with acute renal failure. ● Metronidazole requires cautious use in patients with history or evidence of blood dyscrasia; chemically related compounds are associated with blood dyscrasia.
erythromycin	▶ Inflammatory acne vulgaris. *Adults and children:* apply to affected area b.i.d.	● Mupirocin requires cautious use in patients with burns or impaired renal function.
gentamicin sulfate	▶ Superficial skin infections. *Adults and children over age 1:* rub in small amount gently t.i.d. or q.i.d., with or without gauze dressing.	● Neomycin requires cautious use in patients with extensive dermatologic conditions. ● Nitrofurazone requires cautious use in patients with known or suspected renal impairment.
mafenide acetate	▶ Adjunct treatment of second- and third-degree burns. *Adults and children:* apply ¹⁄₁₆″ thickness of cream daily or b.i.d. to clean, debrided wounds. Reapply p.r.n. to keep burned area covered.	● Mafenide and silver sulfadiazine require cautious use in patients hypersensitive to sulfonamides. ● Tetracycline requires cautious use in patients with hepatic or renal impairment.
metronidazole	▶ Acne rosacea. *Adults:* apply a thin film to affected area b.i.d., a.m. and p.m. Frequency and duration of therapy is adjusted after response is seen. ▶ Bacterial vaginosis. *Adults:* 1 applicatorful b.i.d., a.m. and p.m., for 5 days.	● Clean area before applying (if appropriate), especially areas with crusted or suppurative lesions. ● If the patient exhibits signs of hypersensitivity, withhold the drug and notify the doctor immediately.
mupirocin	▶ Impetigo. *Adults and children:* apply to affected areas t.i.d. for 1 to 2 weeks.	● Be aware that prolonged use of antibacterial drugs may result in overgrowth of nonsusceptible organisms. ● Know that some antibacterial topical agents may need to be supplemented by appropriate systemic medications for all but very superficial infections.
neomycin sulfate	▶ Prevention or treatment of superficial bacterial infections. *Adults and children:* rub into affected area one to three times daily.	*(continued)*

Drug	Indications and dosages	Special considerations

Antibacterial drugs *(continued)*

Drug	Indications and dosages	Special considerations
nitrofurazone	▶ Adjunctive treatment of second- and third-degree burns; prevention of skin allograft infection. *Adults and children:* apply directly to lesion daily or every few days, depending on severity of burn. May also be applied to dressings used to cover affected area.	• Tell the patient to clean the area well before applying (if appropriate), especially areas with crusted or suppurative lesions. • Teach the patient how to apply the prescribed drug. • Instruct the patient to avoid drug contact with the eyes and mouth.
silver sulfadiazine	▶ Prevention and treatment of wound infection in second-and third-degree burns. *Adults and children:* apply 1/16″ thickness to clean debrided burn wound daily or b.i.d.	• Tell the patient to continue using the topical agent for the full treatment period prescribed, even if his condition has improved. • Advise the patient to store the drug at room temperature, away from excessive heat.
tetracycline hydrochloride	▶ Acne vulgaris. *Adults and children over age 12:* rub generously into affected areas b.i.d. until skin is thoroughly covered. ▶ Superficial skin infections. *Adults and children:* apply to affected area once to five times daily.	• Tell the patient not to share medication with family members. • Tell the patient to notify the doctor if no improvement occurs or if his condition worsens.

Topical corticosteroids

Drug	Indications and dosages	Special considerations
alclometasone dipropionate	▶ Inflammation associated with corticosteroid-responsive dermatoses. *Adults:* apply a thin film to affected areas b.i.d. or t.i.d. Gently massage until drug disappears.	• Pregnancy risk category for topical corticosteroids is C. • Topical corticosteroids are contraindicated in patients hypersensitive to the drug or other corticosteroids. • Fluticasone propionate is also contraindicated in patients with viral, fungal, herpetic, or tubercular skin lesions.
amcinonide	▶ Inflammation associated with corticosteroid-responsive dermatoses. *Adults and children:* apply a light film to affected areas b.i.d. or t.i.d. Rub cream in gently and thoroughly until it disappears.	• Gently wash skin before applying. To prevent skin damage, rub medication in gently, leaving a thin coat. When treating hairy sites, part the hair and apply the medication directly to lesions.
betamethasone benzoate	▶ Inflammation associated with corticosteroid-responsive dermatoses. *Adults and children:* clean area; apply sparingly daily to q.i.d.	• Avoid application near eyes, mucous membranes, or in ear canal; topical corticosteroids may be safely used on the face, groin, and armpits and under the breasts.
clobetasol propionate	▶ Inflammation associated with corticosteroid-responsive dermatoses. *Adults:* apply a thin layer to affected skin areas b.i.d., in the morning and evening for a maximum of 14 days. Total dosage should not exceed 50 g weekly.	• If an occlusive dressing is ordered, don't leave it in place longer than 16 hours each day; don't use occlusive dressings on infected or exudative lesions.

Drug	Indications and dosages	Special considerations
Topical corticosteroids (continued)		

Drug	Indications and dosages	Special considerations
desonide	▶ Inflammation associated with corticosteroid-responsive dermatoses. *Adults and children:* clean area; apply sparingly b.i.d. to q.i.d.	• For patients with eczematous dermatitis whose skin may be irritated by adhesive material, hold dressings in place with gauze, elastic bandages, stockings, or stockinette.
desoximetasone	▶ Inflammation associated with corticosteroid-responsive dermatoses. *Adults and children:* clean area; apply sparingly b.i.d.	• Notify the doctor and remove occlusive dressing if fever develops. • Change dressing as ordered. • Discontinue drug and notify the doctor if skin infection, striae, or atrophy occurs.
dexamethasone dexamethasone sodium phosphate	▶ Inflammation associated with corticosteroid-responsive dermatoses. *Adults and children:* clean area; apply sparingly t.i.d. to q.i.d.	• When using an aerosol preparation around the face, cover the patient's eyes and warn against inhalation of the spray. Aerosol preparation contains alcohol and may produce irritation or burning in open lesions. Do not spray longer than 3 seconds or closer than 6″ (15 cm) to avoid freezing of tissues. Apply to dry scalp after shampooing; no need to massage medication into scalp after spraying.
diflorasone diacetate	▶ Inflammation associated with corticosteroid-responsive dermatoses. *Adults and children:* clean area; apply sparingly in a thin film. Apply daily to q.i.d. as determined by severity.	
fluocinolone acetonide	▶ Inflammation associated with corticosteroid-responsive dermatoses. *Adults and children over age 2:* clean area; apply sparingly b.i.d. to q.i.d.	• If antifungal agents or antibiotics are used concomitantly, stop corticosteroids until infection is controlled, as ordered. • Monitor the patient for systemic adverse reactions. Systemic absorption is likely with use of occlusive dressings, prolonged treatment, or extensive body-surface treatment.
fluocinonide	▶ Inflammation associated with corticosteroid-responsive dermatoses. *Adults and children:* clean area; apply sparingly b.i.d. or t.i.d.	• Avoid using plastic pants or tight-fitting diapers on treated areas in young children. Children may absorb larger amounts of drug and be more prone to systemic toxicity.
flurandrenolide	▶ Inflammation associated with corticosteroid-responsive dermatoses. *Adults and children:* clean area; apply sparingly daily to q.i.d. Apply Cordran tape q 12 hours.	• To prevent recurrence, continue treatment for a few days after lesions clear, as ordered. • Know that repeated application for some topical corticosteroids results in diminished effectiveness.
fluticasone propionate	▶ Inflammation associated with corticosteroid-responsive dermatoses. *Adults:* apply sparingly to affected area b.i.d. and rub in gently and completely.	• Stop drug and notify the doctor if the patient develops signs of systemic absorption, skin irritation or ulceration, hypersensitivity, or infection.
halcinonide	▶ Inflammation associated with corticosteroid-responsive dermatoses. *Adults and children:* clean area; apply sparingly b.i.d. or t.i.d.	• Know that the elderly patient is more likely to develop purpura and skin lacerations and should be monitored closely.

(continued)

Drug	Indications and dosages	Special considerations

Topical corticosteroids (continued)

halobetasol propionate	▶ Inflammation associated with corticosteroid-responsive dermatoses. *Adults:* apply sparingly to affected area once daily or b.i.d. and rub in gently and completely. Treatment beyond 2 consecutive weeks is not recommended. Total dosage should not exceed 50 g weekly.	• Be aware that when betamethasone dipropionate is dispensed as Diprolene or Diprolene AF, generic substitution should not be given because other products have different potencies. • Instruct the patient how to apply the drug. Know that children are more likely to develop adrenal suppression, Cushing's syndrome, intracranial hypertension, and growth retardation with improper use of the drug. Ensure that the parents or child (if applying the drug) fully understand frequency and how to apply the drug correctly.
hydrocortisone hydrocortisone acetate hydrocortisone butyrate hydrocortisone valerate	▶ Inflammation associated with corticosteroid-responsive dermatoses; adjunctive topical management of seborrheic dermatitis of scalp. *Adults and children:* clean area; apply cream, gel, lotion, ointment, or topical solution sparingly daily to q.i.d. Spray aerosol onto affected area daily until acute phase is controlled; then reduce dosage to one to three times weekly as needed. ▶ Inflammation associated with proctitis. *Adults:* 1 applicatorful of rectal foam P.R. daily or b.i.d. for 2 to 3 weeks, then every other day as necessary.	• Teach the patient how to apply an occlusive dressing, if ordered. Tell the patient not to leave it on each day for longer than 16 hours and to stop the drug and notify the doctor if a fever occurs. • Tell the patient to stop the drug and notify the doctor if signs of systemic absorption, skin irritation or ulceration, hypersensitivity, or infection occur. • Stress importance of using the drug exactly as directed and not to exceed frequency of application or dosage.
mometasone furoate	▶ Inflammation associated with corticosteroid-responsive dermatoses. *Adults:* apply to affected areas once daily.	• Tell the breast-feeding woman not to apply a topical corticosteroid preparation to her breast before breast-feeding. • If a dose is missed, instruct the patient to apply the drug as soon as possible. However, if it almost time for the next dose, he should skip the missed dose and resume the normal dosing schedule to avoid double dosing.
triamcinolone acetonide	▶ Inflammation associated with corticosteroid-responsive dermatoses. *Adults and children:* clean area; apply cream, lotion, or ointment sparingly b.i.d. to q.i.d., or spray b.i.d. or q.i.d ▶ Inflammation associated with oral lesions. *Adults and children:* apply paste h.s. and, if needed, b.i.d. or t.i.d., preferably after meals. Apply a small amount without rubbing and press to lesion in mouth until a thin film develops.	• Warn the patient that some forms of topical corticosteroids contain alcohol and may cause burning or irritation in open lesions. If burning or irritation persists, tell the patient to notify the doctor. • Tell the patient prescribed the use of Cordran tape not to tear the tape but to cut it with scissors. • Instruct the patient on proper storage of the drug.

Selected ophthalmic drugs

Drug	Indications and dosages	Special considerations
Ophthalmic anti-infectives		
bacitracin	▶ Ocular infections. *Adults and children:* small amount of ointment applied into conjunctival sac once daily to t.i.d.	• Pregnancy risk categories for ophthalmic anti-infective drugs are as follows: – B (erythromycin, polymyxin B sulfate, tobramycin) – C (bacitracin, chloramphenicol, ciprofloxacin, gentamicin, idoxuridine, natamycin, norfloxacin, ofloxacin 0.3%, silver nitrate 1%, sulfacetamide sodium, sulfisoxazole diolamine, trifluridine, vidarabine) • Ophthalmic anti-infectives are contraindicated in patients who are hypersensitive to the drugs. Additional contraindications occur with the following drugs: – Bacitracin is contraindicated in atopic patients. – Ciprofloxacin, norfloxacin, and ofloxacin 0.3% are contraindicated in patients with a history of hypersensitivity to other fluoroquinolone antibiotics. – Ofloxacin 0.3% is also contraindicated in breast-feeding women. – Sulfacetamide sodium and sulfisoxazole diolamine are contraindicated in children younger than age 2 months. – Sulfisoxazole diolamine is also contraindicated in pregnant women who are at term and in breast-feeding women. – Note: Silver nitrate 1% has no contraindications. • Use ciprofloxacin cautiously in breast-feeding women. • Use gentamicin cautiously in patients with history of sensitivity to aminoglycosides; cross-sensitivity may occur. • Before giving, ask the patient about past allergic reactions to the drug. • When using chloramphenicol, reconstitute powder for solution with supplied diluent. Use 5 ml of diluent to make a 0.5% solution, 10 ml of diluent to make a 0.25% solution, or 15 ml to make a 0.16% solution.
chloramphenicol	▶ Surface bacterial Infection involving conjunctiva or cornea. *Adults and children:* 2 drops of solution or a small amount of ointment to affected eye q 3 hours or more frequently, as instructed by the doctor, for the first 48 hours. Then, the interval between applications may be increased. Treatment should continue for 48 hours after the eye appears normal.	
ciprofloxacin hydrochloride	▶ Corneal ulcers. *Adults and children over age 12:* 2 drops in the affected eye q 15 minutes for the first 6 hours; then 2 drops q 30 minutes for the remainder of the first day. On day 2, 2 drops hourly. On days 3 to 14, 2 drops q 4 hours. ▶ Bacterial conjunctivitis. *Adults and children over age 12:* 1 or 2 drops into the conjunctival sac of the affected eye q 2 hours while awake, for the first 2 days. Then 1 or 2 drops q 4 hours while awake, for the next 5 days.	
erythromycin	▶ Acute and chronic conjunctivitis, trachoma, other eye infections. *Adults and children:* 1 cm in length applied directly to the infected eye up to six times daily, depending on the severity of infection. ▶ Ophthalmia neonatorum. *Neonates:* a ribbon of ointment about 1 cm long applied in the lower conjunctival sac of each eye shortly after birth.	

(continued)

Drug	Indications and dosages	Special considerations
Ophthalmic anti-infectives (continued)		
gentamicin sulfate	▶ External ocular infections (conjunctivitis, keratoconjunctivitis, corneal ulcers, blepharitis, blepharoconjunctivitis, meibomianitis, and dacryocystitis). *Adults and children:* 1 or 2 drops instilled in eye q 4 hours. In severe infections, up to 2 drops q hour. Or, ointment applied to lower conjunctival sac b.i.d. or t.i.d.	● Be aware that idoxuridine should not be mixed with other topical eye medications. ● Clean eye area of excessive exudate before application. ● When applying eye drops, apply light finger pressure on lacrimal sac for 1 minute after drops are instilled to help prevent systemic absorption. ● Remember that the patient's eye can hold only one drop at a time. When instilling more than one drop, wait 2 to 3 minutes between drops to avoid losing a drop from tearing or blinking.
idoxuridine	▶ Herpes simplex keratitis. *Adults and children:* 1 drop of solution into conjunctival sac q hour during day and q 2 hours at night until improvement; then decreased to 1 drop q 2 hours during day and q 4 hours at night. If no response occurs in 7 days, drug is discontinued.	
natamycin	▶ Fungal keratitis. *Adults:* 1 drop in conjunctival sac q 1 to 2 hours. After 3 to 4 days, 1 drop six to eight times daily. ▶ Blepharitis or fungal conjunctivitis. *Adults:* 1 drop q 4 to 6 hours.	● Shake suspension forms well before using. ● When two different ophthalmic solutions are used, allow at least 5 minutes before instillation. ● When applying eye ointment, have the patient look upward, then pull down the lower lid with the finger. As the patient continues to look up, apply a thin ribbon of ointment into the conjunctival sac, beginning at the inner canthus.
norfloxacin	▶ Conjunctivitis. *Adults and children 1 year and over:* 1 or 2 drops in affected eye q.i.d. for up to 7 days. If condition warrants, 2 drops q 2 hours during waking hours of first day of treatment.	● To avoid contamination, do not let the tube touch the patient's eye or conjunctiva. At the outer canthus, rotate the tube to detach the ointment. ● Have the patient gently close the eye containing the ointment, but caution him not to squeeze it closed
ofloxacin 0.3%	▶ Conjunctivitis. *Adults and children over age 1:* 1 to 2 drops in conjunctival sac q 2 to 4 hours while awake for first 2 days, and then q.i.d. for 5 days.	● If the patient has more than a superficial infection, anticipate using systemic therapy as well. ● Institute appropriate therapy if superinfection occurs. Prolonged use of
polymyxin B sulfate	▶ Superficial eye infections involving the conjunctiva and cornea. *Adults and children:* 1 to 3 drops of 0.1% to 0.25% (10,000 to 25,000 units/ml) q hour until favorable response occurs. Not to exceed 2 million units daily. Or, apply small amount of ointment q 3 to 4 hours for 7 to 10 days depending on the severity of the infection.	some ophthalmic anti-infectives may result in overgrowth of nonsusceptible organisms, including fungi. ● Store the drug in tightly closed, light-resistant container at room temperature (except for iodoxuridine and trifluridine which must be refrigerated) unless otherwise directed. ● Tell the patient to take the drug as prescribed, even after he is feeling better, because if the drug is stopped too soon the infection may return.
silver nitrate 1%	▶ Gonorrheal ophthalmia neonatorum. *Neonates:* 2 drops of 1% solution into the lower conjunctival sac of each eye at angle of the nasal bridge and eyes, no later than 1 hour after delivery.	

Drug	Indications and dosages	Special considerations
Ophthalmic anti-infectives (continued)		
sulfacetamide sodium 10% sulfacetamide sodium 15% sulfacetamide sodium 30%	▶ Inclusion conjunctivitis, corneal ulcers, trachoma, prophylaxis to ocular infection. *Adults and children:* 1 to 2 drops of 10% solution instilled into lower conjunctival sac q 2 to 3 hours during day, less often at night; or 1 to 2 drops of 15% solution instilled into lower conjunctival sac q 1 to 2 hours initially. Interval increased as condition responds; or 1 drop of 30% solution instilled into lower conjunctival sac q 2 hours. 1.25 to 2.5 cm 10% ointment applied into conjunctival sac q.i.d. and h.s. Ointment may be used at night along with drops during the day.	• Teach the patient how to clean the eye area before application and how to apply the form of the drug prescribed. Tell him to wash his hands before and after administration and caution him not to touch the tip of the tube to the eye or surrounding tissue. • Tell the patient who is using the ointment form of the drug that only a small amount is needed. • Instruct the patient instilling eye drops to apply light finger pressure on the lacrimal sac for 1 minute after drops are instilled. • Tell the patient to wait at least 5 minutes before administering other eye drops.
sulfisoxazole diolamine	▶ Conjunctivitis, corneal ulcers, and other superficial ocular infections; adjunct in systemic sulfonamide therapy of trachoma. *Adults:* 1 to 2 drops instilled in the conjunctival sac q 1 to 4 hours daily.	• Teach the patient who is instilling a suspension form to shake the container well before using. • Caution the patient not to use solutions if they have become discolored. • Tell the patient that if he misses a
tobramycin	▶ External ocular infections. *Adults and children:* in mild to moderate infections, 1 or 2 drops into affected eye q 4 to 6 hours. In severe infections, 2 drops into infected eye q hour until condition improves; then frequency reduced. Or, a thin strip of ointment applied into conjunctival sac t.i.d. or q.i.d.	dose, he should apply the drug as soon as he remembers. However, if it's almost time for his next dose, he should skip the missed dose and go back to his regular dosing schedule. • Warn the patient that ophthalmic anti-infective drugs may cause blurred vision temporarily. Be sure to remind him to take safety precautions until vision clears.
trifluridine	▶ Primary keratoconjunctivitis and recurrent epithelial keratitis caused by herpes simplex virus, types I and II. *Adults:* 1 drop of solution into affected eye q 2 hours while patient is awake, to a maximum of 9 drops daily until corneal ulcer reepithelialization occurs; then 1 drop q 4 hours (minimum 5 drops daily) for an additional 7 days. Trifluridine should not be used for more than 21 days continuously because of the risk of ocular toxicity.	• Advise the patient to watch for signs of sensitivity, such as itching lids, swelling, or constant burning. Encourage a patient who develops such signs to withhold the drug and to notify the doctor immediately. • Advise the patient not to use leftover ophthalmic anti-infective medication for a new eye infection. Adverse reactions may occur, or the drug may have lost its potency. • Tell the patient to discard his medication when therapy has ended. • Advise the patient not to share eye medications, washcloths, or towels with family members. • If anyone in the family develops the same symptoms, the doctor should be notified immediately.

(continued)

Drug	Indications and dosages	Special considerations

Ophthalmic anti-infectives (continued)

vidarabine	▶ Acute keratoconjunctivitis, superficial keratitis, and recurrent epithelial keratitis resulting from herpes simplex type I and II. *Adults and children:* 1 cm ointment applied into lower conjunctival sac five times daily at 3-hour intervals.	• Stress the importance of compliance with recommended therapy, even when the patient is feeling better. • Instruct the patient to notify the doctor if his eye condition does not improve. Advise him to call the doctor if his condition worsens. • Tell the patient to minimize photophobia caused by some ophthalmic anti-infective agents by wearing sunglasses and by avoiding prolonged exposure to sunlight. • Instruct the patient to store the drug in a tightly closed, light-resistant container at room temperature (except for idoxuridine and trifluridine), unless otherwise instructed. • Tell the patient to keep eye medication out of the reach of children.

Ophthalmic anti-inflammatory drugs

dexamethasone dexamethasone sodium phosphate	▶ Uveitis; iridocyclitis; inflammatory conditions of eyelids, conjunctiva, cornea, anterior segment of globe; corneal injury from chemical or thermal burns, or penetration of foreign bodies; allergic conjunctivitis. *Adults and children:* 1 to 2 drops of suspension or solution or 1.25 to 2.5 cm of ointment into conjunctival sac. In severe disease, drops may be used hourly, tapering to discontinuation as condition improves. In mild conditions, drops may be used up to six times daily or ointment applied t.i.d. or q.i.d. As condition improves, dosage tapered to b.i.d., then once daily. Treatment may last up to several weeks.	• Pregnancy risk category for ophthalmic anti-inflammatory agents is C except for diclofenac sodium 0.1% and flurbiprofen sodium, which are B. • Ophthalmic anti-inflammatory agents are contraindicated in patients with known hypersensitivity to the drugs. The following drugs have additional contraindications: – Dexamethasone, dexamethasone sodium phosphate, fluorometholone, medrysone, prednisolone acetate, prednisolone sodium phosphate, and rimexolone are contraindicated in patients with acute superficial herpes simplex (dendritic keratitis), vaccinia, varicella, or other fungal or viral disease of cornea and conjunctiva; ocular tuberculosis; or acute, purulent, untreated infections of the eye. – Diclofenac sodium 0.1% and ketorolac tromethamine are contraindicated in patients wearing soft contact lenses – Diclofenac sodium 0.1% is also contraindicated during late pregnancy. – Suprofen is contraindicated in patients with epithelial herpes simplex keratitis.
diclofenac sodium 0.1%	▶ Postoperative inflammation following removal of cataract. *Adults:* 1 drop in conjunctival sac q.i.d., beginning 24 hours after surgery and continuing for 2 weeks.	
fluorometholone	▶ Inflammation of cornea, conjunctiva, sclera, anterior uvea. *Adults and children:* 1 to 2 drops in conjunctival sac b.i.d. to q.i.d. May be given q hour during first 1 to 2 days or 1.25 cm of ointment to conjunctival sac q 4 hours, decreasing to once to three times daily as inflammation subsides.	

Drug	Indications and dosages	Special considerations

Ophthalmic anti-inflammatory drugs (continued)

flurbiprofen sodium
▶ Inhibition of intraoperative miosis. *Adults:* 1 drop into eye undergoing surgery about every ½ hour, beginning 2 hours before surgery. A total of 4 drops is given.

ketorolac tromethamine
▶ Relief of itching caused by allergic conjunctivitis. *Adults:* 1 drop into conjunctival sac q.i.d.
▶ Treatment of postoperative inflammation in patients who have undergone cataract extraction. *Adults:* 1 drop in the operative eye(s) q.i.d. starting 24 hours after cataract surgery and continued throughout the first 2 weeks.

medrysone
▶ Allergic conjunctivitis, vernal conjunctivitis, episcleritis, ophthalmic epinephrine sensitivity reaction. *Adults and children:* 1 drop in conjunctival sac b.i.d. to q.i.d. May use q hour during first 1 to 2 days.

prednisolone acetate

prednisolone sodium phosphate (solution)
▶ Inflammation of palpebral and bulbar conjunctiva, cornea, and anterior segment of globe. *Adults and children:* 1 to 2 drops instilled in eye. In severe conditions, may be used hourly, tapering to discontinuation as inflammation subsides. In mild conditions, may be used up to six times daily.

rimexolone
▶ Postoperative inflammation following ocular surgery. *Adults:* 1 to 2 drops in the conjunctival sac q.i.d., beginning 24 hours after surgery and continuing throughout the first 2 weeks of the postoperative period.
▶ Anterior uveitis. *Adults:* 1 to 2 drops in the conjunctival sac q hour during waking hours for the first week, 1 drop q 2 hours during waking hours of the second week, and then tapered until uveitis is resolved.

suprofen
▶ Inhibition of intraoperative miosis. *Adults:* 2 drops instilled into the conjunctival sac q 4 hours the day before surgery. On the day of surgery, 2 drops instilled 3 hours, 2 hours, and 1 hour before surgery.

Special considerations

● Ophthalmic anti-inflammatory agents have a variety of precautions. Check the manufacturer's warnings before administering any of these drugs.
● Be aware that corneal viral and fungal infections may be exacerbated by steroid application.
● Know that ophthalmic anti-inflammatory agents are usually not intended for long-term use and may delay wound healing if used.
● Check with the doctor to determine whether an eye pad should be worn after ointment application.
● When administering eye drops, apply light finger pressure on the lacrimal sac for about 1 minute after instillation.
● Notify the doctor immediately if the patient complains of visual disturbances. Also notify the doctor if the patient's eye condition does not improve or becomes worse.
● Teach the patient how to apply the drug. Remind him to wash hands before and after administration; and caution him not to allow the tip of the dropper or tube to contact the eye or surrounding tissue.
● Tell the patient applying eye drops to apply light finger pressure on lacrimal sac for 1 minute after instillation.
● Instruct the patient using a suspension to shake container well before use.
● Warn the patient not to use leftover medication for a new eye inflammation; it may cause serious problems.
● Warn the patient to call doctor immediately and to stop drug if visual acuity changes or visual field diminishes.
● Tell the patient not to share eye medications, washcloths, or towels with family members. If anyone develops similar symptoms, tell the patient to notify the doctor.

Selected otic drugs

Drug	Indications and dosages	Special considerations
acetic acid	▶ External ear canal infection. *Adults and children:* 4 to 6 drops into ear canal q 2 to 3 hours; or insert saturated wick for first 24 hours, then continue with instillations.	● Pregnancy risk category for most topically applied otic drugs is NR; C for carbamide peroxide, chloramphenicol, and triethanolamine polypeptide oleate-condensate.
carbamide peroxide	▶ Impacted cerumen. *Adults and children age 12 and over:* 5 to 10 drops into ear canal b.i.d. for 3 to 4 days. Allow solution to remain in ear canal for 15 to 30 minutes; remove with warm water.	● Otic agents are contraindicated in patients with perforated eardrum. ● Triethanolamine polypeptide oleate-condensate is also contraindicated in patients with otitis media and otitis externa. ● Reculture persistent drainage.
chloramphenicol	▶ External ear canal infection. *Adults and children:* 2 to 3 drops into ear canal t.i.d. or q.i.d.	● Watch for signs of superinfection (continual pain, inflammation, fever). ● Teach the patient or caregiver how to administer the drug.
triethanolamine polypeptide oleate-condensate	▶ Impacted cerumen. *Adults and children:* fill ear canal with solution and insert cotton plug. After 15 to 30 minutes, flush ear with warm water.	● Warn the patient or caregiver to avoid touching the ear with the dropper to prevent reinfection. ● Tell the patient using a cotton plug to moisten it with medication. ● Instruct the patient to keep the container tightly closed and away from moisture and heat.

Table of equivalents

Metric system equivalents

Metric weight		**Metric volume**	
1 kilogram (kg or Kg)	= 1,000 grams (g or gm)	1 liter (l or L)	= 1,000 milliiters (ml)*
1 gram	= 1,000 milligrams (mg)	1 milliliter	= 1,000 microliters (µl)
1 milligram	= 1,000 micrograms (µg or mcg)		
		Household	**Metric**
0.6 g	= 600 mg	1 teaspoon (tsp)	= 5 ml
0.3 g	= 300 mg	1 tablespoon (T or tbs)	= 15 ml
0.1 g	= 100 mg	2 tablespoons	= 30 ml
0.06 g	= 60 mg	1 measuring cupful	= 240 ml
0.03 g	= 30 mg	1 pint (pt)	= 473 ml
0.015 g	= 15 mg	1 quart (qt)	= 946 ml
0.001 g	= 1 mg	1 gallon (gal)	= 3,785 ml

Temperature conversions

Fahrenheit degrees	Centigrade degrees	Fahrenheit degrees	Centigrade degrees	Fahrenheit degrees	Centigrade degrees
106.0	41.1	100.6	38.1	95.2	35.1
105.8	41.0	100.4	38.0	95.0	35.0
105.6	40.9	100.2	37.9	94.8	34.9
105.4	40.8	100.0	37.8	94.6	34.8
105.2	40.7	99.8	37.7	94.4	34.7
105.0	40.6	99.6	37.6	94.2	34.6
104.8	40.4	99.4	37.4	94.0	34.4
104.6	40.3	99.2	37.3	93.8	34.3
104.4	40.2	99.0	37.2	93.6	34.2
104.2	40.1	98.8	37.1	93.4	34.1
104.0	40.0	98.6	37.0	93.2	34.0
103.8	39.9	98.4	36.9	93.0	33.9
103.6	39.8	98.2	36.8	92.8	33.8
103.4	39.7	98.0	36.7	92.6	33.7
103.2	39.6	97.8	36.5	92.4	33.6
103.0	39.4	97.6	36.4	92.2	33.4
102.8	39.3	97.4	36.3	92.0	33.3
102.6	39.2	97.2	36.2	91.8	33.2
102.4	39.1	97.0	36.1	91.6	33.1
102.2	39.0	96.8	36.0	91.4	33.0
102.0	38.9	96.6	35.9	91.2	32.9
101.8	38.8	96.4	35.8	91.0	32.8
101.6	38.7	96.2	35.7	90.8	32.7
101.4	38.6	96.0	35.6	90.6	32.6
101.2	38.4	95.8	35.4	90.4	32.4
101.0	38.3	95.6	35.3	90.2	32.3
100.8	38.2	95.4	35.2	90.0	32.2

Weight conversions

1 oz = 30 g	1 lb = 453.6 g	2.2 lb = 1 kg

*1 ml = 1 cubic centimeter (cc); however, ml is the preferred measurement term today.

Estimating surface area in children

Pediatric drug dosages should be calculated on the basis of body surface area or body weight. If the child is of average size, find his weight and corresponding surface area in the box. Otherwise, to use the nomogram, lay a straightedge on the correct height and weight points for the patient, and observe the point where it intersects on the surface area scale. *Note:* Don't use drug dosages based on body surface area in premature or full-term newborns. Instead, use body weight.

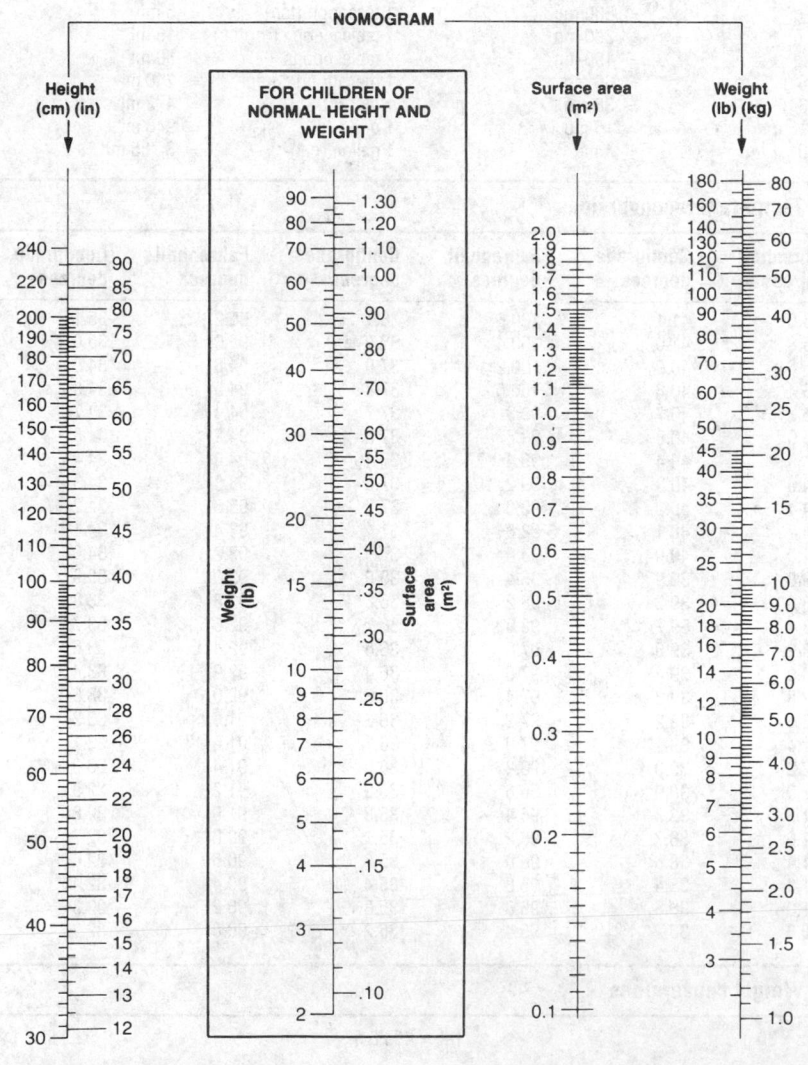

Drug imprint codes

When administering medications, you may come across some pills that are not recognizable by sight. A reliable method for identifying these pills is to check the drug's imprint code found on the tablet or capsule.

Below are drug imprint codes and descriptions for some of the most commonly prescribed tablets and capsules. The drug code in numeric and alphabetical order; the pill's shape, color, type (tablet or capsule), and additional characteristics (C = coated; S = scored); and the generic drug name, trade name, manufacturer, strength, and class are shown.

Code	Color and shape	Drug, strength, therapeutic class
25	round orange tablet, S	levothyroxine (Synthroid/Knoll), 25 mcg, thyroid hormone replacement
25 W 701	shield-shaped peach tablet, S	venlafaxine (Effexor/Wyeth-Ayerst), 25 mg, antidepressant
37.5 W 781	shield-shaped peach tablet, S	venlafaxine (Effexor/Wyeth-Ayerst), 37.5 mg, antidepressant
50	round white tablet, S	levothyroxine (Synthroid/Knoll), 50 mcg, thyroid hormone replacement
50 W 703	shield-shaped peach tablet, S	venlafaxine (Effexor/Wyeth-Ayerst), 50 mg, antidepressant
51 51	oblong pink tablet, S	metoprolol (Lopressor/Novartis), 50 mg, antihypertensive
54 543	round white tablet	acetaminophen/oxycodone (Roxicet/Roxane), 325 mg/5 mg, analgesic
71 71	oblong blue tablet, S	metoprolol (Lopressor/Novartis), 100 mg, antihypertensive
75 W 704	shield-shaped peach tablet, S	venlafaxine (Effexor/Wyeth-Ayerst), 75 mg, antidepressant
93 50	round white tablet, S	acetaminophen/codeine (Teva), 300 mg/15 mg, analgesic
93 152	coral/scarlet capsule	acetaminophen/codeine (Teva), 300 mg/30 mg, analgesic
93 172	brown/gray capsule	acetaminophen/codeine (Teva), 300 mg/60 mg, analgesic
93 490	oblong white tablet, C	acetaminophen/propoxyphene (Teva), 650 mg/100 mg, analgesic
93 541	gray/orange capsule	cephalexin (Teva), 250 mg, antibiotic
93 543	orange capsule	cephalexin (Teva), 500 mg, antibiotic
100	round yellow tablet, S	levothyroxine (Synthroid/Knoll),100 mcg, thyroid hormone replacement

(continued)

Code	Color and shape	Drug, strength, therapeutic class
100 W 705	shield-shaped peach tablet, S	venlafaxine (Effexor/Wyeth-Ayerst), 100 mg, antidepressant
150	round blue tablet, S	levothyroxine (Synthroid/Knoll), 150 mcg, thyroid hormone replacement
200	round pink tablet, S	levothyroxine(Synthroid/Knoll), 200 mcg, thyroid hormone replacement
884 MILES 30	round pink tablet	nifedipine (Adalat CC/Bayer), 30 mg, antihypertensive
885 MILES 60	round salmon tablet	nifedipine (Adalat CC/Bayer), 60 mg, antihypertensive
886 MILES 90	round dark red tablet	nifedipine (Adalat CC/Bayer), 90 mg, antihypertensive
3170	blue/gray capsule	loracarbef (Lorabid/Lilly), 200 mg, antibiotic
5513	round white tablet	carisoprodol (Schein), 350 mg, muscle relaxant
A 49	round white tablet, S	atenolol (Lederle), 50 mg, antihypertensive
A 71	round white tablet	atenolol (Lederle), 100 mg, antihypertensive
A KT KT	oval yellow tablet, C	clarithromycin (Biaxin/Abbott), 250 mg, antibiotic
AMB 5 5401	capsule-shaped pink tablet, C	zolpidem (Ambien/Searle), 5 mg, sedative
AMB 10 5421	capsule-shaped white tablet, C	zolpidem (Ambien/Searle), 10 mg, sedative
A MO	round white tablet; C, S	metoprolol (Toprol-XL/Astra), 50 mg, antihypertensive
A MS	round white tablet; C, S	metoprolol (Toprol-XL/Astra), 100 mg, antihypertensive
A MY	oval white tablet; C, S	metoprolol (Toprol-XL/Astra), 200 mg, antihypertensive
B 11	round light green tablet	ethinyl estradiol/levonorgestrel (Tri-Levlen/Berlex), placebo, oral contraceptive
B 95	round brown tablet	ethinyl estradiol/levonorgestrel (Tri-Levlen/Berlex), 0.030 mg/0.05 mg, oral contraceptive
B 96	round white tablet	ethinyl estradiol/levonorgestrel (Tri-Levlen/Berlex), 0.040 mg/0.075 mg, oral contraceptive
B 97	round light yellow tablet	ethinyl estradiol/levonorgestrel (Tri-Levlen/Berlex), 0.030 mg/0.125 mg, oral contraceptive
BARR 514	gray/orange capsule	cephalexin (Barr), 250 mg, antibiotic
BARR 515	orange capsule	cephalexin (Barr), 500 mg, antibiotic
BARR 545	capsule-shaped orange tablet	cephalexin (Barr), 250 mg, antibiotic
BARR 546	capsule-shaped dark orange tablet	cephalexin (Barr), 500 mg, antibiotic
BIOCRAFT 01	caramel/buff capsule	amoxicillin (Teva), 250 mg, antibiotic
BIOCRAFT 03	buff capsule	amoxicillin (Teva), 500 mg, antibiotic
BIOCRAFT 33	oval white tablet, S	sulfamethoxazole/trimethoprim (Teva), 800 mg/160 mg, antibiotic
BIOCRAFT 115	gray/orange capsule	cephalexin (Teva), 250 mg, antibiotic
BIOCRAFT 117	orange capsule	cephalexin (Teva), 500 mg, antibiotic

Code	Color and shape	Drug, strength, therapeutic class
BL 32	round white tablet, S	sulfamethoxazole/trimethoprim (Teva), 400 mg/80 mg, antibiotic
BMS 7720 250	oval light orange tablet, C	cefprozil (Cefzil/Bristol-Myers Squibb), 250 mg, antibiotic
BMS 7721 500	oval white tablet, C	cefprozil (Cefzil/Bristol-Myers Squibb), 500 mg, antibiotic
BRISTOL 7278	pink/maroon capsule	amoxicillin (Apothecon), 250 mg, antibiotic
BRISTOL 7279	pink/maroon capsule	amoxicillin (Apothecon), 500 mg, antibiotic
C	oval white tablet, S	medroxyprogesterone (Cycrin/ESI Lederle), 2.5 mg, progestin
CIBA 3	round pale green tablet, S	methylphenidate (Ritalin/Novartis), 10 mg, psychotherapeutic
CIBA 7	round yellow tablet	methylphenidate (Ritalin/Novartis), 5 mg, psychotherapeutic
CIBA 34	round pale yellow tablet, S	methylphenidate (Ritalin/Novartis), 20 mg, psychotherapeutic
DAN 5442 DAN	round white tablet, S	prednisone (Geneva), 10 mg, anti-inflammatory
DAN 5443 DAN	round peach tablet, S	prednisone (Danbury), 20 mg, anti-inflammatory
DAN 5490 DAN	round white tablet, S	prednisone (Schein), 50 mg, anti-inflammatory
DP 301	oval white tablet, S	methylprednisolone (Duramed), 4 mg, anti-inflammatory
E 647	yellow capsule	phentermine (Eon Labs), 30 mg, anorexant
EC	rectangular pink tablet	erythromycin base (Ery-Tab/Abbott), 250 mg, antibiotic
ED	oval pink tablet	erythromycin base (Ery-Tab/Abbott), 500 mg, antibiotic
EH	rectangular white tablet	erythromycin base (Ery-Tab/Abbott), 333 mg, antibiotic
ES	round pink tablet, C	erythromycin stearate (Erythrocin/Abbott), 250 mg, antibiotic
ET	oval pink tablet, C	erythromycin stearate (Erythrocin/Abbott), 500 mg, antibiotic
G 0556	round peach tablet	hydrochlorothiazide (Zenith), 25 mg, antihypertensive
G 800	capsule-shaped white tablet, C	ibuprofen (Greenstone), 800 mg, anti-inflammatory
G 3719	oval white tablet, S	alprazolam (Greenstone), 0.25 mg, antianxiety
G 3720	oval peach tablet, S	alprazolam (Greenstone), 0.5 mg, antianxiety
G 3721	oval blue tablet, S	alprazolam (Greenstone), 1 mg, antianxiety
G 3722	oval white tablet, S	alprazolam (Greenstone), 2 mg, antianxiety
G 3725	round white tablet, S	glyburide (Greenstone), 1.25 mg, antidiabetic
G 3726	round pink tablet, S	glyburide (Greenstone), 2.5 mg, antidiabetic
G 3727	round blue tablet, S	glyburide (Greenstone), 5 mg, antidiabetic
G 3740	round orange tablet, S	medroxyprogesterone (Greenstone), 2.5 mg, progestin

(continued)

Code	Color and shape	Drug, strength, therapeutic class
G 3741	hexagonal white tablet, S	medroxyprogesterone (Greenstone), 5 mg, progestin
G 3742	round white tablet, S	medroxyprogesterone (Greenstone), 10 mg, progestin
GG 172	round yellow tablet, S	triamterene/hydrochlorothiazide (Geneva), 75 mg/50 mg, antihypertensive
GG 263	round white tablet; C, S	atenolol (Geneva), 50 mg, antihypertensive
GG 264	round white tablet, C	atenolol (Geneva), 100 mg, antihypertensive
GG 580	red capsule	triamterene/hydrochlorothiazide (Geneva), 50 mg/25 mg, antihypertensive
GG 606	white capsule	triamterene/hydrochlorothiazide (Geneva), 37.5 mg/25 mg, antihypertensive
GL 500	cylindrical white tablet, C	metformin (Glucophage/Bristol-Myers Squibb), 500 mg, antidiabetic
GL 850	cylindrical white tablet, C	metformin (Glucophage/Bristol-Myers Squibb), 850 mg, antidiabetic
GLAXO 387	capsule-shaped light blue tablet, C	cefuroxime axetil (Ceftin/Glaxo Wellcome), 250 mg, antibiotic
GLAXO 394	capsule-shaped dark blue tablet, C	cefuroxime axetil (Ceftin/Glaxo Wellcome), 500 mg, antibiotic
GLAXO 395	capule-shaped white tablet, C	cefuroxime axetil (Ceftin/Glaxo Wellcome), 125 mg, antibiotic
GLYBUR 364 364	round blue tablet	glyburide (Copley), 5 mg, antidiabetic
GLYBUR 433 433	round pink tablet, S	glyburide (Copley), 2.5 mg, antidiabetic
GLYBUR 477 477	round white tablet, S	glyburide (Copley), 1.25 mg, antidiabetic
HH	gray capsule	terazosin (Hytrin/Abbott), 1 mg, antihypertensive
HK	red capsule	terazosin (Hytrin/Abbott), 5 mg, antihypertensive
HN	blue capsule	terazosin (Hytrin/Abbott), 10 mg, antihypertensive
HY	yellow capsule	terazosin (Hytrin/Abbott), 2 mg, antihypertensive
I25	round white tablet, C	sumatriptan (Imitrex/Glaxo Wellcome), 25 mg, antimigraine
IBU 600	oval white tablet, C	ibuprofen (Boots), 600 mg, anti-inflammatory
IBU 800	oval white tablet, C	ibuprofen (Boots), 800 mg, anti-inflammatory
JANSSEN P 10	round white tablet, S	cisapride (Propulsid/Janssen), 10 mg, GI stimulant
JANSSEN P 20	oval blue tablet	cisapride (Propulsid/Janssen), 20 mg, GI stimulant
JANSSEN R 1	oval white tablet, S	risperldone (Risperdal/Janssen), 1 mg, antipsychotic
JANSSEN R 2	oval orange tablet	risperidone (Risperdal/Janssen), 2 mg, antipsychotic
JANSSEN R 3	oval yellow tablet	risperidone (Risperdal/Janssen), 3 mg, antipsychotic
JANSSEN R 4	oval green tablet	risperidone (Risperdal/Janssen), 4 mg, antipsychotic
KL	oval yellow tablet, C	clarithromycin (Biaxin/Abbott), 500 mg, antibiotic

Code	Color and shape	Drug, strength, therapeutic class
KLOR-CON 8	round blue tablet, C	potassium chloride (Klor-Con/Upsher-Smith), 8 mEq, potassium supplement
KLOR-CON 10	round yellow tablet, C	potassium chloride (Klor-Con/Upsher-Smith), 10 mEq, potassium supplement
LANOXIN T9A	round green tablet, S	digoxin (Lanoxin/Glaxo Wellcome), 0.5 mg, antiarrhythmic
LANOXIN X3A	round white tablet, S	digoxin (Lanoxin/Glaxo Wellcome), 0.25 mg, antiarrhythmic
LANOXIN Y3B	round yellow tablet, S antiarrhythmic	digoxin (Lanoxin/Glaxo Wellcome), 0.125 mg,
LASIX HOECHST	oval white tablet	furosemide (Lasix/Hoechst Marion Roussel), 20 mg, diuretic
LL HEART B12	round yellow tablet	hydrochlorothiazide/bisoprolol (Ziac/Lederle), 6.25 mg/2.5 mg, antihypertensive
LL HEART B13	round pink tablet	hydrochlorothiazide/bisoprolol (Ziac/Lederle), 6.25 mg/5 mg, antihypertensive
LL HEART B14	round white tablet	hydrochlorothiazide/bisoprolol (Ziac/Lederle), 6.25 mg/10 mg, antihypertensive
M 32	round pink tablet, S	metoprolol (Mylan), 50 mg, antihypertensive
M 37	round purple tablet	amitriptyline (Mylan), 75 mg, antidepressant
M 47	round blue tablet; C, S	metoprolol (Mylan), 100 mg, antihypertensive
M 53	five-sided green tablet, C	cimetidine (Mylan), 200 mg, antiulcer
M 77	round white tablet, C	amitriptyline (Mylan), 10 mg, antidepressant
M 241	round white tablet, S	atenolol (Mylan), 50 mg, antihypertensive
M 321	round white tablet	lorazepam (Mylan), 0.5 mg, antianxiety
M 537	round blue tablet, C	naproxen (Mylan), 275 mg, anti-inflammatory
M 751	round orange tablet, C	cyclobenzaprine (Mylan), 10 mg, muscle relaxant
M 757	round white tablet	atenolol (Mylan), 100 mg, antihypertensive
MCNEIL 659	capsule-shaped white tablet, C	tramadol (Ultram/Ortho-McNeil), 50 mg, analgesic
MD 530	round green-blue tablet, S	methylphenidate (MD Pharm), 10 mg, psychotherapeutic
MD 531	round yellow tablet	methylphenidate (MD Pharm), 5 mg, psychotherapeutic
MJ 021	round white tablet	estradiol (Estrace/Bristol-Myers Squibb), 0.5 mg, estrogen replacement
MJ 755	round lavender tablet	estradiol (Estrace/Bristol-Myers Squibb), 1 mg, estrogen replacement
MJ 756	round turquoise tablet	estradiol (Estrace/Bristol-Meyers Squibb), 2 mg, estrogen replacement

(continued)

Code	Color and shape	Drug, strength, therapeutic class
MRK 951	teardrop-shaped light green tablet	losartan (Cozaar/Merck), 25 mg, antihypertensive
MRK 952	teardrop-shaped green tablet	losartan (Cozaar/Merck), 50 mg, antihypertensive
MSD 963	U-shaped beige tablet, C	famotidine (Pepcid/Merck), 20 mg, antiulcer
MSD 964	U-shaped light brown tablet, C	famotidine (Pepcid/Merck), 40 mg, antiulcer
MYLAN 130	capsule-shaped reddish orange tablet, C	propoxyphene/acetaminophen (Mylan), 65 mg/650 mg, analgesic
MYLAN 152	round white tablet, S	clonidine (Mylan), 0.1 mg, antihypertensive
MYLAN 185	round white tablet, S	clonidine (Mylan), 0.2 mg, antihypertensive
MYLAN 199	round white tablet, S	clonidine (Mylan), 0.3 mg, antihypertensive
MYLAN 216 40	round white tablet, S	furosemide (Mylan), 40 mg, diuretic
MYLAN 232 80	round white tablet, S	furosemide (Mylan), 80 mg, diuretic
MYLAN 271	round white tablet, S	diazepam (Mylan), 2 mg, antianxiety
MYLAN 345	round orange tablet, S	diazepam (Mylan), 5 mg, antianxiety
MYLAN 457	round white tablet, S	lorazepam (Mylan), 1 mg, antianxiety
MYLAN 477	round green tablet, S	diazepam (Mylan), 10 mg, antianxiety
MYLAN 521	capsule-shaped white tablet	propoxyphene/acetaminophen (Mylan), 100 mg/ 650 mg, analgesic
MYLAN 733	oval light blue tablet, C	naproxen (Mylan), 550 mg, anti-inflammatory
MYLAN 777	round white tablets, S	lorazepam (Mylan), 2 mg, antianxiety
MYLAN 4010	peach capsule	temazepam (Mylan), 15 mg, sedative
MYLAN 5050	yellow capsule	temazepam (Mylan), 30 mg, sedative
MYLAN 7250	pink/white capsule	cefaclor (Mylan), 250 mg, antibiotic
MYLAN 7500	pink/gray capsules	cefaclor (Mylan), 500 mg, antibiotic
MYLAN A	round white tablet, S	alprazolam (Mylan), 0.25 mg, antianxiety
MYLAN A1	round blue tablet, S	alprazolam (Mylan), 1 mg, antianxiety
MYLAN A3	round peach tablet, S	alprazolam (Mylan), 0.5 mg, antianxiety
MYLAN A4	round white tablet, S	alprazolam (Mylan), 2 mg, antianxiety
MYLAN G1	round white tablets, S	glipizide (Mylan), 5 mg, antidiabetic
MYLAN G2	round white tablets, S	glipizide (Mylan), 10 mg, antidiabetic
NR	oval peach tablet	divalproex (Depakote/Abbott), 250 mg, anticonvulsant
NS	oval lavender tablet	divalproex (Depakote/Abbott), 500 mg, anticonvulsant
NT	oval salmon tablet	divalproex (Depakote/Abbott), 125 mg, anticonvulsant
ORTHO 75	round light peach tablet	ethinyl estradiol/norethindrone (Ortho-Novum 7/7/7/Ortho-McNeil), 35 mcg/0.75 mg, oral ontraceptive

Code	Color and shape	Drug, strength, therapeutic class
ORTHO 135	round peach tablet	ethinyl estradiol/norethindrone (Ortho-Novum 7/7/7/Ortho-McNeil), 35 mcg/1 mg, oral contraceptive
ORTHO 180	round white tablet	ethinyl estradiol/norgestimate (Ortho Tri-Cyclen/Ortho-McNeil), 35 mcg/0.18 mg, oral contraceptive
ORTHO 215	round light blue tablet	ethinyl estradiol/norgestimate (Ortho Tri-Cyclen/Ortho-McNeil), 35 mcg/0.215 mg, oral contraceptive
ORTHO 250	round blue tablet	ethinyl estradiol/norgestimate (Ortho Cyclen/Ortho-McNeil), 35 mcg/0.25 mg, oral contraceptive
ORTHO 535	round white tablet	ethinyl estradiol/norethindrone (Ortho-Novum 7/7/7/Ortho-McNeil), 35 mcg/0.5 mg, oral contraceptive
ORTHO D 150	round orange tablet	ethinyl estradiol/desogestrel (Ortho-Cept/Ortho-McNeil), 30 mcg/0.15mg, oral contraceptive
P 57	round white tablet, S	lorazepam (Purpac), 0.5 mg, antianxiety
P 59	round white tablet, S	lorazepam (Purpac), 1 mg, antianxiety
PAR 161 300	round white tablet	ibuprofen (Par), 300 mg, anti-inflammatory
PAR 467	capsule-shaped white tablet, C	ibuprofen (Par), 400 mg, anti-inflammatory
PAR 468	capsule-shaped white tablet, C	ibuprofen (Par), 600 mg, anti-inflammatory
P-D 362	orange-banded white capsule	phenytoin sodium (Dilantin Kapseals/Parke-Davis), 100 mg, anticonvulsant
P-D 365	pink-banded white capsule	phenytoin sodium (Dilantin Kapseals/Parke-Davis), 30 mg, anticonvulsant
P-D 532 20	round brown tablet, C	quinapril (Accupril/Parke-Davis), 20 mg, antihypertensive
P-D 535 40	oval brown tablet, C	quinapril (Accupril/Parke-Davis), 40 mg, antihypertensive
P-D 916	round green tablet	ethinyl estradiol/norethindrone (Loestrin [Fe]/Parke-Davis), 30 mcg/1.5 mg, oral contraceptive
PFIZER 305	red capsule	azithromycin (Zithromax/Pfizer), 250 mg, antibiotic
PFIZER 308	oval white tablet	azithromycin (Zithromax/Pfizer), 600 mg, antibiotic
PFIZER 550	round off-rectangular white tablet, C	cetirizine (Zyrtec/Pfizer), 5 mg, antihistamine
PFIZER 551	round off-rectangular white tablet, C	cetirizine (Zyrtec/Pfizer), 10 mg, antihistamine
PPP 785	oval white tablet, S	cefadroxil (Duricef/Bristol-Myers Squibb), 1000 mg, antibiotic
R 001 3	round white tablet, S	acetaminophen/codeine (Purepac), 300 mg/30 mg, analgesic
R 003 4	round white tablet, S	acetaminophen/codeine (Purepac), 300 mg/60 mg, analgesic
R 027	round white tablet, S	alprazolam (Purepac), 0.25 mg, antianxiety

(continued)

Code	Color and shape	Drug, strength, therapeutic class
R 029	round peach tablet, S	alprazolam (Purepac), 0.5 mg, antianxiety
R 031	round blue tablet, S	alprazolam (Purepac), 1.0 mg, antianxiety
R 063	round white tablet, S	lorazepam (Purepac), 2 mg, antianxiety
RUGBY 3367	blue capsule	dicyclomine (Rugby), 10 mg, antispasmodic
RUGBY 3377	round blue tablet	dicyclomine (Rugby), 20 mg, antispasmodic
SEARLE 151	round white tablet	ethinyl estradiol/ethynodiol diacetate (Demulen 1/35/Searle), 35 mcg/1 mg, oral contraceptive
SGP 1/35	round pale blue tablet	ethinyl estradiol/norethindrone (Genora 1/35/Rugby), 35 mcg/1 mg, oral contraceptive
SQUIBB 181	orange/gray capsule	cephalexin (Apothecon), 250 mg, antibiotic
SQUIBB 239	orange capsule	cephalexin (Apothecon), 500 mg, antibiotic
SQUIBB 603	oblong pink tablet, C	tetracycline (Sumycin/Apothecon), 500 mg, antibiotic
SQUIBB 648	round white tablet, C	penicillin V potassium (Veetids 500/Apothecon), 500 mg, antibiotic
SQUIBB 663	pink tablet, C	tetracycline (Sumycin/Apothecon), 250 mg, antibiotic
SQUIBB 684	round peach tablet, C	penicillin V potassium (Veetids 250/ Apothecon), 250 mg, antibiotic
SQUIBB 971	red/gray capsule	ampicillin (Principen/Apothecon), 250 mg, antibiotic
SQUIBB 974	red/gray capsule	ampicillin (Principen/Apothecon), 500 mg, antibiotic
TR 5/ORGANON	round white tablet	ethinyl estradiol/desogestrel (Desogen/Organon), 30 mcg/0.15 mg, oral contraceptive
W 641	round brown tablet	ethinyl estradiol/levonorgestrel (Triphasil/Wyeth-Ayerst), 30 mcg/0.05 mg, oral contraceptive
W 642	round white tablet	ethinyl estradiol/levonorgestrel (Triphasil/Wyeth-Ayerst), 40 mcg/0.075 mg, oral contraceptive
W 643	round light yellow tablet	ethinyl estradiol/levonorgestrel (Triphasil/Wyeth-Ayerst), 30 mcg/0.125 mg, oral contraceptive
W 650	round light green tablet	ethinyl estradiol/levonorgestrel (Triphasil/Wyeth-Ayerst), placebo, oral contraceptive
WATSON 540	oval blue tablet, S	hydrocodone/acetaminophen (Watson), 10 mg/500 mg, analgesic
WC 084	oval white tablet, C	gemfibrozil (Warner Chilcott), 600 mg, antihyperlipidemic
WYETH 78	round white tablet	ethinyl estradiol/norgestrel (Lo/Ovral/Wyeth-Ayerst), 30 mcg/0.3 mg, oral contraceptive
Z 2984	light blue/white capsule	doxycycline (Zenith), 50 mg, antibiotic
Z 2985	light blue capsule	doxycycline (Zenith), 100 mg, antibiotic
Z 4280	capsule-shaped white tablet; C, S	verapamil (Verapamil SR/Zenith), 240 mg, antihypertensive
Z 4286	oval white tablet; C, S	verapamil (Verapamil SR/Zenith), 180 mg, antihypertensive

Acknowledgments

We would like to thank the following companies for granting us permission to include their drugs in the full-color photoguide.

Abbott Laboratories
Biaxin®
Depakote®
Depakote® Sprinkle
E.E.S.®
Ery-Tab®
Erythrocin Stearate Filmtab®
Erythromycin Base Filmtab®
Hytrin®
PCE®

AstraZeneca LP
Prilosec®
Toprol XL®

Bayer Corporation
Adalat CC®
Cipro®

Bristol-Myers Squibb Company
BuSpar®
Capoten®
Cefzil®
cephalexin
Duricef®
Estrace®
Glucophage®
Pravachol®
Sumycin®
Trimox®
Veetids®

DuPont Pharmaceuticals Company
Coumadin®

Endo Pharmaceuticals, Inc.
Percocet®

ESI Lederle Division of American Home Products Corporation
atenolol

Ethex Corporation
potassium chloride

Forest Pharmaceuticals, Inc.
Lorcet® 10/650

Glaxo Wellcome, Inc.
Ceftin®
Lanoxin®
Zantac®
Zantac® EFFERdose®
Zovirax®

Hoechst Marion Roussel
Allegra®
Altace®
Carafate®
Cardizem®
Cardizem® CD
DiaBeta®
Lasix®
Trental®

Janssen Pharmaceutica, Inc.
Propulsid®
Risperdal®

Jones Pharma
Levoxyl®

Knoll Pharmaceutical Company
E-Mycin®
ibuprofen
Synthroid®
Vicodin®
Vicodin ES®

Eli Lilly and Company
Axid®
Ceclor®
Darvocet-N® 100
Lorabid®
Prozac®

McNeil-PPC, Inc.
Motrin®

Medeva Pharmaceuticals
methylphenidate hydrochloride

Merck & Co., Inc.
Cozaar®
Fosamax®
Mevacor®
Pepcid®
Prinivil®
Sinemet®
Sinemet® CR
Vasotec®
Zocor®

Mylan Pharmaceuticals, Inc.
amitriptyline hydrochloride
cimetidine
cyclobenzaprine hydrochloride
doxepin hydrochloride
furosemide
glipizide
naproxen
propoxyphene napsylate with acetaminophen

Novartis Pharmaceuticals Corporation
Fiorinal® with Codeine
Lotensin®
Pamelor®

Novopharm USA, Inc., Division of Novopharm Limited
amoxicillin trihydrate

Ortho-McNeil Pharmaceutical
Floxin®
Tylenol® with Codeine No. 3
Ultram®

Pfizer, Inc.
Cardura®
Diflucan®
Glucotrol®
Glucotrol XL®
Norvasc®
Procardia XL®
Zithromax®
Zoloft®
Zyrtec®

Pharmacia & Upjohn
Deltasone®
Glynase®
Micronase®
Provera®
Xanax®

**Proctor and Gamble
Pharmaceuticals, Inc.**
Macrobid®

**Rhône-Poulenc Rorer
Pharmaceuticals, Inc.**
Dilacor XR®
Slo-bid™ Gyrocaps®

Roche Laboratories, Inc.
Bumex®
Klonopin®
Naprosyn®
Ticlid®
Toradol®
Valium®

Roxane Laboratories, Inc.
Roxicet ™

Schein Pharmaceutical, Inc.
nortriptyline hydrochloride

**Schering Corporation and
Key Pharmaceuticals, Inc.**
Claritin®
K-Dur®
Theo-Dur®

Schwarz Pharma
Verelan®

G.D. Searle & Company
Ambien®
Calan®
Daypro®

**SmithKline Beecham
Pharmaceuticals**
Amoxil®
Augmentin®
Compazine®
Coreg®
Dyazide®
Paxil®
Relafen®
Tagamet®

Tap Pharmaceuticals, Inc.
Prevacid®

Warner-Lambert Company
Accupril®
Dilantin® Infatabs®
Dilantin® Kapseals®
Lipitor®
Lopid®
Nitrostat®

Watson Laboratories, Inc.
hydrocodone bitartrate and
    acetaminophen

Wyeth-Ayerst Laboratories
Ativan®
Cordarone®
Effexor®
Inderal®
Lodine®
Oruvail®
Premarin®

Zeneca Pharmaceuticals
Nolvadex®
Tenormin®
Zestril®

**Zenith Goldline
Pharmaceuticals**
verapamil hydrochloride

Index

t refers to a table; **boldface** refers to full-color photographs

t refers to a table; **boldface** refers to full-color photographs

t refers to a table; **boldface** refers to full-color photographs

t refers to a table; **boldface** refers to full-color photographs

t refers to a table; **boldface** refers to full-color photographs

t refers to a table; **boldface** refers to full-color photographs

t refers to a table; **boldface** refers to full-color photographs

t refers to a table; **boldface** refers to full-color photographs

t refers to a table; **boldface** refers to full-color photographs

t refers to a table; **boldface** refers to full-color photographs

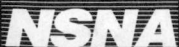

About *PharmDisk 3.0* and www.eDrugInfo.com

PharmDisk 3.0 mini-CD contains:
- Pharmacology Review—a self-paced test complete with rationales for correct and incorrect answers
- Drug Class Challenge—a game that helps you learn to identify drug classes
- Dosage Calculator—a powerful tool for performing dosage calculations
- a direct link to **www.eDrugInfo.com** for drug updates and important drug news.

Minimum system requirements
- Windows 95 or higher
- Pentium 90 or higher
- 16 MB RAM
- 7 MB free hard-disk space
- 256 color-display adapter (16-bit color recommended)
- CD-ROM drive and mouse

Installing and running the program
CAUTION: Do not attempt to use this mini-CD in a floppy disk drive, Zip drive, slot drive, or car stereo.

CAUTION: Do not insert the mini-CD into a CD-ROM drive that requires the mini-CD to be in a vertical position. Placing the CD into such a drive may result in jamming.

Before installing this program, make sure your monitor is set up to display 256 colors or greater. If it isn't, consult your user's manual for instructions about changing the display settings.

To install:
- Place the mini-CD on the inner ring of the CD-ROM drive tray. Close the tray. In a few moments, the CD should automatically start. Once it starts, click the "Install" button to install on your computer.
- Click "Start" and select "Run" if the CD doesn't start automatically.
- Type **d:\setup** (where d:\ is the letter of your CD-ROM drive), and click *OK*. Follow on-screen instructions for installing the CD.

Special note: Before using *PharmDisk 3.0*, read the file *Readme.txt* for important information about operating the program.

For technical support, call toll free 1-877-872-7748, Monday through Friday, 8 am to 5 pm Eastern Standard Time.

For information about obtaining a network license for *PharmDisk 3.0*, call 1-800-346-7844 ext. 1500.

The clinical information and tools in *PharmDisk 3.0* are based on research and consultation with nursing, medical, and legal authorities. To the best of our knowledge, this program reflects currently accepted practice; nevertheless, it can't be considered absolute and universal. For individual application, all recommendations must be considered in light of your institution's policies and procedures, the patient's clinical condition and, before administration of new or infrequently used drugs, in light of the latest package-insert information. The authors and publisher disclaim responsibility for adverse effects resulting directly or indirectly from the suggested procedures, from undetected errors, or from the reader's misunderstanding of the program.